AMERICA'S
TOP DOCTORS®
A CASTLE CONNOLLY GUIDE

7th Edition

America's trusted source for
identifying Top Doctors

For more information, please contact:

Castle Connolly Medical Ltd., 42 West 24th St, New York, New York 10010
212-367-8400x10
E-mail: info@castleconnolly.com
Web site: http://www.castleconnolly.com.

Library of Congress Control Number: 2007922945

| ISBN | 1-883769-79-5; | 978-1-883769-79-6 | (paperback) |
| ISBN | 1-883769-80-9; | 978-1-883769-80-2 | (hardcover) |

Printed in the United States of America

Table of Contents

Table of Contents

Table of Contents

Table of Contents

Table of Contents

Table of Contents

Table of Contents

Table of Contents

Table of Contents

Table of Contents

Table of Contents

Table of Contents

Table of Contents

Table of Contents

Appendices

Indices

About The Publishers

John K. Castle has spent much of the last three decades involved with healthcare institutions and issues. Mr. Castle served as Chairman of the Board of New York Medical College for eleven years, an institution where he served on the Board of Trustees for twenty-two years.

Mr. Castle has been extensively involved in other healthcare and voluntary activities as well. He served for five years as a public commissioner on the Joint Commission on Accreditation of Healthcare Organizations (JCAHO), the body which accredits most public and private hospitals throughout the United States. Mr. Castle has also served as a trustee of five different hospitals in the metropolitan New York region, including New York-Presbyterian Hospital, where he continues to serve.

Mr. Castle is also the Chairman of the Columbia Presbyterian Science Advisory Council and a Director of the Whitehead Institute for Biomedical Research. He is a Fellow of The New York Academy of Medicine and has served as a Trustee of the Academy. He is Chairman of the United Hospital Fund of New York's Capital Campaign. He continues as Director Emeritus of the United Hospital Fund. He is a Life Member of the MIT Corporation, the governing body of the Massachusetts Institute of Technology.

Mr. Castle is the Chairman and Co-Publisher of Castle Connolly Medical Ltd. and affiliated companies which publish *Castle Connolly America's Top Doctors*™ *7th Edition*; *Castle Connolly Top Doctors: New York Metro Area* and other books to help people find the best healthcare.

John J. Connolly, Ed.D. is the President & CEO of Castle Connolly Medical Ltd., and is the nation's foremost authority on identifying top physicians. Dr. Connolly's experience in healthcare is extensive.

For more than a decade he served as President of New York Medical College, the nation's second largest private medical college. He is a Fellow of the New York Academy of Medicine, a Fellow of the New York Academy of Sciences, a Director of the New York Business Group on Health, a member of the President's Council of the United Hospital Fund, and a member of the Board of Advisors of Funding First, a Lasker Foundation initiative. Dr. Connolly has served as a trustee of two hospitals and as Chairman of the Board of one. He is extensively involved in healthcare and community activities and has served on a number of voluntary and corporate boards including the Board of the American Lyme Disease Foundation, of which he is a founder and past chairman, and the Board of Advisors of the Whitehead Institute for Biomedical Research. He is also a Director and Chairman of the Professional Examination Service. He holds a Bachelor of Science degree from Worcester State College, a Master's degree from the University of Connecticut, and a Doctor of Education degree in College and University Administration from Teacher's College, Columbia University.

Dr. Connolly has appeared on or been interviewed by over 100 television and radio stations nationwide including *"Good Morning America"* (ABC-TV), *"The Today Show"* (NBC-TV), *"20/20"* (ABC-TV), *"48 Hours"* (CBS-TV), *"Fox Cable News"* (national), *"Morning News"* (CNN) and *"Weekend Today in New York"* (WNBC-TV). The *New York Times*, the *Chicago Tribune*, the *Daily News* (New York), the *Boston Herald* and other newspapers, as well as many national and regional magazines, have featured Castle Connolly Guides and/or Dr. Connolly in stories.

Medical Advisory Board

Castle Connolly Medical Ltd. is pleased to have associated with a distinguished group of medical leaders who offer invaluable advice and wisdom in our efforts to assist consumers in making good healthcare choices. We thank each member of the Medical Advisory Board for their valuable contributions.

Roger Bulger, M.D.
National Institutes of Health

Harry J. Buncke, M.D.
California Pacific Medical Center

Menard M. Gertler, M.D., D.Sc.
Clinical Prof. of Medicine
Cornell University Medical School

Leo Henikoff, M.D.
President and CEO (retired)
Rush Presbyterian-St. Luke's Medical Center

Yutaka Kikkawa, M.D.
Professor and Chairman Emeritus
Department of Pathology, University of California,
Irvine College of Health Sciences

David Paige, M.D.
Professor
Bloomberg School of Public Health,
Johns Hopkins University

Ronald Pion, M.D.
Chairman and CEO
Medical Telecommunications Associates

Richard L. Reece, M.D.
Editor
Physician Practice Options

Leon G. Smith, M.D.
Chairman of Medicine
St. Michael's Medical Center, N.J.

Helen Smits, M.D.
Former Deputy Director
Health Care Financing Administration (HCFA)

Ralph Snyderman, M.D.
Chairman Emeritus
Duke University Health System

Foreword

The challenge of finding the best healthcare is a formidable one for most Americans and for others who seek medical care in the United States. While this country offers the best medical care in the world, many people are overwhelmed by its complexity and bureaucracy.

While most of us are fortunate and never need to venture beyond our local communities to find medical specialists able to meet our healthcare needs, the needs of many patients cannot be met in their local areas. For them, the search for the top specialists can be as important as life itself!

This great nation is fortunate in possessing some of the world's leading medical centers and specialty hospitals where cutting edge research is conducted and innovative new therapies are practiced daily. These health centers employ and train many of the world's most skilled physicians. The organization which I formerly headed, the Association of Academic Health Centers, serves as a forum of exchange for these centers of medical excellence and, therefore, I know them well. However, I also know well the difficulty and challenges that patients and their families face in identifying and locating the tremendous wealth of medical talent and dedication that lies within the walls of these outstanding facilities.

Castle Connolly Medical Ltd. has dedicated extensive time and resources to identify-ing the best healthcare this nation has to offer. They have done this not to serve physicians or hospitals, but to serve healthcare consumers. Their efforts will be vital and important resources to Americans and others who seek the best medical care available in this country—wherever it is being practiced.

Roger Bulger, M.D.
National Institutes of Health
Washington DC

Introduction

There are times in life when the nature of a disease or medical condition that afflicts you or a loved one warrants identifying the top doctor—the very best specialist anywhere in the nation—to diagnose or treat that particular medical problem. At times like these, you need Castle Connolly America's Top Doctors' 7th Edition, the national guide designed to assist you under just these circumstances.

While the overall quality of medical care throughout the United States is generally of very high quality and in many places is superb, there are still those rare, complex or extremely difficult problems that demand resources beyond the ordinary or that require talents that are exceptional.

This guide identifies those top medical specialists throughout the country who possess the skill and experience to address these problems. Top specialists who provide excellent care tend to be located predominantly, although not exclusively, at major medical centers, specialty hospitals and leading teaching hospitals. These exceptional physicians are acknowledged as such by their peers and are recognized for their expertise by the medical profession.

The top specialists we have identified are not the only excellent physicians who are caring for patients in this nation. Since there are more than 650,000 doctors in the United States, we cannot identify every top specialist. Therefore, we have included narrative to assist those using this guide who may not find the specialist they need within its listings. Clearly, there are many primary care physicians and other well-trained specialists in communities and hospitals throughout the United States.

Most physicians in this guide are board certified not only in a specialty, but also in a subspecialty or in multiple subspecialties. Board or subspecialty certification alone, however, does not distinguish them from excellent specialists at hospitals in your community, many of whom are also board certified in both a specialty and a subspecialty.

However, the majority of physicians included in this guide have trained at the top medical centers under medical pioneers who possess state-of-the-art knowledge in a specific disease or problem and have often devised new techniques and therapeutic approaches, many of which are life-saving procedures or cures. These doctors most often practice their science and art at leading hospitals and, more specifically, in programs at hospitals that are recognized for their excellence in a given field. Many others have been trained at leading centers in other nations since the U.S. is not alone in pioneering new medical knowledge, although its position as the leader in "high-tech" medicine is generally acknowledged.

Another major characteristic distinguishing the majority of physicians in this guide from those at local hospitals is their continued focus and training. Rather than practicing at a community hospital (or even at a leading regional hospital) and developing a general, broad-based practice, these physicians continued their training in a particular disease, syndrome or subspecialty to such a degree that they developed extensive knowledge and unique skills in treating that particular problem.

Often that focused, advanced training is accompanied by active involvement in clinical research. This is an additional reason why the physicians listed in this guide are located at only a few hundred of the more than six thousand hospitals in the United States. It is difficult, although not impossible, to conduct important clinical research in isolation or without an environment supportive of research. It takes time, money, residents, research associates, technicians, equipment and more to produce significant clinical research. Certainly there have been individuals who have made important and lasting contributions to research with little or none of this support, but those instances are rare. Today, for the most part, major advances in medicine occur in the labs and on the floors of major medical centers and specialty hospitals, in medical schools and in clinical labs created and financed for that purpose by commercial enterprises.

How Physicians Were Selected For Inclusion In This Guide

The basis of the Castle Connolly selection process is peer nomination. In some ways, this resembles an enhancement of the process in which a personal physician provides a patient with a referral to another physician for a particular problem. However, if the recommendation of one doctor is good, the recommendation of many doctors is even better. So, we ask many doctors for their recommendations; in fact, more than 230,000 doctors were surveyed during our first effort at building this database.

How do we accomplish this enormous task? Over the years, the Castle Connolly physician-led research team developed its extensive database of physicians across the nation through periodic mail, telephone and email surveys. This cumulative database is systematically maintained and continuously updated. Surveyed physicians nominate top doctors in both their own and related specialties – especially those to whom they would refer their own patients. Each year this database is supplemented by further mail surveys and telephone interviews with leaders in the various medical specialties and leading physicians at major medical centers. In our research for the first edition of this guide, online surveys also were conducted with members of Physicians' Online (POL), the country's largest community of physicians connected through the Internet.

To augment our large mail, telephone and online samplings, additional surveys are conducted among the following carefully selected groups: directors of graduate medical programs; directors of clinical services at member hospitals of the Council of Teaching Hospitals (COTH); board members of medical specialty academies, associations and societies; and deans and chairs of departments at medical schools.

Building on years of prior research, thousands of top doctors included in earlier editions of our guides, as well as a random sample of physicians not listed, are invited to offer their nominations for Castle Connolly *America's Top Doctors®*.

Over 25,000 physicians have been nominated through this process. Extensive biographical forms were sent to those physicians most frequently nominated for completion. After careful review of their professional backgrounds, the Castle Connolly research staff conducted further research to check disciplinary and license histories.

The result is a carefully researched and highly selective list of the top specialists in the nation. This select group of physicians, identified through our extensive research process, constitutes a list of physicians recognized by their peers for their excellence in providing care for specific diseases and problems.

Undoubtedly, there will be comments that we have missed some fine doctors who should be included. That is inevitable, since this guide is designed to identify only those doctors noted for excellence in diagnosing or treating a specific problem or disease.

We do not intentionally include physicians simply because they have important titles. While a position as a chief of service or a department head at a teaching hospital is an important post, such positions are achieved through a combination of many talents including administrative skills, seniority and factors that are not as important for inclusion in this guide as is skill in clinical care. The same is true of leaders of county medical societies, professional associations or even specialty groups. While these are significant positions and acknowledge a leadership among peers, these titles are not essential to clinical skill recognition.

The same perspective applies to research expertise. Many physicians listed in the Guide are engaged in clinical research and make significant contributions to their fields, with some devoting a substantial portion of their time to research. However, we avoided including those physicians who solely conduct research and who do not provide patient care.

The result of this extensive research effort is a list of outstanding, highly skilled physicians who are recognized as among the best in their specialties and in the nation; a list which consumers/patients can use to find the very best specialists to meet their particular needs.

Introduction

Lastly, this book differs from the regional Castle Connolly Guides in two important ways. First, Castle Connolly *America's Top Doctors* 7th Edition is national, not regional, in scope. Second, the regional Guides are based on the generally accurate premise that healthcare is local and most people find their healthcare where they live and work. However, Castle Connolly *America's Top Doctors* 7th Edition is designed to meet the needs of those people who cannot find the right specialists locally but who can and will travel anywhere in the country to be cared for by a top specialist at an outstanding hospital. This guide will assist readers in that important search and, for that reason, does not include primary care physicians.

Using This Guide To Find Top Specialists

This guide is organized and planned to be as user-friendly as possible. Still, as with anything as complex as medical specialties, subspecialties and the myriad of diseases and problems that specialists treat, there needs to be a system to organize the physicians' names, the diseases and problems they manage and their special expertise.

To organize the specialists in this guide, we have followed the American Board of Medical Specialties (ABMS) format. The ABMS is the authoritative body for the recognition of medical specialties. Without the ABMS as the official controlling body there would be hundreds of unregulated medical specialties.

The ABMS recognizes twenty-five specialties and more than ninety subspecialties. The listing of ABMS specialties and subspecialties can be found in Appendix A. In addition to ABMS recognized specialties, there are at least one hundred other groups calling themselves "medical specialists" that are not recognized by the ABMS. Some of these groups are working toward recognition and have exams and other standards for membership. Others are organizations of physicians interested in a particular problem or area of medicine that exist to exchange information but have no intention of seeking ABMS recognition. Some groups calling themselves "boards" really have little authority or meaningful standards. Thus, while a physician may state he/she is, for example, a specialist in cosmetic surgery, there is no ABMS recognized specialty by that name. Therefore, you have no idea whether this physician has any special training and expertise or is simply trying to recruit paying patients to a lucrative aspect of surgical practice.

You can get information on a doctor's credentials from the doctor, from the doctor's hospital (Medical Affairs Office) or from your health plan if a doctor is in the network. You can also get this information from numerous Web sites, including www.castleconnolly.com. You can check on a physician's board certification by calling the ABMS at (866) 275-2267 or by logging on to its Web site at www.abms.org.

If you seek a particular type of specialist or subspecialist, turn to the section of this guide covering that medical specialty or subspecialty. There you will be able to further restrict your search to a specific geographic region or, if you prefer, to search throughout the nation.

To make your search easier, we have organized the specialties and subspecialties into the following regions: New England, Mid Atlantic, Midwest, Southeast, Southwest, Great Plains and Mountains, and West Coast and Pacific. To find an outstanding cardiologist in St. Louis, for example, look under Cardiovascular Disease and then under the Midwest region. (See Page 39 for geographical regions and states.)

A second way to use this guide is to look at the Special Expertise Index, which lists the areas of special expertise of included physicians. This list of special expertise indicates more than 2,000 medical topics including diseases, therapeutic approaches and techniques. You can look up the particular disease, problem or technique you are interested in and locate a physician in that manner. We assume that many people using this guide will know what their particular problem is and will begin their exploration with this index. However, we encourage you to read the entire text since it will help you to better understand how to find the right physician for yourself or a family member, especially if one is not found in this guide.

Choosing An Appropriate Specialist

It may seem that choosing the correct specialist to treat a particular medical problem is simply a matter of finding a top doctor in a specific medical specialty. For treatment of a problem with your vision, you would choose an ophthalmologist. A skin or hair problem would require treatment by a dermatologist and a broken bone would need the care of an orthopaedic surgeon.

Sometimes, however, the type of specialist needed may not be obvious. For example, back surgery may be performed by either an orthopaedic surgeon or a neurosurgeon. Different aspects of sports medicine, as another example, are practiced by orthopaedic surgeons who treat sports-related injuries in both adults and children, pediatricians who treat only children or internists and family practitioners whose focus is on prevention of injuries.

In some cases, several specialists with expertise in different areas of medical practice all become involved in treating the same patient's health problem. For example, a person with diabetes might need care from an endocrinologist, a cardiologist and an ophthalmologist. In other situations, doctors trained in different specialties may use varied approaches or differing therapies to manage a disease or condition. Such is the case, for example, with prostate cancer: a patient could be treated by a urologist, a medical oncologist, or a radiation oncologist. The urologist might provide the patient with a surgical treatment option, while the medical oncologist would treat the patient with chemotherapy and the radiotherapist would use radiation therapy and/or radioactive seed implantation. All approaches could be successful, or one might be preferable to another, depending on the patient and his condition. Therefore, a wise patient will thoroughly explore all options before making a choice.

Finding the right specialist is also important in terms of the quality of your care. For example, many orthopaedic surgeons will operate on hands, but it is clearly preferable to have someone trained and certified specifically in hand surgery (a subspecialty of both orthopaedic surgery and plastic surgery) to perform that delicate surgery. Similarly, a dermatologist may indicate that his/her practice includes cosmetic surgery; however, there is no approved ABMS dermatology subspecialty or fellowship training in cosmetic surgery. While many dermatologists do pursue additional training in cosmetic surgery, it should be understood that dermatologic practice is limited to cutaneous procedures ranging from the removal of skin tumors to laser resurfacing. On the other hand, some board certified otolaryngologists have additional training that enables them to perform cosmetic surgery procedures on the head and neck.

Choosing the right type of specialist is as important as selecting the right doctor. For example, the diagnosis of melanoma, a very serious, potentially life threatening form of skin cancer, is missed in many cases. Therefore, if you have a skin lesion that might possibly be melanoma, you should be certain that the pathologist reading your slides is board certified in the subspecialty of dermatopathology.

These examples illustrate this important principle: always seek the best healthcare. Look for the best-trained doctors, not those who simply can do the job. That doesn't mean that you need to consult a doctor listed in this guide every time you have a health problem. It does mean you should be certain that the physicians who care for you, whether in your community or at a world-class medical center, are trained appropriately and are qualified to provide the care you require. Remember, when it comes to healthcare no one wants second best!

Given this complexity, how do you find the right specialist to provide your care? The first and most important person to look to for guidance is your primary care physician. He/she will assess your medical condition, determine the appropriate type of specialist to recommend and perhaps refer you to a specific doctor or doctors. You should always ask your primary care physician why a particular specialist is being recommended, since that specialist may be a colleague in your doctor's medical group or may be the only (or the most conveniently located) specialist of the type in your health plan. Ask how well your primary care physician knows the specialist, whether they have a long-standing professional relationship and if other patients referred to the specialist had successful outcomes. Be sure to ask for several recommendations, if possible, to provide you with some choice among specialists.

If you do not have a primary care doctor, try to learn as much as you can about your medical problem and the type of specialist best suited to treat it. However, keep in mind that many diseases or conditions present with symptoms that often are indistinguishable from those of other diseases or conditions, making them difficult to diagnose precisely even for physicians armed with the results of diagnostic tests.

Judging The Qualifications Of A Physician

The specialists listed in Castle Connolly America's Top Doctors® 7th Edition are clearly among the best in the nation and have been identified through a rigorous research process and thorough screening by the Castle Connolly research team. Through our extensive surveys and research we have done much of the work in finding a top referral specialist for you. But how do you judge the qualifications of a physician who may not be listed in this Guide? If you are trying to find a specialist on your own, how should you go about it? How can you tell when a physician has the appropriate training in a specialty and how do you distinguish what is meaningful and what is not from among all those plaques and certificates on a doctor's wall?

The following pages will outline that process for you. In fact, what is written here reflects much of the logic that underlies the selection of physicians for this book.

The following material will help you not only in finding a top specialist in this Guide, but it also should be helpful to you in choosing among the many specialists, primary care doctors and other physicians that you will need to consult throughout your life.

The reality is that few of us see only one doctor in our lifetime. Each of us may be cared for by a primary care physician, an ophthalmologist, an orthopaedic surgeon, a dermatologist, a surgeon or a number of other specialists. The choices can be many and they can be among the most important choices that we make in our lives.

Education

Your review of your prospective doctor's education and training should begin with medical school. While you may feel that the institution at which someone earned a bachelor's degree could be an indication of the quality of the doctor, most people in the medical field do not believe it plays a major role. A degree from a highly selective undergraduate college or university will help an aspiring doctor gain admission to a medical school, but once there, all students are peers. However, the information on undergraduate colleges, if important to you, is available in *The Official ABMS Directory of Board Certified Medical Specialists®* and other medical directories.

American medical schools are highly standardized, at least in terms of minimal quality. A group known as the Liaison Committee for Medical Education (LCME) accredits all U.S. medical schools that grant medical degrees (MDs) and osteopathic degrees (DOs). Most also are accredited by the appropriate state agency, if one exists, and by regional accrediting agencies that accredit colleges and universities of all kinds.

Furthermore, U.S. medical schools have universally high standards for admission, including success on the undergraduate level and on the Medical College Admissions Tests (MCATs). Although frequently criticized for being slow to change and for training too many specialists, the system of medical education in the United States has insured high quality in medical practice. One recent positive change is a strong effort in most medical schools to diversify the composition of the student body. While these schools have been less successful in enrolling racial minorities, the number of women in U.S. medical schools has increased to the point that women now make up about 50 percent of most classes. In certain specialties preferred by women medical graduates (pediatrics, for example) it is possible that in coming years the majority of specialists will be female.

Most doctors practicing in the United States are graduates of U.S. medical schools, but there are two other groups of doctors who make up a relatively small portion of the total physician population. They are (1) foreign nationals who graduated from foreign schools and (2) U.S. nationals who graduated from foreign schools. (Canadian medical schools are not considered foreign).

Foreign Medical Graduates

Foreign medical schools vary greatly in quality. Even some of the oldest and finest European schools have become virtually "open door," with huge numbers of unscreened students making teaching and learning difficult. Others are excellent and provided the model for our system of medical education.

The fact that someone graduated from a foreign school does not mean that he/she is a poor doctor. Foreign schools, like U.S. schools, produce good doctors and poor doctors. Foreign medical graduates must pass the same exam taken by U.S. graduates for licensure, but the failure rate for foreign graduates is significantly higher. In the first year of using the new United States Medical Licensing Exam (USMLE), 93 percent of U.S. medical school graduates passed Step II, the clinical exam, as compared with 39 percent of the foreign graduates. It is clear that the quality of foreign schools, if not individual doctors, is not the same as U.S. medical schools, at least as measured by our standards. Nonetheless, many communities and patients have been well served by foreign medical graduates practicing in this country—often in areas where it has been difficult to attract graduates of American schools.

In addition, many foreign medical schools and their teaching hospitals are world renowned for their leadership in medical care, research and teaching and many of the technologies and techniques we utilize in the U.S. today have been developed and perfected in foreign countries.

Residency

Most doctors practicing today have at least three years of postgraduate training (following the MD or DO) in an approved residency program. This not only is an important step in the process of becoming a competent doctor, but it is also a requirement for board (specialty) certification. Most people assume that a prospective doctor needs to complete a three-year residency program to obtain a medical license. That is not an accurate assumption! New York State, for example, requires only one postgraduate year. However, since all approved residencies last at least three years and some, such as those in neurosurgery, general surgery, orthopaedic surgery and urology, may extend for five or more years, it is important to know the details of a doctor's training. Licensure alone is not enough of a basis upon which to make a decision.

Without undertaking extensive and detailed research on every residency program, the best assessment you can make of a doctor's residency program is to see if it took place in a large medical center whose name you recognize. The more prestigious institutions tend to attract the best medical students, sometimes regardless of the quality of the individual residency program. If in doubt about a doctor's training, ask the doctor if the residency he/she completed was in the specialty of the practice; if not, ask why not.

It is also important to be certain that a doctor completed a residency that has been approved by the appropriate governing board of the specialty, such as the American Board of Surgery, the American Board of Radiology, or the American Osteopathic Board of Pediatrics. These board groups are listed in Appendix A. If you are really concerned about a doctor's training, you should call the hospital that offered the residency and ask if the residency program was approved by the appropriate specialty group. If still in doubt, consult the publication *Directory of Graduate Medical Education Programs*, often called the "green book," found in medical school or hospital libraries, which lists all approved residencies.

Board Certification

With an MD or DO degree and a license, an individual may practice in any medical specialty with or without additional training. For example, doctors with a license but no special training may call themselves cardiologists, pediatricians or gynecologists. This is why board certification is such an important factor. The American Board of Medical Specialties (ABMS) recognizes 25 specialties and more than 90 subspecialties. Visit www.abms.org or call 866-275-2267 for more information. Eighteen boards certify in 106 specialties under the aegis of the American Osteopathic Association (AOA). Visit www.osteopathic.org or call 800-621-1773 for more information. Doctors who have qualified for such specialization are called board certified; they have completed an approved residency and passed the board's exam. (See Appendix A for the approved ABMS and AOA lists). While many doctors who are not board certified do call themselves "specialists," board certification is the best standard by which to measure competence and training. Throughout this Guide a description of each specialty and subspecialty is provided as an introduction to the listing of physicians in that specialty.

You can be confident that doctors who are board certified have, at a minimum, the proper training in their specialty and have demonstrated their proficiency through supervision and testing. While there are many non-board certified doctors who are highly competent, it is more difficult to assess the level of their training. While board certification alone does not guarantee competence, it is a standard that reflects successful completion of an appropriate training program. If it is impossible to find a doctor in your area who is board certified in a particular subspecialty, for example, geriatric medicine or sports medicine, at least be certain the physician is board certified in a related specialty such as internal medicine or orthopaedic surgery.

Board certified doctors are referred to as Diplomates of the Board. Some of the colleges of medical specialties (e.g., the American College of Radiology, the American College of Surgeons) have multiple levels of recognition. The first is basic membership and the second, more prestigious and difficult to obtain, is status as a Fellow. Fellowship status in the colleges is meaningful and is based on experience, professional achievement and recognition by one's peers, including extensive experience in patient care. It should be viewed as a significant professional qualification.

Board Eligibility

Many doctors who have been more recently trained are waiting to take the boards. They are sometimes described as "board eligible," a common term that the ABMS advocates abandoning because of its ambiguity. Board eligible means that the doctor has completed an approved residency and is qualified to sit for the related board's exam.

Each member board of the ABMS has its own policy regarding the use and recognition of the board eligible term. Therefore, the description "board eligible" should not be viewed as a genuine qualification, especially if a doctor has been out of medical school long enough to have taken the certification exam. To the boards, a doctor is either board certified or not. Furthermore, most of the specialty boards permit unlimited attempts to pass the exam and, in some cases, doctors who have failed the exam twice or even ten times continue to call themselves board eligible. In osteopathic medicine, the board eligible status is recognized only for the first six years after completion of a residency.

In addition to the approved lists of specialties and subspecialties of the ABMS and AOA, there are a wide variety of other doctors and groups of doctors who call themselves specialists. At present there are at least 100 such groups called "self-designated medical specialties." They range from doctors who are working to create a recognized body of knowledge and subspecialty training to less formal groups interested in a particular approach to the practice of medicine. These groups may or may not have standards for membership. There is no way to determine the true extent of their members' training and neither the ABMS or the AOA recognizes them. While you should be cautious of doctors who claim they are specialists in these areas, many do have advanced training and the groups at least offer a listing of people interested in a particular approach to medical care. Rely on board certification to assure yourself of basic competence, and use membership in one of these groups to indicate strong interest and possible additional training in a particular aspect of medicine. A list of these self-designated medical specialties may be found in Appendix B.

Recertification

A relatively new focus of the specialty boards is the area of recertification. Until recently, board certification lasted for an unlimited time. Now, almost all the boards have put time limits on the certification period. For example, in Internal Medicine and Anesthesiology, the time limit is ten years; in Family Practice, six, and under some circumstances, seven years. These more stringent standards reflect an increasing emphasis on recertification by both the medical boards and state agencies responsible for licensing doctors.

Since the policies of the boards vary widely, it is a good procedure to ask a doctor if certification was awarded and when. If the date was seven to ten years ago, ask if he/she has been recertified. Unfortunately, many boards permit "grandfathering," whereby already certified doctors do not have to be recertified, and recertification requirements apply only to newly certified doctors. Appendix A contains a list of the names and addresses of the boards and the certification period for each board specialty. Even if recertification is not required, it is good professional practice for doctors to undertake the process. It assures you, the patient, that they are attempting to stay current.

Many states have a continuing medical education requirement for doctors. These states typically require a minimum number of continuing medical education (CME) credits for a doctor to maintain a medical license. Seven states require 150 CME credits over a three-year period. Osteopathic doctors are required to take 120 hours of CME credits within three years to maintain certification.

Fellowships

The purpose of a fellowship is to provide advanced training in the clinical techniques and research of a particular specialty. Fellowships usually, but not always, are designed to lead to board certification in a subspecialty such as cardiology, which is a subspecialty of internal medicine. Many physicians listed in this Guide have had fellowship training. In the U.S. there are a variety of fellowship programs available to doctors, which fall into two broad categories: approved and unapproved. Approved fellowships are those that are approved by the appropriate medical specialty board (e.g., the American Board of Radiology) and lead to subspecialty certificates. Fellowship programs that are unapproved are often in the same areas of training as those that are approved, but they do not lead to subspecialty certificates. Unfortunately, all too often, an unapproved fellowship exists only to provide relatively inexpensive labor for the research and/or patient care activities of a clinical department in a medical school or hospital. In such cases, the learning that takes place is secondary and may be a good deal less than in an approved fellowship. On the other hand, any fellowship is better than none at all and some unapproved fellowships have that status for a valid reason that should not reflect negatively on the program. For example, the fellowship may have been recently created, with approval being sought. To check that a fellowship is an approved one, call the hospital where the training took place or call the medical board for that specialty.

Some physicians may have completed more than one fellowship and may be boarded in two or more subspecialties. Also, some physicians may pursue fellowship training and subspecialty certification, but then choose to practice in their primary field of certification. For example, a doctor who is board certified in internal medicine also may have obtained board certification in cardiology, but may choose to practice primarily internal medicine rather than cardiology. For the most part, the physicians in this Guide practice in their subspecialties.

Professional Reputation

There are doctors who meet every professional standard on paper, but who are simply not good doctors. In all probability the medical community has ascertained that and, while the individual may still practice medicine, his/her reputation will reflect that collective assessment. There are also doctors who are outstanding leaders in their fields because of research or professional activities but who are not particularly strong, or perhaps even active, in patient care. It is important to distinguish that kind of professional reputation from a reputation as a competent, caring doctor in delivering patient care, or in the case of this Guide, as an outstanding practitioner in a given specialty.

Hospital Appointment

Most doctors are on the medical staff of one or more hospitals and are known as "attendings;" some are not. If a doctor does not have admitting privileges or is not on the attending staff of a hospital, you may wish to consider choosing a different doctor. It can be very difficult to ascertain whether or not the lack of hospital appointment is for a good reason. For example, it is understandable that some doctors who are raising families or heading toward retirement choose not to meet the demands (meetings, committees, etc.) of being an attending. However, if you need care in a hospital, the lack of such an appointment means that another doctor will have to oversee that care. In some specialties, such as dermatology and psychiatry, doctors may conduct their entire practice in the office and a hospital appointment is not as essential, or as good a criterion for assessment, as in other specialties.

While mistakes are made, most hospitals are quite careful about admissions to their medical staffs. The best hospitals are highly selective, so a degree of screening (or "credentialing") has been done for you. In other words, the best doctors practice at the best hospitals. Since caring for a patient in a hospital is often a team effort involving a number of specialists, the reputation of the hospital to which the doctor admits patients carries special weight. Hospital medical staffs review their colleagues' credentials and authorize performance of specific procedures. In addition, they typically review and reappoint their medical staff every two or three years. In effect, this is an additional screening to protect patients. It is especially true of hospitals that have what are known as closed staffs, where it is impossible to obtain admitting privileges unless there is a vacancy that the administration and medical staff deem necessary to fill. If you are having a surgical procedure and are concerned about the doctor's skill or experience, it may be worthwhile to call the Medical Affairs office at the doctor's hospital to see if he/she is authorized to perform that procedure in that hospital.

The reasons for a hospital's selectivity are easy to understand: no hospital wishes to expose itself to liability and every hospital wants to have the best reputation possible in order to attract patients. Obviously, the quality of the medical staff is immensely important in creating that reputation.

Physicians listed in this guide are primarily on the staffs of major medical centers, usually teaching hospitals, and leading specialty hospitals, e.g. children's, cancer, heart, psychiatric, etc. There are many excellent physicians on the staffs of community hospitals that call themselves "medical centers," but they are not physicians who typically attract complex cases and referrals from outside their area.

To learn about a hospital visit its website. It is also useful to review a hospital's accreditation status under the Joint Commission on the Accreditation of Healthcare Organizations at www.JCAHO.com

A last and very important reason why a hospital appointment is an essential requirement in your choice of doctor is that some states permit doctors to practice without malpractice insurance. If you are injured as a result of a doctor's poor care, you could be without recourse. However, few hospitals permit doctors to practice in them unless they carry malpractice insurance. This not only protects the hospital, but the patient as well.

Medical School Faculty Appointment

Many doctors have appointments on the faculties of medical schools. There is a range of categories from "straight" appointments, meaning full-time appointment as professor, associate professor, assistant professor or instructor, to clinical ranks that may reflect lesser degrees of involvement in teaching or research. If someone carries what is known as a straight academic rank (i.e. "professor of surgery," without clinical in the title), this usually means that the individual is engaged full-time in medical school research, teaching activities and patient care. The title "clinical professor of surgery" usually indicates a less direct involvement in medical school activities such as teaching and research.

Doctors who are full-time academicians may be in the forefront of new techniques and research, but they are not necessarily better doctors. Nonetheless, you would be assured that they have the support of other faculty, residents and medical students.

When you are seeking a subspecialist, a doctor's relationship to a medical school becomes more meaningful since medical school faculties tend to be made up of subspecialists. You are less likely to find large numbers of general or primary care practitioners engaged full-time on a medical school faculty. The newest approaches and techniques in medicine, for the most part, are explored and developed by medical school faculties in their laboratories and clinical practice settings. This is where they practice their subspecialties, as well as teach and conduct research. Such leading specialists are not necessarily better doctors than community doctors; rather, they are trained to provide a different kind of medical care. Obviously the type of medical care users of this guide are seeking is that different kind of care available primarily from top subspecialists at leading hospitals and medical centers.

Medical Society Membership

Most medical society memberships sound very prestigious and some are; however, there are many societies that are not selective and which virtually any doctor can join. In addition, membership in many of the more prestigious societies is based on research and publication or on leadership in the field and may have little to do with direct patient care. While it is clearly an honor to be invited to join these groups, membership may be less than helpful in discerning whether a doctor can deliver the excellent clinical care you require.

Experience

Experience is difficult to assess. Obviously, in most cases, an older doctor has more experience; on the other hand, a younger doctor has been more recently immersed in the challenge of medical school, residency, or even a fellowship, and may be the most up-to-date. If a doctor is board certified, you may assume that assures at least a minimal amount of experience, but since it could be as little as a year, check the date of graduation from medical school or completion of residency to know precisely how long a doctor has been in practice.

There is a good deal of evidence that there is a positive relationship between quantity of experience and quality of care. It may be that, the more a doctor performs a procedure, the better he/she becomes at it. That is why it is important to ask a doctor about his or her experience with the procedure that you need. Does the doctor see and treat similar cases every day, every week or only rarely? Of course, with some rare diseases, rarely is the only possible answer, but it is relative frequency that is critical. Major metropolitan areas, especially New York and San Francisco, became leaders in the treatment of AIDS because of the number of patients seen in those metropolitan areas. Doctors in the suburbs of New York City (especially in New York's Westchester, Nassau and Suffolk counties) and in Fairfield County, Connecticut became leaders in the research and treatment of Lyme disease because that region is the epicenter of the disease.

In some states, data is available on volume or numbers of certain procedures performed at hospitals. For this information in New York you can call the Center for Medical Consumers, a non-profit advocacy organization, or visit its web site at www.medicalconsumers.org. For volume and outcome information in other states, visit the web site of Health Care Choices at www.healthcarechoices.org. The federal government has posted outcome data for hospitals, but for a limited number of procedures, on a website www.healthcarecompare.com. There is a good deal of controversy, however, on the validity and usefulness of such data. Opponents cite the fact that some of the data is produced from Medicare patient records only and, thus, is based solely on an elderly population that does not represent the total activity of a hospital or doctor. Proponents of the use of such volume data agree that it is not perfect, but suggest it can be one useful criterion in selecting the best places to receive care for these specific problems

The one type of experience you should specifically want to know about is that dealing with any special procedure, particularly a surgical one, that has recently been developed and introduced into practice. For example, in the 1980's many doctors using laparoscopic cholecystectomy, a then new surgical technique for removing gallbladders, experienced a high percentage of problems because they were not properly trained. This prompted the American Board of Surgery to announce new standards for the training of surgeons using this technique. Do not hesitate to ask about your doctor's training in a procedure and how frequently and with what degree of success he/she has performed it. Practice may not lead to perfection, but it does improve skills and enhance the probability of success.

In some cases, relatively young doctors have recently completed residency or fellowship training under recognized leaders who have developed new approaches or techniques for dealing with a particular problem. They may have learned the new techniques from their mentors and may be far ahead of the field (and ahead of more senior and distinguished colleagues) in using those approaches. So age and experience must be considered and weighed along with other factors when choosing a physician.

Second Opinions

Second opinions are a valuable medical tool, too infrequently used in many instances and overused in others. Clearly, you do not want to seek another doctor's opinion on every ailment or problem that you face, but a second opinion should be pursued in the following situations:

• before major surgery

• if the diagnosis is serious or life threatening

• if a rare disease is diagnosed

• if a diagnosis is uncertain

• if the number of tests or procedures recommended might be excessive

• if a test result has serious implications (e.g., a positive Pap smear)

• if the treatment suggested is risky or expensive

• if you are uncomfortable with the diagnosis and/or treatment

• if a course of treatment is not successful

• if you question your doctor's competence

• if your insurance company requires it

Most doctors will be supportive if you request a second opinion and many will recommend it. In many cases, insurance companies will pay for second opinions, but check ahead of time to make sure your insurance plan does cover them. In an HMO you may have to be more assertive because one way HMOs control costs is by limiting second opinions. Often, the opinion of a second doctor will confirm the opinion of the first, but the reassurance may be worth the time and extra cost. On the other hand, if the second opinion differs from the first, you have two alternatives: seek the opinion of a third doctor, or educate yourself as much as possible by talking to both doctors, reading up on the problem, and trusting your instincts about which diagnosis is correct.

Office And Practice Arrangements

Although clearly not as important as training or reputation, a specialist's office and practice arrangements often are of significance to patients. Practice arrangements include office hours, office location, billing procedures and accessibility among the many factors that result in how well the office is run.

Some specialists only will see new patients who are referred to them by another doctor. Therefore, you may need to have your treating physician contact the specialist's office to arrange for your initial visit. Your health plan may also require that your primary care doctor provide a referral.

If English is not your first language, it may be advisable to determine whether someone in the specialist's office speaks your primary language or if a translator can be present during appointments. This will ease communication and assure that all questions, responses and instructions are understood.

Accessibility of the specialist's office may be a concern if you are wheelchair-bound, are elderly or cannot climb stairs or negotiate narrow corridors. Convenient parking may also be important to you.

Other arrangements that may need to be made in advance of your first visit or discussed with the specialist's office staff concern payment. You may wish to ask the following:

- Does the specialist accept your health insurance coverage?

- Is the specialist within your plan's network and will you need to pay a co-payment? Or, is the specialist out-of-network and will you have to pay for your care out-of-pocket, meet a deductible or submit a form for reimbursement?

- Are credit cards an acceptable mode of payment?

- Does the specialist accept Medicare, Medicaid or no-fault insurance? Does the specialist treat workers' compensation cases?

- If you are a non-resident of the United States, will you need to arrange for the transfer or exchange of currency to pay the specialist's fee?

When you are choosing a top specialist, these issues may be of lesser or greater importance, depending on the problem and type of care warranted. If you are traveling a great distance to have a specific procedure performed by a top specialist at a major medical center, continuing long-term monitoring or follow-up care by that physician may not be required or may not be feasible and such things as office practice arrangements are of less importance. On the other hand, if you have a chronic problem that needs to be monitored with follow-up care provided by the same top specialist, then such issues as accessibility of the doctor's office, appointment hours, waiting times and courtesy and professionalism of the staff become more significant.

Personal Chemistry

One element of the doctor-patient relationship that we stress in our guides is chemistry between doctor and patient, a part of which is often referred to as a doctor's "bedside manner." While this factor is of major import in a long-term relationship such as one you would have with your primary care physician, it is of less importance when you see a specialist only once or twice. However, since many people using this book may have chronic conditions that require ongoing care, it is important to give the matter some consideration.

It is vital that there is a sense of mutual trust and respect between patient and doctor; a judgment that individuals must make for themselves. Among the many talented doctors listed in this guide, there are very likely some to whom you would relate well and others with whom you may not feel as comfortable.

Patients prefer doctors who listen, demonstrate concern, are responsive to patient needs and spend sufficient time with them. The qualities of physicians in this regard, even the excellent ones in this guide, vary immensely.

You, the patient, are the only one who can assess these qualities because individuals react differently to various personalities. It is important for you to carefully judge your feelings towards a physician, especially if you are embarking on a long-term relationship. You should feel you can be open, trusting and responsive to your physician and that your relationship will be a positive one. Otherwise, find another doctor, since not doing so could adversely affect your care.

Once you have used this guide to identify the top specialist(s) best suited to treat your condition, there is much you can do to maximize the value of your first visit.

Maximizing Your First Appointment With A Top Doctor

After your research is done and you've secured an appointment for an initial consultation with a top doctor known for his/her expertise in the diagnosis or treatment of your particular medical condition, what should you do?

Whether your visit to the specialist's office is a car ride or a plane trip away, there undoubtedly will be arrangements to make before your appointment. You may have to take time off from work, arrange for childcare while you are away and make travel plans and hotel reservations, but there are a number of other important steps to take to assure that you and the specialist make the best use of the time you spend together.

Have you done everything you can to prepare yourself and the specialist for the consultation? The following checklist will help you maximize the value of your visit to the specialist and will go a long way toward focusing you on the task at hand—getting the best advice or treatment for your health problem from one of the top doctors in the medical specialty related to your condition.

Gathering The Facts

- Does the specialist have all the information needed to make a diagnosis of or treatment plan for your condition?

- Have your medical records, test results and X-rays been sent ahead of time to allow for their review by the specialist in advance of your first appointment?

- Have you written out your medical history, including that of your siblings, parents and grandparents, emphasizing the particular problem for which you are visiting this specialist?

- Are you prepared with a written list of questions?

- Do you understand the answers?

A specialist becoming newly involved in your care needs to learn as much as possible about the state of your health in a very limited time. Since top doctors are extremely busy people with many demands on their time, you should make certain that all relevant records and case summaries are obtained and sent to the specialist well in advance of your appointment.

Obtaining Your Records

All healthcare providers, including hospitals, doctors and their staffs, are under legal obligation to maintain the privacy of your medical records. In order to obtain release of those records, you must make a request in writing. If you need to obtain records from a number of providers, you should write one clear and concise letter authorizing release of your records and including your name, address, telephone number, date of birth, identification number and any other identifying information such as a hospital chart number. You then can make photocopies of this letter, but be sure to sign and date each copy as if it were an original. You also may want to specifically name those test results (e.g., pathology slides) or X-ray films (not just written reports or summaries) that must be included in addition to making a general request for your records. It's also a good idea to indicate the date of your appointment so the office staff can respond in a timely manner.

Although state laws require the timely release of medical records, hospital medical records departments and doctors' offices often take several weeks to pull and review patient charts and get them in the mail either to you or to another doctor. In addition to written authorization, you may be asked to pay the costs involved in copying your records, test results and X-ray films because many doctors' offices will not release the originals. Consider placing a call in advance to determine the procedure for releasing your records, how long you can expect it to take and the costs involved so that you can save time by including payment with your release authorization letter. Be sure to allow sufficient time in advance of your consultation appointment for your request to be processed. Since you often must wait several weeks for an appointment with a specialist, allow at least that amount of time to obtain your records.

Even after making your written requests, you should follow up each letter with a telephone call to be sure that your records actually are sent. You should not assume that your request for records will be promptly fulfilled by an often overburdened, although well-intentioned, office staff.

Remember, the more information the specialist has about your condition, the fewer repeat or additional tests or procedures you will need to undergo, the lower the costs of your consultation and, most important, the more expeditiously the specialist will be able to render an opinion.

The Facts And Only The Facts

Be thorough and organized in documenting your personal and familial medical histories, the medications you take and in relaying information about your condition. Even seemingly minor bits of information may provide subtle clues to the nature of your medical problem and the optimal way in which to treat it. It's also advisable to bring a list with you of names, addresses and telephone numbers of all physicians who have cared for you, especially those you have seen regarding your current medical problem.

Even though thoroughness is essential to presenting a clear picture of your medical condition, bear in mind that the specialist needs to get to your core health concerns as quickly as possible. Therefore, if you have a complex medical history, you may want to ask your current doctors to provide treatment summaries in addition to copies of your medical records. Hospital records should include your admission history and physical exam, dictated consultation and operation notes and discharge summaries for all hospitalizations. You may also be able to get a cumulative lab and X-ray summary for your hospital stays.

Unlike X-rays, which can be copied at reasonable cost, original pathology slides must be transported by mail or hand-carried. Your specialist may wish to have the pathologist with whom he/she works speak directly with the pathologist who initially interpreted your slides as part of the process of evaluating your case.

Being Prepared

You are likely to be a bit nervous when you meet with the specialist you have chosen. Anxiety about your health and concern about your future care may cause you to forget information you should provide or miss hearing or understanding important information that the specialist communicates. Therefore, you may want to write down all relevant information so that you do not leave out anything of importance when you meet with the specialist or complete forms in the office. You also may want to write out your questions in advance so you don't forget anything.

To avoid leaving out important details of your condition or past treatment, prepare a concise, chronological summary before your consultation takes place. You may wish to type it and provide a copy to the specialist for inclusion in your chart. Highlight major medical results or significant events in the course of an illness or treatment if these will enlighten the doctor about your condition. Your personal perspective on the state of your health is vital to a full understanding of your medical problem.

It is possible that the specialist will use language that you do not understand or may speak quickly assuming certain knowledge on your part about your condition or its treatment. Don't hesitate to ask for clarification as often or repeatedly as you may need to in order to fully comprehend what you are being told. If you are concerned that you may forget what the doctor tells you, ask the doctor's permission to take notes or ask if you might bring along a tape recorder so you can later replay what was said, especially any instructions you are given. You may prefer to bring along a relative or close friend to serve as a "second set of ears," but, again, seek the doctor's permission to do so in advance of your appointment.

Following this process will assure that you and the specialist you are consulting get the most from your appointment. After all, you both have the same goal: restoring you to optimal health and well being.

What To Do If You Can't Get An Appointment

At times it may be difficult, perhaps even impossible, to secure an appointment with the specific specialist you have identified. There are a number of reasons why this may occur. For example, the specialist may not be taking any new patients or may have such a busy schedule that it takes several weeks or months to get an appointment. He/she may only see patients during very limited hours because of teaching, research or other responsibilities or currently may have other limitations related to the acceptance of new patients.

However, bear in mind that the doctors in this guide are the leaders in their specialties and therefore they work with and train the very best and brightest in their specialties. So, if you are unable to consult with a particular doctor, consider making an appointment with one of his/her outstanding colleagues. You can do this by asking a member of the doctor's office staff to refer you to an associate who is a member of the practice group or to another excellent physician who is specially trained to address your particular medical issue.

You can be comfortable knowing that you will receive high quality care from another specialist who practices in the same top setting.

Utilizing Special Resources

The following information on special resources has been included to meet the needs of healthcare consumers who have extraordinarily difficult or unique health problems, and have been unable to identify the resources to address their problems. These patients and their doctors may need to search for very new, cutting-edge, perhaps even experimental and not yet approved therapies. In such cases the search may lead to clinical trials; tests of new drugs and new medical devices or innovative therapeutic approaches. Fortunately, these situations are rare, but when they do occur, they are critical.

In addition to the outstanding private and public hospitals recognized in this guide, the U.S. government maintains its own unique, expert source of patient care and clinical research at the National Institutes of Health (NIH). In fact, the NIH operates its own hospital at which the care provided is usually related to clinical studies its researchers are undertaking.

In addition to those at the NIH, clinical trials also are conducted at leading medical centers and other organizations throughout the country. These facilities may be testing a new drug therapy, a new use for an existing medication or a medical device to deal with a problem that is not being resolved through the use of more traditional approaches.

This section will guide you in utilizing these special resources.

The Clinical Trial As A Treatment Option

For some patients the best medical treatment may only be available through clinical trials (also called treatment studies), which are designed to develop improved ways to use current medical treatments or to find new medical treatments by studying their effects on humans. Treatments are studied to determine if they are safe, effective and better treatments than conventional or standard therapies. Only if they meet all three of these criteria are they made available to the general public.

Many people are frightened by the term "clinical trial" because it conveys the notion of being a "guinea pig" in an experiment. Contrary to popular belief, however, most new treatments are extensively studied by scientists in the laboratory before they are ever tested by physicians in clinical settings. Among the factors that keep patients from participating in clinical trials are: lack of awareness about clinical trials as a treatment option; fear of side effects or adverse reactions to treatment; refusal of insurance companies to pay for experimental treatments; failure of a physician to inform the patient about clinical trials; difficulty finding suitable clinical trials; unavailability of clinical trials for certain medical problems; distance of the patient from major medical centers conducting clinical trials; disruption of personal and family life; and the decision to stop medical treatment altogether.

Despite these and other obstacles, many people do seek out clinical trials. One of the most pressing reasons to participate is the opportunity to obtain treatment that might not be available otherwise. New medical treatments can offer participants hope for a cure, an extended lifespan, or an improvement in how they feel. Some participants also take comfort in knowing that others may benefit from their contribution to medical knowledge.

Deciding if a clinical trial is the right treatment option for you is no simple matter. Certainly, you will want to talk about it with your doctor(s) and other professionals involved in your care, as well as with family members and friends. But in order to fully benefit from what others have to say — based on either their professional knowledge or personal experience — you need to understand exactly what a clinical trial is and what your role as a volunteer will be.

Understanding Clinical Trials

Clinical trials are conducted for just about every medical condition, including life-threatening diseases such as AIDS or cancer; chronic illnesses such as diabetes and asthma; psychiatric disorders such as depression or anxiety; behavioral problems such as smoking and substance abuse; and even common ailments such as hair loss and acne. Chances are, there is at least one trial (and probably more) that may be appropriate for you.

With more than 100 different types of cancer, it is understandable that a large number of clinical trials are cancer-related. Extensive information about clinical trials for cancer can be found on www.cancer.gov, the Web site of the National Cancer Institute (NCI). NCI is part of the NIH. CenterWatch, an online clinical trials listing service, identifies over 14,000 clinical trials that are actively recruiting patients. Veritas Medicine, another useful online organization, allows individuals to perform personalized searches of its clinical trials database. See Appendix D for "Selected Resources" for more information on clinical trials.

Most clinical trials study new medical treatments, combinations of treatments, or improvements in conventional treatments using drugs, surgery and other medical procedures, medical devices, radiation or other therapies. Newer types of clinical trials, called screening or prevention trials, study how to prevent the incidence or recurrence of disease through the use of medicines, vitamins, minerals or other supplements; and how to screen for disease, especially in its early stages. Another type of trial studies how to improve the quality of life for patients, including both their physical and emotional well-being.

Clinical trials are sponsored both by the federal government (through the National Institutes of Health, the National Cancer Institute and many others) and by private industry through pharmaceutical and biotechnology companies, and through healthcare institutions (hospitals or health maintenance organizations) and community-based physician-investigators. The National Cancer Institute sponsors clinical trials at more than 1000 sites in the United States. Trials are carried out in major medical research centers such as teaching hospitals as well as in community hospitals, specialized medical clinics (for example, those for the treatment of AIDS or Alzheimer's disease) and in doctors' offices.

Though clinical trials often involve hospitalized patients, a fair number of trials are conducted on an outpatient basis. Many trials are part of a cooperative network which may include as few as one or two sites or hundreds of locations, although one center generally assumes responsibility for overall coordination of the research. More than 45 research-oriented institutions, recognized for their scientific excellence, have been designated by the NCI as comprehensive or clinical cancer centers. See Appendix D "Selected Resources" to find out how to locate these centers.

Clinical research is based on a protocol (established rules or procedures) describing who will be studied, how and when medications, procedures and/or treatments will be administered and how long the study will last. Trials that are conducted simultaneously at different sites use the same protocol to ensure that all patients are treated identically and all data are collected uniformly so that study findings can be compared.

Clinical trials generally are conducted in three phases, as outlined in the study protocol. The first phase begins testing of the treatment on a small group of human subjects after rigorous and successful animal testing has been concluded. The interim phase varies, but usually involves a broader test group and is designed to further evaluate the treatment's safety and more accurately determine appropriate dosage, application methods and side effects. In some trials there may be a fourth phase, conducted after the treatment is in widespread use, to monitor the results of long-term use and the occurrence of any serious side effects.

Some clinical trials test one treatment on one group of subjects, while others compare two or more groups of subjects. In such comparison studies participants are divided into two groups: the control group that receives the standard treatment and the experimental or treatment group which receives the new treatment. For example, the control group may undergo a surgical procedure while the experimental or treatment group undergoes a surgical procedure plus radiation to determine which treatment modality is more effective. To ensure that patient characteristics do not unduly influence the study findings, patients may be randomly assigned to either the control or the experimental group, meaning that each patient's assignment is based purely on chance. In cases in which a standard treatment does not exist for a particular disease, the experimental group of patients receives the new treatment and the control group receives no treatment at all, or receives a placebo, an inactive medicine or procedure that has no treatment value and is sometimes called a "dummy" pill or a "sugar" pill. It is important to keep in mind that patients are never put into a control group without any treatment if there is a known treatment that could help them. Also, whether a patient is receiving an investigational drug or a placebo, he/she receives the same level and quality of medical care as those receiving the investigational treatment.

Questions to ask your doctor and the trial's research team if you are considering participating in a clinical trial:

- Who is sponsoring the trial?

- How many patients will be involved?

- Will the trial be testing a single treatment or a combination of treatments?

- Will there be one treatment group or more than one treatment group?

- If more than one treatment group, how are patients assigned to each group?

- Has this treatment been studied in previous clinical trials? What were the findings?

Protecting the Rights of Participants

The safety of those who participate in clinical trials is a serious matter and is the number one priority of medical investigators. All clinical research, regardless of type of sponsorship, is guided by the same ethical and legal codes that govern the medical profession and the practice of medicine. Most clinical research is federally funded or federally regulated (at least in part) with built-in safeguards for patients. According to federal government regulations (and some state laws), every clinical trial in the United States must be approved and monitored by an Institutional Review Board (IRB), which is an independent committee of physicians, statisticians, community advocates and others (representing at least five distinct disciplines) to ensure that the protocol is being followed.

Government regulations require researchers to fully inform participants about all aspects of a clinical trial before they agree to participate through a process called informed consent. To be sure that you understand your role in a clinical trial, you should jot down any questions beforehand so as not to forget them. You should also consider bringing along a friend or family member for support and additional input, and perhaps even tape recording the conversation (after asking permission to do so) to make sure you do not forget or misunderstand anything. Each participant in a clinical trial must be given a written consent form, which should be available in English and other languages. The consent form explains the following:

- Why the research is being done.

- What the researchers hope to accomplish.

- What types of treatment interventions (and other tests or procedures) will be performed.

- How long the study will continue.

- What the expected benefits and the possible risks are.

- What other treatments are available.

- What costs will be covered by the study, by the patient or by third-party payers such as Medicare, Medicaid or private insurance.

Patients also are informed that they may leave the trial, or exclude themselves from any part of it, at any time. Informed consent means exactly what the term implies: you agree to join a clinical trial only after you completely understand exactly what your participation will involve for the duration of the study. By law, each patient must be provided with a copy of the signed consent form, which also must include the name and telephone number of a contact person for questions or additional information. Informed consent is a continuous process, so do not hesitate to ask questions before, during or after the trial.

The investigators must protect the privacy of each participant in a clinical trial by ensuring that all medical records are kept confidential except for inspection by the sponsoring agency, the Food and Drug Administration and other agencies involved in regulating the drug or treatment, and all data are collected anonymously by assigning a numeric code or initials to each individual.

During the course of the trial, participants are regularly seen by members of the research team to monitor their health and well-being. Participants also should be responsible for their own health by following the treatment plan (such as taking the proper dosage of medications on time), keeping all scheduled visits and informing members of the healthcare team about any symptoms that occur. If during the course of the trial, the treatment proves to be ineffective or harmful, the patient is free to leave the study and still obtain conventional care. Conversely, as soon as there is evidence that one treatment modality is better than another, all patients in the trial are given the benefit of the new information.

Questions to ask the sponsors about your rights as a participant in a clinical trial:

- Who is responsible for approving and monitoring this research? Is there an IRB?

- Who informs me about the trial process? Do I sign a consent form? Will I receive a copy?

- May I leave the trial at any time? Have previous patients dropped out? Why?

- Whom do I contact if I am experiencing any difficulty with this trial?

Enrolling In Clinical Trials

Each clinical trial has its own guidelines, called eligibility criteria, for determining who can participate. Treatment studies recruit participants who have a disease or other medical condition, while screening and prevention studies generally recruit healthy volunteers. Inclusion criteria (those that allow you to participate in a study) and exclusion criteria (those that keep you from participating in a study) ensure that the study will answer the research questions posed in the research protocol while maintaining the safety of participants. The disease being studied is a primary factor in selecting suitable patients, but other factors such as the patient's gender, age, treatment history and other diagnosed medical conditions may also be important. Unfortunately, eligibility also may depend upon ability to pay. Many health plans do not cover all of the costs associated with clinical trials because they define these trials as experimental procedures. However, trials sometimes pay volunteers for their time and/or reimburse them for travel, childcare, meals and lodging.

To prevent people who qualify from being excluded from clinical trials for financial reasons, agencies such as the National Cancer Institute are working with health plans to find solutions and a growing number of states require insurance companies to pay for all routine patient care costs in cancer trials. To encourage more senior citizens to participate in cancer trials, Medicare plans to revise its payment policy to cover those trials.

When choosing a clinical trial you should determine the factors that are most important to you. For instance, patients generally prefer to participate in trials near their homes so that they can maintain their usual day-to-day activities, be surrounded by family and friends and avoid travel and lodging costs. If travel or temporary relocation becomes necessary, try to find a trial site that is near to some family member or friend or one that is in a locale similar to your own city or town. Many organizations, such as the National Cancer Institute, will work with patients and their families to identify support networks for them wherever they participate.

Questions to ask the trial's sponsor about eligibility criteria:

- What are the inclusion and exclusion criteria for the clinical trial(s) I am considering?

- How can I improve my chances of being accepted?
  Can I change my health plan to one that will cover the trial's costs?
  Can I relocate to another city or state?

- If I am not eligible for one trial, what other trials are being conducted for my condition?

- Will I be paid for my time or reimbursed for my out-of-pocket expenses?

Participating In A Clinical Trial

Clinical trials are conducted by a research team led by a principal investigator (usually a physician) and are comprised of physicians, nurses and other health professionals such as social workers, psychologists and nutritionists. As a participant you may be required to commit a fair amount of time to a clinical trial, often more than with standard treatment. Initially, you will probably be given a physical examination and asked for your medical history. During the trial, you will have regular or periodic visits to the trial site which may include diagnostic and laboratory tests. You also may be asked to follow fixed schedules for medications and other interventions and to keep detailed records of your symptoms and health condition. Generally, clinical trials last from six to twenty-six weeks, though some (called maintenance trials) can last up to a year to determine if a treatment will prevent the relapse of a medical condition.

Participants in clinical trials should remain under the care of their regular physician(s) since clinical trials tend to provide short-term treatment for a specific medical condition and do not generally provide comprehensive primary care. In fact, some trials require that a patient's regular physician sign a consent form before the patient is enrolled. In addition, your regular physician can collaborate with the research team to make sure there are no adverse reactions between your other medications or treatments and the investigational treatment.

Questions to ask the research team or your physician about your role in a clinical trial:

- Who are the members of the health team?
  Who will be in charge of my care?

- How long will the trial last?

- How does treatment in the trial compare with or differ from the standard treatment?

- Will I be hospitalized? How often? For how long a period of time?

- What will occur during each visit?
  What treatments or procedures will I be given?

- Will I still be able to see my regular physician(s)?
  Will my doctor and the research team collaborate?

- Can I be put in touch with other patients who have participated in this trial?

Weighing The Benefits And Risks Of A Clinical Trial

If you are considering participation in a clinical trial, you need to consider the medical, emotional and financial ramifications of participation. Of course, the obvious benefit of a clinical trial is the chance that a new treatment may improve your health and prognosis. You will have access to drugs and other medical interventions before they are widely available to the public and you will obtain expert and specialized medical care at leading healthcare facilities. Many patients receive an added psychological benefit by taking an active role in their treatment.

It is important to bear in mind that some medical interventions used in clinical trials may carry potential risks depending upon the type of treatment and the patient's condition. While many side effects or adverse reactions are temporary (such as hair loss and nausea caused by some anti-cancer drugs), other more serious reactions can be permanent and even life-threatening (for example, heart, liver or kidney damage).

Deciding whether or not to participate in a clinical trial is often a matter of determining if the trial's potential benefits outweigh its possible risks. This is a highly personal decision that may be difficult to make in situations involving experimental treatment in which limited medical information may be available.

Questions to ask the research team about the benefits and risks of a clinical trial:

- What other treatment option(s) do I have at this time?
  Is there any chance that a more promising treatment may be available soon?

- What are the short and long-term benefits and risks as compared with standard treatment?

- Will I experience any known side effects or adverse reactions?
  Will these be temporary, long-term or permanent?
  Relatively minor or perhaps life-threatening?

- If I am harmed in any way by the new treatment, what other treatments will I be entitled to?
  Who will pay for subsequent treatment?

Getting Information On Clinical Trials

The more information you have about a clinical trial, the easier it will be to make a decision about whether or not it is right for you, and the more confident you will be that you made an appropriate decision. In addition to the "Selected Resources" appendix in this guide, the staff at your local public library, community hospital, or major medical center can assist you in locating the information you need from books, consumer organizations and on the Internet.

Learning About The National Institutes Of Health(NIH)

The National Institutes of Health (NIH) comprise one of the world's leading medical research centers and the Federal government's principal agency for biomedical research. An agency of the United States Department of Health, United States Public Health Service, NIH encompasses 25 separate institutions and centers with its main campus located in Bethesda, Maryland. Research is also conducted at several field units across the country and abroad.

Patient Care At The NIH

The Warren Grant Magnuson Clinical Center, NIH's principal medical research center and hospital located in Bethesda, Maryland, provides medical care only to patients participating in clinical research programs. Two categories of patients participate in the Clinical Center studies: children and adults who wish to improve their own health, such as those with newly diagnosed medical problems, ongoing medical problems or family history of disease; and healthy volunteers wishing to advance knowledge about the causes, progress and treatment of disease. The patient's case must fit into an ongoing NIH research project for which the patient has the precise kind or stage of illness under investigation. General diagnostic and treatment services common to community hospitals are not available.

The Magnuson Clinical Center is the world's largest biomedical research hospital and ambulatory care facility, housing 1,600 laboratories conducting basic and clinical research. There are 1,200 tenured physicians, dentists and researchers on staff along with 660 nurses and 570 allied healthcare professionals (dieticians, imaging technologists, medical technologists, medical records and clerical staff, pharmacists and therapists).

The Center's hospital is specially designed for medical research and accommodates 540 carefully selected patients who are participating in clinical research programs. Its 350-bed facility has 24 inpatient care units to which 7,000 patients are admitted annually. The Center also has an Ambulatory Care Research Facility (ACRF) that serves 68,000 outpatient visits each year. A new facility, called the Mark O. Hatfield Clinical Research Center, which began accepting patients in early 2005, has 242 beds for inpatient care and 90 day-hospital stations for outpatient care. The Mark O. Hatfield Center carries out the latest biomedical research that results in new forms of disease diagnosis, prevention and treatment, which is then incorporated into improved methods of patient care.

This is a fine example of Translational Medicine where excellent research discoveries are translated into new and improved methods of clinical treatment. In other words, the laboratory discoveries are brought to the bedside.

The Clinical Center also maintains a Children's Inn for pediatric outpatients and their families. This family-centered residence operates 24 hours a day, 7 days a week, 365 days a year.

In an effort to bring clinical research to the community, NIH supports approximately 80 General Clinical Research Centers (GCRCs) around the country, located within hospitals of major academic medical centers.

It is important to note that, as part of the federal government, the Warren Grant Magnuson Clinical Center provides treatment in clinical trials at no cost to its patients. In some cases, patients receive a stipend to help cover the costs of traveling to Bethesda for treatment and follow-up care. Travel costs for the initial screening visit, however, are not covered.

Areas Of Clinical Study At The NIH

At the Magnuson Clinical Center alone, NIH physician-scientists conduct nearly 1,000 studies each year. Among the areas of study are cancer and related diseases.

Not all of these clinical areas are under investigation at any given time, however. The Patient Recruitment and Public Liaison Office (PRPL) at the NIH Clinical Center assists patients, their families and their physicians in obtaining information about participation in NIH clinical trials. Trained nurses are available to answer questions about the research programs and admission procedures.

Cancer Care At The Warren Grant Magnuson Clinical Center

The National Cancer Institute (NCI) is the largest of the biomedical research institutes and centers at NIH. There, clinical studies are designed to evaluate new and promising ways to prevent, detect, diagnose and treat cancer. The Warren Grant Magnuson Clinical Center provides a separate outpatient division for cancer patients and also has several designated inpatient units.

If you are interested in entering a cancer study at the Magnuson Clinical Center (or at the General Clinical Research Centers), you should first discuss treatment options with a physician. As a general rule, patients interested in participating in clinical studies must be referred by a physician. However, in some instances, self-referral may be permitted.

Patients with medical problems other than cancer or healthy volunteers who wish to participate in a clinical study should contact the particular NIH institute responsible for the clinical area involved.

Cancer Care At The NCI Clinical Centers And Comprehensive Cancer Centers

You may also obtain clinical oncology services (education, screening, diagnosis or treatment) or participate in clinical trials at one of the 22 Cancer Centers or 39 Comprehensive Cancer Centers designated by the NCI for their scientific excellence and extensive resources devoted to cancer and cancer-related problems. Centers are located in 32 states, with the majority of sites in California, New York and Pennsylvania. You can find out about clinical trials at the NCI-designated centers by contacting NCI's Clinical Studies Support Center (CSSC) or by calling each center directly. Information about other cancer-related services at these centers also may be obtained from the center itself. For more information, you can visit the National Cancer Institute's website at www.cancer.gov.

How To Use This Guide

Locating A Specialist

This guide is organized to make finding the right specialists for you or your loved ones as simple as possible. Physicians' biographies are presented by specialty and are organized by geographic region within each specialty or subspecialty. Thus, you may search for a particular type of specialist or subspecialist in one or more regions or throughout the nation.

A second way to locate the right specialist is to use the "**Special Expertise Index**" beginning on page 1163. This index is organized according to diseases, conditions and procedures or techniques. For example, you can locate a top specialist for diabetes or for Mohs' surgery by looking for those terms in the "**Special Expertise Index**."

If you already know a specialist's name, you can find his/her listing by using the "**Alphabetical Listing of Doctors**" beginning on page 1249.

SAMPLE PHYSICIAN LISTING

Smith, John MD [Ped] - **Spec Exp:** Asthma Allergy; **Hospital:** Children's Hosp (page 120);
Name [Specialty]   Special Expertise(s)   Admitting Hospital & Hospital
                                                      Information Page

Address: 300 Ridge Road Boston, MA 12345; **Phone:** (617) 555-2343; **Board Cert:** Ped 75;
Office Address   Office Phone   Board Certification(s)

Med School: Harvard Med Sch 70; **Resid:** Ped, Children's Hosp 73;
Medical School   Residency(ies)

Fellow: AM, Children's Hosp 74; **Fac Appt:** Assoc Prof Ped, The Med Sch
Fellowship(s)   Faculty Appointment

Geographic Regions And States

To assist you in using Castle Connolly *America's Top Doctors*® in the most efficient and effective manner, the Guide is divided into seven geographic regions. This will help you to locate a specialist in your local or neighboring region. For example, if you live in Mississippi in the Southeast region and you are willing and able to travel to Louisiana in the Southwest region to consult with a specialist in neurology, you can review just those two regions, under the section headed "NEUROLOGY." However, if you prefer to review the information on neurologists throughout the country, you can search the entire neurology section. Or, you can consult the "SPECIAL EXPERTISE INDEX" in the back of this Guide and choose a neurologist who has specific expertise to meet your particular needs.

The geographic regions are as follows:

New England

Mid Atlantic

Southeast

Midwest

Great Plains and Mountains

Southwest

West Coast and Pacific

The states that are included in each region are listed on the following page and a map of the regions is also provided. Please note that not all regions are represented in all specialties. For example, in "Geriatric Psychiatry" there are no listings in the Southwest region.

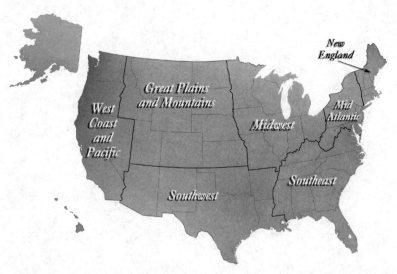

West Coast and Pacific:
Alaska
California
Hawaii
Nevada
Oregon
Washington

Great Plains and Mountains:
Colorado
Idaho
Kansas
Montana
Nebraska
North Dakota
South Dakota
Utah
Wyoming

Southwest:
Arizona
Arkansas
Louisiana
New Mexico
Oklahoma
Texas

Midwest:
Illinois
Indiana
Iowa
Michigan
Minnesota
Missouri
Ohio
Wisconsin

New England:
Connecticut
Maine
Massachusetts
New Hampshire
Rhode Island
Vermont

Mid Atlantic:
Delaware
Maryland
New Jersey
New York
Pennsylvania
Washington, DC
West Virginia

Southeast:
Alabama
Florida
Georgia
Kentucky
Mississippi
North Carolina
South Carolina
Tennessee
Virginia

Medical Specialties

In the pages that follow, each list of doctors in a medical specialty or subspecialty is preceded by a brief description of that specialty (or subspecialty) and the training required for board certification.

Critical Care Medicine has been excluded because in emergency situations there is neither time nor opportunity for choice. A number of other specialities not relevant to most patients (e.g., Forensic Psychiatry) have not been included as well.

The following descriptions of medical specialties and subspecialties were provided by the American Board of Medical Specialties (ABMS), an organization comprised of the 24 medical specialty boards that provide certification in 25 medical specialties. A complete listing of all specialists certified by the ABMS can be found in *The Official ABMS Directory of Board Certified Medical Specialists*, and is published by *Marquis Who's Who*. It is available (either in a multi-volume directory or on CD-ROM) in most public libraries, hospital libraries, university libraries and medical libraries. The ABMS also operates a toll-free phone line at 1-866-275-2267 and a website at www.abms.org to verify the certification status of individual doctors.

The following important policy statement, approved by the ABMS Assembly on March 19, 1987, remains valid.

The Purpose Of Certification

The intent of the certification process, as defined by the member boards of the American Board of Medical Specialties, is to provide assurance to the public that a certified medical specialist has successfully completed an approved educational program and an evaluation, including an examination process designed to assess the knowledge, experience and skills requisite to the provision of high quality patient care in that specialty.

Medical Specialties

Medical Specialty and Subspecialty Descriptions and Abbreviations

The following medical specialties and subspecialties are indicated in the doctors' listings by their abbreviations. Specialties are indicated in bold, subspecialties in italics, and the four primary care specialties in bold capitals. To review the official American Board of Medical Specialties (ABMS) organization of specialties, refer to Appendix A.

Addiction Psychiatry   *AdP*

Deals with habitual psychological and physiological dependence on a substance or practice which is beyond voluntary control.

Adolescent Medicine   *AM*

Involves the primary care treatment of adolescents and young adults.

Allergy & Immunology   **A&I**

Diagnosis and treatment of allergies, asthma, and skin problems such as hives and contact dermatitis.

Anesthesiology   **Anes**

Provides pain relief in maintenance or restoration of a stable condition during and following an operation. Anesthesiologists also diagnose and treat acute and long standing pain problems.

Cardiac Electrophysiology (Clinical)   *CE*

Involves complicated technical procedures to evaluate heart rhythms and determine appropriate treatment for them.

Cardiovascular Disease   *Cv*

Involves the diagnosis and treatment of disorders of the heart, lungs, and blood vessels.

Child & Adolescent Psychiatry   *ChAP*

Deals with the diagnosis and treatment of mental diseases in children and adolescents.

Child Neurology   *ChiN*

Diagnosis and medical treatment of disorders of the brain, spinal cord, and nervous system in children.

Clinical Genetics   **CG**

Deals with identifying the genetic causes of inherited diseases and ailments and preventing, when possible, their occurrence.

Colon and Rectal Surgery   **CRS**

Surgical treatment of diseases of the intestinal tract, colon and rectum, anal canal, and perianal area.

Critical Care Medicine   *CCM*

Involves diagnosing and taking immediate action to prevent death or further injury of a patient. Examples of critical injuries include shock, heart attack, drug overdose, and massive bleeding.

Dermatology   **D**

Diagnosis and treatment of benign and malignant disorders of the skin, mouth, external genitalia, hair and nails, as well as a number of sexually transmitted diseases.

Diagnostic Radiology   *DR*

Involves the study of all modalities of radiant energy in medical diagnoses and therapeutic procedures utilizing radiologic guidance.

Endocrinology, Diabetes & Metabolism   *EDM*

Involves the study and treatment of patients suffering from hormonal and chemical disorders.

FAMILY MEDICINE   **FP**

Deals with and oversees the total healthcare of individual patients and their family members. Family practitioners are more common in rural areas and may perform procedures more commonly performed by specialists (e.g., minor surgery).

Forensic Psychiatry   *FPsy*

Concerns the evaluation of certain diagnostic groups of patients that include those with sexual disorders, antisocial personality disorders, paranoid disorders, and addictive disorders.

Gastroenterology   *Ge*

The study, diagnosis and treatment of diseases of the digestive organs including the stomach, bowels, liver, and gallbladder.

Geriatric Medicine   *Ger*

Deals with diseases of the elderly and the problems associated with aging.

Geriatric Psychiatry   *GerPsy*

Involves the diagnosis, prevention, and treatment of mental illness in the elderly.

Gynecologic Oncology   *GO*

Deals with cancers of the female genital tract and reproductive systems.

Hand Surgery   *HS*

Involves the treatment of injury to the hand through surgical techniques.

Hematology   *Hem*

Involves the diagnosis and treatment of diseases and disorders of the blood, bone marrow, spleen, and lymph glands.

Infectious Disease   *Inf*

The study and treatment of diseases caused by a bacterium, virus, fungus, or animal parasite.

INTERNAL MEDICINE   **IM**

Diagnosis and nonsurgical treatment of diseases, especially those of adults. Internists may act as primary care specialists, highly trained family doctors, or they may subspecialize in specialties such as cardiology or nephrology.

Maternal & Fetal Medicine   *MF*

Involves the care of women with high-risk pregnancies and their unborn fetuses.

Medical Specialties

Medical Oncology   *Onc*

Refers to the study and treatment of tumors and other cancers.

Neonatal-Perinatal Medicine   *NP*

Involves the diagnosis and treatments of infants prior to, during, and one month beyond birth.

Nephrology   *Nep*

Concerned with disorders of the kidneys, high blood pressure, fluid and mineral balance, dialysis of body wastes when the kidneys do not function, and consultation with surgeons about kidney transplantation.

Neurological Surgery   **NS**

Involves surgery of the brain, spinal cord, and nervous system.

Neurology   **N**

Diagnosis and medical treatment of disorders of the brain, spinal cord, and nervous system.

Neuroradiology   *NRad*

Involves the utilization of imaging procedures during diagnosis as they relate to the brain, spine and spinal cord, head, neck, and organs of special sense in adults and children.

Nuclear Medicine   **NuM**

Evaluation of the functions of all the organs in the body and treatment of thyroid disease, benign and malignant tumors, and radiation exposure through the use of radioactive substances.

Nuclear Radiology   *NR*

Involves the use of radioactive substances to diagnose and treat certain functions and diseases of the body.

OBSTETRICS & GYNECOLOGY   **ObG**

Deals with the medical aspects of and intervention in pregnancy and labor and the overall health of the female reproductive system.

Occupational Medicine   *OM*

Concentrates on the effect of the work environment on the health of employees.

Ophthalmology   **Oph**

Diagnosis and treatment of diseases of and injuries to the eye.

Orthopaedic Surgery   **OrS**

Involves operations to correct injuries which interfere with the form and function of the extremities, spine, and associated structures.

Otolaryngology   **Oto**

Explores and treats diseases in the interrelated areas of the ears, nose and throat.

Otology/Neurotology   *ON*

Concentrates on the management, prevention, cure and care of patients with diseases of the ear and temporal bone, including disorders of hearing and balance.

Pain Medicine   PM

Involves providing a high level of care for patients experiencing problems with acute or chronic pain in both hospital and ambulatory settings.

Pediatric Cardiology   PCd

Involves the diagnosis and treatment of heart disease in children.

Pediatric Critical Care Medicine   PCCM

Involves the care of children who are victims of life threatening disorders such as severe accidents, shock, and diabetes acidosis.

Pediatric Dermatology   PD

Diagnosis and treatment of benign and malignant disorders of the skin, mouth, external genitalia, hair and nails in children.

Pediatric Endocrinology   PEn

Involves the study and treatment of children with hormonal and chemical disorders.

Pediatric Gastroenterology   PGe

The study, diagnosis, and treatment of diseases of the digestive tract in children.

Pediatric Hematology-Oncology   PHO

The study and treatment of cancers of the blood and blood-forming parts of the body in children.

Pediatric Infectious Disease   PInf

The study and treatment of diseases caused by a virus, bacterium, fungus, or animal parasite in children.

Pediatric Nephrology   PNep

Deals with the diagnosis and treatment of disorders of the kidneys in children.

Pediatric Otolaryngology   POto

Involves the diagnosis and treatment of disorders of the ear, nose, and throat which affect children.

Pediatric Pulmonology   PPul

Involves the diagnosis and treatment of diseases of the chest, lungs, and chest tissue in children.

Pediatric Radiology   PR

Involves diagnostic imaging as it pertains to the newborn, infant, child, and adolescent.

Pediatric Rheumatology   PRhu

Involves the treatment of diseases of the joints and connective tissues in children.

Pediatric Surgery   PS

Treatment of disease, injury, or deformity in children through surgical techniques.

PEDIATRICS   **Ped**

Diagnosis and treatment of diseases of childhood and monitoring of the growth, development, and well-being of preadolescents.

Physical Medicine & Rehabilitation   **PMR**

The use of physical therapy and physical agents such as water, heat, light electricity, and mechanical manipulations in the diagnosis, treatment, and prevention of disease and body disorders.

Plastic Surgery   **PlS**

Involves reconstructive and cosmetic surgery of the face and other body parts.

Preventive Medicine   **PrM**

A specialty focusing on the prevention of illness and on the health of groups rather than individuals.

Psychiatry   **Psyc**

Examination, treatment, and prevention of mental illness through the use of psychoanalysis and/or drugs.

Public Health & General Preventive Medicine   *PHGPM*

Involves the investigation of the causes of epidemic disease and the prevention of a wide variety of acute and chronic illness.

Pulmonary Disease   *Pul*

Involves the diagnosis and treatment of diseases of the chest, lungs, and airways.

Radiation Oncology   *RadRo*

Involves the use of radiant energy and isotopes in the study and treatment of disease, especially malignant cancer.

Reproductive Endocrinology   *RE*

Deals with the endocrine system (including the pituitary, thyroid, parathyroid, adrenal glands, placenta, ovaries, and testes) and how its failure relates to infertility.

Rheumatology   *Rhu*

Involves the treatment of diseases of the joints, muscles, bones and associated structures.

Sleep Medicine   *Sleep Med*

Involves the investigation and treatment of patients with sleep disorders.

Spinal Cord Injury Medicine   *SpCdInj*

Involves the prevention, diagnosis, treatment and management of traumatic spinal cord injuries.

Sports Medicine   *SM*

Refers to the practice of an orthopaedist or other physician who specializes in injuries to the bone or other soft tissues (muscles, tendons, ligaments) caused by participation in athletic activity.

Surgery   **S**

Treatment of disease, injury, and deformity by surgical procedures.

Surgery of the Hand   *SHd*

Involves providing appropriate care for all structures in the upper extremity directly affecting the hand and wrist function.

Surgical Critical Care   *SCC*

Involves specialized care in the management of the critically ill patient, particularly the trauma victim and postoperative patient in the emergency department, intensive care unit, trauma unit, burn unit, and other similar settings.

Thoracic Surgery (includes open heart surgery)   **TS**

Involves surgery on the heart, lungs, and chest area.

Urology   **U**

Diagnosis and treatment of diseases of the genitals in men and disorders of the urinary tract and bladder in both men and women.

Vascular & Interventional Radiology   *VIR*

Involves diagnosing and treating diseases by percutaneous methods guided by various radiologic imaging modalities.

Vascular Surgery   *VascS*

Involves the operative treatment of disorders of the blood vessels excluding those to the heart, lungs, or brain.

The Training Of A Specialist

Excerpted from "Which Medical Specialist For You?" American Board of Medical Specialties, Evanston, IL, Revised 2000

Everyone knows that a "medical doctor" is a physician who has had years of training to understand the diagnosis, treatment and prevention of disease. The basic training for a physician specialist includes four years of premedical education in a college or university, four years of medical school, and after receiving the M.D. degree, at least three years of specialty training under supervision (called a "residency"). Training in subspecialties can take an additional one to three years.

Some specialists are primary care doctors such as family physicians, general internists and general pediatricians. Other specialists concentrate on certain body systems, specific age groups, or complex scientific techniques developed to diagnose or treat certain types of disorders. Specialties in medicine developed because of the rapidly expanding body of knowledge about health and illness and the constantly evolving new treatment techniques for disease.

A subspecialist is a physician who has completed training in a general medical specialty and then takes additional training in a more specific area of that specialty called a subspecialty. This training increases the depth of knowledge and expertise of the specialist in that particular field. For example, cardiology is a subspecialty of internal medicine, pediatric surgery is a subspecialty of surgery and pediatrics, and child and adolescent psychiatry is a subspecialty of psychiatry. The training of a subspecialist within a specialty requires an additional one or more years of full-time education.

The training, or residency, of a specialist begins after the doctor has received the M.D. degree from a medical school. Resident physicians dedicate themselves for three to seven years to full-time experience in hospital and/or ambulatory care settings, caring for patients under the supervision of experienced specialists. Educational conferences and research experience are often part of that training. In years past, the first year of post-medical school training was called an internship, but is now called residency.

Licensure

The legal privilege to practice medicine is governed by state law and is not designed to recognize the knowledge and skills of a trained specialist. A physician is licensed to practice general medicine and surgery by a state board of medical examiners after passing a state or national licensure examination. Each state or territory has its own procedures to license physicians and sets the general standards for all physicians in that state or territory.

Who Credentials A Specialist And Subspecialist?

Specialty boards certify physicians as having met certain published standards. There are 24 specialty boards that are recognized by the American Board of Medical Specialties (ABMS) and the American Medical Association (AMA). All of the specialties and subspecialties recognized by the ABMS and the AMA are listed in the brief descriptions that follow. Remember, a subspecialist first must be trained and certified as a specialist.

In order to be certified as a medical specialist by one of these recognized boards a physician must complete certain requirements. Generally, these include:

1 Completion of a course of study leading to the M.D. or D.O. (Doctor of Osteopathy) degree from a recognized school of medicine.

2 Completion of three to seven years of full-time training in an accredited residency program designed to train specialists in the field.

3 Many specialty boards require assessments and documentation of individual performance from the residency training director, or from the chief of service in the hospital where the specialist has practiced.

4 All of the ABMS Member Boards require that a person seeking certification have an unrestricted license to practice medicine in order to take the certification examination.

5 Finally, each candidate for certification must pass a written examination given by the specialty board. Fifteen of the 24 specialty boards also require an oral examination conducted by senior specialists in that field. Candidates who have passed the exams and other requirements are then given the status of "Diplomate" and are certified as specialists. A similar process is followed for specialists who want to become subspecialists.

All of the ABMS Member Boards now, or will soon, issue only time-limited certificates which are valid for six to ten years. In order to retain certification, diplomates must become "recertified," and must periodically go through an additional process involving continuing education in the specialty, review of credentials and further examination. Boards that may not yet require recertification have provided voluntary recertification with similar requirements.

How To Determine If A Physician Is A Certified Specialist

Certified specialists are listed in *The Official ABMS Directory of Board Certified Medical Specialists* published by *Marquis Who's Who*. The ABMS Directory can be found in most public libraries, hospital libraries, university libraries and medical libraries, and is also available on CD-ROM. Alternatively, you could ask for that information from your county medical society, the American Board of Medical Specialties, or one of the specialty boards.

The ABMS operates a toll free number (1-866-275-2267) to verify the certification status of individual physicians. Additionally, information about the ABMS organization and links to an electronic directory of certified specialists can be accessed through the ABMS Web site at www.abms.org.

Almost all board certified specialists also are members of their medical specialty societies. These societies are dedicated to furthering standards, practice and professional and public education within individual medical specialties. Some, such as the American College of Surgeons and the American College of Obstetricians and Gynecologists, require board certification for full membership. A physician who has attained full membership is called a "Fellow" of the society and is entitled to use this designation in all formal communications such as certificates, publications, business cards, stationery and signage. Thus, "John Doe, M.D., F.A.C.S." (Fellow of the American College of Surgeons) is a board certified surgeon. Similarly, F.A.A.D. (Fellow of the American Academy of Dermatology) following the M.D. or D.O. in a physician's title would likely indicate board certification in that specialty.

The Partnership For Excellence Program

Among the more than 6,000 acute care and specialty hospitals in the United States, many have extraordinary capabilities for superior patient care. These hospitals, renowned for their use of state-of-the-art equipment and up-to-the-minute technology, also attract outstanding physicians and other healthcare professionals. Many of their physicians are among those in the listings in this Guide.

To assist you in your search for top specialists and to supplement the information contained in the physician listings that follow, we invited a select group of these fine institutions to profile their services, special programs and centers of excellence in the *Partnership for Excellence* program. This special section contains pages sponsored by the included hospitals. This paid sponsorship program is totally separate from the physician selection process, which is based upon nominations by physicians a completely independent review by our physician led research team.

The *Partnership for Excellence* program provides an overview of the programs and services offered by the included hospitals with information related to their accreditation and sponsorship. Most also provide their physician referral numbers, should you wish to ask the hospitals for recommendations of doctors not listed in Castle Connolly *America's Top Doctors®* 7th Edition.

In addition to the *Partnership for Excellence* program, profiled hospitals were also invited to highlight their special programs or services that focus on a particular disease or medical condition. These can be found in the "Centers of Excellence" sections that are interspersed throughout this book following the medical specialties and/or subspecialties to which they relate. Sponsored pages in the centers of excellence sections reflect the depth of commitment of these hospitals, which provide the staff, resources and financial support necessary to develop these special programs.

By visiting our website **www.AmericasTopDoctors.com**, you may also link to the websites of these outstanding hospitals for even more detailed information on their cancer programs. We believe you will find this informaton helpful in your search for the best healthcare—from both physicians and hospitals—through out the United States!

Participating Hospitals

- Bascom Palmer Eye Institute

- Childrens Hospital Los Angeles

- Cleveland Clinic

- Continuum Health Partners

- Fox Chase Cancer Center

- Hospital for Special Surgery

- The Johns Hopkins Hospital

- Lenox Hill Hospital

- Maimonides Medical Center

- Mount Sinai Medical Center

- New York Eye & Ear Infirmary

- New York-Presbyterian Hospital

- NYU Medical Center

- NYU Hospital for Joint Diseases

- Rusk Institute of Rehabilitation Medicine

- St. Francis Hospital -The Heart Center

- University of Pennsylvania Health System

- The University of Texas M.D. Anderson Cancer Center

- Wake Forest University Baptist Medical Center

Bascom Palmer

EYE INSTITUTE

University of Miami Miller School of Medicine
www.bascompalmer.org
(800) 329-7000

Miami	*Naples*	*Plantation*	*Palm Beach Gardens*
900 NW 17th Street	*311 9th Street North*	*1000 South Pine Island Road*	*7101 Fairway Drive*
Miami, FL 33136	*Naples, FL 34102*	*Plantation, FL.33324*	*Palm Beach Gardens, FL. 33418*
(305) 326-6000	*(239) 659-3937*	*(239) 659-3937*	*(561) 515-1500*
(800) 329-7000			

INTERNATIONALLY ACCLAIMED

Bascom Palmer Eye Institute is committed to the protection and preservation of the treasured gift of sight. The Institute's full-time faculty of internationally-respected physicians and scientists are skilled in every ophthalmic subspecialty. Bascom Palmer Eye Institute, which serves as the Department of Ophthalmology for the University of Miami Miller School of Medicine in Miami, Florida, is recognized as one of the world's finest and most progressive centers for ophthalmic care, research and education.

BASCOM PALMER EYE INSTITUTE EARNS TOP RATINGS

Bascom Palmer Eye Institute continues to be rated as one of the nation's best ophthalmic hospitals by board-certified ophthalmologists from across the United States. In 2004, 2005 and 2006 Bascom Palmer was named the #1 eye hospital in the United States by *U.S.News & World Report*. Bascom Palmer has also received the #1 ranking for its Clinical (Patient Care) and Residency programs by *Ophthalmology Times*, which annually ranks the top ophthalmology programs in the United States.

BASCOM PALMER RESEARCHERS ADVANCE OPHTHALMIC CARE AND TREATMENT

Consistent with its mission to resolve diseases and disorders of the eye, the physicians and scientists of Bascom Palmer Eye Institute develop new theories, therapeutic techniques and surgical instruments. Many of the Institute's innovations have advanced the course of ophthalmic practices worldwide, including:
• The first successful vitreous surgery – and invention of miniature surgical instrumentation required for this procedure.
• The identification of the herpes virus as the cause of acute retinal necrosis.
• The introduction of limbal cell transplantation therapy.
• The unraveling the mystery of normal tension glaucoma.
• Establishing predictive tests and new treatments for complicated retinal detachments.
• New, non-toxic treatments for ocular cancer.

Bascom Palmer Eye Institute ranked #1 in USA.

Bascom Palmer Eye Institute has four convenient Florida locations: In Miami, Palm Beach Gardens, Naples, and Plantation. Each of the Institute's 46 internationally respected clinical faculty members specialize in a specific area of ophthalmology and all are board-certified by the American Board of Ophthalmology. In addition to providing care to more than 200,000 patients annually, all physicians have research and teaching responsibilities at the University of Miami Miller School of Medicine.

TO SCHEDULE AN APPOINTMENT PLEASE CALL 1-888-845-0002

598

Childrens Hospital Los Angeles

4650 Sunset Boulevard
Los Angeles, California 90027
www.ChildrensHospitalLA.org

ChildrensHospitalLosAngeles

International Leader in Pediatrics

Founded in 1901, Childrens Hospital Los Angeles has been treating the most seriously ill and injured children in Los Angeles for more than a century. It is acknowledged throughout the United States and around the world for its leadership in pediatric and adolescent health.

Childrens Hospital Los Angeles treats more than 58,000 patients a year in its Emergency Department. It admits more than 11,000 children a year to the hospital. There are more than 285,000 visits a year to its 29 outpatient clinics and laboratories; more than 3,300 visits at community sites through its Division of Adolescent Medicine. Childrens Hospital Los Angeles is able to offer the optimum in multidisciplinary care, with 85 pediatric subspecialties and dozens of special services for children and families.

Training programs at Childrens Hospital Los Angeles include 274 medical students, 83 full-time residents and three chief residents and 73 fellows, who collectively reflect the diversity of the patient population and the city of Los Angeles. The RN Residency in Pediatrics is a six-month program that provides new nursing school graduates with a comprehensive guided clinical experience to prepare them for work in an acute care pediatric environment.

The Saban Research Institute of Childrens Hospital Los Angeles is among the largest and most productive pediatric research facilities in the United States, with 100 investigators engaged in 251 laboratory studies, clinical trials and community-based research and health services. It is one of the few freestanding research centers in the nation to combine scientific inquiry with patient care – dedicated exclusively to children and adolescents. Its decade of scientific inquiry has earned the respect of the National Institutes of Health (NIH) and the Centers for Disease Control and Prevention. Its base of knowledge is widely considered to be among the best in pediatric medicine.

Today, physician-scientists at Childrens Hospital Los Angeles are able to integrate their laboratory experience with their clinical expertise, to move effectively from "bench to bedside," addressing difficult medical questions others might never see or hear. It's these questions and, most importantly, their answers that can lead to changes in the standard of care for children, not only at Childrens Hospital, but also throughout pediatric medicine.

601

Cleveland Clinic

Hospital Overview

One of the largest and busiest health centers in America. Number one in heart care. National leaders in urology and digestive diseases. Treating all illnesses and disorders of the body. Second opinions a specialty.

General Overview

Founded in 1921, Cleveland Clinic is a 1,000-staffed-bed hospital that integrates clinical and hospital care with research and education in a private, non-profit group practice. This group practice model provides an environment that allows our physicians to stay at the cutting edge of medical technology. They pool their expertise and their wisdom for the benefit of the patient and the community.

Vital Statistics

In 2006, more than 1,700 full-time physicians and scientists, representing 120 medical specialties and subspecialties, provided for 3 million outpatient visits, 53,000 hospital admissions and 71,000 surgeries for patients from throughout the United States and more than 80 countries.

One of America's Best

In 2006, Cleveland Clinic was ranked one of the top 3 hospitals in America in the *U.S.News & World Report* annual "America's Best Hospitals" survey. In cardiology and cardiac surgery, we lead the nation. Our heart program has been ranked number one in America for 12 years in a row. Cleveland Clinic's Glickman Urological & Kidney Institute and Digestive Disease Center both are ranked second in the nation. Additional specialties rated among America's best include Cancer, Endocrinology, Gynecology, Nephrology, Neurology and Neurological Surgery, Ophthalmology, Orthopaedics, Otolaryngology, Pediatrics, Psychiatry, Pulmonary, Rehabilitation and Rheumatology.

Global Patient Services

Global Patient Services is a full-service department dedicated to meeting the needs of both our out-of-state and international patients. The National Center and the International Center, which make up Global Patient Services, provide personalized concierge programs and services to welcome patients and add to their comfort before, during and after their stay.

To schedule an appointment or for more information about Cleveland Clinic, call 800.890.2467 or visit www.clevelandclinic.org/topdocs.

Cleveland Clinic | 9500 Euclid Avenue / W14 | Cleveland OH 44195

"Better care of the sick, investigation of their problems and further education of those who serve."

"Patients first"

"Patients First" is the guiding principle of Cleveland Clinic. It declares the primacy of patient care, patient comfort and patient communication in every activity we undertake. It affirms the importance of research and education for their contributions to clinical medicine and the improvement of patient care. At the same time, "Patients First" demands a relentless focus on measurable quality. By setting standards, collecting data and analyzing the results, Cleveland Clinic puts patients first through improved outcomes and better service, providing a healthier future for all.

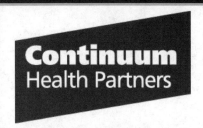

Continuum Health Partners

Phone (800) 420-4004
www.chpnyc.org

Sponsorship: Voluntary Not-for-Profit
Beds: 2,761 certified beds
Accreditation: Joint Commission of Accreditation of Healthcare Organizations (JCAHO). Accreditation
Council for Graduate Medical Education, Medical Society of New York, in conjunction with the
Accreditation Council for Continuing Medical Education

A STRONG PARTNERSHIP WITH A PROUD HERITAGE

Continuum Health Partners, Inc. is a partnership of five venerable health care providers, Beth Israel Medical Center, St. Luke's Hospital, Roosevelt Hospital, Long Island College Hospital, and the New York Eye and Ear Infirmary. Each of the five partner institutions was established more than a century ago by individuals committed to improving health and health care in their communities. Today, the system represents more than 4,000 physicians and dentists and is superbly equipped to respond to the health care needs of the populations we serve. Continuum providers also see patients in group and private practice settings and in ambulatory centers in New York City and Westchester County.

LOCATIONS

Continuum Health Partners has campuses throughout Manhattan and Brooklyn. Beth Israel Medical Center has two divisions: the Milton and Caroll Petrie Division on the East Side, and the Kings Highway Division in Brooklyn. The Phillips Ambulatory Care Center, a state-of-the-art outpatient center, is located at Union Square. St. Luke's Hospital is in Morningside Heights and Roosevelt Hospital is in the Columbus Circle and Lincoln Center neighborhoods on the West Side. Long Island College Hospital is located in the Brooklyn Heights/Cobble Hill section of Brooklyn. The New York Eye and Ear Infirmary is located on Second Avenue and 14th Street.

ACADEMIC AFFILIATIONS

Beth Israel Medical Center is the University Hospital and Manhattan Campus for the Albert Einstein College of Medicine. St. Luke's-Roosevelt Hospital Center is an academic affiliate of the Columbia University College of Physicians and Surgeons. Long Island College Hospital is the primary teaching affiliate of the SUNY-Health Science Center in Brooklyn. The New York Eye and Ear Infirmary is the primary teaching center of the New York Medical College and affiliated teaching hospitals in the areas of ophthalmology and otolaryngology.

Physician Referral For a referral to a doctor in your neighborhood, call (800) 420-4004. Continuum's Referral Service can help you find a primary care physician or specialist affiliated with Beth Israel, St. Luke's, Roosevelt, Long Island College Hospital, or the New York Eye and Ear Infirmary. **Visit our Website at www.chpnyc.org**

827

FOX CHASE
CANCER CENTER

333 Cottman Avenue
Philadelphia, PA 19111-2497
Phone: 1-888-FOX CHASE • Fax: 215-728-2702
www.fccc.edu

Sponsorship	Independent Nonprofit
Beds	100 licensed beds
Accreditation	The Joint Commission; American Hospital Association; American College of Surgeons Commission on Cancer; College of American Pathology; American College of Radiology

U.S. News & World Report has named Fox Chase Cancer Center the leading cancer center serving eastern Pennsylvania, New Jersey and Delaware and 16th in the entire nation. Fox Chase is also the first hospital in Pennsylvania and the nation's first cancer hospital to earn the Magnet Award for Nursing Excellence from the American Nurses Credentialing Center.

Overview

Fox Chase Cancer Center was founded in 1904 in Philadelphia as the nation's first cancer hospital. In 1974, Fox Chase became one of the first institutions designated as a National Cancer Institute Comprehensive Cancer Center. The mission of Fox Chase is to reduce the burden of human cancer through the highest-quality programs in basic, clinical, population and translational research; programs of prevention, detection and treatment of cancer; and community outreach.

- Fox Chase's 100-bed hospital is one of the few in the country devoted entirely to adult cancer care.
- Annual hospital admissions exceed 4,000 and outpatient visits to physicians total more than 68,700 a year.
- Fox Chase's board-certified specialists are recognized nationally and internationally in medical, radiation and surgical oncology, diagnostic imaging, diagnostic pathology, pain management, oncology nursing and oncology social work.
- The multidisciplinary staff provides a coordinated approach to meet the treatment needs of each patient. Special multidisciplinary centers provide consultations and treatment recommendations for specific types of cancer.
- The nursing staff of specially trained oncology nurses provides one of the best nurse-to-patient ratios in the area.
- Fox Chase investigators have received numerous awards and honors, including Nobel Prizes in medicine and chemistry; a Kyoto Prize, a Lasker Clinical Research Award, memberships in the National Academy of Sciences and General Motors Cancer Research Foundation Prizes.
- Fox Chase is a founding member of the National Comprehensive Cancer Network, an alliance of the nation's leading academic cancer centers, and the hub of Fox Chase Cancer Center Partners, which includes nearly 30 community cancer centers.

For more about Fox Chase physicians and services, visit our web site, www.fccc.edu, or call 1-888-FOX CHASE.

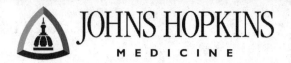

600 North Wolfe Street; Baltimore, MD 21287
www.hopkinsmedicine.org

JOHNS HOPKINS MEDICINE

Johns Hopkins Medicine unites physicians and scientists of The Johns Hopkins University School of Medicine with the organizations, health professionals and facilities of the Johns Hopkins Health System, including the world-renowned Johns Hopkins Hospital. All share a single mission: to improve the health of the community and the world by setting the standard of excellence in medical education, research and clinical care.

We heal. Ranked as America's top hospital year after year, The Johns Hopkins Hospital and its related facilities serve as beacons of hope for thousands of patients in our community, our nation and throughout the world.

We discover. Research is the foundation of clinical care. Hopkins physicians and researchers consistently receive more research grants from the National Institutes of Health than faculty at any other institution. Hopkins has been home to three Nobel laureates, 11 Lasker awardees, 12 National Academy of Sciences members and 32 members of the Institute of Medicine of the National Academy of Sciences.

We teach. The Johns Hopkins University School of Medicine educates and trains medical students, graduate students and postdoctoral fellows from around the world.

Our Centers of Excellence include:

Asthma & Allergy Center
Brady Urologic Institute
Children's Center
Sidney Kimmel Comprehensive Cancer Center
Comprehensive Transplant Center
Heart Institute
Institute of Basic Biomedical Sciences.
Solomon H. Snyder Department of Neuroscience
McKusick-Nathans Institute for Genetic Medicine
Wilmer Eye Institute

The Marburg Pavilion, a special group of patient rooms offering five-star hotel-like accommodations and amenities, is available at The Johns Hopkins Hospital. An executive physical program also is available that offers comprehensive and expedited examinations.

To find a physician (or make an appointment) at Johns Hopkins,
call: 410-955-5464 in Baltimore. For calls outside Baltimore, call 410-847-3582.
For calls outside the United States, call +01-410-847-3580.

855

Maimonides Medical Center

4802 Tenth Avenue • Brooklyn, New York 11219
Phone: (718) 283-6000
Physician Referral: 1-888 MMC DOCS
http://www.maimonidesmed.org

Sponsorship:	Voluntary, Not-for-Profit
Beds:	705 acute, 70 psychiatric
Accreditation:	The Joint Commission
	American College of Surgeons
	American Council of Graduate Medical Education (ACGME)

The nation's third largest independent teaching hospital, Maimonides Medical Center is a conductor of clinical trials for new treatments and therapies. Cited for overall clinical excellence by numerous healthcare report cards and evaluation services, Maimonides is a celebrated leader in the use of information technology to enhance patient care.

Centers of Excellence

Cancer Center

Provides comprehensive cancer services in a state-of-the-art facility. The Cancer Center at Maimonides utilizes the most advanced imaging technology and radiologic treatments for cancer patients.

Cardiac Institute

Renowned for its Catheterization Lab and pioneering new surgical procedures. The Institute includes an electrophysiology (EP) lab, two ICUs, Chest Pain Observation Unit, Advanced Cardiac Care Unit, and Congestive Heart Failure Program.

Stroke Center

One of only 40 Centers in the nation that provide interventional neuroradiology techniques to remove stroke-causing blood clots from the brain – without surgery – significantly reducing the debilitating effects of stroke.

Infants & Children's Hospital

Accredited by the National Association of Children's Hospitals and Related Institutions (NACHRI), Maimonides Infants and Children's Hospital includes Pediatric ICU, Neonatal ICU, Outpatient Pavilion, and Pediatric ER.

Vascular Institute

The world's top technology and advances in testing, surgery and medical care are offered at the Vascular Institute, which includes a Diagnostic Lab, Wound Center, Vascular Surgery Center and Vein Center.

Stella & Joseph Payson Birthing Center

Delivering the most babies in New York State, the Payson Birthing Center offers patients a home like setting with doulas and midwives, combined with advanced technology, including a perinatal testing center with 3-D ultrasound.

Geriatrics Program

Serving one of the oldest populations in New York City, the Maimonides Geriatrics Program includes outstanding inpatient and outpatient services, an ACE Unit (Acute Care for Elders) and home-visiting service.

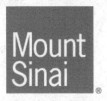

THE MOUNT SINAI MEDICAL CENTER

One Gustave L. Levy Place (Fifth Avenue and 100th Street)
New York, NY 10029
Physician Referral: 1-800-MD-SINAI
www.mountsinai.org

Sponsorship:	Voluntary Not-for-Profit
Beds:	1,171
Accreditation:	Joint Commission on Accreditation of Healthcare Organizations (JACHO), Commission for Accreditation of Rehabilitation Facilities (CARF), Magnet Award for Nursing Excellence

The Mount Sinai Medical Center, located on the Upper East Side in New York City, consists of The Mount Sinai Hospital, a tertiary and quaternary care facility known for excellence in patient care, and Mount Sinai School of Medicine, a leader in medical research and in the education of tomorrow's physicians by internationally known faculty. Founded in 1852, The Mount Sinai Hospital is one of the oldest voluntary teaching hospitals in the country. Today, the patients of Mount Sinai benefit as teams of physicians and scientists work together to rapidly translate laboratory research into new patient treatments. Many of the groundbreaking approaches that result from these collaborations are initially available at only a handful of facilities in the country —some, only at Mount Sinai. These advances make Mount Sinai the first choice for patients with complex medical and surgical needs.

Mount Sinai Heart, under the direction of Valentin Fuster, MD, PhD, combines all of Mount Sinai's world-class resources with innovative thinking, creative programs, and an unwavering commitment to the prevention and treatment of cardiovascular disease. Capitalizing upon the talent and expertise of internationally renowned Mount Sinai physicians David Adams, MD; Michael Marin, MD; Samin Sharma, MD, and a host of other highly regarded cardiac surgeons, interventionalists, and cardiologists, Mount Sinai Heart provides an integrated approach to clinical care utilizing basic and clinical research. With the rapid translation of innovative research concepts into improved preventive, diagnostic, and therapeutic care, patients receive multidisciplinary treatment of unprecedented quality.

The Multidisciplinary Head and Neck Cancer Center, under the leadership of Eric Genden, MD, FACS, provides each patient with a team of nationally recognized physicians and surgeons who work together to provide state-of-the-art curative management of tumors of the oral cavity, larynx, skull-base and thyroid gland.

The Recanati/Miller Transplantation Institute is recognized as a national leader in organ transplantation, and one the few institutes in the country to provide combined organ transplantation. Renowned for its long-term experience in the field, The Mount Sinai Hospital was the site of the first liver transplant in New York State.

Minimally Invasive Surgery at Mount Sinai continues to be at the forefront of providing advanced procedures using state-of-the-art instruments. We also provide specialized and unique expertise in the use of minimally invasive procedures in addition to traditional surgery options.

To find a Mount Sinai physician, surgeon, or specialist, please call
1-800-MD-SINAI or visit www.mountsinai.org
Both services are available 24 hours a day / 7 days a week

607

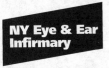

NY Eye & Ear Infirmary

Continuum Health Partners, Inc.

THE NEW YORK EYE AND EAR INFIRMARY

310 East 14th Street
New York, New York 10003
Tel. 212.979.4000   Fax. 212.228.0664
http://www.nyee.edu

BEDS:	34; Operating Rooms: 17; Surgical Cases: 20,000+ a year
Sponsorship:	Voluntary Not-for-Profit
Accreditation:	Joint Commission on the Accreditation of Healthcare Organizations
	College of American Pathologists

GENERAL OVERVIEW

The New York Eye and Ear Infirmary is one of the world's leading facilities for the diagnosis and treatment of diseases of the eyes, ears, nose, throat and related conditions. Founded in 1820, it is the oldest continuously operating specialty hospital in the nation, as well as one of the busiest.

ACADEMIC AND CLINICAL AFFILIATIONS

A voluntary, not-for-profit institution, the Infirmary is a member of Continuum Health Partners, Inc. and an affiliated teaching hospital of New York Medical College. There are highly regarded residency programs in ophthalmology and otolaryngology, plus some two dozen post-graduate fellowship positions.

THE MEDICAL STAFF

The Medical Staff includes more than 500 board-certified attending physicians and surgeons throughout the metropolitan area. Many are renowned for their breakthrough research introducing widely practiced techniques.

SPECIALTIES

Ophthalmology: Within this area are subspecialties of cataract, glaucoma, retina, cornea and refractive surgery, ocular plastic surgery, pediatric ophthalmology and strabismus, neuro-ophthalmology and ocular tumor. Laser, photography, fluorescein angiography and electrophysiological testing are among the most advanced services available anywhere.

Otolaryngology: The department is in the forefront of treatment modalities using highly sophisticated endoscopic and laser equipment. Subspecialties include rhinology, laryngology, head & neck surgery, otology/neurotology, pediatric otolaryngology, audiology, speech therapy and hearing aid dispensing.

Plastic & Reconstructive Surgery: Microsurgical capabilities and premium patient accommodations provide an optimum environment for facial plasty, liposuction and repair of defects from disease or trauma.

RELATED SERVICES

New York Eye Trauma Center: An advanced program for emergency treatment of eye injuries, it also is the Eye Injury Registry of New York State and leading collector of data which will help develop preventative strategies.

Ambulatory Surgery: A comprehensive Ambulatory Surgery Center is designed to expedite admission testing, pre-op preparation and post-op recovery in an efficient and comfortable setting.

Pediatric Specialty Care: Services of eye and ear, nose and throat specialists are coordinated with other professional and support staff especially sensitive to the youngest patients.

RESEARCH AND EDUCATION

The New York Eye and Ear Infirmary is a national and international leader in research in its specialties, achieving many "firsts" in successful surgical procedures and medical treatments. Laboratories include Cell Culture, Ocular Imaging, and Microsurgical Education. Over a hundred studies and clinical trials are currently being conducted.

Physician Referral: Call 1.800.449.HOPE (4673)

⅃ NewYork-Presbyterian
⅂ The University Hospital of Columbia and Cornell

Affiliated with Columbia University College of Physicians and Surgeons and Weill Medical College of Cornell University

NewYork-Presbyterian Hospital	NewYork-Presbyterian Hospital
Weill Cornell Medical Center	Columbia University Medical Center
525 East 68th Street	622 West 168th Street
New York, NY 10021	New York, NY 10032

Sponsorship: Voluntary Not-for-Profit
Beds: 2,335
Accreditation: Joint Commission on Accreditation of Healthcare Organizations (JCAHO), Commission on Accreditation of Rehabilitation Facilities (CARF) and College of American Pathologists (CAP)

The *U.S. News & World Report* has ranked NewYork-Presbyterian Hospital higher in more specialties than any other hospital in the New York area. NewYork-Presbyterian Hospital was named to the *Honor Roll of America's Best Hospitals.*

OVERVIEW:

NewYork-Presbyterian Hospital is the largest hospital in New York and one of the most comprehensive health-care institutions in the world with 5,500 physicians, approximately 96,000 discharges and nearly 1 million out-patient visits annually, and with its affiliated medical schools, more than $330 million in research support.

AMONG ITS RENOWNED CENTERS OF EXCELLENCE ARE:

Morgan Stanley Children's Hospital and the Komansky Center for Children's Health – One of the largest, most comprehensive children's hospitals in the world providing highly sophisticated pediatric medical, surgical and intensive care, including a pediatric cardiovascular center, in a compassionate environment.

NewYork-Presbyterian Cancer Centers – Coordinated, multidisciplinary care and the latest therapeutic options and clinical trials available for all types of cancer.

NewYork-Presbyterian Heart – Expert diagnostic capabilities and medical and surgical innovations for simple to complex heart conditions.

NewYork-Presbyterian Neuroscience Centers – Latest research, diagnosis and treatment capabilities in Alzheimer's disease, Multiple Sclerosis, Parkinson's disease, aneurysms, epilepsy, brain tumors, stokes and other neurological disorders.

NewYork-Presbyterian Psychiatry – World-renowned center of excellence in psychiatric treatment, research and education.

NewYork-Presbyterian Transplant Institute – Adult and pediatric heart, liver, and kidney and adult pancreas and lung transplantation and cutting-edge research.

NewYork-Presbyterian Vascular Care Center – Comprehensive and integrated preventive, diagnostic and treatment program for diverse problems related to arteries and veins throughout the body.

NewYork-Presbyterian Digestive Disease Services – Expert capabilities in the broad range of conditions that affect the organs as well as other components of the digestive system.

William Randolph Hearst Burn Center – Largest and busiest burn center in the nation which also conducts research to improve survival and enhance quality of life for burn victims.

In addition, the Hospital offers extraordinary expertise, comprehensive programs and specialized resources in the fields of AIDS, Complementary Medicine, Gene Therapy, Reproductive Medicine and Infertility, Trauma Center and Women's Health Care.

ACADEMIC AFFILIATIONS:

NewYork-Presbyterian is the only hospital in the world affiliated with two Ivy League medical schools; The Joan and Sanford I Weill Medical College of Cornell University and the Columbia University College of Physicians and Surgeons.

Physician Referral: To find a NewYork-Presbyterian Hospital affiliated physician to meet your needs, call toll free 1-877-NYP-WELL (1-877-697-9355) or visit our website at www.nyp.org

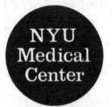

NYU Medical Center

550 First Avenue (at 31st Street)
New York, NY 10016
Physician Referral:
(888)7-NYU-MED (888-769-8633)
www.nyumc.org

Sponsorship:	Private, Not-for-Profit
Beds:	879 beds
Accreditation:	Joint Commission on Accreditation of Healthcare Organizations (JACHO), Commission for Accreditation of Rehabilitation Facilities (CARF) and Magnet Status

A LEADER IN PATIENT CARE

NYU Medical Center is one of the nation's leading academic medical centers, combining excellence in patient care research and medical education. A not-for-profit institution, NYU Medical Center includes Tisch Hospital, a voluntary 705-bed tertiary care facility serving more than 38,000 inpatients annually, and the Rusk Institute of Rehabilitation Medicine, which has 174 beds and serves 3,400 inpatients and more than 53,000 outpatients annually and the NYU Hospital for Joint Diseases, which has 190 beds and is one of the nation's premier hospitals for treating orthopaedic and rheumatological disorders.

SPECIAL PROGRAMS

Cardiac Surgery: A leader in minimally invasive techniques and robotic procedures.

Cardiology: A full range of diagnostic, prognostic and treatment services for patients of all ages.

Epilepsy: The largest facility of its kind on the East Coast.

Pain Management: Specialties: acute cancer and chronic pain management services.

Plastic Surgery: The largest facility of its kind in the world.

Pregnancy (High-Risk): Unparalled diagnostic techniques and surgical innovations for those with trouble conceiving or with special risks.

Skin Disease: Renowned for treating serious and rare skin disorders.

Surgery: Leading the nation in advancement of minimally invasive procedures and surgical techniques.

Transplant: Some of the nation's best patient and graft survival outcomes.

Urology: Leaders in treating prostate disorders and other urological problems.

The Rusk Institute of Rehabilitation Medicine is the world's first and still one of the largest university centers for adult and pediatric rehabilitation, ranked the #1 rehabilitation hospital in New York City by *U.S. News & World Reports* for the last seventeen years.

The NYU Cancer Institute's Clinical Cancer Center meets the outpatient needs of people with cancer and provides the latest cancer prevention, screening, diagnostic, treatment, genetic counseling, and support services in one convenient and comfortable facility.

NYU Hospital for Joint Diseases is one of the nation's leading orthopaedic, rheumatologic, neurologic, and rehabilitation specialty sites dedicated to the prevention and treatment of neuromusculoskeletal diseases. NYUHJD is a voluntary, not-for-profit teaching institution and is part of NYU Medical Center.

Physician Referral (888) 7-NYU-MED-(888)-769-8633) A free telephone referral service staffed by R.N.s trained to access over 1,500 NYU Physicians.

684

NYU Hospital for Joint Diseases

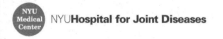 NYU**Hospital for Joint Diseases**

301 East 17th Street (at Second Avenue)
New York, NY 10003
212-598-6000   FAX: 212-260-1203
Website: www.nyuhjd.org

Sponsorship:	NYU Medical Center
Beds:	190
Accreditation:	Joint Commission on Accreditation of Healthcare Organizations (JCAHO), Commission of Accreditation for Rehabilitation Facilities (CARF)

PROFILE

NYU Hospital for Joint Diseases is one of the nation's leading orthopaedic, rheumatologic, rehabilitation and neurologic specialty sites dedicated to the prevention and treatment of neuromusculoskeletal diseases. NYUHJD is a voluntary, not-for-profit teaching institution and is part of NYU Medical Center.

MEDICAL STAFF

NYU Hospital for Joint Diseases has over 500 board certified members of the attending medical staff specializing in orthopaedics, rheumatology, rehabilitation medicine, neurology and anesthesiology.

TEACHING PROGRAMS

NYUHJD sponsors a fully accredited five-year orthopaedic surgery residency program with twelve residents each year. In addition, seven different fellowships are offered in the subspecialty areas of orthopaedics including hand, foot and ankle, spine, sports medicine, shoulder, and total joint replacement..

SPECIAL PROGRAMS

Orthopaedic Surgery: Arthritis and Joint Replacement Center, The Spine Center, Arthroscopic Surgery, Pediatric Orthopaedics, Bone Tumors and Orthopaedic Oncology, Foot and Ankle Surgery, Hand Surgery, Limb Lengthening and Bone Growth, Occupational and Industrial Orthopaedic Care, Sports Medicine, Shoulder and Elbow Service, Center for Neuromuscular and Developmental Disorders, Diabetes Foot and Ankle Center, The Harkness Center for Dance Injuries, and an Orthopaedic Urgent Care Center.

Department of Rheumatology and Medicine: Center for Arthritis & Autoimmunity and the Peter D. Seligman Center for Advanced Therapeutics. Rheumatoid Arthritis, Osteoarthritis, Psoriatic Arthritis, Lupus, Osteoporosis, Fibromyalgia, Scleroderma, Sjogren's Syndrome.

Rehabilitation Medicine: The Rusk Institute of Rehabilitation Medicine at 17th Street offers comprehensive inpatient (orthopaedic and neurological rehabilitation, pain management) and outpatient rehabilitation services at NYUHJD and other locations.

Additional Programs: Orthopaedic Neurology, Initiative for Women with Disabilities, Multiple Sclerosis, Neuroimmunology, Neurosurgery, Comprehensive Pain Treatment Center, Clinical Neurophysiology, Movement Disorders, Infusion Center, and Neurorehabilitation.

OTHER SERVICES

Managed Care Plans: NYU Hospital for Joint Diseases participates in over 44 managed care plans covering 100 different products (i.e., HMO, POS, PPO, Medicare, Medicaid, etc.).

Physician Referral	NYUHJD offers a free telephone physician referral service, Monday-Friday, 8:30 am to 6:00 pm. The physician referral service can be reached at 1-888-HID-DOCS (1-888-453-3627).

690

RUSK INSTITUTE OF REHABILITATION
MEDICINE at NYU Medical Center

400 East 34th Street (between 1st Avenue and FDR Drive)
New York, NY 10016 at NYU Hospital for Joint Diseases
301 East 17th Street (at 2nd Avenue); New York, NY 10003
212-263-6028; www.ruskinstitute.org

Sponsorship:	Private, Not-for-Profit
Beds:	174 (NYUHC) and 46 (NYU Hospital for Joint Disease)
Accreditation:	Joint Commission on Accreditation of Healthcare Organizations (JCAHO) Commission for Accreditation of Rehabilitation Facilities (CARF)

Founded in 1948 by Dr. Howard A. Rusk, the Rusk Institute of Rehabilitation Medicine, the flagship facility of the Rusk Institute of Rehabilitation Network, has been voted the best rehabilitation hospital in New York and among the top ten in the country since 1989, when U.S. News & World Report introduced its annual 'Best Hospitals' ranking. The world's first university-affiliated facility devoted entirely to rehabilitation medicine, the Rusk Institute is the largest center of its kind for the treatment of adults and children with disabilities.

Rusk Institute operates under the auspices of the Department of Rehabilitation Medicine of New York University School of Medicine, one of the nation's foremost medical schools. The relationship between Rusk Institute and other clinical and research units within the Medical Center - including Tisch Hospital, a 726-bed acute-care facility and NYU Hospital for Joint Diseases a 190-bed facility dedicated to the treatment of orthopaedic, rheumatologic, and neurologic disorders provides patients with complete and immediate access to superb tertiary-care and the full range of medical and surgical subspecialty care.

The Rusk Institute of Rehabilitation Network provides patients with access to treatment across a continuum of care depending on their individual medical needs: acute hospital based inpatient programs, sub-acute facilities, and outpatient programs.

Comprehensive and carefully coordinated hospital based rehabilitation services are offered at two inpatient locations: NYU Hospital @ 34th Street and First Avenue and at the Rusk Institute at NYU Hospital for Joint Disease @ 17th Street and Second Avenue.

Brain Injury
Cardiac and Pulmonary Conditions
Chronic Neurological Impairment
Muskuloskeletal Impairment
Pediatric Family-Centered Program
Spinal Cord Injury
Stroke

Patients that can benefit from rehabilitation without requiring the intensity of inpatient or subacute programs participate in a vast array of outpatient programs offered at Rusk:

Aphasia Program	*Lymphedema*	*Swallowing Disorders*
Barrier Free Design	*Muscular Dystrophy Clinic*	*Spasticity Management*
Brain Injury Day Treatment Program	*Multiple Sclerosis Care Center*	*Spine and Sports Therapy*
Cardiopulmonary rehabilitation	*Neuropsychology*	*Vestibular Rehabilitation / Balance Disorders*
Cognitive Rehabilitation	*Parkinson's Disease*	*Vocational Rehabilitation*
Communication Disorders	*Pre/Post Cochlear Implant Speech-Language Pathology Program*	*Visual Perceptional Rehabilitation*
Hand Service	*Pain Management*	*Women's Health Rehabilitation*
Harkness Dance Center	*Pediatric Programs*	*Horticulture therapy*
Recreation Therapy		

688

St. Francis Hospital, The Heart Center®

100 Port Washington Blvd.
Tel. (516) 562-6000
www.stfrancisheartcenter.com

Sponsorship:	Voluntary Not-for-Profit
Beds:	279
Accreditation:	Awarded Accreditation from the Joint Commission on Accreditation of Healthcare Organizations (JCAHO)
Affiliation:	A Member of Catholic Health Services of Long Island

St. Francis Hospital, The Heart Center® is New York State's only specialty designated cardiac center, offering one of the leading cardiac care programs in the nation. Founded in 1922 by the Franciscan Missionaries of Mary, the Hospital is recognized as an innovator in the delivery of specialized cardiovascular services in an environment where excellence and compassion are emphasized. St. Francis also offers a superb program in non-cardiac surgery, including some of the most advanced technology and minimally invasive techniques available for vascular, prostate, ear-nose-throat (ENT), and orthopedic surgery.

Cardiac Diagnostics and Treatment

St. Francis Hospital performs more cardiac procedures than any other hospital in New York State and has been consistently recognized for its outstanding quality of care. In 2007, St. Francis Hospital had more "best doctors" for cardiac care than any other hospital on Long Island according to *New York Magazine.*

Cardiac surgery: In 2006, 1,685 open-heart surgeries were performed at St. Francis Hospital. The hospital's eight cardiothoracic surgeons have the combined experience of over 20,000 open-heart procedures in the last 10 years alone and are experts in all types of heart surgery, from conventional, open-heart bypass to off-pump coronary artery bypass (OPCAB) to the newest, minimally invasive valve procedures, including surgical techniques designed to treat certain cardiac arrhythmias or irregular heart rhythms.

Cardiac catheterization: In 2006, St. Francis interventional cardiologists performed 9,837 cardiac catheterizations and 3,961 percutaneous coronary interventions (angioplasty and insertion of stents). According to the Department of Health, St. Francis had the highest caseload in New York State. The Hospital is also recognized as one of the East Coast's highest volume centers for catheter-based techniques to close atrial septal defects (ASDs) and patent foramen ovale (PFO).

Arrhythmia and Pacemaker Center: St. Francis has a leading national program for pacemaker implantation and the diagnosis and treatment of cardiac rhythm abnormalities. The Center has unparalleled expertise in radiofrequency cardiac ablation, including treatment of atrial fibrillation.

Research and Technology

At the St. Francis Cardiac Research Institute, a team of world-renowned researchers is working with the latest non-invasive imaging technology, including the new 64-slice CT scanner, 3-dimensional echocardiography system, and the area's first dedicated cardiac magnetic resonance (MRI) unit. This multimodality approach to investigating the heart's function and disease processes is aimed at improving methods of diagnosing heart disease.

Prevention and Education

St. Francis Hospital's satellite campus, The DeMatteis Center for Cardiac Research and Education, in Old Brookville, New York, is one of the few freestanding campuses in the U.S. dedicated to the prevention of heart disease. It is the site of community health lectures, as well as the largest medically staffed cardiac fitness and rehabilitation program on Long Island.

Physician referral: 1-888-HEARTNY

UNIVERSITY OF PENNSYLVANIA HEALTH SYSTEM

WE ARE MEDICINE.

Philadelphia, PA 19104
1.800.789.PENN
pennhealth.com

OVERVIEW

For more than two centuries, the University of Pennsylvania Health System has been committed to the highest standards of patient care, education and research. Our commitment has been recognized by our peers and by others throughout the greater Philadelphia region and across the nation.

The University of Pennsylvania Health System ranks second nationally in special grant funding from the National Institutes of Health, with several departments ranking first nationally. *U.S.News & World Report* consistently ranks the University of Pennsylvania Schools of Medicine and Nursing among the nation's best, and ranks all adult specialties at the Hospital of the University of Pennsylvania.

We Are Medicine

Our physicians, nurses and researchers are united in the health system's mission to expand the frontiers of medicine through new discoveries in the detection, treatment and prevention of human disease. Because we develop and test new treatments through clinical trials, our patients gain access to the very latest advances and future generations will benefit from the work we do today.

Penn continues to lead the way in discovering new treatment methods for diseases once considered incurable, including groundbreaking research in cancer, cardiac, neurosciences, orthopaedics, genetics and imaging. Over the past 30 years, Penn physicians and scientists have participated in many important discoveries, including:

- The first general vaccine against pneumonia.

- The introduction of total intravenous feeding.

- The development of cognitive therapy.

- The development of magnetic resonance imaging and other imaging technologies.

- The discovery of the Philadelphia chromosome, which revolutionized cancer research by making the connection between genetic abnormalities and cancer.

- The development of a cure for atrial fibrillation.

Locations
Patients are seen at:
- Hospital of the University of Pennsylvania
- Penn Presbyterian Medical Center
- Pennsylvania Hospital
- Penn Medicine at Bucks County
- Penn Medicine at Cherry Hill
- Penn Medicine at Radnor
- PennCare, our primary care physician network, provides services in the local communities in Bucks, Chester, Delaware, Montgomery and Philadelphia counties in Pennsylvania and in Southern New Jersey.
- Hospice and home care services are provided by Penn Home Care and Hospice Services.

On the Web
Visit pennhealth.com for the latest patient education with explanation of diseases and conditions, surgical procedures and follow-up care, screening tools, drug interactions and descriptions as well as an encyclopedia of health information.

To learn more about Penn physicians or services, call 1-800-789-PENN or visit pennhealth.com

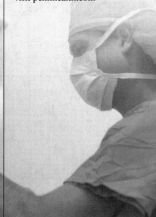

Hospital of the University of Pennsylvania | Penn Presbyterian Medical Center | Pennsylvania Hospital

THE UNIVERSITY OF TEXAS
MD ANDERSON
CANCER CENTER
Making Cancer History®

The University of Texas
M. D. Anderson Cancer Center
1515 Holcombe Blvd.
Houston, Texas 77030-4095
Tel. 713-792-6161 Toll Free 877-MDA-6789
www.mdanderson.org

OUR MISSION

Since 1941, M. D. Anderson Cancer Center has had a single goal – to eliminate cancer. Achieving that goal begins with integrated programs in cancer treatment, clinical trials, education programs and cancer prevention.

More than 60 years of cancer treatment has resulted in unmatched experience in the diagnosis and treatment of all cancer types, as well as expertise in emerging technologies such as proton therapy and robotic surgery. With over 1,600 faculty members, physicians specialize in specific types of cancer while benefiting from collaboration with colleagues in surgery, oncology, pediatrics, and radiation therapy to design individualized treatment plans for every patient.

PATIENT CARE

At M. D. Anderson, we hold ourselves to quality standards higher than the industry requires, and provide a rare breadth of technology, experience, and expertise, all which translate into personalized care and the best outcomes possible.

Our doctors work in teams that include surgeons, medical oncologists, radiation oncologists, and nurses who have expertise in a specific types of cancer. These specialized teams use their experience to create a plan that is individualized for each patient. Therefore, every patient receives the benefit of M. D. Anderson's wide range of cancer expertise combined with personalized care.

CLINICAL RESEARCH

As a federally designated comprehensive cancer center, M. D. Anderson is required to have a strong research program. Many cancer treatments now considered standard had their beginnings at M. D. Anderson, from groundbreaking radiation therapies in the 1950s to designer drugs that target cancer cells today. Patients benefit from M. D. Anderson research through participation in dozens of clinical trials to apply new therapies that may well become tomorrow's standard treatments.

MORE INFORMATION For more information or to make an appointment, call 877-MDA-6789, or visit us online at http://www.mdanderson.org.

83(

Wake Forest University Baptist
MEDICAL CENTER ®
Comprehensive Cancer Center

Medical Center Boulevard • Winston-Salem, NC 27157 • 336-716-2011
Health On-Call® (Patient access) 1-800-446-2255
PAL® (Physician-to-physician calls) 1-800-277-7654
www.wfubmc.edu/cancer/

TOP RANKINGS

The Comprehensive Cancer Center of Wake Forest University Baptist Medical is among an elite group of only 39 U.S. cancer centers designated by the National Cancer Institute as comprehensive, indicating excellence in research, patient care and education. The comprehensive designation was renewed for an additional five years in late 2006.

RESEARCH ADVANTAGES

Wake Forest Baptist offers more cancer-related clinical trials than any other hospital in western N.C. From gene therapy to vitamin and nutrition studies to new surgical and radiological treatments, patients benefit from the leading edge of cancer knowledge and care. Innovative basic science, public health and clinical research promote new discovery about prevention, detection and treatment of cancers. Wake Forest scientists were first in the world to discover cancer resistant cells in mice.

TECHNOLOGY AND TREATMENT STRENGTHS

Wake Forest University Baptist Medical Center is home to North Carolina's first Gamma Knife, a non-invasive, stereotactic radiosurgical tool used to treat malignant and benign brain tumors once considered inoperable. Operated by one of the nation's most experienced treatment teams, the Gamma Knife painlessly bombards tumors with precisely focused beams of gamma energy – sparing normal tissue -- and is performed on an outpatient basis. Extracranial body stereotactic radiosurgery offers new options for other types of cancers.

Wake Forest Baptist offers an integrated brachytherapy unit (IBU) and highly targeted Intensity Modulated Radiation Therapy (IMRT) for treatment of prostate, brain, lung, head and neck, and gynecological cancers. Other treatment innovations include IPHC (intraperitoneal hyperthermic chemotherapy) for abdominal cavity cancers and radiofrequency ablation for liver malignancies.

MULTIDISCIPLINARY EXPERTISE

Expert, subspecialized oncology teams provide patients a consensus opinion on treatment. Multidisciplinary centers include the Thoracic Oncology Program, the Breast Care Center, the Brain Tumor Clinic and the Head and Neck Cancers Multidisciplinary Clinic

To make an appointment or find a specialist, call Health On-Call® at 1-800-446-2255.

HIGHLIGHTS OF EXCELLENCE

- Western North Carolina's only NCI-designated Comprehensive Cancer Center offers the convenience and comfort of a state-of-the-art Outpatient Cancer Center. The nation's first Cancer Patient Support Group was developed here.

- The Cancer Center's Blood and Marrow Transplant Program operates the nation's second-largest collection site.

- The Breast Cancer Risk Assessment Clinic and the Hereditary Cancer Clinic help patients understand their risk profile.

- Minimally invasive treatments include high dose rate (HDR) brachytherapy for prostate cancer. Lymph node mapping increases chance for lymph-sparing breast surgery.

- Clinical trials testing new methods of drug delivery offer patients with brain tumors potentially more effective treatment while minimizing effects on healthy tissue.

KNOWLEDGE MAKES ALL THE DIFFERENCE.

Physician
Listings

Adolescent Medicine

a subspecialty of Pediatrics

An internist or pediatrician who specializes in adolescent medicine is a multidiciplinary healthcare specialist trained in the unique physical, psychological and social characteristics of adolescents, their healthcare problems and needs.

Training Required: Three years in internal medicine OR three years in pediatrics *plus* additional training and examination for certification in adolescent medicine

Adolescent Medicine

New England

Emans, Sarah Jean H MD [AM] - **Spec Exp:** Pediatric Gynecology; Adolescent Gynecology; **Hospital:** Children's Hospital - Boston; **Address:** Childrens Hosp, Dept Adolescent Med, 300 Longwood Ave, Boston, MA 02115-5724; **Phone:** 617-355-7181; **Board Cert:** Pediatrics 1993; Adolescent Medicine 2002; **Med School:** Harvard Med Sch 1970; **Resid:** Pediatrics, Chldns Hosp 1973; **Fellow:** Adolescent Medicine, Chldns Hosp 1974; **Fac Appt:** Prof Ped, Harvard Med Sch

Mid Atlantic

Diaz, Angela MD [AM] - **Spec Exp:** Adolescent Reproductive Health; Abuse/Neglect; **Hospital:** Mount Sinai Med Ctr; **Address:** 320 E 94th St Fl 2, New York, NY 10128-5604; **Phone:** 212-423-2900; **Board Cert:** Pediatrics 1987; Adolescent Medicine 2004; **Med School:** Columbia P&S 1981; **Resid:** Pediatrics, Mt Sinai Med Ctr 1984; **Fellow:** Adolescent Medicine, Mt Sinai Med Ctr 1985; **Fac Appt:** Prof Ped, Mount Sinai Sch Med

Murray, Pamela J MD [AM] - **Spec Exp:** Adolescent Gynecology; **Hospital:** Chldns Hosp of Pittsburgh - UPMC; **Address:** Children's Hosp Pittsburgh, Adolescent Medicine, 3705 Fifth Ave at DeSoto St, Pittsburgh, PA 15213; **Phone:** 412-692-8504; **Board Cert:** Pediatrics 1983; Adolescent Medicine 2002; **Med School:** Med Coll PA 1978; **Resid:** Pediatrics, Children's Hosp 1981; **Fellow:** Public Health, Univ New South Wales 1987; **Fac Appt:** Assoc Prof Ped, Univ Pittsburgh

Slap, Gail MD [AM] - **Spec Exp:** Chronic Illness; Developmental Disorders; **Hospital:** Chldns Hosp of Philadelphia, The; **Address:** Childrens Hosp Philadelphia, Main Bldg - 9412, 34th St & Civic Center Blvd, Philadelphia, PA 19104; **Phone:** 215-590-5868; **Board Cert:** Internal Medicine 1980; Adolescent Medicine 1994; **Med School:** Univ Pennsylvania 1977; **Resid:** Internal Medicine, Hosp Univ Penn 1980; **Fellow:** Adolescent Medicine, Chldns Hosp 1982; **Fac Appt:** Prof Ped, Univ Pennsylvania

Southeast

Ford, Carol Ann MD [AM] - **Hospital:** Univ NC Hosps; **Address:** UNC-Chapel Hill, Dept Ped Adol Med, 130 Mason Farm Rd, Box 7220, Chapel Hill, NC 27599-7220; **Phone:** 919-966-2504; **Board Cert:** Internal Medicine 1987; Pediatrics 1998; Adolescent Medicine 1994; **Med School:** Univ Fla Coll Med 1983; **Resid:** Internal Medicine, North Carolina Meml Hosp 1987; Pediatrics, North Carolina Meml Hosp 1987; **Fellow:** Adolescent Medicine, UCSF Med Ctr 1995; **Fac Appt:** Asst Prof Ped, Univ NC Sch Med

Midwest

Fortenberry, J Dennis MD [AM] - **Spec Exp:** Sexually Transmitted Diseases; **Hospital:** Riley Hosp for Children; **Address:** Indiana Univ - Adolescent Medicine, 410 W 10th, rm 1001, Indianapolis, IN 46202; **Phone:** 317-274-8812; **Board Cert:** Internal Medicine 1983; Adolescent Medicine 2004; **Med School:** Univ Okla Coll Med 1979; **Resid:** Internal Medicine, Univ OK Hlth Sci Ctr 1982; **Fellow:** Adolescent Medicine, Univ OK Hlth Sci Ctr 1983; **Fac Appt:** Prof Med, Indiana Univ

Kokotailo, Patricia K MD [AM] - **Spec Exp:** Adolescent Gynecology; Substance Abuse; **Hospital:** Univ WI Hosp & Clins; **Address:** Univ Wisc Chldns Hosp, Dept Peds-Adol Med, 2870 University Ave, Ste 200, Madison, WI 53705; **Phone:** 608-263-6421; **Board Cert:** Pediatrics 1987; Adolescent Medicine 2002; **Med School:** Northwestern Univ 1982; **Resid:** Pediatrics, Johns Hopkins Hosp 1985; **Fellow:** Adolescent Medicine, Johns Hopkins Hosp 1989; **Fac Appt:** Prof Ped, Univ Wisc

Great Plains and Mountains

Kaplan, David W MD [AM] - **Spec Exp:** Eating Disorders; Depression; Headache; **Hospital:** Chldn's Hosp - Denver, The; **Address:** Chldns Hosp, 1056 E 19th Ave, Box B025, Denver, CO 80218-1088; **Phone:** 303-861-6133; **Board Cert:** Pediatrics 1975; Public Health & Genl Preventive Med 1980; Adolescent Medicine 2002; **Med School:** Case West Res Univ 1970; **Resid:** Pediatrics, Univ Colorado Med Ctr 1972; Pediatrics, Chldns Hosp Med Ctr 1975; **Fellow:** Public Health & Genl Preventive Med, Harvard Sch Pub Hlth 1976; **Fac Appt:** Prof Ped, Univ Colorado

Southwest

Bermudez, Ovidio MD [AM] - **Spec Exp:** Eating Disorders; Obesity; **Hospital:** Laureate Psyc Clinic & Hosp; **Address:** 6655 S Yale Ave, Tulsa, OK 74136; **Phone:** 918-491-3702; **Board Cert:** Pediatrics 2005; Adolescent Medicine 2002; **Med School:** Dominican Republic 1985; **Resid:** Pediatrics, Med Coll Penn 1988; **Fellow:** Adolescent Medicine, Univ of Alabama 1990; **Fac Appt:** Clin Prof Ped, Univ Okla Coll Med

West Coast and Pacific

Anderson, Martin M MD [AM] - **Hospital:** UCLA Med Ctr; **Address:** UCLA Med Ctr, Dept Pediatrics, 10833 Le Conte Ave, Los Angeles, CA 90095; **Phone:** 310-825-0867; **Board Cert:** Pediatrics 1986; Adolescent Medicine 2002; **Med School:** UC Davis 1980; **Resid:** Pediatrics, Mott Chldns Hosp 1983; **Fellow:** Adolescent Medicine, UCSF Med Ctr 1986; **Fac Appt:** Prof Ped, UCLA

Irwin Jr, Charles E MD [AM] - **Spec Exp:** Eating Disorders; Adolescent Gynecology; **Hospital:** UCSF Med Ctr; **Address:** UCSF Chldns Hosp, 400 Parnassus Ave, Box 0503, San Francisco, CA 94143; **Phone:** 415-353-2002; **Board Cert:** Pediatrics 1993; Adolescent Medicine 2002; **Med School:** UCSF 1971; **Resid:** Pediatrics, UCSF Med Ctr 1974; **Fellow:** Adolescent Medicine, UCSF Med Ctr 1977; **Fac Appt:** Prof Ped, UCSF

MacKenzie, Richard G MD [AM] - **Spec Exp:** Eating Disorders; Menstrual Disorders; **Hospital:** Chldns Hosp - Los Angeles (page 56), USC Univ Hosp - R K Eamer Med Plz; **Address:** 5000 Sunset Blvd, Fl 4, Los Angeles, CA 90027-5861; **Phone:** 323-669-2112; **Med School:** McGill Univ 1966; **Resid:** Internal Medicine, Royal Victoria Hosp-Montreal 1969; **Fellow:** Adolescent Medicine, Chidrens Hosp 1970; **Fac Appt:** Assoc Prof Ped, USC Sch Med

Morris, Robert E MD [AM] - **Spec Exp:** Chronic Illness; Teen Behavior Evaluation-High Risk; Juvenile Correctional Health Care; **Hospital:** Santa Monica - UCLA Med Ctr, UCLA Med Ctr; **Address:** UCLA Sch Med, Dept Peds, 10833 Le Conte Ave, Los Angeles, CA 90095-1752; **Phone:** 310-825-9346; **Board Cert:** Pediatrics 1986; Adolescent Medicine 2005; **Med School:** Temple Univ 1971; **Resid:** Pediatrics, Univ Wash 1974; Pediatric Gastroenterology, UCLA Med Ctr 1982; **Fac Appt:** Prof Ped, UCLA

Allergy & Immunology

An allergist-immunologist is trained in evaluation, physical and laboratory diagnosis and management of disorders involving the immune system. Selected examples of such conditions include asthma, anaphylaxis, rhinitis, eczema and adverse reactions to drugs, foods and insect stings as well as immune deficiency diseases (both acquired and congenital), defects in host defense and problems related to autoimmune disease, organ transplantation or malignancies of the immune system. As our understanding of the immune system develops, the scope of this specialty is widening.

Training programs are available at some medical centers to provide individuals with expertise in both allergy/immunology and adult rheumatology, or in both allergy/immunology and pediatric pulmonology. Such individuals are candidates for dual certification.

Training Required: Two years in allergy/immunology OR prior certification in internal medicine or pediatrics *plus* additional training and examination

Allergy & Immunology

New England

MacLean, James A MD [A&I] - **Spec Exp:** Asthma; Allergy; Urticaria; **Hospital:** Mass Genl Hosp, N Shore Med Ctr - Salem Hosp; **Address:** Mass Genl Hosp, 55 Fruit St, Cox 201, Boston, MA 02114-2621; **Phone:** 617-726-3850; **Board Cert:** Internal Medicine 1988; Allergy & Immunology 1991; **Med School:** McGill Univ 1985; **Resid:** Internal Medicine, Royal Victoria Hosp 1989; **Fellow:** Allergy & Immunology, Mass Genl Hosp 1991; Immunopathology, Mass Genl Hosp 1994; **Fac Appt:** Asst Prof A&I, Harvard Med Sch

Umetsu, Dale T MD/PhD [A&I] - **Spec Exp:** Asthma; Immune Deficiency; Eczema; **Hospital:** Children's Hospital - Boston; **Address:** Div Immunology, Children's Hosp, 1 Blackfan Cir, Karp Labs, rm 10127, Boston, MA 02115; **Phone:** 617-919-2439; **Board Cert:** Pediatrics 1984; Allergy & Immunology 1985; **Med School:** NYU Sch Med 1979; **Resid:** Pediatrics, Chldns Hosp 1982; **Fellow:** Allergy & Immunology, Chldns Hosp 1984; **Fac Appt:** Prof Ped, Harvard Med Sch

Wong, Johnson T MD [A&I] - **Spec Exp:** Asthma; Rhinosinusitis; Urticaria; Food Allergy; **Hospital:** Mass Genl Hosp, Newton - Wellesley Hosp; **Address:** 8 Hawthorne Pl, Ste 104, Boston, MA 02114; **Phone:** 617-742-5730; **Board Cert:** Internal Medicine 1983; Allergy & Immunology 1985; **Med School:** UCSF 1980; **Resid:** Internal Medicine, UCLA-Wadsworth VA Hosp 1983; **Fellow:** Allergy & Immunology, Mass Genl Hosp 1986; **Fac Appt:** Asst Prof Med, Harvard Med Sch

Mid Atlantic

Baraniuk, James N MD [A&I] - **Spec Exp:** Asthma; Immune Deficiency; Sinusitis; **Hospital:** Georgetown Univ Hosp; **Address:** 3800 Reservior Rd NW, Kober Cogan Bldg, Ste B100, Washington, DC 20007; **Phone:** 202-687-8233; **Board Cert:** Internal Medicine 1984; Allergy & Immunology 1987; **Med School:** Canada 1981; **Resid:** Internal Medicine, St Thomas Hosp 1984; Internal Medicine, Duke Univ Med Ctr 1985; **Fellow:** Allergy & Immunology, Duke Univ 1989; Allergy & Immunology, Natl Heart Lung Inst 1991; **Fac Appt:** Asst Clin Prof A&I, Georgetown Univ

Buchbinder, Ellen MD [A&I] - **Spec Exp:** Asthma; Allergy; Rhinitis; **Hospital:** Mount Sinai Med Ctr; **Address:** 111B E 88th St, New York, NY 10128; **Phone:** 212-410-3246; **Board Cert:** Internal Medicine 1981; Allergy & Immunology 1983; **Med School:** Tulane Univ 1978; **Resid:** Internal Medicine, New England Deaconess Hosp 1981; **Fellow:** Allergy & Immunology, Mass Genl Hosp 1983; **Fac Appt:** Asst Clin Prof Med, Mount Sinai Sch Med

Chandler, Michael MD [A&I] - **Spec Exp:** Asthma; Sinus Disorders; **Hospital:** Lenox Hill Hosp (page 62), Mount Sinai Med Ctr; **Address:** 115 E 61st St Fl 12, New York, NY 10021-8183; **Phone:** 212-486-6715; **Board Cert:** Internal Medicine 1984; Allergy & Immunology 1987; **Med School:** Wayne State Univ 1981; **Resid:** Internal Medicine, Northwestern Meml Hosp 1984; **Fellow:** Allergy & Immunology, Northwestern Meml Hosp 1986; **Fac Appt:** Asst Clin Prof Med, Mount Sinai Sch Med

Cunningham-Rundles, Charlotte MD/PhD [A&I] - **Spec Exp:** Immunotherapy; Immunodeficiency Disorders; **Hospital:** Mount Sinai Med Ctr; **Address:** 5 E 98th St, New York, NY 10029; **Phone:** 212-659-9268; **Board Cert:** Internal Medicine 1972; **Med School:** Columbia P&S 1969; **Resid:** Internal Medicine, Bellevue Hosp Ctr 1972; **Fellow:** Allergy & Immunology, NYU Med Ctr 1974; **Fac Appt:** Prof Med, Mount Sinai Sch Med

Dattwyler, Raymond MD [A&I] - **Spec Exp:** Allergy; Immune Deficiency; Tick-borne Diseases; Lyme Disease; **Hospital:** Westchester Med Ctr; **Address:** Allergy, Immunology And Rheumatology, NYMC-Munger Pavilion, rm G73, Valhalla, NY 10595; **Phone:** 914-594-4444; **Board Cert:** Internal Medicine 1977; Allergy & Immunology 1979; Clinical & Laboratory Immunology 1986; **Med School:** SUNY Buffalo 1973; **Resid:** Internal Medicine, New England Med Ctr 1977; **Fellow:** Immunology, Mayo Clinic 1976; Clinical Immunology, Mass General Hosp 1978; **Fac Appt:** Prof Med, SUNY Stony Brook

Kaliner, Michael A MD [A&I] - **Spec Exp:** Asthma & Allergy; Sinusitis; Rhinitis; **Hospital:** Washington Hosp Ctr; **Address:** Institute for Asthma and Allergy, 5454 Wisconsin Ave, Ste 700, Chevy Chase, MD 20815; **Phone:** 301-986-9262; **Board Cert:** Internal Medicine 1974; Allergy & Immunology 1993; **Med School:** Univ MD Sch Med 1967; **Resid:** Internal Medicine, UCSF Med Ctr 1970; **Fellow:** Allergy & Immunology, Harvard Univ 1973; **Fac Appt:** Prof Med, Geo Wash Univ

Levinson, Arnold MD [A&I] - **Spec Exp:** Autoimmune Disease; Immune Deficiency; Allergy; **Hospital:** Hosp Univ Penn - UPHS (page 72); **Address:** Hosp Univ Penn, Div A&I, 39th and Market St, Mutch Bldg Fl 5, Philadelphia, PA 19104; **Phone:** 215-662-2425; **Board Cert:** Internal Medicine 1972; Allergy & Immunology 1975; **Med School:** Univ MD Sch Med 1969; **Resid:** Internal Medicine, Baltimore City Hosps 1971; Immunology, Hosp Univ Penn 1972; **Fellow:** Clinical Immunology, UCSF Med Ctr 1973; Allergy & Immunology, Hosp Univ Penn 1975; **Fac Appt:** Prof Med, Univ Pennsylvania

Mazza, David S MD [A&I] - **Spec Exp:** Asthma; Sinus Disorders; Eczema; **Hospital:** St Luke's - Roosevelt Hosp Ctr - Roosevelt Div, St Vincent Cath Med Ctrs - Manhattan; **Address:** 7 Lexington Ave, Ste 3, New York, NY 10010-5517; **Phone:** 212-677-7170; **Board Cert:** Pediatrics 1983; Allergy & Immunology 1999; **Med School:** Univ VT Coll Med 1977; **Resid:** Pediatrics, NYU-Bellevue Hosp 1980; **Fellow:** Pediatrics, Bellevue Hosp 1982; Allergy & Immunology, St Luke's-Roosevelt Hosp Ctr 1989; **Fac Appt:** Assoc Prof Ped, Columbia P&S

Metcalfe, Dean D MD [A&I] - **Spec Exp:** Mast Cell Diseases; Food Allergy; **Hospital:** Natl Inst of Hlth - Clin Ctr; **Address:** Natl Inst Allergy & Infectious Disease, Allergic Disease Lab, 10 Center Drive Bldg 10 - rm 11C205, Bethesda, MD 20892-1881; **Phone:** 301-496-2165; **Board Cert:** Internal Medicine 1975; Allergy & Immunology 1977; Rheumatology 1980; **Med School:** Univ Tenn Coll Med, Memphis 1972; **Resid:** Internal Medicine, Univ Mich Hosps 1974; Allergy & Immunology, Natl Inst Allergy & Infectious Dis-NIH 1977; **Fellow:** Rheumatology, Peter Bent Brigham Hosp 1979

Reisman, Robert E MD [A&I] - **Spec Exp:** Anaphylaxis; Asthma; Insect Allergies; **Hospital:** Buffalo General Hosp, Women's & Chldn's Hosp of Buffalo, The; **Address:** Buffalo Medical Group, 295 Essjay Rd, Williamsville, NY 14221-8216; **Phone:** 716-630-1130; **Board Cert:** Internal Medicine 1969; Allergy & Immunology 1972; **Med School:** SUNY Buffalo 1956; **Resid:** Internal Medicine, Buffalo Genl Hosp 1959; **Fellow:** Allergy & Immunology, Buffalo Genl Hosp 1961; **Fac Appt:** Clin Prof Med, SUNY Buffalo

Shepherd, Gillian M MD [A&I] - **Spec Exp:** Food & Drug Allergy; Rhinosinusitis & Asthma; Urticaria; Insect Allergies; **Hospital:** NY-Presby Hosp/Weill Cornell (page 66), Meml Sloan Kettering Cancer Ctr; **Address:** 235 E 67th St, Ste 203, New York, NY 10021-6040; **Phone:** 212-288-9300; **Board Cert:** Internal Medicine 1979; Allergy & Immunology 1981; **Med School:** NY Med Coll 1976; **Resid:** Internal Medicine, Lenox Hill Hosp 1979; **Fellow:** Allergy & Immunology, New York Hosp-Cornell 1981; **Fac Appt:** Assoc Clin Prof Med, Cornell Univ-Weill Med Coll

Allergy & Immunology

Slankard, Marjorie MD [A&I] - **Spec Exp:** Rhinitis; Asthma; Sinusitis; Food Allergy; **Hospital:** NY-Presby Hosp/Columbia (page 66), Valley Hosp; **Address:** 16 E 60th St, Ste 321, New York, NY 10022-1002; **Phone:** 212-326-8410; **Board Cert:** Internal Medicine 1974; Allergy & Immunology 1977; **Med School:** Univ MO-Columbia Sch Med 1971; **Resid:** Internal Medicine, New York Hosp 1974; Internal Medicine, Rockefeller Univ Hosp 1974; **Fellow:** Immunology, New York Hosp-Cornell 1976; Immunology, Mount Sinai Med Ctr 1980; **Fac Appt:** Clin Prof Med, Columbia P&S

Strober, Warren MD [A&I] - **Spec Exp:** Immune Deficiency; Inflammatory Bowel Disease/Crohn's; **Hospital:** Natl Inst of Hlth - Clin Ctr; **Address:** NIH-Laboratory of Clinical Investigation, Bldg 10-CRC, rm 5-3940, Bethesda, MD 20892-1890; **Phone:** 301-496-6810; **Board Cert:** Internal Medicine 1974; Allergy & Immunology 1977; **Med School:** Univ Rochester 1962; **Resid:** Internal Medicine, Strong Meml Hosp 1964; Allergy & Immunology, Natl Inst Hlth 1972

Southeast

Benenati, Susan MD [A&I] - **Spec Exp:** Asthma; Latex Allergy; Sinus Disorders; **Hospital:** Baptist Hosp of Miami, South Miami Hosp; **Address:** 7000 SW 62nd Ave, Ste 510, South Miami, FL 33143-4721; **Phone:** 305-665-1623; **Board Cert:** Internal Medicine 1988; Allergy & Immunology 1999; **Med School:** Univ S Fla Coll Med 1984; **Resid:** Internal Medicine, Indiana Univ Med Ctr 1988; **Fellow:** Allergy & Immunology, Johns Hopkins Hosp 1990

Bonner, James R MD [A&I] - **Spec Exp:** Asthma; Urticaria; Sinusitis; **Hospital:** Univ of Ala Hosp at Birmingham; **Address:** Univ Alabama Hosp, Allergy/Immunology, 2000 Sixth Ave S, Birmingham, AL 35233-2110; **Phone:** 205-801-8100; **Board Cert:** Internal Medicine 1974; Infectious Disease 1976; Allergy & Immunology 1979; **Med School:** Univ Mich Med Sch 1971; **Resid:** Internal Medicine, Univ Ala Med Ctr 1974; **Fellow:** Allergy & Immunology, Univ Ala Med Ctr 1977; **Fac Appt:** Prof Med, Univ Ala

deShazo, Richard D MD [A&I] - **Spec Exp:** Immunodeficiency Disorders; Allergy; Rheumatology; **Hospital:** Univ Hosps & Clins - Jackson, Baptist Hosp - Jackson; **Address:** Univ Mississippi Med Ctr, Dept Med, 2500 N State St, Jackson, MS 39216-4505; **Phone:** 601-984-5600; **Board Cert:** Internal Medicine 1974; Allergy & Immunology 1977; Rheumatology 1982; Geriatric Medicine 2005; **Med School:** Univ Ala 1971; **Resid:** Internal Medicine, Walter Reed Genl Hosp 1974; **Fellow:** Microbiology, Walter Reed Army Inst Rsch 1975; Clinical Immunology, Walter Reed Genl Hosp 1977; **Fac Appt:** Prof Med, Univ Miss

Fox, Roger W MD [A&I] - **Spec Exp:** Asthma; Rhinosinusitis; Urticaria; **Hospital:** University Comm Hosp, Tampa Genl Hosp; **Address:** 13801 Bruce B Downs Blvd, Ste 505, Tampa, FL 33613; **Phone:** 813-971-9743; **Board Cert:** Internal Medicine 1978; Allergy & Immunology 1981; **Med School:** St Louis Univ 1975; **Resid:** Internal Medicine, Univ S Florida Affil Hosps 1978; **Fellow:** Allergy & Immunology, Univ S Florida Affil Hosps 1980; **Fac Appt:** Assoc Prof Med, Univ S Fla Coll Med

Friedman, Stuart A MD [A&I] - **Spec Exp:** Asthma; Sinus Disorders; Allergy; **Hospital:** Boca Raton Comm Hosp, Delray Med Ctr; **Address:** 5162 Linton Blvd, Ste 201, Delray Beach, FL 33484-6567; **Phone:** 561-495-2580; **Board Cert:** Internal Medicine 1980; Allergy & Immunology 1983; **Med School:** Spain 1976; **Resid:** Internal Medicine, Winthrop Univ Hosp 1980; **Fellow:** Immunology, Univ Cincinnati Med Ctr 1982; **Fac Appt:** Asst Clin Prof Med, Univ Miami Sch Med

Gluck, Joan MD [A&I] - **Spec Exp:** Asthma in Pregnancy; Asthma & Allergy; Food Allergy; **Hospital:** Baptist Hosp of Miami, South Miami Hosp; **Address:** 8970 SW 87th Ct, Ste 100, Miami, FL 33176-2207; **Phone:** 305-279-3366; **Med School:** NYU Sch Med 1972; **Resid:** Pediatrics, Jackson Meml Hosp 1974; **Fellow:** Allergy & Immunology, Jackson Meml Hosp 1976

Kaplan, Allen MD [A&I] - **Spec Exp:** Urticaria; **Hospital:** MUSC Med Ctr; **Address:** 1879 Savage Rd, Charleston, SC 29407; **Phone:** 843-573-9373; **Board Cert:** Internal Medicine 1972; Rheumatology 1972; Allergy & Immunology 1974; Clinical & Laboratory Immunology 1986; **Med School:** SUNY Downstate 1965; **Resid:** Internal Medicine, Strong Meml Hosp 1967; **Fac Appt:** Prof Med, Univ SC Sch Med

Ledford, Dennis MD [A&I] - **Spec Exp:** Asthma; **Hospital:** University Comm Hosp, Tampa Genl Hosp; **Address:** Univ So Florida Coll Med, Dept Allergy & Immunology, 13000 Bruce B Downs Blvd, VAR111D, Tampa, FL 33613-4745; **Phone:** 813-971-9743; **Board Cert:** Internal Medicine 1980; Rheumatology 1984; Allergy & Immunology 1985; Clinical & Laboratory Immunology 1986; **Med School:** Univ Tenn Coll Med, Memphis 1976; **Resid:** Internal Medicine, City of Memphis Hosp 1980; **Fellow:** Rheumatology, NYU Hosp-Bellevue 1982; Allergy & Immunology, Univ S Florida Coll Med 1985; **Fac Appt:** Assoc Prof A&I, Univ S Fla Coll Med

Lieberman, Phillip L MD [A&I] - **Spec Exp:** Asthma; Rhinitis; Anaphylaxis; **Hospital:** Baptist Memorial Hospital - Memphis, Methodist Univ Hosp - Memphis; **Address:** 7205 Wolf River Blvd, Ste 200, Germantown, TN 38138; **Phone:** 901-757-6100; **Board Cert:** Internal Medicine 1970; Allergy & Immunology 2001; **Med School:** Univ Tenn Coll Med, Memphis 1965; **Resid:** Internal Medicine, Memphis City Hosps 1969; **Fellow:** Allergy & Immunology, Northwestern Univ 1971; **Fac Appt:** Clin Prof A&I, Univ Tenn Coll Med, Memphis

Lockey, Richard MD [A&I] - **Spec Exp:** Immune Deficiency; Asthma; Rhinitis; **Hospital:** University Comm Hosp, Tampa Genl Hosp; **Address:** 13801 Bruce B Downs Blvd, Ste 502, Tampa, FL 33613-3946; **Phone:** 813-971-9743; **Board Cert:** Internal Medicine 1970; Allergy & Immunology 1974; **Med School:** Temple Univ 1965; **Resid:** Internal Medicine, Univ Mich Hosp 1968; **Fellow:** Allergy & Immunology, Univ Mich Hosp 1970; **Fac Appt:** Prof Med, Univ S Fla Coll Med

Pacin, Michael P MD [A&I] - **Spec Exp:** Insect Allergies; Asthma; Rhinitis; **Hospital:** Baptist Hosp of Miami, South Miami Hosp; **Address:** 8970 SW 87th Court, Ste 100, Miami, FL 33176-2207; **Phone:** 305-279-3366; **Board Cert:** Internal Medicine 1974; Allergy & Immunology 1979; **Med School:** Washington Univ, St Louis 1969; **Resid:** Internal Medicine, Jewish Hosp 1971; Internal Medicine, Jackson Meml Hosp 1972; **Fellow:** Allergy & Immunology, Long Beach VA Hosp 1974

Stein, Mark R MD [A&I] - **Spec Exp:** Asthma; Immune Deficiency; Gastroesophageal Reflux Disease (GERD); **Hospital:** Good Sam Med Ctr - W Palm Beach, Palm Beach Gardens Med Ctr; **Address:** 840 US Hwy 1, Ste 235, North Palm Beach, FL 33408-3835; **Phone:** 561-626-2006; **Board Cert:** Internal Medicine 1975; Allergy & Immunology 1977; **Med School:** Jefferson Med Coll 1968; **Resid:** Internal Medicine, Letterman Army Med Ctr 1975; **Fellow:** Allergy & Immunology, Fitzsimmons Army Med Ctr 1977

Sullivan, Timothy J MD [A&I] - **Spec Exp:** Drug Allergy; Anaphylaxis; Asthma; **Hospital:** Northside Hosp, St Joseph's Hosp - Atlanta; **Address:** 5555 Peachtree Dunwoody Rd, Ste 125, Atlanta, GA 30342; **Phone:** 404-255-2918; **Board Cert:** Allergy & Immunology 1979; **Med School:** Univ Miami Sch Med 1966; **Resid:** Internal Medicine, Barnes Hosp 1971; **Fellow:** Allergy & Immunology, Barnes Hosp 1973

Allergy & Immunology

Midwest

Baker Jr, James Russell MD [A&I] - **Spec Exp:** Immune Deficiency-Thyroid; **Hospital:** Univ Michigan Hlth Sys; **Address:** Tabuman Ctr-Allergy Div, 1500 E Med Ctr Drive, rm 3918, Box 0380, Ann Arbor, MI 48109-0380; **Phone:** 734-647-2777; **Board Cert:** Internal Medicine 1981; Allergy & Immunology 1983; Clinical & Laboratory Immunology 1986; **Med School:** Loyola Univ-Stritch Sch Med 1978; **Resid:** Internal Medicine, Walter Reed Army Med Ctr 1981; **Fellow:** Allergy & Immunology, Walter Reed Army Med Ctr/NIAID 1984; **Fac Appt:** Prof A&I, Univ Mich Med Sch

Berger, Melvin MD/PhD [A&I] - **Spec Exp:** Immune Deficiency; Asthma & Allergy; Allergy; **Hospital:** Rainbow Babies & Chldns Hosp, Univ Hosps Case Med Ctr; **Address:** Pediatric Immunology, 11100 Euclid Ave, MC 6008B, Cleveland, OH 44106-1736; **Phone:** 216-844-3237; **Board Cert:** Pediatrics 1981; Allergy & Immunology 1981; **Med School:** Case West Res Univ 1976; **Resid:** Pediatrics, Chldns Hosp Med Ctr 1978; **Fellow:** Allergy & Immunology, Natl Inst Allergy & Infect Dis (NIH) 1981; **Fac Appt:** Prof Ped, Case West Res Univ

Busse, William MD [A&I] - **Spec Exp:** Asthma; Autoimmune Disease; Rhinitis; **Hospital:** Univ WI Hosp & Clins; **Address:** 600 Highland Ave, rm B6-242, Madison, WI 53792; **Phone:** 608-263-6180; **Board Cert:** Internal Medicine 1972; Allergy & Immunology 1974; **Med School:** Univ Wisc 1966; **Resid:** Internal Medicine, Cincinnati Genl Hosp 1968; Internal Medicine, Cincinnati Genl Hosp 1971; **Fellow:** Allergy & Immunology, Univ Wisconsin 1973; **Fac Appt:** Prof Med, Univ Wisc

Gewurz, Anita MD [A&I] - **Spec Exp:** Immune Deficiency; Asthma; **Hospital:** Rush Univ Med Ctr; **Address:** Univ Consultants, 1725 W Harrison St, Ste 117, Chicago, IL 60612; **Phone:** 312-942-6296; **Board Cert:** Pediatrics 1976; Allergy & Immunology 1977; **Med School:** Albany Med Coll 1970; **Resid:** Pediatrics, Univ Illinois Med Ctr 1973; Allergy & Immunology, Rush-Presby-St Lukes Hosp 1976; **Fellow:** Allergy & Immunology, Grant Hosp 1977; Allergy & Immunology, Northwestern Univ Med Sch 1985; **Fac Appt:** Prof Med, Rush Med Coll

Grammer, Leslie C MD [A&I] - **Spec Exp:** Asthma; Sinusitis; Drug Allergy; **Hospital:** Northwestern Meml Hosp, Rehab Inst - Chicago; **Address:** Northwestern Med Faculty Fdn-Amb Care Ctr, 675 N St Clair, Fl 18 - Ste 18-250, Chicago, IL 60611-5975; **Phone:** 312-695-8624; **Board Cert:** Internal Medicine 1979; Allergy & Immunology 1981; Clinical & Laboratory Immunology 1986; Occupational Medicine 1989; **Med School:** Northwestern Univ 1976; **Resid:** Internal Medicine, Northwestern Meml Hosp 1979; **Fellow:** Allergy & Immunology, Northwestern Univ 1981; **Fac Appt:** Prof Med, Northwestern Univ

Greenberger, Paul A MD [A&I] - **Spec Exp:** Asthma; Anaphylaxis; Drug Allergy; **Hospital:** Northwestern Meml Hosp, Jesse A Brown VA Med Ctr; **Address:** Northwestern Medical Faculty Fdn, Ambulatory Care Center, 675 N St Clair Fl 18 - Ste 18-250, Chicago, IL 60611; **Phone:** 312-695-8624; **Board Cert:** Internal Medicine 1976; Allergy & Immunology 1979; Diagnostic Lab Immunology 1986; **Med School:** Indiana Univ 1973; **Resid:** Internal Medicine, Jewish Hosp 1976; **Fellow:** Allergy & Immunology, Northwestern Meml Hosp 1978; **Fac Appt:** Prof Med, Northwestern Univ

Kaiser, Harold MD [A&I] - **Spec Exp:** Asthma; Rhinitis; Clinical Trials; **Hospital:** Abbott - Northwestern Hosp, Northern Meml Hlth Care; **Address:** 825 Nicollett Mall, Ste 1149, Minneapolis, MN 55402-2750; **Phone:** 612-338-3333; **Board Cert:** Internal Medicine 1963; Allergy & Immunology 1977; **Med School:** Univ Minn 1956; **Resid:** Internal Medicine, Wadsworth VA Hosp 1958; Allergy & Immunology, VA Hosp-Univ Minn Hosp 1962; **Fellow:** Allergy & Immunology, UCLA Med Ctr 1965; **Fac Appt:** Clin Prof Med, Univ Minn

Korenblat, Phillip E MD [A&I] - **Spec Exp:** Allergy; Asthma; Anaphylaxis; **Hospital:** Barnes-Jewish Hosp, Missouri Baptist Med Ctr; **Address:** 1040 N Mason Rd, Ste 115, St. Louis, MO 63141-6361; **Phone:** 314-542-0606; **Board Cert:** Internal Medicine 1971; Allergy & Immunology 1974; **Med School:** Univ Ark 1960; **Resid:** Internal Medicine, Jewish Hosp 1965; **Fellow:** Allergy & Immunology, Scripps Clin Rsch Fdn 1966; **Fac Appt:** Clin Prof Med, Washington Univ, St Louis

Rosenwasser, Lanny J MD [A&I] - **Spec Exp:** Asthma; Vasculitis; Immunotherapy; **Hospital:** Chldns Mercy Hosps & Clinics, Truman Med Ctr; **Address:** Chldns Mercy Hosps & Clinics, 2401 Gillham Rd, Kansas City, MO 64108; **Phone:** 816-234-3700; **Board Cert:** Internal Medicine 1975; Allergy & Immunology 1977; Clinical & Laboratory Immunology 1990; **Med School:** NYU Sch Med 1972; **Resid:** Internal Medicine, UCSF Afil Hosps 1974; **Fac Appt:** Prof Med, Univ MO-Kansas City

Sanders, Georgiana MD [A&I] - **Spec Exp:** Asthma; Food Allergy & Eczema; Rhinitis; **Hospital:** Univ Michigan Hlth Sys, St Joseph Med Ctr; **Address:** Domino's Farms, 24 Frank Lloyd Wright Dr, Ste H-2100, Ann Arbor, MI 48106; **Phone:** 734-936-5634; **Board Cert:** Pediatrics 1983; Allergy & Immunology 1985; **Med School:** Univ Cincinnati 1975; **Resid:** Pediatrics, Children's Hosp Mich 1978; Pediatrics, Boston City Hospi 1979; **Fellow:** Allergy & Immunology, Univ of Michigan Hosp 1984; **Fac Appt:** Asst Clin Prof Med, Univ Mich Med Sch

Ten, Rosa Maria MD/PhD [A&I] - **Spec Exp:** Immune Deficiency; Asthma; **Hospital:** Riley Hosp for Children; **Address:** Riley Hosp for Children, 702 Barnhill Drive, rm 4270, Indianapolis, IN 46202-5225; **Phone:** 317-274-7208; **Board Cert:** Allergy & Immunology 1997; **Med School:** Spain 1982; **Resid:** Internal Medicine, Mayo Clinic 1994; **Fellow:** Immunology, Inst Pasteur 1991; Allergy & Immunology, Mayo Clinic 1996; **Fac Appt:** Assoc Prof Ped, Indiana Univ

Wood, John A MD [A&I] - **Spec Exp:** Asthma; **Hospital:** St Luke's Hosp - Chesterfield, MO; **Address:** 224 S Woodsmill Rd, Ste 500S, Chesterfield, MO 63017; **Phone:** 314-878-6260; **Board Cert:** Internal Medicine 1972; Pulmonary Disease 1978; Allergy & Immunology 1979; **Med School:** Univ Okla Coll Med 1968; **Resid:** Internal Medicine, Univ Hosp 1970; Internal Medicine, Barnes Hosp-Wash Univ Sch Med 1971; **Fellow:** Pulmonary Disease, Wash Univ Sch Med 1977; Allergy & Immunology, Wash Univ Sch Med 1977; **Fac Appt:** Asst Prof Med, Washington Univ, St Louis

Great Plains and Mountains

Nelson, Harold MD [A&I] - **Spec Exp:** Asthma; Allergy; Rhinitis; **Hospital:** Natl Jewish Med & Rsch Ctr; **Address:** National Jewish Med & Rsch Ctr, 1400 Jackson St, Denver, CO 80206-2762; **Phone:** 303-398-1562; **Board Cert:** Internal Medicine 1963; Allergy & Immunology 1983; **Med School:** Emory Univ 1955; **Resid:** Internal Medicine, Letterman Genl Hosp 1962; **Fellow:** Allergy & Immunology, Univ Mich Med Ctr 1969; **Fac Appt:** Prof Med, Univ Colorado

Southwest

Freeman, Theodore MD [A&I] - **Spec Exp:** Insect Allergies; Asthma; Rhinitis; **Hospital:** SW TX Meth Hosp; **Address:** 8287 Fredericksberg Rd, San Antonio, TX 78229; **Phone:** 210-614-3923; **Board Cert:** Internal Medicine 1983; Allergy & Immunology 1987; Clinical & Laboratory Immunology 1988; **Med School:** Univ S Fla Coll Med 1980; **Resid:** Internal Medicine, Keesler Med Ctr 1983; **Fellow:** Allergy & Immunology, Wilford Hall Med Ctr 1986; Diagnostic Lab Immunology, Mass Genl Hosp 1987; **Fac Appt:** Assoc Prof Med, Uniformed Srvs Univ, Bethesda

Gruchalla, Rebecca S MD/PhD [A&I] - **Spec Exp:** Asthma & Allergy; Drug Allergy; **Hospital:** UT Southwestern Med Ctr - Dallas, Chldns Med Ctr of Dallas; **Address:** Univ Tex SW, Div A&I, 5303 Harry Hines Blvd, Internal Medicine Sub Specialty Clinic, Dallas, TX 75390-8859; **Phone:** 214-648-3004; **Board Cert:** Internal Medicine 1988; Allergy & Immunology 2001; **Med School:** Univ Tex SW, Dallas 1985; **Resid:** Internal Medicine, Hosp Univ Penn 1988; **Fellow:** Allergy & Immunology, Univ Tex SW Med Ctr 1990; **Fac Appt:** Assoc Prof Med, Univ Tex SW, Dallas

Lewis, John C MD [A&I] - **Spec Exp:** Autoimmune Disease; **Hospital:** Mayo Clin Hosp - Scottsdale; **Address:** Mayo Clinic, Div Allergy & Immunology, 13400 E Shea Blvd, ALRG-2B, Scottsdale, AZ 85259-5404; **Phone:** 480-301-8227; **Board Cert:** Internal Medicine 1985; Allergy & Immunology 2001; **Med School:** Loyola Univ-Stritch Sch Med 1982; **Resid:** Internal Medicine, Wilford Hall USAF Med Ctr 1985; **Fellow:** Allergy & Immunology, Mayo Clinic 1990; **Fac Appt:** Prof Med, Mayo Med Sch

Schubert, Mark S MD/PhD [A&I] - **Spec Exp:** Asthma & Allergy; Sinus Disorders; Immunodeficiency Disorders; **Hospital:** Banner Good Samaritan Regl Med Ctr - Phoenix, St Joseph's Hosp & Med Ctr - Phoenix; **Address:** 300 W Clarendon Rd, Ste 120, Phoenix, AZ 85013-2517; **Phone:** 602-277-3337; **Board Cert:** Internal Medicine 1987; Allergy & Immunology 1999; **Med School:** Univ Ariz Coll Med 1983; **Resid:** Neurological Surgery, Barrow Neurological Inst 1985; Internal Medicine, Good Samaritan Med Ctr 1987; **Fellow:** Allergy Immunology & Rheumatology, Stanford Univ Med Ctr 1989; **Fac Appt:** Assoc Clin Prof Med, Univ Ariz Coll Med

West Coast and Pacific

Meltzer, Eli MD [A&I] - **Spec Exp:** Asthma & Allergy; Sinus Disorders; **Hospital:** Rady Children's Hosp - San Diego, Sharp Meml Hosp; **Address:** Allergy & Asthma Medical & Research Ctr, 9610 Granite Ridge Drive, Ste B, San Diego, CA 92123-2661; **Phone:** 858-292-1144; **Board Cert:** Pediatrics 1969; Allergy & Immunology 1972; **Med School:** Jefferson Med Coll 1964; **Resid:** Pediatrics, St Christophers Hosp for Chld 1967; **Fellow:** Pediatric Allergy & Immunology, National Jewish Hosp 1969; **Fac Appt:** Clin Prof Ped, UCSD

Montanaro, Anthony MD [A&I] - **Spec Exp:** Asthma; Allergy; Anaphylaxis; Immunodeficiency Disorders; **Hospital:** OR Hlth & Sci Univ; **Address:** OHSU Div Allergy & Clin Immunology, 3181 SW Sam Jackson Park Rd, rm OP-34, Portland, OR 97239-2098; **Phone:** 503-494-4300; **Board Cert:** Internal Medicine 1981; Allergy & Immunology 1993; Rheumatology 1984; **Med School:** Univ Wash 1978; **Resid:** Internal Medicine, Mercy Med Ctr 1981; **Fellow:** Allergy Immunology & Rheumatology, Oregon Hlth Sci Univ 1983; **Fac Appt:** Prof Med, Oregon Hlth Sci Univ

Ostrom, Nancy K MD [A&I] - **Spec Exp:** Asthma & Allergy; **Hospital:** Rady Children's Hosp - San Diego; **Address:** 9610 Granite Ridge Drive, Ste B, San Diego, CA 92123; **Phone:** 858-292-1144; **Board Cert:** Pediatrics 1984; Allergy & Immunology 1987; **Med School:** Mayo Med Sch 1980; **Resid:** Pediatrics, Mayo Clinic 1983; **Fellow:** Allergy & Immunology, Mayo Clinic 1985; **Fac Appt:** Assoc Clin Prof Ped, UCSD

Tamaroff, Marc A MD [A&I] - **Spec Exp:** Sinus Disorders; Asthma; Rhinitis; **Hospital:** Long Beach Meml Med Ctr, Lakewood Reg Med Ctr; **Address:** 3816 Woodruff Ave, Ste 209, Long Beach, CA 90808-2145; **Phone:** 562-496-4749; **Board Cert:** Internal Medicine 1979; Allergy & Immunology 1983; **Med School:** Univ Ariz Coll Med 1974; **Resid:** Internal Medicine, St Mary Med Ctr 1977; **Fellow:** Allergy & Immunology, UCLA Med Ctr 1979; **Fac Appt:** Assoc Clin Prof Med, UCLA

Wasserman, Stephen MD [A&I] - **Spec Exp:** Asthma; Rhinitis; Sinus Disorders; Urticaria; **Hospital:** UCSD Med Ctr; **Address:** UCSD, MC 0637, Stein Bldg-rm 244, 9500 Gilman Drive, La Jolla, CA 92093-0637; **Phone:** 858-822-4261; **Board Cert:** Internal Medicine 1973; Allergy & Immunology 1975; **Med School:** UCLA 1968; **Resid:** Internal Medicine, Peter Bent Brigham Hosp 1970; **Fellow:** Allergy & Immunology, R Breck-PB Brigham Hosp 1974; **Fac Appt:** Prof Med, UCSD

Cleveland Clinic

Pulmonary, Allergy and Critical Care Medicine

The Section of Allergy/Immunology at Cleveland Clinic is one of the largest allergy and immunology groups in the United States with a national reputation for excellence. Patients have access not only to state-of-the-art medical therapies but also to investigational protocols. From 2002 to 2006, more than 135,000 skin tests were safely performed to identify inhalant, food, drug or venom allergy.

Allergy/immunology diagnosis and treatment takes place in a multidisciplinary fashion that includes close coordination with specialists in other areas.

Asthma

We provide state-of-the-art management for patients whose asthma is not well controlled. This includes assessments of coexisting conditions that make asthma difficult to treat or unresponsive to standard treatment. We offer new medications that may not be available in primary care settings and interventions that may not be provided by asthma specialists in the community.

Aspirin Sensitivity and Desensitization

Individuals who are sensitive to aspirin often experience respiratory reactions, including wheezing, shortness of breath, or skin reactions, such as hives or swelling. We offer a special desensitization program for aspirin-sensitive patients who have respiratory reactions but require aspirin for cardiovascular or rheumatic conditions. This procedure, available at only a few centers in the United States, can permit such patients to take aspirin safely.

Areas of Expertise

- Asthma
- Rhinitis, allergic and non-allergic
- Sinusitis
- Chronic cough
- Aspirin sensitivity
- Urticaria/angioedema
- Atopic dermatitis
- Adverse reactions to medicine, food and bee stings
- Anaphylaxis
- Systemic mastocytosis
- Immunodeficiency

To schedule an appointment or for more information about the Cleveland Clinic Department of Pulmonary, Allergy and Critical Care Medicine call 800.890.2467 or visit www.clevelandclinic.org/allergytopdocs.

Department of Pulmonary, Allergy and Critical Care Medicine
9500 Euclid Avenue / W14 | Cleveland OH 44195

Second Opinion – Online

Use e-Cleveland Clinic's convenient, online second opinion service without leaving home. Call 800.223.2273, ext 43223, or visit www. eclevelandclinic.org.

Assistance for Out-of-Town and International Patients

Get complimentary help scheduling medical appointments and arranging for hotels and transportation.

For out-of-town patients call 800.223.2273, ext. 55580, or visit www. clevelandclinic. org/services. For International patients call 216.444.6404 or visit www.clevelandclinic. org/ic.

Cardiovascular Disease
a subspecialty of Internal Medicine

Cardiovascular Disease: An internist specializing in diseases of the heart, lungs and blood vessels and manages complex cardiac conditions such as heart attacks and life-threatening, abnormal heartbeat rhythms.

Cardiac Electrophysiology: A field of special interest within the subspecialty of cardiovascular disease which involves intricate technical procedures to evaluate heart rhythms and determine appropriate treatment for them.

Interventional Cardiology: An area of medicine within the subspecialty of cardiology which uses specialized imaging and other diagnostic techniques to evaluate blood flow and pressure in the coronary arteries and chambers of the heart, and uses technical procedures and medications to treat abnormalities that impair the function of the heart.

Training Required: Three years in internal medicine *plus* additional training and examination for certification in cardiovascular disease, clinical electrophysiology or interventional cardiology

Cardiovascular Disease

New England

Balady, Gary MD [Cv] - **Spec Exp:** Preventive Cardiology; **Hospital:** Boston Med Ctr; **Address:** Boston Med Ctr, Dept Cardiology, 88 East Newton St, Bldg C8, Boston, MA 02118; **Phone:** 617-638-7490; **Board Cert:** Internal Medicine 1982; Cardiovascular Disease 1985; **Med School:** UMDNJ-Rutgers Med Sch 1979; **Resid:** Internal Medicine, Boston Univ Med Ctr 1982; **Fellow:** Cardiovascular Disease, Boston Univ Med Ctr 1985; **Fac Appt:** Prof Med, Boston Univ

Baughman, Kenneth MD [Cv] - **Spec Exp:** Congestive Heart Failure; Cardiomyopathy; **Hospital:** Brigham & Women's Hosp; **Address:** Brigham & Womens Hosp, Cardiovascular, 75 Francis St Bldg A - rm AB362, Boston, MA 02115; **Phone:** 617-732-8970; **Board Cert:** Internal Medicine 1975; Cardiovascular Disease 1979; **Med School:** Univ MO-Columbia Sch Med 1972; **Resid:** Internal Medicine, Johns Hopkins Hosp 1977; **Fellow:** Cardiovascular Disease, Mass Genl Hosp 1979; **Fac Appt:** Prof Med, Harvard Med Sch

Cabin, Henry S MD [Cv] - **Spec Exp:** Interventional Cardiology; Cardiac Catheterization; **Hospital:** Yale - New Haven Hosp; **Address:** 333 Cedar St, PO Box 208017, New Haven, CT 06520-8017; **Phone:** 203-785-4129; **Board Cert:** Internal Medicine 1978; Cardiovascular Disease 1983; Interventional Cardiology 2000; **Med School:** Yale Univ 1975; **Resid:** Internal Medicine, Yale-New Haven Hosp 1978; **Fellow:** Internal Medicine, Natl Heart Lung and Blood Inst 1981; Cardiovascular Disease, Yale New Haven Hosp 1982; **Fac Appt:** Prof Med, Yale Univ

Cohen, Lawrence S MD [Cv] - **Spec Exp:** Coronary Artery Disease; Heart Valve Disease; Geriatric Cardiology; **Hospital:** Yale - New Haven Hosp; **Address:** Yale Univ Sch Med - Cardiology, 333 Cedar St, Ste FMP 313, Box 208017, New Haven, CT 06520-8017; **Phone:** 203-785-4128; **Board Cert:** Internal Medicine 1966; Cardiovascular Disease 1967; **Med School:** NYU Sch Med 1958; **Resid:** Internal Medicine, Yale-New Haven Hosp 1960; Internal Medicine, Yale-New Haven Hosp 1965; **Fellow:** Research, Peter Bent Brigham Hosp 1964; **Fac Appt:** Prof Med, Yale Univ

Davidoff, Ravin MD [Cv] - **Spec Exp:** Echocardiography; Heart Valve Disease; **Hospital:** Boston Med Ctr; **Address:** Boston Univ Med Ctr, Div Cardiology, 88 E Newton Street, Boston, MA 02118; **Phone:** 617-638-7490; **Board Cert:** Internal Medicine 1985; Cardiovascular Disease 1987; **Med School:** South Africa 1977; **Resid:** Internal Medicine, Boston City Hosp 1985; **Fellow:** Cardiovascular Disease, Mass Genl Hosp 1988; **Fac Appt:** Prof Med, Boston Univ

DeSanctis, Roman MD [Cv] - **Spec Exp:** Coronary Artery Disease; Heart Valve Disease; **Hospital:** Mass Genl Hosp; **Address:** Mass General Hosp, Yawkey Ste 5800, 55 Fruit St, Ste 5700, Boston, MA 02114; **Phone:** 617-726-2889; **Board Cert:** Internal Medicine 1962; Cardiovascular Disease 1971; **Med School:** Harvard Med Sch 1955; **Resid:** Internal Medicine, Mass Genl Hosp 1960; **Fellow:** Cardiovascular Disease, Mass Genl Hosp 1962; **Fac Appt:** Prof Med, Harvard Med Sch

Huang, Paul MD [Cv] - **Spec Exp:** Nutrition & Obesity; Vascular Disease; Hypertension; Stroke; **Hospital:** Mass Genl Hosp; **Address:** Cardiac Unit Associates, 55 Fruit St, Gray Bigelow Bldg Fl 8, Boston, MA 02114-2696; **Phone:** 617-724-9849; **Board Cert:** Internal Medicine 1988; Cardiovascular Disease 2002; **Med School:** Harvard Med Sch 1985; **Resid:** Internal Medicine, Mass Genl Hosp 1988; **Fellow:** Cardiovascular Disease, Mass Genl Hosp 1991; **Fac Appt:** Assoc Prof Med, Harvard Med Sch

Hutter Jr, Adolph M MD [Cv] - **Hospital:** Mass Genl Hosp; **Address:** 32 Fruit St, Yawkey Ctr - 5B, Boston, MA 02114-3139; **Phone:** 617-726-2884; **Board Cert:** Internal Medicine 1969; Cardiovascular Disease 1971; **Med School:** Univ Wisc 1963; **Resid:** Internal Medicine, Strong Meml Hosp 1968; **Fellow:** Cardiovascular Disease, Mass Genl Hosp 1970; **Fac Appt:** Prof Med, Harvard Med Sch

Johnson, Paula A MD [Cv] - **Spec Exp:** Heart Disease in Women; Preventive Cardiology; Congestive Heart Failure; **Hospital:** Brigham & Women's Hosp; **Address:** BWH, Dept Med-Womens Health Div, 75 Francis St, PB-Admin-5, Boston, MA 02115; **Phone:** 617-732-4837; **Board Cert:** Internal Medicine 1988; Cardiovascular Disease 2001; **Med School:** Harvard Med Sch 1985; **Resid:** Internal Medicine, Brigham & Womens Hosp 1988; **Fellow:** Cardiovascular Disease, Brigham & Womens Hosp 1991; **Fac Appt:** Assoc Prof Med, Harvard Med Sch

Josephson, Mark Eric MD [Cv] - **Spec Exp:** Cardiac Electrophysiology; Arrhythmias; **Hospital:** Beth Israel Deaconess Med Ctr - Boston; **Address:** 185 Pilgrim Rd, Baker 4, Boston, MA 02215; **Phone:** 617-632-7457; **Board Cert:** Internal Medicine 1973; Cardiovascular Disease 1975; Cardiac Electrophysiology 2002; **Med School:** Columbia P&S 1969; **Resid:** Internal Medicine, Mt Sinai Med Ctr 1971; **Fellow:** Cardiovascular Disease, Hosp Univ Penn 1975; **Fac Appt:** Prof Med, Harvard Med Sch

Kirshenbaum, James M MD [Cv] - **Spec Exp:** Cardiac Catheterization; Coronary Artery Disease; Congestive Heart Failure; **Hospital:** Brigham & Women's Hosp; **Address:** Brigham & Womens Hosp, Div Cardiology, 75 Francis St, Boston, MA 02115-6110; **Phone:** 617-732-7173; **Board Cert:** Internal Medicine 1982; Cardiovascular Disease 1985; Interventional Cardiology 1999; **Med School:** Harvard Med Sch 1979; **Resid:** Internal Medicine, Peter Bent Brigham Hosp 1982; **Fellow:** Cardiovascular Disease, Brigham & Womens Hosp 1985; **Fac Appt:** Assoc Prof Med, Harvard Med Sch

Konstam, Marvin A MD [Cv] - **Spec Exp:** Transplant Medicine-Heart; Heart Failure; Coronary Angioplasty/Stents; **Hospital:** Tufts-New England Med Ctr, Beth Israel Deaconess Med Ctr - Boston; **Address:** New England Med Ctr, Div Cardiology, 750 Washington St, Boston, MA 02111; **Phone:** 617-636-6293; **Board Cert:** Internal Medicine 1979; Cardiovascular Disease 1981; Diagnostic Radiology 1980; **Med School:** Columbia P&S 1975; **Resid:** Diagnostic Radiology, Mass Genl Hosp 1978; Internal Medicine, Mass Genl Hosp 1979; **Fellow:** Cardiovascular Disease, Brigham & Women's Hosp 1981; **Fac Appt:** Prof Med, Tufts Univ

Liang, Bruce T MD [Cv] - **Spec Exp:** Ischemic Heart Disease; Congestive Heart Failure; **Hospital:** Univ of Conn Hlth Ctr, John Dempsey Hosp; **Address:** Univ Connecticut Health Ctr, Cardiopulmonary & Hypertension Service, 263 Farmington Ave, Farmington, CT 06030-2202; **Phone:** 860-679-3343; **Board Cert:** Internal Medicine 1985; Cardiovascular Disease 1987; **Med School:** Harvard Med Sch 1982; **Resid:** Internal Medicine, Hosp Univ Penn 1985; **Fellow:** Cardiovascular Disease, Brigham & Womens Hosp 1987; **Fac Appt:** Prof Med, Univ Conn

Libby, Peter MD [Cv] - **Spec Exp:** Preventive Cardiology; Coronary Artery Disease; Cholesterol/Lipid Disorders; **Hospital:** Brigham & Women's Hosp; **Address:** Brigham & Women's Hosp, Cardiovasc Div, 75 Francis St, Boston, MA 02115-5822; **Phone:** 617-732-8086; **Board Cert:** Internal Medicine 1976; Cardiovascular Disease 1981; **Med School:** UCSD 1973; **Resid:** Internal Medicine, Peter Bent Brigham Hosp 1976; **Fellow:** Physiology, Harvard Med Sch 1979; Cardiovascular Disease, Brigham & Woman's Hosp 1980; **Fac Appt:** Prof Med, Harvard Med Sch

Cardiovascular Disease

Loscalzo, Joseph MD/PhD [Cv] - **Spec Exp:** Coronary Artery Disease; Peripheral Vascular Disease; **Hospital:** Brigham & Women's Hosp; **Address:** Brigham & Women's Hosp, Div Cardiology, 75 Francis St, Boston, MA 02115; **Phone:** 617-732-6340; **Board Cert:** Internal Medicine 1981; Cardiovascular Disease 1983; **Med School:** Univ Pennsylvania 1978; **Resid:** Internal Medicine, Peter Bent Brigham Hosp. 1981; **Fellow:** Cardiovascular Disease, Brigham & Women's Hosp 1983; **Fac Appt:** Prof Med, Harvard Med Sch

Manning, Warren MD [Cv] - **Spec Exp:** Heart Valve Disease; Echocardiography; **Hospital:** Beth Israel Deaconess Med Ctr - Boston; **Address:** BIDMC, Dept Non-Invasive Cardiology, 330 Brookline Ave, Boston, MA 02215-5400; **Phone:** 617-667-2192; **Board Cert:** Internal Medicine 1986; Cardiovascular Disease 1989; **Med School:** Harvard Med Sch 1983; **Resid:** Internal Medicine, Beth Israel Hosp 1986; **Fellow:** Cardiovascular Disease, Beth Israel Hosp 1989; **Fac Appt:** Prof Med, Harvard Med Sch

O'Gara, Patrick T MD [Cv] - **Spec Exp:** Heart Valve Disease; Coronary Artery Disease; Aortic Diseases & Dissection; **Hospital:** Brigham & Women's Hosp; **Address:** Brigham & Womens Hosp, Cardiovascular Div, 75 Francis St, Boston, MA 02115-6106; **Phone:** 617-732-8380; **Board Cert:** Internal Medicine 1981; Cardiovascular Disease 1983; **Med School:** Northwestern Univ 1978; **Resid:** Internal Medicine, Mass Genl Hosp 1981; **Fellow:** Cardiovascular Disease, Mass Genl Hosp 1983; **Fac Appt:** Assoc Prof Med, Harvard Med Sch

Palacios, Igor F MD [Cv] - **Spec Exp:** Interventional Cardiology; **Hospital:** Mass Genl Hosp; **Address:** Mass Genl Hosp, Cardiac Unit, 55 Fruit St, Bulfinch 105, Boston, MA 02114; **Phone:** 617-726-8424; **Board Cert:** Internal Medicine 1979; Cardiovascular Disease 1981; Interventional Cardiology 1999; **Med School:** Venezuela 1969; **Resid:** Cardiovascular Disease, Hosp Univ de Caracas 1973; **Fellow:** Cardiovascular Disease, Mass Genl Hosp-Harvard 1980; **Fac Appt:** Assoc Prof Med, Harvard Med Sch

Pfeffer, Marc Alan MD [Cv] - **Hospital:** Brigham & Women's Hosp; **Address:** Brigham & Women's Hospital, 75 Francis St, Boston, MA 02115; **Phone:** 617-732-5681; **Board Cert:** Internal Medicine 1979; Cardiovascular Disease 1981; **Med School:** Univ Okla Coll Med 1976; **Resid:** Internal Medicine, Peter Bent Brigham Hosp 1979; **Fellow:** Cardiovascular Disease, Peter Bent Brigham Hosp 1980; **Fac Appt:** Prof Med, Harvard Med Sch

Phillips, Robert A MD/PhD [Cv] - **Spec Exp:** Hypertension; Coronary Artery Disease; Heart Valve Disease; **Hospital:** UMass Memorial Med Ctr; **Address:** U Mass Memorial Cardiovascular Ctr, 55 Lake Ave North, S3-866, Worcester, MA 01655; **Phone:** 508-856-3452; **Board Cert:** Internal Medicine 1983; Cardiovascular Disease 1985; **Med School:** Mount Sinai Sch Med 1980; **Resid:** Internal Medicine, Columbia Presby Med Ctr 1983; **Fellow:** Cardiovascular Disease, Mount Sinai Med Ctr 1985; Hypertension, Mount Sinai Med Ctr 1986; **Fac Appt:** Prof Med, Univ Mass Sch Med

Ridker, Paul M MD [Cv] - **Spec Exp:** Coronary Artery Disease; Preventive Cardiology; **Hospital:** Brigham & Women's Hosp; **Address:** Brigham & Women's Hospital, Div Preventive Medicine, 640 Center St, Jamaica Plains, MA 02130; **Phone:** 617-983-4100; **Board Cert:** Internal Medicine 1989; **Med School:** Harvard Med Sch 1986; **Resid:** Internal Medicine, Brigham-Womens Harvard 1989; **Fellow:** Cardiovascular Disease, Brigham-Womens Harvard 1991; **Fac Appt:** Assoc Prof Med, Harvard Med Sch

Roberts, Barbara H MD [Cv] - **Spec Exp:** Heart Disease in Women; Preventive Cardiology; **Hospital:** Miriam Hosp; **Address:** The Miriam Hosp - Women's Cardiac Ctr, 164 Summit Ave, Fain Hlth Ctrs Fl 2, Providence, RI 02906; **Phone:** 401-793-7870; **Board Cert:** Internal Medicine 1975; Cardiovascular Disease 1975; **Med School:** Case West Res Univ 1968; **Resid:** Internal Medicine, Yale-New Haven Hosp 1971; **Fellow:** Cardiovascular Disease, PB Brigham Hosp-Harvard 1975; **Fac Appt:** Assoc Clin Prof Med, Brown Univ

Simons, Michael MD [Cv] - **Spec Exp:** Ischemic Heart Disease; Nuclear Cardiology; **Hospital:** Dartmouth - Hitchcock Med Ctr; **Address:** Dartmouth Hitchcock Med Ctr, Cardiology, One Medical Center Drive, Lebanon, NH 03756; **Phone:** 603-650-5724; **Board Cert:** Internal Medicine 1987; Cardiovascular Disease 2001; **Med School:** Yale Univ 1984; **Resid:** Internal Medicine, New England Med Ctr 1986; **Fellow:** Cardiology Research, Natl Inst Hlth 1989; Cardiovascular Disease, Beth Israel Hosp 1991; **Fac Appt:** Prof Med, Dartmouth Med Sch

Stevenson, Lynne W MD [Cv] - **Spec Exp:** Heart Failure; Cardiomyopathy; Transplant Medicine-Heart; **Hospital:** Brigham & Women's Hosp; **Address:** Brigham & Women's Hospital, 75 Francis St, Boston, MA 02115; **Phone:** 617-732-4837; **Board Cert:** Internal Medicine 1982; Cardiovascular Disease 1985; **Med School:** Stanford Univ 1979; **Resid:** Internal Medicine, UCLA Med Ctr 1982; **Fellow:** Cardiovascular Disease, UCLA Med Ctr 1984; **Fac Appt:** Assoc Prof Med, Harvard Med Sch

Zaret, Barry L MD [Cv] - **Spec Exp:** Nuclear Cardiology; Heart Failure; Coronary Artery Disease; **Hospital:** Yale - New Haven Hosp; **Address:** 333 Cedar St, 3-FMP, New Haven, CT 06520-8017; **Phone:** 203-785-4127; **Board Cert:** Internal Medicine 1973; Cardiovascular Disease 1973; **Med School:** NYU Sch Med 1966; **Resid:** Internal Medicine, Bellevue Hosp Ctr 1969; **Fellow:** Cardiovascular Disease, Johns Hopkins Hosp 1971; **Fac Appt:** Prof Med, Yale Univ

Zusman, Randall M MD [Cv] - **Spec Exp:** Hypertension; **Hospital:** Mass Genl Hosp; **Address:** Massachusettes Hospital, Yawkey Ctr, 55 Fruit St, Ste 5928, Boston, MA 02114; **Phone:** 617-726-7790; **Board Cert:** Internal Medicine 1976; Cardiovascular Disease 1983; **Med School:** Yale Univ 1973; **Resid:** Internal Medicine, Mass General Hosp 1978; Internal Medicine, Natl Heart, Lung, & Blood Inst (NHBLI) 1977; **Fellow:** Cardiovascular Disease, Mass General Hosp 1979; **Fac Appt:** Assoc Prof Med, Harvard Med Sch

Mid Atlantic

Achuff, Stephen C MD [Cv] - **Spec Exp:** Coronary Artery Disease; Heart Valve Disease; **Hospital:** Johns Hopkins Hosp - Baltimore (page 61); **Address:** 600 N Wolfe St, Carnegie Bldg, rm 568, Baltimore, MD 21287-0005; **Phone:** 410-955-7670; **Board Cert:** Internal Medicine 1974; Cardiovascular Disease 1977; **Med School:** Univ MO-Columbia Sch Med 1969; **Resid:** Internal Medicine, Johns Hopkins Hosp 1971; Internal Medicine, Johns Hopkins Hosp 1974; **Fellow:** Cardiovascular Disease, Johns Hopkins Hosp 1973; Cardiovascular Disease, Royal Infirmary 1975; **Fac Appt:** Prof Med, Johns Hopkins Univ

Blumenthal, David S MD [Cv] - **Spec Exp:** Heart Valve Disease; Preventive Cardiology; Coronary Artery Disease; **Hospital:** NY-Presby Hosp/Weill Cornell (page 66); **Address:** 407 E 70th St, Fl 1, New York, NY 10021-5302; **Phone:** 212-861-3222; **Board Cert:** Internal Medicine 1978; Cardiovascular Disease 1981; **Med School:** Cornell Univ-Weill Med Coll 1975; **Resid:** Internal Medicine, New York Hosp 1978; Internal Medicine, New York Hosp 1981; **Fellow:** Cardiovascular Disease, Johns Hopkins Hosp 1980; **Fac Appt:** Clin Prof Med, Cornell Univ-Weill Med Coll

Cardiovascular Disease

Blumenthal, Roger S MD [Cv] - **Spec Exp:** Preventive Cardiology; Hypertension; Cardiovascular Disease/Young Adult; **Hospital:** Johns Hopkins Hosp - Baltimore (page 61); **Address:** Johns Hopkins Hospital, Div Cardiology, 600 N Wolfe St Blalock Bldg - rm 524C, Baltimore, MD 21287; **Phone:** 410-955-7376; **Board Cert:** Internal Medicine 1988; Cardiovascular Disease 2003; **Med School:** Cornell Univ-Weill Med Coll 1985; **Resid:** Internal Medicine, Johns Hopkins Hosp 1988; **Fellow:** Cardiovascular Disease, Johns Hopkins Hosp 1992; **Fac Appt:** Assoc Prof Med, Johns Hopkins Univ

Borer, Jeffrey MD [Cv] - **Spec Exp:** Heart Valve Disease; Heart Failure; Nuclear Cardiology; **Hospital:** NY-Presby Hosp/Weill Cornell (page 66); **Address:** NY Presby Hosp, Gilman Inst Heart Dis, 525 E 68th St, Box 118, New York, NY 10021-4870; **Phone:** 212-746-4646; **Board Cert:** Internal Medicine 1973; Cardiovascular Disease 1975; **Med School:** Cornell Univ-Weill Med Coll 1969; **Resid:** Internal Medicine, Mass Genl Hosp 1971; **Fellow:** Cardiovascular Disease, Natl Heart, Lung & Blood Inst 1974; Cardiovascular Disease, Guy's Hosp 1975; **Fac Appt:** Prof Med, Cornell Univ-Weill Med Coll

Bove, Alfred A MD/PhD [Cv] - **Spec Exp:** Diving Medicine; Heart Failure; **Hospital:** Temple Univ Hosp; **Address:** Temple Univ Hosp, Div Cardiology, 3401 N Broad St, Parkinson Pavillon, Philadelphia, PA 19140; **Phone:** 215-707-3346; **Board Cert:** Internal Medicine 1971; Cardiovascular Disease 1983; Undersea & Hyperbaric Medicine 2000; **Med School:** Temple Univ 1966; **Resid:** Internal Medicine, Temple Univ Hosp 1970; **Fellow:** Physiology, Temple Univ Hosp 1970; Physiology, Mayo Clinic 1971; **Fac Appt:** Prof Emeritus Med, Temple Univ

Brozena, Susan Celia MD [Cv] - **Spec Exp:** Transplant Medicine-Heart; Congestive Heart Failure; Heart Disease in Women; **Hospital:** Hosp Univ Penn - UPHS (page 72); **Address:** Hosp Univ Penn, Div Cardiovascular Med, 3400 Spruce St, 6 Penn Tower, Philadelphia, PA 19104-4283; **Phone:** 215-615-0800; **Board Cert:** Internal Medicine 1984; Cardiovascular Disease 1987; **Med School:** Temple Univ 1981; **Resid:** Internal Medicine, Temple Univ Hosp 1984; **Fellow:** Cardiovascular Disease, Temple Univ Hosp 1986; **Fac Appt:** Assoc Prof Med, Univ Pennsylvania

Cohen, Howard A MD [Cv] - **Spec Exp:** Interventional Cardiology; **Hospital:** Lenox Hill Hosp (page 62); **Address:** Lenox Hill Hosp, Interv Cardiology, 130 E 77th St Fl 9, New York, NY 10021; **Phone:** 212-434-2606; **Board Cert:** Internal Medicine 1974; Cardiovascular Disease 1977; **Med School:** NYU Sch Med 1970; **Resid:** Internal Medicine, Bellevue Hosp Ctr 1974; **Fellow:** Cardiovascular Disease, Johns Hopkins Hosp 1976

Coppola, John T MD [Cv] - **Spec Exp:** Cardiac Catheterization; Angioplasty; **Hospital:** St Vincent Cath Med Ctrs - Manhattan; **Address:** 275 7th Ave Fl 3, New York, NY 10001; **Phone:** 646-660-9999; **Board Cert:** Internal Medicine 1981; Cardiovascular Disease 1983; Interventional Cardiology 1999; **Med School:** NY Med Coll 1978; **Resid:** Internal Medicine, St Vincent Catholic Med Ctr 1981; **Fellow:** Cardiovascular Disease, St Vincent Catholic Med Ctr 1983

Demopoulos, Laura A MD [Cv] - **Spec Exp:** Heart Disease in Women; Preventive Cardiology; **Hospital:** Hosp Univ Penn - UPHS (page 72); **Address:** Penn Cardiac Care at Radnor, 250 King of Prussia Rd, Ste 2D, Radnor, PA 19087; **Phone:** 610-902-2273; **Board Cert:** Internal Medicine 1989; Cardiovascular Disease 2003; **Med School:** NYU Sch Med 1986; **Resid:** Internal Medicine, NYU/ Bellevue Med Ctr 1989; **Fellow:** Cardiovascular Disease, NYU/Bellevue Med Ctr 1992; Cardiology Research, Albert Einstein Coll Med 1993; **Fac Appt:** Assoc Clin Prof Med, Univ Pennsylvania

Devereux, Richard B MD [Cv] - **Spec Exp:** Marfan's Syndrome; **Hospital:** NY-Presby Hosp/Weill Cornell (page 66); **Address:** 525 E 68th St, rm K-415, New York, NY 10021-4870; **Phone:** 212-746-4655; **Board Cert:** Internal Medicine 1974; Cardiovascular Disease 1977; **Med School:** Univ Pennsylvania 1971; **Resid:** Internal Medicine, New York Hosp 1974; **Fellow:** Cardiovascular Disease, Hosp Univ Penn 1976; **Fac Appt:** Prof Med, Cornell Univ-Weill Med Coll

Eisen, Howard J MD [Cv] - **Spec Exp:** Transplant Medicine-Heart; Congestive Heart Failure; **Hospital:** Hahnemann Univ Hosp; **Address:** Drexel Univ Coll Med, Div Cardiology, 245 N 15th St, MS 1012, Philadelphia, PA 19102; **Phone:** 215-762-3829; **Board Cert:** Internal Medicine 1984; Cardiovascular Disease 1987; **Med School:** Univ Pennsylvania 1981; **Resid:** Internal Medicine, Hosp Univ Penn 1984; **Fellow:** Cardiovascular Disease, Barnes Hosp-Wash Univ 1987; **Fac Appt:** Prof Med, Drexel Univ Coll Med

Follansbee, William MD [Cv] - **Hospital:** UPMC Presby, Pittsburgh; **Address:** UPMC Cardiovascular Inst, 200 Lothrop St, Ste 5B, Pittsburgh, PA 15213; **Phone:** 412-647-6000; **Board Cert:** Internal Medicine 1977; Cardiovascular Disease 1981; **Med School:** Univ Pennsylvania 1974; **Resid:** Internal Medicine, Hosp Univ Penn 1979; **Fellow:** Cardiovascular Disease, Hosp Univ Penn 1978

Fuster, Valentin MD/PhD [Cv] - **Spec Exp:** Coronary Artery Disease; Heart Valve Disease; Congenital Heart Disease; **Hospital:** Mount Sinai Med Ctr; **Address:** One Gustave L Levy Pl, Box 1030, New York, NY 10029-6500; **Phone:** 212-241-7911; **Board Cert:** Internal Medicine 1976; Cardiovascular Disease 1977; **Med School:** Spain 1967; **Resid:** Internal Medicine, Mayo Clinic 1972; Cardiovascular Disease, Mayo Clinic 1974; **Fellow:** Cardiovascular Disease, Univ Edinburgh 1971; **Fac Appt:** Prof Med, Mount Sinai Sch Med

Gliklich, Jerry MD [Cv] - **Spec Exp:** Heart Valve Disease; Arrhythmias; **Hospital:** NY-Presby Hosp/Columbia (page 66); **Address:** 161 Fort Washington Ave, Ste 535, New York, NY 10032-3713; **Phone:** 212-305-5588; **Board Cert:** Internal Medicine 1978; Cardiovascular Disease 1981; **Med School:** Columbia P&S 1975; **Resid:** Internal Medicine, New York Hosp 1978; **Fellow:** Cardiovascular Disease, Columbia-Presby Med Ctr 1981; **Fac Appt:** Clin Prof Med, Columbia P&S

Gottdiener, John S MD [Cv] - **Spec Exp:** Echocardiography; **Hospital:** Univ of MD Med Sys; **Address:** 22 S Greene St, rm S3B08, Baltimore, MD 21201; **Phone:** 410-328-6190; **Board Cert:** Internal Medicine 1975; Cardiovascular Disease 1979; **Med School:** Georgetown Univ 1970; **Resid:** Internal Medicine, Univ NC Hosp 1972; **Fellow:** Cardiovascular Disease, Georgetown Univ Hosp 1976; **Fac Appt:** Prof Med, Univ MD Sch Med

Gottlieb, Stephen Scott MD [Cv] - **Spec Exp:** Heart Failure; Tranplant Medicine-Heart; **Hospital:** Univ of MD Med Sys; **Address:** Univ Maryland Med Ctr, Cardiology, 22 S Greene St, rm S3B08, Baltimore, MD 21201; **Phone:** 410-328-8788; **Board Cert:** Internal Medicine 1984; Cardiovascular Disease 1987; **Med School:** Brown Univ 1981; **Resid:** Internal Medicine, Univ Chicago Hosps 1984; **Fellow:** Cardiovascular Disease, Mt Sinai Hosp 1985; **Fac Appt:** Prof Med, Univ MD Sch Med

Greenberg, Mark MD [Cv] - **Spec Exp:** Interventional Cardiology; Cardiac Catheterization; Cardiac Consultation; Ischemic Heart Disease; **Hospital:** Montefiore Med Ctr; **Address:** 111 E 210th St, Division of Cardiology, Bronx, NY 10467; **Phone:** 718-920-4212; **Board Cert:** Internal Medicine 1973; Cardiovascular Disease 1979; Interventional Cardiology 1999; **Med School:** Univ IL Coll Med 1973; **Resid:** Internal Medicine, Montefiore Hosp Med Ctr 1976; **Fellow:** Cardiovascular Disease, Montefiore Hosp Med Ctr 1978; **Fac Appt:** Clin Prof Med, Albert Einstein Coll Med

Cardiovascular Disease

Halperin, Jonathan L MD [Cv] - **Spec Exp:** Peripheral Vascular Disease; Atrial Fibrillation; **Hospital:** Mount Sinai Med Ctr; **Address:** Fifth Ave at 100th St, New York, NY 10029; **Phone:** 212-241-7243; **Board Cert:** Internal Medicine 1980; Cardiovascular Disease 1981; **Med School:** Boston Univ 1975; **Resid:** Internal Medicine, Mass Genl Hosp 1977; **Fellow:** Vascular Medicine, Boston Univ Med Ctr 1978; Cardiovascular Disease, Boston Univ Med Ctr 1980; **Fac Appt:** Prof Med, Mount Sinai Sch Med

Herling, Irving M MD [Cv] - **Spec Exp:** Cholesterol/Lipid Disorders; Heart Valve Disease; Aortic Diseases & Dissection; Preventive Cardiology; **Hospital:** Hosp Univ Penn - UPHS (page 72); **Address:** Hosp Univ Penn, Div Cardiology, 3400 Spruce St, Ste 800 Penn Tower, Philadelphia, PA 19104; **Phone:** 215-662-6020; **Board Cert:** Internal Medicine 1977; Cardiovascular Disease 1979; **Med School:** Univ Pennsylvania 1974; **Resid:** Internal Medicine, Hosp Univ Penn 1977; **Fellow:** Cardiovascular Disease, Hosp Univ Penn 1979; **Fac Appt:** Assoc Prof Med, Univ Pennsylvania

Hochman, Judith S MD [Cv] - **Spec Exp:** Coronary Artery Disease; **Hospital:** NYU Med Ctr (page 67); **Address:** NYU Medical Ctr, 530 First Ave, rm HCC 1173, New York, NY 10016; **Phone:** 212-263-6927; **Board Cert:** Internal Medicine 1980; Cardiovascular Disease 1983; **Med School:** Harvard Med Sch 1977; **Resid:** Internal Medicine, Peter Bent Brigham Hosp 1979; Internal Medicine, U Mass Med Ctr 1980; **Fellow:** Cardiovascular Disease, Johns Hopkins Hosp 1982; **Fac Appt:** Prof Med, NYU Sch Med

Hsia, Judith A MD [Cv] - **Spec Exp:** Heart Disease in Women; Cholesterol/Lipid Disorders; **Hospital:** G Washington Univ Hosp; **Address:** Geo Washington Univ Faculty Assocs, 2150 Pennsylvania Ave NW, Ste 4 - 414, Washington, DC 20037; **Phone:** 202-741-2323; **Board Cert:** Internal Medicine 1981; Cardiovascular Disease 1987; **Med School:** Univ IL Coll Med 1978; **Resid:** Internal Medicine, Tufts-New England Med Ctr 1981; **Fellow:** Research, Natl Heart, Lung,Blood Inst/NIH 1984; Cardiovascular Disease, George Washington Univ 1986; **Fac Appt:** Prof Med, Geo Wash Univ

Inra, Lawrence A MD [Cv] - **Spec Exp:** Coronary Artery Disease; Heart Valve Disease; Cholesterol/Lipid Disorders; Hypertension; **Hospital:** NY-Presby Hosp/Weill Cornell (page 66), Hosp For Special Surgery (page 60); **Address:** 407 E 70th St, New York, NY 10021; **Phone:** 212-249-1011; **Board Cert:** Internal Medicine 1979; Cardiovascular Disease 1981; **Med School:** Johns Hopkins Univ 1976; **Resid:** Internal Medicine, New York Hosp 1979; **Fellow:** Cardiovascular Disease, Mount Sinai Hosp 1981; **Fac Appt:** Assoc Prof Med, Cornell Univ-Weill Med Coll

Kostis, John B MD [Cv] - **Spec Exp:** Hypertension; Coronary Artery Disease; Cholesterol/Lipid Disorders; **Hospital:** Robert Wood Johnson Univ Hosp - New Brunswick; **Address:** 125 Paterson St, Ste 5200, New Brunswick, NJ 08903-0019; **Phone:** 732-235-7685; **Board Cert:** Internal Medicine 1973; Cardiovascular Disease 1973; **Med School:** Greece 1960; **Resid:** Internal Medicine, Evanglismos Hosp 1964; Internal Medicine, Cumberland Med Ctr 1967; **Fellow:** Cardiovascular Disease, Philadelphia Genl Hosp 1969; **Fac Appt:** Prof Med, UMDNJ-RW Johnson Med Sch

Meller, Jose MD [Cv] - **Spec Exp:** Cardiac Catheterization; Hypertension; Angioplasty; **Hospital:** Mount Sinai Med Ctr; **Address:** 941 Park Ave, New York, NY 10028; **Phone:** 212-988-3772; **Board Cert:** Internal Medicine 1973; Cardiovascular Disease 1975; **Med School:** Chile 1969; **Resid:** Internal Medicine, Elmhurst Hosp 1971; Internal Medicine, Mt Sinai Med Ctr 1972; **Fellow:** Cardiovascular Disease, Mt Sinai Med Ctr 1974; **Fac Appt:** Prof Med, Mount Sinai Sch Med

Mosca, Lori J MD/PhD [Cv] - **Spec Exp:** Preventive Cardiology; **Hospital:** NY-Presby Hosp/Columbia (page 66); **Address:** NY Presby Med Ctr, Div Preventive Cardiology, 622 W 168th St, PH10-203D, New York, NY 10032; **Phone:** 212-305-4866; **Board Cert:** Internal Medicine 1989; **Med School:** SUNY Upstate Med Univ 1984; **Resid:** Internal Medicine, SUNYHealth Sci Ctr 1987; **Fellow:** Cardiovascular Disease, Columbia Presby Med Ctr 1991; Epidemiology, Columbia Presby Med Ctr 1992; **Fac Appt:** Assoc Prof Med, Columbia P&S

Naccarelli, Gerald V MD [Cv] - **Spec Exp:** Cardiac Electrophysiology; Pacemakers; Arrhythmias; **Hospital:** Penn State Milton S Hershey Med Ctr; **Address:** Penn State Coll Med, Cardiovasc Ctr, H042, 500 University Drive, Box 850, Hershey, PA 17033-2360; **Phone:** 717-531-3907; **Board Cert:** Internal Medicine 1979; Cardiovascular Disease 1981; **Med School:** Penn State Univ-Hershey Med Ctr 1976; **Resid:** Internal Medicine, NC Bapt Hosp 1978; Internal Medicine, Hershey Med Ctr 1979; **Fellow:** Cardiovascular Disease, Indiana Univ Med Ctr 1982; **Fac Appt:** Prof Med, Penn State Univ-Hershey Med Ctr

Parmacek, Michael S MD [Cv] - **Spec Exp:** Diabetic Heart Disease; Angiogenesis; **Hospital:** Hosp Univ Penn - UPHS (page 72); **Address:** Hosp U Penn, Div Cardiovascular Medicine, 3400 Spruce St, 9.123 Founders Pavilion, Philadelphia, PA 19104; **Phone:** 215-662-3140; **Board Cert:** Internal Medicine 1984; Cardiovascular Disease 1987; **Med School:** Northwestern Univ 1981; **Resid:** Internal Medicine, Univ Michigan Med Ctr 1984; Cardiovascular Disease, Northwestern Univ 1986; **Fac Appt:** Prof Med, Univ Pennsylvania

Parrillo, Joseph E MD [Cv] - **Spec Exp:** Septic Shock; Cardiogenic shock; Heart Failure; **Hospital:** Cooper Univ Hosp; **Address:** Cooper Medical Ctr, Div Cardiology, 1 Cooper Plaza, Dorrance Bldg, Ste D384, Camden, NJ 08103; **Phone:** 856-342-8349; **Board Cert:** Internal Medicine 1975; Allergy & Immunology 1977; Cardiovascular Disease 1981; Critical Care Medicine 2005; **Med School:** Cornell Univ-Weill Med Coll 1972; **Resid:** Internal Medicine, Mass General Hosp 1975; Allergy & Immunology, NIH 1978; **Fellow:** Cardiovascular Disease, Mass General Hosp 1980; **Fac Appt:** Prof Med, UMDNJ-RW Johnson Med Sch

Plehn, Jonathan MD [Cv] - **Spec Exp:** Echocardiography; Congestive Heart Failure; Heart Valve Disease; **Hospital:** G Washington Univ Hosp, Natl Inst of Hlth - Clin Ctr; **Address:** MFA, Div Cardiology, 2150 Pennsylvania Ave NW, Washington, DC 20037; **Phone:** 202-741-3333; **Board Cert:** Internal Medicine 1981; Cardiovascular Disease 1983; **Med School:** NYU Sch Med 1977; **Resid:** Internal Medicine, Montefiore Hosp 1980; Cardiovascular Disease, Montefiore Hosp 1981; **Fellow:** Cardiovascular Disease, Rush Presby-St Lukes Hosp 1983

Poon, Michael MD [Cv] - **Spec Exp:** Coronary Artery Disease; Pulmonary Hypertension; Cardiac CT Angiography; Cardiac Imaging; **Hospital:** Cabrini Med Ctr, Mount Sinai Med Ctr; **Address:** Cabrini Medical Ctr Bldg B, 227 E 19th St, rm 549, New York, NY 10003; **Phone:** 212-995-6865; **Board Cert:** Cardiovascular Disease 1997; **Med School:** Mount Sinai Sch Med 1987; **Resid:** Internal Medicine, Mount Sinai Med Ctr 1991; **Fellow:** Cardiovascular Disease, Mount Sinai Med Ctr 1993; **Fac Appt:** Assoc Prof Med, Mount Sinai Sch Med

Reis, Steven E MD [Cv] - **Spec Exp:** Heart Disease in Women; Congestive Heart Failure; Syndrome X; **Hospital:** UPMC Presby, Pittsburgh, Magee-Womens Hosp - UPMC; **Address:** Comprehensive Heart Ctr, 120 Lytton Ave, Ste 100B, Pittsburgh, PA 15213; **Phone:** 412-802-3000; **Board Cert:** Internal Medicine 2000; Cardiovascular Disease 2000; **Med School:** Harvard Med Sch 1987; **Resid:** Internal Medicine, Brigham & Womens Hosp 1990; **Fellow:** Cardiovascular Disease, Johns Hopkins Hosp 1994; **Fac Appt:** Assoc Prof Med, Univ Pittsburgh

Cardiovascular Disease

Sacchi, Terrence J MD [Cv] - **Spec Exp:** Arrhythmias; Cardiac Catheterization; Coronary Angioplasty/Stents; **Hospital:** New York Methodist Hosp; **Address:** 506 6th St, Brooklyn, NY 11215; **Phone:** 718-780-7830; **Board Cert:** Internal Medicine 1979; Cardiovascular Disease 1981; Interventional Cardiology 1999; **Med School:** Albany Med Coll 1976; **Resid:** Internal Medicine, St Vincents Hosp 1979; **Fellow:** Cardiovascular Disease, Georgetown Univ Hosp 1981; Interventional Cardiology, Mercy Hospital 1986; **Fac Appt:** Assoc Clin Prof Med, SUNY Downstate

Saunders, Elijah MD [Cv] - **Spec Exp:** Hypertension-Complex; Coronary Disease in Black Populations; **Hospital:** Univ of MD Med Sys; **Address:** Univ MD Med Sch, Div Hypertension, 419 W Redwood St, Ste 620, Baltimore, MD 21201; **Phone:** 410-328-4366; **Med School:** Univ MD Sch Med 1960; **Resid:** Internal Medicine, Univ Maryland Med Ctr; **Fellow:** Cardiovascular Disease, Univ Maryland Med Ctr; **Fac Appt:** Prof Med, Univ MD Sch Med

Schulman, Steven P MD [Cv] - **Hospital:** Johns Hopkins Hosp - Baltimore (page 61); **Address:** 600 N Wolfe St, Carnegie 568, Baltimore, MD 21287; **Phone:** 410-955-7378; **Board Cert:** Internal Medicine 1986; Cardiovascular Disease 1989; **Med School:** Johns Hopkins Univ 1981; **Resid:** Internal Medicine, Johns Hopkins Hosp 1984; **Fellow:** Cardiovascular Disease, Johns Hopkins Hosp 1988; **Fac Appt:** Assoc Prof Med, Johns Hopkins Univ

Schwartz, Allan MD [Cv] - **Spec Exp:** Interventional Cardiology; Cardiac Catheterization; Mitral Valve Disease; **Hospital:** NY-Presby Hosp/Columbia (page 66); **Address:** 161 Ft Washington Ave, Ste 551, New York, NY 10032-3713; **Phone:** 212-305-5367; **Board Cert:** Internal Medicine 1977; Cardiovascular Disease 1979; **Med School:** Columbia P&S 1974; **Resid:** Internal Medicine, Columbia-Presby Med Ctr 1976; **Fellow:** Cardiovascular Disease, Mass Genl Hosp 1978; **Fac Appt:** Clin Prof Med, Columbia P&S

Shlofmitz, Richard A MD [Cv] - **Spec Exp:** Interventional Cardiology; **Hospital:** St Francis Hosp - The Heart Ctr (page 70); **Address:** 100 Port Washington Blvd, Ste 105, Roslyn, NY 11576-1353; **Phone:** 516-390-9640; **Board Cert:** Internal Medicine 1984; Cardiovascular Disease 1987; **Med School:** NYU Sch Med 1980; **Resid:** Internal Medicine, North Shore Univ Hosp 1984; **Fellow:** Cardiovascular Disease, Columbia Presby Med Ctr 1987

Smart, Frank W MD [Cv] - **Spec Exp:** Congestive Heart Failure; Transplant Medicine-Heart; Ventricular Assist Device (LVAD); **Hospital:** Morristown Mem Hosp, Overlook Hosp; **Address:** Morristown Meml Hosp, Dept Cardiology, 100 Madison Ave, Morristown, NJ 07962; **Phone:** 973-971-5597; **Board Cert:** Internal Medicine 1988; Cardiovascular Disease 2001; **Med School:** Louisiana State Univ 1985; **Resid:** Internal Medicine, Ochsner Fdn Hosp 1988; **Fellow:** Cardiovascular Disease, Baylor Coll Med 1991

Sonnenblick, Edmund MD [Cv] - **Spec Exp:** Hypertension; Congestive Heart Failure; Coronary Artery Disease; **Hospital:** Montefiore Med Ctr - Weiler-Einstein Div, Mount Sinai Med Ctr; **Address:** Montefiore Med Ctr-Weiler-Einstein Div, Cardiology, 1825 Eastchester Rd, Bronx, NY 10461-2301; **Phone:** 718-904-2932; **Board Cert:** Internal Medicine 1968; **Med School:** Harvard Med Sch 1958; **Resid:** Internal Medicine, Columbia-Presby Med Ctr 1963; **Fellow:** Cardiovascular Disease, Natl Heart Inst 1967; **Fac Appt:** Prof Med, Albert Einstein Coll Med

Steingart, Richard MD [Cv] - **Spec Exp:** Heart Failure; Nuclear Cardiology; Heart Disease in Cancer Patients; **Hospital:** Meml Sloan Kettering Cancer Ctr; **Address:** Meml Sloan-Kettering Cancer Ctr, Dept Cardiology, 1275 York Ave, New York, NY 10021; **Phone:** 212-639-8488; **Board Cert:** Internal Medicine 1977; Cardiovascular Disease 1979; **Med School:** Mount Sinai Sch Med 1974; **Resid:** Internal Medicine, Yale-New Haven Hosp 1977; **Fellow:** Cardiovascular Disease, Mt Sinai Med Ctr 1979; **Fac Appt:** Prof Med, Cornell Univ-Weill Med Coll

Tenenbaum, Joseph MD [Cv] - **Spec Exp:** Heart Valve Disease; Coronary Artery Disease; Atrial Fibrillation; **Hospital:** NY-Presby Hosp/The Allen Pavilion (page 66); **Address:** 161 Ft Washington Ave, Ste 535, Irving Pavilion, New York, NY 10032-3713; **Phone:** 212-305-5288; **Board Cert:** Internal Medicine 1977; Cardiovascular Disease 1979; **Med School:** Harvard Med Sch 1974; **Resid:** Internal Medicine, Columbia-Presby Med Ctr 1977; **Fellow:** Cardiovascular Disease, Mt Sinai Hosp 1979; **Fac Appt:** Clin Prof Med, Columbia P&S

Waxman, Harvey L MD [Cv] - **Spec Exp:** Arrhythmias; Cardiac Catheterization; Heart Valve Disease; **Hospital:** Penn Presby Med Ctr - UPHS (page 72); **Address:** Penn Presby Med Ctr, Philadelphia Heart Institute, 39th & Market Sts, 4PHI, Philadelphia, PA 19104; **Phone:** 215-662-9000; **Board Cert:** Internal Medicine 1977; Cardiovascular Disease 1979; Cardiac Electrophysiology 2002; **Med School:** Mount Sinai Sch Med 1974; **Resid:** Internal Medicine, Bellevue Hosp 1977; **Fellow:** Cardiovascular Disease, Jackson Meml Hosp 1979; Cardiac Electrophysiology, Hosp Univ Penn 1980; **Fac Appt:** Clin Prof Med, Univ Pennsylvania

Weitz, Howard H MD [Cv] - **Spec Exp:** Preventive Cardiology; **Hospital:** Thomas Jefferson Univ Hosp; **Address:** Jefferson Heart Institute, 925 Chestnut St, Philadelphia, PA 19107; **Phone:** 215-955-4194; **Board Cert:** Internal Medicine 1981; Cardiovascular Disease 1985; **Med School:** Thomas Jefferson Univ 1978; **Resid:** Internal Medicine, Thomas Jefferson Univ Hosp 1982; **Fellow:** Cardiovascular Disease, Thomas Jefferson Univ Hosp 1984; **Fac Appt:** Prof Med, Thomas Jefferson Univ

Southeast

Bashore, Thomas MD [Cv] - **Spec Exp:** Heart Valve Disease; Pulmonary Hypertension; Congenital Heart Disease-Adult; **Hospital:** Duke Univ Med Ctr; **Address:** Duke Univ Med Ctr, PO Box 3012, Durham, NC 27710-0001; **Phone:** 919-684-2407; **Board Cert:** Internal Medicine 1975; Cardiovascular Disease 1977; **Med School:** Ohio State Univ 1972; **Resid:** Internal Medicine, NC Meml Hosp 1975; **Fellow:** Cardiovascular Disease, Duke Univ Med Ctr 1977; **Fac Appt:** Prof Med, Duke Univ

Bass, Theodore Adam MD [Cv] - **Spec Exp:** Interventional Cardiology; **Hospital:** Shands Jacksonville; **Address:** Health Science Center/Jacksonville, 655 W 8th St ACC Bldg Fl 5, Jacksonville, FL 32209; **Phone:** 904-244-2655; **Board Cert:** Internal Medicine 1979; Cardiovascular Disease 1981; Interventional Cardiology 2001; **Med School:** Brown Univ 1976; **Resid:** Internal Medicine, Mayo Clinic 1979; **Fellow:** Cardiovascular Disease, University Hosp 1981; **Fac Appt:** Prof Med, Univ Fla Coll Med

Beller, George A MD [Cv] - **Spec Exp:** Coronary Artery Disease; Nuclear Cardiology; **Hospital:** Univ Virginia Med Ctr; **Address:** UVA Hlth Systems, Cardiology Dept, Box 800158, Charlottesville, VA 22908-0158; **Phone:** 434-924-2134; **Board Cert:** Internal Medicine 1971; Cardiovascular Disease 1977; **Med School:** Univ VA Sch Med 1966; **Resid:** Internal Medicine, Univ Wisconsin Hosps 1968; Cardiovascular Disease, Boston City Hosp 1970; **Fellow:** Cardiovascular Disease, Mass Genl Hosp 1974; **Fac Appt:** Prof Med, Univ VA Sch Med

Cardiovascular Disease

Borzak, Steven MD [Cv] - **Spec Exp:** Coronary Artery Disease; Arrhythmias; Heart Failure; Cholesterol/Lipid Disorders; **Hospital:** JFK Med Ctr - Atlantis, Bethesda Memorial; **Address:** 110 JFK Drive, Ste 110, Atlantis, FL 33462-1146; **Phone:** 561-641-9541; **Board Cert:** Internal Medicine 1987; Cardiovascular Disease 2001; **Med School:** Univ IL Coll Med 1984; **Resid:** Internal Medicine, Michael Reese Hosp 1988; **Fellow:** Cardiovascular Disease, Brigham & Womens Hosp-Harvard Med Sch 1991; **Fac Appt:** Prof Med, Nova SE Univ, Coll Osteo Med

Bourge, Robert Charles MD [Cv] - **Spec Exp:** Heart Failure; Transplant Medicine-Heart; Pulmonary Hypertension; **Hospital:** Univ of Ala Hosp at Birmingham; **Address:** 1900 University Blvd, Bldg 311, Birmingham, AL 35294-0001; **Phone:** 205-934-3624; **Board Cert:** Internal Medicine 1982; Cardiovascular Disease 1985; Nuclear Medicine 1987; **Med School:** Louisiana State Univ 1979; **Resid:** Internal Medicine, Univ Alabama Hosps 1982; Nuclear Medicine, Univ Alabama Hosps 1985; **Fellow:** Cardiovascular Disease, Univ Alabama Hosps 1984; **Fac Appt:** Prof Med, Univ Ala

Byrd III, Benjamin F MD [Cv] - **Spec Exp:** Congenital Heart Disease; Echocardiography; **Hospital:** Vanderbilt Univ Med Ctr; **Address:** Vanderbilt Heart Inst, 1215 21st Ave, MCE S Tower, Ste 5209, Nashville, TN 37232; **Phone:** 615-322-2318; **Board Cert:** Internal Medicine 1981; Cardiovascular Disease 1983; **Med School:** Vanderbilt Univ 1977; **Resid:** Psychiatry, Harvard Univ 1979; Internal Medicine, Vanderbilt Univ Hosp 1981; **Fellow:** Cardiovascular Disease, Vanderbilt Univ Hosp 1983; Cardiovascular Disease, UCSF 1984; **Fac Appt:** Assoc Prof Med, Vanderbilt Univ

Clements Jr, Stephen MD [Cv] - **Spec Exp:** Cardiac Catheterization; Echocardiography; **Hospital:** Emory Univ Hosp; **Address:** Emory Clinic, 1365 Clifton Rd NE Bldg A, Atlanta, GA 30322; **Phone:** 404-778-3468; **Board Cert:** Internal Medicine 1971; Cardiovascular Disease 1975; **Med School:** Med Coll GA 1966; **Resid:** Internal Medicine, Grady Meml Hosp 1970; **Fellow:** Cardiovascular Disease, Emory Univ Hosp 1971; **Fac Appt:** Prof Med, Emory Univ

Conti, Charles Richard MD [Cv] - **Spec Exp:** Angioplasty; Heart Attack; **Hospital:** Shands Hlthcre at Univ of FL; **Address:** Shands Healthcare Univ FL, 1600 SW Archer Rd, Box 100277, Gainesville, FL 32610-0277; **Phone:** 352-265-0457; **Board Cert:** Internal Medicine 1967; Cardiovascular Disease 1971; **Med School:** Johns Hopkins Univ 1960; **Resid:** Internal Medicine, Johns Hopkins Hosp 1965; Internal Medicine, Johns Hopkins Hosp 1968; **Fellow:** Cardiovascular Disease, Johns Hopkins Hosp 1967

Douglas Jr, John S MD [Cv] - **Spec Exp:** Interventional Cardiology; Cardiac Catheterization; Coronary Artery Disease; **Hospital:** Emory Univ Hosp; **Address:** Emory Univ Hosp, 1364 Clifton Rd, rm F606, Atlanta, GA 30322; **Phone:** 404-727-7040; **Board Cert:** Internal Medicine 1972; Cardiovascular Disease 1975; Interventional Cardiology 1999; **Med School:** Washington Univ, St Louis 1967; **Resid:** Internal Medicine, NC Memorial Hosp 1969; Internal Medicine, Grady Memorial Hosp 1972; **Fellow:** Cardiovascular Disease, Emory Affil Hosps 1974; **Fac Appt:** Prof Med, Emory Univ

Dzau, Victor J MD [Cv] - **Spec Exp:** Hypertension; Heart Failure; Vascular Disease; **Hospital:** Duke Univ Med Ctr; **Address:** Duke Univ Med Ctr, 106 Davison Bldg, DUMC Box 3701, Durham, NC 27710; **Phone:** 919-684-2255; **Board Cert:** Internal Medicine 1976; Cardiovascular Disease 1981; **Med School:** McGill Univ 1972; **Resid:** Internal Medicine, PB Brigham Hosp 1976; **Fellow:** Research, Mass Genl Hosp 1978; Cardiovascular Disease, Mass Genl Hosp 1980; **Fac Appt:** Prof Med, Duke Univ

Gandy Jr, Winston MD [Cv] - **Spec Exp:** Echocardiography; Invasive Cardiology; **Hospital:** St Joseph's Hosp - Atlanta; **Address:** Atlanta Cardiology Group, 5665 Peachtee Dunwoody Rd, Ste 172, Atlanta, GA 30342; **Phone:** 404-851-5400; **Board Cert:** Internal Medicine 1989; Cardiovascular Disease 2002; **Med School:** Howard Univ 1986; **Resid:** Internal Medicine, Emory Univ 1989; **Fellow:** Cardiovascular Disease, Univ Alabama 1992

Hare, Joshua M MD [Cv] - **Spec Exp:** Heart Failure; Stem Cell Therapy in Heart Failure; **Hospital:** Univ of Miami Hosp & Clins/Sylvester Comp Canc Ctr; **Address:** University of Miami, Miller School, 1475 NW 12th Ave, Miami, FL 33136; **Phone:** 305-243-1998; **Board Cert:** Cardiovascular Disease 2006; **Med School:** Johns Hopkins Univ 1988; **Resid:** Internal Medicine, Johns Hopkins Hosp 1991; **Fellow:** Cardiovascular Disease, Brigham & Women's Hosp 1993

Harrison, John K MD [Cv] - **Spec Exp:** Interventional Cardiology; Heart Valve Disease; **Hospital:** Duke Univ Med Ctr; **Address:** Duke Univ Med Ctr, PO Box 3331, Durham, NC 27710; **Phone:** 919-681-3763; **Board Cert:** Internal Medicine 1988; Cardiovascular Disease 2001; Interventional Cardiology 2003; **Med School:** NYU Sch Med 1984; **Resid:** Internal Medicine, Johns Hopkins Hosp 1987; **Fellow:** Cardiovascular Disease, Duke Univ Med Ctr 1990; **Fac Appt:** Prof Med, Duke Univ

Iskandrian, Ami E MD [Cv] - **Spec Exp:** Nuclear Cardiology; Coronary Artery Disease; Heart Valve Disease; **Hospital:** Univ of Ala Hosp at Birmingham; **Address:** Univ Alabama Birmingham, 1900 Univ Blvd, rm 311, Birmingham, AL 35294; **Phone:** 205-934-0545; **Board Cert:** Internal Medicine 1974; Cardiovascular Disease 1975; **Med School:** Iraq 1965; **Resid:** Internal Medicine, Univ Baghdad Affil Hosp 1971; Internal Medicine, Hahnemann Univ Hosp 1973; **Fellow:** Cardiovascular Disease, Hahnemann Univ Hosp 1975; **Fac Appt:** Prof Med, Univ Ala

Linton, MacRae F MD [Cv] - **Spec Exp:** Cholesterol/Lipid Disorders; Preventive Cardiology; **Hospital:** Vanderbilt Univ Med Ctr; **Address:** Vanderbilt Heart Inst, 1215 21st Ave, MCE S Tower, Ste 2509, Nashville, TN 37232-8802; **Phone:** 615-322-2318; **Board Cert:** Internal Medicine 1988; **Med School:** Univ Tenn Coll Med, Memphis 1985; **Resid:** Internal Medicine, Vanderbilt Univ Med Ctr 1988; **Fellow:** Endocrinology, UCSF Med Ctr 1991; **Fac Appt:** Prof Med, Vanderbilt Univ

Miller, D Douglas MD [Cv] - **Spec Exp:** Heart Disease in Women; Nuclear Cardiology; **Hospital:** Med Coll of GA Hosp and Clin; **Address:** Dean's Office Sch of Med, 1120 15th St, rm AA152, Augusta, GA 30912-4750; **Phone:** 706-721-2426; **Med School:** McGill Univ 1978; **Resid:** Internal Medicine, Montreal Genl Hosp 1980; **Fellow:** Cardiovascular Disease, Emory Univ 1984; Nuclear Cardiology, Mass Genl Hosp-Harvard; **Fac Appt:** Prof Med, St Louis Univ

Myerburg, Robert MD [Cv] - **Spec Exp:** Cardiac Electrophysiology; Arrhythmias; Pacemakers; Heart Attack; **Hospital:** Jackson Meml Hosp; **Address:** Univ Miami School Med, Div Cardiology, PO Box 016960 (D-39), Miami, FL 33101-6960; **Phone:** 305-585-5523; **Board Cert:** Internal Medicine 1968; Cardiovascular Disease 1970; Cardiac Electrophysiology 1998; **Med School:** Univ MD Sch Med 1961; **Resid:** Internal Medicine, Charity Hosp 1966; **Fellow:** Cardiovascular Disease, Grady Meml Hosp 1968; Cardiac Electrophysiology, Columbia P&S 1970; **Fac Appt:** Prof Med, Univ Miami Sch Med

Cardiovascular Disease

Nocero Jr, Michael MD [Cv] - **Spec Exp:** Nuclear Cardiology; **Hospital:** Florida Hosp - Orlando; **Address:** 1745 N Mills Ave, Orlando, FL 32803; **Phone:** 407-841-7151; **Board Cert:** Internal Medicine 1972; Cardiovascular Disease 1976; **Med School:** NYU Sch Med 1966; **Resid:** Internal Medicine, Bellevue Hosp Ctr NYU 1971; **Fellow:** Cardiovascular Disease, Bellevue Hosp Ctr NYU 1973

O'Neill, William W MD [Cv] - **Spec Exp:** Interventional Cardiology; Heart Valve Disease; **Hospital:** Univ of Miami Hosp & Clins/Sylvester Comp Canc Ctr; **Address:** Univ Miami Dept Medicine, 1600 NW Kent Ave, R-MSB 1122A, Miami, FL 33136; **Phone:** 305-243-9483; **Board Cert:** Internal Medicine 1980; Cardiovascular Disease 1983; Interventional Cardiology 1999; **Med School:** Wayne State Univ 1977; **Resid:** Internal Medicine, Wayne State Univ Affil Hosps 1980; **Fellow:** Cardiovascular Disease, Univ Mich Med Ctr 1982; **Fac Appt:** Prof Med, Univ Miami Sch Med

Oparil, Suzanne MD [Cv] - **Spec Exp:** Hypertension; Heart Disease in Women; **Hospital:** Univ of Ala Hosp at Birmingham; **Address:** Hypertension Program, 115 Comm Hlth Service Bldg, 933 19th St S, Birmingham, AL 35294; **Phone:** 205-934-9281; **Board Cert:** Internal Medicine 1970; **Med School:** Columbia P&S 1965; **Resid:** Internal Medicine, Columbia Presby Med Ctr 1967; Internal Medicine, Mass Genl Hosp 1968; **Fellow:** Cardiovascular Disease, Mass Genl Hosp 1971; **Fac Appt:** Prof Med, Univ Ala

Pepine, Carl J MD [Cv] - **Spec Exp:** Coronary Artery Disease; Hypertension; Heart Disease in Women; **Hospital:** Shands Hlthcre at Univ of FL; **Address:** Univ Florida, Div Cardiovascular Med, 1600 SW Archer Rd, Box 100277, Gainesville, FL 32610-0277; **Phone:** 352-846-0620; **Board Cert:** Internal Medicine 1971; Cardiovascular Disease 1973; **Med School:** UMDNJ-NJ Med Sch, Newark 1966; **Resid:** Internal Medicine, Jefferson Univ Hosp 1968; Internal Medicine, Naval Hosp-Thomas Jefferson Univ 1969; **Fellow:** Cardiovascular Disease, Naval Hosp-Thomas Jeff Univ 1971; **Fac Appt:** Prof Med, Univ Fla Coll Med

Phillips III, Harry R MD [Cv] - **Spec Exp:** Angioplasty; Cardiac Catheterization; **Hospital:** Duke Univ Med Ctr; **Address:** Duke Univ Med Ctr, Box 3126, Durham, NC 27710; **Phone:** 919-681-4804; **Board Cert:** Internal Medicine 1978; Cardiovascular Disease 1979; Interventional Cardiology 2001; **Med School:** Duke Univ 1975; **Resid:** Internal Medicine, Mass General Hosp 1977; **Fellow:** Cardiovascular Disease, Mass General Hosp 1979

Powers, Eric Randall MD [Cv] - **Spec Exp:** Heart Valve Disease; Interventional Cardiology; Coronary Artery Disease; **Hospital:** MUSC Med Ctr; **Address:** Med Univ of South Carolina Med Ctr, 135 Rutledge Ave, Ste 1201, Charleston, SC 29425; **Phone:** 843-792-5817; **Board Cert:** Internal Medicine 1977; Cardiovascular Disease 1979; Interventional Cardiology 2000; **Med School:** Harvard Med Sch 1974; **Resid:** Internal Medicine, Mass Genl Hosp 1976; **Fellow:** Cardiovascular Disease, Mass Genl Hosp 1979; **Fac Appt:** Prof Med, Med Univ SC

Rogers, Joseph MD [Cv] - **Spec Exp:** Congestive Heart Failure; Transplant Medicine-Heart; **Hospital:** Duke Univ Med Ctr; **Address:** DUMC, Box 3034, Durham, NC 27710; **Phone:** 919-681-3398; **Board Cert:** Internal Medicine 1991; Cardiovascular Disease 1995; **Med School:** Univ Nebr Coll Med 1988; **Resid:** Internal Medicine, Univ Nebraska Med Ctr 1991; **Fellow:** Cardiovascular Disease, Wash Univ Med Ctr 1995; **Fac Appt:** Assoc Prof Med, Duke Univ

Smith Jr, Sidney C MD [Cv] - **Spec Exp:** Cholesterol/Lipid Disorders; Coronary Artery Disease; Invasive Cardiology; **Hospital:** Univ NC Hosps; **Address:** UNC Div Cardiology, Burnett Womack Bldg Fl 6th, 099 Manning Dr, CB 7075, Chapel Hill, NC 27599; **Phone:** 919-966-7244; **Board Cert:** Internal Medicine 1972; Cardiovascular Disease 1973; **Med School:** Yale Univ 1967; **Resid:** Internal Medicine, Peter Bent Brigham Hosp 1969; **Fellow:** Cardiovascular Disease, Peter Bent Brigham Hosp 1971; Research, Harvard Med Sch 1971; **Fac Appt:** Prof Med, Univ NC Sch Med

Vaughan, Douglas E MD [Cv] - **Spec Exp:** Bleeding/Coagulation Disorders; Cholesterol/Lipid Disorders; **Hospital:** Vanderbilt Univ Med Ctr; **Address:** Vanderbilt Heart Inst, 1215 21st Ave S, MCE-Ste 5209, South Tower, Nashville, TN 37232; **Phone:** 615-322-2318; **Board Cert:** Internal Medicine 1984; Cardiovascular Disease 1987; **Med School:** Univ Tex SW, Dallas 1980; **Resid:** Internal Medicine, Parkland Meml Hosp 1984; **Fellow:** Cardiovascular Disease, Brigham & Womens Hosp 1987; **Fac Appt:** Prof Med, Vanderbilt Univ

Vetrovec, George MD [Cv] - **Spec Exp:** Interventional Cardiology; **Hospital:** Med Coll of VA Hosp; **Address:** 1200 E Broad St, rm 607, Box 980036, West Hospital, Richmond, VA 23298; **Phone:** 804-628-1215; **Board Cert:** Internal Medicine 1974; Cardiovascular Disease 1977; Interventional Cardiology 1999; **Med School:** Univ VA Sch Med 1970; **Resid:** Internal Medicine, Med Coll Virginia Hosp 1974; **Fellow:** Cardiovascular Disease, Med Coll Virginia Hosp 1976; **Fac Appt:** Prof Med, Med Coll VA

Vignola, Paul MD [Cv] - **Spec Exp:** Interventional Cardiology; **Hospital:** Mount Sinai Med Ctr - Miami; **Address:** Mt Sinai Med Ctr, Greenspan Pavilion, 4300 Alton Rd, Ste 2220, Miami Beach, FL 33140-2800; **Phone:** 305-674-2533; **Board Cert:** Internal Medicine 1974; Cardiovascular Disease 1977; Cardiac Electrophysiology 1999; **Med School:** Yale Univ 1971; **Resid:** Internal Medicine, Yale-New Haven Hosp 1974; **Fellow:** Cardiovascular Disease, Mass Genl Hospital-Harvard 1976; **Fac Appt:** Assoc Clin Prof Med, Univ Miami Sch Med

Midwest

Armstrong, William F MD [Cv] - **Spec Exp:** Echocardiography; Cardiac Consultation; **Hospital:** Univ Michigan Hlth Sys; **Address:** Women's Hosp, 1500 E Med Ctr Drive, rm L3119, Ann Arbor, MI 48108-0273; **Phone:** 734-647-7321; **Board Cert:** Internal Medicine 1979; Cardiovascular Disease 1981; **Med School:** Med Coll VA 1976; **Resid:** Internal Medicine, Med Coll Va Hosp 1979; **Fellow:** Cardiovascular Disease, Indiana Univ Hosp 1982; **Fac Appt:** Prof Med, Univ Mich Med Sch

Bonow, Robert O MD [Cv] - **Spec Exp:** Heart Valve Disease; Coronary Artery Disease; Cardiomyopathy; **Hospital:** Northwestern Meml Hosp; **Address:** Northwestern Cardiovascular Inst, 675 N St Clair St, Galter 19-100, Chicago, IL 60611; **Phone:** 312-695-4965; **Board Cert:** Internal Medicine 1976; Cardiovascular Disease 1981; **Med School:** Univ Pennsylvania 1973; **Resid:** Internal Medicine, Hosp Univ Penn 1976; **Fellow:** Cardiovascular Disease, NIH-NHLBI 1979; **Fac Appt:** Prof Med, Northwestern Univ

Braverman, Alan C MD [Cv] - **Spec Exp:** Marfan's Syndrome; Aortic Diseases & Dissection; **Hospital:** Barnes-Jewish Hosp; **Address:** Wash Univ Med Sch, Div Cardiovascular Disease, 660 S Euclid Ave, Box 8086, St Louis, MO 63110; **Phone:** 314-362-1291; **Board Cert:** Internal Medicine 1988; Cardiovascular Disease 2001; **Med School:** Univ MO-Kansas City 1985; **Resid:** Internal Medicine, Brigham & Womens Hosp 1991; **Fellow:** Cardiovascular Disease, Brigham & Womens Hosp/Harvard 1990; **Fac Appt:** Prof Med, Washington Univ, St Louis

Cardiovascular Disease

Burket, Mark W MD [Cv] - **Spec Exp:** Peripheral Vascular Disease; Coronary Artery Disease; Percutaneous Vascular Interventions; **Hospital:** Univ of Toledo Med Ctr; **Address:** 3000 Arlington Ave, Ste 1192, Toledo, OH 43614; **Phone:** 419-383-3697; **Board Cert:** Internal Medicine 1982; Cardiovascular Disease 1985; Interventional Cardiology 1999; **Med School:** Ohio State Univ 1979; **Resid:** Internal Medicine, Ohio State Univ 1982; **Fellow:** Cardiovascular Disease, Med Coll Ohio 1985; **Fac Appt:** Prof Med, Med Univ Ohio at Toledo

Cerqueira, Manuel MD [Cv] - **Spec Exp:** Cardiac Imaging; Nuclear Cardiology; **Hospital:** Cleveland Clin Fdn (page 57); **Address:** Cleveland Clinic, 9500 Euclid Ave, GB-3, Cleveland, OH 44195; **Phone:** 216-444-2665; **Board Cert:** Internal Medicine 1981; Nuclear Medicine 1984; Cardiovascular Disease 1989; **Med School:** NYU Sch Med 1976; **Resid:** Internal Medicine, Bellevue Hosp Ctr 1980; Cardiovascular Disease, Yale-New Haven Hosp 1982; **Fellow:** Nuclear Medicine, Yale-New Haven Hosp 1983; **Fac Appt:** Prof Med, Cleveland Cl Coll Med/Case West Res

Chaitman, Bernard R MD [Cv] - **Spec Exp:** Nuclear Cardiology; Echocardiography; **Hospital:** St Louis Univ Hosp; **Address:** Univ Club Tower, 1034 S Brentwood Blvd, Ste 1550, St Louis, MO 63117; **Phone:** 314-725-4668; **Board Cert:** Internal Medicine 1973; Cardiovascular Disease 1975; **Med School:** McGill Univ 1969; **Resid:** Internal Medicine, Royal Victoria Hosp 1972; **Fellow:** Cardiovascular Disease, Univ Oregon Hosps 1974; Cardiovascular Disease, Univ of Montreal 1975; **Fac Appt:** Prof Med, St Louis Univ

Connolly, Heidi M MD [Cv] - **Spec Exp:** Congenital Heart Disease; Carcinoid Heart Disease; Heart Disease in Pregnancy; **Hospital:** Mayo Med Ctr & Clin - Rochester; **Address:** Mayo Clinic, 200 First St SW, Gonda 6 Rm 468, Rochester, MN 55905; **Phone:** 507-284-1226; **Board Cert:** Internal Medicine 1989; Cardiovascular Disease 2001; **Med School:** Ireland 1986; **Resid:** Internal Medicine, Mayo Clinic 1989; **Fellow:** Cardiovascular Disease, Mayo Clinic 1991; **Fac Appt:** Assoc Prof Med, Mayo Med Sch

Cooper, Christopher MD [Cv] - **Spec Exp:** Renal Artery Revascularization; Interventional Cardiology; **Hospital:** Univ of Toledo Med Ctr; **Address:** University of Toledo, Cardiovascular Medicine, 3000 Arlington Ave, Toledo, OH 43614-2595; **Phone:** 419-383-3963; **Board Cert:** Internal Medicine 2004; Cardiovascular Disease 2005; Interventional Cardiology 1999; **Med School:** Univ Cincinnati 1988; **Resid:** Internal Medicine, Brigham & Womens Hosp 1991; **Fellow:** Cardiovascular Disease, Brigham & Women's Hosp-Harvard Med Sch 1994; **Fac Appt:** Prof Med, Med Univ Ohio at Toledo

Eagle, Kim A MD [Cv] - **Spec Exp:** Aortic Diseases & Dissection; Acute Coronary Syndromes; Heart Attack; Peripheral Vascular Disease; **Hospital:** Univ Michigan Hlth Sys; **Address:** Dominos Farms, 24 Frank Lloyd Wright Drive, Ann Arbor, MI 48106; **Phone:** 734-998-7400; **Board Cert:** Internal Medicine 1982; Cardiovascular Disease 1987; **Med School:** Tufts Univ 1979; **Resid:** Internal Medicine, Yale New Haven Hosp 1983; **Fellow:** Cardiovascular Disease, Mass Genl Hosp-Harvard 1986; **Fac Appt:** Asst Prof Med, Univ Mich Med Sch

Gardin, Julius Markus MD [Cv] - **Spec Exp:** Echocardiography; Geriatric Cardiology; Preventive Cardiology; **Hospital:** St John Hosp and Med Ctr; **Address:** St John Hosp & Med Ctr, 22201 Moross Rd, PB II, Ste 470, Detroit, MI 48236-2168; **Phone:** 313-343-6390; **Board Cert:** Internal Medicine 1975; Cardiovascular Disease 1977; **Med School:** Univ Mich Med Sch 1972; **Resid:** Internal Medicine, Univ Mich Hosp 1975; **Fellow:** Cardiovascular Disease, Georgetown Univ Hosp 1977; **Fac Appt:** Prof Med, Wayne State Univ

Geltman, Edward M MD [Cv] - **Spec Exp:** Congestive Heart Failure; Transplant Medicine-Heart; Invasive Cardiology; **Hospital:** Barnes-Jewish Hosp; **Address:** Washington Univ Sch of Med, Cardiovascular Div, 660 S Euclid Ave, Box 8086, St Louis, MO 63110; **Phone:** 314-362-1291; **Board Cert:** Internal Medicine 1974; Cardiovascular Disease 1979; **Med School:** NYU Sch Med 1971; **Resid:** Internal Medicine, Bellevue Hosp 1974; **Fellow:** Cardiovascular Disease, Barnes Jewish Hosp 1978; **Fac Appt:** Prof Med, Washington Univ, St Louis

Gibbons, Raymond J MD [Cv] - **Spec Exp:** Nuclear Cardiology; Heart Attack; **Hospital:** Mayo Med Ctr & Clin - Rochester; **Address:** Mayo Clinic, Div Cardiovascular Disease, 200 First St SW, Rochester, MN 55905; **Phone:** 507-284-2541; **Board Cert:** Internal Medicine 1979; Cardiovascular Disease 1981; **Med School:** Harvard Med Sch 1976; **Resid:** Internal Medicine, Mass Genl Hosp 1978; **Fellow:** Cardiovascular Disease, Duke Univ Med Ctr 1981; **Fac Appt:** Prof Med, Mayo Med Sch

Grubb, Blair P MD [Cv] - **Spec Exp:** Autonomic Disorders; Cardiac Electrophysiology; **Hospital:** Univ of Toledo Med Ctr, St Vincent's Mercy Med Ctr - Toledo; **Address:** Med Univ Ohio - Cardiology Clinic, 3000 Arlington Ave, Toledo, OH 43614-2598; **Phone:** 419-383-3963; **Board Cert:** Internal Medicine 1985; Cardiovascular Disease 1987; **Med School:** Dominican Republic 1980; **Resid:** Internal Medicine, Grtr Baltimore Med Ctr 1985; **Fellow:** Cardiovascular Disease, MS Hershey Med Ctr/Penn State 1987; Cardiac Electrophysiology, MS Hershey Med Ctr/Penn State 1988; **Fac Appt:** Prof Med, Univ SD Sch Med

Hayes, Sharonne N MD [Cv] - **Spec Exp:** Heart Disease in Women; Preventive Cardiology; Echocardiography; **Hospital:** Mayo Med Ctr & Clin - Rochester; **Address:** Mayo Clinic Women's Heart Clinic, 200 First St SW Gonda 5 Bldg - rm 368, Rochester, MN 55905; **Phone:** 507-284-8612; **Board Cert:** Internal Medicine 1986; Cardiovascular Disease 1989; **Med School:** Northwestern Univ 1983; **Resid:** Internal Medicine, Mayo Clinic 1986; **Fellow:** Cardiovascular Research, Mayo Clinic 1987; Cardiovascular Disease, Mayo Clinic 1990; **Fac Appt:** Assoc Prof Med, Mayo Med Sch

Heroux, Alain MD [Cv] - **Spec Exp:** Transplant Medicine-Heart; Heart Failure; **Hospital:** Loyola Univ Med Ctr; **Address:** 2160 S 1st Ave Bldg 110 - rm 6217, Maywood, IL 60153; **Phone:** 708-327-2738; **Med School:** Canada 1981; **Resid:** Internal Medicine, Laval Univ Med Ctr 1985; Cardiovascular Disease, Royal Victory Hosp 1987; **Fellow:** Univ Virginia Med Coll 1989; **Fac Appt:** Asst Prof Med, Rush Med Coll

Jaffe, Allan S MD [Cv] - **Spec Exp:** Ischemic Heart Disease; Heart Disease & Depression; **Hospital:** Mayo Med Ctr & Clin - Rochester; **Address:** Mayo Clinic, Div Cardiovasc Dis, 200 First St SW, Gonda 5-468, Rochester, MN 55905; **Phone:** 507-284-3680; **Board Cert:** Internal Medicine 1976; Cardiovascular Disease 1979; **Med School:** Univ MD Sch Med 1973; **Resid:** Internal Medicine, Barnes Hosp 1975; Internal Medicine, Wash Univ 1976; **Fellow:** Cardiovascular Disease, Barnes Hosp 1978; **Fac Appt:** Prof Med, Mayo Med Sch

Johnson, Maryl R MD [Cv] - **Spec Exp:** Congestive Heart Failure; Transplant Medicine-Heart; **Hospital:** Univ WI Hosp & Clins; **Address:** Univ Wisconsin Hosp/Clinics - Cardiology, 600 Highland Ave, Madison, WI 53792-0001; **Phone:** 608-263-0080; **Board Cert:** Internal Medicine 1981; Cardiovascular Disease 1983; **Med School:** Univ Iowa Coll Med 1977; **Resid:** Internal Medicine, Univ Iowa Hosp 1981; **Fellow:** Cardiovascular Disease, Univ Iowa Hosp 1982; **Fac Appt:** Prof Med, Univ Wisc

Cardiovascular Disease

Kereiakes, Dean J MD [Cv] - **Spec Exp:** Coronary Angioplasty/Stents; Cardiomyopathy; Congestive Heart Failure; **Hospital:** Christ Hospital; **Address:** 2123 Auburn Ave, Ste 136, Cincinnati, OH 45219-2966; **Phone:** 513-721-8881; **Board Cert:** Internal Medicine 1981; Cardiovascular Disease 1985; **Med School:** Univ Cincinnati 1978; **Resid:** Internal Medicine, UCSF Med Ctr 1982; Internal Medicine, Mass Genl Hosp 1981; **Fellow:** Cardiovascular Disease, UCSF 1984; Coronary Angioplasty, Sequoia Hospital 1984; **Fac Appt:** Clin Prof Med, Ohio State Univ

Klein, Lloyd MD [Cv] - **Spec Exp:** Coronary Artery Disease; Angiography-Coronary; Interventional Cardiology; **Hospital:** Gottlieb Meml Hosp, Rush Univ Med Ctr; **Address:** Clinical Cardiology Assocs, 675 W North Ave POB Fl 3 - Ste 314, Melrose Park, IL 60160; **Phone:** 708-681-7878; **Board Cert:** Internal Medicine 1980; Cardiovascular Disease 1983; Interventional Cardiology 1999; **Med School:** Univ Cincinnati 1977; **Resid:** Internal Medicine, Einstein-Bronx Muni Hosp 1980; **Fellow:** Cardiovascular Disease, Mt Sinai Hosp 1982; **Fac Appt:** Prof Med, Rush Med Coll

Mehlman, David J MD [Cv] - **Spec Exp:** Echocardiography; Heart Valve Disease; Coronary Artery Disease; **Hospital:** Northwestern Meml Hosp; **Address:** Northwestern Cardiovascular Inst, 675 N St Clair Galter 19-100, Chicago, IL 60611; **Phone:** 312-695-4965; **Board Cert:** Internal Medicine 1976; Cardiovascular Disease 1979; **Med School:** Johns Hopkins Univ 1973; **Resid:** Internal Medicine, Johns Hopkins Hosp 1976; **Fellow:** Cardiovascular Disease, Univ Chicago Hosps 1978; **Fac Appt:** Assoc Prof Med, Northwestern Univ

Messer, Joseph V MD [Cv] - **Spec Exp:** Coronary Artery Disease; Congestive Heart Failure; Preventive Cardiology; Hypertension; **Hospital:** Rush Univ Med Ctr, Weiss Meml Hosp; **Address:** 1725 W Harrison St, Ste 1138, Chicago, IL 60612-3835; **Phone:** 312-563-3233; **Board Cert:** Internal Medicine 1972; **Med School:** Harvard Med Sch 1956; **Resid:** Internal Medicine, Peter Bent Brigham Hosp 1958; Internal Medicine, Peter Bent Brigham Hosp 1961; **Fellow:** Cardiovascular Disease, Peter Bent Brigham Hosp/Harvard Univ 1960; Biochemistry, Brandeis Univ 1964; **Fac Appt:** Prof Med, Rush Med Coll

Moran, John f MD [Cv] - **Spec Exp:** Coronary Artery Disease; Congestive Heart Failure; Cholesterol/Lipid Disorders; **Hospital:** Loyola Univ Med Ctr; **Address:** 2160 S 1st Ave, Bldg 110 - Ste 6210, Maywood, IL 60153; **Phone:** 708-327-2784; **Board Cert:** Internal Medicine 1971; Cardiovascular Disease 1973; **Med School:** Loyola Univ-Stritch Sch Med 1964; **Resid:** Internal Medicine, Univ Illinois Hosps 1967; **Fellow:** Cardiovascular Disease, Univ Chicago Hosps 1969; **Fac Appt:** Prof Med, Loyola Univ-Stritch Sch Med

Nemickas, Rimgaudas MD [Cv] - **Spec Exp:** Coronary Artery Disease; Heart Valve Disease; Cholesterol/Lipid Disorders; **Hospital:** Adv Illinois Masonic Med Ctr, Holy Cross Hosp - Chicago; **Address:** 4901 W 79th St, Ste 7, Burbank, IL 60459; **Phone:** 708-233-5630; **Board Cert:** Internal Medicine 1969; Cardiovascular Disease 1973; **Med School:** Loyola Univ-Stritch Sch Med 1961; **Resid:** Internal Medicine, Univ Illinois Hosp 1967; **Fellow:** Cardiovascular Disease, Cook County Hosp 1963; Cardiovascular Disease, Univ Chicago Hosps 1969; **Fac Appt:** Clin Prof Med, Loyola Univ-Stritch Sch Med

Nishimura, Rick A MD [Cv] - **Spec Exp:** Echocardiography; Cardiomyopathy; Pericardial Disease; **Hospital:** Mayo Med Ctr & Clin - Rochester, St Mary's Hosp - Rochester; **Address:** Mayo Clinic, 200 First St SW Gonda 5 Bldg - rm 368, Rochester, MN 55905; **Phone:** 507-284-8342; **Board Cert:** Internal Medicine 1981; Cardiovascular Disease 1983; **Med School:** Rush Med Coll 1978; **Resid:** Internal Medicine, Mayo Clinic 1980; **Fellow:** Cardiovascular Disease, Mayo Clinic 1983; **Fac Appt:** Prof Med, Mayo Med Sch

Nissen, Steven E MD [Cv] - **Spec Exp:** Cholesterol/Lipid Disorders; Intravascular Ultrasound; Coronary Intensive Care; **Hospital:** Cleveland Clin Fdn (page 57); **Address:** Cleveland Clinic Fdn, 9500 Euclid Ave, MC F15, Cleveland, OH 44195; **Phone:** 216-445-6852; **Board Cert:** Internal Medicine 1981; Cardiovascular Disease 1983; **Med School:** Univ Mich Med Sch 1978; **Resid:** Internal Medicine, UC Davis Medical Ctr 1981; **Fellow:** Cardiovascular Disease, Univ Kentucky-Chandler Med Ctr 1983; **Fac Appt:** Prof Med, Cleveland Cl Coll Med/Case West Res

Rahko, Peter S MD [Cv] - **Spec Exp:** Congestive Heart Failure; Heart Valve Disease; Echocardiography; **Hospital:** Univ WI Hosp & Clins, Meriter Hosp; **Address:** 600 Highland Ave, rm G7-343 CSC, MC 3248, Madison, WI 53792-3248; **Phone:** 608-263-1530; **Board Cert:** Internal Medicine 1982; Cardiovascular Disease 1985; **Med School:** Univ Minn 1979; **Resid:** Internal Medicine, Indiana Univ Med Ctr 1982; **Fellow:** Cardiovascular Disease, Univ Pittsburgh 1985; **Fac Appt:** Assoc Prof Med, Univ Wisc

Reiss, Craig MD [Cv] - **Spec Exp:** Ischemic Heart Disease; Heart Valve Disease; Preventive Cardiology; Cardiomyopathy; **Hospital:** Barnes-Jewish Hosp, Barnes-Jewish West County Hosp; **Address:** Heart Care Institute, 1020 N Mason Rd, Ste 100, St Louis, MO 63141; **Phone:** 314-362-1291; **Board Cert:** Internal Medicine 1986; Cardiovascular Disease 1989; **Med School:** Univ MO-Kansas City 1983; **Resid:** Internal Medicine, Brigham & Women's Hosp 1989; **Fellow:** Cardiovascular Disease, Brigham & Women's Hosp 1988; **Fac Appt:** Assoc Prof Med, Washington Univ, St Louis

Rich, Stuart MD [Cv] - **Spec Exp:** Pulmonary Hypertension; Heart Failure; **Hospital:** Univ of Chicago Hosps; **Address:** 5841 S Maryland Ave, MC 2016, Chicago, IL 60637; **Phone:** 773-702-5589; **Board Cert:** Internal Medicine 1978; Cardiovascular Disease 1981; **Med School:** Loyola Univ-Stritch Sch Med 1974; **Resid:** Internal Medicine, Barnes-Jewish Hosp 1978; **Fellow:** Cardiovascular Disease, Univ Chicago 1980; **Fac Appt:** Prof Med, Rush Med Coll

Rosenbush, Stuart MD [Cv] - **Spec Exp:** Cardiac Catheterization; Coronary Angioplasty/Stents; Heart Failure; Coronary Artery Disease; **Hospital:** Rush Univ Med Ctr; **Address:** Assocs In Cardiology Ltd, 1725 W Harrison St, Ste 1138, Chicago, IL 60612-3835; **Phone:** 312-563-3233; **Board Cert:** Internal Medicine 1979; Cardiovascular Disease 1981; Interventional Cardiology 2000; **Med School:** Univ IL Coll Med 1976; **Resid:** Internal Medicine, Michael Reese Hosp 1979; **Fellow:** Cardiovascular Disease, Rush Presby-St Lukes Med Ctr 1981; **Fac Appt:** Asst Prof Med, Rush Med Coll

Safian, Robert D MD [Cv] - **Spec Exp:** Interventional Cardiology; **Hospital:** William Beaumont Hosp; **Address:** Beaumont Heart Ctr, 3601 W 13 Mile Rd Fl 3, Royal Oak, MI 48073; **Phone:** 248-898-4163; **Board Cert:** Internal Medicine 1983; Cardiovascular Disease 1987; Interventional Cardiology 1999; **Med School:** Univ Fla Coll Med 1979; **Resid:** Pathology, Univ Miami Med Ctr 1981; Internal Medicine, UCSD Med Ctr 1983; **Fellow:** Cardiovascular Disease, Beth Israel Hosp-Harvard 1987

Sanborn, Timothy MD [Cv] - **Spec Exp:** Interventional Cardiology; Gene Therapy-Cardiac Angiogenesis; Heart Valve Disease; Carotid Artery Stent Placement; **Hospital:** Evanston Hosp, Glenbrook Hosp; **Address:** 2650 Ridge Ave, Walgreen Bldg Fl 3, Evanston, IL 60201; **Phone:** 847-570-2250; **Board Cert:** Internal Medicine 1980; Cardiovascular Disease 2003; Interventional Cardiology 1999; **Med School:** Northwestern Univ 1977; **Resid:** Internal Medicine, Boston City Hosp 1980; **Fellow:** Cardiovascular Disease, Boston Univ Med Ctr 1983; **Fac Appt:** Prof Med, Northwestern Univ

Cardiovascular Disease

Seward, James B MD [Cv] - **Spec Exp:** Pediatric Cardiology; Echocardiography; **Hospital:** Mayo Med Ctr & Clin - Rochester, St Mary's Hosp - Rochester; **Address:** Mayo Clinic, Div Cardiovasc Disease, 200 First St SW, Rochester, MN 55905; **Phone:** 507-284-3581; **Board Cert:** Internal Medicine 1974; Cardiovascular Disease 1975; **Med School:** Univ Mich Med Sch 1968; **Resid:** Internal Medicine, Boston City Hosp 1971; Internal Medicine, Mayo Clinic; **Fellow:** Cardiovascular Disease, Mayo Clinic 1975; **Fac Appt:** Prof Ped, Mayo Med Sch

Stein, James H MD [Cv] - **Spec Exp:** Preventive Cardiology; Echocardiography; Cholesterol/Lipid Disorders; **Hospital:** Univ WI Hosp & Clins; **Address:** Univ WI Hosp, Clinic Sci Center, 600 Highland Ave, Ste G7341, MC 3248, Madison, WI 53792; **Phone:** 608-263-9648; **Board Cert:** Internal Medicine 1993; Cardiovascular Disease 1997; **Med School:** Yale Univ 1990; **Resid:** Internal Medicine, U Chicago-Pritzker Sch Med Ctr 1993; **Fellow:** Cardiovascular Disease, Rush-Presby St Lukes Med Ctr 1996; **Fac Appt:** Assoc Prof Med, Univ Wisc

Stewart, William J MD [Cv] - **Spec Exp:** Heart Valve Disease; Echocardiography; **Hospital:** Cleveland Clin Fdn (page 57); **Address:** Cleveland Clinic, Div Cardiovasc Med, 9500 Euclid Ave, Desk F15, Cleveland, OH 44195; **Phone:** 216-444-5923; **Board Cert:** Internal Medicine 1980; Cardiovascular Disease 1983; **Med School:** Univ Cincinnati 1977; **Resid:** Internal Medicine, Univ Mich Hosp 1980; **Fellow:** Cardiovascular Disease, Boston Univ Med Ctr 1982; Cardiovascular Disease, Mass Genl Hosp 1984; **Fac Appt:** Assoc Prof Med, Cleveland Cl Coll Med/Case West Res

Volgman, Annabelle S MD [Cv] - **Spec Exp:** Cardiac Electrophysiology; Heart Disease in Women; Arrhythmias; Atrial Fibrillation; **Hospital:** Rush Univ Med Ctr; **Address:** Rush Heart Inst, 1725 W Harrison St, Ste 1159, Chicago, IL 60612; **Phone:** 312-942-5020; **Board Cert:** Internal Medicine 1993; Cardiac Electrophysiology 1996; Cardiovascular Disease 2006; **Med School:** Columbia P&S 1984; **Resid:** Internal Medicine, Univ Chicago Hosps 1987; **Fellow:** Cardiovascular Disease, Northwestern Meml Hosp 1989; Cardiac Electrophysiology, Northwestern Meml Hosp 1990; **Fac Appt:** Assoc Prof Med, Rush Med Coll

von der Lohe, Elisabeth MD [Cv] - **Spec Exp:** Heart Disease in Women; Interventional Cardiology; **Hospital:** Indiana Univ Hosp, Methodist Hosp - Indianapolis; **Address:** Krannert Inst Cardiology, Womens Heart Clinic, 1800 N Capital Blvd, Ste E400, Indianapolis, IN 46202; **Phone:** 317-962-0560; **Board Cert:** Internal Medicine 2000; Cardiovascular Disease 2001; Interventional Cardiology 2003; **Med School:** Germany 1978; **Resid:** Internal Medicine, Marien Hosp 1981; **Fellow:** Cardiovascular Disease, Klinikum Aachen 1986; **Fac Appt:** Prof Med, Indiana Univ

Wagoner, Lynne E MD [Cv] - **Spec Exp:** Congestive Heart Failure; Heart Disease in Women; Transplant Medicine-Heart; **Hospital:** Univ Hosp - Cincinnati, Christ Hospital; **Address:** Univ Cincinnati, Dept Cardiology, 231 Albert Sabin Way, ML 0542, Cincinnati, OH 45267-0542; **Phone:** 513-558-3487; **Board Cert:** Internal Medicine 1989; Cardiovascular Disease 1993; **Med School:** E Carolina Univ 1986; **Resid:** Internal Medicine, Pitt Co Meml Hosp 1989; **Fellow:** Cardiovascular Disease, Univ Utah 1994; **Fac Appt:** Assoc Prof Med, Univ Cincinnati

Walsh, Mary N MD [Cv] - **Spec Exp:** Heart Disease in Women; Nuclear Cardiology; Congestive Heart Failure; **Hospital:** St Vincent Hosp & Hlth Svcs - Indianapolis; **Address:** Indiana Heart Inst, 8333 Naab Rd, Ste 400, Indianapolis, IN 46260; **Phone:** 317-338-6666; **Board Cert:** Internal Medicine 1986; Cardiovascular Disease 2001; **Med School:** Univ Minn 1983; **Resid:** Internal Medicine, Univ Tex SW Med Ctr 1986; **Fellow:** Cardiovascular Disease, Wash Univ 1989; **Fac Appt:** Asst Clin Prof Med, Indiana Univ

Weaver, W Douglas MD [Cv] - **Spec Exp:** Heart Attack; Angioplasty; Cholesterol/Lipid Disorders; **Hospital:** Henry Ford Hosp; **Address:** Henry Ford Hosp, Div Cardiology, 2799 W Grand Blvd Fl K-14, Detriot, MI 48202-2689; **Phone:** 313-916-4420; **Board Cert:** Internal Medicine 1974; Cardiovascular Disease 1977; **Med School:** Tufts Univ 1971; **Resid:** Internal Medicine, Univ Wash Hosps 1974; **Fellow:** Cardiovascular Disease, Univ Wash Hosps 1976

Williams, Kim A MD [Cv] - **Spec Exp:** Nuclear Cardiology; Coronary Artery Disease; **Hospital:** Univ of Chicago Hosps; **Address:** 5758 S Maryland Ave, MC 9015, Chicago, IL 60637; **Phone:** 773-702-9461; **Board Cert:** Internal Medicine 1982; Cardiovascular Disease 1985; Nuclear Medicine 1986; **Med School:** Univ Chicago-Pritzker Sch Med 1975; **Resid:** Internal Medicine, Emory Univ 1982; **Fellow:** Cardiovascular Disease, Univ Chicago 1984; Nuclear Medicine, Univ Chicago 1986; **Fac Appt:** Assoc Prof Med, Univ Chicago-Pritzker Sch Med

Young, James B MD [Cv] - **Spec Exp:** Transplant Medicine-Heart; Heart Failure; **Hospital:** Cleveland Clin Fdn (page 57); **Address:** Cleveland Clin Fdn, 9500 Euclid Ave, Desk T13, Cleveland, OH 44195; **Phone:** 216-444-2270; **Board Cert:** Internal Medicine 1977; Cardiovascular Disease 1979; **Med School:** Baylor Coll Med 1974; **Resid:** Internal Medicine, Baylor Affil Hosp 1977; Internal Medicine, Methodist Hosp 1980; **Fellow:** Cardiovascular Disease, Baylor Affl Hosp 1979; **Fac Appt:** Prof Med, Cleveland Cl Coll Med/Case West Res

Great Plains and Mountains

Anderson, Jeffrey L MD [Cv] - **Spec Exp:** Arrhythmias; Cholesterol/Lipid Disorders; Cardiac MRI; **Hospital:** LDS Hosp, Salt Lake Regional Med Ctr; **Address:** LDS Hospital, Dept Cardiology, 325 8th Ave, Salt Lake City, UT 84143; **Phone:** 801-408-5552; **Board Cert:** Internal Medicine 1975; Cardiovascular Disease 1979; Cardiac Electrophysiology 2002; **Med School:** Harvard Med Sch 1972; **Resid:** Internal Medicine, Mass Genl Hosp 1974; **Fellow:** Research, Natl Inst Hlth 1976; Cardiovascular Disease, Stanford Univ Med Ctr 1978; **Fac Appt:** Prof Med, Univ Utah

Benjamin, Ivor J MD [Cv] - **Spec Exp:** Arrhythmias; Cardiomyopathy; **Hospital:** Univ Utah Hosps and Clins; **Address:** Univ UT Health Sci Ctr, Div Cardiology, 30 N 1900 E, rm 4A100, Salt Lake City, UT 84132; **Phone:** 801-581-7715; **Board Cert:** Internal Medicine 1985; Cardiovascular Disease 1989; **Med School:** Johns Hopkins Univ 1982; **Resid:** Internal Medicine, Yale-New Haven Hosp 1985; **Fellow:** Cardiology Research, Yale-New Haven Hosp 1988; Echocardiography, Michael Reese Hosp 1989; **Fac Appt:** Prof Med, Univ Utah

Lindenfeld, JoAnn MD [Cv] - **Spec Exp:** Congestive Heart Failure; Transplant Medicine-Heart; Heart Disease in Women; **Hospital:** Univ Colorado Hosp; **Address:** Univ Colorado Hlth Sci Ctr, 4200 E 9th Ave, Box B-130, Denver, CO 80262-0001; **Phone:** 303-315-4410; **Board Cert:** Internal Medicine 1976; Cardiovascular Disease 1979; **Med School:** Univ Mich Med Sch 1973; **Resid:** Internal Medicine, UCSD Med Ctr 1977; **Fellow:** Cardiovascular Disease, Univ Tex Hlth Sci Ctr 1979; **Fac Appt:** Prof Med, Univ Colorado

Cardiovascular Disease

Southwest

Carabello, Blase A MD [Cv] - **Spec Exp:** Heart Valve Disease; **Hospital:** DeBakey VA Med Ctr-Houston; **Address:** Houston VA Medical Ctr, 2002 Holcombe Blvd, MS 111MCL, Houston, TX 77030; **Phone:** 713-794-7070; **Board Cert:** Internal Medicine 1977; Cardiovascular Disease 1979; **Med School:** Temple Univ 1973; **Resid:** Internal Medicine, Mass General Hosp 1976; **Fellow:** Cardiovascular Disease, Peter Bent Brigham Hosp 1978; **Fac Appt:** Prof Med, Baylor Coll Med

Freeman, Gregory L MD [Cv] - **Spec Exp:** Interventional Cardiology; Angioplasty; **Hospital:** Univ Hlth Sys - Univ Hosp; **Address:** Cardiology Clinical Associates, 4411 Medical Drive, Ste 300, San Antonio, TX 78229; **Phone:** 210-614-5400; **Board Cert:** Internal Medicine 1979; Cardiovascular Disease 1983; **Med School:** Loyola Univ-Stritch Sch Med 1976; **Resid:** Internal Medicine, Cook County Hosp 1979; **Fellow:** Cardiovascular Disease, Loyola Univ Med Ctr 1981; Research, UCSD Sch Med 1983; **Fac Appt:** Prof Med, Univ Tex, San Antonio

Gould, K Lance MD [Cv] - **Spec Exp:** Preventive Cardiology; PET Imaging; Cholesterol/Lipid Disorders; **Hospital:** Meml Hermann Hosp - Houston; **Address:** Univ Texas Med Sch - PET Imaging Ctr, 6431 Fannin, Rm 4.256 MSB, Houston, TX 77030-1501; **Phone:** 713-500-6611; **Med School:** Case West Res Univ 1964; **Resid:** Internal Medicine, Univ Wash Med Ctr 1967; Cardiovascular Disease, Univ Wash Med Ctr 1964; **Fellow:** Cardiovascular Disease, Univ Wash Med Ctr 1971; **Fac Appt:** Prof Med, Univ Tex, Houston

Krajcer, Zvonimir MD [Cv] - **Spec Exp:** Peripheral Vascular Disease; **Hospital:** St Luke's Episcopal Hosp - Houston; **Address:** 6624 Fannin St, Ste 2780, Houston, TX 77030; **Phone:** 713-791-4158; **Board Cert:** Internal Medicine 1975; Cardiovascular Disease 1977; **Med School:** Slovenia 1970; **Resid:** Internal Medicine, Northwestern Medical Ctr 1974; **Fellow:** Cardiovascular Disease, St Luke's Episcopal Hosp 1977; **Fac Appt:** Clin Prof Med, Baylor Coll Med

Massin, Edward Krauss MD [Cv] - **Spec Exp:** Congestive Heart Failure; Transplant Medicine-Heart; Coronary Artery Disease; **Hospital:** St Luke's Episcopal Hosp - Houston; **Address:** Cardiology Consultants Houston, 6624 Fannin St, Ste 2310, Houston, TX 77030-2335; **Phone:** 713-796-2668; **Board Cert:** Internal Medicine 1973; Cardiovascular Disease 1973; **Med School:** Washington Univ, St Louis 1965; **Resid:** Internal Medicine, Barnes Hosp 1967; **Fellow:** Cardiovascular Disease, Univ Colo Med Ctr 1971; **Fac Appt:** Clin Prof Med, Baylor Coll Med

McPherson, David D MD [Cv] - **Spec Exp:** Echocardiography; Congenital Heart Disease-Adult; Heart Valve Disease; **Hospital:** Univ Hlth Sys - Univ Hosp; **Address:** 6431 Fannin, Houston, TX 77030; **Phone:** 713-500-6553; **Board Cert:** Internal Medicine 2005; Cardiovascular Disease 1997; **Med School:** Univ Alberta 1978; **Resid:** Internal Medicine, Dalhousie Univ 1981; **Fellow:** Cardiovascular Disease, Dalhousie Univ 1983; Cardiovascular Disease, Iowa Univ Med 1984; **Fac Appt:** Prof Med, Northwestern Univ

Packer, Milton MD [Cv] - **Spec Exp:** Congestive Heart Failure; **Hospital:** UT Southwestern Med Ctr - Dallas; **Address:** UT SW Med Ctr, 5323 Harry Hines Blvd, Dallas, TX 75390-9066; **Phone:** 214-648-0491; **Board Cert:** Internal Medicine 1976; Cardiovascular Disease 1979; **Med School:** Jefferson Med Coll 1973; **Resid:** Internal Medicine, Bronx Muni Hosp Ctr 1976; **Fellow:** Cardiovascular Disease, Mount Sinai Hosp 1978; **Fac Appt:** Prof Med, Univ Tex SW, Dallas

Ramee, Stephen Robert MD [Cv] - **Spec Exp:** Angiography-Coronary; Interventional Cardiology; **Hospital:** Ochsner Fdn Hosp; **Address:** Ochsner Clinic, Cath Lab, 1514 Jefferson Hwy, New Orleans, LA 70121; **Phone:** 504-842-3724; **Board Cert:** Internal Medicine 1983; Cardiovascular Disease 1985; Interventional Cardiology 1999; **Med School:** Geo Wash Univ 1980; **Resid:** Internal Medicine, Letterman Army Med Ctr 1983; **Fellow:** Cardiovascular Disease, Letterman Army Med Ctr 1985

Tajik, A Jamil MD [Cv] - **Spec Exp:** Echocardiography; Heart Valve Disease; **Hospital:** Mayo Clin Hosp - Scottsdale; **Address:** 13400 E Shea Blvd, Scotsdale, AZ 85259; **Phone:** 480-301-4876; **Board Cert:** Internal Medicine 1973; Cardiovascular Disease 1973; **Med School:** Pakistan 1965; **Resid:** Internal Medicine, Mayo Clinic 1970; **Fellow:** Cardiovascular Disease, Mayo Clinic 1972

Thames, Marc D MD [Cv] - **Spec Exp:** Coronary Artery Disease; Congestive Heart Failure; **Hospital:** Scottsdale Hlthcare - Shea; **Address:** 16601 N 40th St, Ste 204, Phoenix, AZ 85032-3356; **Phone:** 602-867-8644; **Board Cert:** Internal Medicine 1974; Cardiovascular Disease 1979; **Med School:** Med Coll VA 1970; **Resid:** Internal Medicine, Peter Bent Brigham Hosp 1974; **Fellow:** Cardiology Research, Peter Bent Brigham Hosp 1975; Cardiovascular Disease, Mayo Clinic 1977

Wilansky, Susan MD [Cv] - **Spec Exp:** Heart Disease in Women; Heart Disease in Pregnancy; Echocardiography; **Hospital:** Mayo Clin Hosp - Scottsdale; **Address:** Mayo Clinic, Dept Cardiology, 13400 E Shea Blvd, Scottsdale, AZ 85259; **Phone:** 480-301-8200; **Board Cert:** Cardiovascular Disease 1989; **Med School:** McMaster Univ 1979; **Resid:** Internal Medicine, Univ Toronto Hosp 1983; **Fellow:** Cardiovascular Disease, Univ Toronto Hosp 1985; Echocardiography, Univ Toronto Hosp 1986; **Fac Appt:** Assoc Prof Med, Mayo Med Sch

Willerson, James T MD [Cv] - **Spec Exp:** Ischemic Heart Disease; Stem Cell Therapy in Heart Failure; **Hospital:** St Luke's Episcopal Hosp - Houston; **Address:** 7000 Fannin St, Ste 1700, Houston, TX 77030; **Phone:** 832-355-3942; **Board Cert:** Internal Medicine 1972; Cardiovascular Disease 1974; **Med School:** Baylor Coll Med 1965; **Resid:** Internal Medicine, Mass Genl Hosp 1967; **Fellow:** Cardiovascular Disease, Mass Genl Hosp 1967; **Fac Appt:** Prof Med, Univ Tex, Houston

West Coast and Pacific

Bairey-Merz, C Noel MD [Cv] - **Spec Exp:** Preventive Cardiology; Heart Disease in Women; **Hospital:** Cedars-Sinai Med Ctr; **Address:** Cedars-Sinai Women's Hlth Program, 444 S San Vicente Blvd, Ste 600, Los Angeles, CA 90048; **Phone:** 310-423-9680; **Board Cert:** Internal Medicine 1984; Cardiovascular Disease 1987; **Med School:** Harvard Med Sch 1981; **Resid:** Internal Medicine, UCSF Med Ctr 1984; **Fellow:** Cardiovascular Disease, Cedars-Sinai Med Ctr 1986; **Fac Appt:** Assoc Clin Prof Med, UCLA

Brindis, Ralph G MD [Cv] - **Spec Exp:** Acute Coronary Syndromes; Interventional Cardiology; **Hospital:** Kaiser Permanente Oakland Med Ctr, Alta Bates Summit Med Ctr - Summit Campus; **Address:** Hospital Bldg Fl 2, 280 W MacArthur Blvd, Oakland, CA 94611; **Phone:** 510-752-6424; **Board Cert:** Internal Medicine 1980; Cardiovascular Disease 1983; Interventional Cardiology 1999; **Med School:** Emory Univ 1977; **Resid:** Internal Medicine, Herbert C Moffitt Hosp 1980; Internal Medicine, Fort Miley VA Hosp 1981; **Fellow:** Cardiovascular Disease, Herbert C Moffitt Hosp 1983; **Fac Appt:** Prof Med, UCSF

Cardiovascular Disease

Budoff, Matthew J MD [Cv] - **Spec Exp:** Cholesterol/Lipid Disorders; Coronary Artery Disease; Cardiac Imaging; **Hospital:** LAC - Harbor - UCLA Med Ctr; **Address:** 1124 W Carson St, Torrance, CA 90502; **Phone:** 310-222-4107; **Board Cert:** Internal Medicine 2003; Cardiovascular Disease 1997; **Med School:** Geo Wash Univ 1990; **Resid:** Internal Medicine, UCLA/Harbor Med Ctr 1993; **Fellow:** Cardiovascular Disease, UCLA/Harbor Med Ctr 1997; **Fac Appt:** Assoc Prof Med, UCLA

Chatterjee, Kanu MD [Cv] - **Spec Exp:** Coronary Artery Disease; Congestive Heart Failure; **Hospital:** UCSF Med Ctr; **Address:** 1182 Moffitt Hospital, 505 Parnassus Ave, Box 0124, San Francisco, CA 94143-0327; **Phone:** 415-476-1326; **Board Cert:** Internal Medicine 1973; Cardiovascular Disease 1975; **Med School:** India 1956; **Resid:** Internal Medicine, Coventry & Warwickshire Hosps 1966; **Fellow:** Cardiovascular Disease, St George's Hosp 1969; Research, Brompton Hosp 1971; **Fac Appt:** Prof Med, UCSF

Dichek, David A MD [Cv] - **Spec Exp:** Gene Therapy; Atherosclerosis; **Hospital:** Univ Wash Med Ctr; **Address:** University of Washington, Dept Cardiology, 1959 NE Pacific St, Box 357710, Seattle, WA 98195; **Phone:** 206-598-4300; **Board Cert:** Internal Medicine 1987; Cardiovascular Disease 2004; **Med School:** UCLA 1984; **Resid:** Internal Medicine, Mass Genl Hosp 1987; **Fellow:** Cardiovascular Disease, NIH/Johns Hopkins Hosp 1992; **Fac Appt:** Prof Med, Univ Wash

Elkayam, Uri MD [Cv] - **Spec Exp:** Congestive Heart Failure; Heart Disease in Pregnancy; Heart Valve Disease; **Hospital:** LAC & USC Med Ctr, USC Univ Hosp - R K Eamer Med Plz; **Address:** LAC & USC Med Ctr, Div Cardiology, 1200 N State St, rm 7621, Los Angeles, CA 90033; **Phone:** 323-226-7541; **Board Cert:** Internal Medicine 1989; **Med School:** Israel 1973; **Resid:** Internal Medicine, Ichilov Hosp 1976; **Fellow:** Cardiovascular Disease, Albert Einstein Hosp 1978; Cardiovascular Disease, Cedars Sinai Med Ctr 1979; **Fac Appt:** Prof Med, USC Sch Med

Fishbein, Daniel P MD [Cv] - **Spec Exp:** Congestive Heart Failure; Transplant Medicine-Heart; **Hospital:** Univ Wash Med Ctr; **Address:** Univ Wash, Div Cardiology, 1959 NE Pacific St, Box 356422, Seattle, WA 98195-6422; **Phone:** 206-221-4507; **Board Cert:** Internal Medicine 1983; Cardiovascular Disease 1987; **Med School:** Albert Einstein Coll Med 1980; **Resid:** Internal Medicine, Univ Wash Med Ctr 1983; **Fellow:** Cardiovascular Disease, Univ Wash Med Ctr 1987; Interventional Cardiology, Univ Wash Med Ctr 1989; **Fac Appt:** Assoc Prof Med, Univ Wash

Fonarow, Gregg C MD [Cv] - **Spec Exp:** Preventive Cardiology; Heart Failure; Cardiomyopathy; Cholesterol/Lipid Disorders; **Hospital:** UCLA Med Ctr; **Address:** UCLA Medical Ctr, Div Cardiology, 10833 Le Conte Ave, CHS BH-307, Los Angeles, CA 90095; **Phone:** 310-206-9112; **Board Cert:** Cardiovascular Disease 2003; **Med School:** UCLA 1987; **Resid:** Internal Medicine, UCLA Med Ctr 1990; **Fellow:** Cardiovascular Disease, UCLA Med Ctr 1993; **Fac Appt:** Prof Med, UCLA

Goodman, Dennis A MD [Cv] - **Spec Exp:** Women's Health; Preventive Cardiology; Complementary Medicine; Cholesterol/Lipid Disorders; **Hospital:** Scripps Meml Hosp - La Jolla; **Address:** 9850 Genesee Ave, Ste 940, La Jolla, CA 92037; **Phone:** 858-457-1234; **Board Cert:** Internal Medicine 1984; Cardiovascular Disease 1989; Interventional Cardiology 2000; **Med School:** South Africa 1979; **Resid:** Internal Medicine, Montefiore Med Ctr 1984; **Fellow:** Cardiovascular Disease, Baylor Coll Med 1987; **Fac Appt:** Assoc Clin Prof Med, UCSD

Hunt, Sharon Ann MD [Cv] - **Spec Exp:** Transplant Medicine-Heart; **Hospital:** Stanford Univ Med Ctr; **Address:** 300 Pasteur Drive CVRB 265 Bldg, Stanford, CA 94305; **Phone:** 650-498-6605; **Board Cert:** Internal Medicine 1977; Cardiovascular Disease 1979; **Med School:** Stanford Univ 1972; **Resid:** Internal Medicine, Stanford Univ Hosp 1974; **Fellow:** Cardiovascular Disease, Stanford Univ Hosp 1976; **Fac Appt:** Prof Med, Stanford Univ

Johnson, Allen D MD [Cv] - **Spec Exp:** Coronary Artery Disease; Heart Valve Disease; Congenital Heart Disease-Adult; Congestive Heart Failure; **Hospital:** Scripps Green Hosp; **Address:** Scripps Clinic-Torrey Pines, 10666 N Torrey Pines Rd, rm SW206, La Jolla, CA 92037; **Phone:** 858-554-8836; **Board Cert:** Internal Medicine 1973; Cardiovascular Disease 1973; **Med School:** Johns Hopkins Univ 1965; **Resid:** Internal Medicine, Johns Hopkins Hosp 1969; **Fellow:** Cardiovascular Disease, UCSD Med Ctr 1972; **Fac Appt:** Clin Prof Med, Univ SD Sch Med

Judelson, Debra R MD [Cv] - **Spec Exp:** Hypertension; Cholesterol/Lipid Disorders; Heart Disease in Women; **Hospital:** Cedars-Sinai Med Ctr, Brotman Med Ctr; **Address:** Women's Heart Institute, Cardiovascular Med Group of S CA, 414 N Camden Drive, Ste 1100, Beverly Hills, CA 90210-4532; **Phone:** 310-278-3400 x155; **Board Cert:** Internal Medicine 1979; Cardiovascular Disease 1981; **Med School:** Harvard Med Sch 1976; **Resid:** Internal Medicine, Kaiser Foundation Hosp 1979; **Fellow:** Cardiovascular Disease, Kaiser Foundation Hosp 1981

Kaul, Sanjiv MD [Cv] - **Spec Exp:** Cardiac Imaging; Echocardiography; **Hospital:** OR Hlth & Sci Univ; **Address:** OHSU Cardiovascular Med, 3181 SW Sam Jackson Park Rd, MC UHN62, Portland, OR 97239; **Phone:** 503-494-8750; **Board Cert:** Internal Medicine 1980; Cardiovascular Disease 1983; **Med School:** India 1975; **Resid:** Internal Medicine, Univ Vermont Med Ctr 1980; Cardiovascular Disease, Wadsworth VA Hosp-UCLA 1982; **Fellow:** Cardiovascular Disease, Mass Genl Hosp 1984; **Fac Appt:** Prof Med, Oregon Hlth Sci Univ

Kobashigawa, Jon Akira MD [Cv] - **Spec Exp:** Transplant Medicine-Heart; **Hospital:** UCLA Med Ctr; **Address:** 100 UCLA Med Plaza, Ste 630, Los Angeles, CA 90095-6988; **Phone:** 310-794-1200; **Board Cert:** Internal Medicine 1983; Cardiovascular Disease 1987; **Med School:** Mount Sinai Sch Med 1980; **Resid:** Internal Medicine, UCLA Med Ctr 1983; **Fellow:** Cardiovascular Disease, UCLA Med Ctr 1986; **Fac Appt:** Clin Prof Med, UCLA

Lewis, Sandra J MD [Cv] - **Spec Exp:** Heart Disease in Women; Preventive Cardiology; Congestive Heart Failure; **Hospital:** Legacy Good Samaritan Hosp and Med Ctr, Legacy Emanuel Hospitals; **Address:** Portland Cardiovascular Inst, 2222 NW Lovejoy St, Ste 606, Portland, OR 97210; **Phone:** 503-229-7554; **Board Cert:** Internal Medicine 1980; Cardiovascular Disease 1985; **Med School:** Stanford Univ 1977; **Resid:** Internal Medicine, Stanford Univ Med Ctr 1980; **Fellow:** Cardiovascular Disease, Stanford Univ 1983; **Fac Appt:** Assoc Clin Prof Med, Oregon Hlth Sci Univ

Redberg, Rita Fran MD [Cv] - **Spec Exp:** Echocardiography; Heart Disease in Women; Preventive Cardiology; **Hospital:** UCSF Med Ctr; **Address:** UCSF Cardiology, 513 Parnassus Ave, Ste 300, San Francisco, CA 94143; **Phone:** 415-353-2873; **Board Cert:** Internal Medicine 1985; Cardiovascular Disease 1989; **Med School:** Univ Pennsylvania 1982; **Resid:** Internal Medicine, Columbia-Presby Med Ctr 1985; **Fellow:** Cardiovascular Disease, Columbia-Presby Med Ctr 1988; **Fac Appt:** Assoc Prof Med, UCSF

Cardiac Electrophysiology

Schnittger, Ingela MD [Cv] - **Spec Exp:** Cardiovascular Imaging; Cardiac Imaging; **Hospital:** Stanford Univ Med Ctr; **Address:** 300 Pasteur Drive, rm H2157, Stanford, CA 94305-5233; **Phone:** 650-723-5196; **Board Cert:** Internal Medicine 1980; Cardiovascular Disease 1983; **Med School:** Sweden 1975; **Resid:** Internal Medicine, Stanford Univ Hosp 1980; **Fellow:** Cardiovascular Disease, Stanford Univ Hosp 1983; **Fac Appt:** Assoc Prof Med, Stanford Univ

Shah, Prediman K MD [Cv] - **Spec Exp:** Coronary Artery Disease; Cholesterol/Lipid Disorders; **Hospital:** Cedars-Sinai Med Ctr; **Address:** Cedars-Sinai Med Ctr, 8700 Beverly Blvd, rm 5531, Los Angeles, CA 90048-1865; **Phone:** 310-423-3884; **Board Cert:** Internal Medicine 1975; Cardiovascular Disease 1977; **Med School:** India 1969; **Resid:** Internal Medicine, All India Inst Med Scis 1971; Internal Medicine, Montefiore Hosp 1974; **Fellow:** Cardiovascular Disease, Montefiore Hosp 1976; **Fac Appt:** Prof Med, UCLA

Cardiac Electrophysiology

New England

Batsford, William P MD [CE] - **Spec Exp:** Arrhythmias; **Hospital:** Yale - New Haven Hosp; **Address:** Yale Univ School Medicine, Section Cardiovascular Medicine, 333 Cedar St, 3 FMP, Box 208017, New Haven, CT 06520-8017; **Phone:** 203-785-4126; **Board Cert:** Internal Medicine 1972; Cardiovascular Disease 1977; **Med School:** Albany Med Coll 1969; **Resid:** Internal Medicine, Hosp Univ Penn 1972; **Fac Appt:** Prof Med, Yale Univ

Buxton, Alfred E MD [CE] - **Spec Exp:** Arrhythmias; **Hospital:** Rhode Island Hosp; **Address:** 2 Dudley St, Ste 360, Providence, RI 02905; **Phone:** 401-444-3020; **Board Cert:** Internal Medicine 1977; Cardiovascular Disease 1981; Cardiac Electrophysiology 2002; **Med School:** Univ Pennsylvania 1973; **Resid:** Internal Medicine, Hosp Univ Penn 1977; **Fac Appt:** Prof Med, Brown Univ

Ruskin, Jeremy N MD [CE] - **Spec Exp:** Arrhythmias; **Hospital:** Mass Genl Hosp; **Address:** Mass General Hosp, Div Cardiology, 55 Fruit St, Boston, MA 02114; **Phone:** 617-726-8514; **Board Cert:** Internal Medicine 1974; Cardiovascular Disease 1975; Cardiac Electrophysiology 2003; **Med School:** Harvard Med Sch 1971; **Resid:** Internal Medicine, Beth Israel Hosp 1974; Cardiovascular Disease, Mass Genl Hosp 1977; **Fac Appt:** Assoc Prof Med, Harvard Med Sch

Stevenson, William G MD [CE] - **Spec Exp:** Arrhythmias; **Hospital:** Brigham & Women's Hosp; **Address:** Brigham-Womens Hosp, Cardiovasc Div, 75 Francis St, Boston, MA 02115; **Phone:** 617-732-7535; **Board Cert:** Internal Medicine 1982; Cardiovascular Disease 1985; Cardiac Electrophysiology 2005; **Med School:** Tulane Univ 1979; **Resid:** Internal Medicine, UCLA Med Ctr 1982; **Fellow:** Cardiovascular Disease, UCLA Med Ctr 1984; Cardiac Electrophysiology, UCLA Med Ctr 1985; **Fac Appt:** Assoc Prof Med, Harvard Med Sch

Mid Atlantic

Callans, David J MD [CE] - **Spec Exp:** Arrhythmias; Pacemakers; **Hospital:** Hosp Univ Penn - UPHS (page 72); **Address:** Penn Cardiac Care at Hosp U Penn, 3400 Spruce St Founders Bldg Fl 9, Philadelphia, PA 19104; **Phone:** 215-662-6052; **Board Cert:** Internal Medicine 1989; Cardiovascular Disease 2005; Cardiac Electrophysiology 2005; **Med School:** Johns Hopkins Univ 1986; **Resid:** Internal Medicine, Hosp U Penn 1989; Cardiovascular Disease, Hosp U Penn 1999; **Fac Appt:** Prof Med, Univ Pennsylvania

Chinitz, Larry MD [CE] - **Spec Exp:** Arrhythmias; Pacemakers; Defibrillators; **Hospital:** NYU Med Ctr (page 67); **Address:** 403 E 34th St Fl 2, New York, NY 10016-6402; **Phone:** 212-263-7149; **Board Cert:** Internal Medicine 1982; Cardiovascular Disease 1985; Cardiac Electrophysiology 1998; **Med School:** NYU Sch Med 1979; **Resid:** Internal Medicine, Bellevue Hosp 1983; **Fellow:** Cardiovascular Disease, NYU Med Ctr/Bellevue 1985; Cardiac Electrophysiology, Montefiore/NYU 1985; **Fac Appt:** Assoc Prof Med, NYU Sch Med

Cohen, Martin B MD [CE] - **Spec Exp:** Interventional Cardiology; Pacemakers; Defibrillators; **Hospital:** Westchester Med Ctr; **Address:** 19 Bradhurst Ave, Ste 700, Hawthorne, NY 10532-2140; **Phone:** 914-593-7800; **Board Cert:** Internal Medicine 1983; Cardiovascular Disease 1985; Cardiac Electrophysiology 2006; Interventional Cardiology 2004; **Med School:** SUNY Downstate 1980; **Resid:** Internal Medicine, Univ Hosp 1983; **Fellow:** Cardiovascular Disease, Univ Hosp 1985; Interventional Cardiology, Westchester Co Med Ctr 1986; **Fac Appt:** Assoc Clin Prof Med, NY Med Coll

Gomes, J Anthony MD [CE] - **Spec Exp:** Arrhythmias; Heart Attack; Atrial Fibrillation; Pacemakers; **Hospital:** Mount Sinai Med Ctr; **Address:** Mount Sinai Medical Ctr, One Gustave L Levy Pl, Box 1030, New York, NY 10029-6500; **Phone:** 212-241-7272; **Board Cert:** Internal Medicine 1974; Cardiovascular Disease 1975; Cardiac Electrophysiology 1994; **Med School:** India 1970; **Resid:** Internal Medicine, Mt Sinai Med Ctr 1973; **Fellow:** Cardiovascular Disease, Mt Sinai Med Ctr 1975; **Fac Appt:** Prof Med, Mount Sinai Sch Med

Lerman, Bruce MD [CE] - **Spec Exp:** Catheter Ablation; Defibrillators; Arrhythmias; **Hospital:** NY-Presby Hosp/Weill Cornell (page 66); **Address:** NY Weill Cornell Med Ctr, 520 E 70th St, Starr 4, New York, NY 10021-9800; **Phone:** 212-746-2169; **Board Cert:** Internal Medicine 1980; Cardiovascular Disease 1985; Cardiac Electrophysiology 2002; **Med School:** Loyola Univ-Stritch Sch Med 1977; **Resid:** Internal Medicine, Northwestern Univ Hosp 1980; Internal Medicine, Univ Michigan Med Ctr 1981; **Fellow:** Cardiovascular Disease, Hosp Univ Penn 1982; Cardiovascular Disease, Johns Hopkins Hosp 1983; **Fac Appt:** Prof Med, Cornell Univ-Weill Med Coll

Levine, Joseph H MD [CE] - **Spec Exp:** Arrhythmias; Sudden Death Prevention; Defibrillators; Pacemakers; **Hospital:** St Francis Hosp - The Heart Ctr (page 70), Good Samaritan Hosp Med Ctr - West Islip; **Address:** 100 Port Washington Blvd, Roslyn, NY 11576; **Phone:** 516-622-1011; **Board Cert:** Internal Medicine 1983; Cardiovascular Disease 1987; Cardiac Electrophysiology 2003; **Med School:** Univ Rochester 1980; **Resid:** Internal Medicine, Yale-New Haven Hosp 1983; **Fellow:** Cardiovascular Disease, Johns Hopkins Hosp 1986; Cardiac Electrophysiology, Hosp Univ Penn 1986

Marchlinski, Francis E MD [CE] - **Spec Exp:** Pacemakers; Arrhythmias; **Hospital:** Hosp Univ Penn - UPHS (page 72), Penn Presby Med Ctr - UPHS (page 72); **Address:** Hosp University Penn, Div Cardiology, 3400 Spruce St Founders Bldg Fl 9, Philadelphia, PA 19104-4206; **Phone:** 215-662-6005; **Board Cert:** Internal Medicine 1979; Cardiovascular Disease 1981; Cardiac Electrophysiology 2002; **Med School:** Univ Pennsylvania 1976; **Resid:** Internal Medicine, Hosp Univ Penn 1979; **Fellow:** Cardiovascular Disease, Hosp Univ Penn 1982; **Fac Appt:** Prof Med, Univ Pennsylvania

Cardiac Electrophysiology

Southeast

Curtis, Anne B MD [CE] - **Spec Exp:** Pacemakers; Arrhythmias; Defibrillators; **Hospital:** Tampa Genl Hosp, VA Hosp - Tampa; **Address:** 4 Columbia Drive, Ste 725, Tampa, FL 33606; **Phone:** 813-259-0600; **Board Cert:** Internal Medicine 1982; Cardiovascular Disease 1985; Cardiac Electrophysiology 2002; **Med School:** Columbia P&S 1979; **Resid:** Internal Medicine, Columbia- Presby Hosp 1982; **Fellow:** Cardiovascular Disease, Duke Univ Med Ctr 1986; **Fac Appt:** Prof Med, Univ S Fla Coll Med

Del Negro, Albert A MD [CE] - **Spec Exp:** Arrhythmias; **Hospital:** Inova Fairfax Hosp, Inova Alexandria Hosp; **Address:** 3020 Hamaker Ct, Ste 401, Fairfax, VA 22031; **Phone:** 703-849-0770; **Board Cert:** Internal Medicine 1979; Cardiovascular Disease 1981; **Med School:** Georgetown Univ 1969; **Resid:** Internal Medicine, DC Genl Hosp 1972; **Fellow:** Cardiovascular Disease, Georgetown Univ Med Ctr 1973; Cardiovascular Disease, VA Med Ctr 1974; **Fac Appt:** Asst Clin Prof Med, Georgetown Univ

DiMarco, John P MD/PhD [CE] - **Spec Exp:** Arrhythmias; Pacemakers; Defibrillators; **Hospital:** Univ Virginia Med Ctr; **Address:** Univ Virginia Hlth Scis Ctr, PO Box 800158, Charlottesville, VA 22908-0158; **Phone:** 434-924-2031; **Board Cert:** Internal Medicine 1978; Cardiovascular Disease 1981; Cardiac Electrophysiology 2005; **Med School:** Case West Res Univ 1975; **Resid:** Internal Medicine, Mass Genl Hosp 1977; Critical Care Medicine, Case West Res Univ 1978; **Fellow:** Cardiovascular Disease, Mass Genl Hosp 1980; Cardiac Electrophysiology, Mass Genl Hosp 1981; **Fac Appt:** Prof Med, Univ VA Sch Med

Ellenbogen, Kenneth A MD [CE] - **Spec Exp:** Arrhythmias; Pacemakers; Defibrillators; **Hospital:** Med Coll of VA Hosp, Henrico Doctors Hosp; **Address:** Med Coll VA/ Electrophysiology, PO Box 980053, Richmond, VA 23298; **Phone:** 804-828-7565; **Board Cert:** Internal Medicine 1983; Cardiovascular Disease 1985; Cardiac Electrophysiology 2005; **Med School:** Johns Hopkins Univ 1980; **Resid:** Internal Medicine, Johns Hopkins Hosp 1983; **Fellow:** Cardiovascular Disease, Duke Univ Med Ctr 1986; **Fac Appt:** Assoc Prof Med, Med Coll VA

Epstein, Andrew Ernest MD [CE] - **Spec Exp:** Arrhythmias; Defibrillators; Catheter Ablation; **Hospital:** Univ of Ala Hosp at Birmingham; **Address:** Univ of Alabama at Birmingham, 1530 3rd Ave S, THT 321, Birmingham, AL 35294-0006; **Phone:** 205-934-7114; **Board Cert:** Internal Medicine 1980; Cardiovascular Disease 1983; Cardiac Electrophysiology 1996; **Med School:** Univ Rochester 1977; **Resid:** Internal Medicine, Barnes Hosp-Wash Univ 1980; **Fellow:** Cardiovascular Disease, Univ Ala Hosp 1982; **Fac Appt:** Prof Med, Univ Ala

Interian Jr, Alberto MD [CE] - **Hospital:** Jackson Meml Hosp, Mercy Hosp - Miami; **Address:** Jackson Memorial Hospital, PO Box 016960, Locator Code D39, Miami, FL 33136; **Phone:** 305-585-5532; **Board Cert:** Internal Medicine 1985; Cardiovascular Disease 1987; Cardiac Electrophysiology 2000; **Med School:** Univ Miami Sch Med 1982; **Resid:** Internal Medicine, Univ Miami Hosps 1985; **Fellow:** Cardiovascular Disease, Univ Miami Hosps 1988; **Fac Appt:** Prof Med, Univ Miami Sch Med

Kay, G Neal MD [CE] - **Spec Exp:** Arrhythmias; Pacemakers; **Hospital:** Univ of Ala Hosp at Birmingham; **Address:** UAB, Div Cardiology, 1530 3rd Ave S, THT, Ste 321-J, Birmingham, AL 35294-0006; **Phone:** 205-934-1335; **Board Cert:** Internal Medicine 1983; Cardiovascular Disease 1989; **Med School:** Univ Mich Med Sch 1979; **Resid:** Internal Medicine, Univ Alabama Hosp 1983; **Fellow:** Cardiovascular Disease, Duke Univ Med Ctr 1986; **Fac Appt:** Prof Med, Univ Ala

Sorrentino, Robert A MD [CE] - **Spec Exp:** Arrhythmias; Defibrillators; Pacemakers; Heart Failure; **Hospital:** Med Coll of GA Hosp and Clin; **Address:** Medical College of Georgia, 1120 15th St BBR Bldg - rm 6518, Augusta, GA 30912-0004; **Phone:** 706-721-4997; **Board Cert:** Internal Medicine 1988; Cardiovascular Disease 2002; Cardiac Electrophysiology 1996; **Med School:** Albany Med Coll 1985; **Resid:** Internal Medicine, Duke Univ Med Ctr 1988; **Fellow:** Cardiovascular Disease, Duke Univ Med Ctr 1991; Cardiac Electrophysiology, Duke Univ Med Ctr 1991; **Fac Appt:** Prof Med, Med Coll GA

Midwest

Anderson, Mark E MD/PhD [CE] - **Spec Exp:** Arrhythmias; **Hospital:** Univ Iowa Hosp & Clinics; **Address:** Univ Iowa-Carver College Medicine, 200 Hawkins Dr, E315, GH, Iowa City, IA 52242-1081; **Phone:** 319-353-7101; **Board Cert:** Internal Medicine 2003; Cardiovascular Disease 2003; Cardiac Electrophysiology 1996; **Med School:** Univ Minn 1989; **Resid:** Internal Medicine, Stanford Univ Med Ctr 1991; **Fellow:** Cardiovascular Disease, Stanford Univ Sch Med 1994; Cardiac Electrophysiology, Stanford Univ Sch Med 1996; **Fac Appt:** Prof Med, Univ Iowa Coll Med

Hammill, Stephen C MD [CE] - **Spec Exp:** Pacemakers; Arrhythmias; **Hospital:** Mayo Med Ctr & Clin - Rochester; **Address:** Mayo Clinic, Div Cardiovasc Disease, 200 First St SW, Rochester, MN 55905; **Phone:** 507-284-4888; **Board Cert:** Internal Medicine 1978; Cardiovascular Disease 1981; Cardiac Electrophysiology 2005; **Med School:** Univ Colorado 1973; **Resid:** Internal Medicine, Univ Colo Hlth Sci Ctr 1977; **Fellow:** Cardiovascular Disease, Duke Univ Med Ctr 1981; **Fac Appt:** Prof Med, Mayo Med Sch

Hayes, David L MD [CE] - **Spec Exp:** Pacemakers; **Hospital:** Mayo Med Ctr & Clin - Rochester; **Address:** Mayo Clinic, 200 1st St SW Gonda 5 Bldg - rm 200, Rochester, MN 55905; **Phone:** 507-284-3684; **Board Cert:** Internal Medicine 1980; Cardiovascular Disease 1982; **Med School:** Univ MO-Kansas City 1977; **Resid:** Internal Medicine, Mayo Clinic 1980; **Fellow:** Cardiovascular Disease, Mayo Clinic 1982; **Fac Appt:** Prof Med, Mayo Med Sch

Lindsay, Bruce D MD [CE] - **Spec Exp:** Arrhythmias; **Hospital:** Barnes-Jewish Hosp; **Address:** Washington Univ Schl Med, Div Cardiology, 660 S Euclid Ave, Box 8086, St Louis, MO 63110; **Phone:** 314-454-7834; **Board Cert:** Internal Medicine 1980; Cardiovascular Disease 1987; Cardiac Electrophysiology 2002; **Med School:** Jefferson Med Coll 1976; **Resid:** Internal Medicine, Univ Michigan Medical Ctr 1980; **Fellow:** Cardiovascular Disease, Barnes-Jewish Hosp 1985; **Fac Appt:** Assoc Prof Med, Univ Wash

Morady, Fred MD [CE] - **Spec Exp:** Arrhythmias; WPW Syndrome; **Hospital:** Univ Michigan Hlth Sys; **Address:** Specialty Electrophysiology, 1500 E Med Ctr Drive, TCB1 226-0311, Ann Arbor, MI 48109; **Phone:** 734-647-7321; **Board Cert:** Internal Medicine 1978; Cardiovascular Disease 1981; Cardiac Electrophysiology 2005; **Med School:** UCSF 1975; **Resid:** Internal Medicine, UCSF Med Ctr 1978; **Fellow:** Cardiovascular Disease, UCSF Med Ctr 1980; **Fac Appt:** Prof Med, Univ Mich Med Sch

Natale, Andrea MD [CE] - **Spec Exp:** Arrhythmias; Atrial Fibrillation; **Hospital:** Cleveland Clin Fdn (page 57); **Address:** Cleveland Clinic, Dept Cardiology, 9500 Euclid Ave, rm F15, Cleveland, OH 44195; **Phone:** 216-444-4293; **Board Cert:** Internal Medicine 1999; Cardiovascular Disease 2000; Cardiac Electrophysiology 2001; **Med School:** Italy 1985; **Resid:** Internal Medicine, Univ Rome bMed Ctr 1989; **Fellow:** Cardiovascular Disease, Univ Western Ontario 1992; Cardiac Electrophysiology, Sinai Samaritan Med Ctr 1994; **Fac Appt:** Prof Med, Ohio State Univ

Cardiac Electrophysiology

Prystowsky, Eric N MD [CE] - **Spec Exp:** Arrhythmias; Catheter Ablation; Atrial Fibrillation; **Hospital:** St Vincent Hosp & Hlth Svcs - Indianapolis; **Address:** 8333 Naab Rd, Ste 400, Indianapolis, IN 46260; **Phone:** 317-338-6024; **Board Cert:** Internal Medicine 1976; Cardiovascular Disease 1979; Cardiac Electrophysiology 2006; **Med School:** Mount Sinai Sch Med 1973; **Resid:** Internal Medicine, Mt Sinai Hosp 1976; **Fellow:** Cardiovascular Disease, Duke Univ Med Ctr 1979; **Fac Appt:** Prof Med, Duke Univ

Schuger, Claudio David MD [CE] - **Spec Exp:** Arrhythmias; Defibrillators; **Hospital:** Henry Ford Hosp; **Address:** Henry Ford Hosp, Div Cardiology, 2799 W Grand Blvd, Ste E235, Detroit, MI 48202; **Phone:** 313-916-2417; **Board Cert:** Cardiac Electrophysiology 1998; Cardiovascular Disease 1997; **Med School:** Argentina 1977; **Resid:** Internal Medicine, Hacarmel Hosp 1982; Cardiovascular Disease, Hacarmel Hosp 1982; **Fellow:** Cardiovascular Disease, Bikur Cholim Hosp 1985; Cardiac Electrophysiology, Harper Hosp-Wayne State Univ 1990; **Fac Appt:** Assoc Prof Med, Wayne State Univ

Tchou, Patrick J MD [CE] - **Spec Exp:** Arrhythmias; **Hospital:** Cleveland Clin Fdn (page 57); **Address:** Cleveland Clinic, Dept Cardiology, 9500 Euclid Ave, rm F15, Cleveland, OH 44195; **Phone:** 216-444-6792; **Board Cert:** Internal Medicine 1982; Cardiovascular Disease 1985; Cardiac Electrophysiology 2002; **Med School:** Case West Res Univ 1979; **Resid:** Internal Medicine, Metro Genl Hosp 1982; **Fellow:** Cardiovascular Disease, Metro Genl Hosp 1984; Cardiac Electrophysiology, Mt Sinai Med Ctr 1985; **Fac Appt:** Prof Med, Ohio State Univ

Waldo, Albert MD [CE] - **Spec Exp:** Arrhythmias; Syncope; Atrial Fibrillation; **Hospital:** Univ Hosps Case Med Ctr; **Address:** Univ Hosps Case Med Ctr-Cardiology, 11100 Euclid Ave, MS LKS-5038, Cleveland, OH 44106-1736; **Phone:** 216-844-7690; **Board Cert:** Internal Medicine 1971; Cardiovascular Disease 1975; **Med School:** SUNY Downstate 1962; **Resid:** Internal Medicine, Baltimore City Hosp 1965; Internal Medicine, Kings Co Hosp 1966; **Fellow:** Cardiovascular Disease, Columbia Presby Med Ctr 1968; Cardiac Electrophysiology, Columbia Presby Med Ctr 1969; **Fac Appt:** Prof Med, Case West Res Univ

Wilber, David James MD [CE] - **Spec Exp:** Atrial Fibrillation; Catheter Ablation; Sudden Death Prevention; **Hospital:** Loyola Univ Med Ctr, Hinsdale Hosp; **Address:** Loyola Univ Med Ctr, Cardiovascular Inst, 2160 S First Ave Bldg 110 - rm 6232, Maywood, IL 60153; **Phone:** 708-216-2642; **Board Cert:** Internal Medicine 1980; Cardiovascular Disease 1985; Cardiac Electrophysiology 2002; **Med School:** Northwestern Univ 1977; **Resid:** Internal Medicine, Northwestern Meml Hosp 1980; **Fellow:** Cardiovascular Disease, Univ Mich Med Sch 1984; Cardiac Electrophysiology, Mass Genl Hosp 1986; **Fac Appt:** Prof Med, Loyola Univ-Stritch Sch Med

Great Plains and Mountains

Lewkowiez, Laurent MD [CE] - **Spec Exp:** Arrhythmias; Ventricular Tachycardia Ablation; Atrial Fibrillation; **Hospital:** Denver Health Med Ctr; **Address:** Denver Health Med Ctr, Div Cardiology, 777 Bannock St, Denver, CO 80204; **Phone:** 303-436-5499; **Board Cert:** Internal Medicine 1996; Cardiovascular Disease 2000; Cardiac Electrophysiology 2003; **Med School:** Univ SC Sch Med 1992; **Resid:** Internal Medicine, Univ Colorado Hlth Sci Ctr 1996; **Fellow:** Nuclear Cardiology, Univ Colorado Hlth Sci Ctr 1998; Cardiac Electrophysiology, Univ Colorado Hlth Sci Ctr 2001; **Fac Appt:** Asst Prof Med, Univ Colorado

Southwest

Jackman, Warren M MD [CE] - **Spec Exp:** Catheter Ablation; Atrial Fibrillation; WPW Syndrome; **Hospital:** OU Med Ctr; **Address:** 1200 Everett Drive, TUH-6E-103, Oklahoma City, OK 73104; **Phone:** 405-271-4985; **Board Cert:** Internal Medicine 1979; Cardiovascular Disease 1981; Cardiac Electrophysiology 2003; **Med School:** Univ Fla Coll Med 1976; **Resid:** Internal Medicine, Wake Fores Univ Hosp 1979; **Fellow:** Cardiac Electrophysiology, Indiana Univ Hosp 1981; **Fac Appt:** Prof Med, Univ Okla Coll Med

West Coast and Pacific

Cannom, David S MD [CE] - **Spec Exp:** Arrhythmias; **Hospital:** Good Samaritan Hosp - Los Angeles; **Address:** 1245 Wilshire Blvd, Ste 703, Los Angeles, CA 90017-4806; **Phone:** 213-977-0419; **Board Cert:** Internal Medicine 1980; Cardiovascular Disease 1975; **Med School:** Univ Minn 1967; **Resid:** Internal Medicine, Yale-New Haven Hosp 1969; **Fellow:** Cardiovascular Disease, Stanford Unv 1973; **Fac Appt:** Clin Prof Med, UCLA

Gang, Eli Shimshon MD [CE] - **Spec Exp:** Arrhythmias; **Hospital:** Cedars-Sinai Med Ctr, Brotman Med Ctr; **Address:** 414 N Camden Drive, Ste 1100, Beverly Hills, CA 90210; **Phone:** 310-278-3400; **Board Cert:** Internal Medicine 1978; Cardiovascular Disease 1981; **Med School:** Columbia P&S 1975; **Resid:** Internal Medicine, Roosevelt Hosp 1978; **Fellow:** Cardiovascular Disease, Columbia Presby Hosp 1979; **Fac Appt:** Clin Prof Med, UCLA

Swerdlow, Charles D MD [CE] - **Spec Exp:** Defibrillators; Arrhythmias; **Hospital:** Cedars-Sinai Med Ctr; **Address:** 8635 W 3rd St, Ste 1190W, Los Angeles, CA 90048-6101; **Phone:** 310-652-4600; **Board Cert:** Internal Medicine 1979; Cardiovascular Disease 1981; Cardiac Electrophysiology 2004; **Med School:** Harvard Med Sch 1976; **Resid:** Internal Medicine, LA Co- Harbor Genl Hosp 1979; **Fellow:** Cardiovascular Disease, Stanford Univ Med Ctr 1981; **Fac Appt:** Clin Prof Med, UCLA

Interventional Cardiology

New England

Diver, Daniel J MD [IC] - **Spec Exp:** Angioplasty; Coronary Artery Disease; **Hospital:** St Francis Hosp & Med Ctr; **Address:** St Francis Hosp - Div Cardiology, 114 Woodland St, Hartford, CT 06105; **Phone:** 860-714-4019; **Board Cert:** Internal Medicine 1984; Cardiovascular Disease 1989; Interventional Cardiology 1999; **Med School:** Johns Hopkins Univ 1981; **Resid:** Internal Medicine, Johns Hopkins Hosp 1984; **Fellow:** Cardiovascular Disease, Beth Israel Hosp/Harvard 1987; **Fac Appt:** Prof Med, Univ Conn

Jacobs, Alice K MD [IC] - **Spec Exp:** Cardiac Catheterization; Heart Disease in Women; Interventional Cardiology; **Hospital:** Boston Med Ctr; **Address:** Boston Univ Med Ctr, Dept Cardiology, 88 E Newton St, Boston, MA 02118; **Phone:** 617-638-8707; **Board Cert:** Internal Medicine 1978; Endocrinology 1979; Cardiovascular Disease 1985; Interventional Cardiology 1999; **Med School:** St Louis Univ 1975; **Resid:** Internal Medicine, St Louis Univ Hosp 1977; **Fellow:** Endocrinology, UCSD Med Ctr 1980; Cardiovascular Disease, Boston Univ Med Ctr 1982; **Fac Appt:** Prof Med, Boston Univ

Laham, Roger MD [IC] - **Spec Exp:** Angioplasty; **Hospital:** Beth Israel Deaconess Med Ctr - Boston; **Address:** Beth Israel Deaconess Med Ctr, 330 Brookline Ave, West Baker 4, Boston, MA 02215; **Phone:** 617-632-9204; **Board Cert:** Internal Medicine 2004; Cardiovascular Disease 2005; Interventional Cardiology 1999; **Med School:** Lebanon 1989; **Resid:** Internal Medicine, Duke Univ Med Ctr 1992; **Fellow:** Cardiovascular Disease, Harvard Med Sch 1995; **Fac Appt:** Assoc Prof Med, Harvard Med Sch

Williams, David O MD [IC] - **Spec Exp:** Interventional Cardiology; **Hospital:** Rhode Island Hosp; **Address:** Rhode Island Hosp, Div Cardiology, 593 Eddy St, rm APC 814, Providence, RI 02903; **Phone:** 401-444-4581; **Board Cert:** Internal Medicine 1972; Cardiovascular Disease 1975; Interventional Cardiology 1999; **Med School:** Hahnemann Univ 1969; **Resid:** Internal Medicine, Hahnemann Univ Hosp 1972; **Fellow:** Cardiovascular Disease, UC Davis Med Ctr 1974; **Fac Appt:** Prof Med, Brown Univ

Mid Atlantic

Abittan, Meyer H MD [IC] - **Spec Exp:** Angiography-Coronary; Preventive Cardiology; **Hospital:** St Francis Hosp - The Heart Ctr (page 70); **Address:** St Francis Hosp, The Heart Ctr, 100 Port Washington Blvd, Ste G-03, Roslyn, NY 11576; **Phone:** 516-365-6444; **Board Cert:** Internal Medicine 1989; Interventional Cardiology 1999; **Med School:** Mount Sinai Sch Med 1986; **Resid:** Internal Medicine, Brookdale Univ Hosp Med Ctr 1989; **Fellow:** Cardiovascular Disease, Mt Sinai Med Ctr 1990

Herrmann, Howard C MD [IC] - **Spec Exp:** Cardiac Catheterization; Angioplasty & Stent Placement; Heart Valve Disease; Atrial Septal Defect Closure; **Hospital:** Hosp Univ Penn - UPHS (page 72), Penn Presby Med Ctr - UPHS (page 72); **Address:** Hosp Univ Penn, Div Cardiovascular Med, 3400 Spruce St, 9.120 Founders Bldg, Philadelphia, PA 19104-4283; **Phone:** 215-662-2180; **Board Cert:** Internal Medicine 1984; Cardiovascular Disease 1987; Interventional Cardiology 1999; **Med School:** Harvard Med Sch 1981; **Resid:** Internal Medicine, Mass General Hosp 1984; **Fellow:** Cardiovascular Disease, Mass General Hosp 1987; **Fac Appt:** Prof Med, Univ Pennsylvania

Leon, Martin MD [IC] - **Hospital:** NY-Presby Hosp/Columbia (page 66); **Address:** 161 Ft Washington Ave Fl 5, New York, NY 10032; **Phone:** 212-305-7060; **Board Cert:** Internal Medicine 1979; Cardiovascular Disease 1983; Interventional Cardiology 1999; **Med School:** Yale Univ 1975; **Resid:** Internal Medicine, Yale-New Haven Hosp 1978; **Fellow:** Cardiovascular Disease, Yale-New Haven Hosp 1980

Moses, Jeffrey W MD [IC] - **Spec Exp:** Angiography-Coronary; Angioplasty & Stent Placement; Heart Valve Disease; **Hospital:** NY-Presby Hosp/Columbia (page 66); **Address:** 161 Fort Washington Fl 5, New York, NY 10032; **Phone:** 212-305-7060; **Board Cert:** Internal Medicine 1977; Cardiovascular Disease 1981; Interventional Cardiology 1999; **Med School:** Univ Pennsylvania 1974; **Resid:** Internal Medicine, Presby Univ Med Ctr 1977; **Fellow:** Cardiovascular Disease, Presby Univ Penn Med Ctr 1980

Pichard, Augusto MD [IC] - **Spec Exp:** Angioplasty & Stent Placement; Cardiac Catheterization; **Hospital:** Washington Hosp Ctr; **Address:** 110 Irving St NW, Ste 4B1, Washington, DC 20010; **Phone:** 202-877-5975; **Board Cert:** Internal Medicine 1975; Cardiovascular Disease 1977; Interventional Cardiology 1999; **Med School:** Chile 1969; **Resid:** Internal Medicine, Univ Chile 1970; Internal Medicine, Catholic Univ 1971; **Fellow:** Cardiovascular Disease, Cleveland Clinic 1973; **Fac Appt:** Clin Prof Med, Geo Wash Univ

Reiner, Jonathan S MD [IC] - **Spec Exp:** Angioplasty & Stent Placement; **Hospital:** G Washington Univ Hosp; **Address:** MFA, Dept Cardiology, 2150 Pennsylvania Ave NW, Washington, DC 20037; **Phone:** 202-741-3333; **Board Cert:** Internal Medicine 1989; Cardiovascular Disease 2004; Interventional Cardiology 1999; **Med School:** Georgetown Univ 1986; **Resid:** Internal Medicine, North Shore Univ Hosp 1989; **Fellow:** Cardiovascular Disease, George Wash Univ Sch Med 1993; **Fac Appt:** Asst Prof Med, Geo Wash Univ

Resar, Jon R MD [IC] - **Spec Exp:** Percutaneous Coronary Intervention; Percutaneous Valvuloplasty; Percutaneous ASD/PFO closure; **Hospital:** Johns Hopkins Hosp - Baltimore (page 61); **Address:** Johns Hopkins Hosp, Dept Cardiology, 600 N Wolfe st, Blalock 524, Baltimore, MD 21287; **Phone:** 410-614-1132; **Board Cert:** Internal Medicine 1988; Cardiovascular Disease 2000; Interventional Cardiology 1999; **Med School:** Med Coll Wisc 1985; **Resid:** Internal Medicine, Johns Hopkins Hosp 1988; **Fellow:** Cardiovascular Disease, Johns Hopkins Hosp 1990; Interventional Cardiology, Johns Hopkins Hosp; **Fac Appt:** Assoc Prof Med, Johns Hopkins Univ

Roubin, Gary MD/PhD [IC] - **Spec Exp:** Coronary Angioplasty/Stents; Carotid Artery Stent Placement; Peripheral Vascular Disease; **Hospital:** Lenox Hill Hosp (page 62); **Address:** 130 E 77th St Fl 9th, New York, NY 10021; **Phone:** 212-434-2606; **Med School:** Australia 1975; **Resid:** Internal Medicine, Royal Prince Albert Hosp 1979; Cardiovascular Disease, Hallstrom Inst of Cardiology 1981; **Fellow:** Cardiology Research, Natl Heart Fdn 1983; Interventional Cardiology, Emory Univ 1985

Shani, Jacob MD [IC] - **Spec Exp:** Cardiac Catheterization; Angioplasty & Stent Placement; Percutaneous Valvuloplasty; **Hospital:** Maimonides Med Ctr (page 63); **Address:** Maimonides Med Ctr, Cardiac Cath Lab, 4802 10th Ave, Brooklyn, NY 11219-2844; **Phone:** 718-283-7480; **Board Cert:** Internal Medicine 1981; Cardiovascular Disease 1983; Interventional Cardiology 1999; **Med School:** Israel 1977; **Resid:** Internal Medicine, Maimonides Med Ctr 1981; **Fellow:** Cardiovascular Disease, Beth Israel Hosp-Harvard 1983; **Fac Appt:** Prof Med, Mount Sinai Sch Med

Shorofsky, Stephen R MD/PhD [IC] - **Spec Exp:** Arrhythmias; **Hospital:** Univ of MD Med Sys; **Address:** Univ Maryland Med Ctr, Div Cardiology, 22 S Greene St, rm N3W77, Baltimore, MD 21201; **Phone:** 410-328-6056; **Board Cert:** Internal Medicine 1988; Cardiovascular Disease 2001; Cardiac Electrophysiology 2004; **Med School:** Univ Chicago-Pritzker Sch Med 1985; **Resid:** Internal Medicine, Univ Chicago Hosps 1988; **Fellow:** Cardiovascular Disease, Univ Chicago Hosps 1991; **Fac Appt:** Assoc Prof Med, Univ MD Sch Med

Stone, Gregg W MD [IC] - **Spec Exp:** Angioplasty & Stent Placement; Coronary Artery Disease; **Hospital:** NY-Presby Hosp/Columbia (page 66); **Address:** Columbia Univ Med Ctr, 161 Fort Washington Ave Fl 5, New York, NY 10032; **Phone:** 212-851-9304; **Board Cert:** Internal Medicine 1985; Cardiovascular Disease 1987; Interventional Cardiology 1999; **Med School:** Johns Hopkins Univ 1982; **Resid:** Internal Medicine, NY Hosp-Cornell Medical Ctr 1985; **Fellow:** Cardiovascular Disease, Cedars-Sinai Medical Ctr 1988; Coronary Angioplasty, Mid-America Heart Inst 1989

Interventional Cardiology

Southeast

Applegate, Robert J MD [IC] - **Spec Exp:** Cardiac Catheterization; Angioplasty; **Hospital:** Wake Forest Univ Baptist Med Ctr (page 73); **Address:** Wake Forest Univ Baptist Med Ctr, Div Cardio, Medical Center Blvd, Winston-Salem, NC 27157-1045; **Phone:** 336-716-3272; **Board Cert:** Internal Medicine 1983; Cardiovascular Disease 1987; Interventional Cardiology 1999; **Med School:** Univ VA Sch Med 1980; **Resid:** Internal Medicine, Oregon Hlth Sci Univ Hosp 1983; **Fellow:** Pharmacology, Univ Texas Hlth Sci Ctr 1984; Cardiovascular Disease, Univ Texas Hlth Sci Ctr 1986; **Fac Appt:** Prof Med, Wake Forest Univ

King III, Spencer MD [IC] - **Spec Exp:** Angioplasty; **Hospital:** Piedmont Hosp; **Address:** 1938 Peachtree Rd NW, Ste 705, Atlanta, GA 30309; **Phone:** 404-605-3567; **Board Cert:** Internal Medicine 1970; Cardiovascular Disease 1971; Interventional Cardiology 1999; **Med School:** Med Coll GA 1963; **Resid:** Internal Medicine, Emory Univ Hosp 1968; **Fellow:** Cardiovascular Disease, Emory Univ Sch Med 1970

Margolis, James MD [IC] - **Spec Exp:** Cardiac Catheterization; Invasive Cardiology; Angioplasty; **Hospital:** Cedars Med Ctr - Miami, Baptist Hosp of Miami; **Address:** Miami Intl Cardiac Consultants, 3801 Biscayne Blvd Fl 3, Miami Beach, FL 33137; **Phone:** 305-674-3117; **Board Cert:** Internal Medicine 1973; Cardiovascular Disease 1975; Interventional Cardiology 1999; **Med School:** Univ IL Coll Med 1968; **Resid:** Internal Medicine, Barnes Hosp 1972; **Fellow:** Cardiovascular Disease, Duke Med Ctr 1974; **Fac Appt:** Clin Prof Med, Univ Miami Sch Med

Matar, Fadi MD [IC] - **Spec Exp:** Angioplasty; **Hospital:** Tampa Genl Hosp, St Joseph's Hosp - Tampa; **Address:** 509 S Armenia Ave, Ste 200, Tampa, FL 33609; **Phone:** 813-353-1515; **Board Cert:** Interventional Cardiology 1999; **Med School:** Lebanon 1987; **Resid:** Internal Medicine, Maryland Genl Hosp 1990; **Fellow:** Cardiovascular Disease, Wash Hosp Ctr 1994; **Fac Appt:** Asst Prof Med, Univ S Fla Coll Med

Morris, Douglas MD [IC] - **Spec Exp:** Interventional Cardiology; **Hospital:** Emory Univ Hosp, Crawford Long Hosp of Emory Univ; **Address:** Heart Center, 1365 Clifton Rd NE A Bldg - Ste A2205, Atlanta, GA 30322; **Phone:** 404-778-5310; **Board Cert:** Internal Medicine 1973; Cardiovascular Disease 1975; Interventional Cardiology 1999; **Med School:** Baylor Coll Med 1968; **Resid:** Internal Medicine, Vanderbilt Univ Med Ctr 1970; Internal Medicine, Vanderbilt Univ Med Ctr 1973; **Fellow:** Cardiovascular Disease, Emory Univ 1975; **Fac Appt:** Prof Med, Emory Univ

Midwest

Ellis, Stephen G MD [IC] - **Spec Exp:** Angioplasty & Stent Placement; Angiogenesis; **Hospital:** Cleveland Clin Fdn (page 57); **Address:** Cleveland Clinic, Div Cardiovasc Med, 9500 Euclid Ave, Desk F25, Cleveland, OH 44195; **Phone:** 216-445-6712; **Board Cert:** Internal Medicine 1981; Cardiovascular Disease 1985; Interventional Cardiology 1999; **Med School:** UCLA 1978; **Resid:** Internal Medicine, Cedars-Sinai Med Ctr 1981; **Fellow:** Cardiovascular Disease, Stanford Univ Med Ctr 1985; Interventional Cardiology, Emory Univ Hosp 1986; **Fac Appt:** Prof Med, Cleveland Cl Coll Med/Case West Res

Feldman, Ted E MD [IC] - **Spec Exp:** Angioplasty; **Hospital:** Evanston Hosp; **Address:** ENH Med Group, Cardiology, 9977 Woods Drive, Skokie, IL 60077-1057; **Phone:** 847-663-8410; **Board Cert:** Internal Medicine 1981; Cardiovascular Disease 1985; Interventional Cardiology 1999; **Med School:** Indiana Univ 1978; **Resid:** Internal Medicine, Rush-Presby-St Lukes Hosp 1982; **Fellow:** Cardiovascular Disease, Univ Chicago 1985; **Fac Appt:** Prof Med, Northwestern Univ

Henry, Timothy D MD [IC] - **Spec Exp:** Acute Coronary Syndromes; Angiogenesis; **Hospital:** Abbott - Northwestern Hosp; **Address:** Minneapolis Heart Inst, 920 E 28th St, Ste 40, Minneapolis, MN 55407; **Phone:** 612-863-3900; **Board Cert:** Internal Medicine 1985; Cardiovascular Disease 1989; Interventional Cardiology 2000; **Med School:** UCSF 1982; **Resid:** Internal Medicine, Univ Colorado Hosp 1985; **Fellow:** Cardiovascular Disease, Univ Minnesota 1990; Interventional Cardiology, Univ Minnesota 1991; **Fac Appt:** Assoc Prof Med, Univ Minn

Holmes Jr, David R MD [IC] - **Spec Exp:** Heart Attack; Acute Coronary Syndromes; Angioplasty & Restenosis; **Hospital:** Mayo Med Ctr & Clin - Rochester; **Address:** Mayo Clinic, Div Cardiovasc Dis, 200 First St SW, Rochester, MN 55905; **Phone:** 507-255-2504; **Board Cert:** Internal Medicine 1974; Cardiovascular Disease 1977; Interventional Cardiology 1999; **Med School:** Med Coll Wisc 1971; **Resid:** Internal Medicine, Mayo Clinic 1974; **Fellow:** Cardiovascular Disease, Mayo Clinic 1977; **Fac Appt:** Prof Med, Mayo Med Sch

Losordo, Douglas W MD [IC] - **Spec Exp:** Stem Cell Therapy in Heart Failure; Angiogenesis; Angioplasty & Stent Placement; Heart Attack; **Hospital:** Northwestern Meml Hosp; **Address:** Feinberg Cardiovascular Research Inst, 303 E Chicago Ave, Tarry 12-703, Chicago, IL 60611; **Phone:** 312-503-2296; **Board Cert:** Internal Medicine 1986; Cardiovascular Disease 1989; Interventional Cardiology 2002; **Med School:** Univ VT Coll Med 1983; **Resid:** Internal Medicine, St Elizabeth's Med Ctr 1986; **Fellow:** Cardiovascular Disease, St Elizabeth's Med Ctr 1989; **Fac Appt:** Prof Med, Northwestern Univ-Feinberg Sch Med

Pitt, Bertram MD [IC] - **Spec Exp:** Heart Failure; Heart Attack; Hypertension; **Hospital:** Univ Michigan Hlth Sys; **Address:** Univ Mich, Div Cardiology, 1500 E Med Ctr, rm 3214 TC, Ann Arbor, MI 48109-0366; **Phone:** 734-936-5260; **Board Cert:** Internal Medicine 1973; Cardiovascular Disease 1975; **Med School:** Switzerland 1959; **Resid:** Internal Medicine, Beth Israel Hosp 1963; **Fellow:** Cardiovascular Disease, Johns Hopkins Hosp 1968; **Fac Appt:** Prof Emeritus Med, Univ Mich Med Sch

Schreiber, Theodore L MD [IC] - **Spec Exp:** Coronary Angioplasty/Stents; Carotid Artery Disease; **Hospital:** Harper Univ Hosp; **Address:** Harper University Hospital, 3990 John R St Webber Bldg - Ste 9370, Detroit, MI 48201; **Phone:** 313-745-7025; **Board Cert:** Internal Medicine 1981; Cardiovascular Disease 1983; Interventional Cardiology 2000; **Med School:** Cornell Univ-Weill Med Coll 1978; **Resid:** Internal Medicine, New Yok Hosp-Cornell Med Ctr 1981; **Fellow:** Cardiovascular Disease, NY Hosp-Cornell Med Ctr 1983; **Fac Appt:** Assoc Prof Med, Wayne State Univ

Whitlow, Patrick MD [IC] - **Spec Exp:** Cardiac Catheterization; **Hospital:** Cleveland Clin Fdn (page 57); **Address:** Cleveland Clinic, Dept Cardiology, 9500 Euclid Ave, MC F25, Cleveland, OH 44195; **Phone:** 216-444-1746; **Board Cert:** Internal Medicine 1979; Cardiovascular Disease 1981; Interventional Cardiology 1999; **Med School:** Duke Univ 1976; **Resid:** Internal Medicine, Parkland Meml Hosp 1979; **Fellow:** Cardiovascular Disease, Univ Alabama Hosp 1981

Southwest

Bailey, Steven R MD [IC] - **Spec Exp:** Coronary Artery Disease; Coronary Angioplasty/Stents; **Hospital:** Univ Hlth Sys - Univ Hosp; **Address:** 7703 Floyd Curl Drive, MC 7872, San Antonio, TX 78229-3900; **Phone:** 210-567-4601; **Board Cert:** Internal Medicine 1981; Cardiovascular Disease 1983; Interventional Cardiology 1999; **Med School:** Oregon Hlth Sci Univ 1978; **Resid:** Internal Medicine, Fitzsimmons AMC 1981; **Fellow:** Cardiovascular Disease, Fitzsimmons AMC 1983; **Fac Appt:** Prof Med, Univ Tex, San Antonio

Interventional Cardiology

Kleiman, Neal Stephen MD [IC] - **Spec Exp:** Angioplasty; **Hospital:** Methodist Hosp - Houston; **Address:** 6550 Fannin, Smith Tower, Ste 1901, Houston, TX 77030; **Phone:** 713-441-1100; **Board Cert:** Internal Medicine 1984; Cardiovascular Disease 1987; Interventional Cardiology 1999; **Med School:** Columbia P&S 1981; **Resid:** Internal Medicine, Baylor Coll Med 1984; **Fellow:** Interventional Cardiology, Baylor Coll Med 1987; **Fac Appt:** Assoc Prof Med, Baylor Coll Med

Perin, Emerson C MD [IC] - **Spec Exp:** Stem Cell Therapy in Heart Failure; Angiogenesis; **Hospital:** St Luke's Episcopal Hosp - Houston; **Address:** Southwest Cardiology Consultants, 6624 Fannin St, Ste 2220, St Lukes Medical Tower Fl 22, Houston, TX 77030-2334; **Phone:** 713-791-9400; **Board Cert:** Internal Medicine 1988; Cardiovascular Disease 1991; Interventional Cardiology 1999; **Med School:** Brazil 1983; **Resid:** Internal Medicine, Jackson Meml Hosp 1988; **Fellow:** Cardiovascular Disease, St Luke's Episcopal Hosp 1991; **Fac Appt:** Asst Prof Med, Baylor Coll Med

Smalling, Richard Warren MD/PhD [IC] - **Spec Exp:** Coronary Artery Disease; Peripheral Vascular Disease; Heart Valve Disease; Congenital Heart Disease; **Hospital:** Meml Hermann Hosp - Houston; **Address:** 6431 Fannin St, MS 1246, Houston, TX 77030-1501; **Phone:** 713-500-6559; **Board Cert:** Internal Medicine 1978; Cardiovascular Disease 1981; Interventional Cardiology 1999; **Med School:** Univ Tex, Houston 1975; **Resid:** Internal Medicine, UCSD Med Ctr 1978; **Fellow:** Cardiovascular Disease, UCSD Med Ctr 1980; **Fac Appt:** Prof Med, Univ Tex, Houston

West Coast and Pacific

Buchbinder, Maurice MD [IC] - **Spec Exp:** Cardiac Catheterization; Peripheral Vascular Disease; **Hospital:** Scripps Meml Hosp - La Jolla; **Address:** 9834 Genesee Ave, Ste 310, La Jolla, CA 92037; **Phone:** 858-625-4488; **Board Cert:** Internal Medicine 1981; Cardiovascular Disease 1983; **Med School:** Canada 1978; **Resid:** Internal Medicine, Jewish Genl Hosp 1980; Internal Medicine, Stanford Univ Hosp 1982; **Fellow:** Cardiovascular Disease, Stanford Univ Hosp 1983

Teirstein, Paul S MD [IC] - **Spec Exp:** Coronary Angioplasty/Stents; Coronary Radiation Therapy; **Hospital:** Scripps Green Hosp; **Address:** Scripps Clinic - Torrey Pines, 10666 N Torrey Pines Rd, La Jolla, CA 92037; **Phone:** 858-554-9905; **Board Cert:** Internal Medicine 1983; Cardiovascular Disease 1987; Interventional Cardiology 1999; **Med School:** Mount Sinai Sch Med 1980; **Resid:** Internal Medicine, Brigham & Womens Hosp 1983; **Fellow:** Cardiovascular Disease, Stanford Univ 1986; Interventional Cardiology, Mid-Amer Heart Inst 1987

Yeung, Alan MD [IC] - **Spec Exp:** Mitral Valve Disease; Coronary Artery Disease; **Hospital:** Stanford Univ Med Ctr; **Address:** Stanford U Medical Ctr, Dept Cardiology, 300 Pasteur Drive, rm H2103, MC 5218, Stanford, CA 94305-5218; **Phone:** 650-723-0180; **Board Cert:** Internal Medicine 1987; Cardiovascular Disease 1989; Interventional Cardiology 2000; **Med School:** Harvard Med Sch 1984; **Resid:** Internal Medicine, Mass General Hosp 1987; **Fellow:** Cardiovascular Disease, Brigham & Women's Hosp 1990; **Fac Appt:** Prof Med, Stanford Univ

ChildrensHospitalLosAngeles

International Leader in Pediatrics

Childrens Hospital Los Angeles

4650 Sunset Boulevard
Los Angeles, California 90027
www.ChildrensHospitalLA.org

Childrens Hospital Los Angeles is acknowledged throughout the United States and around the world for its leadership in pediatric and adolescent health. It is able to offer the very best in multidisciplinary care, with 85 pediatric subspecialties and dozens of special services for children and families. Its physicians are recognized as leaders. Its treatments set the standard of care. Its research is recognized worldwide.

The Heart Institute

The Heart Institute is known throughout the world as a leader in the treatment of pediatric heart disease, offering the most advanced diagnostic and treatment modalities available in cardiology, cardio thoracic surgery, cardio thoracic transplantation and intensive care, as well as innovation in cardiac research. Physicians provide comprehensive care to 8,000 children each year – fetus through adolescent – who have congenital or acquired heart and lung disorders. For information contact (323) 669-4148.

Center for Endocrinology, Diabetes and Metabolism

The Center for Endocrinology, Diabetes and Metabolism is at the forefront of patient care, basic and clinical research in diabetes, obesity, growth, bone metabolism and endocrinology. More than 2,000 children and adolescents with Type 1 and Type 2 diabetes are under the care of its pediatric diabetes specialists, certified diabetes educators and nutritionists – one of the largest programs of its kind in America. For information contact (323) 669-4604.

Childrens Center for Cancer and Blood Diseases

The Childrens Center for Cancer and Blood Diseases is the nation's largest pediatric hematology/oncology program. Physician- scientists integrate their laboratory experience with their clinical expertise in an approach to medical problem-solving that enables them to move effectively from "Bench to Bedside." Breakthroughs in the treatment of childhood cancer, many pioneered at Childrens Hospital Los Angeles, offer children, teenagers and young adults the most advanced treatment available anywhere. For information contact (323) 669-2121.

Childrens Orthopaedic Center

The Childrens Orthopaedic Center is one of the nation's most comprehensive programs dedicated to pediatric musculoskeletal care, education and research. Its Scoliosis and Spine Disorders Program, one of the largest in the country, is the only one of its kind in Los Angeles County devoted exclusively to the pediatric population. Its state-of-the-art Motion Analysis Laboratory is designed to analyze muscle activity and joint movements in children who have difficulty walking, such as those with cerebral palsy, spina bifida and congenital leg conditions. For information contact (323) 669-2142.

602

Cleveland Clinic

Heart and Vascular Institute

America's Best Heart Center

Cleveland Clinic Heart and Vascular Institute, recognized as an international cardiovascular referral center, is one of the largest and busiest heart programs in the United States. Our physicians are leaders in cardiology, cardiovascular surgery and research into the heart and its diseases. No heart program has more experience, more knowledge and better access to technology. *U.S.News & World Report* has ranked the Cleveland Clinic best in the nation for heart care since 1995.

Patients come to the Cleveland Clinic Heart and Vascular Institute from across the United States and around the world. In 2006, institute physicians recorded 234,000 patient visits, completed more than 10,240 surgical procedures and performed more than 3,500 open heart surgeries. These numbers, and the outcomes resulting from numerous procedures used to treat each case of heart disease, distinguish the Heart and Vascular Institute from other institutions.

Clinical Trials and Research

Our Heart and Vascular Institute is a recognized leader in multicenter and international trials. An outstanding clinical infrastructure and strong commitment to basic science allow Cleveland Clinic to remain on the cutting edge of treatment and research in cardiovascular disease. More than 200 clinical research projects and trials currently are under way here, ranging from basic cellular research to the development of a new artificial heart. Cleveland Clinic researchers have recently made history with their confirmation of a specific gene identified as a cause of human coronary heart disease.

Leading the Battle Against Heart Disease

In many cases, Cleveland Clinic Heart and Vascular Institute patients have access to procedures not available elsewhere, and many techniques now in use around the world were first performed here. As a result of this leadership, Cleveland Clinic specialists have accumulated the world's largest volume of experience in many highly specialized interventions and an unmatched breadth and depth of experience in treating cardiovascular disease.

Cleveland Clinic cardiologists and surgeons treat all conditions affecting the structure and functions of the heart including:

- coronary artery disease (including heart attack)
- valve disease
- abnormal heart rhythms
- heart failure
- congenital heart disease
- hypertrophic cardiomyopathy

History of Innovationsse

Cleveland Clinic doctors made two major breakthroughs that catapulted the world into the modern era of heart care: coronary angiography and saphenous vein bypass surgery.

To schedule an appointment or for more information about the Cleveland Clinic Heart and Vascular Institute call 800.890.2467 or visit www.clevelandclinic.org/hearttopdocs

Heart and Vascular Institute | 9500 Euclid Avenue / W14 | Cleveland OH 44195

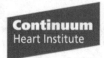

Beth Israel Medical Center
Roosevelt Hospital
St. Luke's Hospital
Long Island College Hospital

Phone (800) 420-4004
www.chpnyc.org

The Continuum Heart Institute combines the strengths of the cardiac programs at Beth Israel Medical Center, Roosevelt Hospital, St. Luke's Hospital and Long Island College Hospital for clinical, technological and innovative excellence. The skill and caliber of its cardiologists, cardiovascular surgeons, and other cardiac specialists is matched only by its state-of-the-art facilities—including the most technologically advanced diagnostic units, catheterization and electrophysiology labs, cardiac surgery suites, and cardiac intensive care units.

The Continuum Heart Institute offers every clinical expertise needed to prevent, diagnose, and treat heart disease, including catheter-based diagnosis and treatment, hypertension diagnosis and treatment, heart failure diagnosis and treatment, leading-edge cardiac surgery, and a hypertrophic cardiomyopathy program. Strong believers in prevention and early detection, the professionals throughout the Continuum Heart Institute also provide complete medical evaluations, echocardiography, nuclear cardiology services, coronary artery disease prevention, treatment centers for obesity and diabetes, smoking cessation programs, and complementary techniques for relaxation and stress reduction, such as massage therapy and therapeutic touch.

Some of the unique features available at the hospitals of the Continuum Heart Institute include a robotic surgical suite for closed-chest coronary artery bypass surgery; a nationally recognized arrhythmia service; and a 64-slice CT scanner used to perform non-invasive cardiac angiograms in less than an hour.

Our cardiac surgery program is recognized by the New York State Department of Health as having one of the lowest mortality rates of any New York City hospital, and is consistently ranked among the best programs in New York State.

CONTINUUM HEART INSTITUTE

The Continuum Heart Institute was established in an effort to bridge the many cardiac care programs of our partner hospitals and provide patients with more streamlined access to our full range of services. This interdisciplinary cardiology, cardiac surgery and cardiac rehabilitation team consists of clinicians, surgeons, nurses and nurse practitioners, physician assistants, social workers, complementary care experts and rehabilitation specialists—all working together to give patients a full range of individualized treatment choices and services.

603

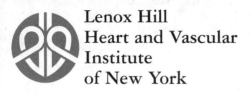

Lenox Hill Heart and Vascular Institute of New York

Lenox Hill Hospital

100 East 77th Street
New York, NY 10021
212-434-4514
www.lenoxhillheartvascular.com

SETTING THE WORLD STANDARD FOR COMPLEX CARDIAC CARE

The Lenox Hill Heart and Vascular Institute is among the leading cardiovascular care programs nationwide. From diagnosis to treatment and recovery, the Institute provides comprehensive care through its distinguished team of cardiologists, interventional cardiologists, electrophysiologists, cardiothoracic and vascular surgeons, and radiologists.

DEPTH OF EXPERIENCE

Lenox Hill Hospital has been a leader in cardiovascular care for decades, developing groundbreaking techniques to minimize heart damage and speed recovery:

1938 -- Lenox Hill Hospital cardiologists performed first angiogram in U.S.

1978 -- First coronary angioplasty in country performed at Lenox Hill Hospital

1991 -- Lenox Hill Hospital doctors implanted first coronary stent in NYC

1994 -- Lenox Hill Hospital surgeons introduced minimally invasive direct coronary artery bypass surgery to nation

2003 -- First FDA approved drug coated stent in the nation was implanted at Lenox Hill Hospital in a procedure our doctors now perform over 3,000 times each year

2004 -- Largest carotid stent program in U.S.

2005 -- Largest minimally invasive hear assist program in tri-state area; second largest nationally

2007 -- Lenox Hill Hospital is five-star rated for coronary interventional procedures and cardiology care by HealthGrades

2007 -- Ranked #15 nationally among top hospitals in Heart and Heart Surgery by U.S. News & World Report

A WIDE RANGE OF TREATMENTS

Physicians at the Institute constantly seek to broaden the understanding of heart and vascular disease and expand the boundaries of care through research and clinical trials. The interventional cardiology team is recognized for leadership in the use of angioplasty to clear clogged arteries. The endovascular specialists are involved in groundbreaking research involving the use of carotid stents to provide lower-risk treatment of arterial blockages without surgery and also perform minimally invasive procedures to treat complex abdominal aneurysms. The Institute's cardiothoracic surgeons are pioneers in "beating heart" surgery, and the use of robotics and minimally invasive procedures including coronary bypass, valve repair, atrial fibrillation surgery, and heart failure surgery. Surgeons specializing in vascular surgery perform surgery on the aorta, and the carotid and lower extremity arteries, including aneurysms. The Institute's electrophysiology specialists perform diagnostic, treatment and curative procedures for abnormal heart rhythms.

2007 was a year of particular distinction for Lenox Hill Hospital. It was ranked #15 nationally in Heart and Heart Surgery by U.S. News & World Report, and was five-star rated for coronary interventional procedures and cardiology care by HealthGrades.

TIME IS MUSCLE

It's a fact. The faster a person is treated for a heart attack, the greater the chances of saving precious heart muscle and making a full recovery. That's why doctors say "time is muscle."

Today, using the most advanced technologies and sophisticated emergency communications from our ambulance directly to our cardiologists, Lenox Hill Hospital doctors have drastically reduced the time it takes for a heart attack patient to get lifesaving treatment. After all, time is muscle – and you know how important that is.

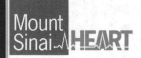

THE MOUNT SINAI MEDICAL CENTER
MOUNT SINAI HEART - CARDIOVASCULAR HEALTH

One Gustave L. Levy Place (Fifth Avenue and 100th Street)
New York, NY 10029-6574
Physician Referral: 1-800-MD-SINAI (637-4624)
www.mountsinai.org

At Mount Sinai Heart, we take a global view of cardiovascular health. Our system of integrated care combines some of the world's most accomplished physicians, research scientists, educators, and professional staff with innovative thinking, creative programs, and an unwavering commitment to the prevention and treatment of cardiovascular disease. With the rapid translation of innovative research concepts into improved preventive, diagnostic, and therapeutic care, patients receive multidisciplinary treatment of unprecedented quality.

In addition to consultative and noninvasive cardiology, cardiac catheterization, heart and lung transplantation, cardiovascular surgery, heart failure, pulmonary hypertension, lipid management, and hypertension, we also specialize in the following areas:

• *Noninvasive diagnostic imaging* - leading techniques for echocardiography, nuclear cardiology, PET, CT, and MRI imaging cardiology;
• *Coronary artery disease* - ranked as the state's safest center for patients undergoing coronary angioplasty and other catheter-based interventions;
• *Cardiac rhythm disturbances* - expert management of all aspects of heart rhythm disorders such as atrial fibrillation and tachycardia, and the insertion of implantable devices including pacemakers and defibrillators;
• *Valvular heart disease* - a wide range of medical and surgical options including a leading program for valve repair and long-term follow-up care;
• *Aortic diseases* - pioneered techniques for stent-graft repair of thoracic and abdominal aortic aneurysms, and for surgical correction of the most complex aortic pathology;
• *Congenital heart disease* - specialists in pediatric cardiology and experts in minimally invasive approaches to the correction of congenital heart defects in children and adults;
• *Cardiac failure and transplantation* - a multidisciplinary team approach to comprehensive, compassionate care for the most advanced forms of heart failure and cardiomyopathy patients;
• *Comprehensive cardiac disease prevention and rehabilitation* - a unique synergism that provides unparalleled patient care, while yielding breakthroughs in the prevention and treatment of cardiovascular disease;
• *Vascular medicine and surgery* - noninvasive diagnostic procedures and an interdisciplinary approach to disease management, from medical, surgical, catheter-based, and gene therapy techniques to arterial obstruction, limb salvage, venous, and lymphatic diseases.

Mount Sinai's Cardiac Catheterization Laboratories offer leading-edge technologies of all kinds, including diagnostic angiography, angioplasty, and biopsy. We study the heart with the greatest precision available. We are pioneering new genetic techniques to help hearts with diseased arteries grow new vessels, and to help a damaged heart muscle repair itself.

MOUNT SINAI HEART

Under the creative direction of internationally renowned cardiologist Valentin Fuster, MD, PhD, Mount Sinai is recognized worldwide for its expertise in evaluating, managing, and preventing cardiovascular disease through the integration of patient care, education, and research. Mount Sinai Heart encompasses The Zena and Michael A. Wiener Cardiovascular Institute and the Marie-Josée and Henry R. Kravis Center for Cardiovascular Health at The Mount Sinai Medical Center, preeminent resources for the study and treatment of heart and blood vessel diseases. Following are some of the cardiac conditions we treat at Mount Sinai Heart: arrhythmia (including atrial fibrillation, pacemakers, defibrillators and other implanted devices), coronary artery disease, heart attack and angina, heart failure and transplantation, hyperlipidemia (cholesterol), hypertension, mitral valve prolapse, myocarditis, pericardial disease, peripheral vascular disease and claudication, pulmonary hypertension, and valvular heart disease.

621

NewYork-Presbyterian

⌐ The University Hospital of Columbia and Cornell
NewYork-Presbyterian Heart

Affiliated with Columbia University College of Physicians and Surgeons and Weill Medical College of Cornell University

NewYork-Presbyterian Hospital
Columbia University Medical Center
622 West 168th Street
New York, NY 10032

NewYork-Presbyterian Hospital
Weill Cornell Medical Center
525 East 68th Street
New York, NY 10021

OVERVIEW:

The NewYork-Presbyterian Heart has a reputation for treating some of the highest risk cases in the world – healing those patients who cannot be helped anywhere else. We are committed to delivering the finest possible care to adult and pediatric patients by:

- combining the finest minds and cutting-edge technology with the most compassionate care

- helping patients make sense of the complex steps involved in treating their heart condition;

- providing them with a full set of appropriate treatment options for consideration after a complete diagnosis;

- listening, guiding and fully informing patients so that together we can confidently choose the best treatment.

The NewYork-Presbyterian Heart has:

- A well-deserved reputation for clinical excellence – the only heart center in the New York area ranked among the nation's best by *U.S. News & World Report*;

- World-renowned expertise in all areas of cardiac care, including transplantation, open-heart surgery, arrhythmia control, left ventricular assist devices (LVAD) and robotics;

- One of the country's largest and most successful pediatric cardiology, cardiology interventional and cardiac surgery programs.

- The latest heart-imaging technology, including such innovative tools as advanced digital equipment for stress echocardiography SPECT, state-of-the-art MRI, intravascular/intracoronary ultrasound, electrophysiologic studies, nuclear scanning and an outstanding cardiac catheterization laboratory;

- A state-of-the-art Interventional Cardiology Center to diagnose and treat heart disease without surgery, on an inpatient or outpatient basis, including: angioplasty, balloon valvuloplasty, stenting, and intracoronary radiation for restenosis.

Physician Referral: For a physician referral or to learn more about the NewYork-Presbyterian Heart call toll free **1-877-NYP-WELL** (1-877-697-9355) visit our website at **www.nypheart.org**

HIGHLIGHTS INCLUDE:

- Performed more heart transplants than any other hospital in the world over the last two decades.

- First Robotics-Assisted Coronary Artery Bypass Surgery in the U.S.

- One of the principal investigators (12 institutions throughout the United States) involved in ongoing FDA clinical trials to explore the use and effectiveness of robotics in cardiac surgery.

- Lead medical center in a three-year landmark study of 129 patients – REMATCH (Randomized Evaluation of Mechanical Assistance for the Treatment of Congestive Heart Failure) — which found that implanted heart pumps can extend and improve the quality of life of terminally ill heart failure patients.

- Participating in FDA-approved randomized clinical trial to evaluate use of drug-coated stents versus regular stents on incidence of reoccurrence of renarrowing inside stent.

NYU Cardiac & Vascular Institute
550 First Avenue (at 31st Street)
New York, NY 10016
Physician Referral:
1-877-4-NYU-CVI

Collaboration with the NYU Cardiac & Vascular Institute brings care full circle.

The skilled, world-class heart and vascular specialists at the NYU Cardiac & Vascular Institute (CVI) never take any patient with cardiovascular disease for granted. Each case is unique. The philosophy has made the NYU CVI a leader in developing new techniques for repairnig heart valves, curing heart rhythem disorders, treating aortic disease and developing care plans for congestive heart failure. Our cardiac and vascular physicians work collaboratively with the cardiac rehabilitation team to move patients seamlessly from treatment into the recovery and maintenance phase of their care. Other programs such as weight management, smoking cesstion and diabetic management focus on prevention. It is total patient experience at NYU that has resulted in so many successes for patients of all ages with cardiovascular hear disease.

Cardiology
NYU's Division of Cardiology is a world-renowned leader in cardiovascular biomedical research. patient care and education, with a long-standing tradition of educating and training some of the brightest and most promising physicians and researchers of the future. Members of the Division of Cardiology are devoted to providing evidence-based, state-of-the-art, compassionate healthcare. Our clinicians and researchers are advancing the field of cardiovascular medicine, and contribute to the reputation of NYU as comprehensive cardiovascular center of excellence.

Cardiac Surgery
NYU's Cardiac surgeons are internationally recognized for pioneering mitral valve repair and minimally invasive cardiac surgery. Our team has performed more than 3,000 minimally invasive valve repairs and replacements, changing the standard of care fore heart surgery and dramatically improving results. NYU's surgeons are widely known for expert care of elderly and high-risk patients, using new technology and less invasive techniques to improve results and lower risks. This expertise is shared with other surgeons from around the world, who come to NYU to study with the cardiac surgical team.

Vascular Surgery
With decades of expertise treating thousands of patients with conditions ranging from life-threatening issues of arterial aneurysms to deep vein thrombosis, as well as carotid stenosis and limb salvage, the Division of Vascular and Endovascular Surgery offers expert patient care with emphasis on minimally invasive diagnostic and treatment approaches. Traditionally cosmetic procedures such as treatment of varicose and spider veins, are performed at the NYU Vein Center with comprehensive, medical approach. Our vascular surgeons are part of the teaching team for NYU School of Medicine and are training the next generation of physicians through a top vascular surgery fellowship program. The Division also holds training courses in minimally invasive vein surgery, endovascular aortic surgery, thoracic aneurysm correction, and abdominal aneurysm interventions for practicing surgeons throughout the world.

Cardiac Catheterization Lab
At the leading edge of interventional cardiology, the Cardiac Cathterterization Lab at NYU continues to set the standard for catheter-based diagnosis and evaluation of cardiac health. Located at Tisch Hospital, the Cath Lab provides a full range of procedures to evaluate how well the heart muscle and valves are working; to detect and measure any narrowing in the coronary arteries; and to recommend appropriate treatment as needed. Our lab is defined by its comprehensive, evidence-based approach to the care of each individual patient.

Electrophysiology—Heart Rhythm Center
With years of research and experience in the causes and treatment of the cardiac arrhythmias, NYU's heart rhythm specialists are nationally recognized leaders who have had great success treating people with a broad range of heart rhythm disorders. Our electrophysiologists care for patients with pacemakers, implantable cardioverter defibrillators and cardiac resynchronization devices.The Heart Rhythm Center is on of the leading programs in the world for treatment of atrial fibillation. The depth and breadth of expertise and expericen in heart rhythm testing and treatment are the reasons why the NYU Heart Rhythm Center has become so widely respected.

Cardiac Rehabilitation Center
Rehabilitation is a necessity for the cardiac patients who have undergone heart procedures. With distinguishes cardiac rehab at NYU Medical Center is its individualized patient care. At the Cardiac Rehab Center, physical rehavilitation takes place in a state-of-the-art facility, where patients work on building both aerobic capacity and strength. Our Cardiac Rehab team works closely with cardiologists, physiatrists, nurses, physical and occupational therapists, psychologists, social workers, exercise physiologists, nutritionists and other healthcare professionals to help patients return, rehabilitated, to their everyday lives.

A Leader in Cardiac Care

St. Francis Hospital, The Heart Center® is New York State's only specialty designated cardiac center and is the busiest heart center in the Northeast. Located in Roslyn, New York, on Long Island's North Shore, St. Francis Hospital has been ranked among the best hospitals in the nation by *U.S. News & World Report* and *Modern Maturity*, and most recently was ranked the best hospital on Long Island for cardiac care by *New York Magazine.*

St. Francis:

• Performs more open-heart surgeries and cardiac interventional procedures than any other hospital in New York State Maintains the highest level of quality of care – according to *New York Magazine,* the hospital has more "Best Doctors" for cardiac care than any other hospital on Long Island
• Offers innovative approaches to cardiac surgery, including minimally-invasive procedures and off-pump coronary artery bypass surgery, designed to minimize trauma and reduce surgical complications
• Performs one of the region's highest volumes of catheter-based techniques to close atrial septal defects (ASDs) and patent foramen ovale (PFO)
• Operates a nationally recognized Arrhythmia and Pacemaker Center staffed with electrophysiologists with extensive experience in radiofrequency ablation, a permanent cure for certain arrhythmias, including atrial fibrillation
• Maintains a high volume center for the implantation of cardiac pacemakers and defibrillators
• Continues leadership in noninvasive imaging, including cardiac MRI, three-dimensional echocardiography, and CT scanning, and was the first Long Island hospital to offer state-of-the-art 64-slice CT scanning for coronary imaging and other applications

St. Francis Hospital has near-perfect patient satisfaction ratings, with over 99 percent of patients saying they would recommend the hospital to family and friends.

"Our large cardiac caseload and our growing research program put us in an excellent position to introduce new techniques that can benefit thousands of people in need each year."
-- Alan D. Guerci, M.D., President and Chief Executive Officer St. Francis Hospital, The Heart Center®

726

PENN CARDIAC CARE

Penn Cardiac Care is comprised of a multidisciplinary team of cardiologists, cardiovascular surgeons, anesthesiologists, and specially trained nurses and technologists, who are experts in preventing, diagnosing and treating a variety of routine and complex conditions related to the heart, including but not limited to:

- Blocked heart arteries (coronary artery disease)
- Congenital heart defects
- Heart failure
- Heart palpitations
- High blood pressure
- High cholesterol
- Valve disease
- Vascular disease

World-Class Heart Care

Penn is recognized as one of the nation's leading heart programs with expertise in heart failure and transplantation, thoracic aortic surgery, mitral valve repair and replacement, endovascular stent graft repair, cardiac electrophysioiogy, interventional cardiology, preventive cardiology and lipid management. Penn is among the nation's top 10 heart transplant centers, performing more than 650 transplants since its opening in 1987.

State-Of-The-Art Technology And Research

- A leader in medicine for more than 230 years, Penn is a pioneer of research, utilizing the latest technologies to ensure the best care for patients.
- Developing progressive medical and surgical technologies, many of which are not available elsewhere and enable patients to avoid surgery.
- Pioneering the most advanced techniques and devices, such as ablation therapy for ventricular tachycardia and atrial fibrillation.
- Offering a full-range of surgical options including minimally invasive robotic, off-pump, port access, and bloodless techniques.

- Conducting numerous medical and surgical clinical studies, such as robotic surgery and mechanical assist devices, percutaneous approaches to treating valvular and structural heart disease and new immunosuppressive therapies.
- Serving as the lead national site for several trials, including endovascular stent graft repair for thoracic aortic aneurysms, being conducted in collaboration with Penn vascular surgeons.
- Performing innovative surgical procedures, such as the temporary total artificial heart, the first transplant of its kind in the North East region.

Regional Referral Center

The Heart Failure and Transplantation Program at Penn provides comprehensive care for patients with heart failure, offering more treatment options than ever before.

Cutting-edge therapy for heart failure includes:
- Drug therapy
- Pacemakers
- Implantable cardioverter defibrillators (ICDs)
- Ablative therapy
- Coronary artery bypass grafting (CABG)
- Heart valve repair or replacement
- Ventricular assist devices (VADs)
- Heart transplantation, including the temporary total artificial heart

In 2006, the Heart Failure and Transplantation Program at the Hospital of the University of Pennsylvania (HUP) performed the largest number of heart transplant procedures in the region.

The Penn Thoracic Aortic Surgery Program is the first comprehensive program of its kind in the region to treat thoracic aortic diseases, including aneurysms and dissections.

Nationally Recognized Expertise

Penn's doctors have been recognized for excellence in cardiology and cardiothoracic services:
- Hospital of the University of Pennsylvania and Pennsylvania Hospital are consistently recognized among the nation's best hospitals for heart care in *U.S.News & World Report*.
- Solucient, Inc. named Penn Presbyterian Medical Center among its *"100 Top Hospitals"* for excellence in heart care for the fifth year in a row.
- *Philadelphia* magazine named the Hospital of the University of Pennsylvania and Penn Presbyterian as centers of excellence for heart care and other specialties.
- *Best Doctors in America®* lists more doctors from the University of Pennsylvania Health System than any other health system in the Philadelphia region.
- The Hospital of the University of Pennsylvania and Penn Presbyterian are recognized by Independence Blue Cross as *"Centers of Blue Distinction"* for excellence in quality standards and patient care.

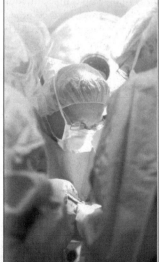

Child Neurology

a subspecialty of Neurology

A neurologist specializes in the diagnosis and treatment of all types of disease or impaired function of the brain, spinal cord, peripheral nerves, muscles and autonomic nervous system, as well as the blood vessels that relate to these structures. A child neurologist has special skills in the diagnosis and management of neurologic disorders of the neonatal period, infancy, early childhood and adolescence.

Training Required: Four years

Child Neurology

Darras, Basil T MD [ChiN] - **Spec Exp:** Neuromuscular Disorders; Cerebral Palsy; **Hospital:** Children's Hospital - Boston; **Address:** 300 Longwood Ave, Childrens Hosp, Neurology, Fegan II, Boston, MA 02115; **Phone:** 617-355-8235; **Board Cert:** Pediatrics 1988; Child Neurology 1992; Clinical Genetics 1987; **Med School:** Greece 1977; **Resid:** Pediatrics, Nassau County Med Ctr 1982; Child Neurology, Tufts-New England Med Ctr 1985; **Fellow:** Clinical Genetics, Yale Univ Sch Med 1988; **Fac Appt:** Prof N, Harvard Med Sch

Holmes, Gregory L MD [ChiN] - **Spec Exp:** Epilepsy/Seizure Disorders; Neurologic Disorders; **Hospital:** Dartmouth - Hitchcock Med Ctr; **Address:** Dartmouth-Hitchcock Med Ctr, Dept Neurology, 1 Medical Center Drive, Lebanon, NH 03756; **Phone:** 603-650-8586; **Board Cert:** Pediatrics 1979; Neurology 1980; **Med School:** Univ VA Sch Med 1974; **Resid:** Pediatrics, Yale-New Haven Hosp 1976; **Fellow:** Pediatric Neurology, Univ Va 1979; **Fac Appt:** Prof N, Dartmouth Med Sch

Mandelbaum, David E MD/PhD [ChiN] - **Spec Exp:** Epilepsy/Seizure Disorders; Brain Tumors-Pediatric; Neonatal Neurology; Autism; **Hospital:** Rhode Island Hosp, Women & Infants Hosp - Rhode Island; **Address:** Dept of Neurology, 110 Lockwood St, Ste 342, Providence, RI 02903; **Phone:** 401-444-4345; **Board Cert:** Neurology 1987; Pediatrics 1987; Clinical Neurophysiology 2003; Neurodevelopmental Disabilities 2001; **Med School:** Columbia P&S 1980; **Resid:** Pediatrics, Yale-New Haven Hosp 1982; Neurology, Neuro Inst-Columbia 1983; **Fellow:** Child Neurology, Neuro Inst-Columbia 1985; **Fac Appt:** Prof Ped, Brown Univ

Novotny, Edward MD [ChiN] - **Spec Exp:** Epilepsy/Seizure Disorders; Neurologic Imaging; Neurophysiology-Pediatric; **Hospital:** Yale - New Haven Hosp; **Address:** Dept of Pediatrics, Yale Sch of Med, P.O. Box 208064, New Haven, CT 06520-8064; **Phone:** 203-785-5730; **Board Cert:** Pediatrics 1986; Child Neurology 1986; Clinical Neurophysiology 2004; **Med School:** St Louis Univ 1979; **Resid:** Pediatrics, Univ CA Daivs Med Ctr 1981; Neurology, Stanford Univ Med Ctr 1984; **Fellow:** Epilepsy, Stanford Univ Med Ctr 1986; Magnetic Resonance Imaging, Yale Univ 1989; **Fac Appt:** Assoc Prof Ped, Yale Univ

Pomeroy, Scott L MD/PhD [ChiN] - **Spec Exp:** Neuro-Oncology; Brain Tumors; **Hospital:** Children's Hospital - Boston, Dana-Farber Cancer Inst; **Address:** Chldns Hosp, Dept Neurology-Fegan 11, 300 Longwood Ave, Boston, MA 02115; **Phone:** 617-355-6386; **Board Cert:** Pediatrics 2003; Child Neurology 1988; **Med School:** Univ Conn 1982; **Resid:** Pediatrics, Chldns Hosp 1984; Neurology, Barnes Hosp/Washington Univ 1985; **Fellow:** Pediatric Neurology, St Louis Chldns Hosp 1987; Neurological Biology, Washington Univ 1989; **Fac Appt:** Prof N, Harvard Med Sch

Riviello Jr, James J MD [ChiN] - **Spec Exp:** Epilepsy/Seizure Disorders; Epilepsy in Tuberous Sclerosis; **Hospital:** Children's Hospital - Boston; **Address:** Children's Hosp Boston, Dept Neurology, 300 Longwood Ave, Fegan 9, Boston, MA 02115; **Phone:** 617-355-2443; **Board Cert:** Pediatrics 1984; Child Neurology 1985; Clinical Neurophysiology 1996; **Med School:** Tulane Univ 1978; **Resid:** Pediatrics, St Christopher Hosp Chldn 1981; Neurology, Temple Univ Hosp 1982; **Fellow:** Pediatric Neurology, St Christopher Hosp Chldn 1983; **Fac Appt:** Prof N, Harvard Med Sch

Shaywitz, Bennett A MD [ChiN] - **Spec Exp:** Learning Disorders; Dyslexia; Headache; **Hospital:** Yale - New Haven Hosp; **Address:** Yale Univ Sch Med, Dept Peds, 333 Cedar St, Box 208064, New Haven, CT 06520-8064; **Phone:** 203-785-4641; **Board Cert:** Pediatrics 1968; Child Neurology 1973; **Med School:** Washington Univ, St Louis 1963; **Resid:** Pediatrics, Bronx Muni Hosp Ctr 1967; **Fellow:** Child Neurology, Albert Einstein Coll Med 1970; **Fac Appt:** Prof Ped, Yale Univ

Volpe, Joseph J MD [ChiN] - **Spec Exp:** Neonatal Neurology; Cerebral Palsy; **Hospital:** Children's Hospital - Boston, Mass Genl Hosp; **Address:** 300 Longwood Ave, Fegan 11, Boston, MA 02115-5724; **Phone:** 617-355-6388; **Board Cert:** Pediatrics 1970; Child Neurology 1974; **Med School:** Harvard Med Sch 1964; **Resid:** Pediatrics, Mass Genl Hosp 1966; Neurology, Mass Genl Hosp 1971; **Fellow:** Research, Natl Inst Child Hlth Human Dev 1968; **Fac Appt:** Prof N, Harvard Med Sch

Mid Atlantic

Allen, Jeffrey MD [ChiN] - **Spec Exp:** Neuro-Oncology; Brain Tumors; **Hospital:** NYU Med Ctr (page 67), St Luke's - Roosevelt Hosp Ctr - Roosevelt Div; **Address:** Hassenfeld Childrens Ctr, 160 E 32nd St, New York, NY 10016; **Phone:** 212-263-6725; **Board Cert:** Child Neurology 1977; **Med School:** Harvard Med Sch 1969; **Resid:** Pediatrics, Montreal Chldns Hosp 1973; Pediatric Neurology, Montreal Neur Inst/McGill 1976; **Fac Appt:** Prof Ped, NYU Sch Med

Aron, Alan MD [ChiN] - **Spec Exp:** Neurofibromatosis; Movement Disorders; Developmental Delay; **Hospital:** Mount Sinai Med Ctr; **Address:** Mt Sinai Hosp, Child Neurology, 5 E 98th St, Box 1206, New York, NY 10029; **Phone:** 212-831-4393; **Board Cert:** Pediatrics 1963; Neurology 1967; Child Neurology 1969; **Med School:** Columbia P&S 1958; **Resid:** Pediatrics, Babies Hosp-Columbia-Presby Hosp 1961; **Fellow:** Pediatric Neurology, Babies Hosp-Columbia Presby Hosp 1964; **Fac Appt:** Prof N, Mount Sinai Sch Med

Chutorian, Abraham MD [ChiN] - **Spec Exp:** Autoimmune Disease; Movement Disorders; Headache; Migraine; **Hospital:** NY-Presby Hosp/Weill Cornell (page 66), Hosp For Special Surgery (page 60); **Address:** 654 Madison Ave, New York, NY 10021; **Phone:** 212-750-2800; **Board Cert:** Pediatrics 1962; Neurology 1964; Child Neurology 1968; **Med School:** Univ Manitoba 1957; **Resid:** Pediatrics, Chldns Hosp 1960; **Fellow:** Neurology, Columbia-Presby Med Ctr 1963; **Fac Appt:** Prof N, Cornell Univ-Weill Med Coll

Crawford, Thomas O MD [ChiN] - **Spec Exp:** Neuromuscular Disorders; Muscular Dystrophy; Ataxia Telangiectasia; **Hospital:** Johns Hopkins Hosp - Baltimore (page 61); **Address:** Pediatric Neurology, 200 N Wolfe St, Ste 2158, Baltimore, MD 21287; **Phone:** 410-955-4259; **Board Cert:** Pediatrics 1986; Child Neurology 1990; Clinical Neurophysiology 1997; **Med School:** USC Sch Med 1980; **Resid:** Pediatrics, LAC-USC Med Ctr 1984; Child Neurology, Childrens Hosp 1987; **Fellow:** Neuromuscular Disease, Johns Hopkins Hosp 1988; **Fac Appt:** Assoc Prof N, Johns Hopkins Univ

De Vivo, Darryl C MD [ChiN] - **Spec Exp:** Metabolic Disorders; Neuromuscular Disorders; Spinal Muscular Atrophy (SMA); **Hospital:** NY-Presby Hosp/Columbia (page 66); **Address:** Neurological Institute, 710 W 168th St, rm 201, New York, NY 10032; **Phone:** 212-305-5244; **Board Cert:** Child Neurology 1972; **Med School:** Univ VA Sch Med 1964; **Resid:** Pediatrics, Mass Genl Hosp 1966; Neurology, Mass Genl Hosp 1967; **Fellow:** Neurology, Natl Inst Hlth 1969; Child Neurology, Children's Hosp 1970; **Fac Appt:** Prof N, Columbia P&S

Child Neurology

Duffner, Patricia K MD [ChiN] - **Spec Exp:** Brain Tumors; Krabbe Disease; Cancer Survivors-Late Effects of Therapy; **Hospital:** Women's & Chldn's Hosp of Buffalo, The; **Address:** Women & Chlds Hosp, Dept Neurology, 219 Bryant St, Buffalo, NY 14222-2006; **Phone:** 716-878-7819; **Board Cert:** Pediatrics 1977; Child Neurology 1979; **Med School:** SUNY Buffalo 1972; **Resid:** Pediatrics, Buffalo Chldns Hosp 1975; **Fellow:** Child Neurology, SUNY Buffalo-Buffalo Chldns Hosp 1978; **Fac Appt:** Prof N, SUNY Buffalo

Eviatar, Lydia MD [ChiN] - **Spec Exp:** Headache; Balance Disorders; Tourette's Syndrome; Cerebral Palsy; **Hospital:** Schneider Chldn's Hosp, Blythedale Children's Hosp; **Address:** 269-01 76th Ave, rm 267, New Hyde Park, NY 11040-1433; **Phone:** 718-470-3450; **Board Cert:** Pediatrics 1968; Child Neurology 1977; **Med School:** Israel 1961; **Resid:** Pediatrics, Tel Hashomer Hosp 1966; **Fellow:** Child Neurology, UCLA Med Ctr 1967; Neurology, UCLA Med Ctr 1969; **Fac Appt:** Prof N, Albert Einstein Coll Med

Maytal, Joseph MD [ChiN] - **Spec Exp:** Epilepsy/Seizure Disorders; Migraine; **Hospital:** Schneider Chldn's Hosp; **Address:** 269-01 76th Ave Fl 2nd - rm 267, New Hyde Park, NY 11040-1434; **Phone:** 718-470-3450; **Board Cert:** Pediatrics 1986; Child Neurology 1988; **Med School:** Israel 1978; **Resid:** Pediatrics, Brookdale Hosp 1983; Child Neurology, Montefiore Med Ctr 1986; **Fellow:** Neurological Physiology, Albert Einstein Med Coll 1987; **Fac Appt:** Clin Prof N, Albert Einstein Coll Med

Packer, Roger MD [ChiN] - **Spec Exp:** Brain Tumors; Neurofibromatosis; **Hospital:** Chldns Natl Med Ctr; **Address:** Childrens Natl Med Ctr, Dept Neurology, 111 Michigan Ave NW, Washington, DC 20010-2978; **Phone:** 202-884-2120; **Board Cert:** Child Neurology 1982; Pediatrics 1982; **Med School:** Northwestern Univ 1976; **Resid:** Pediatrics, Chldns Med Ctr 1978; Neurology, Chldns Hosp-Univ Penn 1981; **Fac Appt:** Prof N, Geo Wash Univ

Phillips, Peter C MD [ChiN] - **Spec Exp:** Brain Tumors; Neuro-Oncology; **Hospital:** Chldns Hosp of Philadelphia, The; **Address:** Childrens Hosp Philadelphia, 34th St & Civic Center Blvd, Philadelphia, PA 19104; **Phone:** 215-590-3015; **Board Cert:** Pediatrics 1985; Child Neurology 1986; **Med School:** Univ Conn 1978; **Resid:** Pediatrics, Chldns Hosp 1980; Pediatric Neurology, Neuro Inst 1983; **Fellow:** Neuro-Oncology, Meml Sloan Kettering Hosp 1986; **Fac Appt:** Prof N, Univ Pennsylvania

Southeast

Fenichel, Gerald M MD [ChiN] - **Spec Exp:** Neuromuscular Disorders; Muscular Dystrophy; **Hospital:** Vanderbilt Univ Med Ctr; **Address:** Vanderbilt Childrens Hosp, Dept Neurology, 2200 Childrens Way, DOT, rm 11244, Nashville, TN 37232-9559; **Phone:** 615-936-2024; **Board Cert:** Neurology 1966; Child Neurology 1968; **Med School:** Yale Univ 1959; **Resid:** Neurology, Natl Inst Neuro Disorders-NIH 1963; Neurology, Yale-New Haven Hosp 1964; **Fac Appt:** Prof N, Vanderbilt Univ

Greenwood, Robert S MD [ChiN] - **Spec Exp:** Neurofibromatosis; Epilepsy; **Hospital:** Univ NC Hosps; **Address:** UNC - Dept Neurology, 3114 Bioinformatics Bldg - CB 7025, Chapel Hill, NC 27599; **Phone:** 919-966-2528; **Board Cert:** Pediatrics 1974; Child Neurology 1979; **Med School:** Univ Tex Med Br, Galveston 1968; **Resid:** Pediatrics, Chldns Hosp 1971; Child Neurology, Chldns Hosp 1975; **Fellow:** Child Neurology, Chldns Hosp 1977; **Fac Appt:** Prof N, Univ NC Sch Med

Turk, William MD [ChiN] - **Spec Exp:** Epilepsy/Seizure Disorders; Headache; Movement Disorders; **Hospital:** Wolfson Chldns Hosp; **Address:** Nemors Children's Clinic, 807 Children's Way, Jacksonville, FL 32207; **Phone:** 904-390-3665; **Board Cert:** Pediatrics 1981; Child Neurology 1984; Clinical Neurophysiology 1997; **Med School:** Case West Res Univ 1976; **Resid:** Pediatrics, NC Meml Hosp 1979; Neurology, Barnes Hospital 1980; **Fellow:** Child Neurology, St Louis Chldns Hosp 1983; **Fac Appt:** Asst Prof N, Mayo Med Sch

Wheless, James W MD [ChiN] - **Spec Exp:** Epilepsy/Seizure Disorders; **Hospital:** Le Bonheur Chldns Med Ctr, St Jude Children's Research Hosp; **Address:** 777 Washington Ave, Ste 240, Memphis, TN 38105; **Phone:** 901-287-5060; **Board Cert:** Pediatrics 1987; Child Neurology 1989; **Med School:** Univ Okla Coll Med 1982; **Resid:** Pediatrics, Univ Oklahoma Med Ctr 1985; **Fellow:** Pediatric Neurology, Children's Meml Hosp 1988; Epilepsy, Med Coll Georgia 1989; **Fac Appt:** Prof N, Univ Tenn Coll Med, Memphis

Midwest

Brunstrom, Janice E MD [ChiN] - **Spec Exp:** Cerebral Palsy; **Hospital:** St Louis Chldns Hosp; **Address:** Washington Univ Sch Med, Dept Ped Neuro, 660 S Euclid Ave, Box 8111, St Louis, MO 63110; **Phone:** 314-454-6120; **Board Cert:** Pediatrics 1992; Child Neurology 1994; **Med School:** Med Coll VA 1987; **Resid:** Neurology, St Louis Chldns Hosp 1989; Neurology, Barnes Jewish Hosp 1990; **Fellow:** Child Neurology, St Louis Chldns Hosp 1995; **Fac Appt:** Asst Prof N, Washington Univ, St Louis

Charnas, Lawrence R MD/PhD [ChiN] - **Spec Exp:** Pediatric Neurology; Genetic Disorders-Nervous System; Neurofibromatosis; **Hospital:** Univ Minn Med Ctr, Fairview - Univ Campus; **Address:** Pediatric Clinical Neuroscience, 420 Delaware St, SE, MMC 486, Minneapolis, MN 55455; **Phone:** 612-625-7466; **Board Cert:** Neurology 1986; Clinical Genetics 1990; Clinical Biochemical Genetics 1990; Child Neurology 1999; **Med School:** Univ Pennsylvania 1981; **Resid:** Neurology, Johns Hopkins Hosp 1985; **Fellow:** Genetics, NIH 1989; Child Neurology, Univ Minn Hosps & Clinics 1998; **Fac Appt:** Assoc Prof N, Univ Minn

Edgar, Terence MD [ChiN] - **Spec Exp:** Neuromuscular Disorders; Cerebral Palsy; Epilepsy; **Hospital:** St Vincent Hosp - Green Bay, Aurora Sinai Med Ctr; **Address:** Prevea Clin-Van Buren, Ped Neur, 835 S Van Buren St, Fl 2, P.O. Box 19070, Green Bay, WI 54307-9070; **Phone:** 920-272-1288; **Board Cert:** Pediatrics 2003; Child Neurology 1997; **Med School:** South Africa 1984; **Resid:** Pediatrics, Univ Wisconsin Hosp & Clin 1995; **Fellow:** Pediatrics, Univ Wisconsin Hosp & Clin 1993; Child Neurology, Univ Wisconsin Hosp & Clin 1996; **Fac Appt:** Assoc Prof N, Univ Wisc

Epstein, Leon G MD [ChiN] - **Spec Exp:** AIDS/HIV; **Hospital:** Children's Mem Hosp; **Address:** Chldns Meml Hosp, Div Neurology, 2300 Childrens Plaza, Box 51, Chicago, IL 60614; **Phone:** 773-880-4352; **Board Cert:** Child Neurology 1979; **Med School:** Wayne State Univ 1973; **Resid:** Neurology, St Josephs Mercy Hosp 1974; Neurology, Univ Arizona Med Ctr 1976; **Fellow:** Neurology, Columbia Presby Med Ctr 1978; **Fac Appt:** Prof Ped, Northwestern Univ

Kotagal, Suresh MD [ChiN] - **Spec Exp:** Sleep Disorders/Apnea; **Hospital:** Mayo Med Ctr & Clin - Rochester, St Mary's Hosp - Rochester; **Address:** Mayo Clinic, 200 First St SW, Rochester, MN 55905-0002; **Phone:** 507-266-0774; **Board Cert:** Pediatrics 1979; Child Neurology 1982; **Med School:** India 1974; **Resid:** Child Neurology, Chldns Hosp Mich 1976; Pediatrics, St Louis Univ 1979; **Fellow:** Sleep Medicine, Stanford Univ 1982; **Fac Appt:** Prof N, Mayo Med Sch

Kovnar, Edward H MD [ChiN] - **Spec Exp:** Epilepsy/Seizure Disorders; Neurophysiology; Developmental Disorders; **Hospital:** Chldns Hosp - Wisconsin; **Address:** Advanced Healthcare, SC, 3003 W Good Hope Rd, Milwaukee, WI 53209-0996; **Phone:** 414-352-8828; **Board Cert:** Pediatrics 1984; Child Neurology 1984; Neurodevelopmental Disabilities 2005; **Med School:** Washington Univ, St Louis 1977; **Resid:** Pediatrics, Chldns Hosp 1979; Neurology, Barnes Hosp 1980; **Fellow:** Pediatric Neurology, Chldns Hosp 1982; Clinical Neurophysiology, Chldns Hosp 1991

Noetzel, Michael MD [ChiN] - **Spec Exp:** Cerebral Palsy; Brain Injury; Movement Disorders; **Hospital:** St Louis Chldns Hosp; **Address:** 660 S Euclid Ave, Box 8111, St Louis, MO 63110; **Phone:** 314-454-6120; **Board Cert:** Child Neurology 1984; Pediatrics 1984; **Med School:** Univ VA Sch Med 1977; **Resid:** Pediatrics, St Louis Chldns Hosp 1979; Neurology, Barnes Hosp 1980; **Fellow:** Child Neurology, St Louis Chldns Hosp 1982; **Fac Appt:** Prof Ped, Washington Univ, St Louis

Nordli Jr, Douglas R MD [ChiN] - **Spec Exp:** Epilepsy; Rasmussen's Syndrome; **Hospital:** Children's Mem Hosp; **Address:** Children's Memorial Hospital, Epilepsy Ctr, 2300 Children's Plaza, Box 29, Chicago, IL 60614-3394; **Phone:** 773-883-6159; **Board Cert:** Child Neurology 1990; Clinical Neurophysiology 1997; **Med School:** Columbia P&S 1984; **Resid:** Pediatrics, Babies Hosp 1986; Child Neurology, Neuro Inst/Columbia-Presby Med Ctr 1989; **Fellow:** Clinical Neurophysiology, Neuro Inst/Columbia-Presby Med Ctr 1990; **Fac Appt:** Assoc Prof N, Northwestern Univ

Patterson, Marc MD [ChiN] - **Spec Exp:** Neurogenetics; Developmental Delay; Metabolic Disorders; **Hospital:** Mayo Med Ctr & Clin - Rochester; **Address:** Mayo Clinic, Dept Neurology, 200 First St SW, Rochester, MN 55905; **Phone:** 507-284-9974; **Board Cert:** Child Neurology 2004; Neurodevelopmental Disabilities 2001; **Med School:** Australia 1981; **Resid:** Neurology, Univ Queenland 1988; Child Neurology, Mayo Clinic 1990; **Fellow:** Metabolic Neurology, Natl Inst Health 1992; Pediatrics, Mayo Cilnic 1993; **Fac Appt:** Prof N, Mayo Med Sch

Prensky, Arthur MD [ChiN] - **Spec Exp:** Headache; **Hospital:** St Louis Chldns Hosp; **Address:** Dept of Ped Neurology, Washington Univ Sch of Medicine, 660 S Euclid Ave, Campus Box 8111, St Louis, MO 63110-1093; **Phone:** 314-454-6120; **Board Cert:** Neurology 1966; Child Neurology 1969; **Med School:** NYU Sch Med 1955; **Resid:** Neurology, Mass Genl Hosp 1963; **Fellow:** Neurology, Mass Genl Hosp 1966; **Fac Appt:** Prof N, Washington Univ, St Louis

Wiznitzer, Max MD [ChiN] - **Hospital:** Rainbow Babies & Chldns Hosp; **Address:** Rainbow Babies & Chldns Hosp, 11100 Euclid Ave, rm 585, MS RBC6090, Cleveland, OH 44106; **Phone:** 216-844-3691; **Board Cert:** Pediatrics 1982; Child Neurology 1986; **Med School:** Northwestern Univ 1977; **Resid:** Pediatrics, Chldns Hosp Med Ctr 1980; **Fellow:** Developmental-Behavioral Pediatrics, Cincinnati Med Ctr 1981; Pediatric Neurology, Chldns Hosp 1984; **Fac Appt:** Assoc Prof Ped, Case West Res Univ

Wyllie, Elaine MD [ChiN] - **Spec Exp:** Epilepsy/Seizure Disorders; **Hospital:** Cleveland Clin Fdn (page 57); **Address:** Cleveland Clinic, Div Ped Neurology, 9500 Euclid Ave, Desk S51, Cleveland, OH 44195; **Phone:** 216-444-2095; **Board Cert:** Pediatrics 1982; Child Neurology 1986; **Med School:** Indiana Univ 1978; **Resid:** Pediatrics, Indiana Univ Med Ctr 1980; Pediatrics, Case West Med Ctr 1981; **Fellow:** Child Neurology, Cleveland Clinic 1984; Clinical Neurophysiology, Cleveland Clinic 1985

Great Plains and Mountains

Bale Jr, James F MD [ChiN] - **Spec Exp:** Infections-Neurologic; Infections-Congenital; **Hospital:** Primary Children's Med Ctr, Univ Utah Hosps and Clins; **Address:** Primary Chldns Med Ctr, Ped Res Office, 100 N Medical Drive, Salt Lake City, UT 84113; **Phone:** 801-587-7575; **Board Cert:** Pediatrics 2003; Child Neurology 1982; **Med School:** Univ Mich Med Sch 1975; **Resid:** Pediatrics, Univ Utah Hosps 1977; Neurology, Univ Utah Hosps 1980; **Fellow:** Infectious Disease, Univ Utah 1981; Neurovirology, UCSF-VA Med Ctr 1982; **Fac Appt:** Prof N, Univ Utah

Southwest

Fishman, Marvin A MD [ChiN] - **Spec Exp:** Seizure Disorders; Epilepsy/Seizure Disorders-Pediatric; Headache; **Hospital:** Texas Chldns Hosp - Houston; **Address:** 6621 Fannin CC1250, Houston, TX 77030; **Phone:** 832-822-5046; **Board Cert:** Pediatrics 1966; Child Neurology 1972; Neurodevelopmental Disabilities 2001; **Med School:** Univ IL Coll Med 1961; **Resid:** Pediatrics, Michael Reese Hosp 1964; Child Neurology, Mass Genl Hosp 1967; **Fellow:** Child Neurology, Chldns Hosp 1969; **Fac Appt:** Prof Ped, Baylor Coll Med

Iannaccone, Susan MD [ChiN] - **Spec Exp:** Neuromuscular Disorders; **Hospital:** UT Southwestern Med Ctr - Dallas, Chldns Med Ctr of Dallas; **Address:** Division of Pediatric Neurology, Ambulatory Care Pavilion in Dallas, 2350 Stemmons Frwy., Ste 5074, Dallas, TX 75207; **Phone:** 214-559-7830; **Board Cert:** Pediatrics 1975; Child Neurology 1976; **Med School:** SUNY Hlth Sci Ctr 1969; **Resid:** Pediatrics, St Louis Chldns Hosp 1972; Neurology, Strong Meml Hosp 1975; **Fellow:** Neurology, Strong Meml Hosp 1975

Sharp, Gregory MD [ChiN] - **Spec Exp:** Epilepsy; **Hospital:** UAMS Med Ctr, Arkansas Chldns Hosp; **Address:** 800 Marshall St, Little Rock, AR 72202; **Phone:** 501-364-1100; **Board Cert:** Pediatrics 2004; Child Neurology 1993; **Med School:** Univ Ark 1984; **Resid:** Pediatrics, Univ AR Chldns Hosp 1987; **Fellow:** Pediatric Neurology, Mayo Clinic 1990; **Fac Appt:** Asst Prof Ped, Univ Ark

Tardo, Carmela L MD [ChiN] - **Spec Exp:** Epilepsy; Clinical Trials; **Hospital:** Children's Hospital - New Orleans; **Address:** 200 Clay Ave, New Orleans, LA 70118; **Phone:** 504-896-9458; **Board Cert:** Pediatrics 1974; Child Neurology 1976; Clinical Neurophysiology 1996; **Med School:** Tulane Univ 1969; **Resid:** Pediatrics, Johns Hopkins Hosp 1971; Pediatrics, UCSF Med Ctr 1972; **Fellow:** Pediatric Neurology, Columbia Univ 1975; **Fac Appt:** Assoc Prof N, Louisiana State Univ

West Coast and Pacific

Ashwal, Stephen MD [ChiN] - **Spec Exp:** Metabolic Disorders; **Hospital:** Loma Linda Univ Med Ctr; **Address:** 2195 Club Center Drive, San Bernadino, CA 92408; **Phone:** 909-558-2383; **Board Cert:** Pediatrics 1975; Child Neurology 1978; **Med School:** NYU Sch Med 1970; **Resid:** Pediatrics, Bellevue Hosp 1973; **Fellow:** Child Neurology, Univ Minn Med Ctr 1976; **Fac Appt:** Prof Ped, Loma Linda Univ

Ferriero, Donna Marie MD [ChiN] - **Spec Exp:** Neuroendocrinology; **Hospital:** UCSF Med Ctr; **Address:** UCSF, Box 0663, 521 Parnassus Ave, San Francisco, CA 94143-0663; **Phone:** 415-353-2525; **Board Cert:** Pediatrics 1986; Child Neurology 1987; **Med School:** UCSF 1979; **Resid:** Pediatrics, Mass Genl Hosp 1982; Child Neurology, UCSF Med Ctr 1985; **Fellow:** Neurological Endocrinology, UCSF Med Ctr 1987; **Fac Appt:** Prof N, UCSF

Child Neurology

Fisher, Paul G MD [ChiN] - **Spec Exp:** Neuro-Oncology; Brain Tumors; **Hospital:** Lucile Packard Chldns Hosp/Stanford Univ Med Ctr; **Address:** Stanford Cancer Ctr-Dept Neurology, 875 Blake Wilbur Drive, rm 2220, Stanford, CA 94305; **Phone:** 650-725-8630; **Board Cert:** Pediatrics 1995; Child Neurology 1998; **Med School:** UCSF 1989; **Resid:** Pediatrics, Johns Hopkins Univ Hosp 1991; Neurology, Johns Hopkins Univ Hosp 1994; **Fellow:** Neuro-Oncology, Children's Hosp 1994; **Fac Appt:** Assoc Prof Ped, Stanford Univ

Haas, Richard H MD [ChiN] - **Spec Exp:** Mitochondrial Disorders; Neurometabolic Disease; **Hospital:** UCSD Med Ctr, Rady Children's Hosp - San Diego; **Address:** UCSD Sch Med, Div Ped Neuro, 9500 Gilman Drive, MC 0935, La Jolla, CA 92093-0935; **Phone:** 858-822-6700; **Board Cert:** Child Neurology 1983; Pediatrics 1985; **Med School:** England 1972; **Resid:** Pediatrics, Univ London 1979; Child Neurology, Univ Colo Hlth Sci Ctr 1981; **Fellow:** Biochemical Mental Retardation, Univ Colo Hlth Sci Ctr 1981; **Fac Appt:** Prof Ped, UCSD

Lott, Ira T MD [ChiN] - **Spec Exp:** Down Syndrome; **Hospital:** UC Irvine Med Ctr, Saddleback Mem Med Ctr; **Address:** UC Irvine Med Ctr, Dept Ped Neur, 101 City Drive S, Orange, CA 92868; **Phone:** 714-456-7011; **Board Cert:** Pediatrics 1975; Child Neurology 1977; **Med School:** Ohio State Univ 1967; **Resid:** Pediatrics, Mass Genl Hosp 1969; **Fellow:** Research, Natl Inst Hlth 1971; Neurology, Harvard-Mass Genl Hosp 1974; **Fac Appt:** Prof N, UC Irvine

Mitchell, Wendy Gayle MD [ChiN] - **Spec Exp:** Epilepsy/Seizure Disorders; Opsoclonus-Ataxia in Children; **Hospital:** Chldns Hosp - Los Angeles (page 56); **Address:** Chldns Hosp Los Angeles, Dept Neuro, 4650 Sunset Blvd, Box 82, Los Angeles, CA 90027-6062; **Phone:** 323-669-2471; **Board Cert:** Pediatrics 1978; Child Neurology 1983; **Med School:** UCSF 1973; **Resid:** Pediatrics, Moffit Hosp-UCSF 1975; Child Neurology, Univ North Carolina 1981; **Fellow:** Behavioral Pediatrics, Mt Zion Hosp 1976; Univ North Carolina 1978; **Fac Appt:** Prof N, USC Sch Med

Mobley, William C MD/PhD [ChiN] - **Hospital:** Stanford Univ Med Ctr; **Address:** 1201 Welch Rd, MSLS Bldg, rm P205, Stanford, CA 94305; **Phone:** 650-723-6424; **Board Cert:** Pediatrics 1983; Child Neurology 1987; **Med School:** Stanford Univ 1976; **Resid:** Pediatrics, Stanford Univ Sch Med 1979; Neurology, Johns Hopkins Hosp 1982; **Fac Appt:** Prof N, UCSF

Roddy, Sarah Marie MD [ChiN] - **Spec Exp:** Tourette's Syndrome; **Hospital:** Loma Linda Chldns Hosp; **Address:** Pediatric Neuroscience Center, 2195 Club Center Drive, Ste A, San Bernadino, CA 92408; **Phone:** 909-835-1810; **Board Cert:** Child Neurology 1987; Pediatrics 1987; **Med School:** Loma Linda Univ 1980; **Resid:** Pediatrics, Loma Linda Univ Med Ctr 1983; **Fellow:** Pediatric Neurology, Loma Linda Univ Med Ctr 1986; **Fac Appt:** Assoc Prof N, Loma Linda Univ

Rosser, Tena L MD [ChiN] - **Spec Exp:** Neurocutaneous Disorders; Neurofibromatosis; Tuberous Sclerosis; **Hospital:** Chldns Hosp - Los Angeles (page 56); **Address:** Chldns Hosp Los Angeles, Dept Neurology, 4650 Sunset Blvd, Los Angeles, CA 90027; **Phone:** 323-669-2471; **Board Cert:** Pediatrics 1999; Child Neurology 2003; **Med School:** Univ NC Sch Med 1996; **Resid:** Pediatrics, Chldns Natl Med Ctr 1999; **Fellow:** Child Neurology, Chldns Natl Med Ctr 2003; **Fac Appt:** Asst Prof N, USC-Keck School of Medicine

Sankar, Raman MD [ChiN] - **Spec Exp:** Epilepsy/Seizure Disorders; Headache; Migraine; **Hospital:** Mattel Chldns Hosp at UCLA, UCLA Med Ctr; **Address:** UCLA Sch Med-Div Ped Neurology, 22-474 MDCC, Box 951752, Los Angeles, CA 90095-1752; **Phone:** 310-825-6196; **Board Cert:** Child Neurology 2005; **Med School:** Tulane Univ 1986; **Resid:** Pediatrics, Chldns Hosp 1988; Neurology, UCLA Med Ctr 1989; **Fellow:** Child Neurology, UCLA Med Ctr 1991; **Fac Appt:** Prof Ped, UCLA

Shields, William Donald MD [ChiN] - **Spec Exp:** Epilepsy/Seizure Disorders; **Hospital:** UCLA Med Ctr; **Address:** UCLA Med Ctr, Dept Ped Neurology, 10833 Le Conte Ave, Los Angeles, CA 90095-1752; **Phone:** 310-825-6196; **Board Cert:** Child Neurology 1977; Pediatrics 1978; **Med School:** Univ Utah 1971; **Resid:** Pediatrics, USC Med Ctr 1973; Neurology, Univ Utah Med Ctr 1976; **Fac Appt:** Prof Ped, UCLA

Trauner, Doris Ann MD [ChiN] - **Spec Exp:** Autism; Speech Disorders; **Hospital:** Rady Children's Hosp - San Diego; **Address:** UCSD Med Ctr, Div Ped Neurology, 9500 Gilman Drive, Dept 0935, La Jolla, CA 92093-0935; **Phone:** 858-966-5819; **Board Cert:** Pediatrics 1978; Child Neurology 1979; Neurodevelopmental Disabilities 2001; **Med School:** Med Coll VA 1972; **Resid:** Pediatrics, UCSD Med Ctr 1974; Neurology, UCSD Med Ctr 1975; **Fellow:** Child Neurology, Univ Chicago 1977; **Fac Appt:** Prof Ped, UCSD

Clinical Genetics

A specialist trained in diagnostic and therapeutic procedures for patients with genetically-linked diseases. This specialist uses modern cytogenetic, radiologic and biochemical testing to assist in specialized genetic counseling, implements needed therapeutic interventions and provides prevention through prenatal diagnosis.

A clinical geneticist demonstrates competence in providing comprehensive diagnostic, management and counseling services for genetic disorders.

A medical geneticist plans and coordinates large scale screening programs for inborn errors of metabolism, hemoglobinopathies, chromosome abnormalities and neural tube defects.

Training Required: Two or four years

Clinical Genetics

New England

Bianchi, Diana MD [CG] - **Spec Exp:** Twin to Twin Transfusion Syndrome (TTTS); Fetal Abnormalities; **Hospital:** Tufts-New England Med Ctr; **Address:** New Engl Med Ctr/Div Med Genetics, 750 Washington St, Box 394, Boston, MA 02111; **Phone:** 617-636-1468; **Board Cert:** Pediatrics 1985; Clinical Genetics 1987; Neonatal-Perinatal Medicine 1987; **Med School:** Stanford Univ 1980; **Resid:** Pediatrics, Childrens Hosp 1983; **Fellow:** Neonatology, Childrens Hosp 1986; Clinical Genetics, Harvard Med Sch 1987; **Fac Appt:** Prof Ped, Tufts Univ

Holmes, Lewis B MD [CG] - **Spec Exp:** Birth Defects; Inherited Disorders; **Hospital:** Mass Genl Hosp; **Address:** Mass Genl Hosp, Dept Pediatrics, 175 Cambridge St, rm 504, Boston, MA 02114; **Phone:** 617-726-1742; **Board Cert:** Pediatrics 1968; Clinical Genetics 1982; **Med School:** Duke Univ 1963; **Resid:** Pediatrics, Mass Genl Hosp 1970; **Fac Appt:** Prof Ped, Harvard Med Sch

Mahoney, Maurice J MD [CG] - **Spec Exp:** Fetal Therapy; Prenatal Diagnosis; **Hospital:** Yale - New Haven Hosp; **Address:** Yale Genetics Consultation Serv, 333 Cedar St, rm WWW330, New Haven, CT 06520-8005; **Phone:** 203-785-2661; **Board Cert:** Pediatrics 1967; Clinical Genetics 1982; Clinical Biochemical Genetics 1982; **Med School:** Univ Pittsburgh 1962; **Resid:** Pediatrics, Johns Hopkins Hosp 1965; Pediatrics, Childrens Hosp 1966; **Fellow:** Clinical Genetics, Yale Univ Sch Med 1970; **Fac Appt:** Prof CG, Yale Univ

Seashore, Margretta MD [CG] - **Spec Exp:** Inherited Metabolic Disorders; **Hospital:** Yale - New Haven Hosp; **Address:** Yale Univ Sch Med, Dept Genetics, 333 Cedar St, rm 305, Box 208005, New Haven, CT 06520-8005; **Phone:** 203-785-2660; **Board Cert:** Pediatrics 1970; Clinical Biochemical Genetics 1982; Clinical Genetics 1982; **Med School:** Yale Univ 1965; **Resid:** Pediatrics, Yale-New Haven Hosp 1968; **Fellow:** Clinical Genetics, Yale-New Haven Hosp 1970; **Fac Appt:** Prof CG, Yale Univ

Mid Atlantic

Anyane-Yeboa, Kwame MD [CG] - **Spec Exp:** Dysmorphology; Prenatal Diagnosis; **Hospital:** NYPresby-Morgan Stanley Children's Hosp, St Luke's - Roosevelt Hosp Ctr - Roosevelt Div; **Address:** Morgan Stanley Children's Hospital of NY, 3959 Broadway Fl 6N - rm 601A, New York, NY 10032; **Phone:** 212-305-6731; **Board Cert:** Pediatrics 1979; Clinical Genetics 1982; **Med School:** Ghana 1972; **Resid:** Pediatrics, Harlem Hosp 1977; **Fellow:** Clinical Genetics, Babies Hosp-Columbia Presby 1980; **Fac Appt:** Assoc Prof Ped, Columbia P&S

Bialer, Martin G MD/PhD [CG] - **Spec Exp:** Marfan's Syndrome; Neurofibromatosis; Metabolic Genetic Disorders; **Hospital:** Schneider Chldn's Hosp, Long Island Jewish Med Ctr; **Address:** 1554 Northern Blvd, Ste 204, Manhasset, NY 11030; **Phone:** 516-365-3996; **Board Cert:** Clinical Genetics 1990; Clinical Biochemical Genetics 1990; Clinical Molecular Genetics 1990; Pediatrics 1987; **Med School:** Med Univ SC 1983; **Resid:** Pediatrics, N Shore Univ Hosp 1986; **Fellow:** Clinical Genetics, Univ VA Hlth Sci Ctr 1989; **Fac Appt:** Clin Prof Ped, NYU Sch Med

Davis, Jessica G MD [CG] - **Spec Exp:** Marfan's Syndrome; Mental Retardation; Neurofibromatosis; Ehlers-Danlos Syndrome; **Hospital:** NY-Presby Hosp/Weill Cornell (page 66), Hosp For Special Surgery (page 60); **Address:** 525 E 68th St, Box 128, New York, NY 10021-4870; **Phone:** 212-746-1496; **Board Cert:** Clinical Genetics 1984; **Med School:** Columbia P&S 1959; **Resid:** Pediatrics, St Luke's Hosp 1962; Clinical Genetics, Albert Einstein Coll Med 1965; **Fellow:** Cytogenetics, Albert Einstein Coll Med 1966; Pediatrics, Albert Einstein Col Med 1968; **Fac Appt:** Assoc Clin Prof Ped, Cornell Univ-Weill Med Coll

Desnick, Robert J MD/PhD [CG] - **Spec Exp:** Inherited Metabolic Disorders; Fabry's Disease; Gaucher Disease; Porphyria; **Hospital:** Mount Sinai Med Ctr, Elmhurst Hosp Ctr; **Address:** Mt Sinai Sch Med, Box 1498, Fifth Ave @ 100th St, New York, NY 10029; **Phone:** 212-241-6947; **Board Cert:** Clinical Genetics 1982; Clinical Molecular Genetics 1999; Clinical Biochemical Genetics 1982; **Med School:** Univ Minn 1971; **Resid:** Pediatrics, Univ Minn Hosps 1973; **Fac Appt:** Prof CG, Mount Sinai Sch Med

Desposito, Franklin MD [CG] - **Spec Exp:** Birth Defects; Genetic Disorders; **Hospital:** UMDNJ-Univ Hosp-Newark; **Address:** 90 Bergen St, Ste 5400, Newark, NJ 07103; **Phone:** 973-972-3300; **Board Cert:** Pediatrics 1986; Clinical Genetics 1982; Clinical Cytogenetics 1990; Clinical Molecular Genetics 2006; **Med School:** Ros Franklin Univ/Chicago Med Sch 1957; **Resid:** Pediatrics, Long Island Jewish Hosp 1961; **Fellow:** Hematology, Univ Wisc Sch Med 1963; **Fac Appt:** Prof Ped, UMDNJ-NJ Med Sch, Newark

Driscoll, Deborah A MD [CG] - **Spec Exp:** Prenatal Genetic Diagnosis; Fetal Abnormalities; Adolescent Gynecology; **Hospital:** Hosp Univ Penn - UPHS (page 72); **Address:** Chldns Hosp of Philadelphia, Clin Genetics Ctr, 34th St and Civic Ctr Blvd, rm 9S20, Philadelphia, PA 19104; **Phone:** 215-662-3232; **Board Cert:** Obstetrics & Gynecology 2005; Clinical Genetics 1990; Clinical Molecular Genetics 1993; **Med School:** NYU Sch Med 1983; **Resid:** Obstetrics & Gynecology, Hosp Univ Penn 1987; **Fellow:** Clinical Genetics, Hosp Univ Penn 1989; **Fac Appt:** Assoc Prof ObG, Univ Pennsylvania

Marion, Robert MD [CG] - **Spec Exp:** Spina Bifida; Williams Syndrome; Marfan's Syndrome; Down Syndrome; **Hospital:** Montefiore Med Ctr, Blythedale Children's Hosp; **Address:** Montefiore Med Ctr, Dept Pediatrics, 111 E 210th St, Bronx, NY 10467-2401; **Phone:** 718-741-2323; **Board Cert:** Pediatrics 1985; Clinical Genetics 1987; **Med School:** Albert Einstein Coll Med 1979; **Resid:** Pediatrics, Montefiore Med Ctr 1982; **Fellow:** Clinical Genetics, Montefiore Med Ctr 1984; **Fac Appt:** Prof Ped, Albert Einstein Coll Med

Ostrer, Harry MD [CG] - **Spec Exp:** Genetic Disorders; Hereditary Cancer; **Hospital:** NYU Med Ctr (page 67); **Address:** NYU Medical Ctr, 550 1st Ave, rm MSB136, New York, NY 10016; **Phone:** 212-263-5746; **Board Cert:** Clinical Genetics 1984; Pediatrics 1985; Clinical Cytogenetics 1990; Clinical Molecular Genetics 2004; **Med School:** Columbia P&S 1976; **Resid:** Pediatrics, Johns Hopkins Hosp 1978; Clinical Genetics, Natl Inst Health 1981; **Fellow:** Molecular Genetics, Johns Hopkins Hosp 1983; **Fac Appt:** Prof Ped, NYU Sch Med

Pyeritz, Reed E MD/PhD [CG] - **Spec Exp:** Marfan's Syndrome; Hereditary Hemorrhagic Telangiectasia; Inherited Disorders; **Hospital:** Hosp Univ Penn - UPHS (page 72), Chldns Hosp of Philadelphia, The; **Address:** Univ Penn, Div Medical Genetics, 3400 Spruce St, 538 Maloney Bldg, Philadelphia, PA 19104; **Phone:** 215-662-4740; **Board Cert:** Internal Medicine 1978; Clinical Genetics 2004; **Med School:** Harvard Med Sch 1975; **Resid:** Internal Medicine, Peter Bent Brigham Hosp 1977; Clinical Genetics, Johns Hopkins Hosp 1978; **Fac Appt:** Prof Med, Univ Pennsylvania

Clinical Genetics

Rosenbaum, Kenneth MD [CG] - **Spec Exp:** Birth Defects; **Hospital:** Chldns Natl Med Ctr; **Address:** Chldns Natl Med Ctr, Dept Med Genetics, 111 Michigan Ave NW, rm 1950, Washington, DC 20010; **Phone:** 202-884-2187; **Board Cert:** Pediatrics 1976; Clinical Genetics 1982; Clinical Cytogenetics 1982; **Med School:** Univ Louisville Sch Med 1971; **Resid:** Pediatrics, Childrens Natl Med Ctr 1974; **Fellow:** Clinical Genetics, Johns Hopkins Hosp 1977; **Fac Appt:** Assoc Prof Ped, Geo Wash Univ

Shapiro, Lawrence R MD [CG] - **Spec Exp:** Dysmorphology; Prenatal Diagnosis; Hereditary Cancer; Developmental Disorders; **Hospital:** Westchester Med Ctr; **Address:** Regional Med Genetics Ctr, 19 Bradhurst Ave, Ste 1600, Hawthorne, NY 10532-2140; **Phone:** 914-593-8900; **Board Cert:** Pediatrics 1967; Clinical Genetics 1982; Clinical Cytogenetics 1982; **Med School:** NYU Sch Med 1962; **Resid:** Pediatrics, Chldns Hosp 1964; Pediatrics, Bellevue Hosp 1965; **Fellow:** Clinical Genetics, Mount Sinai Med Ctr 1968; **Fac Appt:** Prof Ped, NY Med Coll

Willner, Judith P MD [CG] - **Spec Exp:** Prenatal Diagnosis; Dysmorphology; Metabolic Genetic Disorders; **Hospital:** Mount Sinai Med Ctr, Englewood Hosp & Med Ctr; **Address:** Mt Sinai Med Ctr, Dept Clinical Genetics, 1 Gustave Levy Pl, Box 1497, New York, NY 10029-6500; **Phone:** 212-241-6947; **Board Cert:** Pediatrics 1977; Clinical Genetics 1982; **Med School:** NYU Sch Med 1971; **Resid:** Pediatrics, Chldns Hosp Natl Med Ctr 1973; **Fellow:** Clinical Genetics, Mount Sinai Hosp 1977; **Fac Appt:** Prof CG, Mount Sinai Sch Med

Zackai, Elaine MD [CG] - **Spec Exp:** Craniosynostosis; Cytogenetic Disorders; **Hospital:** Chldns Hosp of Philadelphia, The; **Address:** Childrens Hosp Philadelphia, Dept Clinical Genetics, 34th St & Civic Center Blvd, rm 9S20, Philadelphia, PA 19104; **Phone:** 215-590-2920; **Board Cert:** Pediatrics 1977; Clinical Genetics 1982; Clinical Cytogenetics 1982; **Med School:** NYU Sch Med 1968; **Resid:** Pediatrics, Chldns Hosp 1970; **Fellow:** Clinical Genetics, Chldns Hosp 1971; Clinical Genetics, Yale Univ Med Sch 1972; **Fac Appt:** Prof Ped, Univ Pennsylvania

Southeast

Driscoll, Daniel J MD/PhD [CG] - **Spec Exp:** Prader-Willi Syndrome; Obesity; Angelman Syndrome; **Hospital:** Shands Hlthcre at Univ of FL; **Address:** Univ Florida-Pediatric Genetics, 1600 SW Archer Rd, Box 100296, Gainesville, FL 32610-0296; **Phone:** 352-392-4104; **Board Cert:** Pediatrics 1987; Clinical Genetics 1990; Clinical Cytogenetics 1990; Clinical Molecular Genetics 2004; **Med School:** Albany Med Coll 1983; **Resid:** Pediatrics, Johns Hopkins Hosp 1986; **Fellow:** Clinical Genetics, Johns Hopkins Hosp 1989; **Fac Appt:** Prof Ped, Univ Fla Coll Med

Fernhoff, Paul M MD [CG] - **Spec Exp:** Birth Defects; Metabolic Genetic Disorders; **Hospital:** Chldns Hlthcare Atlanta - Scottish Rite, Emory Univ Hosp; **Address:** Emory Univ Sch Med, Div Med Genetics, 2165 N Decatur Rd, Decatur, GA 30033-5307; **Phone:** 404-778-8500; **Board Cert:** Pediatrics 1976; Clinical Genetics 1983; **Med School:** Jefferson Med Coll 1971; **Resid:** Pediatrics, Children's Hosp 1974; **Fellow:** Clinical Genetics, Emory Univ Hosp 1979; **Fac Appt:** Assoc Prof Ped, Emory Univ

Korf, Bruce MD/PhD [CG] - **Spec Exp:** Inherited Disorders; Neuro-Genetics; Neurofibromatosis; **Hospital:** Univ of Ala Hosp at Birmingham; **Address:** Univ Alabama-KAUL 230, 720 20th St S, Birmingham, AL 35294-0024; **Phone:** 205-934-9411; **Board Cert:** Clinical Genetics 1984; Child Neurology 1986; Pediatrics 1988; Clinical Molecular Genetics 2004; **Med School:** Cornell Univ-Weill Med Coll 1980; **Resid:** Pediatrics, Chldns Hosp 1982; Child Neurology, Chldns Hosp 1985; **Fellow:** Clinical Genetics, Chldns Hosp 1985; **Fac Appt:** Prof CG, Univ Ala

Saul, Robert MD [CG] - **Spec Exp:** Birth Defects; Neurofibromatosis; **Hospital:** Self Regional Healthcare; **Address:** Greenwood Genetic Ctr, 101 Gregor Mendel Cir, Greenwood, SC 29646-2307; **Phone:** 864-941-8100; **Board Cert:** Pediatrics 1981; Clinical Genetics 1982; **Med School:** Univ Colorado 1976; **Resid:** Pediatrics, Duke Med Ctr 1979; **Fellow:** Clinical Genetics, Greenwood Genetics Ctr 1981; **Fac Appt:** Clin Prof Ped, Univ SC Sch Med

Stevenson, Roger E MD [CG] - **Spec Exp:** Birth Defects; Mental Retardation; **Hospital:** Self Regional Healthcare; **Address:** Greenwood Genetic Ctr, 101 Gregor Mendel Cir, Greenwood, SC 29646; **Phone:** 864-941-8100; **Board Cert:** Pediatrics 1971; Clinical Genetics 1982; Clinical Cytogenetics 1984; **Med School:** Wake Forest Univ 1966; **Resid:** Pediatrics, Johns Hopkins Hosp 1969; **Fellow:** Clinical Genetics, Johns Hopkins Hosp 1972

Midwest

Charrow, Joel MD [CG] - **Spec Exp:** Biochemical Genetics; Lysosomal Diseases; Neurofibromatosis; **Hospital:** Children's Mem Hosp; **Address:** Chldns Meml Hosp-Div Genetics, 2300 Chldn Plaza, MS 59, Chicago, IL 60614-3318; **Phone:** 773-880-4462; **Board Cert:** Pediatrics 1980; Clinical Genetics 1982; Clinical Biochemical Genetics 1987; **Med School:** Mount Sinai Sch Med 1976; **Resid:** Pediatrics, Chldns Meml Hosp 1979; **Fellow:** Clinical Genetics, Chldns Meml Hosp-Northwestern Univ 1981; **Fac Appt:** Prof Ped, Northwestern Univ

Martin, Rick A MD [CG] - **Spec Exp:** Dysmorphology; **Hospital:** St Louis Chldns Hosp; **Address:** Washington Univ, Div Med Genetics, 660 S Euclid St, Campus Box 8116, St Louis, MO 63110; **Phone:** 314-454-6093; **Board Cert:** Pediatrics 2005; Clinical Genetics 2006; **Med School:** Univ Utah 1987; **Resid:** Pediatrics, UCSD Med Ctr 1990; **Fellow:** Clinical Genetics, UCSD Med Ctr 1992; **Fac Appt:** Assoc Prof CG, Washington Univ, St Louis

Pergament, Eugene MD/PhD [CG] - **Spec Exp:** Prenatal Genetic Diagnosis; Down Syndrome; Genetic Preimplantation Diagnosis; **Hospital:** Northwestern Meml Hosp; **Address:** 680 N Lake Shore Drive, Ste 1230, Chicago, IL 60611; **Phone:** 312-981-4360; **Board Cert:** Clinical Genetics 1982; Clinical Cytogenetics 1984; **Med School:** Univ Chicago-Pritzker Sch Med 1970; **Resid:** Pediatrics, Univ Chicago 1972; **Fac Appt:** Prof ObG, Northwestern Univ

Saal, Howard MD [CG] - **Spec Exp:** Craniofacial Disorders; Cleft Palate/Lip; Neurofibromatosis; **Hospital:** Cincinnati Chldns Hosp Med Ctr; **Address:** Chldns Hosp Med Ctr, Div Human Genetics, 3333 Burnet Ave Bldg E5 - rm 5430, MC 4006, Cinncinnati, OH 45229-3039; **Phone:** 513-636-4760; **Board Cert:** Clinical Genetics 1984; Clinical Cytogenetics 1984; Pediatrics 1985; **Med School:** Wayne State Univ 1979; **Resid:** Pediatrics, Univ Conn Hlth Ctr 1982; **Fellow:** Medical Genetics, Univ Washington 1984; **Fac Appt:** Prof Ped, Univ Cincinnati

Weaver, David D MD [CG] - **Spec Exp:** Bone Disorders-Inherited; Genetic Disorders; Inherited Disorders; Birth Defects; **Hospital:** Riley Hosp for Children, Indiana Univ Hosp; **Address:** 975 W Walnut St IB Bldg - Ste 130, Indianapolis, IN 46202-5251; **Phone:** 317-274-1057; **Board Cert:** Pediatrics 1978; Clinical Genetics 1982; **Med School:** Oregon Hlth Sci Univ 1966; **Resid:** Pediatrics, Oregon Hlth Scis Univ Sch Med 1972; **Fellow:** Clinical Genetics, Univ Washington Sch Med 1974; Metabolic Diseases, Oregon Health Scis Med Ctr 1976; **Fac Appt:** Prof Emeritus CG, Indiana Univ

Clinical Genetics

Whelan, Alison MD [CG] - **Spec Exp:** Gynecologic Cancer Risk Assessment; Colon & Rectal Cancer Risk Assessment; Hereditary Cancer; **Hospital:** Barnes-Jewish Hosp, St Louis Chldns Hosp; **Address:** Washington Univ Sch Med, 660 S Euclid Ave, Campus Box 8073, St Louis, MO 63110; **Phone:** 314-454-6093; **Board Cert:** Clinical Genetics 1996; **Med School:** Washington Univ, St Louis 1986; **Resid:** Internal Medicine, Barnes Hosp 1989; Pediatrics, Wash Univ Sch Med 1994; **Fellow:** Research, Wash Univ Sch Med 1991; Clinical Genetics, Wash Univ Sch Med 1994; **Fac Appt:** Prof Med, Washington Univ, St Louis

Great Plains and Mountains

Carey, John C MD [CG] - **Spec Exp:** Neurofibromatosis; Birth Defects; Deafness; Hearing Loss; **Hospital:** Primary Children's Med Ctr, Univ Utah Hosps and Clins; **Address:** Univ Utah Med Ctr-Div of Med Gen, 50 N Med Drive Bldg SOM - rm 2C412, Salt Lake City, UT 84132; **Phone:** 801-581-8943; **Board Cert:** Pediatrics 1979; Clinical Genetics 1982; **Med School:** Georgetown Univ 1972; **Resid:** Pediatrics, UCSF Med Ctr 1975; **Fellow:** Clinical Genetics, UCSF Med Ctr 1979; **Fac Appt:** Prof Ped, Univ Utah

Southwest

Beaudet, Arthur L MD [CG] - **Spec Exp:** Genetic Biochemical Disorders; **Hospital:** Texas Chldns Hosp - Houston; **Address:** Texas Children's Hosp, 6621 Fannin St, MC CC1560, Houston, TX 77030; **Phone:** 832-822-4280; **Board Cert:** Pediatrics 1973; Clinical Genetics 1982; Clinical Biochemical Genetics 1982; Clinical Molecular Genetics 2004; **Med School:** Yale Univ 1967; **Resid:** Pediatrics, Johns Hopkins Hosp 1969; **Fellow:** Biochemical Genetics, Natl Inst Hlth 1971; **Fac Appt:** Prof CG, Baylor Coll Med

Craigen, William MD [CG] - **Spec Exp:** Biochemical Genetics; Mitochondrial Disorders; **Hospital:** Texas Chldns Hosp - Houston, Ben Taub General Hosp; **Address:** Texas Children's Hosp, 6621 Fannin St, MC CC1560, Houston, TX 77030; **Phone:** 832-822-4280; **Board Cert:** Pediatrics 1992; Clinical Genetics 1993; Clinical Biochemical Genetics 1993; **Med School:** Baylor Coll Med 1988; **Resid:** Pediatrics, Baylor Coll Med 1990; Pediatrics, Baylor Coll Med 1992; **Fellow:** Clinical Genetics, Baylor Coll Med 1990; **Fac Appt:** Assoc Prof CG, Baylor Coll Med

Cunniff, Christopher MD [CG] - **Spec Exp:** Birth Defects; **Hospital:** Univ Med Ctr - Tucson; **Address:** Univ Ariz Coll Med, Dept Ped Genetics, 1501 N Campbell Ave, Tucson, AZ 85724; **Phone:** 520-626-5175; **Board Cert:** Pediatrics 2003; Clinical Genetics 1990; **Med School:** Univ Ala 1984; **Resid:** Pediatrics, MC Hosp Vermont 1987; **Fellow:** Dysmorphology, UCSD Med Ctr 1989; **Fac Appt:** Assoc Prof Ped, Univ Ariz Coll Med

Mulvihill, John J MD [CG] - **Spec Exp:** Genetic Disorders; Neurofibromatosis; Fertility in Cancer Survivors; **Hospital:** Chldns Hosp OU Med Ctr; **Address:** Childrens Hosp, 940 NE 13th St, rm 2B2418, Oklahoma City, OK 73104; **Phone:** 405-271-8685; **Board Cert:** Pediatrics 1975; Clinical Genetics 1982; **Med School:** Univ Wash 1969; **Resid:** Pediatrics, Johns Hopkins Hosp 1974; **Fellow:** Research, NCI-Natl Inst Hlth 1972; **Fac Appt:** Prof CG, Univ Okla Coll Med

Northrup, Hope MD [CG] - **Spec Exp:** Biochemical Genetics; Neuro-Genetics; Dysmorphology; **Hospital:** Meml Hermann Hosp - Houston, LBJ General Hosp; **Address:** Univ TX Med Sch, Dept Peds-Div Med Genetics, rm MSB-3.144, Box 20708, Houston, TX 77225-0708; **Phone:** 713-500-5760; **Board Cert:** Pediatrics 1988; Clinical Genetics 1990; Clinical Biochemical Genetics 1990; **Med School:** Med Univ SC 1983; **Resid:** Pediatrics, Chldns Med Ctr-Univ Tex SW 1986; **Fellow:** Clinical Genetics, Inst Molec Gene-Baylor Coll Med 1989; **Fac Appt:** Prof Ped, Univ Tex, Houston

West Coast and Pacific

Boles, Richard G MD [CG] - **Spec Exp:** Mitochondrial Disorders; Vomiting-Cyclic; **Hospital:** Chldns Hosp - Los Angeles (page 56); **Address:** 4650 Sunset Blvd, MS 90, Los Angeles, CA 90027; **Phone:** 323-669-2178; **Board Cert:** Clinical Genetics 2004; Clinical Biochemical Genetics 2004; Pediatrics 2002; **Med School:** UCLA 1987; **Resid:** Pediatrics, Harbor-UCLA Med Ctr 1990; **Fellow:** Genetics and Metabolism, Yale Univ Sch Med 1993; **Fac Appt:** Assoc Prof Ped, USC Sch Med

Cassidy, Suzanne MD [CG] - **Spec Exp:** Prader-Willi Syndrome; Connective Tissue Disorders; Neurocutaneous Disorders; **Hospital:** UCSF Med Ctr; **Address:** 533 Parnassus Ave, rm U-100A, Box 0706, San Francisco, CA 94143; **Phone:** 415-476-2757; **Board Cert:** Pediatrics 1982; Clinical Genetics 1983; **Med School:** Vanderbilt Univ 1976; **Resid:** Pediatrics, Univ Wash Affil Prgms 1979; **Fellow:** Clinical Genetics, Univ Wash 1981; **Fac Appt:** Prof Ped, UC Irvine

Cederbaum, Stephen D MD [CG] - **Spec Exp:** Inborn Errors of Metabolism; **Hospital:** UCLA Med Ctr; **Address:** 635 Charles E Young Drive S, rm 347, Los Angeles, CA 90095-7332; **Phone:** 310-825-0402; **Board Cert:** Clinical Genetics 1982; Clinical Biochemical Genetics 1982; **Med School:** NYU Sch Med 1964; **Resid:** Internal Medicine, Barnes Hosp 1966; **Fellow:** Clinical Genetics, Univ Wash 1970; **Fac Appt:** Prof Ped, UCLA

Curry, Cynthia J MD [CG] - **Hospital:** Chldns Hosp Central California, Comm Med Ctr - Fresno; **Address:** Genetic Medicine Central California, 351 E Barstow, Ste 106, Fresno, CA 93710-6073; **Phone:** 559-227-4472; **Board Cert:** Pediatrics 1973; Clinical Genetics 1982; **Med School:** Yale Univ 1967; **Resid:** Pediatrics, Univ Wash Orth Chldns Hosp 1969; Pediatrics, Univ Minn Hosp 1970; **Fellow:** Dysmorphology, UCSF Med Ctr 1976; **Fac Appt:** Prof CG, UCSF

Falk, Rena Ellen MD [CG] - **Spec Exp:** Prenatal Diagnosis; Mental Retardation; Prenatal Genetic Diagnosis; **Hospital:** Cedars-Sinai Med Ctr; **Address:** 444 S San Vicente Blvd, Ste 1001, Los Angeles, CA 90048; **Phone:** 310-423-9914; **Board Cert:** Pediatrics 1976; Clinical Genetics 1982; Clinical Cytogenetics 1984; **Med School:** UCLA 1971; **Resid:** Pediatrics, Cedars-Sinai Med Ctr 1973; **Fellow:** Clinical Genetics, UCLA Med Schl 1975; UCLA 1977; **Fac Appt:** Prof Ped, UCLA

Graham Jr, John M MD [CG] - **Spec Exp:** Dysmorphology; Craniofacial Disorders; Mental Retardation; **Hospital:** Cedars-Sinai Med Ctr; **Address:** 8700 Beverly Blvd, Ste 1152, Cedars Sinai Medical Center, Los Angeles, CA 90048; **Phone:** 310-423-9914; **Board Cert:** Pediatrics 1982; Clinical Genetics 1982; **Med School:** Med Univ SC 1975; **Resid:** Pediatrics, Boston Chldns Hosp-Harvard 1977; **Fellow:** Developmental-Behavioral Pediatrics, Boston Chldns Hosp 1978; Dysmorphology, Univ Wash 1980; **Fac Appt:** Prof Ped, UCLA

Grody, Wayne W MD/PhD [CG] - **Spec Exp:** Genetic Disorders; Hereditary Cancer; **Hospital:** UCLA Med Ctr; **Address:** UCLA School Medicine, Division of Genetic Molecular Pathology, 10833 Le Conte Ave, #37-121CHS Ave, Los Angeles, CA 90095-1732; **Phone:** 310-825-5648; **Board Cert:** Clinical Genetics 1990; Anatomic & Clinical Pathology 1987; Clinical Biochemical Genetics 1990; Molecular Genetic Pathology 2001; **Med School:** Baylor Coll Med 1977; **Resid:** Pathology, UCLA Med Ctr 1986; **Fellow:** Clinical Genetics, UCLA Med Ctr 1987; **Fac Appt:** Prof CG, UCLA

Clinical Genetics

Hoyme, H Eugene MD [CG] - **Spec Exp:** Fetal Alcohol Syndrome; Cytogenetic Disorders; Dysmorphology; **Hospital:** Stanford Univ Med Ctr; **Address:** Stanford Univ Med Ctr, Dept Peds-Med Genetics, 300 Pasteur Drive, rm H315, Stanford, CA 94305-5208; **Phone:** 650-723-6858; **Board Cert:** Pediatrics 1980; Clinical Genetics 1984; Clinical Cytogenetics 1987; **Med School:** Univ Chicago-Pritzker Sch Med 1976; **Resid:** Pediatrics, UCSD Med Ctr 1979; **Fellow:** Dysmorphology, UCSD Med Ctr 1981; **Fac Appt:** Prof Ped, Stanford Univ

Hudgins, Louanne MD [CG] - **Spec Exp:** Congenital Anomalies-Limb; **Hospital:** Stanford Univ Med Ctr; **Address:** Stanford Univ Med Ctr, Dept Peds-Med Genetics, 300 Pasteur Drive, rm H315, Stanford, CA 94305-5208; **Phone:** 650-723-6858; **Board Cert:** Pediatrics 1997; Clinical Genetics 1993; **Med School:** Univ Kans 1984; **Resid:** Pediatrics, Univ Conn Hlth Ctr 1987; **Fellow:** Clinical Genetics, Univ Conn Hlth Ctr 1990; **Fac Appt:** Assoc Prof Ped, Stanford Univ

Jonas, Adam J MD [CG] - **Spec Exp:** Biochemical Genetics; Inherited Disorders; **Hospital:** LAC - Harbor - UCLA Med Ctr; **Address:** Harbor-UCLA Med Ctr, Div Med Genetics, 1000 W Carson St, Box 17, Torrance, CA 90509-2910; **Phone:** 310-222-2301; **Board Cert:** Pediatrics 1982; Clinical Biochemical Genetics 1987; Clinical Genetics 1990; **Med School:** UCSD 1976; **Resid:** Pediatrics, Chldns Ortho Hosp 1978; Pediatrics, Univ Hosp 1979; **Fellow:** Genetics and Metabolism, UCSD Sch Med 1982; **Fac Appt:** Prof Ped, UCLA

Jones, Marilyn MD [CG] - **Spec Exp:** Dysmorphology; Craniofacial Disorders; **Hospital:** Rady Children's Hosp - San Diego, UCSD Med Ctr; **Address:** 3020 Children's Way, MC 5031, San Diego, CA 92123-2746; **Phone:** 858-966-5840; **Board Cert:** Pediatrics 1979; Clinical Genetics 1982; **Med School:** Columbia P&S 1974; **Resid:** Internal Medicine, UCSD Med Ctr 1977; Pediatrics, UCSD Med Ctr 1978; **Fellow:** Dysmorphology, UCSD Med Ctr 1979

Morris, Colleen A MD [CG] - **Spec Exp:** Williams Syndrome; Inherited Disorders; Fetal Alcohol Syndrome; **Hospital:** Univ Med Ctr - Las Vegas; **Address:** Univ Nevada Sch Medicine, Dept Pediatrics/Genetics, 2040 W Charleston Blvd, Ste 401, Las Vegas, NV 89102; **Phone:** 702-671-2200; **Board Cert:** Pediatrics 1986; Clinical Genetics 1987; **Med School:** Loyola Univ-Stritch Sch Med 1981; **Resid:** Pediatrics, Phoenix Hosp 1984; **Fellow:** Clinical Genetics, Univ Utah Sch Med 1986; **Fac Appt:** Prof Ped, Univ Nevada

Nussbaum, Robert MD [CG] - **Spec Exp:** Genetic Disorders; **Hospital:** UCSF Med Ctr; **Address:** Institute of Human Genetics, 513 Parnassus Ave, Box 0794, rm HSE901E, San Francisco, CA 94143-0794; **Phone:** 415-476-1127; **Board Cert:** Internal Medicine 1978; Clinical Genetics 1982; Clinical Molecular Genetics 2004; **Med School:** Harvard Med Sch 1975; **Resid:** Internal Medicine, Barnes Hosp 1978; **Fellow:** Clinical Genetics, Baylor Univ 1983

Pagon, Roberta Anderson MD [CG] - **Spec Exp:** Eye Diseases-Hereditary; Sexual Differentiation Disorders; **Hospital:** Chldns Hosp and Regl Med Ctr - Seattle; **Address:** Chldns Hosp & Reg Med Ctr, PO Box 5371, MS M2-9, Seattle, WA 98105-3901; **Phone:** 206-987-2056; **Board Cert:** Pediatrics 1978; Clinical Genetics 1982; **Med School:** Harvard Med Sch 1972; **Resid:** Pediatrics, Univ Wash Affil Hosp 1975; **Fellow:** Clinical Genetics, Univ Wash 1979; **Fac Appt:** Prof Ped, Univ Wash

Randolph, Linda M MD [CG] - **Spec Exp:** Dysmorphology; Neurocutaneous Disorders; Prenatal Diagnosis; **Hospital:** Chldns Hosp - Los Angeles (page 56); **Address:** Chldns Hosp Los Angeles-Div Med Genetics, 4650 Sunset Blvd, MS 90, Los Angeles, CA 90027; **Phone:** 323-669-2178; **Board Cert:** Pediatrics 1987; Clinical Genetics 1987; Clinical Cytogenetics 1990; **Med School:** Geo Wash Univ 1982; **Resid:** Pediatrics, Chldns Natl Med Ctr 1985; **Fellow:** Clinical Molecular Genetics, Harbor-UCLA Med Ctr 1989; **Fac Appt:** Asst Prof Ped, USC-Keck School of Medicine

Rimoin, David L MD/PhD [CG] - **Spec Exp:** Skeletal Dysplasia; Marfan's Syndrome; Birth Defects; **Hospital:** Cedars-Sinai Med Ctr; **Address:** Cedars-Sinai Med Ctr, Med Genetics Inst, 8700 Beverly Blvd, Ste 665W, Los Angeles, CA 90048; **Phone:** 310-423-4461; **Board Cert:** Internal Medicine 1968; Clinical Genetics 1984; **Med School:** McGill Univ 1961; **Resid:** Internal Medicine, Royal Victoria Hosp 1963; Internal Medicine, Johns Hopkins Hosp 1964; **Fellow:** Clinical Genetics, Johns Hopkins Hosp 1967; **Fac Appt:** Prof Ped, UCLA

Seaver, Laurie H MD [CG] - **Spec Exp:** Birth Defects; Fetal Alcohol Syndrome; Dysmorphology; **Hospital:** Kapiolani Med Ctr for Women & Chldn, Queen's Med Ctr - Honolulu; **Address:** Hawaii Community Genetics, 1441 Kapiolani Blvd, Ste 1800, Honolulu, HI 96814; **Phone:** 808-973-3403; **Board Cert:** Pediatrics 1998; Clinical Genetics 2004; **Med School:** Univ Ariz Coll Med 1987; **Resid:** Pediatrics, Univ Ariz 1990; **Fellow:** Clinical Genetics, Univ Ariz Coll Med 1993

Weitzel, Jeffrey N MD [CG] - **Spec Exp:** Breast Cancer; Ovarian Cancer; Hereditary Cancer; **Hospital:** City of Hope Natl Med Ctr & Beckman Rsch; **Address:** City of Hope Cancer Ctr, 1500 E Duarte Rd, Duarte, CA 91010; **Phone:** 626-256-8662; **Board Cert:** Internal Medicine 1986; Medical Oncology 1989; Clinical Genetics 1996; **Med School:** Univ Minn 1983; **Resid:** Internal Medicine, Univ Minn Hosps 1986; Hematology, Hammersmith Hosp 1987; **Fellow:** Hematology & Oncology, Tufts -New England Med Ctr 1992; Clinical Genetics, Tufts-New England Med Ctr 1996; **Fac Appt:** Assoc Clin Prof Med, USC Sch Med

Wilcox, William MD [CG] - **Spec Exp:** Inborn Errors of Metabolism; Skeletal Dysplasia; **Hospital:** Cedars-Sinai Med Ctr; **Address:** Cedars Sinai Med Ctr, Dept Med Genetics, 8700 Beverly Blvd, Ste SSB 122, Los Angeles, CA 90048; **Phone:** 310-423-9914; **Board Cert:** Clinical Genetics 2006; Clinical Biochemical Genetics 2007; Clinical Molecular Genetics 2007; **Med School:** UCLA 1988; **Resid:** Pediatrics, UCLA Med Ctr 1991; **Fellow:** Clinical Genetics, Cedars-Sinai Med Ctr 1994; **Fac Appt:** Assoc Prof Ped, UCLA

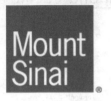

CLINICAL GENETICS

The Clinical Genetics Program at NYU Medical Center offers a comprehensive program of genetic evaluation, counseling, and testing, supported by vital, ongoing research efforts and active treatment protocols. Our integrated team approach includes centralized, easy access to medical geneticists and genetic counselors. We are nationally known for groundbreaking work identifying genetic markers for breast, colorectal, ovarian, and prostate cancer, and assessing cancer risks.

BREAST AND OVARIAN CANCER - a leading participant in the New York Breast Cancer Study and the National Ovarian Cancer Early Detection Program; latest blood test can help identify early indications of ovarian cancer.

COLORECTAL CANCER - diagnostic evaluations followed by tests for identifying high-risk individuals.

PROSTATE CANCER - the latest research and ongoing protocols.

EARLY DETECTION - in the absence of a targeted test, we provide screening tests to identify high-risk patients in need of follow-up care.

COUNSELING - personalized, confidential insight into matters related to prevention, surveillance, and early diagnosis and treatment in a non-judgmental atmosphere.

725

Colon & Rectal Surgery

A colon and rectal surgeon is trained to diagnose and treat various diseases of the intestinal tract, colon, rectum, anal canal and perianal area by medical and surgical means. This specialist also deals with other organs and tissues (such as the liver, urinary and female reproductive system) involved with primary intestinal disease.

Colon and rectal surgeons have the expertise to diagnose and often manage anorectal conditions such as hemorrhoids, fissures (painful tears in the anal lining), abscesses and fistulae (infections located around the anus and rectum) in the office setting. They also treat problems of the intestine and colon and perform endoscopic procedures to evaluate and treat problems such as cancer, polyps (precancerous growths) and inflammatory conditions.

Training Required: Six years (including general surgery)

Colon & Rectal Surgery

New England

Bleday, Ronald MD [CRS] - **Spec Exp:** Colon & Rectal Cancer; **Hospital:** Brigham & Women's Hosp, Dana-Farber Cancer Inst; **Address:** Brigham & Women's Hosp, Dept Genl Surg, 75 Francis St, ASB II, Boston, MA 02115; **Phone:** 617-732-8460; **Board Cert:** Surgery 1999; Colon & Rectal Surgery 2003; **Med School:** McGill Univ 1982; **Resid:** Surgery, Rhode Island Hosp 1989; Surgical Oncology, Brigham & Womens Hosp 1986; **Fellow:** Endoscopy, Mass Genl Hosp 1990; Colon & Rectal Surgery, Univ Minn 1991; **Fac Appt:** Assoc Prof S, Harvard Med Sch

Coller, John MD [CRS] - **Spec Exp:** Colon Cancer; Laparoscopic Surgery; Incontinence-Fecal; Sacral Stimulation/Fecal Incontinence; **Hospital:** Lahey Clin; **Address:** Lahey Clinic-Colon & Rectal Surg, 41 Mall Rd, Burlington, MA 01805; **Phone:** 781-744-8581; **Board Cert:** Surgery 1973; Colon & Rectal Surgery 1973; **Med School:** Univ Pennsylvania 1965; **Resid:** Surgery, Hosp Univ Penn 1972; **Fellow:** Colon & Rectal Surgery, Lahey Clinic Fdn 1973; **Fac Appt:** Asst Clin Prof S, Tufts Univ

Harnsberger, Jeffrey R MD [CRS] - **Spec Exp:** Inflammatory Bowel Disease; Colon & Rectal Cancer; **Hospital:** Dartmouth - Hitchcock Med Ctr; **Address:** Dartmouth-Hitchcock Manchester, 100 Hitchcock Way, Manchester, NH 03104; **Phone:** 603-695-2840; **Board Cert:** Surgery 2001; Colon & Rectal Surgery 2005; **Med School:** Med Coll OH 1987; **Resid:** Surgery, Dartamouth-Hitchkock Med Ctr 1992; **Fellow:** Colon & Rectal Surgery, St Louis Univ Med Ctr 1993; **Fac Appt:** Asst Prof S, Dartmouth Med Sch

Longo, Walter E MD [CRS] - **Spec Exp:** Colon & Rectal Cancer; Gastrointestinal Surgery; Inflammatory Bowel Disease; **Hospital:** Yale - New Haven Hosp; **Address:** Yale Univ School Medicine, Dept Surgery/Gastroenterology, Box 208062, New Haven, CT 06520-8062; **Phone:** 203-785-2616; **Board Cert:** Surgery 2001; Colon & Rectal Surgery 2006; **Med School:** NY Med Coll 1984; **Resid:** Surgery, Yale-New Haven Hosp 1990; **Fellow:** Research, Yale-New Haven Hosp 1988; Colon & Rectal Surgery, Cleveland Clinic 1991; **Fac Appt:** Prof S, Yale Univ

Nagle, Deborah A MD [CRS] - **Hospital:** Beth Israel Deaconess Med Ctr - Boston; **Address:** Beth Israel Deaconess Med Ctr, 330 Brookline Ave Stoneman Bldg - rm 932, Boston, MA 02215; **Phone:** 617-667-4170; **Board Cert:** Colon & Rectal Surgery 2006; Surgery 2004; **Med School:** Thomas Jefferson Univ 1988; **Resid:** Surgery, Thos Jefferson U Hosp 1993; Colon & Rectal Surgery, Thos Jefferson U Hosp 1994

Roberts, Patricia L MD [CRS] - **Spec Exp:** Diverticulitis; Colon & Rectal Cancer; Inflammatory Bowel Disease; **Hospital:** Lahey Clin; **Address:** 41 Mall Rd, Burlington, MA 01805; **Phone:** 781-744-8243; **Board Cert:** Surgery 1996; Colon & Rectal Surgery 2003; **Med School:** Boston Univ 1981; **Resid:** Surgery, Boston City Hosp 1986; **Fellow:** Colon & Rectal Surgery, Lahey Clinic 1988; **Fac Appt:** Assoc Prof S, Tufts Univ

Schoetz, David MD [CRS] - **Spec Exp:** Inflammatory Bowel Disease/Crohn's; Colon & Rectal Cancer; Incontinence-Fecal; Anorectal Disorders; **Hospital:** Lahey Clin; **Address:** Lahey Clinic Med Ctr, Dept Colon & Rectal Surg, 41 Mall Rd, Burlington, MA 01805-0001; **Phone:** 781-744-8889; **Board Cert:** Surgery 2001; Colon & Rectal Surgery 1983; **Med School:** Med Coll Wisc 1974; **Resid:** Surgery, Boston Univ Med Ctr 1981; **Fellow:** Colon & Rectal Surgery, Lahey Clin Med Ctr 1982; **Fac Appt:** Prof S, Tufts Univ

Shellito, Paul C MD [CRS] - **Spec Exp:** Colon & Rectal Cancer; Ulcerative Colitis; Anorectal Disorders; **Hospital:** Mass Genl Hosp; **Address:** 15 Parkman St, Ste 460, Boston, MA 02114-3117; **Phone:** 617-724-0365; **Board Cert:** Surgery 1992; Colon & Rectal Surgery 1994; **Med School:** Harvard Med Sch 1977; **Resid:** Surgery, Mass Genl Hosp 1983; Surgery, Auckland Univ Med Sch 1981; **Fellow:** Colon & Rectal Surgery, Univ Minn 1985; **Fac Appt:** Asst Prof S, Harvard Med Sch

Mid Atlantic

Fry, Robert D MD [CRS] - **Spec Exp:** Colon & Rectal Cancer; Inflammatory Bowel Disease/Crohn's; **Hospital:** Pennsylvania Hosp (page 72), Hosp Univ Penn - UPHS (page 72); **Address:** Pennsylvania Hospital, Div Colon & Rectal Surgery, 700 Spruce St, Ste 305, Philadelphia, PA 19106; **Phone:** 215-829-5333; **Board Cert:** Surgery 1996; Colon & Rectal Surgery 1998; **Med School:** Washington Univ, St Louis 1972; **Resid:** Surgery, Barnes Jewish Hosp 1977; **Fellow:** Colon & Rectal Surgery, Cleveland Clinic 1978; **Fac Appt:** Prof S, Univ Pennsylvania

Gingold, Bruce S MD [CRS] - **Spec Exp:** Colostomy Avoidance; Inflammatory Bowel Disease/Crohn's; Colonoscopy; **Hospital:** St Vincent Cath Med Ctrs - Manhattan, Beth Israel Med Ctr - Petrie Division; **Address:** 36 7th Ave, Ste 522, New York, NY 10011-6600; **Phone:** 212-675-2997; **Board Cert:** Colon & Rectal Surgery 1976; Surgery 1977; **Med School:** Jefferson Med Coll 1970; **Resid:** Surgery, St Vincent's Hosp & Med Ctr 1975; **Fellow:** Colon & Rectal Surgery, Cleveland Clinic 1976; **Fac Appt:** Assoc Clin Prof S, NY Med Coll

Gorfine, Stephen MD [CRS] - **Spec Exp:** Anal Disorders & Reconstruction; Hemorrhoids; Rectal Cancer; Anal Cancer; **Hospital:** Mount Sinai Med Ctr, Lenox Hill Hosp (page 62); **Address:** 25 E 69th St, New York, NY 10021-4925; **Phone:** 212-517-8600; **Board Cert:** Internal Medicine 1981; Surgery 1996; Colon & Rectal Surgery 1988; **Med School:** Univ Mass Sch Med 1978; **Resid:** Internal Medicine, Mount Sinai Hosp 1981; Surgery, Mount Sinai Hosp 1985; **Fellow:** Colon & Rectal Surgery, Ferguson Hosp 1987; **Fac Appt:** Clin Prof S, Mount Sinai Sch Med

Guillem, Jose MD [CRS] - **Spec Exp:** Colon & Rectal Cancer; Rectal Cancer/Sphincter Preservation; Minimally Invasive Surgery; Colon & Rectal Cancer-Familial Polyposis; **Hospital:** Meml Sloan Kettering Cancer Ctr; **Address:** Meml Sloan Kettering Cancer Ctr, 1275 York Ave, rm C1077, New York, NY 10021; **Phone:** 212-639-8278; **Board Cert:** Colon & Rectal Surgery 2004; Surgery 2004; **Med School:** Yale Univ 1983; **Resid:** Surgery, Columbia-Presby Med Ctr 1990; **Fellow:** Colon & Rectal Surgery, Lahey Clinic 1991; **Fac Appt:** Prof CRS, Cornell Univ-Weill Med Coll

Medich, David MD [CRS] - **Spec Exp:** Colon & Rectal Cancer; Ulcerative Colitis; Inflammatory Bowel Disease/Crohn's; **Hospital:** Allegheny General Hosp; **Address:** Allegheny General Hosp, South Tower, 320 E North Ave Fl 5, Pittsburgh, PA 15212; **Phone:** 412-359-3901; **Board Cert:** Surgery 2004; Colon & Rectal Surgery 2006; **Med School:** Ohio State Univ 1987; **Resid:** Surgery, Univ Pittsburgh Med Ctr 1990; **Fellow:** Research, Univ Pittsburgh 1993; Colon & Rectal Surgery, Cleveland Clin Fdn 1994; **Fac Appt:** Assoc Prof CRS, Drexel Univ Coll Med

Milsom, Jeffrey W MD [CRS] - **Spec Exp:** Inflammatory Bowel Disease; Laparoscopic Surgery; Colon & Rectal Cancer; Crohn's Disease; **Hospital:** NY-Presby Hosp/Columbia (page 66); **Address:** NY Cornell Med Ctr, Div Colorectal Surgery, 1315 York Ave Fl 2, New York, NY 10021-4870; **Phone:** 212-746-6030; **Board Cert:** Colon & Rectal Surgery 1986; **Med School:** Univ Pittsburgh 1979; **Resid:** Surgery, Roosevelt Hosp 1981; Surgery, Univ Virginia Med Ctr 1984; **Fellow:** Colon & Rectal Surgery, Ferguson Hosp 1985; **Fac Appt:** Prof S, Columbia P&S

Rombeau, John L MD [CRS] - **Spec Exp:** Colon & Rectal Cancer; Crohn's Disease; Ulcerative Colitis; **Hospital:** Temple Univ Hosp; **Address:** Department of Surgery, 3401 N Broad St, Parkinson Pavilion Fl 4, Philadelphia, PA 19104; **Phone:** 215-707-3133; **Board Cert:** Colon & Rectal Surgery 1977; **Med School:** Loma Linda Univ 1967; **Resid:** Surgery, Good Samaritan Hosp 1971; Surgery, LAC-USC Med Ctr 1975; **Fellow:** Colon & Rectal Surgery, Cleveland Clinic 1976; **Fac Appt:** Prof S, Temple Univ

Smith, Lee MD [CRS] - **Spec Exp:** Colon & Rectal Cancer; Inflammatory Bowel Disease/Crohn's; Anorectal Disorders; **Hospital:** Washington Hosp Ctr, Georgetown Univ Hosp; **Address:** 106 Irving St NW, Ste 2100, Washington, DC 20010-2975; **Phone:** 202-877-8484; **Board Cert:** Surgery 1971; Colon & Rectal Surgery 1973; **Med School:** UCSF 1962; **Resid:** Surgery, Naval Hosp 1970; Colon & Rectal Surgery, Univ Minn 1973; **Fac Appt:** Prof S, Georgetown Univ

Steinhagen, Randolph MD [CRS] - **Spec Exp:** Colostomy Avoidance; Colon & Rectal Cancer; Inflammatory Bowel Disease/Crohn's; **Hospital:** Mount Sinai Med Ctr; **Address:** Div Colon & Rectal Surgery, 5 E 98th St Fl 14, Box 1259, New York, NY 10029-6501; **Phone:** 212-241-3547; **Board Cert:** Surgery 2002; Colon & Rectal Surgery 1985; **Med School:** Wayne State Univ 1977; **Resid:** Surgery, Mount Sinai Hosp 1982; **Fellow:** Colon & Rectal Surgery, Cleveland Clinic 1983; **Fac Appt:** Assoc Prof S, Mount Sinai Sch Med

Whelan, Richard L MD [CRS] - **Spec Exp:** Laparoscopic Surgery; Colon & Rectal Cancer; **Hospital:** NY-Presby Hosp/Columbia (page 66); **Address:** 161 Ft Washington Ave, rm 820, New York, NY 10032; **Phone:** 212-342-1155; **Board Cert:** Surgery 1997; Colon & Rectal Surgery 1989; **Med School:** Columbia P&S 1982; **Resid:** Surgery, Columbia Presby Hosp 1987; **Fellow:** Colon & Rectal Surgery, Univ Minn Med Ctr 1988; **Fac Appt:** Assoc Clin Prof S, Columbia P&S

Wong, W Douglas MD [CRS] - **Spec Exp:** Rectal Cancer/Sphincter Preservation; Colon & Rectal Cancer; Anal Disorders & Reconstruction; **Hospital:** Meml Sloan Kettering Cancer Ctr; **Address:** Meml Sloan Kettering Cancer Ctr, 1275 York Ave, rm C-1067, New York, NY 10021-6094; **Phone:** 212-639-5117; **Board Cert:** Surgery 1997; Colon & Rectal Surgery 2004; **Med School:** Canada 1972; **Resid:** Surgery, Univ Manitoba Hosp 1977; **Fellow:** Colon & Rectal Surgery, Univ Minn Med Ctr 1984; **Fac Appt:** Prof S, Cornell Univ-Weill Med Coll

Southeast

Foley, Eugene F MD [CRS] - **Spec Exp:** Colon & Rectal Cancer; Ulcerative Colitis; **Hospital:** Univ Virginia Med Ctr; **Address:** Univ Va Hlth Sys, Dept Surg, PO Box 800709, Charlottesville, VA 22908-0709; **Phone:** 434-924-9304; **Board Cert:** Surgery 1993; Colon & Rectal Surgery 1994; **Med School:** Harvard Med Sch 1985; **Resid:** Surgery, New England Deaconess Hosp 1991; **Fellow:** Colon & Rectal Surgery, Lahey Clinic 1993; **Fac Appt:** Assoc Prof S, Univ VA Sch Med

Galandiuk, Susan MD [CRS] - **Spec Exp:** Colon & Rectal Cancer; Inflammatory Bowel Disease/Crohn's; **Hospital:** Univ of Louisville Hosp, Norton Hosp; **Address:** 601 S Floyd St, Ste 700, Louisville, KY 40202; **Phone:** 502-583-8303; **Board Cert:** Surgery 1998; Colon & Rectal Surgery 1999; **Med School:** Germany 1982; **Resid:** Surgery, Cleveland Clinic Fdn 1988; **Fellow:** Research, Univ Louisville Hosp 1989; Colon & Rectal Surgery, Mayo Clinic 1990; **Fac Appt:** Prof CRS, Univ Louisville Sch Med

Golub, Richard MD [CRS] - **Spec Exp:** Colon & Rectal Cancer; Laparoscopic Surgery; Hemorrhoids; **Hospital:** Sarasota Meml Hosp, Doctors Hosp - Sarasota; **Address:** Sarasota Memorial Hospital, 3333 Cattlemen Rd, Ste 206, Sarasota, FL 34232; **Phone:** 941-341-0042; **Board Cert:** Surgery 2000; Colon & Rectal Surgery 2003; **Med School:** Albert Einstein Coll Med 1984; **Resid:** Surgery, Univ Hosp Stony Brook 1990; **Fellow:** Colon & Rectal Surgery, Grant Medical Center 1991

Hartmann, Rene MD [CRS] - **Spec Exp:** Laparoscopic Surgery; Rectovaginal Fistula; Colon Cancer; Inflammatory Bowel Disease; **Hospital:** Baptist Hosp of Miami, Doctors' Hosp; **Address:** 3661 S Miami Ave, Ste 301, Miami, FL 33133; **Phone:** 305-285-2787; **Board Cert:** Colon & Rectal Surgery 1994; **Med School:** Venezuela 1971; **Resid:** Surgery, Jackson Meml Hosp 1976; Surgery, Orange Meml Hosp 1977; **Fellow:** Colon & Rectal Surgery, Grant Hosp 1978; **Fac Appt:** Assoc Clin Prof S, Univ Miami Sch Med

Ludwig, Kirk A MD [CRS] - **Spec Exp:** Colon & Rectal Cancer & Surgery; Pelvic Organ Prolapse; Rectal Cancer/Sphincter Preservation; Incontinence-Fecal; **Hospital:** Duke Univ Med Ctr; **Address:** Duke University Medical Ctr-Dept Surgery, Box 3262, Durham, NC 27710; **Phone:** 919-681-3977; **Board Cert:** Colon & Rectal Surgery 1998; Surgery 2005; **Med School:** Univ Cincinnati 1988; **Resid:** Surgery, Med Coll Wisc 1994; **Fellow:** Colon & Rectal Surgery, Cleveland Clinic 1996; **Fac Appt:** Asst Prof S, Duke Univ

Marcet, Jorge MD [CRS] - **Spec Exp:** Colon & Rectal Cancer; **Hospital:** H Lee Moffitt Cancer Ctr & Research Inst, Tampa Genl Hosp; **Address:** H Lee Moffitt Cancer Ctr, Ste F145, Box 1289, Tampa, FL 33601; **Phone:** 813-844-4545; **Board Cert:** Colon & Rectal Surgery 2003; Surgery 2001; **Med School:** Cornell Univ-Weill Med Coll 1985; **Resid:** Surgery, St Luke's-Roosevelt Hospt Ctr 1990; **Fellow:** Colon & Rectal Surgery, Columbia Presbyterian Hosp 1990; Colon & Rectal Surgery, St Luke's-Roosevelt Hosp Ctr 1991; **Fac Appt:** Assoc Prof S, Univ S Fla Coll Med

Nogueras, Juan J MD [CRS] - **Spec Exp:** Colon & Rectal Cancer; Inflammatory Bowel Disease/Crohn's; Incontinence-Fecal; **Hospital:** Cleveland Clin - Weston (page 57); **Address:** Cleveland Clinic, Dept Colorectal Surgery, 2950 Cleveland Clinic Blvd, Weston, FL 33331; **Phone:** 954-659-5251; **Board Cert:** Surgery 1997; Colon & Rectal Surgery 2003; **Med School:** Jefferson Med Coll 1982; **Resid:** Surgery, Columbia Presby Med Ctr 1987; **Fellow:** Colon & Rectal Surgery, Univ Minn Med Ctr 1991

Vernava III, Anthony M MD [CRS] - **Spec Exp:** Colon & Rectal Cancer; Incontinence-Fecal; Inflammatory Bowel Disease; **Hospital:** Physicians Regl Med Ctr; **Address:** Medical Surgical Specialists, 6101 Pine Ridge Rd, Naples, FL 34119; **Phone:** 239-348-4000; **Board Cert:** Surgery 1997; Colon & Rectal Surgery 1989; **Med School:** St Louis Univ 1982; **Resid:** Surgery, St Louis Univ Med Ctr 1988; Colon & Rectal Surgery, Univ Minnesota Med Ctr 1989; **Fellow:** Colon & Rectal Surgery, St Marks Hosp 1990

Wexner, Steven MD [CRS] - **Spec Exp:** Colon & Rectal Cancer; Inflammatory Bowel Disease/Crohn's; Laparoscopic Surgery; **Hospital:** Cleveland Clin - Weston (page 57); **Address:** 2950 Cleveland Clinic Blvd, Weston, FL 33331-3609; **Phone:** 954-659-5278; **Board Cert:** Surgery 2005; Colon & Rectal Surgery 2006; **Med School:** Cornell Univ-Weill Med Coll 1982; **Resid:** Surgery, Roosevelt Hosp 1987; **Fellow:** Colon & Rectal Surgery, Univ Minn 1988; **Fac Appt:** Prof S, Cleveland Cl Coll Med/Case West Res

Colon & Rectal Surgery

Midwest

Abcarian, Herand MD [CRS] - **Spec Exp:** Rectal Cancer/Sphincter Preservation; Inflammatory Bowel Disease; Anorectal Disorders; Incontinence-Fecal; **Hospital:** Univ of IL Med Ctr at Chicago, Gottlieb Meml Hosp; **Address:** 675 W North Ave, Ste 406, Melrose Park, IL 60160; **Phone:** 708-450-5075; **Board Cert:** Surgery 1972; Colon & Rectal Surgery 1972; **Med School:** Iran 1965; **Resid:** Surgery, Cook County Hosp 1971; Colon & Rectal Surgery, Cook County Hosp 1972; **Fac Appt:** Prof S, Univ IL Coll Med

Delaney, Conor P MD/PhD [CRS] - **Spec Exp:** Laparoscopic Surgery; Colon & Rectal Cancer; Inflammatory Bowel Disease/Crohn's; **Hospital:** Univ Hosps Case Med Ctr; **Address:** Univ Hosp of Cleveland, 11100 Euclid Ave, MS 5047, Cleveland, OH 44106-5047; **Phone:** 216-844-8087; **Board Cert:** Surgery 1998; Colon & Rectal Surgery 1998; **Med School:** Ireland 1989; **Resid:** Surgery, Univ Hosp 1993; Surgery, Univ Hosp 1999; **Fellow:** Research, Univ of Pittsburgh 1995; Colon & Rectal Surgery, Cleveland Clinic 2000; **Fac Appt:** Prof S, Cleveland Cl Coll Med/Case West Res

Fleshman, James MD [CRS] - **Spec Exp:** Colon & Rectal Cancer; Laparoscopic Surgery; Inflammatory Bowel Disease; **Hospital:** Barnes-Jewish Hosp, Barnes-Jewish West County Hosp; **Address:** Wash Univ Sch Med, Div Col Rectal Surgery, 660 S Euclid Ave, Box 8109, St Louis, MO 63110; **Phone:** 314-454-7177; **Board Cert:** Colon & Rectal Surgery 1988; Surgery 1996; **Med School:** Washington Univ, St Louis 1980; **Resid:** Surgery, Jewish Hospital 1986; **Fellow:** Colon & Rectal Surgery, Univ Toronto 1987; **Fac Appt:** Prof S, Washington Univ, St Louis

Kodner, Ira J MD [CRS] - **Spec Exp:** Colon & Rectal Cancer; Inflammatory Bowel Disease/Crohn's; Laparoscopic Surgery; **Hospital:** Barnes-Jewish Hosp; **Address:** Wash Univ Sch Med, Div Col Rectal Surgery, 660 S Euclid Ave, Box 8109, St. Louis, MO 63110; **Phone:** 314-454-7177; **Board Cert:** Surgery 1975; Colon & Rectal Surgery 1975; **Med School:** Washington Univ, St Louis 1967; **Resid:** Surgery, Barnes-Jewish Hosp 1974; **Fellow:** Colon & Rectal Surgery, Cleveland Clinic 1975; **Fac Appt:** Prof S, Washington Univ, St Louis

Lavery, Ian C MD [CRS] - **Spec Exp:** Colon & Rectal Cancer; Inflammatory Bowel Disease; Pediatric Gastrointestinal Surgery; **Hospital:** Cleveland Clin Fdn (page 57); **Address:** Cleveland Clinic, Desk A30, 9500 Euclid Ave, Cleveland, OH 44195; **Phone:** 216-444-6930; **Board Cert:** Colon & Rectal Surgery 1998; **Med School:** Australia 1967; **Resid:** Surgery, Princess Alexandra Hosp 1974; Colon & Rectal Surgery, Cleveland Clinic 1977; **Fac Appt:** Prof S, Case West Res Univ

Lowry, Ann C MD [CRS] - **Spec Exp:** Anal Sphincter Repair; Rectovaginal Fistula; Inflammatory Bowel Disease; **Hospital:** Abbott - Northwestern Hosp, Fairview Southdale Hosp; **Address:** 6363 France Ave S, Ste 212, Edina, MN 55435; **Phone:** 651-312-1700; **Board Cert:** Surgery 1993; Colon & Rectal Surgery 1988; **Med School:** Tufts Univ 1977; **Resid:** Surgery, New Eng Med Ctr Hosps 1982; **Fellow:** Colon & Rectal Surgery, Univ Minn Affil Hosps 1987; **Fac Appt:** Clin Prof S, Univ Minn

MacKeigan, John MD [CRS] - **Spec Exp:** Rectal Cancer; Anal Surgery; Ulcerative Colitis; **Hospital:** Spectrum Hlth Blodgett Campus, Spectrum Hlth Butterworth Campus; **Address:** The Ferguson Clinic, 4100 Lake SE, Ste 205, Grand Rapids, MI 49546-8292; **Phone:** 616-356-4100; **Board Cert:** Colon & Rectal Surgery 1974; **Med School:** Dalhousie Univ 1969; **Resid:** Surgery, Dalhousie Univ 1973; Colon & Rectal Surgery, Ferguson Hosp 1974; **Fac Appt:** Assoc Prof S, Mich State Univ

Madoff, Robert D MD [CRS] - **Spec Exp:** Colon & Rectal Cancer; Inflammatory Bowel Disease; Incontinence/Pelvic Floor Disorders; **Hospital:** Univ Minn Med Ctr, Fairview - Univ Campus; **Address:** 420 Delaware St SE, MMC 450, Minneapolis, MN 55455; **Phone:** 612-624-9708; **Board Cert:** Surgery 1995; Colon & Rectal Surgery 2002; **Med School:** Columbia P&S 1979; **Resid:** Surgery, Univ Minn Hosps 1987; **Fellow:** Colon & Rectal Surgery, Univ Minn Hosps 1988; **Fac Appt:** Prof S, Univ Minn

Nelson, Heidi MD [CRS] - **Spec Exp:** Colon & Rectal Cancer; Gastrointestinal Cancer; **Hospital:** Mayo Med Ctr & Clin - Rochester, Rochester Meth Hosp; **Address:** Mayo Clinic, Div Colon & Rectal Surg, 200 First St SW, Rochester, MN 55905; **Phone:** 507-284-3329; **Board Cert:** Surgery 1995; Colon & Rectal Surgery 1989; **Med School:** Univ Wash 1981; **Resid:** Surgery, Oregon Hlth Sci Univ Hosp 1987; Colon & Rectal Surgery, Oregon Hlth Sci Univ Hosp 1985; **Fellow:** Colon & Rectal Surgery, Mayo Clinic 1988; **Fac Appt:** Prof S, Mayo Med Sch

Pemberton, John MD [CRS] - **Spec Exp:** Rectal Surgery; Inflammatory Bowel Disease/Crohn's; Colon & Rectal Cancer; **Hospital:** St Mary's Hosp - Rochester, Rochester Meth Hosp; **Address:** Mayo Clinic, Div Colon & Rectal Surg, 200 First St SW, Gonda 9-S, Rochester, MN 55905; **Phone:** 507-284-2359; **Board Cert:** Surgery 2001; Colon & Rectal Surgery 1985; **Med School:** Tulane Univ 1976; **Resid:** Surgery, Mayo Clinic 1983; **Fellow:** Colon & Rectal Surgery, Mayo Clinic 1984; **Fac Appt:** Prof S, Mayo Med Sch

Rafferty, Janice F MD [CRS] - **Spec Exp:** Colon & Rectal Cancer; Ulcerative Colitis; Crohn's Disease; Anal Disorders & Reconstruction; **Hospital:** Univ Hosp - Cincinnati; **Address:** U of Cincinnati, Colon & Rectal Surgery, 2123 Auburn Ave, Ste 524, Cincinnati, OH 45219; **Phone:** 513-929-0104; **Board Cert:** Colon & Rectal Surgery 2007; Surgery 2004; **Med School:** Ohio State Univ 1988; **Resid:** Surgery, Univ CincinnatiHosp 1995; Colon & Rectal Surgery, Barnes Jewish Hosp 1996; **Fac Appt:** Assoc Prof S, Univ Cincinnati

Rothenberger, David A MD [CRS] - **Spec Exp:** Colon & Rectal Cancer; **Hospital:** Univ Minn Med Ctr, Fairview - Univ Campus; **Address:** Dept Surg, 420 Delaware St SE, MMC 195, Minneapolis, MN 55455; **Phone:** 612-626-6666; **Board Cert:** Colon & Rectal Surgery 2005; **Med School:** Tufts Univ 1973; **Resid:** Surgery, St Paul-Ramsey Med Ctr 1978; **Fellow:** Colon & Rectal Surgery, Univ Minnesota Hosps 1979; **Fac Appt:** Prof S, Univ Minn

Saclarides, Theodore J MD [CRS] - **Spec Exp:** Rectal Cancer/Sphincter Preservation; Incontinence-Fecal; Inflammatory Bowel Disease; **Hospital:** Rush Univ Med Ctr, Rush N Shore Med Ctr; **Address:** University Surgeons, 1725 W Harrison St, Ste 810, Chicago, IL 60612-3832; **Phone:** 312-942-6543; **Board Cert:** Surgery 1996; Colon & Rectal Surgery 1989; **Med School:** Univ Miami Sch Med 1982; **Resid:** Surgery, Rush Presby-St Luke's Hosp 1987; **Fellow:** Colon & Rectal Surgery, Mayo Clinic 1988; **Fac Appt:** Prof S, Rush Med Coll

Senagore, Anthony MD [CRS] - **Spec Exp:** Laparoscopic Surgery; Colon & Rectal Cancer; Anorectal Disorders; Inflammatory Bowel Disease/Crohn's; **Hospital:** Spectrum Hlth Blodgett Campus; **Address:** Spectrum Health, 100 Michigan St NE, MC 005, Grand Rapids, MI 49503; **Phone:** 616-391-2467; **Board Cert:** Surgery 1995; Colon & Rectal Surgery 2001; **Med School:** Mich State Univ 1981; **Resid:** Surgery, Butterworth Hosp 1987; Colon & Rectal Surgery, Ferguson Hosp 1989; **Fac Appt:** Prof S, Med Univ Ohio at Toledo

Colon & Rectal Surgery

Stryker, Steven J MD [CRS] - **Spec Exp:** Colon & Rectal Cancer; Inflammatory Bowel Disease; Laparoscopic Surgery; **Hospital:** Northwestern Meml Hosp; **Address:** 676 N Saint Clair St, Ste 1525A, Chicago, IL 60611-2862; **Phone:** 312-943-5427; **Board Cert:** Surgery 2004; Colon & Rectal Surgery 1986; **Med School:** Northwestern Univ 1978; **Resid:** Surgery, Northwestern Meml Hosp 1983; **Fellow:** Colon & Rectal Surgery, Mayo Clinic 1985; **Fac Appt:** Clin Prof S, Northwestern Univ

Wolff, Bruce G MD [CRS] - **Spec Exp:** Inflammatory Bowel Disease; Crohn's Disease; Colon & Rectal Cancer; **Hospital:** Mayo Med Ctr & Clin - Rochester; **Address:** Mayo Clinic, Div Colon & Rectal Surg, 200 First St SW, Rochester, MN 55905; **Phone:** 507-284-0800; **Board Cert:** Surgery 2000; Colon & Rectal Surgery 2001; **Med School:** Duke Univ 1973; **Resid:** Surgery, NY Hosp-Cornell Med Ctr 1981; **Fellow:** Colon & Rectal Surgery, Mayo Clinic 1982; **Fac Appt:** Prof S, Mayo Med Sch

Great Plains and Mountains

Thorson, Alan MD [CRS] - **Spec Exp:** Colon & Rectal Cancer; Laparoscopic Surgery; Incontinence-Fecal; **Hospital:** Nebraska Meth Hosp, Archbishop Bergen Mercy Med Ctr; **Address:** 9850 Nicholas St, Ste 100, Omaha, NE 68114-2191; **Phone:** 402-343-1122; **Board Cert:** Surgery 1994; Colon & Rectal Surgery 1999; **Med School:** Univ Nebr Coll Med 1979; **Resid:** Surgery, Univ Nebraska 1984; Colon & Rectal Surgery, Univ Minn 1985; **Fac Appt:** Assoc Clin Prof S, Creighton Univ

Southwest

Adkins, Terrance P MD [CRS] - **Spec Exp:** Colon & Rectal Cancer; Inflammatory Bowel Disease; **Hospital:** Tucson Med Ctr; **Address:** Southwestern Surgery Assoc, 1951 N Wilmot Rd Bldg 2, Tucson, AZ 85712; **Phone:** 520-795-5845; **Board Cert:** Surgery 2001; Colon & Rectal Surgery 2004; **Med School:** Univ Tex SW, Dallas 1985; **Resid:** Surgery, Univ Utah Med Ctr 1991; **Fellow:** Colon & Rectal Surgery, Univ Texas Med Ctr 1992; **Fac Appt:** Asst Clin Prof S, Univ Ariz Coll Med

Bailey, Harold Randolph MD [CRS] - **Spec Exp:** Rectal Cancer/Sphincter Preservation; Inflammatory Bowel Disease; Incontinence-Fecal; Endometriosis-Intestine; **Hospital:** Methodist Hosp - Houston, St Luke's Episcopal Hosp - Houston; **Address:** Colon & Rectal Clinic, Smith Twr, 6550 Fannin St, Ste 2307, Houston, TX 77030-2717; **Phone:** 713-790-9250; **Board Cert:** Surgery 1974; Colon & Rectal Surgery 2004; **Med School:** Univ Tex SW, Dallas 1968; **Resid:** Surgery, Hermann Hosp-Univ Tex Med Sch 1973; **Fellow:** Colon & Rectal Surgery, Ferguson-Droste Hosp 1974; **Fac Appt:** Clin Prof S, Univ Tex, Houston

Beck, David E MD [CRS] - **Spec Exp:** Colon & Rectal Cancer; Minimally Invasive Surgery; Inflammatory Bowel Disease; **Hospital:** Ochsner Fdn Hosp, Summit Hosp-Baton Rouge; **Address:** Ochsner Clinic Fdn, Colorectal Surgery, 1514 Jefferson Hwy, 4th Fl, rm 04 East, New Orleans, LA 70121; **Phone:** 504-842-4060; **Board Cert:** Colon & Rectal Surgery 1987; **Med School:** Univ Miami Sch Med 1979; **Resid:** Surgery, Wilford Hall USAF Med Ctr 1984; **Fellow:** Colon & Rectal Surgery, Cleveland Clinic Fdn 1986; **Fac Appt:** Assoc Clin Prof S, Louisiana State Univ

Efron, Jonathan E MD [CRS] - **Spec Exp:** Colon & Rectal Cancer; Incontinence-Fecal; Inflammatory Bowel Disease; Anorectal Disorders; **Hospital:** Mayo Clin Hosp - Scottsdale; **Address:** Mayo Clinic, Concourse B, 13400 E Shea Blvd, Scottsdale, AZ 85259; **Phone:** 480-342-2697; **Board Cert:** Surgery 1999; Colon & Rectal Surgery 2000; **Med School:** Univ MD Sch Med 1993; **Resid:** Surgery, LIJ Medical Ctr 1999; **Fellow:** Colon & Rectal Surgery, Cleveland Clinic 2000; Research, Cleveland Clinic 2001; **Fac Appt:** Assoc Prof S, Mayo Med Sch

Heppell, Jacques P MD [CRS] - **Spec Exp:** Colon & Rectal Cancer; Inflammatory Bowel Disease; Anorectal Disorders; **Hospital:** Mayo - Phoenix; **Address:** Mayo Clinic, ATTN: GENS/CB/Distribution 13, 5777 E Mayo Blvd, Phoenix, AZ 85259-5404; **Phone:** 480-342-2697; **Board Cert:** Surgery 2004; Colon & Rectal Surgery 1995; **Med School:** Univ Montreal 1974; **Resid:** Surgery, Univ Montreal Med Ctr 1979; **Fellow:** Colon & Rectal Surgery, Mayo Clinic 1983; **Fac Appt:** Prof S, Mayo Med Sch

Huber Jr, Philip J MD [CRS] - **Spec Exp:** Colon & Rectal Cancer; Inflammatory Bowel Disease; **Hospital:** Med City Dallas Hosp, Presby Hosp of Dallas; **Address:** 7777 Forest Lane, Ste C-760, Dallas, TX 75230; **Phone:** 972-566-8039; **Board Cert:** Surgery 1997; Colon & Rectal Surgery 1993; **Med School:** Columbia P&S 1972; **Resid:** Surgery, Parkland Hosp 1977; Colon & Rectal Surgery, Presby Hosp 1978

West Coast and Pacific

Beart Jr, Robert W MD [CRS] - **Spec Exp:** Colon & Rectal Cancer; Inflammatory Bowel Disease/Crohn's; **Hospital:** USC Norris Comp Cancer Ctr, USC Univ Hosp - R K Eamer Med Plz; **Address:** USC Comprehensive Cancer Center, Topping Tower Suite 7418, 1441 Eastlake Ave, Los Angeles, CA 90033; **Phone:** 323-865-3690; **Board Cert:** Surgery 1993; Colon & Rectal Surgery 1995; **Med School:** Harvard Med Sch 1971; **Resid:** Surgery, Univ Colo Med Ctr 1976; Colon & Rectal Surgery, Mayo Clinic 1978; **Fellow:** Transplant Surgery, Univ Colo Med Ctr 1975; **Fac Appt:** Prof S, USC Sch Med

Coutsoftides, Theodore MD [CRS] - **Spec Exp:** Laparoscopic Surgery; Inflammatory Bowel Disease; Anal Sphincter Repair; **Hospital:** St Joseph's Hosp - Orange; **Address:** 1310 W Stewart, Ste 605, Orange, CA 92868-3857; **Phone:** 714-532-2544; **Board Cert:** Colon & Rectal Surgery 1977; **Med School:** Israel 1970; **Resid:** Surgery, Cleveland Clinic 1973; Surgery, Royal Victoria Hosp 1976; **Fellow:** Colon & Rectal Surgery, Cleveland Clinic 1977; **Fac Appt:** Assoc Prof S, UC Irvine

Stamos, Michael J MD [CRS] - **Spec Exp:** Rectal Cancer/Sphincter Preservation; Laparoscopic Surgery; Inflammatory Bowel Disease; Colon & Rectal Cancer; **Hospital:** UC Irvine Med Ctr; **Address:** UC Irvine Med Ctr, Div Colon & Rectal Surg, 333 City Blvd W, Ste 850, Orange, CA 92868; **Phone:** 714-456-8511; **Board Cert:** Surgery 2000; Colon & Rectal Surgery 2003; **Med School:** Case West Res Univ 1985; **Resid:** Surgery, Jackson Meml Hosp 1990; Colon & Rectal Surgery, Ochsner Clinic 1991; **Fac Appt:** Prof S, UC Irvine

Volpe, Peter A MD [CRS] - **Spec Exp:** Colon Cancer; Colonoscopy; Anorectal Disorders; **Hospital:** CA Pacific Med Ctr - Pacific Campus, St Mary's Med Ctr - San Fran; **Address:** 3838 California St, Ste 616, San Francisco, CA 94118; **Phone:** 415-668-0411; **Board Cert:** Surgery 1970; Colon & Rectal Surgery 1971; **Med School:** Ohio State Univ 1961; **Resid:** Surgery, UCSF Hosps 1969; Colon & Rectal Surgery, ABCRS Preceptorship 1971; **Fac Appt:** Clin Prof S, UCSF

Welton, Mark L MD [CRS] - **Spec Exp:** Ulcerative Colitis; Crohn's Disease; Colon & Rectal Cancer; Anal Cancer; **Hospital:** Stanford Univ Med Ctr; **Address:** Stanford Univ - Colon & Rectal Surgery, 300 Pasteur Drive, rm H 3680, Stanford, CA 94305-5655; **Phone:** 650-723-5461; **Board Cert:** Surgery 2000; Colon & Rectal Surgery 2005; **Med School:** UCLA 1984; **Resid:** Surgery, UCLA Med Ctr 1992; **Fellow:** Colon & Rectal Surgery, Barnes Jewish Hosp 1993; **Fac Appt:** Assoc Prof S, Stanford Univ

Wong, Ronald J MD [CRS] - **Spec Exp:** Laparoscopic Surgery; **Hospital:** Queen's Med Ctr - Honolulu; **Address:** Queen's Physicians' Office Bldg 1, 1380 Lusitana St, Ste 614, Honolulu, HI 96813; **Phone:** 808-524-1856; **Board Cert:** Surgery 1997; **Med School:** Univ Hawaii JA Burns Sch Med 1981; **Resid:** Surgery, Univ Hawaii 1985; Surgery, Catholic Med Ctr 1987; **Fellow:** Colon & Rectal Surgery, Suburban Hosp 1989; Research, Cornell Univ Med Ctr 1988; **Fac Appt:** Clin Prof S, Univ Hawaii JA Burns Sch Med

Worsey, M Jonathan MD [CRS] - **Spec Exp:** Colon & Rectal Cancer; Inflammatory Bowel Disease; **Hospital:** Scripps Meml Hosp - La Jolla; **Address:** Advanced Surgical Associates, 9850 Genesee Ave, Ste 640, La Jolla, CA 92037; **Phone:** 858-558-2272; **Board Cert:** Surgery 1998; Colon & Rectal Surgery 1999; **Med School:** England 1985; **Resid:** Surgery, Bristol Royal Infirm & Royal Gwent Hosp 1989; Surgery, U Pittsburgh Med Ctr 1997; **Fellow:** Colon & Rectal Surgery, Cleveland Clinic 1998

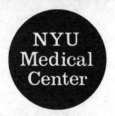

550 First Avenue (at 31st Street)
New York, NY 10016
Physician Referral:
(888)7-NYU-MED (888-769-8633)
www.nyumc.org

COLON AND RECTAL SURGERY

The gastrointestinal surgery program is a division of the Department of Surgery, whose surgeons perform over 5,000 outpatient and inpatient procedures each year using laser, laparoscopic, endoscopic, and other minimally invasive techniques. It maintains a nationally-regarded residency training program in Surgery through the NYU School of Medicine. Candidates for gastrointestinal surgery receive same-day care that includes imaging, radiation, and nutritional support.

The program provides an integrated team approach based on communication between surgeons and caregivers. The result is cancer care in a full service environment that offers a complete, patient-centered approach.

Virtual colonoscopies – a noninvasive method of cancer screening that uses the same techniques as a CT scan

Laparoscopic techniques – surgeons use tiny incisions to remove a segment of the colon; this dramatically speeds recovery and reduces the need for pain medication

Liver lesions – these are effectively treated using painless radiofrequency ablation

Specialists at the NCI-designated NYU Cancer Institute seek to enhance and coordinate the extensive resources of NYU Medical Center to optimize research, treatment, and the ultimate control of cancer.

Our new NYU Clinical Cancer Center is located at 160 East 34th Street. This state-of-the-art 13-level, 85,000-square-foot building serves as "home base" for patients, by providing the latest cancer prevention, screening, diagnostic treatment, genetic counseling, and support services in one central location. The NYU Clinical Cancer Center stands to dramatically improve the lives of people with cancer. As part of NYU Medical Center, patients can access a variety of other non-cancer services throughout the institution.

Physician Referral
1-888-7-NYU-MED
(1-888-769-8633)
www.nyumc.org
www.nyuci.org

695

Dermatology

A dermatologist is trained to diagnose and treat pediatric and adult patients with benign and malignant disorders of the skin, mouth, external genitalia, hair and nails, as well as a number of sexually transmitted diseases. The dermatologist has had additional training and experience in the diagnosis and treatment of skin cancers, melanomas, moles and other tumors of the skin, the management of contact dermatitis and other allergic and nonallergic skin disorders, and in the recognition of the skin manifestations of systemic (including internal malignancy) and infectious diseases. Dermatologists have special training in dermatopathology and in the surgical techniques used in dermatology. They also have expertise in the management of cosmetic disorders of the skin such as hair loss and scars, and the skin changes associated with aging.

Training Required: Four years.

Certification in the following subspecialties requires additional training and examination.

Dermatopathology: A dermatopathologist has the expertise to diagnose and monitor diseases of the skin including infectious, immunologic, degenerative and neoplastic diseases. This entails the examination and interpretation of specially prepared tissue sections, cellular scrapings and smears of skin lesions by means of routine and special (electron and fluorescent) microscopes.

Pediatric Dermatology: A dermatologist trained to diagnose and treat pediatric patients with dermatologic diseases.

Dermatology

New England

Anderson, Richard Rox MD [D] - **Spec Exp:** Skin Laser Surgery; Cosmetic Dermatology; Skin Cancer; **Hospital:** Mass Genl Hosp; **Address:** Dermatology Laser Center, 50 Staniford St, Ste 250, Boston, MA 02114; **Phone:** 617-724-6960; **Board Cert:** Dermatology 2001; **Med School:** Harvard Med Sch 1984; **Resid:** Dermatology, Mass Genl Hosp 1991; **Fellow:** Dermatologic Research, Mass Genl Hosp 1988; **Fac Appt:** Assoc Prof D, Harvard Med Sch

Arndt, Kenneth MD [D] - **Spec Exp:** Skin Laser Surgery; Cosmetic Dermatology; **Hospital:** Beth Israel Deaconess Med Ctr - Boston, New England Bapt Hosp; **Address:** Skincare Phys of Chestnut Hill, 1244 Boylston St, Ste 302, Chestnut Hill, MA 02467; **Phone:** 617-731-1600; **Board Cert:** Dermatology 1966; **Med School:** Yale Univ 1961; **Resid:** Dermatology, Mass Genl Hosp 1965; **Fellow:** Dermatology, Harvard Med Sch 1965; **Fac Appt:** Clin Prof D, Harvard Med Sch

Braverman, Irwin MD [D] - **Spec Exp:** Psoriasis; Lupus/SLE; Cutaneous Lymphoma; **Hospital:** Yale - New Haven Hosp; **Address:** Yale Dermatology, 2 Church St S, Ste 305, New Haven, CT 06519; **Phone:** 203-789-1249; **Board Cert:** Dermatology 1963; Dermatopathology 1982; **Med School:** Yale Univ 1955; **Resid:** Internal Medicine, Yale-New Haven Hosp 1956; Internal Medicine, Yale-New Haven Hosp 1959; **Fellow:** Dermatology, Yale-New Haven Hosp 1962; **Fac Appt:** Prof D, Yale Univ

Del Giudice, Stephen M MD [D] - **Spec Exp:** Skin Cancer; Phototherapy in Skin Disease; Psoriasis; Acne; **Hospital:** Concord Hospital; **Address:** Dartmouth Hitchcock Concord - Dermatology, 253 Pleasant St, Concord, NH 03301; **Phone:** 603-226-6119; **Board Cert:** Dermatology 1987; **Med School:** Tufts Univ 1981; **Resid:** Dermatology, Yale-New Haven Hosp 1987

Dover, Jeffrey MD [D] - **Spec Exp:** Skin Laser Surgery; Cosmetic Dermatology; Phototherapy in Skin Disease; **Hospital:** Beth Israel Deaconess Med Ctr - Boston, New England Bapt Hosp; **Address:** 1244 Boylston St, Ste 302, Chestnut Hill, MA 02467; **Phone:** 617-731-1600; **Board Cert:** Dermatology 1985; **Med School:** Univ Ottawa 1981; **Resid:** Dermatology, Univ Toronto 1984; Dermatology, St Johns Hosp 1985; **Fellow:** Dermatology, Mass Genl Hosp-Harvard 1987; **Fac Appt:** Assoc Prof D, Dartmouth Med Sch

Edelson, Richard L MD [D] - **Spec Exp:** Cutaneous Lymphoma; Immune Deficiency-Skin Disorders; **Hospital:** Yale - New Haven Hosp; **Address:** 2 Church St S, Ste 305, New Haven, CT 06519; **Phone:** 203-789-1249; **Board Cert:** Dermatology 1977; **Med School:** Yale Univ 1970; **Resid:** Dermatology, Mass Genl Hosp 1972; Dermatology, Natl Inst Hlth 1975; **Fac Appt:** Prof D, Yale Univ

Falanga, Vincent MD [D] - **Spec Exp:** Wound Healing/Care; Collagen Vascular Diseases; Scleroderma; **Hospital:** Roger Williams Hosp; **Address:** Roger Williams Med Ctr, Dept Dermatology, 50 Maude St Elmhurst Bldg, Providence, RI 02908; **Phone:** 401-456-2521; **Board Cert:** Internal Medicine 1980; Dermatology 1982; **Med School:** Harvard Med Sch 1977; **Resid:** Internal Medicine, Univ Miami 1980; **Fellow:** Dermatology, Univ Penn 1982; **Fac Appt:** Prof D, Boston Univ

Fewkes, Jessica L MD [D] - **Spec Exp:** Mohs' Surgery; Skin Cancer-Head & Neck; Melanoma-Head & Neck; **Hospital:** Mass Eye & Ear Infirmary; **Address:** Mass Eye & Ear Infirmary, 243 Charles St Fl 9, Boston, MA 02114; **Phone:** 617-573-3789; **Board Cert:** Dermatology 1982; **Med School:** UCSF 1978; **Resid:** Dermatology, Mass General Hosp 1982; **Fellow:** Mohs Surgery, Duke Univ Med Ctr 1983; **Fac Appt:** Asst Prof D, Harvard Med Sch

Gilchrest, Barbara MD [D] - **Spec Exp:** Photoaging; Melanoma; Skin Cancer; **Hospital:** Boston Med Ctr; **Address:** 609 Albany St Bldg J - Ste 507, Boston, MA 02118-2394; **Phone:** 617-638-5538; **Board Cert:** Internal Medicine 1975; Dermatology 1978; **Med School:** Harvard Med Sch 1971; **Resid:** Internal Medicine, Boston City Hosp 1973; Dermatology, Harvard Med Sch 1976; **Fellow:** Photo Biology, Harvard Med Sch 1975; **Fac Appt:** Prof D, Boston Univ

Leffell, David J MD [D] - **Spec Exp:** Mohs' Surgery; Melanoma; Skin Cancer; Skin Laser Surgery; **Hospital:** Yale - New Haven Hosp, Hosp of St Raphael; **Address:** New Haven Hosp-Dept Dermatology, 40 Temple St, Ste 5A, PO Box 208059, New Haven, CT 06520; **Phone:** 203-785-3466; **Board Cert:** Internal Medicine 1984; Dermatology 1987; **Med School:** McGill Univ 1981; **Resid:** Internal Medicine, New York Hosp 1984; Dermatology, Yale-New Haven Hosp 1986; **Fellow:** Dermatology, Yale-New Haven Hosp 1987; Dermatologic Surgery, Univ Michigan Med Ctr 1988; **Fac Appt:** Prof D, Yale Univ

Maloney, Mary MD [D] - **Spec Exp:** Mohs' Surgery; Skin Laser Surgery; **Hospital:** UMass Memorial Med Ctr; **Address:** Univ Mass Med Ctr, Dept Derm, 281 Lincoln St Fl 4, Worcester, MA 01605; **Phone:** 508-334-5962; **Board Cert:** Dermatology 1982; **Med School:** Univ VT Coll Med 1977; **Resid:** Internal Medicine, Hartford Hospital 1979; Dermatology, Dartmouth-Hitchcock Med Ctr 1982; **Fellow:** Dermatologic Surgery, UCSF Med Ctr 1983; **Fac Appt:** Prof D, Univ Mass Sch Med

McDonald, Charles J MD [D] - **Spec Exp:** Cutaneous Lymphoma; Autoimmune Disease; Psoriasis; **Hospital:** Rhode Island Hosp; **Address:** Rhode Island Hosp, Dept Dermatology, 593 Eddy St, APC-10, Providence, RI 02903-4923; **Phone:** 401-444-7959; **Board Cert:** Dermatology 1966; **Med School:** Howard Univ 1960; **Resid:** Internal Medicine, Hosp St Raphael 1963; Dermatology, Yale New Haven Hosp 1965; **Fellow:** Clinical Oncology, Yale New Haven Hosp 1966; **Fac Appt:** Prof D, Brown Univ

Mihm Jr, Martin C MD [D] - **Spec Exp:** Melanoma; Vascular Birthmarks; Dermatopathology; **Hospital:** Mass Genl Hosp; **Address:** Mass General Hosp, 55 Fruit St, Warren Bldg 827, Boston, MA 02114-2926; **Phone:** 617-724-1350; **Board Cert:** Dermatology 1969; Dermatopathology 1974; Anatomic Pathology 1974; **Med School:** Univ Pittsburgh 1961; **Resid:** Internal Medicine, Mt Sinai Hosp 1964; Dermatology, Mass Genl Hosp 1967; **Fellow:** Anatomic Pathology, Mass Genl Hosp 1972; **Fac Appt:** Clin Prof Path, Harvard Med Sch

Sober, Arthur MD [D] - **Spec Exp:** Melanoma; Skin Cancer; **Hospital:** Mass Genl Hosp; **Address:** Mass General Hospital, 50 Staniford St, Ste 200, Boston, MA 02114; **Phone:** 617-726-2914; **Board Cert:** Dermatology 1975; Internal Medicine 1974; **Med School:** Geo Wash Univ 1968; **Resid:** Internal Medicine, Beth Israel Hosp 1970; Dermatology, Mass General Hosp 1974; **Fellow:** Immunology, Peter Bent Brigham Hosp 1976; **Fac Appt:** Prof D, Harvard Med Sch

Dermatology

Mid Atlantic

Ackerman, A Bernard MD [D] - **Spec Exp:** Dermatopathology; Melanoma Consultation; Inflammatory Diseases of Skin; **Hospital:** SUNY Downstate Med Ctr; **Address:** 145 E 32nd St Fl 10, New York, NY 10016; **Phone:** 212-889-6225; **Board Cert:** Dermatology 1970; Dermatopathology 1974; **Med School:** Columbia P&S 1962; **Resid:** Dermatology, Columbia Presby Hosp 1964; Dermatology, Univ Penn Hosp 1967; **Fellow:** Dermatopathology, Mass Genl Hosp 1969

Alster, Tina MD [D] - **Spec Exp:** Cosmetic Dermatology; Scar Revision; Hemangiomas/Birthmarks; **Hospital:** Georgetown Univ Hosp; **Address:** 1430 K St NW Fl 2, Washington, DC 20005; **Phone:** 202-628-8855; **Board Cert:** Dermatology 1990; **Med School:** Duke Univ 1986; **Resid:** Dermatology, Yale Univ 1989; **Fellow:** Dermatologic Laser Surgery, Boston Univ Hosp 1990; **Fac Appt:** Clin Prof D, Georgetown Univ

Anhalt, Grant J MD [D] - **Spec Exp:** Blistering Diseases; Pemphigus; Autoimmune Disease; **Hospital:** Johns Hopkins Hosp - Baltimore (page 61); **Address:** 7401 Osler Drive, Ste 107, Towson, MD 21204; **Phone:** 410-321-5900; **Board Cert:** Dermatology 1980; Clinical & Laboratory Dematologic Immunology 1987; **Med School:** Canada 1975; **Resid:** Internal Medicine, Hlth Scis Ctr 1977; Dermatology, Univ Mich Med Ctr 1980; **Fellow:** Immunology, Univ Mich Med Ctr 1981; **Fac Appt:** Prof D, Johns Hopkins Univ

Bernstein, Robert M MD [D] - **Spec Exp:** Hair Restoration/Transplant; **Hospital:** NY-Presby Hosp/Columbia (page 66), Englewood Hosp & Med Ctr; **Address:** 110 E 55th St, New York, NY 10022; **Phone:** 212-826-2400; **Board Cert:** Dermatology 1982; Hair Restoration Surgery 1998; **Med School:** UMDNJ-NJ Med Sch, Newark 1978; **Resid:** Dermatology, Albert Einstein Med Ctr 1982; **Fac Appt:** Assoc Clin Prof D, Columbia P&S

Bystryn, Jean Claude MD [D] - **Spec Exp:** Melanoma; Blistering Diseases; Skin Cancer; Hair loss; **Hospital:** NYU Med Ctr (page 67); **Address:** 530 1st Ave, Ste 7F, New York, NY 10016; **Phone:** 212-889-3846; **Board Cert:** Dermatology 1970; Clinical & Laboratory Dematologic Immunology 1985; **Med School:** NYU Sch Med 1962; **Resid:** Internal Medicine, Montefiore Hosp 1964; Dermatology, NYU Med Ctr 1969; **Fellow:** Immunology, New York Univ 1972; **Fac Appt:** Prof D, NYU Sch Med

Cotsarelis, George MD [D] - **Spec Exp:** Hair loss; Scalp Disorders; **Hospital:** Hosp Univ Penn - UPHS (page 72); **Address:** Penn Medicine at Radnor, Dermatology, 250 King of Prussia Rd, Radnor, PA 19087; **Phone:** 610-902-2400; **Board Cert:** Dermatology 2001; **Med School:** Univ Pennsylvania 1987; **Resid:** Dermatology, Hosp Univ Penn 1992; **Fellow:** Dermatology, Hosp Univ Penn; **Fac Appt:** Asst Prof D, Univ Pennsylvania

Deleo, Vincent A MD [D] - **Spec Exp:** Photosensitive Skin Diseases; Facial Rejuvenation; Eczema; **Hospital:** St Luke's - Roosevelt Hosp Ctr - Roosevelt Div, Beth Israel Med Ctr - Petrie Division; **Address:** 425 W 59th St, Ste 5C, New York, NY 10019-1104; **Phone:** 212-523-6003; **Board Cert:** Dermatology 1976; **Med School:** Louisiana State Univ 1969; **Resid:** Dermatology, Columbia-Presby Med Ctr 1976; **Fac Appt:** Assoc Prof D, Columbia P&S

Dzubow, Leonard MD [D] - **Spec Exp:** Mohs' Surgery; Skin Laser Surgery; **Hospital:** Bryn Mawr Hosp, Riddle Meml Hosp; **Address:** 101 Chesley Drive, Media, PA 19063; **Phone:** 484-621-0082; **Board Cert:** Internal Medicine 1978; Dermatology 1980; **Med School:** Univ Pennsylvania 1975; **Resid:** Internal Medicine, Hosp Univ Penn 1978; Dermatology, NYU-Skin Cancer Unit 1980; **Fellow:** Mohs Surgery, NYU-Skin Cancer Unit; **Fac Appt:** Clin Prof D, Univ Pennsylvania

Franks Jr, Andrew G MD [D] - **Spec Exp:** Lupus/SLE; Raynaud's Disease; Scleroderma; **Hospital:** NYU Med Ctr (page 67), Lenox Hill Hosp (page 62); **Address:** 60 Gramercy Park N, Ste 1N, New York, NY 10010-5429; **Phone:** 212-475-2312; **Board Cert:** Internal Medicine 1975; Dermatology 1977; Rheumatology 1978; **Med School:** NYU Sch Med 1971; **Resid:** Internal Medicine, Beth Israel Med Ctr 1974; Dermatology, Columbia-Presby Med Ctr 1975; **Fellow:** Rheumatology, Columbia-Presby Med Ctr 1977; **Fac Appt:** Prof D, NYU Sch Med

Geronemus, Roy MD [D] - **Spec Exp:** Skin Laser Surgery; Cosmetic Dermatology; Mohs' Surgery; Skin Cancer; **Hospital:** NYU Med Ctr (page 67), New York Eye & Ear Infirm (page 65); **Address:** 317 E 34 St, Ste 11N, New York, NY 10016-4974; **Phone:** 212-686-7306; **Board Cert:** Dermatology 1983; **Med School:** Univ Miami Sch Med 1979; **Resid:** Dermatology, NYU-Skin Cancer Unit 1983; **Fellow:** Mohs Surgery, NYU-Skin Cancer Unit 1984; **Fac Appt:** Clin Prof D, NYU Sch Med

Gordon, Marsha MD [D] - **Spec Exp:** Cosmetic Dermatology; Botox Therapy; **Hospital:** Mount Sinai Med Ctr; **Address:** 5 E 98th St Fl 5, New York, NY 10029-6501; **Phone:** 212-241-9728; **Board Cert:** Dermatology 1988; **Med School:** Univ Pennsylvania 1984; **Resid:** Dermatology, Mount Sinai Hosp 1988; **Fac Appt:** Clin Prof D, Mount Sinai Sch Med

Granstein, Richard D MD [D] - **Spec Exp:** Autoimmune Disease; Skin Cancer; Psoriasis; **Hospital:** NY-Presby Hosp/Weill Cornell (page 66); **Address:** 520 E 70th St Fl 3 - Ste 326, New York, NY 10021; **Phone:** 212-746-2007; **Board Cert:** Dermatology 1983; Clinical & Laboratory Dematologic Immunology 1985; **Med School:** UCLA 1978; **Resid:** Dermatology, Mass Genl Hosp 1981; **Fellow:** Research, Natl Cancer Inst 1982; Dermatology, Mass Genl Hosp 1983; **Fac Appt:** Prof D, Cornell Univ-Weill Med Coll

Grossman, Melanie MD [D] - **Spec Exp:** Skin Laser Surgery; Laser Resurfacing; Facial Rejuvenation; Botox Therapy; **Hospital:** NY-Presby Hosp/Columbia (page 66); **Address:** 161 Madison Ave, Ste 4NW, New York, NY 10016-5405; **Phone:** 212-725-8600; **Board Cert:** Dermatology 1999; **Med School:** NYU Sch Med 1988; **Resid:** Internal Medicine, Yale-New Haven Hosp 1989; Dermatology, Columbia-Presby Med Ctr 1992; **Fellow:** Laser Surgery, Mass Genl Hosp 1995; **Fac Appt:** Asst Clin Prof D, Columbia P&S

Halpern, Allan C MD [D] - **Spec Exp:** Skin Cancer; Melanoma; Melanoma Early Detection/Prevention; **Hospital:** Meml Sloan Kettering Cancer Ctr; **Address:** 160 E 53rd St, New York, NY 10022; **Phone:** 212-610-0766; **Board Cert:** Internal Medicine 1984; Dermatology 1988; **Med School:** Albert Einstein Coll Med 1981; **Resid:** Dermatology, Hosp Univ Penn 1988; **Fellow:** Epidemiology, Hosp Univ Penn 1989; **Fac Appt:** Assoc Prof Med, Cornell Univ-Weill Med Coll

James, William D MD [D] - **Spec Exp:** Contact Dermatitis; Acne; Rosacea; **Hospital:** Hosp Univ Penn - UPHS (page 72); **Address:** U Penn Health Serices, Dermatology, 3600 Spruce St, 2 Maloney, Philadelphia, PA 19104; **Phone:** 215-662-4282; **Board Cert:** Dermatology 1981; Diagnostic Lab Immunology 1985; **Med School:** Indiana Univ 1975; **Resid:** Dermatology, Letterman Army Med Ctr 1981; **Fac Appt:** Prof D, Univ Pennsylvania

Katz, Stephen MD [D] - **Spec Exp:** Immune Deficiency-Skin Disorders; Fibromyalgia; **Hospital:** Natl Inst of Hlth - Clin Ctr; **Address:** NIH- Dermatology Branch, 31 Center Drive, MSC 2350, Bldg 31 - rm 4632, Bethesda, MD 20892; **Phone:** 301-496-2481; **Board Cert:** Dermatology 1971; Clinical & Laboratory Dematologic Immunology 1985; **Med School:** Tulane Univ 1966; **Resid:** Dermatology, Jackson Meml Hosp 1970; **Fellow:** Research 1974

Dermatology

Kriegel, David MD [D] - **Spec Exp:** Mohs' Surgery; Botox Therapy; Skin Laser Surgery; Cosmetic Dermatology; **Hospital:** Mount Sinai Med Ctr; **Address:** 250 W 57th St, Ste 825, New York, NY 10107; **Phone:** 212-489-6669; **Board Cert:** Dermatology 2003; **Med School:** Boston Univ 1987; **Resid:** Dermatology, New England Med Ctr 1991; **Fellow:** Mohs Surgery, Stony Brook Univ Hosp 1993; **Fac Appt:** Assoc Prof D, Mount Sinai Sch Med

Lebwohl, Mark MD [D] - **Spec Exp:** Skin Cancer; Cutaneous Lymphoma; Psoriasis; **Hospital:** Mount Sinai Med Ctr; **Address:** 5 E 98th St Fl 5, New York, NY 10029-6501; **Phone:** 212-241-9728; **Board Cert:** Internal Medicine 1981; Dermatology 1983; **Med School:** Harvard Med Sch 1978; **Resid:** Internal Medicine, Mount Sinai Hosp 1981; **Fellow:** Dermatology, Mount Sinai Hosp 1983; **Fac Appt:** Prof D, Mount Sinai Sch Med

Lessin, Stuart R MD [D] - **Spec Exp:** Melanoma; Skin Cancer; Cutaneous Lymphoma; Melanoma Risk Assessment; **Hospital:** Fox Chase Cancer Ctr (page 59); **Address:** Fox Chase Cancer Ctr, Dept Dermatology, 333 Cottman Ave, Philadelphia, PA 19111; **Phone:** 215-728-2570; **Board Cert:** Dermatology 1986; **Med School:** Temple Univ 1982; **Resid:** Dermatology, Hosp Univ Penn 1986; **Fac Appt:** Prof D, Temple Univ

Miller, Stanley MD [D] - **Spec Exp:** Dermatologic Surgery; Skin Cancer; Mohs' Surgery; **Hospital:** Johns Hopkins Hosp - Baltimore (page 61); **Address:** Charles Towson Bldg, Ste 201, 1104 Kenilworth Drive, Ste 201, Towson, MD 21204; **Phone:** 443-279-0340; **Board Cert:** Dermatology 1989; **Med School:** Univ VT Coll Med 1984; **Resid:** Dermatology, UCSD Med Ctr 1989; **Fellow:** Dermatologic Surgery, Hosp Univ Penn 1991; **Fac Appt:** Prof D, Johns Hopkins Univ

Nigra, Thomas P MD [D] - **Spec Exp:** Hair loss; Psoriasis; Skin Cancer; Vitiligo; **Hospital:** Washington Hosp Ctr; **Address:** Washington Hosp Ctr, Derm Assocs, 110 Irving St NW, 2B44, Washington, DC 20010; **Phone:** 202-877-6227; **Board Cert:** Dermatology 1973; **Med School:** Univ Pennsylvania 1967; **Resid:** Dermatology, Mass Genl Hosp 1973; Dermatology, Natl Insts of Health 1971; **Fac Appt:** Clin Prof D, Geo Wash Univ

Orlow, Seth MD/PhD [D] - **Spec Exp:** Pediatric Dermatology; Hemangiomas/Birthmarks; Psoriasis/Eczema; **Hospital:** NYU Med Ctr (page 67); **Address:** 530 1st Ave, Ste 7R, New York, NY 10016-6402; **Phone:** 212-263-5889; **Board Cert:** Dermatology 1990; Pediatric Dermatology 2004; **Med School:** Albert Einstein Coll Med 1986; **Resid:** Pediatrics, Mt Sinai Hosp 1987; Dermatology, Yale-New Haven Hosp 1989; **Fellow:** Dermatology, Yale-New Haven Hosp 1990; **Fac Appt:** Prof D, NYU Sch Med

Ramsay, David L MD [D] - **Spec Exp:** Cutaneous Lymphoma; Skin Cancer; **Hospital:** NYU Med Ctr (page 67); **Address:** 530 1st Ave, Ste 7G, New York, NY 10016-6402; **Phone:** 212-683-6283; **Board Cert:** Dermatology 1974; **Med School:** Indiana Univ 1969; **Resid:** Dermatology, New York Univ Med Ctr 1973; **Fellow:** Dermatology, Univ Ill Hosp 1973; **Fac Appt:** Clin Prof D, NYU Sch Med

Rigel, Darrell S MD [D] - **Spec Exp:** Melanoma; Skin Cancer; Cosmetic Dermatology; **Hospital:** NYU Med Ctr (page 67), Mount Sinai Med Ctr; **Address:** 35 E 35th Street, Ste 208, New York, NY 10016-3823; **Phone:** 212-684-5964; **Board Cert:** Dermatology 1983; **Med School:** Geo Wash Univ 1978; **Resid:** Dermatology, NYU Med Ctr 1982; **Fellow:** Dermatologic Surgery, NYU Med Ctr 1983; **Fac Appt:** Clin Prof D, NYU Sch Med

Robins, Perry MD [D] - **Spec Exp:** Mohs' Surgery; Skin Cancer; Melanoma; **Hospital:** NYU Med Ctr (page 67), Bellevue Hosp Ctr; **Address:** 530 First Ave, Ste 7H, New York, NY 10016; **Phone:** 212-263-7222; **Med School:** Germany 1961; **Resid:** Dermatology, VA Med Ctr 1964; **Fellow:** Dermatology, NYU Med Ctr 1967; **Fac Appt:** Prof D, NYU Sch Med

Rook, Alain H MD [D] - **Spec Exp:** Cutaneous Lymphoma; Immune Deficiency-Skin Disorders; Mycosis Fungoides; **Hospital:** Hosp Univ Penn - UPHS (page 72); **Address:** Hosp Univ Penn, Dept Dermatology, 3400 Spruce St Rhoades Bldg, Philadelphia, PA 19104; **Phone:** 215-662-7610; **Board Cert:** Internal Medicine 1979; Nephrology 1980; Dermatology 2001; **Med School:** Univ Mich Med Sch 1975; **Resid:** Internal Medicine, McGill Univ Med Ctr 1977; Dermatology, Hosp Univ Penn 1989; **Fellow:** Nephrology, McGill Univ Med Ctr 1979; Immunology, NIH 1986; **Fac Appt:** Prof D, Univ Pennsylvania

Safai, Bijan MD [D] - **Spec Exp:** Dermatologic Surgery; Skin Cancer; Skin Laser Surgery; **Hospital:** Metropolitan Hosp Ctr - NY, Westchester Med Ctr; **Address:** 625 Park Ave, New York, NY 10021-6545; **Phone:** 212-988-8918; **Board Cert:** Dermatology 1974; **Med School:** Iran 1965; **Resid:** Internal Medicine, VA Med Ctr 1970; Dermatology, NYU Med Ctr 1973; **Fellow:** Immunology, Mem Sloan-Kettering Cancer Ctr 1974; **Fac Appt:** Prof D, NY Med Coll

Shalita, Alan MD [D] - **Spec Exp:** Acne; Rosacea; **Hospital:** SUNY Downstate Med Ctr; **Address:** SUNY Downstate Med Ctr, 450 Clarkson Ave, Dermatology, Box 46, Brooklyn, NY 11203-2012; **Phone:** 718-270-1230; **Board Cert:** Dermatology 1971; **Med School:** Wake Forest Univ 1964; **Resid:** Dermatology, NYU Med Ctr 1970; **Fellow:** Dermatologic Research, NYU Med Ctr 1973; **Fac Appt:** Prof D, SUNY Downstate

Shupack, Jerome L MD [D] - **Spec Exp:** Rare Skin Disorders; Psoriasis; **Hospital:** NYU Med Ctr (page 67); **Address:** 530 1st Ave, New York, NY 10016-6402; **Phone:** 212-263-7344; **Board Cert:** Dermatology 1970; **Med School:** Columbia P&S 1963; **Resid:** Internal Medicine, Mt Sinai Hosp 1965; Dermatology, NYU Med Ctr 1970; **Fac Appt:** Prof D, NYU Sch Med

Soter, Nicholas A MD [D] - **Spec Exp:** Urticaria; Psoriasis; Vasculitis; **Hospital:** NYU Med Ctr (page 67); **Address:** 530 1st Ave, Ste 7R, New York, NY 10016-6402; **Phone:** 212-263-5889; **Board Cert:** Dermatology 1970; Diagnostic Lab Immunology 1985; **Med School:** Univ Tex SW, Dallas 1965; **Resid:** Dermatology, Baylor Med Ctr 1968; Dermatology, Mass Genl Hosp 1969; **Fellow:** Immunology, Harvard 1973; **Fac Appt:** Prof D, NYU Sch Med

Stanley, John R MD [D] - **Spec Exp:** Blistering Diseases; Pemphigus; **Hospital:** Hosp Univ Penn - UPHS (page 72); **Address:** Univ of Pennsylvania, Dept Dermatology, 3400 Spruce St, 2 Rhoads Pavilion, Philadelphia, PA 19104; **Phone:** 215-662-2737; **Board Cert:** Dermatology 1978; Clinical & Laboratory Dematologic Immunology 1985; **Med School:** Harvard Med Sch 1974; **Resid:** Dermatology, NYU Med Ctr 1978; **Fac Appt:** Prof D, Univ Pennsylvania

Vonderheid, Eric C MD [D] - **Spec Exp:** Cutaneous Lymphoma; Skin Cancer; **Hospital:** Johns Hopkins Hosp - Baltimore (page 61); **Address:** Johns Hopkins Dept Dermatology, 550 N Broadway, Ste 1002, Baltimore, MD 21205; **Phone:** 410-955-5933; **Board Cert:** Dermatology 1976; **Med School:** Temple Univ 1968; **Resid:** Internal Medicine, St Louis Univ Med Ctr 1972; Dermatology, Temple Univ Med Ctr 1975; **Fac Appt:** Prof D, Johns Hopkins Univ

Werth, Victoria P MD [D] - **Spec Exp:** Autoimmune Disease; Lupus/SLE; Connective Tissue Disorders; Blistering Diseases; **Hospital:** Hosp Univ Penn - UPHS (page 72); **Address:** Univ Penn Health Services, 3600 Spruce St, 2 Rhoads Pavilion, Philadelphia, PA 19104; **Phone:** 215-662-2737; **Board Cert:** Internal Medicine 1983; Dermatology 1986; Diagnostic Lab Immunology 1989; **Med School:** Johns Hopkins Univ 1980; **Resid:** Internal Medicine, Northwestern Meml Hosp 1983; Dermatology, NYU Med Ctr 1986; **Fellow:** Immunological Dermatology, NYU Sch Med 1988; **Fac Appt:** Assoc Prof D, Univ Pennsylvania

Dermatology

Yan, Albert C MD [D] - **Spec Exp:** Pediatric Dermatology; **Hospital:** Chldns Hosp of Philadelphia, The; **Address:** Children's Hosp of Philadelphia, Dept Dermatology, 34th & Civic Ctr Blvd, Philadelphia, PA 19104; **Phone:** 215-590-2169; **Board Cert:** Dermatology 1999; Pediatrics 2004; Pediatric Dermatology 2004; **Med School:** Univ Pennsylvania 1993; **Resid:** Pediatrics, Children's Hosp 1996; Dermatology, Hosp U Penn 1999; **Fac Appt:** Asst Prof D, Univ Pennsylvania

Zitelli, John MD [D] - **Spec Exp:** Mohs' Surgery; Skin Cancer; Melanoma; **Hospital:** UPMC Shadyside, Jefferson Hosp - Pittsburgh; **Address:** Shadyside Med Ctr, 5200 Centre Ave, Ste 303, Pittsburgh, PA 15232-1312; **Phone:** 412-681-9400; **Board Cert:** Dermatology 1980; **Med School:** Univ Pittsburgh 1976; **Resid:** Dermatology, Univ Hlth Ctr Hosp 1979; **Fellow:** Mohs Surgery, Univ Wisconsin 1980; **Fac Appt:** Assoc Clin Prof D, Univ Pittsburgh

Southeast

Amonette, Rex A MD [D] - **Spec Exp:** Skin Cancer; Mohs' Surgery; **Hospital:** Methodist Univ Hosp - Memphis, Baptist Memorial Hospital - Memphis; **Address:** Memphis Dermatology Clinic, 1455 Union Ave, Memphis, TN 38104-6727; **Phone:** 901-726-6655; **Board Cert:** Dermatology 1974; **Med School:** Univ Ark 1966; **Resid:** Dermatology, Univ Tenn Med Ctr 1971; **Fellow:** Mohs Surgery, NYU Med Ctr 1972; **Fac Appt:** Clin Prof D, Univ Tenn Coll Med, Memphis

Brandt, Fredric S MD [D] - **Spec Exp:** Botox Therapy; **Address:** 4425 Ponce de Leon Blvd, Ste 200, Coral Gables, FL 33146; **Phone:** 305-443-6606; **Board Cert:** Internal Medicine 1978; Dermatology 1981; **Med School:** Hahnemann Univ 1975; **Resid:** Internal Medicine, VA Hosp 1981; Dermatology, Univ Miami Hosps 1983

Brody, Harold J MD [D] - **Spec Exp:** Cosmetic Dermatology; Cosmetic Surgery; **Hospital:** Crawford Long Hosp of Emory Univ; **Address:** 1218 W Paces Ferry Rd NE, Ste 200, Atlanta, GA 30327; **Phone:** 404-525-7409; **Board Cert:** Dermatology 1978; **Med School:** Med Univ SC 1974; **Resid:** Dermatology, Emory Affil Hosps 1978; **Fac Appt:** Clin Prof D, Emory Univ

Burton III, Claude S MD [D] - **Spec Exp:** Leg Ulcers; Wound Healing/Care; Hemangiomas; **Hospital:** Duke Univ Med Ctr; **Address:** DUMC, Box 3511, Durham, NC 27710; **Phone:** 919-681-5442; **Board Cert:** Internal Medicine 1982; Dermatology 1984; **Med School:** Duke Univ 1979; **Resid:** Internal Medicine, Duke Univ Med Ctr 1982; Dermatology, Duke Univ Med Ctr 1984; **Fac Appt:** Assoc Prof Med, Duke Univ

Callen, Jeffrey P MD [D] - **Spec Exp:** Lupus/SLE; Dermatomyositis; Vasculitis; **Hospital:** Univ of Louisville Hosp, Jewish Hosp HlthCre Svcs Inc; **Address:** 310 E Broadway, Ste 200, Louisville, KY 40202; **Phone:** 502-583-1749; **Board Cert:** Internal Medicine 1975; Dermatology 1999; **Med School:** Univ Mich Med Sch 1972; **Resid:** Internal Medicine, Univ Mich Med Ctr 1975; Dermatology, Univ Mich Med Ctr 1977; **Fac Appt:** Prof Med, Univ Louisville Sch Med

Camisa, Charles MD [D] - **Spec Exp:** Psoriasis; Oral Dermatology; Lichen Planus; **Hospital:** Physicians Regl Med Ctr; **Address:** 6101 Pine Ridge Rd, Naples, FL 34119; **Phone:** 239-348-4335; **Board Cert:** Dermatology 1981; Clinical & Laboratory Dematologic Immunology 1987; **Med School:** Mount Sinai Sch Med 1977; **Resid:** Dermatology, NYU Med Ctr 1981; **Fac Appt:** Assoc Prof D, Univ S Fla Coll Med

Cohen, Bernard H MD [D] - **Spec Exp:** Hair Restoration/Transplant; Cosmetic Dermatology; Botox Therapy; **Hospital:** Jackson Meml Hosp; **Address:** 4425 Ponce de Leon Blvd, Ste 230, Coral Gables, FL 33146; **Phone:** 305-476-9544; **Board Cert:** Dermatology 1972; **Med School:** Columbia P&S 1967; **Resid:** Dermatology, NYU Med Ctr 1971; **Fac Appt:** Clin Prof D, Univ Miami Sch Med

Eichler, Craig MD [D] - **Spec Exp:** Skin Cancer; Dermatologic Surgery; **Hospital:** Physicians Regl Med Ctr; **Address:** 6101 Pine Ridge Rd, Naples, FL 34119-3900; **Phone:** 239-348-4335; **Board Cert:** Dermatology 2003; **Med School:** Univ Fla Coll Med 1989; **Resid:** Dermatology, Univ Texas Med Branch 1993

Elmets, Craig A MD [D] - **Spec Exp:** Psoriasis/Eczema; Phototherapy in Skin Disease; Skin Cancer; **Hospital:** Univ of Ala Hosp at Birmingham, VA Med Ctr; **Address:** Univ of Alabama-Birmingham-Derm Dept, 1530 Third Ave S, EFH 414, Birmingham, AL 35294; **Phone:** 205-996-7546; **Board Cert:** Dermatology 1980; Internal Medicine 1978; Clinical & Laboratory Immunology 1989; **Med School:** Univ Iowa Coll Med 1975; **Resid:** Internal Medicine, Kansas Med Ctr 1978; Dermatology, Univ Iowa Hosps 1980; **Fellow:** Immunological Dermatology, Univ Texas Hlth Sci Ctr 1982; **Fac Appt:** Prof D, Univ Ala

Fenske, Neil A MD [D] - **Spec Exp:** Skin Cancer; Melanoma; Psoriasis; **Hospital:** H Lee Moffitt Cancer Ctr & Research Inst, Tampa Genl Hosp; **Address:** 12901 Bruce B Downs Blvd, MDC-79, Tampa, FL 33612-4742; **Phone:** 813-974-2920; **Board Cert:** Dermatology 1977; Dermatopathology 1984; **Med School:** St Louis Univ 1973; **Resid:** Dermatology, Wisconsin Hlth Sci Ctr 1977; **Fac Appt:** Prof Med, Univ S Fla Coll Med

Flowers, Franklin P MD [D] - **Spec Exp:** Mohs' Surgery; Dermatopathology; **Hospital:** Shands Hlthcre at Univ of FL; **Address:** Shands Healthcare, PO Box 100383, Gainesville, FL 32610; **Phone:** 352-265-8001; **Board Cert:** Dermatology 1976; Dermatopathology 1981; **Med School:** Univ Fla Coll Med 1971; **Resid:** Dermatology, Ohio State Univ 1975; **Fellow:** Mohs Surgery, Univ Alabama 1993; **Fac Appt:** Prof Med, Univ Fla Coll Med

Green, Howard MD [D] - **Spec Exp:** Mohs' Surgery; Skin Cancer; **Hospital:** St Mary's Med Ctr - W Palm Bch, JFK Med Ctr - Atlantis; **Address:** 120 Butler St, Ste A, West Palm Beach, FL 33407-6106; **Phone:** 561-659-1510; **Board Cert:** Internal Medicine 1988; Dermatology 2004; **Med School:** Boston Univ 1985; **Resid:** Internal Medicine, Jefferson Univ Hosp 1988; Dermatology, Harvard Med Sch 1992; **Fellow:** Mohs Surgery, Boston Univ Med Ctr 1993

Johr, Robert MD [D] - **Spec Exp:** Pigmented Lesions; Melanoma; Pediatric Dermatology; **Hospital:** Univ of Miami Hosp & Clins/Sylvester Comp Canc Ctr, Boca Raton Comm Hosp; **Address:** 1050 NW 15th St, Ste 201A, Boca Raton, FL 33486-1341; **Phone:** 561-368-4545; **Board Cert:** Dermatology 1981; **Med School:** Mexico 1975; **Resid:** Dermatology, Roswell Park Cancer Ctr 1977; Dermatology, Metro Med Ctr/Case Western Reserve 1979; **Fac Appt:** Clin Prof D, Univ Miami Sch Med

Jorizzo, Joseph L MD [D] - **Spec Exp:** Rheumatologic Dermatology; Immune Deficiency-Skin Disorders; **Hospital:** Wake Forest Univ Baptist Med Ctr (page 73); **Address:** Wake Forest Univ Sch Med, Dept Derm, Med Ctr Blvd, Winston-Salem, NC 27157-0001; **Phone:** 336-716-3926; **Board Cert:** Dermatology 1979; **Med School:** Boston Univ 1975; **Resid:** Dermatology, Univ North Carolina Hosps 1979; **Fellow:** Dermatology, Dermatology Inst 1980; **Fac Appt:** Prof D, Wake Forest Univ

Dermatology

Leshin, Barry MD [D] - **Spec Exp:** Skin Cancer; Mohs' Surgery; Dermatologic Surgery; **Address:** 125 Sunnynoll Ct, Ste 100, Winston-Salem, NC 27106; **Phone:** 336-724-2434; **Board Cert:** Dermatology 1985; **Med School:** Univ Tex, Houston 1981; **Resid:** Dermatology, Univ Iowa Hosp 1985; **Fellow:** Dermatologic Surgery, Univ Iowa Hosp 1986; **Fac Appt:** Clin Prof PlS, Wake Forest Univ

Olsen, Elise A MD [D] - **Spec Exp:** Hair loss; Hirsutism; Cutaneous Lymphoma; **Hospital:** Duke Univ Med Ctr; **Address:** Duke Univ Med Ctr, Box 3294, Durham, NC 27710; **Phone:** 919-684-3432; **Board Cert:** Dermatology 1983; **Med School:** Baylor Coll Med 1978; **Resid:** Internal Medicine, Univ NC Meml Hosp 1980; Dermatology, Duke Univ Med Ctr 1983; **Fac Appt:** Prof D, Duke Univ

Sherertz, Elizabeth F MD [D] - **Spec Exp:** Eczema; Contact Dermatitis; Occupational Skin Diseases; **Hospital:** Wake Forest Univ Baptist Med Ctr (page 73); **Address:** 125 Sunnynoll Ct, Ste 100, Winston Salem, NC 27106; **Phone:** 336-724-2434; **Board Cert:** Dermatology 1982; **Med School:** Univ VA Sch Med 1978; **Resid:** Dermatology, Duke Univ Med Ctr 1982; **Fac Appt:** Clin Prof D, Wake Forest Univ

Sobel, Stuart MD [D] - **Spec Exp:** Skin Cancer; Cosmetic Dermatology; **Hospital:** Meml Regl Hosp - Hollywood, Joe Di Maggio Chldns Hosp; **Address:** 4340 Sheridan St, Ste 101, Hollywood, FL 33021-3511; **Phone:** 954-983-5533; **Board Cert:** Dermatology 1977; **Med School:** Tufts Univ 1972; **Resid:** Dermatology, Mt Sinai Hosp 1976

Sokoloff, Daniel MD [D] - **Spec Exp:** Skin Cancer; Cosmetic Dermatology; **Hospital:** St Mary's Med Ctr - W Palm Bch, Good Sam Med Ctr - W Palm Beach; **Address:** Palm Beach Dermatology, 1000 45th St, Ste 1, West Palm Beach, FL 33407-2416; **Phone:** 561-863-1000; **Board Cert:** Dermatology 1982; **Med School:** Geo Wash Univ 1977; **Resid:** Dermatology, Baylor Coll Med 1982

Thiers, Bruce H MD [D] - **Spec Exp:** Cutaneous Lymphoma; Skin Cancer; Psoriasis; **Hospital:** MUSC Med Ctr; **Address:** MUSC Dept Dermatology, 135 Rutledge Ave Fl 11, Box 250578, Charleston, SC 29425; **Phone:** 843-792-5858; **Board Cert:** Dermatology 1978; **Med School:** SUNY Buffalo 1974; **Resid:** Dermatology, SUNY Buffalo Med Ctr 1978; **Fac Appt:** Prof D, Med Univ SC

Midwest

Bailin, Philip L MD [D] - **Spec Exp:** Mohs' Surgery; Skin Laser Surgery; Skin Cancer; **Hospital:** Cleveland Clin Fdn (page 57); **Address:** Cleveland Clinic Fdn, 9500 Euclid Ave, Desk A61, Cleveland, OH 44195-5032; **Phone:** 216-444-2115; **Board Cert:** Dermatology 1975; **Med School:** Northwestern Univ 1968; **Resid:** Dermatology, Cleveland Clin Fdn 1974; **Fellow:** Dermatopathology, Armed Forces Inst Pathology 1975; Mohs Surgery, Univ Wisc Hosp & Clin

Cornelius, Lynn A MD [D] - **Spec Exp:** Melanoma; **Hospital:** Barnes-Jewish Hosp, St Louis Chldns Hosp; **Address:** 660 S Euclid, Box 8123, St Louis, MO 63110; **Phone:** 314-362-8187; **Board Cert:** Dermatology 1989; **Med School:** Univ MO-Columbia Sch Med 1984; **Resid:** Dermatology, Barnes Jewish Hosp-Wash Univ 1989; **Fellow:** Immunological Dermatology, Emory Univ Med Ctr 1992; **Fac Appt:** Assoc Prof D, Washington Univ, St Louis

Fivenson, David MD [D] - **Spec Exp:** Blistering Diseases; Wound Healing/Care; Lupus/SLE; **Hospital:** St Joseph Mercy Hosp - Ann Arbor; **Address:** 25 Research Drive, Ann Arbor, MI 48103; **Phone:** 734-222-9630; **Board Cert:** Dermatology 1989; Clinical & Laboratory Dematologic Immunology 1991; **Med School:** Univ Mich Med Sch 1984; **Resid:** Dermatology, Univ Cincinnati Med Ctr 1989; **Fellow:** Immunological Dermatology, UCSD Med Ctr 1986

Garden, Jerome M MD [D] - **Spec Exp:** Skin Laser Surgery; Skin Rejuvenation; Vascular Birthmarks; Skin Rejuvenation; **Hospital:** Northwestern Meml Hosp, Children's Mem Hosp; **Address:** 150 E Huron St, Ste 1200, Chicago, IL 60611-2946; **Phone:** 312-280-0890; **Board Cert:** Dermatology 1984; **Med School:** Northwestern Univ 1980; **Resid:** Internal Medicine, Northwestern Univ 1981; Dermatology, Northwestern Univ 1984; **Fac Appt:** Prof D, Northwestern Univ

Hanke, C William MD [D] - **Spec Exp:** Mohs' Surgery; Skin Laser Surgery; Cosmetic Dermatology; Photodynamic Therapy; **Hospital:** St Vincent Carmel Hosp, Clarian Hlth Ptrs; **Address:** Laser & Skin Surgery Ctr of Indiana, 13450 N Meridian St, Ste 355, Carmel, IN 46032-1486; **Phone:** 317-582-8484; **Board Cert:** Dermatology 1978; Dermatopathology 1982; **Med School:** Univ Iowa Coll Med 1971; **Resid:** Dermatology, Cleveland Clinic 1978; Dermatopathology, Indiana Univ 1982; **Fellow:** Cutaneous Oncology, Cleveland Clinic 1979; **Fac Appt:** Clin Prof D, Indiana Univ

Hruza, George J MD [D] - **Spec Exp:** Skin Laser Surgery; Mohs' Surgery; Cosmetic Surgery; **Hospital:** St Luke's Hosp - Chesterfield, MO, St Louis Univ Hosp; **Address:** Laser & Derm Surg Ctr, 14377 Woodlake Drive, Ste 111, St. Louis, MO 63017-5735; **Phone:** 314-878-3839; **Board Cert:** Dermatology 1986; **Med School:** NYU Sch Med 1982; **Resid:** Dermatology, NYU Med Ctr-Skin Cancer Unit 1986; **Fellow:** Laser Surgery, Mass Genl Hosp-Harvard 1987; Surgery, Univ Wisc 1988; **Fac Appt:** Assoc Clin Prof D, St Louis Univ

Johnson, Timothy M MD [D] - **Spec Exp:** Melanoma; Mohs' Surgery; **Hospital:** Univ Michigan Hlth Sys; **Address:** Univ Michigan Hlth System, Dept Dermatology, 1910 Taubman Ctr, Ann Arbor, MI 48109-0314; **Phone:** 734-936-4190; **Board Cert:** Dermatology 1988; **Med School:** Univ Tex, Houston 1984; **Resid:** Dermatology, Univ Texas Med Ctr 1988; **Fellow:** Cutaneous Oncology, Univ Mich Med Ctr 1989; Mohs Surgery, Univ Oregon Hlth Sci Ctr 1990; **Fac Appt:** Prof D, Univ Mich Med Sch

Lim, Henry W MD [D] - **Spec Exp:** Phototherapy of Skin Disease; Vitiligo; Cutaneous Lymphoma; Skin Cancer; **Hospital:** Henry Ford Hosp; **Address:** Henry Ford Hosp, Dept Derm, 3031 W Grand Blvd, Ste 800, Detroit, MI 48202-3141; **Phone:** 313-916-4060; **Board Cert:** Dermatology 2005; Clinical & Laboratory Dematologic Immunology 1985; **Med School:** SUNY Downstate 1975; **Resid:** Dermatology, NYU Med Ctr 1979; **Fellow:** Immunological Dermatology, NYU Med Ctr 1980; **Fac Appt:** Prof Path, Wayne State Univ

Lucky, Anne W MD [D] - **Spec Exp:** Pediatric Dermatology; Acne; **Hospital:** Cincinnati Chldns Hosp Med Ctr; **Address:** Derm Assocs Cincinnati, 7691 Five Mile Rd, Cincinnati, OH 45230; **Phone:** 513-232-3332; **Board Cert:** Pediatrics 1975; Pediatric Endocrinology 1978; Dermatology 1981; Pediatric Dermatology 2004; **Med School:** Yale Univ 1970; **Resid:** Pediatrics, Boston Chldns Hosp 1973; Dermatology, Yale-New Haven Hosp 1981; **Fellow:** Pediatric Endocrinology, Natl Inst Hlth 1976; **Fac Appt:** Prof D, Univ Cincinnati

Dermatology

Neuburg, Marcelle MD [D] - **Spec Exp:** Mohs' Surgery; Skin Cancer; Pigmented Lesions; **Hospital:** Froedtert Meml Lutheran Hosp; **Address:** Dept Dermatology, 9200 W Wisconsin Ave, Milwaukee, WI 53226; **Phone:** 414-805-5300; **Board Cert:** Internal Medicine 1985; Dermatology 1988; **Med School:** Oregon Hlth Sci Univ 1982; **Resid:** Internal Medicine, Georgetown Univ Hosp 1985; Dermatology, Boston Univ Sch Med Ctr 1988; **Fellow:** Mohs Surgery, Tufts New England Med Ctr 1990; **Fac Appt:** Assoc Prof D, Med Coll Wisc

Paller, Amy S MD [D] - **Spec Exp:** Genetic Disorders-Skin; Immune Deficiency-Skin Disorders; Atopic Dermatitis; **Hospital:** Children's Mem Hosp; **Address:** Chldns Meml Hosp, 2300 Chldns Plaza #107, Chicago, IL 60614-3394; **Phone:** 773-327-3446; **Board Cert:** Pediatrics 1982; Dermatology 1983; Pediatric Dermatology 2004; **Med School:** Stanford Univ 1978; **Resid:** Pediatrics, Chldns Meml Hosp 1981; Dermatology, Northwestern Meml Hosp 1983; **Fellow:** Research, Univ NC Hosp 1984; **Fac Appt:** Prof D, Northwestern Univ

Treadwell, Patricia MD [D] - **Spec Exp:** Pediatric Dermatology; Vascular Birthmarks; **Hospital:** Riley Hosp for Children, Wishard Hlth Srvs; **Address:** 1001 W 10th St Bryce Bldg, Fl 2 - rm B2100, Indianapolis, IN 46202; **Phone:** 317-630-7396; **Board Cert:** Pediatrics 1982; Dermatology 1983; **Med School:** Cornell Univ-Weill Med Coll 1977; **Resid:** Pediatrics, James Whitcomb Riley Hosp 1980; Dermatology, Indiana Univ Med Ctr 1983; **Fac Appt:** Prof D, Indiana Univ

Voorhees, John MD [D] - **Spec Exp:** Psoriasis; Photoaging; **Hospital:** Univ Michigan Hlth Sys; **Address:** Univ Michigan, Dept Dermatology, 1500 E Med Ctr Drive, rm 1910 Taubman Ctr, Ann Arbor, MI 48109-0314; **Phone:** 734-936-4054; **Board Cert:** Dermatology 1970; **Med School:** Univ Mich Med Sch 1963; **Resid:** Dermatology, Univ Mich Hosp 1969; **Fac Appt:** Prof D, Univ Mich Med Sch

Wheeland, Ronald MD [D] - **Spec Exp:** Skin Laser Surgery; Mohs' Surgery; Cosmetic Dermatology; **Hospital:** Univ of Missouri Hosp & Clins; **Address:** Univ Missouri, Dept Dermatology, One Hospital Drive, Columbia, MO 65212; **Phone:** 573-884-6415; **Board Cert:** Dermatology 1977; Dermatopathology 1978; **Med School:** Univ Ariz Coll Med 1973; **Resid:** Dermatology, Univ Ok Hlth Sci Ctr 1977; **Fellow:** Dermatopathology, Univ Ok Hlth Sci Ctr 1978; Dermatologic Surgery, Cleveland Clin Fnd 1984; **Fac Appt:** Prof D, Univ MO-Columbia Sch Med

Wood, Gary S MD [D] - **Spec Exp:** Cutaneous Lymphoma; Melanoma; Skin Cancer; **Hospital:** Univ WI Hosp & Clins, VA Hospital, Madison; **Address:** Univ Wisconsin Health, Dept Dermatology, 1 S Park St Fl 7, Madison, WI 53715-1375; **Phone:** 608-287-2620; **Board Cert:** Anatomic Pathology 1983; Dermatology 1986; Dermatopathology 1987; **Med School:** Univ IL Coll Med 1979; **Resid:** Anatomic Pathology, Stanford Univ Med Ctr 1983; Dermatology, Stanford Univ Med Ctr 1985; **Fellow:** Immunopathology, Stanford Univ Med Ctr 1981; **Fac Appt:** Prof D, Univ Wisc

Zelickson, Brian D MD [D] - **Spec Exp:** Skin Laser Surgery; **Hospital:** Abbott - Northwestern Hosp, Fairview Southdale Hosp; **Address:** 825 Nicollet Mall, Med Arts Bldg - Ste 1002, Minneapolis, MN 55402; **Phone:** 612-338-0711; **Board Cert:** Dermatology 1999; **Med School:** Mayo Med Sch 1986; **Resid:** Dermatology, Mayo Clinic 1990; **Fac Appt:** Asst Prof D, Univ Minn

Great Plains and Mountains

Belsito, Donald V MD [D] - **Spec Exp:** Contact Dermatitis; Cutaneous Lymphoma; Immune Deficiency-Skin Disorders; Skin Cancer; **Hospital:** Univ of Kansas Hosp; **Address:** American Dermatology Assocs, 6333 Long Ave, Shawnee, KS 66216; **Phone:** 913-631-6330; **Board Cert:** Internal Medicine 1979; Dermatology 1983; Clinical & Laboratory Dematologic Immunology 1985; **Med School:** Cornell Univ-Weill Med Coll 1976; **Resid:** Internal Medicine, Case West Res Univ Hosps 1979; Dermatology, NYU Med Ctr 1982

Krueger, Gerald MD [D] - **Spec Exp:** Psoriasis; **Hospital:** Univ Utah Hosps and Clins; **Address:** Univ Utah Hlth Sci Ctr, Dept Derm, 30 N 1900 E, Ste 4B454, Salt Lake City, UT 84132; **Phone:** 801-581-6465; **Board Cert:** Dermatology 1973; **Med School:** Loma Linda Univ 1966; **Resid:** Dermatology, Univ Colorado Med Ctr 1972; **Fac Appt:** Prof D, Univ Utah

Weston, William L MD [D] - **Spec Exp:** Lupus/SLE; Erythema Multiforme; Atopic Dermatitis; **Hospital:** Univ Colorado Hosp, Chldn's Hosp - Denver, The; **Address:** Univ Hosp, Anschutz Cancer Pavilion, PO Box 6510, MS F703, Aurora, CO 80045-0510; **Phone:** 720-848-0500; **Board Cert:** Pediatrics 1970; Dermatology 1973; Clinical & Laboratory Dematologic Immunology 1985; **Med School:** Univ Colorado 1965; **Resid:** Pediatrics, Univ Colorado Med Ctr 1968; Dermatology, Univ Colorado Med Ctr 1972; **Fac Appt:** Prof D, Univ Colorado

Southwest

Butler, David F MD [D] - **Spec Exp:** Skin Cancer; **Hospital:** Scott & White Mem Hosp; **Address:** Scott White Meml Hosp, Dept Dermatology, 409 W Adams St, Temple, TX 76501; **Phone:** 254-742-3724; **Board Cert:** Dermatology 1985; **Med School:** Univ Tex Med Br, Galveston 1980; **Resid:** Dermatology, Walter Reed Army Med Ctr 1985; **Fac Appt:** Assoc Prof D, Texas Tech Univ

Carney, John M MD [D] - **Spec Exp:** Mohs' Surgery; Skin Cancer; **Hospital:** UAMS Med Ctr; **Address:** Southwest Med Arts Bldg, 11321 Interstate 30, Ste 201, Little Rock, AR 72209; **Phone:** 501-455-4700; **Board Cert:** Dermatology 1984; **Med School:** Northwestern Univ 1979; **Resid:** Dermatology, Univ Hosps 1984; **Fellow:** Physiology, Harvard Med Sch 1985; Dermatologic Surgery, Univ Tenn Med Ctr 1986; **Fac Appt:** Clin Prof D, Univ Ark

Cockerell, Clay J MD [D] - **Spec Exp:** Dermatopathology; **Hospital:** UT Southwestern Med Ctr - Dallas; **Address:** Dermatopath Labs, 2330 Butler St, Ste 115, Dallas, TX 75235; **Phone:** 214-638-2222; **Board Cert:** Dermatology 1999; Dermatopathology 1986; **Med School:** Baylor Coll Med 1981; **Resid:** Dermatology, NYU Med Ctr 1985; **Fellow:** Dermatopathology, NYU Med Ctr 1986; **Fac Appt:** Prof DP, Univ Tex SW, Dallas

Duvic, Madeleine MD [D] - **Spec Exp:** Cutaneous Lymphoma; Skin Cancer; Alopecia Areata; **Hospital:** UT MD Anderson Cancer Ctr (page 71); **Address:** MD Anderson Cancer Ctr, Dept Dermatology, 1515 Holcombe Blvd, Unit 434, Houston, TX 77030; **Phone:** 713-745-1113; **Board Cert:** Dermatology 1981; Internal Medicine 1982; **Med School:** Duke Univ 1977; **Resid:** Dermatology, Duke Univ Med Ctr 1980; Internal Medicine, Duke Univ Med Ctr 1982; **Fellow:** Geriatric Medicine, Duke Univ Med Ctr 1984; **Fac Appt:** Prof D, Univ Tex, Houston

Dermatology

Hansen, Ronald MD [D] - **Spec Exp:** Pediatric Dermatology; **Hospital:** Phoenix Children's Hosp; **Address:** Phoenix Childrens Hosp, Dept Dermatology, 1919 E Thomas Rd, Phoenix, AZ 85016-7710; **Phone:** 602-546-0895; **Board Cert:** Pediatrics 1974; Dermatology 1980; **Med School:** Univ Iowa Coll Med 1968; **Resid:** Pediatrics, Childrens Hosp 1970; Pediatrics, Stanford Univ Med Ctr 1972; **Fellow:** Dermatology, Univ Medical Ctr 1980; **Fac Appt:** Prof D, Univ Ariz Coll Med

Horn, Thomas D MD [D] - **Spec Exp:** Skin Cancer; Graft vs Host Disease; **Hospital:** UAMS Med Ctr; **Address:** UAMS, Dept Derm, 4301 W Markham Street, Slot 576, Little Rock, AR 72205; **Phone:** 501-686-5110; **Board Cert:** Dermatology 2001; Dermatopathology 1988; **Med School:** Univ VA Sch Med 1982; **Resid:** Dermatology, Univ Maryland Med Ctr 1987; **Fellow:** Dermatopathology, Johns Hopkins Hosp 1989; **Fac Appt:** Prof D, Univ Ark

Levy, Moise L MD [D] - **Spec Exp:** Pediatric Dermatology; Vascular Malformations; **Hospital:** Texas Chldns Hosp - Houston; **Address:** 6701 Fannin, MC CC620.16, Houston, TX 77030; **Phone:** 832-822-3718; **Board Cert:** Pediatrics 1985; Dermatology 1986; **Med School:** Univ Tex, Houston 1979; **Resid:** Pediatrics, Univ Tex Affil Hosp 1983; Dermatology, Baylor Coll Med 1986; **Fac Appt:** Prof D, Baylor Coll Med

Menter, M Alan MD [D] - **Spec Exp:** Psoriasis; Cosmetic Dermatology; **Hospital:** Baylor Univ Medical Ctr; **Address:** 5310 Harvest Hill Rd, Ste 260, Dallas, TX 75230-5811; **Phone:** 972-386-7546 x400; **Board Cert:** Dermatology 1978; **Med School:** South Africa 1966; **Resid:** Dermatology, Pretoria Genl Hosp 1971; Dermatology, Guys Hosp 1972; **Fellow:** Dermatology, St Johns Hosp 1973; Dermatology, Univ Texas SW 1979; **Fac Appt:** Clin Prof D, Univ Tex SW, Dallas

Sontheimer, Richard MD [D] - **Spec Exp:** Immune Deficiency-Skin Disorders; Lupus/SLE; **Hospital:** OU Med Ctr, VA Med Ctr - Oklahoma City; **Address:** 619 NE 13th St, Oklahoma City, OK 73104; **Phone:** 405-271-6110; **Board Cert:** Internal Medicine 1976; Dermatology 1979; Clinical & Laboratory Dematologic Immunology 1985; **Med School:** Univ Tex SW, Dallas 1972; **Resid:** Internal Medicine, Univ Utah Affil Hosps 1976; Dermatology, Parkland Meml Hosp 1979; **Fellow:** Research, Southwestern Med Sch 1978; **Fac Appt:** Prof D, Univ Iowa Coll Med

Taylor, R Stan MD [D] - **Spec Exp:** Mohs' Surgery; Melanoma; Skin Cancer; **Hospital:** UT Southwestern Med Ctr - Dallas, Parkland Meml Hosp - Dallas; **Address:** Univ Tex SW Med Sch, Dept Derm, 5323 Harry Hines Blvd, MC 9192, Dallas, TX 75390-9192; **Phone:** 214-645-8950; **Board Cert:** Dermatology 1989; **Med School:** Univ Tex Med Br, Galveston 1985; **Resid:** Dermatology, Univ Mich Med Ctr 1989; **Fellow:** Immunological Dermatology, Univ Mich 1990; Mohs Surgery, Oregon Hlth Sci Univ 1991; **Fac Appt:** Prof D, Univ Tex SW, Dallas

West Coast and Pacific

Bennett, Richard G MD [D] - **Spec Exp:** Mohs' Surgery; Skin Cancer; **Hospital:** UCLA Med Ctr, USC Univ Hosp - R K Eamer Med Plz; **Address:** 1301 20th St, Ste 570, Santa Monica, CA 90404-2080; **Phone:** 310-315-0171; **Board Cert:** Dermatology 1975; **Med School:** Case West Res Univ 1970; **Resid:** Dermatology, Hosp Univ Penn 1974; **Fellow:** Chemosurgery, NYU Med Ctr 1977; **Fac Appt:** Clin Prof D, UCLA

Berg, Daniel MD [D] - **Spec Exp:** Skin Laser Surgery; Skin Cancer; **Hospital:** Univ Wash Med Ctr; **Address:** 4225 Roosevelt Way NE, Seattle, WA 98105; **Phone:** 206-598-6647; **Board Cert:** Dermatology 1999; **Med School:** Univ Toronto 1985; **Resid:** Internal Medicine, Sunnybrook Med Ctr 1988; Dermatology, Duke Univ Med Ctr 1991; **Fellow:** Dermatologic Surgery, Univ Toronto 1993; Dermatologic Surgery, Univ British Columbia 1994; **Fac Appt:** Prof D, Univ Wash

Conant, Marcus A MD [D] - **Spec Exp:** AIDS/HIV-Kaposi's Sarcoma; **Hospital:** UCSF Med Ctr, CA Pacific Med Ctr; **Address:** 470 Castro St, Ste 202, San Francisco, CA 94114; **Phone:** 415-575-7500; **Board Cert:** Dermatology 1969; **Med School:** Duke Univ 1961; **Resid:** Dermatology, UCSF Med Ctr 1967; **Fac Appt:** Clin Prof D, UCSF

Eichenfield, Lawrence F MD [D] - **Spec Exp:** Eczema; Acne; Vascular Birthmarks; Pediatric Dermatology; **Hospital:** Rady Children's Hosp - San Diego, UCSD Med Ctr; **Address:** Chldns Hosp, Ped & Adolescent Dermatology, 8010 Frost St, Ste 602, San Diego, CA 92123-4204; **Phone:** 858-966-6795; **Board Cert:** Dermatology 1999; Pediatrics 1998; **Med School:** Mount Sinai Sch Med 1984; **Resid:** Pediatrics, Chldns Hosp 1987; Dermatology, Hosp Univ Penn 1991; **Fac Appt:** Prof Ped, UCSD

Fitzpatrick, Richard MD [D] - **Spec Exp:** Cosmetic Dermatology; Skin Laser Surgery-Resurfacing; Hair Restoration/Transplant; **Hospital:** Scripps Meml Hosp - La Jolla; **Address:** 9850 Genesee St, Ste 480, La Jolla, CA 90237; **Phone:** 858-452-2066; **Board Cert:** Dermatology 2003; **Med School:** Emory Univ 1970; **Resid:** Dermatology, UCLA Med Ctr 1978; **Fac Appt:** Assoc Clin Prof D, UCSD

Frieden, Ilona J MD [D] - **Spec Exp:** Pediatric Dermatology; Vascular Birthmarks; Hemangiomas; **Hospital:** UCSF - Mt Zion Med Ctr; **Address:** UCSF, Dept Dermatology, 1701 Divisadero St, Box 0316, San Francisco, CA 94143-0316; **Phone:** 415-353-7800; **Board Cert:** Dermatology 2005; Pediatrics 1983; Pediatric Dermatology 2004; **Med School:** UCSF 1977; **Resid:** Pediatrics, UCSF Med Ctr 1980; Dermatology, UCSF Med Ctr 1983; **Fac Appt:** Clin Prof D, UCSF

Glogau, Richard G MD [D] - **Spec Exp:** Cosmetic Dermatology; Skin Laser Surgery; Mohs' Surgery; Botox Therapy; **Hospital:** UCSF Med Ctr; **Address:** 350 Parnassus Ave, Ste 400, San Francisco, CA 94117; **Phone:** 415-564-1261; **Board Cert:** Dermatology 1978; Dermatopathology 1982; **Med School:** Harvard Med Sch 1973; **Resid:** Dermatology, UCSF Med Ctr 1977; **Fellow:** Chemosurgery, UCSF Med Ctr 1978; **Fac Appt:** Clin Prof D, UCSF

Greenway, Hubert T MD [D] - **Spec Exp:** Skin Cancer; Mohs' Surgery; Melanoma; **Hospital:** Scripps Green Hosp; **Address:** Scripps Clinic, Dept Mohs' Surgery, 10666 N Torrey Pines Rd, MS 112A, La Jolla, CA 92037; **Phone:** 858-554-8646; **Board Cert:** Dermatology 1982; **Med School:** Med Coll GA 1974; **Resid:** Dermatology, Naval Hosp 1982; **Fellow:** Chemosurgery, Univ Wisconsin Med Ctr 1983

Grimes, Pearl E MD [D] - **Spec Exp:** Pigmented Lesions; **Hospital:** UCLA Med Ctr; **Address:** 5670 Wilshire Blvd, Ste 650, Los Angeles, CA 90036; **Phone:** 323-467-4389; **Board Cert:** Dermatology 1979; **Med School:** Washington Univ, St Louis 1974; **Resid:** Dermatology, Howard Univ 1979; **Fac Appt:** Clin Prof D, UCLA

Hanifin, Jon M MD [D] - **Spec Exp:** Atopic Dermatitis; **Hospital:** OR Hlth & Sci Univ; **Address:** Oregon Hlth & Sci Univ, Dept Derm, 3303 SW Bond Ave, MC CH16D, Portland, OR 97239; **Phone:** 503-418-3376; **Board Cert:** Dermatology 1970; **Med School:** Univ Wisc 1965; **Resid:** Dermatology, UCSF Med Ctr 1969; **Fac Appt:** Prof D, Oregon Hlth Sci Univ

Kilmer, Suzanne L MD [D] - **Spec Exp:** Skin Laser Surgery-Resurfacing; Skin Rejuvenation; **Hospital:** Mercy General Hosp - Sacramento; **Address:** 3835 J St, Sacramento, CA 95816-5520; **Phone:** 916-456-0400; **Board Cert:** Dermatology 1999; **Med School:** UC Davis 1987; **Resid:** Dermatology, UC Davis Med Ctr 1991; **Fellow:** Laser Surgery, Mass Genl Hosp 1992; **Fac Appt:** Asst Clin Prof D, UC Davis

Kim, Youn-Hee MD [D] - **Spec Exp:** Cutaneous Lymphoma; Skin Cancer; **Hospital:** Stanford Univ Med Ctr; **Address:** 900 Blake Wilbur Drive, rm W0010, MC 5334, Stanford Univ Med Ctr, Dept Dermatology, Stanford, CA 94305-5334; **Phone:** 650-723-6316; **Board Cert:** Dermatology 1989; **Med School:** Stanford Univ 1985; **Resid:** Dermatology, Metropolitan Hospital 1989

Klein, Arnold W MD [D] - **Spec Exp:** Cosmetic Dermatology; Botox Therapy; **Hospital:** UCLA Med Ctr, Cedars-Sinai Med Ctr; **Address:** 435 N Roxbury Dr, Ste 204, Beverly Hills, CA 90210-5027; **Phone:** 310-275-5136; **Board Cert:** Dermatology 1976; **Med School:** Univ Pennsylvania 1971; **Resid:** Dermatology, Hosp Univ Penn 1973; Dermatology, UCLA Med Ctr 1975; **Fac Appt:** Prof D, UCLA

Koo, John Ying Ming MD [D] - **Spec Exp:** Psoriasis/Eczema; Photosensitive Skin Disorders; Psychodermatology; **Hospital:** UCSF Med Ctr; **Address:** Psoriasis Day Treatment Ctr, 515 Spruce St, San Francisco, CA 94118; **Phone:** 415-476-4701; **Board Cert:** Dermatology 1988; Psychiatry 1988; **Med School:** Harvard Med Sch 1981; **Resid:** Psychiatry, UCLA Neur Psyc Inst 1985; Dermatology, UCSF Med Ctr 1988; **Fac Appt:** Prof D, UCSF

Lask, Gary P MD [D] - **Spec Exp:** Skin Laser Surgery-Resurfacing; Cosmetic Dermatology; **Hospital:** UCLA Med Ctr; **Address:** 16260 Ventura Blvd, Ste 530, Encino, CA 91436; **Phone:** 818-788-4022; **Board Cert:** Dermatology 1983; **Med School:** Mexico 1977; **Resid:** Dermatology, Martin Luther King Jr Hosp 1983; **Fac Appt:** Clin Prof D, UCLA

Rubin, Mark G MD [D] - **Spec Exp:** Skin Laser Surgery; Cosmetic Dermatology; **Hospital:** UCSD Med Ctr; **Address:** 153 S Lasky Drive, Ste 1, Beverly Hills, CA 90212; **Phone:** 310-556-0119; **Board Cert:** Dermatology 1985; **Med School:** Jefferson Med Coll 1981; **Resid:** Dermatology, Henry Ford Hosp 1985; **Fac Appt:** Assoc Prof D, UCSD

Swanson, Neil MD [D] - **Spec Exp:** Skin Cancer; Cosmetic Dermatology; **Hospital:** OR Hlth & Sci Univ, VA Medical Center - Portland; **Address:** Oregon HSU, Center for Health & Healing, 3303 SW Bond Ave, CH16D, Portland, OR 97239; **Phone:** 503-418-3376; **Board Cert:** Dermatology 1980; **Med School:** Univ Rochester 1976; **Resid:** Dermatology, Univ Michigan Med Ctr 1979; **Fellow:** Dermatology, UCSF Med Ctr 1980; **Fac Appt:** Prof D, Oregon Hlth Sci Univ

Swetter, Susan M MD [D] - **Spec Exp:** Melanoma; Melanoma Early Detection/Prevention; Skin Cancer; **Hospital:** VA Hlth Care Sys - Palo Alto, Stanford Univ Med Ctr; **Address:** Stanford U Medical Ctr, Dept Dermatology, 900 Blake Wilbur Dr, W0069, Stanford, CA 94305; **Phone:** 650-852-3494; **Board Cert:** Dermatology 2001; **Med School:** Univ Pennsylvania 1990; **Resid:** Dermatology, Stanford U Med Ctr 1994; **Fac Appt:** Assoc Prof D, Stanford Univ

Tabak, Brian MD [D] - **Spec Exp:** Skin Cancer; **Hospital:** Long Beach Meml Med Ctr; **Address:** 3918 Long Beach Blvd, Ste 200, Long Beach, CA 90807; **Phone:** 562-989-5512; **Board Cert:** Dermatology 1981; **Med School:** McGill Univ 1977; **Resid:** Dermatology, USC Med Ctr 1981; **Fac Appt:** Asst Clin Prof Med, USC Sch Med

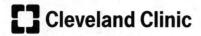 **Cleveland Clinic**

Dermatology

Cleveland Clinic Department of Dermatology offers a full array of subspecialized care for adult and pediatric patients. Our physicians diagnose and treat all disorders of the skin, hair and nails, whether primary or related to an underlying systemic illness, including industrial-related conditions.

Cleveland Clinic Dermatologist offer expert diagnostic and management options including:

- Skin Cancer and Mohs Surgery
- Psoriasis
- Varicose Veins and Spider Veins
- Phototherapy
- Pediatric Dermatology
- Industrial Dermatology
- Cosmetic Dermatology
- Laser Surgery

Dermatologic Surgery

The department offers a full range of procedures in the subspecialty area of dermatologic surgery. These include Mohs micrographic surgery for high-risk skin cancers (including local tissue reconstruction), laser surgery, chemical peels, soft tissue augmentation, botox injections, hair transplant and liposuction. Additionally, our Cutaneous Care Center provides outpatient treatment, rather than hospitalization, for patients with extensive, severe or chronic skin diseases utilizing phototherapy and excimer laser treatment.

Staff dermatologists and residents are involved in research, either institutionally or through industrial support of clinical trials.

To schedule an appointment or for more information about the Cleveland Clinic Department of Dermatology call 800.890.2467 or visit www.clevelandclinic.org/dermtopdocs.

Second Opinion-Online

Use e-Cleveland Clinic's convenient, online second opinion service without leaving home. Call 800.223.2273, ext 43223, or visit www.eclevelandclinic.org.

Assistance for Out-of-Town and International Patients

Get complimentary help scheduling medical appointments and arranging for hotels and transportation. For out-of-town patients call 800.223.2273, ext. 55580, or visit www.clevelandclinic.org/services. For International patients call 216.444.6404 or visit www.clevelandclinic.org/ic.

Department of Dermatology | 9500 Euclid Avenue / W14 | Cleveland OH 44195

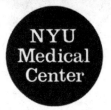

NYU Medical Center

550 First Avenue (at 31st Street)
New York, NY 10016
Physician Referral:
(888)7-NYU-MED (888-769-8633)
www.nyumc.org

DERMATOLOGY
State-of-the-Art Care of Skin Problems

With a history dating back to 1882, the Ronald O. Perelman Department of Dermatology at NYU Medical Center is recognized nationally and internationally as a leader in dermatology. Through the Charles C. Harris Skin and Cancer Pavilion, in the offices of Dermatologic Associates, and in the general and specialty clinics at affiliated hospital facilities, the staff members of the Department provide primary and consultative dermatologic care for over 100,000 ambulatory and hospitalized patients yearly. In addition, faculty members of the Department conduct major research projects aimed at the most significant dermatologic problems of our day including major efforts aimed at prevention, detection and therapy of melanoma and other skin cancers.

The expertise of NYU Medical Center's dermatologists encompasses all facets of medical, surgical, pediatric and cosmetic dermatology, including diseases of the hair, nails, and mucuous membranes. Laser surgery is performed for a wide variety of skin and hair problems, and Mohs micrographic surgery and is available for skin cancers. Dermatologists at NYU Medical Center work closely with researchers trying to better understand and help alleviate dermatologic conditions, so their care of even the most common dermatological problems such as acne, eczema, psoriasis, and warts takes advantage of the most up-to-date breakthroughs in medicine and science. Research in the Department is carried out in a variety of settings, and the Deopartment of Dermatology's Cutaneous Biology Research Program encompasses an entire floor of the new Smilow Translational Research Building.

Research for the purpose of discovering the causes of and developing new treatments for skin diseases goes hand in hand with patient care and teaching. The Department conducts a strong and diversified research program in the basic and applied sciences, studying fundamental processes which have a bearing on clinical practice, as well as new and different methods of therapy. Over 25 members of the full-time faculty are engaged in laboratory and clinical research and active participation in their research projects forms an integral part of the educational program for the many young dermatologists trained in the Department .

Areas of Basic and Clinical Research

AIDS: Kaposi's sarcoma and skin infections

Bullous Diseases: Pemphigus and bullous pemphigoid

Congenital and Genetic Skin Diseases

Contact Dermatitis and Occupational Dermatitis

Dermatopharmacology: clinical trials of the latest therapeutic agents and diagnostic devices

Dermatopathology: study of the microscopic diagnosis of skin disease

Pediatric Dermatology: Hemangiomas, eczema,psoriasis, birthmarks

Epithelial Biology: Psoriasis and Ichthyosis

Allergic Diseases: Hives and Vasculitis

Viral Diseases: AIDS and Herpes

Laser: Birthmarks, skin tumors, pigmentary disorders

Mycology: Superficial and deep fungal infections

Oncology: Melanoma, basal cell carcinoma, squamous cell carcinoma, cutaneous lymphoma

Photomedicine: Psoriasis, vitiligo

Surgery: Cosmetic and cancer surgery

Hair: Alopecia and Hirsutism

Physician Referral
(888) 7-NYU-MED
(888-769-8633)
www.med.nyu.edu

Endocrinology, Diabetes & Metabolism

a subspecialty of Internal Medicine

An internist who concentrates on disorders of the internal (endocrine) glands such as the thyroid and adrenal glands. This specialist also deals with disorders such as diabetes, metabolic and nutritional disorders, pituitary diseases, menstrual and sexual problems.

Training Required: Three years in internal medicine *plus* additional training and examination for certification in endocrinology, diabetes and metabolism.

Endocrinology, Diabetes & Metabolism

New England

Abrahamson, Martin J MD [EDM] - **Spec Exp:** Diabetes; **Hospital:** Beth Israel Deaconess Med Ctr - Boston; **Address:** Joslin Diabetes Clinic, 1 Joslin Pl, Boston, MA 02215; **Phone:** 617-732-2501; **Board Cert:** Internal Medicine 2005; Endocrinology, Diabetes & Metabolism 2005; **Med School:** South Africa 1977; **Resid:** Internal Medicine, Groote Schuuer Hosp-Univ Cape Town 1983; **Fellow:** Endocrinology, Diabetes & Metabolism, Groote Schuuer Hosp-Univ Cape Town 1985; Research, Univ Cape Town 1987; **Fac Appt:** Assoc Prof Med, Harvard Med Sch

Axelrod, Lloyd MD [EDM] - **Spec Exp:** Diabetes; Geriatric Endocrinology; **Hospital:** Mass Genl Hosp; **Address:** 50 Staniford St Fl 3 - Ste 340, Boston, MA 02114; **Phone:** 617-726-8722; **Board Cert:** Internal Medicine 1973; Endocrinology, Diabetes & Metabolism 1973; **Med School:** Harvard Med Sch 1967; **Resid:** Internal Medicine, Peter Bent Brigham Hosp 1969; Internal Medicine, Mass Genl Hosp 1971; **Fellow:** Endocrinology, Diabetes & Metabolism, Peter Bent Brigham Hosp 1970; Endocrinology, Diabetes & Metabolism, Mass Genl Hosp 1972; **Fac Appt:** Assoc Prof Med, Harvard Med Sch

Biller, Beverly M K MD [EDM] - **Spec Exp:** Pituitary Disorders; Cushing's Syndrome; Acromegaly; **Hospital:** Mass Genl Hosp; **Address:** Neuroendocrine Clinic Center, Zero Emerson Pl, Ste 112, Boston, MA 02114-3117; **Phone:** 617-726-3870; **Board Cert:** Internal Medicine 1986; Endocrinology 1989; **Med School:** Univ Okla Coll Med 1983; **Resid:** Internal Medicine, Beth Israel Deaconness Hosp 1986; **Fellow:** Endocrinology, Diabetes & Metabolism, Mass Genl Hosp 1989; **Fac Appt:** Assoc Prof Med, Harvard Med Sch

Comi, Richard J MD [EDM] - **Spec Exp:** Diabetes; Hypoglycemia; Thyroid Disorders; Pituitary Disorders; **Hospital:** Dartmouth - Hitchcock Med Ctr; **Address:** Dartmouth-Hitchcock Med Ctr, Endocrinology, One Medical Ctr Drive, Lebanon, NH 03756; **Phone:** 603-650-8630; **Board Cert:** Internal Medicine 1983; Endocrinology 1987; **Med School:** Harvard Med Sch 1980; **Resid:** Internal Medicine, Mass Genl Hosp 1983; **Fellow:** Endocrinology & Diabetes, Natl Inst Hlth 1986

Daniels, Gilbert MD [EDM] - **Spec Exp:** Thyroid Disorders; Parathyroid Disease; Adrenal Disorders; **Hospital:** Mass Genl Hosp; **Address:** 15 Parkman St, Bldg WACC - Ste 730, Boston, MA 02114; **Phone:** 617-726-8430; **Board Cert:** Internal Medicine 1972; Endocrinology, Diabetes & Metabolism 1975; **Med School:** Harvard Med Sch 1966; **Resid:** Internal Medicine, Mass Genl Hosp 1972; **Fellow:** Biochemistry, Natl Inst Hlth 1970; Endocrinology, Diabetes & Metabolism, UCSF Med Ctr 1971; **Fac Appt:** Prof Med, Harvard Med Sch

Godine, John E MD/PhD [EDM] - **Spec Exp:** Diabetes; **Hospital:** Mass Genl Hosp; **Address:** 50 Staniford St Fl 3 - Ste 340, Boston, MA 02114; **Phone:** 617-726-8722; **Board Cert:** Internal Medicine 1979; Endocrinology, Diabetes & Metabolism 1981; **Med School:** Harvard Med Sch 1976; **Resid:** Internal Medicine, Mass Genl Hosp 1978; **Fellow:** Endocrinology, Diabetes & Metabolism, Mass Genl Hosp 1981; **Fac Appt:** Asst Prof Med, Harvard Med Sch

Inzucchi, Silvio E MD [EDM] - **Spec Exp:** Diabetes; Pituitary Disorders; Growth Hormone Therapy-Adult; **Hospital:** Yale - New Haven Hosp; **Address:** Yale Univ Sch Med, Div Endocrinology, Box 208020, New Haven, CT 06520-8020; **Phone:** 203-737-1932; **Board Cert:** Internal Medicine 1988; **Med School:** Harvard Med Sch 1985; **Resid:** Internal Medicine, Yale-New Haven Hosp 1988; **Fellow:** Endocrinology, Diabetes & Metabolism, Yale-New Haven Hosp 1994; **Fac Appt:** Prof Med, Yale Univ

Klibanski, Anne MD [EDM] - **Spec Exp:** Pituitary Disorders; Prolactin Disorders; Acromegaly; **Hospital:** Mass Genl Hosp; **Address:** Neuroendocrine Clinic Ctr, Zero Emerson Pl, Ste 112, Boston, MA 02114; **Phone:** 617-726-7948; **Board Cert:** Internal Medicine 1978; Endocrinology, Diabetes & Metabolism 1981; **Med School:** NYU Sch Med 1975; **Resid:** Internal Medicine, Bellevue Hosp Ctr 1978; **Fellow:** Endocrinology, Mass Genl Hosp 1981; **Fac Appt:** Prof Med, Harvard Med Sch

LeBoff, Meryl S MD [EDM] - **Spec Exp:** Osteoporosis; Metabolic Bone Disease; Women's Health; Endocrinology; **Hospital:** Brigham & Women's Hosp; **Address:** 221 Longwood Ave, Boston, MA 02115; **Phone:** 617-732-5666; **Board Cert:** Internal Medicine 1979; Endocrinology, Diabetes & Metabolism 1981; **Med School:** UMDNJ-NJ Med Sch, Newark 1975; **Resid:** Internal Medicine, USC Med Ctr 1979; **Fellow:** Endocrinology, Brigham & Womens Hosp 1982; **Fac Appt:** Assoc Prof Med, Harvard Med Sch

Lechan, Ronald MD/PhD [EDM] - **Spec Exp:** Pituitary Disorders; Hypothalamic Dysfunction; Islet Cell Tumors; **Hospital:** Tufts-New England Med Ctr; **Address:** New England Med Ctr, 750 Washington St, Box 268, Boston, MA 02111; **Phone:** 617-636-5689; **Board Cert:** Internal Medicine 1979; Endocrinology, Diabetes & Metabolism 1981; **Med School:** Univ VT Coll Med 1976; **Resid:** Internal Medicine, Beth Israel Hosp 1978; **Fellow:** Endocrinology, Diabetes & Metabolism, Tufts-New England Med Ctr 1981; **Fac Appt:** Prof Med, Tufts Univ

Levine, Robert A MD [EDM] - **Spec Exp:** Thyroid Cancer; Growth/Development Disorders; Metabolic Bone Disease; Thyroid Disorders; **Hospital:** St Joseph Hosp; **Address:** Thyroid Center of New Hampshire, 5 Coliseum Ave, Nashua, NH 03060; **Phone:** 603-881-7141; **Board Cert:** Internal Medicine 1984; Endocrinology, Diabetes & Metabolism 1987; **Med School:** Univ Conn 1981; **Resid:** Internal Medicine, Mt Auburn Hosp 1984; **Fellow:** Endocrinology, Yale Univ 1987

Seely, Ellen Wells MD [EDM] - **Spec Exp:** Pregnancy & Endocrine Disorders; Diabetes in Pregnancy; Osteoporosis; **Hospital:** Brigham & Women's Hosp; **Address:** Brigham & Womens Hosp, Endocrine Div, 221 Longwood Ave, rm 277, Boston, MA 02115-5804; **Phone:** 617-732-5661; **Board Cert:** Internal Medicine 1984; Endocrinology, Diabetes & Metabolism 1987; **Med School:** Columbia P&S 1981; **Resid:** Internal Medicine, Brigham & Womens Hosp 1984; **Fellow:** Endocrinology, Diabetes & Metabolism, Brigham & Womens Hosp 1987; **Fac Appt:** Assoc Prof Med, Harvard Med Sch

Sherwin, Robert MD [EDM] - **Spec Exp:** Diabetes; **Hospital:** Yale - New Haven Hosp; **Address:** Yale Univ Sch Med, Sect Endocrinology, 333 Cedar St, Box 208020, New Haven, CT 06520-8020; **Phone:** 203-785-4183; **Board Cert:** Internal Medicine 1972; **Med School:** Albert Einstein Coll Med 1967; **Resid:** Internal Medicine, Mt Sinai Hosp 1969; Internal Medicine, Mt Sinai Hosp 1972; **Fellow:** Metabolism, Yale-New Haven Hosp 1973; **Fac Appt:** Prof Med, Yale Univ

Williams, Gordon H MD [EDM] - **Spec Exp:** Hypertension; Pituitary Disorders; **Hospital:** Brigham & Women's Hosp; **Address:** 221 Longwood Ave, Boston, MA 02115-5817; **Phone:** 617-732-5666; **Board Cert:** Internal Medicine 1970; Endocrinology, Diabetes & Metabolism 1975; **Med School:** Harvard Med Sch 1963; **Resid:** Internal Medicine, Peter Bent Brigham Hosp 1967; **Fellow:** Endocrinology, Diabetes & Metabolism, Peter Bent Brigham Hosp 1970; **Fac Appt:** Prof Med, Harvard Med Sch

Endocrinology, Diabetes & Metabolism

Mid Atlantic

Bergman, Donald MD [EDM] - **Spec Exp:** Osteoporosis; Thyroid Disorders; Calcium Disorders; **Hospital:** Mount Sinai Med Ctr; **Address:** 1199 Park Ave, Ste 1F, New York, NY 10128; **Phone:** 212-876-7333; **Board Cert:** Internal Medicine 1975; Endocrinology, Diabetes & Metabolism 1977; **Med School:** Jefferson Med Coll 1971; **Resid:** Obstetrics & Gynecology, Mount Sinai Hosp 1972; Internal Medicine, Mount Sinai Hosp 1975; **Fellow:** Endocrinology, Diabetes & Metabolism, Mount Sinai Hosp 1977; **Fac Appt:** Clin Prof Med, Mount Sinai Sch Med

Bilezikian, John P MD [EDM] - **Spec Exp:** Osteoporosis; Bone Disorders-Metabolic; Parathyroid Disease; **Hospital:** NY-Presby Hosp/Columbia (page 66); **Address:** NY Presby Hosp, Metabolic Bone Diseases, Harkness Pavilion, 180 Ft Washington Ave Fl 9 - Ste 920, New York, NY 10032; **Phone:** 212-305-2663; **Board Cert:** Internal Medicine 1975; Endocrinology, Diabetes & Metabolism 1977; **Med School:** Columbia P&S 1969; **Resid:** Internal Medicine, Columbia-Presby Hosp 1975; **Fellow:** Endocrinology, Diabetes & Metabolism, Natl Inst Health 1977; **Fac Appt:** Prof Med, Columbia P&S

Blum, Conrad MD [EDM] - **Spec Exp:** Cholesterol/Lipid Disorders; Thyroid Disorders; Diabetes; **Hospital:** NY-Presby Hosp/Columbia (page 66); **Address:** 16 E 60th St, Ste 320, New York, NY 10022-1002; **Phone:** 212-326-8421; **Board Cert:** Internal Medicine 1976; Endocrinology, Diabetes & Metabolism 1977; **Med School:** Northwestern Univ 1971; **Resid:** Internal Medicine, Brigham Hosp 1976; **Fellow:** Endocrinology, Diabetes & Metabolism, Northwestern Univ Med Sch 1977; **Fac Appt:** Clin Prof Med, Columbia P&S

Bockman, Richard MD/PhD [EDM] - **Spec Exp:** Bone Disorders-Metabolic; Osteoporosis; Thyroid Disorders; **Hospital:** Hosp For Special Surgery (page 60), NY-Presby Hosp/Weill Cornell (page 66); **Address:** 519 E 72nd St, New York, NY 10021; **Phone:** 212-606-1458; **Board Cert:** Internal Medicine 1975; **Med School:** Yale Univ 1968; **Resid:** Internal Medicine, NYU Med Ctr 1975; **Fellow:** Internal Medicine, NY-Cornell Med Ctr 1973; **Fac Appt:** Prof Med, Cornell Univ-Weill Med Coll

Cooper, David S MD [EDM] - **Spec Exp:** Thyroid Disorders; **Hospital:** Sinai Hosp - Baltimore, Johns Hopkins Hosp - Baltimore (page 61); **Address:** Sinai Hospital, Div Endocrinology, 2435 W Belvedere Ave, Ste 25, Baltimore, MD 21215; **Phone:** 410-601-5961; **Board Cert:** Internal Medicine 1987; Endocrinology, Diabetes & Metabolism 1979; **Med School:** Tufts Univ 1973; **Resid:** Internal Medicine, Barnes Hosp 1976; **Fellow:** Endocrinology, Mass Genl Hosp 1978; **Fac Appt:** Prof Med, Johns Hopkins Univ

Davies, Terry MD [EDM] - **Spec Exp:** Thyroid Disorders; Graves' Disease; Hashimoto's Disease; **Hospital:** Mount Sinai Med Ctr; **Address:** 5 E 98th St, Box 1055, New York, NY 10029-6500; **Phone:** 212-241-7975; **Med School:** England 1971; **Resid:** Internal Medicine, Univ Newcastle 1975; **Fellow:** Endocrinology, Diabetes & Metabolism, Univ Newcastle 1977; Endocrinology, Diabetes & Metabolism, Natl Inst Hlth 1979; **Fac Appt:** Prof Med, Mount Sinai Sch Med

Dobs, Adrian Sandra MD [EDM] - **Spec Exp:** Hormonal Disorders; Hypogonadism; Diabetes; Metabolic Disorders; **Hospital:** Johns Hopkins Hosp - Baltimore (page 61); **Address:** Johns Hopkins Hosp, 1830 E Monument St, Fl 3 - Ste 328, Baltimore, MD 21287; **Phone:** 410-955-2130; **Board Cert:** Internal Medicine 1981; Endocrinology 1987; **Med School:** Albany Med Coll 1978; **Resid:** Internal Medicine, Montefiore Hosp 1982; **Fellow:** Endocrinology, Johns Hopkins Hosp 1984; **Fac Appt:** Prof Med, Johns Hopkins Univ

Felig, Philip MD [EDM] - **Spec Exp:** Diabetes; Thyroid Disorders; Osteoporosis; **Hospital:** Lenox Hill Hosp (page 62), Beth Israel Med Ctr - Petrie Division; **Address:** 1056 5th Ave, New York, NY 10028-0112; **Phone:** 212-534-5900; **Board Cert:** Internal Medicine 1968; **Med School:** Yale Univ 1961; **Resid:** Internal Medicine, Yale-New Haven Hosp 1967; **Fellow:** Endocrinology, Diabetes & Metabolism, Peter Bent Brigham Hosp 1969

Fleischer, Norman MD [EDM] - **Spec Exp:** Thyroid Disorders; Adrenal Disorders; Pituitary Disorders; **Hospital:** Montefiore Med Ctr - Weiler-Einstein Div; **Address:** 1575 Blondell Ave, Ste 200, Bronx, NY 10461-2601; **Phone:** 718-405-8260; **Board Cert:** Internal Medicine 1968; Endocrinology, Diabetes & Metabolism 1973; **Med School:** Vanderbilt Univ 1961; **Resid:** Internal Medicine, Bronx Muni Hosp Ctr 1964; **Fellow:** Endocrinology, Diabetes & Metabolism, Vanderbilt Univ 1966; **Fac Appt:** Prof Med, Albert Einstein Coll Med

Greene, Loren Wissner MD [EDM] - **Spec Exp:** Diabetes; Thyroid Disorders; Osteoporosis; **Hospital:** NYU Med Ctr (page 67), NY Downtown Hosp; **Address:** 530 1st Ave, Ste 4B, New York, NY 10016-6402; **Phone:** 212-263-7449; **Board Cert:** Internal Medicine 1978; Endocrinology, Diabetes & Metabolism 1981; **Med School:** NYU Sch Med 1975; **Resid:** Internal Medicine, Bellevue Hosp Ctr-NYU 1978; **Fellow:** Endocrinology, Diabetes & Metabolism, Bellevue Hosp Ctr-NYU 1980; **Fac Appt:** Assoc Clin Prof Med, NYU Sch Med

Greenspan, Susan L MD [EDM] - **Spec Exp:** Osteoporosis; **Hospital:** UPMC Presby, Pittsburgh; **Address:** Univ Pittsburgh, Osteoporosis Ctr, 3471 Fifth Ave, Kaufmann Bldg - Ste 1110, Pittsburgh, PA 15213; **Phone:** 412-692-2220; **Board Cert:** Internal Medicine 1982; Endocrinology, Diabetes & Metabolism 1987; Geriatric Medicine 1998; **Med School:** Harvard Med Sch 1979; **Resid:** Internal Medicine, Beth Israel Hosp 1982; **Fellow:** Endocrinology, Mass Genl Hosp 1985; **Fac Appt:** Prof Med, Univ Pittsburgh

Jacobs, Thomas MD [EDM] - **Spec Exp:** Adrenal Disorders; Pituitary Disorders; Calcium Disorders; **Hospital:** NY-Presby Hosp/Columbia (page 66); **Address:** 161 Fort Washington Ave, rm 210, New York, NY 10032-3713; **Phone:** 212-305-5578; **Board Cert:** Internal Medicine 1973; Endocrinology, Diabetes & Metabolism 1975; **Med School:** Johns Hopkins Univ 1968; **Resid:** Internal Medicine, Columbia Presby Hosp 1973; **Fellow:** Endocrinology, Diabetes & Metabolism, Univ Wash Med Ctr 1975; **Fac Appt:** Clin Prof Med, Columbia P&S

Kleinberg, David MD [EDM] - **Spec Exp:** Neuroendocrinology; Pituitary Disorders; **Hospital:** NYU Med Ctr (page 67); **Address:** 530 1st Ave, Ste 4C, New York, NY 10016; **Phone:** 212-263-6772; **Board Cert:** Internal Medicine 1972; Endocrinology 1975; **Med School:** Univ Miami Sch Med 1966; **Resid:** Internal Medicine, Maimonides Med Ctr 1968; Internal Medicine, Columbia-Presby Med Ctr 1971; **Fellow:** Endocrinology, Diabetes & Metabolism, Columbia-Presby Med Ctr 1970; **Fac Appt:** Prof Med, NYU Sch Med

Korytkowski, Mary T MD [EDM] - **Spec Exp:** Diabetes; Polycystic Ovarian Syndrome; Thyroid Disorders; **Hospital:** UPMC Presby, Pittsburgh; **Address:** Univ Pittsburgh Physicians - Div Endocrinology, 3601 Fifth Ave, Falk Bldg, Ste 2B, Pittsburgh, PA 15213-3403; **Phone:** 412-586-9714; **Board Cert:** Internal Medicine 1985; Endocrinology 1989; **Med School:** Univ NC Sch Med 1982; **Resid:** Internal Medicine, Francis Scott Key Med Ctr 1985; **Fellow:** Endocrinology, Diabetes & Metabolism, Sinai Hosp/Johns Hopkins Hosp 1988; **Fac Appt:** Prof Med, Univ Pittsburgh

Endocrinology, Diabetes & Metabolism

Ladenson, Paul W MD [EDM] - **Spec Exp:** Thyroid Disorders; Thyroid Cancer; **Hospital:** Johns Hopkins Hosp - Baltimore (page 61); **Address:** Johns Hopkins-Div Endocrinology & Metabolism, 1830 E Monument St, rm 333, Baltimore, MD 21287; **Phone:** 410-955-3663; **Board Cert:** Internal Medicine 1978; Endocrinology, Diabetes & Metabolism 1981; **Med School:** Harvard Med Sch 1975; **Resid:** Internal Medicine, Mass Genl Hosp 1978; **Fellow:** Endocrinology, Diabetes & Metabolism, Mass Genl Hosp 1980; **Fac Appt:** Prof Med, Johns Hopkins Univ

Mahler, Richard J MD [EDM] - **Spec Exp:** Thyroid Disorders; Diabetes; **Hospital:** NY-Presby Hosp/Weill Cornell (page 66); **Address:** 220 E 69th St, New York, NY 10021-5737; **Phone:** 212-879-4073; **Board Cert:** Internal Medicine 1987; **Med School:** NY Med Coll 1959; **Resid:** Internal Medicine, NY Med-Metro Med 1962; Endocrinology, Diabetes & Metabolism, NY Med Coll 1963; **Fellow:** Endocrinology, Diabetes & Metabolism, Univ Durham/Univ New Castle 1964; **Fac Appt:** Assoc Clin Prof Med, Cornell Univ-Weill Med Coll

Mandel, Susan MD [EDM] - **Spec Exp:** Thyroid Disorders; Calcium Disorders; **Hospital:** Hosp Univ Penn - UPHS (page 72); **Address:** Hosp Univ Penn, Div Endocrinology, 3400 Spruce St, 1 Maloney, Philadelphia, PA 19104; **Phone:** 215-662-2300; **Board Cert:** Internal Medicine 1989; Endocrinology 2001; **Med School:** Columbia P&S 1986; **Resid:** Internal Medicine, Columbia Presby Med Ctr 1989; **Fellow:** Endocrinology, Brigham & Womens Hosp 1992; **Fac Appt:** Assoc Prof Med, Univ Pennsylvania

McConnell, Robert John MD [EDM] - **Spec Exp:** Thyroid Disorders; Thyroid Ultrasound; **Hospital:** NY-Presby Hosp/Columbia (page 66); **Address:** 161 Fort Washington Ave, Ste 210, New York, NY 10032-3713; **Phone:** 212-305-5579; **Board Cert:** Internal Medicine 1978; Endocrinology, Diabetes & Metabolism 1981; **Med School:** Columbia P&S 1973; **Resid:** Internal Medicine, Barnes Hosp 1975; **Fellow:** Endocrinology, Diabetes & Metabolism, Columbia-Presby Hosp 1978; **Fac Appt:** Prof Med, Columbia P&S

Mersey, James H MD [EDM] - **Spec Exp:** Diabetes; **Hospital:** Greater Baltimore Med Ctr, St Joseph Med Ctr; **Address:** 6535 N Charles St, Ste 400, Towson, MD 21204; **Phone:** 410-828-7417; **Board Cert:** Internal Medicine 1975; Endocrinology, Diabetes & Metabolism 1977; **Med School:** Johns Hopkins Univ 1972; **Resid:** Internal Medicine, Johns Hopkins Hosp 1977; **Fellow:** Endocrinology, Diabetes & Metabolism, Peter Bent Brigham Hosp 1976; **Fac Appt:** Asst Prof Med, Johns Hopkins Univ

Ratner, Robert E MD [EDM] - **Spec Exp:** Diabetes in Pregnancy; Thyroid Disorders; Diabetes; Cholesterol/Lipid Disorders; **Hospital:** Washington Hosp Ctr, Georgetown Univ Hosp; **Address:** MedStar Clinical Research Ctr, 650 Pennsylvania Ave SE, Ste 50, Washington, DC 20003; **Phone:** 202-787-5320; **Board Cert:** Internal Medicine 1980; Endocrinology, Diabetes & Metabolism 1983; **Med School:** Baylor Coll Med 1977; **Resid:** Internal Medicine, Baylor Affil Hosps 1980; **Fellow:** Endocrinology, Diabetes & Metabolism, Lahey Clin/Joslin Clin 1982; **Fac Appt:** Prof Med, Georgetown Univ

Saudek, Christopher D MD [EDM] - **Spec Exp:** Diabetes; **Hospital:** Johns Hopkins Hosp - Baltimore (page 61); **Address:** 600 N Wolfe St, Osler 575, Baltimore, MD 21287; **Phone:** 410-955-2132; **Board Cert:** Internal Medicine 1972; **Med School:** Cornell Univ-Weill Med Coll 1967; **Resid:** Internal Medicine, Presby-St Lukes Hosp 1969; Internal Medicine, Boston City Hosp 1970; **Fellow:** Endocrinology, Diabetes & Metabolism, Thorndale Lab-Harvard 1972; **Fac Appt:** Prof Med, Johns Hopkins Univ

Schwartz, Stanley S MD [EDM] - **Spec Exp:** Diabetes; **Hospital:** Hosp Univ Penn - UPHS (page 72); **Address:** Hosp Univ Penn, EDM Div, 3400 Spruce St, 9-Penn Twr, Philadelphia, PA 19104; **Phone:** 215-662-2518; **Board Cert:** Internal Medicine 1976; Endocrinology, Diabetes & Metabolism 1979; **Med School:** Univ Chicago-Pritzker Sch Med 1973; **Resid:** Internal Medicine, Hosp Univ Penn 1976; **Fellow:** Endocrinology, Diabetes & Metabolism, Univ Chicago Hosps 1978; **Fac Appt:** Assoc Clin Prof Med, Univ Pennsylvania

Shuldiner, Alan R MD [EDM] - **Spec Exp:** Diabetes; Eating Disorders/Obesity; **Hospital:** Univ of MD Med Sys; **Address:** Univ MD Sch Med, Div Endocrinology, 660 W Redwood St, rm HH-494, Baltimore, MD 21201; **Phone:** 410-706-1623; **Board Cert:** Internal Medicine 1988; Endocrinology 1989; **Med School:** Harvard Med Sch 1984; **Resid:** Internal Medicine, Columbia-Presby Hosp 1986; **Fellow:** Endocrinology, Diabetes & Metabolism, Natl Inst Hlth 1990; **Fac Appt:** Prof Med, Univ MD Sch Med

Siris, Ethel MD [EDM] - **Spec Exp:** Osteoporosis; Paget's Disease of Bone; Bone Disorders-Metabolic; **Hospital:** NY-Presby Hosp/Columbia (page 66); **Address:** 180 Ft Washington Ave, Harkness Bldg - Ste 904, New York, NY 10032-3710; **Phone:** 212-305-9531; **Board Cert:** Internal Medicine 1974; Endocrinology, Diabetes & Metabolism 1977; **Med School:** Columbia P&S 1971; **Resid:** Internal Medicine, Columbia-Presby Med Ctr 1974; **Fellow:** Endocrinology, Diabetes & Metabolism, Natl Inst Hlth 1976; Endocrinology, Diabetes & Metabolism, Columbia-Presby Med Ctr 1977; **Fac Appt:** Prof Med, Columbia P&S

Snyder, Peter J MD [EDM] - **Spec Exp:** Pituitary Tumors; Reproductive Endocrinology-Male; **Hospital:** Hosp Univ Penn - UPHS (page 72); **Address:** Univ Pennsylvania Med Group, 3400 Spruce St, Philadelphia, PA 19104; **Phone:** 215-898-0208; **Board Cert:** Internal Medicine 1972; Endocrinology, Diabetes & Metabolism 1972; **Med School:** Harvard Med Sch 1965; **Resid:** Internal Medicine, Beth Israel Hosp 1967; Internal Medicine, Beth Israel Hosp 1970; **Fellow:** Endocrinology, Diabetes & Metabolism, Hosp Univ Penn 1971; **Fac Appt:** Prof Med, Univ Pennsylvania

Surks, Martin MD [EDM] - **Spec Exp:** Thyroid Disorders; **Hospital:** Montefiore Med Ctr, N Central Bronx Hosp; **Address:** 3400 Bainbridge Ave Fl 2, Bronx, NY 10467; **Phone:** 866-633-8255; **Board Cert:** Internal Medicine 1967; Endocrinology, Diabetes & Metabolism 1977; **Med School:** NYU Sch Med 1960; **Resid:** Internal Medicine, Montefiore Hosp Med Ctr 1962; Internal Medicine, VA Hosp 1964; **Fellow:** Research, Natl Inst Arthritis-Metabolic Disease 1964; **Fac Appt:** Prof Med, Albert Einstein Coll Med

Tuttle, Robert Michael MD [EDM] - **Spec Exp:** Thyroid Cancer; Nuclear Medicine; **Hospital:** Meml Sloan Kettering Cancer Ctr; **Address:** Memorial Sloane Kettering Cancer Ctr, 1275 York St, Box 419, New York, NY 10021; **Phone:** 212-639-6042; **Board Cert:** Endocrinology, Diabetes & Metabolism 2004; **Med School:** Univ Louisville Sch Med 1987; **Resid:** Internal Medicine, DD Eisenhower Army Med Ctr 1990; **Fellow:** Endocrinology, Diabetes & Metabolism, Madigan Army Med Ctr 1993; **Fac Appt:** Assoc Prof Med, Cornell Univ-Weill Med Coll

Wartofsky, Leonard MD [EDM] - **Spec Exp:** Thyroid Cancer; Thyroid Disorders; **Hospital:** Washington Hosp Ctr; **Address:** 110 Irving St NW, Ste 2A62, Washington, DC 20010-2975; **Phone:** 202-877-3109; **Board Cert:** Internal Medicine 1971; Endocrinology, Diabetes & Metabolism 1972; **Med School:** Geo Wash Univ 1964; **Resid:** Internal Medicine, Barnes Hosp 1966; Internal Medicine, Bronx Muni Hosp Ctr 1967; **Fellow:** Endocrinology, Diabetes & Metabolism, Boston City Hosp 1969; **Fac Appt:** Prof Med, Georgetown Univ

Endocrinology, Diabetes & Metabolism

Young, Iven MD [EDM] - **Spec Exp:** Thyroid Disorders; Osteoporosis; Pituitary Disorders; **Hospital:** St Vincent Cath Med Ctrs - Manhattan; **Address:** 130 W 12th St, Ste 7D, New York, NY 10011-8250; **Phone:** 212-675-9332; **Board Cert:** Internal Medicine 1966; Endocrinology, Diabetes & Metabolism 1973; **Med School:** NYU Sch Med 1959; **Resid:** Internal Medicine, VA Med Ctr 1963; **Fellow:** Endocrinology, NYU Med Ctr 1966; **Fac Appt:** Assoc Clin Prof Med, NY Med Coll

Southeast

Barrett, Eugene J MD [EDM] - **Spec Exp:** Diabetes; Cholesterol/Lipid Disorders; **Hospital:** Univ Virginia Med Ctr; **Address:** Univ Virginia, Div Endocrinology, PO Box 801410, Charlottesville, VA 22908; **Phone:** 434-924-1175; **Board Cert:** Internal Medicine 1978; Endocrinology, Diabetes & Metabolism 1995; **Med School:** Univ Rochester 1975; **Resid:** Internal Medicine, Strong Meml Hosp 1977; **Fellow:** Endocrinology, Diabetes & Metabolism, Yale Univ 1980; **Fac Appt:** Prof Med, Univ VA Sch Med

Bell, David S H MD [EDM] - **Spec Exp:** Diabetes; Diabetes-Insulin Pump Therapy; Diabetic Heart Disease; **Hospital:** Univ of Ala Hosp at Birmingham; **Address:** 1020 26th St S, Birmingham, AL 35205; **Phone:** 205-933-2667; **Board Cert:** Internal Medicine 1987; Endocrinology, Diabetes & Metabolism 1981; **Med School:** Ireland 1970; **Resid:** Internal Medicine, Royal Victoria Hosp 1973; Endocrinology, Diabetes & Metabolism, Univ Saskatchewan Hosp 1975; **Fellow:** Endocrinology, Diabetes & Metabolism, Greater Baltimore Med Ctr 1976; **Fac Appt:** Prof Med, Univ Ala

Clore, John MD [EDM] - **Spec Exp:** Diabetes; Hypoglycemia; **Hospital:** Med Coll of VA Hosp; **Address:** PO Box 980155, Richmond, VA 23298; **Phone:** 804-828-2161; **Board Cert:** Internal Medicine 1985; Endocrinology, Diabetes & Metabolism 1989; **Med School:** Med Coll VA 1982; **Resid:** Internal Medicine, Med Coll Virginia 1985; **Fellow:** Endocrinology, Diabetes & Metabolism, Med Coll Virginia 1988; **Fac Appt:** Assoc Prof Med, Va Commonwealth Univ

Dalkin, Alan Craig MD [EDM] - **Spec Exp:** Bone Disorders-Metabolic; Osteoporosis; **Hospital:** Univ Virginia Med Ctr; **Address:** Univ VA Hlth Sys, Div Endocrinology, PO Box 801412, Charlottesville, VA 22908; **Phone:** 434-243-2603; **Board Cert:** Internal Medicine 1987; Endocrinology 1989; **Med School:** Univ Mich Med Sch 1984; **Resid:** Internal Medicine, Univ Chicago Hosps 1987; **Fellow:** Endocrinology, Diabetes & Metabolism, Univ Mich Med Ctr 1990; **Fac Appt:** Assoc Prof Med, Univ VA Sch Med

Earp III, H Shelton MD [EDM] - **Spec Exp:** Cancer-Hormonal Influences; **Hospital:** Univ NC Hosps; **Address:** UNC Lineberger Comprehensive Cancer Center, 102 Mason Farm Rd, CB 7295, Chapel Hill, NC 27599-7295; **Phone:** 919-966-3036; **Board Cert:** Internal Medicine 1976; Endocrinology, Diabetes & Metabolism 1977; **Med School:** Univ NC Sch Med 1970; **Resid:** Internal Medicine, NC Memorial Hosp 1975; **Fellow:** Endocrinology, Diabetes & Metabolism, Univ North Carolina Hosp 1977; **Fac Appt:** Prof Med, Univ NC Sch Med

Feinglos, Mark MD [EDM] - **Spec Exp:** Diabetes; **Hospital:** Duke Univ Med Ctr; **Address:** Duke Univ Med Ctr, Box 3921, Durham, NC 27710-0001; **Phone:** 919-684-4005; **Board Cert:** Internal Medicine 1976; Endocrinology, Diabetes & Metabolism 1977; **Med School:** McGill Univ 1973; **Resid:** Internal Medicine, Duke Univ Med Ctr 1975; **Fellow:** Endocrinology, Diabetes & Metabolism, Duke Univ Med Ctr 1977; **Fac Appt:** Prof Med, Duke Univ

Marshall, John C MD/PhD [EDM] - **Spec Exp:** Pituitary Disorders; Neuroendocrinology; Polycystic Ovarian Syndrome; **Hospital:** Univ Virginia Med Ctr; **Address:** Univ VA Hlth System, Hospital Dr, Box 800612, Charlottesville, VA 22908-0001; **Phone:** 434-924-2431; **Board Cert:** Internal Medicine 1978; Endocrinology, Diabetes & Metabolism 1981; **Med School:** England 1965; **Resid:** Neurology, Natl Hosp Queen Square 1968; Cardiovascular Disease, Natl Heart Hosp 1969; **Fellow:** Endocrinology, Diabetes & Metabolism, Hammersmith Hosp 1972; Endocrinology, Diabetes & Metabolism, UCLA 1974; **Fac Appt:** Prof Med, Univ VA Sch Med

Nestler, John E MD [EDM] - **Spec Exp:** Polycystic Ovarian Syndrome; Diabetes; **Hospital:** Med Coll of VA Hosp; **Address:** Med Coll Va, Div Endocrinology, Box 980111, Richmond, VA 23298-0111; **Phone:** 804-828-2161; **Board Cert:** Internal Medicine 1982; Endocrinology 1985; **Med School:** Univ Pennsylvania 1979; **Resid:** Internal Medicine, Med Coll Virginia 1983; **Fellow:** Endocrinology, Hosp Univ Penn 1985; **Fac Appt:** Prof Med, Med Coll VA

Ontjes, David A MD [EDM] - **Spec Exp:** Osteoporosis; Thyroid Disorders; Adrenal Disorders; Pituitary Disorders; **Hospital:** Univ NC Hosps; **Address:** UNC-Chapel Hill, 257 MacNider Bldg, Chapel Hill, NC 27599-7527; **Phone:** 919-966-3336; **Board Cert:** Internal Medicine 1972; Endocrinology, Diabetes & Metabolism 1972; **Med School:** Harvard Med Sch 1964; **Resid:** Internal Medicine, Boston City Hosp 1966; **Fac Appt:** Prof Med, Univ NC Sch Med

Ovalle, Fernando MD [EDM] - **Spec Exp:** Diabetes; Polycystic Ovarian Syndrome; Hypoglycemia; **Hospital:** Univ of Ala Hosp at Birmingham; **Address:** UAB Sch Med, 510 20th St S FOT Bldg Fl 7 - Ste 702, Birmingham, AL 35294; **Phone:** 205-975-2422; **Board Cert:** Endocrinology, Diabetes & Metabolism 1997; **Med School:** Mexico 1989; **Resid:** Internal Medicine, Henry Ford Hosp 1995; **Fellow:** Endocrinology, Diabetes & Metabolism, Barnes Jewish Hosp 1997; **Fac Appt:** Assoc Prof Med, Univ Ala

Powers, Alvin C MD [EDM] - **Spec Exp:** Diabetes; Thyroid Disorders; **Hospital:** Vanderbilt Univ Med Ctr; **Address:** Vanderbilt Univ Med Ctr, Div Endo, 2220 Pierce Ave, rm 715 PRB, Nashville, TN 37232-0021; **Phone:** 615-936-1653; **Board Cert:** Internal Medicine 1982; Endocrinology, Diabetes & Metabolism 1985; **Med School:** Univ Tenn Coll Med, Memphis 1979; **Resid:** Internal Medicine, Duke Univ Med Ctr 1982; **Fellow:** Endocrinology, Diabetes & Metabolism, Joslin Diabetes Ctr 1983; Endocrinology, Diabetes & Metabolism, Mass Genl Hosp 1985; **Fac Appt:** Prof Med, Vanderbilt Univ

Quinn, Suzanne Lorraine MD [EDM] - **Hospital:** Shands Hlthcre at Univ of FL, VA Med Ctr - Gainesville; **Address:** Shands Univ Florida, Dept Endocrinology, 2000 SW Archer Rd, Gainesville, FL 32610; **Phone:** 352-265-8230; **Board Cert:** Internal Medicine 1988; Endocrinology, Diabetes & Metabolism 2003; **Med School:** Univ Fla Coll Med 1985; **Resid:** Internal Medicine, Univ Fla Coll Med 1988; **Fellow:** Endocrinology, Diabetes & Metabolism, Univ Fla Coll Med 1992; **Fac Appt:** Assoc Prof Med, Univ Fla Coll Med

Skyler, Jay S MD [EDM] - **Spec Exp:** Diabetes; **Hospital:** Jackson Meml Hosp, Univ of Miami Hosp & Clins/Sylvester Comp Canc Ctr; **Address:** Diabetes Research Inst, 1450 NW 10th Ave, Ste 3054, Miami, FL 33136; **Phone:** 305-243-6146; **Board Cert:** Internal Medicine 1972; Endocrinology, Diabetes & Metabolism 1973; **Med School:** Jefferson Med Coll 1969; **Resid:** Internal Medicine, Duke Med Ctr 1971; **Fellow:** Endocrinology, Diabetes & Metabolism, Duke Med Ctr 1973; **Fac Appt:** Prof Med, Univ Miami Sch Med

Endocrinology, Diabetes & Metabolism

Vance, Mary Lee MD [EDM] - **Spec Exp:** Pituitary Disorders; Adrenal Disorders; **Hospital:** Univ Virginia Med Ctr; **Address:** Univ Virginia Hlth Sys, PO Box 800601, Charlottesville, VA 22908-0601; **Phone:** 434-924-2284; **Board Cert:** Internal Medicine 1980; **Med School:** Louisiana State Univ 1977; **Resid:** Internal Medicine, Baylor Univ Med Ctr 1980; **Fellow:** Endocrinology, Univ Virginia Med Ctr 1983; **Fac Appt:** Prof Med, Univ VA Sch Med

Weissman, Peter MD [EDM] - **Spec Exp:** Diabetes; **Hospital:** Baptist Hosp of Miami; **Address:** 7867 N Kendall Drive, Ste 80, Miami, FL 33156; **Phone:** 305-595-0777; **Board Cert:** Internal Medicine 1972; Endocrinology, Diabetes & Metabolism 1972; **Med School:** NYU Sch Med 1966; **Resid:** Internal Medicine, Barnes Hosp/Wash Univ 1968; **Fellow:** Geriatric Medicine, Gerontology Rsch Ctr 1970; Endocrinology, Diabetes & Metabolism, Univ Mich Hosp 1972; **Fac Appt:** Assoc Clin Prof Med, Univ Miami Sch Med

Midwest

Bahn, Rebecca Sue MD [EDM] - **Spec Exp:** Thyroid Disorders; Graves' Disease; **Hospital:** Mayo Med Ctr & Clin - Rochester; **Address:** Mayo Clinic, Div Endocrinology, 200 First St SW, Rochester, MN 55905; **Phone:** 507-284-1600; **Board Cert:** Internal Medicine 1985; Endocrinology, Diabetes & Metabolism 1987; **Med School:** Mayo Med Sch 1981; **Resid:** Internal Medicine, Mayo Clinic 1984; **Fellow:** Endocrinology, Diabetes & Metabolism, Mayo Clinic 1986; **Fac Appt:** Prof Med, Mayo Med Sch

Brennan, Michael Desmond MD [EDM] - **Spec Exp:** Thyroid Disorders; Diabetes; **Hospital:** Mayo Med Ctr & Clin - Rochester; **Address:** Mayo Clinic, Div Endocrinology, 200 First St SW, Rochester, MN 55905; **Phone:** 507-284-3707; **Board Cert:** Internal Medicine 1975; Endocrinology, Diabetes & Metabolism 1977; **Med School:** Ireland 1969; **Resid:** Internal Medicine, Mayo Clinic 1975; Internal Medicine, Henry Ford Hosp 1972; **Fellow:** Endocrinology, Diabetes & Metabolism, Mayo Clinic 1977; **Fac Appt:** Assoc Prof Med, Mayo Med Sch

Clutter, William E MD [EDM] - **Spec Exp:** Endocrine Cancers; Calcium Disorders; Metabolic Bone Disease; **Hospital:** Barnes-Jewish Hosp; **Address:** Barnes Jewish Hosp, Dept Internal Medicine, 4921 Parkview Pl Fl 5 - Ste B, St Louis, MO 63110; **Phone:** 314-362-3500; **Board Cert:** Internal Medicine 1978; Endocrinology, Diabetes & Metabolism 1981; **Med School:** Ohio State Univ 1975; **Resid:** Internal Medicine, Barnes Jewish Hosp 1978; **Fellow:** Endocrinology, Diabetes & Metabolism, Barnes Jewish Hosp 1980; **Fac Appt:** Prof Med, Washington Univ, St Louis

Cryer, Philip E MD [EDM] - **Spec Exp:** Diabetes; Hypoglycemia; **Hospital:** Barnes-Jewish Hosp, St Louis Chldns Hosp; **Address:** Wash Univ Sch Med, Div Endo, Metab & Lipid Rsch, 660 S Euclid Ave, Box 8127, St Louis, MO 63110-1093; **Phone:** 314-362-7635; **Board Cert:** Internal Medicine 1972; Endocrinology, Diabetes & Metabolism 1972; **Med School:** Northwestern Univ 1965; **Resid:** Internal Medicine, Barnes Jewish Hosp 1972; **Fellow:** Endocrinology, Diabetes & Metabolism, Wash Univ Sch Med 1968; **Fac Appt:** Prof Med, Washington Univ, St Louis

Econs, Michael J MD [EDM] - **Spec Exp:** Osteoporosis; Paget's Disease of Bone; Metabolic Bone Disease-Inherited; **Hospital:** Indiana Univ Hosp; **Address:** 541 N Clinical Dr, CL 459, Indianapolis, IN 46202; **Phone:** 317-274-1339; **Board Cert:** Internal Medicine 1986; Endocrinology, Diabetes & Metabolism 1989; **Med School:** UCSF 1983; **Resid:** Internal Medicine, Univ Maryland Hosp 1986; **Fellow:** Endocrinology, Duke Univ Med Ctr 1989; **Fac Appt:** Prof Med, Indiana Univ

Ehrmann, David A MD [EDM] - **Spec Exp:** Polycystic Ovarian Syndrome; Diabetes; **Hospital:** Univ of Chicago Hosps; **Address:** Univ Chicago, Div Endocrinology, 5758 S Maryland Ave, Ste 5A, MC 1027, Chicago, IL 60637; **Phone:** 773-702-6138; **Board Cert:** Internal Medicine 1985; Endocrinology, Diabetes & Metabolism 1987; **Med School:** Univ Mich Med Sch 1982; **Resid:** Internal Medicine, Univ Mich Med Ctr 1985; **Fellow:** Endocrinology, Diabetes & Metabolism, Univ Chicago Hosps 1987; **Fac Appt:** Assoc Prof Med, Univ Chicago-Pritzker Sch Med

Emanuele, Mary Ann MD [EDM] - **Spec Exp:** Diabetes; **Hospital:** Loyola Univ Med Ctr; **Address:** Loyola Univ Med Ctr, Dept Endocrinology, 2160 S 1st Ave Bldg 54 - rm 137A, Maywood, IL 60153-3304; **Phone:** 708-216-0160; **Board Cert:** Internal Medicine 1978; Endocrinology, Diabetes & Metabolism 1983; **Med School:** Loyola Univ-Stritch Sch Med 1975; **Resid:** Internal Medicine, Univ Hawaii Med Ctr 1978; **Fellow:** Endocrinology, Edward Hines Jr VA Hosp 1980; **Fac Appt:** Prof Med, Loyola Univ-Stritch Sch Med

Emanuele, Nicholas V MD [EDM] - **Hospital:** Loyola Univ Med Ctr, VA Med Ctr - N Chicago, IL; **Address:** Loyola Univ Med Ctr, Dept Endocrinology, 2160 S First Ave Bldg 54 - rm 137A, Maywood, IL 60153-3304; **Phone:** 708-216-0160; **Board Cert:** Internal Medicine 1975; Endocrinology 1979; **Med School:** Northwestern Univ 1967; **Resid:** Internal Medicine, Hines VA Hosp 1974; **Fellow:** Endocrinology, Northwestern Univ 1976

Herman, William H MD [EDM] - **Spec Exp:** Diabetes; **Hospital:** Univ Michigan Hlth Sys; **Address:** 1500 E Medical Center Drive, 3920 TC, Ann Arbor, MI 48109-0354; **Phone:** 734-647-5922; **Board Cert:** Internal Medicine 1982; Endocrinology, Diabetes & Metabolism 1989; **Med School:** Boston Univ 1979; **Resid:** Internal Medicine, Univ Mich Med Ctr 1982; Preventive Medicine, Ctrs Dis Control 1985; **Fellow:** Endocrinology, Diabetes & Metabolism, Univ Mich Med Ctr 1988; **Fac Appt:** Prof Med, Univ Mich Med Sch

Hoogwerf, Byron MD [EDM] - **Spec Exp:** Diabetes; Cholesterol/Lipid Disorders; Clinical Trials; Preventive Cardiology; **Hospital:** Cleveland Clin Fdn (page 57); **Address:** Cleveland Clinic Fdn, Div Endocrinology, 9500 Euclid Ave, Desk A-53, Cleveland, OH 44195-0001; **Phone:** 216-444-8347; **Board Cert:** Internal Medicine 1978; Endocrinology, Diabetes & Metabolism 1981; **Med School:** Univ Minn 1971; **Resid:** Internal Medicine, Hennepin Co Med Ctr 1978; **Fellow:** Endocrinology, Diabetes & Metabolism, Univ Minn Hosps 1981; **Fac Appt:** Prof Med, Ohio State Univ

Jensen, Michael D MD [EDM] - **Spec Exp:** Eating Disorders/Obesity; Diabetes; **Hospital:** Mayo Med Ctr & Clin - Rochester; **Address:** Mayo Clinic, Div Endocrinology, 200 W First St SW Fl 18, Rochester, MN 55905; **Phone:** 507-284-2462; **Board Cert:** Internal Medicine 1982; Endocrinology, Diabetes & Metabolism 1985; **Med School:** Univ MO-Kansas City 1979; **Resid:** Internal Medicine, Mayo Clinic 1982; **Fellow:** Endocrinology, Diabetes & Metabolism, Mayo Clinic 1985; **Fac Appt:** Prof Med, Mayo Med Sch

Khosla, Sundeep MD [EDM] - **Spec Exp:** Osteoporosis; Bone Disorders-Metabolic; **Hospital:** Mayo Med Ctr & Clin - Rochester; **Address:** Mayo Clinic, Div Endocrinology, 200 First St SW, Rochester, MN 55905; **Phone:** 507-284-1600; **Board Cert:** Internal Medicine 1985; Endocrinology 1987; **Med School:** Harvard Med Sch 1982; **Resid:** Internal Medicine, Mass Genl Hosp 1985; **Fellow:** Endocrinology, Diabetes & Metabolism, Mass Genl Hosp 1988; **Fac Appt:** Asst Prof Med, Mayo Med Sch

Endocrinology, Diabetes & Metabolism

Kloos, Richard MD [EDM] - **Spec Exp:** Thyroid Cancer; **Hospital:** Ohio St Univ Med Ctr; **Address:** 446 McCampbell Hall, 1581 Dodd Drive, Columbus, OH 43210; **Phone:** 614-292-3800; **Board Cert:** Nuclear Medicine 2005; Internal Medicine 2002; Endocrinology, Diabetes & Metabolism 2005; **Med School:** Case West Res Univ 1989; **Resid:** Internal Medicine, MetroHealth MC 1992; **Fellow:** Endocrinology, Diabetes & Metabolism, Univ Michigan 1995; Nuclear Medicine, Univ Michigan 1996; **Fac Appt:** Assoc Prof Med, Ohio State Univ

Kopp, Peter A MD [EDM] - **Spec Exp:** Thyroid Cancer; Pituitary Disorders; Parathyroid Disease; Diabetes; **Hospital:** Northwestern Meml Hosp; **Address:** Northwestern Meml Hospital, 675 N St Clair St, Ste 14-100, Chicago, IL 60611; **Phone:** 312-695-7970; **Board Cert:** Internal Medicine 2003; Endocrinology, Diabetes & Metabolism 2004; **Med School:** Switzerland 1985; **Resid:** Internal Medicine, Regl Hosp 1992; Endocrinology, Diabetes & Metabolism, Univ Berne 1990; **Fellow:** Endocrinology, Diabetes & Metabolism, Northwestern Univ Hosp 1997; **Fac Appt:** Assoc Prof Med, Northwestern Univ-Feinberg Sch Med

Licata, Angelo A MD [EDM] - **Spec Exp:** Bone Disorders-Metabolic; Osteoporosis; Calcium Disorders; **Hospital:** Cleveland Clin Fdn (page 57); **Address:** Cleveland Clinic, Div Endocrinology, 9500 Euclid Ave, Desk A53, Cleveland, OH 44195; **Phone:** 216-444-6248; **Board Cert:** Internal Medicine 1983; **Med School:** Univ Rochester 1973; **Resid:** Internal Medicine, Washington Univ Hosp 1974; Internal Medicine, Georgetown Univ Hosp 1978; **Fellow:** Endocrinology, Diabetes & Metabolism, Natl Inst Hlth 1976; **Fac Appt:** Asst Clin Prof Med, Case West Res Univ

Mazzone, Theodore MD [EDM] - **Spec Exp:** Cholesterol/Lipid Disorders; Diabetes; **Hospital:** Univ of IL Med Ctr at Chicago; **Address:** Univ Illinois Chicago, Div Diabetes & Metabolism, 1819 W Polk St, Chicago, IL 60612-7333; **Phone:** 312-355-4426; **Board Cert:** Internal Medicine 1980; Endocrinology, Diabetes & Metabolism 1983; **Med School:** Northwestern Univ 1977; **Resid:** Internal Medicine, UCLA Med Ctr 1980; **Fellow:** Endocrinology, Diabetes & Metabolism, Univ Wash Med Ctr 1983; **Fac Appt:** Prof Med, Univ IL Coll Med

McGill, Janet B MD [EDM] - **Spec Exp:** Diabetes; **Hospital:** Barnes-Jewish Hosp; **Address:** 4921 Parkview Pl, Box 8015, St Louis, MO 63110-1010; **Phone:** 314-362-3500; **Board Cert:** Internal Medicine 1983; Endocrinology, Diabetes & Metabolism 1987; **Med School:** Mich State Univ 1979; **Resid:** Internal Medicine, William Beaumont Hosp 1984; Endocrinology, Diabetes & Metabolism, William Beaumont Hosp 1985; **Fellow:** Diabetes, Washington Univ 1987; **Fac Appt:** Assoc Prof Med, Washington Univ, St Louis

McMahon, M Molly MD [EDM] - **Spec Exp:** Nutrition; Diabetes; **Hospital:** Mayo Med Ctr & Clin - Rochester; **Address:** Mayo Clinic, Div Endocrinology, 200 First St SW, Rochester, MN 55905; **Phone:** 507-284-2463; **Board Cert:** Internal Medicine 1985; Endocrinology, Diabetes & Metabolism 1987; **Med School:** Univ Wisc 1981; **Resid:** Internal Medicine, Med Coll Wisc 1984; **Fellow:** Endocrinology, Diabetes & Metabolism, Mayo Clinic 1987; Nutrition, New Eng Deaconess Hosp 1988

Polonsky, Kenneth S MD [EDM] - **Spec Exp:** Diabetes; **Hospital:** Barnes-Jewish Hosp; **Address:** Wash Univ School Medicine, Div Endo, Metab, & Lipid Rsch, 660 S Euclid Ave, Campus Box 8066, St Louis, MO 63110-1010; **Phone:** 314-362-8061; **Board Cert:** Internal Medicine 1978; **Med School:** South Africa 1973; **Resid:** Internal Medicine, Michael Reese Hosp & Med Ctr 1976; Internal Medicine, VA Hosp 1976; **Fellow:** Internal Medicine, Univ Chicago 1978; **Fac Appt:** Prof Med, Washington Univ, St Louis

Rizza, Robert Alan MD [EDM] - **Spec Exp:** Diabetes; Cholesterol/Lipid Disorders; **Hospital:** St Mary's Hosp - Rochester, Rochester Meth Hosp; **Address:** Mayo Clinic - Div Endo, 200 First St SW, Fl W18B, Rochester, MN 55905-0002; **Phone:** 507-284-1600; **Board Cert:** Internal Medicine 1976; Endocrinology, Diabetes & Metabolism 1979; **Med School:** Univ Fla Coll Med 1971; **Resid:** Internal Medicine, Johns Hopkins Hosp 1973; **Fellow:** Endocrinology, Mayo Clinic 1979; **Fac Appt:** Prof Med, Mayo Med Sch

Semenkovich, Clay F MD [EDM] - **Spec Exp:** Cholesterol/Lipid Disorders; Diabetes; Endocrinology; **Hospital:** Barnes-Jewish Hosp; **Address:** Wash Univ Sch Med, Div Endo, Metab & Lipid Rsch, 660 S Euclid Ave, Box 8127, St Louis, MO 63110; **Phone:** 314-362-7617; **Board Cert:** Internal Medicine 1984; Endocrinology, Diabetes & Metabolism 1987; **Med School:** Washington Univ, St Louis 1981; **Resid:** Internal Medicine, Barnes Hosp 1984; **Fellow:** Endocrinology, Diabetes & Metabolism, Wash Univ 1986; **Fac Appt:** Prof Med, Washington Univ, St Louis

Service, Frederick J MD/PhD [EDM] - **Spec Exp:** Hypoglycemia; Diabetes; **Hospital:** Mayo Med Ctr & Clin - Rochester; **Address:** Mayo Clinic, Div Endocrinology, 200 1st St SW, Rochester, MN 55905-0001; **Phone:** 507-284-5643; **Board Cert:** Internal Medicine 1977; Endocrinology, Diabetes & Metabolism 1972; **Med School:** McGill Univ 1962; **Resid:** Internal Medicine, Royal Victoria Hosp 1965; **Fellow:** Endocrinology, Diabetes & Metabolism, Mayo Grad Sch 1969; **Fac Appt:** Prof Med, Mayo Med Sch

Sowers, James R MD [EDM] - **Spec Exp:** Diabetes; Hypertension; Cholesterol/Lipid Disorders; **Hospital:** Univ of Missouri Hosp & Clins; **Address:** UMC, Dept Internal Med, One Hospital Drive, rm MA 410, Columbia, MO 65212; **Phone:** 573-884-2194; **Board Cert:** Internal Medicine 1974; Endocrinology, Diabetes & Metabolism 1977; **Med School:** Univ MO-Columbia Sch Med 1971; **Resid:** Internal Medicine, St Johns Mercy Med Ctr 1974; **Fellow:** Endocrinology, Wadsworth VA Hosp Ctr-UCLA 1976; **Fac Appt:** Prof Med, Univ MO-Columbia Sch Med

Veldhuis, Johannes D MD [EDM] - **Spec Exp:** Reproductive Endocrinology; Pituitary Disorders; Adrenal Disorders; Hypogonadism; **Hospital:** Mayo Med Ctr & Clin - Rochester; **Address:** Mayo Clinic, Div Endocrinology, 200 First St Sw, Joseph 5-194, Rochester, MN 55905; **Phone:** 507-284-3915; **Board Cert:** Internal Medicine 1977; Endocrinology 1979; **Med School:** Penn State Univ-Hershey Med Ctr 1974; **Resid:** Internal Medicine, Mayo Grad Sch Med 1977; **Fellow:** Endocrinology, Diabetes & Metabolism, Penn State Univ Hosp 1978; **Fac Appt:** Prof Med, Mayo Med Sch

Watts, Nelson B MD [EDM] - **Spec Exp:** Osteoporosis; Metabolic Bone Disease; Paget's Disease of Bone; **Hospital:** Univ Hosp - Cincinnati; **Address:** Univ Bone Health & Osteoporosis Ctr, 222 Piedmont Ave, Ste 4300, Cincinnati, OH 45219; **Phone:** 513-475-7400; **Board Cert:** Internal Medicine 1972; Endocrinology, Diabetes & Metabolism 1985; **Med School:** Univ NC Sch Med 1969; **Resid:** Internal Medicine, Charlotte Meml Hosp 1972; **Fellow:** Endocrinology, Diabetes & Metabolism, NC Meml Hosp 1971; **Fac Appt:** Prof Med, Univ Cincinnati

Werner, Phillip L MD [EDM] - **Spec Exp:** Diabetes; **Hospital:** Adv Luth Genl Hosp; **Address:** 1775 Ballard Rd, Nesset Pavilion, Park Ridge, IL 60068; **Phone:** 847-318-2400; **Board Cert:** Internal Medicine 1975; Endocrinology 1977; **Med School:** Univ IL Coll Med 1972; **Resid:** Internal Medicine, Univ Illinois Affl Hosp 1975; **Fellow:** Endocrinology, Diabetes & Metabolism, Univ Wash 1977; **Fac Appt:** Prof Med, Ros Franklin Univ/Chicago Med Sch

Endocrinology, Diabetes & Metabolism

Great Plains and Mountains

Eckel, Robert H MD [EDM] - **Spec Exp:** Cholesterol/Lipid Disorders; Eating Disorders/Obesity; Diabetes; **Hospital:** Univ Colorado Hosp; **Address:** Univ Colorado Hlth Scis Ctr, PO Box 6510, MS F732, Aurora, CO 80045; **Phone:** 303-315-8443; **Board Cert:** Internal Medicine 1976; Endocrinology, Diabetes & Metabolism 1979; **Med School:** Univ Cincinnati 1973; **Resid:** Internal Medicine, Univ Wisconsin Hosps 1976; **Fellow:** Endocrinology, Diabetes & Metabolism, Univ Washington 1979; **Fac Appt:** Prof Med, Univ Colorado

Recker, Robert MD [EDM] - **Spec Exp:** Osteoporosis; Diabetes; Endocrinology; **Hospital:** Creighton Univ Med Ctr, VA Medical Ctr - Omaha; **Address:** Creighton Univ School Med, Div Endocrinology, 601 N 30th St, Ste 5766, Omaha, NE 68131; **Phone:** 402-280-4470; **Board Cert:** Internal Medicine 1971; **Med School:** Creighton Univ 1963; **Resid:** Internal Medicine, Creighton Affil Hosps 1969; **Fellow:** Endocrinology, Diabetes & Metabolism, Creighton Univ 1971; **Fac Appt:** Prof Med, Creighton Univ

Ridgway, E Chester MD [EDM] - **Spec Exp:** Thyroid Cancer; Thyroid Disorders; Pituitary Disorders; **Hospital:** Univ Colorado Hosp, VA Med Ctr; **Address:** UCHSC at Fitzsimons, Endocrinology, 1635 N Ursula St, Box 6510, MS F732, Aurora, CO 80045; **Phone:** 720-848-2650; **Board Cert:** Internal Medicine 1972; Endocrinology 1973; **Med School:** Univ Colorado 1968; **Resid:** Internal Medicine, Mass Genl Hosp 1970; **Fellow:** Endocrinology, Mass Genl Hosp 1972; **Fac Appt:** Prof Med, Univ Colorado

Southwest

Cunningham, Glenn R MD [EDM] - **Spec Exp:** Diabetes; Hypogonadism; Erectile Dysfunction; **Hospital:** St Luke's Episcopal Hosp - Houston; **Address:** 6624 Fannin St, Ste 1240, Houston, TX 77030; **Phone:** 832-355-7208; **Board Cert:** Internal Medicine 1972; Endocrinology, Diabetes & Metabolism 1972; **Med School:** Univ Okla Coll Med 1966; **Resid:** Internal Medicine, Duke Univ Med Ctr 1970; **Fellow:** Endocrinology, Duke Univ Med Ctr 1971; **Fac Appt:** Prof Med, Baylor Coll Med

Gagel, Robert F MD [EDM] - **Spec Exp:** Thyroid Cancer; **Hospital:** UT MD Anderson Cancer Ctr (page 71); **Address:** MD Anderson Cancer Ctr, 1515 Holcombe Blvd, Unit 433, Houston, TX 77030; **Phone:** 713-792-6517; **Board Cert:** Internal Medicine 1975; Endocrinology 1977; **Med School:** Ohio State Univ 1971; **Resid:** Internal Medicine, New England Med Ctr 1973; **Fellow:** Endocrinology, New England Med Ctr 1975; Research, Harvard Med Sch 1981; **Fac Appt:** Prof Med, Univ Tex, Houston

Lavis, Victor Ralph MD [EDM] - **Spec Exp:** Diabetes; **Hospital:** UT MD Anderson Cancer Ctr (page 71), Meml Hermann Hosp - Houston; **Address:** MD Anderson Cancer Ctr, 1515 Holcombe Blvd, Ste 435, Houston, TX 77050; **Phone:** 713-792-2841; **Board Cert:** Internal Medicine 1969; Endocrinology, Diabetes & Metabolism 1998; **Med School:** Stanford Univ 1962; **Resid:** Internal Medicine, Boston Cty Hosp 1964; Internal Medicine, UCLA Med Ctr 1967; **Fellow:** Endocrinology, Diabetes & Metabolism, Univ Washington 1970; **Fac Appt:** Prof Med, Univ Tex, Houston

Levy, Philip MD [EDM] - **Spec Exp:** Diabetes; Thyroid Disorders; **Hospital:** Banner Good Samaritan Regl Med Ctr - Phoenix, St Joseph's Hosp & Med Ctr - Phoenix; **Address:** 1300 N 12th St, Ste 600, Phoenix, AZ 85006-2850; **Phone:** 602-252-3699; **Board Cert:** Internal Medicine 1963; Endocrinology 1972; Nuclear Medicine 1976; **Med School:** Univ Pittsburgh 1956; **Resid:** Internal Medicine, Michael Reese Hosp 1960; Endocrinology, Diabetes & Metabolism, Guys Hosp Med Sch 1962; **Fellow:** Endocrinology, Diabetes & Metabolism, Michael Reese Hosp 1961; **Fac Appt:** Clin Prof Med, Univ Ariz Coll Med

Raskin, Philip MD [EDM] - **Spec Exp:** Diabetes; **Hospital:** Parkland Meml Hosp - Dallas, UT Southwestern Med Ctr - Dallas; **Address:** Univ Tex SW Med Ctr, 5323 Harry Hines Blvd, Ste G5.238, Dallas, TX 75390-8858; **Phone:** 214-645-2800; **Board Cert:** Internal Medicine 1972; Endocrinology 1973; **Med School:** Univ Pittsburgh 1966; **Resid:** Internal Medicine, Hlth Ctr Hosps-Univ Pittsburgh 1968; **Fellow:** Endocrinology, Diabetes & Metabolism, UT SW Med Sch 1972; **Fac Appt:** Prof Med, Univ Tex SW, Dallas

Reasner, Charles A MD [EDM] - **Spec Exp:** Thyroid Disorders; **Hospital:** Univ Hlth Sys - Univ Hosp; **Address:** Texas Diabetes Inst, 701 S Zarzamora St, MS 12-5, San Antonio, TX 78207; **Phone:** 210-358-7402; **Board Cert:** Internal Medicine 1983; Endocrinology 1985; **Med School:** Loma Linda Univ 1979; **Resid:** Internal Medicine, USAF Med Ctr 1983; **Fellow:** Endocrinology, Diabetes & Metabolism, Wilford Hall Med Ctr 1985; **Fac Appt:** Assoc Prof Med, Univ Tex, San Antonio

West Coast and Pacific

Berkson, Richard Alan MD [EDM] - **Spec Exp:** Diabetes; Thyroid Disorders; **Hospital:** St Mary Med Ctr - Long Beach, CA, Long Beach Meml Med Ctr; **Address:** 1868 Pacific Ave, Long Beach, CA 90806-6113; **Phone:** 562-595-4718; **Board Cert:** Internal Medicine 1975; Endocrinology, Diabetes & Metabolism 1977; **Med School:** SUNY Buffalo 1972; **Resid:** Internal Medicine, SUNY Buffalo Affil Hosp 1975; **Fellow:** Endocrinology, Diabetes & Metabolism, Joslin Clinic 1976; Endocrinology, Diabetes & Metabolism, UCLA Med Ctr 1977; **Fac Appt:** Assoc Clin Prof Med, UCLA

Chait, Alan MD [EDM] - **Spec Exp:** Cholesterol/Lipid Disorders; Diabetes; Nutrition & Cancer/Disease Prevention; **Hospital:** Univ Wash Med Ctr; **Address:** Univ Washington Med Ctr, 1959 NE Pacific St, Box 356166, Seattle, WA 98195; **Phone:** 206-598-4615; **Med School:** South Africa 1967; **Resid:** Internal Medicine, Hammersmith Hosp 1971; **Fellow:** Endocrinology, Diabetes & Metabolism, Hammersmith Hosp 1973; Endocrinology, Diabetes & Metabolism, Univ Washington 1977; **Fac Appt:** Prof Med, Univ Wash

Chopra, Inder Jit MD [EDM] - **Spec Exp:** Thyroid Disorders; Endocrine Disorders; **Hospital:** UCLA Med Ctr; **Address:** UCLA Sch Med, Div Endocrinology, 900 Veteran Ave, Ste 24-130, Los Angeles, CA 90095-7073; **Phone:** 310-825-2346; **Board Cert:** Internal Medicine 1972; Endocrinology, Diabetes & Metabolism 1973; **Med School:** India 1961; **Resid:** Internal Medicine, All India Inst Med Sci 1965; Internal Medicine, Queens Med Ctr 1968; **Fellow:** Endocrinology, Diabetes & Metabolism, LAC-Harbor-UCLA Med Ctr 1971; **Fac Appt:** Prof Med, UCLA

Darwin, Christine H MD [EDM] - **Spec Exp:** Pituitary Tumors; Diabetes; **Hospital:** UCLA Med Ctr; **Address:** 200 UCLA Medical Plaza, Ste 365 C1, Box 951693, Los Angeles, CA 90095-7065; **Phone:** 310-794-5584; **Board Cert:** Geriatric Medicine 1994; Endocrinology, Diabetes & Metabolism 1997; **Med School:** India 1980; **Resid:** Internal Medicine, UC Irvine Med Ctr 1987; **Fellow:** Endocrinology, VA Hosp 1988; Endocrinology, USC Med Ctr 1993; **Fac Appt:** Assoc Prof Med, UCLA

Fitzgerald, Paul Anthony MD [EDM] - **Spec Exp:** Diabetes; Thyroid Cancer; Pituitary Tumors; Thyroid Disorders; **Hospital:** UCSF Med Ctr; **Address:** 350 Parnassus Ave, Ste 710, San Francisco, CA 94117; **Phone:** 415-665-1136; **Board Cert:** Internal Medicine 1975; Endocrinology, Diabetes & Metabolism 1981; **Med School:** Jefferson Med Coll 1972; **Resid:** Internal Medicine, Presby Med Ctr-Univ Colo 1975; **Fellow:** Endocrinology, Diabetes & Metabolism, UCSF Med Ctr 1978; **Fac Appt:** Clin Prof Med, UCSF

Endocrinology, Diabetes & Metabolism

Heber, David MD [EDM] - **Spec Exp:** Nutrition & Cancer Prevention; Nutrition & Disease Prevention/Control; Nutrition & Obesity; **Hospital:** UCLA Med Ctr; **Address:** 900 Veteran Ave, Rm 12-217, UCLA Center for Human Nutrition, Los Angeles, CA 90095-1742; **Phone:** 310-206-1987; **Board Cert:** Internal Medicine 1976; Endocrinology, Diabetes & Metabolism 1977; **Med School:** Harvard Med Sch 1973; **Resid:** Internal Medicine, LA Co Harbor Genl Hosp 1975; **Fellow:** Endocrinology, Diabetes & Metabolism, LA Co Harbor Genl Hosp 1978; **Fac Appt:** Prof Med, UCLA

Hoffman, Andrew R MD [EDM] - **Spec Exp:** Pituitary Disorders; Pituitary Tumors; Neuroendocrinology; **Hospital:** Stanford Univ Med Ctr, VA Hlth Care Sys - Palo Alto; **Address:** 300 Pastur Drive Boswell Bldg - rm A-175, Stanford, CA 94305; **Phone:** 650-723-6961; **Board Cert:** Internal Medicine 1979; Endocrinology 1981; **Med School:** Stanford Univ 1976; **Resid:** Internal Medicine, Mass Genl Hosp 1978; **Fellow:** Pharmacology, Mass Genl Hosp 1980; Endocrinology, Diabetes & Metabolism, Mass Genl Hosp 1982; **Fac Appt:** Prof Med, Stanford Univ

Hsueh, Willa Ann MD [EDM] - **Spec Exp:** Diabetes; Hypertension; **Hospital:** UCLA Med Ctr; **Address:** 900 Veteran Ave, Ste 24-130, Los Angeles, CA 90095; **Phone:** 310-794-7555; **Board Cert:** Internal Medicine 1976; Endocrinology, Diabetes & Metabolism 1977; **Med School:** Ohio State Univ 1973; **Resid:** Internal Medicine, Johns Hopkins Hosp 1975; **Fellow:** Endocrinology, Diabetes & Metabolism, Johns Hopkins Hosp 1976; **Fac Appt:** Prof Med, UCLA

Ipp, Eli MD [EDM] - **Spec Exp:** Diabetes; **Hospital:** LAC - Harbor - UCLA Med Ctr; **Address:** 21840 S Normandy Ave, Ste 700, Torrance, CA 90502; **Phone:** 310-222-5101; **Board Cert:** Internal Medicine 1979; Endocrinology, Diabetes & Metabolism 1981; **Med School:** South Africa 1968; **Resid:** Internal Medicine, Tel Hashomer Hosp 1974; **Fellow:** Endocrinology, Diabetes & Metabolism, Univ Tex SW Med Ctr 1978; **Fac Appt:** Prof Med, UCLA

Kamdar, Vikram V MD [EDM] - **Spec Exp:** Diabetes; Diabetic Leg/Foot; Thyroid Disorders; **Hospital:** Santa Monica - UCLA Med Ctr, UCLA Med Ctr; **Address:** 1801 Wilshire Blvd, Ste 100, Santa Monica, CA 90403; **Phone:** 310-828-7172; **Board Cert:** Internal Medicine 1978; Endocrinology, Diabetes & Metabolism 1979; **Med School:** India 1971; **Resid:** Internal Medicine, Lemuel Shattuck Hosp; Endocrinology, Diabetes & Metabolism, Cedars-Sinai Med Ctr 1977; **Fellow:** Endocrinology, Diabetes & Metabolism, LA Co-USC Med Ctr 1975; **Fac Appt:** Assoc Clin Prof Med, UCLA

Melmed, Shlomo MD [EDM] - **Spec Exp:** Pituitary Tumors; Acromegaly; Pituitary Function/Hormones; **Hospital:** Cedars-Sinai Med Ctr; **Address:** Cedars Sinai Med Ctr, 8700 Beverly Blvd, Ste 2015, Los Angeles, CA 90048; **Phone:** 310-423-4691; **Board Cert:** Internal Medicine 1979; Endocrinology, Diabetes & Metabolism 1983; **Med School:** South Africa 1970; **Resid:** Internal Medicine, Sheba Med Ctr 1976; **Fellow:** Endocrinology, Diabetes & Metabolism, Wadsworth VA Hosp 1980; **Fac Appt:** Prof Med, UCLA

Orwoll, Eric S MD [EDM] - **Spec Exp:** Osteoporosis; Osteoporosis in Men; **Hospital:** OR Hlth & Sci Univ; **Address:** Oregon Hlth & Sci Univ, Bone/Mineral Unit, 3181 SW Sam Jackson Park Rd, MC OPO5, Portland, OR 97239; **Phone:** 503-494-3273; **Board Cert:** Internal Medicine 1977; Endocrinology, Diabetes & Metabolism 1979; **Med School:** Univ MD Sch Med 1974; **Resid:** Internal Medicine, Providence Med Ctr 1977; **Fellow:** Endocrinology, Diabetes & Metabolism, Univ Oregon Hlth Sci Ctr 1979; **Fac Appt:** Prof Med, Oregon Hlth Sci Univ

Riddle, Matthew Casey MD [EDM] - **Spec Exp:** Diabetes; Clinical Trials; **Hospital:** OR Hlth & Sci Univ; **Address:** Oregon Hlth & Sci Univ, Div Endo, 3181 SW Sam Jackson Park Rd, MC L-345, Portland, OR 97239-3011; **Phone:** 503-494-3273; **Board Cert:** Internal Medicine 1972; Endocrinology, Diabetes & Metabolism 1972; **Med School:** Harvard Med Sch 1964; **Resid:** Internal Medicine, Rush-Presby-St Lukes Hosp 1969; **Fellow:** Endocrinology, Diabetes & Metabolism, Rush Presby-St Lukes Hosp 1971; Endocrinology, Diabetes & Metabolism, Univ Washington 1973; **Fac Appt:** Prof Med, Oregon Hlth Sci Univ

Singer, Peter A MD [EDM] - **Spec Exp:** Thyroid Disorders; **Hospital:** USC Univ Hosp - R K Eamer Med Plz; **Address:** 1520 San Pablo St, Ste 1000, Los Angeles, CA 90033; **Phone:** 323-442-5100; **Board Cert:** Internal Medicine 1972; Endocrinology, Diabetes & Metabolism 1973; **Med School:** UCSF 1965; **Resid:** Internal Medicine, LAC-USC Med Ctr 1971; **Fellow:** Endocrinology, Diabetes & Metabolism, LAC-USC Med Ctr 1973; **Fac Appt:** Clin Prof Med, USC Sch Med

Swerdloff, Ronald Sherwin MD [EDM] - **Spec Exp:** Reproductive Endocrinology-Male; Pituitary Disorders; **Hospital:** LAC - Harbor - UCLA Med Ctr; **Address:** 1000 W Carson St, Box 446, Torrance, CA 90509-2910; **Phone:** 310-222-1867; **Board Cert:** Internal Medicine 1968; Endocrinology 1972; **Med School:** UCSF 1962; **Resid:** Internal Medicine, Univ Washington Hosp 1964; Endocrinology, Diabetes & Metabolism, NIH Gerontology Branch 1966; **Fellow:** Endocrinology, Diabetes & Metabolism, Harbor-UCLA Med Ctr 1969; **Fac Appt:** Prof Med, UCLA

Woeber, Kenneth A MD [EDM] - **Spec Exp:** Thyroid Disorders; Adrenal Disorders; **Hospital:** UCSF Med Ctr; **Address:** 1600 Divisadero St Fl 4 - rm C-432, San Francisco, CA 94115-3010; **Phone:** 415-885-7574; **Board Cert:** Internal Medicine 1980; Endocrinology, Diabetes & Metabolism 1973; **Med School:** South Africa 1957; **Resid:** Internal Medicine, Jackson Meml Hosp 1962; **Fellow:** Endocrinology, Diabetes & Metabolism, Harvard/Boston City Hosp 1964; **Fac Appt:** Prof Med, UCSF

Childrens Hospital Los Angeles

4650 Sunset Boulevard
Los Angeles, California 90027
www.ChildrensHospitalLA.org

Childrens Hospital Los Angeles is acknowledged throughout the United States and around the world for its leadership in pediatric and adolescent health. It is able to offer the very best in multidisciplinary care, with 85 pediatric subspecialties and dozens of special services for children and families. Its physicians are recognized as leaders. Its treatments set the standard of care. Its research is recognized worldwide.

The Heart Institute

The Heart Institute is known throughout the world as a leader in the treatment of pediatric heart disease, offering the most advanced diagnostic and treatment modalities available in cardiology, cardio thoracic surgery, cardio thoracic transplantation and intensive care, as well as innovation in cardiac research. Physicians provide comprehensive care to 8,000 children each year – fetus through adolescent – who have congenital or acquired heart and lung disorders. For information contact (323) 669-4148.

Center for Endocrinology, Diabetes and Metabolism

The Center for Endocrinology, Diabetes and Metabolism is at the forefront of patient care, basic and clinical research in diabetes, obesity, growth, bone metabolism and endocrinology. More than 2,000 children and adolescents with Type 1 and Type 2 diabetes are under the care of its pediatric diabetes specialists, certified diabetes educators and nutritionists – one of the largest programs of its kind in America. For information contact (323) 669-4604.

Childrens Center for Cancer and Blood Diseases

The Childrens Center for Cancer and Blood Diseases is the nation's largest pediatric hematology/oncology program. Physician- scientists integrate their laboratory experience with their clinical expertise in an approach to medical problem-solving that enables them to move effectively from "Bench to Bedside." Breakthroughs in the treatment of childhood cancer, many pioneered at Childrens Hospital Los Angeles, offer children, teenagers and young adults the most advanced treatment available anywhere. For information contact (323) 669-2121.

Childrens Orthopaedic Center

The Childrens Orthopaedic Center is one of the nation's most comprehensive programs dedicated to pediatric musculoskeletal care, education and research. Its Scoliosis and Spine Disorders Program, one of the largest in the country, is the only one of its kind in Los Angeles County devoted exclusively to the pediatric population. Its state-of-the-art Motion Analysis Laboratory is designed to analyze muscle activity and joint movements in children who have difficulty walking, such as those with cerebral palsy, spina bifida and congenital leg conditions. For information contact (323) 669-2142.

602

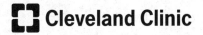
Cleveland Clinic

Endocrinology, Diabetes and Metabolism

Cleveland Clinic Department of Endocrinology treats patients in all the major disease categories such as, diabetes, thyroid disorders, sexual hormone disorders, metabolism, pituitary disorders and more. In addition, the department has several specialty clinics dedicated to:

- Pancreases Transplant Clinic/Post Transplant Diabetes Mellitus
- Cardiovascular risk reduction
- Type 1 Diabetes
- Pituitary
- Thyroid
- Transition Clinic (Pediatrics to Adult)
- Intensive Diabetic Care- DM2 Clinic

Patients with difficult-to-control diabetes or high risk patients with diabetes (i.e. diabetics who recently experienced a heart attack or underwent bypass surgery), can be treated at the Diabetes Mellitus Disease Management (DM2) Clinic for seamless, intensive management of their disease. The goal is to stabilize patients within six months, and return them back to their primary care providers within twelve months.

Second Opinion-Online

Use e-Cleveland Clinic's convenient, online second opinion service without leaving home. Call 800.223.2273, ext 43223, or visit www.eclevelandclinic.org.

Assistance for Out-of-Town and International Patients

Get complimentary help scheduling medical appointments and arranging for hotels and transportation. For out-of-town patients call 800.223.2273, ext. 55580, or visit www.clevelandclinic.org/services. For International patients call 216.444.6404 or visit www.clevelandclinic.org/ic.

Thyroid Biopsy

The department has been a leader in incorporating fine needle aspirations and ultrasounds into the realm of endocrinology. Our fellowship program was one of the first in the nation to train fellows in ultrasound-guided biopsy techniques of the thyroid.

Pituitary Clinic

Pituitary care at Cleveland Clinic is a collaborative approach between endocrinologist, neurosurgeons and radiation oncologists, resulting in national recognition. Cleveland Clinic is one of the top centers in the U.S. for volume of pituitary surgeries at an institution.

Center for Osteoporosis and Metabolic Bone Disease

A joint effort between the Departments of Endocrinology and Rheumatology, the Center for Osteoporosis and Metabolic Bone Disease is devoted to the evaluation and treatment of patients with osteoporosis and other forms of diseases that affect bones. The Center's goal is to evaluate patients at an early stage to prevent complications and treat patients at the earliest possible stage to prevent additional disease manifestations.

To schedule an appointment or for more information about the Cleveland Clinic Department of Endocrinology, Diabetes and Metabolism call 800.890.2467 or visit www.clevelandclinic.org/endotopdocs .

Department of Endocrinology, Diabetes and Metabolism
9500 Euclid Avenue / W14 | Cleveland OH 44195

Gastroenterology
a subspecialty of Internal Medicine

An internist who specializes in diagnosis and treatment of diseases of the digestive organs including the stomach, bowels, liver and gallbladder. This specialist treats conditions such as abdominal pain, ulcers, diarrhea, cancer and jaundice and performs complex diagnostic and therapeutic procedures using endoscopes to see internal organs.

Training Required: Three years in internal medicine *plus* additional training and examination for certification in gastroenterology.

Gastroenterology

New England

Banks, Peter Alan MD [Ge] - **Spec Exp:** Inflammatory Bowel Disease/Crohn's; Pancreatic Disease; **Hospital:** Brigham & Women's Hosp; **Address:** Brigham & Women's Hosp, Div Gastro, 45 Francis St, ASB II Fl 2, Boston, MA 02115; **Phone:** 617-732-6389; **Board Cert:** Internal Medicine 1968; Gastroenterology 1970; **Med School:** Columbia P&S 1961; **Resid:** Internal Medicine, Beth Israel Hosp 1963; **Fellow:** Gastroenterology, Mt Sinai Hosp 1967; **Fac Appt:** Prof Med, Harvard Med Sch

Bonkovsky, Herbert MD [Ge] - **Spec Exp:** Liver Disease; Hepatitis; Iron & Porphyrin Metabolism Disorders; **Hospital:** Univ of Conn Hlth Ctr, John Dempsey Hosp; **Address:** 263 Farmington Ave, Farmington, CT 06030-1111; **Phone:** 860-679-3238; **Board Cert:** Internal Medicine 1973; Gastroenterology 1977; **Med School:** Case West Res Univ 1967; **Resid:** Internal Medicine, MetroHealth Med Ctr 1969; Internal Medicine, Dartmouth-Hitchcock Med Ctr 1973; **Fellow:** Gastroenterology, Dartmouth Med Sch 1973; Hepatology, Yale Univ Sch Med 1974; **Fac Appt:** Prof Med, Univ Conn

Carr-Locke, David L MD [Ge] - **Spec Exp:** Pancreatic/Biliary Endoscopy (ERCP); Pancreatic & Biliary Disease; Endoscopy; **Hospital:** Brigham & Women's Hosp; **Address:** Brigham & Women's Hosp-Endoscopy Ctr, 45 Francis St, Boston, MA 02115-6106; **Phone:** 617-732-7414; **Board Cert:** Internal Medicine 1974; **Med School:** England 1972; **Resid:** Obstetrics & Gynecology, Orsett Hosp 1974; Internal Medicine, Leicester Hosp 1976; **Fellow:** Gastroenterology, Leicester Hosp 1978; Research, New Eng Baptist Hosp 1979; **Fac Appt:** Assoc Prof Med, Harvard Med Sch

Chung, Raymond T MD [Ge] - **Spec Exp:** Transplant Medicine-Liver; Liver Disease; Hepatitis C; **Hospital:** Mass Genl Hosp; **Address:** Mass Genl Hosp, 55 Fruit St Warren Bldg Fl 10, Boston, MA 02114; **Phone:** 617-724-7562; **Board Cert:** Internal Medicine 1989; **Med School:** Yale Univ 1986; **Resid:** Internal Medicine, Johns Hopkins Hosp 1989; **Fac Appt:** Assoc Prof Med, Harvard Med Sch

Dienstag, Jules L MD [Ge] - **Spec Exp:** Liver Disease; Hepatitis; Transplant Medicine-Liver; **Hospital:** Mass Genl Hosp; **Address:** Mass Genl Hosp, GI Unit, 55 Fruit St Warren Bldg Fl 10, Boston, MA 02114-2622; **Phone:** 617-724-7562; **Board Cert:** Internal Medicine 1975; **Med School:** Columbia P&S 1972; **Resid:** Internal Medicine, Univ Chicago-Billings Hosp 1974; **Fellow:** Infectious Disease, Natl Inst Hlth 1976; Gastroenterology, Mass Genl Hosp 1978; **Fac Appt:** Prof Med, Harvard Med Sch

Friedman, Lawrence S MD [Ge] - **Spec Exp:** Liver Disease; **Hospital:** Newton - Wellesley Hosp, Mass Genl Hosp; **Address:** Newton-Wellesley Hospital, Dept Medicine, 2014 Washington St, Newton, MA 02462; **Phone:** 617-243-5480; **Board Cert:** Internal Medicine 1981; Gastroenterology 1983; **Med School:** Johns Hopkins Univ 1978; **Resid:** Internal Medicine, Johns Hopkins Hosp 1981; **Fellow:** Gastroenterology, Mass Genl Hosp 1984; **Fac Appt:** Prof Med, Harvard Med Sch

Levine, Joel B MD [Ge] - **Spec Exp:** Colon & Rectal Cancer Detection; Colonoscopy; Gastroesophageal Reflux Disease (GERD); **Hospital:** Univ of Conn Hlth Ctr, John Dempsey Hosp; **Address:** Univ Connecticut, Colon Cancer Prevention Program, 263 Farmington Ave, Farmington, CT 06030-2813; **Phone:** 860-679-4567; **Board Cert:** Internal Medicine 1973; Gastroenterology 1977; **Med School:** SUNY Downstate 1969; **Resid:** Internal Medicine, Univ Chicago Hosps 1971; Internal Medicine, Mass Genl Hosp 1974; **Fellow:** Gastroenterology, Mass Genl Hosp 1977; **Fac Appt:** Prof Med, Univ Conn

Mason, Joel B MD [Ge] - **Spec Exp:** Nutrition in Acute Illness; Nutrition in Bowel Disorders; Nutrition & Cancer Prevention; **Hospital:** Tufts-New England Med Ctr; **Address:** Tufts-New England Med Ctr, Div Gastroenterology, 750 Washington St, Boston, MA 02111; **Phone:** 617-636-1621; **Board Cert:** Internal Medicine 1984; Gastroenterology 1987; **Med School:** Univ Chicago-Pritzker Sch Med 1981; **Resid:** Internal Medicine, Univ Iowa Hosps 1984; **Fellow:** Gastroenterology, Univ Chicago Hosps 1986; Nutrition, Univ Chicago Hosps 1986; **Fac Appt:** Assoc Prof Med, Tufts Univ

Peppercorn, Mark A MD [Ge] - **Spec Exp:** Crohn's Disease-2nd opinion only; Ulcerative Colitis-2nd opinion only; **Hospital:** Beth Israel Deaconess Med Ctr - Boston; **Address:** Beth Israel Deaconess Med Ctr, 330 Brookline Ave, Boston, MA 02215; **Phone:** 617-667-9355; **Board Cert:** Internal Medicine 1974; Gastroenterology 1977; **Med School:** Harvard Med Sch 1968; **Resid:** Internal Medicine, Beth Israel Hosp 1974; Metabolic Diseases, Natl Inst Hlth 1972; **Fellow:** Gastroenterology, Beth Israel Hosp 1973; **Fac Appt:** Prof Med, Harvard Med Sch

Podolsky, Daniel K MD [Ge] - **Spec Exp:** Irritable Bowel Syndrome; **Hospital:** Mass Genl Hosp; **Address:** Mass Genl Hosp, GI Unit, 55 Fruit St Warren Bldg Fl 10, Boston, MA 02114; **Phone:** 617-724-7562; **Board Cert:** Internal Medicine 1981; Gastroenterology 1983; **Med School:** Harvard Med Sch 1978; **Resid:** Internal Medicine, Mass Genl Hosp 1981; **Fac Appt:** Prof Med, Harvard Med Sch

Rothstein, Richard I MD [Ge] - **Spec Exp:** Gastroesophageal Reflux Disease (GERD); Swallowing Disorders; Barrett's Esophagus; **Hospital:** Dartmouth - Hitchcock Med Ctr; **Address:** Dartmouth-Hitchcock Medical Center, Div Gastroenterology, 1 Medical Center Drive, Lebanon, NH 03756; **Phone:** 603-653-8343; **Board Cert:** Internal Medicine 1983; Gastroenterology 1987; **Med School:** Boston Univ 1980; **Resid:** Internal Medicine, Univ Mass Med Ctr 1983; **Fellow:** Gastroenterology, Dartmouth-Hitchcock Med Ctr 1985; **Fac Appt:** Prof Med, Dartmouth Med Sch

Wolfe, M Michael MD [Ge] - **Hospital:** Boston Med Ctr; **Address:** 650 Albany St, Ste 504, Boston, MA 02118; **Phone:** 617-638-7440; **Board Cert:** Internal Medicine 1979; Gastroenterology 1981; **Med School:** Ohio State Univ 1976; **Resid:** Internal Medicine, Med Coll Penn Hosp 1979; **Fellow:** Gastroenterology, Univ Florida Hosps 1982; **Fac Appt:** Prof Med, Boston Univ

Mid Atlantic

Abreu, Maria T MD [Ge] - **Spec Exp:** Inflammatory Bowel Disease/Crohn's; Ulcerative Colitis; **Hospital:** Mount Sinai Med Ctr; **Address:** 5 East 98th Street, Box 1625, New York, NY 10029-6501; **Phone:** 212-241-4299; **Board Cert:** Gastroenterology 2005; **Med School:** Univ Miami Sch Med 1990; **Resid:** Internal Medicine, Brigham & Women's Hosp 1992; **Fellow:** Gastroenterology, UCLA Med Ctr 1995; **Fac Appt:** Assoc Prof Med, Mount Sinai Sch Med

Albert, Michael B MD [Ge] - **Spec Exp:** Inflammatory Bowel Disease; Ulcerative Colitis; **Hospital:** G Washington Univ Hosp; **Address:** 2141 K St NW, Ste 208, Washington, DC 20037; **Phone:** 202-223-5544; **Board Cert:** Internal Medicine 1985; Gastroenterology 1987; **Med School:** Johns Hopkins Univ 1982; **Resid:** Internal Medicine, Mayo Clinic 1984; Internal Medicine, Duke Univ Med Ctr 1985; **Fellow:** Gastroenterology, G Washington Univ Med Ctr 1987; **Fac Appt:** Prof Med, Geo Wash Univ

Gastroenterology

Aronchick, Craig A MD [Ge] - **Spec Exp:** Barrett's Esophagus; Pancreatic/Biliary Endoscopy (ERCP); **Hospital:** Pennsylvania Hosp (page 72); **Address:** 230 W Washington Square, Farm Journal Bldg, Fl 4, Philadelphia, PA 19106; **Phone:** 215-829-3561; **Board Cert:** Internal Medicine 1981; Gastroenterology 1983; **Med School:** Temple Univ 1978; **Resid:** Internal Medicine, Temple Univ Hosp 1981; **Fellow:** Gastroenterology, Hosp Univ Penn 1983; **Fac Appt:** Assoc Clin Prof Med, Univ Pennsylvania

Bayless, Theodore MD [Ge] - **Spec Exp:** Inflammatory Bowel Disease/Crohn's; Ulcerative Colitis; Malabsorption Syndrome; **Hospital:** Johns Hopkins Hosp - Baltimore (page 61); **Address:** 600 N Wolfe St, Blalock Bldg - Ste 461, C/O Johns Hopkins Hosp, Baltimore, MD 21287-0005; **Phone:** 410-955-4916; **Board Cert:** Internal Medicine 1966; **Med School:** Ros Franklin Univ/Chicago Med Sch 1957; **Resid:** Internal Medicine, Cornell-Bellevue Hosp 1958; Internal Medicine, Meml Sloan Kettering Hosp 1960; **Fellow:** Gastroenterology, Johns Hopkins Hosp 1962; **Fac Appt:** Prof Med, Johns Hopkins Univ

Bodenheimer Jr, Henry C MD [Ge] - **Spec Exp:** Hepatitis; Transplant Medicine-Liver; Liver & Biliary Disease; **Hospital:** Beth Israel Med Ctr - Petrie Division; **Address:** Beth Israel Med Ctr, Div Digestive Diseases, 1st Ave @ 16th St, New York, NY 10003; **Phone:** 212-420-4015; **Board Cert:** Internal Medicine 1978; Gastroenterology 1981; **Med School:** Tufts Univ 1975; **Resid:** Internal Medicine, Mount Sinai Hosp 1978; **Fellow:** Gastroenterology, Mount Sinai Hosp 1979; Gastroenterology, Rhode Island Hosp 1981; **Fac Appt:** Prof Med, Albert Einstein Coll Med

Borum, Marie L MD [Ge] - **Spec Exp:** Liver Disease; AIDS/HIV-Gastrointestinal Complications; Women's Health; **Hospital:** G Washington Univ Hosp; **Address:** MFA, 2150 Pennsylvania Ave NW, Ste 3-410, Washington, DC 20037; **Phone:** 202-741-3333; **Board Cert:** Internal Medicine 1988; Gastroenterology 2001; **Med School:** UMDNJ-Rutgers Med Sch 1985; **Resid:** Internal Medicine, G Washington Univ Med Ctr 1988; **Fellow:** Gastroenterology, G Washington Univ Med Ctr 1991; **Fac Appt:** Prof Med, Geo Wash Univ

Brandt, Lawrence MD [Ge] - **Spec Exp:** Geriatric Gastroenterology; Ischemic Bowel Disease; Inflammatory Bowel Disease; **Hospital:** Montefiore Med Ctr; **Address:** 3400 Bainbridge Ave Fl 2, Bronx, NY 10467-2401; **Phone:** 866-633-8255; **Board Cert:** Internal Medicine 1972; Gastroenterology 1975; **Med School:** SUNY Downstate 1968; **Resid:** Internal Medicine, Mount Sinai Hosp 1972; **Fellow:** Gastroenterology, Mount Sinai Hosp 1972; **Fac Appt:** Prof Med, Albert Einstein Coll Med

Cohen, Jonathan MD [Ge] - **Spec Exp:** Pancreatic/Biliary Endoscopy (ERCP); Pancreatic Disease; Liver Disease; Colonoscopy; **Hospital:** NYU Med Ctr (page 67); **Address:** 232 E 30th St, New York, NY 10016-8202; **Phone:** 212-889-5544; **Board Cert:** Internal Medicine 1993; Gastroenterology 1995; **Med School:** Harvard Med Sch 1990; **Resid:** Internal Medicine, Beth Israel Hosp 1993; **Fellow:** Gastroenterology, UCLA Med Ctr 1995; Endoscopy, Wellesley Hosp 1995; **Fac Appt:** Clin Prof Med, NYU Sch Med

Cohen, Lawrence B MD [Ge] - **Spec Exp:** Gastroesophageal Reflux Disease (GERD); Esophageal Disorders; Colon & Rectal Cancer; **Hospital:** Mount Sinai Med Ctr; **Address:** 311 E 79th St, Ste A, New York, NY 10021-0903; **Phone:** 212-996-6633; **Board Cert:** Internal Medicine 1981; Gastroenterology 1983; **Med School:** Hahnemann Univ 1978; **Resid:** Internal Medicine, Mount Sinai Hosp 1981; **Fellow:** Gastroenterology, Mount Sinai Hosp 1983; **Fac Appt:** Assoc Clin Prof Med, Mount Sinai Sch Med

Deren, Julius J MD [Ge] - **Spec Exp:** Inflammatory Bowel Disease/Crohn's; Diarrheal Diseases; **Hospital:** Penn Presby Med Ctr - UPHS (page 72), Hosp Univ Penn - UPHS (page 72); **Address:** Penn-Presbyterian Med Ctr, Wright-Saunders Bldg, Ste 218, 39th & Market St, Philadelphia, PA 19104; **Phone:** 215-662-8900; **Board Cert:** Internal Medicine 1968; Gastroenterology 1970; **Med School:** SUNY Downstate 1958; **Resid:** Internal Medicine, Maimonides Hosp 1961; Gastroenterology, Boston City Hosp 1962; **Fellow:** Physiology, Harvard Univ 1964; **Fac Appt:** Prof Med, Univ Pennsylvania

Dieterich, Douglas MD [Ge] - **Spec Exp:** Hepatitis; AIDS/HIV-Gastrointestinal Complications; Liver Disease; Endoscopy; **Hospital:** Mount Sinai Med Ctr, NYU Med Ctr (page 67); **Address:** 5 E 98th St Fl 11, New York, NY 10029; **Phone:** 212-241-7270; **Board Cert:** Internal Medicine 1981; Gastroenterology 1987; **Med School:** NYU Sch Med 1978; **Resid:** Internal Medicine, Bellevue Hosp Ctr-NYU 1981; **Fellow:** Gastroenterology, Bellevue Hosp Ctr-NYU 1983; **Fac Appt:** Prof Med, Mount Sinai Sch Med

DiMarino, Anthony J MD [Ge] - **Spec Exp:** Celiac Disease; Gastroesophageal Reflux Disease (GERD); Ulcerative Colitis; Irritable Bowel Syndrome; **Hospital:** Thomas Jefferson Univ Hosp; **Address:** T Jefferson Univ, Div Gastroenterology, 132 S 10th St, Ste 480, Philadelphia, PA 19107; **Phone:** 215-955-2728; **Board Cert:** Internal Medicine 1977; Gastroenterology 1972; **Med School:** Hahnemann Univ 1968; **Resid:** Internal Medicine, Hahnemann Univ Hosp 1970; Hosp Univ Penn 1971; **Fellow:** Gastroenterology, Hosp Univ Penn 1973; **Fac Appt:** Prof Med, Thomas Jefferson Univ

Farmer, Richard G MD [Ge] - **Spec Exp:** Inflammatory Bowel Disease/Crohn's; **Hospital:** Univ of Rochester Strong Meml Hosp; **Address:** Univ Rochester Med Ctr, 601 Elmwood Ave, Box 646, Rochester, NY 14642; **Phone:** 585-275-7432; **Board Cert:** Internal Medicine 1963; Gastroenterology 1968; **Med School:** Univ MD Sch Med 1956; **Resid:** Internal Medicine, Mayo Clinic 1960; **Fellow:** Gastroenterology, Mayo Clinic 1960; **Fac Appt:** Prof Med, Univ Rochester

Gerdes, Hans MD [Ge] - **Spec Exp:** Endoscopy; Endoscopic Ultrasound; Barrett's Esophagus; Gastrointestinal Cancer; **Hospital:** Meml Sloan Kettering Cancer Ctr; **Address:** 1275 York Ave, rm Howard 504, New York, NY 10021-6007; **Phone:** 212-639-7108; **Board Cert:** Internal Medicine 1987; Gastroenterology 1989; **Med School:** Cornell Univ-Weill Med Coll 1983; **Resid:** Internal Medicine, New York Hosp 1986; **Fellow:** Gastroenterology, Meml Sloan Kettering Cancer Ctr 1989

Ginsberg, Gregory G MD [Ge] - **Spec Exp:** Pancreatic/Biliary Endoscopy (ERCP); Endoscopy; Endoscopic Ultrasound; **Hospital:** Hosp Univ Penn - UPHS (page 72); **Address:** Clinical Practices of U Pennsylvania, 3400 Spruce St 3 Dulles Bldg, Philadelphia, PA 19104; **Phone:** 215-349-8222; **Board Cert:** Internal Medicine 2000; Gastroenterology 2000; **Med School:** Jefferson Med Coll 1987; **Resid:** Internal Medicine, Georgetown Univ Med Ctr 1990; **Fellow:** Gastroenterology, Georgetown Univ Med Ctr 1992; **Fac Appt:** Prof Med, Univ Pennsylvania

Green, Peter MD [Ge] - **Spec Exp:** Celiac Disease; Endoscopy; Colonoscopy; Malabsorption; **Hospital:** NY-Presby Hosp/Columbia (page 66); **Address:** Celiac Disease Ctr, Harkness Bldg, 180 Fort Washington Ave, rm 956, New York, NY 10032-3713; **Phone:** 212-305-5590; **Med School:** Australia 1970; **Resid:** Internal Medicine, North Shore Med Ctr 1974; **Fellow:** Gastroenterology, North Shore Med Ctr 1976; Gastroenterology, Beth Israel Hosp 1977; **Fac Appt:** Clin Prof Med, Columbia P&S

Gastroenterology

Greenwald, Bruce D MD [Ge] - **Spec Exp:** Endoscopic Ultrasound; Barrett's Esophagus; Gastroesophageal Reflux Disease (GERD); Clinical Trials; **Hospital:** Univ of MD Med Sys; **Address:** Univ of Maryland Hosp, Gastroenterology, 22 S Greene St Fl 3 - rm N3W62, Baltimore, MD 21201-1595; **Phone:** 410-328-8731; **Board Cert:** Internal Medicine 2000; Gastroenterology 2000; **Med School:** Univ MD Sch Med 1987; **Resid:** Internal Medicine, Univ of Virginia Hosp 1990; **Fellow:** Gastroenterology, Univ of Maryland Hosp 1992; **Fac Appt:** Assoc Prof Med, Univ MD Sch Med

Haluszka, Oleh MD [Ge] - **Spec Exp:** Pancreatic/Biliary Endoscopy (ERCP); Gastrointestinal Cancer; Endoscopic Ultrasound; Endoscopy; **Hospital:** Fox Chase Cancer Ctr (page 59); **Address:** Fox Chase Cancer Ctr, 333 Cottman Ave, Ste C307, Philadelphia, PA 19111; **Phone:** 215-214-1424; **Board Cert:** Internal Medicine 1987; Gastroenterology 2001; **Med School:** Uniformed Srvs Univ, Bethesda 1982; **Resid:** Internal Medicine, US Naval Hosp 1987; **Fellow:** Gastroenterology, US Naval Hosp 1990; Endoscopy, Med Coll Wisconsin 1993; **Fac Appt:** Assoc Clin Prof Med, Temple Univ

Hoops, Timothy C MD [Ge] - **Spec Exp:** Gastrointestinal Cancer; Esophageal Disorders; Endoscopy; **Hospital:** Penn Presby Med Ctr - UPHS (page 72); **Address:** Penn Presbyterian Medical Ctr, 51 N 39th St, Ste 218, Philadelphia, PA 19104; **Phone:** 215-662-8900; **Board Cert:** Internal Medicine 1984; Gastroenterology 1987; **Med School:** Univ IL Coll Med 1981; **Resid:** Internal Medicine, U Colorado Hlth Sci Ctr 1984; **Fellow:** Gastroenterology, U Colorado Hlth Sci Ctr 1986; **Fac Appt:** Assoc Clin Prof Med, Univ Pennsylvania

Jacobson, Ira MD [Ge] - **Spec Exp:** Liver Disease; Pancreatic/Biliary Endoscopy (ERCP); Colonoscopy; Hepatitis; **Hospital:** NY-Presby Hosp/Weill Cornell (page 66); **Address:** 450 E 69th St, New York, NY 10021-5016; **Phone:** 212-746-2115; **Board Cert:** Internal Medicine 1982; Gastroenterology 1985; **Med School:** Columbia P&S 1979; **Resid:** Internal Medicine, UCSF Med Ctr 1982; **Fellow:** Gastroenterology, Mass Genl Hosp 1984; **Fac Appt:** Prof Med, Cornell Univ-Weill Med Coll

Kalloo, Anthony N MD [Ge] - **Spec Exp:** Endoscopy; Pancreatic Disease; **Hospital:** Johns Hopkins Hosp - Baltimore (page 61); **Address:** Cancer Research Bldg II, 1550 Orleans St, 1-M12, Baltimore, MD 21231; **Phone:** 410-955-9697; **Board Cert:** Internal Medicine 1985; Gastroenterology 1987; **Med School:** Jamaica 1979; **Resid:** Internal Medicine, Howard Univ Hosp 1985; **Fellow:** Gastroenterology, VA Med Ctr/Georgetown Univ Hosp 1987; **Fac Appt:** Assoc Prof Med, Johns Hopkins Univ

Kantsevoy, Sergey V MD/PhD [Ge] - **Spec Exp:** Pancreatic Disease; Endoscopic Ultrasound; Pancreatic/Biliary Endoscopy (ERCP); **Hospital:** Johns Hopkins Hosp - Baltimore (page 61); **Address:** Johns Hopkins Gastroenterology, 1830 E Mmonument St, rm 426, Baltimore, MD 21287; **Phone:** 410-614-6798; **Board Cert:** Internal Medicine 1997; Gastroenterology 2000; **Med School:** Russia 1983; **Resid:** Internal Medicine, Bronx-Lebanon Hosp Ctr 1995; Internal Medicine, Washington Hosp Ctr 1997; **Fellow:** Gastroenterology, Johns Hopkins Hosp 2000; **Fac Appt:** Asst Prof Med, Johns Hopkins Univ

Katz, Philip O MD [Ge] - **Spec Exp:** Gastroesophageal Reflux Disease (GERD); Swallowing Disorders; Barrett's Esophagus; Chest Pain-Non Cardiac; **Hospital:** Albert Einstein Med Ctr; **Address:** 5501 Old York Rd, Klein Bldg - Ste 363, Philadelphia, PA 19141; **Phone:** 215-456-8210; **Board Cert:** Internal Medicine 1981; Gastroenterology 1987; **Med School:** Bowman Gray 1978; **Resid:** Internal Medicine, NC Baptist Hosp 1981; **Fellow:** Gastroenterology, NC Baptist Hosp 1986; **Fac Appt:** Clin Prof Med, Thomas Jefferson Univ

Kochman, Michael L MD [Ge] - **Spec Exp:** Endoscopy; Pancreatic/Biliary Endoscopy (ERCP); Gastrointestinal Cancer; **Hospital:** Hosp Univ Penn - UPHS (page 72); **Address:** Hosp Univ Penn, Div Gastroenterology, 3400 Spruce St, 3 Dulles, Philadelphia, PA 19104-4206; **Phone:** 215-349-8222; **Board Cert:** Internal Medicine 1989; Gastroenterology 2003; **Med School:** Univ IL Coll Med 1986; **Resid:** Internal Medicine, Univ Illinois Med Ctr 1990; **Fellow:** Gastroenterology, Univ Michigan Med Ctr 1993; **Fac Appt:** Prof Med, Univ Pennsylvania

Korelitz, Burton I MD [Ge] - **Spec Exp:** Inflammatory Bowel Disease; Ulcerative Colitis; Crohn's Disease; **Hospital:** Lenox Hill Hosp (page 62); **Address:** 115 E 57th St, Ste 510, New York, NY 10022; **Phone:** 212-988-3800; **Board Cert:** Internal Medicine 1958; Gastroenterology 1961; **Med School:** Boston Univ 1951; **Resid:** Internal Medicine, VA Hosp 1953; Gastroenterology, Beth Israel Hosp 1954; **Fellow:** Gastroenterology, Mt Sinai Hosp 1956; **Fac Appt:** Clin Prof Med, NYU Sch Med

Korsten, Mark A MD [Ge] - **Spec Exp:** Constipation; Gastrointestinal Motility Disorders; Spinal Cord Injury & Colonic Motility; Liver Disease; **Hospital:** Mount Sinai Med Ctr, VA Med Ctr - Bronx; **Address:** 130 W Kingsbridge Rd, Bronx, NY 10468-3904; **Phone:** 718-584-9000 x6753; **Board Cert:** Internal Medicine 1973; Gastroenterology 1975; **Med School:** Yale Univ 1970; **Resid:** Internal Medicine, Mt Sinai Hosp 1973; **Fellow:** Gastroenterology, Mt Sinai Hosp 1975; **Fac Appt:** Prof Med, Mount Sinai Sch Med

Kotler, Donald P MD [Ge] - **Spec Exp:** Esophageal Disorders; Nutrition & AIDS; **Hospital:** St Luke's - Roosevelt Hosp Ctr - St Luke's Hosp; **Address:** 1111 Amsterdam Ave, SR 12, New York, NY 10025; **Phone:** 212-523-3670; **Board Cert:** Internal Medicine 1976; Gastroenterology 1979; **Med School:** Albert Einstein Coll Med 1973; **Resid:** Internal Medicine, Jacobi Med Ctr 1976; **Fellow:** Gastroenterology, Hosp Univ Penn 1978; **Fac Appt:** Assoc Prof Med, Columbia P&S

Kurtz, Robert C MD [Ge] - **Spec Exp:** Gastrointestinal Cancer; Pancreatic Cancer; Endoscopy; Nutrition & Cancer Prevention/Control; **Hospital:** Meml Sloan Kettering Cancer Ctr; **Address:** Meml Sloan Kettering Cancer Ctr, 1275 York Ave, rm H510, New York, NY 10021-6007; **Phone:** 212-639-7620; **Board Cert:** Internal Medicine 1971; Gastroenterology 1977; **Med School:** Jefferson Med Coll 1968; **Resid:** Internal Medicine, NY Hosp/Meml Sloan Kettering Cancer Ctr 1971; **Fellow:** Gastroenterology, Meml Sloan Kettering Cancer Ctr 1973; **Fac Appt:** Prof Med, Cornell Univ-Weill Med Coll

Lebwohl, Oscar MD [Ge] - **Spec Exp:** Endoscopy; Inflammatory Bowel Disease/Crohn's; Ulcerative Colitis; **Hospital:** NY-Presby Hosp/Columbia (page 66); **Address:** 161 Fort Washington Ave, New York, NY 10032-3713; **Phone:** 212-305-5363; **Board Cert:** Internal Medicine 1975; Gastroenterology 1977; **Med School:** Harvard Med Sch 1972; **Resid:** Internal Medicine, Mt Sinai Med Ctr 1975; **Fellow:** Gastroenterology, Columbia-Presby Med Ctr 1976; Hepatology, Mt Sinai Med Ctr 1977; **Fac Appt:** Clin Prof Med, Columbia P&S

Lichtenstein, Gary R MD [Ge] - **Spec Exp:** Inflammatory Bowel Disease; **Hospital:** Hosp Univ Penn - UPHS (page 72); **Address:** Univ Penn, Div Gastroenterology, 3400 Spruce St, 3 Ravdin Bldg, Philadelphia, PA 19104-4283; **Phone:** 215-349-8222; **Board Cert:** Internal Medicine 1987; Gastroenterology 1989; **Med School:** Mount Sinai Sch Med 1984; **Resid:** Internal Medicine, Duke Univ Med Ctr 1987; **Fellow:** Gastroenterology, Hosp Univ Penn 1990; **Fac Appt:** Assoc Prof Med, Univ Pennsylvania

Gastroenterology

Lightdale, Charles MD [Ge] - **Spec Exp:** Barrett's Esophagus; Gastrointestinal Cancer; Endoscopic Ultrasound; **Hospital:** NY-Presby Hosp/Columbia (page 66); **Address:** Columbia-Presby Med Ctr, Irving Pavilion, 161 Fort Washington Ave, rm 812, New York, NY 10032-3713; **Phone:** 212-305-3423; **Board Cert:** Internal Medicine 1972; Gastroenterology 1973; **Med School:** Columbia P&S 1966; **Resid:** Internal Medicine, Yale-New Haven Hosp 1968; Internal Medicine, New York Hosp 1969; **Fellow:** Gastroenterology, New York Hosp-Cornell 1973; **Fac Appt:** Prof Med, Columbia P&S

Lipshutz, William H MD [Ge] - **Spec Exp:** Inflammatory Bowel Disease/Crohn's; Colon Cancer; Esophageal Disorders; Gastroesophageal Reflux Disease (GERD); **Hospital:** Pennsylvania Hosp (page 72); **Address:** 230 W Washington Sq, Farm Journal Bldg, Fl 4, Philadelphia, PA 19106; **Phone:** 215-829-3561; **Board Cert:** Internal Medicine 1972; Gastroenterology 1973; **Med School:** Univ Pennsylvania 1967; **Resid:** Internal Medicine, Pennsylvania Hosp 1972; **Fellow:** Gastroenterology, Hosp Univ Penn 1971; **Fac Appt:** Clin Prof Med, Univ Pennsylvania

Magun, Arthur MD [Ge] - **Spec Exp:** Hepatitis; Ulcerative Colitis; Endoscopy; Inflammatory Bowel Disease/Crohn's; **Hospital:** NY-Presby Hosp/Columbia (page 66); **Address:** 161 Fort Washington Ave, rm 338, New York, NY 10032-3713; **Phone:** 212-305-5287; **Board Cert:** Internal Medicine 1980; Gastroenterology 1983; **Med School:** Mount Sinai Sch Med 1977; **Resid:** Internal Medicine, Columbia-Presby Med Ctr 1980; **Fellow:** Gastroenterology, Columbia-Presby Med Ctr 1983; **Fac Appt:** Clin Prof Med, Columbia P&S

Markowitz, David MD [Ge] - **Spec Exp:** Gastroesophageal Reflux Disease (GERD); Esophageal Disorders; Endoscopy; **Hospital:** NY-Presby Hosp/Columbia (page 66); **Address:** 161 Ft Washington Ave, Ste 853, New York, NY 10032; **Phone:** 212-305-1024; **Board Cert:** Internal Medicine 1988; Gastroenterology 2001; **Med School:** Columbia P&S 1985; **Resid:** Internal Medicine, Columbia-Presby Hosp 1988; **Fellow:** Gastroenterology, Columbia-Presby Hosp 1991; **Fac Appt:** Asst Clin Prof Med, Columbia P&S

Martin, Paul MD [Ge] - **Spec Exp:** Liver Disease; Hepatitis; Transplant Medicine-Liver; **Hospital:** Mount Sinai Med Ctr; **Address:** 5 E 98th St Fl 11, New York, NY 10029; **Phone:** 212-241-0034; **Board Cert:** Internal Medicine 1984; Gastroenterology 1987; **Med School:** Ireland 1978; **Resid:** Internal Medicine, St Vincent's Hosp 1982; Internal Medicine, Univ Alberta 1984; **Fellow:** Gastroenterology, Queen Univ 1986; Hepatology, Natl Inst Hlth 1989; **Fac Appt:** Prof Med, Mount Sinai Sch Med

Mayer, Lloyd MD [Ge] - **Spec Exp:** Inflammatory Bowel Disease/Crohn's; Ulcerative Colitis; **Hospital:** Mount Sinai Med Ctr; **Address:** 1425 Madison Ave, rm 11-20, Box 1089, New York, NY 10029; **Phone:** 212-659-9266; **Board Cert:** Internal Medicine 1979; Gastroenterology 1981; **Med School:** Mount Sinai Sch Med 1976; **Resid:** Internal Medicine, Bellevue Hosp 1979; **Fellow:** Gastroenterology, Mount Sinai Hosp 1981; **Fac Appt:** Prof Med, Mount Sinai Sch Med

Metz, David C MD [Ge] - **Spec Exp:** Peptic Acid Disorders; Neuroendocrine Tumors; Gastroesophageal Reflux Disease (GERD); Gastrointestinal Motility Disorders; **Hospital:** Hosp Univ Penn - UPHS (page 72); **Address:** Hosp Univ Penn, Div Gastroenterology, 3400 Spruce St, 3 Ravdin, Philadelphia, PA 19104; **Phone:** 215-662-4279; **Board Cert:** Internal Medicine 1989; Gastroenterology 2001; **Med School:** South Africa 1982; **Resid:** Internal Medicine, Albert Einstein Med Ctr 1988; **Fellow:** Gastroenterology, Natl Inst Hlth 1991; **Fac Appt:** Prof Med, Univ Pennsylvania

Miskovitz, Paul MD [Ge] - **Spec Exp:** Endoscopy; Liver Disease; **Hospital:** NY-Presby Hosp/Weill Cornell (page 66); **Address:** 635 Madison Ave Fl 17, New York, NY 10022; **Phone:** 212-717-4966; **Board Cert:** Internal Medicine 1978; Gastroenterology 1981; **Med School:** Cornell Univ-Weill Med Coll 1975; **Resid:** Internal Medicine, NY Hosp 1978; **Fellow:** Gastroenterology, NY Hosp 1980; **Fac Appt:** Clin Prof Med, Cornell Univ-Weill Med Coll

Pochapin, Mark B MD [Ge] - **Spec Exp:** Pancreatic Cancer; Endoscopic Ultrasound; Colon & Rectal Cancer Detection; Diarrheal Diseases; **Hospital:** NY-Presby Hosp/Weill Cornell (page 66); **Address:** The Jay Monahan Ctr for GI Hlth, 1315 York Ave, New York, NY 10022; **Phone:** 212-746-4014; **Board Cert:** Gastroenterology 2004; **Med School:** Cornell Univ-Weill Med Coll 1988; **Resid:** Internal Medicine, NY Hosp-Cornell Med Ctr 1991; **Fellow:** Gastroenterology, Montefiore Med Ctr 1993; **Fac Appt:** Assoc Clin Prof Med, Cornell Univ-Weill Med Coll

Present, Daniel MD [Ge] - **Spec Exp:** Inflammatory Bowel Disease/Crohn's; Ulcerative Colitis; Crohn's Disease; **Hospital:** Mount Sinai Med Ctr; **Address:** 12 E 86th St, New York, NY 10028-0506; **Phone:** 212-861-2000; **Board Cert:** Internal Medicine 1966; Gastroenterology 1970; **Med School:** SUNY Downstate 1959; **Resid:** Internal Medicine, Mount Sinai Hosp 1964; **Fellow:** Gastroenterology, Mount Sinai Hosp 1966; **Fac Appt:** Clin Prof Med, Mount Sinai Sch Med

Ravich, William J MD [Ge] - **Spec Exp:** Swallowing Disorders; Gastroesophageal Reflux Disease (GERD); Barrett's Esophagus; **Hospital:** Johns Hopkins Hosp - Baltimore (page 61), Greater Baltimore Med Ctr; **Address:** 10751 Falls Rd, Ste 401, Lutherville, MD 21093; **Phone:** 410-616-2840; **Board Cert:** Internal Medicine 1978; Gastroenterology 1981; **Med School:** Ros Franklin Univ/Chicago Med Sch 1975; **Resid:** Internal Medicine, Montefiore Hosp 1978; **Fellow:** Gastroenterology, Johns Hopkins Hosp 1981; **Fac Appt:** Assoc Prof Med, Johns Hopkins Univ

Reddy, K Rajender MD [Ge] - **Spec Exp:** Liver Disease; Hepatitis; Transplant Medicine-Liver; **Hospital:** Hosp Univ Penn - UPHS (page 72); **Address:** Hosp U Penn, Gastroenterology, 3 Dulles, 3400 Spruce St, Philadelphia, PA 19104; **Phone:** 215-349-8222; **Board Cert:** Internal Medicine 1980; Gastroenterology 1983; **Med School:** India 1972; **Resid:** Internal Medicine, NY Med Coll Hosps 1980; **Fellow:** Gastroenterology, E Tenn State U Hosp 1982; Hepatology, U Miami Hosps 1983; **Fac Appt:** Prof Med, Univ Pennsylvania

Richter, Joel E MD [Ge] - **Spec Exp:** Gastroesophageal Reflux Disease (GERD); Esophageal Disorders; **Hospital:** Temple Univ Hosp; **Address:** Temple Univ Hospital, Parkinson Pavilion, 8401 N Broad St, rm 800, Philadelphia, PA 19140; **Phone:** 215-707-5069; **Board Cert:** Internal Medicine 1978; Gastroenterology 1981; **Med School:** Univ Tex SW, Dallas 1975; **Resid:** Internal Medicine, Natl Naval Med Ctr 1978; **Fellow:** Gastroenterology, Natl Naval Med Ctr 1980; **Fac Appt:** Prof Med, Temple Univ

Sachar, David MD [Ge] - **Spec Exp:** Crohn's Disease; Ulcerative Colitis; Inflammatory Bowel Disease; **Hospital:** Mount Sinai Med Ctr; **Address:** One Gustave L Levy Pl, Box 1069, New York, NY 10029-6501; **Phone:** 212-241-4299; **Board Cert:** Internal Medicine 1969; Gastroenterology 1972; **Med School:** Harvard Med Sch 1963; **Resid:** Internal Medicine, Beth Israel Hosp 1965; Internal Medicine, Beth Israel Hosp 1968; **Fellow:** Gastroenterology, Mount Sinai Hosp 1970; **Fac Appt:** Clin Prof Med, Mount Sinai Sch Med

Gastroenterology

Shike, Moshe MD [Ge] - **Spec Exp:** Gastrointestinal Cancer; Nutrition & Cancer Prevention; Endoscopy; **Hospital:** Meml Sloan Kettering Cancer Ctr, NY-Presby Hosp/Weill Cornell (page 66); **Address:** 1275 York Ave, rm S-536, New York, NY 10021; **Phone:** 212-639-7230; **Board Cert:** Internal Medicine 1977; Gastroenterology 1981; **Med School:** Israel 1975; **Resid:** Internal Medicine, Mt Auburn Hosp 1977; **Fellow:** Gastroenterology, Toronto Genl Hosp 1981; **Fac Appt:** Prof Med, Cornell Univ-Weill Med Coll

Tobias, Hillel MD [Ge] - **Spec Exp:** Liver Disease; Hepatitis B & C; Liver & Biliary Disease; **Hospital:** NYU Med Ctr (page 67); **Address:** 232 E 30th St, New York, NY 10016-8202; **Phone:** 212-889-5544; **Board Cert:** Internal Medicine 1967; Gastroenterology 1979; **Med School:** Washington Univ, St Louis 1960; **Resid:** Internal Medicine, Bellevue Hosp 1963; **Fellow:** Hepatology, Royal Free Hosp 1965; Hepatology, Mount Sinai Hosp 1967; **Fac Appt:** Prof Med, NYU Sch Med

Waye, Jerome MD [Ge] - **Spec Exp:** Endoscopy; Colon Cancer; Colonoscopy; **Hospital:** Mount Sinai Med Ctr, Lenox Hill Hosp (page 62); **Address:** 650 Park Ave, New York, NY 10021-6115; **Phone:** 212-439-7779; **Board Cert:** Internal Medicine 1965; Gastroenterology 1970; **Med School:** Boston Univ 1958; **Resid:** Internal Medicine, Mount Sinai Hosp 1961; **Fellow:** Gastroenterology, Mount Sinai Hosp 1962; **Fac Appt:** Clin Prof Med, Mount Sinai Sch Med

Winawer, Sidney J MD [Ge] - **Spec Exp:** Colonoscopy; Colon Cancer; Cancer Prevention; **Hospital:** Meml Sloan Kettering Cancer Ctr; **Address:** 1275 York Ave, Box 90, New York, NY 10021-6094; **Phone:** 212-639-7678; **Board Cert:** Internal Medicine 1965; Gastroenterology 1973; **Med School:** SUNY Downstate 1956; **Resid:** Internal Medicine, VA Hosp 1961; Internal Medicine, Maimonides Hosp 1962; **Fellow:** Gastroenterology, Boston City Hosp 1964; **Fac Appt:** Prof Med, Cornell Univ-Weill Med Coll

Southeast

Barkin, Jamie S MD [Ge] - **Spec Exp:** Pancreatic & Biliary Disease; Gastrointestinal Cancer; Endoscopy; **Hospital:** Mount Sinai Med Ctr - Miami, Univ of Miami Hosp & Clins/Sylvester Comp Canc Ctr; **Address:** Mount Sinai Medical Center, Gumenick Bldg, 4300 Alton Rd, Ste 2522, Miami Beach, FL 33140-2800; **Phone:** 305-674-2240; **Board Cert:** Internal Medicine 1973; Gastroenterology 1975; **Med School:** Univ Miami Sch Med 1970; **Resid:** Internal Medicine, Univ Miami Hosp 1973; **Fellow:** Gastroenterology, Univ Miami Hosp 1975; **Fac Appt:** Prof Med, Univ Miami Sch Med

Bloomer, Joseph MD [Ge] - **Spec Exp:** Porphyria; Liver Disease; Transplant Medicine-Liver; **Hospital:** Univ of Ala Hosp at Birmingham; **Address:** Univ of Ala at Birmingham, 284 MCLM, 1918 University Blvd, Birmingham, AL 35294-0005; **Phone:** 205-975-9699; **Board Cert:** Internal Medicine 1972; **Med School:** Case West Res Univ 1966; **Resid:** Internal Medicine, UCSF Med Ctr 1968; **Fellow:** Hepatology, Yale School of Med 1972; **Fac Appt:** Prof Med, Univ Ala

Boyce Jr, H Worth MD [Ge] - **Spec Exp:** Esophageal Disorders; Barrett's Esophagus; Esophageal Cancer; **Hospital:** H Lee Moffitt Cancer Ctr & Research Inst, Tampa Genl Hosp; **Address:** Ctr for Swallowing Disorders, 12901 Bruce B Downs Blvd, MDC 72, Tampa, FL 33612-4742; **Phone:** 813-974-3374; **Board Cert:** Internal Medicine 1977; Gastroenterology 1965; **Med School:** Wake Forest Univ 1955; **Resid:** Internal Medicine, Brooke Army Hosp 1959; Gastroenterology, Brooke Army Hosp 1960; **Fac Appt:** Prof Med, Univ S Fla Coll Med

Brazer, Scott R MD [Ge] - **Spec Exp:** Gastroesophageal Reflux Disease (GERD); Chest Pain-Non Cardiac; Colonoscopy; **Hospital:** Durham Regional Hosp; **Address:** 249 E Highway 54, Durham, NC 27713; **Phone:** 919-806-8322; **Board Cert:** Internal Medicine 1984; Gastroenterology 1987; **Med School:** Case West Res Univ 1981; **Resid:** Internal Medicine, Duke Univ 1984; Internal Medicine, Duke Univ 1988; **Fellow:** Gastroenterology, Duke Unic 1987

Castell, Donald O MD [Ge] - **Spec Exp:** Esophageal Disorders; Gastroesophageal Reflux Disease (GERD); Gastrointestinal Motility Disorders; **Hospital:** MUSC Med Ctr; **Address:** MUSC Digestive Disease Ctr, 96 Jonathan Lucas St, Box 250327, Charleston, SC 29425; **Phone:** 843-792-7522; **Board Cert:** Internal Medicine 1977; Gastroenterology 1970; **Med School:** Geo Wash Univ 1960; **Resid:** Internal Medicine, US Naval Hosp 1965; **Fellow:** Gastroenterology, Tufts Univ 1969; **Fac Appt:** Prof Med, Univ SC Sch Med

Cominelli, Fabio MD/PhD [Ge] - **Spec Exp:** Inflammatory Bowel Disease/Crohn's; Ulcerative Colitis; **Hospital:** Univ Virginia Med Ctr; **Address:** Univ VA Hlth Sys, Div Gastroenterology, PO Box 800708, Charlottesville, VA 22908; **Phone:** 434-243-6400; **Med School:** Italy 1983; **Resid:** Gastroenterology, Careggi Hosp-Univ Italy 1986; **Fellow:** Gastroenterology, Harbor-UCLA Med Ctr 1989; **Fac Appt:** Prof Med, Univ VA Sch Med

Cotton, Peter MD [Ge] - **Spec Exp:** Pancreatic Disease; Biliary Disease; Pancreatic/Biliary Endoscopy (ERCP); **Hospital:** MUSC Med Ctr; **Address:** MUSC, Digestive Disease Center - 210 CSB, 96 Jonathan Lucas St, Box 250327, Charleston, SC 29425; **Phone:** 843-792-6865; **Med School:** England 1963; **Resid:** Internal Medicine, St Thomas' Hosp 1970; Gastroenterology, St Thomas' Hosp 1973; **Fac Appt:** Prof Med, Med Univ SC

DeVault, Kenneth MD [Ge] - **Spec Exp:** Gastroesophageal Reflux Disease (GERD); **Hospital:** Mayo - Jacksonville, St Luke's Hosp - Jacksonville; **Address:** Mayo Clinic, Davis Bldg, 6th Fl, 4500 San Pablo Rd S, Jacksonville, FL 32224-1865; **Phone:** 904-953-2254; **Board Cert:** Internal Medicine 1989; Gastroenterology 2003; **Med School:** Bowman Gray 1986; **Resid:** Internal Medicine, Vanderbilt Univ Med Ctr 1989; **Fellow:** Gastroenterology, Jefferson Univ Med Ctr 1992; **Fac Appt:** Assoc Prof Med, Mayo Med Sch

Drossman, Douglas A MD [Ge] - **Spec Exp:** Gastrointestinal Motility Disorders; Pain-Abdominal/Functional; Gastrointestinal Functional Disorders; **Hospital:** Univ NC Hosps; **Address:** Univ NC, Div Digestive Diseases, 4150 Bio Informatics Bldg, Campus Box 7080, Chapel Hill, NC 27599-7080; **Phone:** 919-966-0141; **Board Cert:** Internal Medicine 1973; Gastroenterology 1979; **Med School:** Albert Einstein Coll Med 1970; **Resid:** Internal Medicine, NC Meml Hosp 1972; Internal Medicine, Bellevue Hosp Ctr-NYU 1973; **Fellow:** Psychiatry, Univ Rochester 1976; Gastroenterology, NC Meml Hosp-UNC 1978; **Fac Appt:** Prof Med, Univ NC Sch Med

Fallon, Michael B MD [Ge] - **Spec Exp:** Liver Disease; Hepatitis C; **Hospital:** Univ of Ala Hosp at Birmingham; **Address:** University of Alabama Scool of Medicine, 1530 S 3rd Ave, MCLM 290, Birmingham, AL 35294; **Phone:** 205-975-5676; **Board Cert:** Internal Medicine 1988; Gastroenterology 2001; **Med School:** W VA Univ 1984; **Resid:** Internal Medicine, Yale-New Haven Hosp 1988; **Fellow:** Gastroenterology, Yale-New Haven Hosp 1990; **Fac Appt:** Assoc Prof Med, Univ Ala

Gastroenterology

Forsmark, Christopher MD [Ge] - **Spec Exp:** AIDS/HIV-Gastrointestinal Complications; Colonoscopy; Pancreatic Disease; Pancreatic/Biliary Endoscopy (ERCP); **Hospital:** Shands Hlthcre at Univ of FL; **Address:** University of Florida, 1600 SW Archer Rd, Box 100214, Gainesville, FL 32610; **Phone:** 352-392-2877; **Board Cert:** Internal Medicine 1986; Gastroenterology 1989; **Med School:** Johns Hopkins Univ 1983; **Resid:** Internal Medicine, UCSF Med Ctr 1987; **Fellow:** Gastroenterology, USCF Med Ctr 1990; **Fac Appt:** Prof Med, Univ Fla Coll Med

Hawes, Robert H MD [Ge] - **Spec Exp:** Endoscopic Ultrasound; Pancreatic/Biliary Endoscopy (ERCP); Pancreatic Disease; **Hospital:** MUSC Med Ctr; **Address:** 96 Jonathan Lucas St, Ste 210, Box 250327, Charleston, SC 29425; **Phone:** 843-792-7896; **Board Cert:** Internal Medicine 1985; Gastroenterology 1987; **Med School:** Indiana Univ 1980; **Fac Appt:** Prof Med, Med Univ SC

Hoffman, Brenda J MD [Ge] - **Spec Exp:** Liver & Biliary Disease; Endoscopic Ultrasound; Gastrointestinal Cancer; Colon & Rectal Cancer-Familial Polyposis; **Hospital:** MUSC Med Ctr; **Address:** Digestive Disease Center, 210 CSB, 96 Jonathan Lucas St, Box 250327, Charleston, SC 29425; **Phone:** 843-792-6999; **Board Cert:** Internal Medicine 1986; Gastroenterology 1989; **Med School:** Univ KY Coll Med 1983; **Resid:** Internal Medicine, MUSC Med Ctr 1987; **Fellow:** Gastroenterology, MUSC Med Ctr 1989; **Fac Appt:** Prof Med, Univ SC Sch Med

Lambiase, Louis MD [Ge] - **Spec Exp:** Pancreatic Disease; Endoscopic Ultrasound; **Hospital:** Shands Jacksonville, Naval Hosp - Jacksonville; **Address:** 4555 Emerson Expressway Fl 3 - Ste 300, Jacksonville, FL 32207; **Phone:** 904-244-3273; **Board Cert:** Internal Medicine 2000; Gastroenterology 1993; **Med School:** Univ Miami Sch Med 1987; **Resid:** Internal Medicine, Univ Pittsburgh-Presby/ VA Hosps 1990; **Fellow:** Gastroenterology, Univ Fla Coll Med 1993; **Fac Appt:** Assoc Prof Med, Univ Fla Coll Med

Liddle, Rodger Alan MD [Ge] - **Spec Exp:** Gastrointestinal Cancer; Pancreatic Disease; Hormone Secreting Tumors; **Hospital:** Duke Univ Med Ctr, VA Med Ctr - Durham; **Address:** Duke Univ Med Ctr, Div Gastroenterology, Box 3913, Durham, NC 27710; **Phone:** 919-681-6380; **Board Cert:** Internal Medicine 1981; Gastroenterology 1983; **Med School:** Vanderbilt Univ 1978; **Resid:** Internal Medicine, UCSF Med Ctr 1981; **Fellow:** Gastroenterology, UCSF Med Ctr 1984; **Fac Appt:** Prof Med, Duke Univ

Lind, Christopher D MD [Ge] - **Spec Exp:** Gastroesophageal Reflux Disease (GERD); Swallowing Disorders; Biliary Disease; **Hospital:** Vanderbilt Univ Med Ctr; **Address:** Vanderbilt Univ Med Ctr, Div GI, 1660 TVC GI Clinic, Nashville, TN 37232-5280; **Phone:** 615-322-0128; **Board Cert:** Internal Medicine 1984; Gastroenterology 1987; **Med School:** Vanderbilt Univ 1981; **Resid:** Internal Medicine, Univ Virginia Hosps 1985; **Fellow:** Gastroenterology, Shands/Univ Florida 1986; Gastroenterology, Univ Virginia Hosps 1988; **Fac Appt:** Prof Med, Vanderbilt Univ

Mertz, Howard MD [Ge] - **Spec Exp:** Irritable Bowel Syndrome; Endoscopic Ultrasound; Inflammatory Bowel Disease; **Hospital:** Saint Thomas Hosp - Nashville; **Address:** 4230 Harding Rd, Ste 309W, Nashville, TN 37205; **Phone:** 615-383-0165; **Board Cert:** Internal Medicine 1989; Gastroenterology 2002; **Med School:** Baylor Coll Med 1986; **Resid:** Internal Medicine, Johns Hopkins Hosp 1989; **Fellow:** Gastroenterology, UCLA Med Ctr 1991; **Fac Appt:** Assoc Prof Med, Vanderbilt Univ

Raiford, David S MD [Ge] - **Spec Exp:** Liver Disease; Drug Toxicity in Liver; Liver Tumors; Transplant Medicine-Liver; **Hospital:** Vanderbilt Univ Med Ctr; **Address:** Vanderbilt Hepatology, 1660 The Vanderbilt Clinic, Nashville, TN 37232-5280; **Phone:** 615-322-0128; **Board Cert:** Internal Medicine 1989; Gastroenterology 2001; **Med School:** Johns Hopkins Univ 1985; **Resid:** Internal Medicine, Johns Hopkins Hosp 1988; **Fellow:** Hepatology, Johns Hopkins Hosp 1991; **Fac Appt:** Prof Med, Vanderbilt Univ

Roche, James K MD/PhD [Ge] - **Spec Exp:** Inflammatory Bowel Disease/Crohn's; Diarrheal Diseases; **Hospital:** Univ Virginia Med Ctr; **Address:** Univ VA Hlth Sys, Div Gastroenterology, Box 801317, Charlottesville, VA 22908-1317; **Phone:** 434-924-9922; **Board Cert:** Internal Medicine 1975; **Med School:** Univ Pennsylvania 1969; **Resid:** Internal Medicine, Univ Hlth Ctr 1971; Internal Medicine, Duke Univ Med Ctr 1974; **Fellow:** Gastroenterology, Duke Univ Med Ctr 1977; **Fac Appt:** Assoc Prof Med, Univ VA Sch Med

Sartor, R Balfour MD [Ge] - **Spec Exp:** Inflammatory Bowel Disease; **Hospital:** Univ NC Hosps; **Address:** Univ NC Sch Med, Div Gastroenterology/Hepatology, Biomolecular Bldg- rm 7309, Box 7032, Chapel Hill, NC 27599-7032; **Phone:** 919-966-0140; **Board Cert:** Internal Medicine 1978; Gastroenterology 1981; **Med School:** Baylor Coll Med 1974; **Resid:** Internal Medicine, Baylor Affil Hosp 1977; **Fellow:** Gastroenterology, Univ NC Hosps 1981; **Fac Appt:** Prof Med, Univ NC Sch Med

Schiff, Eugene MD [Ge] - **Spec Exp:** Hepatitis C; Liver Disease; **Hospital:** Cedars Med Ctr - Miami, Jackson Meml Hosp; **Address:** Sylvester Cancer Ctr, 1500 NW 12th Ave, Miami, FL 33136; **Phone:** 305-243-5787; **Board Cert:** Internal Medicine 1980; Gastroenterology 1972; **Med School:** Columbia P&S 1962; **Resid:** Internal Medicine, Cincinnati Genl Hosp 1964; Internal Medicine, Parkland Meml Hosp 1967; **Fellow:** Gastroenterology, Univ Tex SW Med Ctr 1969; **Fac Appt:** Prof Med, Univ Miami Sch Med

Scudera, Peter MD [Ge] - **Spec Exp:** Transplant Medicine-Liver; Pancreatic/Biliary Endoscopy (ERCP); Hepatitis C; **Hospital:** Inova Fair Oaks Hosp, Inova Fairfax Hosp; **Address:** 3700 Joseph Siewick Dr, Ste 308, Fairfax, VA 22033; **Phone:** 703-716-8700; **Board Cert:** Internal Medicine 1987; Gastroenterology 1989; **Med School:** Cornell Univ-Weill Med Coll 1984; **Resid:** Internal Medicine, New York Hosp 1987; **Fellow:** Gastroenterology, New York Hosp-Cornell 1989

Shiffman, Mitchell MD [Ge] - **Spec Exp:** Transplant Medicine-Liver; Hepatitis C; **Hospital:** Med Coll of VA Hosp; **Address:** VCU Health Systems, Div Hepatology, Box 980341, Richmond, VA 23298-0341; **Phone:** 804-828-4060; **Board Cert:** Internal Medicine 1986; Gastroenterology 1989; **Med School:** SUNY Upstate Med Univ 1983; **Resid:** Internal Medicine, Med Coll Va Hosp 1986; **Fellow:** Gastroenterology, Med Coll Va Hosp 1988; **Fac Appt:** Prof Med, Med Coll VA

Toskes, Phillip MD [Ge] - **Spec Exp:** Nutrition; Malabsorption Syndrome; Pancreatic Disease; **Hospital:** Shands Hlthcre at Univ of FL; **Address:** Univ Florida, Div Gastroenterolgy, Box 100214, Gainesville, FL 32610-0214; **Phone:** 352-392-2877; **Board Cert:** Internal Medicine 1970; Gastroenterology 1973; **Med School:** Univ MD Sch Med 1965; **Resid:** Internal Medicine, Univ Maryland Hosp 1968; **Fellow:** Gastroenterology, Hosp Univ Penn 1970; **Fac Appt:** Prof Med, Univ Fla Coll Med

Wilcox, Charles M MD [Ge] - **Spec Exp:** AIDS/HIV-Gastrointestinal Complications; Endoscopy; Pancreatic & Biliary Disease; **Hospital:** Univ of Ala Hosp at Birmingham; **Address:** Univ Alabama Hosp, 703 S 19th St, rm 633 ZRB, Birmingham, AL 35294-0007; **Phone:** 205-975-4958; **Board Cert:** Internal Medicine 1986; Gastroenterology 1989; **Med School:** Med Coll GA 1983; **Resid:** Internal Medicine, Univ Alabama Hosps 1986; **Fellow:** Gastroenterology, UCSF Med Ctr 1990; **Fac Appt:** Prof Med, Univ Ala

Gastroenterology

Midwest

Achkar, Edgar MD [Ge] - **Spec Exp:** Esophageal Disorders; Gastrointestinal Motility Disorders; **Hospital:** Cleveland Clin Fdn (page 57); **Address:** 9500 Euclid Ave, Desk A30, Cleveland, OH 44195; **Phone:** 216-444-6523; **Board Cert:** Internal Medicine 1978; Gastroenterology 1979; **Med School:** Lebanon 1964; **Resid:** Internal Medicine, Lahey Clin 1967; **Fellow:** Gastroenterology, Lahey Clin 1968; Gastroenterology, Clevland Clin 1969; **Fac Appt:** Prof Med, Cleveland Cl Coll Med/Case West Res

Bacon, Bruce MD [Ge] - **Spec Exp:** Hepatitis C; Hepatic Iron Metabolism; Liver Disease; **Hospital:** St Louis Univ Hosp, SSM St Mary's Hlth Ctr - St Louis; **Address:** 3660 Vista Ave, Ste 308, St Louis, MO 63110-2540; **Phone:** 314-977-6150; **Board Cert:** Internal Medicine 1978; Gastroenterology 1983; **Med School:** Case West Res Univ 1975; **Resid:** Internal Medicine, Metro Genl Hosp 1979; **Fellow:** Gastroenterology, Metro Genl Hosp 1982; **Fac Appt:** Prof Med, St Louis Univ

Baron, Todd H MD [Ge] - **Spec Exp:** Endoscopy; Pancreatic/Biliary Endoscopy (ERCP); **Hospital:** Mayo Med Ctr & Clin - Rochester; **Address:** Mayo Clinic, 200 First St SW, Charleton 8, Rochester, MN 55905; **Phone:** 507-266-6931; **Board Cert:** Internal Medicine 1989; Gastroenterology 2003; **Med School:** Univ Fla Coll Med 1986; **Resid:** Internal Medicine, Univ Alabama Med Ctr 1990; **Fellow:** Gastroenterology, Univ Alabama Med Ctr 1993; **Fac Appt:** Assoc Prof Med, Univ Ariz Coll Med

Blei, Andres T MD [Ge] - **Spec Exp:** Hepatitis C; Liver Disease; **Hospital:** Northwestern Meml Hosp; **Address:** 675 N St Clair St Fl 14 - Ste 100, Chicago, IL 60611; **Phone:** 312-695-4837; **Board Cert:** Internal Medicine 1981; Gastroenterology 1985; **Med School:** Argentina 1973; **Resid:** Internal Medicine, Police Posadas 1976; Hepatology, Yale Univ Sch Med 1978; **Fellow:** Gastroenterology, Univ Chicago Hosp 1980; **Fac Appt:** Prof Med, Northwestern Univ

Brown, Kimberly A MD [Ge] - **Spec Exp:** Liver Disease; Transplant Medicine-Liver; Hepatitis C; Liver Cancer; **Hospital:** Henry Ford Hosp; **Address:** Henry Ford Hosp, Dept Gastroenterology, 2799 W Grand Blvd Bldg K Fl 7, Detroit, MI 48202-2608; **Phone:** 313-916-8632; **Board Cert:** Internal Medicine 1988; Gastroenterology 2002; **Med School:** Wayne State Univ 1985; **Resid:** Internal Medicine, Univ Michigan Med Ctr 1989; **Fellow:** Gastroenterology, Univ Michigan Med Ctr 1992

Chari, Suresh T MD [Ge] - **Spec Exp:** Pancreatic Disease; **Hospital:** Mayo Med Ctr & Clin - Rochester; **Address:** Mayo Clinic, 200 First St SW Gonda Bldg Fl 9, Rochester, MN 55905; **Phone:** 507-266-4347; **Board Cert:** Internal Medicine 1996; Gastroenterology 1999; **Med School:** India 1982; **Resid:** Internal Medicine, Univ Arizona Hlth Sci Ctr 1996; **Fellow:** Gastroenterology, Mayo Clinic 1999; **Fac Appt:** Prof Med, Mayo Med Sch

Clouse, Ray E MD [Ge] - **Spec Exp:** Gastroesophageal Reflux Disease (GERD); Esophageal Disorders; Gastrointestinal Functional Disorders; **Hospital:** Barnes-Jewish Hosp; **Address:** Washington Univ Sch Med, 4921 Park View Pl Fl 8, St Louis, MO 63110; **Phone:** 314-747-2066; **Board Cert:** Internal Medicine 1979; **Med School:** Indiana Univ 1976; **Resid:** Internal Medicine, Barnes Hosp/Wash Univ Sch Med 1978; **Fellow:** Gastroenterology, Barnes Hosp/Wash Univ Sch Med 1979; **Fac Appt:** Prof Med, Washington Univ, St Louis

Craig, Robert M MD [Ge] - **Spec Exp:** Inflammatory Bowel Disease/Crohn's; Liver Disease; Swallowing Disorders; Diarrheal Diseases; **Hospital:** Northwestern Meml Hosp; **Address:** 233 E Erie St, Ste 206, Chicago, IL 60611-5938; **Phone:** 312-908-9644; **Board Cert:** Internal Medicine 1972; Gastroenterology 1975; **Med School:** Northwestern Univ 1967; **Resid:** Internal Medicine, VA Rsch Hosp 1969; Internal Medicine, VA Rsch Hosp 1972; **Fellow:** Gastroenterology, Northwestern Univ Med Ctr 1974; **Fac Appt:** Prof Med, Northwestern Univ

Crippin, Jeffrey S MD [Ge] - **Spec Exp:** Transplant Medicine-Liver; Liver Disease; Liver Failure; Gastrointestinal Cancer; **Hospital:** Barnes-Jewish Hosp; **Address:** Barnes Jewish Hosp, Div Gastroenterology, 660 S Euclid Ave Campus Box 8124, St Louis, MO 63110; **Phone:** 314-454-8160; **Board Cert:** Internal Medicine 1987; Gastroenterology 2001; **Med School:** Univ Kans 1984; **Resid:** Internal Medicine, Kansas Univ Med Ctr 1988; **Fellow:** Gastroenterology, Mayo Clinic 1991; **Fac Appt:** Assoc Prof Med, Washington Univ, St Louis

Di Bisceglie, Adrian Michael MD [Ge] - **Spec Exp:** Hepatitis C; Hepatitis; Liver Cancer; **Hospital:** St Louis Univ Hosp; **Address:** St Louis Univ Hosp, Dept. Gastroenterology, 3635 Vista Ave, PO Box 15250, St. Louis, MO 63110-0250; **Phone:** 314-577-8764; **Board Cert:** Internal Medicine 2002; Gastroenterology 2002; **Med School:** South Africa 1977; **Resid:** Internal Medicine, Baragwanath Hosp 1984; **Fellow:** Hepatology, Natl Inst Hlth 1988; **Fac Appt:** Prof Med, St Louis Univ

Edmundowicz, Steven MD [Ge] - **Spec Exp:** Endoscopy; Biliary Disease; Pancreatic Disease; **Hospital:** Barnes-Jewish Hosp; **Address:** Washington Univ Sch Med, Div Gastroenterology, 660 S Euclid Ave, Box 8124, St Louis, MO 63110; **Phone:** 314-747-2066; **Board Cert:** Internal Medicine 1986; Gastroenterology 1989; **Med School:** Jefferson Med Coll 1983; **Resid:** Internal Medicine, Barnes Hosp/Wash Univ 1986; **Fellow:** Gastroenterology, Barnes Hosp/Wash Univ 1989; **Fac Appt:** Assoc Prof Med, Washington Univ, St Louis

Elliott, David MD [Ge] - **Spec Exp:** Celiac Disease; Inflammatory Bowel Disease/Crohn's; Intestinal Parasites; **Hospital:** Univ Iowa Hosp & Clinics; **Address:** Univ Iowa Hosp, Digestive Disease, 200 Hawkins Drive, rm 4611-JCP, Iowa City, IA 52242; **Phone:** 319-356-4060; **Board Cert:** Internal Medicine 1991; Gastroenterology 1993; **Med School:** Wayne State Univ 1988; **Resid:** Internal Medicine, Johns Hopkins Hosp 1991; **Fellow:** Gastroenterology, Univ Iowa Hosps 1993; **Fac Appt:** Assoc Prof Med, Univ Iowa Coll Med

Elta, Grace H MD [Ge] - **Spec Exp:** Biliary Disease; Inflammatory Bowel Disease/Crohn's; **Hospital:** Univ Michigan Hlth Sys; **Address:** Univ Michigan Health System, Taubman Center, 1500 E Medical Ctr Drive, rm 3912, Ann Arbor, MI 48109-0362; **Phone:** 888-229-7408; **Board Cert:** Internal Medicine 1980; Gastroenterology 1983; **Med School:** Univ Mich Med Sch 1977; **Resid:** Internal Medicine, New England Med Ctr 1980; **Fellow:** Gastroenterology, New England Med Ctr 1982; **Fac Appt:** Prof Med, Univ Mich Med Sch

Goldberg, Michael J MD [Ge] - **Spec Exp:** Colon Cancer; Inflammatory Bowel Disease; Pancreatic & Biliary Disease; Pancreatic/Biliary Endoscopy (ERCP); **Hospital:** Evanston Hosp, Glenbrook Hosp; **Address:** 2650 Ridge Ave, Ste G-208, Evanston, IL 60201; **Phone:** 847-657-1900; **Board Cert:** Internal Medicine 1978; Gastroenterology 1981; **Med School:** Univ IL Coll Med 1975; **Resid:** Internal Medicine, Univ Illinois Hosp 1978; **Fellow:** Gastroenterology, Tufts-New England Med Ctr 1980; **Fac Appt:** Assoc Clin Prof Med, Northwestern Univ

Gastroenterology

Gostout, Christopher John MD [Ge] - **Spec Exp:** Gastroscopy; Endoscopy; **Hospital:** Mayo Med Ctr & Clin - Rochester; **Address:** Mayo Clinic, Div GI, 200 First St SW, Charleton 8, Rochester, MN 55905; **Phone:** 507-266-6932; **Board Cert:** Internal Medicine 1979; Gastroenterology 1981; **Med School:** SUNY Downstate 1976; **Resid:** Internal Medicine, Mayo Clinic 1979; **Fellow:** Gastroenterology, Mayo Clinic 1981

Hanauer, Stephen MD [Ge] - **Spec Exp:** Inflammatory Bowel Disease/Crohn's; Crohn's Disease; Ulcerative Colitis; Clinical Trials; **Hospital:** Univ of Chicago Hosps; **Address:** Univ Chicago Hosps, 5841 S Maryland Ave, MC 4076, Chicago, IL 60637-1426; **Phone:** 773-702-1466; **Board Cert:** Internal Medicine 1980; Gastroenterology 1983; **Med School:** Univ IL Coll Med 1977; **Resid:** Internal Medicine, Univ Chicago Hosps 1980; **Fellow:** Gastroenterology, Univ Chicago Hosps 1982; **Fac Appt:** Prof Med, Univ Chicago-Pritzker Sch Med

Jensen, Donald M MD [Ge] - **Spec Exp:** Transplant Medicine-Liver; Hepatitis C; Liver & Biliary Disease; Liver Cancer; **Hospital:** Univ of Chicago Hosps; **Address:** Univ of Chicago, Ctr for Liver Disease, 5841 S Maryland Ave, MC 7120, Chicago, IL 60637; **Phone:** 773-702-2300; **Board Cert:** Internal Medicine 1975; Gastroenterology 1981; **Med School:** Univ IL Coll Med 1972; **Resid:** Internal Medicine, Rush Presby St Lukes Hosp 1975; Gastroenterology, Rush Presby St Lukes Hosp 1976; **Fellow:** Gastroenterology, King's College Hosp 1978; **Fac Appt:** Prof Med, Univ Chicago-Pritzker Sch Med

Kahrilas, Peter J MD [Ge] - **Spec Exp:** Esophageal Disorders; Swallowing Disorders; **Hospital:** Northwestern Meml Hosp; **Address:** 675 N St Clair, Fl 17 - Ste 250, Chicago, IL 60611; **Phone:** 312-695-0606; **Board Cert:** Internal Medicine 1982; Gastroenterology 1987; **Med School:** Univ Rochester 1979; **Resid:** Internal Medicine, Univ Hosp 1982; **Fellow:** Gastroenterology, Northwestern Univ 1984; Research, Med Coll Wisconsin 1986; **Fac Appt:** Prof Med, Northwestern Univ

Konicek, Frank MD [Ge] - **Spec Exp:** Endoscopy; Inflammatory Bowel Disease/Crohn's; Pancreatic Disease; Liver Disease; **Hospital:** Swedish Covenant Hosp, Sherman Hosp; **Address:** 3004 N Ashland Ave, Chicago, IL 60657-3012; **Phone:** 773-871-4600; **Board Cert:** Internal Medicine 1977; Gastroenterology 1975; **Med School:** Loyola Univ-Stritch Sch Med 1963; **Resid:** Internal Medicine, St Francis Hosp 1965; Internal Medicine, Hines VA Hosp 1969; **Fellow:** Gastroenterology, Hines VA Hosp 1971; **Fac Appt:** Clin Prof Med, Loyola Univ-Stritch Sch Med

Kwo, Paul Y MD [Ge] - **Spec Exp:** Hepatitis B & C; Transplant Medicine-Liver; **Hospital:** Indiana Univ Hosp; **Address:** 975 W Walnut St, IB327, Indianapolis, IN 46202-5181; **Phone:** 317-274-3090; **Board Cert:** Gastroenterology 2005; Transplant Hepatology 2006; **Med School:** Wayne State Univ 1988; **Resid:** Internal Medicine, Univ Maryland Med Ctr 1991; **Fellow:** Gastroenterology, Mayo Clinic 1995; **Fac Appt:** Clin Prof Med, Indiana Univ

La Russo, Nicholas F MD [Ge] - **Spec Exp:** Transplant Medicine-Liver; Liver & Biliary Disease; **Hospital:** Mayo Med Ctr & Clin - Rochester; **Address:** Mayo Clinic, Div Gastroenterology, 200 First St SW, Rochester, MN 55905-0001; **Phone:** 507-284-8700; **Board Cert:** Internal Medicine 1972; Gastroenterology 1979; **Med School:** NY Med Coll 1969; **Resid:** Internal Medicine, Mayo Clinic 1972; **Fellow:** Gastroenterology, Mayo Clinic 1975; **Fac Appt:** Prof Med, Mayo Med Sch

Lashner, Bret A MD [Ge] - **Spec Exp:** Inflammatory Bowel Disease; **Hospital:** Cleveland Clin Fdn (page 57); **Address:** 9500 Euclid Ave, Desk A30, Cleveland, OH 44195; **Phone:** 216-444-6523; **Board Cert:** Internal Medicine 1983; Gastroenterology 1985; **Med School:** NYU Sch Med 1980; **Resid:** Internal Medicine, Temple Univ Hosp 1983; **Fellow:** Gastroenterology, Univ Chicago Hosps 1986; **Fac Appt:** Assoc Prof Med, Case West Res Univ

Levitan, Ruven MD [Ge] - **Spec Exp:** Malabsorption Syndrome; Inflammatory Bowel Disease; Esophageal Disorders; **Hospital:** Adv Luth Genl Hosp, Rush N Shore Med Ctr; **Address:** 4711 Golf Rd, Ste 500, Skokie, IL 60076; **Phone:** 847-677-1170; **Board Cert:** Internal Medicine 1980; Gastroenterology 1968; **Med School:** Israel 1953; **Resid:** Internal Medicine, Mount Sinai Med Ctr 1957; Gastroenterology, Beth Israel Hosp 1959; **Fellow:** Internal Medicine, Mem Sloan Kettering Cancer Ctr 1958; Gastroenterology, Mass General Hosp 1963; **Fac Appt:** Clin Prof Med, Univ IL Coll Med

Lindor, Keith Douglas MD [Ge] - **Spec Exp:** Liver Disease; Biliary Disease; **Hospital:** Mayo Med Ctr & Clin - Rochester; **Address:** Mayo Clinic, Div GI, 200 First St SW, Rochester, MN 55905; **Phone:** 507-284-4823; **Board Cert:** Internal Medicine 1983; Gastroenterology 1987; **Med School:** Mayo Med Sch 1979; **Resid:** Internal Medicine, N Carolina Baptist Hosp 1982; **Fellow:** Gastroenterology, Mayo Clinic 1986; **Fac Appt:** Prof Med, Mayo Med Sch

Lucey, Michael R MD [Ge] - **Spec Exp:** Liver Disease; Transplant Medicine-Liver; **Hospital:** Univ WI Hosp & Clins; **Address:** Univ Wisc Hosps & Clins, 600 Highland Ave, H6-516 CSC, Madison, WI 53792; **Phone:** 608-263-7322; **Board Cert:** Internal Medicine 2001; Gastroenterology 2001; **Med School:** Ireland 1980; **Resid:** Internal Medicine, Fed Dublin Vol Hosps 1979; Gastroenterology, St Bartholomews Hosp/Kings Coll Hosp 1985; **Fellow:** Gastroenterology, Univ Michigan Med Ctr 1987; **Fac Appt:** Prof Med, Univ Wisc

Luxon, Bruce MD/PhD [Ge] - **Spec Exp:** Liver Disease; Hepatitis C; Autoimmune Liver Disease; **Hospital:** Univ Iowa Hosp & Clinics; **Address:** 4607 JCP UIHC, 200 Hawkins Drive, Iowa City, IA 52242; **Phone:** 319-356-4060; **Board Cert:** Internal Medicine 1989; Gastroenterology 2001; **Med School:** Univ MO-Columbia Sch Med 1985; **Resid:** Internal Medicine, Univ MO-Columbia Sch Med 1989; **Fellow:** Gastroenterology, UCSF Med Ctr 1992; **Fac Appt:** Prof Med, St Louis Univ

Meiselman, Mick Scott MD [Ge] - **Spec Exp:** Colonoscopy; Pancreatic & Biliary Disease; Gastroesophageal Reflux Disease (GERD); **Hospital:** Evanston Hosp, Glenbrook Hosp; **Address:** 506 Green Bay Rd, Kenilworth, IL 60043-1002; **Phone:** 847-256-3495; **Board Cert:** Internal Medicine 1982; Gastroenterology 1985; **Med School:** Northwestern Univ 1979; **Resid:** Internal Medicine, Cedars-Sinai/UCLA 1982; **Fellow:** Gastroenterology, UCSF Med Ctr 1984; **Fac Appt:** Assoc Clin Prof Med, Northwestern Univ

Murray, Joseph A MD [Ge] - **Spec Exp:** Celiac Disease; Esophageal Disorders; **Hospital:** Mayo Med Ctr & Clin - Rochester; **Address:** Mayo Clinic, Div Gastroenterology, 200 1st St SW, Rochester, MN 55905; **Phone:** 507-284-2631; **Board Cert:** Internal Medicine 1999; Gastroenterology 2000; **Med School:** Ireland 1983; **Resid:** Internal Medicine, St Laurences Hosp 1986; Gastroenterology, Beaumont Hosp 1988; **Fellow:** Gastroenterology, Univ Iowa Hosps & Clins 1990; **Fac Appt:** Prof Med, Mayo Med Sch

Gastroenterology

Owyang, Chung MD [Ge] - **Spec Exp:** Gastrointestinal Motility Disorders; Digestive Disorders; **Hospital:** Univ Michigan Hlth Sys; **Address:** Univ Mich, Div Gastroenterology, 1500 E Med Ctr Dr, Rm 3912 Taubman Ctr, Ann Arbor, MI 48109-0362; **Phone:** 734-936-4785; **Board Cert:** Internal Medicine 1976; Gastroenterology 1981; **Med School:** McGill Univ 1972; **Resid:** Internal Medicine, Montreal Genl Hosp 1975; **Fellow:** Gastroenterology, Mayo Grad Sch 1978; **Fac Appt:** Prof Med, Univ Mich Med Sch

Rao, Satish S C MD [Ge] - **Spec Exp:** Constipation; Incontinence-Fecal; Chest Pain-Non Cardiac; **Hospital:** Univ Iowa Hosp & Clinics; **Address:** Univ Iowa Coll Med, Div Gastroenterology, 4612 JCP, 200 Hawkins Drive, Iowa City, IA 52242; **Phone:** 319-353-6602; **Board Cert:** Internal Medicine 1996; Gastroenterology 1998; **Med School:** India 1978; **Resid:** Internal Medicine, Sunderland Hosps 1982; Internal Medicine, York Dist Hosp 1984; **Fellow:** Royal Hallamshire Hosp 1986; Gastroenterology, Royal Liverpool Hosp 1988; **Fac Appt:** Prof Med, Univ Iowa Coll Med

Reichelderfer, Mark MD [Ge] - **Spec Exp:** Endoscopy; Inflammatory Bowel Disease; **Hospital:** Univ WI Hosp & Clins; **Address:** 600 Highland Ave, H6/516, Madison, WI 53792-5124; **Phone:** 608-263-8094; **Board Cert:** Internal Medicine 1977; Gastroenterology 1979; **Med School:** Columbia P&S 1974; **Resid:** Internal Medicine, Mary Imogene Bassett Hosp 1977; **Fellow:** Gastroenterology, Univ Wisc Hosps & Clin 1979; **Fac Appt:** Prof Med, Univ Wisc

Rex, Douglas K MD [Ge] - **Spec Exp:** Endoscopy; Endoscopic Ultrasound; **Hospital:** Indiana Univ Hosp; **Address:** 550 N University Blvd, Ste 4100, Indianapolis, IN 46202; **Phone:** 317-278-9763; **Board Cert:** Internal Medicine 1985; Gastroenterology 1987; **Med School:** Indiana Univ 1980; **Resid:** Internal Medicine, Indiana Univ Med Ctr 1982; Internal Medicine, Indiana Univ Hosp 1985; **Fellow:** Gastroenterology, Indiana Univ Med Ctr 1984; **Fac Appt:** Prof Med, Indiana Univ

Sandborn, William J MD [Ge] - **Spec Exp:** Inflammatory Bowel Disease/Crohn's; Ulcerative Colitis; Crohn's Disease; **Hospital:** Mayo Med Ctr & Clin - Rochester; **Address:** Mayo Clinic, Div GI, 200 First St SW, Rochester, MN 55905; **Phone:** 507-284-0959; **Board Cert:** Internal Medicine 1990; Gastroenterology 2003; **Med School:** Loma Linda Univ 1987; **Resid:** Internal Medicine, Loma Linda Univ 1990; **Fellow:** Gastroenterology, Mayo Clinic 1993; **Fac Appt:** Assoc Prof Med, Mayo Med Sch

Schmidt, Warren N MD [Ge] - **Spec Exp:** Liver Disease; **Hospital:** Univ Iowa Hosp & Clinics; **Address:** UIHC, Dept Gastroenterology, 200 Hawkins Drive, rm 4553-JCP, Iowa City, IA 52242; **Phone:** 319-356-4060; **Board Cert:** Internal Medicine 1993; Gastroenterology 1997; **Med School:** Univ Tenn Coll Med, Memphis 1989; **Resid:** Internal Medicine, Univ Tenn Ctr Hlth Sci 1992; **Fellow:** Gastroenterology, Univ Iowa Hosp & Clin 1992; **Fac Appt:** Assoc Prof Med, Univ Iowa Coll Med

Schulze, Konrad S MD [Ge] - **Spec Exp:** Gastroesophageal Reflux Disease (GERD); Peptic Acid Disorders; Gastroparesis; **Hospital:** Univ Iowa Hosp & Clinics; **Address:** UIHC, Digestive Disease Clinic, 200 Hawkins Drive, rm 4551-JCP, Iowa City, IA 52242; **Phone:** 319-356-4060; **Board Cert:** Internal Medicine 1987; Gastroenterology 1975; **Med School:** Germany 1968; **Resid:** Psychiatry, Boston City Hosp 1971; Internal Medicine, Montreal Genl Hosp 1974; **Fellow:** Gastroenterology, Univ Iowa 1977; **Fac Appt:** Prof Med, Univ Iowa Coll Med

Seidner, Douglas MD [Ge] - **Spec Exp:** Nutrition; Inflammatory Bowel Disease; Endoscopy; **Hospital:** Cleveland Clin Fdn (page 57); **Address:** Cleveland Clinic, Gastroenterology & Hepatology, 9500 Euclid Ave, Desk A30, Cleveland, OH 44195; **Phone:** 216-444-6510; **Board Cert:** Internal Medicine 1986; Gastroenterology 2000; **Med School:** SUNY Upstate Med Univ 1983; **Resid:** Internal Medicine, Beth Israel Deaconess Med Ctr 1986; **Fellow:** Nutrition & Metabolism, Beth Israel Deaconess Med Ctr 1987; Gastroenterology, George Washington Univ Med Ctr 1989

Semrad, Carol E MD [Ge] - **Spec Exp:** Celiac Disease; Diarrheal Diseases; Malabsorption Syndrome; Nutrition; **Hospital:** Univ of Chicago Hosps; **Address:** 5841 S Maryland Ave, MC 4080.S401, Chicago, IL 60637; **Phone:** 773-702-6921; **Board Cert:** Internal Medicine 1985; Gastroenterology 1987; **Med School:** Columbia P&S 1982; **Resid:** Internal Medicine, Columbia-Presby Med Ctr 1985; **Fellow:** Gastroenterology, Columbia-Presby Med Ctr 1986; **Fac Appt:** Assoc Prof Med, Univ Chicago-Pritzker Sch Med

Shaker, Reza MD [Ge] - **Spec Exp:** Swallowing Disorders; Gastrointestinal Motility Disorders; Gastroesophageal Reflux Disease (GERD); Pancreatic/Biliary Endoscopy (ERCP); **Hospital:** Froedtert Meml Lutheran Hosp; **Address:** Froedtert Memorial Lutheran Hosp, 9200 W Wisconsin Ave, rm E4510, Milwaukee, WI 53226; **Phone:** 414-456-6840; **Med School:** Iran 1975; **Resid:** Internal Medicine, Kingsbrook Jewish Med Ctr 1985; **Fellow:** Gastroenterology, Med Coll Wisconsin 1988; **Fac Appt:** Prof Med, Univ Wisc

Sherman, Stuart MD [Ge] - **Spec Exp:** Pancreatic & Biliary Disease; Endoscopy; Pancreatic/Biliary Endoscopy (ERCP); **Hospital:** Indiana Univ Hosp; **Address:** Indiana Univ Medical Ctr, 550 N University Blvd, Ste 4100, Indianapolis, IN 46202; **Phone:** 317-274-0925; **Board Cert:** Internal Medicine 1985; Gastroenterology 1989; **Med School:** Washington Univ, St Louis 1982; **Resid:** Internal Medicine, Presby Univ Hosp 1985; **Fellow:** Gastroenterology, UCLA Med Ctr 1989; **Fac Appt:** Clin Prof Med, Indiana Univ

Silverman, William B MD [Ge] - **Spec Exp:** Pancreatic/Biliary Endoscopy (ERCP); **Hospital:** Univ Iowa Hosp & Clinics; **Address:** UIHC, Div GI/Hepatology, 200 Hawkins Drive, rm 4553-JCP, Iowa City, IA 52242; **Phone:** 319-356-4060; **Board Cert:** Internal Medicine 1988; Gastroenterology 1997; **Med School:** Belgium 1984; **Resid:** Internal Medicine, Lutheran General Hosp 1987; **Fellow:** Gastroenterology, Case Western Res Univ 1989; Gastroenterology, Indiana Univ Hosp 1990; **Fac Appt:** Prof Med, Univ Iowa Coll Med

Tremaine, William J MD [Ge] - **Spec Exp:** Inflammatory Bowel Disease/Crohn's; Ulcerative Colitis; Irritable Bowel Syndrome; **Hospital:** Mayo Med Ctr & Clin - Rochester, St Mary's Hosp - Rochester; **Address:** Mayo Clinic, Div GI, 200 First St SW, Rochester, MN 55905-0002; **Phone:** 507-284-2468; **Board Cert:** Internal Medicine 1979; Gastroenterology 1981; **Med School:** Univ Miss 1976; **Resid:** Internal Medicine, Mayo Clinic 1980; **Fellow:** Gastroenterology, Mayo Clinic 1981; **Fac Appt:** Prof Med, Mayo Med Sch

Van Thiel, David MD [Ge] - **Spec Exp:** Transplant Medicine-Liver; Hepatitis; Liver Disease; **Hospital:** Rush Univ Med Ctr; **Address:** Rush Univ Hepatologists, 1725 W Harrison Rd, Ste 158, Chicago, IL 60612; **Phone:** 312-942-8910; **Board Cert:** Internal Medicine 1972; Gastroenterology 1975; **Med School:** UCLA 1967; **Resid:** Internal Medicine, NY Hosp 1969; Internal Medicine, Univ Hosp 1972; **Fellow:** Gastroenterology, Univ Hosp 1974; Research, NIH 1976; **Fac Appt:** Prof Med, Loyola Univ-Stritch Sch Med

Gastroenterology

Vege, Santhi S MD [Ge] - **Spec Exp:** Pancreatic Disease; **Hospital:** Mayo Med Ctr & Clin - Rochester; **Address:** Mayo Clinic, 200 First St SW Gonda Bldg Fl 9, Rochester, MN 55905; **Phone:** 507-284-2478; **Board Cert:** Internal Medicine 1997; **Med School:** India 1975; **Resid:** Internal Medicine, Govt Genl Hosp 1978; Internal Medicine, Mayo Clinic 1997; **Fellow:** Gastroenterology, Post Grad Inst 1981; Gastroenterology, Mayo Clinic 1998; **Fac Appt:** Prof Med, Mayo Med Sch

Wald, Arnold MD [Ge] - **Spec Exp:** Constipation; Gastrointestinal Motility Disorders; Irritable Bowel Syndrome; **Hospital:** Univ WI Hosp & Clins; **Address:** Univ Wisconsin Hosp & Clinics, 600 Highland Ave, H6/516 CSC, Madison, WI 57392-2451; **Phone:** 608-263-8094; **Board Cert:** Internal Medicine 1972; Gastroenterology 1975; **Med School:** SUNY Downstate 1968; **Resid:** Internal Medicine, SUNY - Downstate Med Ctr 1971; **Fellow:** Gastroenterology, Johns Hopkins Hosp 1975; **Fac Appt:** Prof Med, Univ Wisc

Waxman, Irving MD [Ge] - **Spec Exp:** Gastrointestinal Cancer; Pancreatic Cancer; Endoscopy; **Hospital:** Univ of Chicago Hosps; **Address:** University of Chicago Hospitals, 5758 S Maryland Ave, MC 9028, Chicago, IL 60637; **Phone:** 773-702-1459; **Board Cert:** Internal Medicine 1988; Gastroenterology 2003; **Med School:** Mexico 1986; **Resid:** Internal Medicine, New England Deaconess Hosp 1988; **Fellow:** Gastroenterology, Georgetown Univ Med Ctr 1991; Endoscopy, Academic Med Ctr-Univ Amsterdam 1991; **Fac Appt:** Prof Med, Univ Chicago-Pritzker Sch Med

Wiesner, Russell MD [Ge] - **Spec Exp:** Transplant Medicine-Liver; **Hospital:** Mayo Med Ctr & Clin - Rochester; **Address:** Mayo Clinic, Div GI, 200 First St SW, Rochester, MN 55905; **Phone:** 507-284-8714; **Board Cert:** Internal Medicine 1978; Gastroenterology 1981; **Med School:** Med Coll Wisc 1975; **Resid:** Internal Medicine, Mayo Clinic 1978

Winans, Charles S MD [Ge] - **Spec Exp:** Esophageal Disorders; Gastroesophageal Reflux Disease (GERD); Swallowing Disorders; **Hospital:** Univ of Chicago Hosps; **Address:** 5758 S Maryland Ave, MC 9028, Chicago, IL 60637-1426; **Phone:** 773-834-4180; **Board Cert:** Internal Medicine 1968; Gastroenterology 1970; **Med School:** Case West Res Univ 1961; **Resid:** Internal Medicine, Univ Hosp 1964; **Fellow:** Gastroenterology, Boston Univ Med Ctr 1966; **Fac Appt:** Prof Med, Univ Chicago-Pritzker Sch Med

Great Plains and Mountains

Bjorkman, David MD [Ge] - **Spec Exp:** Peptic Acid Disorders; Endoscopy; **Hospital:** Univ Utah Hosps and Clins; **Address:** 30 N Medical Drive, 1900 E, Salt Lake City, UT 84132; **Phone:** 801-581-6436; **Board Cert:** Internal Medicine 1983; Gastroenterology 1985; **Med School:** Univ Utah 1980; **Resid:** Internal Medicine, Brigham & Women's Harvard 1983; **Fellow:** Gastroenterology, Brigham & Women's Harvard 1985; **Fac Appt:** Prof Med, Univ Utah

Burt, Randall W MD [Ge] - **Spec Exp:** Colon Cancer; Colon & Rectal Cancer-Familial Polyposis; **Hospital:** Univ Utah Hosps and Clins; **Address:** Huntsman Cancer Institute, 2000 Circle of Hope, Salt Lake City, UT 84112; **Phone:** 801-585-3281; **Board Cert:** Internal Medicine 1977; Gastroenterology 1979; **Med School:** Univ Utah 1974; **Resid:** Internal Medicine, Barnes Hosp 1977; **Fellow:** Gastroenterology, Univ Utah Med Ctr 1979; **Fac Appt:** Prof Med, Univ Utah

Everson, Gregory T MD [Ge] - **Spec Exp:** Liver Disease; Hepatitis; Transplant Medicine-Liver; **Hospital:** Univ Colorado Hosp; **Address:** Univ Colorado Hlth Sci Ctr, Div Hepatology, 4200 E 9th Ave, Box B154, Denver, CO 80262; **Phone:** 303-372-8866; **Board Cert:** Internal Medicine 1979; Gastroenterology 1983; **Med School:** Cornell Univ-Weill Med Coll 1976; **Resid:** Internal Medicine, Creighton Univ Med Ctr 1979; **Fellow:** Gastroenterology, Univ Colorado Health Sci Ctr 1982; **Fac Appt:** Prof Med, Univ Colorado

Fang, John C MD [Ge] - **Spec Exp:** Endoscopy; Esophageal Disorders; Irritable Bowel Syndrome; Barrett's Esophagus; **Hospital:** Univ Utah Hosps and Clins; **Address:** 1525 W 2100 S, Salt Lake City, UT 84119; **Phone:** 801-213-9900; **Board Cert:** Gastroenterology 1998; **Med School:** Washington Univ, St Louis 1989; **Resid:** Internal Medicine, Temple Univ Hosp 1992; **Fellow:** Gastroenterology, Univ VA Hlth Sci Ctr 1995; **Fac Appt:** Assoc Prof Med, Univ Utah

Hunter, Ellen B MD [Ge] - **Spec Exp:** Hepatitis; **Hospital:** St. Luke's Reg Med Ctr - Boise; **Address:** 425 W Vannock, Boise, ID 83702; **Phone:** 208-343-6458; **Board Cert:** Internal Medicine 1986; Gastroenterology 1989; **Med School:** Georgetown Univ 1983; **Resid:** Internal Medicine, Vanderbilt Univ Med Ctr 1986; **Fellow:** Gastroenterology, Mayo Clinic 1989

O'Brien, John J MD [Ge] - **Spec Exp:** Esophageal Disorders; Liver Disease; **Hospital:** Creighton Univ Med Ctr; **Address:** Creighton Univ Med Ctr, Div Gastroenterology, 601 N 30th St, Ste 5730, Omaha, NE 68131; **Phone:** 402-449-4692; **Board Cert:** Internal Medicine 1988; Gastroenterology 1993; **Med School:** Univ MO-Columbia Sch Med 1981; **Resid:** Internal Medicine, St Lukes Hosp 1984; Gastroenterology, Univ KY Med Ctr 1986; **Fellow:** Gastroenterology, Johns Hopkins Hosp 1989; **Fac Appt:** Prof Med, Creighton Univ

Sorrell, Michael MD [Ge] - **Spec Exp:** Transplant Medicine-Liver; Hepatitis; Liver Tumors; **Hospital:** Nebraska Med Ctr; **Address:** 983285 Nebraska Medical Ctr, Omaha, NE 68198-3285; **Phone:** 402-559-7912; **Board Cert:** Internal Medicine 1972; **Med School:** Univ Nebr Coll Med 1959; **Resid:** Internal Medicine, Univ Nebraska Hosp 1968; Gastroenterology, Univ Nebraska Hosp 1969; **Fellow:** Hepatology, New Jersey Coll Med 1971; **Fac Appt:** Prof Med, Univ Nebr Coll Med

Southwest

Anderson, Karl MD [Ge] - **Spec Exp:** Porphyria; Liver Disease; **Hospital:** UT Med Br Hosp at Galveston; **Address:** Univ Tex Med Ctr-Ewing Hall 3.102, 700 Harborside Dr, Galveston, TX 77555-1109; **Phone:** 409-747-7500; **Board Cert:** Internal Medicine 1972; Gastroenterology 1972; **Med School:** Johns Hopkins Univ 1965; **Resid:** Internal Medicine, Vanderbilt Univ Hosp 1967; Internal Medicine, New York Hosp-Cornell Med Ctr 1968; **Fellow:** Gastroenterology, New York Hosp-Cornell Med Ctr 1970; **Fac Appt:** Prof Med, Univ Tex Med Br, Galveston

Balart, Luis A MD [Ge] - **Spec Exp:** Hepatitis C; **Hospital:** Ochsner Baptist Med Ctr, L Boggs Med Ctr; **Address:** 2820 Napoleon Ave, Ste 700, New Orleans, LA 70115; **Phone:** 504-899-8411; **Board Cert:** Internal Medicine 1976; Gastroenterology 1981; **Med School:** Cuba 1972; **Resid:** Internal Medicine, Naval Regl Med Ctr; **Fac Appt:** Assoc Clin Prof Med, Louisiana State Univ

Gastroenterology

Boyer, Thomas D MD [Ge] - **Spec Exp:** Liver Disease; Hepatitis; **Hospital:** Univ Med Ctr - Tucson; **Address:** Liver Research Inst, 1501 N Campbell Ave, Box 245136, Tucson, AZ 85724; **Phone:** 520-626-5952; **Board Cert:** Internal Medicine 1975; Gastroenterology 1977; **Med School:** USC Sch Med 1969; **Resid:** Internal Medicine, LAC-USC Med Ctr 1974; **Fellow:** Hepatology, John Wesley Co Hosp-USC Med Ctr 1976; **Fac Appt:** Prof Med, Univ Ariz Coll Med

Brady III, Charles E MD [Ge] - **Spec Exp:** Esophageal Disorders; **Hospital:** Univ Hlth Sys - Univ Hosp; **Address:** Univ Tex Hlth Sci Ctr, Div GI, 7703 Floyd Curl Drive, MC 7878, San Antonio, TX 78229-3900; **Phone:** 210-567-4879; **Board Cert:** Internal Medicine 1974; Gastroenterology 1977; **Med School:** Med Coll VA 1971; **Resid:** Internal Medicine, Wilford Hall Med Ctr 1974; **Fellow:** Gastroenterology, Univ Tex 1976; **Fac Appt:** Assoc Prof Med, Univ Tex, San Antonio

Bresalier, Robert MD [Ge] - **Spec Exp:** Gastrointestinal Cancer; Peptic Acid Disorders; **Hospital:** UT MD Anderson Cancer Ctr (page 71); **Address:** MD Anderson Canc Ctr, GI Med & Nutrition, 1515 Holcombe Blvd - Unit 436, Houston, TX 77030-4009; **Phone:** 713-745-4340; **Board Cert:** Internal Medicine 1981; Gastroenterology 1983; **Med School:** Univ Chicago-Pritzker Sch Med 1978; **Resid:** Internal Medicine, Barnes Hosp-Washington Univ 1981; **Fellow:** Gastroenterology, UCSF Med Ctr 1983; **Fac Appt:** Prof Med, Univ Tex, Houston

Cunningham, John MD [Ge] - **Spec Exp:** Biliary Disease; Pancreatic Disease; **Hospital:** Univ Med Ctr - Tucson; **Address:** Univ Arizona, Div Gastroenterology, 1501 N Campbell Ave, PO Box 245028, Tuscon, AZ 85724-5028; **Phone:** 520-626-6119; **Board Cert:** Internal Medicine 1975; Gastroenterology 1977; **Med School:** Med Coll VA 1970; **Resid:** Internal Medicine, Med Univ South Carolina 1975; **Fellow:** Gastroenterology, Med Univ South Carolina 1977; **Fac Appt:** Prof Med, Univ Ariz Coll Med

Das, Ananya MD [Ge] - **Spec Exp:** Endoscopy; Endoscopic Ultrasound; Pancreatic/Biliary Endoscopy (ERCP); **Hospital:** Mayo Clin Hosp - Scottsdale; **Address:** Mayo Clinic, Div Gastroenterology, 13400 E Shea Blvd, Scottsdale, AZ 85259; **Phone:** 480-301-6990; **Board Cert:** Internal Medicine 1996; Gastroenterology 1998; **Med School:** India 1987; **Resid:** Internal Medicine, SUNY Hlth Sci Ctr 1996; **Fellow:** Gastroenterology, Cleveland Clinic 1998; Endoscopy, Cleveland Clinic 2000; **Fac Appt:** Assoc Prof Med, Mayo Med Sch

Davis, Gary L MD [Ge] - **Spec Exp:** Liver Disease; Hepatitis; Transplant Medicine-Liver; **Hospital:** Baylor Univ Medical Ctr; **Address:** 3500 Gaston Ave, 4 Roberts, Transplant Services Department, Dallas, TX 75246; **Phone:** 214-820-8500; **Board Cert:** Internal Medicine 1979; Gastroenterology 1983; **Med School:** Univ Minn 1976; **Resid:** Internal Medicine, Mayo Clinic 1979; **Fellow:** Gastroenterology, Mayo Clinic 1981; Hepatology, Natl Inst Hlth 1984; **Fac Appt:** Prof Med, Baylor Coll Med

Feldman, Mark MD [Ge] - **Spec Exp:** Peptic Acid Disorders; **Hospital:** Presby Hosp of Dallas; **Address:** 8200 Walnut Hill Ln, Dept Internal Med, Dallas, TX 75231; **Phone:** 214-345-7881; **Board Cert:** Internal Medicine 1976; Gastroenterology 1989; **Med School:** Temple Univ 1972; **Resid:** Internal Medicine, Temple Univ 1977; **Fellow:** Gastroenterology, Univ SW Texas 1976; **Fac Appt:** Prof Med, Univ Tex SW, Dallas

Fitz, J Gregory MD [Ge] - **Spec Exp:** Liver Disease; Hepatitis; Transplant Medicine-Liver; Digestive Disorders; **Hospital:** UT Southwestern Med Ctr - Dallas; **Address:** Univ Texas SW Medical School, 5323 Harry Hines Blvd, Dallas, TX 75390-9030; **Phone:** 214-648-3486; **Board Cert:** Internal Medicine 1982; Gastroenterology 1985; **Med School:** Duke Univ 1979; **Resid:** Internal Medicine, UCSF Med Ctr 1982; **Fellow:** Gastroenterology, UCSF Med Ctr 1985; **Fac Appt:** Prof Med, Univ Tex SW, Dallas

Fleischer, David MD [Ge] - **Spec Exp:** Barrett's Esophagus; Esophageal Cancer; **Hospital:** Mayo Clin Hosp - Scottsdale; **Address:** Mayo Clinic - Scottsdale, 13400 E Shea Blvd, Div Gastroenterology 2A, Scottsdale, AZ 85259; **Phone:** 480-301-8484; **Board Cert:** Internal Medicine 1975; Gastroenterology 1977; **Med School:** Vanderbilt Univ 1970; **Resid:** Internal Medicine, Metro General Hosp 1975; **Fellow:** Gastroenterology, LA Co Harbor-UCLA Med Ctr 1977; **Fac Appt:** Prof Med, Mayo Med Sch

Fordtran, John MD [Ge] - **Spec Exp:** Malabsorption Syndrome; Diarrheal Diseases; **Hospital:** Baylor Univ Medical Ctr; **Address:** Baylor Univ Med Ctr, Dept Med, 3500 Gaston Ave, Jonsson 500.0, Dallas, TX 75246; **Phone:** 214-820-2672; **Med School:** Tulane Univ 1956; **Resid:** Internal Medicine, Parkland Hosp 1958; **Fellow:** Gastroenterology, Mass Meml Hosp 1962

Galati, Joseph Steven MD [Ge] - **Spec Exp:** Liver Disease; Transplant Medicine-Liver; Hepatitis C; **Hospital:** St Luke's Episcopal Hosp - Houston, Meml Hermann Hosp - Houston; **Address:** 6624 Fannin St, Ste 1990, Houston, TX 77030; **Phone:** 713-794-0700; **Board Cert:** Gastroenterology 2005; **Med School:** Grenada 1987; **Resid:** Internal Medicine, SUNY Hlth Sci Ctr-Kings Co Hosp 1991; **Fellow:** Gastroenterology, Univ Nebraska 1994; **Fac Appt:** Asst Prof Med, Univ Tex, Houston

Glombicki, Alan Paul MD [Ge] - **Spec Exp:** Hepatitis; Transplant Medicine-Liver; Digestive Disorders; **Hospital:** St Luke's Episcopal Hosp - Houston, Meml Hermann Hosp - Houston; **Address:** 7737 SW Freeway, Ste 840, Houston, TX 77074; **Phone:** 713-777-2555; **Board Cert:** Internal Medicine 1986; Gastroenterology 1987; **Med School:** Univ IL Coll Med 1981; **Resid:** Internal Medicine, Baylor Coll Med 1984; Hepatology, Baylor Coll Med 1987; **Fellow:** Gastroenterology, Baylor Coll Med 1986; **Fac Appt:** Asst Clin Prof Med, Univ Tex, Houston

Hodges, David S MD [Ge] - **Spec Exp:** Inflammatory Bowel Disease/Crohn's; Irritable Bowel Syndrome; Gastrointestinal Functional Disorders; **Hospital:** Univ Med Ctr - Lubbock; **Address:** Tex Tech Med Ctr, Dept Int Med, 3601 4th St, MC 9410, Lubbock, TX 79430; **Phone:** 806-743-3155; **Board Cert:** Internal Medicine 1986; Gastroenterology 1989; **Med School:** Texas Tech Univ 1983; **Resid:** Internal Medicine, Lubbock Genl Hosp 1986; **Fellow:** Gastroenterology, Lubbock Genl Hosp 1989; **Fac Appt:** Assoc Prof Med, Texas Tech Univ

Levin, Bernard MD [Ge] - **Spec Exp:** Gastrointestinal Cancer; Colon & Rectal Cancer; Cancer Prevention; **Hospital:** UT MD Anderson Cancer Ctr (page 71); **Address:** Univ Tex MD Anderson Cancer Ctr, 1515 Holcombe Blvd Unit #1370, Houston, TX 77030-4095; **Phone:** 713-792-3900; **Board Cert:** Internal Medicine 1972; Gastroenterology 1972; **Med School:** South Africa 1964; **Resid:** Internal Medicine, Rush Presby-St Lukes Hosp 1968; **Fellow:** Pathology, Univ Chicago 1970; Gastroenterology, Univ Chicago 1972

Maddrey, Willis C MD [Ge] - **Spec Exp:** Hepatitis B & C; Liver Disease-Drug Induced; Liver Disease-Alcohol Related; **Hospital:** UT Southwestern Med Ctr - Dallas; **Address:** Univ Tex SW Med Ctr, 5323 Harry Hines Blvd, MC 8570, Dallas, TX 75390-8570; **Phone:** 214-648-2024; **Board Cert:** Internal Medicine 1971; **Med School:** Johns Hopkins Univ 1964; **Resid:** Internal Medicine, Johns Hopkins Hosp 1970; Internal Medicine, Johns Hopkins Hosp 1966; **Fellow:** Hepatology, Yale-New Haven Hosp 1971; **Fac Appt:** Prof Med, Univ Tex SW, Dallas

Gastroenterology

Olden, Kevin W MD [Ge] - **Spec Exp:** Psychiatry in Gastrointestinal Illness; Pain-Abdominal/Functional; Vomiting-Chronic; **Hospital:** UAMS Med Ctr; **Address:** Univ Arkansas, Dept Medicine, 4301 W Markham, Slot 567, Little Rock, AR 72205; **Phone:** 501-686-8000; **Board Cert:** Internal Medicine 1982; Gastroenterology 1989; Psychiatry 1989; Addiction Psychiatry 2002; **Med School:** SUNY Downstate 1976; **Resid:** Internal Medicine, UCLA Med Ctr 1979; Psychiatry, Mass Genl Hosp 1981; **Fellow:** Addiction Psychiatry, Stanford Univ Med Ctr 1983; Endoscopy, VA Med Ctr 1989; **Fac Appt:** Prof Med, Univ Ark

Pasricha, Pankaj MD [Ge] - **Spec Exp:** Swallowing Disorders-Botox Therapy; Gastrointestinal Motility Disorders; Pancreatic Disease; **Hospital:** UT Med Br Hosp at Galveston; **Address:** Univ Texas Medical Branch, 301 University Blvd, 4.106 McCullough Bldg, Galveston, TX 77555-0764; **Phone:** 409-772-5615; **Board Cert:** Internal Medicine 1988; **Med School:** India 1983; **Resid:** Internal Medicine, DC Genl Hosp 1988; **Fellow:** Pulmonary Disease, New England Med Ctr 1990; Gastroenterology, Johns Hopkins Hosp 1992; **Fac Appt:** Prof Med, Univ Tex Med Br, Galveston

Speeg, Kermit V MD/PhD [Ge] - **Spec Exp:** Transplant Medicine-Liver; **Hospital:** Univ Hlth Sys - Univ Hosp; **Address:** Univ Tex Hlth Sci Ctr, Div GI, 7703 Floyd Curl Drive, MC 7878, San Antonio, TX 78229-3900; **Phone:** 210-567-4879; **Board Cert:** Internal Medicine 1976; **Med School:** Univ Tex SW, Dallas 1972; **Resid:** Internal Medicine, Vanderbilt Univ Hosp 1974; **Fellow:** Gastroenterology, Vanderbilt Univ Hosp 1977; **Fac Appt:** Prof Med, Univ Tex, San Antonio

Vierling, John M MD [Ge] - **Spec Exp:** Liver Disease; Transplant Medicine-Liver; Autoimmune Liver Disease; Hepatitis; **Hospital:** Methodist Hosp - Houston, St Luke's Episcopal Hosp - Houston; **Address:** Dept of Med, Baylor College of Med, 1709 Dryden, Ste 500, Houston, TX 77030; **Phone:** 713-798-8070; **Board Cert:** Internal Medicine 1975; Gastroenterology 1979; **Med School:** Stanford Univ 1972; **Resid:** Internal Medicine, Strong Meml Hosp 1974; Hepatology, Natl Inst Hlth 1977; **Fellow:** Gastroenterology, UCSF Med Ctr 1978; **Fac Appt:** Prof Med, Baylor Coll Med

West Coast and Pacific

Cello, John P MD [Ge] - **Spec Exp:** Endoscopy; Colonoscopy; Capsule Endoscopy; Pancreatic/Biliary Endoscopy (ERCP); **Hospital:** San Francisco Genl Hosp, UCSF Med Ctr; **Address:** San Francisco Genl Hosp-Univ California, 1001 Potrero Ave, Ste NH3D, San Francisco, CA 94110; **Phone:** 415-206-4746; **Board Cert:** Internal Medicine 1972; Gastroenterology 1977; **Med School:** Harvard Med Sch 1969; **Resid:** Internal Medicine, Peter Bent Brigham Hosp 1972; **Fellow:** Gastroenterology, UCSF Med Ctr 1977; **Fac Appt:** Prof Med, UCSF

Chang, Kenneth J MD [Ge] - **Spec Exp:** Gastrointestinal Cancer; Endoscopic Ultrasound; **Hospital:** UC Irvine Med Ctr; **Address:** UC Irvine Medical Ctr, 101 The City Drive Bldg 23 - rm 106, Orange, CA 92868; **Phone:** 714-456-8440; **Board Cert:** Internal Medicine 1988; Gastroenterology 2001; **Med School:** Brown Univ 1985; **Resid:** Internal Medicine, Rhode Island Hosp 1988; **Fellow:** Gastroenterology, UC-Irvine Med Ctr 1990

Ellis, Jonathan C MD [Ge] - **Spec Exp:** Colonoscopy; Endoscopy; Inflammatory Bowel Disease; **Hospital:** Cedars-Sinai Med Ctr; **Address:** 9090 Wilshire Blvd, Ste 101, Beverly Hills, CA 90211; **Phone:** 310-550-0400; **Board Cert:** Internal Medicine 1985; Gastroenterology 1989; **Med School:** Stanford Univ 1982; **Resid:** Internal Medicine, Cedars Sinai Med Ctr 1986; **Fellow:** Gastroenterology, UCLA 1988; **Fac Appt:** Assoc Prof Med, UCLA

Fennerty, Brian MD [Ge] - **Spec Exp:** Gastroesophageal Reflux Disease (GERD); **Hospital:** OR Hlth & Sci Univ; **Address:** Digestive Hlth, Ctr for Hlth & Healing, 3303 SW Bond Ave, Portland, OR 97239; **Phone:** 503-494-4373; **Board Cert:** Internal Medicine 1984; Gastroenterology 1989; **Med School:** Creighton Univ 1980; **Resid:** Internal Medicine, Naval Hospital; **Fellow:** Gastroenterology, Arizona Hlth Sci Ctr; **Fac Appt:** Prof Med, Oregon Hlth Sci Univ

Hillebrand, Donald J MD [Ge] - **Spec Exp:** Transplant Medicine-Liver; Liver Failure; **Hospital:** Scripps Green Hosp; **Address:** Scripps Green Hospital, 10666 N Torrey Pines Rd, MC 203N, La Jolla, CA 92037; **Phone:** 858-554-8055; **Board Cert:** Internal Medicine 2004; Gastroenterology 2006; **Med School:** Univ Iowa Coll Med 1990; **Resid:** Internal Medicine, Univ Iowa Hosps 1993; **Fellow:** Gastroenterology, Univ Iowa Hosps 1994

Keeffe, Emmet B MD [Ge] - **Spec Exp:** Hepatitis B & C; Liver Disease; Transplant Medicine-Liver; **Hospital:** Stanford Univ Med Ctr; **Address:** 750 Welch Rd, Ste 210, Palo Alto, CA 94304-1509; **Phone:** 650-498-5691; **Board Cert:** Internal Medicine 1972; Gastroenterology 1975; **Med School:** Creighton Univ 1969; **Resid:** Internal Medicine, Oreg Hlth Sci Univ 1973; Gastroenterology, Oreg Hlth Sci Univ 1974; **Fellow:** Gastroenterology, UCSF Med Ctr 1979; **Fac Appt:** Prof Med, Stanford Univ

Kimmey, Michael B MD [Ge] - **Spec Exp:** Pancreatic/Biliary Endoscopy (ERCP); Endoscopy; Endoscopic Ultrasound; **Hospital:** St Joseph Med Ctr - Tacoma, Tacoma Genl Hosp; **Address:** 1112 6th Ave, Ste 200, Tacoma, WA 98405; **Phone:** 253-272-8664; **Board Cert:** Internal Medicine 1982; Gastroenterology 1987; **Med School:** Washington Univ, St Louis 1979; **Resid:** Internal Medicine, Univ Wash Med Ctr 1982; **Fellow:** Gastroenterology, Univ Wash Med Ctr 1987; **Fac Appt:** Clin Prof Med, Univ Wash

Kozarek, Richard MD [Ge] - **Spec Exp:** Pancreatic/Biliary Endoscopy (ERCP); Inflammatory Bowel Disease; Pancreatic Disease; **Hospital:** Virginia Mason Med Ctr, Swedish Med Ctr - Seattle; **Address:** 1100 9th Ave, Seattle, WA 98101-2756; **Phone:** 206-223-6934; **Board Cert:** Internal Medicine 1977; Gastroenterology 1979; **Med School:** Univ Wisc 1973; **Resid:** Internal Medicine, Good Samaritan Hosp 1976; **Fellow:** Gastroenterology, Univ Arizona/ VA Hosp 1978; **Fac Appt:** Clin Prof Med, Univ Wash

Ostroff, James Warren MD [Ge] - **Spec Exp:** Pancreatic/Biliary Endoscopy (ERCP); Colonoscopy; **Hospital:** UCSF Med Ctr, UCSF - Mt Zion Med Ctr; **Address:** 350 Parnassus Ave, Ste 410, San Francisco, CA 94117-3608; **Phone:** 415-502-2112; **Board Cert:** Internal Medicine 1980; Gastroenterology 1983; **Med School:** Cornell Univ-Weill Med Coll 1977; **Resid:** Internal Medicine, NY Hosp-Cornell Med Ctr 1980; **Fellow:** Gastroenterology, UCSF Hosps 1982; **Fac Appt:** Prof Med, UCSF

Pimstone, Neville R MD [Ge] - **Spec Exp:** Porphyria; Hepatitis C; **Hospital:** VA Med Ctr - W Los Angeles; **Address:** 11301 Wilshire Blvd, rm 4045B, Los Angeles, CA 90073; **Phone:** 916-734-3751; **Med School:** South Africa 1960; **Resid:** Internal Medicine, Groote Schuur Hosp 1968; **Fellow:** Gastroenterology, Moffit Hosp-UCSF 1970; **Fac Appt:** Prof Med, UC Davis

Roth, Bennett E MD [Ge] - **Spec Exp:** Gastroesophageal Reflux Disease (GERD); Inflammatory Bowel Disease/Crohn's; Irritable Bowel Syndrome; **Hospital:** UCLA Med Ctr; **Address:** 200 UCLA Med Plaza, Ste 365A, Los Angeles, CA 90095; **Phone:** 310-825-1597; **Board Cert:** Internal Medicine 1972; Gastroenterology 1975; **Med School:** Hahnemann Univ 1968; **Resid:** Internal Medicine, Hosp Univ Penn 1971; **Fellow:** Gastroenterology, UCLA Med Ctr 1974; **Fac Appt:** Prof Med, UCLA

Surawicz, Christina MD [Ge] - **Spec Exp:** Clostridium Difficile Disease; Infectious Diarrhea; **Hospital:** Harborview Med Ctr, Univ Wash Med Ctr; **Address:** 325 9th Ave, Box 359773, Seattle, WA 98104-2420; **Phone:** 206-731-5021; **Board Cert:** Internal Medicine 1976; Gastroenterology 1979; **Med School:** Univ KY Coll Med 1973; **Resid:** Internal Medicine, Univ Washington Med Ctr 1976; **Fellow:** Gastroenterology, Univ Washington Med Ctr 1979; **Fac Appt:** Prof Med, Univ Wash

Targan, Stephan R MD [Ge] - **Spec Exp:** Inflammatory Bowel Disease; Crohn's Disease; **Hospital:** Cedars-Sinai Med Ctr; **Address:** Cedars-Sinai IBD Ctr, 110 George Burns Rd, Bldg 4063, Los Angeles, CA 90048; **Phone:** 310-423-4100; **Board Cert:** Internal Medicine 1974; Infectious Disease 1976; Gastroenterology 1979; **Med School:** Johns Hopkins Univ 1971; **Resid:** Internal Medicine, Harbor-UCLA Med Ctr 1976; **Fellow:** Infectious Disease, Harbor-UCLA Med Ctr 1976; Gastroenterology, UCLA Med Ctr 1978; **Fac Appt:** Prof Med, UCLA

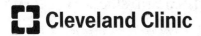

Cleveland Clinic

Digestive Disease Center

A National Leader in Digestive Disease

Cleveland Clinic's Digestive Disease Center is one of the largest in the country and one of the first to fully integrate its departments of Colorectal Surgery and Gastroenterology & Hepatology. Combining these disciplines in one location facilitates unprecedented patient care, multidisciplinary education and collaborative research.

One of the largest U.S. specialty centers for swallowing and esophageal disorders is part of the Digestive Disease Center, as is the largest registry for inherited forms of colorectal cancer. Additionally, the center is a leader in minimally invasive colorectal surgery, averaging more than 15 cases per week and training surgeons from around the world in laparoscopic techniques. The hepatology section supports the transplant program, which performs 130 liver transplants annually, and conducts groundbreaking research in fatty liver disease, viral hepatitis and nutrition. The Center is also a recognized leader in the endoscopic diagnosis and treatment of disorders of the bile duct and pancreas. In the treatment of digestive diseases, the center is a recognized leader in many areas, including pelvic pouch procedures. Cleveland Clinic colorectal surgeons have performed more than 3,500 pelvic pouch procedures and are the established leaders in pouch salvage. Inflammatory Bowel Disease specialists are at the forefront of testing new medications to treat IBD and examining biomarkers to predict the development of cancer in IBD patients.

> **Special Service for Out-of-State Patients**
>
> Global Patient Services is a full-service department dedicated to meeting the needs and requirements of both out-of-state and international patients who receive their care at Cleveland Clinic. That National Center and the International Center, which make up Global Patient Services, provide personalized concierge programs and services to welcome patients and add to their comfort before, during and after their stay. Call 800.223.2273, ext. 55580, or send an e-mail to medicalconcierge@ccf.org.

Over the years, the staff of the Digestive Disease Center has pioneered many new technologies and procedures, including: continent ileostomy/stapled pouch to valve, stapled pelvic pouch procedures, capsule endoscopy, diagnostic tests for fatty liver, laparoscopic bowel operations, cryotherapy for Barrett's Esophagus, endoscopic pancreatic function test, endoscopic management of anastamotic and inflammatory strictures, Bravo system for monitoring esophageal pH level, surgery for ostomy complications, genetic testing for inherited colorectal cancer, extracorporeal shock wave lithotripsy of pancreatic stones, surgery for fecal incontinence, advancement flap/ sleeves for perianal fistulas and Crohn's disease, endoscopic diagnosis and treatment of pancreatic cystic disorders, coloplasty for enhanced function after rectal resection, strictureplasty for Crohn's disease, cholangioscopy, artificial sphincter for bowel incontinence, salvage surgery for "apparently" failed ileal pelvic (J) pouches, balloon enteroscopy for the diagnosis and management of small bowel disorders

Cleveland Clinic Digestive Disease Center is ranked second in the nation by *U.S.News & World Report's* 2006 "America's Best Hospitals" Survey.

To schedule an appointment or for more information about the Cleveland Clinic Digestive Disease Center call 800.890.2467 or visit www.clevelandclinic.org/gastrotopdocs.

Cleveland Clinic Digestive Disease Center
9500 Euclid Avenue / W14 | Cleveland OH 44195

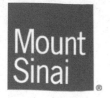

THE MOUNT SINAI MEDICAL CENTER
GASTROINTESTINAL AND SURGICAL SPECIALTIES

One Gustave L. Levy Place (Fifth Avenue and 100th Street)
New York, NY 10029-6574
Physician Referral: 1-800-MD-SINAI (637-4624)
www.mountsinai.org

Mount Sinai's *Divisions of Gastroenterology, Colon and Rectal Surgery, Liver Diseases,* and *Pediatric Gastroenterology, Nutrition*, and *Liver Diseases* are renowned for their delivery of patient care, research, and education in diseases of the gastrointestinal tract. In 2000, the National Institutes of Health (NIH) recognized the importance of Mount Sinai as a research center with a grant for GI/Liver fellowship training, making Mount Sinai the only medical school in New York City to earn this prestigious award.

Successes within the *Division of Gastroenterology* include breakthroughs in the medical and surgical management of inflammatory bowel disease (IBD) (ulcerative colitis and Crohn's disease). Mount Sinai spearheaded novel therapies for treating severe IBD, and helped establish the role of colonoscopy for preventing colon cancer by removing precancerous polyps. More recent innovations include employing a tiny camera within a swallowable capsule to capture images in the stomach and intestines. Mount Sinai's small intestine transplantation program is one of only four such programs in the country. Mount Sinai's IBD Center, Women's GI Health Center, and GI Cancer Center offer patients the latest comprehensive, interdisciplinary care, newer agents through clinical trials, and services such as psychologists and nutritionists.

Mount Sinai surgeons have a distinguished history in the surgical treatment of gastrointestinal disorders, and today surgeons in the *Division of Colon and Rectal Surgery* continue that tradition, focusing on surgical therapies for all diseases involving the colon, rectum, and anus. With special expertise in the treatment of Crohn's disease (which was first described at Mount Sinai in 1932), ulcerative colitis, colon and rectal cancer and diverticulitis, we specialize in the newer techniques of rectal surgery with special emphasis on colostomy avoidance. The newest minimally invasive techniques are offered as well as other cutting-edge technologies for the treatment of such disorders as hemorrhoids, fistulas, and rectal tumors.

Mount Sinai's *Division of Liver Diseases* has a long history of outstanding clinical care and scientific investigation, with a tradition of excellence in several clinical areas, including liver transplantation; diagnosis and treatment of viral hepatitis; treatment of scarring, or fibrosis; management of primary biliary cirrhosis, an autoimmune disease of bile ducts; treatment of liver cancer; and diagnosis and treatment of genetic liver diseases, including Wilson's disease (copper overload) and hemachromatosis (iron overload). With a steadily growing research budget, Mount Sinai carries out a diverse portfolio of research projects.

The Division of Pediatric Gastroenterology, Nutrition, and *Liver Diseases* provides consultative services and treatment for the full range of children's digestive and nutritional diseases. The Children's IBD Center is the only multidisciplinary center for pediatric patients with Crohn's disease and ulcerative colitis in the tri-state area and receives referrals from all over the country. The Transplant Program is one of the largest in the nation and was the first program in New York to perform liver transplants, and later small bowel transplants. The Division is active in clinical research in IBD, focusing on issues of genetic factors, psychosocial interactions, and drug trials. Several NIH grants support research in the areas of biliary atresia, bile salt absorption, and outcome analysis in children with liver failure.

Mount Sinai provides a comprehensive center, uniting the medical disciplines of gastroenterology and its related surgical specialties, as well as an array of minimally invasive surgical programs. The Center houses renowned programs for the treatment of IBD and colorectal diseases, as well as reconstructive and laparoscopic surgery programs through the *Division of Laparoscopic Surgery*, which is internationally known for pioneering a number of minimally invasive procedures for the treatment of Crohn's disease and ulcerative colitis.

608

⌐ NewYork-Presbyterian
⌐ The University Hospital of Columbia and Cornell
NewYork-Presbyterian Digestive Disease Services

Affiliated with Columbia University College of Physicians and Surgeons and Weill Medical College of Cornell University

NewYork-Presbyterian Hospital
Weill Cornell Medical Center
525 East 68th Street
New York, NY 10021

NewYork-Presbyterian Hospital
Columbia University Medical Center
622 West 168th Street
New York, NY 10032

OVERVIEW:

The Digestive Disease Services of NewYork-Presbyterian Hospital provide expert capabilities in research, education and clinical care of patients with gastrointestinal, liver and bile duct, pancreatic and nutritional disorders.

The Hospital offers a wide range of diagnostic tests including,
- Routine procedures, such as endoscopy, capsule endoscopy, colonoscopy and flexible sigmoidoscopy.

- Endoscopic retrograde cholangiopancreatography (ERCP) to evaluate the ducts of the gallbladder, pancreas and liver

- Endoscopic ultrasonography (EUS)to provide detailed images of the upper and lower gastrointestinal tract and for the staging of patients with esophageal, gastric and rectal cancers. The Hospital is one of the few centers using EUS for needle aspiration of pancreatic cysts and tumors.

- Laparoscopy for direct examination of the liver, gallbladder and spleen and in the diagnosis, staging and treatment of pancreatic, gastric, esophageal and colorectal cancer.

The Hospital is a leader in treating gastrointestinal (GI) conditions. For example,
- The Minimal Access Surgery Center (MASC) is at the forefront of developing and applying new technologies, such as robotics, computerized image processing and enhanced optics. It is improving the outcomes of GI surgical patients and speeding their recovery from conditions such as GERD, gallbladder disease, and benign and malignant colon and rectal disease.

- Our surgeons also perform endoscopic sewing (endocinch) and radiofrequency treatment (Stretta procedure) for GERD.

- Our surgeons are internationally renowned in the use of laparoscopic methods for cancer and other colorectal conditions. They are highly experienced with the Whipple procedure to remove a pancreas tumor, which improves the survival rates and life expectancies of patients with pancreatic cancer and other less common pancreas problems.

Additionally, our physicians are involved in numerous clinical trials, (including studies on Cox-2 inhibitors) for preventing colorectal cancer and familial polyposis (a precursor to colorectal cancer), and antiviral therapy for chronic hepatitis C.

Physician Referral: For a physician referral or to learn more about the NewYork-Presbyterian Digestive Disease Services call toll free **1-877-NYP-WELL** (1-877-697-9355) or visit our website at **www.nypdigestive.org**

COMPREHENSIVE CARE

Patients benefit from the collaboration of gastroenterologists, hepatologists, surgeons and diagnostic and pathology experts who develop optimal treatment plans. Areas of expertise include:

- GI Cancer, including esophageal, colorectal, liver, pancreatic and gastric tumors

- Inflammatory Bowel Diseases (Ulcerative Colitis and Crohn's Disease)

- Liver Diseases. The Hospital has a comprehensive Hepatitis C Center and the Center for Liver Disease and Transplantation

- Esophageal Disorders, including gastroesophageal reflux disease (GERD) and Barrett's esophagus

- Pancreatic and Biliary Disorders

- Celiac Disease

- Polyps of the Colon

- Peptic Ulcer Disease/Helicobacter Pylori Infections

- Gallbladder and Bile Duct Disorders

- Restorative surgery to avoid colostomies in diseases like rectal cancer, Crohn's disease, ulcerative colitis, and incontinence

- Anal diseases, such as hemorrhoids, fistulas, vascular tumors, abscesses and others

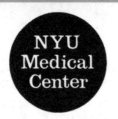

NYU Medical Center

550 First Avenue (at 31st Street)
New York, NY 10016
Physician Referral:
(888)7-NYU-MED (888-769-8633)
www.nyumc.org

GASTROENTEROLOGY

The mission of the Division of Gastroenterology at NYU Medical Center is excellence in the delivery of patient care, research, and education in diseases of the gastrointestinal tract. Its physicians bring with them a rich body of knowledge in the diagnosis and management of inflammatory bowel disease, peptic ulcer disease, esophageal disorders, gastrointestinal cancer, and liver, biliary, and pancreatic diseases. Their multidisciplinary approach insures the greatest possible patient care at NYU's three acclaimed, academically integrated teaching hospitals: Tisch Hospital (New York University Hospital), Bellevue Hospitals Center, and the New York Harbor Health Care System (Manhattan Veterans Hospital).

Members of the Division of Gastroenterology are nationally recognized leaders who are involved in numerous studies in the field of gastroenterology and hepatology, including clinical research in liver diseases (especially hepatitis C), endoscopy, colon cancer screening, acute and chronic GI bleeding, and Helicobacter pylori.

Always at the forefront of new technologies, NYU's gastroenterologists work side-by-side with radiologists to perform virtual colonoscopies, a new minimally invasive technique for finding early-stage cancers in the colon.

Virtual colonoscopy is a new screening test in which a radiologist uses a CAT (Computer Assisted Tomography) scanner and sophisticated image processing computers to actually recreate and evaluate the inner surface of the colon. The CAT scanner provides the x-ray images; the image-processing computers create the 3-D display for the final interpretation by the referring gastroenterologist. The study gives a complete evaluation of the entire surface of the colon and can be performed quickly, with little discomfort and extremely accurate readings.

NYU MEDICAL CENTER

The colon and the rectum are the final sections of the large intestine. In the United States, approximately 150,000 people are diagnosed with colorectal cancer every year and of these, approximately 55,000 will die of the disease. Cancer of the colon is the second leading cause of cancer death in the United States. Most experts agree that it is preventable, and NYU is on the cutting edge of 21st century research into quicker, safer, and more accurate diagnosis and treatment, with its advanced video colonoscopy and noninvasive radiologic techniques.

**Physician Referral
(888) 7-NYU-MED
(888-769-8633)
www.nyumc.org**

696

Geriatric Medicine

a subspecialty of Internal Medicine or Family Practice

An internist or family physician with special knowledge of the aging process and special skills in the diagnostic, therapeutic, preventive and rehabilitative aspects of illness in the elderly.   This specialist cares for geriatric patients in the patient's home, the office, long-term care settings such as nursing homes and the hospital.

Family Medicine

A family physician is concerned with the total healthcare of the individual and the family, and is trained to diagnose and treat a wide variety of ailments in patients of all ages. The family physician receives a broad range of training that includes internal medicine, pediatrics, obstetrics and gynecology, psychiatry and geriatrics. Special emphasis is placed on prevention and the primary care of entire families, utilizing consultations and community resources when appropriate.

Training Required: Three years in internal medicine or family practice *plus* additional training and examination for certification in geriatric medicine.

Geriatric Medicine

New England

Cooney Jr, Leo M MD [Ger] - **Spec Exp:** Rheumatology; **Hospital:** Yale - New Haven Hosp; **Address:** 20 York St, Tompkins 17, New Haven, CT 06520; **Phone:** 203-688-2204; **Board Cert:** Internal Medicine 1974; Rheumatology 1978; Geriatric Medicine 2000; **Med School:** Yale Univ 1969; **Resid:** Internal Medicine, Boston City Hosp 1971; Internal Medicine, Boston City Hosp 1974; **Fellow:** Rheumatology, Boston Med Ctr 1975; **Fac Appt:** Prof Med, Yale Univ

Lipsitz, Lewis Arnold MD [Ger] - **Spec Exp:** Falls & Fractures; Fainting Disorders; **Hospital:** Beth Israel Deaconess Med Ctr - Boston; **Address:** Beth Israel Med Ctr, Gerontology, 110 Francis St, LMOB 1B, Boston, MA 02215; **Phone:** 617-632-8696; **Board Cert:** Internal Medicine 1980; Geriatric Medicine 1999; **Med School:** Univ Pennsylvania 1977; **Resid:** Internal Medicine, Beth Israel Hosp 1980; **Fellow:** Geriatric Medicine, Harvard Univ 1983; **Fac Appt:** Prof Med, Harvard Med Sch

Minaker, Kenneth MD [Ger] - **Spec Exp:** Aging; Neuroendocrinology; Cardiovascular Disease; **Hospital:** Mass Genl Hosp, Brigham & Women's Hosp; **Address:** Charles River Plaza, Ste 502, 165 Cambridge St, Boston, MA 02114-2723; **Phone:** 617-726-4600; **Board Cert:** Internal Medicine 1979; Geriatric Medicine 1985; **Med School:** Univ Toronto 1972; **Resid:** Internal Medicine, Univ Toronto 1981; **Fellow:** Geriatric Medicine, Mass Gen Hosp-Harvard 1983; **Fac Appt:** Assoc Prof Med, Harvard Med Sch

Tinetti, Mary E MD [Ger] - **Spec Exp:** Falls in the Elderly; Geriatric Functional Assessment; **Hospital:** Yale - New Haven Hosp; **Address:** Yale-New Haven Hosp, Adler Geriatric Ctr, 200 York St, New Haven, CT 06510; **Phone:** 203-688-6361; **Board Cert:** Internal Medicine 1981; Geriatric Medicine 1988; **Med School:** Univ Mich Med Sch 1978; **Resid:** Internal Medicine, Univ Minnesota 1981; **Fellow:** Geriatric Medicine, Univ Rochester 1984; **Fac Appt:** Prof Med, Yale Univ

Mid Atlantic

Bloom, Patricia A MD [Ger] - **Spec Exp:** Dementia; Geriatric Functional Assessment; Osteoporosis; **Hospital:** Mount Sinai Med Ctr; **Address:** 1470 Madison Ave, New York, NY 10029-6542; **Phone:** 212-659-8552; **Board Cert:** Internal Medicine 1978; Geriatric Medicine 1998; **Med School:** Univ Minn 1975; **Resid:** Internal Medicine, Montefiore Hosp 1978; **Fac Appt:** Assoc Prof Med, Mount Sinai Sch Med

Burton, John R MD [Ger] - **Hospital:** Johns Hopkins Hosp - Baltimore (page 61); **Address:** Division of Geriatric Medicine, 5505 Hopkins Bayview Cir, Baltimore, MD 21224; **Phone:** 410-550-0520; **Board Cert:** Internal Medicine 1980; Geriatric Medicine 1990; Nephrology 1974; **Med School:** McGill Univ 1965; **Resid:** Internal Medicine, Baltimore City Hosp 1971; **Fellow:** Nephrology, Mass Genl Hosp 1972; **Fac Appt:** Prof Med, Johns Hopkins Univ

Finucane, Thomas E MD [Ger] - **Spec Exp:** Pain Management; Swallowing Disorders; Ethics; **Hospital:** Johns Hopkins Bayview Med Ctr (page 61), Johns Hopkins Hosp - Baltimore (page 61); **Address:** 5505 Hopkins Bayview Cir, Level 01, Baltimore, MD 21224; **Phone:** 410-550-0925; **Board Cert:** Internal Medicine 1982; Geriatric Medicine 1998; **Med School:** Emory Univ 1978; **Resid:** Internal Medicine, George Washington Univ Hosp 1982; **Fac Appt:** Prof Med, Johns Hopkins Univ

Freedman, Michael L MD [Ger] - **Spec Exp:** Alzheimer's Disease; Anemia; Nutrition; **Hospital:** NYU Med Ctr (page 67), Bellevue Hosp Ctr; **Address:** 530 First Ave, Ste 4J, New York, NY 10016-6402; **Phone:** 212-263-7043; **Board Cert:** Internal Medicine 1971; Hematology 1974; Geriatric Medicine 1998; **Med School:** Tufts Univ 1963; **Resid:** Internal Medicine, Bellevue Hosp 1965; Internal Medicine, Bellevue Hosp 1969; **Fellow:** Hematology, Natl Inst Hlth-NCI 1968; **Fac Appt:** Prof Med, NYU Sch Med

Gambert, Steven MD [Ger] - **Spec Exp:** Endocrinology; Osteoporosis; Aging; **Hospital:** Sinai Hosp - Baltimore; **Address:** Sinai Hosp Baltimore Hoffberger Bldg, 2401 W Belvedere Ave, Ste 56, Baltimore, MD 21215; **Phone:** 410-601-6340; **Board Cert:** Internal Medicine 1978; **Med School:** Columbia P&S 1975; **Resid:** Internal Medicine, Dartmouth Affl Hosp 1977; **Fellow:** Geriatric Medicine, Beth Israel Hosp-Harvard 1979; Endocrinology, Beth Israel Hosp-Harvard 1979; **Fac Appt:** Prof Med, Johns Hopkins Univ

Lachs, Mark MD [Ger] - **Spec Exp:** Abuse/Neglect; **Hospital:** NY-Presby Hosp/Weill Cornell (page 66); **Address:** Irving Sherwood Wright Center on Aging, 1484 First Ave, New York, NY 10021; **Phone:** 212-746-7000; **Board Cert:** Internal Medicine 1988; Geriatric Medicine 2002; **Med School:** NYU Sch Med 1985; **Resid:** Internal Medicine, Hosp Univ Penn 1988; **Fellow:** Geriatric Medicine, Yale Univ 1990; **Fac Appt:** Assoc Prof Med, Cornell Univ-Weill Med Coll

Libow, Leslie MD [Ger] - **Spec Exp:** Diagnostic Problems; **Hospital:** Mount Sinai Med Ctr; **Address:** 1470 Madison Ave, New York, NY 10029; **Phone:** 212-659-8552; **Board Cert:** Internal Medicine 1977; Geriatric Medicine 1988; **Med School:** Ros Franklin Univ/Chicago Med Sch 1958; **Resid:** Internal Medicine, Bronx VA Hosp 1960; Internal Medicine, Mt Sinai Hosp 1964; **Fac Appt:** Prof Med, Mount Sinai Sch Med

Meier, Diane MD [Ger] - **Spec Exp:** Palliative Care; **Hospital:** Mount Sinai Med Ctr; **Address:** Mt Sinai School Medicine, Box 1070, New York, NY 10029-6501; **Phone:** 212-241-1446; **Board Cert:** Internal Medicine 1981; Geriatric Medicine 1999; **Med School:** Northwestern Univ 1977; **Resid:** Internal Medicine, Oregon Hlth Sci Univ 1981; **Fellow:** Geriatric Medicine, VA Med Ctr 1983; **Fac Appt:** Prof Med, Mount Sinai Sch Med

Resnick, Neil M MD [Ger] - **Spec Exp:** Voiding Dysfunction; Incontinence; **Hospital:** UPMC Presby, Pittsburgh, UPMC Shadyside; **Address:** 3471 5th Ave, Kaufmann Bldg, Ste 500, Pittsburgh, PA 15213-3313; **Phone:** 412-692-2364; **Board Cert:** Internal Medicine 1980; Geriatric Medicine 1998; **Med School:** Stanford Univ 1977; **Resid:** Internal Medicine, Beth Israel Hosp 1980; **Fellow:** Geriatric Medicine, Harvard Univ 1982; Urodynamics, Harvard Univ 1984; **Fac Appt:** Prof Med, Univ Pittsburgh

Studenski, Stephanie A MD [Ger] - **Spec Exp:** Balance Disorders; Mobility Evaluation & Treatment; Falls in the Elderly; **Hospital:** UPMC Presby, Pittsburgh; **Address:** 4 East Montefiore, 200 Lothrop St, Pittsburgh, PA 15213; **Phone:** 412-692-4200; **Board Cert:** Internal Medicine 1982; Rheumatology 1984; Geriatric Medicine 2002; **Med School:** Univ Kans 1979; **Resid:** Internal Medicine, Duke Univ Med Ctr 1982; **Fellow:** Rheumatology, Duke Univ Med Ctr 1984; Geriatric Medicine, Duke Univ Med Ctr 1986; **Fac Appt:** Prof Med, Univ Pittsburgh

Geriatric Medicine

Southeast

Ciocon, Jerry MD [Ger] - **Spec Exp:** Chronic Fatigue-Elderly; Pain-Musculoskeletal; Memory Disorders; **Hospital:** Cleveland Clin - Weston (page 57); **Address:** Cleveland Clinic, Div Geriatrics, 2950 Cleveland Clinic Blvd, Weston, FL 33331-3609; **Phone:** 954-659-5867; **Board Cert:** Internal Medicine 1985; Geriatric Medicine 2000; **Med School:** Philippines 1980; **Resid:** Internal Medicine, Mercy Hosp 1985; **Fellow:** Geriatric Medicine, LI Jewish Med Ctr 1987; **Fac Appt:** Asst Clin Prof Med, Ohio State Univ

Greganti, Mac Andrew MD [Ger] - **Spec Exp:** Diagnostic Problems; Dementia; **Hospital:** Univ NC Hosps; **Address:** Univ North Carolina Hosp, Dept Med, 125 MacNider Bldg, Chapel Hill, NC 27599-7005; **Phone:** 919-966-3063; **Board Cert:** Internal Medicine 1987; Geriatric Medicine 1988; **Med School:** Univ Miss 1972; **Resid:** Internal Medicine, Strong Meml Hosp 1975; **Fac Appt:** Prof Med, Univ NC Sch Med

Groene, Linda A MD [Ger] - **Spec Exp:** Osteoporosis; Sleep Disorders/Apnea; Dementia; **Hospital:** Imperial Point Med Ctr, Holy Cross Hosp - Fort Lauderdale; **Address:** 6405 N Federal Hwy, Ste 102, Ft Lauderdale, FL 33308; **Phone:** 954-772-0062; **Board Cert:** Internal Medicine 1986; Geriatric Medicine 2000; **Med School:** Louisiana State Univ 1981; **Resid:** Pathology, Jackson Meml Hosp 1983; Internal Medicine, Mt Sinai Med Ctr 1986

Hanson, Laura C MD [Ger] - **Spec Exp:** Frailty Syndrome; Palliative Care; **Hospital:** Univ NC Hosps; **Address:** UNC Sch Med, MacNider Bldg, CB 7550, Chapel Hill, NC 27599; **Phone:** 919-966-5945 x251; **Board Cert:** Internal Medicine 1989; Geriatric Medicine 2002; **Med School:** Harvard Med Sch 1986; **Resid:** Internal Medicine, Brigham & Womens Hosp 1988; Internal Medicine, Univ North Carolina Hosp 1989; **Fellow:** Geriatric Medicine, Univ North Carolina Hosp 1991; **Fac Appt:** Assoc Prof Med, Univ NC Sch Med

Lyles, Kenneth W MD [Ger] - **Spec Exp:** Bone Disorders-Metabolic; Tumoral Calcinosis; Parathyroid Disease; **Hospital:** Duke Univ Med Ctr, VA Med Ctr - Durham; **Address:** Duke Univ Med Center, Box 3881, Durham, NC 27710; **Phone:** 919-660-7520; **Board Cert:** Internal Medicine 1977; Endocrinology 1979; Geriatric Medicine 2000; **Med School:** Med Coll VA 1974; **Resid:** Internal Medicine, Med Coll VA 1977; **Fellow:** Endocrinology, Diabetes & Metabolism, Duke Univ Med Ctr 1979; Geriatric Medicine, Duke Univ/VA Med Ctr 1981; **Fac Appt:** Prof Med, Duke Univ

Ouslander, Joseph G MD [Ger] - **Spec Exp:** Incontinence; Urinary Tract Disorders; **Hospital:** Emory Univ Hosp; **Address:** Wesley Woods Center of Emory University, 1821 Clifton Rd NE, Atlanta, GA 30329; **Phone:** 404-728-6363; **Board Cert:** Internal Medicine 1980; Geriatric Medicine 2000; **Med School:** Case West Res Univ 1977; **Resid:** Internal Medicine, Univ Hosp 1979; Internal Medicine, Sepulveda Med Ctr 1980; **Fellow:** Geriatric Medicine, UCLA Med Ctr 1982

Snustad, Diane G MD [Ger] - **Spec Exp:** Osteoporosis; Dementia; **Hospital:** Univ Virginia Med Ctr; **Address:** Colonnades Med Assocs, 100 Colonnades Hill Drive, Charlottesville, VA 22901-2121; **Phone:** 434-924-1212; **Board Cert:** Internal Medicine 1982; Geriatric Medicine 1998; **Med School:** Univ Minn 1979; **Resid:** Internal Medicine, West Virginia Univ 1982; **Fac Appt:** Assoc Prof Med, Univ VA Sch Med

Tenover, Joyce S MD/PhD [Ger] - **Spec Exp:** Menopause-Male; Prostate Disease; Polypharmacology (Excess Medications); Hormonal Disorders; **Hospital:** Wesley Woods Ger Hosp, Emory Univ Hosp; **Address:** Wesley Woods Hlth Ctr, Div Geriatrics/Gerontology, 1841 Clifton Rd NE Fl 5, Atlanta, GA 30329; **Phone:** 404-728-6331; **Board Cert:** Internal Medicine 1983; Geriatric Medicine 1997; **Med School:** Geo Wash Univ 1980; **Resid:** Internal Medicine, Univ Wash Alffil Hosp 1983; Internal Medicine, VA Med Ctr 1984; **Fellow:** Geriatric Medicine, VA Med Ctr 1987; **Fac Appt:** Prof Med, Emory Univ

Midwest

Carr, David B MD [Ger] - **Spec Exp:** Polypharmacology (Excess Medications); Alzheimer's Disease; **Hospital:** Barnes-Jewish Hosp; **Address:** Wash Univ Sch Med, Div Geriatrics, 660 S Euclid Ave, Box 8303, St Louis, MO 63110; **Phone:** 314-286-2700; **Board Cert:** Internal Medicine 1989; Geriatric Medicine 2000; **Med School:** Univ MO-Columbia Sch Med 1985; **Resid:** Internal Medicine, Mich State Assoc Hosps 1988; **Fellow:** Geriatric Medicine, Duke Univ 1990; **Fac Appt:** Prof Med, Washington Univ, St Louis

Dale, Lowell C MD [Ger] - **Spec Exp:** Nicotine Dependence; Nutrition; **Hospital:** Mayo Med Ctr & Clin - Rochester; **Address:** Mayo Clinic, 200 First St SW, Colonial 3-10, Rochester, MN 55905; **Phone:** 507-266-1093; **Board Cert:** Internal Medicine 1984; **Med School:** Univ Minn 1981; **Resid:** Internal Medicine, Mayo Clinic 1984; **Fellow:** Internal Medicine, Mayo Clinic 1985; **Fac Appt:** Asst Prof Med, Mayo Med Sch

Duthie, Edmund H MD [Ger] - **Spec Exp:** Geriatric Functional Assessment; **Hospital:** Froedtert Meml Lutheran Hosp, Clement J Zablocki VA Med Ctr; **Address:** 9200 W Wisconsin Ave, Milwaukee, WI 53226; **Phone:** 414-456-7070; **Board Cert:** Internal Medicine 1979; Geriatric Medicine 1998; **Med School:** Georgetown Univ 1976; **Resid:** Internal Medicine, Med Coll Wisc Hosps 1979; **Fellow:** Geriatric Medicine, Jewish Inst Geri Care-SUNY 1980; **Fac Appt:** Prof Med, Med Coll Wisc

Gorbien, Martin MD [Ger] - **Spec Exp:** Dementia; Alzheimer's Disease; Geriatric Functional Assessment; **Hospital:** Rush Univ Med Ctr; **Address:** 1725 W Harrison St, Ste 955, Chicago, IL 60612; **Phone:** 312-942-7030; **Board Cert:** Internal Medicine 1996; Geriatric Medicine 1998; **Med School:** Mexico 1983; **Resid:** Internal Medicine, Mercy Hosp & Med Ctr 1987; **Fellow:** Geriatric Medicine, UCLA Med Ctr 1989; **Fac Appt:** Assoc Prof Med, Rush Med Coll

Halter, Jeffrey Brian MD [Ger] - **Spec Exp:** Endocrinology; Diabetes; **Hospital:** Univ Michigan Hlth Sys; **Address:** Univ Mich Turner Geriatric Ctr, 4260 Plymouth Rd, Ann Arbor, MI 48109; **Phone:** 734-764-6831; **Board Cert:** Internal Medicine 1974; Endocrinology 1977; **Med School:** Univ Minn 1969; **Resid:** Internal Medicine, LA Co Harbor Gen Hosp 1971; Internal Medicine, Univ Wash Affil Hosp 1974; **Fellow:** Geriatric Medicine, VA Hosp 1977; **Fac Appt:** Prof Med, Univ Mich Med Sch

Morley, John MD [Ger] - **Spec Exp:** Nutrition; Endocrinology; Menopause-Male; Alzheimer's Disease; **Hospital:** St Louis Univ Hosp; **Address:** St Louis Univ Hlth Sci Ctr, Div Ger Med, 1402 S Grand Blvd, rm M 238, St Louis, MO 63104-1004; **Phone:** 314-977-6055; **Board Cert:** Internal Medicine 1978; Geriatric Medicine 1998; Endocrinology 1981; **Med School:** South Africa 1972; **Resid:** Internal Medicine, Johannesburg Genl Hosp 1974; Internal Medicine, Baragwanath Hosp 1976; **Fellow:** Endocrinology, Diabetes & Metabolism, Wadsworth VA Hosp-UCLA 1979; **Fac Appt:** Prof Med, St Louis Univ

Geriatric Medicine

Olson, Jack Conrad MD [Ger] - **Spec Exp:** Dementia; Depression; **Hospital:** Rush Univ Med Ctr; **Address:** 1725 W Harrison St, Ste 955, Chicago, IL 60612-3836; **Phone:** 312-942-7030; **Board Cert:** Internal Medicine 1987; Geriatric Medicine 2000; **Med School:** Univ Mich Med Sch 1984; **Resid:** Internal Medicine, Univ Wisc Med Sch 1987; **Fellow:** Geriatric Medicine, Univ Wisc Med Sch 1989; **Fac Appt:** Asst Prof Med, Univ Chicago-Pritzker Sch Med

Palmer, Robert M MD [Ger] - **Spec Exp:** Geriatric Functional Assessment; Dementia; **Hospital:** Cleveland Clin Fdn (page 57); **Address:** 9500 Euclid Ave, MC A-91, Cleveland, OH 44195-0001; **Phone:** 216-444-8091; **Board Cert:** Internal Medicine 1975; Geriatric Medicine 1998; **Med School:** Univ Mich Med Sch 1971; **Resid:** Internal Medicine, LA County Med Ctr 1975; **Fellow:** Geriatric Medicine, UCLA Med Ctr 1986; **Fac Appt:** Assoc Clin Prof Med, Case West Res Univ

Sachs, Greg A MD [Ger] - **Spec Exp:** Memory Disorders; Alzheimer's Disease; **Hospital:** Univ of Chicago Hosps; **Address:** Univ Chicago, Dept Med-Sect Geriatrics, 5841 S Maryland Ave, MC-6098, Chicago, IL 60637; **Phone:** 773-702-8840; **Board Cert:** Internal Medicine 1988; Geriatric Medicine 2000; **Med School:** Yale Univ 1985; **Resid:** Internal Medicine, Univ Chicago Hosps 1987; **Fellow:** Geriatric Medicine, Univ Chicago Hosps 1990; **Fac Appt:** Assoc Prof Med, Univ Chicago-Pritzker Sch Med

Sheehan, Myles MD [Ger] - **Spec Exp:** Dementia; Geriatric Functional Assessment; **Hospital:** Loyola Univ Med Ctr; **Address:** Loyola Univ Med Ctr, 2160 S 1st Ave , Bldg 120 - rm 310, Maywood, IL 60153; **Phone:** 708-216-8887; **Board Cert:** Internal Medicine 1984; Geriatric Medicine 2002; **Med School:** Dartmouth Med Sch 1981; **Resid:** Internal Medicine, Beth Israel Deaconess Med Ctr 1984; **Fellow:** Geriatric Medicine, Beth Israel Deaconess Med Ctr 1991; **Fac Appt:** Assoc Prof Med, Loyola Univ-Stritch Sch Med

Von Sternberg, Thomas MD [Ger] - **Spec Exp:** Dementia; **Hospital:** Northern Meml Hlth Care; **Address:** Hlth Partners Riverside Clin, Adult Med, 2220 Riverside Ave S Fl 1, Minneapolis, MN 55454; **Phone:** 952-967-7175; **Board Cert:** Family Medicine 1997; Geriatric Medicine 1998; **Med School:** Ohio State Univ 1980; **Resid:** Family Medicine, Fairview-Univ Med Ctr 1983; **Fellow:** Geriatric Medicine, Westminster Med Sch

Great Plains and Mountains

Schwartz, Robert S MD [Ger] - **Spec Exp:** Diabetes; Exercise Therapy; Hormonal Disorders; **Hospital:** Univ Colorado Hosp, VA Med Ctr; **Address:** Univ Colorado at Denver & Health Sci Ctr, 4200 E Ninth Ave, Box B179, Denver, CO 80262-0001; **Phone:** 303-319-7891; **Board Cert:** Internal Medicine 1977; Endocrinology 1981; Geriatric Medicine 2000; **Med School:** Ohio State Univ 1974; **Resid:** Internal Medicine, Univ Wash Med Ctr 1977; **Fellow:** Endocrinology, Diabetes & Metabolism, Univ Wash Med Ctr 1980; **Fac Appt:** Prof Med, Univ Colorado

Supiano, Mark A MD [Ger] - **Spec Exp:** Hypertension; Geriatric Functional Assessment; **Hospital:** Univ Utah Hosps and Clins; **Address:** Univ Utah, Geriatrics Div, 30 N 1900 E, SOM AB 193, Salt Lake City, UT 84132; **Phone:** 801-587-9103; **Board Cert:** Internal Medicine 1985; Geriatric Medicine 1998; **Med School:** Univ Wisc 1982; **Resid:** Internal Medicine, Univ Mich Med Ctr 1985; **Fellow:** Geriatric Medicine, Univ Mich Med Ctr 1987; **Fac Appt:** Prof Med, Univ Utah

Southwest

Carter, William Jerry MD [Ger] - **Spec Exp:** Geriatric Endocrinology; **Hospital:** John L McClellan VA Med Ctr; **Address:** 2200 Fort Roots Drive, Geriatric Clinic 3B, North Little Rock, AR 72114; **Phone:** 501-257-2061; **Board Cert:** Internal Medicine 1974; Endocrinology, Diabetes & Metabolism 1975; Geriatric Medicine 2005; **Med School:** Univ Ark 1963; **Resid:** Internal Medicine, Univ Ark Med Scis 1967; **Fellow:** Endocrinology, Diabetes & Metabolism, Univ Ark Med Scis 1971; **Fac Appt:** Prof Med, Univ Ark

Dyer, Carmel B MD [Ger] - **Spec Exp:** Elder Abuse; **Hospital:** Meml Hermann Hosp - Houston, LBJ General Hosp; **Address:** 6431 Fannin St, rm MSB-4.200, Houston, TX 77030; **Phone:** 713-500-6290; **Board Cert:** Internal Medicine 2000; Geriatric Medicine 2000; **Med School:** Baylor Coll Med 1988; **Resid:** Internal Medicine, Baylor Affil Hosps 1991; **Fellow:** Geriatric Medicine, Baylor Affil Hosps 1993; **Fac Appt:** Assoc Prof Med, Baylor Coll Med

Liem, Pham MD [Ger] - **Spec Exp:** Dementia; Alzheimer's Disease; Delirium; **Hospital:** UAMS Med Ctr, Cent Ark Vet Hlthcare Sys; **Address:** Univ Hosp Arkansas Med Sci, 4301 W Markham #748, Little Rock, AR 72205-7101; **Phone:** 501-686-5944; **Board Cert:** Family Medicine 1999; Geriatric Medicine 1998; **Med School:** Vietnam 1973; **Resid:** Family Medicine, Univ Ark Med Sch 1980; **Fellow:** Geriatric Medicine, Univ Ark Med Sch 1982; **Fac Appt:** Prof Med, Univ Ark

Lipschitz, David A MD/PhD [Ger] - **Spec Exp:** Nutrition; **Hospital:** UAMS Med Ctr; **Address:** Univ Arkansas Med Sci, 4301 W Markham St, MS 748, Little Rock, AR 72205-7101; **Phone:** 501-686-6219; **Board Cert:** Internal Medicine 1975; Hematology 1976; **Med School:** South Africa 1966; **Resid:** Internal Medicine, Johannesburg Genl Hosp 1972; **Fellow:** Hematology, Univ Washington 1974; Internal Medicine, Montefiore Hosp 1975; **Fac Appt:** Prof Med, Univ Ark

Vicioso, Belinda Angelica MD [Ger] - **Hospital:** Parkland Meml Hosp - Dallas, UT Southwestern Med Ctr - Dallas; **Address:** 5323 Harry Hines Blvd, Dallas, TX 75390-8889; **Phone:** 214-648-9012; **Board Cert:** Internal Medicine 1989; Geriatric Medicine 2000; **Med School:** Dominican Republic 1979; **Resid:** Internal Medicine, St Francis Med Ctr 1983; **Fellow:** Geriatric Medicine, Univ Penn Med Sch 1986; **Fac Appt:** Assoc Prof Med, Univ Tex SW, Dallas

Wei, Jeanne MD/PhD [Ger] - **Spec Exp:** Cardiovascular Disease; **Hospital:** UAMS Med Ctr, John L McClellan VA Med Ctr; **Address:** Donald W Reynolds Ctr on Aging, 4301 W Markham St, Slot 748, Little Rock, AR 72205; **Phone:** 501-296-1000; **Board Cert:** Internal Medicine 1978; Cardiovascular Disease 1979; Geriatric Medicine 2001; **Med School:** Univ IL Coll Med 1975; **Resid:** Internal Medicine, Johns Hopkins Hosp 1977; **Fellow:** Cardiovascular Disease, Johns Hopkins Hosp 1979; Research, Natl Inst Aging 1979; **Fac Appt:** Prof Med, Univ Ark

West Coast and Pacific

Abrass, Itamar MD [Ger] - **Spec Exp:** Endocrinology; Diabetes; **Hospital:** Harborview Med Ctr, Univ Wash Med Ctr; **Address:** Harborview Medical Ctr, 325 9th Ave Fl 5 - rm 5043, Box 359755, Seattle, WA 98104-2499; **Phone:** 206-744-9100; **Board Cert:** Internal Medicine 1974; Endocrinology, Diabetes & Metabolism 1975; Geriatric Medicine 1988; **Med School:** UCSF 1966; **Resid:** Internal Medicine, Columbia-Pesby Med Ctr 1968; **Fellow:** Endocrinology, Diabetes & Metabolism, UCSD Med Ctr 1971; **Fac Appt:** Prof Med, Univ Wash

Davis Jr, James W MD [Ger] - **Hospital:** UCLA Med Ctr; **Address:** 200 UCLA Medical Plaza, Ste 420, Los Angeles, CA 90095; **Phone:** 310-206-8272; **Board Cert:** Internal Medicine 1979; Geriatric Medicine 2000; **Med School:** Med Univ SC 1975; **Resid:** Internal Medicine, Mount Zion Med Ctr; Geriatric Medicine, Mount Zion Med Ctr

Landefeld, Charles Seth MD [Ger] - **Spec Exp:** Cardiovascular Disease; **Hospital:** UCSF Med Ctr, VA Med Ctr - San Francisco; **Address:** 3333 California St, Ste 380, San Francisco, CA 94118; **Phone:** 415-750-6625; **Board Cert:** Internal Medicine 1982; **Med School:** Yale Univ 1979; **Resid:** Internal Medicine, UCSF Med Ctr 1983; **Fellow:** Geriatric Medicine, Brigham-Womens Hosp 1985; **Fac Appt:** Prof Med, UCSF

McCormick, Wayne MD [Ger] - **Spec Exp:** Dementia; AIDS/HIV; **Hospital:** Univ Wash Med Ctr, Harborview Med Ctr; **Address:** Harborview Medical Ctr, 325 9th Ave, Box 359860, Seattle, WA 98104; **Phone:** 206-731-4191; **Board Cert:** Internal Medicine 1986; Geriatric Medicine 1992; Public Health & Genl Preventive Med 1992; **Med School:** Washington Univ, St Louis 1983; **Resid:** Internal Medicine, Michael Reese Hosp 1987; **Fellow:** Geriatric Medicine, Univ Wash Med Ctr 1990; **Fac Appt:** Asst Prof Med, Univ Wash

Reuben, David MD [Ger] - **Spec Exp:** Aging; **Hospital:** Santa Monica - UCLA Med Ctr, UCLA Med Ctr; **Address:** UCLA Sch Med, Div Geriatrics, 10945 Le Conte Ave, Ste 2339, Los Angeles, CA 90095; **Phone:** 310-206-8272; **Board Cert:** Internal Medicine 1980; Geriatric Medicine 2005; **Med School:** Emory Univ 1977; **Resid:** Internal Medicine, Rhode Island Hosp 1980; **Fellow:** Geriatric Medicine, UCLA Med Ctr 1987; **Fac Appt:** Prof Med, UCLA

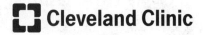
Cleveland Clinic

Geriatric Medicine

Cleveland Clinic's Section of Geriatric Medicine specializes in diagnosing and treating frail, elderly patients with complex medical conditions and social problems.

Cleveland Clinic's Section of Geriatric Medicine consists of an interdisciplinary team of health care professionals dedicated to creating comprehensive, coordinated care plans for all patients. The Section of Geriatric Medicine fulfills its "patients first" mission through clinical, educational and research activities with an emphasis on improving the quality of life of older patients. The Section of Geriatric Medicine is an integral part of Cleveland Clinic, a not-for-profit multispecialty academic medical center.

Cleveland Clinic and the Section of Geriatric Medicine offer several specialized programs to help ensure older patients receive the full scope of care necessary for optimal outcomes. These programs include:

Geriatric Evaluation and Management (GEM) Program
Cleveland Clinic's GEM Program is the cornerstone of the comprehensive care offered to older patients and their families. It takes an in-depth look at a patient's physical and psychological health, including the person's medical history, current status, recent changes and special concerns. Cleveland Clinic specialists from all disciplines are consulted as needed. After the evaluation is complete, the patient and invited family meet with the assessment team to discuss how best to care for the patient, using the most appropriate medications, therapies, community programs and other resources. The Section of Geriatric Medicine also operates a similar comprehensive Geriatric Assessment Program at Euclid Hospital, a Cleveland Clinic community hospital.

Geriatric Oncology Clinic
Cleveland Clinic's Geriatric Oncology Clinic combines the expertise of geriatricians, oncologists, nutritionists, physical therapists and other experts to ensure that older cancer patients receive the comprehensive care necessary for their special needs. Benefits of a geriatric oncology assessment include prediction of the benefits and risks of chemotherapy, prediction of the relationship of other existing medical conditions, identification of patients at higher risk of early and long-term mortality, and identification of patients most likely to benefit from physical rehabilitation.

Aging Brain Clinic
Cleveland Clinic's Aging Brain Clinic brings together a medical team that includes physicians who specialize in geriatric medicine, neurology and neurosurgery. Experts in other medical specialties, such as urology and vascular medicine, as well as professionals in social work, nutrition, psychiatry and neuropsychology, are involved as needed.

Fall Prevention Program
Cleveland Clinic's Fall Prevention Program screens inpatients and makes recommendations to help them avoid falls and the serious, sometimes life-threatening injuries that can accompany falls. Each patient is assessed by nurse specialists for risk factors that include balance, gait, cognitive impairment and muscle weakness. A pharmacist also reviews all medications to help prevent drug-related falls.

To schedule an appointment or for more information about the Cleveland Clinic Section of Geriatric Medicine, call 800.890.2467 or visit www.clevelandclinic.org/geriatrictopdocs.

Section of Geriatric Medicine | 9500 Euclid Avenue / W14 | Cleveland OH 44195

Maimonides serves one of the oldest populations in New York City, with one in ten of our patients over the age of 85. The Geriatrics Program at Maimonides is fully equipped to meet the special needs of this growing segment of the population. Directed by Barbara Paris, MD, the program encompasses inpatient and outpatient services, featuring the Acute Care for Elderly (ACE) Unit. The staff of this unit is focused on the continuity, coordination, quality and dignity of care provided.

Patient Evaluation
ACE Unit services focus on acute medical care and account for the complex needs of hospitalized elderly patients. Special attention is given to the assessment of memory loss and understanding the underlying causes of geriatric syndromes such as incontinence, falls and frailty. Psychosocial issues affecting elderly patients such as loneliness and end-of-life care are also addressed.

Wound Care
Because patients can have wounds that do not heal easily, we provide special attention through our wound care team.

Discharge & Medical Care at Home
Caregiver support groups are initiated while patients are in the hospital and are available after discharge. Once at home, if indicated, patients can receive a home visit from a member of our geriatric team, ensuring the coordination and continuity of their care.

Community & Nursing Home Liaison
The ACE Unit team serves as a bridge between hospital and community health care providers. Discharged patients are given a comprehensive plan that, if needed, includes a one-time home visit by our nurse practitioner, continued follow-up by geriatric specialists and referrals to community services. Maimonides has long established relationships with many nursing and rehabilitation facilities in Brooklyn.

Outpatient Geriatric Services
Our geriatric team offers comprehensive assessment and primary care services throughout Southern Brooklyn.

Physicians at Maimonides are among the eight percent in the US who use computers to enter patient orders, thereby reducing the risk of errors, increasing efficiency, and speeding the healing process. Maimonides has appeared on the American Hospital Association's "Most Wired" and "Most Wireless" lists more often than any other healthcare institution in the metropolitan area. Advanced technology allows our doctors to focus more attention on caring for their patients.

Maimonides Medical Center – Passionate about medicine, compassionate about people.

www.maimonidesmed.org/geriatrics

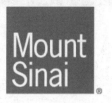

THE MOUNT SINAI MEDICAL CENTER
GERIATRICS AND ADULT DEVELOPMENT
One Gustave L. Levy Place (Fifth Avenue and 100th Street)
New York, NY 10029-6574
Physician Referral: 1-800-MD-SINAI (637-4624)
www.mountsinai.org

THE BEST IN CLINICAL CARE

In recognition of the care offered to older patients, Mount Sinai specialists are cited time and time again as the finest in the nation. In its 2007 "Best Graduate Schools" issue, *US News & World Report* ranked Mount Sinai School of Medicine at number 27 for research and ranked its geriatrics specialty second in the nation.

We offer a full spectrum of patient care, including a specialized care unit for the elderly (to minimize complications sometimes associated with an older person's hospital stay), a primary care geriatrics practice for older adults living in the community, a hospital-based consultation service for patients throughout Mount Sinai, a number of community-linked programs and partnerships, and a palliative care team dedicated to assuring quality care and support for patients and families facing serious illnesses.

The Martha Stewart Center for Living, a new modern facility designed by renowned architect I.M. Pei, provides clinical care and education for patients and serves as a training ground for physicians.

GROUNDBREAKING RESEARCH

Mount Sinai's researchers continue to advance the understanding, prevention, and treatment of age-related disorders.
The extensive research on aging conducted by the Department includes studies on health services, medical decision making and ethical dilemmas, palliative care, neurobiology of aging, and clinical interventions to promote independence in old age. The Department's expertise serves as a renowned educational resource for all Mount Sinai affiliates and other institutions in teaching geriatrics and gerontology to medical students, medical residents, geriatrics fellows, established physicians, and health profession trainees in other disciplines.

HISTORY OF EXCELLENCE

The Mount Sinai Medical Center is a pioneer in geriatric medicine. In 1909, a Mount Sinai physician coined the term "geriatrics," and in 1914, wrote the first textbook on medical care for older adults.

Today, the Brookdale Department of Geriatrics and Adult Development continues to break new ground, offering comprehensive care, disease prevention, and the promotion of healthy and productive aging. The Department's enhanced expertise in assessing and managing patients with dementia greatly complements its established, interdisciplinary approach to patient care, in which medical staff and social workers address patients' needs as a team.

THE MOUNT SINAI MEDICAL CENTER

Mount Sinai's Brookdale Department of Geriatrics and Adult Development was the first freestanding department of geriatrics established by a US medical school, and it continues to be one of the very best. It offers unparalleled inpatient and outpatient care and numerous treatment programs designed to meet the unique needs of older adults. Mount Sinai is also home to world-class researchers dedicated to advancing our understanding of Alzheimer's disease and other common geriatric conditions. At the Department's heart are our patients. The geriatricians of The Mount Sinai Medical Center work hard to improve life and longevity for New York's elderly.

865

550 First Avenue (at 31st Street)
New York, NY 10016
Physician Referral:
(888)7-NYU-MED (888-769-8633)
www.nyumc.org

GERIATRIC MEDICINE
CARING FOR THE ELDERLY

The goal of geriatrics is to keep us all-and for as long as possible- healthy, functional, and vital members of our families and communities.

NYU has a distinguished history in this increasingly important specialty, as a federally designated research center and, since 1973, a leader in the care of older patients. Finding new answers and applying them to patient care are equally important. Among NYU's accomplishments in the care of the elderly are:

• The Silberstein Aging and Dementia Research Center, one of the largest in the nation and designated a center of excellence in Alzheimer's treatment by the National Institute on Aging.

•The Belfer Geriatrics Center, a multidisciplinary approach to the care of people over 65. Geriatrics, home care, neurology, orthopedics, dentistry, geropsychiatry, and many other disciplines are available to the Center's patients, whether referred from NYU, Bellevue, or the Manhattan Veteran's Administration Hospital.

•Inpatient Geriatrics Service at NYU Hospitals Center, a team approach to inpatient care. A senior geriatrician leads the team of nurses, pharmacists, geropsychiatrists, rehabilitation experts, and fellowship trainees in caring for geriatric patients with complex conditions.

•The NYU Geriatric Falls Prevention Program, an initiative across the NYU affiliated hospitals to address this major risk to life and independence in the elderly.

NYU MEDICAL CENTER

The William and Sylvia Silberstein Aging and Dementia Research Center provides:

• comprehensive diagnostic evaluations to determine if memory loss is "normal" or more serious

• a memory enhancement program for age-related memory decline

• pharmaceutical clinical trials for mild memory loss and for Alzheimer's treatment

• state-of-the-art brain imaging techniques

• methods to prevent excess disability in Alzheimer's disease patients

• and comprehensive, on-going counseling and support groups for patients, caregivers and family members. Its longitudinal study of Alzheimer's patients is the most comprehensive ongoing study of its kind in the world.

697

Gynecologic Oncology

a subspecialty of
Obstetrics & Gynecology

An obstetrician/gynecologist who provides consultation and comprehensive management of patients with gynecologic cancer, including those diagnostic and therapeutic procedures necessary for the total care of the patient with gynecologic cancer and resulting complications.

Training Required: Four years *plus* two years in clinical practice before certification in obstetrics and gynecology is complete *plus* additional training and examination in gynecologic oncology.

Gynecologic Oncology

New England

Berkowitz, Ross S MD [GO] - **Spec Exp:** Gynecologic Cancer; **Hospital:** Brigham & Women's Hosp, Dana-Farber Cancer Inst; **Address:** Brigham & Women's Hosp, Dept OB/GYN, 75 Francis St, Boston, MA 02115-6110; **Phone:** 617-732-8843; **Board Cert:** Obstetrics & Gynecology 1981; Gynecologic Oncology 1982; **Med School:** Boston Univ 1973; **Resid:** Obstetrics & Gynecology, Boston Hosp for Women 1978; Surgery, Peter Bent Brigham Hosp 1975; **Fellow:** Gynecologic Oncology, Boston Hosp for Women 1980; **Fac Appt:** Prof ObG, Harvard Med Sch

Currie, John L MD [GO] - **Spec Exp:** Gynecologic Cancer; Pelvic Reconstruction; Gynecologic Problems of Obesity; **Hospital:** Hartford Hosp; **Address:** Hartford Hospital, 85 Seymour St Fl 7 - Ste 705, Box 5037, Hartford, CT 06106; **Phone:** 860-545-4341; **Board Cert:** Obstetrics & Gynecology 1991; Gynecologic Oncology 1982; **Med School:** Univ NC Sch Med 1967; **Resid:** Gynecologic Oncology, Hosp Univ Penn 1972; **Fellow:** Gynecologic Oncology, Duke Univ Med Ctr 1980; **Fac Appt:** Prof ObG, Univ Conn

Goodman, Annekathryn MD [GO] - **Spec Exp:** Gynecologic Cancer; Gynecologic Surgery-Complex; Acupuncture; **Hospital:** Mass Genl Hosp; **Address:** 55 Fruit St, Boston, MA 02114; **Phone:** 617-724-4800; **Board Cert:** Obstetrics & Gynecology 2003; Gynecologic Oncology 2003; **Med School:** Tufts Univ 1983; **Resid:** Obstetrics & Gynecology, Tufts New England Med Ctr 1987; **Fellow:** Gynecologic Oncology, Mass Genl Hosp 1990; **Fac Appt:** Assoc Prof ObG, Harvard Med Sch

Muto, Michael G MD [GO] - **Spec Exp:** Ovarian Cancer; Cervical Cancer; Vulvar & Vaginal Cancer; **Hospital:** Dana-Farber Cancer Inst; **Address:** Dana Farber Cancer Inst, 44 Binney St Fl 9, Boston, MA 02115; **Phone:** 617-582-7931; **Board Cert:** Gynecologic Oncology 2005; Obstetrics & Gynecology 2005; **Med School:** Univ Mass Sch Med 1983; **Resid:** Obstetrics & Gynecology, Brigham & Women's Hosp 1987; **Fellow:** Gynecologic Oncology, Brigham & Women's Hosp 1990; **Fac Appt:** Assoc Prof ObG, Harvard Med Sch

Rutherford, Thomas MD [GO] - **Spec Exp:** Ovarian Cancer; Uterine Cancer; Ovarian Cancer-Early Detection; Cervical Cancer; **Hospital:** Yale - New Haven Hosp; **Address:** Yale Univ Sch Med Dept Ob-Gyn, 333 Cedar St, Box 208063, New Haven, CT 06520; **Phone:** 203-785-6301; **Board Cert:** Obstetrics & Gynecology 1997; Gynecologic Oncology 2000; **Med School:** Med Coll OH 1989; **Resid:** Obstetrics & Gynecology, Cooper Hosp 1993; **Fellow:** Gynecologic Oncology, Yale-New Haven Hosp 1995; **Fac Appt:** Assoc Prof ObG, Yale Univ

Schwartz, Peter E MD [GO] - **Spec Exp:** Ovarian Cancer; Uterine Cancer; Gynecologic Surgery-Complex; Cervical Cancer; **Hospital:** Yale - New Haven Hosp, Hosp of St Raphael; **Address:** Yale Univ Sch Med, Dept Ob/Gyn, 333 Cedar St, rm FMB-316, New Haven, CT 06510-3289; **Phone:** 203-785-4014; **Board Cert:** Obstetrics & Gynecology 1973; Gynecologic Oncology 1979; **Med School:** Albert Einstein Coll Med 1966; **Resid:** Obstetrics & Gynecology, Yale-New Haven Hosp 1970; **Fellow:** Gynecologic Oncology, MD Anderson Cancer Ctr 1975; **Fac Appt:** Prof ObG, Yale Univ

Tarraza, Hector MD [GO] - **Spec Exp:** Gynecologic Cancer; **Hospital:** Maine Med Ctr; **Address:** 102 Campus Drive, rm 116, Scarborough, ME 04074; **Phone:** 207-883-0069; **Board Cert:** Obstetrics & Gynecology 1998; Gynecologic Oncology 1998; **Med School:** Harvard Med Sch 1981; **Resid:** Obstetrics & Gynecology, Mass Genl Hosp 1985; **Fellow:** Gynecologic Oncology, Mass Genl Hosp 1987; **Fac Appt:** Prof ObG, Univ VT Coll Med

Mid Atlantic

Abu-Rustum, Nadeem R MD [GO] - **Spec Exp:** Ovarian Cancer; Uterine Cancer; Cervical Cancer; Vulvar Disease/Cancer; **Hospital:** Meml Sloan Kettering Cancer Ctr; **Address:** Meml Sloan Kettering Cancer Ctr, 1275 York Ave, rm H-1308, New York, NY 10021; **Phone:** 212-639-7051; **Board Cert:** Obstetrics & Gynecology 1998; Gynecologic Oncology 2000; **Med School:** Lebanon 1990; **Resid:** Obstetrics & Gynecology, Greater Baltimore Med Ctr 1994; **Fellow:** Gynecologic Oncology, Meml Sloan Kettering Cancer Ctr 1997; **Fac Appt:** Assoc Prof ObG, Cornell Univ-Weill Med Coll

Barakat, Richard MD [GO] - **Spec Exp:** Laparoscopic Surgery; Ovarian Cancer; Uterine Cancer; **Hospital:** Meml Sloan Kettering Cancer Ctr; **Address:** Memorial Sloan Kettering Cancer Ctr, 1275 York Ave, rm H4135, New York, NY 10021; **Phone:** 212-639-2453; **Board Cert:** Obstetrics & Gynecology 1992; Gynecologic Oncology 1994; **Med School:** SUNY Hlth Sci Ctr 1985; **Resid:** Obstetrics & Gynecology, Bellevue Hosp 1989; **Fellow:** Gynecologic Oncology, Meml Sloan Kettering Cancer Ctr 1991; **Fac Appt:** Assoc Prof ObG, Cornell Univ-Weill Med Coll

Barnes, Willard MD [GO] - **Spec Exp:** Pelvic Tumors; Gynecologic Cancer; **Hospital:** Georgetown Univ Hosp, Virginia Hosp Ctr - Arlington; **Address:** Lombardi Cancer Ctr, Dept Gyn Oncology, 3800 Reservoir Rd NW, Washington, DC 20007-2194; **Phone:** 202-444-2114; **Board Cert:** Obstetrics & Gynecology 1997; Gynecologic Oncology 1997; **Med School:** Univ Miss 1979; **Resid:** Obstetrics & Gynecology, Univ Miss Med Ctr 1983; **Fellow:** Gynecologic Oncology, Georgetown Univ Med Ctr 1985; **Fac Appt:** Assoc Prof ObG, Georgetown Univ

Barter, James MD [GO] - **Spec Exp:** Laparoscopic Surgery; Ovarian Cancer; Gynecologic Cancer; **Hospital:** Holy Cross Hospital - Silver Spring, Suburban Hosp - Bethesda; **Address:** 6301 Executive Blvd, Rockville, MD 20852; **Phone:** 301-770-4967; **Board Cert:** Obstetrics & Gynecology 1997; Gynecologic Oncology 1997; **Med School:** Univ VA Sch Med 1977; **Resid:** Internal Medicine, Univ Kentucky Med Ctr 1979; Obstetrics & Gynecology, Duke Univ Med Ctr 1983; **Fellow:** Gynecologic Oncology, Univ Alabama 1986; **Fac Appt:** Clin Prof ObG, Georgetown Univ

Bristow, Robert E MD [GO] - **Spec Exp:** Ovarian Cancer; Cervical Cancer; Uterine Cancer; **Hospital:** Johns Hopkins Hosp - Baltimore (page 61); **Address:** Johns Hopkins Hosp, 601 Caroline St Fl 8, Baltimore, MD 21287; **Phone:** 410-955-6700; **Board Cert:** Obstetrics & Gynecology 1999; Gynecologic Oncology 2003; **Med School:** USC Sch Med 1991; **Resid:** Obstetrics & Gynecology, Johns Hopkins Hosp 1995; **Fellow:** Gynecologic Oncology, UCLA Med Ctr 1998; **Fac Appt:** Assoc Prof ObG, Johns Hopkins Univ

Caputo, Thomas A MD [GO] - **Spec Exp:** Cervical Cancer; Ovarian Cancer; Uterine Cancer; **Hospital:** NY-Presby Hosp/Weill Cornell (page 66); **Address:** 525 E 68th St, Ste J130, New York, NY 10021; **Phone:** 212-746-3179; **Board Cert:** Obstetrics & Gynecology 1993; Gynecologic Oncology 1977; **Med School:** UMDNJ-NJ Med Sch, Newark 1965; **Resid:** Obstetrics & Gynecology, Martland Hosp 1969; **Fellow:** Gynecologic Oncology, Emory Univ Hosp 1974; **Fac Appt:** Clin Prof ObG, Cornell Univ-Weill Med Coll

Gynecologic Oncology

Carlson, John A MD [GO] - **Spec Exp:** Gynecologic Cancer; Ovarian Cancer; Gynecologic Surgery-Complex; **Hospital:** St Peter's Univ Hosp; **Address:** St Peter's Univ Hosp, 254 Easton Ave, New Brunswick, NJ 08901; **Phone:** 732-937-6003; **Board Cert:** Obstetrics & Gynecology 1981; Gynecologic Oncology 1982; **Med School:** Georgetown Univ 1974; **Resid:** Obstetrics & Gynecology, Hosp Univ Penn 1978; **Fellow:** Gynecologic Oncology, MD Anderson Hosp 1980; **Fac Appt:** Prof ObG, Drexel Univ Coll Med

Chalas, Eva MD [GO] - **Spec Exp:** Gynecologic Cancer; Ovarian Cancer; Cervical Cancer; **Hospital:** Stony Brook Univ Med Ctr, Winthrop - Univ Hosp; **Address:** 1077 W Jericho Tpke, Smithtown, NY 11787; **Phone:** 631-864-5440; **Board Cert:** Obstetrics & Gynecology 2006; Gynecologic Oncology 2006; **Med School:** SUNY Stony Brook 1981; **Resid:** Obstetrics & Gynecology, Univ Hosp 1985; **Fellow:** Gynecologic Oncology, Meml Sloan Kettering Cancer Ctr 1987; **Fac Appt:** Prof ObG, SUNY Stony Brook

Cohen, Carmel MD [GO] - **Spec Exp:** Ovarian Cancer; Cervical Cancer; Pelvic Tumors; **Hospital:** NY-Presby Hosp/Columbia (page 66); **Address:** Columbia Presby Med Ctr, Div Gyn Oncol, 161 Ft Washington Ave Fl 8th - rm 837, New York, NY 10032; **Phone:** 212-305-3410; **Board Cert:** Obstetrics & Gynecology 2006; Gynecologic Oncology 2006; **Med School:** Tulane Univ 1958; **Resid:** Obstetrics & Gynecology, Mount Sinai Hosp 1964; **Fellow:** Gynecologic Oncology, Mount Sinai Hosp 1965; **Fac Appt:** Prof ObG, Columbia P&S

Curtin, John P MD [GO] - **Spec Exp:** Uterine Cancer; Ovarian Cancer; Laparoscopic Surgery; **Hospital:** NYU Med Ctr (page 67); **Address:** NYU Clinical Cancer Ctr, 160 E 34th St Fl 4, New York, NY 10016-6402; **Phone:** 212-731-5345; **Board Cert:** Obstetrics & Gynecology 1996; Gynecologic Oncology 1996; **Med School:** Creighton Univ 1979; **Resid:** Obstetrics & Gynecology, Univ Minn Med Ctr 1984; **Fellow:** Gynecologic Oncology, Meml Sloan-Kettering Cancer Ctr 1988; **Fac Appt:** Prof ObG, NYU Sch Med

Dottino, Peter R MD [GO] - **Spec Exp:** Laparoscopic Surgery; Gynecologic Cancer; **Hospital:** Mount Sinai Med Ctr, Hackensack Univ Med Ctr; **Address:** 800-A 5th Ave, Ste 405, New York, NY 10021-7215; **Phone:** 212-888-8439; **Board Cert:** Obstetrics & Gynecology 1996; Gynecologic Oncology 1996; **Med School:** Georgetown Univ 1979; **Resid:** Obstetrics & Gynecology, SUNY Downstate Med Ctr 1983; **Fellow:** Gynecologic Oncology, Mount Sinai Hosp 1985

Fishman, David A MD [GO] - **Spec Exp:** Ovarian Cancer; Ovarian Cancer-Early Detection; Gynecologic Cancer; **Hospital:** NYU Med Ctr (page 67); **Address:** NYU Clinical Cancer Ctr, 160 E 34 St Fl 4, New York, NY 10016; **Phone:** 212-731-5345; **Board Cert:** Obstetrics & Gynecology 2005; Gynecologic Oncology 2005; **Med School:** Texas Tech Univ 1988; **Resid:** Obstetrics & Gynecology, Yale-New Haven Hosp 1992; **Fellow:** Gynecologic Oncology, Yale-New Haven Hosp 1994; **Fac Appt:** Prof ObG, NYU Sch Med

Herzog, Thomas J MD [GO] - **Spec Exp:** Cervical Cancer; Gynecologic Cancer; Laparoscopic Surgery; Ovarian Cancer; **Hospital:** NY-Presby Hosp/Columbia (page 66); **Address:** Herbert Irving Pavilion, 161 Fort Washington Ave, 8-837, New York, NY 10032; **Phone:** 212-305-3410; **Board Cert:** Obstetrics & Gynecology 2006; Gynecologic Oncology 2006; **Med School:** Univ Cincinnati 1986; **Resid:** Obstetrics & Gynecology, Good Samaritan Hosp 1990; **Fellow:** Gynecologic Oncology, Barnes Jewish Hosp 1993; **Fac Appt:** Assoc Prof ObG, Columbia P&S

Kelley III, Joseph L MD [GO] - **Spec Exp:** Breast Cancer; Gynecologic Cancer; **Hospital:** Magee-Womens Hosp - UPMC; **Address:** Magee-Womens Hosp Dept OB/GYN, 300 Halket St, Pittsburgh, PA 15213; **Phone:** 412-641-5411; **Board Cert:** Obstetrics & Gynecology 2005; Gynecologic Oncology 2005; **Med School:** St Louis Univ 1985; **Resid:** Obstetrics & Gynecology, Magee-Womens Hosp 1988; **Fellow:** Gynecologic Oncology, MD Anderson Cancer Ctr 1991; **Fac Appt:** Assoc Prof ObG, Univ Pittsburgh

Morgan, Mark A MD [GO] - **Spec Exp:** Laparoscopic Surgery; Gynecologic Surgery-Complex; Gynecologic Cancer; Uro-Gynecology; **Hospital:** Fox Chase Cancer Ctr (page 59); **Address:** Fox Chase Cancer Ctr-Chief, Gyne Oncology, 333 Cottman Ave, Philadelphia, PA 19111; **Phone:** 215-214-1430; **Board Cert:** Obstetrics & Gynecology 2005; Gynecologic Oncology 2005; **Med School:** SUNY Downstate 1982; **Resid:** Obstetrics & Gynecology, Hosp Univ Penn 1986; **Fellow:** Gynecologic Oncology, Hosp Univ Penn 1988

Rosenblum, Norman G MD/PhD [GO] - **Spec Exp:** Ovarian Cancer; Uterine Cancer; Vulvar Disease/Cancer; **Hospital:** Thomas Jefferson Univ Hosp; **Address:** 834 Chesnut St, Ste 300, Philadelphia, PA 19107-5127; **Phone:** 215-955-6200; **Board Cert:** Obstetrics & Gynecology 2005; Gynecologic Oncology 2005; **Med School:** Jefferson Med Coll 1978; **Resid:** Obstetrics & Gynecology, Hosp Univ Penn 1982; **Fellow:** Gynecologic Oncology, Hosp Univ Penn 1984; **Fac Appt:** Prof ObG, Jefferson Med Coll

Rubin, Stephen C MD [GO] - **Spec Exp:** Gynecologic Cancer; Ovarian Cancer; Cervical Cancer; **Hospital:** Hosp Univ Penn - UPHS (page 72); **Address:** Hosp Univ Penn, Gynecologic Oncology, 3400 Spruce St, 1000 Courtyard Bldg, Philadelphia, PA 19104-4283; **Phone:** 215-662-3318; **Board Cert:** Obstetrics & Gynecology 2006; Gynecologic Oncology 2006; **Med School:** Univ Pennsylvania 1976; **Resid:** Obstetrics & Gynecology, Hosp Univ Penn 1980; **Fellow:** Gynecologic Oncology, Hosp Univ Penn 1982; **Fac Appt:** Prof ObG, Univ Pennsylvania

Wallach, Robert C MD [GO] - **Spec Exp:** Vulvar & Vaginal Cancer; Ovarian Cancer; Cervical Cancer; Uterine Cancer; **Hospital:** NYU Med Ctr (page 67); **Address:** NYU Clinical Cancer Ctr, 160 E 34th St, New York, NY 10016; **Phone:** 212-735-5345; **Board Cert:** Obstetrics & Gynecology 1967; Gynecologic Oncology 1974; **Med School:** Yale Univ 1960; **Resid:** Obstetrics & Gynecology, Beth Israel Med Ctr 1965; **Fellow:** Gynecologic Oncology, SUNY Downstate Med Ctr 1966; **Fac Appt:** Prof ObG, NYU Sch Med

Southeast

Alleyn, James MD [GO] - **Spec Exp:** Cervical Cancer; Ovarian Cancer; Uterine Cancer; **Hospital:** Mercy Hosp - Miami, Baptist Hosp of Miami; **Address:** 3661 S Miami Ave, Ste 308, Miami, FL 33133-4232; **Phone:** 305-854-3603; **Board Cert:** Obstetrics & Gynecology 1978; **Med School:** Indiana Univ 1972; **Resid:** Obstetrics & Gynecology, Miami-Jackson Meml Hosp 1976; **Fellow:** Gynecologic Oncology, Miami-Jackson Meml Hosp 1978; **Fac Appt:** Asst Clin Prof ObG, Univ Miami Sch Med

Alvarez, Ronald D MD [GO] - **Spec Exp:** Gynecologic Cancer; Ovarian Cancer; **Hospital:** Univ of Ala Hosp at Birmingham, Brookwood Med Ctr; **Address:** Univ Alabama, Div Gyn Oncology, 619 19th St S, OHB 538, Birmingham, AL 35249-7333; **Phone:** 205-934-4986; **Board Cert:** Obstetrics & Gynecology 2006; Gynecologic Oncology 2006; **Med School:** Louisiana State Univ 1983; **Resid:** Obstetrics & Gynecology, Univ Alabama Hosp 1987; **Fellow:** Gynecologic Oncology, Univ Alabama Hosp 1990; **Fac Appt:** Assoc Prof ObG, Univ Ala

Gynecologic Oncology

Berchuck, Andrew MD [GO] - **Spec Exp:** Ovarian Cancer; Uterine Cancer; **Hospital:** Duke Univ Med Ctr; **Address:** Duke Univ Med Center, DUMC Box 3079, Durham, NC 27710; **Phone:** 919-684-3765; **Board Cert:** Obstetrics & Gynecology 1998; Gynecologic Oncology 1998; **Med School:** Case West Res Univ 1980; **Resid:** Obstetrics & Gynecology, Case Western Resrv 1984; **Fellow:** Gynecology, UT Southwestern 1985; Gynecologic Oncology, Meml Sloan-Kettering 1987; **Fac Appt:** Prof ObG, Duke Univ

Clarke-Pearson, Daniel L MD [GO] - **Spec Exp:** Pelvic Reconstruction; Gynecologic Surgery-Complex; Gynecologic Cancer; **Hospital:** Univ NC Hosps, Wesley Long Comm Hosp; **Address:** Univ of North Carolina, CB #7570, Chapel Hill, NC 27599; **Phone:** 919-966-5280; **Board Cert:** Obstetrics & Gynecology 2006; Gynecologic Oncology 2006; **Med School:** Case West Res Univ 1975; **Resid:** Obstetrics & Gynecology, Duke Univ Med Ctr 1979; **Fellow:** Gynecologic Oncology, Duke Univ Med Ctr 1981; **Fac Appt:** Prof ObG, Univ NC Sch Med

DePriest, Paul D MD [GO] - **Spec Exp:** Ovarian Cancer-Early Detection; Cervical Cancer; Pap Smear Abnormalities; **Hospital:** Univ of Kentucky Chandler Hosp; **Address:** Univ Kentucky Med Ctr, Dept Ob/Gyn, Whiteney Hendrickson Bldg, 800 Rose St, rm 331E1, Lexington, KY 40536-0084; **Phone:** 859-323-5277; **Board Cert:** Obstetrics & Gynecology 2005; Gynecologic Oncology 2005; **Med School:** Univ KY Coll Med 1985; **Resid:** Obstetrics & Gynecology, Univ Kentucky Med Ctr 1989; **Fellow:** Gynecologic Oncology, Univ Kentucky Med Ctr 1991; **Fac Appt:** Assoc Prof ObG, Univ KY Coll Med

Finan, Michael A MD [GO] - **Spec Exp:** Ovarian Cancer; Cervical Cancer; Uterine Cancer; **Hospital:** Mobile Infirmary Med Ctr, USA Children & Women's Hospital; **Address:** 1700 Springhill Ave, Ste 100, Mobile, AL 36604; **Phone:** 251-435-1200; **Board Cert:** Obstetrics & Gynecology 2005; Gynecologic Oncology 2005; **Med School:** Louisiana State Univ 1986; **Resid:** Obstetrics & Gynecology, Univ South Fla Affil Hosps 1990; **Fellow:** Gynecologic Oncology, H Lee Moffitt Cancer Ctr 1992; **Fac Appt:** Prof ObG, Univ S Ala Coll Med

Fiorica, James V MD [GO] - **Spec Exp:** Gynecologic Cancer; Breast Cancer; Cervical Cancer; **Hospital:** Sarasota Meml Hosp; **Address:** 118 Hillview St, Sarasota, FL 34239; **Phone:** 941-917-8383; **Board Cert:** Obstetrics & Gynecology 2005; Gynecologic Oncology 2005; **Med School:** Tufts Univ 1982; **Resid:** Obstetrics & Gynecology, Univ South Fla Affil Hosp 1986; **Fellow:** Gynecologic Oncology, Univ South Fla Affil Hosp 1989; Breast Disease, Tufts Univ 1990; **Fac Appt:** Clin Prof ObG, Univ S Fla Coll Med

Fowler Jr, Wesley C MD [GO] - **Spec Exp:** Vulvar Disease/Cancer; DES-Exposed Females; **Hospital:** Univ NC Hosps; **Address:** U NC Chapel Hill, Div of Ob/Gyn, Campus Box 7570, Chapel Hill, NC 27599-7570; **Phone:** 919-966-1196; **Board Cert:** Obstetrics & Gynecology 1991; Gynecologic Oncology 1979; **Med School:** Univ NC Sch Med 1966; **Resid:** Obstetrics & Gynecology, NC Memorial Hosp 1971; **Fac Appt:** Prof ObG, Univ NC Sch Med

Horowitz, Ira R MD [GO] - **Spec Exp:** Laparoscopic Surgery; Ovarian Cancer; Cervical Cancer; **Hospital:** Emory Univ Hosp, Crawford Long Hosp of Emory Univ; **Address:** Emory Clinic, 1365 Clifton Rd NE A Bldg Fl 4, Atlanta, GA 30322; **Phone:** 404-778-4416; **Board Cert:** Obstetrics & Gynecology 1997; Gynecologic Oncology 1997; **Med School:** Baylor Coll Med 1980; **Resid:** Obstetrics & Gynecology, Baylor Coll Med 1984; **Fellow:** Gynecologic Oncology, Johns Hopkins Hosp 1987; **Fac Appt:** Prof ObG, Emory Univ

Jones III, Howard Wilbur MD [GO] - **Spec Exp:** Pap Smear Abnormalities; Cervical Cancer; Uterine Cancer; **Hospital:** Vanderbilt Univ Med Ctr; **Address:** Vanderbilt Univ Med Ctr, Medical Center North, rm B1100, Nashville, TN 37232-2519; **Phone:** 615-322-2114; **Board Cert:** Obstetrics & Gynecology 1999; Gynecologic Oncology 1999; **Med School:** Duke Univ 1968; **Resid:** Obstetrics & Gynecology, Univ Colo Med Ctr 1972; **Fellow:** Gynecologic Oncology, Univ Tex-MD Anderson Hosp 1974; **Fac Appt:** Prof ObG, Vanderbilt Univ

Kohler, Matthew MD [GO] - **Spec Exp:** Pelvic Reconstruction; **Hospital:** MUSC Med Ctr; **Address:** MUSC Med Ctr- Women's Hlth Ob/Gyn, 96 Jonathan Lucas St, Box 250619, Charleston, SC 29425; **Phone:** 843-792-9300; **Board Cert:** Obstetrics & Gynecology 1995; Gynecologic Oncology 1997; **Med School:** Duke Univ 1987; **Resid:** Obstetrics & Gynecology, Duke University Med Ctr 1991; **Fellow:** Gynecologic Oncology, Duke University Med Ctr 1993; **Fac Appt:** Assoc Prof ObG, Med Univ SC

Lancaster, Johnathan M MD/PhD [GO] - **Spec Exp:** Ovarian Cancer; Cancer Genetics; Genee Therapy; **Hospital:** H Lee Moffitt Cancer Ctr & Research Inst; **Address:** H Lee Moffitt Cancer Ctr - Gyn Oncology, 12902 Magnolia Drive, Tampa, FL 33612; **Phone:** 813-745-7272; **Board Cert:** Obstetrics & Gynecology 2005; **Med School:** Wales 1992; **Resid:** Obstetrics & Gynecology, Duke Univ Med Ctr 2000; **Fellow:** Gynecologic Oncology, Duke Univ Med Ctr 2003; **Fac Appt:** Asst Prof ObG, Univ S Fla Coll Med

Partridge, Edward E MD [GO] - **Spec Exp:** Ovarian Cancer; **Hospital:** Univ of Ala Hosp at Birmingham; **Address:** Univ Alabama, Div Gyn Oncology, 619 19th St S, OHB 538, Birmingham, AL 35249-7333; **Phone:** 205-934-4986; **Board Cert:** Obstetrics & Gynecology 1993; Gynecologic Oncology 1981; **Med School:** Univ Ala 1973; **Resid:** Obstetrics & Gynecology, Univ Alabama Hosp 1977; **Fellow:** Gynecologic Oncology, Univ Alabama Hosp 1979; **Fac Appt:** Prof ObG, Univ Ala

Penalver, Manuel A MD [GO] - **Spec Exp:** Gynecologic Cancer; Cervical Cancer; Pelvic Tumors; **Hospital:** Doctors' Hosp, Baptist Hosp of Miami; **Address:** South Florida Gyn Oncology, 5000 University Drive, Ste 3300, Coral Gables, FL 33146; **Phone:** 305-663-7001; **Board Cert:** Obstetrics & Gynecology 1997; Gynecologic Oncology 1997; **Med School:** Univ Miami Sch Med 1977; **Resid:** Obstetrics & Gynecology, Univ Miami/Jackson Meml Hosp 1982; **Fellow:** Gynecologic Oncology, Univ Miami/Jackson Meml Hosp 1984

Poliakoff, Steven MD [GO] - **Spec Exp:** Ovarian Cancer; Minimally Invasive Surgery; Cancer Genetics; **Hospital:** Mount Sinai Med Ctr - Miami, South Miami Hosp; **Address:** 6280 Sunset Dr, Ste 502, South Miami, FL 33143-4870; **Phone:** 305-596-0870; **Board Cert:** Obstetrics & Gynecology 1983; **Med School:** Univ NC Sch Med 1975; **Resid:** Obstetrics & Gynecology, Johns Hopkins Hosp 1979; **Fellow:** Gynecologic Oncology, Jackson Meml Hosp/Univ Miami 1981

Rice, Laurel W MD [GO] - **Spec Exp:** Ovarian Cancer; Uterine Cancer; Cervical Cancer; **Hospital:** Univ Virginia Med Ctr; **Address:** UVA Health System, Div Gyn-Onc, PO Box 800712, Charlottesville, VA 22908; **Phone:** 434-924-5100; **Board Cert:** Obstetrics & Gynecology 2005; Gynecologic Oncology 2005; **Med School:** Univ Colorado 1983; **Resid:** Obstetrics & Gynecology, Brigham-Womens Hosp 1987; **Fellow:** Obstetrics & Gynecology, Brigham-Womens Hosp 1989; **Fac Appt:** Assoc Prof ObG, Univ VA Sch Med

Gynecologic Oncology

Soper, John T MD [GO] - **Spec Exp:** Gynecologic Cancer; **Hospital:** Univ NC Hosps; **Address:** Univ North Carolina, Dept OB/GYN, 5017 Old Clinic Bldg, Chapel Hill, NC 27599; **Phone:** 919-966-1194; **Board Cert:** Obstetrics & Gynecology 1996; Gynecologic Oncology 1996; **Med School:** Univ Iowa Coll Med 1978; **Resid:** Obstetrics & Gynecology, Univ Utah Med Ctr 1982; **Fellow:** Gynecologic Oncology, Duke Univ Med Ctr 1985; **Fac Appt:** Prof ObG, Univ NC Sch Med

Spann Jr, Cyril O MD [GO] - **Spec Exp:** Gynecologic Cancer; Ovarian Cancer; **Hospital:** Emory Univ Hosp; **Address:** Emory Clinic Crawford Long, 550 Peachtree St, Ste 900, Atlanta, GA 30308; **Phone:** 404-616-3540; **Board Cert:** Obstetrics & Gynecology 2005; Gynecologic Oncology 2005; **Med School:** Meharry Med Coll 1981; **Resid:** Obstetrics & Gynecology, Emory Univ Med Ctr 1985; **Fellow:** Gynecologic Oncology, Univ NC Meml Hosp 1989; **Fac Appt:** Prof ObG, Emory Univ

Taylor Jr, Peyton T MD [GO] - **Spec Exp:** Gynecologic Surgery-Complex; Gynecologic Cancer; **Hospital:** Univ Virginia Med Ctr; **Address:** Univ VA Hlth Sys, Dept Ob/Gyn, PO Box 800712, Charlottesville, VA 22908; **Phone:** 434-924-9933; **Board Cert:** Obstetrics & Gynecology 1994; Gynecologic Oncology 1981; **Med School:** Univ Ala 1968; **Resid:** Obstetrics & Gynecology, Univ VA Hosp 1970; Obstetrics & Gynecology, Univ VA Hosp 1975; **Fellow:** Surgical Oncology, Natl Cancer Inst 1972; Gynecologic Oncology, Univ Va Hosp 1977; **Fac Appt:** Prof ObG, Univ VA Sch Med

Van Nagell Jr, John R MD [GO] - **Spec Exp:** Ovarian Cancer; Cervical Cancer; **Hospital:** Univ of Kentucky Chandler Hosp; **Address:** UKMC, Dept Ob/Gyn, 800 Rose St, Lexington, KY 40536-0001; **Phone:** 859-323-5553; **Board Cert:** Obstetrics & Gynecology 1973; Gynecologic Oncology 1976; **Med School:** Univ Pennsylvania 1967; **Resid:** Obstetrics & Gynecology, Kentucky Med Ctr 1971; **Fac Appt:** Prof ObG, Univ KY Coll Med

Midwest

Belinson, Jerome L MD [GO] - **Spec Exp:** Ovarian Cancer; Cervical Cancer; **Hospital:** Cleveland Clin Fdn (page 57); **Address:** 9500 Euclid Ave, Desk A81, Cleveland, OH 44195; **Phone:** 216-444-7933; **Board Cert:** Obstetrics & Gynecology 1998; Gynecologic Oncology 1980; **Med School:** Univ MO-Columbia Sch Med 1968; **Resid:** Obstetrics & Gynecology, Columbia Presby Med Ctr 1973; **Fellow:** Gynecologic Oncology, Jackson Meml Hosp 1977; **Fac Appt:** Prof ObG, Ohio State Univ

Copeland, Larry J MD [GO] - **Spec Exp:** Ovarian Cancer; Uterine Cancer; Gynecologic Cancer; **Hospital:** Arthur G James Cancer Hosp & Research Inst, Ohio St Univ Med Ctr; **Address:** 1654 Upham Drive, Ste 505, Columbus, OH 43210-1250; **Phone:** 614-293-8697; **Board Cert:** Obstetrics & Gynecology 1991; Gynecologic Oncology 1981; **Med School:** Univ Western Ontario 1973; **Resid:** Obstetrics & Gynecology, McMaster Univ Affil Hosps 1977; **Fellow:** Gynecologic Oncology, MD Anderson Cancer Ctr-Univ Tex 1979; **Fac Appt:** Prof ObG, Ohio State Univ

De Geest, Koen MD [GO] - **Spec Exp:** Ovarian Cancer; Cervical Cancer; Clinical Trials; **Hospital:** Univ Iowa Hosp & Clinics; **Address:** Univ Iowa, Div Gynecological Oncology, 200 Hawkins Drive, rm 4630 JCP, Iowa City, IA 52242; **Phone:** 319-356-2015; **Board Cert:** Obstetrics & Gynecology 1997; Gynecologic Oncology 1997; **Med School:** Belgium 1977; **Resid:** Obstetrics & Gynecology, Univ Ghent 1982; **Fellow:** Gynecologic Oncology, Penn State/Hershey Med Ctr 1990; **Fac Appt:** Prof ObG, Univ Iowa Coll Med

Johnston, Carolyn Marie MD [GO] - **Spec Exp:** Gynecologic Surgery-Complex; **Hospital:** Univ Michigan Hlth Sys; **Address:** Womens Hosp-Div Gyn Onc, 1500 E Med Ctr Drive, rm L4510, Ann Arbor, MI 48109-0276; **Phone:** 734-647-8906; **Board Cert:** Obstetrics & Gynecology 2000; Gynecologic Oncology 2000; **Med School:** Yale Univ 1984; **Resid:** Obstetrics & Gynecology, Univ Chicago Hosp 1988; **Fellow:** Gynecologic Oncology, Mt Sinai Hosp 1990; **Fac Appt:** Assoc Clin Prof ObG, Univ Mich Med Sch

Kim, Woo Shin MD [GO] - **Spec Exp:** Ovarian Cancer; Uterine Cancer; Gestational Trophoblastic Disease; **Hospital:** Henry Ford Hosp; **Address:** 3031 W Grand Blvd, Ste 800, Detroit, MI 48202-2608; **Phone:** 313-916-2465; **Board Cert:** Obstetrics & Gynecology 1977; Gynecologic Oncology 1979; **Med School:** South Korea 1966; **Resid:** Obstetrics & Gynecology, Boston City Hosp 1973; **Fellow:** Gynecologic Oncology, Meml Sloan-Kettering Cancer Ctr 1976; **Fac Appt:** Assoc Clin Prof ObG, Wayne State Univ

Look, Katherine Y MD [GO] - **Spec Exp:** Ovarian Cancer; Uterine Cancer; **Hospital:** Indiana Univ Hosp, Methodist Hosp - Indianapolis; **Address:** 535 Barnhill Drive, Ste 434, Indianapolis, IN 46202; **Phone:** 317-274-2130; **Board Cert:** Obstetrics & Gynecology 2005; Gynecologic Oncology 2005; **Med School:** Univ Mich Med Sch 1979; **Resid:** Obstetrics & Gynecology, Univ Illinois Med Ctr 1983; **Fellow:** Gynecologic Oncology, Meml Sloan Kettering Cancer Ctr 1986; **Fac Appt:** Prof ObG, Indiana Univ

Lurain, John R MD [GO] - **Spec Exp:** Gestational Trophoblastic Disease; Uterine Cancer; Ovarian Cancer; **Hospital:** Northwestern Meml Hosp; **Address:** Northwestern Univ Feinberg Sch Med, 333 E Superior St, Chicago, IL 60611-3056; **Phone:** 312-926-7365; **Board Cert:** Obstetrics & Gynecology 1977; Gynecologic Oncology 1981; **Med School:** Univ NC Sch Med 1972; **Resid:** Obstetrics & Gynecology, Univ Pittsburgh Med Ctr 1975; **Fellow:** Gynecologic Oncology, Roswell Park Cancer Inst 1979; **Fac Appt:** Prof ObG, Northwestern Univ

Mutch, David MD [GO] - **Spec Exp:** Gynecologic Cancer; Pelvic Reconstruction; **Hospital:** Barnes-Jewish Hosp; **Address:** 4911 Barnes Jewish Hospital Plaza, St. Louis, MO 63110; **Phone:** 314-362-3181; **Board Cert:** Obstetrics & Gynecology 2003; Gynecologic Oncology 2003; **Med School:** Washington Univ, St Louis 1980; **Resid:** Obstetrics & Gynecology, Barnes Hosp-Wash Univ 1984; **Fellow:** Gynecologic Oncology, Duke Univ Med Ctr 1987; **Fac Appt:** Prof ObG, Washington Univ, St Louis

Podratz, Karl C MD/PhD [GO] - **Spec Exp:** Pelvic Tumors; **Hospital:** Mayo Med Ctr & Clin - Rochester; **Address:** Mayo Clinic SW, 200 1st St SW, Rochester, MN 55905-0001; **Phone:** 507-266-7712; **Board Cert:** Obstetrics & Gynecology 1993; Gynecologic Oncology 1993; **Med School:** St Louis Univ 1974; **Resid:** Obstetrics & Gynecology, Univ Chicago Hosps 1977; **Fellow:** Gynecologic Oncology, Mayo Clinic 1979; **Fac Appt:** Prof ObG, Mayo Med Sch

Potkul, Ronald MD [GO] - **Spec Exp:** Ovarian Cancer; Cervical Cancer; **Hospital:** Loyola Univ Med Ctr, Elmhurst Meml Hosp; **Address:** Loyola Univ Med Ctr, 2160 S 1st Ave Bldg 112 - rm 267, Maywood, IL 60153; **Phone:** 708-327-3500; **Board Cert:** Obstetrics & Gynecology 1997; Gynecologic Oncology 1997; **Med School:** Univ Chicago-Pritzker Sch Med 1981; **Resid:** Obstetrics & Gynecology, Univ Chicago Hosps 1985; **Fellow:** Gynecologic Oncology, Georgetown Univ 1988; **Fac Appt:** Prof ObG, Loyola Univ-Stritch Sch Med

Gynecologic Oncology

Reynolds, R Kevin MD [GO] - **Hospital:** Univ Michigan Hlth Sys; **Address:** Women's Hosp, Div Gyn Onc, 1500 E Med Ctr Drive, rm L4510, Ann Arbor, MI 48109-0276; **Phone:** 734-764-9106; **Board Cert:** Obstetrics & Gynecology 1998; Gynecologic Oncology 1994; **Med School:** Univ New Mexico 1982; **Resid:** Obstetrics & Gynecology, Univ Vt Hosp 1986; **Fellow:** Gynecologic Oncology, Univ Mich Med Ctr 1991; **Fac Appt:** Asst Prof ObG, Univ Mich Med Sch

Rose, Peter G MD [GO] - **Spec Exp:** Cervical Cancer; Ovarian Cancer; **Hospital:** Cleveland Clin Fdn (page 57), MetroHealth Med Ctr; **Address:** Cleveland Clinic Fdn, 9500 Euclid Ave A-81, Cleveland, OH 44195; **Phone:** 216-444-1712; **Board Cert:** Obstetrics & Gynecology 1999; Gynecologic Oncology 1990; **Med School:** Boston Univ 1981; **Resid:** Surgery, Vanderbilt Med Ctr 1983; Obstetrics & Gynecology, Ohio State Univ Med Ctr 1986; **Fellow:** Gynecologic Oncology, Roswell Park Med Ctr 1988; **Fac Appt:** Prof ObG, Case West Res Univ

Rotmensch, Jacob MD [GO] - **Spec Exp:** Gynecologic Cancer; Ovarian Cancer; Cervical Cancer; **Hospital:** Rush Univ Med Ctr; **Address:** Gyn Oncology Assocs, 1725 W Harrison St, Ste 842, Chicago, IL 60612; **Phone:** 312-942-6300; **Board Cert:** Obstetrics & Gynecology 1986; Gynecologic Oncology 1990; **Med School:** Meharry Med Coll 1977; **Resid:** Obstetrics & Gynecology, Johns Hopkins Hosp 1981; **Fellow:** Gynecologic Oncology, Johns Hopkins Hosp 1984; **Fac Appt:** Prof ObG, Rush Med Coll

Schink, Julian C MD [GO] - **Spec Exp:** Ovarian Cancer; **Hospital:** Northwestern Meml Hosp; **Address:** 675 N St Clair St, Fl 21 - Ste 100, Chicago, IL 60611; **Phone:** 312-695-0990; **Board Cert:** Obstetrics & Gynecology 2000; Gynecologic Oncology 2000; **Med School:** Univ Tex, San Antonio 1982; **Resid:** Obstetrics & Gynecology, Northwestern Univ Med Sch 1986; **Fellow:** Gynecologic Oncology, UCLA Med Ctr 1988; **Fac Appt:** Prof ObG, Northwestern Univ

Smith, Donna Marie MD [GO] - **Spec Exp:** Cervical Cancer; Ovarian Cancer; **Hospital:** Loyola Univ Med Ctr; **Address:** Cardinal Bernardin Cancer Ctr, Clinic A, 2160 S 1st Ave Bldg 112 - rm 267, Maywood, IL 60153; **Phone:** 708-327-3500; **Board Cert:** Obstetrics & Gynecology 1997; Gynecologic Oncology 1997; **Med School:** Univ MO-Kansas City 1980; **Resid:** Obstetrics & Gynecology, Emory Univ Hosp 1984; **Fellow:** Gynecologic Oncology, Georgetown Univ Med Ctr 1987; **Fac Appt:** Assoc Prof ObG, Loyola Univ-Stritch Sch Med

Stehman, Frederick B MD [GO] - **Spec Exp:** Clinical Trials; Gynecologic Cancer; **Hospital:** Indiana Univ Hosp, Wishard Hlth Srvs; **Address:** Indiana Univ Hosp, Dept ObGyn, 550 N University Blvd, rm 2440, Indianapolis, IN 46202; **Phone:** 317-274-8609; **Board Cert:** Obstetrics & Gynecology 2005; Gynecologic Oncology 2003; **Med School:** Univ Mich Med Sch 1972; **Resid:** Obstetrics & Gynecology, Univ Kansas Med Ctr 1975; Surgery, Univ Kansas Med Ctr 1977; **Fellow:** Gynecologic Oncology, UCLA Med Ctr 1979; **Fac Appt:** Prof ObG, Indiana Univ

Waggoner, Steven MD [GO] - **Spec Exp:** Ovarian Cancer; Cervical Cancer; Uterine Cancer; **Hospital:** Univ Hosps Case Med Ctr; **Address:** Dept Ob/Gyn, Div Gyn Oncology, 11100 Euclid Ave, MC 5034, Cleveland, OH 44106; **Phone:** 216-844-3954; **Board Cert:** Obstetrics & Gynecology 2002; Gynecologic Oncology 2002; **Med School:** Univ Wash 1984; **Resid:** Obstetrics & Gynecology, Univ Chicago Hosps 1988; **Fellow:** Gynecologic Oncology, Georgetown Univ 1991; **Fac Appt:** Prof ObG, Case West Res Univ

Great Plains and Mountains

Davidson, Susan MD [GO] - **Spec Exp:** Gynecologic Cancer; **Hospital:** Univ Colorado Hosp; **Address:** Univ Colorado Hosp, Dept OB/GYN, 4200 E Ninth Ave, Box B198, Denver, CO 80262; **Phone:** 303-315-7897; **Board Cert:** Obstetrics & Gynecology 2005; Gynecologic Oncology 2005; **Med School:** Univ Tex, San Antonio 1984; **Resid:** Obstetrics & Gynecology, Univ Texas Med Ctr 1988; **Fellow:** Gynecologic Oncology, Meml Sloan Kettering Cancer Ctr 1990; **Fac Appt:** Assoc Prof ObG, Univ Colorado

Remmenga, Steven W MD [GO] - **Spec Exp:** Ovarian Cancer; **Hospital:** Nebraska Med Ctr; **Address:** Univ NE Med Ctr, Dept Ob/Gyn, 983255 NE Med Ctr, Omaha, NE 68198; **Phone:** 402-559-5068; **Board Cert:** Obstetrics & Gynecology 1998; Gynecologic Oncology 1998; **Med School:** Univ Nebr Coll Med 1981; **Resid:** Obstetrics & Gynecology, Naval Hospital 1986; **Fellow:** Gynecologic Oncology, Walter Reed Army Med Ctr 1990; **Fac Appt:** Assoc Prof ObG, Univ Nebr Coll Med

Soisson, Andrew MD [GO] - **Spec Exp:** Cervical Cancer; **Hospital:** LDS Hosp, Univ Utah Hosps and Clins; **Address:** Univ Utah, Div Gyn Oncology, 1950 Circle of Hope, Salt Lake City, UT 84112; **Phone:** 801-585-0100; **Board Cert:** Obstetrics & Gynecology 2002; Gynecologic Oncology 2002; **Med School:** Georgetown Univ 1981; **Resid:** Obstetrics & Gynecology, Madigan AMC 1985; **Fellow:** Gynecologic Oncology, Duke Univ Med Ctr 1990; **Fac Appt:** Assoc Prof ObG, Univ Utah

Southwest

Chambers, Setsuko K MD [GO] - **Spec Exp:** Gynecologic Cancer; Breast Cancer; Ovarian Cancer; **Hospital:** Univ Med Ctr - Tucson; **Address:** 1515 N Campbell Ave, rm 1968, Tucson, AZ 85724; **Phone:** 520-626-9285; **Board Cert:** Obstetrics & Gynecology 1997; Gynecologic Oncology 1997; **Med School:** Brown Univ 1980; **Resid:** Obstetrics & Gynecology, Yale-New Haven Hosp 1984; **Fellow:** Gynecologic Oncology, Yale-New Haven Hosp 1986; **Fac Appt:** Prof ObG, Univ Ariz Coll Med

Follen-Mitchell, Michele MD/PhD [GO] - **Spec Exp:** Gynecologic Cancer; Clinical Trials; **Hospital:** UT MD Anderson Cancer Ctr (page 71); **Address:** MD Anderson Cancer Ctr, 1515 Holcombe Blvd, Unit 193, Houston, TX 77030; **Phone:** 713-745-2564; **Board Cert:** Obstetrics & Gynecology 1999; Gynecologic Oncology 1999; **Med School:** Univ Mich Med Sch 1980; **Resid:** Obstetrics & Gynecology, Columbia-Presby Med Ctr 1983; **Fellow:** Gynecologic Oncology, MD Anderson Cancer Ctr 1986; **Fac Appt:** Prof ObG, Univ Tex, Houston

Gershenson, David M MD [GO] - **Spec Exp:** Ovarian Cancer & Borderline Tumors; Peritoneal Carcinomatosis; Fertility Preservation in Cancer; **Hospital:** UT MD Anderson Cancer Ctr (page 71), St Luke's Episcopal Hosp - Houston; **Address:** Univ Tex MD Anderson Cancer Ctr, PO Box 301439, Houston, TX 77030-1439; **Phone:** 713-745-2565; **Board Cert:** Obstetrics & Gynecology 1991; Gynecologic Oncology 1981; **Med School:** Vanderbilt Univ 1971; **Resid:** Obstetrics & Gynecology, Yale-New Haven Hosp 1975; **Fellow:** Gynecologic Oncology, MD Anderson Cancer Ctr 1979

Hatch, Kenneth MD [GO] - **Spec Exp:** Cervical Cancer; Uro-Gynecology; Pelvic Organ Prolapse; **Hospital:** Univ Med Ctr - Tucson, NW Med Ctr; **Address:** Univ Arizona College of Medicine, 1515 N Campbell Ave, rm 1968, Tucson, AZ 85724; **Phone:** 520-626-9285; **Board Cert:** Obstetrics & Gynecology 1993; Gynecologic Oncology 1981; **Med School:** Univ Nebr Coll Med 1971; **Resid:** Obstetrics & Gynecology, Univ AL Med Ctr Birmingham 1976; **Fellow:** Gynecologic Oncology, Univ AL Med Ctr Birmingham 1978; **Fac Appt:** Prof ObG, Univ Ariz Coll Med

Gynecologic Oncology

Magrina, Javier MD [GO] - **Spec Exp:** Gynecologic Cancer; Endometriosis; Hysterectomy Alternatives; Robotic Surgery; **Hospital:** Mayo Clin Hosp - Scottsdale; **Address:** Mayo Clinic, 13400 E Shea Blvd, Scottsdale, AZ 85259-5404; **Phone:** 480-342-2668; **Board Cert:** Obstetrics & Gynecology 1994; Gynecologic Oncology 1982; **Med School:** Spain 1972; **Resid:** Obstetrics & Gynecology, Mayo Clinic 1977; **Fellow:** Gynecologic Oncology, Kansas Med Ctr 1980; **Fac Appt:** Prof ObG, Mayo Med Sch

Roman-Lopez, Juan J MD [GO] - **Spec Exp:** Vulvar Disease/Cancer; Bladder Problems Post-Hysterectomy; Gynecologic Cancer; **Hospital:** UAMS Med Ctr; **Address:** 4301 W Markham St, Slot 793, Little Rock, AR 72205-7199; **Phone:** 501-296-1099; **Board Cert:** Obstetrics & Gynecology 1971; **Med School:** Univ Puerto Rico 1963; **Resid:** Obstetrics & Gynecology, San Juan City Hosp 1967; Obstetrics & Gynecology, Tulane-Charity Hosp 1969; **Fellow:** Gynecologic Oncology, Tulane-LSU Med Ctr 1970; **Fac Appt:** Assoc Clin Prof ObG, Univ Ark

Smith, Harriet O MD [GO] - **Spec Exp:** Uterine Cancer; Pelvic Reconstruction; Ovarian Cancer; **Hospital:** Univ NM Hlth & Sci Ctr; **Address:** 1 University of New Mexico NE, MS 105580, Albuquerque, NM 87131; **Phone:** 505-272-3392; **Board Cert:** Obstetrics & Gynecology 1995; Gynecologic Oncology 2005; **Med School:** Med Coll GA 1981; **Resid:** Obstetrics & Gynecology, Med Coll Georgia 1985; Gynecologic Oncology, MD Anderson 1988; **Fellow:** Reconstructive Pelvic Surgery, Emory Univ Hosp 1989; Gynecologic Oncology, Albert Einstein Coll Med 1990; **Fac Appt:** Prof ObG, Univ New Mexico

West Coast and Pacific

Berek, Jonathan S MD [GO] - **Spec Exp:** Ovarian Cancer; Uterine Cancer; Cervical Cancer; **Hospital:** Stanford Univ Med Ctr; **Address:** Stanford Univ School of Medicine, 300 Pasteur Dr, HH333, Stanford, CA 94305-5317; **Phone:** 650-498-5618; **Board Cert:** Obstetrics & Gynecology 2005; Gynecologic Oncology 2005; **Med School:** Johns Hopkins Univ 1975; **Resid:** Obstetrics & Gynecology, Brigham & Womans Hosp 1979; **Fellow:** Gynecologic Oncology, UCLA Sch Med 1981; **Fac Appt:** Prof ObG, Stanford Univ

Berman, Michael L MD [GO] - **Spec Exp:** Gynecologic Cancer; **Hospital:** UC Irvine Med Ctr, Long Beach Meml Med Ctr; **Address:** Cho Family Comprehensive Cancer Ctr, 101 The City Drive Bldg 56 - Ste 260, Orange, CA 92868-3201; **Phone:** 714-456-8020; **Board Cert:** Obstetrics & Gynecology 2005; Gynecologic Oncology 2005; **Med School:** Geo Wash Univ 1967; **Resid:** Obstetrics & Gynecology, GW Univ Hosp 1969; Obstetrics & Gynecology, Los Angeles Co-Harbor 1974; **Fellow:** Gynecologic Oncology, UCLA Med Ctr 1976; **Fac Appt:** Prof ObG, UC Irvine

Cain, Joanna MD [GO] - **Spec Exp:** Ovarian Cancer; Breast Cancer Risk Assessment; Uterine Cancer; Ovarian Cancer-Early Detection; **Hospital:** OR Hlth & Sci Univ; **Address:** 3181 SW Sam Jackson Park Rd, MC L-466, Portland, OR 97239; **Phone:** 503-494-2999; **Board Cert:** Obstetrics & Gynecology 2005; Gynecologic Oncology 2005; **Med School:** Creighton Univ 1978; **Resid:** Obstetrics & Gynecology, Univ Washington Med Ctr 1981; **Fellow:** Gynecologic Oncology, Meml Sloan Kettering Cancer Ctr 1983; **Fac Appt:** Prof ObG, Oregon Hlth Sci Univ

Goff, Barbara MD [GO] - **Spec Exp:** Ovarian Cancer; Uterine Cancer; Cervical Cancer; **Hospital:** Univ Wash Med Ctr; **Address:** Univ Washington, Dept ObGyn, Box 356460, Seattle, WA 98195; **Phone:** 206-543-3669; **Board Cert:** Obstetrics & Gynecology 2004; Gynecologic Oncology 2004; **Med School:** Univ Pennsylvania 1986; **Resid:** Obstetrics & Gynecology, Mass Genl Hosp/Brigham & Womens Hosp 1990; **Fellow:** Gynecologic Oncology, Mass Genl Hosp 1993; **Fac Appt:** Assoc Prof ObG, Univ Wash

Greer, Benjamin MD [GO] - **Spec Exp:** Gynecologic Cancer; **Hospital:** Univ Wash Med Ctr; **Address:** Univ Wash, Dept OB/GYN, Box 356460, Seattle, WA 98195; **Phone:** 206-543-3669; **Board Cert:** Obstetrics & Gynecology 2002; Gynecologic Oncology 2002; **Med School:** Univ Pennsylvania 1966; **Resid:** Obstetrics & Gynecology, Univ Colorado Med Ctr 1970; **Fac Appt:** Prof ObG, Univ Wash

Karlan, Beth Young MD [GO] - **Spec Exp:** Ovarian Cancer; Gynecologic Cancer; **Hospital:** Cedars-Sinai Med Ctr, UCLA Med Ctr; **Address:** 8700 Beverly Blvd, Ste 290W, Los Angeles, CA 90048; **Phone:** 310-423-3302; **Board Cert:** Obstetrics & Gynecology 1998; Gynecologic Oncology 1998; **Med School:** Harvard Med Sch 1982; **Resid:** Obstetrics & Gynecology, Yale-New Haven Hosp 1986; **Fellow:** Gynecologic Oncology, UCLA Med Sch 1989; **Fac Appt:** Prof ObG, UCLA

Powell, Catherine Bethan MD [GO] - **Spec Exp:** Gynecologic Cancer; Cancer Genetics; Complementary Medicine; **Hospital:** UCSF - Mt Zion Med Ctr; **Address:** UCSF Comp Cancer Ctr, 1600 Divisadero St Fl 4, San Francisco, CA 94143; **Phone:** 415-353-9838; **Board Cert:** Obstetrics & Gynecology 2005; Gynecologic Oncology 2005; **Med School:** Univ Pennsylvania 1982; **Resid:** Obstetrics & Gynecology, Pennsylvania Hosp 1987; **Fellow:** Gynecologic Oncology, Wash Univ 1990; **Fac Appt:** Asst Clin Prof ObG, UCSF

Smith, Lloyd H MD [GO] - **Spec Exp:** Ovarian Cancer; Uterine Cancer; Vulvar Disease/Cancer; Vaginal Cancer; **Hospital:** UC Davis Med Ctr, Sutter Mem Hospital - Sacramento; **Address:** UC Davis Med Ctr, Dept Ob/Gyn, 4860 Y St, Ste 2500, Sacramento, CA 95817; **Phone:** 916-734-6946; **Board Cert:** Obstetrics & Gynecology 1998; Gynecologic Oncology 1998; **Med School:** UC Davis 1981; **Resid:** Obstetrics & Gynecology, UC Davis Med Ctr 1985; **Fellow:** Gynecologic Oncology, Stanford Univ Hosp 1988; **Fac Appt:** Prof ObG, UC Davis

Spirtos, Nicola Michael MD [GO] - **Spec Exp:** Gynecologic Cancer; Ovarian Cancer; **Hospital:** Univ Med Ctr - Las Vegas; **Address:** 3131 La Canada St, Ste 110, Las Vegas, NV 89109; **Phone:** 650-988-8421; **Board Cert:** Obstetrics & Gynecology 1998; Gynecologic Oncology 1998; **Med School:** Northwestern Univ 1980; **Resid:** Obstetrics & Gynecology, Women's Hosp LAC-USC Med Ctr 1984; **Fellow:** Gynecologic Oncology, Stanford Univ 1987

Stern, Jeffrey L MD [GO] - **Spec Exp:** Laparoscopic Surgery; Vulvar Disease/Cancer; **Hospital:** Alta Bates Summit Med Ctr; **Address:** Womens Cancer Ctr Northern Calif, 2500 Malvia St, Ste 224, Berkley, CA 94704; **Phone:** 510-540-8235; **Board Cert:** Obstetrics & Gynecology 1983; Gynecologic Oncology 1984; **Med School:** SUNY Upstate Med Univ 1976; **Resid:** Obstetrics & Gynecology, Johns Hopkins Hosp 1980; **Fellow:** Gynecologic Oncology, USC Med Ctr 1982

Teng, Nelson NH MD/PhD [GO] - **Spec Exp:** Ovarian Cancer; Clinical Trials; **Hospital:** Stanford Univ Med Ctr; **Address:** Stanford Univ Sch Med, Dept Gyn Oncology, 300 Pasteur Drive, Ste HH333, Stanford, CA 94305-5317; **Phone:** 650-498-8080; **Board Cert:** Obstetrics & Gynecology 1985; Gynecologic Oncology 1987; **Med School:** Univ Miami Sch Med 1977; **Resid:** Obstetrics & Gynecology, UCLA Med Ctr 1981; **Fellow:** Gynecologic Oncology, Stanford Univ Sch Med 1984; **Fac Appt:** Assoc Prof ObG, Stanford Univ

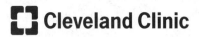

Obstetrics and Gynecology

Reproductive Endocrinology and Infertility
Our Reproductive Endocrinology and Infertility Program involves close collaboration among male and female infertility specialists, andrologists and embryologists, as well as our colleagues in the Minimally Invasive Surgery Center. Cleveland Clinic reproductive surgeons were among the first to routinely remove advanced endometriosis laparoscopically. Many procedures today are performed with robotic assistance.

Urogynecology and Reconstructive Pelvic Surgery
This Center offers cutting-edge and traditional surgery for urinary incontinence and pelvic organ prolapse, along with medical and behavioral therapy

Center for Female Pelvic Medicine and Reconstructive Surgery
Cleveland Clinic urogynecologists established the Center for Female Pelvic Medicine and Reconstructive Surgery in conjunction with Cleveland Clinic urologists and colo-rectal surgeons. The sub specialists on this team treat incontinence and prolapse via the abdominal, vaginal and laparoscopic routes.

Maternal-Fetal Medicine/Obstetrics
Cleveland Clinic maternal-fetal medicine specialists provide overall management of complicated pregnancies, beginning with genetic counseling for high-risk patients.

The Fetal Care Center
The Fetal Care Center involves a multidisciplinary team of perinatologists, neonatologists, pediatric surgeons and other specialists. Through collaboration and communication, we provide prenatal diagnosis using state-of-the-art techniques such as high-resolution ultrasound, fetal MRI and fetoscopy. We then apply this information as we develop a management plan for pregnancy, delivery and newborn care.

Menstrual Disorders, Fibroids and Hysteroscopic Services
This Center offers unified and streamlined consultations, workups and treatment for menstrual dysfunction and uterine fibroids in the least invasive manner, so as to preserve a woman's reproductive potential.

Gynecologic Oncology
Our gynecologic oncologists have garnered national and international recognition for expertise in complex reproductive cancers, clinical and basic research, and preventive oncology. Cleveland Clinic gynecologists were among the first to treat early cervical and endometrial cancers laparoscopically. In performing less invasive surgical procedures, we always weigh curative potential against preservation of fertility. We offer oocyte, embryo and ovarian tissue cryopreservation for cancer patients.

Women's Health Center
The Cleveland Clinic Women's Health Center offers a full range of specialized women's health services in one location. We manage menopause, hormone therapy, vulvar disorders, and premenstrual dysthymic disorder and hormonally exacerbated. We offer evaluation and treatment for women with urinary incontinence, osteoporosis or breast concerns. Breast specialists evaluate and treat breast cancer as well as benign breast disease in our center.

To schedule an appointment or for more information about Cleveland Clinic Department of Obstetrics and Gynecology call 800.890.2467 or visit www.clevelandclinic.org/obgyntopdocs

Department of Obstetrics and Gynecology | 9500 Euclid Avenue / W14 | Cleveland OH 44195

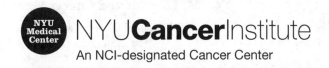

GYNECOLOGIC ONCOLOGY

Over 1,200 new patients come from around the world each year to M. D. Anderson's Gynecologic Oncology Center which specializes in diagnosis, early detection, prevention and treatment of cancers of the vagina, cervix, uterus, ovaries, vulva and fallopian tubes.

ROBOTIC AND MINIMALLY INVASIVE SURGERY

Advanced technology in the hands of cancer experts gives patients the best opportunity for a positive outcome. The DaVinci Robot is one of the latest additions to our surgical artillery against cancer. Our surgeons use laparoscopic, harmonic scalpel, and endoscopic surgical techniques to maximize outcomes. As a result, patients experience less bleeding, less scarring and pain, and enjoy faster recovery and return to normal activities.
M. D. Anderson cancer surgeons use minimally invasive surgery to treat gynecologic cancers as well as prostate, lung, and head and neck cancers.

MORE INFORMATION
For more information or to make an appointment, call 877-MDA-6789, or visit us online at http://www.mdanderson.org.

838

Sponsored Page

Hand Surgery

a subspecialty of Orthopaedics, Surgery or Plastic Surgery

A specialist trained in the investigation, preservation and restoration by medical, surgical and rehabilitative means of all structures of the upper extremity directly affecting the form and function of the hand and wrist.

For more information about the mentioned specialties or those physicians, see **Orthopaedic Surgery, Surgery** or **Plastic Surgery** section(s).

Training Required: Five years (including general surgery) in orthopaedics *plus* two years in clinical practice before final certification is achieved *plus* additional training and examination in hand surgery OR five to seven years in plastic surgery *plus* additional training and examination in hand surgery.

Hand Surgery

New England

Akelman, Edward MD [HS] - **Spec Exp:** Carpal Tunnel Syndrome; Arthritis; Wrist/Hand Injuries; **Hospital:** Rhode Island Hosp; **Address:** 2 Dudley St, Ste 200, Providence, RI 02905; **Phone:** 401-457-1510; **Board Cert:** Orthopaedic Surgery 1998; Hand Surgery 1998; **Med School:** Dartmouth Med Sch 1978; **Resid:** Surgery, Peter Bent Brigham Hosp 1980; Orthopaedic Surgery, Yale-New Haven Hosp 1984; **Fellow:** Hand Surgery, Roosevelt Hosp 1985; **Fac Appt:** Prof OrS, Brown Univ

Belsky, Mark R MD [HS] - **Spec Exp:** Arthritis; Nerve Disorders/Surgery; Elbow Surgery; **Hospital:** Newton - Wellesley Hosp; **Address:** 2000 Washington St, Green - Ste 563, Newton, MA 02462-1629; **Phone:** 617-965-4263; **Board Cert:** Orthopaedic Surgery 1982; Hand Surgery 2001; **Med School:** Tufts Univ 1974; **Resid:** Surgery, Peter Bent Brigham Hosp 1976; Orthopaedic Surgery, Tufts-New England Med Ctr 1979; **Fellow:** Hand Surgery, Roosevelt Hosp 1980; **Fac Appt:** Clin Prof OrS, Tufts Univ

Sampson, Christian E MD [HS] - **Spec Exp:** Hand Injuries; Hand & Fingers Vascular Surgery; **Hospital:** Brigham & Women's Hosp; **Address:** Brigham & Women's Hosp, Div Plastic Surg, 75 Francis St, Boston, MA 02115; **Phone:** 617-732-6297; **Board Cert:** Plastic Surgery 2004; Hand Surgery 2003; **Med School:** Boston Univ 1986; **Resid:** Surgery, Boston Univ Med Ctr 1991; Plastic Surgery, Brigham & Women's Hosp 1993; **Fellow:** Hand Surgery, Roosevelt Hosp 1994

Waters, Peter Michael MD [HS] - **Spec Exp:** Brachial Plexus Palsy; Hand-Congenital Anomaly; **Hospital:** Children's Hospital - Boston; **Address:** Chldns Hosp, Dept Ortho Surg, 300 Longwood Ave, Hunnewell - 2, Boston, MA 02115-5724; **Phone:** 617-355-6021; **Board Cert:** Orthopaedic Surgery 2001; Hand Surgery 2004; **Med School:** Tufts Univ 1981; **Resid:** Pediatrics, Mass Genl Hosp 1983; Orthopaedic Surgery, Harvard Combined Prog 1988; **Fellow:** Hand Surgery, Brigham/Chldns Hosp 1989; **Fac Appt:** Assoc Prof OrS, Harvard Med Sch

Weiss, Arnold P MD [HS] - **Spec Exp:** Carpal Tunnel Syndrome; Wrist Surgery; Elbow Replacement; **Hospital:** Rhode Island Hosp; **Address:** Univ Orthopedics Inc, 2 Dudley St, Ste 200, Providence, RI 02905-3248; **Phone:** 401-457-1520; **Board Cert:** Orthopaedic Surgery 2004; Hand Surgery 2004; **Med School:** Johns Hopkins Univ 1985; **Resid:** Orthopaedic Surgery, Johns Hopkins Hosp 1990; **Fellow:** Hand Surgery, Indiana Hand Ctr 1991; **Fac Appt:** Prof OrS, Brown Univ

Mid Atlantic

Athanasian, Edward MD [HS] - **Spec Exp:** Bone & Soft Tissue Tumors; Hand & Upper Extremity Tumors; Hand & Upper Extremity Fractures; **Hospital:** Hosp For Special Surgery (page 60), Meml Sloan Kettering Cancer Ctr; **Address:** Hospital for Special Surgery, 535 E 72th St, New York, NY 10021; **Phone:** 212-606-1962; **Board Cert:** Orthopaedic Surgery 1997; Hand Surgery 1999; **Med School:** Columbia P&S 1988; **Resid:** Surgery, Beth Israel Hosp 1989; Orthopaedic Surgery, Hosp Special Surgery 1993; **Fellow:** Hand Surgery, Mayo Clinic 1994; Orthopaedic Oncology, Meml Sloan Kettering Cancer Ctr 1995; **Fac Appt:** Asst Prof OrS, Cornell Univ-Weill Med Coll

Culp, Randall MD [HS] - **Spec Exp:** Microsurgery; Hand & Upper Extremity Surgery; **Hospital:** Thomas Jefferson Univ Hosp; **Address:** 700 S Henderson Rd, Ste 200, King of Prussia, PA 19406; **Phone:** 610-768-4474; **Board Cert:** Orthopaedic Surgery 2001; Hand Surgery 2001; **Med School:** Penn State Univ-Hershey Med Ctr 1982; **Resid:** Orthopaedic Surgery, Hosp Univ Penn 1987; **Fellow:** Hand Surgery, Hosp Univ Penn 1988; **Fac Appt:** Assoc Prof OrS, Jefferson Med Coll

Glickel, Steven MD [HS] - **Spec Exp:** Hand & Wrist Surgery; Elbow Surgery; Peripheral Nerve Surgery; **Hospital:** St Luke's - Roosevelt Hosp Ctr - Roosevelt Div; **Address:** 1000 10th Ave Fl 3, New York, NY 10019-1147; **Phone:** 212-523-7590; **Board Cert:** Orthopaedic Surgery 1985; Hand Surgery 2000; **Med School:** Harvard Med Sch 1976; **Resid:** Surgery, Columbia Presby Hosp 1978; Orthopaedic Surgery, Harvard Comb Ortho 1981; **Fellow:** Hand Surgery, St Luke's-Roosevelt Hosp Ctr 1983; Research, Columbia Presby Hosp 1982; **Fac Appt:** Assoc Clin Prof OrS, Columbia P&S

Graham, Thomas J MD [HS] - **Spec Exp:** Hand & Wrist Surgery; Elbow Surgery; Sports Injuries; Wrist/Hand Injuries; **Hospital:** Union Meml Hosp - Baltimore; **Address:** Curtis National Hand Ctr, 3333 N Calvert St Fl 2, Baltimore, MD 21218; **Phone:** 410-235-5405; **Board Cert:** Orthopaedic Surgery 1996; Hand Surgery 1997; **Med School:** Univ Cincinnati 1988; **Resid:** Orthopaedic Surgery, Univ Michigan Med Ctr 1993; **Fellow:** Hand Surgery, Indiana Hand Ctr 1994; Elbow Surgery, Mayo Clinic 1994; **Fac Appt:** Assoc Clin Prof OrS, Johns Hopkins Univ

Imbriglia, Joseph E MD [HS] - **Spec Exp:** Arthritis; Carpal Tunnel Syndrome; Shoulder Surgery; **Hospital:** UPMC Passavant-Cranberry, UPMC Passavant; **Address:** 6001 Stonewood Drive, Wexford, PA 15090-7380; **Phone:** 724-933-3850; **Board Cert:** Orthopaedic Surgery 1977; Hand Surgery 2000; **Med School:** Hahnemann Univ 1970; **Resid:** Surgery, Univ Pittsburgh Med Ctr 1972; Orthopaedic Surgery, Columbia Presby Med Ctr 1975; **Fellow:** Hand Surgery, Columbia Presby Med Ctr 1976; **Fac Appt:** Clin Prof OrS, Univ Pittsburgh

Kozin, Scott H MD [HS] - **Spec Exp:** Congenital Hand Deformities; Brachial Plexus Palsy-Pediatric; Spinal Cord Injury-Pediatric; **Hospital:** Philadelphia Shriners Hosp; **Address:** Shriners Hosp for Children, 3551 N Broad St, Philadelphia, PA 19140; **Phone:** 215-430-4074; **Board Cert:** Orthopaedic Surgery 2005; Hand Surgery 2005; **Med School:** Hahnemann Univ 1986; **Resid:** Orthopaedic Surgery, Albert Einstein Med Ctr 1991; **Fellow:** Hand Surgery, Mayo Clinic 1992; **Fac Appt:** Assoc Prof OrS, Temple Univ

Kulick, Roy G MD [HS] - **Spec Exp:** Carpal Tunnel Syndrome; Arthritis; Tendon Surgery; **Hospital:** Montefiore Med Ctr - Weiler-Einstein Div, Westchester Med Ctr; **Address:** The Tower at Montefiore Medical Park, 1695 Eastchester Rd, Bronx, NY 10461; **Phone:** 718-920-2060; **Board Cert:** Orthopaedic Surgery 1980; Hand Surgery 2001; **Med School:** Cornell Univ-Weill Med Coll 1973; **Resid:** Surgery, St Lukes-Roosevelt Hosp 1975; Orthopaedic Surgery, Columbia Presbyterian Hosp 1978; **Fellow:** Hand Surgery, Hosp for Special Surgery 1979; **Fac Appt:** Assoc Prof OrS, Albert Einstein Coll Med

Lane, Lewis B MD [HS] - **Spec Exp:** Carpal Tunnel Syndrome; Arthritis; Sports Injuries; **Hospital:** N Shore Univ Hosp at Manhasset, St Francis Hosp - The Heart Ctr (page 70); **Address:** 600 Northern Blvd, Ste 300, Great Neck, NY 11021; **Phone:** 516-627-8717; **Board Cert:** Orthopaedic Surgery 1981; Hand Surgery 2000; **Med School:** Columbia P&S 1974; **Resid:** Surgery, NY Hosp 1975; Orthopaedic Surgery, Hosp for Special Surg 1979; **Fellow:** Research, Hosp for Special Surg 1976; Hand Surgery, St Luke's-Roosevelt Hosp Ctr 1980; **Fac Appt:** Assoc Clin Prof OrS, Albert Einstein Coll Med

Hand Surgery

Lee, W P Andrew MD [HS] - **Spec Exp:** Reconstructive Surgery; Cartilage Damage; Transplant-Hand; Pediatric Hand Surgery; **Hospital:** UPMC Presby, Pittsburgh, Chldns Hosp of Pittsburgh - UPMC; **Address:** Univ Pittsburgh, Scaife Hall 6B, 3550 Terrace St, Pittsburgh, PA 15261; **Phone:** 412-648-9670; **Board Cert:** Hand Surgery 1996; Plastic Surgery 1995; **Med School:** Johns Hopkins Univ 1983; **Resid:** Surgery, Johns Hopkins Univ Hosp 1989; Plastic Surgery, Mass General Hosp 1991; **Fellow:** Microsurgery, Johns Hopkins Hosp 1987; Hand Surgery, Indiana Hand Ctr 1993; **Fac Appt:** Prof S, Univ Pittsburgh

Lubahn, John D MD [HS] - **Spec Exp:** Microsurgery; **Hospital:** Hamot Med Ctr, St Vincent Hlth Ctr; **Address:** 300 State St, Ste 205, Erie, PA 16507; **Phone:** 814-456-6022; **Board Cert:** Orthopaedic Surgery 1992; Hand Surgery 1998; **Med School:** Case West Res Univ 1975; **Resid:** Surgery, Univ Rochester Med Ctr 1977; Orthopaedic Surgery, Univ Rochester Med Ctr 1980; **Fellow:** Hand Surgery, Univ Louisville Hosp 1981

Melone Jr, Charles P MD [HS] - **Spec Exp:** Arthritis; Wrist Surgery; Fractures; **Hospital:** Beth Israel Med Ctr - Petrie Division; **Address:** 321 E 34th St, New York, NY 10016; **Phone:** 212-340-0000; **Board Cert:** Orthopaedic Surgery 1976; Hand Surgery 2004; **Med School:** Georgetown Univ 1969; **Resid:** Surgery, Nassau Co Med Ctr 1971; Orthopaedic Surgery, Nassau Co Med Ctr 1974; **Fellow:** Hand Surgery, NYU Med Ctr 1975; **Fac Appt:** Clin Prof OrS, Albert Einstein Coll Med

Osterman Jr, A Lee MD [HS] - **Spec Exp:** Upper Extremity Surgery; Wrist Surgery; Neuromuscular Disorders; **Hospital:** Thomas Jefferson Univ Hosp, Chldns Hosp of Philadelphia, The; **Address:** Philadelphia Hand Ctr, 700 S Henderson Rd, Ste 200, King of Prussia, PA 19406-4207; **Phone:** 610-265-3135; **Board Cert:** Orthopaedic Surgery 1980; Hand Surgery 2001; **Med School:** Univ Pennsylvania 1973; **Resid:** Orthopaedic Surgery, Hosp Univ Penn 1978; **Fellow:** Hand Surgery, Hosp Univ Penn 1979; Microvascular Surgery, Duke Univ Med Ctr 1980; **Fac Appt:** Prof OrS, Jefferson Med Coll

Patel, Mukund MD [HS] - **Spec Exp:** Arthritis; Carpal Tunnel Syndrome; Fractures; **Hospital:** Long Island Coll Hosp, Richmond Univ Med Ctr; **Address:** Comprehensive Hand Surgery, 4901 Fort Hamilton Pkwy, Brooklyn, NY 11219; **Phone:** 718-435-4944; **Board Cert:** Orthopaedic Surgery 1972; Hand Surgery 2000; **Med School:** India 1967; **Resid:** Orthopaedic Surgery, Maimonides Med Ctr 1970; **Fellow:** Hand Surgery, Mass Genl Hosp 1971; **Fac Appt:** Assoc Clin Prof S, SUNY Hlth Sci Ctr

Raskin, Keith MD [HS] - **Spec Exp:** Wrist/Hand Injuries; Arthritis; Carpal Tunnel Syndrome; **Hospital:** NYU Med Ctr (page 67), Hosp For Joint Diseases (page 68); **Address:** 317 E 34th St, Fl 3, New York, NY 10016; **Phone:** 212-263-4263; **Board Cert:** Orthopaedic Surgery 2002; Hand Surgery 2002; **Med School:** Geo Wash Univ 1983; **Resid:** Orthopaedic Surgery, NYU Med Ctr 1988; **Fellow:** Hand Surgery, Union Mem Hosp 1989; **Fac Appt:** Assoc Clin Prof OrS, NYU Sch Med

Rosenwasser, Melvin MD [HS] - **Spec Exp:** Carpal Tunnel Syndrome; Hand Surgery; Sports Medicine-Hand; Elbow Surgery; **Hospital:** NY-Presby Hosp/Columbia (page 66); **Address:** 622 W 168th St, PH 11, rm 1119, New York, NY 10032; **Phone:** 212-305-4565; **Board Cert:** Orthopaedic Surgery 1999; Hand Surgery 1999; **Med School:** Columbia P&S 1976; **Resid:** Surgery, Roosevelt Hosp 1979; Orthopaedic Surgery, Columbia Presby Hosp 1982; **Fellow:** Hand Surgery, Columbia Presby Hosp 1983; **Fac Appt:** Prof OrS, Columbia P&S

Strauch, Robert MD [HS] - **Spec Exp:** Hand Reconstruction; Hand & Elbow Nerve Disorders; Hand & Wrist Injuries; Elbow Surgery; **Hospital:** NY-Presby Hosp/Columbia (page 66); **Address:** 622 W 168th St, rm PH-11, New York, NY 10032; **Phone:** 212-305-4272; **Board Cert:** Orthopaedic Surgery 2005; Hand Surgery 2005; **Med School:** Columbia P&S 1986; **Resid:** Orthopaedic Surgery, Columbia-Presby Hosp 1991; **Fellow:** Hand Surgery, Indiana Hand Center 1992; **Fac Appt:** Assoc Prof OrS, Columbia P&S

Weiland, Andrew J MD [HS] - **Spec Exp:** Wrist/Hand Injuries; Hand Reconstruction; **Hospital:** Hosp For Special Surgery (page 60), NY-Presby Hosp/Weill Cornell (page 66); **Address:** 535 E 70th St, New York, NY 10021-4872; **Phone:** 212-606-1575; **Board Cert:** Hand Surgery 1989; Orthopaedic Surgery 1992; **Med School:** Wake Forest Univ 1968; **Resid:** Surgery, Univ Michigan Med Ctr 1970; Orthopaedic Surgery, Johns Hopkins Hosp 1975; **Fellow:** Hand Surgery, Kleinert Hosp 1975; **Fac Appt:** Prof OrS, Cornell Univ-Weill Med Coll

Wolfe, Scott W MD [HS] - **Spec Exp:** Wrist Surgery; Nerve Disorders/Surgery; Fractures; **Hospital:** Hosp For Special Surgery (page 60), St Vincent's Med Ctr - Bridgeport; **Address:** Hand & Upper Extremity Surgery, 535 E 70 St, New York, NY 10021; **Phone:** 212-606-1529; **Board Cert:** Orthopaedic Surgery 2003; Hand Surgery 2003; **Med School:** Cornell Univ-Weill Med Coll 1984; **Resid:** Orthopaedic Surgery, Hosp Special Surg 1989; **Fellow:** Hand & Microvascular Surgery, Columbia Presby Med Ctr 1990; **Fac Appt:** Prof OrS, Cornell Univ-Weill Med Coll

Southeast

Breidenbach, Warren C MD [HS] - **Spec Exp:** Transplant-Hand; **Hospital:** Jewish Hosp HlthCre Svcs Inc; **Address:** 225 Abraham Flexner Way, Ste 700, Louisville, KY 40202; **Phone:** 502-561-4263; **Board Cert:** Plastic Surgery 1988; Hand Surgery 1992; **Med School:** Univ Calgary 1975; **Resid:** Plastic Surgery, McGill Univ 1982; **Fellow:** Microsurgery, Eastern Va Med Sch 1982; Hand Surgery, Univ Med Ctr 1983; **Fac Appt:** Asst Clin Prof PlS, Univ Louisville Sch Med

Carneiro, Ronaldo D S MD [HS] - **Spec Exp:** Carpal Tunnel Syndrome; Wrist Surgery; Arthritis; **Hospital:** Physicians Regl Med Ctr; **Address:** 6101 Pine Ridge Rd, Naples, FL 34119-3900; **Phone:** 239-348-4040; **Board Cert:** Plastic Surgery 1990; Hand Surgery 1994; **Med School:** Brazil 1970; **Resid:** Surgery, Union Meml Hosp 1975; Plastic Surgery, Allentown & Sacred Heart Hosp Ctr 1977; **Fellow:** Hand Surgery, Jackson Meml Hosp-Univ Miami Hosp 1977; Plastic Surgery, Univ Miami Sch Med 1978; **Fac Appt:** Assoc Clin Prof PlS, Univ S Fla Coll Med

Greene, Thomas L MD [HS] - **Spec Exp:** Arthritis; Peripheral Nerve Surgery; Arthroscopic Surgery; Tendon Surgery; **Hospital:** Tampa Genl Hosp, St Joseph's Hosp - Tampa; **Address:** 2727 W Dr Martin Luther King Jr Blvd, Ste 560, Tampa, FL 33607-6009; **Phone:** 813-873-0337; **Board Cert:** Orthopaedic Surgery 1983; Hand Surgery 2000; **Med School:** Ohio State Univ 1975; **Resid:** Surgery, Univ Michigan Med Ctr 1977; Orthopaedic Surgery, Univ Michigan Med Ctr 1980; **Fellow:** Hand Surgery, St Vincent's Hosp 1981

Hunt III, Thomas R MD [HS] - **Spec Exp:** Hand & Wrist Surgery; Hand & Wrist Sports Injuries; Arthritis; **Hospital:** Univ of Ala Hosp at Birmingham; **Address:** Univ of Alabama Hosp, Div Ortho Surg, 510 20th St S FOT Bldg - Ste 930, Birmingham, AL 35294-3409; **Phone:** 205-996-2688; **Board Cert:** Orthopaedic Surgery 2006; Hand Surgery 2006; **Med School:** Vanderbilt Univ 1986; **Resid:** Orthopaedic Surgery, Univ Kansas Med Ctr 1992; **Fellow:** Hand Surgery, Hosp Univ Penn 1993; **Fac Appt:** Prof S, Univ Ala

Hand Surgery

Koman, L Andrew MD [HS] - **Spec Exp:** Pediatric Hand Surgery; Vascular Disorders-Upper Extremity; Pain-Nerve Injury; **Hospital:** Wake Forest Univ Baptist Med Ctr (page 73); **Address:** WFU Hlth Sci, Medical Center Blvd, Dept Orthopaedic Surgery, Winston-Salem, NC 27157-1070; **Phone:** 336-716-8094; **Board Cert:** Orthopaedic Surgery 1981; Hand Surgery 2000; **Med School:** Duke Univ 1974; **Resid:** Surgery, Duke Univ Med Ctr. 1975; Orthopaedic Surgery, Duke Univ Med Ctr. 1979; **Fellow:** Hand Surgery, Duke Univ Med Ctr 1980; **Fac Appt:** Prof OrS, Wake Forest Univ

Tsai, Tsu Min MD [HS] - **Spec Exp:** Microsurgery; Carpal Tunnel Syndrome; Cubital Tunnel Syndrome; **Hospital:** Jewish Hosp HlthCre Svcs Inc, Univ of Louisville Hosp; **Address:** 225 Abraham Flexner Way, Ste 800, Louisville, KY 40202-1846; **Phone:** 502-561-4246; **Board Cert:** Orthopaedic Surgery 1984; Hand Surgery 2001; **Med School:** Taiwan 1961; **Resid:** Surgery, Natl Taiwan Univ Hosp 1970; Orthopaedic Surgery, Univ Louisville Hosp 1979; **Fellow:** Hand Surgery, Univ Louisville Hosp 1976; **Fac Appt:** Clin Prof OrS, Univ Louisville Sch Med

Midwest

Bishop, Allen T MD [HS] - **Spec Exp:** Microsurgery; Brachial Plexus Palsy; **Hospital:** Mayo Med Ctr & Clin - Rochester; **Address:** Mayo Clinic, Div Hand Surgery, 200 First St SW, Rochester, MN 55905; **Phone:** 507-284-4149; **Board Cert:** Orthopaedic Surgery 2000; Hand Surgery 2000; **Med School:** Mayo Med Sch 1981; **Resid:** Orthopaedic Surgery, Mayo Clinic 1986; **Fellow:** Hand Surgery, St Vincent Hosp 1987; **Fac Appt:** Prof OrS, Mayo Med Sch

Carroll, Charles MD [HS] - **Spec Exp:** Carpal Tunnel Syndrome; Upper Extremity Surgery; Shoulder & Elbow Surgery; **Hospital:** Northwestern Meml Hosp, Evanston NW Hlthcare; **Address:** 676 N St Clair, Ste 450, Chicago, IL 60611-2983; **Phone:** 312-943-7850; **Board Cert:** Orthopaedic Surgery 2001; Hand Surgery 2001; **Med School:** Univ MD Sch Med 1982; **Resid:** Surgery, Johns Hopkins Hosp 1984; Orthopaedic Surgery, Johns Hopkins Hosp 1987; **Fellow:** Hand Surgery, Indiana Univ Med Ctr 1988; Shoulder Surgery, Univ Western Ontario 1988; **Fac Appt:** Assoc Clin Prof OrS, Northwestern Univ

Chung, Kevin Chi MD [HS] - **Spec Exp:** Reconstructive Surgery; Hand & Microvascular Surgery; Upper Extremity Trauma; Nail Surgery; **Hospital:** Univ Michigan Hlth Sys; **Address:** University of Michigan, 2130 Taubman Health Ctr, 1500 E Medical Ctr Drive, Box 0340, Ann Arbor, MI 48109; **Phone:** 734-936-5885; **Board Cert:** Hand Surgery 1997; Plastic Surgery 1997; **Med School:** Emory Univ 1987; **Resid:** Plastic Surgery, Univ Michigan Hosp & Hlth Ctr 1994; Hand Surgery, Union Meml Hosp 1995; **Fac Appt:** Assoc Prof S, Univ Mich Med Sch

Cohen, Mark S MD [HS] - **Spec Exp:** Hand Surgery; Wrist Surgery; Elbow Surgery; **Hospital:** Rush Univ Med Ctr; **Address:** 1725 W Harrison St, Ste 1063, Chicago, IL 60612-3841; **Phone:** 312-243-4244; **Board Cert:** Orthopaedic Surgery 2006; Hand Surgery 2006; **Med School:** Harvard Med Sch 1986; **Resid:** Orthopaedic Surgery, UCSD Med Ctr 1992; **Fellow:** Hand Surgery, Indiana Hand Ctr 1993; **Fac Appt:** Prof OrS, Rush Med Coll

Derman, Gordon Harris MD [HS] - **Spec Exp:** Carpal Tunnel Syndrome; Tendon Surgery; Repetitive Motion Injuries; Nerve Disorders/Surgery; **Hospital:** Rush Univ Med Ctr, Evanston NW Hlthcare; **Address:** 1725 W Harrison St, Ste 740, Chicago, IL 60612; **Phone:** 312-432-9200; **Board Cert:** Plastic Surgery 1984; Hand Surgery 1996; **Med School:** Rush Med Coll 1975; **Resid:** Surgery, Loyola Univ Med Ctr 1981; Plastic Surgery, Univ Mich Hosp 1983; **Fellow:** Microsurgery, Rush/Presby St Luke's Med Ctr 1976; **Fac Appt:** Asst Prof S, Rush Med Coll

Failla, Joseph M MD [HS] - **Spec Exp:** Hand Surgery; Hand Reconstruction; **Hospital:** Providence Hosp - Southfield, Huron Valley-Sinai Hosp; **Address:** Farmbrook Med Complex One Bldg - Ste 201, 29829 Telegraph Rd, Southfield, MI 48034; **Phone:** 248-352-4263; **Board Cert:** Orthopaedic Surgery 2001; Hand Surgery 2001; **Med School:** SUNY Buffalo 1982; **Resid:** Orthopaedic Surgery, SUNY-Buffalo 1987; **Fellow:** Hand Surgery, Mayo Clinic 1988

Fischer, Thomas J MD [HS] - **Spec Exp:** Microsurgery; Elbow Reconstruction; **Hospital:** St Vincent Hosp & Hlth Svcs - Indianapolis, Methodist Hosp - Indianapolis; **Address:** 8501 Harcourt Rd, Indianapolis, IN 46280-0434; **Phone:** 317-875-9105; **Board Cert:** Orthopaedic Surgery 2000; Hand Surgery 2000; **Med School:** Indiana Univ 1979; **Resid:** Orthopaedic Surgery, Univ Wash Affil Hosp 1984; **Fellow:** Hand Surgery, Hand Surg Assocs 1985; Hand Surgery, Duke Univ Med Ctr; **Fac Appt:** Assoc Clin Prof OrS, Indiana Univ

Gelberman, Richard MD [HS] - **Spec Exp:** Tendon Surgery; Peripheral Nerve Surgery; **Hospital:** Barnes-Jewish Hosp; **Address:** Wash Univ Sch Med, Dept Ortho Surg, 660 S Euclid Ave, Box 8233, St Louis, MO 63110; **Phone:** 314-747-2500; **Board Cert:** Orthopaedic Surgery 1997; Hand Surgery 1996; **Med School:** Univ Tenn Coll Med, Memphis 1969; **Resid:** Surgery, Univ Wisc Med Ctr 1975; **Fellow:** Hand Surgery, Duke Univ Med Ctr 1977; Pediatric Orthopaedic Surgery, Chldns Hosp-Harvard 1986; **Fac Appt:** Prof OrS, Washington Univ, St Louis

Hastings II, Hill MD [HS] - **Spec Exp:** Wrist Surgery; Elbow Reconstruction; Fractures & Tendon Transfers; Arthritis; **Hospital:** St Vincent Hosp & Hlth Svcs - Indianapolis; **Address:** 8501 Harcourt Rd, Indianapolis, IN 46280-0434; **Phone:** 317-875-9105; **Board Cert:** Orthopaedic Surgery 1982; Hand Surgery 2000; **Med School:** USC Sch Med 1974; **Resid:** Surgery, Univ Colorado Med Ctr 1976; Orthopaedic Surgery, Mass Genl Hosp 1980; **Fellow:** Hand Surgery, St Vincent Hosp 1981; **Fac Appt:** Clin Prof OrS, Indiana Univ

Idler, Richard S MD [HS] - **Spec Exp:** Upper Extremity Surgery; **Hospital:** St Vincent Hosp & Hlth Svcs - Indianapolis, Indiana Univ Hosp; **Address:** 8501 Harcourt Rd, Indianapolis, IN 46260; **Phone:** 317-875-9105; **Board Cert:** Orthopaedic Surgery 1985; Hand Surgery 2000; **Med School:** Dartmouth Med Sch 1975; **Resid:** Surgery, UCLA Med Ctr 1977; Plastic Surgery, UCLA Med Ctr 1978; **Fellow:** Orthopaedic Surgery, Mass Genl Hosp-Harvard 1981; Hand Surgery, St Vincent Hosp 1982; **Fac Appt:** Asst Clin Prof OrS, Indiana Univ

Kleinman, William B MD [HS] - **Spec Exp:** Arthritis; Congenital Hand Deformities; **Hospital:** St Vincent Hosp & Hlth Svcs - Indianapolis; **Address:** 8501 Harcourt Rd, Indianapolis, IN 46280; **Phone:** 317-875-9105; **Board Cert:** Orthopaedic Surgery 1979; Hand Surgery 2000; **Med School:** Cornell Univ-Weill Med Coll 1972; **Resid:** Surgery, Univ Colorado 1974; Orthopaedic Surgery, NY Orthopaedic Hosp/Columbia 1977; **Fellow:** Hand Surgery, Columbia-Presby Med Ctr 1978; Microvascular Surgery, Duke Univ; **Fac Appt:** Clin Prof OrS, Indiana Univ

Light, Terry MD [HS] - **Spec Exp:** Hand-Congenital Anomaly; Hand Injuries-Pediatric; Arthritis; **Hospital:** Loyola Univ Med Ctr, Chicago Shriners Hosp; **Address:** Loyola Univ Med Ctr, Dept Ortho, 2160 S First Ave Maguire Bldg - rm 1700, Maywood, IL 60153-5590; **Phone:** 708-216-4570; **Board Cert:** Orthopaedic Surgery 1979; Hand Surgery 2000; **Med School:** Ros Franklin Univ/Chicago Med Sch 1973; **Resid:** Orthopaedic Surgery, Yale-New Haven Hosp 1977; **Fellow:** Hand Surgery, Hartford Combined Prog 1977; **Fac Appt:** Prof OrS, Loyola Univ-Stritch Sch Med

Hand Surgery

Louis, Dean MD [HS] - **Spec Exp:** Hand-Congenital Anomaly; Wrist Surgery; Arthritis; Carpal Tunnel Syndrome; **Hospital:** Univ Michigan Hlth Sys; **Address:** 2098 S Main St, Ann Arbor, MI 48103; **Phone:** 734-936-5200; **Board Cert:** Orthopaedic Surgery 1998; Hand Surgery 1998; **Med School:** Univ VT Coll Med 1962; **Resid:** Orthopaedic Surgery, Univ Michigan Med Ctr 1970; **Fellow:** Hand Surgery, Columbia Presby Hosp 1971; **Fac Appt:** Prof OrS, Univ Mich Med Sch

Manske, Paul MD [HS] - **Spec Exp:** Congenital Hand Deformities; Pediatric Hand Surgery; **Hospital:** Barnes-Jewish Hosp; **Address:** Wash Univ Sch Med, Dept Ortho Surg, 4921 Parkview Pl, Box 8605, St. Louis, MO 63110-1032; **Phone:** 314-747-2500; **Board Cert:** Orthopaedic Surgery 1974; Hand Surgery 2000; **Med School:** Washington Univ, St Louis 1964; **Resid:** Surgery, Univ Wash Med Ctr 1966; Orthopaedic Surgery, Barnes Hosp-Wash Univ 1972; **Fellow:** Hand Surgery, Univ Louisville Hosp 1971; **Fac Appt:** Prof OrS, Washington Univ, St Louis

Mass, Daniel MD [HS] - **Spec Exp:** Tendon Surgery; Shoulder Reconstruction; Elbow Reconstruction; Wrist Surgery; **Hospital:** Univ of Chicago Hosps; **Address:** 5841 S Maryland Ave, MC 3079, Chicago, IL 60637-1448; **Phone:** 773-834-3531; **Board Cert:** Orthopaedic Surgery 1994; Hand Surgery 2000; **Med School:** Univ Chicago-Pritzker Sch Med 1975; **Resid:** Orthopaedic Surgery, Univ Chicago Hosp 1979; **Fellow:** Hand Surgery, St Francis Hosp 1980; **Fac Appt:** Prof S, Univ Chicago-Pritzker Sch Med

Mih, Alexander MD [HS] - **Spec Exp:** Microsurgery; **Hospital:** Indiana Univ Hosp, St Vincent Hosp & Hlth Svcs - Indianapolis; **Address:** Indiana Hand Center, 541 Clinical Drive, rm 600, Indianapolis, IN 46202; **Phone:** 317-274-5648; **Board Cert:** Orthopaedic Surgery 2003; Hand Surgery 2003; **Med School:** Johns Hopkins Univ 1984; **Resid:** Orthopaedic Surgery, Mayo Clinic 1989; **Fellow:** Hand Surgery, Indiana Ctr for Hand Surg 1990; **Fac Appt:** Assoc Prof OrS, Indiana Univ

Nagle, Daniel J MD [HS] - **Spec Exp:** Wrist Surgery; Carpal Tunnel Syndrome; **Hospital:** Northwestern Meml Hosp, Children's Mem Hosp; **Address:** 737 N Michigan Ave, Ste 700, Chicago, IL 60611-7108; **Phone:** 312-337-6960; **Board Cert:** Orthopaedic Surgery 1997; Hand Surgery 1997; **Med School:** Belgium 1978; **Resid:** Orthopaedic Surgery, Northwestern Univ Med Sch 1983; **Fellow:** Hand Surgery, Christine Kleinert 1984; **Fac Appt:** Prof OrS, Northwestern Univ

Putnam, Matthew D MD [HS] - **Spec Exp:** Wrist Surgery; Fracture Deformities/Arm; Arthritis; **Hospital:** Univ Minn Med Ctr, Fairview - Univ Campus, Univ Minn Med Ctr, Fairview - Riverside Campus; **Address:** 2450 Riverside Ave S, Ste R200, Minneapolis, MN 55454; **Phone:** 612-273-9400; **Board Cert:** Orthopaedic Surgery 1998; Hand Surgery 2001; **Med School:** Dartmouth Med Sch 1977; **Resid:** Surgery, Roosevelt Hosp 1979; Orthopaedic Surgery, Univ Pittsburgh 1984; **Fellow:** Hand Surgery, NVOH 1985; **Fac Appt:** Prof OrS, Univ Minn

Schenck, Robert Roy MD [HS] - **Spec Exp:** Carpal Tunnel Syndrome; Dupuytren's Contracture; Finger Fractures; **Hospital:** Rush Univ Med Ctr; **Address:** 1725 W Harrison St, Ste 319, Chicago, IL 60612-3841; **Phone:** 312-738-3426; **Board Cert:** Plastic Surgery 1973; Hand Surgery 1998; **Med School:** Univ IL Coll Med 1955; **Resid:** Surgery, Western Penn Hosp 1969; Plastic Surgery, Columbia-Presby Hosp 1971; **Fellow:** Hand Surgery, Roosevelt Hosp 1972; **Fac Appt:** Assoc Prof S, Rush Med Coll

Seitz, William H MD [HS] - **Spec Exp:** Hand & Upper Extremity Surgery; Shoulder Surgery; **Hospital:** Cleveland Clin Fdn (page 57), Lutheran Med Ctr - Cleveland (page 57); **Address:** Cleveland Clinic, Beachwood Family Hlth Surg Ctr, 26900 Cedar Rd, Ste 305S, Beachwood, OH 44122-1148; **Phone:** 216-839-3700; **Board Cert:** Orthopaedic Surgery 1998; Hand Surgery 1998; **Med School:** Columbia P&S 1979; **Resid:** Surgery, St Vincents Med Ctr 1981; Orthopaedic Surgery, Columbia-Presby Med Ctr 1984; **Fellow:** Hand & Microvascular Surgery, Columbia-Presby Med Ctr 1985; **Fac Appt:** Assoc Clin Prof OrS, Case West Res Univ

Steichen, James B MD [HS] - **Spec Exp:** Microvascular Surgery; **Hospital:** St Vincent Hosp & Hlth Svcs - Indianapolis; **Address:** 8501 Harcourt Rd, Indianapolis, IN 46280-0434; **Phone:** 317-875-9105; **Board Cert:** Orthopaedic Surgery 1973; **Med School:** Univ IL Coll Med 1967; **Resid:** Orthopaedic Surgery, Indiana Univ Hosps 1972; **Fellow:** Hand Surgery, Indiana Univ Hosps 1974; Microvascular Surgery, Davies Med Ctr-Franklin Hosp; **Fac Appt:** Clin Prof OrS, Indiana Univ

Stern, Peter MD [HS] - **Spec Exp:** Hand & Wrist Surgery; Microsurgery; **Hospital:** Good Samaritan Hosp - Cincinnati, Univ Hosp - Cincinnati; **Address:** Hand Surg Specialists, 538 Oak St, Ste 200, Cincinnati, OH 45219; **Phone:** 513-961-4263; **Board Cert:** Orthopaedic Surgery 1993; Hand Surgery 2000; **Med School:** Washington Univ, St Louis 1970; **Resid:** Surgery, Beth Israel Hosp 1972; Orthopaedic Surgery, Harvard Combined Prgm 1977; **Fellow:** Hand Surgery, Univ Louisville Hosps 1979; **Fac Appt:** Prof OrS, Univ Cincinnati

Southwest

Ezaki, Marybeth MD [HS] - **Spec Exp:** Hand-Congenital Anomaly; Hand Reconstruction-Pediatric; **Hospital:** Texas Scottish Rite Hosp for Chldn; **Address:** 2222 Welborn St, Ste 131, Dallas, TX 75219; **Phone:** 214-559-7842; **Board Cert:** Orthopaedic Surgery 1993; Hand Surgery 2000; **Med School:** Yale Univ 1977; **Resid:** Orthopaedic Surgery, Univ Tex SW Med Ctr 1982; **Fellow:** Hand Surgery, Weyham Pk Hosp 1982; **Fac Appt:** Assoc Prof OrS, Univ Tex SW, Dallas

Moneim, Moheb S MD [HS] - **Spec Exp:** Hand Surgery; **Hospital:** Univ NM Hlth & Sci Ctr; **Address:** Univ of New Mexico, Dept Orthopedics, MSC 10 5600, Albuquerque, NM 87131-0001; **Phone:** 505-272-4107; **Board Cert:** Orthopaedic Surgery 1998; Hand Surgery 1998; **Med School:** Egypt 1963; **Resid:** Orthopaedic Surgery, Duke Univ Med Ctr 1975; **Fellow:** Hand Surgery, Hosp for Spec Surgery 1976; **Fac Appt:** Prof OrS, Univ New Mexico

Rayan, Ghazi M MD [HS] - **Spec Exp:** Microsurgery; Congenital Limb Deformities; Arthritis; **Hospital:** Intergris Baptist Med Ctr - OK, OU Med Ctr; **Address:** 3366 Northwest Expressway, Ste 700, Oklahoma City, OK 73112-4439; **Phone:** 405-945-4888; **Board Cert:** Orthopaedic Surgery 2000; Hand Surgery 2000; **Med School:** Egypt 1973; **Resid:** Surgery, S Baltimore Genl Hosp 1977; Orthopaedic Surgery, Union Meml Hosp 1980; **Fellow:** Hand & Microvascular Surgery, Union Meml Hosp 1980; **Fac Appt:** Clin Prof OrS, Univ Okla Coll Med

Hand Surgery

West Coast and Pacific

Atkinson, Robert E MD [HS] - **Spec Exp:** Arthritis; Arthroscopic Surgery; Nerve Disorders/Surgery; **Hospital:** Queen's Med Ctr - Honolulu, Kapiolani Med Ctr @ Pali Momi; **Address:** Queen's Physicians' Office Bldg 1, 1380 Lusitana St, Ste 604, Honolulu, HI 96813; **Phone:** 808-521-8128; **Board Cert:** Orthopaedic Surgery 1985; **Med School:** Jefferson Med Coll 1977; **Resid:** Orthopaedic Surgery, Hosp Special Surgery 1982; **Fellow:** Hand Surgery, Mass Genl Hosp 1983; **Fac Appt:** Clin Prof OrS, Univ Hawaii JA Burns Sch Med

Godzik, Cathleen MD [HS] - **Spec Exp:** Congenital Hand Deformities; Sports Injuries; Dupuytren's Contracture; **Hospital:** California Hosp Med Ctr, Good Samaritan Hosp - Los Angeles; **Address:** 1414 S Grand Ave, Ste 300, Los Angeles, CA 90015; **Phone:** 213-742-9708; **Board Cert:** Orthopaedic Surgery 2001; Hand Surgery 2001; **Med School:** NY Med Coll 1981; **Resid:** Surgery, Brown Univ Sch Med 1983; Orthopaedic Surgery, Univ Conn Sch Med 1984; **Fellow:** Hand Surgery, Joseph Boyes Hand Fell-USC 1987

Hanel, Douglas P MD [HS] - **Spec Exp:** Reconstructive Microvascular Surgery; Hand-Congenital Anomaly; Elbow Reconstruction; **Hospital:** Univ Wash Med Ctr; **Address:** Harborview Medical Ctr, 325 9th Ave, Box 359798, Seattle, WA 98104-2420; **Phone:** 206-731-3462; **Board Cert:** Orthopaedic Surgery 1997; Hand Surgery 1997; **Med School:** St Louis Univ 1977; **Resid:** Orthopaedic Surgery, St Louis Univ Hosp 1982; **Fellow:** Hand Surgery, Univ Louisville Hosp 1983; Microsurgery, Univ Louisville Hosp 1983; **Fac Appt:** Prof OrS, Univ Wash

Hentz, Vincent R MD [HS] - **Spec Exp:** Hand Plastic Surgery; **Hospital:** Stanford Univ Med Ctr; **Address:** 1000 Welch Rd, Ste 100, Palto Alto, CA 94304; **Phone:** 650-723-5256; **Board Cert:** Plastic Surgery 1977; **Med School:** Univ Fla Coll Med 1968; **Resid:** Plastic Surgery, Stanford Univ Hosp 1974; **Fellow:** Hand Surgery, Roosevelt Hosp 1975; **Fac Appt:** Prof S, Stanford Univ

Jones, Neil MD [HS] - **Spec Exp:** Hand Reconstruction-Pediatric; Nerve Disorders/Surgery; Tendon Surgery; Toe-to-Hand Transfer; **Hospital:** UCLA Med Ctr, Los Angeles Shriners Hosp; **Address:** 10945 Leconte Ave, Ste 3355, Los Angeles, CA 90095; **Phone:** 310-794-7784; **Board Cert:** Plastic Surgery 1985; **Med School:** England 1974; **Resid:** Surgery, Radcliffe Infirmary 1979; Plastic Surgery, Univ Mich Med Ctr 1981; **Fellow:** Plastic Surgery, St Bartholomew's Hosp 1982; Hand & Microvascular Surgery, Mass Gen Hosp/Harvard 1983; **Fac Appt:** Prof PlS, UCLA

Meals, Roy Allen MD [HS] - **Hospital:** UCLA Med Ctr; **Address:** 100 UCLA Medical Plaza, Ste 305, Los Angeles, CA 90024; **Phone:** 310-206-6337; **Board Cert:** Orthopaedic Surgery 1980; Hand Surgery 2000; **Med School:** Vanderbilt Univ 1971; **Resid:** Surgery, Johns Hopkins Hosp 1973; Orthopaedic Surgery, Johns Hopkins Hosp 1978; **Fellow:** Hand Surgery, Mass Genl Hosp 1979; **Fac Appt:** Clin Prof S, UCLA

Szabo, Robert M MD [HS] - **Spec Exp:** Peripheral Nerve Surgery; Hand Injuries; Hand & Upper Extremity Tumors; **Hospital:** UC Davis Med Ctr, Mercy General Hosp - Sacramento; **Address:** UC Davis, Dept Orthopaedics, 4860 Y St, Ste 3800, Sacramento, CA 95817-2307; **Phone:** 916-734-3678; **Board Cert:** Orthopaedic Surgery 1998; Hand Surgery 1998; **Med School:** SUNY Buffalo 1977; **Resid:** Surgery, Mt Sinai Hosp 1979; Orthopaedic Surgery, Mt Sinai Hosp 1982; **Fellow:** Hand Surgery, UCSD Med Ctr 1983; Epidemiology, UC Berkeley 1995; **Fac Appt:** Prof OrS, UC Davis

Trumble, Thomas MD [HS] - **Spec Exp:** Nerve Disorders/Surgery; Upper Extremity Trauma; Biomechanics-Arms; **Hospital:** Univ Wash Med Ctr, Harborview Med Ctr; **Address:** Harborview Med Ctr, 325 9th Ave, Box 359798, Seattle, WA 98104; **Phone:** 206-731-3462; **Board Cert:** Orthopaedic Surgery 1999; Hand Surgery 1999; **Med School:** Yale Univ 1979; **Resid:** Orthopaedic Surgery, Yale-New Haven Hosp 1984; **Fellow:** Microvascular Surgery, Duke Univ Med Ctr 1984; Hand Surgery, Mass Genl Hosp 1985; **Fac Appt:** Prof S, Univ Wash

Cleveland Clinic

Hand and Upper Extremity Center

Cleveland Clinic Hand and Upper Extremity Center, a division of the Department of Orthopaedic Surgery, provides a centralized, comprehensive and diagnostic treatment center for problems affecting the hand, wrist, elbow and shoulder. If you are among the millions of Americans experiencing hand and upper extremity problems each year, finding expert care is all-important. For the past several years, *U.S.News & World Report* has consistently ranked the Department of Orthopaedic Surgery among the nation's top five orthopaedic programs.

Our surgeons treat all disorders of the upper extremity. The following is a list of many of the injuries and disorders we treat. We encourage you to ask about our experience with your particular problem.

Shoulder
Fractures and dislocations
Arthritis
instability
Chronic instability
Rotator cuff tears
Brachial plexus injuries

Wrist
Fractures and nonunions
Dislocations and

Carpal tunnel syndrom
Tendinitis
Rheumatoid wrist

Elbow
Fractures and dislocations
Tennis and golfer's elbow
Arthritis
Throwing elbow

Hand
Fractures and dislocations
Trigger finger
Cysts and tumors
Burns

Surgery of the Hand and Upper Extremity
Our surgeons are experts in the operative care of a wide array of upper extremity disorders. For some injuries, this includes the newest surgical techniques, such as microsurgery and minimally invasive surgery.

Work-Related Disorders
Acute injuries and chronic problems of the hand and upper extremity can result from occupational activity. Our surgeons are expert in determining whether a disorder is work-related and at determining a treatment course that will help you meet the physical demands of your job.

To schedule an appointment or for more information about the Cleveland Clinic Hand and upper Extremity Center call 800.890.2467 or visit www.clevelandclinic.org/orthotopdocs.

Hand and Upper Extremity Center | 9500 Euclid Avenue / W14 | Cleveland OH 44195

Second Opinion-Online

Use e-Cleveland Clinic's convenient, online second opinion service without leaving home. Call 800.223.2273, ext 43223, or visit www.eclevelandclinic.org.

Assistance for Out-of-Town and International Patients

Get complimentary help scheduling medical appointments and arranging for hotels and transportation.

For out-of-town patients call 800.223.2273, ext. 55580, or visit www.clevelandclinic.org/services. For International patients call 216.444.6404 or visit www.clevelandclinic.org/ic.

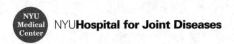
NYU**Hospital for Joint Diseases**

NYU Medical Center

550 First Avenue (at 31st Street)
New York, NY 10016
Physician Referral:
(888)7-NYU-MED (888-769-8633)
www.nyumc.org

HAND SURGERY

The NYU Hospital for Joint Diseases provides provides comprehensive care of patients with hand and wrist disorders, including:

- Fractures
- Congenital anomalies
- Soft tissue and skeletal trauma
- Degenerative and rheumatoid arthritis
- Sports-related injuries of the hand and wrist
- Vascular disorders
- Tumors
- Occupational hand and wrist disorders

Care is provided by 16 specialists encompassing all aspects of diagnosis and treatment of the full spectrum of problems that affect the hand and wrist.

Specific emphases include fractures of the wrist and distal radius and reconstructive aspects of hand surgery, as reflected by the large volume of cases involving post traumatic, arthritis, congenital, neuromuscular, and neoplastic conditions.

The research focus of the **NYUHJD Hand Service** is on a variety of clinical problems, including wrist fractures, non-unions of the scaphoid, avascular necrosis of the lunate (Kienböck's disease), intercarpal subluxations, and neuropathies of the upper extremity.

After surgery, the **Rusk Institute of Rehabilitation Medicine's Hand Therapy Unit** helps surgical patients recover full or partial use of their hands, providing comprehensive rehabilitation for a variety of ailments associated with the hand and upper body. The Hand Therapy Unit specializes in fractures, traumatic injuries, tendonitis, sports injuries, work-related injuries, repetitive stress injuries, carpal tunnel syndrome, tendon and nerve repairs, and arthritis. It is staffed by licensed occupational therapists who specialize in the treatment of the hand and upper extremities.

NYU HOSPITAL FOR JOINT DISEASES MEDICAL CENTER

Optimal care of hands requires a specialist who has advanced training in the entire spectrum of hand and wrist disorders including rehabilitation techniques.

At NYU Hospital for Joint Diseases, world-class hand surgery and rehabilitation are brought together ensuring patients and their families have a positive outcome.

**Physician Referral
(888) HJD-DOCS
(888-453-3627)
www.nyuhjd.org**

698

Hematology &
Medical Oncology
a subspecialty of Internal Medicine

Hematology: An internist with additional training who specializes in diseases of the blood, spleen and lymph glands. This specialist treats conditions such as anemia, clotting disorders, sickle cell disease, hemophilia, leukemia and lymphoma.

Medical Oncology: An internist who specializes in the diagnosis and treatment of all types of cancer and other benign and malignant tumors. This specialist decides on and administers chemotherapy for malignancy, as well as consulting with surgeons and radiotherapists on other treatments for cancer.

Training Required: Three years in internal medicine *plus* additional training and examination for certification in hematology or medical oncology.

Hematology

New England

Benz Jr, Edward MD [Hem] - **Spec Exp:** Anemias & Red Cell Disorders; Bone Marrow Transplant; **Hospital:** Brigham & Women's Hosp, Children's Hospital - Boston; **Address:** 44 Binney St, rm D-1628, Boston, MA 02115; **Phone:** 617-632-2159; **Board Cert:** Internal Medicine 1979; Hematology 1982; **Med School:** Harvard Med Sch 1973; **Resid:** Internal Medicine, Peter Bent Brigham Hosp 1975; Hematology, Yale New Haven Hosp 1980; **Fellow:** Hematology, Natl Inst of Hlth 1978; **Fac Appt:** Prof Med, Harvard Med Sch

Duffy, Thomas P MD [Hem] - **Spec Exp:** Mast Cell Diseases; Leukemia; Lymphoma; **Hospital:** Yale - New Haven Hosp; **Address:** Yale Univ, Sect Hematology, 333 Cedar St, rm 403-WWW, Box 208021, New Haven, CT 06520-8021; **Phone:** 203-785-4744; **Board Cert:** Internal Medicine 1972; Hematology 1974; **Med School:** Johns Hopkins Univ 1962; **Resid:** Internal Medicine, Johns Hopkins Hosp 1965; **Fellow:** Hematology, Johns Hopkins Hosp 1970; **Fac Appt:** Prof Med, Yale Univ

Groopman, Jerome E MD [Hem] - **Spec Exp:** AIDS/HIV; AIDS Related Cancers; **Hospital:** Beth Israel Deaconess Med Ctr - Boston; **Address:** Beth Israel Deaconess Medical Ctr, 330 Brookline Ave, Boston, MA 02215; **Phone:** 617-667-0070; **Board Cert:** Internal Medicine 1979; Medical Oncology 1981; Hematology 1984; **Med School:** Columbia P&S 1976; **Resid:** Internal Medicine, Mass Genl Hosp 1978; **Fellow:** Hematology & Oncology, UCLA Med Ctr 1979; Research, Dana Farber Cancer Ctr 1980; **Fac Appt:** Prof Med, Harvard Med Sch

Miller, Kenneth B MD [Hem] - **Spec Exp:** Bone Marrow Transplant; Leukemia; **Hospital:** Beth Israel Deaconess Med Ctr - Boston; **Address:** 330 Brookline Ave, Kirstein Bldg, rm 121, Boston, MA 02215; **Phone:** 617-667-9920 x2; **Board Cert:** Internal Medicine 1976; Hematology 1980; **Med School:** NY Med Coll 1972; **Resid:** Internal Medicine, NYU Med Ctr/VA Hosp 1976; Internal Medicine, NYU Med Ctr 1976; **Fellow:** Hematology, New England Med Ctr 1979; **Fac Appt:** Assoc Prof Med, Harvard Med Sch

Spitzer, Thomas R MD [Hem] - **Spec Exp:** Bone Marrow Transplant; Leukemia; **Hospital:** Mass Genl Hosp; **Address:** Mass Genl Hosp-Bone Marrow Tranplant Program, 55 Fruit St, Ste 118, Boston, MA 02114; **Phone:** 617-724-1124; **Board Cert:** Internal Medicine 1977; Medical Oncology 1983; Hematology 1984; **Med School:** Univ Rochester 1974; **Resid:** Internal Medicine, NYew York Hosp-Cornell Med Ctr 1977; **Fellow:** Hematology & Oncology, Case West Res Univ 1983; **Fac Appt:** Prof Med, Harvard Med Sch

Stone, Richard M MD [Hem] - **Spec Exp:** Leukemia; **Hospital:** Dana-Farber Cancer Inst, Brigham & Women's Hosp; **Address:** Dana Farber Cancer Inst, Adult Leukemia Prog, 44 Binney St, Ste M1B17, Boston, MA 02115-6084; **Phone:** 617-632-2214; **Board Cert:** Internal Medicine 1984; Medical Oncology 1987; Hematology 1988; **Med School:** Harvard Med Sch 1981; **Resid:** Internal Medicine, Brigham & Womens Hosp 1984; **Fellow:** Medical Oncology, Dana Farber Cancer Inst 1987; **Fac Appt:** Assoc Prof Med, Harvard Med Sch

Mid Atlantic

Abrams, Charles S MD [Hem] - **Spec Exp:** Bleeding/Coagulation Disorders; Thrombotic Disorders; **Hospital:** Hosp Univ Penn - UPHS (page 72); **Address:** Univ Penn, Dept Hem/Onc, 421 Curie Blvd, Bio Medical Research Bldg 2/3, Philadelphia, PA 19104-6160; **Phone:** 215-573-3288; **Board Cert:** Internal Medicine 1987; Medical Oncology 1989; Hematology 1990; **Med School:** Yale Univ 1984; **Resid:** Internal Medicine, Hosp U Penn 1987; **Fellow:** Hematology & Oncology, Hosp U Penn 1988; **Fac Appt:** Assoc Prof Med, Univ Pennsylvania

Cheson, Bruce D MD [Hem] - **Spec Exp:** Leukemia; Hematologic Malignancies; **Hospital:** Georgetown Univ Hosp; **Address:** GUMC - Lombardi Cancer Ctr, 3800 Reservoir Rd NW, Podium A, Washington, DC 20007; **Phone:** 202-444-2223; **Board Cert:** Internal Medicine 1974; Hematology 1976; **Med School:** Tufts Univ 1971; **Resid:** Internal Medicine, Univ Virginia Hosp 1974; **Fellow:** Hematology, New England Med Ctr Hosp 1976

Coller, Barry MD [Hem] - **Spec Exp:** Glanzmann's Thrombasthenia; **Hospital:** Rockefeller Univ, Mount Sinai Med Ctr; **Address:** Rockefeller Univ, 1230 York Ave, New York, NY 10021; **Phone:** 212-327-7490; **Board Cert:** Internal Medicine 1973; Hematology 1975; **Med School:** NYU Sch Med 1970; **Resid:** Internal Medicine, Bellevue Hosp 1972; **Fellow:** Hematology, Natl Inst Hlth Clin Ctr 1974; **Fac Appt:** Clin Prof Med, Mount Sinai Sch Med

Diuguid, David L MD [Hem] - **Spec Exp:** Bleeding/Coagulation Disorders; **Hospital:** NY-Presby Hosp/Columbia (page 66); **Address:** 161 Ft Washington Ave, Rm 862, New York, NY 10032; **Phone:** 212-305-0527; **Board Cert:** Internal Medicine 1982; Hematology 1986; Medical Oncology 1985; **Med School:** Cornell Univ-Weill Med Coll 1979; **Resid:** Internal Medicine, Boston Univ Med Ctr 1983; **Fellow:** Hematology & Oncology, New England Med Ctr 1986; **Fac Appt:** Assoc Prof Med, Columbia P&S

Emerson, Stephen G MD/PhD [Hem] - **Spec Exp:** Leukemia; Lymphoma; **Hospital:** Hosp Univ Penn - UPHS (page 72); **Address:** Hospital U Penn, 510 Maloney Bldg, 3400 Spruce St, Philadelphia, PA 19104; **Phone:** 215-573-4137; **Board Cert:** Internal Medicine 1983; Hematology 1986; Medical Oncology 1987; **Med School:** Yale Univ 1980; **Resid:** Internal Medicine, Mass Genl Hosp 1982; **Fellow:** Hematology & Oncology, Brigham & Women's Hosp 1986; **Fac Appt:** Prof Med, Univ Pennsylvania

Fruchtman, Steven M MD [Hem] - **Spec Exp:** Myeloproliferative Disorders; Polycythemia Rubra Vera; Stem Cell Transplant; **Hospital:** Mount Sinai Med Ctr; **Address:** 1111 Park Ave, New York, NY 10029; **Phone:** 212-427-7700; **Board Cert:** Internal Medicine 1980; Hematology 1984; **Med School:** NY Med Coll 1977; **Resid:** Internal Medicine, Univ Hosp 1981; **Fellow:** Hematology, Mount Sinai Med Ctr 1984; Hematology, Meml Sloan Kettering Cancer Ctr 1985; **Fac Appt:** Assoc Prof Med, NY Med Coll

Gewirtz, Alan M MD [Hem] - **Spec Exp:** Leukemia; Gene Therapy; **Hospital:** Hosp Univ Penn - UPHS (page 72); **Address:** Univ Penn - Div Hem/Onc, 421 Curie Blvd, 716BRB, Philadelphia, PA 19104; **Phone:** 215-662-3914; **Board Cert:** Internal Medicine 1979; Hematology 1982; Medical Oncology 1981; **Med School:** SUNY Buffalo 1976; **Resid:** Internal Medicine, Mt Sinai Hosp 1979; **Fellow:** Medical Oncology, Yale-New Haven Hosp 1981; **Fac Appt:** Prof Med, Univ Pennsylvania

Goldberg, Jack MD [Hem] - **Spec Exp:** Bleeding/Coagulation Disorders; Leukemia & Lymphoma; Solid Tumors; **Hospital:** Penn Presby Med Ctr - UPHS (page 72), Virtua West Jersey Hosp - Voorhees (page 59); **Address:** 409 Route 70 E, Cherry Hill, NJ 08034; **Phone:** 856-429-1519; **Board Cert:** Internal Medicine 1976; Hematology 1980; Medical Oncology 1989; **Med School:** SUNY Upstate Med Univ 1973; **Resid:** Internal Medicine, Boston Univ Hosp 1975; **Fellow:** Hematology & Oncology, SUNY Syracuse Med Ctr 1977; **Fac Appt:** Clin Prof Med, Univ Pennsylvania

Kempin, Sanford Jay MD [Hem] - **Spec Exp:** Bleeding/Coagulation Disorders; Leukemia; Lymphoma; **Hospital:** St Vincent Cath Med Ctrs - Manhattan; **Address:** St Vincents Cancer Ctr, 325 W 15th St, New York, NY 10011; **Phone:** 212-604-6010; **Board Cert:** Internal Medicine 1976; Medical Oncology 1977; Hematology 1978; **Med School:** Belgium 1971; **Resid:** Internal Medicine, Lemuel Shattuck Hosp 1972; **Fellow:** Hematology, St Jude Chldns Hosp 1975; Medical Oncology, Meml Sloan Kettering Cancer Ctr 1976

Kessler, Craig M MD [Hem] - **Spec Exp:** Bleeding/Coagulation Disorders; Hemophilia; Hematologic Malignancies; **Hospital:** Georgetown Univ Hosp; **Address:** GUMC, Lombardi Cancer Ctr, 3800 Reservoir Rd NW, Washington, DC 20007; **Phone:** 202-444-7094; **Board Cert:** Internal Medicine 1976; Hematology 1980; **Med School:** Tulane Univ 1973; **Resid:** Internal Medicine, Ochsner Fdn Hosp 1976; **Fellow:** Hematology, Johns Hopkins Hosp 1978; **Fac Appt:** Prof Med, Georgetown Univ

Millenson, Michael M MD [Hem] - **Spec Exp:** Leukemia & Lymphoma; Thromboembolic Disorders; **Hospital:** Fox Chase Cancer Ctr (page 59); **Address:** Fox Chase Cancer Center, 7701 Burholme Ave, Ste C307, Philadelphia, PA 19111; **Phone:** 215-728-2600; **Board Cert:** Medical Oncology 2000; Hematology 2000; **Med School:** Temple Univ 1984; **Resid:** Internal Medicine, Temple Univ Hosp 1987; **Fellow:** Hematology & Oncology, Beth Israel Hosp 1991

Nimer, Stephen D MD [Hem] - **Spec Exp:** Bone Marrow Transplant; Myelodysplastic Syndromes; Leukemia; Stem Cell Transplant; **Hospital:** Meml Sloan Kettering Cancer Ctr; **Address:** Memorial Sloan Kettering Cancer Ctr, 1275 York Ave, Box 575, New York, NY 10021; **Phone:** 212-639-7871; **Board Cert:** Internal Medicine 1982; Hematology 1986; Medical Oncology 1985; **Med School:** Univ Chicago-Pritzker Sch Med 1979; **Resid:** Internal Medicine, UCLA Med Ctr 1982; **Fellow:** Hematology & Oncology, UCLA Med Ctr 1986; **Fac Appt:** Prof Med, Cornell Univ-Weill Med Coll

Porter, David L MD [Hem] - **Spec Exp:** Leukemia; Bone Marrow Transplant; **Hospital:** Hosp Univ Penn - UPHS (page 72); **Address:** Hosp Univ Penn, Div Hem/Oncology, 3400 Spruce St, 16 Penn Twr, Philadelphia, PA 19104; **Phone:** 215-662-7909; **Board Cert:** Internal Medicine 1990; Medical Oncology 1993; Hematology 1994; **Med School:** Brown Univ 1987; **Resid:** Internal Medicine, Univ Hosp 1990; **Fellow:** Hematology & Oncology, Brigham & Womens Hosp 1992; **Fac Appt:** Assoc Prof Med, Univ Pennsylvania

Rai, Kanti MD [Hem] - **Spec Exp:** Leukemia; Lymphoma; Multiple Myeloma; **Hospital:** Long Island Jewish Med Ctr; **Address:** 270-05 76th Ave, New Hyde Park, NY 11040-1433; **Phone:** 718-470-7135; **Board Cert:** Pediatrics 1961; **Med School:** India 1955; **Resid:** Pediatrics, Lincoln Hosp 1958; Pediatrics, North Shore Univ Hosp 1959; **Fellow:** Hematology, LI Jewish Med Ctr 1960; **Fac Appt:** Prof Med, Albert Einstein Coll Med

Rand, Jacob H MD [Hem] - **Spec Exp:** Bleeding/Coagulation Disorders; Pregnancy-Hematologic Complications; Thrombotic Disorders; **Hospital:** Montefiore Med Ctr; **Address:** Montefiore Medical Ctr, 111 E 210th St, N8 Silverzone, Bronx, NY 10467-2401; **Phone:** 718-920-4481; **Board Cert:** Internal Medicine 1977; Hematology 1978; **Med School:** Albert Einstein Coll Med 1973; **Resid:** Pathology, Montefiore Med Ctr 1974; Internal Medicine, Mount Sinai Hosp 1976; **Fellow:** Hematology, Montefiore Med Ctr 1978; **Fac Appt:** Prof Med, Albert Einstein Coll Med

Raphael, Bruce MD [Hem] - **Spec Exp:** Lymphoma; Leukemia; Multiple Myeloma; **Hospital:** NYU Med Ctr (page 67), NY Downtown Hosp; **Address:** 160 E 34th Street Ave Fl 7, NYU Clinical Cancer Ctr, New York, NY 10016-6402; **Phone:** 212-731-5185; **Board Cert:** Internal Medicine 1978; Hematology 1980; Medical Oncology 1981; **Med School:** McGill Univ 1975; **Resid:** Internal Medicine, Jewish Genl Hosp 1977; **Fellow:** Medical Oncology, Meml Sloan Kettering Cancer Ctr 1978; Hematology, NYU Med Ctr 1980; **Fac Appt:** Assoc Prof Med, NYU Sch Med

Roodman, G David MD [Hem] - **Spec Exp:** Multiple Myeloma; **Hospital:** UPMC Shadyside, VA Pittsburgh Hlth Care Sys; **Address:** VA Pittsburgh Healthcare System, 151-U, rm 2E113, University Drive C, Pittsburgh, PA 15240; **Phone:** 412-688-6571; **Board Cert:** Internal Medicine 1978; Hematology 1980; **Med School:** Univ KY Coll Med 1973; **Resid:** Internal Medicine, Univ Minnesota Hosp 1978; **Fellow:** Hematology, Univ Minnesota Hosp 1980; **Fac Appt:** Prof Med, Univ Pittsburgh

Savage, David G MD [Hem] - **Spec Exp:** Stem Cell Transplant; Multiple Myeloma; Lymphoma; **Hospital:** NY-Presby Hosp/Columbia (page 66); **Address:** 177 Fort Washington Ave, Millstein Bldg Fl 6 - rm 435, New York, NY 10032; **Phone:** 212-305-9783; **Board Cert:** Internal Medicine 1977; Hematology 1982; Medical Oncology 1985; **Med School:** Columbia P&S 1971; **Resid:** Internal Medicine, Harlem Hosp/Columbia Presby Med Ctr 1975; **Fellow:** Hematology & Oncology, Harlem Hosp/Columbia Presby Med Ctr 1977; **Fac Appt:** Assoc Prof Med, Columbia P&S

Schuster, Michael W MD [Hem] - **Spec Exp:** Bone Marrow Transplant; **Hospital:** NY-Presby Hosp/Weill Cornell (page 66); **Address:** NY Weill Cornell Medical Ctr, 525 E 68th St, Starr 341, New York, NY 10021; **Phone:** 212-746-2119; **Board Cert:** Internal Medicine 1984; Hematology 1986; **Med School:** Dartmouth Med Sch 1980; **Resid:** Internal Medicine, New England Deaconess Hosp 1983; **Fellow:** Hematology & Oncology, Beth Israel Med Ctr 1987; **Fac Appt:** Assoc Prof Med, Cornell Univ-Weill Med Coll

Spivak, Jerry L MD [Hem] - **Spec Exp:** Myeloproliferative Disorders; Polycythemia Rubra Vera; Leukemia; **Hospital:** Johns Hopkins Hosp - Baltimore (page 61); **Address:** 720 Rutland Ave Bldg Ross - Ste 1025, Baltimore, MD 21205; **Phone:** 410-614-0167; **Board Cert:** Internal Medicine 1971; Hematology 1974; **Med School:** Cornell Univ-Weill Med Coll 1964; **Resid:** Internal Medicine, Johns Hopkins Hosp 1966; Internal Medicine, Johns Hopkins Hosp 1972; **Fellow:** Hematology, Natl Cancer Inst 1968; Hematology, Johns Hopkins Hosp 1971; **Fac Appt:** Prof Med, Johns Hopkins Univ

Wisch, Nathaniel MD [Hem] - **Spec Exp:** Lymphoma; Breast Cancer; Leukemia; **Hospital:** Lenox Hill Hosp (page 62), Mount Sinai Med Ctr; **Address:** 12 E 86th St, New York, NY 10028-0506; **Phone:** 212-861-6660; **Board Cert:** Internal Medicine 1965; Hematology 1972; Medical Oncology 1977; **Med School:** Northwestern Univ 1958; **Resid:** Internal Medicine, VA Hosp 1960; Internal Medicine, Montefiore Hosp 1961; **Fellow:** Hematology, Mount Sinai Hosp 1962; **Fac Appt:** Clin Prof Med, Mount Sinai Sch Med

Hematology

Zalusky, Ralph MD [Hem] - **Spec Exp:** Anemia; Leukemia; Lymphoma; **Hospital:** Beth Israel Med Ctr - Petrie Division; **Address:** Beth Israel Med Ctr, First Ave at 16th St, New York, NY 10003; **Phone:** 212-420-4185; **Board Cert:** Internal Medicine 1964; Hematology 1972; **Med School:** Boston Univ 1957; **Resid:** Internal Medicine, Duke Univ Med Ctr 1962; **Fellow:** Hematology, Boston Med Ctr 1961; **Fac Appt:** Prof Med, Albert Einstein Coll Med

Southeast

Bigelow, Carolyn L MD [Hem] - **Spec Exp:** Bone Marrow Transplant; Sickle Cell Disease; **Hospital:** Univ Hosps & Clins - Jackson; **Address:** Univ Mississippi Med Ctr-Div Hematology, 2500 N State St, Jackson, MS 39216; **Phone:** 601-984-5615; **Board Cert:** Internal Medicine 1982; Hematology 1988; **Med School:** Univ Miss 1979; **Resid:** Internal Medicine, Univ Mississippi Med Ctr 1982; **Fellow:** Hematology & Oncology, Univ Washington Med Ctr 1987; **Fac Appt:** Prof Med, Univ Miss

Buadi, Francis K MD [Hem] - **Spec Exp:** Lymphoma; Stem Cell Transplant; **Hospital:** Univ of Tennesee Mem Hosp; **Address:** UT Cancer Inst, 1331 Union Ave, Ste 800, Memphis, TN 38104; **Phone:** 901-725-1785; **Board Cert:** Internal Medicine 1999; Hematology 2002; Medical Oncology 2003; **Med School:** Ghana 1991; **Resid:** Internal Medicine, St Agnes Hosp 1997; **Fellow:** Hematology & Oncology, Univ Maryland Hosp 1999; Bone Marrow Transplant, Mayo Clinic 2001

Files, Joe C MD [Hem] - **Spec Exp:** Bone Marrow Transplant; Stem Cell Transplant; Leukemia; **Hospital:** Univ Hosps & Clins - Jackson; **Address:** Univ Miss Med Ctr-Div Hematology, 2500 N State St, Jackson, MS 39216; **Phone:** 601-984-5615; **Board Cert:** Internal Medicine 1976; Hematology 1980; **Med School:** Univ Miss 1972; **Resid:** Internal Medicine, Univ Miss Med Ctr 1976; **Fellow:** Hematology, Univ Wash Sch Med 1979; **Fac Appt:** Prof Med, Univ Miss

Greer, John P MD [Hem] - **Spec Exp:** Leukemia & Lymphoma; Myelodysplastic Syndromes; Stem Cell Transplant; **Hospital:** Vanderbilt Univ Med Ctr; **Address:** 2665 The Vanderbilt Clinic, 1301 22nd Ave S, Nashville, TN 37232-5505; **Phone:** 615-936-1803; **Board Cert:** Pediatrics 1985; Internal Medicine 1979; Hematology 1984; Medical Oncology 1985; **Med School:** Vanderbilt Univ 1976; **Resid:** Internal Medicine, Tulane Univ Med Ctr 1979; Pediatrics, Med Coll Virginia 1981; **Fellow:** Hematology & Oncology, Vanderbilt Univ Med Ctr 1984; **Fac Appt:** Prof Med, Vanderbilt Univ

Lin, Weei-Chin MD/PhD [Hem] - **Spec Exp:** Hematologic Malignancies; Bleeding/Coagulation Disorders; **Hospital:** Univ of Ala Hosp at Birmingham; **Address:** Univ of Alabama, 1530 3rd Ave S, Ste 520A, Birmingham, AL 35294; **Phone:** 205-934-3980; **Board Cert:** Internal Medicine 1996; Hematology 1999; Medical Oncology 1999; **Med School:** Taiwan 1986; **Resid:** Internal Medicine, Duke Univ Med Ctr 1996; **Fellow:** Hematology & Oncology, Duke Univ Med Ctr 1999

List, Alan F MD [Hem] - **Spec Exp:** Myelodysplastic Syndromes; Leukemia; **Hospital:** H Lee Moffitt Cancer Ctr & Research Inst; **Address:** 12902 Magnolia Drive, SRB 4, Tampa, FL 33612-9497; **Phone:** 813-745-6086; **Board Cert:** Internal Medicine 1983; Medical Oncology 1985; Hematology 1986; **Med School:** Univ Pennsylvania 1980; **Resid:** Internal Medicine, Good Samaritan Hosp 1983; Oncology, Vanderbilt Univ Med Ctr 1985; **Fellow:** Hematology, Vanderbilt Univ Med Ctr 1986

Lutcher, Charles MD [Hem] - **Spec Exp:** Hemophilia-Adult; **Hospital:** Med Coll of GA Hosp and Clin; **Address:** Med Coll of Georgia Hosp, Dept Hem/Onc, 1120 15th St, rm BAA-5407, Augusta, GA 30912; **Phone:** 706-721-2505; **Board Cert:** Internal Medicine 1987; Hematology 1974; **Med School:** Washington Univ, St Louis 1961; **Resid:** Internal Medicine, St Louis City Hosp 1963; Hematology, Univ Oregon Hosp 1964; **Fellow:** Hematology, Univ Oregon Hosp 1966; **Fac Appt:** Prof Med, Med Coll GA

Ortel, Thomas L MD/PhD [Hem] - **Spec Exp:** Bleeding/Coagulation Disorders; Hemophilia; **Hospital:** Duke Univ Med Ctr; **Address:** Duke Medical Ctr, Box 3422, Durham, NC 27710; **Phone:** 919-684-5530; **Board Cert:** Internal Medicine 1988; Hematology 2002; **Med School:** Indiana Univ 1985; **Resid:** Internal Medicine, Duke Univ Med Ctr 1988; **Fellow:** Hematology & Oncology, Duke Univ Med Ctr 1989; **Fac Appt:** Prof Med, Duke Univ

Powell, Bayard L MD [Hem] - **Spec Exp:** Leukemia; Myelodysplastic Syndromes; **Hospital:** Wake Forest Univ Baptist Med Ctr (page 73); **Address:** Wake Forest Univ Baptist Med Ctr, Med Ctr Blvd-Cancer Center, Winston-Salem, NC 27157; **Phone:** 336-716-7970; **Board Cert:** Internal Medicine 1983; Medical Oncology 1985; **Med School:** Univ NC Sch Med 1980; **Resid:** Internal Medicine, NC Baptist Hospital 1983; **Fellow:** Hematology & Oncology, Wake Forest Univ Sch Med 1986; **Fac Appt:** Prof Med, Wake Forest Univ

Rosenblatt, Joseph D MD [Hem] - **Spec Exp:** Lymphoma; Leukemia; Multiple Myeloma; **Hospital:** Univ of Miami Hosp & Clins/Sylvester Comp Canc Ctr, Jackson Meml Hosp; **Address:** Sylvester Comprehensive Cancer Ctr, 1475 NW 12th Ave, D8-4, Ste 3300, Miami, FL 33136; **Phone:** 305-243-4909; **Board Cert:** Internal Medicine 1983; Hematology 1990; Medical Oncology 1985; **Med School:** UCLA 1980; **Resid:** Internal Medicine, UCLA Medical Ctr 1983; **Fellow:** Hematology & Oncology, UCLA Medical Ctr 1986; **Fac Appt:** Prof Med, Univ Miami Sch Med

Schwartzberg, Lee S MD [Hem] - **Spec Exp:** Breast Cancer; Lung Cancer; Stem Cell Transplant; **Hospital:** Baptist Hosp - Nashville; **Address:** The West Clinic, 100 N Humphreys Blvd, Memphis, TN 38120; **Phone:** 901-683-0055; **Board Cert:** Internal Medicine 1983; Hematology 1986; Medical Oncology 1985; **Med School:** NY Med Coll 1980; **Resid:** Internal Medicine, North Shore Univ Hosp 1983; Internal Medicine, Meml Sloan Kettering Cancer Ctr 1985; **Fellow:** Hematology & Oncology, Meml Sloan Kettering Cancer Ctr 1984; Hematology & Oncology, Meml Sloan Kettering Cancer Ctr 1987; **Fac Appt:** Assoc Prof Med, Univ Tenn Coll Med, Memphis

Solberg, Lawrence MD/PhD [Hem] - **Spec Exp:** Bone Marrow Transplant; Myeloproliferative Disorders; Porphyria; **Hospital:** Mayo - Jacksonville, St Luke's Hosp - Jacksonville; **Address:** Mayo Clinic-Dept Hem-Onc, 4500 San Pablo Rd Fl 8, Jacksonville, FL 32224; **Phone:** 904-953-7292; **Board Cert:** Internal Medicine 1978; Hematology 1980; **Med School:** St Louis Univ 1975; **Resid:** Internal Medicine, Mayo Clinic 1978; **Fellow:** Hematology, Mayo Clinic 1980; **Fac Appt:** Prof Med, Mayo Med Sch

Telen, Marilyn J MD [Hem] - **Spec Exp:** Transfusion Medicine; Anemia & Red Cell Disorders; Sickle Cell Disease; **Hospital:** Duke Univ Med Ctr; **Address:** Duke Univ Med Ctr, Box 2615, Durham, NC 27710; **Phone:** 919-684-5426; **Board Cert:** Internal Medicine 1980; Hematology 1984; **Med School:** NYU Sch Med 1977; **Resid:** Internal Medicine, Erie Co Med Cr 1980; **Fellow:** Hematology, Duke Univ Med Ctr 1983; **Fac Appt:** Prof Med, Duke Univ

Zuckerman, Kenneth S MD [Hem] - **Spec Exp:** Myeloproliferative Disorders; Myelodysplastic Syndromes; Leukemia; Lymphoma; **Hospital:** H Lee Moffitt Cancer Ctr & Research Inst, Tampa Genl Hosp; **Address:** H Lee Moffitt Cancer Ctr, 12902 Magnolia Drive, MS SRB 4, Tampa, FL 33612-9416; **Phone:** 813-745-8090; **Board Cert:** Internal Medicine 1975; Hematology 1978; **Med School:** Ohio State Univ 1972; **Resid:** Internal Medicine, Ohio State Univ Hosps 1975; **Fellow:** Hematology, Brigham Hosp/Harvard Univ 1978; **Fac Appt:** Prof Med, Univ S Fla Coll Med

Midwest

Baron, Joseph M MD [Hem] - **Spec Exp:** Bleeding/Coagulation Disorders; Lymphoma; Myeloproliferative Disorders; **Hospital:** Univ of Chicago Hosps; **Address:** 5841 S Maryland Ave, MC 2115, Chicago, IL 60637-1463; **Phone:** 773-702-6149; **Board Cert:** Internal Medicine 1969; Hematology 1972; Medical Oncology 1975; **Med School:** Univ Chicago-Pritzker Sch Med 1962; **Resid:** Internal Medicine, Univ Chicago Hosps 1964; **Fellow:** Hematology, Univ Chicago Hosps 1968; **Fac Appt:** Assoc Prof Med, Univ Chicago-Pritzker Sch Med

Blinder, Morey MD [Hem] - **Spec Exp:** Bleeding/Coagulation Disorders; Anemia; Sickle Cell Disease; **Hospital:** Barnes-Jewish Hosp; **Address:** Barnes Jewish Hospital, Div Hematology, 660 S Euclid Ave, Box 8125, St. Louis, MO 63110; **Phone:** 314-362-8808; **Board Cert:** Internal Medicine 1984; Hematology 1988; Medical Oncology 1987; **Med School:** St Louis Univ 1981; **Resid:** Internal Medicine, Univ Illinois Hosp 1984; **Fellow:** Hematology & Oncology, Univ Wash Med Ctr 1986; **Fac Appt:** Assoc Prof Med, Washington Univ, St Louis

Bockenstedt, Paula MD [Hem] - **Spec Exp:** Bleeding/Coagulation Disorders; Leukemia; Von Willebrand's Disease; **Hospital:** Univ Michigan Hlth Sys; **Address:** Div Hematology, 1500 E Med Ctr Dr, MIB, rm C-344, Ann Arbor, MI 48109-8048; **Phone:** 734-647-8921; **Board Cert:** Internal Medicine 1981; Hematology 1984; **Med School:** Harvard Med Sch 1978; **Resid:** Internal Medicine, Brigham-Womens Hosp 1981; **Fellow:** Hematology, Brigham-Womens Hosp 1984; **Fac Appt:** Assoc Clin Prof Med, Univ Mich Med Sch

Flynn, Patrick MD [Hem] - **Spec Exp:** Hematologic Malignancies; Colon & Rectal Cancer; Clinical Trials; **Hospital:** Abbott - Northwestern Hosp, Fairview Southdale Hosp; **Address:** 800 E 28th St, Piper Bldg, Ste 405, Minneapolis, MN 55407; **Phone:** 612-863-8585; **Board Cert:** Internal Medicine 1978; Medical Oncology 1981; Hematology 1982; **Med School:** Univ Minn 1975; **Resid:** Internal Medicine, Hennepin Co Med Ctr 1978; **Fellow:** Hematology & Oncology, Univ Minnesota Hosp 1981

Gaynor, Ellen MD [Hem] - **Spec Exp:** Lymphoma; Genitourinary Cancer; Breast Cancer; **Hospital:** Loyola Univ Med Ctr; **Address:** Loyola Univ Med Ctr, Dept Hematology, 2160 S First Ave Bldg 112 - rm 108, Maywood, IL 60153; **Phone:** 708-327-3214; **Board Cert:** Internal Medicine 1982; Hematology 1986; Medical Oncology 1985; **Med School:** Univ Wisc 1978; **Resid:** Internal Medicine, Loyola Univ Med Ctr 1982; **Fellow:** Medical Oncology, Loyola Univ Med Ctr 1981; Hematology & Oncology, Univ Chicago Hosp 1984; **Fac Appt:** Prof Med, Loyola Univ-Stritch Sch Med

Gertz, Morris MD [Hem] - **Spec Exp:** Multiple Myeloma; Amyloidosis; Waldenstrom's Macroglobulinemia; Plasma Cell Disorders; **Hospital:** Mayo Med Ctr & Clin - Rochester, Rochester Meth Hosp; **Address:** 200 SW 1st St Fl W10, Rochester, MN 55905; **Phone:** 507-284-2511; **Board Cert:** Internal Medicine 1979; Hematology 1982; Medical Oncology 1983; **Med School:** Loyola Univ-Stritch Sch Med 1975; **Resid:** Internal Medicine, St Lukes Hosp 1979; **Fellow:** Hematology & Oncology, Mayo Clin 1982; **Fac Appt:** Prof Med, Mayo Med Sch

Godwin, John MD [Hem] - **Spec Exp:** Thrombotic Disorders; Leukemia in Elderly; **Hospital:** St John's Hosp - Springfield; **Address:** Southern IL University Med Ctr, Carol Jo Vecchie Center, PO Box 19678, Springfield, IL 62794; **Phone:** 217-545-5817; **Board Cert:** Internal Medicine 1981; Hematology 1986; **Med School:** Univ Ala 1978; **Resid:** Internal Medicine, Baylor Coll Med 1981; Internal Medicine, Baylor Coll Med 1982; **Fellow:** Hematology, Baylor Coll Med 1983; Hematology, North Carolina Meml Hosp 1985; **Fac Appt:** Prof Med, Southern IL Univ

Gordon, Leo I MD [Hem] - **Spec Exp:** Lymphoma, Non-Hodgkin's; Hodgkin's Disease; Bone Marrow Transplant; **Hospital:** Northwestern Meml Hosp; **Address:** 675 N St Clair St, Ste 850, Chicago, IL 60611-3124; **Phone:** 312-695-0990; **Board Cert:** Internal Medicine 1976; Hematology 1978; Medical Oncology 1979; **Med School:** Univ Cincinnati 1973; **Resid:** Internal Medicine, Univ Chicago Hosps 1976; **Fellow:** Hematology, Univ Minnesota Hosps 1978; Hematology & Oncology, Univ Chicago Hosps 1979; **Fac Appt:** Prof Med, Northwestern Univ

Gregory, Stephanie A MD [Hem] - **Spec Exp:** Lymphoma; Leukemia; Plasma Cell Disorders; Multiple Myeloma; **Hospital:** Rush Univ Med Ctr; **Address:** 1725 W Harrison St, Ste 834, Rush Professional Office Building, Chicago, IL 60612-3861; **Phone:** 312-563-2320; **Board Cert:** Internal Medicine 1972; Hematology 1972; **Med School:** Med Coll PA Hahnemann 1965; **Resid:** Internal Medicine, Rush/Presby-St Luke's Med Ctr 1969; **Fellow:** Hematology, Rush/Presby-St Luke's Med Ctr 1972; **Fac Appt:** Prof Med, Rush Med Coll

Greipp, Philip R MD [Hem] - **Spec Exp:** Multiple Myeloma; **Hospital:** Mayo Med Ctr & Clin - Rochester; **Address:** Mayo Clinic, Div Hematology, 200 First St SW Bldg Mayo Fl W-10, Rochester, MN 55905-0001; **Phone:** 507-284-3159; **Board Cert:** Internal Medicine 1974; Hematology 1994; **Med School:** Georgetown Univ 1968; **Resid:** Internal Medicine, Mayo Clinic 1973; **Fellow:** Hematology, Mayo Clinic 1975; **Fac Appt:** Prof Med, Mayo Med Sch

Grever, Michael R MD [Hem] - **Spec Exp:** Hematologic Malignancies; Leukemia; Drug Development; Clinical Trials; **Hospital:** Ohio St Univ Med Ctr; **Address:** 215 Means Hall, 1654 Upham Drive, Columbus, OH 43210; **Phone:** 614-293-8724; **Board Cert:** Internal Medicine 1975; Hematology 1988; Medical Oncology 1979; **Med School:** Univ Pittsburgh 1971; **Resid:** Internal Medicine, Presby-Univ Hosp 1974; **Fellow:** Hematology & Oncology, Ohio State Univ 1978; **Fac Appt:** Prof Med, Ohio State Univ

Kraut, Eric H MD [Hem] - **Spec Exp:** Hematologic Malignancies; Leukemia; Drug Development; Clinical Trials; **Hospital:** Ohio St Univ Med Ctr; **Address:** B405 Starling Loving Hall, 320 W 10th Ave, Columbus, OH 43210; **Phone:** 614-293-8726; **Board Cert:** Internal Medicine 1975; Hematology 1978; Medical Oncology 1977; **Med School:** Temple Univ 1972; **Resid:** Internal Medicine, Univ Pittsburgh 1975; **Fellow:** Hematology & Oncology, Ohio State Univ Hosp 1977; **Fac Appt:** Prof Med, Ohio State Univ

Kuzel, Timothy M MD [Hem] - **Spec Exp:** Kidney Cancer; Testicular Cancer; Bladder Cancer; Lymphoma; **Hospital:** Northwestern Meml Hosp; **Address:** Northwestern Meml Hosp, 676 N St Clair, Ste 100, Chicago, IL 60611; **Phone:** 312-695-8697; **Board Cert:** Internal Medicine 1987; Hematology 2000; Medical Oncology 1989; **Med School:** Univ Mich Med Sch 1984; **Resid:** Internal Medicine, McGraw MC-Northwestern Univ 1987; **Fellow:** Hematology & Oncology, McGraw MC-Northwestern Univ 1990; **Fac Appt:** Prof Med, Northwestern Univ

Hematology

Larson, Richard A MD [Hem] - **Spec Exp:** Leukemia & Lymphoma; Bone Marrow Transplant; Myelodysplastic Syndromes; **Hospital:** Univ of Chicago Hosps; **Address:** Univ Chicago Hospitals, 5841 S Maryland Ave, MC 2115, Chicago, IL 60637; **Phone:** 773-702-6149; **Board Cert:** Internal Medicine 1980; Hematology 1982; Medical Oncology 1983; **Med School:** Stanford Univ 1977; **Resid:** Internal Medicine, Univ Chicago Hosps 1980; **Fellow:** Hematology & Oncology, Univ Chicago Hosps 1983; **Fac Appt:** Prof Med, Univ Chicago-Pritzker Sch Med

Lazarus, Hillard M MD [Hem] - **Spec Exp:** Bone Marrow Transplant; Stem Cell Transplant; Leukemia; **Hospital:** Univ Hosps Case Med Ctr; **Address:** Univ Hosp Med Ctr, 11100 Euclid Ave, Cleveland, OH 44106-5065; **Phone:** 216-844-3629; **Board Cert:** Internal Medicine 1977; Medical Oncology 1979; Hematology 1980; **Med School:** Univ Rochester 1974; **Resid:** Internal Medicine, Univ Hosps 1977; **Fellow:** Hematology & Oncology, Univ Hosps 1979; **Fac Appt:** Prof Med, Case West Res Univ

Litzow, Mark Robert MD [Hem] - **Spec Exp:** Bone Marrow Transplant; Leukemia; **Hospital:** Mayo Med Ctr & Clin - Rochester; **Address:** Mayo Clinic, Div Hematology, 200 First St SW, Rochester, MN 55905; **Phone:** 507-284-0923; **Board Cert:** Internal Medicine 1983; Hematology 1988; Medical Oncology 1989; **Med School:** Univ Chicago-Pritzker Sch Med 1980; **Resid:** Internal Medicine, Mayo Clinic 1984; **Fellow:** Medical Oncology, Mayo Clinic 1990; **Fac Appt:** Asst Prof Med, Mayo Med Sch

Maciejewski, Jaroslow P MD/PhD [Hem] - **Spec Exp:** Anemia-Aplastic; Hematologic Malignancies; Stem Cell Transplant; **Hospital:** Cleveland Clin Fdn (page 57); **Address:** Cleveland Clinic, 9500 Euclid Ave, Desk R40, Cleveland, OH 44195; **Phone:** 216-445-5962; **Board Cert:** Internal Medicine 1999; Hematology 2001; **Med School:** Germany 1987; **Resid:** Internal Medicine, Univ Nevada Med Ctr 1997; **Fellow:** Hematology, Natl Inst Hlth 2000

McGlave, Philip B MD [Hem] - **Spec Exp:** Leukemia; Bone Marrow Transplant; **Hospital:** Univ Minn Med Ctr, Fairview - Univ Campus; **Address:** Univ Minn, Dept Med - Div Hem/Onc, 420 Delaware St SE, MMC 480, Minneapolis, MN 55455; **Phone:** 612-626-2446; **Board Cert:** Internal Medicine 1977; Hematology 1980; **Med School:** Univ IL Coll Med 1974; **Resid:** Internal Medicine, Univ Minn 1977; **Fellow:** Hematology & Oncology, Univ Minn 1980; **Fac Appt:** Prof Med, Univ Minn

Mosher, Deane F MD [Hem] - **Hospital:** Univ WI Hosp & Clins; **Address:** Univ Wisc Hosp, Dept Hematology, 600 Highland Ave Fl 5, Madison, WI 53792; **Phone:** 608-263-7022; **Board Cert:** Internal Medicine 1973; Hematology 1980; **Med School:** Harvard Med Sch 1968; **Resid:** Internal Medicine, Beth Israel Hosp 1970; **Fellow:** Hematology, Harvard Med Sch 1972; **Fac Appt:** Prof Med, Univ Wisc

Nand, Sucha MD [Hem] - **Spec Exp:** Myelodysplastic Syndromes; Myeloproliferative Disorders; Leukemia; **Hospital:** Loyola Univ Med Ctr; **Address:** Cardinal Bernardin Cancer Ctr, 2160 S First Ave Bldg 112 - rm 342, Maywood, IL 60153-3304; **Phone:** 708-327-3217; **Board Cert:** Internal Medicine 1979; Medical Oncology 1981; Hematology 1982; **Med School:** India 1971; **Resid:** Physical Medicine & Rehabilitation, Northwestern Meml Hosp 1976; Internal Medicine, North Chicago VA Hosp 1978; **Fellow:** Medical Oncology, Northwestern Meml Hosp 1981; **Fac Appt:** Prof Med, Loyola Univ-Stritch Sch Med

Palascak, Joseph E MD [Hem] - **Spec Exp:** Hemophilia; Bleeding/Coagulation Disorders; Thrombotic Disorders; **Hospital:** Univ Hosp - Cincinnati; **Address:** Univ Cincinnati, Div Hem/Onc, 231 Albert Sabin Way, Box 670562, Cincinnati, OH 45267-0562; **Phone:** 513-584-1937; **Board Cert:** Internal Medicine 1975; Hematology 1978; **Med School:** Jefferson Med Coll 1968; **Resid:** Internal Medicine, Thomas Jefferson Univ Hosp 1971; **Fellow:** Hematology, Thomas Jefferson Univ Hosp 1976; **Fac Appt:** Prof Med, Univ Cincinnati

Silverstein, Roy L MD [Hem] - **Spec Exp:** Thrombotic Disorders; Bleeding/Coagulation Disorders; **Hospital:** Cleveland Clin Fdn (page 57); **Address:** Cleveland Clinic, Dept Cell Biology, 9500 Euclid Ave, NC10, Cleveland, OH 44195; **Phone:** 216-444-5520; **Board Cert:** Internal Medicine 1982; Hematology 1984; Medical Oncology 1985; **Med School:** Emory Univ 1979; **Resid:** Internal Medicine, New York Hosp-Cornell Med Ctr 1982; Hematology & Oncology, New York Hosp-Cornell Med Ctr 1984; **Fac Appt:** Prof Med, Cleveland Cl Coll Med/Case West Res

Stiff, Patrick J MD [Hem] - **Spec Exp:** Bone Marrow Transplant; Lymphoma, Non-Hodgkin's; Leukemia; **Hospital:** Loyola Univ Med Ctr; **Address:** Cardinal Bernadin Cancer Ctr, 2160 S First Ave Bldg 112 - rm 342, Maywood, IL 60153; **Phone:** 708-327-3216; **Board Cert:** Internal Medicine 1978; Medical Oncology 1981; Hematology 1982; **Med School:** Loyola Univ-Stritch Sch Med 1975; **Resid:** Internal Medicine, Cleveland Clinic 1978; **Fellow:** Hematology & Oncology, Meml Sloan Kettering Cancer Ctr 1981; **Fac Appt:** Prof Med, Loyola Univ-Stritch Sch Med

Tallman, Martin S MD [Hem] - **Spec Exp:** Bone Marrow Transplant; Leukemia; Lymphoma; **Hospital:** Northwestern Meml Hosp; **Address:** 675 N St Clair St, Ste 21-100, Chicago, IL 60611; **Phone:** 312-695-0990; **Board Cert:** Internal Medicine 1983; Medical Oncology 1987; Hematology 1988; **Med School:** Ros Franklin Univ/Chicago Med Sch 1980; **Resid:** Internal Medicine, Evanston Hosp 1983; **Fellow:** Medical Oncology, Fred Hutchinson Cancer Ctr 1987; **Fac Appt:** Prof Med, Northwestern Univ

van Besien, Koen W MD [Hem] - **Spec Exp:** Lymphoma; Stem Cell Transplant; **Hospital:** Univ of Chicago Hosps; **Address:** Univ Chicago Stem Cell Transplant Program, 5841 S Maryland Ave, MC 2115, Chicago, IL 60637; **Phone:** 773-702-4400; **Board Cert:** Internal Medicine 2005; Medical Oncology 2005; Hematology 1996; **Med School:** Belgium 1984; **Resid:** Internal Medicine, Univ Leuven Med Ctr 1987; **Fellow:** Hematology & Oncology, Indiana Univ Med Ctr 1990; **Fac Appt:** Prof Med, Univ Chicago-Pritzker Sch Med

Winter, Jane N MD [Hem] - **Spec Exp:** Lymphoma, Non-Hodgkin's; Hodgkin's Disease; Bone Marrow Transplant; **Hospital:** Northwestern Meml Hosp; **Address:** Northwestern Univ - Div Hem/Oncology, 675 N St Clair St, Ste 21-100, Chicago, IL 60611; **Phone:** 312-695-0990; **Board Cert:** Internal Medicine 1980; Hematology 1982; Medical Oncology 1983; **Med School:** Univ Pennsylvania 1977; **Resid:** Internal Medicine, Univ Chicago Hosps 1980; **Fellow:** Hematology & Oncology, Columbia Presby Hosp 1981; Hematology & Oncology, Northwestern Univ 1983; **Fac Appt:** Prof Med, Northwestern Univ

Great Plains and Mountains

Walters, Theodore MD [Hem] - **Spec Exp:** Bleeding/Coagulation Disorders; Myeloproliferative Disorders; Lymphoma; **Hospital:** St. Luke's Reg Med Ctr - Boise, St Alphonsus Regl Med Ctr; **Address:** 520 S Eagle Rd, Lower Level, Meridian, ID 83642; **Phone:** 208-706-5651; **Board Cert:** Internal Medicine 1972; Hematology 1976; **Med School:** Oregon Hlth Sci Univ 1963; **Resid:** Internal Medicine, Univ Oregon Med Ctr 1970; **Fellow:** Hematology, Univ Oregon Med Ctr 1972; **Fac Appt:** Asst Clin Prof Med, Univ Wash

Hematology

Southwest

Barlogie, Bart MD/PhD [Hem] - **Spec Exp:** Bone Marrow Transplant; Plasma Cell Disorders; Multiple Myeloma; **Hospital:** UAMS Med Ctr; **Address:** UAMS-Myeloma Inst Rsch & Therapy, 4301 West Markham St, Slot 816, Little Rock, AR 72205; **Phone:** 501-603-1583; **Med School:** Germany 1969; **Resid:** Internal Medicine, Univ Muenster Med Sch; **Fellow:** Medical Oncology, MD Anderson Cancer Ctr-Tumor Inst 1976; **Fac Appt:** Prof Med, Univ Ark

Champlin, Richard E MD [Hem] - **Spec Exp:** Bone Marrow Transplant; Stem Cell Transplant; Leukemia & Lymphoma; **Hospital:** UT MD Anderson Cancer Ctr (page 71); **Address:** MD Anderson Cancer Ctr, Div Hematology, 1515 Holcombe Blvd, Box 0423, Houston, TX 77030; **Phone:** 713-792-3618; **Board Cert:** Internal Medicine 1978; Hematology 1980; Medical Oncology 1981; **Med School:** Univ Chicago-Pritzker Sch Med 1975; **Resid:** Internal Medicine, LA Co Harbor/UCLA Med Ctr 1978; **Fellow:** Hematology & Oncology, LA Co Harbor/UCLA Med Ctr 1980; **Fac Appt:** Prof Med, Univ Tex, Houston

Cobos, Everardo MD [Hem] - **Spec Exp:** Bone Marrow Transplant; Bleeding/Coagulation Disorders; **Hospital:** Univ Med Ctr - Lubbock; **Address:** Texas Tech Univ Med Sch, Dept Med, 3601 4th St, MS 9410, Lubbock, TX 79430; **Phone:** 806-743-3155; **Board Cert:** Internal Medicine 1985; Medical Oncology 1987; Hematology 1988; **Med School:** Univ Tex, San Antonio 1981; **Resid:** Internal Medicine, Letterman Army Med Ctr 1985; **Fellow:** Hematology & Oncology, Letterman Army Med Ctr 1988; **Fac Appt:** Prof Med, Texas Tech Univ

Cooper, Barry MD [Hem] - **Spec Exp:** Leukemia; Lymphoma; Bleeding/Coagulation Disorders; **Hospital:** Baylor Univ Medical Ctr; **Address:** 3535 Worth St, Ste 200, Dallas, TX 75246-2096; **Phone:** 214-370-1002; **Board Cert:** Internal Medicine 1974; Medical Oncology 1977; Hematology 1978; **Med School:** Johns Hopkins Univ 1971; **Resid:** Internal Medicine, Johns Hopkins Hosp 1973; **Fellow:** Metabolism, Natl Inst of Health 1975; Hematology, Peter Bent Brigham Hosp 1977; **Fac Appt:** Clin Prof Med, Univ Tex SW, Dallas

Kantarjian, Hagop M MD [Hem] - **Spec Exp:** Leukemia; **Hospital:** UT MD Anderson Cancer Ctr (page 71); **Address:** 1400 Holcombe Blvd, Unit 428, Houston, TX 77030; **Phone:** 713-792-7026; **Board Cert:** Internal Medicine 1983; Medical Oncology 1985; **Med School:** Lebanon 1979; **Resid:** Internal Medicine, Univ Tex MD Anderson Cancer Ctr 1983; **Fellow:** Hematology & Oncology, Univ Tex MD Anderson Cancer Ctr 1983; **Fac Appt:** Prof Med, Univ Tex, Houston

Keating, Michael MD [Hem] - **Spec Exp:** Leukemia; **Hospital:** UT MD Anderson Cancer Ctr (page 71); **Address:** MD Anderson Cancer Ctr, 1515 Holcombe Blvd, Box 428, Houston, TX 77030; **Phone:** 713-745-2376; **Med School:** Australia 1966; **Resid:** Internal Medicine, St Vincents Hosp 1973; **Fellow:** Hematology, MD Anderson Cancer Ctr 1975; **Fac Appt:** Prof Med, Univ Tex, Houston

Lyons, Roger M MD [Hem] - **Spec Exp:** Leukemia & Lymphoma; Multiple Myeloma; Bleeding/Coagulation Disorders; Platelet Disorders; **Hospital:** SW TX Meth Hosp, Methodist Spec & Transpl Hosp; **Address:** 4411 Medical Drive, Ste 100, San Antonio, TX 78229-3325; **Phone:** 210-595-5300; **Board Cert:** Internal Medicine 1981; Hematology 1982; **Med School:** Canada 1967; **Resid:** Internal Medicine, Winnipeg Genl Hosp 1969; Internal Medicine, Barnes-Wohl Hosps 1972; **Fellow:** Hematology, Washington Univ Hosps 1975; **Fac Appt:** Clin Prof Med, Univ Tex, San Antonio

Maddox, Anne Marie MD [Hem] - **Spec Exp:** Hematologic Malignancies; Lung Cancer; Head & Neck Cancer; Clinical Trials; **Hospital:** UAMS Med Ctr; **Address:** Univ Arkansas Med Ctr, 4301 W Markham St, Slot 74-5, Little Rock, AR 72205; **Phone:** 501-686-8530; **Board Cert:** Internal Medicine 1979; Medical Oncology 1985; Hematology 2004; **Med School:** Dalhousie Univ 1975; **Resid:** Internal Medicine, Univ Toronto 1978; **Fellow:** Medical Oncology, MD Anderson Cancer Ctr 1982; **Fac Appt:** Prof, Univ Ark

Miro-Quesada, Miguel MD [Hem] - **Hospital:** Meml Hermann Hosp - Houston, St Luke's Episcopal Hosp - Houston; **Address:** 920 Frostwood, Ste 780, Houston, TX 77030; **Phone:** 713-827-9525; **Board Cert:** Internal Medicine 1972; Hematology 1974; Medical Oncology 1985; **Med School:** Johns Hopkins Univ 1969; **Resid:** Internal Medicine, Northwestern Univ Hosp 1971; Internal Medicine, Rush-Presby-St Luke's Med Ctr 1972; **Fellow:** Hematology, Montefiore Hosp 1974

Strauss, James F MD [Hem] - **Spec Exp:** Bleeding/Coagulation Disorders; Leukemia; Lymphoma; **Hospital:** Presby Hosp of Dallas; **Address:** Texas Oncology, Professional Bldg 2, 8220 Walnut Hill Ln, Ste 700, Dallas, TX 75231; **Phone:** 214-739-4175; **Board Cert:** Internal Medicine 1976; Hematology 1978; Medical Oncology 1981; **Med School:** NYU Sch Med 1972; **Resid:** Internal Medicine, Baylor Univ Medical Ctr 1976; **Fellow:** Hematology, Univ Texas SW Medical Ctr 1977

Yeager, Andrew M MD [Hem] - **Spec Exp:** Bone Marrow & Stem Cell Transplant; Graft vs Host Disease; Leukemia; **Hospital:** Univ Med Ctr - Tucson; **Address:** Arizona Cancer Ctr, 1515 N Campbell Ave, Ste 2956, Tuscon, AZ 85724-0001; **Phone:** 520-626-0662; **Board Cert:** Pediatrics 1979; Pediatric Hematology-Oncology 1980; **Med School:** Johns Hopkins Univ 1975; **Resid:** Pediatrics, Johns Hopkins Hosp 1978; **Fellow:** Pediatric Hematology-Oncology, Johns Hopkins Hosp 1980; **Fac Appt:** Prof Med, Univ Ariz Coll Med

West Coast and Pacific

Damon, Lloyd E MD [Hem] - **Spec Exp:** Multiple Myeloma; Hematologic Malignancies; Stem Cell Transplant; **Hospital:** UCSF Med Ctr; **Address:** UCSF Comprehensive Cancer Ctr, 400 Parnassus Ave, Ste A502, San Francisco, CA 94143; **Phone:** 415-353-2421; **Board Cert:** Internal Medicine 1985; Hematology 1988; Medical Oncology 1987; **Med School:** Univ Mich Med Sch 1982; **Resid:** Internal Medicine, UCSF Med Ctr 1985; **Fellow:** Hematology & Oncology, UCSF Med Ctr 1988; **Fac Appt:** Clin Prof Med, UCSF

Feinstein, Donald I MD [Hem] - **Spec Exp:** Bleeding/Coagulation Disorders; Hematologic Malignancies; **Hospital:** USC Norris Comp Cancer Ctr, USC Univ Hosp - R K Eamer Med Plz; **Address:** USC Keck Sch Med, Topping Tower, 1441 Eastlake Ave, Ste 3436, Los Angeles, CA 90033-9172; **Phone:** 323-865-3964; **Board Cert:** Internal Medicine 1965; Hematology 1974; **Med School:** Stanford Univ 1958; **Resid:** Internal Medicine, LAC-USC Med Ctr 1962; **Fellow:** Hematology, NYU Med Ctr 1966; **Fac Appt:** Prof Med, USC Sch Med

Forman, Stephen J MD [Hem] - **Spec Exp:** Lymphoma; Leukemia; Bone Marrow Transplant; **Hospital:** City of Hope Natl Med Ctr & Beckman Rsch; **Address:** City Hope National Medical Ctr, 1500 E Duarte Rd, rm 3002, Duarte, CA 91010-3012; **Phone:** 626-256-4673 x62403; **Board Cert:** Internal Medicine 1977; **Med School:** USC Sch Med 1974; **Resid:** Internal Medicine, LAC-Harbor-UCLA Med Ctr 1976; **Fellow:** Hematology, LAC-USC Med Ctr 1978; Hematology, City of Hope Med Ctr 1979; **Fac Appt:** Clin Prof Med, USC Sch Med

Hematology

Kaushansky, Kenneth MD [Hem] - **Spec Exp:** Platelet Disorders; **Hospital:** UCSD Med Ctr; **Address:** UCSD, Dept Medicine, 402 Dickinson St, Ste 380, San Diego, CA 92103-8811; **Phone:** 619-543-6170; **Board Cert:** Internal Medicine 1982; Hematology 1984; **Med School:** UCLA 1979; **Resid:** Internal Medicine, Univ Wash Med Ctr 1982; **Fellow:** Hematology, Univ Wash Med Ctr 1986; **Fac Appt:** Prof Med, UCSD

Leung, Lawrence L MD [Hem] - **Spec Exp:** Thrombotic Disorders; **Hospital:** Stanford Univ Med Ctr, VA Hlth Care Sys - Palo Alto; **Address:** Stanford Univ Med Ctr, Dept Hem, 269 Campus Drive CCSR Bldg - rm 1155, Stanford, CA 94305-5156; **Phone:** 650-723-9729; **Board Cert:** Internal Medicine 1978; Hematology 1980; Medical Oncology 1981; **Med School:** Columbia P&S 1975; **Resid:** Internal Medicine, NY Hosp/Cornell Med Ctr 1978; **Fellow:** Hematology & Oncology, NY Hosp/Cornell Med Ctr 1981; **Fac Appt:** Prof Med, Stanford Univ

Levine, Alexandra M MD [Hem] - **Spec Exp:** Leukemia & Lymphoma; AIDS Related Cancers; AIDS/HIV; **Hospital:** City of Hope Natl Med Ctr & Beckman Rsch; **Address:** 1500 E Duarte Rd, Needleman 213, Duarte, CA 91010; **Phone:** 626-256-4673; **Med School:** USC Sch Med 1971; **Resid:** Internal Medicine, LAC-USC Med Ctr 1974; **Fellow:** Hematology & Oncology, Grady Meml Hosp-Emory Univ 1975; Hematology, LAC-USC Med Ctr 1978; **Fac Appt:** Prof Med, USC Sch Med

Linenberger, Michael MD [Hem] - **Spec Exp:** Bone Marrow Transplant; Leukemia & Lymphoma; Multiple Myeloma; **Hospital:** Univ Wash Med Ctr; **Address:** 825 Eastlake Ave E, MS G6-800, Seattle, WA 98109; **Phone:** 206-288-1260; **Board Cert:** Internal Medicine 1985; Hematology 1988; **Med School:** Univ Kans 1982; **Resid:** Internal Medicine, Rhode Island Hosp 1985; **Fellow:** Hematology, Univ Wash Med Ctr 1989; **Fac Appt:** Assoc Prof Med, Univ Wash

Linker, Charles A MD [Hem] - **Spec Exp:** Leukemia; Bone Marrow Transplant; Multiple Myeloma; **Hospital:** UCSF Med Ctr, St Francis Memorial Hosp; **Address:** 400 Parnassus Ave, Ste A502, San Francisco, CA 94143; **Phone:** 415-353-2421; **Board Cert:** Internal Medicine 1978; Hematology 1980; Medical Oncology 1981; **Med School:** Stanford Univ 1974; **Resid:** Internal Medicine, Stanford Univ Hosp 1978; **Fellow:** Hematology & Oncology, UCSF Med Ctr 1981; **Fac Appt:** Clin Prof Med, UCSF

Negrin, Robert S MD [Hem] - **Spec Exp:** Bone Marrow Transplant; **Hospital:** Stanford Univ Med Ctr; **Address:** BMT Program, 300 Pasteur Drive, rm H3249, MC 5623, Stanford, CA 94305; **Phone:** 650-723-0822; **Board Cert:** Internal Medicine 1987; Hematology 1992; **Med School:** Harvard Med Sch 1984; **Resid:** Internal Medicine, Stanford Univ Hosp 1987; **Fellow:** Hematology, Stanford Univ Hosp 1990; **Fac Appt:** Prof Med, Stanford Univ

Saven, Alan MD [Hem] - **Spec Exp:** Leukemia; Lymphoma; **Hospital:** Scripps Green Hosp; **Address:** Scripps Green Hosp, 10666 N Torrey Pines Rd, MS 217, La Jolla, CA 92037; **Phone:** 858-554-9489; **Board Cert:** Internal Medicine 1987; Medical Oncology 1989; Hematology 1990; **Med School:** South Africa 1982; **Resid:** Internal Medicine, Albert Einstein Med Ctr 1986; **Fellow:** Hematology & Oncology, Scripps Clinic 1987

Schiller, Gary J MD [Hem] - **Spec Exp:** Leukemia; **Hospital:** UCLA Med Ctr; **Address:** UCLA Med Ctr, 10833 Le Conte Ave, rm 42-121 CHS, Los Angeles, CA 90095; **Phone:** 310-825-5513; **Board Cert:** Internal Medicine 1987; Hematology 2000; Medical Oncology 1989; **Med School:** USC Sch Med 1984; **Resid:** Internal Medicine, UCLA Med Ctr 1987; **Fellow:** Hematology & Oncology, UCLA Med Ctr 1990; **Fac Appt:** Prof Med, UCLA

Medical Oncology

New England

Anderson, Kenneth C MD [Onc] - **Spec Exp:** Multiple Myeloma; **Hospital:** Dana-Farber Cancer Inst, Brigham & Women's Hosp; **Address:** Dana Farber Cancer Inst, 44 Binney St Mayer Bldg - rm 557, Boston, MA 02115; **Phone:** 617-632-2144; **Board Cert:** Internal Medicine 1980; **Med School:** Johns Hopkins Univ 1977; **Resid:** Internal Medicine, Johns Hopkins Hosp 1980; **Fellow:** Hematology & Oncology, Dana Farber Cancer Inst 1983; **Fac Appt:** Prof Med, Harvard Med Sch

Antin, Joseph Harry MD [Onc] - **Spec Exp:** Bone Marrow Transplant; Stem Cell Transplant; Leukemia; **Hospital:** Brigham & Women's Hosp, Dana-Farber Cancer Inst; **Address:** 44 Binney St, rm D1B12, Boston, MA 02115-6013; **Phone:** 617-632-3667; **Board Cert:** Internal Medicine 1981; Medical Oncology 1983; Hematology 1984; **Med School:** Cornell Univ-Weill Med Coll 1978; **Resid:** Internal Medicine, Peter Bent Brigham Hosp 1981; **Fellow:** Hematology & Oncology, Brigham & Womens Hosp/Dana Farber 1984; **Fac Appt:** Prof Med, Harvard Med Sch

Atkins, Michael B MD [Onc] - **Spec Exp:** Melanoma; Kidney Cancer; Immunotherapy; **Hospital:** Beth Israel Deaconess Med Ctr - Boston; **Address:** Beth Israel Deaconess Med Ctr, Cancer Clinical Trials, 330 Brookline Ave, E-157, Boston, MA 02215; **Phone:** 617-667-1930; **Board Cert:** Internal Medicine 1983; Medical Oncology 1987; **Med School:** Tufts Univ 1980; **Resid:** Internal Medicine, New England Med Ctr 1983; **Fellow:** Hematology & Oncology, New England Med Ctr 1987; **Fac Appt:** Prof Med, Harvard Med Sch

Canellos, George P MD [Onc] - **Spec Exp:** Lymphoma; Leukemia; Breast Cancer; **Hospital:** Dana-Farber Cancer Inst, Brigham & Women's Hosp; **Address:** 44 Binney St, Boston, MA 02115; **Phone:** 617-632-3470; **Board Cert:** Internal Medicine 1967; Hematology 1972; Medical Oncology 1973; **Med School:** Columbia P&S 1960; **Resid:** Internal Medicine, Mass Genl Hosp 1963; Internal Medicine, Mass Genl Hosp 1966; **Fellow:** Medical Oncology, Natl Cancer Inst 1965; Hematology, Hammersmith Hosp 1967; **Fac Appt:** Prof Med, Harvard Med Sch

Come, Steven E MD [Onc] - **Spec Exp:** Breast Cancer; Hodgkin's Disease; **Hospital:** Beth Israel Deaconess Med Ctr - Boston, Dana-Farber Cancer Inst; **Address:** Beth Israel Deaconess Hosp, 330 Brookline Ave, Boston, MA 02215-5400; **Phone:** 617-667-4599; **Board Cert:** Internal Medicine 1975; Medical Oncology 1979; **Med School:** Harvard Med Sch 1972; **Resid:** Internal Medicine, Beth Israel Hosp 1977; **Fellow:** Medical Oncology, Natl Cancer Inst 1976; **Fac Appt:** Assoc Prof Med, Harvard Med Sch

Demetri, George D MD [Onc] - **Spec Exp:** Sarcoma; **Hospital:** Dana-Farber Cancer Inst; **Address:** Dana Farber Cancer Inst, 44 Binney St, Shields-Warren 530, Boston, MA 02115; **Phone:** 617-632-3985; **Board Cert:** Internal Medicine 1986; Medical Oncology 1989; **Med School:** Stanford Univ 1983; **Resid:** Internal Medicine, Univ Wash Med Ctr 1986; **Fellow:** Medical Oncology, Dana Farber Cancer Inst 1989; **Fac Appt:** Assoc Prof Med, Harvard Med Sch

DeVita Jr, Vincent T MD [Onc] - **Spec Exp:** Lymphoma Consultation; Hodgkin's Disease Consultation; **Hospital:** Yale - New Haven Hosp; **Address:** Yale Cancer Ctr, 333 Cedar St, rm WWW-211B, New Haven, CT 06520-8028; **Phone:** 203-737-1010; **Board Cert:** Internal Medicine 1974; Hematology 1972; Medical Oncology 1973; **Med School:** Geo Wash Univ 1961; **Resid:** Internal Medicine, Geo Wash Hosp 1963; Internal Medicine, Yale-New Haven Hosp 1966; **Fellow:** Medical Oncology, Natl Cancer Inst 1965; **Fac Appt:** Prof Med, Yale Univ

Garber, Judy E MD [Onc] - **Spec Exp:** Breast Cancer; **Hospital:** Dana-Farber Cancer Inst; **Address:** Dana Farber Cancer Inst, 44 Binney St, Smith 209, Boston, MA 02115; **Phone:** 617-632-5770; **Board Cert:** Internal Medicine 1984; Medical Oncology 1987; Hematology 1988; **Med School:** Yale Univ 1981; **Resid:** Internal Medicine, Brigham & Womens Hosp 1984; **Fellow:** Medical Oncology, Dana Farber Cancer Inst 1988; Epidemiology, Dana Farber Cancer Inst 1990; **Fac Appt:** Assoc Prof Med, Harvard Med Sch

Garnick, Marc B MD [Onc] - **Spec Exp:** Prostate Cancer; Urologic Cancer; **Hospital:** Beth Israel Deaconess Med Ctr - Boston; **Address:** Beth Israel Deaconess Medical Ctr, SCC9, 330 Brookline Ave, Boston, MA 02215; **Phone:** 617-667-9187; **Board Cert:** Internal Medicine 1976; Medical Oncology 1979; **Med School:** Univ Pennsylvania 1972; **Resid:** Internal Medicine, Univ Penn Hosp 1974; **Fellow:** Research, Natl Inst Hlth 1976; Medical Oncology, Dana-Farber Cancer Inst 1978; **Fac Appt:** Clin Prof Med, Harvard Med Sch

Haluska, Frank G MD/PhD [Onc] - **Spec Exp:** Melanoma; **Hospital:** Tufts-New England Med Ctr; **Address:** Tufts-New England Med Ctr, 750 Washington St, Box 245, Boston, MA 02111; **Phone:** 617-636-5147; **Board Cert:** Internal Medicine 2002; Medical Oncology 1995; **Med School:** Univ Pennsylvania 1989; **Resid:** Internal Medicine, Mass Genl Hosp 1991; **Fellow:** Medical Oncology, Dana-Farber Cancer Inst 1994; **Fac Appt:** Prof Med, Tufts Univ

Johnson, Bruce E MD [Onc] - **Spec Exp:** Lung Cancer; Thoracic Cancers; Merkel Cell Carcinoma; **Hospital:** Dana-Farber Cancer Inst, Brigham & Women's Hosp; **Address:** Lowe Ctr Thoracic Oncology, 44 Binney St, Ste D-1234, Boston, MA 02115; **Phone:** 617-632-4790; **Board Cert:** Internal Medicine 1982; Medical Oncology 1985; **Med School:** Univ Minn 1979; **Resid:** Internal Medicine, Univ Chicago Hosps 1982; **Fellow:** Medical Oncology, Natl Cancer Inst 1985; **Fac Appt:** Assoc Prof Med, Harvard Med Sch

Kaelin, William G MD [Onc] - **Spec Exp:** Drug Discovery & Development; **Hospital:** Dana-Farber Cancer Inst; **Address:** Dana Farber Cancer Inst, 44 Binney St, rm MA-457, Boston, MA 02115; **Phone:** 617-632-4747; **Board Cert:** Internal Medicine 1987; Medical Oncology 1989; **Med School:** Duke Univ 1982; **Resid:** Internal Medicine, Johns Hopkins Hosp 1986; **Fellow:** Medical Oncology, Dana Farber Cancer Inst 1989; **Fac Appt:** Prof Med, Harvard Med Sch

Kantoff, Philip W MD [Onc] - **Spec Exp:** Genitourinary Cancer; Prostate Cancer; **Hospital:** Dana-Farber Cancer Inst, Brigham & Women's Hosp; **Address:** 44 Binney St, Ste D-1230, Boston, MA 02115; **Phone:** 617-632-3466; **Board Cert:** Internal Medicine 1982; Medical Oncology 1989; **Med School:** Brown Univ 1979; **Resid:** Internal Medicine, NYU/Bellevue Hosp 1983; **Fellow:** Gene Therapy Research, NIH 1986; **Fac Appt:** Prof Med, Harvard Med Sch

Kaufman, Peter A MD [Onc] - **Spec Exp:** Breast Cancer; Clinical Trials; **Hospital:** Dartmouth - Hitchcock Med Ctr; **Address:** Dartmouth-Hitchcock Med Ctr, Dept Hem/Onc, One Medical Center Drive, Lebanon, NH 03756; **Phone:** 603-653-6181; **Board Cert:** Internal Medicine 1986; Medical Oncology 1989; **Med School:** NYU Sch Med 1983; **Resid:** Internal Medicine, Duke Univ Med Ctr 1986; **Fellow:** Hematology & Oncology, Duke Univ Med Ctr 1989; **Fac Appt:** Assoc Prof Med, Dartmouth Med Sch

Lynch, Thomas MD [Onc] - **Spec Exp:** Lung Cancer; Thoracic Cancers; **Hospital:** Mass Genl Hosp; **Address:** Mass Genl Hosp, Dept Hem/Onc, 55 Fruit St, Yawkey Bldg - Ste 7B, Boston, MA 02114-2617; **Phone:** 617-724-1136; **Board Cert:** Internal Medicine 1989; Medical Oncology 2003; **Med School:** Yale Univ 1986; **Resid:** Internal Medicine, Mass Genl Hosp 1989; **Fellow:** Medical Oncology, Dana-Farber Cancer Inst 1991; **Fac Appt:** Asst Prof Med, Harvard Med Sch

Mayer, Robert J MD [Onc] - **Spec Exp:** Colon & Rectal Cancer; Gastrointestinal Cancer; **Hospital:** Dana-Farber Cancer Inst, Brigham & Women's Hosp; **Address:** Dana Farber Cancer Inst, 44 Binney St, rm D1608, Boston, MA 02115-6084; **Phone:** 617-632-3474; **Board Cert:** Internal Medicine 1973; Medical Oncology 1975; Hematology 1976; **Med School:** Harvard Med Sch 1969; **Resid:** Internal Medicine, Mt Sinai Hosp 1971; Hematology & Oncology, Natl Cancer Inst 1974; **Fellow:** Dana Farber Cancer Inst 1976; **Fac Appt:** Prof Med, Harvard Med Sch

Muss, Hyman B MD [Onc] - **Spec Exp:** Breast Cancer; **Hospital:** FAHC - Med Ctr Campus; **Address:** Fletcher Allen Health Care-UHC Campus, 1 S Prospect St, Joseph 3, Burlington, VT 05401-1429; **Phone:** 802-847-3827; **Board Cert:** Internal Medicine 1973; Hematology 1974; Medical Oncology 1975; **Med School:** SUNY Downstate 1968; **Resid:** Internal Medicine, Peter Bent Brigham Hosp 1970; **Fellow:** Hematology & Oncology, Peter Bent Brigham Hosp 1974; **Fac Appt:** Prof Med, Univ VT Coll Med

Nadler, Lee M MD [Onc] - **Spec Exp:** Lymphoma; **Hospital:** Dana-Farber Cancer Inst, Brigham & Women's Hosp; **Address:** Dana Farber Cancer Inst, 44 Binney St, SM 339, Boston, MA 02115; **Phone:** 617-632-3331; **Board Cert:** Internal Medicine 1976; **Med School:** Harvard Med Sch 1973; **Resid:** Internal Medicine, Columbia-Presby Hosp 1975; **Fellow:** Medical Oncology, Natl Cancer Inst 1977; Medical Oncology, Dana-Farber Cancer Inst 1978; **Fac Appt:** Prof Med, Harvard Med Sch

Schnipper, Lowell E MD [Onc] - **Spec Exp:** Breast Cancer; **Hospital:** Beth Israel Deaconess Med Ctr - Boston; **Address:** Beth Israel Deaconess Med Ctr, 330 Brookline Ave, Boston, MA 02215; **Phone:** 617-667-1198; **Board Cert:** Internal Medicine 1973; Medical Oncology 1983; **Med School:** SUNY Downstate 1968; **Resid:** Internal Medicine, Yale-New Haven Hosp 1970; Medical Oncology, Natl Cancer Inst 1973; **Fellow:** Hematology & Oncology, Barnes Jewish Hosp 1974; **Fac Appt:** Prof Med, Harvard Med Sch

Shulman, Lawrence N MD [Onc] - **Spec Exp:** Breast Cancer; Lymphoma; **Hospital:** Dana-Farber Cancer Inst; **Address:** Dana-Farber Cancer Inst, 44 Binney St, rm Dana-1608, Boston, MA 02115; **Phone:** 617-632-2277; **Board Cert:** Internal Medicine 1978; Medical Oncology 1981; Hematology 1982; **Med School:** Harvard Med Sch 1975; **Resid:** Internal Medicine, Beth Israel Hosp 1977; **Fellow:** Hematology & Oncology, Beth Israel Hosp 1980; **Fac Appt:** Assoc Prof Med, Harvard Med Sch

Medical Oncology

Treon, Steven P MD/PhD [Onc] - **Spec Exp:** Waldenstrom's Macroglobulinemia; Multiple Myeloma; **Hospital:** Dana-Farber Cancer Inst; **Address:** Dana-Farber Cancer Inst, 44 Binney St, Mayer 548B, Boston, MA 02115; **Phone:** 617-632-2681; **Board Cert:** Internal Medicine 1995; Medical Oncology 1997; **Med School:** Boston Univ 1993; **Resid:** Internal Medicine, Boston Univ Med Ctr 1995; **Fellow:** Hematology & Oncology, Mass Genl Hosp 1996; Research, Dana Farber Cancer Inst 1997; **Fac Appt:** Asst Prof Med, Harvard Med Sch

Weisberg, Tracey MD [Onc] - **Spec Exp:** Breast Cancer; **Hospital:** Maine Med Ctr; **Address:** 100 Campus Drive, Unit 108, Scarborough, ME 04074; **Phone:** 207-885-7600; **Board Cert:** Internal Medicine 1987; Medical Oncology 1989; **Med School:** SUNY Stony Brook 1983; **Resid:** Internal Medicine, Mount Sinai Hosp 1985; Internal Medicine, Hartford Hosp 1986; **Fellow:** Medical Oncology, Yale Univ Hosp 1988

Winer, Eric P MD [Onc] - **Spec Exp:** Breast Cancer; **Hospital:** Dana-Farber Cancer Inst, Brigham & Women's Hosp; **Address:** Dana Farber Cancer Inst, 44 Binney St, Mayer 2, Boston, MA 02115; **Phone:** 617-632-2175; **Board Cert:** Internal Medicine 1987; Medical Oncology 1989; **Med School:** Yale Univ 1983; **Resid:** Internal Medicine, Yale-New Haven Hosp 1987; **Fellow:** Hematology & Oncology, Duke Univ 1989; **Fac Appt:** Assoc Prof Med, Harvard Med Sch

Mid Atlantic

Abeloff, Martin MD [Onc] - **Spec Exp:** Breast Cancer; **Hospital:** Johns Hopkins Hosp - Baltimore (page 61); **Address:** 401 N Broadway, Ste 1100, Baltimore, MD 21231; **Phone:** 410-955-8822; **Board Cert:** Internal Medicine 1973; Medical Oncology 1973; **Med School:** Johns Hopkins Univ 1966; **Resid:** Internal Medicine, Beth Israel Hosp 1970; **Fellow:** Hematology, New England Med Ctr 1971; **Fac Appt:** Prof Med, Johns Hopkins Univ

Ahlgren, James D MD [Onc] - **Spec Exp:** Gastrointestinal Cancer; **Hospital:** G Washington Univ Hosp; **Address:** Geo Wash Univ Med Ctr, Div Hem/Oncology, 2150 Pennsylvania Ave NW, Ste 3-428, Washington, DC 20037-3201; **Phone:** 202-741-2478; **Board Cert:** Internal Medicine 1980; Medical Oncology 1989; **Med School:** Georgetown Univ 1977; **Resid:** Internal Medicine, Georgetown Univ Hosp 1979; **Fellow:** Medical Oncology, Georgetown Univ Hosp 1981; **Fac Appt:** Prof Med, Geo Wash Univ

Aisner, Joseph MD [Onc] - **Spec Exp:** Lung Cancer; Solid Tumors; **Hospital:** Robert Wood Johnson Univ Hosp - New Brunswick; **Address:** Cancer Inst of New Jersey, 195 Little Albany St, rm 2012, New Brunswick, NJ 08903-2681; **Phone:** 732-235-6777; **Board Cert:** Internal Medicine 1973; Medical Oncology 1975; **Med School:** Wayne State Univ 1970; **Resid:** Internal Medicine, Georgetown Univ Hosp 1972; **Fellow:** Medical Oncology, Natl Cancer Inst 1975

Algazy, Kenneth M MD [Onc] - **Spec Exp:** Lung Cancer; Mesothelioma; Hematologic Malignancies; **Hospital:** Hosp Univ Penn - UPHS (page 72), VA Med Ctr; **Address:** Hosp Univ Pennsylvania, 3400 Spruce St, 12 Penn Tower, Philadelphia, PA 19104; **Phone:** 215-614-1858; **Board Cert:** Internal Medicine 1972; Hematology 1974; Medical Oncology 1979; **Med School:** Temple Univ 1969; **Resid:** Internal Medicine, Univ Rochester-Strong Meml Hosp 1972; **Fellow:** Hematology & Oncology, Johns Hopkins Med Ctr 1974; **Fac Appt:** Clin Prof Med, Univ Pennsylvania

Ambinder, Richard F MD/PhD [Onc] - **Spec Exp:** Lymphoma; Hodgkin's Disease; AIDS Related Cancers; **Hospital:** Johns Hopkins Hosp - Baltimore (page 61); **Address:** Cancer Research Bldg, 1650 Orleans St, rm CRB 389, Baltimore, MD 21231; **Phone:** 410-955-8964; **Board Cert:** Internal Medicine 1982; Medical Oncology 1985; **Med School:** Johns Hopkins Univ 1979; **Resid:** Internal Medicine, Johns Hopkins Hosp 1981; **Fellow:** Internal Medicine, Johns Hopkins Hosp 1982; Medical Oncology, Johns Hopkins Hosp 1985; **Fac Appt:** Prof Med, Johns Hopkins Univ

Belani, Chandra MD [Onc] - **Spec Exp:** Lung Cancer; Drug Discovery; **Hospital:** UPMC Shadyside, UPMC Presby, Pittsburgh; **Address:** UPMC Cancer Pavilion, 5150 Centre Ave Fl 5, Pittsburgh, PA 15232; **Phone:** 412-648-6619; **Board Cert:** Internal Medicine 1986; Medical Oncology 1987; **Med School:** India 1978; **Resid:** Internal Medicine, SMS Med Hosp 1981; Internal Medicine, Good Samaritan/Univ MD Hosp 1984; **Fellow:** Hematology & Oncology, Univ Maryland Hosp 1987; **Fac Appt:** Prof Med, Univ Pittsburgh

Bosl, George MD [Onc] - **Spec Exp:** Testicular Cancer; Head & Neck Cancer; **Hospital:** Meml Sloan Kettering Cancer Ctr; **Address:** 1275 York Ave, rm C1289, New York, NY 10021; **Phone:** 212-639-8473; **Board Cert:** Internal Medicine 1976; Medical Oncology 1979; **Med School:** Creighton Univ 1973; **Resid:** Internal Medicine, New York Hosp 1975; Internal Medicine, Memorial Sloan-Kettering Cancer Ctr 1977; **Fellow:** Medical Oncology, Univ Minn Hosps 1979; **Fac Appt:** Prof Med, Cornell Univ-Weill Med Coll

Chapman, Paul MD [Onc] - **Spec Exp:** Melanoma; Immunotherapy; Vaccine Therapy; **Hospital:** Meml Sloan Kettering Cancer Ctr; **Address:** 1275 York Ave, New York, NY 10021; **Phone:** 646-888-2378; **Board Cert:** Internal Medicine 1984; Medical Oncology 1987; **Med School:** Cornell Univ-Weill Med Coll 1981; **Resid:** Internal Medicine, Univ Chicago Hosps 1984; **Fellow:** Medical Oncology, Meml Sloan-Kettering Cancer Ctr 1987; **Fac Appt:** Prof Med, Cornell Univ-Weill Med Coll

Cohen, Philip MD [Onc] - **Spec Exp:** Breast Cancer; **Hospital:** Georgetown Univ Hosp; **Address:** Georgetown Univ Hosp, Lombardi Cancer Ctr, 3800 Reservoir Rd NW, Washington, DC 20007; **Phone:** 202-444-2198; **Board Cert:** Internal Medicine 1973; Medical Oncology 1975; Hematology 1976; **Med School:** Harvard Med Sch 1970; **Resid:** Internal Medicine, Mass Genl Hosp 1972; **Fellow:** Medical Oncology, Natl Cancer Inst 1974; **Fac Appt:** Assoc Prof Med, Geo Wash Univ

Cohen, Roger MD [Onc] - **Spec Exp:** Drug Discovery & Development; Clinical Trials; **Hospital:** Fox Chase Cancer Ctr (page 59); **Address:** Fox Chase Cancer Ctr, 333 Cottman Ave, Ste C307, Philadelphia, PA 19111; **Phone:** 215-728-2570; **Board Cert:** Internal Medicine 1984; Medical Oncology 1993; Hematology 1986; **Med School:** Harvard Med Sch 1980; **Resid:** Internal Medicine, Mt Sinai Hosp 1982; **Fellow:** Research, Sloan Kettering Cancer Inst 1985; Hematology, Mt Sinai Hosp 1986

Cohen, Seymour M MD [Onc] - **Spec Exp:** Melanoma; Breast Cancer; Lung Cancer; Merkel Cell Carcinoma; **Hospital:** Mount Sinai Med Ctr; **Address:** 1045 5th Ave, New York, NY 10028-0138; **Phone:** 212-249-9141; **Board Cert:** Internal Medicine 1971; Medical Oncology 1973; **Med School:** Univ Pittsburgh 1962; **Resid:** Internal Medicine, Montefiore Med Ctr 1964; Internal Medicine, Mount Sinai Med Ctr 1965; **Fellow:** Hematology, Mount Sinai Med Ctr 1966; Hematology & Oncology, LI Jewish Hosp 1969; **Fac Appt:** Assoc Clin Prof Med, Mount Sinai Sch Med

Medical Oncology

Coleman, Morton MD [Onc] - **Spec Exp:** Lymphoma; Hodgkin's Disease; Multiple Myeloma; Waldenstrom's Macroglobulinemia; **Hospital:** NY-Presby Hosp/Weill Cornell (page 66); **Address:** 407 E 70th St, FL 3, New York, NY 10021-5302; **Phone:** 212-517-5900; **Board Cert:** Internal Medicine 1971; Hematology 1972; Medical Oncology 1973; **Med School:** Med Coll VA 1963; **Resid:** Internal Medicine, Grady Meml Hosp-Emory 1965; Internal Medicine, New York Hosp-Cornell 1968; **Fellow:** Hematology & Oncology, New York Hosp-Cornell 1970; **Fac Appt:** Clin Prof Med, Cornell Univ-Weill Med Coll

Comis, Robert L MD [Onc] - **Spec Exp:** Lung Cancer; **Hospital:** Hahnemann Univ Hosp; **Address:** 1818 Market St, Ste 1100, Philadelphia, PA 19103; **Phone:** 215-789-3609; **Board Cert:** Internal Medicine 1975; Medical Oncology 1977; **Med School:** SUNY Upstate Med Univ 1971; **Resid:** Internal Medicine, SUNY Upstate Med Ctr 1975; **Fac Appt:** Prof Med, Drexel Univ Coll Med

Cullen, Kevin MD [Onc] - **Spec Exp:** Head & Neck Cancer; **Hospital:** Univ of MD Med Sys; **Address:** Univ Md Greenbaum Cancer Ctr, 22 S Greene St, rm N9E22, Baltimore, MD 21201; **Phone:** 410-328-5506; **Board Cert:** Internal Medicine 1986; Medical Oncology 1989; **Med School:** Harvard Med Sch 1983; **Resid:** Internal Medicine, Beth Israel Hosp 1986; Internal Medicine, Hammersmith Hosp; **Fellow:** Medical Oncology, Natl Cancer Inst 1988

Daly, Mary B MD/PhD [Onc] - **Spec Exp:** Breast Cancer; Breast Cancer Risk Assessment; Cancer Prevention; Ovarian Cancer Risk Assessment; **Hospital:** Fox Chase Cancer Ctr (page 59); **Address:** Fox Chase Cancer Ctr, 333 Cottman Ave, P1054, Philadelphia, PA 19111; **Phone:** 215-728-2791; **Board Cert:** Internal Medicine 1981; Medical Oncology 1983; **Med School:** Univ NC Sch Med 1978; **Resid:** Internal Medicine, Univ Texas Hlth Sci Ctr 1981; **Fellow:** Medical Oncology, Univ Texas Hlth Sci Ctr 1983; **Fac Appt:** Clin Prof Med, Temple Univ

Davidson, Nancy E MD [Onc] - **Spec Exp:** Breast Cancer; **Hospital:** Johns Hopkins Hosp - Baltimore (page 61); **Address:** Johns Hopkins Oncology Center, 1650 Orleans St, Baltimore, MD 21231-1000; **Phone:** 410-955-8964; **Board Cert:** Internal Medicine 1982; Medical Oncology 1985; **Med School:** Harvard Med Sch 1979; **Resid:** Internal Medicine, Johns Hopkins Hosp 1982; **Fellow:** Medical Oncology, Natl Cancer Inst 1986; **Fac Appt:** Prof Med, Johns Hopkins Univ

Donehower, Ross Carl MD [Onc] - **Spec Exp:** Pancreatic Cancer; Colon Cancer; Prostate Cancer; **Hospital:** Johns Hopkins Hosp - Baltimore (page 61); **Address:** Hopkins Kimmel Cancer Ctr, 1650 Orleans St, CRB-187, Baltimore, MD 21231-1000; **Phone:** 410-955-8838; **Board Cert:** Internal Medicine 1977; Medical Oncology 1979; **Med School:** Univ Minn 1974; **Resid:** Internal Medicine, Johns Hopkins Hosp 1976; **Fellow:** Medical Oncology, Natl Inst Hlth 1980; **Fac Appt:** Prof Med, Johns Hopkins Univ

Doroshow, James H MD [Onc] - **Spec Exp:** Drug Discovery & Development; Colon Cancer; Breast Cancer; **Hospital:** Natl Inst of Hlth - Clin Ctr; **Address:** National Cancer Institute, Div Cancer Treatment & Diagnosis, 31 Center, Bldg 31-rm 3A44, Bethesda, MD 20892; **Phone:** 301-496-4291; **Board Cert:** Internal Medicine 1976; Medical Oncology 1977; **Med School:** Harvard Med Sch 1973; **Resid:** Internal Medicine, Mass Genl Hosp 1975; **Fellow:** Medical Oncology, Natl Cancer Inst 1978

Eisenberger, Mario MD [Onc] - **Spec Exp:** Prostate Cancer; **Hospital:** Johns Hopkins Hosp - Baltimore (page 61); **Address:** 1650 Orleans St, rm 1M51, Baltimore, MD 21231; **Phone:** 410-614-3511; **Board Cert:** Internal Medicine 1976; Medical Oncology 1979; **Med School:** Brazil 1972; **Resid:** Internal Medicine, Michael Reese Hosp 1975; **Fellow:** Hematology, Michael Reese Hosp 1976; Medical Oncology, Jackson Meml Hosp/Univ Miami 1979; **Fac Appt:** Prof Med, Johns Hopkins Univ

Ettinger, David S MD [Onc] - **Spec Exp:** Lung Cancer; Sarcoma; Clinical Trials; **Hospital:** Johns Hopkins Hosp - Baltimore (page 61); **Address:** Bunting Blaustein Cancer Rsrch Bldg, 1650 Orleans St, rm G88, Baltimore, MD 21231-1000; **Phone:** 410-955-8847; **Board Cert:** Internal Medicine 1976; Medical Oncology 1977; **Med School:** Univ Louisville Sch Med 1967; **Resid:** Internal Medicine, Mayo Grad Schl 1971; **Fellow:** Medical Oncology, Johns Hopkins Hosp 1975; **Fac Appt:** Prof Med, Johns Hopkins Univ

Fine, Robert MD [Onc] - **Spec Exp:** Pancreatic Cancer; Drug Development; Brain Tumors; Clinical Trials; **Hospital:** NY-Presby Hosp/Columbia (page 66); **Address:** Columbia Univ Comprehensive Cancer Ctr, 650 W 168th St, rm BB 20-05, New York, NY 10032; **Phone:** 212-305-1168; **Board Cert:** Internal Medicine 1983; Medical Oncology 1985; **Med School:** Univ Chicago-Pritzker Sch Med 1979; **Resid:** Internal Medicine, Stanford Univ Med Ctr 1982; **Fellow:** Medical Oncology, National Cancer Inst 1988; **Fac Appt:** Assoc Prof Med, Columbia P&S

Fisher, Richard I MD [Onc] - **Spec Exp:** Lymphoma; Hodgkin's Disease; **Hospital:** Univ of Rochester Strong Meml Hosp; **Address:** James P Wilmot Cancer Ctr, 601 Elmwood Ave, Box 704, Rochester, NY 14642; **Phone:** 585-275-5823; **Board Cert:** Internal Medicine 1973; Medical Oncology 1977; **Med School:** Harvard Med Sch 1970; **Resid:** Internal Medicine, Mass Genl Hosp 1972; **Fac Appt:** Prof Med, Univ Rochester

Flomenberg, Neal MD [Onc] - **Spec Exp:** Bone Marrow Transplant; Stem Cell Transplant; Leukemia & Lymphoma; **Hospital:** Thomas Jefferson Univ Hosp; **Address:** Thomas Jefferson Univ Hosp, 125 S 9th St, Ste 801, Philadelphia, PA 19107; **Phone:** 215-955-0356; **Board Cert:** Internal Medicine 1979; Medical Oncology 1981; Hematology 1982; **Med School:** Jefferson Med Coll 1976; **Resid:** Internal Medicine, Montefiore Med Ctr 1979; **Fellow:** Hematology & Oncology, Meml Sloan Kettering Cancer Ctr 1982; **Fac Appt:** Clin Prof Med, Thomas Jefferson Univ

Forastiere, Arlene A MD [Onc] - **Spec Exp:** Esophageal Cancer; Head & Neck Cancer; **Hospital:** Johns Hopkins Hosp - Baltimore (page 61); **Address:** Bunting Blaustein Cancer Research Bldg, 1650 Orleans St, rm G90, Baltimore, MD 21231; **Phone:** 410-955-8964; **Board Cert:** Internal Medicine 1978; Medical Oncology 1981; **Med School:** NY Med Coll 1975; **Resid:** Internal Medicine, Albert Einstein Med Ctr 1977; Internal Medicine, Univ Conn Health Ctr 1978; **Fellow:** Medical Oncology, Meml Sloan Kettering Cancer Ctr 1980; **Fac Appt:** Prof Med, NY Med Coll

Fox, Kevin R MD [Onc] - **Spec Exp:** Breast Cancer; **Hospital:** Hosp Univ Penn - UPHS (page 72); **Address:** 3400 Spruce St, 14 Penn Tower, Philadelphia, PA 19104; **Phone:** 215-662-7469; **Board Cert:** Internal Medicine 1985; Medical Oncology 1987; **Med School:** Johns Hopkins Univ 1981; **Resid:** Internal Medicine, Johns Hopkins Hosp 1984; **Fellow:** Hematology & Oncology, Hosp Univ Penn 1987; **Fac Appt:** Prof Med, Univ Pennsylvania

Medical Oncology

Gabrilove, Janice MD [Onc] - **Spec Exp:** Myelodysplastic Syndromes; Leukemia; **Hospital:** Mount Sinai Med Ctr; **Address:** Mount Sinai Med Ctr, Box 1129, One Gustave Levy Pl, New York, NY 10029-6574; **Phone:** 212-241-9650; **Board Cert:** Internal Medicine 1980; Medical Oncology 1983; **Med School:** Mount Sinai Sch Med 1977; **Resid:** Internal Medicine, Columbia-Presby Med Ctr 1980; **Fellow:** Hematology & Oncology, Meml Sloan-Kettering Cancer Ctr 1983; **Fac Appt:** Prof Med, Mount Sinai Sch Med

Gelmann, Edward P MD [Onc] - **Spec Exp:** Prostate Cancer; Testicular Cancer; **Hospital:** Georgetown Univ Hosp; **Address:** Lombardi Cancer Ctr, Podium A, 3800 Reservoir Rd NW, Washington, DC 20007; **Phone:** 202-444-7303; **Board Cert:** Internal Medicine 1979; Medical Oncology 1981; **Med School:** Stanford Univ 1976; **Resid:** Internal Medicine, Univ Chicago Hosps 1978; **Fellow:** Medical Oncology, National Cancer Inst 1981; **Fac Appt:** Prof Med, Georgetown Univ

Geyer Jr, Charles E MD [Onc] - **Spec Exp:** Breast Cancer; **Hospital:** Allegheny General Hosp; **Address:** Allegheny Cancer Ctr, 320 E North Ave Fl 5, Pittsburgh, PA 15212; **Phone:** 412-359-6147; **Board Cert:** Internal Medicine 1983; Medical Oncology 1987; **Med School:** Texas Tech Univ 1980; **Resid:** Internal Medicine, Baylor Affil Hosps 1983; **Fellow:** Medical Oncology, Baylor Affil Hosps 1985

Glick, John H MD [Onc] - **Spec Exp:** Breast Cancer; Hodgkin's Disease; Lymphoma, Non-Hodgkin's; **Hospital:** Hosp Univ Penn - UPHS (page 72); **Address:** Abramson Cancer Ctr of Univ Penn, 3400 Spruce St, 1218 Penn Tower, Philadelphia, PA 19104; **Phone:** 215-662-6065; **Board Cert:** Internal Medicine 1973; Medical Oncology 1975; **Med School:** Columbia P&S 1969; **Resid:** Internal Medicine, Presbyterian Hosp 1971; **Fellow:** Medical Oncology, Natl Cancer Inst 1973; Medical Oncology, Stanford Univ 1974; **Fac Appt:** Prof Med, Univ Pennsylvania

Goldstein, Lori J MD [Onc] - **Spec Exp:** Breast Cancer; **Hospital:** Fox Chase Cancer Ctr (page 59); **Address:** Fox Chase Cancer Ctr, Dept Med Oncology, 333 Cottman Ave, Philadelphia, PA 19111; **Phone:** 215-728-2689; **Board Cert:** Internal Medicine 1985; Medical Oncology 2002; **Med School:** SUNY Upstate Med Univ 1982; **Resid:** Internal Medicine, Presby Univ Hosp 1985; **Fellow:** Medical Oncology, Natl Cancer Inst/NIH 1990

Grossbard, Michael L MD [Onc] - **Spec Exp:** Lymphoma; Breast Cancer; Gastrointestinal Cancer; **Hospital:** St Luke's - Roosevelt Hosp Ctr - Roosevelt Div, Beth Israel Med Ctr - Petrie Division; **Address:** 1000 10th Ave Fl 11 - Ste C02, New York, NY 10019; **Phone:** 212-523-5419; **Board Cert:** Internal Medicine 1989; Medical Oncology 2001; **Med School:** Yale Univ 1986; **Resid:** Internal Medicine, Mass Genl Hosp 1989; **Fellow:** Medical Oncology, Dana Farber Cancer Inst 1991; **Fac Appt:** Clin Prof Med, Columbia P&S

Grossman, Stuart MD [Onc] - **Spec Exp:** Brain Tumors; Neuro-Oncology; Pain-Cancer; **Hospital:** Johns Hopkins Hosp - Baltimore (page 61); **Address:** 550 N Broadway, Ste 1001, Baltimore, MD 21205; **Phone:** 410-955-8837; **Board Cert:** Internal Medicine 1976; Medical Oncology 1983; **Med School:** Univ Rochester 1973; **Resid:** Internal Medicine, Strong Meml Hosp 1976; **Fellow:** Medical Oncology, Johns Hopkins Hosp 1981; **Fac Appt:** Prof Med, Johns Hopkins Univ

Hait, William MD/PhD [Onc] - **Spec Exp:** Breast Cancer; **Hospital:** Robert Wood Johnson Univ Hosp - New Brunswick; **Address:** Cancer Inst of NJ, 195 Little Albany St, New Brunswick, NJ 08901-1914; **Phone:** 732-235-8064; **Board Cert:** Internal Medicine 1982; Medical Oncology 1987; **Med School:** Med Coll PA 1978; **Resid:** Internal Medicine, Yale-New Haven Hosp 1982; **Fellow:** Medical Oncology, Yale-New Haven Hosp 1983; **Fac Appt:** Prof Med, UMDNJ-RW Johnson Med Sch

Haller, Daniel G MD [Onc] - **Spec Exp:** Gastrointestinal Cancer; Colon & Rectal Cancer; Cancer Prevention; **Hospital:** Hosp Univ Penn - UPHS (page 72); **Address:** Hosp Univ Penn, Div Hematology/Oncology, 3400 Spruce St, 12 Penn Tower, Philadelphia, PA 19104; **Phone:** 215-662-7666; **Board Cert:** Internal Medicine 1976; Medical Oncology 1979; **Med School:** Univ Pittsburgh 1973; **Resid:** Internal Medicine, Georgetown Univ Hosp 1976; **Fellow:** Medical Oncology, Georgetown Univ Hosp 1978; **Fac Appt:** Prof Med, Univ Pennsylvania

Hochster, Howard S MD [Onc] - **Spec Exp:** Gastrointestinal Cancer; Gynecologic Cancer; Colon & Rectal Cancer; **Hospital:** NYU Med Ctr (page 67); **Address:** NYU Cancer Institute, 160 E 34 St Fl 9, New York, NY 10016; **Phone:** 212-731-5100; **Board Cert:** Internal Medicine 1983; Medical Oncology 1985; Hematology 1986; **Med School:** Yale Univ 1980; **Resid:** Internal Medicine, NYU Med Ctr 1983; **Fellow:** Hematology & Oncology, NYU Med Ctr 1985; Medical Oncology, Jules Bordet Inst 1986; **Fac Appt:** Prof Med, NYU Sch Med

Holland, James F MD [Onc] - **Spec Exp:** Breast Cancer; Colon Cancer; Lung Cancer; **Hospital:** Mount Sinai Med Ctr; **Address:** Ruttenberg Cancer Ctr, Div Med Oncology, 1 Gustave L Levy Pl, Box 1129, New York, NY 10029-6500; **Phone:** 212-241-4495; **Board Cert:** Internal Medicine 1955; **Med School:** Columbia P&S 1947; **Resid:** Internal Medicine, Columbia-Presby Hosp 1949; **Fellow:** Medical Oncology, Francis Delafield Hosp 1953; **Fac Appt:** Prof Med, Mount Sinai Sch Med

Hudes, Gary R MD [Onc] - **Spec Exp:** Prostate Cancer; Genitourinary Cancer; Kidney Cancer; **Hospital:** Fox Chase Cancer Ctr (page 59); **Address:** Fox Chase Cancer Ctr, 333 Cottman Ave, rm C307, Philadelphia, PA 19111; **Phone:** 215-728-3889; **Board Cert:** Internal Medicine 1982; Hematology 1984; Medical Oncology 1985; **Med School:** SUNY Downstate 1979; **Resid:** Internal Medicine, Graduate Hosp 1982; **Fellow:** Hematology & Oncology, Presby-Univ Penn Med Ctr 1985

Hudis, Clifford A MD [Onc] - **Spec Exp:** Breast Cancer; **Hospital:** Meml Sloan Kettering Cancer Ctr; **Address:** Meml Sloan Kettering Cancer Ctr, 205 E 64th St, New York, NY 10021; **Phone:** 212-639-5449; **Board Cert:** Internal Medicine 1986; Medical Oncology 2001; **Med School:** Med Coll PA Hahnemann 1983; **Resid:** Internal Medicine, Hosp Med Coll Penn 1986; **Fellow:** Medical Oncology, Meml Sloan Kettering Cancer Ctr 1991; **Fac Appt:** Assoc Prof Med, Cornell Univ-Weill Med Coll

Isaacs, Claudine J MD [Onc] - **Spec Exp:** Breast Cancer; Breast Cancer Risk Assessment; **Hospital:** Georgetown Univ Hosp; **Address:** Lombardi Cancer Ctr, Podium B, 3800 Reservoir Rd NW, Washington, DC 20007; **Phone:** 202-444-3677; **Board Cert:** Internal Medicine 2002; Medical Oncology 2003; **Med School:** McGill Univ 1987; **Resid:** Internal Medicine, Montreal General Hosp 1990; Hematology & Oncology, McGill Univ Hosp 1992; **Fellow:** Medical Oncology, Georgetown Univ Med Ctr 1993; **Fac Appt:** Assoc Prof Med, Georgetown Univ

Karp, Judith MD [Onc] - **Spec Exp:** Leukemia; Clinical Trials; Myelodysplastic Syndromes; **Hospital:** Johns Hopkins Hosp - Baltimore (page 61); **Address:** 1650 Orleans St, rm 289, Baltimore, MD 21231; **Phone:** 410-502-7726; **Board Cert:** Internal Medicine 1976; **Med School:** Stanford Univ 1971; **Resid:** Internal Medicine, John Hopkins Hosp 1974; **Fellow:** Medical Oncology, John Hopkins Hosp 1977; **Fac Appt:** Prof Med, Johns Hopkins Univ

Medical Oncology

Kelsen, David MD [Onc] - **Spec Exp:** Gastrointestinal Cancer; Neuroendocrine Tumors; Unknown Primary Cancer; Merkel Cell Carcinoma; **Hospital:** Meml Sloan Kettering Cancer Ctr; **Address:** Gastrointestinal Oncology Svc, 1275 York Ave Howard Bldg Fl 9 - rm 918, New York, NY 10021; **Phone:** 212-639-8470; **Board Cert:** Internal Medicine 1976; Medical Oncology 1979; **Med School:** Hahnemann Univ 1972; **Resid:** Internal Medicine, Temple Univ Hosp 1976; **Fellow:** Medical Oncology, Meml Sloan Kettering Cancer Ctr 1978; **Fac Appt:** Prof Med, Cornell Univ-Weill Med Coll

Kemeny, Nancy MD [Onc] - **Spec Exp:** Colon Cancer; Rectal Cancer; Liver Cancer; **Hospital:** Meml Sloan Kettering Cancer Ctr; **Address:** Meml Sloan Kettering Cancer Ctr, 1275 York Ave, Ste Howard 916, New York, NY 10021; **Phone:** 212-639-8068; **Board Cert:** Internal Medicine 1974; Medical Oncology 1981; **Med School:** UMDNJ-NJ Med Sch, Newark 1971; **Resid:** Internal Medicine, St Luke's Hosp 1974; **Fellow:** Medical Oncology, Mem Sloan Kettering Cancer Ctr 1976; **Fac Appt:** Prof Med, Cornell Univ-Weill Med Coll

Kirkwood, John M MD [Onc] - **Spec Exp:** Melanoma; Immunotherapy; **Hospital:** UPMC Presby, Pittsburgh, UPMC Shadyside; **Address:** Hillman Cancer Research Pavilion, 5117 Centre Ave, Ste 1.32, Pittsburgh, PA 15213-1862; **Phone:** 412-623-7707; **Board Cert:** Internal Medicine 1976; Medical Oncology 1981; **Med School:** Yale Univ 1973; **Resid:** Internal Medicine, Yale-New Haven Hosp 1976; **Fellow:** Medical Oncology, Dana Farber Cancer Inst 1979; **Fac Appt:** Prof Med, Univ Pittsburgh

Kris, Mark G MD [Onc] - **Spec Exp:** Lung Cancer; Mediastinal Tumors; Thymoma; Thoracic Cancers; **Hospital:** Meml Sloan Kettering Cancer Ctr; **Address:** Memorial Sloan Kettering Cancer Ctr, 1275 York Ave, Howard H1018, New York, NY 10021; **Phone:** 212-639-7590; **Board Cert:** Internal Medicine 1980; Medical Oncology 1983; **Med School:** Cornell Univ-Weill Med Coll 1977; **Resid:** Internal Medicine, New York Hosp 1980; **Fellow:** Medical Oncology, Meml Sloan Kettering Cancer Ctr 1983; **Fac Appt:** Prof Med, Cornell Univ-Weill Med Coll

Langer, Corey J MD [Onc] - **Spec Exp:** Lung Cancer; Head & Neck Cancer; Mesothelioma; **Hospital:** Fox Chase Cancer Ctr (page 59); **Address:** Fox Chase Cancer Ctr, 333 Cottman Ave, Philadelphia, PA 19111-2412; **Phone:** 215-728-2985; **Board Cert:** Internal Medicine 1984; Hematology 1986; Medical Oncology 1987; **Med School:** Boston Univ 1981; **Resid:** Internal Medicine, Graduate Hosp 1984; Hematology & Oncology, Presby Hosp 1986; **Fellow:** Medical Oncology, Fox Chase Cancer Ctr 1987; **Fac Appt:** Assoc Prof Med, Temple Univ

Levine, Ellis MD [Onc] - **Spec Exp:** Breast Cancer; Urologic Cancer; **Hospital:** Roswell Park Cancer Inst; **Address:** Roswell Park Cancer Inst, Elm & Carlton St, Buffalo, NY 14263-0001; **Phone:** 716-845-8547; **Board Cert:** Internal Medicine 1982; Medical Oncology 1985; **Med School:** Univ Pittsburgh 1979; **Resid:** Internal Medicine, Univ Minn Hosps 1982; **Fellow:** Medical Oncology, Univ Minn Hosps 1984; **Fac Appt:** Assoc Prof Med, SUNY Buffalo

Levy, Michael H MD/PhD [Onc] - **Spec Exp:** Pain Management; Palliative Care; Pain-Cancer; Ethics; **Hospital:** Fox Chase Cancer Ctr (page 59); **Address:** Fox Chase Cancer Ctr, Dept Medical Oncology, 333 Cottman Ave, Ste C307, Philadelphia, PA 19111; **Phone:** 215-728-3637; **Board Cert:** Internal Medicine 1979; Medical Oncology 1981; **Med School:** Jefferson Med Coll 1976; **Resid:** Internal Medicine, Mt Sinai Med Ctr 1978; Internal Medicine, Hosp Univ Penn 1979; **Fellow:** Hematology & Oncology, Hosp Univ Penn 1981

Livingston, Philip MD [Onc] - **Spec Exp:** Melanoma; Vaccine Therapy; Immunotherapy; **Hospital:** Meml Sloan Kettering Cancer Ctr; **Address:** 1275 York Ave, New York, NY 10021-6007; **Phone:** 646-888-2376; **Board Cert:** Internal Medicine 1980; Allergy & Immunology 1974; Rheumatology 1974; Medical Oncology 1981; **Med School:** Harvard Med Sch 1969; **Resid:** Internal Medicine, N Shore Hosp-Cornell Med Ctr 1971; **Fellow:** Immunology, NYU Med Ctr 1973; Medical Oncology, Meml Sloan Kettering Cancer Inst 1977; **Fac Appt:** Prof Med, Cornell Univ-Weill Med Coll

Lyman, Gary H MD [Onc] - **Spec Exp:** Breast Cancer; **Hospital:** Univ of Rochester Strong Meml Hosp; **Address:** Univ of Rochester Strong Meml Hosp, 601 Elmwood Ave, Box 704, Rochester, NY 14642-8704; **Phone:** 585-275-3335; **Board Cert:** Internal Medicine 1987; Medical Oncology 1977; Hematology 1979; **Med School:** SUNY Buffalo 1972; **Resid:** Internal Medicine, Univ North Carolina Hosp 1974; **Fellow:** Medical Oncology, Roswell Park Meml Inst 1976; Biostatistics, Harvard Med Sch 1982; **Fac Appt:** Prof Med, Univ Rochester

Macdonald, John S MD [Onc] - **Spec Exp:** Colon Cancer; Gastrointestinal Cancer; Pancreatic Cancer; **Hospital:** St Vincent Cath Med Ctrs - Manhattan; **Address:** 325 W 15th St, New York, NY 10011-5903; **Phone:** 212-604-6011; **Board Cert:** Internal Medicine 1973; Medical Oncology 1975; **Med School:** Harvard Med Sch 1969; **Resid:** Internal Medicine, Beth Israel Hosp 1971; **Fellow:** Hematology & Oncology, Natl Cancer Inst 1974; **Fac Appt:** Prof Med, NY Med Coll

Marks, Stanley M MD [Onc] - **Spec Exp:** Leukemia; Lymphoma; **Hospital:** UPMC Shadyside; **Address:** 5115 Centre Ave, Fl 3, Pittsburgh, PA 15232; **Phone:** 412-235-1020; **Board Cert:** Internal Medicine 1976; Hematology 1978; **Med School:** Univ Pittsburgh 1973; **Resid:** Internal Medicine, Presby Univ Hosp 1976; **Fellow:** Hematology, Peter Bent Brigham Hosp 1978; **Fac Appt:** Assoc Clin Prof Med, Drexel Univ Coll Med

Marshall, John L MD [Onc] - **Spec Exp:** Gastrointestinal Cancer; Drug Development; **Hospital:** Georgetown Univ Hosp; **Address:** Lombardi Cancer Ctr, Podium A, 3800 Reservoir Rd NW, Washington, DC 20007; **Phone:** 202-444-7064; **Board Cert:** Internal Medicine 2001; Medical Oncology 2003; **Med School:** Univ Louisville Sch Med 1988; **Resid:** Internal Medicine, Georgetown Univ Hosp 1991; **Fellow:** Medical Oncology, Georgetown Univ Hosp 1993; **Fac Appt:** Assoc Prof Med, Georgetown Univ

Masters, Gregory A MD [Onc] - **Spec Exp:** Lung Cancer; Esophageal Cancer; Thoracic Cancers; **Hospital:** Christiana Hospital; **Address:** Med Onc-Hem Consultants, Graham Cancer Ctr, 4701 Ogletown-Stanton Rd, Ste 2200, Newark, DE 19713; **Phone:** 302-366-1200; **Board Cert:** Internal Medicine 2003; Medical Oncology 2005; **Med School:** Northwestern Univ 1990; **Resid:** Internal Medicine, Hosp Univ Penn 1993; **Fellow:** Medical Oncology, Univ Chicago Hosps 1995; **Fac Appt:** Assoc Prof Med, Thomas Jefferson Univ

McGuire III, William P MD [Onc] - **Spec Exp:** Gynecologic Cancer; Ovarian Cancer; Breast Cancer; **Hospital:** Franklin Square Hosp; **Address:** Harry & Jeanette Weinberg Cancer Inst, 9103 Franklin Square Drive, Ste 2200, Baltimore, MD 21287; **Phone:** 443-777-7826; **Board Cert:** Internal Medicine 1974; Medical Oncology 1981; **Med School:** Baylor Coll Med 1971; **Resid:** Internal Medicine, Yale-New Haven Hosp 1973; **Fac Appt:** Clin Prof Med, Univ MD Sch Med

Medical Oncology

Meropol, Neal J MD [Onc] - **Spec Exp:** Gastrointestinal Cancer; **Hospital:** Fox Chase Cancer Ctr (page 59); **Address:** Fox Chase Cancer Ctr, Medical Oncology, 333 Cottman Ave, Philadelphia, PA 19111; **Phone:** 215-728-2450; **Board Cert:** Internal Medicine 1988; Medical Oncology 2001; **Med School:** Vanderbilt Univ 1985; **Resid:** Internal Medicine, Univ Hosps/Case West Res 1988; **Fellow:** Hematology & Oncology, Hosp Univ Penn 1992; **Fac Appt:** Prof Med, Temple Univ

Moore, Anne MD [Onc] - **Spec Exp:** Breast Cancer; **Hospital:** NY-Presby Hosp/Weill Cornell (page 66); **Address:** New York Presbyterian Hosp, 428 E 72nd St, Ste 300, New York, NY 10021-4873; **Phone:** 212-746-2085; **Board Cert:** Internal Medicine 1973; Hematology 1976; Medical Oncology 1977; **Med School:** Columbia P&S 1969; **Resid:** Internal Medicine, Cornell Univ Med Ctr 1973; **Fellow:** Medical Oncology, Rockefeller Univ 1973; **Fac Appt:** Prof Med, Cornell Univ-Weill Med Coll

Motzer, Robert J MD [Onc] - **Spec Exp:** Kidney Cancer; Testicular Cancer; Prostate Cancer; **Hospital:** Meml Sloan Kettering Cancer Ctr; **Address:** 1275 York Ave, Box 239, New York, NY 10021; **Phone:** 646-422-4312; **Board Cert:** Internal Medicine 1984; Medical Oncology 1987; **Med School:** Univ Mich Med Sch 1981; **Resid:** Internal Medicine, Meml Sloan Kettering Cancer Ctr 1984; **Fellow:** Medical Oncology, Meml Sloan Kettering Cancer Ctr 1987; **Fac Appt:** Assoc Prof Med, Cornell Univ-Weill Med Coll

Nissenblatt, Michael MD [Onc] - **Spec Exp:** Breast Cancer; Colon Cancer; Hereditary Cancer; Familial Cancer; **Hospital:** Robert Wood Johnson Univ Hosp - New Brunswick, St Peter's Univ Hosp; **Address:** 205 Easton Ave, New Brunswick, NJ 08901-1722; **Phone:** 732-828-9570; **Board Cert:** Internal Medicine 1976; Medical Oncology 1979; **Med School:** Columbia P&S 1973; **Resid:** Internal Medicine, Johns Hopkins Hosp 1976; **Fellow:** Medical Oncology, Johns Hopkins Hosp 1978; **Fac Appt:** Clin Prof Med, Robert W Johnson Med Sch

Norton, Larry MD [Onc] - **Spec Exp:** Breast Cancer; **Hospital:** Meml Sloan Kettering Cancer Ctr; **Address:** 205 E 64th St, New York, NY 10021; **Phone:** 212-639-5438; **Board Cert:** Internal Medicine 1975; Medical Oncology 1977; **Med School:** Columbia P&S 1972; **Resid:** Internal Medicine, Bronx Muni Hosp 1974; **Fac Appt:** Prof Med, Cornell Univ-Weill Med Coll

O'Reilly, Eileen M MD [Onc] - **Spec Exp:** Pancreatic Cancer; Clinical Trials; Biliary Cancer; Neuroendocrine Tumors; **Hospital:** Meml Sloan Kettering Cancer Ctr; **Address:** 1275 York Ave, Box 324, New York, NY 10021; **Phone:** 212-639-6672; **Med School:** Ireland 1990; **Resid:** Internal Medicine, St Vincent's Hosp 1994; **Fellow:** Hematology, St Vincent's Hosp 1995; Medical Oncology, Memorial-Sloan Kettering Cancer Ctr 1997; **Fac Appt:** Asst Prof Med, Cornell Univ-Weill Med Coll

Offit, Kenneth MD [Onc] - **Spec Exp:** Cancer Genetics; Breast Cancer; Lymphoma; **Hospital:** Meml Sloan Kettering Cancer Ctr; **Address:** 1275 York Ave, Box 295, New York, NY 10021-6094; **Phone:** 212-434-5149; **Board Cert:** Internal Medicine 1985; Medical Oncology 1987; **Med School:** Harvard Med Sch 1982; **Resid:** Internal Medicine, Lenox Hill Hosp 1985; **Fellow:** Hematology & Oncology, Meml Sloan Kettering Cancer Ctr 1988; **Fac Appt:** Prof Med, Cornell Univ-Weill Med Coll

Oster, Martin W MD [Onc] - **Spec Exp:** Breast Cancer; Gastrointestinal Cancer; Lung Cancer; **Hospital:** NY-Presby Hosp/Columbia (page 66); **Address:** NY Presby Hosp-Columbia Presby Med Ctr, 161 Fort Washington Ave, New York, NY 10032-3713; **Phone:** 212-305-8231; **Board Cert:** Internal Medicine 1974; Medical Oncology 1975; **Med School:** Columbia P&S 1971; **Resid:** Internal Medicine, Mass Genl Hosp 1973; **Fellow:** Medical Oncology, Natl Cancer Inst/NIH 1976; **Fac Appt:** Assoc Clin Prof Med, Columbia P&S

Ozols, Robert R MD/PhD [Onc] - **Spec Exp:** Ovarian Cancer; **Hospital:** Fox Chase Cancer Ctr (page 59); **Address:** Fox Chase Cancer Ctr, 333 Cottman Ave, rm P 2051, Philadelphia, PA 19111; **Phone:** 215-728-2570; **Board Cert:** Internal Medicine 1977; Medical Oncology 1979; **Med School:** Univ Rochester 1974; **Resid:** Internal Medicine, Dartmouth-Hitchcock Hosp 1976; **Fellow:** Medical Oncology, Natl Cancer Inst 1979; **Fac Appt:** Prof Med, Temple Univ

Pasmantier, Mark MD [Onc] - **Spec Exp:** Lung Cancer; Ovarian Cancer; **Hospital:** NY-Presby Hosp/Weill Cornell (page 66); **Address:** 407 E 70th St, FL 3, New York, NY 10021-5302; **Phone:** 212-517-5900; **Board Cert:** Internal Medicine 1972; Hematology 1974; Medical Oncology 1975; **Med School:** NYU Sch Med 1966; **Resid:** Internal Medicine, Harlem Hosp 1970; **Fellow:** Hematology, Montefiore Hosp Med Ctr 1971; Medical Oncology, New York Hosp 1972; **Fac Appt:** Clin Prof Med, Cornell Univ-Weill Med Coll

Pecora, Andrew L MD [Onc] - **Spec Exp:** Stem Cell Transplant; Myelodysplastic Syndromes; Melanoma; Immunotherapy; **Hospital:** Hackensack Univ Med Ctr; **Address:** The Cancer Ctr at Hackensack Univ Med Ctr, 20 Prospect Ave, Ste 400, Hackensack, NJ 07601; **Phone:** 201-996-5900; **Board Cert:** Internal Medicine 1986; Hematology 1988; Medical Oncology 1989; **Med School:** UMDNJ-NJ Med Sch, Newark 1983; **Resid:** Internal Medicine, New York Hosp-Cornell Med Ctr 1986; **Fellow:** Hematology & Oncology, Meml Sloan Kettering Cancer Ctr 1988; **Fac Appt:** Prof Med, UMDNJ-NJ Med Sch, Newark

Petrylak, Daniel P MD [Onc] - **Spec Exp:** Genitourinary Cancer; Prostate Cancer; Bladder Cancer; **Hospital:** NY-Presby Hosp/Columbia (page 66); **Address:** 161 Fort Washington Ave, New York, NY 10032-3713; **Phone:** 212-305-1731; **Board Cert:** Internal Medicine 2001; Medical Oncology 2003; **Med School:** Case West Res Univ 1985; **Resid:** Internal Medicine, Jacobi Med Ctr 1988; **Fellow:** Oncology, Meml-Sloan Kettering Cancer Ctr 1991; **Fac Appt:** Assoc Prof Med, Columbia P&S

Saltz, Leonard B MD [Onc] - **Spec Exp:** Colon & Rectal Cancer; Gastrointestinal Cancer & Rare Tumors; Liver Cancer; Neuroendocrine Tumors; **Hospital:** Meml Sloan Kettering Cancer Ctr; **Address:** Memorial Sloan Kettering Cancer Ctr, 1275 York Ave, Howard 917, New York, NY 10021; **Phone:** 212-639-2501; **Board Cert:** Internal Medicine 1986; Hematology 1988; Medical Oncology 1989; **Med School:** Yale Univ 1983; **Resid:** Internal Medicine, New York Hosp-Cornell Med Ctr 1986; **Fellow:** Hematology & Oncology, New York Hosp-Cornell Med Ctr/Rockefeller Univ 1987; **Fac Appt:** Prof Med, Cornell Univ-Weill Med Coll

Scheinberg, David MD/PhD [Onc] - **Spec Exp:** Leukemia; Immunotherapy; Vaccine Therapy; **Hospital:** Meml Sloan Kettering Cancer Ctr; **Address:** 1275 York Ave, New York, NY 10021-6007; **Phone:** 646-888-2668; **Board Cert:** Internal Medicine 1986; Medical Oncology 1995; **Med School:** Johns Hopkins Univ 1983; **Resid:** Internal Medicine, New York Hosp/Cornell 1985; **Fellow:** Medical Oncology, Meml Sloan Kettering Cancer Ctr 1987; **Fac Appt:** Prof Med, Cornell Univ-Weill Med Coll

Scher, Howard MD [Onc] - **Spec Exp:** Genitourinary Cancer; Prostate Cancer; Bladder Cancer; **Hospital:** Meml Sloan Kettering Cancer Ctr; **Address:** 1275 York Ave, New York, NY 10021; **Phone:** 646-422-4330; **Board Cert:** Internal Medicine 1979; Medical Oncology 1985; **Med School:** NYU Sch Med 1976; **Resid:** Internal Medicine, Bellevue Hosp 1980; **Fellow:** Medical Oncology, Meml Sloan Kettering Cancer Ctr 1983; **Fac Appt:** Prof Med, Cornell Univ-Weill Med Coll

Schilder, Russell J MD [Onc] - **Spec Exp:** Gynecologic Cancer; Hematologic Malignancies; Drug Development; Clinical Trials; **Hospital:** Fox Chase Cancer Ctr (page 59); **Address:** Fox Chase Cancer Center, 333 Cottman Ave, Philadelphia, PA 19111; **Phone:** 215-728-4300; **Board Cert:** Internal Medicine 1986; Hematology 1988; Medical Oncology 1989; **Med School:** Univ Miami Sch Med 1983; **Resid:** Internal Medicine, Temple Univ Hosp 1986; **Fellow:** Hematology & Oncology, Fox Chase Cancer Ctr 1989; **Fac Appt:** Prof Med, Temple Univ

Schuchter, Lynn M MD [Onc] - **Spec Exp:** Melanoma; Breast Cancer; Clinical Trials; **Hospital:** Hosp Univ Penn - UPHS (page 72); **Address:** Univ Penn/Abramson Cancer Ctr, 3400 Spruce St, 12 Penn Tower, Philadelphia, PA 19104; **Phone:** 215-662-7907; **Board Cert:** Internal Medicine 1985; Medical Oncology 1989; **Med School:** Ros Franklin Univ/Chicago Med Sch 1982; **Resid:** Internal Medicine, Michael Reese Hosp 1985; **Fellow:** Medical Oncology, Johns Hopkins Hosp 1989; **Fac Appt:** Assoc Prof Med, Univ Pennsylvania

Sidransky, David MD [Onc] - **Spec Exp:** Head & Neck Cancer; **Hospital:** Johns Hopkins Hosp - Baltimore (page 61); **Address:** Johns Hopkins Hospital, 1550 Orleans St, rm 5-N03, Baltimore, MD 21231; **Phone:** 410-502-5153; **Board Cert:** Internal Medicine 1988; **Med School:** Baylor Coll Med 1984; **Resid:** Internal Medicine, Baylor Coll Medicine 1988; **Fellow:** Medical Oncology, Johns Hopkins Hosp 1992; **Fac Appt:** Prof Oto, Johns Hopkins Univ

Smith, Mitchell R MD/PhD [Onc] - **Spec Exp:** Lymphoma; Leukemia; Multiple Myeloma; Hematologic Malignancies; **Hospital:** Fox Chase Cancer Ctr (page 59); **Address:** Fox Chase Cancer Center, 333 Cottman Ave, Ste C307, Philadelphia, PA 19111; **Phone:** 215-728-2570; **Board Cert:** Internal Medicine 1985; Hematology 1988; Medical Oncology 1987; **Med School:** Case West Res Univ 1979; **Resid:** Pathology, Barnes Jewish Hosp 1983; Internal Medicine, Barnes Jewish Hosp 1984; **Fellow:** Medical Oncology, Meml Sloan-Ketter Cancer Ctr 1988

Speyer, James MD [Onc] - **Spec Exp:** Ovarian Cancer; Breast Cancer; Cardiac Toxicity in Cancer Therapy; **Hospital:** NYU Med Ctr (page 67); **Address:** NYU Clinical Cancer Center, 160 E 34th St, New York, NY 10016-4750; **Phone:** 212-731-5432; **Board Cert:** Internal Medicine 1977; Hematology 1978; Medical Oncology 1979; **Med School:** Johns Hopkins Univ 1974; **Resid:** Internal Medicine, Columbia-Presby Med Ctr 1976; Hematology, Columbia-Presby Med Ctr 1977; **Fellow:** Medical Oncology, Natl Cancer Inst 1979; **Fac Appt:** Clin Prof Med, NYU Sch Med

Spriggs, David MD [Onc] - **Spec Exp:** Ovarian Cancer; Drug Development; Uterine Cancer; **Hospital:** Meml Sloan Kettering Cancer Ctr; **Address:** 1275 York Ave, Box 67, New York, NY 10021-6007; **Phone:** 212-639-2203; **Board Cert:** Internal Medicine 1981; Medical Oncology 1985; **Med School:** Univ Wisc 1977; **Resid:** Internal Medicine, Columbia-Presby Hosp 1981; **Fellow:** Medical Oncology, Dana-Farber Cancer Inst 1985; **Fac Appt:** Prof Med, Cornell Univ-Weill Med Coll

Stadtmauer, Edward A MD [Onc] - **Spec Exp:** Bone Marrow & Stem Cell Transplant; Leukemia; Multiple Myeloma; **Hospital:** Hosp Univ Penn - UPHS (page 72); **Address:** Univ Penn Cancer Ctr, 3400 Spruce St, 16 Penn Tower, Philadelphia, PA 19104; **Phone:** 215-662-7909; **Board Cert:** Internal Medicine 1986; Hematology 1988; Medical Oncology 1989; **Med School:** Univ Pennsylvania 1983; **Resid:** Internal Medicine, Bronx Muni Hosp 1986; **Fellow:** Hematology & Oncology, Hosp Univ Penn 1989; **Fac Appt:** Assoc Prof Med, Univ Pennsylvania

Stoopler, Mark MD [Onc] - **Spec Exp:** Lung Cancer; Esophageal Cancer; Unknown Primary Cancer; **Hospital:** NY-Presby Hosp/Columbia (page 66); **Address:** 161 Fort Washington Ave, Ste 936, New York, NY 10032-3713; **Phone:** 212-305-8230; **Board Cert:** Internal Medicine 1978; Medical Oncology 1981; **Med School:** Cornell Univ-Weill Med Coll 1975; **Resid:** Internal Medicine, North Shore Univ Hosp 1978; Internal Medicine, Memorial Hosp 1978; **Fellow:** Medical Oncology, Meml-Sloan Kettering Cancer Ctr 1980; **Fac Appt:** Assoc Clin Prof Med, Columbia P&S

Straus, David J MD [Onc] - **Spec Exp:** Lymphoma; Multiple Myeloma; **Hospital:** Meml Sloan Kettering Cancer Ctr; **Address:** 1275 York Ave, New York, NY 10021-6007; **Phone:** 212-639-8365; **Board Cert:** Internal Medicine 1972; Hematology 1976; Medical Oncology 1977; **Med School:** Marquette Sch Med 1969; **Resid:** Internal Medicine, Montefiore Med Ctr 1972; Medical Oncology, Meml Sloan Kettering Cancer Ctr 1977; **Fellow:** Hematology, Beth Israel Hosp 1973; **Fac Appt:** Prof Med, Cornell Univ-Weill Med Coll

Vogel, Victor G MD [Onc] - **Spec Exp:** Breast Cancer; Cancer Genetics; Drug Development; Clinical Trials; **Hospital:** Magee-Womens Hosp - UPMC; **Address:** Magee-Womens Hosp, Breast Cancer Prevention, 300 Halket St, rm 3524, Pittsburgh, PA 15213-3180; **Phone:** 412-641-6500; **Board Cert:** Internal Medicine 1984; Medical Oncology 2003; Public Health & Genl Preventive Med 1993; **Med School:** Temple Univ 1978; **Resid:** Internal Medicine, Baltimore City Hosp 1981; **Fellow:** Medical Oncology, Johns Hopkins Hosp 1986; Epidemiology, Johns Hopkins Hosp 1986; **Fac Appt:** Prof Med, Univ Pittsburgh

von-Mehren, Margaret MD [Onc] - **Spec Exp:** Sarcoma; Melanoma; Immunotherapy; Gastrointestinal Stromal Tumors; **Hospital:** Fox Chase Cancer Ctr (page 59); **Address:** Fox Chase Cancer Ctr, Dept Med Oncology, 333 Cottman Ave, Philadelphia, PA 19111-2434; **Phone:** 215-728-2570; **Board Cert:** Medical Oncology 1997; **Med School:** Albany Med Coll 1989; **Resid:** Internal Medicine, NYU Med Ctr 1993; **Fellow:** Hematology & Oncology, Fox Chase Cancer Ctr 1996; **Fac Appt:** Assoc Prof Med, Temple Univ

Weiner, Louis M MD [Onc] - **Spec Exp:** Gastrointestinal Cancer; Immunotherapy; Thoracic Cancers; Immunotherapy; **Hospital:** Fox Chase Cancer Ctr (page 59), Jeanes Hosp; **Address:** Fox Chase Cancer Ctr, 333 Cottman Ave, rm C315, Philadelphia, PA 19111; **Phone:** 215-728-2480; **Board Cert:** Internal Medicine 1980; Medical Oncology 1985; **Med School:** Mount Sinai Sch Med 1977; **Resid:** Internal Medicine, Med Ctr Hosp Vermont 1981; **Fellow:** Hematology & Oncology, New England Med Ctr 1984; **Fac Appt:** Prof Med, Temple Univ

Zelenetz, Andrew D MD/PhD [Onc] - **Spec Exp:** Lymphoma; **Hospital:** Meml Sloan Kettering Cancer Ctr; **Address:** Meml Sloan-Kettering Cancer Ctr, 1275 York Ave, New York, NY 10021; **Phone:** 212-639-2656; **Board Cert:** Internal Medicine 1992; Medical Oncology 1993; **Med School:** Harvard Med Sch 1984; **Resid:** Internal Medicine, Stanford Univ Med Ctr 1986; **Fellow:** Medical Oncology, Stanford Univ Med Ctr 1991; **Fac Appt:** Asst Prof Med, Cornell Univ-Weill Med Coll

Medical Oncology

Southeast

Balducci, Lodovico MD [Onc] - **Spec Exp:** Genitourinary Cancer; Breast Cancer; **Hospital:** H Lee Moffitt Cancer Ctr & Research Inst, Tampa Genl Hosp; **Address:** H Lee Moffitt Cancer Ctr, 12902 Magnolia Drive, Tampa, FL 33612; **Phone:** 813-745-8658; **Board Cert:** Internal Medicine 1987; Hematology 1978; Medical Oncology 1979; **Med School:** Italy 1968; **Resid:** Internal Medicine, Univ Miss Med Ctr 1976; Hematology & Oncology, Univ Miss Med Ctr 1979; **Fellow:** Internal Medicine, A Gemelli Genl Hosp 1970; **Fac Appt:** Prof Med, Univ S Fla Coll Med

Benedetto, Pasquale W MD [Onc] - **Spec Exp:** Genitourinary Cancer; Bladder Cancer; Kidney Cancer; Pancreatic Cancer; **Hospital:** Univ of Miami Hosp & Clins/Sylvester Comp Canc Ctr, Jackson Meml Hosp; **Address:** Sylvester Comp Cancer Ctr, Med Oncology, 1475 NW 12th Ave, Ste 3310, Locator D8-4, Miami, FL 33136; **Phone:** 305-243-4909; **Board Cert:** Internal Medicine 1979; Medical Oncology 1981; Hematology 1982; **Med School:** Cornell Univ-Weill Med Coll 1976; **Resid:** Internal Medicine, Johns Hopkins Hosp 1979; **Fellow:** Medical Oncology, Meml Sloan Kettering Cancer Ctr 1981; **Fac Appt:** Prof Med, Univ Miami Sch Med

Bolger, Graeme B MD [Onc] - **Spec Exp:** Prostate Cancer; Testicular Cancer; **Hospital:** Univ of Ala Hosp at Birmingham; **Address:** 1530 3rd Ave S, Ste FOT-1105, Birmingham, AL 35294; **Phone:** 205-975-0088; **Board Cert:** Internal Medicine 1984; Medical Oncology 2000; **Med School:** McGill Univ 1980; **Resid:** Internal Medicine, Johns Hopkins Hosp 1984; **Fellow:** Medical Oncology, Fred Hutchinson Cancer Rsch 1985; Oncology, Meml Sloan-Kettering Cancer Ctr 1992; **Fac Appt:** Assoc Prof Med, Univ Ala

Boston, Barry MD [Onc] - **Spec Exp:** Gastrointestinal Cancer; Genitourinary Cancer; Prostate Cancer; **Hospital:** St Francis Hosp - Memphis, Methodist Univ Hosp - Memphis; **Address:** Univ of Tennessee Cancer Inst, 7945 Wolf River Blvd, Ste 300, Germantown, TN 38138; **Phone:** 901-752-6131; **Board Cert:** Internal Medicine 1974; Medical Oncology 1977; **Med School:** Louisiana State Univ 1971; **Resid:** Internal Medicine, Univ Tenn Hosp-VA Hosp 1973; Hematology, Univ Tenn Hosp-VA Hosp 1973; **Fellow:** Medical Oncology, Yale-New Haven Hosp 1975; **Fac Appt:** Assoc Prof Med, Univ Tenn Coll Med, Memphis

Burris III, Howard A MD [Onc] - **Spec Exp:** Drug Development; Drug Discovery; Breast Cancer; **Hospital:** Centennial Med Ctr, Baptist Hosp - Nashville; **Address:** 250 25th Ave N Bldg Atrium - Ste 100, Nashville, TN 37203; **Phone:** 615-329-7276; **Board Cert:** Internal Medicine 1988; Medical Oncology 2001; **Med School:** Univ S Ala Coll Med 1985; **Resid:** Internal Medicine, Brooke Army Med Ctr 1988; **Fellow:** Medical Oncology, Brooke Army Med Ctr 1991

Carbone, David MD [Onc] - **Spec Exp:** Lung Cancer; **Hospital:** Vanderbilt Univ Med Ctr; **Address:** Vanderbilt-Ingram Cancer Ctr, 685 Preston Rsch Bldg, 2200 Pierce Ave, Nashville, TN 37232-6838; **Phone:** 615-936-3524; **Board Cert:** Internal Medicine 1988; Medical Oncology 2001; **Med School:** Johns Hopkins Univ 1985; **Resid:** Internal Medicine, Johns Hopkins Hosp 1988; **Fellow:** Oncology, Natl Cancer Inst 1991; **Fac Appt:** Prof Med, Vanderbilt Univ

Chao, Nelson Jen An MD [Onc] - **Spec Exp:** Bone Marrow Transplant; Lymphoma; Leukemia; **Hospital:** Duke Univ Med Ctr; **Address:** Duke Univ Med Ctr, Box 3961, Durham, NC 27710; **Phone:** 919-668-1002; **Board Cert:** Internal Medicine 1984; Medical Oncology 1987; **Med School:** Yale Univ 1981; **Resid:** Internal Medicine, Stanford Univ Med Ctr 1984; **Fellow:** Oncology, Stanford Univ Med Ctr 1987; **Fac Appt:** Prof Med, Duke Univ

Crawford, Jeffrey MD [Onc] - **Spec Exp:** Lung Cancer; **Hospital:** Duke Univ Med Ctr; **Address:** Duke Univ Med Ctr, Box 3476, 400 Trent Drive 25167A Bldg, Morris Cancer Bldg, Durham, NC 27710-0001; **Phone:** 919-668-6688; **Board Cert:** Internal Medicine 1977; Hematology 1980; Medical Oncology 1981; **Med School:** Ohio State Univ 1974; **Resid:** Internal Medicine, Duke Univ Med Ctr 1977; **Fellow:** Hematology & Oncology, Duke Univ Med Ctr 1981; **Fac Appt:** Prof Med, Duke Univ

Daud, Adil I MD [Onc] - **Spec Exp:** Melanoma; Skin Cancer; Drug Development; **Hospital:** H Lee Moffitt Cancer Ctr & Research Inst; **Address:** H Lee Moffitt Cancer Ctr & Rsch Inst, 12902 Magnolia Drive, Tampa, FL 33612; **Phone:** 813-745-8581; **Board Cert:** Internal Medicine 1997; Hematology 2000; Medical Oncology 2000; **Med School:** India 1987; **Resid:** Internal Medicine, Indiana Univ; **Fellow:** Hematology & Oncology, Meml Sloan Kettering Cancer Ctr

De Simone, Philip MD [Onc] - **Spec Exp:** Colon Cancer; Pancreatic Cancer; **Hospital:** Univ of Kentucky Chandler Hosp; **Address:** UKMC Markey Cancer Ctr, CC-160, 800 Rose St, Lexington, KY 40536; **Phone:** 859-323-6448; **Board Cert:** Internal Medicine 1972; Hematology 1974; **Med School:** Univ VT Coll Med 1967; **Resid:** Internal Medicine, Univ Kentucky Hosp 1972; **Fellow:** Hematology & Oncology, Univ Kentucky Hosp 1974; **Fac Appt:** Prof Med, Univ KY Coll Med

Flinn, Ian MD/PhD [Onc] - **Spec Exp:** Hematologic Malignancies; Lymphoma; Bone Marrow Transplant; Clinical Trials; **Hospital:** Centennial Med Ctr; **Address:** Tennessee Oncology, 250 25th Ave N, Ste 110, Nashville, TN 37203; **Phone:** 615-320-5090; **Board Cert:** Hematology 1996; Medical Oncology 1997; **Med School:** Johns Hopkins Univ 1990; **Resid:** Internal Medicine, Univ Michigan Med Ctr 1993; **Fellow:** Medical Oncology, Johns Hopkins Univ Hosps 1993

Garst, Jennifer L MD [Onc] - **Spec Exp:** Lung Cancer; **Hospital:** Duke Univ Med Ctr; **Address:** Duke Univ Med Ctr, 25176 Morris Bldg, Box 3198, Durham, NC 27710; **Phone:** 919-668-6688; **Board Cert:** Medical Oncology 1997; **Med School:** Med Coll GA 1990; **Resid:** Internal Medicine, Univ Texas Hosp 1993; **Fellow:** Hematology & Oncology, Duke Univ Med Ctr 1996; **Fac Appt:** Prof Med, Duke Univ

Gockerman, Jon Paul MD [Onc] - **Spec Exp:** Leukemia; Lymphoma; **Hospital:** Duke Univ Med Ctr; **Address:** Duke Univ Med Ctr, 1 Trent Drive, rm 25153, Box 3872, Morris Bldg, Durham, NC 27710; **Phone:** 919-684-8964; **Board Cert:** Internal Medicine 1972; Hematology 1974; Medical Oncology 1973; **Med School:** Univ Chicago-Pritzker Sch Med 1967; **Resid:** Internal Medicine, Duke Univ Med Ctr 1969; **Fellow:** Hematology & Oncology, Duke Univ Med Ctr 1971

Goldberg, Richard M MD [Onc] - **Spec Exp:** Stomach Cancer; Esophageal Cancer; Colon & Rectal Cancer; Pancreatic Cancer; **Hospital:** Univ NC Hosps; **Address:** Division of Hematology/Oncology, CB 7305, 3009 Old Clinic Bldg SW, Chapel Hill, NC 27599-0001; **Phone:** 919-843-7711; **Board Cert:** Internal Medicine 1982; Medical Oncology 1985; **Med School:** SUNY Upstate Med Univ 1979; **Resid:** Internal Medicine, Emory Univ Med Ctr 1982; **Fellow:** Medical Oncology, Georgetown Univ Med Ctr 1984; **Fac Appt:** Prof Med, Univ NC Sch Med

Graham, Mark MD [Onc] - **Spec Exp:** Breast Cancer; Breast Cancer Genetics; **Hospital:** WakeMed Cary; **Address:** Waverly Hematology/Oncology, 300 Ashville Ave, Ste 310, Cary, NC 27511; **Phone:** 919-233-8585; **Board Cert:** Internal Medicine 1989; **Med School:** Mayo Med Sch 1982; **Resid:** Internal Medicine, Duke Univ Med Ctr 1985; **Fellow:** Medical Oncology, Univ CO Hlth Sci Ctr 1990; Medical Oncology, Mayo Clinic; **Fac Appt:** Assoc Clin Prof Med, Univ NC Sch Med

Medical Oncology

Greco, F Anthony MD [Onc] - **Spec Exp:** Lung Cancer; Unknown Primary Cancer; **Hospital:** Centennial Med Ctr; **Address:** Sarah Cannon Research Inst, 250 25th Ave N Atrium Bldg - Ste 100, Nashville, TN 37203; **Phone:** 615-320-5090; **Board Cert:** Internal Medicine 1975; Medical Oncology 1977; **Med School:** W VA Univ 1972; **Resid:** Internal Medicine, Univ West Virginia Hosp 1974; **Fellow:** Medical Oncology, Natl Cancer Inst 1976

Grosh, William W MD [Onc] - **Spec Exp:** Melanoma; Sarcoma; Neuroendocrine Tumors; **Hospital:** Univ Virginia Med Ctr; **Address:** UVA Health System, Div Hem/Oncology, PO Box 800716, Charlottesville, VA 22908; **Phone:** 434-924-1904; **Board Cert:** Internal Medicine 1978; Medical Oncology 1985; **Med School:** Columbia P&S 1974; **Resid:** Internal Medicine, Vanderbilt Univ Med Ctr 1977; **Fellow:** Medical Oncology, Vanderbilt Univ Med Ctr 1983; **Fac Appt:** Assoc Prof Med, Univ VA Sch Med

Hande, Kenneth MD [Onc] - **Spec Exp:** Drug Discovery; Sarcoma; Carcinoid Tumors; **Hospital:** Vanderbilt Univ Med Ctr, VA Med Ctr - Nashville; **Address:** Vanderbilt Univ Med Ctr, 777 Preston Research Building, Nashville, TN 37232-6307; **Phone:** 615-322-4967; **Board Cert:** Internal Medicine 1975; Medical Oncology 1977; **Med School:** Johns Hopkins Univ 1972; **Resid:** Internal Medicine, Barnes Hosp 1974; **Fellow:** Medical Oncology, Natl Cancer Inst 1977; **Fac Appt:** Prof Med, Vanderbilt Univ

Jillella, Anand MD [Onc] - **Spec Exp:** Bone Marrow Transplant; Leukemia; Lymphoma; Multiple Myeloma; **Hospital:** Med Coll of GA Hosp and Clin; **Address:** Med Coll Ga - BMT Program, 1120 15th St, BAA 5407, Augusta, GA 30912-3125; **Phone:** 706-721-2505; **Board Cert:** Internal Medicine 1992; Medical Oncology 1997; **Med School:** India 1985; **Resid:** Internal Medicine, Med Coll Georgia 1992; **Fellow:** Medical Oncology, Yale-New Haven Hosp 1996; **Fac Appt:** Prof Med, Med Coll GA

Johnson, David H MD [Onc] - **Spec Exp:** Lung Cancer; Breast Cancer; Drug Development; **Hospital:** Vanderbilt Univ Med Ctr; **Address:** Vanderbilt Univ Med Ctr, Div Med Onc, 2220 Pierce Ave, 777 PRB, Nashville, TN 37232; **Phone:** 615-322-6053; **Board Cert:** Internal Medicine 1979; Medical Oncology 1983; **Med School:** Med Coll GA 1976; **Resid:** Internal Medicine, Univ South Alabama Med Ctr 1979; Internal Medicine, Med Coll Georgia Hosps 1980; **Fellow:** Medical Oncology, Vanderbilt Univ Med Ctr 1983; **Fac Appt:** Prof Med, Vanderbilt Univ

Kraft, Andrew S MD [Onc] - **Spec Exp:** Prostate Cancer; Sarcoma; Drug Development; Clinical Trials; **Hospital:** MUSC Med Ctr; **Address:** 86 Jonathan Lucas St, PO BOX 250955, Charleston, SC 29425; **Phone:** 843-792-8284; **Board Cert:** Internal Medicine 1980; Medical Oncology 1985; **Med School:** Univ Pennsylvania 1975; **Resid:** Internal Medicine, Mt Sinai Hosp 1979; **Fellow:** Medical Oncology, Natl Cancer Inst 1983; **Fac Appt:** Prof Med, Med Univ SC

Kvols, Larry K MD [Onc] - **Spec Exp:** Gastrointestinal Cancer; Carcinoid Tumors; Neuroendocrine Tumors; **Hospital:** H Lee Moffitt Cancer Ctr & Research Inst; **Address:** H Lee Moffitt Cancer Ctr & Research Inst, 12902 Magnolia Drive, Ste WCBIGI, Tampa, FL 33612-9497; **Phone:** 813-972-8324; **Board Cert:** Internal Medicine 1976; Medical Oncology 1977; **Med School:** Baylor Coll Med 1970; **Resid:** Internal Medicine, Johns Hopkins Hosp 1972; **Fellow:** Hematology & Oncology, Johns Hopkins Hosp 1973; **Fac Appt:** Prof Med, Mayo Med Sch

Lossos, Izidore MD [Onc] - **Spec Exp:** Lymphoma; Hodgkin's Disease; Leukemia; **Hospital:** Univ of Miami Hosp & Clins/Sylvester Comp Canc Ctr, Jackson Meml Hosp; **Address:** Univ Miami - Sylvester Comp Cancer Ctr, 1475 NW 12th Ave, D8-4, Miami, FL 33136; **Phone:** 305-243-4785; **Med School:** Israel 1987; **Resid:** Internal Medicine, Hadassah Univ Hosp 1995; **Fellow:** Hematology & Oncology, Hadassah Univ Hosp 1997; Medical Oncology, Stanford Univ 2001; **Fac Appt:** Assoc Prof Med, Univ Miami Sch Med

Lyckholm, Laurel Jean MD [Onc] - **Spec Exp:** Neuro-Oncology; **Hospital:** Med Coll of VA Hosp; **Address:** Med Coll of VA, Div Hem/Onc, PO Box 980230, Richmond, VA 23298; **Phone:** 804-828-9723; **Board Cert:** Internal Medicine 1989; Medical Oncology 1993; Hematology 1994; **Med School:** Creighton Univ 1985; **Resid:** Internal Medicine, Creighton Univ 1989; **Fellow:** Hematology & Oncology, Univ IA Coll Med 1992; **Fac Appt:** Assoc Prof Med, Med Coll VA

Marcom, Paul K MD [Onc] - **Spec Exp:** Breast Cancer; Clinical Trials; Cancer Genetics; **Hospital:** Duke Univ Med Ctr; **Address:** Duke Univ Med Ctr, Morris Cancer Bldg, rm 25167, Box 3115, Durham, NC 27710; **Phone:** 919-684-3877; **Board Cert:** Internal Medicine 2003; Medical Oncology 2005; **Med School:** Baylor Coll Med 1989; **Resid:** Internal Medicine, Duke Univ Med Ctr 1992; Hematology & Oncology, Duke Univ Med Ctr 1995; **Fac Appt:** Assoc Prof Med, Duke Univ

Nabell, Lisle M MD [Onc] - **Spec Exp:** Breast Cancer; Head & Neck Cancer; **Hospital:** Univ of Ala Hosp at Birmingham; **Address:** Univ of Alabama, 1530 3rd Ave S, Ste WTI237, Birmingham, AL 35294; **Phone:** 205-934-3061; **Board Cert:** Internal Medicine 2000; Medical Oncology 2000; **Med School:** Univ NC Sch Med 1987; **Resid:** Internal Medicine, Univ Alabama Hosp 1990; **Fellow:** Hematology & Oncology, Univ Alabama Hosp 1992; **Fac Appt:** Assoc Prof Med, Univ Ala

Orlowski, Robert Z MD/PhD [Onc] - **Spec Exp:** Multiple Myeloma; Lymphoma, Non-Hodgkin's; Leukemia; Clinical Trials; **Hospital:** Univ NC Hosps; **Address:** UNC Cancer Hosp, M0041 Gravely Bldg, Campus Box 7218, 101 Manning Drive, Chapel Hill, NC 27599; **Phone:** 919-966-7782; **Board Cert:** Medical Oncology 1997; **Med School:** Yale Univ 1991; **Resid:** Internal Medicine, Barnes Hosp/Wash Univ 1994; **Fellow:** Hematology & Oncology, Johns Hopkins Hosp 1998; **Fac Appt:** Assoc Prof Med, Univ NC Sch Med

Perez, Edith A MD [Onc] - **Spec Exp:** Breast Cancer; Breast Cancer Risk Assessment; Clinical Trials; **Hospital:** Mayo - Jacksonville; **Address:** Mayo Clinic, 4500 San Pablo Rd Davis Bldg Fl 8, Jacksonville, FL 32224; **Phone:** 904-953-7283; **Board Cert:** Internal Medicine 1983; Hematology 1986; Medical Oncology 1987; **Med School:** Univ Puerto Rico 1979; **Resid:** Internal Medicine, Loma Linda Univ Med Ctr 1982; **Fellow:** Hematology & Oncology, Martinez VA Hosp/UC Davis 1987; **Fac Appt:** Prof Med, Mayo Med Sch

Robert, Nicholas J MD [Onc] - **Spec Exp:** Breast Cancer; **Hospital:** Inova Fairfax Hosp; **Address:** 8503 Arlington Blvd, Ste 400, Fairfax, VA 22031; **Phone:** 703-280-5390; **Board Cert:** Internal Medicine 1978; Anatomic Pathology 1979; Medical Oncology 1981; Hematology 1984; **Med School:** McGill Univ 1974; **Resid:** Internal Medicine, Royal Victoria Hosp 1976; Pathology, Mass Genl Hosp 1979; **Fellow:** Hematology, Peter Bent Brigham Hosp 1980; Medical Oncology, Dana Farber Cancer Inst 1981

Medical Oncology

Romond, Edward H MD [Onc] - **Spec Exp:** Breast Cancer; Hemophilia; **Hospital:** Univ of Kentucky Chandler Hosp; **Address:** Univ Kentucky Med Ctr, Div Hematology/Oncology, CC413 Roach Facility Markey Ctr 0093 St, Lexington, KY 40536-0093; **Phone:** 859-323-8043; **Board Cert:** Internal Medicine 1980; Hematology 1984; Medical Oncology 1983; **Med School:** Univ KY Coll Med 1977; **Resid:** Internal Medicine, Michigan State Univ Hosps 1980; **Fellow:** Hematology & Oncology, Michigan State Univ 1983; **Fac Appt:** Prof Med, Univ KY Coll Med

Roth, Bruce J MD [Onc] - **Spec Exp:** Prostate Cancer; Bladder Cancer; Testicular Cancer; **Hospital:** Vanderbilt Univ Med Ctr; **Address:** Vanderbilt Ingram Cancer Center, 777 Preston Research Bldg, Nashville, TN 37232-6307; **Phone:** 615-343-4070; **Board Cert:** Internal Medicine 1983; Medical Oncology 1985; **Med School:** St Louis Univ 1980; **Resid:** Internal Medicine, Indiana Univ Med Ctr 1983; **Fellow:** Hematology & Oncology, Indiana Univ Med Ctr 1986; **Fac Appt:** Prof Med, Vanderbilt Univ

Rothenberg, Mace MD [Onc] - **Spec Exp:** Pancreatic Cancer; Colon & Rectal Cancer; Clinical Trials; **Hospital:** Vanderbilt Univ Med Ctr; **Address:** Vanderbilt Ingram Cancer Center, 777 Preston Research Bldg, Nashville, TN 37232-6307; **Phone:** 615-322-4967; **Board Cert:** Internal Medicine 1985; Medical Oncology 1987; **Med School:** NYU Sch Med 1982; **Resid:** Internal Medicine, Vanderbilt Univ Med Ctr 1985; **Fellow:** Medical Oncology, Natl Cancer Inst 1988; **Fac Appt:** Prof Med, Vanderbilt Univ

Schwartz, Michael A MD [Onc] - **Spec Exp:** Breast Cancer; Lymphoma; Colon Cancer; **Hospital:** Mount Sinai Med Ctr - Miami, Miami Heart Inst; **Address:** Oncology Hematology Associates, 4306 Alton Rd Fl 3, Miami Beach, FL 33140; **Phone:** 305-535-3310; **Board Cert:** Internal Medicine 1989; Medical Oncology 2004; Hematology 2004; **Med School:** UMDNJ-RW Johnson Med Sch 1986; **Resid:** Internal Medicine, Mt Sinai Medical Ctr 1989; **Fellow:** Hematology & Oncology, Meml Sloan Kettering Cancer Ctr 1992; **Fac Appt:** Asst Clin Prof Med, Univ Miami Sch Med

Serody, Jonathan S MD [Onc] - **Spec Exp:** Breast Cancer Vaccine Therapy; Clinical Trials; Lymphoma; **Hospital:** Univ NC Hosps; **Address:** Lineberger Comprehensive Cancer Ctr, Univ NC Sch Medicine CB# 7295, Chapel Hill, NC 27599-7295; **Phone:** 919-966-8644; **Board Cert:** Internal Medicine 1989; Hematology 1996; **Med School:** Univ VA Sch Med 1986; **Resid:** Internal Medicine, Univ NC Med Ctr 1989; **Fellow:** Hematology, Univ NC Med Ctr 1992; Bone Marrow Transplant, Fred Hutchinson Transplant Program; **Fac Appt:** Assoc Prof Med, Univ NC Sch Med

Shea, Thomas MD [Onc] - **Spec Exp:** Bone Marrow Transplant; Lymphoma; Leukemia; **Hospital:** Univ NC Hosps; **Address:** Univ N Carolina, Dept Medicine, 3009 Old Clinic Bldg , Box 7305, Chapel Hill, NC 27599; **Phone:** 919-966-7746; **Board Cert:** Internal Medicine 1982; Hematology 1984; Medical Oncology 1985; **Med School:** Univ NC Sch Med 1978; **Resid:** Internal Medicine, Beth Israel Deaconess Med Ctr 1982; **Fellow:** Hematology & Oncology, Beth Israel Deaconess Med Ctr 1985; Bone Marrow Transplant, Dana Farber Cancer Inst 1988; **Fac Appt:** Prof Med, Univ NC Sch Med

Sherman, Carol A MD [Onc] - **Spec Exp:** Lung Cancer; Thoracic Cancers; **Hospital:** MUSC Med Ctr; **Address:** 96 Jonathan Lucas St, Ste CSB-903, Charleston, SC 29425; **Phone:** 843-792-9621; **Board Cert:** Internal Medicine 1987; Medical Oncology 1989; **Med School:** Univ Mass Sch Med 1984; **Resid:** Internal Medicine, Univ Mass Med Ctr 1987; **Fellow:** Hematology & Oncology, Univ Mass Med Ctr 1989; **Fac Appt:** Assoc Prof Med, Med Univ SC

Shin, Dong Moon MD [Onc] - **Spec Exp:** Head & Neck Cancer; Cancer Prevention; Mesothelioma; Thymoma; **Hospital:** Emory Univ Hosp; **Address:** Emory Winship Cancer Inst, 1365 C Clifton Rd NE, Ste 3090, Atlanta, GA 30322; **Phone:** 404-778-5990; **Board Cert:** Internal Medicine 1985; Medical Oncology 1989; **Med School:** South Korea 1975; **Resid:** Internal Medicine, Cook Co Hosp 1985; **Fellow:** Medical Oncology, Univ Texas MD Anderson Cancer Ctr 1986; **Fac Appt:** Prof Med, Emory Univ

Smith, Thomas Joseph MD [Onc] - **Spec Exp:** Breast Cancer; Palliative Care; **Hospital:** Med Coll of VA Hosp; **Address:** Med Coll Va, Div Hem/Onc, PO Box 980230, Richmond, VA 23298-0230; **Phone:** 804-828-9992; **Board Cert:** Internal Medicine 1982; Medical Oncology 1987; **Med School:** Yale Univ 1979; **Resid:** Internal Medicine, Hosp Univ Penn 1982; **Fellow:** Medical Oncology, Med Coll Virginia 1987; **Fac Appt:** Prof Med, Med Coll VA

Socinski, Mark A MD [Onc] - **Spec Exp:** Lung Cancer; **Hospital:** Univ NC Hosps; **Address:** UNC Chapel Hill, Div Hem/Onc, 3009 Old Clinic Bldg, Campus Box 7305, Chapel Hill, NC 27599-7305; **Phone:** 919-966-4431; **Board Cert:** Internal Medicine 1988; Medical Oncology 1991; **Med School:** Univ VT Coll Med 1984; **Resid:** Internal Medicine, Beth Israel Hosp 1986; **Fellow:** Medical Oncology, Dana-Farber Cancer Inst 1989; **Fac Appt:** Assoc Prof Med, Univ NC Sch Med

Stone, Joel MD [Onc] - **Spec Exp:** Lung Cancer; Breast Cancer; **Hospital:** St Vincent's Med Ctr - Jacksonville; **Address:** St Vincent's Med Ctr, 1801 Barrs St, Ste 800, Jacksonville, FL 32204; **Phone:** 904-388-2619; **Board Cert:** Internal Medicine 1977; Medical Oncology 1979; **Med School:** Univ VA Sch Med 1974; **Resid:** Internal Medicine, Univ KY Med Ctr 1977; **Fellow:** Hematology & Oncology, Emory Univ 1979

Sutton, Linda Marie MD [Onc] - **Spec Exp:** Breast Cancer; Palliative Care; **Hospital:** Duke Univ Med Ctr; **Address:** Duke Univ Med Ctr, 3100 Tower Blvd, Ste 600, Durham, NC 27707; **Phone:** 919-419-5005; **Board Cert:** Internal Medicine 2002; Medical Oncology 2003; **Med School:** Univ Mass Sch Med 1987; **Resid:** Internal Medicine, Montefiore Med Ctr 1990; **Fellow:** Hematology & Oncology, Duke Univ Med Ctr 1993

Torti, Frank M MD [Onc] - **Spec Exp:** Prostate Cancer; Urologic Cancer; **Hospital:** Wake Forest Univ Baptist Med Ctr (page 73); **Address:** Wake Forest Med Ctr-Comp Cancer Ctr, Medical Center Blvd, Winston-Salem, NC 27157-1082; **Phone:** 336-716-7971; **Board Cert:** Internal Medicine 1976; Medical Oncology 1978; **Med School:** Harvard Med Sch 1974; **Resid:** Internal Medicine, Beth Israel Hosp 1976; **Fellow:** Medical Oncology, Stanford Univ Med Ctr 1979; **Fac Appt:** Prof Med, Wake Forest Univ

Troner, Michael MD [Onc] - **Spec Exp:** Head & Neck Cancer; Urologic Cancer; **Hospital:** Baptist Hosp of Miami; **Address:** 8940 N Kendall Drive, Ste 300, East Tower, Miami, FL 33176-2132; **Phone:** 305-595-2141; **Board Cert:** Internal Medicine 1972; Medical Oncology 1973; **Med School:** SUNY Downstate 1968; **Resid:** Internal Medicine, Univ Maryland Hosp 1971; **Fellow:** Medical Oncology, Univ Miami Med Ctr 1973; **Fac Appt:** Assoc Clin Prof Med, Univ Miami Sch Med

Weiss, Geoffrey R MD [Onc] - **Spec Exp:** Gastrointestinal Cancer; Genitourinary Cancer; Melanoma; **Hospital:** Univ Virginia Med Ctr; **Address:** Univ Virginia Hlth System, Div Hem/Onc, PO Box 800716, Charlottesville, VA 22908-0716; **Phone:** 434-243-0066; **Board Cert:** Internal Medicine 1977; Medical Oncology 1981; **Med School:** St Louis Univ 1974; **Resid:** Internal Medicine, Temple Univ Hosp 1978; **Fellow:** Medical Oncology, Dana Farber Cancer Inst 1982; **Fac Appt:** Prof Med, Univ VA Sch Med

Medical Oncology

Williams, Michael MD [Onc] - **Spec Exp:** Lymphoma; Multiple Myeloma; Leukemia; **Hospital:** Univ Virginia Med Ctr; **Address:** UVA Hlth System, Div Hem/Oncology, PO Box 800716, Charlottesville, VA 22908-0716; **Phone:** 434-924-9637; **Board Cert:** Internal Medicine 1982; Medical Oncology 1987; Hematology 1988; **Med School:** Univ Cincinnati 1979; **Resid:** Internal Medicine, Univ Virginia Med Ctr 1983; **Fellow:** Hematology & Oncology, Univ Virginia Med Ctr 1986; **Fac Appt:** Prof Med, Univ VA Sch Med

Wingard, John R MD [Onc] - **Spec Exp:** Bone Marrow Transplant; Leukemia; Multiple Myeloma; **Hospital:** Shands Hlthcre at Univ of FL; **Address:** 1376 Mowry Rd, Ste 145, Box 103633, Gainesville, FL 32610; **Phone:** 352-273-8010; **Board Cert:** Internal Medicine 1977; Medical Oncology 1981; **Med School:** Johns Hopkins Univ 1973; **Resid:** Internal Medicine, Memphis City Hosps 1976; Internal Medicine, VA Hosp 1977; **Fellow:** Medical Oncology, Johns Hopkins Hosp 1979; **Fac Appt:** Prof Med, Univ Fla Coll Med

Midwest

Albain, Kathy MD [Onc] - **Spec Exp:** Breast Cancer; Lung Cancer; Cancer Survivors-Late Effects of Therapy; **Hospital:** Loyola Univ Med Ctr; **Address:** Loyola Univ Med Ctr, 2160 S First Ave, Bldg 112 - Ste 109, Maywood, IL 60153-5590; **Phone:** 708-327-3102; **Board Cert:** Internal Medicine 1981; Medical Oncology 1983; **Med School:** Univ Mich Med Sch 1978; **Resid:** Internal Medicine, Univ Illinois Med Ctr 1981; **Fellow:** Hematology & Oncology, Univ Chicago Hosps 1984; **Fac Appt:** Prof Med, Loyola Univ-Stritch Sch Med

Anderson, Joseph M MD [Onc] - **Spec Exp:** Breast Cancer; Palliative Care; Neuro-Oncology; **Hospital:** Henry Ford Hosp; **Address:** 2799 W Grand Blvd, Ste K13, Detroit, MI 48202; **Phone:** 313-916-1854; **Board Cert:** Internal Medicine 1985; Medical Oncology 1989; **Med School:** Univ Mich Med Sch 1982; **Resid:** Internal Medicine, Henry Ford Hosp 1986; **Fellow:** Medical Oncology, Henry Ford Hosp 1988

Benson III, Al B MD [Onc] - **Spec Exp:** Colon Cancer; Carcinoid Tumors; Pancreatic Cancer; **Hospital:** Northwestern Meml Hosp, Jesse A Brown VA Med Ctr; **Address:** 675 N St Clair, Ste 21-100, Chicago, IL 60611; **Phone:** 312-695-0990; **Board Cert:** Internal Medicine 1979; Medical Oncology 1983; **Med School:** SUNY Buffalo 1976; **Resid:** Internal Medicine, Univ Wisc Hosps 1979; **Fellow:** Medical Oncology, Univ Wisc Hosps 1984; **Fac Appt:** Prof Med, Northwestern Univ

Bitran, Jacob MD [Onc] - **Spec Exp:** Breast Cancer; Bone Marrow Transplant; Lung Cancer; **Hospital:** Adv Luth Genl Hosp, Rush N Shore Med Ctr; **Address:** Lutheran Genl Cancer Care Specialists, 1700 Luther Lane, Park Ridge, IL 60068-1270; **Phone:** 847-268-8200; **Board Cert:** Internal Medicine 1974; Hematology 1986; Medical Oncology 1977; **Med School:** Univ IL Coll Med 1971; **Resid:** Pathology, Rush Presby St Luke's Hosp 1973; Internal Medicine, Michael Reese Hosp 1973; **Fellow:** Hematology & Oncology, Univ Chicago Hosps 1977; **Fac Appt:** Prof Med, Ros Franklin Univ/Chicago Med Sch

Bolwell, Brian J MD [Onc] - **Spec Exp:** Bone Marrow Transplant; Hematologic Malignancies; **Hospital:** Cleveland Clin Fdn (page 57); **Address:** Cleveland Clinic Fdn, 9500 Euclid Ave, rm R32, Cleveland, OH 44195; **Phone:** 216-444-6922; **Board Cert:** Internal Medicine 1985; Medical Oncology 1987; **Med School:** Case West Res Univ 1981; **Resid:** Internal Medicine, Univ Hosp 1984; **Fellow:** Hematology & Oncology, Hosp Univ Penn 1987; **Fac Appt:** Prof Med, Cleveland Cl Coll Med/Case West Res

Bonomi, Philip MD [Onc] - **Spec Exp:** Lung Cancer; Thymoma; Mesothelioma; **Hospital:** Rush Univ Med Ctr; **Address:** 1725 W Harrison St, Ste 821, Chicago, IL 60612; **Phone:** 312-942-3312; **Board Cert:** Internal Medicine 1975; Medical Oncology 1977; **Med School:** Univ IL Coll Med 1970; **Resid:** Internal Medicine, Geisinger Med Ctr 1972; Internal Medicine, Geisinger Med Ctr 1975; **Fellow:** Medical Oncology, Rush Presby-St Luke's Med Ctr 1977; **Fac Appt:** Prof Med, Rush Med Coll

Borden, Ernest C MD [Onc] - **Spec Exp:** Melanoma; Immunotherapy; Sarcoma; Vaccine Therapy; **Hospital:** Cleveland Clin Fdn (page 57); **Address:** Cleveland Clinic Fdn, Desk R40, 9500 Euclid Ave, Cleveland, OH 44195; **Phone:** 216-444-8183; **Board Cert:** Internal Medicine 1973; Medical Oncology 1975; **Med School:** Duke Univ 1966; **Resid:** Internal Medicine, Hosp Univ Penn 1968; **Fellow:** Medical Oncology, Johns Hopkins Hosp 1973; **Fac Appt:** Prof Med, Cleveland Cl Coll Med/Case West Res

Bricker, Leslie J MD [Onc] - **Spec Exp:** Palliative Care; **Hospital:** Henry Ford Hosp; **Address:** Henry Ford Hospital, 2799 W Grand Blvd, CFP 5, Detroit, MI 48202; **Phone:** 313-916-1859; **Board Cert:** Internal Medicine 1980; Hematology 1982; Medical Oncology 1983; **Med School:** Wayne State Univ 1977; **Resid:** Internal Medicine, Sinai Hosp 1980; **Fellow:** Hematology & Oncology, Univ Mich Hosp 1983; **Fac Appt:** Assoc Prof Med, Wayne State Univ

Budd, George T MD [Onc] - **Spec Exp:** Breast Cancer; **Hospital:** Cleveland Clin Fdn (page 57); **Address:** Cleveland Clinic, Taussig Cancer Ctr, 9500 Euclid Ave, Desk R35, Cleveland, OH 44195; **Phone:** 216-444-6480; **Board Cert:** Internal Medicine 1980; Medical Oncology 1983; **Med School:** Univ Kans 1976; **Resid:** Internal Medicine, Cleveland Clinic 1980; **Fellow:** Hematology & Oncology, Cleveland Clinic 1982

Bukowski, Ronald M MD [Onc] - **Spec Exp:** Kidney Cancer; **Hospital:** Cleveland Clin Fdn (page 57); **Address:** Cleveland Clinic, Taussig Cancer Ctr, 9500 Euclid Ave, Desk R35, Cleveland, OH 44195-0001; **Phone:** 216-444-6825; **Board Cert:** Internal Medicine 1974; Medical Oncology 1975; Hematology 1976; **Med School:** Northwestern Univ 1967; **Resid:** Internal Medicine, Cleveland Clin Fdn 1969; Internal Medicine, Cleveland Clin Fdn 1973; **Fellow:** Hematology, Cleveland Clin Fdn 1975; **Fac Appt:** Prof Med, Cleveland Cl Coll Med/Case West Res

Burt, Richard K MD [Onc] - **Spec Exp:** Stem Cell Transplant in Lupus/Crohn's; Stem Cell Transplant in MS; Autoimmune Disease; **Hospital:** Northwestern Meml Hosp; **Address:** Northwestern Univ, 750 N Lakeshore Drive, Ste 649, Chicago, IL 60611; **Phone:** 312-908-0059; **Board Cert:** Internal Medicine 1989; Medical Oncology 1993; **Med School:** St Louis Univ 1984; **Resid:** Internal Medicine, Baylor Coll Med 1988; **Fellow:** Medical Oncology, Natl Inst Hlth Clin Ctr 1991; Hematology, Nat Inst Hlth Clin Ctr 1993; **Fac Appt:** Assoc Prof Med, Northwestern Univ

Byrd, John C MD [Onc] - **Spec Exp:** Leukemia-Chronic Lymphocytic; **Hospital:** Arthur G James Cancer Hosp & Research Inst; **Address:** Bl02 Starling-Loving Hall, 320 W 10th Ave, Columbus, OH 43210; **Phone:** 614-293-3196; **Board Cert:** Medical Oncology 1997; **Med School:** Univ Ark 1991; **Resid:** Internal Medicine, Walter Reed AMC 1994; **Fellow:** Hematology & Oncology, Walter Reed AMC 1997; **Fac Appt:** Assoc Prof Med, Ohio State Univ

Medical Oncology

Chitambar, Christopher R MD [Onc] - **Spec Exp:** Lymphoma; Leukemia; Breast Cancer; **Hospital:** Froedtert Meml Lutheran Hosp; **Address:** Med Coll Wisconsin, Div Neoplastic Disease, 9200 W Wisconsin Ave, Milwaukee, WI 53226-3522; **Phone:** 414-805-4600; **Board Cert:** Internal Medicine 1980; Hematology 1982; Medical Oncology 1983; **Med School:** India 1977; **Resid:** Internal Medicine, Brackenridge Hosp 1980; **Fellow:** Hematology & Oncology, Univ Colo Hlth Sci Ctr 1983; **Fac Appt:** Prof Med, Med Coll Wisc

Cobleigh, Melody A MD [Onc] - **Spec Exp:** Breast Cancer; **Hospital:** Rush Univ Med Ctr; **Address:** Rush Univ Med Ctr, 1725 W Harrison St, Ste 855, Chicago, IL 60612-3828; **Phone:** 312-942-5904; **Board Cert:** Internal Medicine 1979; Medical Oncology 1981; **Med School:** Rush Med Coll 1976; **Resid:** Internal Medicine, Rush Presby-St Lukes Med Ctr 1979; **Fellow:** Medical Oncology, Indiana Univ 1981; **Fac Appt:** Prof Med, Rush Med Coll

Di Persio, John MD/PhD [Onc] - **Spec Exp:** Bone Marrow Transplant; Hematologic Malignancies; Leukemia; **Hospital:** Barnes-Jewish Hosp; **Address:** Wash Univ Sch Med, Sect BMT & Leukemia, 660 S Euclid Ave, Box 8007, St Louis, MO 63110; **Phone:** 314-454-8306; **Board Cert:** Internal Medicine 1984; Medical Oncology 1987; Hematology 1988; **Med School:** Univ Rochester 1980; **Resid:** Internal Medicine, Parkland Meml Hosp 1984; **Fellow:** Hematology & Oncology, UCLA Sch Med 1987; **Fac Appt:** Prof Med, Washington Univ, St Louis

Dreicer, Robert MD [Onc] - **Spec Exp:** Breast Cancer; Prostate Cancer; **Hospital:** Cleveland Clin Fdn (page 57); **Address:** Cleveland Clinic, Taussig Cancer Ctr, 9500 Euclid Ave, Desk R35, Cleveland, OH 44195; **Phone:** 216-445-4623; **Board Cert:** Internal Medicine 1986; Medical Oncology 1989; **Med School:** Univ Tex, Houston 1983; **Resid:** Internal Medicine, Ind Univ Med Ctr 1986; **Fellow:** Medical Oncology, Univ Wisconsin Hosp & Clins 1989

Einhorn, Lawrence MD [Onc] - **Spec Exp:** Testicular Cancer; Lung Cancer; Urologic Cancer; **Hospital:** Indiana Univ Hosp; **Address:** 535 Barnhill Drive, rm 473, Indianapolis, IN 46202; **Phone:** 317-274-0920; **Board Cert:** Internal Medicine 1972; Medical Oncology 1975; **Med School:** UCLA 1967; **Resid:** Internal Medicine, Indiana Univ Hosp 1969; **Fellow:** Medical Oncology, Indiana Univ Hosp 1972; **Fac Appt:** Prof Med, Indiana Univ

Ensminger, William D MD/PhD [Onc] - **Spec Exp:** Gastrointestinal Cancer; Liver Cancer; Clinical Trials; **Hospital:** Univ Michigan Hlth Sys; **Address:** Upjohn Center, rm 3709, 1310 E Catherine, Ann Arbor, MI 48109-0504; **Phone:** 734-764-5468; **Board Cert:** Internal Medicine 1976; Medical Oncology 1979; **Med School:** Harvard Med Sch 1973; **Resid:** Internal Medicine, Beth Israel Hosp 1975; **Fellow:** Medical Oncology, Dana Farber Cancer Inst 1977; **Fac Appt:** Prof Med, Univ Mich Med Sch

Fracasso, Paula M MD/PhD [Onc] - **Spec Exp:** Ovarian Cancer; Gynecologic Cancer; Breast Cancer; **Hospital:** Barnes Jewish Hosp; **Address:** Washington Univ Sch Med, 660 N Euclid, Box 8056, St Louis, MO 63110-1002; **Phone:** 314-454-8817; **Board Cert:** Internal Medicine 1987; Medical Oncology 2003; **Med School:** Yale Univ 1984; **Resid:** Internal Medicine, Beth Israel Hosp 1987; **Fellow:** Cancer Research, Mass Inst Tech 1989; Hematology & Oncology, Tufts-New England Med Ctr 1991; **Fac Appt:** Assoc Prof Med, Washington Univ, St Louis

Gerson, Stanton MD [Onc] - **Spec Exp:** Leukemia; Lymphoma, Non-Hodgkin's; Stem Cell Transplant; **Hospital:** Univ Hosps Case Med Ctr; **Address:** Case Comprehensive Cancer Ctr, 11000 Euclid Ave, 1 WEARN 151, Cleveland, OH 44106-5065; **Phone:** 216-844-8562; **Board Cert:** Internal Medicine 1980; Medical Oncology 1983; Hematology 1982; **Med School:** Harvard Med Sch 1977; **Resid:** Internal Medicine, Hosp Univ Penn 1980; **Fellow:** Hematology & Oncology, Hosp Univ Penn 1983; **Fac Appt:** Prof Med, Case West Res Univ

Hartmann, Lynn Carol MD [Onc] - **Spec Exp:** Breast Cancer; Ovarian Cancer; **Hospital:** Mayo Med Ctr & Clin - Rochester; **Address:** Mayo Clinic Gonda 10 South, 200 First St SW, Rochester, MN 55905; **Phone:** 507-284-3903; **Board Cert:** Internal Medicine 1986; Medical Oncology 1989; **Med School:** Northwestern Univ 1983; **Resid:** Internal Medicine, Univ Ia Hosps/Clinics 1986; **Fellow:** Medical Oncology, Mayo Clinic 1989; **Fac Appt:** Prof Med, Mayo Med Sch

Hayes, Daniel F MD [Onc] - **Spec Exp:** Breast Cancer; **Hospital:** Univ Michigan Hlth Sys; **Address:** Univ Michigan Comprehensive Cancer Ctr, 1500 E Med Ctr Drive, rm 6312, Box 0942, Ann Arbor, MI 48109-0942; **Phone:** 734-615-6725; **Board Cert:** Internal Medicine 1982; Medical Oncology 1985; **Med School:** Indiana Univ 1979; **Resid:** Internal Medicine, Parkland Meml Hosp 1982; **Fellow:** Medical Oncology, Dana Farber Cancer Inst 1985; **Fac Appt:** Prof Med, Univ Mich Med Sch

Ingle, James N MD [Onc] - **Spec Exp:** Breast Cancer; **Hospital:** Rochester Meth Hosp; **Address:** Mayo Clinic, 200 First St SW, 12 East, Rochester, MN 55905; **Phone:** 507-284-8432; **Board Cert:** Internal Medicine 1974; Medical Oncology 1975; **Med School:** Johns Hopkins Univ 1971; **Resid:** Internal Medicine, Johns Hopkins Hosp 1976; Medical Oncology, Natl Cancer Inst 1975; **Fac Appt:** Prof Med, Mayo Med Sch

Kalaycio, Matt E MD [Onc] - **Spec Exp:** Leukemia; **Hospital:** Cleveland Clin Fdn (page 57); **Address:** Taussig Cancer Ctr, 9500 Euclid Ave, Desk R35, Cleveland, OH 44195; **Phone:** 216-444-3705; **Board Cert:** Internal Medicine 2002; Hematology 2004; Medical Oncology 1995; **Med School:** W VA Univ 1988; **Resid:** Internal Medicine, Mercy Hosp 1991; **Fellow:** Hematology & Oncology, Cleveland Clinic 1994; **Fac Appt:** Assoc Prof Med, Cleveland Cl Coll Med/Case West Res

Kaminski, Mark S MD [Onc] - **Spec Exp:** Lymphoma; Bone Marrow Transplant; Drug Development; Clinical Trials; **Hospital:** Univ Michigan Hlth Sys; **Address:** Univ Michigan Cancer Ctr, 1500 E Medical Ctr Drive, rm 4316, Ann Arbor, MI 48109-0936; **Phone:** 734-936-5310; **Board Cert:** Internal Medicine 1981; Medical Oncology 1983; **Med School:** Stanford Univ 1978; **Resid:** Internal Medicine, Barnes Hosp 1981; **Fellow:** Medical Oncology, Stanford Univ Med Ctr 1985; **Fac Appt:** Prof Med, Univ Mich Med Sch

Kosova, Leonard MD [Onc] - **Spec Exp:** Breast Cancer; Lymphoma; Lung Cancer; **Hospital:** Adv Luth Genl Hosp; **Address:** 8915 W Golf Rd, Ste 3, Niles, IL 60714-5825; **Phone:** 847-827-9060; **Board Cert:** Internal Medicine 1974; Hematology 1972; Medical Oncology 1975; **Med School:** Univ IL Coll Med 1961; **Resid:** Internal Medicine, Hines VA Hosp 1964; **Fellow:** Hematology & Oncology, Hektoen Inst-Cook Cty Hosp 1965

Lippman, Marc E MD [Onc] - **Spec Exp:** Breast Cancer; **Hospital:** Univ Michigan Hlth Sys; **Address:** Univ Mich Health System, 3101 Taubman Ctr, 1500 E Medical Ctr Dr, Ann Arbor, MI 48109-0368; **Phone:** 734-936-4495; **Board Cert:** Internal Medicine 1987; Endocrinology 1975; Medical Oncology 1977; **Med School:** Yale Univ 1968; **Resid:** Internal Medicine, Johns Hopkins Hosp 1970; **Fellow:** Medical Oncology, Natl Cancer Inst 1973; Endocrinology, Yale-New Haven Hosp 1974; **Fac Appt:** Prof Med, Univ Mich Med Sch

Locker, Gershon Y MD [Onc] - **Spec Exp:** Gastrointestinal Cancer; Ovarian Cancer; Breast Cancer; Cancer Genetics; **Hospital:** Evanston Hosp, Northwestern Meml Hosp; **Address:** Evanston Hospital-Kellog Cancer Ctr, 2650 Ridge Ave, rm 5134, Evanston, IL 60201-1781; **Phone:** 847-570-2515; **Board Cert:** Internal Medicine 1976; Medical Oncology 1977; **Med School:** Harvard Med Sch 1973; **Resid:** Internal Medicine, Univ Chicago Hosps 1975; **Fellow:** Medical Oncology, Natl Cancer Inst 1978; **Fac Appt:** Prof Med, Northwestern Univ

Loehrer, Patrick J MD [Onc] - **Spec Exp:** Gastrointestinal Cancer; Thymoma; Genitourinary Cancer; **Hospital:** Indiana Univ Hosp; **Address:** Indiana Cancer Pavilion, 535 Barnhill Drive, rm 473, Indianapolis, IN 46202-5112; **Phone:** 317-278-7418; **Board Cert:** Internal Medicine 1981; Medical Oncology 2006; **Med School:** Rush Med Coll 1978; **Resid:** Internal Medicine, Rush-Presby-St Lukes Hosp 1981; **Fellow:** Medical Oncology, Indiana Univ 1983; **Fac Appt:** Prof Med, Indiana Univ

Loprinzi, Charles L MD [Onc] - **Spec Exp:** Breast Cancer; **Hospital:** Mayo Med Ctr & Clin - Rochester; **Address:** Mayo Clinic, Dept Med Oncology, 200 First St SW, Rochester, MN 55905-0001; **Phone:** 507-284-4137; **Board Cert:** Internal Medicine 1982; Medical Oncology 1985; **Med School:** Oregon Hlth Sci Univ 1979; **Resid:** Internal Medicine, Maricopa Co Hosp 1982; **Fellow:** Medical Oncology, Univ Wisconsin Med Ctr 1984; **Fac Appt:** Prof Med, Mayo Med Sch

Markowitz, Sanford D MD [Onc] - **Spec Exp:** Colon & Rectal Cancer; Hereditary Cancer; **Hospital:** Univ Hosps Case Med Ctr; **Address:** Ireland Cancer Ctr, 11000 Euclid Ave Fl 6, Cleveland, OH 44106; **Phone:** 216-844-3127; **Board Cert:** Internal Medicine 1984; Medical Oncology 1987; **Med School:** Yale Univ 1980; **Resid:** Internal Medicine, Univ Chicago Hosp 1984; **Fellow:** Medical Oncology, Natl Cancer Inst 1986; **Fac Appt:** Prof Med, Case West Res Univ

Olopade, Olufunmilayo I F MD [Onc] - **Spec Exp:** Breast Cancer; Hereditary Cancer; Cancer Genetics; **Hospital:** Univ of Chicago Hosps; **Address:** Univ Chicago Hospital, 5758 S Maryland Ave, MC 9015, Chicago, IL 60637-1470; **Phone:** 773-702-6149; **Board Cert:** Internal Medicine 1986; Hematology 2001; Medical Oncology 1989; **Med School:** Nigeria 1980; **Resid:** Internal Medicine, Cook Co Hosp 1986; **Fellow:** Hematology & Oncology, Univ Chicago Hosps 1991; **Fac Appt:** Prof Med, Univ Chicago-Pritzker Sch Med

Perry, Michael MD [Onc] - **Spec Exp:** Lung Cancer; Breast Cancer; **Hospital:** Univ of Missouri Hosp & Clins; **Address:** Ellis Fischel Cancer Ctr, 115 Business Loop 70 W, DC 116.71, rm 524, Columbia, MO 65203-3299; **Phone:** 573-882-4979; **Board Cert:** Internal Medicine 1987; Hematology 1974; Medical Oncology 1975; **Med School:** Wayne State Univ 1970; **Resid:** Internal Medicine, Mayo Grad Sch 1972; **Fellow:** Hematology, Mayo Grad Sch 1974; Medical Oncology, Mayo Grad Sch 1975; **Fac Appt:** Prof Med, Univ MO-Columbia Sch Med

Pienta, Kenneth J MD [Onc] - **Spec Exp:** Prostate Cancer; **Hospital:** Univ Michigan Hlth Sys; **Address:** Cancer Center/Geriatrics Center, 1500 E Medical Center Drive, rm 7303 CCGC, Ann Arbor, MI 48109-0946; **Phone:** 734-647-3421; **Board Cert:** Internal Medicine 2001; Medical Oncology 2001; **Med School:** Johns Hopkins Univ 1986; **Resid:** Internal Medicine, Univ Chicago Hosps 1988; **Fellow:** Medical Oncology, Johns Hopkins Hosp 1991; **Fac Appt:** Prof Med, Univ Mich Med Sch

Raghavan, Derek MD/PhD [Onc] - **Spec Exp:** Prostate Cancer; Testicular Cancer; Bladder Cancer; **Hospital:** Cleveland Clin Fdn (page 57); **Address:** Cleveland Clinic Taussig Cancer Ctr, 9500 Euclid Ave, MC R35, Cleveland, OH 44195; **Phone:** 216-445-6888; **Med School:** Australia 1974; **Resid:** Internal Medicine, Royal Prince Alfred Hosp 1977; **Fellow:** Medical Oncology, Royal Prince Alfred Hosp 1979; Medical Oncology, Royal Marsden Hosp; **Fac Appt:** Prof Med, Cleveland Cl Coll Med/Case West Res

Ratain, Mark J MD [Onc] - **Spec Exp:** Solid Tumors; Drug Discovery & Development; **Hospital:** Univ of Chicago Hosps; **Address:** 5841 S Maryland Ave, MC 2115, Chicago, IL 60637; **Phone:** 773-702-6149; **Board Cert:** Internal Medicine 1983; Hematology 1986; Medical Oncology 1985; **Med School:** Yale Univ 1980; **Resid:** Internal Medicine, Johns Hopkins Hosp 1983; **Fellow:** Hematology & Oncology, Univ Chicago 1986; **Fac Appt:** Prof Med, Univ Chicago-Pritzker Sch Med

Richards, Jon MD/PhD [Onc] - **Spec Exp:** Testicular Cancer; Prostate Cancer; Melanoma; **Hospital:** Adv Luth Genl Hosp, Rush N Shore Med Ctr; **Address:** Cancer Care Ctr, 1700 Luther Ln Fl 2, Park Ridge, IL 60068; **Phone:** 847-268-8200; **Board Cert:** Internal Medicine 1998; **Med School:** Cornell Univ-Weill Med Coll 1983; **Resid:** Internal Medicine, Univ Chicago Hosp 1985; **Fellow:** Hematology & Oncology, Univ Chicago Hosp 1988; **Fac Appt:** Asst Prof Med, Univ IL Coll Med

Rosen, Steven T MD [Onc] - **Spec Exp:** Hematologic Malignancies; Breast Cancer; Lymphoma; **Hospital:** Northwestern Meml Hosp; **Address:** Northwestern Univ, 303 E Chicago Ave, Lurie 3-125, Chicago, IL 60611-3013; **Phone:** 312-695-1153; **Board Cert:** Internal Medicine 1979; Medical Oncology 1981; Hematology 1984; **Med School:** Northwestern Univ 1976; **Resid:** Internal Medicine, Northwestern Univ Hosp 1979; **Fellow:** Medical Oncology, Natl Cancer Inst 1981; **Fac Appt:** Prof Med, Northwestern Univ

Ruckdeschel, John C MD [Onc] - **Spec Exp:** Lung Cancer; Mesothelioma; **Hospital:** Karmanos Cancer Inst; **Address:** Karmanos Cancer Inst-Excutive Offices, 4100 John R Fl 2, Detroit, MI 48201; **Phone:** 313-526-8621; **Board Cert:** Internal Medicine 1976; Medical Oncology 1977; **Med School:** Albany Med Coll 1971; **Resid:** Internal Medicine, Johns Hopkins Hosp 1972; Internal Medicine, Beth Israel Hosp 1976; **Fellow:** Medical Oncology, Natl Cancer Inst 1975; **Fac Appt:** Prof Med, Wayne State Univ

Salgia, Ravi MD/PhD [Onc] - **Spec Exp:** Lung Cancer; Mesothelioma; Thoracic Cancers; **Hospital:** Univ of Chicago Hosps; **Address:** University of Chicago Hospitals, 5841 S Maryland Ave, MC 2115, Chicago, IL 60637; **Phone:** 773-702-6149; **Board Cert:** Medical Oncology 2006; **Med School:** Loyola Univ-Stritch Sch Med 1987; **Resid:** Internal Medicine, Johns Hopkins Hospital 1990; **Fellow:** Medical Oncology, Dana-Farber Cancer Inst 1993; **Fac Appt:** Assoc Prof Med, Univ IL Coll Med

Saroja, Kurubarahalli MD [Onc] - **Spec Exp:** Neutron Therapy for Advanced Cancer; Head & Neck Cancer; Sarcoma; Prostate Cancer; **Hospital:** Delnor - Comm Hosp, Central DuPage Hosp; **Address:** Raymond G Scott Cancer Care Center, 304 Randall, Geneva, IL 60134; **Phone:** 630-262-8554; **Board Cert:** Pediatrics 1978; Radiation Oncology 1987; Neonatal-Perinatal Medicine 1981; **Med School:** India 1967; **Resid:** Pediatrics, Cook Co Hosp 1976; Radiation Oncology, Rush-Presby St Lukes 1985; **Fellow:** Neonatal-Perinatal Medicine, Milwaukee Co Med Comp 1978

Medical Oncology

Schiffer, Charles A MD [Onc] - **Spec Exp:** Leukemia; Lymphoma; Multiple Myeloma; **Hospital:** Karmanos Cancer Inst, Harper Univ Hosp; **Address:** Karmanos Cancer Inst, Cancer Research Ctr, 4100 John R, 4-Hudson Webber, Detroit, MI 48201; **Phone:** 313-576-8737; **Board Cert:** Internal Medicine 1972; Medical Oncology 1973; **Med School:** NYU Sch Med 1968; **Resid:** Internal Medicine, Bellevue-NY VA Hosp-NYU 1972; **Fellow:** Medical Oncology, Natl Cancer Inst 1974; **Fac Appt:** Prof Med, Wayne State Univ

Schilsky, Richard MD [Onc] - **Spec Exp:** Gastrointestinal Cancer; Pancreatic Cancer; Drug Development; **Hospital:** Univ of Chicago Hosps; **Address:** Univ Chicago- Bio Sciences Div, 5841 S Maryland Ave, MC 7132, Chicago, IL 60637; **Phone:** 773-834-3914; **Board Cert:** Internal Medicine 1978; Medical Oncology 1979; **Med School:** Univ Chicago-Pritzker Sch Med 1975; **Resid:** Internal Medicine, Univ Texas 1977; **Fac Appt:** Prof Med, Univ Chicago-Pritzker Sch Med

Schwartz, Burton S MD [Onc] - **Spec Exp:** Lymphoma; Breast Cancer; **Hospital:** Abbott - Northwestern Hosp; **Address:** 800 E 28th St, Piper Bldg, Ste 405, Minneapolis, MN 55407; **Phone:** 612-863-8585; **Board Cert:** Internal Medicine 1980; Hematology 1976; Medical Oncology 1977; **Med School:** Meharry Med Coll 1968; **Resid:** Internal Medicine, Michael Reese Hosp 1971; **Fellow:** Hematology, Univ Minn Hosp 1976; **Fac Appt:** Clin Prof Med, Univ Minn

Shapiro, Charles L MD [Onc] - **Spec Exp:** Breast Cancer; **Hospital:** Arthur G James Cancer Hosp & Research Inst; **Address:** Starling Loving Hall, rm B405, 320 W 10th Ave, Columbus, OH 43210; **Phone:** 614-293-6401; **Board Cert:** Internal Medicine 1987; Medical Oncology 2005; **Med School:** SUNY Buffalo 1984; **Resid:** Internal Medicine, Temple Univ Hosp 1987; **Fellow:** Medical Oncology, Dana Farber Cancer Inst 1991; **Fac Appt:** Assoc Prof Med, Ohio State Univ

Sledge Jr, George W MD [Onc] - **Spec Exp:** Breast Cancer; **Hospital:** Indiana Univ Hosp; **Address:** 535 Barnhill Drive, rm 473, Indianapolis, IN 46202; **Phone:** 317-274-0920; **Board Cert:** Internal Medicine 1980; Medical Oncology 1983; **Med School:** Tulane Univ 1977; **Resid:** Internal Medicine, St Louis Univ 1980; **Fellow:** Medical Oncology, Univ Texas 1983; **Fac Appt:** Prof Med, Indiana Univ

Stadler, Walter M MD [Onc] - **Spec Exp:** Kidney Cancer; Prostate Cancer; Bladder Cancer; **Hospital:** Univ of Chicago Hosps; **Address:** Univ Chicago Hosps, Div Hem/Onc, 5758 S Maryland Ave, MC 9015, Chicago, IL 60637; **Phone:** 773-834-7424; **Board Cert:** Internal Medicine 2002; Medical Oncology 2003; **Med School:** Yale Univ 1988; **Resid:** Internal Medicine, Michael Reese Hosp 1991; **Fellow:** Medical Oncology, Univ Chicago Hosps 1994; **Fac Appt:** Prof Med, Univ Chicago-Pritzker Sch Med

Todd III, Robert F MD/PhD [Onc] - **Spec Exp:** Gastrointestinal Cancer; Lung Cancer; **Hospital:** Univ Michigan Hlth Sys; **Address:** Univ Michigan Cancer Ctr, 7216CCGC, 1500 E Med Ctr Dr, Box 0948, Ann Arbor, MI 48109; **Phone:** 734-647-8903; **Board Cert:** Internal Medicine 1979; Medical Oncology 1981; **Med School:** Duke Univ 1976; **Resid:** Internal Medicine, Peter Bent Brigham Hosp 1978; **Fellow:** Medical Oncology, Dana Farber Cancer Inst 1981; **Fac Appt:** Prof Med, Univ Mich Med Sch

Urba, Susan G MD [Onc] - **Spec Exp:** Head & Neck Cancer; **Hospital:** Univ Michigan Hlth Sys; **Address:** Comp Cancer Ctr & Geriatrics Ctr, 1500 E Med Ctr Drive, rm 4214, Ann Arbor, MI 48109-0922; **Phone:** 734-647-8902; **Board Cert:** Internal Medicine 1986; Medical Oncology 1991; **Med School:** Univ Mich Med Sch 1983; **Resid:** Internal Medicine, Univ Mich Med Ctr 1986; **Fellow:** Hematology & Oncology, Univ Mich Med Ctr 1988; **Fac Appt:** Assoc Prof Med, Univ Mich Med Sch

Vokes, Everett E MD [Onc] - **Spec Exp:** Lung Cancer; Head & Neck Cancer; Esophageal Cancer; **Hospital:** Univ of Chicago Hosps; **Address:** Univ Chicago Hosps, 5841 S Maryland Ave, MC 2115, Chicago, IL 60637-1470; **Phone:** 773-834-3093; **Board Cert:** Internal Medicine 1983; Medical Oncology 1985; **Med School:** Germany 1980; **Resid:** Internal Medicine, Ravenswood Hosp-Univ Illinois 1982; Internal Medicine, USC Med Ctr 1983; **Fellow:** Medical Oncology, Univ Chicago 1986; **Fac Appt:** Prof Med, Univ Chicago-Pritzker Sch Med

Wicha, Max S MD [Onc] - **Spec Exp:** Breast Cancer; Stem Cell Transplant; **Hospital:** Univ Michigan Hlth Sys; **Address:** Comp Cancer Ctr & Geriatrics Ctr, 1500 E Med Ctr Dr, rm 6302 CCGC, Box 0942, Ann Arbor, MI 48109-0942; **Phone:** 734-936-1831; **Board Cert:** Internal Medicine 1977; Medical Oncology 1983; **Med School:** Stanford Univ 1974; **Resid:** Internal Medicine, Univ Chicago Hosp 1977; **Fellow:** Medical Oncology, Natl Inst Hlth 1980; **Fac Appt:** Prof Med, Univ Mich Med Sch

Wilding, George MD [Onc] - **Spec Exp:** Prostate Cancer; Kidney Cancer; Genitourinary Cancer; Drug Discovery & Development; **Hospital:** Univ WI Hosp & Clins; **Address:** UWCCC, Clinical Science Ctr, K4-614, 600 Highland Ave, MC 6164, Madison, WI 53792; **Phone:** 608-263-8610; **Board Cert:** Internal Medicine 1983; Medical Oncology 1985; **Med School:** Univ Mass Sch Med 1980; **Resid:** Internal Medicine, Univ Mass Med Ctr 1983; **Fellow:** Medical Oncology, Natl Cancer Inst 1985

Williams, Stephen D MD [Onc] - **Spec Exp:** Testicular Cancer; Gynecologic Cancer; Genitourinary Cancer; **Hospital:** Indiana Univ Hosp; **Address:** Indiana University Cancer Ctr, 535 Barnhill Drive, rm 473, Inianapolis, IN 46202; **Phone:** 317-274-0920; **Board Cert:** Internal Medicine 1976; Medical Oncology 1979; **Med School:** Indiana Univ 1971; **Resid:** Internal Medicine, Indiana Univ Hosp 1975; **Fellow:** Medical Oncology, Indiana Univ Hosp 1978; **Fac Appt:** Prof Med, Indiana Univ

Great Plains and Mountains

Akerley, Wallace MD [Onc] - **Spec Exp:** Lung Cancer; Clinical Trials; **Hospital:** Univ Utah Hosps and Clins; **Address:** Huntsman Cancer Inst, 2000 Circle of Hope, rm 2165, Salt Lake City, UT 84112; **Phone:** 801-585-0100; **Board Cert:** Internal Medicine 1984; Medical Oncology 1987; Hematology 1988; **Med School:** Brown Univ 1981; **Resid:** Internal Medicine, USC Medical Ctr 1985; **Fellow:** Medical Oncology, USC Medical Ctr 1986; Hematology, Norris Cotton Cancer Ctr/Dartmouth 1988; **Fac Appt:** Prof Med, Univ Utah

Armitage, James MD [Onc] - **Spec Exp:** Lymphoma; Bone Marrow Transplant; **Hospital:** Nebraska Med Ctr; **Address:** 987680 Nebraska Medical Center, Omaha, NE 68198-7680; **Phone:** 402-559-7290; **Board Cert:** Internal Medicine 1976; Medical Oncology 1977; Hematology 1984; **Med School:** Univ Nebr Coll Med 1973; **Resid:** Internal Medicine, Univ Nebraska Med Ctr 1975; **Fellow:** Hematology & Oncology, Univ Iowa Hosp 1977; **Fac Appt:** Prof Med, Univ Nebr Coll Med

Bunn Jr, Paul MD [Onc] - **Spec Exp:** Lung Cancer; Lymphoma; **Hospital:** Univ Colorado Hosp; **Address:** Univ Colorado Cancer Ctr, Box 6510, MS F-704, Aurora, CO 80045-0510; **Phone:** 720-848-0300; **Board Cert:** Internal Medicine 1974; Medical Oncology 1975; **Med School:** Cornell Univ-Weill Med Coll 1971; **Resid:** Internal Medicine, Moffitt Hosp/ UCSF Med Ctr 1973; **Fellow:** Medical Oncology, Natl Cancer Inst 1976; **Fac Appt:** Prof Med, Univ Colorado

Buys, Saundra S MD [Onc] - **Spec Exp:** Breast Cancer; Breast Cancer Risk Assessment; Breast Cancer Genetics; **Hospital:** Univ Utah Hosps and Clins; **Address:** Huntsman Cancer Institute, 2000 Circle of Hope, Ste 210, Salt Lake City, UT 84112; **Phone:** 801-585-3525; **Board Cert:** Internal Medicine 1982; Medical Oncology 1985; Hematology 1984; **Med School:** Tufts Univ 1979; **Resid:** Internal Medicine, Univ of Utah Hosps and Clinics 1982; **Fellow:** Hematology & Oncology, Univ Utah Hosps and Clinics 1985; **Fac Appt:** Prof Med, Univ Utah

Ebbert, Larry P MD [Onc] - **Spec Exp:** Breast Cancer; Mesothelioma; **Hospital:** Rapid City Reg Hosp; **Address:** Rapid City Regional Hosp, Dept Med Oncology, 353 Fairmont Blvd, Rapid City, SD 57701; **Phone:** 605-719-2301; **Board Cert:** Internal Medicine 1973; Hematology 1974; Medical Oncology 1975; **Med School:** Ohio State Univ 1969; **Resid:** Internal Medicine, Univ Missouri Med Ctr 1971; **Fellow:** Hematology & Oncology, Duke Univ Med Ctr 1973; **Fac Appt:** Asst Clin Prof Med, Univ SD Sch Med

Eckhardt, S Gail MD [Onc] - **Spec Exp:** Gastrointestinal Cancer; Drug Development; **Hospital:** Univ Colorado Hosp; **Address:** Univ Colorado Hospital, Box 6510, MS F-704, Aurora, CO 80045-0510; **Phone:** 720-848-0300; **Board Cert:** Internal Medicine 1988; Medical Oncology 1993; **Med School:** Univ Tex Med Br, Galveston 1985; **Resid:** Internal Medicine, Univ Virginia Med Ctr 1988; **Fellow:** Research, Scripps Clinic 1989; Medical Oncology, UCSD Med Ctr 1992; **Fac Appt:** Prof Med, Univ Colorado

Fabian, Carol J MD [Onc] - **Spec Exp:** Breast Cancer; Breast Cancer Risk Assessment; **Hospital:** Univ of Kansas Hosp; **Address:** Univ Kansas Med Ctr, Div Clinical Oncology, 3901 Rainbow Blvd, Ste 1347 Bell, Kansas City, KS 66160-7418; **Phone:** 913-588-7791; **Board Cert:** Internal Medicine 1976; Medical Oncology 1977; **Med School:** Univ Kans 1972; **Resid:** Internal Medicine, Wesley Med Ctr 1975; **Fellow:** Medical Oncology, Univ Kansas Med Ctr 1977; **Fac Appt:** Prof Med, Univ Kans

Glode, L Michael MD [Onc] - **Spec Exp:** Prostate Cancer; Genitourinary Cancer; **Hospital:** Univ Colorado Hosp; **Address:** U Colo Hlth Scis Ctr, Div Med Oncology, PO Box 6510, MS F710, Aurora, CO 80045-0510; **Phone:** 720-848-0170; **Board Cert:** Internal Medicine 1975; Medical Oncology 1981; **Med School:** Washington Univ, St Louis 1972; **Resid:** Internal Medicine, Univ Texas SW Med Sch 1973; Immunology, Natl Inst Hlth 1976; **Fellow:** Medical Oncology, Dana Farber Cancer Inst 1978; **Fac Appt:** Prof Med, Univ Colorado

Samuels, Brian L MD [Onc] - **Spec Exp:** Sarcoma; **Hospital:** Kootenai Med Ctr; **Address:** North Idaho Cancer Center, 700 W Ironwood Drive, Ste 103, Coeur D'Alene, ID 83814; **Phone:** 208-666-3800; **Board Cert:** Internal Medicine 1984; Medical Oncology 1987; **Med School:** Zimbabwe 1976; **Resid:** Internal Medicine, Albert Einstein Med Ctr 1981; Internal Medicine, Albert Einstein Med Ctr 1984; **Fellow:** Hematology & Oncology, Univ Chicago Hosps 1988

Ward, John H MD [Onc] - **Spec Exp:** Breast Cancer; Gastrointestinal Cancer; **Hospital:** Univ Utah Hosps and Clins; **Address:** Huntsman Cancer Inst, 2000 Circle of Hope, Ste 2100, Salt Lake City, UT 84112-5550; **Phone:** 801-585-0255; **Board Cert:** Internal Medicine 1979; Medical Oncology 1981; Hematology 1982; **Med School:** Univ Utah 1976; **Resid:** Internal Medicine, Duke Univ Med Ctr 1979; **Fellow:** Hematology & Oncology, Univ Utah 1982; **Fac Appt:** Prof Med, Univ Utah

Southwest

Abbruzzese, James L MD [Onc] - **Spec Exp:** Gastrointestinal Cancer; Pancreatic Cancer; Clinical Trials; **Hospital:** UT MD Anderson Cancer Ctr (page 71); **Address:** Univ Tex MD Anderson Cancer Ctr, 1515 Holcombe Blvd, Unit 426, Houston, TX 77030; **Phone:** 713-792-2828; **Board Cert:** Internal Medicine 1981; Medical Oncology 1983; **Med School:** Univ Chicago-Pritzker Sch Med 1978; **Resid:** Internal Medicine, Johns Hopkins Hosp 1981; **Fellow:** Medical Oncology, Dana-Farber Cancer Inst 1983; **Fac Appt:** Assoc Prof Med, Univ Tex, Houston

Ahmann, Frederick R MD [Onc] - **Spec Exp:** Prostate Cancer; Testicular Cancer; Bladder Cancer; **Hospital:** Univ Med Ctr - Tucson; **Address:** Arizona Cancer Ctr, 1515 N Campbell Ave, Box 245024, Tucson, AZ 85724; **Phone:** 520-694-2873; **Board Cert:** Internal Medicine 1977; Medical Oncology 1981; **Med School:** Univ MO-Columbia Sch Med 1974; **Resid:** Internal Medicine, Georgetown Univ Med Ctr 1977; **Fellow:** Medical Oncology, Univ Med Ctr 1980; **Fac Appt:** Prof Med, Univ Ariz Coll Med

Benjamin, Robert S MD [Onc] - **Spec Exp:** Sarcoma; **Hospital:** UT MD Anderson Cancer Ctr (page 71); **Address:** UT MD Anderson Cancer Ctr, 1515 Holcombe Blvd, Unit 450, Houston, TX 77030; **Phone:** 713-792-3626; **Board Cert:** Internal Medicine 1973; Medical Oncology 1973; **Med School:** NYU Sch Med 1968; **Resid:** Internal Medicine, Bellevue Hosp Ctr-NYU 1970; **Fellow:** Medical Oncology, Baltimore Cancer Rsch Ctr 1972; **Fac Appt:** Prof Med, Univ Tex, Houston

Buzdar, Aman U MD [Onc] - **Spec Exp:** Breast Cancer; **Hospital:** UT MD Anderson Cancer Ctr (page 71); **Address:** UT MD Anderson Canc Ctr, 1155 Pressler St, Unit 1354, Houston, TX 77030-4009; **Phone:** 713-792-2817; **Board Cert:** Internal Medicine 1975; Medical Oncology 1979; **Med School:** Pakistan 1967; **Resid:** Internal Medicine, Norwalk Hosp 1973; Internal Medicine, Lakewood Hosp 1971; **Fellow:** Hematology, Norwalk Hosp 1974; Oncology, MD Anderson Cancer Ctr 1975; **Fac Appt:** Prof Med, Univ Tex, Houston

Camoriano, John MD [Onc] - **Spec Exp:** lymphoma; Breast Cancer; Bone Marrow Transplant; Castleman's Disease; **Hospital:** Mayo Clin Hosp - Scottsdale; **Address:** 13400 E Shea, Scottsdale, AZ 85259; **Phone:** 480-301-8335; **Board Cert:** Internal Medicine 1985; Medical Oncology 1989; Hematology 1988; **Med School:** Univ Nebr Coll Med 1982; **Resid:** Internal Medicine, Univ OK 1985; **Fellow:** Hematology & Oncology, Mayo Grad Sch Med 1989; **Fac Appt:** Asst Prof Med, Mayo Med Sch

Fossella, Frank V MD [Onc] - **Spec Exp:** Lung Cancer; **Hospital:** UT MD Anderson Cancer Ctr (page 71); **Address:** Dept Thoracic Head/Neck Med Oncol, Unit 432, Box 301402, Houston, TX 77230-1402; **Phone:** 713-792-6363; **Board Cert:** Internal Medicine 1985; Medical Oncology 1987; **Med School:** Baylor Coll Med 1982; **Resid:** Internal Medicine, Baylor Coll Med 1985; **Fellow:** Medical Oncology, Baylor Coll Med 1987; **Fac Appt:** Prof Med, Univ Tex, Houston

Glisson, Bonnie S MD [Onc] - **Spec Exp:** Head & Neck Cancer; Lung Cancer; **Hospital:** UT MD Anderson Cancer Ctr (page 71); **Address:** 1515 Holcombe Blvd, Unit 432, Houston, TX 77030; **Phone:** 713-792-6363; **Board Cert:** Internal Medicine 1982; Medical Oncology 1985; **Med School:** Ohio State Univ 1979; **Resid:** Internal Medicine, Univ Va Med Ctr 1982; **Fellow:** Medical Oncology, Univ Fla Health Sci Ctr 1985; **Fac Appt:** Prof Med, Univ Tex, Houston

Medical Oncology

Herbst, Roy S MD/PhD [Onc] - **Spec Exp:** Lung Cancer; Head & Neck Cancer; Breast Cancer; Drug Development; **Hospital:** UT MD Anderson Cancer Ctr (page 71); **Address:** Thoracic/Head & Neck Med Onc - Unit 432, UT MD Anderson Cancer Ctr, PO Box 301402, Houston, TX 77230-1402; **Phone:** 713-792-6363; **Board Cert:** Internal Medicine 1994; Medical Oncology 1997; **Med School:** Cornell Univ-Weill Med Coll 1991; **Resid:** Internal Medicine, Brigham & Women's Hosp 1994; **Fellow:** Medical Oncology, Dana Farber Cancer Inst 1996; **Fac Appt:** Assoc Prof Med, Univ Tex, Houston

Hong, Waun Ki MD [Onc] - **Spec Exp:** Lung Cancer; Head & Neck Cancer; Thoracic Cancers; **Hospital:** UT MD Anderson Cancer Ctr (page 71); **Address:** 1515 Holcombe Blvd, Unit 421, Houston, TX 77030; **Phone:** 713-745-6791; **Board Cert:** Internal Medicine 1976; Medical Oncology 1979; **Med School:** South Korea 1967; **Resid:** Internal Medicine, Boston VA Hosp 1973; **Fellow:** Medical Oncology, Meml Sloan-Kettering Cancer Ctr 1975; **Fac Appt:** Prof Med, Univ Tex, Houston

Hortobagyi, Gabriel N MD [Onc] - **Spec Exp:** Breast Cancer; **Hospital:** UT MD Anderson Cancer Ctr (page 71); **Address:** UT MD Anderson Cancer Ctr, Dept Breast Oncology, PO Box 301429, Unit 1354, Houston, TX 77030-1439; **Phone:** 713-792-2817; **Board Cert:** Internal Medicine 1975; Medical Oncology 1977; **Med School:** Colombia 1970; **Resid:** Internal Medicine, St Lukes Hosp 1974; **Fellow:** Medical Oncology, MD Anderson Cancer Ctr 1976; **Fac Appt:** Prof Med, Univ Tex, Houston

Hutchins, Laura MD [Onc] - **Spec Exp:** Breast Cancer; Melanoma; **Hospital:** UAMS Med Ctr; **Address:** Univ Arkansas Med Scis, Dept Hem/Onc, 4301 W Markham St, MS 508, Little Rock, AR 72205-7101; **Phone:** 501-686-8511; **Board Cert:** Internal Medicine 1980; Hematology 1984; Medical Oncology 1987; **Med School:** Univ Ark 1977; **Resid:** Internal Medicine, Univ Ark Med Scis 1980; **Fellow:** Hematology & Oncology, Univ Ark Med Scis 1983; **Fac Appt:** Prof Med, Univ Ark

Jones, Stephen E MD [Onc] - **Spec Exp:** Breast Cancer; **Hospital:** Baylor Univ Medical Ctr; **Address:** Baylor-Sammons Cancer Ctr, 3535 Worth St, Ste 600, Dallas, TX 75246; **Phone:** 214-370-1000; **Board Cert:** Internal Medicine 1972; Medical Oncology 1973; **Med School:** Case West Res Univ 1966; **Resid:** Internal Medicine, Stanford Univ Hosp 1968; **Fellow:** Medical Oncology, Stanford Univ Hosp 1972; **Fac Appt:** Prof Med, Baylor Coll Med

Karp, Daniel D MD [Onc] - **Spec Exp:** Lung Cancer; **Hospital:** UT MD Anderson Cancer Ctr (page 71); **Address:** 1515 Holcombe Blvd, Unit 432, Houston, TX 77030-4009; **Phone:** 713-792-6363; **Board Cert:** Internal Medicine 1976; Hematology 1980; Medical Oncology 1981; **Med School:** Duke Univ 1973; **Resid:** Internal Medicine, Dartmouth-Hitchcock Med Ctr 1976; **Fellow:** Hematology, Dartmouth-Hitchcock Med Ctr 1978; Medical Oncology, Dana Farber Cancer Inst 1979; **Fac Appt:** Prof Med, Univ Tex, Houston

Kies, Merrill S MD [Onc] - **Spec Exp:** Head & Neck Cancer; Lung Cancer; **Hospital:** UT MD Anderson Cancer Ctr (page 71); **Address:** Dept Thoracic, Head & Neck Oncology, 1515 Holcombe Blvd, Unit 432, Houston, TX 77030; **Phone:** 713-792-6363; **Board Cert:** Internal Medicine 1976; Medical Oncology 1979; **Med School:** Loyola Univ-Stritch Sch Med 1973; **Resid:** Internal Medicine, Walter Reed AMC 1976; **Fellow:** Medical Oncology, Brooke AMC 1978; **Fac Appt:** Prof Med, Univ Tex, Houston

Kwak, Larry W MD/PhD [Onc] - **Spec Exp:** Lymphoma; Multiple Myeloma; Vaccine Therapy; Immunotherapy; **Hospital:** UT MD Anderson Cancer Ctr (page 71); **Address:** MD Anderson Cancer Ctr, Dept Lymphoma/Myeloma, 1515 Holcombe Blvd, Ste 429, Houston, TX 77030; **Phone:** 713-745-4244; **Board Cert:** Internal Medicine 1987; Medical Oncology 1989; **Med School:** Northwestern Univ 1982; **Resid:** Internal Medicine, Stanford Univ Hosp 1987; **Fellow:** Oncology, Stanford Univ Hosp 1989

Legha, Sewa Singh MD [Onc] - **Spec Exp:** Melanoma; Breast Cancer; Endocrine Cancers; Sarcoma; **Hospital:** St Luke's Episcopal Hosp - Houston, Methodist Hosp - Houston; **Address:** 6624 Fannin, Ste 1440, Houston, TX 77030; **Phone:** 713-797-9711; **Board Cert:** Internal Medicine 1987; Medical Oncology 1977; **Med School:** India 1970; **Resid:** Internal Medicine, Milwaukee Co Genl Hosp/Med Coll Wisc 1974; Medical Oncology, Natl Cancer Inst 1976; **Fellow:** Medical Oncology, MD Anderson Hosp 1977; **Fac Appt:** Clin Prof Med, Baylor Coll Med

Lippman, Scott M MD [Onc] - **Spec Exp:** Cancer Prevention; Lung Cancer; Head & Neck Cancer; **Hospital:** UT MD Anderson Cancer Ctr (page 71); **Address:** UTMD Anderson Cancer Ctr, Unit 432, 1515 Holcombe Blvd, P.O.Box 301439, Houston, TX 77230-1439; **Phone:** 713-745-5439; **Board Cert:** Internal Medicine 1987; Hematology 1988; Medical Oncology 1989; **Med School:** Johns Hopkins Univ 1981; **Resid:** Internal Medicine, Harbor-UCLA Med Ctr 1983; **Fellow:** Hematology, Stanford Univ Med Ctr 1985; Hematology & Oncology, Univ Ariz Hlth Scis Ctr 1987; **Fac Appt:** Prof Med, Univ Tex, Houston

Livingston, Robert B MD [Onc] - **Spec Exp:** Bone Marrow Transplant; Breast Cancer; Lung Cancer; **Hospital:** Univ Med Ctr - Tucson; **Address:** University Medical Center, 3838 N Campbell Ave, Tucson, AZ 85724; **Phone:** 520-694-2873; **Board Cert:** Internal Medicine 1972; Medical Oncology 1973; **Med School:** Univ Okla Coll Med 1965; **Resid:** Internal Medicine, Univ Oklahoma Med Ctr 1971; **Fellow:** Medical Oncology, Univ Texas Cancer Ctr 1973; **Fac Appt:** Prof Med, Univ Wash

Logothetis, Christopher J MD [Onc] - **Spec Exp:** Prostate Cancer; Bladder Cancer; **Hospital:** UT MD Anderson Cancer Ctr (page 71); **Address:** UT MD Anderson Cancer Ctr, Dept GU Onc, Unit 1374, Box 301439, Houston, TX 77230-1439; **Phone:** 713-792-2830; **Board Cert:** Internal Medicine 1978; Medical Oncology 1981; **Med School:** Greece 1974; **Resid:** Internal Medicine, Univ Texas 1979; **Fellow:** Hematology & Oncology, Univ Tex-MD Anderson Cancer Ctr 1981; **Fac Appt:** Prof Med, Univ Tex, Houston

Markman, Maurie MD [Onc] - **Spec Exp:** Ovarian Cancer; Gynecologic Cancer; Drug Development; Palliative Care; **Hospital:** UT MD Anderson Cancer Ctr (page 71); **Address:** Univ Texas MD Anderson Cancer Ctr, 1515 Holcombe Blvd, Box 121, Houston, TX 77030-4009; **Phone:** 713-745-7140; **Board Cert:** Internal Medicine 1977; Hematology 1982; Medical Oncology 1981; **Med School:** NYU Sch Med 1974; **Resid:** Internal Medicine, Bellevue Hosp Ctr 1978; **Fellow:** Medical Oncology, Johns Hopkins Hosp 1980; **Fac Appt:** Prof Med, Univ Tex, Houston

Millikan, Randall MD/PhD [Onc] - **Spec Exp:** Bladder Cancer; Genitourinary Cancer; Clinical Trials; **Hospital:** UT MD Anderson Cancer Ctr (page 71); **Address:** 1155 Pressler Ln, Box 1374, Bellaire, TX 77030; **Phone:** 713-792-2830; **Board Cert:** Internal Medicine 1991; Medical Oncology 1995; **Med School:** Univ Miami Sch Med 1988; **Resid:** Internal Medicine, Mayo Clinic 1991; **Fellow:** Medical Oncology, Mayo Clinic 1994; **Fac Appt:** Assoc Prof Med, Univ Tex, Houston

Medical Oncology

Northfelt, Donald W MD [Onc] - **Spec Exp:** Breast Cancer; Colon & Rectal Cancer; Lung Cancer; **Hospital:** Mayo Clin Hosp - Scottsdale; **Address:** Mayo Clinic Scottsdale, 13400 E Shea Blvd, Scottsdale, AZ 85259; **Phone:** 480-301-8335; **Board Cert:** Internal Medicine 1988; Medical Oncology 2001; **Med School:** Univ Minn 1985; **Resid:** Internal Medicine, UCLA Med Ctr 1988; **Fellow:** Hematology & Oncology, UCSF 1991; **Fac Appt:** Assoc Prof Med, Mayo Med Sch

O'Brien, Susan M MD [Onc] - **Spec Exp:** Leukemia; Lymphoma; **Hospital:** UT MD Anderson Cancer Ctr (page 71); **Address:** Univ Texas MD Anderson Cancer Ctr, Dept Leukemia, Unit 428, Box 301439, Houston, TX 77230; **Phone:** 713-792-7305; **Board Cert:** Internal Medicine 1983; Medical Oncology 1987; **Med School:** UMDNJ-NJ Med Sch, Newark 1980; **Resid:** Internal Medicine, UMDNJ Med Ctr 1983; **Fellow:** Medical Oncology, Univ TX MD Anderson Med Ctr 1987; **Fac Appt:** Prof Med, Univ Tex, Houston

O'Shaughnessy, Joyce A MD [Onc] - **Spec Exp:** Breast Cancer; **Hospital:** Baylor Univ Medical Ctr; **Address:** US Oncology, 3535 Worth St, Ste 600, Dallas, TX 75246; **Phone:** 214-370-1000; **Board Cert:** Internal Medicine 1985; Medical Oncology 1987; **Med School:** Yale Univ 1982; **Resid:** Internal Medicine, Mass Genl Hosp 1985; **Fellow:** Medical Oncology, National Cancer Inst 1988

Osborne, Charles K MD [Onc] - **Spec Exp:** Breast Cancer; **Hospital:** Methodist Hosp - Houston; **Address:** 1 Baylor Plaza, MS BCM600, Houston, TX 77030; **Phone:** 713-798-1641; **Board Cert:** Internal Medicine 1975; Medical Oncology 1977; **Med School:** Univ MO-Columbia Sch Med 1972; **Resid:** Internal Medicine, Johns Hopkins Hosp 1974; **Fellow:** Medical Oncology, Natl Cancer Inst 1977; **Fac Appt:** Prof Med, Baylor Coll Med

Papadopoulos, Nicholas E MD [Onc] - **Spec Exp:** Melanoma; **Hospital:** UT MD Anderson Cancer Ctr (page 71); **Address:** 1515 Holcombe Blvd, Unit 430, Houston, TX 77030; **Phone:** 713-792-2821; **Med School:** Greece 1966; **Resid:** Internal Medicine, Baylor Coll Med 1976; **Fellow:** Medical Oncology, MD Anderson Cancer Ctr 1978; **Fac Appt:** Assoc Prof Med, Univ Tex, Houston

Patt, Yehuda Z MD [Onc] - **Spec Exp:** Liver Cancer; Biliary Cancer; Colon & Rectal Cancer; **Hospital:** Univ NM Hlth & Sci Ctr; **Address:** Univ New Mexico CRTC, Div Hem/Onc, 900 Camino de Salud NE, MSC 084630, Albuquerque, NM 87131-0001; **Phone:** 505-272-5837; **Board Cert:** Internal Medicine 1982; Medical Oncology 1987; **Med School:** Israel 1967; **Resid:** Internal Medicine, Tel Aviv-Sheba Med Ctr 1974; **Fellow:** Medical Oncology, UT MD Anderson Cancer Ctr 1977; **Fac Appt:** Prof Med, Univ New Mexico

Pisters, Katherine M W MD [Onc] - **Spec Exp:** Lung Cancer; **Hospital:** UT MD Anderson Cancer Ctr (page 71); **Address:** UT MD Anderson Cancer Ctr, PO Box 301402 Unit 432, Houston, TX 77030-1402; **Phone:** 713-792-6363; **Board Cert:** Internal Medicine 1988; Medical Oncology 2002; **Med School:** Univ Western Ontario 1985; **Resid:** Internal Medicine, N Shore Univ Hosp 1988; **Fellow:** Medical Oncology, Meml Sloan Kettering Cancer Ctr 1991; **Fac Appt:** Prof Med, Univ Tex, Houston

Saiki, John H MD [Onc] - **Hospital:** Univ NM Hlth & Sci Ctr; **Address:** Univ of New Mexico Cancer Ctr, 900 Camino de Salud NE, MSC 084630, Albuquerque, NM 87131-0001; **Phone:** 505-272-5837; **Board Cert:** Internal Medicine 1970; Medical Oncology 1973; **Med School:** McGill Univ 1961; **Resid:** Internal Medicine, Univ New Mexico 1968; Hematology, Univ New Mexico 1969; **Fellow:** Medical Oncology, MD Anderson Hosp 1970; **Fac Appt:** Prof Med, Univ New Mexico

Salem, Philip A MD [Onc] - **Spec Exp:** Breast Cancer; Lymphoma; Lung Cancer; **Hospital:** St Luke's Episcopal Hosp - Houston; **Address:** 6624 Fannin St, Ste 1630, Houston, TX 77030; **Phone:** 713-796-1221; **Med School:** Lebanon 1965; **Resid:** Medical Oncology, Meml Sloan Kettering Cancer Ctr 1970; **Fellow:** Oncology Research, MD Anderson Cancer Ctr 1972; **Fac Appt:** Clin Prof Med, Univ Tex, Houston

Schiller, Joan H MD [Onc] - **Spec Exp:** Lung Cancer; **Hospital:** UT Southwestern Med Ctr - Dallas; **Address:** Univ Texas SW, 5323 Harry Hines Blvd, Dallas, TX 75390-8852; **Phone:** 214-648-4180; **Board Cert:** Internal Medicine 1983; Medical Oncology 1987; **Med School:** Univ IL Coll Med 1980; **Resid:** Internal Medicine, Northwestern Meml Hosp 1983; **Fellow:** Medical Oncology, Univ Wisconsin Hosp 1986; **Fac Appt:** Prof Med, Univ Wisc

Stopeck, Alison MD [Onc] - **Spec Exp:** Breast Cancer; Breast Cancer Risk Assessment; **Hospital:** Univ Med Ctr - Tucson; **Address:** 1515 N Campbell Ave, P.O. Box 245024, Tucson, AZ 85724; **Phone:** 520-694-2816; **Board Cert:** Internal Medicine 1988; Medical Oncology 2002; Hematology 2002; **Med School:** Columbia P&S 1985; **Resid:** Internal Medicine, Columbia-Presbyterian Med Ctr 1988; **Fellow:** Hematology & Oncology, New York Hospital 1991; **Fac Appt:** Assoc Prof Med, Univ Ariz Coll Med

Takimoto, Chris Hidemi M MD/PhD [Onc] - **Spec Exp:** Gastrointestinal Cancer; **Hospital:** Univ Hlth Sys - Univ Hosp; **Address:** Inst for Drug Dvlpmt-Cancer Rsch Ctr, 7979 Wurzbach Rd Zeller Bldg Fl 4, San Antonio, TX 78229; **Phone:** 210-562-1725; **Board Cert:** Internal Medicine 1989; Medical Oncology 2005; **Med School:** Yale Univ 1986; **Resid:** Internal Medicine, UCSF Med Ctr 1989; **Fac Appt:** Assoc Prof Med, Univ Tex, San Antonio

Valero, Vicente MD [Onc] - **Spec Exp:** Breast Cancer; **Hospital:** UT MD Anderson Cancer Ctr (page 71), LBJ General Hosp; **Address:** Univ Texas MD Anderson Cancer Ctr, 1515 Holcombe Blvd, Unit 1354, Houston, TX 77030; **Phone:** 713-792-2817; **Board Cert:** Internal Medicine 1985; Hematology 1988; Medical Oncology 1987; **Med School:** Mexico 1980; **Resid:** Internal Medicine, Univ Cincinnati Med Ctr 1985; Hematology & Oncology, Univ Cincinnati Med Ctr 1987; **Fellow:** Hematology & Oncology, Univ Texas Med Br 1988; **Fac Appt:** Prof Med, Univ Tex, Houston

Verschraegen, Claire F MD [Onc] - **Spec Exp:** Ovarian Cancer; Drug Discovery; Mesothelioma; **Hospital:** Univ NM Hlth & Sci Ctr; **Address:** UNM Cancer Research & Treatment Ctr, 900 Camino de Salud NE, rm MS C084630, Albuquerque, NM 87131-0001; **Phone:** 505-272-6760; **Board Cert:** Internal Medicine 2000; Medical Oncology 2000; **Med School:** Belgium 1982; **Resid:** Internal Medicine, Bordet 1985; Internal Medicine, Univ Texas 1991; **Fellow:** Cancer Research, Stehlin Fdn for Cancer Research 1988; Oncology, MD Anderson Cancer Ctr 1994; **Fac Appt:** Prof Med, Univ New Mexico

West Coast and Pacific

Abrams, Donald I MD [Onc] - **Spec Exp:** AIDS Related Cancers; **Hospital:** San Francisco Genl Hosp; **Address:** Positive Hlth Program-SF Genl Hosp, 995 Potrero Ave, Bldg 80, Ward 84, San Francisco, CA 94110; **Phone:** 415-476-4082 x444; **Board Cert:** Internal Medicine 1980; Medical Oncology 1983; **Med School:** Stanford Univ 1977; **Resid:** Internal Medicine, Kaiser Fdn Hosp 1980; **Fellow:** Medical Oncology, UCSF Cancer Rsch 1982; **Fac Appt:** Clin Prof Med, UCSF

Appelbaum, Frederick R MD [Onc] - **Spec Exp:** Bone Marrow Transplant; Leukemia; **Hospital:** Univ Wash Med Ctr; **Address:** 1100 Fairview Ave N, rm D5-310, PO Box 19024, Seattle, WA 98109; **Phone:** 206-288-1024; **Board Cert:** Internal Medicine 1975; Medical Oncology 1977; **Med School:** Tufts Univ 1972; **Resid:** Internal Medicine, Univ Michigan Med Ctr 1974; **Fellow:** Medical Oncology, Natl Cancer Inst 1976; **Fac Appt:** Prof Med, Univ Wash

Ball, Edward D MD [Onc] - **Spec Exp:** Bone Marrow & Stem Cell Transplant; Leukemia & Lymphoma; Multiple Myeloma; **Hospital:** UCSD Med Ctr; **Address:** 3855 Health Sciences Dr, #0960, La Jolla, CA 92093; **Phone:** 858-822-6600; **Board Cert:** Internal Medicine 1979; Medical Oncology 1983; Hematology 2000; **Med School:** Case West Res Univ 1976; **Resid:** Internal Medicine, Hartford Hosp 1979; **Fellow:** Hematology & Oncology, Univ Hosps Cleveland 1981; Hematology & Oncology, Dartmouth-Hitchcock Hosp 1982; **Fac Appt:** Prof Med, UCSD

Beer, Tomasz MD [Onc] - **Spec Exp:** Prostate Cancer; **Hospital:** OR Hlth & Sci Univ; **Address:** 3303 SW Bond Ave, CH7M, Portland, OR 97239; **Phone:** 503-494-6594; **Board Cert:** Internal Medicine 1995; Medical Oncology 2000; **Med School:** Johns Hopkins Univ 1991; **Resid:** Internal Medicine, Oreg Hlth Scis Univ 1994; Internal Medicine, Oreg Hlth Scis Univ 1996; **Fellow:** Hematology & Oncology, Oreg Hlth Scis Univ 1999; **Fac Appt:** Assoc Prof Med, Oregon Hlth Sci Univ

Carlson, Robert Wells MD [Onc] - **Spec Exp:** Breast Cancer; **Hospital:** Stanford Univ Med Ctr; **Address:** Dept Medicine, 875 Blake Wilbur Drive, Stanford, CA 94305; **Phone:** 650-723-7621; **Board Cert:** Internal Medicine 1981; Medical Oncology 1983; **Med School:** Stanford Univ 1978; **Resid:** Internal Medicine, Barnes Hosp Group 1980; Internal Medicine, Stanford Univ Hosp 1981; **Fellow:** Medical Oncology, Stanford Univ Hosp 1983; **Fac Appt:** Prof Med, Stanford Univ

Chap, Linnea MD [Onc] - **Spec Exp:** Breast Cancer; **Hospital:** St John's Hlth Ctr, Santa Monica; **Address:** Premier Oncology, 2020 Santa Monica Blvd, Ste 600, Santa Monica, CA 90404-2023; **Phone:** 310-633-8400; **Board Cert:** Internal Medicine 1991; Hematology 1994; Medical Oncology 1995; **Med School:** Univ Chicago-Pritzker Sch Med 1988; **Resid:** Internal Medicine, Northwestern Meml Hosp 1991; **Fellow:** Hematology & Oncology, UCLA Med Ctr 1992

Chlebowski, Rowan T MD/PhD [Onc] - **Spec Exp:** Breast Cancer; Women's Health; **Hospital:** LAC - Harbor - UCLA Med Ctr; **Address:** 1124 W Carson St J3 Bldg, Torrance, CA 90502; **Phone:** 310-222-2218; **Board Cert:** Internal Medicine 1980; Medical Oncology 1981; **Med School:** Case West Res Univ 1974; **Resid:** Internal Medicine, MetroHealth Med Ctr 1976; Medical Oncology, LAC-USC Med Ctr 1979; **Fac Appt:** Prof Med, UCLA

Chow, Warren Allen MD [Onc] - **Spec Exp:** Sarcoma; Bone Cancer; **Hospital:** City of Hope Natl Med Ctr & Beckman Rsch; **Address:** 1500 E Duarte Rd, Duarte, CA 91010; **Phone:** 626-359-8111; **Board Cert:** Hematology 2004; Medical Oncology 2003; **Med School:** Ros Franklin Univ/Chicago Med Sch 1986; **Resid:** Internal Medicine, Cedars-Sinai Med Ctr 1990; **Fellow:** Hematology & Oncology, City of Hope 1992; Molecular Genetics, City of Hope 1994; **Fac Appt:** Assoc Prof Med

Deeg, H. Joachim MD [Onc] - **Spec Exp:** Bone Marrow Failure Disorders; Hematologic Malignancies; **Hospital:** Univ Wash Med Ctr; **Address:** Fred Hutchinson Cancer Research Center, 1100 Fairview Avenue N, D1-100, Box 19024, Seattle, WA 98109-1024; **Phone:** 206-667-5985; **Board Cert:** Internal Medicine 1976; Medical Oncology 1979; **Med School:** Germany 1972; **Fac Appt:** Prof Med, Univ Wash

Disis, Mary Lenora MD [Onc] - **Spec Exp:** Breast Cancer; Ovarian Cancer; Clinical Trials; **Hospital:** Univ Wash Med Ctr; **Address:** Univ Washington, Ctr Translational Medicine Women's Hlth, 815 Mercer St Fl 2, Seattle, WA 98109; **Phone:** 206-616-1823; **Board Cert:** Internal Medicine 1989; Medical Oncology 1997; **Med School:** Univ Nebr Coll Med 1986; **Resid:** Internal Medicine, Univ Illinois Med Ctr 1990; **Fellow:** Medical Oncology, Fred Hutchinson Cancer Ctr 1993; **Fac Appt:** Assoc Prof Med, Univ Wash

Druker, Brian MD [Onc] - **Spec Exp:** Leukemia; **Hospital:** OR Hlth & Sci Univ; **Address:** 3181 SW Sam Jackson Park Rd, MC L592, Portland, OR 97239-3098; **Phone:** 503-494-5058; **Board Cert:** Internal Medicine 1984; Medical Oncology 1987; **Med School:** UCSD 1981; **Resid:** Internal Medicine, Barnes Jewish Hosp 1984; **Fellow:** Medical Oncology, Dana-Farber Cancer Inst 1987; **Fac Appt:** Prof Med, Oregon Hlth Sci Univ

Ellis, Georgiana K MD [Onc] - **Spec Exp:** Breast Cancer; Clinical Trials; **Hospital:** Univ Wash Med Ctr; **Address:** Univ Washington Med Ctr, 1959 NE Pacific St, Seattle, WA 98195-6043; **Phone:** 206-288-2048; **Board Cert:** Internal Medicine 1985; Medical Oncology 1987; **Med School:** Univ Wash 1982; **Resid:** Internal Medicine, Univ Washington 1985; **Fellow:** Medical Oncology, Univ Washington 1988; **Fac Appt:** Assoc Prof Med, Univ Wash

Figlin, Robert A MD [Onc] - **Spec Exp:** Urologic Cancer; Kidney Cancer; Immunotherapy; **Hospital:** City of Hope Natl Med Ctr & Beckman Rsch, UCLA Med Ctr; **Address:** City of Hope Natl Med Ctr, Med Oncology & Therapeutics Research, 1500 E Duarte Rd, Duarte, CA 91010; **Phone:** 626-256-4673; **Board Cert:** Internal Medicine 1979; Medical Oncology 1983; **Med School:** Med Coll PA Hahnemann 1976; **Resid:** Internal Medicine, Cedars Sinai Med Ctr 1980; **Fellow:** Hematology & Oncology, UCLA Ctr Hlth Sci 1982; **Fac Appt:** Prof Med, UCLA

Ford, James M MD [Onc] - **Spec Exp:** Gastrointestinal Cancer; Colon & Rectal Cancer; Cancer Genetics; **Hospital:** Stanford Univ Med Ctr; **Address:** Stanford Comp Cancer Ctr, 875 Blake Wilbur Drive, Ste Clinic B, Stanford, CA 94305-5820; **Phone:** 650-723-7621; **Board Cert:** Internal Medicine 1996; Medical Oncology 2005; **Med School:** Yale Univ 1989; **Resid:** Internal Medicine, Stanford Univ Med Ctr 1991; **Fellow:** Medical Oncology, Stanford Univ Med Ctr 1994; **Fac Appt:** Assoc Prof Med, Stanford Univ

Gandara, David R MD [Onc] - **Spec Exp:** Lung Cancer; **Hospital:** UC Davis Med Ctr; **Address:** UC Davis Cancer Ctr, 4501 X St, Ste 3016, Sacramento, CA 95817; **Phone:** 916-734-5959; **Board Cert:** Internal Medicine 1976; Medical Oncology 1979; **Med School:** Univ Tex Med Br, Galveston 1973; **Resid:** Internal Medicine, Madigan Med Ctr 1976; **Fellow:** Hematology & Oncology, Letterman AMC 1978; **Fac Appt:** Asst Prof Med, UC Davis

Ganz, Patricia A MD [Onc] - **Spec Exp:** Breast Cancer; Cancer Survivors-Late Effects of Therapy; **Hospital:** UCLA Med Ctr; **Address:** UCLA, Cancer Prev/Control Rsch, A2-125 CHS, 650 Charles Young Drive S, Box 956900, Los Angeles, CA 90095-6900; **Phone:** 310-206-1404; **Board Cert:** Internal Medicine 1976; Medical Oncology 1979; **Med School:** UCLA 1973; **Resid:** Internal Medicine, UCLA Med Ctr 1976; **Fellow:** Hematology, UCLA Med Ctr 1978; **Fac Appt:** Prof Med, UCLA

Glaspy, John A MD [Onc] - **Spec Exp:** Breast Cancer; Melanoma; Lymphoma; **Hospital:** UCLA Med Ctr; **Address:** 100 UCLA Medical Plaza Plaza, Ste 550, Los Angeles, CA 90095; **Phone:** 310-794-4955; **Board Cert:** Internal Medicine 1982; Medical Oncology 1985; Hematology 1986; **Med School:** UCLA 1979; **Resid:** Internal Medicine, UCLA Med Ctr 1982; **Fellow:** Hematology & Oncology, UCLA Med Ctr 1984; **Fac Appt:** Prof Med, UCLA

Medical Oncology

Gralow, Julie MD [Onc] - **Spec Exp:** Breast Cancer; **Hospital:** Univ Wash Med Ctr; **Address:** Seattle Cancer Care Alliance-UW, 825 Eastlake Ave E, Box 358081, MS G4-83, Seattle, WA 98109; **Phone:** 206-288-7722; **Board Cert:** Medical Oncology 2005; **Med School:** USC Sch Med 1988; **Resid:** Internal Medicine, Brigham & Women's Hosp 1991; **Fellow:** Oncology, Univ Wash Med Ctr 1994; **Fac Appt:** Assoc Prof Med, Univ Wash

Horning, Sandra J MD [Onc] - **Spec Exp:** Hodgkin's Disease; Bone Marrow & Stem Cell Transplant; Lymphoma; **Hospital:** Stanford Univ Med Ctr; **Address:** Stanford Cancer Center, 875 Blake Wilbur Drive, Stanford, CA 94305; **Phone:** 650-723-7621; **Board Cert:** Internal Medicine 1978; Medical Oncology 1981; **Med School:** Univ Iowa Coll Med 1975; **Resid:** Internal Medicine, Strong Meml Hosp 1978; **Fellow:** Medical Oncology, Stanford Univ 1980; **Fac Appt:** Prof Med, Stanford Univ

Jacobs, Charlotte D MD [Onc] - **Spec Exp:** Sarcoma; Unknown Primary Cancer; **Hospital:** Stanford Univ Med Ctr; **Address:** 875 Blake Wilbur Drive, Stanford, CA 94305; **Phone:** 650-723-7621 x2; **Board Cert:** Internal Medicine 1975; Medical Oncology 1977; **Med School:** Washington Univ, St Louis 1972; **Resid:** Internal Medicine, Barnes Hosp 1974; Internal Medicine, UCSF Med Ctr 1975; **Fellow:** Medical Oncology, Stanford Univ 1977; **Fac Appt:** Prof Med, Stanford Univ

Jahan, Thierry Marie MD [Onc] - **Spec Exp:** Endocrine Tumors; Lung Cancer; Mesothelioma; Thyroid Cancer; **Hospital:** UCSF Med Ctr; **Address:** UCSF Comprehensive Cancer Center, 1600 Divisadero St, San Francisco, CA 94115; **Phone:** 415-353-9888; **Board Cert:** Hematology 1994; Medical Oncology 1995; Internal Medicine 1990; **Med School:** Geo Wash Univ 1987; **Resid:** Internal Medicine, Cedars-Sinai Med Ctr 1990; **Fac Appt:** Asst Clin Prof Med, UCSF

Kaplan, Lawrence D MD [Onc] - **Spec Exp:** AIDS Related Cancers; Lymphoma; **Hospital:** UCSF Med Ctr; **Address:** UCSF Medical Center, 400 Parnassus Ave, rm A502, San Francisco, CA 94143-0324; **Phone:** 415-353-2737; **Board Cert:** Internal Medicine 1983; Medical Oncology 1985; **Med School:** UCLA 1980; **Resid:** Internal Medicine, Boston City Hosp 1983; **Fellow:** Hematology & Oncology, UCSF Med Ctr 1985; **Fac Appt:** Clin Prof Med, UCSF

Maloney, David G MD/PhD [Onc] - **Spec Exp:** Lymphoma; Bone Marrow & Stem Cell Transplant; Vaccine Therapy; **Hospital:** Univ Wash Med Ctr; **Address:** FHCRC-MS D1-100, 1100 Fairview Ave N, Box 19024, Seattle, WA 98109-1024; **Phone:** 206-667-5616; **Board Cert:** Internal Medicine 1988; Medical Oncology 2005; **Med School:** Stanford Univ 1985; **Resid:** Internal Medicine, Brigham & Women's Hosp 1988; **Fellow:** Medical Oncology, Stanford Univ Med Ctr 1994; **Fac Appt:** Prof Med, Univ Wash

Mitchell, Beverly MD [Onc] - **Spec Exp:** Hematologic Malignancies; Leukemia; Lymphoma; **Hospital:** Stanford Univ Med Ctr; **Address:** Stanford Cancer Center, 800 Welch Rd, Stanford, CA 94305-5402; **Phone:** 650-725-9621; **Board Cert:** Internal Medicine 1973; Hematology 1978; **Med School:** Harvard Med Sch 1969; **Resid:** Internal Medicine, Univ Washington Med Ctr 1972; **Fellow:** Metabolism, Univ Zurich 1975; Hematology & Oncology, Univ Michigan 1977; **Fac Appt:** Prof Med, Stanford Univ

Mortimer, Joanne MD [Onc] - **Spec Exp:** Breast Cancer; Clinical Trials; **Hospital:** UCSD Med Ctr; **Address:** Moores UCSD Cancer Ctr, 3855 Health Sciences Drive, MC 0987, La Jolla, CA 92093-1503; **Phone:** 858-822-6135; **Board Cert:** Internal Medicine 1980; Medical Oncology 1983; **Med School:** Loyola Univ-Stritch Sch Med 1977; **Resid:** Internal Medicine, Cleveland Clinic 1980; **Fellow:** Medical Oncology, Cleveland Clinic 1982; **Fac Appt:** Prof Med, UCSD

Natale, Ronald B MD [Onc] - **Spec Exp:** Lung Cancer; **Hospital:** Cedars-Sinai Med Ctr; **Address:** Cedars-Sinai Comp Cancer Ctr, 8700 Beverly Blvd, Ste C2000, Los Angeles, CA 90048; **Phone:** 310-423-1101; **Board Cert:** Internal Medicine 1977; Medical Oncology 1979; **Med School:** Wayne State Univ 1974; **Resid:** Internal Medicine, Wayne State Univ 1977; **Fellow:** Hematology & Oncology, Meml Sloan Kettering 1980; **Fac Appt:** Prof Med, Univ Mich Med Sch

Nichols, Craig R MD [Onc] - **Spec Exp:** Testicular Cancer; Hodgkin's Disease; Lymphoma; **Hospital:** OR Hlth & Sci Univ; **Address:** Oregon Cancer Center, 3303 SW Bond Ave Fl 7th, MC CH7M, Portland, OR 97239-3098; **Phone:** 503-494-6594; **Board Cert:** Internal Medicine 1981; Medical Oncology 1985; **Med School:** Oregon Hlth Sci Univ 1978; **Resid:** Internal Medicine, Oschner Foundation Hosp 1981; **Fellow:** Medical Oncology, Indiana Univ 1985; **Fac Appt:** Prof Med, Oregon Hlth Sci Univ

O'Day, Steven J MD [Onc] - **Spec Exp:** Melanoma; Melanoma-Advanced; **Hospital:** St John's Hlth Ctr, Santa Monica; **Address:** The Angeles Clinic & Research Inst, 11818 Wilshire Blvd, Ste 200, Los Angeles, CA 90025; **Phone:** 310-231-2178; **Board Cert:** Internal Medicine 1991; Medical Oncology 1993; **Med School:** Johns Hopkins Univ 1988; **Resid:** Internal Medicine, Johns Hopkins Hosp 1991; **Fellow:** Medical Oncology, Dana Farber Cancer Inst 1992; **Fac Appt:** Assoc Clin Prof Med, USC-Keck School of Medicine

Picozzi Jr, Vincent J MD [Onc] - **Spec Exp:** Pancreatic Cancer; **Hospital:** Virginia Mason Med Ctr; **Address:** Virginia Mason Med Ctr, Div Hem/Onc, MS C2-Hem, Seattle, WA 98111; **Phone:** 206-223-6193; **Board Cert:** Internal Medicine 1981; Hematology 1986; Medical Oncology 1987; **Med School:** Stanford Univ 1978; **Resid:** Internal Medicine, Peter Bent Brigham Med Ctr 1981; **Fellow:** Hematology, Stanford Univ Med Ctr 1983; Medical Oncology, Stanford Univ MEd Ctr 1984; **Fac Appt:** Clin Prof Med, Univ Wash

Prados, Michael MD [Onc] - **Spec Exp:** Neuro-Oncology; Brain Tumors; **Hospital:** UCSF Med Ctr; **Address:** UCSF Med Ctr, Div Neuro-Oncology, 400 Parnassus Ave, rm A-808, San Francisco, CA 94143; **Phone:** 415-353-2966; **Board Cert:** Internal Medicine 1977; **Med School:** Louisiana State Univ 1974; **Resid:** Internal Medicine, Earl K Long Hosp 1977; **Fac Appt:** Prof NS, UCSF

Press, Oliver W MD/PhD [Onc] - **Spec Exp:** Lymphoma; Bone Marrow Transplant; **Hospital:** Univ Wash Med Ctr; **Address:** 1100 Fairview Ave N, MS D3-190, Seattle, WA 98109; **Phone:** 206-667-1864; **Board Cert:** Internal Medicine 1982; Medical Oncology 1985; **Med School:** Univ Wash 1979; **Resid:** Internal Medicine, Mass Genl Hosp 1982; Internal Medicine, Univ Hosp 1983; **Fellow:** Medical Oncology, Univ Washington 1985; **Fac Appt:** Prof Med, Univ Wash

Ross, Helen Jane MD [Onc] - **Spec Exp:** Lung Cancer; Esophageal Cancer; Chest Wall Tumors; Clinical Trials; **Hospital:** Providence Portland Med Ctr; **Address:** Oregon Clinic-Cardiothoracic Surgery, 1111 NE 99th Ave, Ste 201, Portland, OR 97220; **Phone:** 503-215-5696; **Board Cert:** Internal Medicine 1987; Medical Oncology 1989; **Med School:** UCLA 1984; **Resid:** Internal Medicine, Cedars Sinai Med Ctr 1987; **Fellow:** Medical Oncology, UCLA Med Ctr 1989; **Fac Appt:** Assoc Prof Med, Oregon Hlth Sci Univ

Russell, Christy A MD [Onc] - **Spec Exp:** Breast Cancer; **Hospital:** USC Univ Hosp - R K Eamer Med Plz; **Address:** Norris Cancer Ctr, The Breast Ctr, 1441 Eastlake Ave, Los Angeles, CA 90033; **Phone:** 323-865-3371; **Board Cert:** Internal Medicine 1983; Medical Oncology 1985; **Med School:** Med Coll PA Hahnemann 1980; **Fac Appt:** Assoc Prof Med, USC Sch Med

Small, Eric J MD [Onc] - **Spec Exp:** Prostate Cancer; Vaccine Therapy; Genitourinary Cancer; **Hospital:** UCSF Med Ctr; **Address:** UCSF Urologic Oncology Practice, 1600 Divisadero St, San Francisco, CA 94115; **Phone:** 415-353-7171; **Board Cert:** Internal Medicine 1988; Medical Oncology 2001; **Med School:** Case West Res Univ 1985; **Resid:** Internal Medicine, Beth Israel Hosp 1988; **Fellow:** Hematology & Oncology, Cancer Research Inst/UCSF 1991; **Fac Appt:** Prof Med, UCSF

Stewart, Forrest Marc MD [Onc] - **Spec Exp:** Unknown Primary Cancer; Sarcoma; **Hospital:** Univ Wash Med Ctr; **Address:** Fred Hutchinson Cancer Rsch Ctr, 825 Eastlake Ave E, Box 19023, Seattle, WA 98109; **Phone:** 206-288-7222; **Board Cert:** Internal Medicine 1980; Hematology 1982; Medical Oncology 1985; **Med School:** Indiana Univ 1977; **Resid:** Internal Medicine, Indiana Univ Med Ctr 1980; Medical Oncology, Indiana Univ Med Ctr 1981; **Fellow:** Hematology, Univ Virginia Med Ctr 1983; **Fac Appt:** Prof Med, Univ Wash

Stockdale, Frank E MD/PhD [Onc] - **Spec Exp:** Breast Cancer; **Hospital:** Stanford Univ Med Ctr; **Address:** Stanford University Medical Ctr, 875 Lake Wilbur Drive, Stanford, CA 94305-5826; **Phone:** 650-723-6449; **Med School:** Univ Pennsylvania 1963; **Resid:** Internal Medicine, Stanford Univ Med Ctr 1967; **Fellow:** Hematology & Oncology, Natl Inst Hlth; **Fac Appt:** Prof Emeritus Med, Stanford Univ

Tempero, Margaret MD [Onc] - **Spec Exp:** Pancreatic Cancer; Gastrointestinal Cancer; **Hospital:** UCSF Med Ctr; **Address:** UCSF, Multi-Disciplinary Practice, 1600 Divisadero St, Box 1705, San Francisco, CA 94115; **Phone:** 415-353-9888; **Board Cert:** Internal Medicine 1980; Hematology 1984; Medical Oncology 1983; **Med School:** Univ Nebr Coll Med 1977; **Resid:** Internal Medicine, Univ Nebraska Hosp 1980; **Fellow:** Medical Oncology, Univ Nebraska 1982

Urba, Walter J MD [Onc] - **Spec Exp:** Breast Cancer; **Hospital:** Providence Portland Med Ctr; **Address:** Oregon Clinic, Div of Medical Oncology, 5050 NE Hoyt, Ste 611, Portland, OR 97213; **Phone:** 503-215-5696; **Board Cert:** Internal Medicine 1985; Medical Oncology 1987; **Med School:** Univ Miami Sch Med 1981; **Resid:** Internal Medicine, Morristown Meml Hosp 1983; **Fellow:** Medical Oncology, Natl Cancer Inst 1986; **Fac Appt:** Assoc Clin Prof Med, Oregon Hlth Sci Univ

Vescio, Robert A MD [Onc] - **Spec Exp:** Multiple Myeloma; Amyloidosis; **Hospital:** Cedars-Sinai Med Ctr; **Address:** Cedars Sinai Med Ctr, Dept Hem/Oncology, 8700 Beverly Blvd, Los Angeles, CA 90048; **Phone:** 310-423-1825; **Board Cert:** Internal Medicine 1989; Hematology 2004; Medical Oncology 2003; **Med School:** UCSD 1986; **Resid:** Internal Medicine, UCSD Med Ctr 1989; **Fellow:** Hematology & Oncology, UCLA Med Ctr 1993; **Fac Appt:** Assoc Prof Med, UCLA

Vogelzang, Nicholas MD [Onc] - **Spec Exp:** Prostate Cancer; Mesothelioma; Kidney Cancer; **Hospital:** Univ Med Ctr - Las Vegas, Summerlin Hosp Med Ctr; **Address:** Nevada Cancer Institute, One Breakthrough Way, Las Vegas, NV 89135; **Phone:** 702-822-5100; **Board Cert:** Internal Medicine 1978; Medical Oncology 1981; **Med School:** Univ IL Coll Med 1974; **Resid:** Internal Medicine, Rush-Presby St Luke's Med Ctr 1978; **Fellow:** Medical Oncology, Univ Minn Med Ctr 1981; **Fac Appt:** Prof Med, Univ Nevada

Volberding, Paul Arthur MD [Onc] - **Spec Exp:** AIDS Related Cancers; **Hospital:** UCSF Med Ctr; **Address:** 4150 Clemens St, VAMC 111, San Francisco, CA 94121; **Phone:** 415-750-2203; **Board Cert:** Internal Medicine 1978; Medical Oncology 1981; **Med School:** Univ Minn 1975; **Resid:** Internal Medicine, Univ Utah Med Ctr 1978; **Fellow:** Medical Oncology, UCSF Med Ctr 1981; **Fac Appt:** Prof Med, UCSF

Yen, Yun MD [Onc] - **Spec Exp:** Liver Cancer; Biliary Cancer; **Hospital:** City of Hope Natl Med Ctr & Beckman Rsch; **Address:** City of Hope Comprehensive Cancer Ctr, 1500 E Duarte Rd, Duarte, CA 91010; **Phone:** 626-359-8111 x62307; **Board Cert:** Internal Medicine 1990; Medical Oncology 2003; **Med School:** Taiwan 1982; **Resid:** Internal Medicine, St Luke's Hosp 1990; **Fellow:** Hematology & Oncology, Yale-New Haven Hosp 1993; **Fac Appt:** Prof Med, USC Sch Med

ChildrensHospitalLosAngeles

International Leader in Pediatrics

Childrens Hospital Los Angeles

4650 Sunset Boulevard
Los Angeles, California 90027
www.ChildrensHospitalLA.org

Childrens Hospital Los Angeles is acknowledged throughout the United States and around the world for its leadership in pediatric and adolescent health. It is able to offer the very best in multidisciplinary care, with 85 pediatric subspecialties and dozens of special services for children and families. Its physicians are recognized as leaders. Its treatments set the standard of care. Its research is recognized worldwide.

The Heart Institute

The Heart Institute is known throughout the world as a leader in the treatment of pediatric heart disease, offering the most advanced diagnostic and treatment modalities available in cardiology, cardio thoracic surgery, cardio thoracic transplantation and intensive care, as well as innovation in cardiac research. Physicians provide comprehensive care to 8,000 children each year – fetus through adolescent – who have congenital or acquired heart and lung disorders. For information contact (323) 669-4148.

Center for Endocrinology, Diabetes and Metabolism

The Center for Endocrinology, Diabetes and Metabolism is at the forefront of patient care, basic and clinical research in diabetes, obesity, growth, bone metabolism and endocrinology. More than 2,000 children and adolescents with Type 1 and Type 2 diabetes are under the care of its pediatric diabetes specialists, certified diabetes educators and nutritionists – one of the largest programs of its kind in America. For information contact (323) 669-4604.

Childrens Center for Cancer and Blood Diseases

The Childrens Center for Cancer and Blood Diseases is the nation's largest pediatric hematology/oncology program. Physician- scientists integrate their laboratory experience with their clinical expertise in an approach to medical problem-solving that enables them to move effectively from "Bench to Bedside." Breakthroughs in the treatment of childhood cancer, many pioneered at Childrens Hospital Los Angeles, offer children, teenagers and young adults the most advanced treatment available anywhere. For information contact (323) 669-2121.

Childrens Orthopaedic Center

The Childrens Orthopaedic Center is one of the nation's most comprehensive programs dedicated to pediatric musculoskeletal care, education and research. Its Scoliosis and Spine Disorders Program, one of the largest in the country, is the only one of its kind in Los Angeles County devoted exclusively to the pediatric population. Its state-of-the-art Motion Analysis Laboratory is designed to analyze muscle activity and joint movements in children who have difficulty walking, such as those with cerebral palsy, spina bifida and congenital leg conditions. For information contact (323) 669-2142.

602

■ Cleveland Clinic

Taussig Cancer Center

Each day, a team of cancer experts at Cleveland Clinic's Taussig Cancer Center pushes the limits of medicine – within the region, across the country and around the world. The quality and innovation of our programs has led to a ranking as one of the nation's top cancer centers by *U.S.News & World Report*.

The Taussig Cancer Center provides care for more than 180,000 patient visits annually. A team of 250 cancer specialists cares for patients with breast, lung, urologic, endocrine, gastrointestinal, gynecologic, head and neck, musculoskeletal and ophthalmic cancers; cancers of the brain and spinal cord; skin cancer and melanoma, hematologic malignancies and a world renowned palliative care program.

- State-of-the-art patient care is provided in the context of major clinical and translational research programs. For pediatric cancer patients, clinical-trials research has led to a high rate of cure, as well as the development of safer treatments for all persons with cancer. Bench-to-bedside research allows patients with resistant cancers to have access to the latest experimental therapies.
- Our Bone Marrow Transplant program consistently achieves excellent outcomes. We have one of the most experienced teams in the nation, having performed over 2,700 bone marrow transplant procedures since 1977.
- In our multidisciplinary clinics, subspecialists bring their expertise to bear on specific tumor types and aspects of treatment and recovery. Medical, surgical and radiation oncologists collaborate closely with pathologists, radiologists, oncology nurses and social workers. These interactions enhance effective communication and optimize the options for individual patients with complex problems. In 2006, Taussig Cancer Center introduced a Late Effects Clinic for cancer survivors. This multidisciplinary clinic helps to address health problems that can arise as late effects of successful cancer treatment.
- The center also is one of just a few hospitals in the region to offer technologies for administering stereotactic radiosurgery. Novalis is used for extracranial lesions, and Gamma Knife is used to treat primary and metastatic brain tumors.

Cancer Genetics at the Center for Personalized Genetic Healthcare

It has long been recognized that people in some families are prone to developing cancer. The last few decades of genetic research have provided us with the ability to identify some of the genetic risk factors that underlie this predisposition. At the Cleveland Clinic's Center for Personalized Genetic Healthcare, we specialize in the evaluation and management of high risk families. Our goal is to prevent cancer by identifying individuals who have a high risk for developing cancer and offering personalized medical management to them and their family members. For more information or to schedule an appointment, call 800.998.4785.

To stay at the forefront of cancer research, Cleveland Clinic continues to recruit world-renowned investigators, maintaining a focus on discovery and innovation. Cleveland Clinic cancer care is available at 10 additional Northeast Ohio locations.

To schedule an appointment or for more information about the Cleveland Clinic Taussig Cancer Center, call 800.890.2467 or visit www.clevelandclinic.org/cancertopdocs.

Taussig Cancer Center | 9500 Euclid Avenue / W14 | Cleveland OH 44195

Continuum Cancer Centers of New York

Continuum Cancer Centers

Beth Israel Medical Center
Roosevelt Hospital
St. Luke's Hospital
Long Island College Hospital
New York Eye and Ear Infirmary

Continuum Cancer Centers of New York

Phone: (212) 844-6027

The hospitals of Continuum – Beth Israel Medical Center, St. Luke's and Roosevelt Hospitals, Long Island College Hospital and the New York Eye and Ear Infirmary – are leading providers of cancer care through Continuum Cancer Centers of New York. Our integrated system allows us to build on the clinical strengths found at each of our partner hospitals.

The goal – and result – is delivery of care in ways that are more efficient, more attractive and more convenient for patients. Specifically, it means that cancer patients at any Continuum hospital can benefit from system-wide cancer expertise, facilities and resources. Continuum Cancer Centers feature world-renowned cancer specialists, including top-rated surgeons, medical oncologists, radiation oncologists, radiologists, pathologists, and oncology nurses.

Comprehensive diagnostic and treatment services are available for breast cancer, prostate cancer, head and neck and thyroid cancers, skin cancer, lung cancer, colorectal and other gastrointestinal cancers, lymphoma/Hodgkin's Disease, gynecological cancers, and cancers of the brain and central nervous system. Delivered efficiently in a friendly and supportive environment, our services include prevention programs – such as community education, screenings and early detection – expert diagnosis, outpatient treatment, inpatient services and home care. In addition, our Research Program offers patients access to investigational protocols through a wide number of clinical trials. Our physicians are leaders in both non-invasive and minimally invasive cancer treatments that focus on maximizing both the cure rate and the quality of life.

Support services play an important role at Continuum Cancer Centers.

Nurses, social workers, psychiatrists, chaplains, pharmacists, rehabilitation therapists and nutritionists all have specialized knowledge and expertise in the field of oncology.

In February 2007, Continuum Cancer Centers of New York received a full three year accreditation with commendation from the American College of Surgeons, Commission on Cancer (CoC). Continuum is the first hospital system in New York State to earn this network accreditation; fewer than 25 networks in the entire United States are so accredited by the Commission.

For help finding the services and care you need, please call us at (212) 844-6027.

536

Maimonides Cancer Center offers a fully integrated approach to cancer care that includes prevention, education, screening, diagnostics, treatment, palliative care and clinical research – all in one location. Staffed by a multidisciplinary team of leading oncologists, nurses, social workers and treatment specialists, the Maimonides Cancer Center provides compassionate, patient-centered, state-of-the-art care that is both accessible and comfortable. This freestanding, 50,000 square foot facility contains the following specialty centers:

Radiation Oncology Center: equipped with state-of-the art imaging and treatment delivery technologies; offers patients the most precise treatments available, yet does so in an airy, life-affirming environment.

Medical Oncology Center: provides oral drug therapies, intravenous chemotherapy infusions, transfusions, intravenous hydration, and antibiotics.

Pediatric Oncology Center: treats children with cancer in a child-friendly environment, and features special areas set aside for parent conferences.

Surgical Oncology Center: provides a convenient location for minor surgical procedures relating to cancer, including biopsies; and pre- and post-surgical care for the most complex cases.

Women's Center: provides mammography, sonography, computerized interpretation, biopsy procedures, same-day reading of results, treatment plans tailored for each patient.

Resource Center: offers access to integrative (complementary) oncology services, a library with Internet resources, social services, and dietary advice.

Research Center: conducts clinical trials that not only help advance science but also offer appropriately screened patients, who wish to volunteer, new therapies and medications.

Physicians at Maimonides are among the eight percent in the US who use computers to enter patient orders, thereby reducing the risk of errors, increasing efficiency, and speeding the healing process. Maimonides has appeared on the American Hospital Association's "Most Wired" and "Most Wireless" lists more often than any other healthcare institution in the metropolitan area. Advanced technology allows our doctors to focus more attention on caring for their patients.

Maimonides Medical Center – Passionate about medicine, compassionate about people.

www.maimonidesmed.org/cancer

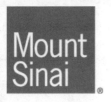

THE MOUNT SINAI MEDICAL CENTER
ONCOLOGY / CANCER CARE

One Gustave L. Levy Place (Fifth Avenue and 100th Street)
New York, NY 10029-6574
Physician Referral: 1-800-MD-SINAI (637-4624)
www.mountsinai.org

A TRADITION OF COMMITMENT AND DEDICATION
Mount Sinai has dedicated itself to one of the most widespread lifethreatening diseases.

SUPERB CARE
In an atmosphere of learning, clinical excellence, and superb patient care, Mount Sinai coordinates a full-service diagnostic and treatment program for cancer patients.

A WIDE RANGE OF PROGRAMS
Programs include medical chemotherapy, radiation, surgery, bone marrow and stem cell transplants, clinical trials for adults and children, and palliative care.

ADVANCED TECHNIQUES
Mount Sinai specialists use the most recent advances in the diagnosis and treatment of all cancers, and especially breast, colorectal, liver, lung, prostate, head and neck, gynecological and genitourinary cancers, and cancers of the blood and lymph systems.

TEAMWORK
Using a multidisciplinary approach, specialists in Medical Oncology, Radiation Oncology, Radiology, Surgery, Pathology, and other areas work together to treat the wide spectrum of types and locations of cancer.

INNOVATION
In addition, the Medical Center takes innovative approaches to the treatment of cancer patients: minimal access, local therapy for endocrine tumors, high risk screening, genetics of breast cancer, multi-modality therapy for gastrointestinal cancer, melanoma screening, vaccine program, and minimal access surgery for cancer in the elderly. In addition, with the knowledge gained through the Human Genome Project, Mount Sinai researchers are working on a gene therapy program for colon, prostate and breast cancer.

CENTER FOR MYELOPROLIFERATIVE DISORDERS
The newly created Center for Myeloproliferative Disorders (MPD) at The Mount Sinai Medical Center is already earning its place as a leader in patient care and research for these conditions. Myeloproliferative Disorders are a group of slow-growing blood cancers, including chronic myelogenous leukemia, in which large numbers of abnormal red blood cells, white blood cells, or platelets grow and spread in the bone marrow and the peripheral blood. Mount Sinai is the lead institution for a large multinational consortium for the study of MPD.

THE RUTTENBERG TREATMENT CENTER

The mission of the Ruttenberg Treatment Center at The Mount Sinai Medical Center is to reduce the burden of human cancer through its outstanding interdisciplinary programs in patient care and research, including cancer prevention, treatment, early detection, and education. Oncologists, surgeons, and specialists from across the medical spectrum work together to provide the highest quality care to all cancer patients.

The members of the Center–scientists and physicians–are developing cancer therapies and prevention strategies to improve cancer care. Patients of the Center often have access to these treatments before they are available anywhere else in the world.

614

⌐ NewYork-Presbyterian
⌐ The University Hospital of Columbia and Cornell
NewYork-Presbyterian Cancer Centers

Affiliated with Columbia University College of Physicians and Surgeons and Weill Medical College of Cornell University

Herbert Irving Comprehensive Cancer Center
At NewYork-Presbyterian Hospital
Columbia University Medical Center
161 Fort Washington Avenue
New York, NY 10032

Weill Cornell Cancer Center
At NewYork-Presbyterian Hospital
Weill Cornell Medical Center
525 East 68th Street
New York, NY 10021

OVERVIEW:

NewYork-Presbyterian Cancer Centers are dedicated to reducing cancer morbidity and mortality by providing
- a full continuum of multidisciplinary, state-of-the-art screening, diagnostic, treatment and support services for all phases of the disease process;
- cutting-edge basic, clinical, and public health research;
- full range of cancer-related educational programs and resources to clinicians, scientists, patients and survivors, families, and the cancer prevention community.

The Cancer Centers, which treat over 6,000 new patients annually, draw on the innovation and excellence of the NCI- designated Herbert Irving Comprehensive Cancer Center at NewYork-Presbyterian Hospital/Columbia University Medical Center and oncology services at NewYork-Presbyterian Hospital/Weill Cornell Medical Center. Programs include:
- AIDS-related Malignancies
- Bone Marrow Transplant
- Breast Cancer
- Dermatologic/Skin Cancer
- Gastrointestinal Cancers
- Genitourinary Cancers
- Gynecologic Cancers
- Head and Neck Cancers
- Hematologic Malignancies, such as lymphoma, myeloma and leukemias
- Lung Cancer
- Neurologic Cancer
- Ophthalmic Cancer
- Pediatric Hematology/Oncology
- Urologic Cancers, including bladder, kidney and prostate cancer
- Sarcomas and Mesotheiliomas

The Centers are frequent recipients of major grants and gifts to support research programs. Recent highlights include:
- Avon Products Foundation $10 million award to NewYork-Presbyterian Hospital/Columbia University Medical Center and Columbia University for establishment of the Avon Products Breast Center to support basic, clinical and public health research in breast cancer;
- The Leukemia and Lymphoma Society five-year $7.5 million grant to NewYork-Presbyterian Hospital/Weill Cornell Medical Center to study fundamental causes of multiple myeloma

Physician Referral: For a physician referral call toll free **1-877-NYP-WELL** (1-877-697-9355) to learn more about our Cancer Centers visit our website at **www.nypcancer.org**

COMPREHENSIVE SERVICES INCLUDE:

- Access to over 400 clinical trials supported by the National Institutes of Health and many prominent pharmaceutical companies.

- Bone marrow and blood stem cell transplant, including New York State approval to perform transplants using unrelated donors for patients with hematologic malignancies

- CT screening for early lung cancer detection

- Sentinel node biopsy to assess spread of breast cancer

- Skin-sparing mastectomy and reconstruction

- Laparoscopic surgery for colon cancer

- Intraoperative brachytherapy for GI, prostate and other cancers

- Stereotactic biopsies for breast cancer and brain cancer

- Stereotactic gamma radiation for brain tumors

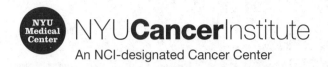

NYUCancerInstitute
An NCI-designated Cancer Center

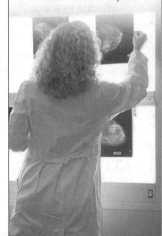

Infectious Disease

a subspecialty of Internal Medicine

An internist who deals with infectious diseases of all types and in all organs. Conditions requiring selective use of antibiotics call for this special skill. This physician often diagnoses and treats AIDS patients and patients with fevers which have not been explained. Infectious disease specialists may also have expertise in preventive medicine and conditions associated with travel.

Training Required: Three years in internal medicine *plus* additional training and examination for certification in infectious disease.

Infectious Disease

New England

Craven, Donald Edward MD [Inf] - **Spec Exp:** AIDS/HIV; Hepatitis C; Hospital Acquired Infections; Pneumonia; **Hospital:** Lahey Clin; **Address:** Lahey Clin Med Ctr, Infectious Diseases, 41 Mall Rd, Burlington, MA 01803; **Phone:** 781-744-8608; **Board Cert:** Internal Medicine 1973; Infectious Disease 1982; **Med School:** Albany Med Coll 1970; **Resid:** Internal Medicine, Royal Victoria Hosp-McGill 1973; Internal Medicine, Royal Victoria Hosp 1974; **Fellow:** Infectious Disease, Boston Univ Hosp 1976; NIH/Bureau of Biologics 1979; **Fac Appt:** Prof Med, Tufts Univ

Flanigan, Timothy MD [Inf] - **Spec Exp:** AIDS/HIV; **Hospital:** Miriam Hosp, Rhode Island Hosp; **Address:** 164 Summit Ave Fain Bldg - Ste E, Providence, RI 02906; **Phone:** 401-793-2928; **Board Cert:** Internal Medicine 1986; Infectious Disease 1988; **Med School:** Cornell Univ-Weill Med Coll 1983; **Resid:** Internal Medicine, Hosp Univ Penn 1986; **Fellow:** Infectious Disease, Case West Res Univ 1987; **Fac Appt:** Prof Med, Brown Univ

Longworth, David L MD [Inf] - **Hospital:** Baystate Med Ctr; **Address:** Baystate Medical Ctr, 759 Chestnut St, Springfield, MA 01199; **Phone:** 413-794-4319; **Board Cert:** Internal Medicine 1981; Infectious Disease 1984; **Med School:** Cornell Univ-Weill Med Coll 1978; **Resid:** Internal Medicine, UCSF-HC Moffitt Hosp 1981; **Fellow:** Infectious Disease, Brigham & Womens Hosp 1983; Research, Harvard Med School 1985; **Fac Appt:** Prof Med, Tufts Univ

Quagliarello, Vincent MD [Inf] - **Spec Exp:** Meningitis; Pneumonia; Endocarditis; **Hospital:** Yale - New Haven Hosp; **Address:** Yale Univ Sch Med, TAC S169A, 300 Cedar St, New Haven, CT 06520-8022; **Phone:** 203-785-7570; **Board Cert:** Internal Medicine 1985; Infectious Disease 1989; **Med School:** Washington Univ, St Louis 1980; **Resid:** Internal Medicine, Yale-New Haven Hosp 1984; **Fellow:** Infectious Disease, Univ VA Hlth Sci Ctr 1987; **Fac Appt:** Prof Med, Yale Univ

Rubin, Robert H MD [Inf] - **Spec Exp:** Infections-Transplant; **Hospital:** Brigham & Women's Hosp; **Address:** Brigham & Women's Hospital, Div Infectious Disease, 75 Francis St, Boston, MA 02115; **Phone:** 617-732-8881; **Board Cert:** Internal Medicine 1972; Infectious Disease 1974; **Med School:** Harvard Med Sch 1966; **Resid:** Internal Medicine, Peter Bent Brigham Hosp 1970; **Fellow:** Infectious Disease, Mass Genl Hosp 1972; **Fac Appt:** Prof Med, Harvard Med Sch

Sax, Paul E MD [Inf] - **Spec Exp:** AIDS/HIV; **Hospital:** Brigham & Women's Hosp; **Address:** Brigham & Women's Hospital, Div Infectious Disease, 75 Francis St, Boston, MA 02115; **Phone:** 617-732-8881; **Board Cert:** Internal Medicine 2000; Infectious Disease 2002; **Med School:** Harvard Med Sch 1987; **Resid:** Internal Medicine, Brigham & Womens Hosp 1990; **Fellow:** Infectious Disease, Mass Genl Hosp 1992

Mid Atlantic

Auwaerter, Paul MD [Inf] - **Spec Exp:** Lyme Disease; Ehrlichiosis; Tick-borne Diseases; Fevers of Unknown Origin; **Hospital:** Johns Hopkins Hosp - Baltimore (page 61); **Address:** 10753 Falls Rd, Ste 325, Lutherville, MD 21093; **Phone:** 410-583-2774; **Board Cert:** Internal Medicine 2002; Infectious Disease 1994; **Med School:** Columbia P&S 1988; **Resid:** Internal Medicine, Johns Hopkins Med Ctr 1992; **Fellow:** Infectious Disease, Johns Hopkins Med Ctr 1996; **Fac Appt:** Assoc Prof Med, Johns Hopkins Univ

Castle Connolly America's Top Doctors® **7th Edition**

Bartlett, John G MD [Inf] - **Spec Exp:** AIDS/HIV; Fevers of Unknown Origin; Pseudomembranous Colitis; **Hospital:** Johns Hopkins Hosp - Baltimore (page 61); **Address:** 1830 E Monument St, Ste 439, Baltimore, MD 21205; **Phone:** 410-955-7634; **Board Cert:** Internal Medicine 1972; **Med School:** SUNY Upstate Med Univ 1963; **Resid:** Internal Medicine, Peter Bent Brigham Hosp 1965; Internal Medicine, Univ Hosp Birmingham 1968; **Fellow:** Infectious Disease, Wadsworth VA Hosp 1970

Berkowitz, Leonard B MD [Inf] - **Spec Exp:** AIDS/HIV; **Hospital:** Brooklyn Hosp Ctr-Downtown; **Address:** 121 DeKalb Ave, Brooklyn, NY 11201-5425; **Phone:** 718-250-6922; **Board Cert:** Internal Medicine 1980; Infectious Disease 1984; **Med School:** SUNY Downstate 1977; **Resid:** Internal Medicine, Kings Co Med Ctr 1981; **Fellow:** Infectious Disease, Kings Co Med Ctr 1983; **Fac Appt:** Asst Clin Prof Med, SUNY Hlth Sci Ctr

Blaser, Martin J MD [Inf] - **Spec Exp:** Fevers of Unknown Origin; Infections-Gastrointestinal; Diarrheal Diseases; **Hospital:** NYU Med Ctr (page 67), Bellevue Hosp Ctr; **Address:** 550 1st Ave, OBV-A606, New York, NY 10016-6402; **Phone:** 212-263-6394; **Board Cert:** Internal Medicine 1977; Infectious Disease 1980; **Med School:** NYU Sch Med 1973; **Resid:** Internal Medicine, Univ Colorado Med Ctr 1977; **Fellow:** Infectious Disease, Univ Colorado Med Ctr 1979; **Fac Appt:** Prof Med, NYU Sch Med

Brause, Barry MD [Inf] - **Spec Exp:** Bone/Joint Infections; Skin/Soft Tissue Infection; Infections in Prosthetic Devices; **Hospital:** Hosp For Special Surgery (page 60), NY-Presby Hosp/Weill Cornell (page 66); **Address:** 535 E 70th St, New York, NY 10021-5718; **Phone:** 212-774-7411; **Board Cert:** Internal Medicine 1973; Infectious Disease 1976; **Med School:** Univ Pittsburgh 1970; **Resid:** Internal Medicine, New York Hosp 1973; **Fellow:** Infectious Disease, New York Hosp 1975; **Fac Appt:** Clin Prof Med, Cornell Univ-Weill Med Coll

Chaisson, Richard E MD [Inf] - **Spec Exp:** AIDS/HIV; Tuberculosis; **Hospital:** Johns Hopkins Hosp - Baltimore (page 61); **Address:** 1503 E Jefferson St, Ste 1104, Baltimore, MD 21231; **Phone:** 410-955-1755; **Board Cert:** Internal Medicine 1985; **Med School:** Univ Mass Sch Med 1982; **Resid:** Internal Medicine, UCSF Med Ctr 1985; **Fellow:** Infectious Disease, UCSF Med Ctr 1987; **Fac Appt:** Assoc Prof Med, Johns Hopkins Univ

Cunha, Burke A MD [Inf] - **Spec Exp:** Infections in Immunocompromised Patients; Fevers of Unknown Origin; Pneumonia; Chronic Fatigue Syndrome; **Hospital:** Winthrop - Univ Hosp; **Address:** 222 Station Plz N, Ste 432, Mineola, NY 11501; **Phone:** 516-663-2507; **Board Cert:** Internal Medicine 1977; Infectious Disease 1978; **Med School:** Penn State Univ-Hershey Med Ctr 1972; **Resid:** Internal Medicine, Hartford Hosp 1975; **Fellow:** Infectious Disease, Hartford Hosp 1977; **Fac Appt:** Prof Med, SUNY Stony Brook

Fauci, Anthony S MD [Inf] - **Spec Exp:** AIDS/HIV; Immunotherapy; **Hospital:** Natl Inst of Hlth - Clin Ctr; **Address:** NIAID , Bldg 31 - rm 7A03, 31 Center Drive   MSC 2520, Bethesda, MD 20892-2520; **Phone:** 301-496-2263; **Board Cert:** Internal Medicine 1972; Allergy & Immunology 1974; Infectious Disease 1974; **Med School:** Cornell Univ-Weill Med Coll 1966; **Resid:** Internal Medicine, New York Hosp Cornell Med Ctr 1972; **Fellow:** Infectious Disease, Natl Inst Infectious Disease NIH 1971

Frank, Ian MD [Inf] - **Spec Exp:** AIDS/HIV; **Hospital:** Hosp Univ Penn - UPHS (page 72); **Address:** Hosp Univ Penn, Div Infectious Disease, 3400 Spruce St, Silverstein Bldg, Fl 3 - Ste D, Philadelphia, PA 19104; **Phone:** 215-662-6932; **Board Cert:** Internal Medicine 1983; Infectious Disease 1992; **Med School:** Dartmouth Med Sch 1980; **Resid:** Internal Medicine, Graduate Hosp 1983; **Fellow:** Infectious Disease, Hosp Univ Penn; **Fac Appt:** Assoc Prof Med, Univ Pennsylvania

Gumprecht, Jeffrey Paul MD [Inf] - **Spec Exp:** AIDS/HIV; Travel Medicine; Infections-Surgical; **Hospital:** Mount Sinai Med Ctr; **Address:** 1100 Park Ave, New York, NY 10128; **Phone:** 212-427-9550; **Board Cert:** Internal Medicine 1987; Infectious Disease 2003; **Med School:** Albany Med Coll 1983; **Resid:** Internal Medicine, Mount Sinai Hosp 1987; **Fellow:** Infectious Disease, Montefiore Med Ctr 1990; **Fac Appt:** Prof Med, Mount Sinai Sch Med

Hammer, Glenn MD [Inf] - **Spec Exp:** AIDS/HIV; Hospital Acquired Infections; Infections-Surgical; **Hospital:** Mount Sinai Med Ctr; **Address:** 1100 Park Ave, New York, NY 10128-1202; **Phone:** 212-427-9550; **Board Cert:** Infectious Disease 1974; Internal Medicine 1973; **Med School:** NYU Sch Med 1969; **Resid:** Internal Medicine, Mount Sinai Hosp 1972; **Fellow:** Infectious Disease, Mount Sinai Hosp 1974; **Fac Appt:** Asst Clin Prof Med, Mount Sinai Sch Med

Hammer, Scott M MD [Inf] - **Spec Exp:** AIDS/HIV; **Hospital:** NY-Presby Hosp/Columbia (page 66); **Address:** 622 W 168th St, PH Bldg - rm 876 West, New York, NY 10032; **Phone:** 212-305-7185; **Board Cert:** Internal Medicine 1975; Infectious Disease 1980; **Med School:** Columbia P&S 1972; **Resid:** Internal Medicine, Columbia-Presby Hosp 1975; Internal Medicine, Stanford Univ Hosp 1976; **Fellow:** Infectious Disease, Mass Genl Hosp 1981; **Fac Appt:** Prof Med, Columbia P&S

Hartman, Barry Jay MD [Inf] - **Spec Exp:** Endocarditis; Infections-Surgical; Parasitic Infections; **Hospital:** NY-Presby Hosp/Weill Cornell (page 66); **Address:** 407 E 70th St, Fl 4, New York, NY 10021-5302; **Phone:** 212-744-4882; **Board Cert:** Internal Medicine 1976; Infectious Disease 1980; **Med School:** Penn State Univ-Hershey Med Ctr 1973; **Resid:** Internal Medicine, New York Hosp /Cornell Med Ctr 1976; **Fellow:** Infectious Disease, New York Hosp/ Cornell Med Ctr 1981; **Fac Appt:** Clin Prof Med, Cornell Univ-Weill Med Coll

Johnson, Warren MD [Inf] - **Spec Exp:** Travel Medicine; Parasitic Infections; **Hospital:** NY-Presby Hosp/Weill Cornell (page 66); **Address:** 1300 York Ave, Ste A-421, New York, NY 10021-4805; **Phone:** 212-746-6320; **Board Cert:** Internal Medicine 1971; Infectious Disease 1974; **Med School:** Columbia P&S 1962; **Resid:** Internal Medicine, NY Hosp-Cornell Med Ctr 1964; Internal Medicine, NY Hosp-Cornell Med Ctr 1969; **Fellow:** Infectious Disease, NY Hosp-Cornell Med Ctr 1968; **Fac Appt:** Prof Med, Cornell Univ-Weill Med Coll

Klotman, Mary E MD [Inf] - **Spec Exp:** AIDS/HIV; **Hospital:** Mount Sinai Med Ctr; **Address:** Mt Sinai Medical Ctr, One Gustave L Levy Pl, Box 1090, New York, NY 10029-6500; **Phone:** 212-241-2950; **Board Cert:** Internal Medicine 1984; Infectious Disease 1986; **Med School:** Duke Univ 1980; **Resid:** Internal Medicine, Duke Univ Med Ctr 1983; **Fellow:** Infectious Disease, Duke Univ Med Ctr 1985; **Fac Appt:** Prof Med, Mount Sinai Sch Med

Masur, Henry MD [Inf] - **Spec Exp:** Critical Care; AIDS/HIV; **Hospital:** Natl Inst of Hlth - Clin Ctr; **Address:** National Institutes of Health, 10 Center Drive, Clinical Ctr 7D43, Bethesda, MD 20892; **Phone:** 301-496-9320; **Board Cert:** Internal Medicine 1975; Infectious Disease 1978; **Med School:** Cornell Univ-Weill Med Coll 1972; **Resid:** Internal Medicine, New York Hosp 1974; Internal Medicine, Johns Hopkins Hosp 1975; **Fellow:** Infectious Disease, New York Hosp-Cornell 1977

Mildvan, Donna MD [Inf] - **Spec Exp:** AIDS/HIV; Clinical Trials; **Hospital:** Beth Israel Med Ctr - Petrie Division; **Address:** Beth Israel Med Ctr, Div Infectious Dis, 1st Ave at 16th St, 19BH17, New York, NY 10003; **Phone:** 212-420-4005; **Board Cert:** Internal Medicine 1972; Infectious Disease 1972; **Med School:** Johns Hopkins Univ 1967; **Resid:** Internal Medicine, Mount Sinai Hosp 1970; **Fellow:** Infectious Disease, Mount Sinai Hosp 1972; **Fac Appt:** Prof Med, Albert Einstein Coll Med

Nahass, Ronald MD [Inf] - **Spec Exp:** Hepatitis B & C; Wound Healing/Care; **Hospital:** Robert Wood Johnson Univ Hosp - New Brunswick, Univ Med Ctr - Princeton; **Address:** 411 Courtyard Drive, Hillsborough, NJ 08844-4254; **Phone:** 908-725-2522; **Board Cert:** Internal Medicine 1985; Infectious Disease 1988; **Med School:** UMDNJ-RW Johnson Med Sch 1982; **Resid:** Internal Medicine, RWJ Univ Hosp 1986; **Fellow:** Infectious Disease, RWJ Univ Hosp 1988; **Fac Appt:** Clin Prof Med, UMDNJ-RW Johnson Med Sch

Perlman, David MD [Inf] - **Spec Exp:** AIDS/HIV; Lyme Disease; Travel Medicine; **Hospital:** Beth Israel Med Ctr - Petrie Division, Lenox Hill Hosp (page 62); **Address:** Beth Israel Med Ctr, 1st Ave at 16th St, New York, NY 10003; **Phone:** 212-420-4470; **Board Cert:** Internal Medicine 1986; Infectious Disease 1988; **Med School:** Albert Einstein Coll Med 1983; **Resid:** Internal Medicine, New York Hosp/Meml Sloan Kettering 1986; **Fellow:** Infectious Disease, Montefiore Hosp 1988; **Fac Appt:** Prof Med, Albert Einstein Coll Med

Polsky, Bruce MD [Inf] - **Spec Exp:** AIDS/HIV; Viral Infections; Infections in Cancer Patients; AIDS Related Cancers; **Hospital:** St Luke's - Roosevelt Hosp Ctr - Roosevelt Div; **Address:** 1111 Amsterdam Ave, New York, NY 10025; **Phone:** 212-523-2525; **Board Cert:** Internal Medicine 1983; Infectious Disease 1986; **Med School:** Wayne State Univ 1980; **Resid:** Internal Medicine, Montefiore Hosp 1983; **Fellow:** Infectious Disease, Meml Sloan Kettering Cancer Ctr 1986; **Fac Appt:** Prof Med, Columbia P&S

Rahal, James MD [Inf] - **Spec Exp:** West Nile Virus; Antibiotic Resistance; Hospital Acquired Infections; **Hospital:** NY Hosp Queens; **Address:** NY Hosp Queens, Div Infectious Disease, 56-45 Main St, Flushing, NY 11355-5095; **Phone:** 718-670-1525; **Board Cert:** Internal Medicine 1967; Infectious Disease 1972; **Med School:** Tufts Univ 1959; **Resid:** Internal Medicine, Bellevue Hosp Ctr 1961; Internal Medicine, New England Ctr Hosp 1964; **Fellow:** Infectious Disease, New England Ctr Hosp 1965; **Fac Appt:** Prof Med, Cornell Univ-Weill Med Coll

Rao, Nalini MD [Inf] - **Spec Exp:** Bone/Joint Infections; Tropical Diseases; Travel Medicine; **Hospital:** UPMC Presby, Pittsburgh, UPMC Shadyside; **Address:** Centre Commons, Suite 510, 5750 Centre Ave, Pittsburgh, PA 15206-3721; **Phone:** 412-661-1633; **Board Cert:** Internal Medicine 1975; Infectious Disease 1980; **Med School:** India 1970; **Resid:** Internal Medicine, Geo Wash Univ Hosp 1974; **Fellow:** Infectious Disease, Baylor Coll Med 1975; Infectious Disease, Univ Pittsburgh Sch Med 1977; **Fac Appt:** Clin Prof Med, Univ Pittsburgh

Sepkowitz, Kent MD [Inf] - **Spec Exp:** Tuberculosis; Infections in Cancer Patients; Fungal Infections; **Hospital:** Meml Sloan Kettering Cancer Ctr; **Address:** 1275 York Ave, New York, NY 10021-0033; **Phone:** 212-639-2441; **Board Cert:** Internal Medicine 1983; Infectious Disease 2000; **Med School:** Univ Okla Coll Med 1980; **Resid:** Internal Medicine, Roosevelt Hosp 1984; **Fellow:** Infectious Disease, Meml Sloan Kettering Cancer Ctr 1991; **Fac Appt:** Prof Med, Cornell Univ-Weill Med Coll

Welch, Peter MD [Inf] - **Spec Exp:** Lyme Disease; Tick-borne Diseases; **Hospital:** Northern Westchester Hosp; **Address:** 16 Orchard Drive, Armonk, NY 10504; **Phone:** 914-273-3404; **Board Cert:** Internal Medicine 1977; Infectious Disease 1980; **Med School:** SUNY Buffalo 1974; **Resid:** Internal Medicine, New York Hosp 1977; **Fellow:** Infectious Disease, New York Hosp 1979

Wormser, Gary MD [Inf] - **Spec Exp:** Lyme Disease; AIDS/HIV; Diagnostic Problems; **Hospital:** Westchester Med Ctr; **Address:** New York Medical College, Munger Pavilion, rm 245, Valhalla, NY 10595; **Phone:** 914-493-8865; **Board Cert:** Internal Medicine 1978; Infectious Disease 1982; **Med School:** Johns Hopkins Univ 1972; **Resid:** Internal Medicine, Mount Sinai Hosp 1975; **Fellow:** Infectious Disease, Mount Sinai Hosp 1977; **Fac Appt:** Prof Med, NY Med Coll

Yancovitz, Stanley MD [Inf] - **Spec Exp:** Lyme Disease; AIDS/HIV; **Hospital:** Beth Israel Med Ctr - Petrie Division; **Address:** 1st Ave at 16th St, Ste 17 BH10, New York, NY 10003; **Phone:** 212-420-2600; **Board Cert:** Internal Medicine 1973; Infectious Disease 1976; **Med School:** SUNY Downstate 1967; **Resid:** Internal Medicine, Metropolitan Hosp 1969; Internal Medicine, Beth Israel Med Ctr 1972; **Fellow:** Infectious Disease, Mount Sinai Hosp 1975; **Fac Appt:** Assoc Prof Med, Albert Einstein Coll Med

Yu, Victor L MD [Inf] - **Spec Exp:** Legionnaire's Disease; Pneumonia; Staphylococcal Infections; **Hospital:** VA Pittsburgh Hlth Care Sys, UPMC Presby, Pittsburgh; **Address:** VA Med Ctr, Div Infectious Disease, University Drive C, Rm 2A-137, Pittsburgh, PA 15240; **Phone:** 412-688-6645; **Board Cert:** Internal Medicine 1978; Infectious Disease 1982; **Med School:** Univ Minn 1970; **Resid:** Internal Medicine, Univ Colo Med Ctr 1972; Internal Medicine, Stanford Univ Med Ctr 1975; **Fellow:** Infectious Disease, Stanford Univ Med Ctr 1977; **Fac Appt:** Prof Med, Univ Pittsburgh

Southeast

Alvarez-Elcoro, Salvador MD [Inf] - **Spec Exp:** Tuberculosis; Travel Medicine; Infections-Transplant; **Hospital:** St Luke's Hosp - Jacksonville; **Address:** Mayo Clinic, Div Infectious Disease, 4500 San Pablo Rd, Jacksonville, FL 32224; **Phone:** 904-953-2419; **Board Cert:** Internal Medicine 1977; Infectious Disease 1982; **Med School:** Mexico 1972; **Resid:** Internal Medicine, Charity Hosp 1977; **Fellow:** Infectious Disease, Boston City Hosp 1979; **Fac Appt:** Prof Med, Univ Fla Coll Med

Archer, Gordon Lee MD [Inf] - **Spec Exp:** Staphylococcal Infections; **Hospital:** Med Coll of VA Hosp; **Address:** Med Coll VA, Div Inf Dis, 1101 E Marshall St, Box 980565, Richmond, VA 23298-0565; **Phone:** 804-828-0673; **Board Cert:** Internal Medicine 1972; Infectious Disease 1976; **Med School:** Univ VA Sch Med 1969; **Resid:** Internal Medicine, Univ Mich Hosps 1972; **Fellow:** Infectious Disease, Univ Mich Hosps 1974; **Fac Appt:** Prof Med, Med Coll VA

Blumberg, Henry MD [Inf] - **Spec Exp:** Tuberculosis; **Hospital:** Grady Hlth Sys, Emory Univ Hosp; **Address:** Emory Univ, Div Infectious Diseases, 49 Jesse Hill Jr Drive, Atlanta, GA 30303; **Phone:** 404-616-6145; **Board Cert:** Internal Medicine 1986; Infectious Disease 2000; **Med School:** Vanderbilt Univ 1983; **Resid:** Internal Medicine, Emory Univ Affil Hosps 1986; Internal Medicine, Crawford-Long Hosp 1988; **Fellow:** Infectious Disease, Emory Univ Affil Hosps 1992; **Fac Appt:** Prof Med, Emory Univ

Cancio, Margarita MD [Inf] - **Spec Exp:** AIDS/HIV; **Hospital:** Tampa Genl Hosp; **Address:** 4 Columbia Dr, Ste 820, Tampa, FL 33606; **Phone:** 813-251-8444; **Board Cert:** Infectious Disease 1988; Internal Medicine 1985; **Med School:** Univ S Fla Coll Med 1982; **Resid:** Internal Medicine, Univ S Florida Affil Hosps 1985; **Fellow:** Infectious Disease, Univ S Florida Affil Hosps 1988; **Fac Appt:** Assoc Prof Med, Univ S Fla Coll Med

Chapman, Stanley W MD [Inf] - **Spec Exp:** Fungal Infections (Systemic Mycoses); **Hospital:** Univ Hosps & Clins - Jackson; **Address:** Univ Mississippi Med Ctr, Div Infectious Disease, 2500 N State St, Jackson, MS 39216; **Phone:** 601-984-5560; **Board Cert:** Internal Medicine 1975; Allergy & Immunology 1977; Infectious Disease 1980; **Med School:** Univ Rochester 1972; **Resid:** Internal Medicine, Emory Affil Hosps 1974; **Fellow:** Allergy & Immunology, NIAID-NIH 1977; Infectious Disease, Univ Rochester Med Ctr 1979; **Fac Appt:** Prof Med, Univ Miss

Cohen, Myron S MD [Inf] - **Spec Exp:** Infections in Immunocompromised Patients; **Hospital:** Univ NC Hosps; **Address:** UNC-Chapel Hill, Div Infectious Disease, 130 Mason Farm Rd, Ste 3115, Box 7030, Chapel Hill, NC 27599-7030; **Phone:** 919-966-7199; **Board Cert:** Internal Medicine 1977; Infectious Disease 1982; **Med School:** Rush Med Coll 1974; **Resid:** Internal Medicine, Univ Mich Hlth Ctr 1977; **Fellow:** Infectious Disease, Yale-New Haven Hosp 1979; **Fac Appt:** Prof Med, Univ NC Sch Med

Corey, G Ralph MD [Inf] - **Spec Exp:** Tropical Diseases; Travel Medicine; **Hospital:** Duke Univ Med Ctr; **Address:** 2400 Pratt St, rm 7021, Durham, NC 27710; **Phone:** 919-668-7174; **Board Cert:** Internal Medicine 1977; Infectious Disease 1980; **Med School:** Baylor Coll Med 1973; **Resid:** Internal Medicine, Duke Univ Med Ctr 1978; **Fellow:** Infectious Disease, Duke Univ Med Ctr 1980; **Fac Appt:** Prof Med, Duke Univ

Dismukes, William E MD [Inf] - **Spec Exp:** Fungal Infections; Endocarditis; Pneumonia; **Hospital:** Univ of Ala Hosp at Birmingham; **Address:** UAB, Dept Med-Div Infectious Disease, 1900 Univ Blvd, rm 229THT, Brimingham, AL 35294-0006; **Phone:** 205-934-5191; **Board Cert:** Internal Medicine 1977; Infectious Disease 1972; **Med School:** Univ Ala 1964; **Resid:** Internal Medicine, Peter Bent Brigham Hosp 1966; Internal Medicine, Peter Bent Brigham Hosp 1969; **Fellow:** Infectious Disease, Mass Genl Hosp 1971; **Fac Appt:** Prof Med, Univ Ala

Droller, David G MD [Inf] - **Spec Exp:** AIDS/HIV; Bone Infections; Infections-Surgical; **Hospital:** Broward General Med Ctr, Imperial Point Med Ctr; **Address:** 5333 N Dixie Hwy, Ste 208, Fort Lauderdale, FL 33334-3454; **Phone:** 954-771-7988; **Board Cert:** Internal Medicine 1977; Infectious Disease 1980; **Med School:** NYU Sch Med 1974; **Resid:** Internal Medicine, Univ Miami Affil Hosps 1977; **Fellow:** Infectious Disease, Univ Miami Affil Hosps 1979; **Fac Appt:** Assoc Prof Med, Univ Miami Sch Med

Gorensek, Margaret MD [Inf] - **Spec Exp:** AIDS/HIV; Infections-Transplant; Chronic Fatigue Syndrome; **Hospital:** Cleveland Clin - Weston (page 57), Broward General Med Ctr; **Address:** Cleveland Clinic Florida, 2950 Cleveland Clinic Blvd, Weston, FL 33331-3609; **Phone:** 954-659-5165; **Board Cert:** Internal Medicine 1985; Pediatrics 1986; Infectious Disease 1988; Pediatric Infectious Disease 2002; **Med School:** Case West Res Univ 1981; **Resid:** Internal Medicine & Pediatrics, Cleveland Clinic Fdn 1985; **Fellow:** Infectious Disease, Cleveland Clinic Fdn 1987; Pediatric Infectious Disease, Chldns Med Ctr 1988; **Fac Appt:** Asst Clin Prof Med, Univ Miami Sch Med

Guerrant, Richard MD [Inf] - **Spec Exp:** Tropical Diseases; Infectious Diarrhea; Travel Medicine; **Hospital:** Univ Virginia Med Ctr; **Address:** Ctr Global Hlth, PO Box 801379, Charlottesville, VA 22908-1379; **Phone:** 434-924-5242; **Board Cert:** Infectious Disease 1976; Internal Medicine 1973; **Med School:** Univ VA Sch Med 1968; **Resid:** Internal Medicine, Boston City Hosp 1970; Internal Medicine, Univ Virginia Hosp 1973; **Fellow:** Infectious Disease, Johns Hopkins 1972; Infectious Disease, Univ Virginia Hosp 1974; **Fac Appt:** Prof Med, Univ VA Sch Med

Katner, Harold MD [Inf] - **Spec Exp:** AIDS/HIV; **Hospital:** Med Ctr of Central GA; **Address:** Mercer Univ Sch Med, Dept Internal Med, 707 Pine St, Macon, GA 31201; **Phone:** 478-301-5809; **Board Cert:** Internal Medicine 1983; Infectious Disease 1986; **Med School:** Louisiana State Univ 1980; **Resid:** Internal Medicine, Univ Med Ctr 1983; **Fellow:** Infectious Disease, Ochsner Fdn Hosp 1986; **Fac Appt:** Prof Med, Mercer Univ Sch Med

Pearson, Richard D MD [Inf] - **Spec Exp:** Tropical Diseases; Travel Medicine; Infectious Disease; **Hospital:** Univ Virginia Med Ctr; **Address:** Univ VA Sch Med, Dept Internal Med, McKin Hall, Box 800739, Charlottesville, VA 22908-0001; **Phone:** 434-924-5579; **Board Cert:** Internal Medicine 1976; Infectious Disease 1980; **Med School:** Univ Mich Med Sch 1973; **Resid:** Internal Medicine, Strong Meml Hosp 1976; **Fellow:** Infectious Disease, Strong Meml Hosp-Univ Rochester 1979; **Fac Appt:** Prof Med, Univ VA Sch Med

Pegram, Paul S MD [Inf] - **Spec Exp:** AIDS/HIV; **Hospital:** Wake Forest Univ Baptist Med Ctr (page 73); **Address:** Wake Forest Baptist Med Ctr, Medical Ctr Blvd, ID Dept, Winston Salem, NC 27157-1042; **Phone:** 336-716-2700; **Board Cert:** Infectious Disease 1978; Internal Medicine 1976; **Med School:** Wake Forest Univ 1970; **Resid:** Internal Medicine, NC Baptist Hosp 1975; **Fellow:** Infectious Disease, NC Baptist Hosp 1978; **Fac Appt:** Prof Med, Wake Forest Univ

Ratzan, Kenneth MD [Inf] - **Spec Exp:** AIDS/HIV; **Hospital:** Mount Sinai Med Ctr - Miami, Miami Heart Inst; **Address:** Mount Sinai Medical Ctr, 4300 Alton Rd, Ste 450, Miami Beach, FL 33140-2800; **Phone:** 305-673-5490; **Board Cert:** Internal Medicine 1971; Infectious Disease 1974; **Med School:** Harvard Med Sch 1965; **Resid:** Internal Medicine, Columbia Presby Med Ctr 1967; Infectious Disease, Tufts New England Med Ctr 1972; **Fellow:** Infectious Disease, Tufts New England Med Ctr 1971; **Fac Appt:** Prof Med, Univ Miami Sch Med

Rein, Michael F MD [Inf] - **Spec Exp:** Sexually Transmitted Diseases; Vaginitis; **Hospital:** Univ Virginia Med Ctr; **Address:** U Va Hlth Scis Ctr, Div of Infectious Disease, Box 800592, Charlottesville, VA 22908-0592; **Phone:** 434-924-9668; **Board Cert:** Internal Medicine 1972; Infectious Disease 1980; **Med School:** Harvard Med Sch 1969; **Resid:** Internal Medicine, Mt Sinai Hosp 1971; Internal Medicine, Univ Va Med Ctr 1972; **Fellow:** Infectious Disease, Univ Va Med Ctr 1973; **Fac Appt:** Prof Med, Univ VA Sch Med

Saag, Michael S MD [Inf] - **Spec Exp:** AIDS/HIV; **Hospital:** Univ of Ala Hosp at Birmingham; **Address:** Community Care Bldg, 908 20th St S, Birmingham, AL 35294; **Phone:** 205-934-1917; **Board Cert:** Internal Medicine 1985; Infectious Disease 1988; **Med School:** Univ Louisville Sch Med 1981; **Resid:** Internal Medicine, Univ Ala Hosp 1984; **Fellow:** Infectious Disease, Univ Ala Hosp 1987

Scheld, William Michael MD [Inf] - **Spec Exp:** Meningitis; Septic Shock; AIDS/HIV; **Hospital:** Univ Virginia Med Ctr; **Address:** Univ VA Hlth Sci Ctr, PO Box 801342, Charlottesville, VA 22908; **Phone:** 434-924-5991; **Board Cert:** Internal Medicine 1976; Infectious Disease 1978; **Med School:** Cornell Univ-Weill Med Coll 1973; **Resid:** Internal Medicine, Univ VA Med Ctr 1976; **Fellow:** Infectious Disease, Univ VA Med Ctr 1979; **Fac Appt:** Prof Med, Univ VA Sch Med

Sparling, P Frederick MD [Inf] - **Spec Exp:** Sexually Transmitted Diseases; **Hospital:** Univ NC Hosps; **Address:** UNC-Chapel Hill Div Infectious Disease, 130 Mason Farm Rd, Ste 2115, Box 7030, Chapel Hill, NC 27599-7031; **Phone:** 919-966-7199; **Board Cert:** Internal Medicine 1970; Infectious Disease 1976; **Med School:** Harvard Med Sch 1962; **Resid:** Internal Medicine, Mass Genl Hosp 1964; **Fellow:** Infectious Disease, Mass Genl Hosp 1969; **Fac Appt:** Prof Med, Univ NC Sch Med

van der Horst, Charles MD [Inf] - **Spec Exp:** AIDS/HIV; Fungal Infections; Viral Infections; **Hospital:** Univ NC Hosps; **Address:** Univ NC-Dept Med, Box CB3368, Chapel Hill, NC 27599-0001; **Phone:** 919-843-4375; **Board Cert:** Internal Medicine 1982; Infectious Disease 1986; **Med School:** Harvard Med Sch 1979; **Resid:** Internal Medicine, Montefiore Hosp 1982; **Fellow:** Infectious Disease, NC Meml Hosp 1985; **Fac Appt:** Prof Med, Univ NC Sch Med

Wallace, Mark R MD [Inf] - **Spec Exp:** Fever in Returning Travelers; Travel Medicine; Valley Fever; **Hospital:** Orlando Regl Med Ctr; **Address:** 1626 Eagle Nest Cir, Winter Springs, FL 32708; **Board Cert:** Internal Medicine 1984; Infectious Disease 2000; **Med School:** St Louis Univ 1981; **Resid:** Internal Medicine, Univ Washington Hosp 1984; **Fellow:** Infectious Disease, Naval Hosp 1989; **Fac Appt:** Prof Med, Uniformed Srvs Univ, Bethesda

Midwest

Bakken, Johan S MD/PhD [Inf] - **Spec Exp:** Human Granulocytic Anaplasmosis; Tick-borne Diseases; Antibiotic Resistance; Ehrlichiosis; **Hospital:** St Luke's Hosp - Duluth, St Mary's Med Ctr - Duluth; **Address:** 1001 E Superior St, Ste L201, Duluth, MN 55802; **Phone:** 218-249-7990; **Board Cert:** Internal Medicine 1999; **Med School:** Univ Wash 1972; **Resid:** Internal Medicine, Univ Wash Hosps 1977; Internal Medicine, Lillehammer Fylkessykehus 1981; **Fellow:** Infectious Disease, Ulleval Hosp 1986; Microbiology, Creighton Univ 1988; **Fac Appt:** Assoc Clin Prof FMed, Univ Minn

Campbell, J William MD [Inf] - **Spec Exp:** AIDS/HIV; **Hospital:** St Luke's Hosp - Chesterfield, MO, Barnes-Jewish Hosp; **Address:** 222 S Woods Mill Rd, Ste 750N, Chesterfield, MO 63017; **Phone:** 314-205-6600; **Board Cert:** Infectious Disease 1982; Internal Medicine 1980; **Med School:** Washington Univ, St Louis 1977; **Resid:** Internal Medicine, Barnes Hosp-Wash Univ 1980; **Fellow:** Infectious Disease, Univ Tex Hlth Sci Ctr 1981; Infectious Disease, Wash Univ 1982; **Fac Appt:** Clin Prof Med, Washington Univ, St Louis

Kazanjian Jr, Powel H MD [Inf] - **Spec Exp:** AIDS/HIV; **Hospital:** Univ Michigan Hlth Sys; **Address:** Infect Dis Clinic, TC Level 3, Reception D, 1500 E Med Ctr Drive, Ann Arbor, MI 48109-0999; **Phone:** 734-647-5899; **Board Cert:** Internal Medicine 1982; Infectious Disease 1986; **Med School:** Tufts Univ 1979; **Resid:** Internal Medicine, Univ Chicago Hosp 1982; **Fellow:** Infectious Disease, Brigham & Womens Hosp 1984; **Fac Appt:** Assoc Prof Med, Univ Mich Med Sch

Maki, Dennis G MD [Inf] - **Spec Exp:** Urinary Tract Infections; Critical Care; **Hospital:** Univ WI Hosp & Clins; **Address:** 600 Highland Ave, H4/572, Madison, WI 53792-5158; **Phone:** 608-263-0946; **Board Cert:** Internal Medicine 1972; Infectious Disease 1974; **Med School:** Univ Wisc 1967; **Resid:** Infectious Disease, Mass Genl Hosp 1972; Internal Medicine, Harvard-Boston City Hosp 1973; **Fellow:** Infectious Disease, Mass Genl Hosp 1974; **Fac Appt:** Prof Med, Univ Wisc

Slama, Thomas MD [Inf] - **Spec Exp:** Fungal Infections; Bone Infections; Infective Endocarditis; **Hospital:** St Vincent Hosp & Hlth Svcs - Indianapolis; **Address:** 8240 Naab Rd, Ste 300, Indianapolis, IN 46260; **Phone:** 317-870-1970; **Board Cert:** Internal Medicine 1976; Infectious Disease 1978; **Med School:** India 1973; **Resid:** Internal Medicine, Indianapolis Meth Hosp 1976; **Fellow:** Infectious Disease, Ohio State Univ Hosps 1978; **Fac Appt:** Clin Prof Med, Indiana Univ

Sobel, Jack MD [Inf] - **Spec Exp:** Sexually Transmitted Diseases; Vaginitis; Fungal Infections; Urinary Tract Infections; **Hospital:** Harper Univ Hosp, Detroit Receiving Hospital; **Address:** 4201 St Antoine, POD 7B, Detroit, MI 48201; **Phone:** 313-745-9035; **Board Cert:** Internal Medicine 1978; Infectious Disease 1982; **Med School:** South Africa 1965; **Resid:** Internal Medicine 1970; **Fellow:** Infectious Disease, Univ Penn Hosps 1977; Research, Natl Inst Hlth 1978; **Fac Appt:** Prof Med, Wayne State Univ

Infectious Disease

Trenholme, Gordon MD [Inf] - **Spec Exp:** Fevers of Unknown Origin; Malaria; Tropical Diseases; **Hospital:** Rush Univ Med Ctr; **Address:** Rush/Presby-St Luke's Med Ctr, 600 S Paulina, Ste 143AAC, Chicago, IL 60612-3809; **Phone:** 312-942-3665; **Board Cert:** Internal Medicine 1972; Infectious Disease 1976; **Med School:** Med Coll Wisc 1970; **Resid:** Internal Medicine, Univ Chicago Hosp 1972; **Fellow:** Infectious Disease, Rush/Presby-St Luke's Med Ctr 1975; **Fac Appt:** Prof Med, Rush Med Coll

Wilson, Walter Ray MD [Inf] - **Spec Exp:** Musculoskeletal Infections; **Hospital:** Mayo Med Ctr & Clin - Rochester; **Address:** Mayo Clinic, Div Infectious Disease, 200 First St SW, Rochester, MN 55905; **Phone:** 507-255-7761; **Board Cert:** Internal Medicine 1973; Infectious Disease 1974; Medical Microbiology 1975; **Med School:** Baylor Coll Med 1967; **Resid:** Internal Medicine, Methodist Hosp 1968; Internal Medicine, Mayo Clinic 1973; **Fellow:** Infectious Disease, Mayo Clinic 1974; Microbiology, Mayo Clinic 1975; **Fac Appt:** Prof Med, Mayo Med Sch

Great Plains and Mountains

Cohn, David MD [Inf] - **Spec Exp:** Tuberculosis; AIDS/HIV; **Hospital:** Denver Health Med Ctr; **Address:** Denver Public Health, 605 Bannock Street, Denver, CO 80204-4507; **Phone:** 303-436-7204; **Board Cert:** Internal Medicine 1978; Infectious Disease 1982; **Med School:** Univ IL Coll Med 1975; **Resid:** Internal Medicine, Univ Wisconsin Hosp 1978; **Fellow:** Infectious Disease, Univ Colorado Hosp 1981; **Fac Appt:** Prof Med, Univ Colorado

Huitt, Gwen A MD [Inf] - **Spec Exp:** Tuberculosis; Cystic Fibrosis-Adult; Mycobacterial Infections; **Hospital:** Natl Jewish Med & Rsch Ctr; **Address:** Natl Jewish Med & Research Ctr, 1400 Jackson St, rm J222, Denver, CO 80206; **Phone:** 303-398-1700; **Board Cert:** Internal Medicine 2003; Infectious Disease 2004; **Med School:** Univ Colorado 1988; **Resid:** Internal Medicine, Univ Colorado Hlth Sci Ctr 1991; **Fellow:** Infectious Disease, Univ Colorado Hlth Sci Ctr 1993; **Fac Appt:** Assoc Prof Med, Univ Colorado

Southwest

DuPont, Herbert L MD [Inf] - **Spec Exp:** Tropical Diseases; Diarrheal Diseases; Travel Medicine; **Hospital:** St Luke's Episcopal Hosp - Houston; **Address:** 6720 Bertner Ave, MC 1-164, Houston, TX 77030-1602; **Phone:** 832-355-4122; **Board Cert:** Internal Medicine 1972; **Med School:** Emory Univ 1965; **Resid:** Internal Medicine, Univ Minn Hosps 1967; **Fellow:** Infectious Disease, Univ Maryland Hosp 1969; **Fac Appt:** Prof Med, Baylor Coll Med

Keiser, Philip MD [Inf] - **Spec Exp:** AIDS/HIV; **Hospital:** UT Southwestern Med Ctr - Dallas; **Address:** 1936 Amelia, Dallas, TX 75235-9173; **Phone:** 214-590-5647; **Board Cert:** Internal Medicine 1989; Infectious Disease 1992; **Med School:** Univ MD Sch Med 1986; **Resid:** Internal Medicine, Francis Scott Key Med Ctr 1989; **Fellow:** Infectious Disease, Univ Maryland 1989; **Fac Appt:** Assoc Prof Med, Univ Tex SW, Dallas

Kimbrough, Robert MD [Inf] - **Spec Exp:** Fungal Infections; Endocarditis; Bone Infections; **Hospital:** Univ Med Ctr - Lubbock; **Address:** Tex Tech Univ Hlth Scis Ctr, Dept IM Div Inf Dis- 3601 4th St, Lubbock, TX 79430-0001; **Phone:** 806-743-3155; **Board Cert:** Internal Medicine 1977; Infectious Disease 1978; **Med School:** Univ Kans 1969; **Resid:** Internal Medicine, Baylor Affil Hosp 1973; **Fellow:** Infectious Disease, Baylor Univ 1974; Infectious Disease, Oreg Hlth Sci Univ 1975; **Fac Appt:** Prof Med, Texas Tech Univ

Luby, James P MD [Inf] - **Spec Exp:** Viral Infections; **Hospital:** Parkland Meml Hosp - Dallas, UT Southwestern Med Ctr - Dallas; **Address:** Univ Tex SW Med Ctr, Div Inf Dis, 5323 Harry Hines Blvd, Y7.218A, Dallas, TX 75390-9113; **Phone:** 214-648-3480; **Board Cert:** Internal Medicine 1968; Infectious Disease 1972; **Med School:** Northwestern Univ 1961; **Resid:** Internal Medicine, Northwestern Univ 1964; **Fac Appt:** Prof Med, Univ Tex SW, Dallas

Patterson, Jan E Evans MD [Inf] - **Spec Exp:** Hospital Acquired Infections; Antibiotic Resistance; **Hospital:** Univ Hlth Sys - Univ Hosp; **Address:** Univ Tex Hlth Sci Ctr, Dept Med, 7703 Floyd Curl Drive, San Antonio, TX 78229-3900; **Phone:** 210-592-0340; **Board Cert:** Internal Medicine 1985; Infectious Disease 1988; **Med School:** Univ Tex, Houston 1982; **Resid:** Internal Medicine, Vanderbilt Univ Hosp 1985; **Fellow:** Infectious Disease, Yale-New Haven Hosp 1988; **Fac Appt:** Prof Med, Univ Tex, San Antonio

Patterson, Thomas F MD [Inf] - **Spec Exp:** Fungal Infections; **Hospital:** Univ Hlth Sys - Univ Hosp; **Address:** Univ Texas HSC, Dept Medicine, Div Infectious Dis, 7703 Floyd Curl Drive, MC 7881, San Antonio, TX 78229-3900; **Phone:** 210-567-4823; **Board Cert:** Internal Medicine 1986; Infectious Disease 1988; **Med School:** Univ Tex, Houston 1983; **Resid:** Internal Medicine, Vanderbilt Univ Hosp 1985; Internal Medicine, Yale-New Haven Hosp 1986; **Fellow:** Infectious Disease, Yale-New Haven Hosp 1989; **Fac Appt:** Prof Med, Univ Tex, San Antonio

Wallace Jr, Richard James MD [Inf] - **Spec Exp:** Non Tuberculous Mycobacteria; Nocardia Infection; **Hospital:** UT Hlth Ctr at Tyler; **Address:** University of Texas Health Ctr, 11937 US Hwy 271, Tyler, TX 75708; **Phone:** 903-877-5122; **Board Cert:** Internal Medicine 1975; Infectious Disease 1976; **Med School:** Baylor Coll Med 1972; **Resid:** Internal Medicine, Boston City Hosp 1974; **Fellow:** Infectious Disease, Boston City Hosp 1975; Infectious Disease, Baylor Coll Med 1977

Westerman, Eric L MD [Inf] - **Spec Exp:** Rickettsial Diseases; Bone/Joint Infections; Staphylococcal Infections; **Hospital:** Methodist Hosp - Houston, St Luke's Episcopal Hosp - Houston; **Address:** 6550 Fannin St, Ste 1001, Smith Tower, Houston, TX 77030; **Phone:** 713-441-6360; **Board Cert:** Internal Medicine 1975; Infectious Disease 1980; **Med School:** Baylor Coll Med 1972; **Resid:** Internal Medicine, Baylor Affil Hosps 1974; **Fellow:** Infectious Disease, Methodist Hosp 1976; **Fac Appt:** Assoc Prof Med, Baylor Coll Med

West Coast and Pacific

Ballon-Landa, Gonzalo MD [Inf] - **Spec Exp:** Hospital Acquired Infections; AIDS/HIV; Travel Medicine; **Hospital:** Scripps Mercy Hosp & Med Ctr; **Address:** 4136 Bachman Pl, San Diego, CA 92103; **Phone:** 619-298-1443; **Board Cert:** Internal Medicine 1980; Infectious Disease 1984; **Med School:** Northwestern Univ 1977; **Resid:** Internal Medicine, Evanston Hosp 1981; **Fellow:** Infectious Disease, UCSD Med Ctr 1983

Bayer, Arnold Sander MD [Inf] - **Spec Exp:** Infective Endocarditis; Arthritis-Septic; Coccidioidomycosis; **Hospital:** LAC - Harbor - UCLA Med Ctr, UCLA Med Ctr; **Address:** 1124 W Carson St Bldg RB2 Fl 2, Torrance, CA 90502; **Phone:** 310-222-3813; **Board Cert:** Internal Medicine 1973; Infectious Disease 1978; **Med School:** Temple Univ 1970; **Resid:** Internal Medicine, Thomas Jefferson Univ Hosp 1972; Internal Medicine, LAC-Harbor UCLA Med Ctr 1974; **Fellow:** Infectious Disease, VA Med Ctr 1976; Infectious Disease, LAC-Harbor UCLA Med Ctr 1977; **Fac Appt:** Prof Med, UCLA

Infectious Disease

Corey, Lawrence MD [Inf] - **Spec Exp:** Viral Infections; AIDS/HIV; **Hospital:** Univ Wash Med Ctr; **Address:** Fred Hutchinson Cancer Ctr, 1100 Fairview Ave N, Ste LE-500, Seattle, WA 98109; **Phone:** 206-667-6702; **Board Cert:** Internal Medicine 1974; **Med School:** Univ Mich Med Sch 1971; **Resid:** Internal Medicine, Univ Mich Med Ctr 1973; **Fellow:** Infectious Disease, Univ Wash Hosp 1977; **Fac Appt:** Prof Med, Univ Wash

Edwards Jr, John Ellis MD [Inf] - **Spec Exp:** Fungal Infections; Infections in Immunocompromised Patients; **Hospital:** LAC - Harbor - UCLA Med Ctr; **Address:** 1124 W Carson St RB2 Bldg Fl 2, Torrance, CA 90502; **Phone:** 310-222-3813; **Board Cert:** Internal Medicine 1980; Infectious Disease 1974; **Med School:** UC Irvine 1968; **Resid:** Internal Medicine, Harbor-UCLA Med Ctr 1971; **Fellow:** Infectious Disease, Harbor-UCLA Med Ctr 1973; **Fac Appt:** Prof Med, UCLA

Hollander, Harry MD [Inf] - **Spec Exp:** AIDS/HIV; **Hospital:** UCSF Med Ctr; **Address:** 400 Parnassus Ave Fl 4th, Box 0378, San Francisco, CA 94143; **Phone:** 415-353-2119; **Board Cert:** Internal Medicine 1983; Infectious Disease 1988; **Med School:** Univ Pennsylvania 1980; **Resid:** Internal Medicine, UCSF Med Ctr 1983; **Fac Appt:** Clin Prof Med, UCSF

Holmes, King K MD [Inf] - **Spec Exp:** AIDS/HIV; Sexually Transmitted Diseases; **Hospital:** Harborview Med Ctr; **Address:** Harborview Med Ctr, 325 Ninth Ave, Box 359931, Seattle, WA 98104; **Phone:** 206-731-4239; **Board Cert:** Internal Medicine 1971; Infectious Disease 1974; **Med School:** Cornell Univ-Weill Med Coll 1963; **Resid:** Internal Medicine, Univ Wash Med Ctr 1969; **Fellow:** Infectious Disease, Univ Wash Med Ctr 1970; **Fac Appt:** Prof Med, Univ Wash

Richman, Douglas MD [Inf] - **Spec Exp:** AIDS/HIV; **Hospital:** VA San Diego Hlthcre Sys, UCSD Med Ctr; **Address:** UCSD-Stein Clin Rsch Bldg, 9500 Gilman, MC 0679, La Jolla, CA 92093-0679; **Phone:** 858-552-7439; **Board Cert:** Internal Medicine 1973; Infectious Disease 1976; **Med School:** Stanford Univ 1970; **Resid:** Internal Medicine, Stanford Univ Hosp 1972; **Fellow:** Infectious Disease, NIAID/NIH 1975; Infectious Disease, Beth Israel/Chldns Hosp-Harvard 1976; **Fac Appt:** Prof Med, UCSD

Schooley, Robert T MD [Inf] - **Spec Exp:** AIDS/HIV; Infectious Disease; **Hospital:** UCSD Med Ctr; **Address:** UCSD - Stein Rsch Bldg, rm 401, MC 071, 9500 Gilman Drive, La Jolla, CA 92023-0665; **Phone:** 858-822-0216; **Board Cert:** Internal Medicine 1977; **Med School:** Johns Hopkins Univ 1974; **Resid:** Internal Medicine, Johns Hopkins Hosp 1976; **Fellow:** Infectious Disease, Natl Inst Hlth 1979; Infectious Disease, Mass Genl Hosp 1981; **Fac Appt:** Prof Med, UCSD

Wiviott, Lory David MD [Inf] - **Spec Exp:** AIDS/HIV; **Hospital:** CA Pacific Med Ctr - Pacific Campus, CA Pacific Med Ctr - Davies Campus; **Address:** 2100 Webster St, Ste 400, San Francisco, CA 94115; **Phone:** 415-923-3883; **Board Cert:** Internal Medicine 1986; Infectious Disease 2000; **Med School:** Albert Einstein Coll Med 1982; **Resid:** Internal Medicine, Columbia Presby Med Ctr 1985; **Fellow:** Infectious Disease, UCSF Med Ctr 1989; **Fac Appt:** Asst Clin Prof Med, UCSF

Yoshikawa, Thomas T MD [Inf] - **Spec Exp:** Infections in the Elderly; **Hospital:** LAC - King/Drew Med Ctr; **Address:** 12012 S Compton Ave, Ste 3-212, Los Angeles, CA 90059; **Phone:** 310-668-4967; **Board Cert:** Internal Medicine 1971; Infectious Disease 1974; **Med School:** Univ Mich Med Sch 1966; **Resid:** Internal Medicine, Harbor Genl Hosp 1970; **Fellow:** Infectious Disease, Harbor Genl Hosp 1972; **Fac Appt:** Prof Med, Charles Drew Univ Med & Sci

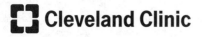
Cleveland Clinic

Infectious Disease

The mission of the Cleveland Clinic Department of Infectious Disease is to provide all patients with the most technologically advanced, compassionate medical care available anywhere. We diagnose and treat patients with a wide range of both opportunistic and acquired infections. The Department is an integral part of Cleveland Clinic, a not-for-profit multispecialty academic medical center ranked by *U.S.News & World Report* as one of the nation's best hospitals.

We provide around-the-clock inpatient care, including three general infectious disease consultation services as well as dedicated solid organ transplant, bone marrow transplant, cardiothoracic intensive care and medical/surgical intensive infectious disease services. The Department also operates several specialty outpatient clinics. Both services are designed to provide patients with optimal care, while supporting research and education initiatives. The Department's outpatient subspecialty clinics include:

Granuloma Clinic

Granulomas are tumor-like masses often caused by tissue infections. One of the most common types of infections that cause granulomatous disease in Northeast Ohio is histoplasmosis. Granulomas are non-cancerous, but many types require special care because they can spread from person to person. Tuberculosis is an example of a contagious and potentially fatal granuloma. Other conditions treated by Cleveland Clinic's Granuloma Clinic include coccidoidmycosis, cyptococcosis and mycobacterial avium-intracellulare complex.

Endocarditis Clinic

Endocarditis is an inflammation of the endocardium, or the inner lining of the heart and the heart valves. The disease is most commonly caused by a bacterial pathogen but can be due to fungal pathogens as well. Major symptoms of bacterial endocarditis include fever, fatigue, heart murmur, enlarged spleen and areas of tissue death. In addition to bacterial endocarditis, Cleveland Clinic's Endocarditis Clinic also treats infections of the endocardium caused by cardiac devices, grafts or implants.

HIV/AIDS Clinic

This specialty clinic provides care and support for patients infected with the human immunodeficiency virus, or HIV. This virus attacks the immune system, weakening a person's ability to fight infections and cancer.

International Traveler's Health Clinic

This specialty clinic provides pre-travel health and safety advice to anyone planning to journey abroad. All vaccinations and prescription medications necessary to facilitate safe travel are administered or prescribed. The International Traveler's Health Clinic also provides a comprehensive itinerary review, developing individualized packets of information for every client. Post-travel evaluation is available as needed.

Outpatient Parenteral Antimicrobal Therapy Program

This program works with patients receiving intravenous treatments for serious infections while living at home or outside a hospital setting. We play an integral role in the managing this program, which has one of the highest volumes of any center in the United States.

To schedule an appointment or for more information about the Cleveland Clinic Department of Infectious Disease, call 800.890.2467 or visit www.clevelandclinic.org/infectioustopdocs.

Department of Infectious Disease | 9500 Euclid Avenue / W14 | Cleveland OH 44195

NYU Medical Center

550 First Avenue (at 31st Street)
New York, NY 10016
Physician Referral:
(888)7-NYU-MED (888-769-8633)
www.nyumc.org

INFECTIOUS DISEASES

Developing effective treatment for infectious diseases is among the miracles of last century's science, but today we are faced with deadly new infections and old ones that were never tamed. These and the rapidly emerging problem of resistance to antobiotics place the study and treatment of infectious diseases (ID) at the forefront of modern medicine.

NYU's ID doctors are actively engaged in research at the laboratory bench and in clinical trials of new antibiotics and other anti-infective strategies..

• A novel program, Population Biology of Infectious Diseases, combines these laboratory and clinical studies with epidemiology and genetics

• The NYU AIDS Clinical Trials Unit is one of the most productive among the 35 such centers nationally. Supported by the National Institutes of Health the NYU unit has played a leading role in drug development and delivering the very latest care to patients with this increasingly controllable infection.

• NYU doctors are deeply involved in local and international research into the early diagnosis, treatment and prevention of such chronic infections as tuberculosis and Helicobacter (the bacteria associated with stomach ulcers)..

• Using lessons learned in their research, NYU ID doctors are actively involved in management of complicated bone and joint infections, prevention of infection in cancer and transplant patients, and developing strategies for managing hepatitis B and C.

• NYU's Department of Medical and Molecular Parasitology, working alongside the Division of Infectious Diseases, is active internationally in bringing malaria and other parasitic diseases under control.

Internal Medicine

A personal physician who provides long-term, comprehensive care in the office and the hospital, managing both common and complex illness of adolescents, adults and the elderly. Internists are trained in the diagnosis and treatment of cancer, infections and diseases affecting the heart, blood, kidneys, joints and digestive, respiratory and vascular systems. They are also trained in the essentials of primary care internal medicine which incorporates an understanding of disease prevention, wellness, substance abuse, mental health and effective treatment of common problems of the eyes, ears, skin, nervous system and reproductive organs.

Note: *Internal Medicine normally includes many primary care physicians. However, for purposes of this directory, no primary care physicians are included.*

Training Required: Three years

Internal Medicine

New England

Barry, Michele MD [IM] - **Spec Exp:** Travel Medicine; Tropical Diseases; **Hospital:** Yale - New Haven Hosp; **Address:** 333 Cedar St, PO Box 208025, New Haven, CT 06520-8025; **Phone:** 203-688-2476; **Board Cert:** Internal Medicine 1980; **Med School:** Albert Einstein Coll Med 1977; **Resid:** Internal Medicine, Yale-New Haven Hosp 1981; **Fellow:** Rheumatology, Yale-New Haven Hosp 1981; Tropical Medicine, Walter Reed AMC 1981; **Fac Appt:** Prof Med, Yale Univ

Beaser, Richard S MD [IM] - **Spec Exp:** Diabetes; Endocrinology; **Hospital:** Beth Israel Deaconess Med Ctr - Boston; **Address:** Joslin Clinic, 1 Joslin Pl, Boston, MA 02215; **Phone:** 617-732-2675; **Board Cert:** Internal Medicine 1980; **Med School:** Boston Univ 1977; **Resid:** Internal Medicine, Mass Med Ctr 1980; **Fellow:** Endocrinology, Diabetes & Metabolism, Joslin Clinic 1981; **Fac Appt:** Assoc Clin Prof Med, Harvard Med Sch

Billings, J Andrew MD [IM] - **Spec Exp:** Palliative Care; Pain Management; **Hospital:** Mass Genl Hosp; **Address:** 55 Fruit St, FND 600, Boston, MA 02114; **Phone:** 617-724-9197; **Board Cert:** Internal Medicine 1975; **Med School:** Harvard Med Sch 1972; **Resid:** Internal Medicine, Univ California Hosps 1975; **Fellow:** Internal Medicine, Mass Genl Hosp 1977; **Fac Appt:** Assoc Prof Med, Harvard Med Sch

Mid Atlantic

Braunstein, Seth N MD/PhD [IM] - **Spec Exp:** Diabetes; **Hospital:** Hosp Univ Penn - UPHS (page 72); **Address:** Hosp of Univ Penn, Diabetes Ctr, 3400 Spruce St, 4 Penn Twr, Philadelphia, PA 19104-4219; **Phone:** 215-662-2468; **Board Cert:** Internal Medicine 1975; **Med School:** NYU Sch Med 1972; **Resid:** Internal Medicine, Hosp Univ Penn 1975; **Fac Appt:** Assoc Prof Med, Univ Pennsylvania

Cirigliano, Michael D MD [IM] - **Spec Exp:** Complementary Medicine; Women's Health; **Hospital:** Hosp Univ Penn - UPHS (page 72); **Address:** Penn Internal Med Practice, UPHS, 3701 Market St, Ste 741, Philadelphia, PA 19104; **Phone:** 215-349-5200; **Board Cert:** Internal Medicine 2005; **Med School:** Univ Pennsylvania 1990; **Resid:** Internal Medicine, Hosp Univ Penn 1993; **Fac Appt:** Assoc Prof Med, Univ Pennsylvania

Fisher, Laura MD [IM] - **Spec Exp:** Preventive Medicine; Lyme Disease; Women's Health; **Hospital:** NY-Presby Hosp/Weill Cornell (page 66); **Address:** 1385 York Ave, New York, NY 10021; **Phone:** 212-717-5920; **Board Cert:** Internal Medicine 1987; **Med School:** Brown Univ 1984; **Resid:** Internal Medicine, NY Hosp-Cornell Med Ctr 1987; **Fellow:** Infectious Disease, Mass Genl Hosp 1989; **Fac Appt:** Asst Clin Prof Med, Cornell Univ-Weill Med Coll

Galland, Leopold MD [IM] - **Spec Exp:** Nutrition; Chronic Disease; **Address:** 133 E 73rd St, Ste 308, New York, NY 10021-3556; **Phone:** 212-772-3077; **Board Cert:** Internal Medicine 1972; **Med School:** NYU Sch Med 1968; **Resid:** Internal Medicine, Bellevue Hosp 1972; **Fellow:** Behavioral Medicine, Univ Conn Hlth Ctr 1981

Legato, Marianne J MD [IM] - **Spec Exp:** Cardiovascular Disease; Women's Health; Gender Specific Medicine; **Hospital:** NY-Presby Hosp/Columbia (page 66), St Luke's - Roosevelt Hosp Ctr - Roosevelt Div; **Address:** 962 Park Ave, New York, NY 10028-2433; **Phone:** 212-737-5663; **Board Cert:** Internal Medicine 2003; **Med School:** NYU Sch Med 1962; **Resid:** Internal Medicine, Columbia-Presby Med Ctr 1965; **Fellow:** Cardiovascular Disease, Columbia-Presby Med Ctr 1968; **Fac Appt:** Prof Emeritus Med, Columbia P&S

Nash, David B MD [IM] - **Spec Exp:** Preventive Medicine; **Hospital:** Thomas Jefferson Univ Hosp; **Address:** Thomas Jefferson Univ Hospital, 1015 Walnut St Curtis Bldg - rm 115, Philadelphia, PA 19107; **Phone:** 215-955-6180; **Board Cert:** Internal Medicine 1985; **Med School:** Univ Rochester 1981; **Resid:** Internal Medicine, Grady Hosp 1984; **Fellow:** RWJoghnson Rfd Clin 1986; **Fac Appt:** Prof Med, Thomas Jefferson Univ

Rader, Daniel J MD [IM] - **Spec Exp:** Cholesterol/Lipid Disorders; Preventive Cardiology; Metabolic Disorders; **Hospital:** Hosp Univ Penn - UPHS (page 72), Penn Presby Med Ctr - UPHS (page 72); **Address:** Univ Penn-UPHS, 52 N 39th St, PHI-2A, Philadelphia, PA 19104; **Phone:** 215-662-9993; **Board Cert:** Internal Medicine 1987; **Med School:** Med Coll PA Hahnemann 1984; **Resid:** Internal Medicine, Yale-New Haven Hosp 1987; **Fellow:** Research, Natl Inst Hlth 1992; **Fac Appt:** Prof Med, Univ Pennsylvania

Rivlin, Richard S MD [IM] - **Spec Exp:** Cancer Prevention; Nutrition & Cancer Prevention; Endocrinology & Thyroid Disease; **Hospital:** NY-Presby Hosp/Weill Cornell (page 66); **Address:** Anne Fisher Nutrition Ctr, Strang Cancer Prevention Ctr, 428 E 72nd St, Ste 600, New York, NY 10021; **Phone:** 212-794-4900 x152; **Board Cert:** Internal Medicine 1969; **Med School:** Harvard Med Sch 1959; **Resid:** Internal Medicine, Bellevue Hosp 1960; Internal Medicine, Johns Hopkins Hosp 1961; **Fellow:** Endocrinology, Diabetes & Metabolism, Natl Inst Hlth 1963; Biochemistry, Johns Hopkins Hosp 1966; **Fac Appt:** Prof Med, Cornell Univ-Weill Med Coll

Selwyn, Peter MD [IM] - **Spec Exp:** AIDS/HIV; Addiction/Substance Abuse; Palliative Care; **Hospital:** Montefiore Med Ctr; **Address:** Montfiore Med Ctr, 3544 Jerome Ave, Bronx, NY 10467; **Phone:** 718-920-4678; **Board Cert:** Family Medicine 1998; **Med School:** Harvard Med Sch 1981; **Resid:** Family Medicine, Montefiore Med Ctr 1984; **Fac Appt:** Prof Med, Albert Einstein Coll Med

Yaffe, Bruce MD [IM] - **Spec Exp:** Gastroscopy; Colonoscopy; **Hospital:** Lenox Hill Hosp (page 62); **Address:** 201 E 65th St, New York, NY 10021-6701; **Phone:** 212-879-4700; **Board Cert:** Internal Medicine 1979; Gastroenterology 1981; **Med School:** Geo Wash Univ 1976; **Resid:** Internal Medicine, Mount Sinai Hosp 1979; Hepatology, Mount Sinai Hosp 1980; **Fellow:** Gastroenterology, Lenox Hill Hosp 1982

Southeast

Carey, Timothy S MD [IM] - **Hospital:** Univ NC Hosps; **Address:** Cecil G Sheps Ctr for Hlth Svcs, 725 Martin Luther King Blvd, CB-7590, Chapel Hill, NC 27599-7590; **Phone:** 919-966-7100; **Board Cert:** Internal Medicine 1979; **Med School:** Univ VT Coll Med 1976; **Resid:** Internal Medicine, Pacific Med Ctr 1979; **Fellow:** Internal Medicine, Univ NC Hosp 1985; **Fac Appt:** Prof Med, Univ NC Sch Med

Corbett Jr, Eugene C MD [IM] - **Spec Exp:** Nutrition; Diabetes; **Hospital:** Univ Virginia Med Ctr; **Address:** Univ VA Hlth Sys, Dept Med, PO Box 800901, Charlottesville, VA 22908; **Phone:** 434-924-1685; **Board Cert:** Internal Medicine 1987; **Med School:** Univ Chicago-Pritzker Sch Med 1970; **Resid:** Internal Medicine, Baltimore City Hosp 1975; **Fellow:** Research, Johns Hopkins Hosp 1975; **Fac Appt:** Assoc Prof Med, Univ VA Sch Med

Cushman, William C MD [IM] - **Spec Exp:** Hypertension; Preventive Cardiology; Cholesterol/Lipid Disorders; **Hospital:** VA Med Ctr - Memphis; **Address:** VA Medical Ctr, 1030 Jefferson Ave, MC 111Q, Memphis, TN 38104-2127; **Phone:** 901-523-8990 x6605; **Board Cert:** Internal Medicine 1977; **Med School:** Univ Miss 1974; **Resid:** Internal Medicine, Univ Mississippi Med Ctr 1977; **Fac Appt:** Prof Med, Univ Tenn Coll Med, Memphis

Heimburger, Douglas C MD [IM] - **Spec Exp:** Nutrition & Disease Prevention/Control; Nutrition & Cancer Prevention; **Hospital:** Univ of Ala Hosp at Birmingham, VA Med Ctr; **Address:** Univ Alabama, Dept Nutrition Sci & Med, 1675 University Blvd, Webb 439, Birmingham, AL 35294-3360; **Phone:** 205-934-7058; **Board Cert:** Internal Medicine 1981; **Med School:** Vanderbilt Univ 1978; **Resid:** Internal Medicine, Washington Univ Hosps 1981; **Fellow:** Nutrition, Univ Alabama Med Ctr 1982

Midwest

Sarosi, George MD [IM] - **Spec Exp:** Infections-Respiratory; Fungal Lung Disease; Diagnostic Problems; **Hospital:** VA Med Ctr - Indianapolis; **Address:** VA Medical Center, ATTN: Medicine 111, 1481 W 10th St, Indianapolis, IN 46202-2803; **Phone:** 317-988-2501; **Board Cert:** Internal Medicine 1970; **Med School:** Harvard Med Sch 1964; **Resid:** Internal Medicine, Univ Minnesota Hosp 1968; **Fac Appt:** Prof Med, Indiana Univ

Weder, Alan B MD [IM] - **Spec Exp:** Hypertension; Renovascular Disease; Peripheral Vascular Disease; Carotid Artery Disease; **Hospital:** Univ Michigan Hlth Sys; **Address:** Univ Mich, Div Cardiovascular Med, 24 Frank Lloyd Wright Drive, Box 322, Ann Arbor, MI 48106-0739; **Phone:** 734-998-7956; **Board Cert:** Internal Medicine 1978; **Med School:** Hahnemann Univ 1975; **Resid:** Internal Medicine, Univ Chicago Hosp 1978; **Fac Appt:** Prof Med, Univ Mich Med Sch

Wright Jr, Jackson T MD [IM] - **Spec Exp:** Hypertension; **Hospital:** Univ Hosps Case Med Ctr; **Address:** Univ Hosps of Cleveland, Div Hypertension, 11100 Euclid Ave, Bolwell Bldg Fl 2nd - rm 2200, Cleveland, OH 44106; **Phone:** 216-844-5174; **Board Cert:** Internal Medicine 1980; **Med School:** Univ Pittsburgh 1976; **Resid:** Internal Medicine, Univ Michigan Hosps 1987; **Fellow:** Pharmacology, Univ Health Ctr 1980; **Fac Appt:** Prof Med, Case West Res Univ

Great Plains and Mountains

Mehler, Philip S MD [IM] - **Spec Exp:** Eating Disorders; Substance Abuse; Preventive Medicine; **Hospital:** Denver Health Med Ctr; **Address:** Denver Health Med Ctr, 777 Bannock St, MC 0278, Denver, CO 80204; **Phone:** 303-436-3234; **Board Cert:** Internal Medicine 1989; **Med School:** Univ Colorado 1983; **Resid:** Internal Medicine, Univ Colorado Affil Hosp 1987; **Fac Appt:** Prof Med, Univ Colorado

Southwest

Wolff, Robert A MD [IM] - **Spec Exp:** Gastrointestinal Cancer; Pancreatic Cancer; Colon & Rectal Cancer; Clinical Trials; **Hospital:** UT MD Anderson Cancer Ctr (page 71); **Address:** MD Anderson Cancer Ctr, Faculty Center Unit 426, Box 301402, Houston, TX 77230; **Phone:** 713-745-5476; **Board Cert:** Internal Medicine 1989; **Med School:** Albany Med Coll 1986; **Resid:** Internal Medicine, Duke Univ Med Ctr 1989; **Fellow:** Hematology & Oncology, Duke Univ Med Ctr 1992; **Fac Appt:** Assoc Prof Med, Univ Tenn Coll Med, Memphis

West Coast and Pacific

Bissell Jr, Dwight M MD [IM] - **Spec Exp:** Porphyria; **Hospital:** UCSF Med Ctr; **Address:** UCSF Med Ctr, Dept Gastroenterology, 350 Parnassus Ave, rm 410, Box 0657, San Francisco, CA 94143; **Phone:** 415-353-2318; **Board Cert:** Internal Medicine 1974; **Med School:** Harvard Med Sch 1967; **Resid:** Internal Medicine, Boston City Hosp-Harvard 1970; **Fellow:** Gastroenterology, UCSF Med Ctr 1973; **Fac Appt:** Prof Med, UCSF

Daar, Eric S MD [IM] - **Spec Exp:** AIDS/HIV; Infectious Disease; **Hospital:** LAC - Harbor - UCLA Med Ctr; **Address:** 1000 W Carson St, Box 449, Torrance, CA 90502; **Phone:** 310-222-2467; **Board Cert:** Internal Medicine 1988; **Med School:** Georgetown Univ 1985; **Resid:** Internal Medicine, Cedars-Sinai Med Ctr 1988; **Fellow:** Infectious Disease, Cedars-Sinai Med Ctr 1991

NYU Medical Center

550 First Avenue (at 31st Street)
New York, NY 10016
Physician Referral:
(888)7-NYU-MED (888-769-8633)
www.nyumc.org

INTERNAL MEDICINE

Famous equally for cutting-edge research and for nurturing lifelong physician-patient relationships, the Internal Medicine physicians of NYU are dedicated to treating the whole patient. NYU internists meet the highest standards of the medical profession, addressing physical, social, and psychological aspects of health and disease. Here, experts in very specialized areas of medicine provide state-of-the-art care that brings the latest developments from the laboratory to the care of patients with rare or difficult diseases. In addition, the Division of General Medicine attracts internists whose passion is the care of patients with multiple problems and who specialize in keeping people healthy. The research interests of our doctors span molecular biology, and the social aspects of medicine such as epidemiology and behavioral medicine that guide good clinical decision-making. These and other skills are actively brought to the service of patient care every day.

Below are just a few of the many services offered by the NYU team:

• Primary health care, including physical examinations.
• Specialized care of illnesses involving the heart, lungs gastrointestinal tract, joints, bones, muscles, endocrine organs, and kidneys.
• Comprehensive womenís health care, from obstetric and gynecologic needs to osteoporosis prevention and treatment
• Geriatric care by experts with special interest and training in the particular circumstances of older people
• A wide range of laboratory, imaging, and advanced diagnostic testingófrom a something as simple as a throat culture to complex mapping of the electrical surface of the heart.
• Guidance and treatment for substance abuse, eating disorders and obesity, and high cholesterol.

NYU MEDICAL CENTER

The physicians of the Division of Internal Medicine at NYU Medical Center treat the full spectrum of conditions, from addiction to rheumatoid arthritis, in an environment that is steeped in NYU's tradition of excellence and a dedication to state-of-the-art patient care and research. This application of world-class science to bedside medicine is enhanced by interdisciplinary collaboration between departments and physicians, demonstrative of NYU Medical Center's professionalism and dedication to teamwork and collegiality.

Physician Referral
(888) 7-NYU-MED
(888-769-8633)
www.nyumc.org

691

Sponsored Page

Maternal & Fetal Medicine

a subspecialty of Obstetrics & Gynecology

An obstetrician/gynecologist possesses special knowledge, skills and professional capability in the medical and surgical care of the female reproductive system and associated disorders. This physician serves as a consultant to other physicians and as a primary physician for women.

Training Required: Four years *plus* two years in clinical practice before certification in obstetrics and gynecology is complete *plus* additional training and examination in maternal-fetal medicine.

Maternal & Fetal Medicine

New England

Acker, David B MD [MF] - **Spec Exp:** Multiple Gestation; Pregnancy-High Risk; **Hospital:** Brigham & Women's Hosp; **Address:** Brigham & Womens Hosp, Dept Ob/Gyn, 75 Francis St, ASB1-3, Boston, MA 02115-6110; **Phone:** 617-732-5445; **Board Cert:** Obstetrics & Gynecology 2005; Maternal & Fetal Medicine 2005; **Med School:** NYU Sch Med 1968; **Resid:** Obstetrics & Gynecology, Einstein Affil Hosp 1971; Obstetrics & Gynecology, Vanderbilt Univ Affil Hosp 1974; **Fellow:** Maternal & Fetal Medicine, Boston Lying-In Hosp 1979; **Fac Appt:** Assoc Prof ObG, Harvard Med Sch

Baker, Emily MD [MF] - **Spec Exp:** Ultrasound; **Hospital:** Dartmouth - Hitchcock Med Ctr; **Address:** Darthmouth-Hitchcock Med Ctr, Dept Ob/Gyn, One Medical Center Drive, Desk 5L, Lebanon, NH 03756; **Phone:** 603-653-9306; **Board Cert:** Obstetrics & Gynecology 2003; Maternal & Fetal Medicine 2003; **Med School:** Stanford Univ 1986; **Resid:** Obstetrics & Gynecology, Univ Chicago Hosps 1990; Maternal & Fetal Medicine, Univ Washington Med Ctr 1991; **Fellow:** Maternal & Fetal Medicine, St Margaret's Hosp-Tufts Univ 1992; **Fac Appt:** Assoc Prof ObG, Dartmouth Med Sch

Copel, Joshua MD [MF] - **Spec Exp:** Prenatal Diagnosis; Fetal Echocardiography; Pregnancy-High Risk; **Hospital:** Yale - New Haven Hosp; **Address:** Yale Univ Sch Med, Dept OB/GYN, 333 Cedar St, Box 208063, New Haven, CT 06520-3206; **Phone:** 203-785-5862; **Board Cert:** Obstetrics & Gynecology 2006; Maternal & Fetal Medicine 2006; **Med School:** Tufts Univ 1979; **Resid:** Obstetrics & Gynecology, Pennsylvania Hosp 1983; **Fellow:** Maternal & Fetal Medicine, Yale-New Haven Hosp 1985; **Fac Appt:** Prof ObG, Yale Univ

Frigoletto, Fredric D MD [MF] - **Spec Exp:** Ultrasound; Prenatal Diagnosis; Pregnancy-High Risk; **Hospital:** Mass Genl Hosp; **Address:** 55 Fruit St, Bldg FND416, Boston, MA 02114; **Phone:** 617-724-3775; **Board Cert:** Maternal & Fetal Medicine 1975; Obstetrics & Gynecology 1969; **Med School:** Boston Univ 1962; **Resid:** Surgery, Boston City Hosp 1964; Obstetrics & Gynecology, Boston Women's Hosp 1967; **Fac Appt:** Prof ObG, Harvard Med Sch

Greene, Michael F MD [MF] - **Spec Exp:** Pregnancy-High Risk; Multiple Gestation; Seizure Disorders & Pregnancy; **Hospital:** Mass Genl Hosp; **Address:** Mass Genl Hosp, Dept Ob/Gyn, 55 Fruit St Yawkey Bldg - rm 4F, Boston, MA 02114; **Phone:** 617-724-2229; **Board Cert:** Obstetrics & Gynecology 1997; Maternal & Fetal Medicine 1997; **Med School:** SUNY Downstate 1976; **Resid:** Obstetrics & Gynecology, Boston Hosp Women 1980; **Fellow:** Maternal & Fetal Medicine, Brigham Hosp Women 1982; **Fac Appt:** Prof ObG, Harvard Med Sch

Heffner, Linda MD/PhD [MF] - **Spec Exp:** Pregnancy-Advanced Maternal Age; Pregnancy-High Risk; **Hospital:** Boston Med Ctr, Brigham & Women's Hosp; **Address:** 85 E Concord St Fl 6, Boston, MA 02118; **Phone:** 617-414-5175; **Board Cert:** Obstetrics & Gynecology 1998; Maternal & Fetal Medicine 1998; **Med School:** Johns Hopkins Univ 1977; **Resid:** Obstetrics & Gynecology, Hosp Univ Penn 1983; **Fellow:** Maternal & Fetal Medicine, Brigham-Womens Hosp 1987; **Fac Appt:** Prof ObG, Boston Univ

Lockwood, Charles MD [MF] - **Spec Exp:** Prematurity Prevention; Miscarriage-Recurrent; Multiple Gestation; **Hospital:** Yale - New Haven Hosp; **Address:** Yale Univ Sch Med, Dept Ob-Gyn, 333 Cedar St, rm FMB 335, New Haven, CT 06520-8063; **Phone:** 203-737-2970; **Board Cert:** Obstetrics & Gynecology 1997; Maternal & Fetal Medicine 1997; **Med School:** Univ Pennsylvania 1981; **Resid:** Obstetrics & Gynecology, Pennsylvania Hosp 1985; **Fellow:** Maternal & Fetal Medicine, Yale-New Haven Hosp 1987; Thrombosis, Mt Sinai Med Ctr 1991; **Fac Appt:** Prof ObG, Yale Univ

Riley, Laura MD [MF] - **Spec Exp:** AIDS/HIV in Pregnancy; Infectious Disease in Pregnancy; **Hospital:** Mass Genl Hosp; **Address:** Mass Genl Hosp, Yawkey Bldg, 32 Fruit St, Ste 4200, Boston, MA 02114; **Phone:** 617-724-2229; **Board Cert:** Obstetrics & Gynecology 2003; Maternal & Fetal Medicine 2003; **Med School:** Univ Pittsburgh 1985; **Resid:** Obstetrics & Gynecology, Univ Pittsburgh Med Ctr 1988; **Fellow:** Maternal & Fetal Medicine, Brigham & Womens Hosp 1990; **Fac Appt:** Asst Prof ObG, Harvard Med Sch

Mid Atlantic

Bardeguez, Arlene D MD [MF] - **Spec Exp:** AIDS/HIV in Pregnancy; Pregnancy-High Risk; **Hospital:** UMDNJ-Univ Hosp-Newark, Columbus Hosp; **Address:** 140 Bergen St, Sea Level, Newark, NJ 07103; **Phone:** 973-972-2700; **Board Cert:** Obstetrics & Gynecology 1998; Maternal & Fetal Medicine 1998; **Med School:** Univ Puerto Rico 1981; **Resid:** Obstetrics & Gynecology, Catholic Med Ctr 1985; **Fellow:** Maternal & Fetal Medicine, Nassau Co Med Ctr 1987; Maternal & Fetal Medicine, Columbia Univ 2001; **Fac Appt:** Prof ObG, UMDNJ-NJ Med Sch, Newark

Berkowitz, Richard MD [MF] - **Spec Exp:** Fetal Therapy; Multiple Gestation; Pregnancy & Hematologic Abnormalities; **Hospital:** NY-Presby Hosp/Columbia (page 66); **Address:** 16 E 60th St Fl 4, New York, NY 10022; **Phone:** 212-326-8952; **Board Cert:** Obstetrics & Gynecology 1974; Maternal & Fetal Medicine 1979; **Med School:** NYU Sch Med 1965; **Resid:** Obstetrics & Gynecology, NY Hosp-Cornell Univ 1972; **Fac Appt:** Prof ObG, Columbia P&S

Chervenak, Francis A MD [MF] - **Spec Exp:** Ultrasound; Pregnancy-High Risk; Ethics; **Hospital:** NY-Presby Hosp/Weill Cornell (page 66); **Address:** 525 E 68th St, Ste J-130, New York, NY 10021-4870; **Phone:** 212-746-3184; **Board Cert:** Obstetrics & Gynecology 1984; Maternal & Fetal Medicine 1985; **Med School:** Jefferson Med Coll 1976; **Resid:** Obstetrics & Gynecology, NY Med Coll-Flower Fifth Ave Hosp 1979; Obstetrics & Gynecology, St Lukes Hosp 1981; **Fellow:** Maternal & Fetal Medicine, Yale-New Haven Hosp 1983; **Fac Appt:** Prof ObG, Cornell Univ-Weill Med Coll

Collea, Joseph Vincent MD [MF] - **Spec Exp:** Multiple Gestation; Obstetric Ultrasound; **Hospital:** Georgetown Univ Hosp; **Address:** GUMC PHC Bldg Fl 3, 3800 Reservoir Rd NW, Washington, DC 20007-2194; **Phone:** 202-444-8531; **Board Cert:** Obstetrics & Gynecology 1974; Maternal & Fetal Medicine 1981; **Med School:** SUNY Upstate Med Univ 1966; **Resid:** Obstetrics & Gynecology, Johns Hopkins Hosp 1972; **Fellow:** Perinatal Medicine, LAC-USC Medical Center 1976; **Fac Appt:** Prof ObG, Georgetown Univ

D'Alton, Mary Elizabeth MD [MF] - **Spec Exp:** Pregnancy-High Risk; Multiple Gestation; Prenatal Diagnosis; **Hospital:** NY-Presby Hosp/Columbia (page 66); **Address:** 16 E 60th St, Ste 480, New York, NY 10032; **Phone:** 212-326-8951; **Board Cert:** Obstetrics & Gynecology 2001; Maternal & Fetal Medicine 2001; **Med School:** Ireland 1976; **Resid:** Obstetrics & Gynecology, Univ Ottawa Med Ctr 1982; **Fellow:** Maternal & Fetal Medicine, New England Med Ctr 1984; **Fac Appt:** Clin Prof ObG, Columbia P&S

Maternal & Fetal Medicine

Edersheim, Terri MD [MF] - **Spec Exp:** Pregnancy-High Risk; Multiple Gestation; Prenatal Diagnosis; **Hospital:** NY-Presby Hosp/Weill Cornell (page 66); **Address:** 523 E 72nd St, FL 9, New York, NY 10021; **Phone:** 212-472-5340; **Board Cert:** Obstetrics & Gynecology 1997; Maternal & Fetal Medicine 1997; **Med School:** Albert Einstein Coll Med 1980; **Resid:** Obstetrics & Gynecology, New York Hosp 1984; **Fellow:** Maternal & Fetal Medicine, New York Hosp 1986; **Fac Appt:** Asst Clin Prof ObG, Cornell Univ-Weill Med Coll

Fox, Harold E MD [MF] - **Spec Exp:** Pregnancy-High Risk; Prematurity Prevention; Multiple Gestation; **Hospital:** Johns Hopkins Hosp - Baltimore (page 61); **Address:** 600 N Wolfe St Phipps Bldg - rm 264, Baltimore, MD 21287; **Phone:** 410-614-0178; **Board Cert:** Obstetrics & Gynecology 2005; Maternal & Fetal Medicine 2005; **Med School:** Univ Rochester 1972; **Resid:** Obstetrics & Gynecology, Strong Meml Hosp 1975; **Fellow:** Maternal & Fetal Medicine, Univ Rochester Hosps 1977; **Fac Appt:** Prof ObG, Johns Hopkins Univ

Landy, Helain Jody MD [MF] - **Spec Exp:** Pregnancy-High Risk; Miscarriage-Recurrent; Multiple Gestation; **Hospital:** Georgetown Univ Hosp; **Address:** GUMC-Pasquerilla Hlthcare Ctr, Dept OB/GYN, 3800 Reservoir Rd NW, Ste 3, Washington, DC 20007-2113; **Phone:** 202-444-8531; **Board Cert:** Obstetrics & Gynecology 1998; Maternal & Fetal Medicine 1998; **Med School:** Northwestern Univ 1982; **Resid:** Obstetrics & Gynecology, Penn Hosp 1986; **Fellow:** Maternal & Fetal Medicine, Geo Washington Univ Med Ctr 1988; **Fac Appt:** Assoc Prof ObG, Georgetown Univ

Pinckert, Thomas L MD [MF] - **Spec Exp:** Pregnancy-High Risk; **Hospital:** Shady Grove Adven Hosp, Holy Cross Hospital - Silver Spring; **Address:** Greater Washington Maternal-Fetal Medicine, 9707 Medical Ctr Drive, Ste 230, Rockville, MD 20850; **Phone:** 301-279-6060; **Board Cert:** Obstetrics & Gynecology 1985; Clinical Genetics 1990; Maternal & Fetal Medicine 2001; **Med School:** Oregon Hlth Sci Univ 1979; **Resid:** Obstetrics & Gynecology, David Grant Med Ctr 1983; **Fellow:** Maternal & Fetal Medicine, UCSF Med Ctr 1989; Clinical Genetics, UCSF Med Ctr 1990

Wapner, Ronald MD [MF] - **Spec Exp:** Perinatal Medicine; Genetic Disorders; Multiple Gestation; Vomiting-Cyclic; **Hospital:** NY-Presby Hosp/Columbia (page 66); **Address:** Division of Maternal/Fetal Medicine, 216 N Broad St Fl 4, Philadelphia, PA 19102-1192; **Phone:** 215-762-3609; **Board Cert:** Obstetrics & Gynecology 2000; Maternal & Fetal Medicine 2000; Clinical Genetics 2006; **Med School:** Jefferson Med Coll 1972; **Resid:** Obstetrics & Gynecology, Jefferson Univ Hosp 1976; **Fellow:** Maternal & Fetal Medicine, Jefferson Med Coll 1978; **Fac Appt:** Prof ObG, Columbia P&S

Southeast

Abuhamad, Alfred Z MD [MF] - **Spec Exp:** Twin to Twin Transfusion Syndrome (TTTS); Prenatal Diagnosis; Prenatal Ultrasound; **Hospital:** Sentara Norfolk Genl Hosp; **Address:** E VA Med Sch, Div Mat Fetal Med, 825 Fairfax Ave, Ste 310, Norfolk, VA 23507; **Phone:** 757-446-7900; **Board Cert:** Obstetrics & Gynecology 2002; Maternal & Fetal Medicine 2002; **Med School:** Amer Univ Beirut 1985; **Resid:** Obstetrics & Gynecology, Jackson Meml Hosp 1989; **Fellow:** Maternal & Fetal Medicine, Jackson Meml Hosp-Univ Miami 1991; Ultrasound, Yale Univ; **Fac Appt:** Prof ObG, Eastern VA Med Sch

Boehm, Frank H MD [MF] - **Spec Exp:** Pregnancy-High Risk; **Hospital:** Vanderbilt Univ Med Ctr; **Address:** Vanderbilt Univ Med Ctr, Dept ObGyn, Medical Center North, rm B1100, Nashville, TN 37232-2519; **Phone:** 615-343-7994; **Board Cert:** Obstetrics & Gynecology 1973; Maternal & Fetal Medicine 1976; **Med School:** Vanderbilt Univ 1965; **Resid:** Obstetrics & Gynecology, Yale-New Haven Hosp 1970; **Fac Appt:** Prof ObG, Vanderbilt Univ

Bruner, Joseph P MD [MF] - **Spec Exp:** Fetal Surgery; Spina Bifida; **Hospital:** Fort Sanders Reg Med Ctr; **Address:** Trustees Tower, 501 19th St, Box #304, Knoxville, TN 37916; **Phone:** 865-541-2020; **Board Cert:** Obstetrics & Gynecology 2003; Maternal & Fetal Medicine 2003; **Med School:** Univ Nebr Coll Med 1979; **Resid:** Obstetrics & Gynecology, Letterman AMC 1983; **Fellow:** Maternal & Fetal Medicine, Hosp U Penn 1988; **Fac Appt:** Assoc Prof ObG, Vanderbilt Univ

Chescheir, Nancy C MD [MF] - **Spec Exp:** Ultrasound; Fetal Surgery; Pregnancy-High Risk; **Hospital:** Vanderbilt Univ Med Ctr; **Address:** Vanderbilt University Medical Ctr, R1217 Medical Ctr North, Nashville, TN 37232-2521; **Phone:** 615-322-3385; **Board Cert:** Obstetrics & Gynecology 2005; Maternal & Fetal Medicine 2005; **Med School:** Univ NC Sch Med 1982; **Resid:** Obstetrics & Gynecology, UNC Hosps 1986; **Fellow:** Maternal & Fetal Medicine, NC Meml Hosp-UNC 1988; **Fac Appt:** Prof ObG, Vanderbilt Univ

Ferguson II, James E MD [MF] - **Spec Exp:** Pregnancy-High Risk; Ultrasound; **Hospital:** Univ of Kentucky Chandler Hosp; **Address:** Univ KY Medical Ctr, Dept Ob/Gyn, 800 Rose St, rm C-375, Lexington, KY 40536-0293; **Phone:** 859-323-6434; **Board Cert:** Obstetrics & Gynecology 2005; Maternal & Fetal Medicine 2005; **Med School:** Wake Forest Univ 1977; **Resid:** Obstetrics & Gynecology, Stanford Univ Med Ctr 1980; **Fellow:** Maternal & Fetal Medicine, Stanford Univ Med Ctr 1984; **Fac Appt:** Prof ObG, Univ KY Coll Med

Gabbe, Steven G MD [MF] - **Spec Exp:** Pregnancy-High Risk; Diabetes in Pregnancy; **Hospital:** Vanderbilt Univ Med Ctr; **Address:** Vanderbilt Univ Medical Ctr, 1161 21st Ave S Bldg Med Ctr N - rm D3300, Nashville, TN 37232-2104; **Phone:** 615-322-5191; **Board Cert:** Obstetrics & Gynecology 1998; Maternal & Fetal Medicine 1998; **Med School:** Cornell Univ-Weill Med Coll 1969; **Resid:** Obstetrics & Gynecology, Boston Hosp Women 1974; **Fellow:** Reproductive Medicine, Boston Lying-In Hosp 1974; **Fac Appt:** Prof ObG, Vanderbilt Univ

McLaren, Rodney A MD [MF] - **Spec Exp:** Prenatal Diagnosis; Amniocentesis; Pregnancy-High Risk; **Hospital:** Virginia Hosp Ctr - Arlington, Georgetown Univ Hosp; **Address:** VA Hosp Ctr, Dept Maternal & Fetal Med, 1701 N George Mason Drive, Ste 190, Arlington, VA 22205-3698; **Phone:** 703-558-6077; **Board Cert:** Obstetrics & Gynecology 2003; Maternal & Fetal Medicine 2003; **Med School:** Tufts Univ 1983; **Resid:** Obstetrics & Gynecology, LI Coll Hosp 1987; **Fellow:** Maternal & Fetal Medicine, Georgetown Univ 1989

Miller, Franklin C MD [MF] - **Spec Exp:** Pregnancy-High Risk; Fetal Assessment; **Hospital:** Univ of Kentucky Chandler Hosp; **Address:** Univ Kentucky Med Ctr, Div High Risk Obstetrics, 800 Rose St, Ste C358, Lexington, KY 40536-0084; **Phone:** 859-257-5158; **Board Cert:** Obstetrics & Gynecology 1999; Maternal & Fetal Medicine 1999; **Med School:** Univ Louisville Sch Med 1962; **Resid:** Obstetrics & Gynecology, Tripler General Hosp 1969; **Fellow:** Maternal & Fetal Medicine, USC Medical Ctr 1974; **Fac Appt:** Prof ObG, Univ KY Coll Med

Thorp Jr, John M MD [MF] - **Spec Exp:** Multiple Gestation; Premature Labor; **Hospital:** Univ NC Hosps; **Address:** UNC-Chapel Hill, 101 Manning Drive, Box 7600, Chapel Hill, NC 27599; **Phone:** 919-966-2496; **Board Cert:** Obstetrics & Gynecology 2004; Maternal & Fetal Medicine 2004; **Med School:** E Carolina Univ 1983; **Resid:** Obstetrics & Gynecology, Univ NC Hosp 1987; **Fellow:** Maternal & Fetal Medicine, Univ NC Hosp 1989; **Fac Appt:** Prof ObG, Univ NC Sch Med

Maternal & Fetal Medicine

Van Dorsten, J Peter MD [MF] - **Spec Exp:** Pregnancy-High Risk; **Hospital:** MUSC Med Ctr; **Address:** MUSC Med Ctr, Dept ObGyn, 96 Jonathan Lucas St, Charleston, SC 29425; **Phone:** 843-792-4509; **Board Cert:** Obstetrics & Gynecology 2004; Maternal & Fetal Medicine 2004; **Med School:** Univ NC Sch Med 1971; **Resid:** Obstetrics & Gynecology, Med Univ SC Hosp 1976; **Fellow:** Maternal & Fetal Medicine, USC-LAC Hosp 1981; **Fac Appt:** Prof ObG, Med Univ SC

Midwest

Bahado-Singh, Ray O MD [MF] - **Spec Exp:** Pregnancy-High Risk; Genetic Disorders; Obstetric Ultrasound; Twin to Twin Transfusion Syndrome (TTTS); **Hospital:** Hutzel Hosp - Detroit; **Address:** University Womens Care, 3750 Woodward Ave, Ste 200C, Detroit, MI 48201; **Phone:** 313-993-4645; **Board Cert:** Obstetrics & Gynecology 1997; Maternal & Fetal Medicine 1997; Clinical Genetics 2004; **Med School:** Jamaica 1979; **Resid:** Obstetrics & Gynecology, Metropolitan Hosp 1985; **Fellow:** Perinatal Medicine, UC-Irvine 1987; Clinical Genetics, Yale Univ 1993

Bartelsmeyer, James MD [MF] - **Spec Exp:** Pregnancy-High Risk; Multiple Gestation; **Hospital:** St John's Mercy Med Ctr - St Louis; **Address:** 621 S New Ballas Rd, Ste 2007B, St Louis, MO 63141; **Phone:** 314-991-5000; **Board Cert:** Obstetrics & Gynecology 2001; Maternal & Fetal Medicine 1995; **Med School:** Univ IL Coll Med 1985; **Resid:** Obstetrics & Gynecology, Univ Ill Coll Med Hosps 1989; **Fellow:** Maternal & Fetal Medicine, Barnes Hosp-Univ Wash 1991; **Fac Appt:** Assoc Prof ObG, Washington Univ, St Louis

Dooley, Sharon L MD [MF] - **Spec Exp:** Fetal Abnormalities; Pregnancy-High Risk; Multiple Gestation; **Hospital:** Northwestern Meml Hosp; **Address:** 333 E Superior St, Ste 400, Chicago, IL 60611; **Phone:** 312-695-7542; **Board Cert:** Obstetrics & Gynecology 1989; Maternal & Fetal Medicine 1981; **Med School:** Univ VA Sch Med 1973; **Resid:** Obstetrics & Gynecology, Northwestern Meml Hosp 1977; **Fac Appt:** Prof ObG, Northwestern Univ

Gianopoulos, John MD [MF] - **Spec Exp:** Perinatal Medicine; Premature Labor; Critical Care; **Hospital:** Loyola Univ Med Ctr; **Address:** Loyola Univ Med Ctr, 2160 S 1st Ave, Bldg 103 - Ste 1019, Maywood, IL 60153; **Phone:** 708-216-5423; **Board Cert:** Obstetrics & Gynecology 2004; Maternal & Fetal Medicine 2004; **Med School:** Loyola Univ-Stritch Sch Med 1977; **Resid:** Obstetrics & Gynecology, Loyola Univ Med Ctr 1981; **Fellow:** Maternal & Fetal Medicine, Loyola Univ Med Ctr 1983; **Fac Appt:** Prof ObG, Loyola Univ-Stritch Sch Med

Hibbard, Judith MD [MF] - **Spec Exp:** Pregnancy-High Risk; Heart Disease in Pregnancy; Prenatal Ultrasound; **Hospital:** Univ of IL Med Ctr at Chicago; **Address:** Univ Illinois at Chicago, Dept OB-GYN, 820 S Wood St, MS 808, Chicago, IL 60612; **Phone:** 312-996-7300; **Board Cert:** Obstetrics & Gynecology 1999; Maternal & Fetal Medicine 1999; **Med School:** Loyola Univ-Stritch Sch Med 1982; **Resid:** Obstetrics & Gynecology, Univ Chicago Hosps 1986; **Fellow:** Maternal & Fetal Medicine, Univ Chicago Hosps 1988; **Fac Appt:** Prof ObG, Univ IL Coll Med

Hussey, Michael J MD [MF] - **Spec Exp:** Perinatal Medicine; Congenital Anomalies; Multiple Gestation; **Hospital:** Rush Univ Med Ctr; **Address:** 1725 W Harrison St, Ste 408, Chicago, IL 60612; **Phone:** 312-997-2229; **Board Cert:** Obstetrics & Gynecology 2005; Maternal & Fetal Medicine 2005; **Med School:** Univ IL Coll Med 1986; **Resid:** Obstetrics & Gynecology, Loyola Univ Med Ctr 1993; **Fellow:** Maternal & Fetal Medicine, Rush-Presby-St Lukes Hosp 1995; Ultrasound, Univ Col Hlth Sci Ctr 1996; **Fac Appt:** Asst Prof ObG, Rush Med Coll

Ismail, Mahmoud MD [MF] - **Spec Exp:** Pregnancy-High Risk; Perinatal Medicine; Infections-Neonatal; Infections in Pregnancy; **Hospital:** Univ of Chicago Hosps; **Address:** 5841 S Maryland Ave, MC 2050, Chicago, IL 60637-1463; **Phone:** 773-702-5200; **Board Cert:** Obstetrics & Gynecology 1997; Maternal & Fetal Medicine 1997; **Med School:** Egypt 1970; **Resid:** Obstetrics & Gynecology, Wayne St Univ Affil Hosps 1977; **Fellow:** Maternal & Fetal Medicine, Univ Chicago Hosps 1982; **Fac Appt:** Prof ObG, Univ Chicago-Pritzker Sch Med

Johnson, Timothy R B MD [MF] - **Spec Exp:** Fetal Assessment; Prenatal Diagnosis; **Hospital:** Univ Michigan Hlth Sys; **Address:** Univ Mich, Dept Ob/Gyn, 1500 E Med Ctr Dr, rm L4000, Box 0276, Ann Arbor, MI 48109; **Phone:** 734-764-8123; **Board Cert:** Obstetrics & Gynecology 2001; Maternal & Fetal Medicine 2001; **Med School:** Univ VA Sch Med 1975; **Resid:** Obstetrics & Gynecology, Univ Michigan Med Ctr 1979; **Fellow:** Maternal & Fetal Medicine, Johns Hopkins Hosp 1981; **Fac Appt:** Prof ObG, Univ Mich Med Sch

Macones, George A MD [MF] - **Spec Exp:** Pregnancy-High Risk; **Hospital:** Barnes-Jewish Hosp, St Louis Chldns Hosp; **Address:** University of Washington Medical Ctr, 660 S Euclid Ave, Box 8064, St Louis, MO 63110; **Phone:** 314-362-7139; **Board Cert:** Obstetrics & Gynecology 2004; Maternal & Fetal Medicine 2004; **Med School:** Jefferson Med Coll 1988; **Resid:** Obstetrics & Gynecology, Pennsylvania Hosp 1992; **Fellow:** Maternal & Fetal Medicine, Jefferson Univ Hosp 1994; **Fac Appt:** Prof ObG, Univ Wash

Philipson, Elliot MD [MF] - **Spec Exp:** Pregnancy-High Risk; Amniocentesis; **Hospital:** Hillcrest Hosp-Mayfield Hts (page 57), Cleveland Clin Fdn (page 57); **Address:** Hillcrest Hosp, Dept OB/Gyn, 6770 Mayfield Rd, Ste 336, Mayfield Heights, OH 44124; **Phone:** 440-312-7774; **Board Cert:** Obstetrics & Gynecology 2004; Maternal & Fetal Medicine 2004; **Med School:** Italy 1975; **Resid:** Obstetrics & Gynecology, Albany Med Ctr 1980; **Fellow:** Maternal & Fetal Medicine, Metro Genl Hosp 1982; **Fac Appt:** Assoc Prof ObG, Cleveland Cl Coll Med/Case West Res

Socol, Michael MD [MF] - **Spec Exp:** Diabetes in Pregnancy; Multiple Gestation; Premature Labor; **Hospital:** Northwestern Meml Hosp; **Address:** Prentice Womens Hosp, 333 E Superior St, Ste 410, Chicago, IL 60611-3056; **Phone:** 312-695-7542; **Board Cert:** Obstetrics & Gynecology 1989; Maternal & Fetal Medicine 1981; **Med School:** Univ IL Coll Med 1974; **Resid:** Obstetrics & Gynecology, Univ Illinois Med Ctr 1977; **Fellow:** Maternal & Fetal Medicine, USC Med Ctr 1979; **Fac Appt:** Prof ObG, Northwestern Univ

Strassner, Howard T MD [MF] - **Spec Exp:** Pregnancy-High Risk; Amniocentesis; Obstetric Ultrasound; **Hospital:** Rush Univ Med Ctr, Resurrection Hlth Care St Joseph Hosp; **Address:** 1725 W Harrison St, Ste 408-West, Chicago, IL 60612; **Phone:** 312-997-2229; **Board Cert:** Obstetrics & Gynecology 2005; Maternal & Fetal Medicine 2005; **Med School:** Univ Chicago-Pritzker Sch Med 1974; **Resid:** Obstetrics & Gynecology, Columbia Presby Med Ctr 1978; **Fellow:** Maternal & Fetal Medicine, LA Co-USC Med Ctr 1980; **Fac Appt:** Prof ObG, Rush Med Coll

Treadwell, Marjorie Clarke MD [MF] - **Spec Exp:** Obstetric Ultrasound; Pregnancy-High Risk; Fetal Diagnosis & Therapy; **Hospital:** Univ Michigan Hlth Sys; **Address:** 1500 E Medical Center Drive, F4835 MOTT, Ann Arbor, MI 48109-0264; **Phone:** 734-936-7573; **Board Cert:** Obstetrics & Gynecology 2000; Maternal & Fetal Medicine 2000; **Med School:** Univ Mich Med Sch 1984; **Resid:** Obstetrics & Gynecology, Wayne State Univ 1988; **Fellow:** Maternal & Fetal Medicine, Wayne State Univ 1990; **Fac Appt:** Prof ObG, Wayne State Univ

Maternal & Fetal Medicine

Wilkins, Isabelle MD [MF] - **Spec Exp:** Multiple Gestation; Congenital Anomalies; Prenatal Ultrasound; **Hospital:** Univ of IL Med Ctr at Chicago; **Address:** Univ Illinois Med Ctr at Chicago, 820 S Wood St, MS 808, Chicago, IL 60612; **Phone:** 312-413-7500; **Board Cert:** Obstetrics & Gynecology 1996; Maternal & Fetal Medicine 1996; **Med School:** Duke Univ 1980; **Resid:** Obstetrics & Gynecology, Mount Sinai Med Ctr 1984; **Fellow:** Maternal & Fetal Medicine, Mount Sinai Med Ctr 1986; **Fac Appt:** Prof ObG, Univ IL Coll Med

Winn, Hung MD [MF] - **Spec Exp:** Multiple Gestation; Pregnancy-High Risk; **Hospital:** Univ of Missouri Hosp & Clins; **Address:** 3401 Berrywood Drive, Ste 203, Columbia, MO 65201; **Phone:** 573-882-6361; **Board Cert:** Obstetrics & Gynecology 2000; Maternal & Fetal Medicine 1992; **Med School:** Univ IL Coll Med 1982; **Resid:** Obstetrics & Gynecology, Univ Ill Hosp 1986; **Fellow:** Maternal & Fetal Medicine, Yale-New Haven Hosp 1988; **Fac Appt:** Prof ObG, Univ MO-Columbia Sch Med

Great Plains and Mountains

Dugoff, Lorraine MD [MF] - **Spec Exp:** Pregnancy-High Risk; Prenatal Diagnosis; Ultrasound; **Hospital:** Univ Colorado Hosp; **Address:** Maternal Fetal Medicine, 4200 E Ninth Ave, Box B198, Denver, CO 80220; **Phone:** 303-372-6695; **Board Cert:** Maternal & Fetal Medicine 1999; Obstetrics & Gynecology 1997; **Med School:** Georgetown Univ 1989; **Resid:** Obstetrics & Gynecology, Philadelphia Hosp 1990; Obstetrics & Gynecology, U Colorado Hlth Sci Ctr 1993; **Fellow:** Maternal & Fetal Medicine, U Colorado Hlth Sci Ctr 1995; Clinical Genetics, U Colorado Hlth Sci Ctr 1996; **Fac Appt:** Assoc Prof ObG, Univ Colorado

Gibbs, Ronald S MD [MF] - **Spec Exp:** Infectious Disease; **Hospital:** Univ Colorado Hosp; **Address:** 4200 E 9th Ave, Box B198, Denver, CO 80262; **Phone:** 720-848-1600; **Board Cert:** Obstetrics & Gynecology 1989; Maternal & Fetal Medicine 1981; **Med School:** Univ Pennsylvania 1969; **Resid:** Obstetrics & Gynecology, Hosp Univ Penn 1974; **Fellow:** Maternal & Fetal Medicine, Univ Tex Hlth Sci Ctr 1978; **Fac Appt:** Prof ObG, Univ Colorado

Tomich, Paul MD [MF] - **Spec Exp:** Pregnancy-High Risk; Prenatal Ultrasound; **Hospital:** Nebraska Med Ctr; **Address:** 983255 Nebraska Medical Center, Omaha, NE 68198-3255; **Phone:** 402-559-6150; **Board Cert:** Obstetrics & Gynecology 2004; Maternal & Fetal Medicine 2004; **Med School:** Loyola Univ-Stritch Sch Med 1973; **Resid:** Obstetrics & Gynecology, Mayo Clinic 1978; **Fellow:** Maternal & Fetal Medicine, Barnes Hosp-Wash Univ 1980; **Fac Appt:** Prof ObG, Univ Nebr Coll Med

Southwest

Clewell, William H MD [MF] - **Spec Exp:** Fetal Hydrocephalus; Fetal Surgery; **Hospital:** Banner Good Samaritan Regl Med Ctr - Phoenix, Banner Desert Med Ctr; **Address:** 3877 N 7th St, Ste 400, Phoenix, AZ 85014; **Phone:** 602-257-8118; **Board Cert:** Obstetrics & Gynecology 1977; Maternal & Fetal Medicine 1981; **Med School:** Stanford Univ 1970; **Resid:** Obstetrics & Gynecology, Stanford Univ Hosp 1974; **Fellow:** Perinatal Medicine, Univ Colorado Med Ctr 1976; **Fac Appt:** Clin Prof ObG, Univ Ariz Coll Med

Elliott, John P MD [MF] - **Spec Exp:** Twin to Twin Transfusion Syndrome (TTTS); Multiple Gestation; Premature Labor; **Hospital:** Banner Good Samaritan Regl Med Ctr - Phoenix, Banner Desert Med Ctr; **Address:** 3877 N 7th St, Ste 400, Phoenix, AZ 85014-5072; **Phone:** 602-257-8118; **Board Cert:** Obstetrics & Gynecology 1980; Maternal & Fetal Medicine 1982; **Med School:** Univ Colorado 1972; **Resid:** Obstetrics & Gynecology, Fitzsimmons Army Med Ctr 1976; **Fellow:** Maternal & Fetal Medicine, Long Beach Meml Hosp/UC Irvine 1980; **Fac Appt:** Clin Prof ObG, Univ Ariz Coll Med

Hankins, Gary D V MD [MF] - **Spec Exp:** Pregnancy-High Risk; **Hospital:** UT Med Br Hosp at Galveston; **Address:** Univ Texas Medical Branch at Galveston, 301 University Blvd, Galveston, TX 77555-0587; **Phone:** 409-772-1957; **Board Cert:** Obstetrics & Gynecology 1994; Maternal & Fetal Medicine 2000; **Med School:** Med Coll VA 1977; **Resid:** Obstetrics & Gynecology, Wilford Hall Med Ctr 1981; **Fellow:** Critical Care Medicine, Wilford Hall Med Ctr 1982; Maternal & Fetal Medicine, Parkland Hosp 1984; **Fac Appt:** Prof ObG, Univ Tex Med Br, Galveston

Reed, Kathryn L MD [MF] - **Spec Exp:** Prenatal Diagnosis; Ultrasound; Fetal Echocardiography; **Hospital:** Univ Med Ctr - Tucson; **Address:** Arizona Hlth Sci Center, 8325, Box 245078, Tuscon, AZ 85724; **Phone:** 520-694-6010; **Board Cert:** Obstetrics & Gynecology 1994; Maternal & Fetal Medicine 1987; **Med School:** Univ Ariz Coll Med 1977; **Resid:** Obstetrics & Gynecology, Ariz Hlth Scis Ctr 1981; Maternal & Fetal Medicine, Ariz Hlth Scis Ctr 1983; **Fac Appt:** Prof ObG, Univ Ariz Coll Med

West Coast and Pacific

Benedetti, Thomas J MD [MF] - **Spec Exp:** Prematurity Prevention; Fetal Macrosomia; **Hospital:** Univ Wash Med Ctr, Yakima Valley Mem Hosp; **Address:** 1959 NE Pacific St, Box 356460, Seattle, WA 98195; **Phone:** 206-543-3729; **Board Cert:** Obstetrics & Gynecology 1980; Maternal & Fetal Medicine 1981; **Med School:** Univ Wash 1973; **Resid:** Obstetrics & Gynecology, LAC-USC Med Ctr 1977; **Fellow:** Maternal & Fetal Medicine, LAC-USC Med Ctr 1979; **Fac Appt:** Prof ObG, Univ Wash

Druzin, Maurice L MD [MF] - **Spec Exp:** Lupus/SLE in Pregnancy; Fetal Electronic Monitors; Miscarriage-Recurrent; **Hospital:** Stanford Univ Med Ctr; **Address:** Stanford Univ, Dept Ob/Gyn, 300 Pasteur Drive, rm HH333, MC 5317, Stanford, CA 94305-5317; **Phone:** 650-725-8617; **Board Cert:** Obstetrics & Gynecology 2001; Maternal & Fetal Medicine 2001; **Med School:** South Africa 1970; **Resid:** Obstetrics & Gynecology, Rose Med Ctr-Univ Colo 1977; **Fellow:** Maternal & Fetal Medicine, LAC-USC Med Ctr 1979; **Fac Appt:** Prof ObG, Stanford Univ

Goldberg, James D MD [MF] - **Spec Exp:** Prenatal Diagnosis; Fetal Diagnosis & Therapy; **Hospital:** CA Pacific Med Ctr - Pacific Campus; **Address:** San Francisco Perinatal Assoc, One Daniel Burnham Ct, Ste 230C, San Francisco, CA 94109; **Phone:** 415-202-1200; **Board Cert:** Obstetrics & Gynecology 1994; Clinical Genetics 1987; **Med School:** Univ Minn 1979; **Resid:** Obstetrics & Gynecology, UCSF Med Ctr 1983; **Fellow:** Maternal & Fetal Medicine, Mt Sinai Hosp 1985; Clinical Genetics, Mt Sinai Hosp 1985

Gravett, Michael Glen MD [MF] - **Spec Exp:** Infectious Disease; **Hospital:** Univ Wash Med Ctr; **Address:** Univ Washington, Dept OB/GYN, Box 356460, Seattle, WA 98195-6460; **Phone:** 206-598-4070; **Board Cert:** Obstetrics & Gynecology 1985; Maternal & Fetal Medicine 1987; **Med School:** UCLA 1977; **Resid:** Obstetrics & Gynecology, Univ Wash Med Ctr 1981; **Fellow:** Maternal & Fetal Medicine, Univ Wash Med Ctr 1983; **Fac Appt:** Prof ObG, Univ Wash

Hobel, Calvin John MD [MF] - **Spec Exp:** Prematurity Prevention; Fetal Diagnosis & Therapy; **Hospital:** Cedars-Sinai Med Ctr; **Address:** 8635 W Third St, #160W, Los Angeles, CA 90048; **Phone:** 310-423-3365; **Board Cert:** Obstetrics & Gynecology 1971; Maternal & Fetal Medicine 1975; **Med School:** Univ Nebr Coll Med 1963; **Resid:** Obstetrics & Gynecology, Harbor Genl Hosp 1968; **Fellow:** Maternal & Fetal Medicine, Natl Womens Hosp 1967; **Fac Appt:** Prof ObG, UCLA

Koos, Brian John MD [MF] - **Spec Exp:** Pregnancy-High Risk; Fetal Diagnosis & Therapy; Heart Disease in Pregnancy; **Hospital:** UCLA Med Ctr; **Address:** UCLA Medical Ctr, 10833 Le Conte Ave, MC 3075, Los Angeles, CA 90095-3075; **Phone:** 310-794-7852; **Board Cert:** Obstetrics & Gynecology 1999; Maternal & Fetal Medicine 1999; **Med School:** Loma Linda Univ 1974; **Resid:** Obstetrics & Gynecology, Brigham & Women's Hosp 1979; **Fellow:** Maternal & Fetal Medicine, Women's Hosp 1983; **Fac Appt:** Prof ObG, UCLA

Landers, Daniel V MD [MF] - **Spec Exp:** Infectious Disease; **Hospital:** Sharp Mary Birch Hosp for Wmn; **Address:** 8010 Frost St, Ste 300, San Diego, CA 92123; **Phone:** 858-939-6880; **Board Cert:** Obstetrics & Gynecology 1998; Maternal & Fetal Medicine 1991; **Med School:** UCSF 1980; **Resid:** Obstetrics & Gynecology, UCSF Med Ctr 1984; **Fellow:** Maternal & Fetal Medicine, UCSF Med Ctr 1986; Infectious Disease, UCSF Med Ctr 1988; **Fac Appt:** Prof ObG, Univ Minn

Moore, Thomas R MD [MF] - **Spec Exp:** Diabetes in Pregnancy; Fetal Diagnosis & Therapy; **Hospital:** UCSD Med Ctr; **Address:** 200 W Arbor Drive, MC 8433, San Diego, CA 92103; **Phone:** 619-543-7900; **Board Cert:** Obstetrics & Gynecology 1995; Maternal & Fetal Medicine 1995; **Med School:** Yale Univ 1979; **Resid:** Obstetrics & Gynecology, Naval Hosp 1983; **Fellow:** Maternal & Fetal Medicine, UCSD 1985; **Fac Appt:** Prof ObG, UCSD

Platt, Lawrence D MD [MF] - **Spec Exp:** Maternal & Fetal Medicine; Ultrasound; Prenatal Diagnosis; **Hospital:** Cedars-Sinai Med Ctr, St John's Hlth Ctr, Santa Monica; **Address:** 6310 W San Vincente Blvd, Ste 520, Los Angeles, CA 90048; **Phone:** 323-857-1952; **Board Cert:** Obstetrics & Gynecology 1979; Maternal & Fetal Medicine 1981; **Med School:** Wayne State Univ 1972; **Resid:** Obstetrics & Gynecology, Sinai Hosp 1976; **Fellow:** Maternal & Fetal Medicine, USC Med Ctr 1978; **Fac Appt:** Prof ObG, UCLA

Tabsh, Khalil M A MD [MF] - **Spec Exp:** Pregnancy-High Risk; **Hospital:** UCLA Med Ctr, Santa Monica - UCLA Med Ctr; **Address:** 200 Medical Plaza, Ste 430, Los Angeles, CA 90095; **Phone:** 310-208-4492; **Board Cert:** Obstetrics & Gynecology 1981; Maternal & Fetal Medicine 1982; **Med School:** Lebanon 1974; **Resid:** Obstetrics & Gynecology, American Univ Beirut Med Ctr 1976; Obstetrics & Gynecology, Yale-New Haven Hosp 1978; **Fellow:** Maternal & Fetal Medicine, UCLA 1979; **Fac Appt:** Clin Prof ObG, UCLA-David Geffen Sch Med

The Birthing Center at Maimonides is ranked among the best hospitals in the nation for maternity care by HealthGrades, the nation's leading source for independent healthcare quality information. More babies were delivered at Maimonides Medical Center in 2006 than at any other hospital in New York State.

The Maimonides Birthing Center features private suites with hardwood floors and a homelike environment. At the same time, physician coverage is provided 24/7 in our advanced Neonatal Intensive Care Unit. Our 36 obstetricians and 26 midwives have found that most families appreciate having the best of both worlds available to them.

Maimonides provides other unique services to its maternity patients. The largest doula program in the metropolitan area can be found at Maimonides. These fully-trained childbirth assistants are available to patients before, during and after delivery at no cost to families. And the maternity units utilize an electronic patient record that sets industry standards for patient safety and hospital efficiency.

This combination of family-centered services and advanced technology continues to have enormous appeal to the women we serve – over 6,700 of them last year alone. Our highly trained staff includes the finest nurses, physicians, midwives and specialists to ensure the safety and comfort of our patients. Several physicians specialize in high-risk pregnancy, including the Chairman of Obstetrics and Gynecology, Howard Minkoff, MD.

In recognition of its excellence in obstetrics and pediatrics, Maimonides was designated a Regional Perinatal Center by the New York State Department of Health. Women who give birth at Maimonides also have a variety of other services available to them, including:

- A Perinatal Testing Center, directed by Shoshana Haberman, MD,offering amniocentesis, 3-D ultrasound, fetal echocardiograms and other diagnostic exams.

- Neonatologists onsite around-the-clock. This vital service is always available during high-risk deliveries, working closely with the obstetrician. The Norma Sutton Center for Neonatology adjoins the Payson Birthing Center and provides the most sophisticated care in a family-friendly environment.

Physicians at Maimonides are among the eight percent in the US who use computers to enter patient orders, thereby reducing the risk of errors, increasing efficiency, and speeding the healing process. Maimonides has appeared on the American Hospital Association's "Most Wired" and "Most Wireless" lists more often than any other healthcare institution in the metropolitan area. Advanced technology allows our doctors to focus more attention on caring for their patients.

Maimonides Medical Center – Passionate about medicine, compassionate about people.

www.maimonidesmed.org/obgyn

NYU Medical Center

550 First Avenue (at 31st Street)
New York, NY 10016
Physician Referral:
(888)7-NYU-MED (888-769-8633)
www.nyumc.org

MATERNAL-FETAL MEDICINE

The NYU Medical Center Program for Maternal Fetal Medicine offers prenatal care for high-risk pregnancies as well as detailed consultations before, during, and after pregnancy. Special attention is given to multifetal pregnancies and to women who have other medical conditions that complicate their pregnancy, like diabetes, heart problems, high blood pressure, and lupus, among others.

The Program's primary concern is making sure each patient delivers a healthy baby. Many of the patients referred to the specialists at NYU are able to conceive but have difficulty carrying babies to term. In response to their particular needs, NYU Medical has conducted extensive research into the causes of recurrent miscarriage and pre-term delivery, with impressive results.

Of course, the ideal time to correct fetal problems is when infants are still in the womb. Using minimally invasive tecniques, doctors at NYU Medical Center are able to repair a number of life-threatening conditions in a child before it is even born. These techniques reduce the risks of pre-term labor and the need for cesarean births.

The program's high success rates are testimony to the immediate impact research has on treatment at NYU Medical Center. This program has generated numerous new treatment modalities for high-risk obstetrics around the nation and around the world.

The Program for Maternal Fetal Medicine enjoys a close, synergistic relationship with the Prenatal Diagnostic Unit. Several of the perinatologists from the Maternal Fetal Medicine Practice provide coverage at the ultrasound unit, and refer patients for sonography and other procedures. From this partnership, our physicians use state-of-the-art techniques for in-utero diagnosis and treatment, and our experienced physicians gain immediate access to the latest findings.

700

NYU MEDICAL CENTER

Maternal-Fetal Medicine at NYU Medical Center

• Specialized care to women with high-risk pregnancies by highly-trained Perinatologists

• Genetic counseling to provide education and genetic tests to evaluate family history

• Tests to help predict patients at risk for preterm labor and delivery, and medications for the mother

• Screening for complications, including preeclampsia, pregnancy-induced hypertension

• Nutritional counseling and education for gestational diabetes, diabetes discovered during pregnancy

Physician Referral
(888) 7-NYU-MED
(888-769-8633)
www.nyumc.edu

Neonatal-Perinatal Medicine

a subspecialty of Pediatrics

A subspecialist in neonatal-perinatal medicine is a pediatrician who is the principal care provider for sick newborn infants. Clinical expertise is used for direct patient care and for consulting with obstetrical colleagues to plan for the care of mothers who have high-risk pregnancies.

Training Required: Three years in pediatrics *plus* additional training and examination.

Neonatal-Perinatal Medicine

New England

Cloherty, John MD [NP] - **Spec Exp:** Neonatology; **Hospital:** Children's Hospital - Boston, Brigham & Women's Hosp; **Address:** 319 Longwood Ave, Fl 4, Boston, MA 02115; **Phone:** 617-277-7320; **Board Cert:** Pediatrics 1986; Neonatal-Perinatal Medicine 1986; **Med School:** Boston Univ 1962; **Resid:** Pediatrics, Mass Genl Hosp 1969; **Fellow:** Neonatal-Perinatal Medicine, Chldns Hosp; **Fac Appt:** Assoc Clin Prof Ped, Harvard Med Sch

Cole, Cynthia H MD [NP] - **Spec Exp:** Retinopathy of Prematurity; Neonatal Chronic Lung Disease (CLD); **Hospital:** Beth Israel Deaconess Med Ctr - Boston; **Address:** BIDMC, Dept Neonatology, 330 Brookline Ave, Boston, MA 02215; **Phone:** 617-667-3276; **Board Cert:** Pediatrics 1981; Neonatal-Perinatal Medicine 1983; **Med School:** Univ Tenn Coll Med, Memphis 1973; **Resid:** Pediatrics, Johns Hopkins Hosp 1981; **Fellow:** Neonatology, Johns Hopkins Hosp 1982; **Fac Appt:** Assoc Prof Ped, Tufts Univ

Ehrenkranz, Richard MD [NP] - **Spec Exp:** Neonatal Critical Care; Nutrition; **Hospital:** Yale - New Haven Hosp; **Address:** Yale Univ-Dept Ped, PO Box 208064, New Haven, CT 06520-8064; **Phone:** 203-688-2320; **Board Cert:** Neonatal-Perinatal Medicine 1979; Pediatrics 1977; **Med School:** SUNY Downstate 1972; **Resid:** Pediatrics, Yale-New Haven Hosp 1974; **Fellow:** Neonatal-Perinatal Medicine, Yale-New Haven Hosp 1978; **Fac Appt:** Prof Ped, Yale Univ

Gross, Ian MD [NP] - **Spec Exp:** Breathing Disorders; Critical Care; **Hospital:** Yale - New Haven Hosp; **Address:** Yale Sch Med, Dept Peds, 333 Cedar St, PO Box 208064, New Haven, CT 06520-8064; **Phone:** 203-688-2320; **Board Cert:** Pediatrics 1974; Neonatal-Perinatal Medicine 1977; **Med School:** South Africa 1967; **Resid:** Pediatrics, Univ Witwatersrand Affil Hosps 1971; Pediatrics, Chldns Hosp Med Ctr 1972; **Fellow:** Pediatrics, Mass Genl Hosp 1973; Neonatal-Perinatal Medicine, Yale-New Haven Hosp 1974; **Fac Appt:** Prof Ped, Yale Univ

Horbar, Jeffrey D MD [NP] - **Hospital:** FAHC - Med Ctr Campus; **Address:** Vermont Oxford Mutual, 33 Kilburn St, Burlington, VT 05401; **Phone:** 802-865-4814; **Board Cert:** Pediatrics 1982; Neonatal-Perinatal Medicine 1983; **Med School:** SUNY Downstate 1977; **Resid:** Pediatrics, Med Ctr Hosp Vermont 1979; **Fellow:** Obstetrics & Gynecology, Med Ctr Hosp Vermont 1981; **Fac Appt:** Assoc Prof Ped, Univ VT Coll Med

Van Marter, Linda J MD [NP] - **Spec Exp:** Neonatal Chronic Lung Disease (CLD); Lung Disease in Newborns; Pulmonary Hypertension of Newborn (PPHN); **Hospital:** Brigham & Women's Hosp, Children's Hospital - Boston; **Address:** 300 Longwood Ave, Hunnewell 430 - Newborn Med, Boston, MA 02115; **Phone:** 617-355-6027; **Board Cert:** Pediatrics 1985; Neonatal-Perinatal Medicine 1985; **Med School:** Univ Pittsburgh 1980; **Resid:** Pediatrics, Childrens Hosp Med Ctr 1983; **Fellow:** Neonatology, Harvard Med Sch 1986; **Fac Appt:** Assoc Prof Ped, Harvard Med Sch

Mid Atlantic

Davidson, Dennis MD [NP] - **Spec Exp:** Lung Disease in Newborns; **Hospital:** Schneider Chldn's Hosp; **Address:** Schneider Chldns Hosp, Neonatal Div, 269-01 76th Ave, Ste 344, New Hyde Park, NY 11040; **Phone:** 718-470-3440; **Board Cert:** Pediatrics 1980; Neonatal-Perinatal Medicine 1981; **Med School:** Loyola Univ-Stritch Sch Med 1974; **Resid:** Pediatrics, Babies Hosp-Columbia Univ 1978; **Fellow:** Neonatal-Perinatal Medicine, Babies Hosp-Columbia Univ 1981; **Fac Appt:** Assoc Prof Ped, Albert Einstein Coll Med

Delivoria-Papadopoulos, Maria MD [NP] - **Spec Exp:** Neonatology; **Hospital:** St Christopher's Hosp for Chldn, Hahnemann Univ Hosp; **Address:** St Christopher's Hosp for Children, Erie Ave at Front St, Ste 2212, Neonatology, Philadelphia, PA 19134; **Phone:** 215-427-5202; **Board Cert:** Pediatrics 1971; Neonatal-Perinatal Medicine 1975; **Med School:** Greece 1957; **Resid:** Pediatrics, Chldns Hosp 1959; Psychiatry, Colo State Hosp 1962; **Fellow:** Neonatology, Hosp Sick Chldn 1964; **Fac Appt:** Prof Ped

Hendricks-Munoz, Karen MD [NP] - **Spec Exp:** Breathing Disorders; Neonatal Neurology; Retinopathy of Prematurity; **Hospital:** NYU Med Ctr (page 67), Bellevue Hosp Ctr; **Address:** NYU Med Ctr, Dept Neonatology, 530 1st Ave, Ste HCC-7A, New York, NY 10016-6402; **Phone:** 212-263-7477; **Board Cert:** Pediatrics 1985; Neonatal-Perinatal Medicine 1987; **Med School:** Yale Univ 1978; **Resid:** Pediatrics, Yale-New Haven Hosp 1981; **Fellow:** Neonatology, Strong Meml Hosp 1984; **Fac Appt:** Assoc Prof Ped, NYU Sch Med

Holzman, Ian MD [NP] - **Spec Exp:** Neonatal Nutrition; Necrotizing Enterocolitis; Prematurity/Low Birth Weight Infants; **Hospital:** Mount Sinai Med Ctr; **Address:** Newborn Assocs, 1 Gustave L Levy Pl, Box 1508, New York, NY 10029-6500; **Phone:** 212-241-5446; **Board Cert:** Pediatrics 1975; Neonatal-Perinatal Medicine 1977; **Med School:** Univ Pittsburgh 1971; **Resid:** Pediatrics, Chldns Hosp 1975; **Fellow:** Neonatal-Perinatal Medicine, Univ Colorado Hosp 1977; **Fac Appt:** Prof Ped, Mount Sinai Sch Med

Hurt, Hallam MD [NP] - **Hospital:** Chldns Hosp of Philadelphia, The, Hosp Univ Penn - UPHS (page 72); **Address:** Chldns Hosp of Philadelphia, 3535 Market St, rm 1509, Philadelphia, PA 19104; **Phone:** 215-590-0560; **Board Cert:** Pediatrics 1976; Neonatal-Perinatal Medicine 2002; **Med School:** Univ VA Sch Med 1971; **Resid:** Pediatrics, Univ Virginia Hosp 1974; **Fellow:** Neonatal-Perinatal Medicine, Univ Virginia Hosp 1976; **Fac Appt:** Prof Ped, Temple Univ

La Gamma, Edmund F MD [NP] - **Spec Exp:** Neonatal Infections; Prematurity/Low Birth Weight Infants; Necrotizing Enterocolitis; **Hospital:** Westchester Med Ctr; **Address:** Maria Fareri Chldns Hosp, Grasslands Rd Fl 2, Valhalla, NY 10595-0001; **Phone:** 914-493-8558; **Board Cert:** Pediatrics 1981; Neonatal-Perinatal Medicine 1981; **Med School:** NY Med Coll 1976; **Resid:** Pediatrics, NY Hosp-Cornell Med Ctr 1978; **Fellow:** Neonatal-Perinatal Medicine, NY Hosp-Cornell Med Ctr 1980; Cardiovascular Disease, UCSF Med Ctr 1981; **Fac Appt:** Prof Ped, NY Med Coll

Lambert, George MD [NP] - **Spec Exp:** Environmental Toxicology-Autism; Neonatal Critical Care; **Hospital:** Robert Wood Johnson Univ Hosp - New Brunswick; **Address:** UMDNJ, 1 Robert Johnson Pl, rm MEB 394, New Brunswick, NJ 08903; **Phone:** 732-235-7900; **Board Cert:** Pediatrics 1979; Neonatal-Perinatal Medicine 1979; **Med School:** Univ IL Coll Med 1972; **Resid:** Pediatrics, Johns Hopkins Hosp 1974; **Fellow:** Pharmacology, Natl Inst Hlth 1976; Neonatal-Perinatal Medicine, Chldns Hosp 1978; **Fac Appt:** Assoc Prof Ped, UMDNJ-RW Johnson Med Sch

Lawson, Edward E MD [NP] - **Spec Exp:** Neonatal Critical Care; Breathing Disorders; Prematurity/Low Birth Weight Infants; **Hospital:** Johns Hopkins Hosp - Baltimore (page 61), Johns Hopkins Bayview Med Ctr (page 61); **Address:** Johns Hopkins Chldns Ctr, 600 N Wolfe St, Nelson 2-133, Baltimore, MD 21287; **Phone:** 410-955-5259; **Board Cert:** Pediatrics 1990; Neonatal-Perinatal Medicine 1997; **Med School:** Northwestern Univ 1972; **Resid:** Pediatrics, Chldns Hosp Med Ctr 1975; **Fellow:** Neonatal-Perinatal Medicine, Harvard Med Sch 1977; **Fac Appt:** Prof Ped, Johns Hopkins Univ

Nogee, Lawrence M MD [NP] - **Spec Exp:** Lung Disease in Newborns-Genetic; **Hospital:** Johns Hopkins Hosp - Baltimore (page 61); **Address:** Johns Hopkins Hosp, Div Neonatolgy, 600 N Wolfe St, Nelson 2-133, Baltimore, MD 21287-3200; **Phone:** 410-955-5259; **Board Cert:** Pediatrics 1986; Neonatal-Perinatal Medicine 1987; **Med School:** Johns Hopkins Univ 1981; **Resid:** Pediatrics, Johns Hopkins Hosp 1984; **Fellow:** Neonatal-Perinatal Medicine, Chldns Hosp Med Ctr 1986; **Fac Appt:** Assoc Prof Ped, Johns Hopkins Univ

Perlman, Jeffrey M MD [NP] - **Spec Exp:** Neonatal Critical Care; Prematurity/Low Birth Weight Infants; Neonatal Neurology; **Hospital:** NY-Presby Hosp/Weill Cornell (page 66); **Address:** 525 E 68th St, Ste N 506, New York, NY 10021; **Phone:** 212-746-3530; **Board Cert:** Pediatrics 1983; Neonatal-Perinatal Medicine 1983; **Med School:** South Africa 1974; **Resid:** Pediatrics, Johannesburg Chlds Hosp 1979; Pediatrics, St Louis Chldns Hosp 1981; **Fellow:** Neonatology, St Louis Chldns Hosp 1983; **Fac Appt:** Prof Ped, Cornell Univ-Weill Med Coll

Polin, Richard MD [NP] - **Spec Exp:** Neonatal Infections; **Hospital:** NYPresby-Morgan Stanley Children's Hosp; **Address:** Morgan Stanley Chlds Hosp of NY-Presby, 3959 Broadway, CHC 115, New York, NY 10032; **Phone:** 212-305-5827; **Board Cert:** Pediatrics 1975; Neonatal-Perinatal Medicine 1977; **Med School:** Temple Univ 1970; **Resid:** Pediatrics, Chldns Meml Hosp 1972; Pediatrics, Babies Hosp-Columbia Presby 1975; **Fellow:** Neonatal-Perinatal Medicine, Babies Hosp-Columbia Presby 1974; **Fac Appt:** Prof Ped, Columbia P&S

Sison, Joseph MD [NP] - **Hospital:** Englewood Hosp & Med Ctr, Mount Sinai Med Ctr; **Address:** 350 Engle St, Englewood, NJ 07631-1808; **Phone:** 201-894-3321; **Board Cert:** Pediatrics 2000; Neonatal-Perinatal Medicine 1997; **Med School:** Philippines 1984; **Resid:** Pediatrics, Jersey Shore Med Ctr 1992; Neonatal-Perinatal Medicine, Vanderbilt Univ Hosp 1993; **Fellow:** Neonatal-Perinatal Medicine, New York Hosp 1995; **Fac Appt:** Clin Prof Ped, Mount Sinai Sch Med

Sola, Augusto MD [NP] - **Hospital:** Morristown Mem Hosp; **Address:** Mid-Atlantic Neonatology Assocs, 100 Madison Ave, Box 85, Morristown, NJ 07962; **Phone:** 973-971-5488; **Board Cert:** Pediatrics 1979; Neonatal-Perinatal Medicine 1979; **Med School:** Argentina 1973; **Resid:** Pediatrics, St Vincents Hosp 1976; Pediatrics, Univ Mass Meml Med Ctr 1977; **Fellow:** Neonatal-Perinatal Medicine, Univ Mass Meml Med Ctr 1978

Southeast

Bancalari, Eduardo MD [NP] - **Spec Exp:** Neonatology; **Hospital:** Jackson Meml Hosp; **Address:** Dept Pediatrics (R-131), PO Box 016960, Miami, FL 33101; **Phone:** 305-585-2328; **Board Cert:** Neonatal-Perinatal Medicine 1993; Pediatrics 1993; **Med School:** Chile 1966; **Resid:** Pediatrics, Hosp Luis Calvo Mackenna 1969; **Fellow:** Pediatric Cardiology, Univ Miami Med Ctr; **Fac Appt:** Prof Ped, Univ Miami Sch Med

Boyle, Robert J MD [NP] - **Spec Exp:** Neonatology; Ethics; **Hospital:** Univ Virginia Med Ctr; **Address:** UVA Hlth Sci Ctr, Dept Peds, PO Box 800386, Charlottesville, VA 22908; **Phone:** 434-924-5429; **Board Cert:** Pediatrics 1978; Neonatal-Perinatal Medicine 1979; **Med School:** Johns Hopkins Univ 1973; **Resid:** Pediatrics, Rainbow Babies Chldns Hosp 1976; **Fellow:** Neonatal-Perinatal Medicine, Women & Infants Hosp 1978; **Fac Appt:** Prof Ped, Univ VA Sch Med

Bucciarelli, Richard L MD [NP] - **Spec Exp:** Neonatal Cardiology; **Hospital:** Shands Hlthcre at Univ of FL; **Address:** Shands Healthcare, 1600 SW Archer Rd, rm M105, Gainesville, FL 32610; **Phone:** 352-273-5329; **Board Cert:** Pediatrics 1977; Neonatal-Perinatal Medicine 1977; Pediatric Cardiology 1977; **Med School:** Univ Mich Med Sch 1972; **Resid:** Pediatrics, Shands Hosp-Univ Fla 1975; **Fellow:** Neonatal-Perinatal Medicine, Shands Hosp-Univ Fla 1977; **Fac Appt:** Prof Ped, Univ Fla Coll Med

Holtzman, Ronald B MD [NP] - **Spec Exp:** Neonatology; Lung Disease in Newborns; **Hospital:** Gaston Meml Hosp; **Address:** Gaston Meml Hosp, NICU Office, 2525 Court Drive, Gastonia, NC 28054-2140; **Phone:** 704-834-3390; **Board Cert:** Pediatrics 1987; Neonatal-Perinatal Medicine 2004; **Med School:** Rush Med Coll 1983; **Resid:** Pediatrics, Chldns Meml/Northwestern Univ 1986; **Fellow:** Neonatal-Perinatal Medicine, Chldns Meml/Northwestern Univ 1986

Kattwinkel, John MD [NP] - **Spec Exp:** Lung Disorders of Prematurity; Sudden Infant Death Syndrome (SIDS); **Hospital:** Univ Virginia Med Ctr; **Address:** Univ Va Hosp, Div Neonatology, Dept Peds, PO Box 800386, Charlottesville, VA 22908-0386; **Phone:** 434-924-5428; **Board Cert:** Pediatrics 1986; Neonatal-Perinatal Medicine 1986; **Med School:** Harvard Med Sch 1968; **Resid:** Pediatrics, Duke Univ Med Ctr 1970; **Fellow:** Neonatology, Case-West Res Univ 1974; **Fac Appt:** Prof Ped, Univ VA Sch Med

Neu, Josef MD [NP] - **Spec Exp:** Neonatal Nutrition; Neonatal Gastroenterology; **Hospital:** Shands Hlthcre at Univ of FL; **Address:** Shands Healthcare-Univ Fla, 1600 SW Archer Rd, rm HD513, Gainesville, FL 32610; **Phone:** 352-392-3020; **Board Cert:** Pediatrics 1980; Neonatal-Perinatal Medicine 1981; **Med School:** Univ Wisc 1975; **Resid:** Pediatrics, Johns Hopkins Hosp 1978; **Fellow:** Neonatal-Perinatal Medicine, Stanford Univ 1980; **Fac Appt:** Prof Ped, Univ Fla Coll Med

Stiles, Alan MD [NP] - **Spec Exp:** Neonatology; **Hospital:** Univ NC Hosps; **Address:** 130 Mason Farm Rd, CB7220, Chapel Hill, NC 27599-7220; **Phone:** 919-966-4427; **Board Cert:** Pediatrics 1984; Neonatal-Perinatal Medicine 1985; **Med School:** Univ NC Sch Med 1977; **Resid:** Pediatrics, North Carolina Meml Hosp 1982; **Fellow:** Neonatal-Perinatal Medicine, Chldns Hosp/Brigham Hosp 1985; **Fac Appt:** Prof Ped, Univ NC Sch Med

Midwest

Bell, Edward F MD [NP] - **Spec Exp:** Neonatal Critical Care; Prematurity/Low Birth Weight Infants; **Hospital:** Univ Iowa Hosp & Clinics, Genesis Med Ctr; **Address:** Univ Iowa Hosps, Dept Pediatrics, 200 Hawkins Drive, rm 8811 JPP, Iowa City, IA 52242; **Phone:** 319-356-4006; **Board Cert:** Pediatrics 1978; Neonatal-Perinatal Medicine 1995; **Med School:** Columbia P&S 1973; **Resid:** Pediatrics, Babies Hosp-Columbia Presby 1976; **Fellow:** Neonatology, McMaster Univ Med Ctr 1977; Neonatology, Women & Infants Hosp-Brown Univ 1979; **Fac Appt:** Prof Ped, Univ Iowa Coll Med

Cole, Francis Sessions MD [NP] - **Spec Exp:** Neonatal Chronic Lung Disease (CLD); Respiratory Distress Syndrome (RDS); Surfactant Biology; Prematurity/Low Birth Weight Infants; **Hospital:** St Louis Chldns Hosp, Barnes-Jewish Hosp; **Address:** St Louis Chldns Hosp, 1 Children's Pl, Box 8116/NWT, St Louis, MO 63110; **Phone:** 314-454-6148; **Board Cert:** Pediatrics 1980; Neonatal-Perinatal Medicine 1983; **Med School:** Yale Univ 1973; **Resid:** Pediatrics, Chldns Hosp Med Ctr 1978; **Fellow:** Neonatology, Brigham & Womens Hosp 1981; **Fac Appt:** Prof Ped, Washington Univ, St Louis

Neonatal-Perinatal Medicine

Donn, Steven M MD [NP] - **Spec Exp:** Breathing Disorders; Respiratory Distress Syndrome (RDS); Pulmonary Hypertension of Newborn (PPHN); Surfactant Biology; **Hospital:** Mott Chldns Hosp; **Address:** F5790 Mott Hosp/ 0254, 1500 E Med Ctr Drive, Ann Arbor, MI 48109-0999; **Phone:** 734-763-4109; **Board Cert:** Pediatrics 1981; Neonatal-Perinatal Medicine 1981; **Med School:** Tulane Univ 1974; **Resid:** Pediatrics, Univ Vermont Med Ctr 1978; **Fellow:** Neonatology, Univ Michigan 1980; **Fac Appt:** Prof Ped, Univ Mich Med Sch

Gewolb, Ira MD [NP] - **Spec Exp:** Breathing Disorders; **Hospital:** Mich State Univ-Sparrow Hos; **Address:** Sparrow Hosp, Div Neonatology, 1215 E Michigan Ave, Lansing, MI 48912; **Phone:** 517-364-2670; **Board Cert:** Pediatrics 1980; Neonatal-Perinatal Medicine 1981; **Med School:** Yale Univ 1976; **Resid:** Pediatrics, Childrens Hosp Med Ctr 1979; **Fellow:** Neonatology, Yale Univ 1981; **Fac Appt:** Prof Ped, Mich State Univ

Hamvas, Aaron MD [NP] - **Spec Exp:** Lung Disease in Newborns-Genetic; **Hospital:** St Louis Chldns Hosp, Barnes-Jewish Hosp; **Address:** St Louis Chldns Hosp, One Childrens Place, NICU-5th Fl, St Louis, MO 63110; **Phone:** 314-454-6148; **Board Cert:** Pediatrics 1989; Neonatal-Perinatal Medicine 2006; **Med School:** Washington Univ, St Louis 1981; **Resid:** Pediatrics, St Louis Chldns Hosp 1984; **Fellow:** Neonatology, St Louis Chldns Hosp 1990; **Fac Appt:** Prof Ped, Washington Univ, St Louis

Jobe, Alan H MD/PhD [NP] - **Spec Exp:** Surfactant Biology; Respiratory Distress Syndrome (RDS); Neonatal Chronic Lung Disease (CLD); **Hospital:** Cincinnati Chldns Hosp Med Ctr; **Address:** Chldns Hosp Med Ctr, Div Pulm Biology, 3333 Burnett Ave, Cincinnati, OH 45229-3039; **Phone:** 513-636-8603; **Board Cert:** Pediatrics 1978; Neonatal-Perinatal Medicine 2000; **Med School:** UCSD 1973; **Resid:** Pediatrics, UCSD Med Ctr 1975; **Fellow:** Neonatal-Perinatal Medicine, UCSD Med Ctr 1977; **Fac Appt:** Prof Ped, Univ Cincinnati

Lemons, James A MD [NP] - **Spec Exp:** Nutrition; Ethics; **Hospital:** Riley Hosp for Children, Indiana Univ Hosp; **Address:** 699 West Drive, RR-208, Indianapolis, IN 46202-5119; **Phone:** 317-274-4716; **Board Cert:** Pediatrics 1993; Neonatal-Perinatal Medicine 1993; **Med School:** Northwestern Univ 1969; **Resid:** Pediatrics, Univ Mich Med Sch 1972; **Fellow:** Neonatal-Perinatal Medicine, Univ Colo Med Ctr 1975; **Fac Appt:** Prof Ped, Indiana Univ

Martin, Richard J MD [NP] - **Spec Exp:** Breathing Disorders; **Hospital:** Rainbow Babies & Chldns Hosp; **Address:** 11100 Euclid Ave, Cleveland, OH 44106-6010; **Phone:** 216-844-3387; **Board Cert:** Pediatrics 1976; Neonatal-Perinatal Medicine 1977; **Med School:** Australia 1970; **Resid:** Pediatrics, Univ Missouri 1973; **Fellow:** Neonatal-Perinatal Medicine, Case West Res Univ 1975; **Fac Appt:** Prof Ped, Case West Res Univ

Meadow, William MD [NP] - **Spec Exp:** Infections-Neonatal; Ethics; **Hospital:** Univ of Chicago Hosps; **Address:** 5841 S Maryland Ave, MC-6060, Chicago, IL 60637; **Phone:** 773-702-6210; **Board Cert:** Pediatrics 1979; Neonatal-Perinatal Medicine 1981; **Med School:** Univ Pennsylvania 1974; **Resid:** Pediatrics, Chldns Meml Hosp 1978; **Fellow:** Neonatology, Wyler Chldns Hosp 1981; Infectious Disease, Wyler Chldns Hosp 1981; **Fac Appt:** Prof Ped, Univ Chicago-Pritzker Sch Med

Muraskas, Jonathan MD [NP] - **Spec Exp:** Prematurity/Low Birth Weight Infants; Multiple Gestation; Conjoined Twins; Ethics; **Hospital:** Loyola Univ Med Ctr; **Address:** Loyola University Medical Ctr, Bldg 107, 2160 S First Ave, rm 5811, Maywood, IL 60153-5500; **Phone:** 708-216-1067; **Board Cert:** Pediatrics 1987; Neonatal-Perinatal Medicine 1987; **Med School:** Loyola Univ-Stritch Sch Med 1982; **Resid:** Pediatrics, Loyola Univ Med Ctr 1985; **Fellow:** Neonatal-Perinatal Medicine, Loyola Univ Med Ctr 1987; **Fac Appt:** Prof Ped, Loyola Univ-Stritch Sch Med

Steinhorn, Robin H MD [NP] - **Spec Exp:** Pulmonary Hypertension; Neonatology; **Hospital:** Children's Mem Hosp, Northwestern Meml Hosp; **Address:** 2300 Children's Plaza, Box 45, Chicago, IL 60614; **Phone:** 773-880-4142; **Board Cert:** Pediatrics 2000; Neonatal-Perinatal Medicine 2002; **Med School:** Washington Univ, St Louis 1980; **Resid:** Obstetrics & Gynecology, Barnes Hosp 1983; Pediatrics, Univ Minn 1986; **Fellow:** Neonatal-Perinatal Medicine, Univ Minn 1988; **Fac Appt:** Prof Ped, Northwestern Univ

Whitsett, Jeffrey A MD [NP] - **Spec Exp:** Lung Disease in Newborns-Genetic; **Hospital:** Cincinnati Chldns Hosp Med Ctr, Good Samaritan Hosp - Cincinnati; **Address:** Cincinnati Chldns Hosp, Div Neonatalogy, 3333 Burnet Ave, Cincinnati, OH 45229-3039; **Phone:** 513-636-4830; **Board Cert:** Pediatrics 1979; Neonatal-Perinatal Medicine 1979; **Med School:** Columbia P&S 1973; **Resid:** Pediatrics, Mt Sinai Hosp 1976; **Fellow:** Neonatology, Chldns Hosp Med Ctr 1977; **Fac Appt:** Prof Ped, Univ Cincinnati

Great Plains and Mountains

Milley, J Ross MD/PhD [NP] - **Spec Exp:** Nutrition; **Hospital:** Primary Children's Med Ctr, Univ Utah Hosps and Clins; **Address:** Univ Utah - Dept Pediatrics/Neonatology, Williams Bldg, PO Box 581289, Salt Lake City, UT 84158; **Phone:** 801-581-7085; **Board Cert:** Pediatrics 1980; Neonatal-Perinatal Medicine 1981; **Med School:** Univ Chicago-Pritzker Sch Med 1975; **Resid:** Pediatrics, Johns Hopkins Hosp 1978; **Fellow:** Neonatology, Johns Hopkins Hosp 1980; **Fac Appt:** Prof Ped, Univ Utah

Southwest

Adams, James M MD [NP] - **Spec Exp:** Lung Disease in Newborns; **Hospital:** Texas Chldns Hosp - Houston; **Address:** 6621 Fannin St, MC WT-6104, Houston, TX 77030; **Phone:** 832-826-1380; **Board Cert:** Pediatrics 1975; Neonatal-Perinatal Medicine 1975; **Med School:** Baylor Coll Med 1969; **Resid:** Pediatrics, Baylor Affil Hosps 1973; **Fellow:** Neonatal-Perinatal Medicine, Baylor Affil Hosps 1975; **Fac Appt:** Prof Ped, Baylor Coll Med

Denson, Susan Ellen MD [NP] - **Spec Exp:** Neonatology; **Hospital:** Meml Hermann Hosp - Houston, LBJ General Hosp; **Address:** Univ Tex Houston Med Sch, Dept Peds, 6431 Fannin, Ste 3.256, Houston, TX 77030; **Phone:** 713-500-5727; **Board Cert:** Pediatrics 1978; Neonatal-Perinatal Medicine 1979; **Med School:** Univ Tex SW, Dallas 1972; **Resid:** Pediatrics, Univ Ariz 1974; **Fellow:** Neonatal-Perinatal Medicine, Univ Ariz 1975; Neonatal-Perinatal Medicine, Univ Tex Med Sch 1976; **Fac Appt:** Prof Ped, Univ Tex, Houston

Escobedo, Marilyn B MD [NP] - **Spec Exp:** Neonatology; Nutrition; **Hospital:** Chldns Hosp OU Med Ctr; **Address:** 1200 Everett Dr, 7th Fl, North Pavilion, Oklahoma City, OK 73104; **Phone:** 405-271-5215; **Board Cert:** Pediatrics 1986; Neonatal-Perinatal Medicine 2004; **Med School:** Washington Univ, St Louis 1970; **Resid:** Pediatrics, Chldns Hosp 1972; Neonatal-Perinatal Medicine, Chldns Hosp 1973; **Fellow:** Neonatal-Perinatal Medicine, Vanderbilt Univ 1976; **Fac Appt:** Prof Ped, Univ Okla Coll Med

Garcia-Prats, Joseph MD [NP] - **Spec Exp:** Lung Disease in Newborns; Neonatology; **Hospital:** Texas Chldns Hosp - Houston, Ben Taub General Hosp; **Address:** 6621 Fannin St, MC WT-6104, Houston, TX 77030-1608; **Phone:** 832-826-1380; **Board Cert:** Pediatrics 1977; Neonatal-Perinatal Medicine 1977; **Med School:** Tulane Univ 1972; **Resid:** Pediatrics, Baylor Affil Hosp 1975; **Fellow:** Neonatal-Perinatal Medicine, Baylor Affil Hosp 1977; **Fac Appt:** Prof Ped, Baylor Coll Med

Neonatal-Perinatal Medicine

Malloy, Michael H MD [NP] - **Spec Exp:** Epidemiology; Sudden Infant Death Syndrome (SIDS); **Hospital:** UT Med Br Hosp at Galveston; **Address:** Univ Texas Med Br, Dept Pediatric Neonatology, 301 University Blvd, Galveston, TX 77555-0526; **Phone:** 409-772-2815; **Board Cert:** Pediatrics 1986; Neonatal-Perinatal Medicine 1995; **Med School:** Univ Tex Med Br, Galveston 1973; **Resid:** Pediatrics, Univ Texas Med Br 1976; **Fellow:** Neonatology, Univ Texas Med Sch 1978; **Fac Appt:** Prof Ped, Univ Tex Med Br, Galveston

Odom, Michael W MD [NP] - **Spec Exp:** Neonatology; **Hospital:** Univ Hlth Sys - Univ Hosp; **Address:** Dept Peds, 7703 Floyd Curl Drive, MC 7812, San Antonio, TX 78229-3900; **Phone:** 210-567-5225; **Board Cert:** Pediatrics 1987; Neonatal-Perinatal Medicine 1997; **Med School:** Univ Tex SW, Dallas 1983; **Resid:** Pediatrics, Vanderbilt Univ Affil Hosps 1986; **Fellow:** Neonatal-Perinatal Medicine, Mt Zion Med Ctr-UCSF 1989; **Fac Appt:** Assoc Prof Ped, Univ Tex, San Antonio

Seidner, Steven R MD [NP] - **Spec Exp:** Neonatal Chronic Lung Disease (CLD); Respiratory Distress Syndrome (RDS); Pulmonary Hypertension of Newborn (PPHN); **Hospital:** Univ Hlth Sys - Univ Hosp; **Address:** Univ Texas Hlth Sci Ctr, Dept Peds, 7703 Floyd Curl Drive, MC 7812, San Antonio, TX 78229-3901; **Phone:** 210-567-5229; **Board Cert:** Pediatrics 1987; Neonatal-Perinatal Medicine 1987; **Med School:** Univ Ariz Coll Med 1982; **Resid:** Pediatrics, Harbor-UCLA Med Ctr 1985; **Fellow:** Neonatal-Perinatal Medicine, Harbor-UCLA Med Ctr 1988; **Fac Appt:** Prof Ped, Univ Tex, San Antonio

Tyson, Jon Edward MD [NP] - **Spec Exp:** Neonatology; Epidemiology; **Hospital:** Meml Hermann Hosp - Houston; **Address:** Univ Tex, Ctr Clin Rsch, 6431 Fannin St, Ste 2.106, Houston, TX 77030; **Phone:** 713-500-5651; **Board Cert:** Pediatrics 1973; Neonatal-Perinatal Medicine 1975; **Med School:** Tulane Univ 1968; **Resid:** Pediatrics, Univ Tenn/Memphis Hosp 1971; **Fellow:** Neonatology, McMaster Univ 1975; **Fac Appt:** Prof Ped, Univ Tex, Houston

West Coast and Pacific

Ariagno, Ronald L MD [NP] - **Spec Exp:** Sudden Infant Death Syndrome (SIDS); Breathing Disorders; **Hospital:** Stanford Univ Med Ctr; **Address:** Stanford Univ, Div Neonatology, 750 Welch Rd, Ste 315, Palo Alto, CA 94304; **Phone:** 650-723-5711; **Board Cert:** Pediatrics 1973; Neonatal-Perinatal Medicine 1975; **Med School:** Univ IL Coll Med 1968; **Resid:** Pediatrics, Presby-St Lukes Hosp 1971; **Fellow:** Neonatology, Chldns Hosp, UCSF 1975; **Fac Appt:** Prof Ped, Stanford Univ

Stevenson, David K MD [NP] - **Spec Exp:** Neonatology; **Hospital:** Lucile Packard Chldns Hosp/Stanford Univ Med Ctr; **Address:** 750 Welch Rd, Ste 315, Palo Alto, CA 94304-1510; **Phone:** 650-723-5711; **Board Cert:** Pediatrics 1979; Neonatal-Perinatal Medicine 2004; **Med School:** Univ Wash 1975; **Resid:** Pediatrics, Univ Washington 1977; **Fellow:** Neonatal-Perinatal Medicine, Stanford Univ 1979; **Fac Appt:** Prof Ped, Stanford Univ

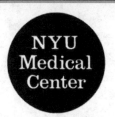

NYU Medical Center

550 First Avenue (at 31st Street)
New York, NY 10016
Physician Referral:
(888)7-NYU-MED (888-769-8633)
www.nyumc.org

PEDIATRIC CRITICAL CARE

When children experience medical problems, they deserve the most compassionate, state-of-the-art medical care possible. Yet, pediatric patients have needs, medical and emotional, that are unique and different from those of adults. To better meet these needs, Tisch Hospital at NYU Medical Center has recently completed a major expansion and improvement of its Pediatric Intensive Care Unit (PICU).

In most hospitals, pediatric patients recover in specialized areas annexed to the adult units for their particular ailment. For example, children recovering from neurosurgery would have awakened in a pediatric section of the neurosurgery unit to find a crowded and noisy recovery room that did not cater to their unique physical and emotional needs. At NYU, they recover in an environment developed especially for them, with a multidisciplinary staff assembled just for them.

The PICU at NYU Medical Center has the added advantage of being a real resource to referring physicians, providing them with the technology, expertise and time-saving procedures that can help them save lives.

At NYU Medical Center, parents are viewed as integral members of the healthcare team because each child's recovery is strongly influenced by continued family involvement. In recognition of this, each room has a rollaway sofa or chair so one parent can spend the night in close proximity to the child for the duration of their stay. In addition, there is a special family room that was created to give families a quiet place to gather together. Of course, the PICU staff also strives to keep children in contact with their parents and to keep parents informed throughout their child's stay.

NYU MEDICAL CENTER

Understanding that healthcare concerns and pediatric emergencies may occur at any time, the PICU staff is available around the clock to provide a second opinion, consult on a specific case, or help expedite a patients' admission. Social services are also available, and there is an on-site pharmacy within the unit.

The new PICU has been equipped with state-of-the-art monitors, dialysis machines, ventilators, and an isolation room. Special capabilities are available to monitor patients who have had surgery for epilepsy.

For children who stay in the PICU for more than a week, physician and occupational therapists will help develop a postdischarge rehabilitation plan. In addition, PICU patients are assigned a social worker, when necessary, to provide referrals for home care and other services.

Nephrology

a subspecialty of Internal Medicine

An internist who treats disorders of the kidney, high blood pressure, fluid and mineral balance and dialysis of body wastes when the kidneys do not function. This specialist consults with surgeons about kidney transplantation.

Training Required: Three years in internal medicine *plus* additional training and examination for certification in nephrology.

Nephrology

New England

Aronson, Peter S MD [Nep] - **Spec Exp:** Fluid/Electrolyte Balance; Kidney Stones; **Hospital:** Yale - New Haven Hosp, VA Conn Hlthcre Sys; **Address:** Yale Sch Med, Dept Medicine, PO Box 208029, New Haven, CT 06520-8029; **Phone:** 203-785-4186; **Board Cert:** Internal Medicine 1973; Nephrology 1976; **Med School:** NYU Sch Med 1970; **Resid:** Internal Medicine, NC Meml Hosp 1972; **Fellow:** Nephrology, Yale Univ Sch Med 1977; **Fac Appt:** Prof Med, Yale Univ

Bazari, Hasan MD [Nep] - **Spec Exp:** Kidney Failure-Acute; Nephrotic Syndrome; Hypertension; **Hospital:** Mass Genl Hosp; **Address:** Renal Assocs, Mass Genl Hospital, 55 Fruit St Gray Bldg - Ste 1003, Boston, MA 02114; **Phone:** 617-726-5050; **Board Cert:** Internal Medicine 1986; Nephrology 1988; **Med School:** Albert Einstein Coll Med 1983; **Resid:** Internal Medicine, Mass Genl Hosp 1986; **Fellow:** Nephrology, Mass Genl Hosp 1988

Brenner, Barry M MD [Nep] - **Spec Exp:** Hypertension; Diabetic Kidney Disease; Kidney Failure-Acute; Kidney Failure-Chronic; **Hospital:** Brigham & Women's Hosp; **Address:** Brigham & Women's Hosp, Renal Div, 75 Francis St, Boston, MA 02115; **Phone:** 617-732-5850; **Med School:** Univ Pittsburgh 1962; **Resid:** Internal Medicine, Albert Einstein Coll Med 1966; **Fellow:** Nephrology, Nat Inst Health 1969; **Fac Appt:** Prof Med, Harvard Med Sch

Coggins, Cecil MD [Nep] - **Spec Exp:** Kidney Disease; Hypertension; **Hospital:** Mass Genl Hosp; **Address:** 100 Charles River Plaza, Ste 501, Boston, MA 02114-2712; **Phone:** 617-726-4900; **Board Cert:** Internal Medicine 1965; Nephrology 1974; **Med School:** Harvard Med Sch 1958; **Resid:** Internal Medicine, Stanford Univ Med Ctr 1965; Internal Medicine; **Fellow:** Nephrology, Stanford Univ Med Ctr 1963; Nephrology, Mass Genl Hosp 1967; **Fac Appt:** Assoc Prof Med, Harvard Med Sch

Kliger, Alan MD [Nep] - **Spec Exp:** Kidney Disease; Kidney Disease-Metabolic; **Hospital:** Hosp of St Raphael; **Address:** 136 Sherman Ave, New Haven, CT 06511-5238; **Phone:** 203-787-0117 x307; **Board Cert:** Internal Medicine 1973; Nephrology 1976; **Med School:** SUNY Upstate Med Univ 1970; **Resid:** Internal Medicine, SUNY Upstate Med Ctr 1973; **Fellow:** Nephrology, Georgetown Univ Hosp 1975; **Fac Appt:** Clin Prof Med, Yale Univ

Perrone, Ronald MD [Nep] - **Spec Exp:** Kidney Disease-Chronic; Kidney Failure-Acute; Polycystic Kidney Disease; **Hospital:** Tufts-New England Med Ctr; **Address:** Tufts-New Eng Med Ctr, Div Nephrology, 750 Washington St, Box 391, Boston, MA 02111; **Phone:** 617-636-5866; **Board Cert:** Internal Medicine 1979; Nephrology 1982; **Med School:** Hahnemann Univ 1975; **Resid:** Internal Medicine, Grady Meml Hosp 1978; **Fellow:** Nephrology, Boston Med Ctr 1982; **Fac Appt:** Prof Med, Tufts Univ

Salant, David MD [Nep] - **Spec Exp:** Kidney Disease-Glomerular; Kidney Disease-Autoimmune; Lupus Nephritis; **Hospital:** Boston Med Ctr; **Address:** 720 Harrison Ave, Boston, MA 02118-2371; **Phone:** 617-638-7480; **Board Cert:** Internal Medicine 1978; Nephrology 1980; **Med School:** South Africa 1969; **Resid:** Internal Medicine, Johannesburg Genl Hosp 1973; **Fellow:** Nephrology, Boston Univ Med Ctr 1978; **Fac Appt:** Prof Med, Boston Univ

Seifter, Julian L MD [Nep] - **Spec Exp:** Diabetic Kidney Disease; Kidney Failure-Chronic; Kidney Stones; **Hospital:** Brigham & Women's Hosp; **Address:** Brigham & Women's Hosp, Div Renal Med, 75 Francis St, MRB-4, Boston, MA 02115; **Phone:** 617-732-5850; **Board Cert:** Internal Medicine 1978; Nephrology 1980; **Med School:** Albert Einstein Coll Med 1975; **Resid:** Internal Medicine, Bronx Muni Hosp Ctr 1981; **Fellow:** Nephrology, Yale-New Haven Hosp 1982; **Fac Appt:** Assoc Prof Med, Harvard Med Sch

Tolkoff-Rubin, Nina MD [Nep] - **Spec Exp:** Transplant Medicine-Kidney; Hypertension; Kidney Failure-Acute; **Hospital:** Mass Genl Hosp; **Address:** 55 Fruit St, GRB 103, Boston, MA 02114; **Phone:** 617-726-3706; **Board Cert:** Nephrology 1974; Internal Medicine 1972; **Med School:** Harvard Med Sch 1968; **Resid:** Internal Medicine, Mass Genl Hosp 1970; Internal Medicine, Mass Genl Hosp 1972; **Fellow:** Nephrology, Mass Genl Hosp 1971; **Fac Appt:** Assoc Prof Med, Harvard Med Sch

Mid Atlantic

Appel, Gerald MD [Nep] - **Spec Exp:** Glomerulonephritis; Lupus Nephritis; Nephrotic Syndrome; **Hospital:** NY-Presby Hosp/Columbia (page 66); **Address:** 622 W 168th St, Ste PH4-124, New York, NY 10032-3720; **Phone:** 212-305-3273; **Board Cert:** Internal Medicine 1975; Nephrology 1978; **Med School:** Albert Einstein Coll Med 1972; **Resid:** Internal Medicine, Columbia Presby Hosp 1975; **Fellow:** Nephrology, Columbia Presby Hosp 1976; Nephrology, Yale-New Haven Hosp 1978; **Fac Appt:** Clin Prof Med, Columbia P&S

August, Phyllis MD [Nep] - **Spec Exp:** Hypertension; Hypertension in Pregnancy; **Hospital:** NY-Presby Hosp/Weill Cornell (page 66); **Address:** 525 E 68th St, Ste L-1, New York, NY 10021-4870; **Phone:** 212-746-2210; **Board Cert:** Internal Medicine 1980; Nephrology 1982; **Med School:** Yale Univ 1977; **Resid:** Internal Medicine, NY Hosp-Cornell Med Ctr 1980; **Fellow:** Nephrology, NY Hosp-Cornell Med Ctr 1983; **Fac Appt:** Prof Med, Cornell Univ-Weill Med Coll

Blumenfeld, Jon D MD [Nep] - **Spec Exp:** Hypertension; Polycystic Kidney Disease; Adrenal Disorders; **Hospital:** NY-Presby Hosp/Weill Cornell (page 66), Rockefeller Univ; **Address:** The Rogosin Institute, 505 E 70th St, rm HT230, New York, NY 10021; **Phone:** 212-746-1495; **Board Cert:** Internal Medicine 1984; Nephrology 1986; **Med School:** Yale Univ 1981; **Resid:** Internal Medicine, NY Hosp-Cornell Med Ctr 1984; **Fellow:** Nephrology, Brigham & Womens Hosp 1988; **Fac Appt:** Prof Med, Cornell Univ-Weill Med Coll

Cohen, David J MD [Nep] - **Spec Exp:** Transplant Medicine-Kidney; Glomerulonephritis; **Hospital:** NY-Presby Hosp/Columbia (page 66); **Address:** Columbia Univ Med Ctr, 622 W 168th St, rm PH 4-124, New York, NY 10032-3720; **Phone:** 212-305-3273; **Board Cert:** Internal Medicine 1980; Nephrology 1984; **Med School:** Albert Einstein Coll Med 1977; **Resid:** Internal Medicine, Mount Sinai Hosp 1980; **Fellow:** Nephrology, Columbia Presby Med Ctr 1981; Transplant Immunobiology, Brigham & Women's Hosp 1983; **Fac Appt:** Assoc Prof Med, Columbia P&S

Dosa, Stefan MD [Nep] - **Spec Exp:** Transplant Medicine-Kidney; Lupus Nephritis; Hypertension; **Hospital:** Washington Hosp Ctr, G Washington Univ Hosp; **Address:** 730 24th St NW, Ste 17, Washington, DC 20037; **Phone:** 202-337-7660; **Board Cert:** Internal Medicine 1980; Nephrology 1982; **Med School:** Czech Republic 1967; **Resid:** Internal Medicine, Manchester Royal Infirmary 1977; **Fellow:** Nephrology, Univ Cincinnati 1979; **Fac Appt:** Clin Prof Med, Geo Wash Univ

Johnston, James R MD [Nep] - **Spec Exp:** Diabetic Kidney Disease; Hypertension; **Hospital:** UPMC Presby, Pittsburgh; **Address:** Univ Pittsburgh Physicians, Renal Div, 3550 Terrace St, Scaife Hall, rm A915, Pittsburgh, PA 15261; **Phone:** 412-647-7157; **Board Cert:** Internal Medicine 1982; Nephrology 1984; **Med School:** Univ Pittsburgh 1979; **Resid:** Internal Medicine, Montefiore Hosp 1982; **Fellow:** Nephrology, Univ Pittsburgh Med Ctr 1983; Nephrology, Brigham & Women's Hosp 1986; **Fac Appt:** Prof Med, Univ Pittsburgh

Klotman, Paul E MD [Nep] - **Spec Exp:** AIDS/HIV Related Kidney Disease; **Hospital:** Mount Sinai Med Ctr; **Address:** Mt Sinai Medical Ctr, One Gustave L Levy Pl, Box 1118, New York, NY 10029; **Phone:** 212-241-8007; **Board Cert:** Internal Medicine 1979; Nephrology 1984; **Med School:** Indiana Univ 1976; **Resid:** Internal Medicine, Duke Univ Med Ctr 1981; **Fellow:** Nephrology, Duke Univ Med Ctr 1982; **Fac Appt:** Prof Med, Mount Sinai Sch Med

Kobrin, Sidney M MD [Nep] - **Spec Exp:** Diabetic Kidney Disease; Kidney Failure; Hypertension; **Hospital:** Hosp Univ Penn - UPHS (page 72); **Address:** Hosp Univ Pennsylvania, 3400 Spruce St 210 White Bldg, Philadelphia, PA 19104; **Phone:** 215-662-2638; **Board Cert:** Internal Medicine 1990; Nephrology 2002; **Med School:** South Africa 1978; **Resid:** Internal Medicine, Johannesburg Tchg Hosp 1984; **Fellow:** Nephrology, Einstein Med Ctr 1988; **Fac Appt:** Assoc Prof Med, Univ Pennsylvania

Madaio, Michael P MD [Nep] - **Spec Exp:** Lupus Nephritis; Kidney Disease-Glomerular; **Hospital:** Temple Univ Hosp; **Address:** Nephrology and Kidney Transplantation, 3401 N Broad St, Ste 580, Parkinson Pavilion, Philadelphia, PA 19140; **Phone:** 215-707-3381; **Board Cert:** Internal Medicine 1977; Nephrology 1980; **Med School:** Albany Med Coll 1974; **Resid:** Internal Medicine, Med Coll Va Hosp 1978; **Fellow:** Nephrology, Boston Univ 1981; Tufts Univ 1982; **Fac Appt:** Prof Med, Temple Univ

Piraino, Beth Marie MD [Nep] - **Spec Exp:** Kidney Failure; Hypertension; **Hospital:** UPMC Presby, Pittsburgh; **Address:** 3504 Fifth Ave, Ste 200, Pittsburgh, PA 15213; **Phone:** 412-383-4899; **Board Cert:** Internal Medicine 1980; Nephrology 1982; **Med School:** Med Coll PA Hahnemann 1977; **Resid:** Internal Medicine, Presby Univ Hosp 1980; **Fellow:** Nephrology, Presby Univ Hosp 1982; **Fac Appt:** Prof Med, Univ Pittsburgh

Rudnick, Michael R MD [Nep] - **Spec Exp:** Hypertension; Kidney Disease; **Hospital:** Penn Presby Med Ctr - UPHS (page 72); **Address:** Presbyterian Medical Ctr, Medical Office Bldg, 39th and Market Sts, Ste 240, Philadelphia, PA 19104; **Phone:** 215-662-8730; **Board Cert:** Internal Medicine 1975; Nephrology 1976; **Med School:** Hahnemann Univ 1972; **Resid:** Internal Medicine, Hahnemann U Med Ctr 1974; **Fellow:** Nephrology, Hosp U Penn 1976; **Fac Appt:** Assoc Prof Med, Univ Pennsylvania

Scheel Jr, Paul J MD [Nep] - **Spec Exp:** Kidney Failure; Renovascular Disease; Glomerulonephritis; **Hospital:** Johns Hopkins Hosp - Baltimore (page 61); **Address:** 1830 E Monument St, Ste 416, Baltimore, MD 21205; **Phone:** 410-955-5268; **Board Cert:** Internal Medicine 1990; Nephrology 1997; **Med School:** Georgetown Univ 1987; **Resid:** Internal Medicine, Johns Hopkins Hosp 1990; **Fellow:** Nephrology, Johns Hopkins Hosp 1992; **Fac Appt:** Assoc Prof Med, Johns Hopkins Univ

Scheinman, Steven J MD [Nep] - **Spec Exp:** Kidney Stones; Bartter's Syndrome; Gitelman's Syndrome; **Hospital:** Univ. Hosp.- SUNY Upstate, Crouse Hosp; **Address:** SUNY Upstate Med Univ, Office of the Dean, 750 E Adams St, Syracuse, NY 13210; **Phone:** 315-464-9720; **Board Cert:** Internal Medicine 1980; Nephrology 1984; **Med School:** Yale Univ 1977; **Resid:** Internal Medicine, Yale New Haven Hosp 1990; Internal Medicine, Upstate Med Ctr 1981; **Fellow:** Nephrology, Upstate Med Ctr 1983; Nephrology, Yale New Haven Hosp 1984; **Fac Appt:** Prof Med, SUNY Upstate Med Univ

Townsend, Raymond R MD [Nep] - **Spec Exp:** Hypertension-Complex; Renal Artery Stenosis; **Hospital:** Hosp Univ Penn - UPHS (page 72); **Address:** Renal Electrolyte/Hypertension Div, 3400 Spruce St White Bldg - Ste 210, Philadelphia, PA 19104; **Phone:** 215-662-2638; **Board Cert:** Internal Medicine 1982; Nephrology 1984; **Med School:** Hahnemann Univ 1979; **Resid:** Internal Medicine, Allegheny Genl Hosp 1982; **Fellow:** Nephrology, Temple Univ Hosp 1984; **Fac Appt:** Assoc Prof Med, Univ Pennsylvania

Umans, Jason MD/PhD [Nep] - **Spec Exp:** Hypertension/Kidney Disease in Pregnancy; Kidney Disease; Hypertension; **Hospital:** Georgetown Univ Hosp, Washington Hosp Ctr; **Address:** 3800 Reservoir Rd NW, PHC Bldg- Fl 6, Washington, DC 20007; **Phone:** 202-444-9183; **Board Cert:** Internal Medicine 1988; Nephrology 2000; **Med School:** Cornell Univ-Weill Med Coll 1984; **Resid:** Internal Medicine, Univ Chicago Hosps 1987; **Fellow:** Nephrology, Univ Chicago Hosps 1988; **Fac Appt:** Assoc Prof Med, Georgetown Univ

Wilcox, Christopher S MD [Nep] - **Spec Exp:** Hypertension-Renovascular; Hypertension-Drug Resistent; **Hospital:** Georgetown Univ Hosp; **Address:** Georgetown Univ Med Ctr, 3800 Reservoir Rd NW, PHC Fl 6th, Washington, DC 20007-2113; **Phone:** 202-444-9183; **Board Cert:** Internal Medicine 1983; Nephrology 1986; **Med School:** England 1968; **Resid:** Internal Medicine, Middlesex Hosp 1971; Nephrology, Middlesex Hosp 1972; **Fellow:** Nephrology, Middlesex Hosp 1975; **Fac Appt:** Prof Med, Georgetown Univ

Williams, Gail S MD [Nep] - **Spec Exp:** Kidney Failure-Chronic; Transplant Medicine-Kidney; Critical Care; **Hospital:** NY-Presby Hosp/Columbia (page 66); **Address:** 161 Fort Washington Ave, Ste 351, New York, NY 10032; **Phone:** 212-305-5376; **Board Cert:** Internal Medicine 1972; Nephrology 1974; **Med School:** Columbia P&S 1968; **Resid:** Internal Medicine, Columbia Presby Hosp 1973; **Fellow:** Nephrology, Columbia Presby Hosp 1974; **Fac Appt:** Assoc Clin Prof Med, Columbia P&S

Southeast

Allon, Michael MD [Nep] - **Spec Exp:** Dialysis Care; **Hospital:** Univ of Ala Hosp at Birmingham; **Address:** 1530 3rd Ave S, PB226, Birmingham, AL 35294; **Phone:** 205-975-9676; **Board Cert:** Internal Medicine 1985; Nephrology 1988; **Med School:** Univ Mich Med Sch 1982; **Resid:** Internal Medicine, Emory Univ Hosp 1985; **Fellow:** Nephrology, Emory Univ 1987; **Fac Appt:** Prof Med, Univ Ala

Bolton, W Kline MD [Nep] - **Spec Exp:** Kidney Disease-Glomerular; Kidney Disease-Chronic; **Hospital:** Univ Virginia Med Ctr; **Address:** Univ VA Hlth Scis Ctr, Box 800 133, Charlottesville, VA 22908-0001; **Phone:** 434-924-5125; **Board Cert:** Internal Medicine 1972; Nephrology 1974; **Med School:** Univ VA Sch Med 1969; **Resid:** Internal Medicine, Boston City Hosp 1971; **Fellow:** Nephrology, Univ Chicago 1973; **Fac Appt:** Prof Med, Univ VA Sch Med

Coffman, Thomas M MD [Nep] - **Spec Exp:** Transplant Medicine-Kidney; Hypertension; **Hospital:** Duke Univ Med Ctr; **Address:** Duke Univ Med Center, Box 3014, Durham, NC 27710; **Phone:** 919-286-6947; **Board Cert:** Internal Medicine 1983; Nephrology 1988; **Med School:** Ohio State Univ 1980; **Resid:** Internal Medicine, Duke Univ Med Ctr 1983; **Fellow:** Nephrology, Duke Univ Med Ctr 1985; **Fac Appt:** Prof Med, Duke Univ

Nephrology

Falk, Ronald J MD [Nep] - **Spec Exp:** Glomerulonephritis; Lupus Nephritis; Wegener's Granulomatosis; Vasculitis; **Hospital:** Univ NC Hosps; **Address:** Univ North Carolina Kidney Ctr, 7023 Burnett Womack Bldg CB #7155, Chapel Hill, NC 27599-7155; **Phone:** 919-966-2561; **Board Cert:** Internal Medicine 1980; Nephrology 1982; **Med School:** Univ NC Sch Med 1977; **Resid:** Internal Medicine, Univ North Carolina Hosps 1980; Nephrology, Univ NC 1981; **Fellow:** Research, Univ Minn 1983; **Fac Appt:** Prof Med, Univ NC Sch Med

Helderman, J Harold MD [Nep] - **Spec Exp:** Transplant Medicine-Kidney; Kidney Disease; **Hospital:** Vanderbilt Univ Med Ctr; **Address:** Div Nephrology & Hypertension, 1161 21st Ave S, S-3223 MCN, Nashville, TN 37232-2372; **Phone:** 615-322-2150; **Board Cert:** Internal Medicine 1974; **Med School:** SUNY Downstate 1971; **Resid:** Internal Medicine, Johns Hopkins Hosp 1973; **Fellow:** Nephrology, Brigham & Womens Hosp-Harvard 1976; **Fac Appt:** Prof Med, Vanderbilt Univ

Hoffman, David MD [Nep] - **Spec Exp:** Kidney Disease; Dialysis Care; **Hospital:** Baptist Hosp of Miami; Cedars Med Ctr - Miami; **Address:** 7900 SW 57th Ave, Ste 21, South Miami, FL 33143-5546; **Phone:** 305-662-3984; **Board Cert:** Internal Medicine 1976; Nephrology 1978; **Med School:** Univ Tenn Coll Med, Memphis 1971; **Resid:** Internal Medicine, Jackson Meml Hosp 1975; **Fellow:** Nephrology, Jackson Meml Hosp/Univ Miami 1977

Okusa, Mark D MD [Nep] - **Spec Exp:** Kidney Failure-Chronic; Nephrotic Syndrome; Kidney Failure-Acute; **Hospital:** Univ Virginia Med Ctr; **Address:** Univ VA Hlth Sci Ctr, Div Nephrology, Lee St, Box 800-133, Charlottesville, VA 22908-0001; **Phone:** 434-924-5125; **Board Cert:** Internal Medicine 1985; Nephrology 1988; **Med School:** Med Coll VA 1982; **Resid:** Internal Medicine, Med Coll Virginia 1985; **Fellow:** Nephrology, Yale Univ Sch Med 1988; **Fac Appt:** Prof Med, Univ VA Sch Med

Rakowski, Thomas A MD [Nep] - **Spec Exp:** Polycystic Kidney Disease; Kidney Disease-Glomerular; **Hospital:** Virginia Hosp Ctr - Arlington, Inova Fairfax Hosp; **Address:** 1635 N George Mason Drive, Ste 215, Arlington, VA 22205; **Phone:** 703-841-0707; **Board Cert:** Internal Medicine 1972; Nephrology 1974; **Med School:** Hahnemann Univ 1969; **Resid:** Internal Medicine, Georgetown Univ 1971; **Fellow:** Nephrology, Georgetown Univ 1972; **Fac Appt:** Assoc Prof Med, Georgetown Univ

Roth, David MD [Nep] - **Spec Exp:** Transplant Medicine-Kidney; Kidney Failure-Chronic; **Hospital:** Jackson Meml Hosp, Univ of Miami Hosp & Clins/Sylvester Comp Canc Ctr; **Address:** Nephrology & Hypertension, PO Box 016960 (R-126), Miami, FL 33101; **Phone:** 305-243-6251; **Board Cert:** Internal Medicine 1980; Nephrology 1982; **Med School:** SUNY Downstate 1977; **Resid:** Internal Medicine, Jackson Meml Hosp 1980; **Fellow:** Nephrology, Jackson Meml Hosp 1982; **Fac Appt:** Prof Med, Univ Miami Sch Med

Warnock, David G MD [Nep] - **Spec Exp:** Liddle's Syndrome; Kidney Stones; Nephrotic Syndrome; **Hospital:** Univ of Ala Hosp at Birmingham; **Address:** Univ Alabama Birmingham, Dept Med, 1530 3rd Ave S, THT 647, Birmingham, AL 35294-0006; **Phone:** 205-934-3585; **Board Cert:** Internal Medicine 1973; Nephrology 2000; **Med School:** UCSF 1970; **Resid:** Internal Medicine, UCSF Med Ctr 1973; **Fellow:** Nephrology, Natl Inst Hlth 1975; **Fac Appt:** Prof Med, Univ Ala

Weiner, I David MD [Nep] - **Spec Exp:** Kidney Disease; Fluid/Electrolyte Balance; Kidney Stones; Hypertension; **Hospital:** Shands Hlthcre at Univ of FL; **Address:** Shands at Univ Florida, Dept Nephrology, PO Box 100224, Gainesville, FL 32610-0224; **Phone:** 352-392-4008; **Board Cert:** Internal Medicine 1987; Nephrology 1990; **Med School:** Vanderbilt Univ 1984; **Resid:** Internal Medicine, Univ Texas Hlth Sci Ctr 1987; **Fellow:** Nephrology, Wash Univ-St Louis 1990; **Fac Appt:** Assoc Prof Med, Univ Fla Coll Med

Midwest

Brennan, Daniel C MD [Nep] - **Spec Exp:** Transplant Medicine-Kidney; **Hospital:** Barnes-Jewish Hosp; **Address:** Wash Univ School Med, Div Renal Diseases, 660 S Euclid Ave, Box 8126, St Louis, MO 63110; **Phone:** 314-362-7603; **Board Cert:** Internal Medicine 1988; Nephrology 2002; **Med School:** Univ Iowa Coll Med 1985; **Resid:** Internal Medicine, U Iowa Hosps 1988; **Fellow:** Nephrology, Brigham & Womens Hosp 1992; **Fac Appt:** Assoc Prof Med, Washington Univ, St Louis

Coe, Fredric MD [Nep] - **Spec Exp:** Kidney Stones; Fluid/Electrolyte Balance; **Hospital:** Univ of Chicago Hosps; **Address:** 5841 S Maryland Ave, MC 5100, Chicago, IL 60637-1463; **Phone:** 773-702-1475; **Board Cert:** Internal Medicine 1968; **Med School:** Univ Chicago-Pritzker Sch Med 1961; **Resid:** Internal Medicine, Michael Reese Hosp 1965; **Fellow:** Renal Disease, Univ Texas SW 1969; **Fac Appt:** Prof Med, Univ Chicago-Pritzker Sch Med

Delmez, James Albert MD [Nep] - **Spec Exp:** Kidney Disease; **Hospital:** Barnes-Jewish Hosp, Washington Univ Med Ctr; **Address:** Wash Univ Sch Med, Div Renal Dis, 660 S Euclid Ave, Box 8126, St Louis, MO 63110; **Phone:** 314-362-7603; **Board Cert:** Internal Medicine 1976; Nephrology 1982; **Med School:** Univ Rochester 1973; **Resid:** Internal Medicine, Barnes Hosp 1976; **Fellow:** Nephrology, Barnes Hosp 1978; **Fac Appt:** Prof Med, Washington Univ, St Louis

Hruska, Keith A MD [Nep] - **Spec Exp:** Kidney Disease-Pediatric & Adult; Kidney Stones; Bone Disorders; **Hospital:** St Louis Chldns Hosp, Barnes-Jewish Hosp; **Address:** St Louis Chldn's Hospital, Dept Peds, 660 S Euclid Ave Fl 5, Box 8208, MC MPR, St Louis, MO 63110-1010; **Phone:** 314-286-2772; **Board Cert:** Internal Medicine 1972; Nephrology 1976; **Med School:** Creighton Univ 1969; **Resid:** Internal Medicine, New York Hosp-Cornell 1971; Internal Medicine, Barnes Hosp-Wash Univ 1972; **Fellow:** Nephrology, Barnes Hosp-Wash Univ 1974; **Fac Appt:** Prof Ped, Washington Univ, St Louis

Josephson, Michelle A MD [Nep] - **Spec Exp:** Transplant Medicine-Kidney; Hypertension; **Hospital:** Univ of Chicago Hosps; **Address:** Univ Chicago, Div Nephrology, 5841 S Maryland Ave, MC 5100, Chicago, IL 60637; **Phone:** 773-702-6134; **Board Cert:** Internal Medicine 1986; Nephrology 2000; **Med School:** Univ Pennsylvania 1983; **Resid:** Internal Medicine, Univ Chicago Hosps 1986; **Fellow:** Nephrology, Univ Chicago 1991; **Fac Appt:** Assoc Clin Prof Med, Univ Chicago-Pritzker Sch Med

Kasiske, Bertram MD [Nep] - **Spec Exp:** Transplant Medicine-Kidney; Kidney Disease-Geriatric; **Hospital:** Hennepin Cnty Med Ctr; **Address:** 701 Park Ave, Minneapolis, MN 55415; **Phone:** 612-347-6088; **Board Cert:** Internal Medicine 1980; Nephrology 1982; **Med School:** Univ Iowa Coll Med 1976; **Resid:** Internal Medicine, Hennepin Co Med Ctr 1980; **Fellow:** Nephrology, Hennepin Co Med Ctr 1983; **Fac Appt:** Prof Med, Univ Minn

Nephrology

Lewis, Edmund J MD [Nep] - **Spec Exp:** Lupus Nephritis; Diabetic Kidney Disease; Glomerulonephritis; **Hospital:** Rush Univ Med Ctr; **Address:** 1426 W Washington Blvd, Chicago, IL 60607; **Phone:** 312-850-8434; **Board Cert:** Internal Medicine 1969; **Med School:** Univ British Columbia Fac Med 1962; **Resid:** Internal Medicine, Johns Hopkins Hosp 1965; **Fellow:** Nephrology, Peter Bent Brigham Hosp 1966; Research, Peter Bent Brigham Hosp 1970; **Fac Appt:** Prof Med, Rush Med Coll

Paganini, Emil MD [Nep] - **Spec Exp:** Kidney Failure-Chronic; Kidney Failure-Acute; **Hospital:** Cleveland Clin Fdn (page 57); **Address:** Cleveland Clinic, Division Nephrology & Hypertension, 9500 Euclid Ave, Desk M82, Cleveland, OH 44195; **Phone:** 216-444-5792; **Board Cert:** Internal Medicine 1977; **Med School:** Italy 1973; **Resid:** Internal Medicine, Winthrop Univ Hosp 1977; **Fellow:** Nephrology, Cleveland Clin Fdn 1979

Pohl, Marc MD [Nep] - **Spec Exp:** Hypertension; Kidney Disease; Diabetes; **Hospital:** Cleveland Clin Fdn (page 57); **Address:** Cleveland Clinic, Div Nephrology & Hypertension, 9500 Euclid Ave, Desk A51, Cleveland, OH 44195; **Phone:** 216-444-6776; **Board Cert:** Internal Medicine 1972; Nephrology 1978; **Med School:** Case West Res Univ 1966; **Resid:** Internal Medicine, Univ Hosps 1968; Internal Medicine, Mass Genl Hosp 1971; **Fellow:** Nephrology, Boston City Hosp-Boston Univ 1972; Nephrology, Mass Genl Hosp 1973

Schwartz, Gary Lee MD [Nep] - **Spec Exp:** Hypertension; Hypotension; Diabetic Kidney Disease; **Hospital:** St Mary's Hosp - Rochester, Methodist Hosp - Minnesota; **Address:** Mayo Clinic, 200 1st St SW, Rochester, MN 55905-0002; **Phone:** 507-284-4083; **Board Cert:** Internal Medicine 1980; Nephrology 1982; **Med School:** Univ Wisc 1977; **Resid:** Internal Medicine, Mayo Clinic 1980; **Fellow:** Nephrology, Mayo Clinic 1982; **Fac Appt:** Assoc Clin Prof Med, Mayo Med Sch

Somerville, James MD [Nep] - **Hospital:** Fairview Southdale Hosp, Fairview Ridges Hosp; **Address:** 6363 France Ave S, Ste 400, Edina, MN 55435; **Phone:** 952-920-2070; **Board Cert:** Internal Medicine 1978; Nephrology 1982; **Med School:** Univ MD Sch Med 1975; **Resid:** Internal Medicine, Hennepin Co Med Ctr 1978; **Fellow:** Nephrology, Hennepin Co Med Ctr 1980

Swartz, Richard D MD [Nep] - **Spec Exp:** Kidney Failure; Dialysis Care; **Hospital:** Univ Michigan Hlth Sys; **Address:** Univ Mich, Div Nephrology, 1500 E Med Ctr Drive, 3914 Taubman Ctr, Ann Arbor, MI 48109-0364; **Phone:** 734-647-9342; **Board Cert:** Internal Medicine 1975; Nephrology 1977; **Med School:** Univ Mich Med Sch 1970; **Resid:** Internal Medicine, Boston City Hosp 1975; Nephrology, Beth Israel Hosp-Harvard 1977; **Fac Appt:** Prof Med, Univ Mich Med Sch

Textor, Stephen C MD [Nep] - **Spec Exp:** Transplant Medicine-Kidney; Hypertension; Renal Artery Stenosis; **Hospital:** Mayo Med Ctr & Clin - Rochester; **Address:** Mayo Clinic, Div Nephrology, 200 First St SW Fl W9A, Rochester, MN 55905; **Phone:** 507-284-4841; **Board Cert:** Internal Medicine 1977; Nephrology 1980; **Med School:** UCLA 1973; **Resid:** Internal Medicine, Boston City Hosp 1977; **Fellow:** Nephrology, Boston Univ 1978; Hypertension, Fogarty Inst 1980; **Fac Appt:** Prof Med, Mayo Med Sch

Torres, Vicente Esbarranch MD [Nep] - **Spec Exp:** Polycystic Kidney Disease; **Hospital:** Mayo Med Ctr & Clin - Rochester; **Address:** Mayo Clinic, Eisenberg Bldg-Rm SL 24, 200 First St SW, Rochester, MN 55905; **Phone:** 507-266-7093; **Board Cert:** Internal Medicine 1977; Nephrology 1980; **Med School:** Spain 1969; **Resid:** Internal Medicine, Mayo Grad Sch Med 1977; **Fellow:** Nephrology, Mayo Grad Sch Med 1979; **Fac Appt:** Prof Med, Mayo Med Sch

Venkat, K K MD [Nep] - **Spec Exp:** Transplant Medicine-Kidney; Kidney Disease; **Hospital:** Henry Ford Hosp; **Address:** Henry Ford Hosp, Div Nephrology, 2799 W Grand Blvd, rm CFP5, Detroit, MI 48202-2689; **Phone:** 313-916-2702; **Board Cert:** Internal Medicine 1977; Nephrology 1978; **Med School:** India 1970; **Resid:** Internal Medicine, Henry Ford Hosp 1976; **Fellow:** Nephrology, Henry Ford Hosp 1978

Zimmerman, Stephen W MD [Nep] - **Spec Exp:** Transplant Medicine-Kidney; Kidney Failure-Chronic; **Hospital:** St Mary's Hosp-Madison, Meriter Hosp; **Address:** Madison Area Renal Spec, 2840 Index Rd, Madison, WI 53713; **Phone:** 608-229-7221; **Board Cert:** Internal Medicine 1972; Nephrology 1972; **Med School:** Univ Wisc 1966; **Resid:** Internal Medicine, Univ Wisc 1969; **Fellow:** Nephrology, Univ Wisc 1970; Research, Univ Wisc 1974; **Fac Appt:** Prof Med, Univ Wisc

Great Plains and Mountains

Berl, Tomas MD [Nep] - **Spec Exp:** Fluid/Electrolyte Balance; Kidney Failure-Chronic; **Hospital:** Univ Colorado Hosp; **Address:** Univ Colo Med Ctr, Dept Med, Renal Div, 4200 E 9th Ave, rm C281, Denver, CO 80262; **Phone:** 303-372-8069; **Board Cert:** Internal Medicine 1972; Nephrology 1976; **Med School:** NYU Sch Med 1968; **Resid:** Internal Medicine, Bronx Municipal Hosp 1970; **Fellow:** Renal Disease, Moffit Hosp-UCSF 1971

Schrier, Robert W MD [Nep] - **Spec Exp:** Hypertension; Polycystic Kidney Disease; **Hospital:** Univ Colorado Hosp; **Address:** Univ Colorado Med Ctr-Dept Medicine, 4200 E 9th Ave, Ste B 173, Denver, CO 80262; **Phone:** 303-315-7297; **Board Cert:** Internal Medicine 1969; **Med School:** Indiana Univ 1962; **Resid:** Internal Medicine, Univ Wash Hosp 1965; **Fellow:** Research, PB Brigham Hosp/Harvard 1966; **Fac Appt:** Prof Med, Univ Colorado

Southwest

Barcenas, Camilo Gustavo MD [Nep] - **Spec Exp:** Transplant Medicine-Kidney; **Hospital:** St Luke's Episcopal Hosp - Houston; **Address:** 6624 Fannin St, Ste 2510, Houston, TX 77030; **Phone:** 713-791-2648; **Board Cert:** Internal Medicine 1973; Nephrology 1974; **Med School:** Nicaragua 1968; **Resid:** Internal Medicine, Baylor Med Coll 1972; **Fellow:** Nephrology, UT SW Hosps 1974; **Fac Appt:** Clin Prof Med, Baylor Coll Med

Brennan, Stephen MD [Nep] - **Spec Exp:** Transplant Medicine-Kidney; Kidney Stones; Kidney Failure-Chronic; **Hospital:** Methodist Hosp - Houston, St Luke's Episcopal Hosp - Houston; **Address:** 1415 La Concha Ln, Houston, TX 77054; **Phone:** 713-790-9080; **Board Cert:** Internal Medicine 1983; Nephrology 1988; **Med School:** Loyola Univ-Stritch Sch Med 1979; **Resid:** Internal Medicine, Loyola Univ Med Ctr 1983; **Fellow:** Nephrology, Univ Wash-Barnes Hosp 1986; **Fac Appt:** Assoc Clin Prof Med, Baylor Coll Med

Hura, Claudia E MD [Nep] - **Spec Exp:** Transplant Medicine-Kidney; Glomerulonephritis; Lupus Nephritis; **Hospital:** Methodist Spec & Transpl Hosp, SW TX Meth Hosp; **Address:** 8042 Wurzbach St, Physician Plaza 2, Ste 500, San Antonio, TX 78229; **Phone:** 210-692-7228; **Board Cert:** Internal Medicine 1982; Nephrology 1986; **Med School:** Ohio State Univ 1979; **Resid:** Internal Medicine, Indiana Univ Med Ctr 1983; **Fellow:** Nephrology, Univ Tex Hlth Sci Ctr 1986; **Fac Appt:** Assoc Clin Prof Med, Univ Tex, San Antonio

Kasinath, Balakuntalam S MD [Nep] - **Spec Exp:** Glomerulonephritis; Diabetic Kidney Disease; **Hospital:** Univ Hlth Sys - Univ Hosp, Audie L Murphy Meml Vets Hosp; **Address:** Univ Tex Hlth Sci Ctr, Dept Med/Div Neph, 7703 Floyd Curl Drive, MC 7882, San Antonio, TX 78229-3901; **Phone:** 210-567-4707; **Board Cert:** Internal Medicine 1980; Nephrology 1982; **Med School:** India 1975; **Resid:** Internal Medicine, Ill Masonic Med Ctr 1980; **Fellow:** Nephrology, Univ Chicago Hosp 1983; **Fac Appt:** Prof Med, Univ Tex, San Antonio

Mitch, William MD [Nep] - **Spec Exp:** Nutrition; Hypertension; Kidney Failure; **Hospital:** Baylor Univ Medical Ctr; **Address:** Baylor College of Medicine, Nephrology Div, MIS:BCM 285, One Baylor Plaza, Ste N-620, Houston, TX 77030; **Phone:** 713-798-8350; **Board Cert:** Internal Medicine 1972; Nephrology 1978; **Med School:** Harvard Med Sch 1967; **Resid:** Internal Medicine, Brigham & Women's Hosp 1974; Nat Cancer Inst-NIH 1972; **Fellow:** Nephrology, Johns Hopkins Hosp 1973; **Fac Appt:** Prof Med, Baylor Coll Med

Olivero, Juan J MD [Nep] - **Spec Exp:** Kidney Failure; Fluid/Electrolyte Balance; **Hospital:** Methodist Hosp - Houston; **Address:** 6560 Fannin St, Scurlock Twr, Ste 2206, Houston, TX 77030; **Phone:** 713-790-4615; **Board Cert:** Internal Medicine 1974; Nephrology 1976; **Med School:** Guatemala 1970; **Resid:** Internal Medicine, Baylor Affil Hosps 1973; Internal Medicine, Ben Taub Genl Hosp 1974; **Fellow:** Nephrology, Baylor Affil Hosps 1975; **Fac Appt:** Clin Prof Med, Baylor Coll Med

Suki, Wadi MD [Nep] - **Spec Exp:** Transplant Medicine-Kidney; Hypertension; Lupus Nephritis; **Hospital:** Methodist Hosp - Houston, St Luke's Episcopal Hosp - Houston; **Address:** 1415 La Concha Ln, Houston, TX 77054; **Phone:** 713-790-9080; **Board Cert:** Internal Medicine 1967; Nephrology 1972; **Med School:** Sudan 1959; **Resid:** Internal Medicine, Parkland Meml Hosp 1963; **Fellow:** Nephrology, Univ Tex SW Med Ctr 1961; Nephrology, Univ Tex SW Med Ctr 1965; **Fac Appt:** Clin Prof Med, Baylor Coll Med

Toto, Robert D MD [Nep] - **Spec Exp:** Hypertension/Kidney Disease; Dialysis Care; Diabetic Kidney Disease; Kidney Failure-Acute; **Hospital:** UT Southwestern Med Ctr - Dallas; **Address:** UT Southwestern Medical Ctr, 5323 Harry Hines Blvd, MC 8856, Dallas, TX 75390-8856; **Phone:** 214-648-3442; **Board Cert:** Internal Medicine 1980; Nephrology 1982; Critical Care Medicine 1997; **Med School:** Univ IL Coll Med 1976; **Resid:** Internal Medicine, Univ Michigan Med Ctr 1979; Internal Medicine, Baylor Univ Med Ctr 1980; **Fellow:** Nephrology, US Public Health Service Hosp 1981; Nephrology, UTSW Med Ctr 1983; **Fac Appt:** Prof Med, Univ Tex SW, Dallas

West Coast and Pacific

Ahmad, Suhail MD [Nep] - **Spec Exp:** Hypertension; Kidney Failure-Chronic; Kidney Stones; **Hospital:** Univ Wash Med Ctr; **Address:** 2150 N 107th St, Ste 160, Seattle, WA 98133; **Phone:** 206-363-5090; **Med School:** India 1968; **Resid:** Internal Medicine, Univ Allahabad 1971; **Fellow:** Nephrology, Univ Washington 1978; **Fac Appt:** Assoc Prof Med, Univ Wash

Bennett, William M MD [Nep] - **Spec Exp:** Polycystic Kidney Disease; Transplant Medicine-Kidney; Drug Toxicity-Kidneys; **Hospital:** Legacy Good Samaritan Hosp and Med Ctr, Legacy Emanuel Hospitals; **Address:** Legacy Good Samaritan Hosp, Transplant Svcs, 1040 NW 22nd, Ste 480, Portland, OR 97210; **Phone:** 503-413-6555; **Board Cert:** Internal Medicine 2003; Nephrology 2003; **Med School:** Northwestern Univ 1963; **Resid:** Internal Medicine, Northwestern Univ 1965; Internal Medicine, Ore Hlth Sci Univ 1966; **Fellow:** Nephrology, Mass Genl Hosp 1970

Ellison, David H MD [Nep] - **Spec Exp:** Bartter's Syndrome; Gitelman's Syndrome; Hypertension; **Hospital:** OR Hlth & Sci Univ, VA Medical Center - Portland; **Address:** Oregon Hlth Scis Univ - Div Nephrology, 3314 SW Veteran's Hospital Rd, MC PP262, Portland, OR 97239-3098; **Phone:** 503-494-8490; **Board Cert:** Internal Medicine 1981; Nephrology 1986; **Med School:** Rush Med Coll 1978; **Resid:** Internal Medicine, Oregon Hlth Scis Univ 1981; **Fellow:** Research, Oregon Hlth Scis Univ 1982; Nephrology, Yale Univ 1985; **Fac Appt:** Prof Med, Oregon Hlth Sci Univ

Gluck, Stephen L MD [Nep] - **Spec Exp:** Kidney Disease; Fluid/Electrolyte Balance; Hypertension; Kidney Stones; **Hospital:** UCSF Med Ctr; **Address:** UCSF, Div Nephrology, HSE 672, 513 Parnassus Ave, Box 0532, San Francisco, CA 94143-0532; **Phone:** 415-476-2173; **Board Cert:** Internal Medicine 1980; Nephrology 1984; **Med School:** UCLA 1977; **Resid:** Internal Medicine, Columbia Presby Med Ctr 1980; **Fellow:** Nephrology, Columbia Presby Med Ctr 1983; **Fac Appt:** Prof Med, UCSF

Kaysen, George Alan MD/PhD [Nep] - **Spec Exp:** Kidney Disease-Metabolic; Kidney Failure-Chronic; **Hospital:** UC Davis Med Ctr; **Address:** UC Davis Med Ctr, Div Nephr, 451 Health Sciences Dr, GBSF, Ste 6300, Davis, CA 95616; **Phone:** 530-752-4010; **Board Cert:** Internal Medicine 1975; Nephrology 1980; **Med School:** Albert Einstein Coll Med 1972; **Resid:** Internal Medicine, Bronx Muni Hosp 1975; **Fellow:** Renal Disease, Bronx Muni Hosp 1977; **Fac Appt:** Prof Med, UC Davis

King, Andrew J MD [Nep] - **Spec Exp:** Kidney Disease-Chronic; Hypertension; Dialysis Care; **Hospital:** Scripps Green Hosp; **Address:** Scripps Green Hospital, 10666 N Torrey Pines Rd, MC N239, La Jolla, CA 92037-1027; **Phone:** 858-554-9765; **Board Cert:** Internal Medicine 1986; Nephrology 1988; **Med School:** Northwestern Univ 1983; **Resid:** Internal Medicine, Northwestern Meml Hosp 1986; **Fellow:** Nephrology, Brigham & Women's Hosp 1990; **Fac Appt:** Clin Prof Med, UCSD

Riordan, John William MD [Nep] - **Hospital:** CA Pacific Med Ctr - Pacific Campus; **Address:** 2100 Webster St, Ste 412, San Francisco, CA 94115; **Phone:** 415-923-3815; **Board Cert:** Nephrology 2005; **Med School:** Univ Tex Med Br, Galveston 1987; **Resid:** Internal Medicine, Univ Texas Hlth Sci Ctr 1990; **Fellow:** Nephrology, UCSF Med Ctr 1995

Scandling Jr, John David MD [Nep] - **Spec Exp:** Transplant Medicine-Kidney; **Hospital:** Stanford Univ Med Ctr; **Address:** 750 Welch Rd, Ste 200, Palo Alto, CA 94304-1509; **Phone:** 650-725-9891; **Board Cert:** Internal Medicine 1981; Nephrology 1984; **Med School:** Med Coll VA 1978; **Resid:** Internal Medicine, West Virginia Univ Hosp 1981; **Fellow:** Nephrology, Univ Rochester 1983; **Fac Appt:** Prof Med, Stanford Univ

Cleveland Clinic

Nephrology & Hypertension

The Department of Nephrology and Hypertension provides comprehensive diagnostic and therapeutic services for patients with kidney disease and hypertension. The department participates in an active kidney transplant program, all modalities of dialysis care, and clinical research studies of diabetic and other glomerular disease. In addition to unique diagnostic capabilities, the department is renowned for its expertise in the areas of renovascular hypertension, primary aldosteronism and pheochromocytoma.

Intensive Care Nephrology Services

The Department of Nephrology and Hypertension is a major participant in the intensive care setting. Cleveland Clinic nephrologists are leaders in research into the risk factors for acute renal failure after surgeries and in evaluations of different techniques for treatment of acute renal failure such as slow continuous ultrafiltration, continuous arteriovenous hemofiltration and venovenous hemofiltration.

Research and Clinical Trials

The Cleveland Clinic Department of Nephrology and Hypertension is actively involved in clinical and basic research. Its legacy of excellence in hypertension research began in 1945.

For more than 30 years, the Clinic has received support from the National Institutes of Health (NIH) for its research into the causes of hypertension.

Kidney/Kidney-Pancreas Transplant

Cleveland Clinic's kidney transplant program dates to January 1963. Since then, more than 3,000 kidney transplants have been performed here. Each year, between 75 and 100 kidney transplants are performed.

To schedule an appointment or for more information about the Cleveland Clinic Department of Nephrology & Hypertension call 800.890.2467 or visit www.clevelandclinic.org/nephrologytopdocs.

Department of Nephrology & Hypertension
9500 Euclid Avenue / W14 | Cleveland OH 44195

Second Opinion-Online

Use e-Cleveland Clinic's convenient, online second opinion service without leaving home. Call 800.223.2273, ext 43223, or visit www.eclevelandclinic.org.

Special Service for Out-of-State Patients

Global Patient Services is a full-service department dedicated to meeting the needs and requirements of both out-of-state and international patients who receive their car at Cleveland Clinic. That National Center and the International Center, which make up global Patient Services, provide personalized concierge programs and services to welcome patients and add to their comfort before, during and after their stay. Call 800.223.2273, ext. 55580, or send an e-mail to medicalconcierge@ccf.org.

Neurological Surgery

A neurological surgeon provides the operative and non-operative management (i.e., prevention, diagnosis, evaluation, treatment, critical care and rehabilitation) of disorders of the central, peripheral and autonomic nervous systems, including their supporting structures and vascular supply; the evaluation and treatment of pathological processes which modify function or activity of the nervous system; and the operative and non-operative management of pain. A neurological surgeon treats patients with disorders of the nervous system; disorders of the brain, meninges, skull and their blood supply, including the extracranial carotid and vertebral arteries; disorders of the pituitary gland; disorders of the spinal cord, meninges and vertebral column, including those which may require treatment by spinal fusion or instrumentation; and disorders of the cranial and spinal nerves throughout their distribution.

Training Required: Seven years (including general surgery)

The American Board of Pediatric Neurological Surgery (ABPNS) is not a recognized ABMS subspecialty. However, this designation has been included because the certification process is meaningful and rigorous. It is awarded to those doctors who hold a current ABMS certification in Neurological Surgery, have completed a fully accredited one year, post-graduate fellowship in pediatric neurological surgery, and have submitted surgical logs indicating a practice of pediatric neurological surgery for one year, followed by a written examination.

Neurological Surgery

New England

Black, Peter MD/PhD [NS] - **Spec Exp:** Brain Tumors; Pituitary Tumors; Seizure Disorders; **Hospital:** Brigham & Women's Hosp, Children's Hospital - Boston; **Address:** Brigham & Women's Hosp, Dept Neurosurg, 75 Francis St, Boston, MA 02115; **Phone:** 617-732-6810; **Board Cert:** Neurological Surgery 1984; **Med School:** McGill Univ 1970; **Resid:** Surgery, Mass Genl Hosp 1972; Neurological Surgery, Mass Genl Hosp 1980; **Fellow:** Neurosurgical Oncology, Mass Genl Hosp 1976; **Fac Appt:** Prof NS, Harvard Med Sch

Borges, Lawrence F MD [NS] - **Spec Exp:** Spinal Surgery; Spinal Tumors; **Hospital:** Mass Genl Hosp; **Address:** Mass Genl Hosp, Div Neurosurg, 32 Fruit St, Boston, MA 02114-2620; **Phone:** 617-726-6156; **Board Cert:** Neurological Surgery 1986; **Med School:** Johns Hopkins Univ 1977; **Resid:** Neurological Surgery, Mass Genl Hosp 1983; **Fac Appt:** Assoc Prof S, Harvard Med Sch

Chapman, Paul H MD [NS] - **Spec Exp:** Pediatric Neurosurgery; Brain & Spinal Tumors-Pediatric; Congenital Anomalies; **Hospital:** Mass Genl Hosp; **Address:** MGH Gray 5, 55 Fruit St, rm GRB-502, Boston, MA 02114-2622; **Phone:** 617-726-3887; **Board Cert:** Neurological Surgery 1976; Pediatric Neurological Surgery 1996; **Med School:** Harvard Med Sch 1964; **Resid:** Surgery, Mass Genl Hosp 1966; Neurological Surgery, Mass Genl Hosp 1972; **Fellow:** Neurological Surgery, Hosp Sick Chldn; **Fac Appt:** Prof S, Harvard Med Sch

Cosgrove, G Rees MD [NS] - **Spec Exp:** Epilepsy/Seizure Disorders; Brain Tumors; **Hospital:** Lahey Clin, Emerson Hosp; **Address:** Lahey Clinic, 41 Mall Rd, Burlington, MA 01805; **Phone:** 781-744-1990; **Board Cert:** Neurological Surgery 1989; **Med School:** Queens Univ 1980; **Resid:** Neurological Surgery, Montreal Neur Inst 1986; **Fac Appt:** Prof NS, Tufts Univ

David, Carlos MD [NS] - **Spec Exp:** Cerebrovascular Surgery; Skull Base Tumors & Surgery; **Hospital:** Lahey Clin, Emerson Hosp; **Address:** Lahey Clinic, Dept Neurosurgery, 41 Mall Rd, Burlington, MA 01805; **Phone:** 781-744-8643; **Board Cert:** Neurological Surgery 2001; **Med School:** Univ Miami Sch Med 1990; **Resid:** Neurological Surgery, Jackson Memorial Hosp 1995; **Fellow:** Cerebrovascular & Skull Base Surgery, Barrow Neuro Inst 1997; **Fac Appt:** Assoc Clin Prof NS, Tufts Univ

Day, Arthur L MD [NS] - **Spec Exp:** Cerebrovascular Surgery; Orbital Tumors/Cancer; Carotid Artery Surgery; Skull Base Tumors; **Hospital:** Brigham & Women's Hosp, St Elizabeth's Med Ctr; **Address:** Brigham & Womens Hosp, Dept Neurosurgery, 75 Francis St, Boston, MA 02115; **Phone:** 617-525-7777; **Board Cert:** Neurological Surgery 1980; **Med School:** Louisiana State Univ 1972; **Resid:** Neurological Surgery, Shands-Univ Florida Hosp 1977; **Fellow:** Neurological Pathology, Shands-Univ Florida Hosp 1978; **Fac Appt:** Prof NS, Harvard Med Sch

Duhaime, Ann Christine MD [NS] - **Spec Exp:** Pediatric Neurosurgery; Brain Tumors; Epilepsy; Craniofacial Surgery; **Hospital:** Dartmouth - Hitchcock Med Ctr; **Address:** Chldns Hosp at Dartmouth-Hitchcock Med Ctr, One Medical Center Drive, Lebanon, NH 03756; **Phone:** 603-653-9880; **Board Cert:** Neurological Surgery 1990; Pediatric Neurological Surgery 1996; **Med School:** Univ Pennsylvania 1981; **Resid:** Neurological Surgery, Hosp Univ Penn 1987; **Fellow:** Pediatric Neurological Surgery, Chldns Hosp 1987; **Fac Appt:** Prof S, Dartmouth Med Sch

Duncan, John A MD/PhD [NS] - **Spec Exp:** Pediatric Neurosurgery; Epilepsy/Seizure Disorders; Neuro-Oncology; Brain Tumors; **Hospital:** Rhode Island Hosp; **Address:** Neurosurgery Foundation Inc., 55 Claverick St, Ste 100, Providence, RI 02903; **Phone:** 401-444-8716; **Board Cert:** Neurological Surgery 1998; Pediatric Neurological Surgery 2001; **Med School:** UMDNJ-RW Johnson Med Sch 1986; **Resid:** Neuropathology, Stanford Univ Sch of Med 1987; Neurological Surgery, Stanford Univ Sch of Med 1992; **Fellow:** Neurology, Neurology Natl Hosp 1989; Pediatric Neurological Surgery, Hosp for Sick Chldn 1993; **Fac Appt:** Assoc Prof NS, Brown Univ

Heilman, Carl B MD [NS] - **Spec Exp:** Skull Base Surgery; Pediatric Neurosurgery; **Hospital:** Tufts-New England Med Ctr; **Address:** Tufts-NE Med Ctr, Dept Neurosurgery, 750 Washington St, Box 178, Bsoton, MA 02111; **Phone:** 617-636-5858; **Board Cert:** Neurological Surgery 1996; **Med School:** Univ Pennsylvania 1986; **Resid:** Neurological Surgery, Tufts New England Med Ctr 1993; **Fellow:** Skull Base Surgery, Baptist Meml Hosp 1993; **Fac Appt:** Assoc Prof NS, Tufts Univ

Madsen, Joseph MD [NS] - **Spec Exp:** Pediatric Neurosurgery; Epilepsy/Seizure Disorders; **Hospital:** Children's Hospital - Boston; **Address:** 300 Longwood Ave, Bader 3, Boston, MA 02115; **Phone:** 617-355-6005; **Board Cert:** Neurological Surgery 1994; Pediatric Neurological Surgery 1997; **Med School:** Harvard Med Sch 1981; **Resid:** Neurological Surgery, Mass Genl Hosp 1989; **Fellow:** Research, Beth Israel Hosp 1983; **Fac Appt:** Assoc Prof NS, Harvard Med Sch

Martuza, Robert L MD [NS] - **Spec Exp:** Brain Tumors; Acoustic Neuroma; Skull Base Surgery; **Hospital:** Mass Genl Hosp; **Address:** Mass General Hosp, 55 Fruit St, White Bldg, rm 502, Boston, MA 02114; **Phone:** 617-726-8581; **Board Cert:** Neurological Surgery 1983; **Med School:** Harvard Med Sch 1973; **Resid:** Neurological Surgery, Mass Genl Hosp 1980; **Fac Appt:** Prof NS, Harvard Med Sch

Penar, Paul MD [NS] - **Spec Exp:** Brain & Spinal Tumors; Epilepsy/Seizure Disorders; Movement Disorders; Stereotactic Radiosurgery; **Hospital:** FAHC - Med Ctr Campus; **Address:** Div Neurosurgery, Fletcher 5, 111 Colchester Ave, Burlington, VT 05401; **Phone:** 802-847-3072; **Board Cert:** Neurological Surgery 1989; **Med School:** Univ Mich Med Sch 1981; **Resid:** Neurological Surgery, Yale-New Haven Hosp 1987

Piepmeier, Joseph MD [NS] - **Spec Exp:** Neuro-Oncology; Brain & Spinal Cord Tumors; **Hospital:** Yale - New Haven Hosp; **Address:** Yale Sch Med, Dept Neurosurgery, 333 Cedar St Fl TMP-410, New Haven, CT 06520; **Phone:** 203-785-2791; **Board Cert:** Neurological Surgery 1984; **Med School:** Univ Tenn Coll Med, Memphis 1975; **Resid:** Neurological Surgery, Yale-New Haven Hosp 1982; **Fac Appt:** Prof NS, Yale Univ

Spencer, Dennis D MD [NS] - **Spec Exp:** Epilepsy/Seizure Disorders; Brain Tumors; **Hospital:** Yale - New Haven Hosp, Hosp of St Raphael; **Address:** Yale Univ Sch Med, Dept Neurosurgery, 333 Cedar St, TMP-4, New Haven, CT 06520; **Phone:** 203-785-4891; **Board Cert:** Neurological Surgery 1980; **Med School:** Washington Univ, St Louis 1971; **Resid:** Surgery, Barnes Hosp 1972; Neurological Surgery, Yale-New Haven Hosp 1976; **Fac Appt:** Prof NS, Yale Univ

Neurological Surgery

Mid Atlantic

Adelson, P David MD [NS] - **Spec Exp:** Pediatric Neurosurgery; Brain Injury; Epilepsy/Seizure Disorders; Spinal Cord Injury; **Hospital:** Chldns Hosp of Pittsburgh - UPMC, UPMC Presby, Pittsburgh; **Address:** Children's Hosp Pittsburgh, Dept Neurosurgery, 3705 Fifth Ave, Pittsburgh, PA 15213-2583; **Phone:** 412-692-5090; **Board Cert:** Neurological Surgery 1997; Pediatric Neurological Surgery 1998; **Med School:** Columbia P&S 1986; **Resid:** Neurological Surgery, UCLA Med Ctr 1992; **Fellow:** Pediatric Neurological Surgery, Children's Hosp 1994; **Fac Appt:** Prof NS, Univ Pittsburgh

Andrews, David MD [NS] - **Spec Exp:** Brain Tumors; Neuro-Endoscopy; Stereotactic Radiosurgery; **Hospital:** Thomas Jefferson Univ Hosp; **Address:** Thom Jefferson Univ Hosp, Dept Neurosurg, 909 Walnut St Fl 2, Philadelphia, PA 19107-5109; **Phone:** 215-503-7005; **Board Cert:** Neurological Surgery 1992; **Med School:** Univ Colorado 1983; **Resid:** Neurological Surgery, NY Presby Hos-Cornell Med Ctr 1989; **Fellow:** Neuro-Oncology, Meml Sloan Kettering Cancer Ctr 1987; **Fac Appt:** Prof NS, Thomas Jefferson Univ

Baltuch, Gordon MD/PhD [NS] - **Spec Exp:** Movement Disorders; Parkinson's Disease; Epilepsy/Seizure Disorders; **Hospital:** Hosp Univ Penn - UPHS (page 72), Pennsylvania Hosp (page 72); **Address:** Penn Neurological Institute, 3400 Spruce St, Silverstein Bldg Fl 3, Philadelphia, PA 19104; **Phone:** 215-662-7788; **Board Cert:** Neurological Surgery 1998; **Med School:** McGill Univ 1986; **Resid:** Surgery, Montreal Genl Hosp 1988; Neurological Surgery, Montreal Neuro Inst 1994; **Fellow:** Neurological Surgery, Centre Hospitalier Univ Vaudois 1995; **Fac Appt:** Assoc Prof NS, Univ Pennsylvania

Benjamin, Vallo MD [NS] - **Spec Exp:** Spinal Surgery; Skull Base Surgery; Acoustic Neuroma; **Hospital:** NYU Med Ctr (page 67); **Address:** 530 First Ave, Ste 7W, New York, NY 10016; **Phone:** 212-263-5013 x1; **Board Cert:** Neurological Surgery 1967; **Med School:** Iran 1958; **Resid:** Neurological Surgery, Bellevue Hosp 1964; **Fellow:** Neurological Surgery, NYU Med Ctr 1966; **Fac Appt:** Prof NS, NYU Sch Med

Bilsky, Mark H MD [NS] - **Spec Exp:** Spinal Tumors; Skull Base Tumors; Brain Tumors; Spinal Reconstructive Surgery; **Hospital:** Meml Sloan Kettering Cancer Ctr, NY-Presby Hosp/Weill Cornell (page 66); **Address:** Memorial Sloan Kettering Cancer Ctr, 1275 York Ave, rm C705, New York, NY 10021; **Phone:** 212-639-8526; **Board Cert:** Neurological Surgery 1999; **Med School:** Emory Univ 1988; **Resid:** Neurological Surgery, NY Hosp-Cornell Med Ctr 1994; **Fellow:** Neuro-Oncology, Louisville Univ Med Ctr 1995; **Fac Appt:** Assoc Prof NS, Cornell Univ-Weill Med Coll

Brem, Henry MD [NS] - **Spec Exp:** Brain & Spinal Cord Tumors; Skull Base Tumors; Pituitary Tumors; **Hospital:** Johns Hopkins Hosp - Baltimore (page 61), Johns Hopkins Bayview Med Ctr (page 61); **Address:** Johns Hopkins Med Ctr-Dept NeuroSurgery, 600 N Wolfe St Bldg Meyer 7-113, Baltimore, MD 21287; **Phone:** 410-955-2248; **Board Cert:** Neurological Surgery 1986; **Med School:** Harvard Med Sch 1978; **Resid:** Neurological Surgery, Columbia-Presby Med Ctr 1984; **Fellow:** Neurological Surgery, Johns Hopkins Hosp 1980; **Fac Appt:** Prof NS, Johns Hopkins Univ

Bruce, Jeffrey MD [NS] - **Spec Exp:** Brain Tumors; Pituitary Tumors; Skull Base Surgery; **Hospital:** NY-Presby Hosp/Columbia (page 66); **Address:** NY Presby Hosp, Dept Neurosurgery, 710 W 168th St N1 Bldg Fl 4 - rm 434, New York, NY 10032; **Phone:** 212-305-7346; **Board Cert:** Neurological Surgery 1993; **Med School:** UMDNJ-RW Johnson Med Sch 1983; **Resid:** Neurological Surgery, Columbia-Presby Med Ctr 1990; **Fellow:** Neurological Surgery, Nat Inst Health 1985; **Fac Appt:** Prof NS, Columbia P&S

Camins, Martin B MD [NS] - **Spec Exp:** Spinal Surgery; Brain Tumors; Microsurgery; **Hospital:** Mount Sinai Med Ctr, Lenox Hill Hosp (page 62); **Address:** 205 E 68th St, Ste T1C, New York, NY 10021-5735; **Phone:** 212-570-0100; **Board Cert:** Neurological Surgery 1980; **Med School:** Ros Franklin Univ/Chicago Med Sch 1969; **Resid:** Neurology, Neuro Inst-Columbia-Presby Med Ctr 1971; Neurological Surgery, Neuro Inst-Columbia Presb Med Ctry 1975; **Fellow:** Neurological Surgery, National Hosp 1974; Neurological Surgery, NYU Med Ctr 1978; **Fac Appt:** Clin Prof NS, Mount Sinai Sch Med

Campbell, James N MD [NS] - **Spec Exp:** Spinal Tumors; Pain-Chronic; Nerve Disorders/Surgery; Spinal Disorders; **Hospital:** Johns Hopkins Hosp - Baltimore (page 61); **Address:** Johns Hopkins Hospital, 600 N Wolfe St Meyer Bldg - Ste 5-109, Baltimore, MD 21287-7509; **Phone:** 410-955-2058; **Board Cert:** Neurological Surgery 1982; **Med School:** Yale Univ 1973; **Resid:** Neurological Surgery, Johns Hopkins Hosp 1979; **Fellow:** Neurological Surgery, Johns Hopkins 1977; **Fac Appt:** Prof NS, Johns Hopkins Univ

Caputy, Anthony J MD [NS] - **Spec Exp:** Epilepsy/Seizure Disorders; Spinal Surgery; **Hospital:** G Washington Univ Hosp, Inova Fairfax Hosp; **Address:** Geo Wash Univ, Dept Neurosurgery, 2150 Pennsylvania Ave NW, Ste 7-420, Washington, DC 20037; **Phone:** 202-741-2735; **Board Cert:** Neurological Surgery 1989; **Med School:** Univ VA Sch Med 1980; **Resid:** Neurological Surgery, Georgetown Univ Hosp 1986; **Fac Appt:** Prof NS, Geo Wash Univ

Carmel, Peter MD [NS] - **Spec Exp:** Brain Tumors-Pediatric; Skull Base Surgery; Pediatric Neurosurgery; **Hospital:** UMDNJ-Univ Hosp-Newark; **Address:** 90 Bergen St, Ste 8100, Newark, NJ 07104; **Phone:** 973-972-2323; **Board Cert:** Neurological Surgery 1969; Pediatric Neurological Surgery 1996; **Med School:** NYU Sch Med 1960; **Resid:** Neurological Surgery, Neuro Inst/Columbia Presby Med Ctr 1967; **Fac Appt:** Prof NS, UMDNJ-NJ Med Sch, Newark

Carson, Benjamin S MD [NS] - **Spec Exp:** Brain Injury; Brain & Spinal Cord Tumors; Pediatric Neurosurgery; Rasmussen's Syndrome; **Hospital:** Johns Hopkins Hosp - Baltimore (page 61); **Address:** 600 N Wolfe St, Harvey 811, Baltimore, MD 21287-8811; **Phone:** 410-955-7888; **Board Cert:** Neurological Surgery 1988; Pediatric Neurological Surgery ; **Med School:** Univ Mich Med Sch 1977; **Resid:** Neurological Surgery, Johns Hopkins Hosp 1983; **Fellow:** Pediatric Neurological Surgery, Queen Elizabeth II Med Ctr 1984; **Fac Appt:** Assoc Prof NS, Johns Hopkins Univ

Chen, Chun Siang MD [NS] - **Spec Exp:** Skull Base Tumors; Skull Base Surgery; Microsurgery; **Hospital:** Mount Sinai Med Ctr; **Address:** Mount Sinai Med Ctr, Annenberg Bldg, One Gustave L Levy Pl Fl 8 - rm 10, New York, NY 10029; **Phone:** 212-241-8480; **Med School:** Brazil 1978; **Resid:** Neurological Surgery, Santa Casa de Misericordia of Sao Paulo Med Sch 1983; Neurological Surgery, Mount Sinai Med Ctr 2005; **Fellow:** Skull Base Surgery, St. Lukes Roosevelt Hosp 2006; **Fac Appt:** Asst Prof NS, Mount Sinai Sch Med

de Lotbiniere, Alain MD [NS] - **Spec Exp:** Movement Disorders; Pain Management; Brain Tumors; Pituitary Tumors; **Hospital:** Northern Westchester Hosp; **Address:** Brain & Spine Surgeons of New York, 244 Westchester Ave, Ste 310, White Plains, NY 10603; **Phone:** 914-948-6688; **Board Cert:** Neurological Surgery 1994; **Med School:** McGill Univ 1981; **Resid:** Surgery, Royal Victoria Hosp 1983; Neurological Surgery, Royal Victoria Hosp 1988; **Fellow:** Neurological Surgery, Univ of Cambridge 1989

Neurological Surgery

Di Giacinto, George V MD [NS] - **Spec Exp:** Spinal Surgery; Brain Tumors; Pain Management; **Hospital:** St Luke's - Roosevelt Hosp Ctr - Roosevelt Div; **Address:** 425 W 59th St, Ste 4E, New York, NY 10019; **Phone:** 212-523-8500; **Board Cert:** Neurological Surgery 1981; **Med School:** Harvard Med Sch 1970; **Resid:** Neurological Surgery, Columbia-Presby Hosp 1978

Eisenberg, Howard M MD [NS] - **Spec Exp:** Acoustic Neuroma; Parkinson's Disease/Movement Disorders; Epilepsy/Seizure Disorders; **Hospital:** Univ of MD Med Sys, Greater Baltimore Med Ctr; **Address:** Univ MD Sch Med, Dept Neurosurg, 22 S Greene St, Ste S-12-D, Baltimore, MD 21201-1544; **Phone:** 410-328-3514; **Board Cert:** Neurological Surgery 1973; **Med School:** SUNY Downstate 1964; **Resid:** Surgery, New York Hosp 1966; Neurological Surgery, Peter Bent Brigham Hosp/Chldns Hosp 1970; **Fellow:** Harvard Univ 1970; **Fac Appt:** Prof NS, Univ MD Sch Med

Feldstein, Neil A MD [NS] - **Spec Exp:** Pediatric Neurosurgery; Chiari's Deformity; Brain Tumors-Pediatric; Spinal Cord Surgery-Pediatric; **Hospital:** NY-Presby Hosp/Columbia (page 66); **Address:** Neurological Inst, 710 W 168th St Fl 2 - rm 213, New York, NY 10032; **Phone:** 212-305-1396; **Board Cert:** Neurological Surgery 1995; Pediatric Neurological Surgery 1995; **Med School:** NYU Sch Med 1984; **Resid:** Neurological Surgery, Baylor Coll Med 1989; **Fellow:** Pediatric Neurological Surgery, NYU Med Ctr 1991; **Fac Appt:** Asst Prof NS, Columbia P&S

Flamm, Eugene S MD [NS] - **Spec Exp:** Aneurysm-Cerebral; Brain Tumors; Cerebrovascular Surgery; **Hospital:** Montefiore Med Ctr; **Address:** Montefiore Med Ctr, 111 E 210th St, Bronx, NY 10467-2841; **Phone:** 718-920-2339; **Board Cert:** Neurological Surgery 1973; **Med School:** SUNY Buffalo 1962; **Resid:** Surgery, New York Hosp 1964; Neurological Surgery, NYU Med Ctr 1970; **Fellow:** Neurological Surgery, Univ Zurich 1971; **Fac Appt:** Prof NS, Albert Einstein Coll Med

Goodman, Robert R MD/PhD [NS] - **Spec Exp:** Parkinson's Disease; Epilepsy; Trigeminal Neuralgia; **Hospital:** NY-Presby Hosp/Columbia (page 66); **Address:** 710 W 168th St, rm 426, New York, NY 10032-2603; **Phone:** 212-305-3774; **Board Cert:** Neurological Surgery 1993; **Med School:** Johns Hopkins Univ 1982; **Resid:** Neurological Surgery, Columbia-Presby Med Ctr 1989; **Fac Appt:** Assoc Prof NS, Columbia P&S

Goodrich, James T MD [NS] - **Spec Exp:** Craniofacial Surgery/Reconstruction; Spina Bifida; Brain Tumors-Pediatric; Pediatric Neurosurgery; **Hospital:** Montefiore Med Ctr, Jacobi Med Ctr; **Address:** Montefiore Med Ctr, Dept Ped Neurosurgery, 111 E 210th St, Bronx, NY 10467-2401; **Phone:** 718-920-4197; **Board Cert:** Neurological Surgery 1989; Pediatric Neurological Surgery 1996; **Med School:** Columbia P&S 1980; **Resid:** Neurological Surgery, NY Neurological Inst 1986; **Fac Appt:** Prof NS, Albert Einstein Coll Med

Grady, M Sean MD [NS] - **Spec Exp:** Skull Base Tumors; Pituitary Tumors; Meningioma; **Hospital:** Hosp Univ Penn - UPHS (page 72), Pennsylvania Hosp (page 72); **Address:** Hosp Univ Penn, Dept Neurosurgery, 3400 Spruce St, Silverstein Bldg Fl 3, Philadelphia, PA 19104; **Phone:** 215-662-3483; **Board Cert:** Neurological Surgery 1990; **Med School:** Georgetown Univ 1981; **Resid:** Neurological Surgery, Univ Virginia Hosp 1987; **Fac Appt:** Prof NS, Univ Pennsylvania

Gutin, Philip MD [NS] - **Spec Exp:** Brain Tumors; Meningioma; Acoustic Neuroma; **Hospital:** Meml Sloan Kettering Cancer Ctr, NY-Presby Hosp/Weill Cornell (page 66); **Address:** Meml Sloan Kettering Cancer Ctr, Dept Neurosurgery, 1275 York Ave, rm C703, New York, NY 10021-6007; **Phone:** 212-639-8556; **Board Cert:** Neurological Surgery 1981; **Med School:** Univ Pennsylvania 1971; **Resid:** Neurological Surgery, UCSF Med Ctr 1979; **Fellow:** Natl Cancer Inst 1976; **Fac Appt:** Prof NS, Cornell Univ-Weill Med Coll

Harbaugh, Robert E MD [NS] - **Spec Exp:** Carotid Artery Surgery; Aneurysm-Cerebral; Arteriovenous Malformations; **Hospital:** Penn State Milton S Hershey Med Ctr; **Address:** Penn State-Hershey Med Ctr, H110 Neurosurg, C3830-Biomed Rsch Bldg, 500 University Drive, Hershey, PA 17033-0850; **Phone:** 717-531-4383; **Board Cert:** Neurological Surgery 1989; **Med School:** Penn State Univ-Hershey Med Ctr 1978; **Resid:** Surgery, Dartmouth-Hitchcock Med Ctr 1980; Neurological Surgery, Dartmouth-Hitchcock Med Ctr 1985; **Fac Appt:** Prof NS, Penn State Univ-Hershey Med Ctr

Hodge Jr, Charles J MD [NS] - **Spec Exp:** Vascular Neurosurgery; **Hospital:** Upstate Med Univ Hosp; **Address:** 725 Irving Ave, Ste 503, Syracuse, NY 13210; **Phone:** 315-464-4470; **Board Cert:** Neurological Surgery 1977; **Med School:** Columbia P&S 1967; **Resid:** Surgery, Yale-New Haven Hosp 1969; Neurological Surgery, SUNY Upstate Med Ctr 1974; **Fac Appt:** Prof NS, SUNY Upstate Med Univ

Hopkins, Leo Nelson MD [NS] - **Spec Exp:** Cerebrovascular Disease; Endovascular Surgery; **Hospital:** Millard Fillmore Gates Cir Hosp; **Address:** Millard Fillmore Hosp, Dept Neurosurgery, 3 Gates Cir, Buffalo, NY 14209; **Phone:** 716-887-5210; **Board Cert:** Neurological Surgery 1977; **Med School:** Albany Med Coll 1969; **Resid:** Neurological Surgery, SUNY Buffalo Med Ctr 1975; **Fac Appt:** Prof NS, SUNY Buffalo

Jho, Hae-Dong MD/PhD [NS] - **Spec Exp:** Minimally Invasive Neurosurgery; **Hospital:** Allegheny General Hosp; **Address:** Institute for Minimally Invasive Neurosurgery, 320 E North Ave, Snyder Pavilion, Fl 7, Pittsburgh, PA 15212-4746; **Phone:** 412-359-6110; **Board Cert:** Neurological Surgery 1991; **Med School:** Korea 1971; **Resid:** Neurological Surgery, Hanyang Univ Hosp 1979; Neurological Surgery, Univ Pittsburgh 1989; **Fellow:** Microsurgery, Univ Pittsburgh 1983; **Fac Appt:** Prof NS, Drexel Univ Coll Med

Judy, Kevin MD [NS] - **Spec Exp:** Brain Tumors; **Hospital:** Hosp Univ Penn - UPHS (page 72), Pennsylvania Hosp (page 72); **Address:** Hosp Univ Penn-Dept Neurosurg, 3400 Spruce St, 3 Silverstein, Philadelphia, PA 19104; **Phone:** 215-662-7854; **Board Cert:** Neurological Surgery 1997; **Med School:** Univ Pittsburgh 1984; **Resid:** Surgery, Mercy Hosp 1986; Neurological Surgery, Johns Hopkins Hosp 1992; **Fellow:** Neurological Surgery, Johns Hopkins Hosp 1991; **Fac Appt:** Assoc Prof NS, Univ Pennsylvania

Kassam, Amin MD [NS] - **Spec Exp:** Skull Base Tumors & Surgery; Cranial Nerve Disorders; Cerebrovascular Surgery; Endoscopic Surgery; **Hospital:** UPMC Presby, Pittsburgh; **Address:** Univ Pittsburgh Med Ctr, Dept Neurosurgery, 200 Lothrop St, Ste B400, Pittsburgh, PA 15213; **Phone:** 412-647-3685; **Med School:** Univ Toronto 1991; **Resid:** Neurological Surgery, Univ Ottawa Med Ctr 1997; **Fac Appt:** Assoc Prof NS, Univ Pittsburgh

Kelly, Patrick J MD [NS] - **Spec Exp:** Brain Tumors; Movement Disorders; Gliomas; **Hospital:** NYU Med Ctr (page 67), Lenox Hill Hosp (page 62); **Address:** NYU Med Ctr, Dept Neurological Surgery, 530 1st Ave, Ste 8R, New York, NY 10016; **Phone:** 212-263-8002; **Board Cert:** Neurological Surgery 1978; **Med School:** SUNY Buffalo 1966; **Resid:** Neurological Surgery, Northwestern Univ Hosp 1972; Neurological Surgery, Univ Texas Med Br Hosp 1974; **Fellow:** Neurological Surgery, St Anne Hosp 1977; **Fac Appt:** Prof NS, NYU Sch Med

Khan, Agha S MD [NS] - **Spec Exp:** Skull Base Surgery; Spinal Surgery; **Hospital:** Sinai Hosp - Baltimore; **Address:** 2411 W Belvedere Ave, Ste 402, Baltimore, MD 21215; **Phone:** 410-601-8314; **Board Cert:** Neurological Surgery 1995; **Med School:** Pakistan 1979; **Resid:** Neurological Surgery, Univ Wisconsin Hosp 1990; **Fellow:** Surgical Oncology, Roswell Park Meml Inst 1982; Neurological Surgery, Allegheny Genl Hosp 1991

Neurological Surgery

Kobrine, Arthur MD/PhD [NS] - **Spec Exp:** Spinal Cord Surgery; Brain & Spinal Cord Tumors; **Hospital:** Sibley Mem Hosp, Georgetown Univ Hosp; **Address:** 2440 M St NW, Ste 315, Washington, DC 20037-1404; **Phone:** 202-293-7136; **Board Cert:** Neurological Surgery 1976; **Med School:** Northwestern Univ 1968; **Resid:** Neurological Surgery, Northwestern Univ Hosp 1970; Neurological Surgery, Walter Reed Army Hosp 1973; **Fellow:** Physiology, Geo Wash Univ 1979; **Fac Appt:** Clin Prof NS, Georgetown Univ

Kondziolka, Douglas MD [NS] - **Spec Exp:** Brain Tumors-Adult & Pediatric; Brain Tumors-Metastatic; Stereotactic Radiosurgery; Movement Disorders; **Hospital:** UPMC Presby, Pittsburgh, Chldns Hosp of Pittsburgh - UPMC; **Address:** Univ Pittsburgh Med Ctr, Dept Neurological Surgery, 200 Lothrop St, Ste B400, Pittsburgh, PA 15213; **Phone:** 412-647-9990; **Board Cert:** Neurological Surgery 1994; **Med School:** Univ Toronto 1985; **Resid:** Neurological Surgery, Univ Toronto 1991; **Fellow:** Stereo Neurological Surgery, UPMC Presby Med Ctr 1991; **Fac Appt:** Prof NS, Univ Pittsburgh

Lavyne, Michael H MD [NS] - **Spec Exp:** Spinal Surgery; Spinal Tumors; Spinal Disorders; **Hospital:** NY-Presby Hosp/Weill Cornell (page 66), Hosp For Special Surgery (page 60); **Address:** 110 E 55th St Fl 9, New York, NY 10022; **Phone:** 212-486-9100; **Board Cert:** Neurological Surgery 1982; **Med School:** Cornell Univ-Weill Med Coll 1972; **Resid:** Neurological Surgery, Mass Genl Hosp 1979; **Fellow:** Neurology, Beth Israel Hosp 1974; **Fac Appt:** Clin Prof NS, Cornell Univ-Weill Med Coll

Loftus, Christopher M MD [NS] - **Spec Exp:** Cerebrovascular Surgery; Brain Tumors; Spinal Disorders-Cervical; **Hospital:** Temple Univ Hosp; **Address:** Temple Univ School Med, 3401 N Broad St, Parkinson Pavilion 540, Philadelphia, PA 19140, **Phone:** 215-707-9747; **Board Cert:** Neurological Surgery 1987; **Med School:** SUNY Downstate 1979; **Resid:** Neurological Surgery, Columbia-Presby Med Ctr 1985; **Fac Appt:** Prof NS, Temple Univ

Long, Donlin M MD/PhD [NS] - **Spec Exp:** Skull Base Tumors; Acoustic Neuroma; Spinal Surgery; **Hospital:** Johns Hopkins Hosp - Baltimore (page 61); **Address:** 600 N Wolfe St Carnegie Bldg - rm 466, Baltimore, MD 21287; **Phone:** 410-955-2251; **Board Cert:** Neurological Surgery 1968; **Med School:** Univ MO-Columbia Sch Med 1959; **Resid:** Neurological Surgery, Univ Minnesota Hosp 1964; Neurological Surgery, Boston Chldn's Hosp & Peter Bent Brigham Hosp 1965; **Fellow:** Neurological Pathology, Natl Insts of Health 1968; **Fac Appt:** Prof NS, Johns Hopkins Univ

Lunsford, L Dade MD [NS] - **Spec Exp:** Brain Tumors; Stereotactic Radiosurgery; Movement Disorders; **Hospital:** UPMC Presby, Pittsburgh, Chldns Hosp of Pittsburgh - UPMC; **Address:** UPMC Presbyterian Hosp, 200 Lothrop St, Ste B400, Pittsburgh, PA 15213-2536; **Phone:** 412-647-3685; **Board Cert:** Neurological Surgery 1983; **Med School:** Columbia P&S 1974; **Resid:** Neurological Surgery, Univ Pittsburgh Med Ctr 1980; **Fellow:** Stereo Neurological Surgery, Karolinska Hospital 1981; **Fac Appt:** Prof NS, Univ Pittsburgh

Maroon, Joseph C MD [NS] - **Spec Exp:** Minimally Invasive Surgery; Microdiscectomy; Brain Injury-Traumatic; **Hospital:** UPMC Presby, Pittsburgh; **Address:** UPMC Presbyterian, Dept Neurological Surgery, 200 Lothrop St, Ste 5-C, Pittsburgh, PA 15213; **Phone:** 412-647-3604; **Board Cert:** Neurological Surgery 1973; **Med School:** Indiana Univ 1965; **Resid:** Surgery, Georgetown Univ Hosp 1967; Neurological Surgery, Indiana Univ Med Ctr 1971; **Fellow:** Neurological Surgery, Radcliffe Infirm/Oxford Univ 1969; Microsurgery, Univ Vermont 1972; **Fac Appt:** Clin Prof NS, Univ Pittsburgh

McCormick, Paul C MD [NS] - **Spec Exp:** Spinal Surgery; Spinal Tumors; **Hospital:** NY-Presby Hosp/Columbia (page 66), Valley Hosp; **Address:** 710 W 168th St, Ste 406, New York, NY 10032-2603; **Phone:** 212-305-7976; **Board Cert:** Neurological Surgery 1993; **Med School:** Columbia P&S 1982; **Resid:** Neurological Surgery, Columbia Presby Med Ctr 1989; **Fellow:** Neurological Surgery, Natl Inst Hlth 1984; Spinal Surgery, Med Coll Wisconsin 1990; **Fac Appt:** Prof NS, Columbia P&S

Milhorat, Thomas H MD [NS] - **Spec Exp:** Chiari's Deformity; Syringomyelia & Spinal Cord Diseases; Hydrocephalus; **Hospital:** N Shore Univ Hosp at Manhasset, Schneider Chldn's Hosp; **Address:** N Shore Univ Hosp, Dept Neurosurgery, 300 Community Drive, Ste 2-DSU, Manhasset, NY 11030-3616; **Phone:** 516-562-3020; **Board Cert:** Neurological Surgery 1972; **Med School:** Cornell Univ-Weill Med Coll 1961; **Resid:** Surgery, NY Hosp-Cornel Med Ctr 1963; Neurological Surgery, NY Hosp-Cornel Med Ctr 1969; **Fellow:** Neurological Surgery, Natl Inst Hlth 1965; **Fac Appt:** Prof NS, NYU Sch Med

Murali, Raj MD [NS] - **Spec Exp:** Trigeminal Neuralgia; Skull Base Surgery; Aneurysm-Cerebral; Pituitary Tumors; **Hospital:** Westchester Med Ctr, St Vincent Cath Med Ctrs - Manhattan; **Address:** Westchester Med Ctr, Dept Neurosurgery, Munger Pavilion, Ste 329, Valhalla, NY 10595; **Phone:** 914-493-8392; **Board Cert:** Neurological Surgery 1982; **Med School:** India 1968; **Resid:** Neurological Surgery, Royal Infirm-Univ Edinburgh 1974; Neurological Surgery, NYU Med Ctr 1979; **Fac Appt:** Prof NS, NY Med Coll

O'Rourke, Donald MD [NS] - **Spec Exp:** Neuro-Oncology; Brain Tumors; Spinal Disorders-Cervical; **Hospital:** Hosp Univ Penn - UPHS (page 72); **Address:** Hosp Univ Penn - Dept Neurosurg, 3400 Spruce St, 3 Silverstein, Philadelphia, PA 19104; **Phone:** 215-662-3490; **Board Cert:** Neurological Surgery 1998; **Med School:** Univ Pennsylvania 1987; **Resid:** Neurological Surgery, Hosp Univ Penn 1994; **Fac Appt:** Assoc Prof NS, Univ Pennsylvania

Pollack, Ian MD [NS] - **Spec Exp:** Pediatric Neurosurgery; Brain Tumors; Craniofacial Surgery; **Hospital:** Chldns Hosp of Pittsburgh - UPMC, UPMC Presby, Pittsburgh; **Address:** Chldns Hosp Pittsburgh, Div Neurosurgery, 3705 Fifth Ave, Ste 3670A, Pittsburgh, PA 15213-2524; **Phone:** 412-692-5881; **Board Cert:** Neurological Surgery 1996; Pediatric Neurological Surgery 1997; **Med School:** Johns Hopkins Univ 1984; **Resid:** Neurological Surgery, Univ Pittsburgh Med Ctr 1991; **Fellow:** Pediatric Neurological Surgery, Hosp Sick Chldn 1992; **Fac Appt:** Prof NS, Univ Pittsburgh

Post, Kalmon MD [NS] - **Spec Exp:** Pituitary Tumors; Acoustic Neuroma; Meningioma; **Hospital:** Mount Sinai Med Ctr; **Address:** 5 E 98th St, Fl 7, New York, NY 10029-6501; **Phone:** 212-241-0933; **Board Cert:** Neurological Surgery 1978; **Med School:** NYU Sch Med 1967; **Resid:** Surgery, Bellevue Hosp 1969; Neurological Surgery, Bellevue Hosp-NYU 1975; **Fac Appt:** Prof NS, Mount Sinai Sch Med

Rigamonti, Daniele MD [NS] - **Spec Exp:** Hydrocephalus-Adult; Brain Tumors; Spinal Disorders; Vascular Neurosurgery; **Hospital:** Johns Hopkins Hosp - Baltimore (page 61); **Address:** Johns Hopkins Hosp, Dept Neurosurgery, 600 N Wolfe St, Phipps 100, Baltimore, MD 21287; **Phone:** 410-955-2259; **Board Cert:** Neurological Surgery 1988; **Med School:** Italy 1976; **Resid:** Neurological Surgery, Mt Sinai Hosp Med Ctr 1984; **Fellow:** Neurological Vascular Surgery, Barrow Neuro Inst 1987; **Fac Appt:** Prof NS, Johns Hopkins Univ

Rosenwasser, Robert H MD [NS] - **Spec Exp:** Aneurysm-Cerebral; Cerebrovascular Surgery; Neuro-Oncology; **Hospital:** Thomas Jefferson Univ Hosp; **Address:** Thomas Jefferson University Hospital, 909 Walnut St Fl 2, Philadelphia, PA 19107; **Phone:** 215-955-7000; **Board Cert:** Neurological Surgery 1987; **Med School:** Louisiana State Univ 1979; **Resid:** Neurological Surgery, Temple Univ Hosp 1984; **Fellow:** Neurological Vascular Surgery, Univ West Ontarion 1985; Interventional Neuroradiology, NYU Med Ctr 1993; **Fac Appt:** Prof NS, Thomas Jefferson Univ

Sen, Chandranath MD [NS] - **Spec Exp:** Brain Tumors; Skull Base Tumors; Skull Base Surgery; **Hospital:** St Luke's - Roosevelt Hosp Ctr - Roosevelt Div; **Address:** St Lukes Roosevelt Hosp Ctr, Dept Neurosurgery, 1000 10th Ave, Ste 5G-80, New York, NY 10019; **Phone:** 212-523-6720; **Board Cert:** Neurological Surgery 1989; **Med School:** India 1976; **Resid:** Surgery, Univ Wisconsin Hosps 1980; Neurological Surgery, Univ Wisconsin Hosps 1985; **Fellow:** Microsurgery, Univ Pittsburgh Med Ctr 1986

Solomon, Robert A MD [NS] - **Spec Exp:** Aneurysm-Cerebral; Arteriovenous Malformations; **Hospital:** NY-Presby Hosp/Columbia (page 66); **Address:** 710 W 168th St, Ste 439, New York, NY 10032; **Phone:** 212-305-4118; **Board Cert:** Neurological Surgery 1988; **Med School:** Johns Hopkins Univ 1980; **Resid:** Neurological Surgery, Neuro Inst-Columbia Univ 1986; **Fac Appt:** Prof NS, Columbia P&S

Stieg, Philip E MD/PhD [NS] - **Spec Exp:** Cerebrovascular Surgery; Acoustic Neuroma; Skull Base Surgery; Meningioma; **Hospital:** NY-Presby Hosp/Weill Cornell (page 66); **Address:** 525 E 68th St, STARR 651, New York, NY 10021-9800; **Phone:** 212-746-4684; **Board Cert:** Neurological Surgery 1992; **Med School:** Med Coll Wisc 1983; **Resid:** Neurological Surgery, Dallas Chldns Hosp/Parkland Meml Hosp 1988; **Fellow:** Neurological Biology, Karolinska Inst 1988; **Fac Appt:** Prof NS, Cornell Univ-Weill Med Coll

Sutton, Leslie N MD [NS] - **Spec Exp:** Brain Tumors-Pediatric; Fetal Neurosurgery; Hydrocephalus; **Hospital:** Chldns Hosp of Philadelphia, The; **Address:** Childrens Hosp of Phila -Div Neurosurgery, 34th St & Civic Ctr Blvd Wood 6 Bldg, Philadelphia, PA 19104; **Phone:** 215-590-2780; **Board Cert:** Neurological Surgery 1984; Pediatric Neurological Surgery 1996; **Med School:** Univ Pennsylvania 1975; **Resid:** Neurological Surgery, Hosp Univ Penn 1981; **Fac Appt:** Prof NS, Univ Pennsylvania

Tamargo, Rafael J MD [NS] - **Spec Exp:** Vascular Neurosurgery; Skull Base Surgery; **Hospital:** Johns Hopkins Hosp - Baltimore (page 61); **Address:** Johns Hopkins Hosp, Dept Neurosurgery, 600 N Wolfe St, Meyer 8-181, Baltimore, MD 21287; **Phone:** 410-614-1533; **Board Cert:** Neurological Surgery 1995; **Med School:** Columbia P&S 1984; **Resid:** Neurological Surgery, Johns Hopkins Hosps 1992; **Fac Appt:** Prof NS, Johns Hopkins Univ

Whiting, Donald M MD [NS] - **Spec Exp:** Movement Disorders; Pain & Spasticity; Spinal Disorders; **Hospital:** Allegheny General Hosp, Washington Hosp, The; **Address:** 380 West Chestnut St, Washington, PA 15301-4657; **Phone:** 724-228-1414; **Board Cert:** Neurological Surgery 1995; **Med School:** Jefferson Med Coll 1985; **Resid:** Surgery, Geisinger Med Ctr 1986; Neurological Surgery, Cleveland Clin Fdn 1991; **Fellow:** Neurological Trauma, Allegheny Gen Hosp 1990; **Fac Appt:** Assoc Prof NS, Drexel Univ Coll Med

Wisoff, Jeffrey H MD [NS] - **Spec Exp:** Pediatric Neurosurgery; Brain Tumors-Pediatric; Hydrocephalus; **Hospital:** NYU Med Ctr (page 67), Maimonides Med Ctr (page 63); **Address:** 317 E 34th St, Ste 1002, New York, NY 10016-4974; **Phone:** 212-263-6419; **Board Cert:** Neurological Surgery 1990; Pediatric Neurological Surgery 1996; **Med School:** Geo Wash Univ 1978; **Resid:** Neurological Surgery, NYU Med Ctr/Bellevue Hosp 1984; **Fellow:** Pediatric Neurological Surgery, NYU Med Ctr 1985; **Fac Appt:** Assoc Prof NS, NYU Sch Med

Southeast

Boop, Frederick A MD [NS] - **Spec Exp:** Pediatric Neurosurgery; Epilepsy; Brain Tumors; **Hospital:** Le Bonheur Chldns Med Ctr, Methodist Univ Hosp - Memphis; **Address:** Semmes Murphy Clinic, 1211 Union Ave, Ste 200, Memphis, TN 38104; **Phone:** 901-259-5340; **Board Cert:** Neurological Surgery 1993; **Med School:** Univ Ark 1983; **Resid:** Neurological Surgery, Univ Tex Hlth Sci Ctr 1989; Neurological Surgery, Inst Neur/Hosp Sick Chldn 1987; **Fellow:** Epilepsy, Univ Minn 1989; Pediatric Neurological Surgery, Ark Chldns Hosp 1990; **Fac Appt:** Assoc Prof NS, Univ Tenn Coll Med, Memphis

Branch Jr, Charles L MD [NS] - **Spec Exp:** Spinal Reconstructive Surgery; Minimally Invasive Spinal Surgery; Stereotactic Radiosurgery; **Hospital:** Wake Forest Univ Baptist Med Ctr (page 73), Forsyth Med Ctr; **Address:** WFU Baptist Med Ctr, Medical Center Blvd, Winston Salem, NC 27157-1029; **Phone:** 336-716-4083; **Board Cert:** Neurological Surgery 1991; **Med School:** Univ Tex SW, Dallas 1981; **Resid:** Neurological Surgery, NC Baptist Hosp 1987; **Fac Appt:** Prof NS, Wake Forest Univ

Brem, Steven MD [NS] - **Spec Exp:** Brain Tumors; Pituitary Tumors; Clinical Trials; **Hospital:** H Lee Moffitt Cancer Ctr & Research Inst; **Address:** H. Lee Moffitt Cancer Ctr/ Neurosurgery, 12902 Magnolia Drive, Tampa, FL 33612-9497; **Phone:** 813-745-3063; **Board Cert:** Neurological Surgery 1983; **Med School:** Harvard Med Sch 1972; **Resid:** Neurological Surgery, Massachusetts Genl Hosp 1981; **Fellow:** Oncology, Natl Cancer Inst 1976; **Fac Appt:** Prof NS, Univ S Fla Coll Med

Freeman, Thomas B MD [NS] - **Spec Exp:** Parkinson's Disease; Nerve Surgery & Transplantation; Spinal Surgery; **Hospital:** Tampa Genl Hosp; **Address:** Harborside Medical Tower, 4 Columbia Dr, Ste 730, Tampa, FL 33606; **Phone:** 813-259-0889; **Board Cert:** Neurological Surgery 1993; **Med School:** Johns Hopkins Univ 1981; **Resid:** Neurological Surgery, NYU Med Ctr 1988; **Fac Appt:** Prof NS, Univ S Fla Coll Med

Friedman, Allan H MD [NS] - **Spec Exp:** Brain Tumors; Skull Base Tumors; Cerebrovascular Surgery; **Hospital:** Duke Univ Med Ctr; **Address:** Duke Univ Med Ctr, DUMC 3807, Durham, NC 27710; **Phone:** 919-681-6421; **Board Cert:** Neurological Surgery 1983; **Med School:** Univ IL Coll Med 1974; **Resid:** Neurological Surgery, Duke Univ Med Ctr 1980; **Fellow:** Vascular Surgery, Univ Western Ontario 1981; **Fac Appt:** Prof S, Duke Univ

Green, Barth MD [NS] - **Spec Exp:** Spinal Surgery; **Hospital:** Jackson Meml Hosp, VA Med Ctr - Miami, FL; **Address:** 1095 NW 14th Terr Fl 2, Miami, FL 33136; **Phone:** 305-243-6946; **Board Cert:** Neurological Surgery 1978; **Med School:** Indiana Univ 1969; **Resid:** Neurological Surgery, Northwestern Univ Sch Med 1975; **Fac Appt:** Prof NS, Univ Miami Sch Med

Neurological Surgery

Guthrie, Barton L MD [NS] - **Spec Exp:** Brain Tumors; Stereotactic Radiosurgery; Parkinson's Disease/Movement Disorders; **Hospital:** Univ of Ala Hosp at Birmingham; **Address:** Univ Alabama, Div Neurosurg, 510 20th St S, FOT 1038, Birmingham, AL 35294; **Phone:** 205-934-8136; **Board Cert:** Neurological Surgery 1992; **Med School:** Univ Ala 1980; **Resid:** Neurological Surgery, Mayo Clinic 1988; **Fellow:** Neurological Surgery, Stanford Univ Med Ctr 1988; **Fac Appt:** Assoc Prof NS, Univ Ala

Hadley, Mark N MD [NS] - **Spec Exp:** Spinal Surgery; Spinal Disorders-Degenerative; **Hospital:** Univ of Ala Hosp at Birmingham; **Address:** UAB Sch Med, Div Neurosurgery, 510 20th St S, Ste FOT 1030, Birmingham, AL 35294-3410; **Phone:** 205-934-1439; **Board Cert:** Neurological Surgery 1992; **Med School:** Albany Med Coll 1982; **Resid:** Neurological Surgery, St Josephs Hosp Med Ctr 1988; **Fac Appt:** Prof NS, Univ Ala

Haid Jr, Regis MD [NS] - **Spec Exp:** Spinal Surgery; Minimally Invasive Spinal Surgery; Spinal Disc Replacement; Microdiscectomy; **Hospital:** Piedmont Hosp; **Address:** Atlanta Brain & Spine Care, 2001 Peachtree Rd NE, Ste 645, Atlanta, GA 30309; **Phone:** 404-350-0106; **Board Cert:** Neurological Surgery 2000; **Med School:** W VA Univ 1982; **Resid:** Surgery, W Va Univ Hosps 1983; Neurological Surgery, W Va Univ Hosps 1988; **Fellow:** Spinal Surgery, Univ Fl Affil Hosps 1989; **Fac Appt:** Assoc Prof NS, Emory Univ

Heros, Roberto MD [NS] - **Spec Exp:** Cerebrovascular Surgery; Skull Base Surgery; Brain Tumors; **Hospital:** Jackson Meml Hosp; **Address:** Univ Miami, Dept Neurosurgery, 1095 NW 14th Terrace, Miami, FL 33136; **Phone:** 305-243-4572; **Board Cert:** Neurological Surgery 1979; **Med School:** Univ Tenn Coll Med, Memphis 1968; **Resid:** Surgery, Mass Genl Hosp 1970; Neurological Surgery, Mass Genl Hosp 1976, **Fac Appt:** Prof NS, Univ Miami Sch Med

Morrison, Glenn MD [NS] - **Spec Exp:** Pediatric Neurosurgery; Epilepsy; Craniofacial Surgery; Spinal Cord Tumors; **Hospital:** Miami Children's Hosp, Jackson Meml Hosp; **Address:** Medical Arts Bldg, 3215 SW 62nd Ave, Ste 3109, Miami, FL 33155; **Phone:** 305-662-8386; **Board Cert:** Neurological Surgery 1976; Pediatric Neurological Surgery 1996; **Med School:** Case West Res Univ 1967; **Resid:** Neurological Surgery, Case Western Univ Hosp 1974; **Fac Appt:** Prof NS, Univ Miami Sch Med

Oakes, W Jerry MD [NS] - **Spec Exp:** Pediatric Neurosurgery; Chiari's Deformity; Occult Spinal Dysraphism (OSD); **Hospital:** Children's Hospital - Birmingham; **Address:** Children's Hosp Alabama, 1600 7th Ave S, ACC, rm 400, Birmingham, AL 35233; **Phone:** 205-939-9653; **Board Cert:** Neurological Surgery 1981; Pediatric Neurological Surgery 1996; **Med School:** Duke Univ 1972; **Resid:** Neurological Surgery, Duke Univ Hosp 1978; **Fellow:** Neurological Surgery, Hosp for Sick Chldn 1975; Neurological Surgery, Great Ormond St Hosp 1979; **Fac Appt:** Prof NS, Univ Ala

Patel, Sunil J MD [NS] - **Spec Exp:** Brain Tumors; Skull Base Surgery; Pain-Facial; Trigeminal Neuralgia; **Hospital:** MUSC Med Ctr; **Address:** MUSC - Department of Neurosciences, Division of Neurosurgery, CSB, Ste 428, Charleston, SC 29425; **Phone:** 843-792-7700; **Board Cert:** Neurological Surgery 1996; **Med School:** Med Univ SC 1985; **Resid:** Neurology, Univ South Carolina 1991; **Fellow:** Neurology, Nagoya Univ Med School 1991; Skull Base Surgery, Univ Pittsburgh 1993; **Fac Appt:** Assoc Prof NS, Med Univ SC

Rodts Jr, Gerald E MD [NS] - **Spec Exp:** Spinal Surgery; **Hospital:** Crawford Long Hosp of Emory Univ, Emory Univ Hosp; **Address:** Emory Spine Center, 59 Executive Park South, Ste 3000, Atlanta, GA 30329; **Phone:** 404-778-6227; **Board Cert:** Neurological Surgery 1998; **Med School:** Columbia P&S 1987; **Resid:** Neurological Surgery, UCLA Med Ctr 1994; **Fellow:** Spinal Surgery, Emory Univ Hosp 1995; **Fac Appt:** Prof NS, Emory Univ

Sanford, Robert A MD [NS] - **Spec Exp:** Pediatric Neurosurgery; Brain Tumors-Pediatric; **Hospital:** Le Bonheur Chldns Med Ctr, St Jude Children's Research Hosp; **Address:** 6325 Humphreys Blvd, Memphis, TN 38120; **Phone:** 901-522-7762; **Board Cert:** Neurological Surgery 1976; Pediatric Neurological Surgery 1980; **Med School:** Univ Ark 1967; **Resid:** Neurological Surgery, Univ Minneapolis Med Ctr 1973; **Fac Appt:** Prof NS, Univ Tenn Coll Med, Memphis

Shaffrey, Christopher I MD [NS] - **Spec Exp:** Spinal Surgery; Spinal Surgery-Pediatric; **Hospital:** Univ Virginia Med Ctr; **Address:** Univ Virg, Dept Neurosurg, Hosp Drive, Private Clinic 3rd Fl, Rm 3508, Charlottesville, VA 22908; **Phone:** 434-243-7026; **Board Cert:** Neurological Surgery 1997; Orthopaedic Surgery 1997; **Med School:** Univ VA Sch Med 1986; **Resid:** Neurological Surgery, Univ Virginia Med Ctr 1992; Orthopaedic Surgery, Univ Virginia Med Ctr 1995; **Fellow:** Spinal Surgery, Univ Virginia Med Ctr 1996; **Fac Appt:** Prof NS, Univ VA Sch Med

Swaid, Swaid N MD [NS] - **Spec Exp:** Stereotactic Radiosurgery; **Hospital:** Healthsouth Med Ctr - Birmingham; **Address:** 513 Brookwood Blvd, Ste 372, Birmingham, AL 35209; **Phone:** 205-802-6844; **Board Cert:** Neurological Surgery 1983; **Med School:** Univ Ala 1976; **Resid:** Neurological Surgery, Univ Alabama 1981; **Fac Appt:** Assoc Prof NS, Univ Ala

Tatter, Stephen MD/PhD [NS] - **Spec Exp:** Brain Tumors; Pituitary Tumors; Stereotactic Radiosurgery; **Hospital:** Wake Forest Univ Baptist Med Ctr (page 73); **Address:** Wake Forest Univ Sch Med, Dept Neurosurg, Medical Center Blvd, Winston-Salem, NC 27157-1029; **Phone:** 336-716-4047; **Board Cert:** Neurological Surgery 2004; **Med School:** Cornell Univ-Weill Med Coll 1990; **Resid:** Neurological Surgery, Mass Genl Hosp 1996; **Fellow:** Neurological Surgery, Mass Genl Hosp 1997; **Fac Appt:** Assoc Prof NS, Wake Forest Univ

Tiel, Robert L MD [NS] - **Hospital:** Univ Hosps & Clins - Jackson; **Address:** Univ Mississippi Med Ctr, 2500 N State St, Jackson, MS 39216-4505; **Phone:** 601-984-6445; **Board Cert:** Neurological Surgery 1991; **Med School:** Univ Minn 1980; **Resid:** Neurological Surgery, Henry Ford Hosp 1986; **Fac Appt:** Prof NS, Univ Miss

Tulipan, Noel B MD [NS] - **Spec Exp:** Pediatric Neurosurgery; Fetal Neurosurgery; Spina Bifida; **Hospital:** Vanderbilt Univ Med Ctr; **Address:** Vanderbilt Chldns Hosp, Dept Neurosurg, 9226 Doctors Office Tower, Nashville, TN 37232-9557; **Phone:** 615-322-6875; **Board Cert:** Neurological Surgery 1989; Pediatric Neurological Surgery 1997; **Med School:** Johns Hopkins Univ 1977; **Resid:** Neurological Surgery, Johns Hopkins Hosp 1984; **Fac Appt:** Prof NS, Vanderbilt Univ

Van Loveren, Harry R MD [NS] - **Spec Exp:** Trigeminal Neuralgia; Skull Base Surgery; **Hospital:** Tampa Genl Hosp; **Address:** Harbourside Medical Tower, 4 Columbia Drive, Ste 650, Tampa, FL 33606; **Phone:** 813-259-0929; **Board Cert:** Neurological Surgery 1988; **Med School:** Univ Cincinnati 1979; **Resid:** Neurological Surgery, Good Samaritan Hosp 1984; **Fellow:** Neurological Surgery, Universitatspital 1985; **Fac Appt:** Prof NS, Univ S Fla Coll Med

Neurological Surgery

Wharen Jr, Robert E MD [NS] - **Spec Exp:** Parkinson's Disease; Brain Tumors; Epilepsy; **Hospital:** St Luke's Hosp - Jacksonville; **Address:** Mayo Clinic, Dept Neurosurgery, 4500 San Pablo Rd, Jacksonville, FL 32224-1865; **Phone:** 904-953-2103; **Board Cert:** Neurological Surgery 1988; **Med School:** Penn State Univ-Hershey Med Ctr 1979; **Resid:** Neurological Surgery, Mayo Clinic 1985; **Fac Appt:** Prof NS, Mayo Med Sch

Wilson, John A MD [NS] - **Spec Exp:** Cerebrovascular Surgery; Skull Base Surgery; Spinal Surgery; **Hospital:** Wake Forest Univ Baptist Med Ctr (page 73); **Address:** Wake Forest Univ Medical Ctr, Medical Center Blvd, Box 1029, Winston-Salem, NC 27157-1029; **Phone:** 336-716-4020; **Board Cert:** Neurological Surgery 1996; **Med School:** Jefferson Med Coll 1982; **Resid:** Surgery, Allegheny Gen Hosp 1985; Neurological Surgery, NYU Med Ctr 1986; **Fellow:** Neurological Surgery, New England Med Ctr 1990; **Fac Appt:** Assoc Prof NS, Wake Forest Univ

Young, A Byron MD [NS] - **Spec Exp:** Brain Tumors; Stereotactic Radiosurgery; Parkinson's Disease; **Hospital:** Univ of Kentucky Chandler Hosp; **Address:** Univ Kentucky Med Ctr, MS 101, Div Neurosurgery, 800 Rose St, Lexington, KY 40536-0298; **Phone:** 859-323-5861; **Board Cert:** Neurological Surgery 1974; **Med School:** Univ KY Coll Med 1965; **Resid:** Surgery, Vanderbilt Hosp 1967; Neurological Surgery, Vanderbilt Hosp 1971; **Fac Appt:** Prof S, Univ KY Coll Med

Midwest

Albright, A Leland MD [NS] - **Spec Exp:** Pediatric Neurosurgery; Spasticity & Movement Disorders; Brain Tumors; **Hospital:** Univ WI Hosp & Clins; **Address:** UW Hosp & Clinics, 600 Highland Ave, rm K4/836, Madison, WI 53792; **Phone:** 608-263-9651; **Board Cert:** Neurological Surgery 1981; Pediatric Neurological Surgery 1996; **Med School:** Louisiana State Univ 1969; **Resid:** Surgery, Wash Hosps 1971; Neurological Surgery, Univ Pittsburgh Med Ctr 1978; **Fellow:** Neurological Surgery, Natl Inst Hlth 1974; Immunopathology, Univ Pittsburgh Med Ctr 1978; **Fac Appt:** Prof NS, Univ Wisc

Atkinson, John MD [NS] - **Spec Exp:** Pituitary Surgery; Stroke; Cerebrovascular Disease; **Hospital:** Mayo Med Ctr & Clin - Rochester; **Address:** Mayo Clinic, Dept Neurosurgery, 200 First St SW, Rochester, MN 55905; **Phone:** 507-284-2376; **Board Cert:** Neurological Surgery 1992; **Med School:** Univ Ala 1984; **Resid:** Neurological Surgery, Mayo Clinic 1990; **Fac Appt:** Assoc Prof NS, Mayo Med Sch

Bakay, Roy A. E. MD [NS] - **Spec Exp:** Parkinson's Disease/Movement Disorders; Epilepsy; Brain Tumors; **Hospital:** Rush Univ Med Ctr; **Address:** Rush Univ Med Ctr, 1725 W Harrison St, Ste 970, Chicago, IL 60612; **Phone:** 312-942-6644; **Board Cert:** Neurological Surgery 1985; **Med School:** Northwestern Univ 1975; **Resid:** Neurological Surgery, Univ Washington Sch Med 1981; **Fellow:** Neuronal Plasticity, Natl Inst Hlth 1982; **Fac Appt:** Prof NS, Rush Med Coll

Barnett, Gene H MD [NS] - **Spec Exp:** Brain Tumors; Stereotactic Radiosurgery; **Hospital:** Cleveland Clin Fdn (page 57); **Address:** Cleveland Clinic Brain Tumor Inst, 9500 Euclid Ave, Desk R20, Cleveland, OH 44195; **Phone:** 216-444-5381; **Board Cert:** Neurological Surgery 1990; **Med School:** Case West Res Univ 1980; **Resid:** Neurological Surgery, Cleveland Clinic 1986; **Fellow:** Neurology, Cleveland Clinic 1982; Research, Mass Genl Hosp-Harvard 1987; **Fac Appt:** Prof NS, Cleveland Cl Coll Med/Case West Res

Batjer, Hunt MD [NS] - **Spec Exp:** Aneurysm-Cerebral; Arteriovenous Malformations; Stroke; **Hospital:** Northwestern Meml Hosp, Evanston Hosp; **Address:** 675 N St Clair, Ste 20-750, Chicago, IL 60611; **Phone:** 312-695-8143; **Board Cert:** Neurological Surgery 1986; **Med School:** Univ Tex SW, Dallas 1977; **Resid:** Neurological Surgery, Parkland Meml Hosp 1981; **Fellow:** Neurological Surgery, Univ West Ontario 1982; **Fac Appt:** Prof NS, Northwestern Univ

Bauer, Jerry MD [NS] - **Spec Exp:** Pain-Back & Neck; Brain Tumors; Spinal Surgery; Minimally Invasive Spinal Surgery; **Hospital:** Adv Luth Genl Hosp; **Address:** Ctr Brain & Spine Surg-Parkside Ctr, 1875 Dempster St, Ste 605, Park Ridge, IL 60068-1168; **Phone:** 847-698-1088; **Board Cert:** Neurological Surgery 1982; **Med School:** Univ IL Coll Med 1974; **Resid:** Neurological Surgery, Univ Illinios Med Ctr 1979; **Fac Appt:** Asst Clin Prof NS, Univ IL Coll Med

Benzel, Edward C MD [NS] - **Spec Exp:** Spinal Surgery; **Hospital:** Cleveland Clin Fdn (page 57); **Address:** 9500 Euclid, Ste S80, Cleveland, OH 44195; **Phone:** 216-445-5514; **Board Cert:** Neurological Surgery 1986; **Med School:** Univ Wisc 1974; **Resid:** Neurological Surgery, Med Coll Wisc Clins 1980; **Fellow:** Spinal Cord Injury Medicine, Wood VA Med Ctr 1981; **Fac Appt:** Prof NS, Case West Res Univ

Bierbrauer, Karin S MD [NS] - **Spec Exp:** Pediatric Neurosurgery; Spina Bifida; Craniosynostosis; Hydrocephalus; **Hospital:** Cincinnati Chldns Hosp Med Ctr; **Address:** Cincinnati Children's Hospital, 3333 Burnet Ave, MC 2016, Cincinnati, OH 45229; **Phone:** 513-636-7124; **Board Cert:** Neurological Surgery 1994; Pediatric Neurological Surgery 1995; **Med School:** Med Univ SC 1984; **Resid:** Neurological Surgery, Emory Univ Hosp 1990; **Fellow:** Pediatric Neurological Surgery, Chldns Meml Hosp 1991; **Fac Appt:** Assoc Clin Prof NS, Ohio State Univ

Brown, Frederick D MD [NS] - **Spec Exp:** Minimally Invasive Spinal Surgery; Spinal Surgery; Pain-Chronic; **Hospital:** Univ of Chicago Hosps; **Address:** Univ Chicago Hosp, Dept Neurosurgery, 5841 S Maryland Ave, MC 3026, Chicago, IL 60637; **Phone:** 773-702-2123; **Board Cert:** Neurological Surgery 1982; **Med School:** Ohio State Univ 1972; **Resid:** Neurological Surgery, Univ Chicago Hosps 1978; **Fac Appt:** Assoc Prof NS, Univ Chicago-Pritzker Sch Med

Chandler, William F MD [NS] - **Spec Exp:** Pituitary Surgery; Brain Tumors; **Hospital:** Univ Michigan Hlth Sys; **Address:** 1500 E Med Center Drive, Ste 3470, Tauban Center, Ann Arbor, MI 48109; **Phone:** 734-936-5020; **Board Cert:** Neurological Surgery 1980; **Med School:** Univ Mich Med Sch 1971; **Resid:** Neurological Surgery, Michigan Hosp 1977; **Fac Appt:** Prof NS, Univ Mich Med Sch

Chiocca, E Antonio MD [NS] - **Spec Exp:** Brain Tumors; Spinal Cord Tumors; **Hospital:** Arthur G James Cancer Hosp & Research Inst, Ohio St Univ Med Ctr; **Address:** OSU Med Ctr, Dept Neurosurgery, 410 W 10th Ave, 1021-N Doan Hall, Columbus, OH 43210; **Phone:** 614-293-9312; **Board Cert:** Neurological Surgery 2000; **Med School:** Univ Tex, Houston 1988; **Resid:** Neurological Surgery, Mass Genl Hosp 1995; **Fac Appt:** Prof NS, Ohio State Univ

Cohen, Alan R MD [NS] - **Spec Exp:** Pediatric Neurosurgery; Brain & Spinal Tumors-Pediatric; Minimally Invasive Neurosurgery; **Hospital:** Rainbow Babies & Chldns Hosp, Univ Hosps Case Med Ctr; **Address:** Rainbow Babies & Chldns Hosp, 11100 Euclid Ave, Ste B501, Cleveland, OH 44106; **Phone:** 216-844-5741; **Board Cert:** Neurological Surgery 1991; Pediatric Neurological Surgery 1997; **Med School:** Cornell Univ-Weill Med Coll 1978; **Resid:** Surgery, NYU Medical Ctr 1980; Neurological Surgery, NYU Medical Ctr 1987; **Fellow:** Neurology, Natl Hosp Queen's Square 1982; **Fac Appt:** Prof NS, Case West Res Univ

Neurological Surgery

Dacey Jr, Ralph G MD [NS] - **Spec Exp:** Cerebrovascular Surgery; Aneurysm-Cerebral; Brain Tumors; **Hospital:** Barnes-Jewish Hosp, Barnes-Jewish West County Hosp; **Address:** Wash Univ Sch Med, Dept Neurosurgery, 660 S Euclid Ave, Box 8057, St. Louis, MO 63110; **Phone:** 314-362-3577; **Board Cert:** Internal Medicine 1978; Neurological Surgery 1985; **Med School:** Univ VA Sch Med 1974; **Resid:** Internal Medicine, Strong Meml Hosp 1977; Neurological Surgery, Univ Virginia Med Ctr 1983; **Fac Appt:** Prof NS, Washington Univ, St Louis

Dempsey, Robert J MD [NS] - **Spec Exp:** Vascular Neurosurgery; Aneurysm-Cerebral; Stroke; **Hospital:** Univ WI Hosp & Clins; **Address:** Univ Wisc Hosp, Dept Neurosurgery, 600 Highland Ave, rm K4-822, Madison, WI 53792; **Phone:** 608-263-9585; **Board Cert:** Neurological Surgery 1985; **Med School:** Univ Chicago-Pritzker Sch Med 1977; **Resid:** Neurological Surgery, Univ Mich Hosps 1983; **Fac Appt:** Prof NS, Univ Wisc

Diaz, Fernando G MD/PhD [NS] - **Spec Exp:** Arteriovenous Malformations; Spinal Surgery; **Hospital:** Providence Hosp - Southfield, Harper Univ Hosp; **Address:** Michigan Head & Spine Institute, 29275 Northwestern Hwy, Ste 100, Southfield, MI 48034; **Phone:** 248-784-3667; **Board Cert:** Neurological Surgery 1980; **Med School:** Mexico 1968; **Resid:** Surgery, Univ Kansas Med Ctr 1973; Neurological Surgery, Univ Minn Med Ctr 1978; **Fellow:** Cerebrovascular Disease, Univ Minn Med Ctr 1979; **Fac Appt:** Prof NS, Wayne State Univ

Fessler, Richard G MD/PhD [NS] - **Spec Exp:** Skull Base Surgery; Spinal Surgery; Minimally Invasive Spinal Surgery; **Hospital:** Univ of Chicago Hosps; **Address:** Univ Chicago, Dept Neurosurgery, 5841 S Maryland Ave, MC 3026, Chicago, IL 60637; **Phone:** 773-702-9385; **Board Cert:** Neurological Surgery 1992; **Med School:** Univ Chicago-Pritzker Sch Med 1983; **Resid:** Neurological Surgery, Univ Chicago Hosp 1989; **Fac Appt:** Prof NS, Univ Chicago-Pritzker Sch Med

Frim, David M MD/PhD [NS] - **Spec Exp:** Pediatric Neurosurgery; Hydrocephalus; Brain & Spinal Tumors; Brain & Spinal Malformations; **Hospital:** Univ of Chicago Hosps; **Address:** Univ of Chicago Hosps-Pediatric Neurosurgery, 5841 S Maryland Ave, MC 4066, Chicago, IL 60637-1463; **Phone:** 773-702-2475; **Board Cert:** Neurological Surgery 1998; Pediatric Neurological Surgery 1998; **Med School:** Harvard Med Sch 1988; **Resid:** Neurological Surgery, Mass Genl Hosp 1995; **Fellow:** Pediatric Neurological Surgery, Children's Hosp 1996; **Fac Appt:** Assoc Prof S, Univ Chicago-Pritzker Sch Med

Greene Jr, Clarence S MD [NS] - **Spec Exp:** Pediatric Neurosurgery; Congenital Nervous System Malformations; Brain Tumors; **Hospital:** Chldns Mercy Hosps & Clinics; **Address:** 2401 Gillham Rd, Kansas City, MO 64108; **Phone:** 816-234-3000; **Board Cert:** Neurological Surgery 1984; Pediatric Neurological Surgery 1997; **Med School:** Howard Univ 1974; **Resid:** Neurological Surgery, Chldns Hosp 1981; Neurological Surgery, Peter Bent Brigham Hosp 1981; **Fellow:** Pediatric Neurological Surgery, Chldns Hosp 1985; **Fac Appt:** Assoc Clin Prof NS, UC Irvine

Grubb Jr, Robert L MD [NS] - **Spec Exp:** Brain Tumors; Acoustic Neuroma; Trigeminal Neuralgia; Skull Base Tumors; **Hospital:** Barnes-Jewish Hosp, St Louis Chldns Hosp; **Address:** Wash Univ Sch Med, Dept Neurosurgery, 660 S Euclid Ave, Box 8057, St Louis, MO 63110; **Phone:** 314-362-3577; **Board Cert:** Neurological Surgery 1976; **Med School:** Univ NC Sch Med 1965; **Resid:** Surgery, Barnes Jewish Hosp 1967; Neurological Surgery, Barnes Jewish Hosp 1973; **Fellow:** Neurological Surgery, National Inst Health 1969; **Fac Appt:** Prof NS, Washington Univ, St Louis

Guthikonda, Murali MD [NS] - **Spec Exp:** Skull Base Tumors; Pituitary Tumors; Aneurysm-Cerebral; Spinal Tumors; **Hospital:** Detroit Med Ctr, Harper Univ Hosp; **Address:** Univ Neurologic Surgeons, 4160 John R, Ste 930, Detroit, MI 48201; **Phone:** 313-831-0777; **Board Cert:** Neurological Surgery 1982; **Med School:** India 1971; **Resid:** Surgery, St Elizabeth Hosp 1976; Neurological Surgery, Med Ctr Hosp VT 1980; **Fellow:** Skull Base Surgery, Univ Cincinnati 1993; **Fac Appt:** Assoc Prof NS, Wayne State Univ

Gutierrez, Francisco A MD [NS] - **Spec Exp:** Brain Tumors; Cerebrovascular Surgery; Spinal Surgery; **Hospital:** Northwestern Meml Hosp, Resurrection Med Ctr; **Address:** 201 E Huron St, Ste 9-160, Gaulter Pavilion, Chicago, IL 60611; **Phone:** 312-926-3490; **Board Cert:** Neurological Surgery 1976; **Med School:** Colombia 1965; **Resid:** Neurological Surgery, San Juan de Dios Hosp 1967; Neurological Surgery, Northwestern Meml Hosp 1973; **Fac Appt:** Assoc Prof NS, Northwestern Univ

Kaufman, Bruce A MD [NS] - **Spec Exp:** Pediatric Neurosurgery; Brain & Spinal Cord Tumors; Spasticity & Movement Disorders; **Hospital:** Chldns Hosp - Wisconsin; **Address:** Chldns Hosp, Dept Neurosurg, 999 N 92nd St, Box 310, Milwaukee, WI 53226; **Phone:** 414-266-6435; **Board Cert:** Neurological Surgery 1992; Pediatric Neurological Surgery ; **Med School:** Case West Res Univ 1982; **Resid:** Neurological Surgery, Univ Hosp Cleveland/Case West Res 1988; **Fellow:** Pediatric Neurological Surgery, Chldns Meml Hosp/Northwestern Univ 1989; **Fac Appt:** Prof NS, Med Coll Wisc

Kranzler, Leonard I MD [NS] - **Spec Exp:** Brain Tumors; **Hospital:** Adv Illinois Masonic Med Ctr, Resurrection Hlth Care St Joseph Hosp; **Address:** 3000 N Halstead St, Ste 701, Chicago, IL 60657; **Phone:** 773-296-6666; **Board Cert:** Neurological Surgery 1974; **Med School:** Northwestern Univ 1963; **Resid:** Neurological Surgery, Northwestern Univ 1969; Neurological Surgery, Chldns Meml Hosp 1967; **Fellow:** Neurological Surgery; **Fac Appt:** Assoc Clin Prof NS, Univ Chicago-Pritzker Sch Med

Levy, Robert M MD/PhD [NS] - **Spec Exp:** Stereotactic Radiosurgery; Brain Tumors; Pain-Chronic; **Hospital:** Northwestern Meml Hosp; **Address:** 675 N Saint Clair St, Ste 2210, Gaulter Pavilion, Chicago, IL 60611-2922; **Phone:** 312-695-8143; **Board Cert:** Neurological Surgery 1991; **Med School:** Stanford Univ 1981; **Resid:** Neurological Surgery, UCSF Med Ctr 1987; **Fellow:** Neurological Surgery, UCSF Med Ctr 1986; **Fac Appt:** Prof NS, Northwestern Univ

Link, Michael J MD [NS] - **Spec Exp:** Skull Base Tumors; Brain Tumors; Cerebrovascular Surgery; **Hospital:** Mayo Med Ctr & Clin - Rochester; **Address:** Mayo Clinic, Dept Neurosurgery, 200 First St SW, Rochester, MN 55905; **Phone:** 507-284-8008; **Board Cert:** Neurological Surgery 2000; **Med School:** Mayo Med Sch 1990; **Resid:** Neurological Surgery, Mayo Clinic 1996; **Fellow:** Cerebrovascular & Skull Base Surgery, Univ Cincinnati/Mayfield Clinic 1998; **Fac Appt:** Assoc Prof NS, Mayo Med Sch

Luken, Martin MD [NS] - **Spec Exp:** Brain Tumors; Spinal Surgery; Chiari's Deformity; **Hospital:** Ingalls Meml Hosp, Rush Univ Med Ctr; **Address:** 71 W 156th St, Ste 208, Harvey, IL 60426; **Phone:** 708-331-6669; **Board Cert:** Neurological Surgery 1983; **Med School:** Columbia P&S 1973; **Resid:** Surgery, Univ Illinois Med Ctr 1976; Neurological Surgery, Neurological Inst-Columbia Presby 1980; **Fac Appt:** Asst Prof NS, Rush Med Coll

Macdonald, R Loch MD/PhD [NS] - **Spec Exp:** Cerebrovascular Surgery; Brain & Spinal Cord Tumors; **Hospital:** Univ of Chicago Hosps; **Address:** Univ Chicago Hospitals, 5841 S Maryland Ave, MC 3026, Chicago, IL 60637; **Phone:** 773-702-2123; **Board Cert:** Neurological Surgery 1995; **Med School:** Canada 1985; **Resid:** Neurological Surgery, Univ Toronto Med Ctr 1993; **Fac Appt:** Prof S, Univ Chicago-Pritzker Sch Med

Malik, Ghaus MD [NS] - **Spec Exp:** Trigeminal Neuralgia; Cerebrovascular Surgery; Brain & Spinal Cord Tumors; **Hospital:** Henry Ford Hosp, William Beaumont Hosp; **Address:** Henry Ford Hosp, Dept Neurosurg, 2799 W Grand Blvd, Detroit, MI 48202; **Phone:** 313-916-1093; **Board Cert:** Neurological Surgery 1978; **Med School:** Pakistan 1968; **Resid:** Surgery, Henry Ford Hosp 1971; Neurological Surgery, Henry Ford Hosp 1975

Menezes, Arnold MD [NS] - **Spec Exp:** Pediatric Neurosurgery; Craniocervical Disorders; Spinal Surgery-Pediatric; **Hospital:** Univ Iowa Hosp & Clinics; **Address:** Univ Iowa Hosp, Dept Neurosurgery, 200 Hawkins Drive, rm 3006BT, Iowa City, IA 52242; **Phone:** 319-356-2768; **Board Cert:** Neurological Surgery 1976; Pediatric Neurological Surgery 1997; **Med School:** India 1967; **Resid:** Surgery, Univ Iowa Hosps 1970; Neurological Surgery, Univ Iowa Hosps 1974; **Fellow:** Child Neurology, Univ Iowa Hosps; **Fac Appt:** Prof NS, Univ Iowa Coll Med

Nagib, Mahmoud MD [NS] - **Spec Exp:** Pediatric Neurosurgery; Skull Base Surgery; **Hospital:** Chldns Hosp and Clinics - Minneapolis, Abbott - Northwestern Hosp; **Address:** 305 Piper Bldg, 800 E 28th Street, Minneapolis, MN 55407-3723; **Phone:** 612-871-7278; **Board Cert:** Neurological Surgery 1985; **Med School:** Egypt 1973; **Resid:** Neurological Surgery, Univ Minn Hosps 1982; **Fellow:** Neurological Physiology, Univ Oslo 1976; **Fac Appt:** Asst Clin Prof NS, Univ Minn

Ondra, Stephen MD [NS] - **Spec Exp:** Spinal Surgery; **Hospital:** Northwestern Meml Hosp; **Address:** Neurological Surgery, 676 N St. Clair St, Ste 2210, Chicago, IL 60611; **Phone:** 312-695-6282; **Board Cert:** Neurological Surgery 1994; **Med School:** Rush Med Coll 1984; **Resid:** Neurological Surgery, Walter Reed Army Med Ctr 1990; **Fac Appt:** Assoc Prof NS, Northwestern Univ

Origitano, Thomas MD/PhD [NS] - **Spec Exp:** Skull Base Tumors & Surgery; Cerebrovascular Surgery; Brain Tumors; **Hospital:** Loyola Univ Med Ctr; **Address:** Loyola Univ Medical Ctr, Dept Neurosurgery, 2160 S First Ave Bldg 105 - rm 1900, Maywood, IL 60153-3304; **Phone:** 708-216-8920; **Board Cert:** Neurological Surgery 1995; **Med School:** Loyola Univ-Stritch Sch Med 1984; **Resid:** Neurological Surgery, Loyola Univ Med Ctr 1990; **Fac Appt:** Prof NS, Loyola Univ-Stritch Sch Med

Park, Tae Sung MD [NS] - **Spec Exp:** Pediatric Neurosurgery; Cerebral Palsy-Select Dorsal Rhizotomy; Chiari's Deformity; Neuro-Oncology; **Hospital:** St Louis Chldns Hosp; **Address:** St Louis Children's Hospital, 1 Children's Place, Ste 4-S20, St Louis, MO 63110; **Phone:** 314-454-4629; **Board Cert:** Neurological Surgery 1985; Pediatric Neurological Surgery 1988; **Med School:** Korea 1971; **Resid:** Neurological Surgery, Univ Virginia Hosp 1980; **Fellow:** Neuropathology, Mass General; Pediatric Neurological Surgery, Hospital for Sick Children; **Fac Appt:** Prof NS, St Louis Univ

Piepgras, David MD [NS] - **Spec Exp:** Cardiovascular Neurosurgery; Minimally Invasive Spinal Surgery; Neuralgias-Facial; **Hospital:** Mayo Med Ctr & Clin - Rochester, St Mary's Hosp - Rochester; **Address:** Mayo Clinic, Dept Neuro Surg, 200 First St SW, Rochester, MN 55905; **Phone:** 507-284-3331; **Board Cert:** Neurological Surgery 1977; **Med School:** Univ Minn 1965; **Resid:** Surgery, Hennipin Co Genl Hosp 1970; Neurological Surgery, Mayo Clinic 1974; **Fac Appt:** Prof NS, Mayo Med Sch

Raffel, Corey MD/PhD [NS] - **Spec Exp:** Pediatric Neurosurgery; Brain Tumors; Medulloblastoma; **Hospital:** Mayo Med Ctr & Clin - Rochester; **Address:** Mayo Clinic, Dept Neurosurgery, 200 1st St SW, Rochester, MN 55905; **Phone:** 507-284-8008; **Board Cert:** Neurological Surgery 1990; Pediatric Neurological Surgery 1996; **Med School:** UCSD 1980; **Resid:** Neurological Surgery, UCSF Med Ctr 1986; **Fellow:** Pediatric Neurological Surgery, Hosp Sick Chldn 1988; **Fac Appt:** Prof NS, Mayo Med Sch

Rezai, Ali R MD [NS] - **Spec Exp:** Parkinson's Disease; Pain-Chronic; **Hospital:** Cleveland Clin Fdn (page 57); **Address:** 9500 Euclid Ave, Desk S31, Cleveland, OH 44195; **Phone:** 216-444-2210; **Board Cert:** Neurological Surgery 2003; **Med School:** USC Sch Med 1990; **Resid:** Neurological Surgery, NYU Med Ctr 1997; **Fellow:** Stereo Neurological Surgery, Univ Toronto Med Ctr 1998; Neurological Surgery, Karolinska Inst; **Fac Appt:** Assoc Prof NS, Cleveland Cl Coll Med/Case West Res

Rich, Keith M MD [NS] - **Spec Exp:** Brain Tumors; Neurovascular Surgery; Stereotactic Radiosurgery; **Hospital:** Barnes-Jewish Hosp; **Address:** Washington University School of Medicine, 660 S Euclid Ave, Box 8057, St Louis, MO 63110; **Phone:** 314-362-3577; **Board Cert:** Neurological Surgery 1987; **Med School:** Indiana Univ 1977; **Resid:** Neurological Surgery, Barnes Jewish Hosp 1982; **Fellow:** Neurological Pharmacology, Barnes Jewish Hosp 1984; **Fac Appt:** Assoc Prof NS, Washington Univ, St Louis

Rosenblum, Mark L MD [NS] - **Spec Exp:** Brain Tumors; Spinal Surgery; Infections-Neurologic; Neuro-Oncology; **Hospital:** Henry Ford Hosp, William Beaumont Hosp; **Address:** Henry Ford Hospital, K11, 2799 W Grand Blvd, Detroit, MI 48202; **Phone:** 313-916-1340; **Board Cert:** Neurological Surgery 1982; **Med School:** NY Med Coll 1969; **Resid:** Surgery, UCLA Med Ctr 1973; Neurological Surgery, UCSF Med Ctr 1979; **Fellow:** Neuro-Oncology, Natl Cancer Inst 1972; **Fac Appt:** Prof NS, Case West Res Univ

Ruge, John MD [NS] - **Spec Exp:** Pediatric Neurosurgery; Brain Tumors; Hydrocephalus; **Hospital:** Adv Luth Genl Hosp; **Address:** 1875 Dempster St, Ste 605, Park Ridge, IL 60068; **Phone:** 847-698-1088; **Board Cert:** Neurological Surgery 1993; **Med School:** Northwestern Univ 1983; **Resid:** Neurological Surgery, Northwestern Meml Hosp 1989; **Fellow:** Pediatric Neurological Surgery, Childrens Hosp 1990; **Fac Appt:** Asst Prof S, Rush Med Coll

Ryken, Timothy MD [NS] - **Spec Exp:** Brain Tumors; Spinal Surgery; **Hospital:** Univ Iowa Hosp & Clinics; **Address:** Univ Iowa Hosps & Clinics, Div Neurosurg, 200 Hawkins Drive, rm 1844 JPP, Iowa City, IA 52242; **Phone:** 319-356-2237; **Board Cert:** Neurological Surgery 1998; **Med School:** Univ Iowa Coll Med 1988; **Resid:** Neurological Surgery, Univ Iowa 1995; **Fellow:** Cambridge Univ 1996; **Fac Appt:** Assoc Prof NS, Univ Iowa Coll Med

Selman, Warren R MD [NS] - **Spec Exp:** Stroke; Pituitary Surgery; Aneurysm-Cerebral; Microsurgery; **Hospital:** Univ Hosps Case Med Ctr; **Address:** Univ Hosps of Cleveland, Dept Neurosurg, 11100 Euclid Ave, Cleveland, OH 44106; **Phone:** 216-844-5745; **Board Cert:** Neurological Surgery 1986; **Med School:** Case West Res Univ 1977; **Resid:** Neurological Surgery, Univ Hosps 1984; **Fellow:** Research, Univ Hosps 1980; Neurological Surgery, Mayo Clinic 1984; **Fac Appt:** Prof NS, Case West Res Univ

Neurological Surgery

Shapiro, Scott A MD [NS] - **Spec Exp:** Brain Tumors; Aneurysm-Cerebral; Spinal Cord Injury; Pituitary Tumors; **Hospital:** Indiana Univ Hosp; **Address:** Inidiana Univ, Wishard Memorial Hosp, 1001 W 10th St, Ste EOP323, Indianapolis, IN 46202; **Phone:** 317-630-7625; **Board Cert:** Neurological Surgery 1990; **Med School:** Indiana Univ 1981; **Resid:** Neurological Surgery, Indiana Univ Med Ctr 1987; **Fac Appt:** Prof NS, Indiana Univ

Thompson, B Gregory MD [NS] - **Spec Exp:** Acoustic Neuroma; Neurovascular Surgery; Skull Base Tumors & Surgery; Aneurysm-Cerebral; **Hospital:** Univ Michigan Hlth Sys; **Address:** Dept Neurosurgery, 3552 Taubman, 1500 E Medical Center Drive, Ann Arbor, MI 48109; **Phone:** 734-936-7493; **Board Cert:** Neurological Surgery 1998; **Med School:** Univ Kans 1986; **Resid:** Neurological Surgery, Univ Pittsburgh 1993; Research, Natl Inst Hlth 1992; **Fellow:** Neurological Surgery, Barrow Neuro Inst 1994; Interventional Radiology, Thomas Jefferson Univ 2005

Tomita, Tadanori MD [NS] - **Spec Exp:** Pediatric Neurosurgery; Brain Tumors-Pediatric; Hydrocephalus; **Hospital:** Children's Mem Hosp, Northwestern Meml Hosp; **Address:** Chldns Meml Hosp, Div Ped Neurosurg, 2300 Children's Plaza, Box 28, Chicago, IL 60614-3318; **Phone:** 773-880-4373; **Board Cert:** Neurological Surgery 1984; Pediatric Neurological Surgery 1996; **Med School:** Japan 1970; **Resid:** Neurological Surgery, Kobe Univ 1974; Neurological Surgery, Northwestern Meml Hosp 1980; **Fellow:** Surgery, Meml Sloan Kettering Canc Ctr 1981; **Fac Appt:** Prof NS, Northwestern Univ

Traynelis, Vincent C MD [NS] - **Spec Exp:** Spinal Surgery; **Hospital:** Univ Iowa Hosp & Clinics; **Address:** Univ Iowa Hosp, Dept Neurosurgery, 200 Hawkins Drive, rm 3005BT, Iowa City, IA 52242; **Phone:** 319-356-2774; **Board Cert:** Neurological Surgery 1992; **Med School:** W VA Univ 1983; **Resid:** Neurological Surgery, Univ West Virginia Med Ctr 1989; **Fac Appt:** Prof NS, Univ Iowa Coll Med

Warnick, Ronald E MD [NS] - **Spec Exp:** Neuro-Oncology; Brain Tumors; **Hospital:** Univ Hosp - Cincinnati, Good Samaritan Hosp - Cincinnati; **Address:** 222 Piedmont Ave, Ste 3100, Cincinnati, OH 45219; **Phone:** 513-475-8629; **Board Cert:** Neurological Surgery 1995; **Med School:** Univ Rochester 1982; **Resid:** Neurological Surgery, NYU Med Ctr 1989; **Fellow:** Neuro-Oncology, UCSF Med Ctr 1991; **Fac Appt:** Prof NS, Univ Cincinnati

Great Plains and Mountains

Apfelbaum, Ronald I MD [NS] - **Spec Exp:** Spinal Surgery; **Hospital:** Univ Utah Hosps and Clins; **Address:** Univ Utah Hosp, Dept Neurosurgery, 30 N 1900 E, Ste 3B-409, Salt Lake City, UT 84132-2303; **Phone:** 801-585-6040; **Board Cert:** Neurological Surgery 1976; **Med School:** Hahnemann Univ 1965; **Resid:** Surgery, Montefiore Med Ctr 1969; Neurological Surgery, Montefiore Med Ctr 1974; **Fac Appt:** Prof NS, Univ Utah

Cherny, W Bruce MD [NS] - **Spec Exp:** Pediatric Neurosurgery; Brain Tumors; Spina Bifida; **Hospital:** St. Luke's Reg Med Ctr - Boise; **Address:** 100 E Idaho St, Ste 202, Boise, ID 83712; **Phone:** 208-381-7360; **Board Cert:** Neurological Surgery 2000; **Med School:** Univ Ariz Coll Med 1987; **Resid:** Neurological Surgery, Barrow Neuro Inst/St Joseph's Med Ctr 1994; **Fellow:** Pediatric Neurological Surgery, Primary Chldns Hosp 1995

Couldwell, William MD/PhD [NS] - **Spec Exp:** Brain Tumors; Epilepsy/Movement Disorders; Parkinson's Disease; Pituitary Tumors; **Hospital:** Univ Utah Hosps and Clins; **Address:** Univ Utah, Dept Neurological Surgery, 175 N Medical Drive E, Salt Lake City, UT 84132-2303; **Phone:** 801-581-6908; **Board Cert:** Neurological Surgery 1994; **Med School:** McGill Univ 1984; **Resid:** Neurological Surgery, LAC/USC Med Ctr 1989; **Fellow:** Neurological Immunology, Montreal Neur Inst/McGill Univ 1991; Neurological Surgery, CHUV; **Fac Appt:** Prof NS, Univ Utah

Johnson, Stephen D MD [NS] - **Spec Exp:** Skull Base Tumors & Surgery; **Hospital:** Presby - St Luke's Med Ctr; **Address:** Western Neurological Group, 1601 E 19th Ave, Ste 4400, Denver, CO 80218; **Phone:** 303-861-2266; **Board Cert:** Neurological Surgery 1988; **Med School:** Univ Tenn Coll Med, Memphis 1974; **Resid:** Neurological Surgery, Virginia Mason Med Ctr; Neurological Surgery, New York Hosp; **Fellow:** Neurological Surgery, Univ Tennessee; **Fac Appt:** Assoc Prof NS, Univ Colorado

Kestle, John RW MD [NS] - **Spec Exp:** Pediatric Neurosurgery; Epilepsy/Seizure Disorders; **Hospital:** Primary Children's Med Ctr; **Address:** 100 N Medical Drive, Ste 2400, Salt Lake City, UT 84113; **Phone:** 801-662-5340; **Board Cert:** Neurological Surgery 2002; **Med School:** Canada 1984; **Resid:** Neurology, Univ Toronto 1990; **Fellow:** Pediatric Neurological Surgery, Hosp Sick Chldn/Univ Toronto 1992; **Fac Appt:** Assoc Prof NS, Univ Utah

Krauth, Lee E MD [NS] - **Spec Exp:** Aneurysm-Cerebral; Skull Base Surgery; **Hospital:** Regional West Med Ctr; **Address:** 2 W 42nd St, Ste 2550, Scottsbluff, NE 69361; **Phone:** 308-630-1947; **Board Cert:** Neurological Surgery 1983; **Med School:** Duke Univ 1975; **Resid:** Neurological Surgery, Univ Colorado Med Ctr 1980; **Fac Appt:** Clin Prof NS, Univ Colorado

Nazzaro, Jules M MD [NS] - **Spec Exp:** Parkinson's Disease; Movement Disorders; Stereotactic Radiosurgery; **Hospital:** Univ of Kansas Hosp; **Address:** Kansas University Medical Ctr, 3901 Rainbow Blvd, MS 3021, Kansas City, KS 66160; **Phone:** 913-588-5129; **Board Cert:** Neurological Surgery 1996; **Med School:** Albert Einstein Coll Med 1984; **Resid:** Neurological Surgery, NYU Med Ctr 1991; **Fellow:** Neurosurgical Oncology, Meml Sloan-Kettering Cancer Ctr 1992; **Fac Appt:** Assoc Prof NS, Univ Kans

Walker, Marion L MD [NS] - **Spec Exp:** Pediatric Neurosurgery; Spasticity & Movement Disorders; Hydrocephalus; Brain Tumors; **Hospital:** Primary Children's Med Ctr, Univ Utah Hosps and Clins; **Address:** Primary Children's Med Ctr, Div Ped Neurosurgery, 100 N Medical, Ste 1475, Salt Lake City, UT 84113-1103; **Phone:** 801-662-5340; **Board Cert:** Neurological Surgery 1979; Pediatric Neurological Surgery 1996; **Med School:** Univ Tenn Coll Med, Memphis 1969; **Resid:** Surgery, St Joseph's Hosp 1971; Neurological Surgery, St Joseph's Hosp-Barrow Neuro Inst 1976; **Fellow:** Pediatric Neurological Surgery, Hosp for Sick Chldn 1973; **Fac Appt:** Prof NS, Univ Utah

Winston, Ken R MD [NS] - **Spec Exp:** Pediatric Neurosurgery; Craniosynostosis; Epilepsy/Seizure Disorders; **Hospital:** Chldn's Hosp - Denver, The, Univ Colorado Hosp; **Address:** 1056 E 19th Ave, Box B330, Denver, CO 80218; **Phone:** 303-861-6100; **Board Cert:** Neurological Surgery 1973; **Med School:** Univ Tenn Coll Med, Memphis 1963; **Resid:** Surgery, Colorado Genl Hosp 1967; Neurological Surgery, Colorado Genl Hosp 1971; **Fac Appt:** Prof NS, Univ Colorado

Neurological Surgery

Southwest

Al-Mefty, Ossama MD [NS] - **Spec Exp:** Skull Base Surgery; Brain Tumors; Cerebrovascular Surgery; **Hospital:** UAMS Med Ctr, Arkansas Chldns Hosp; **Address:** Univ Hosp of Arkansas for Med Scis, 4301 W Markham Slot 507, Little Rock, AR 72205; **Phone:** 501-686-8757; **Board Cert:** Neurological Surgery 1980; **Med School:** Syria 1972; **Resid:** Surgery, Med Coll Ohio 1974; Neurological Surgery, West Va Med Ctr 1978; **Fac Appt:** Prof NS, Univ Ark

De Monte, Franco MD [NS] - **Spec Exp:** Skull Base Tumors & Surgery; Neuro-Oncology; **Hospital:** UT MD Anderson Cancer Ctr (page 71); **Address:** UT MD Anderson Cancer Ctr, Dept Neurosurgery, 1515 Holcombe Blvd, Ste 442, Houston, TX 77030; **Phone:** 713-792-2400; **Board Cert:** Neurological Surgery 1995; **Med School:** Canada 1985; **Resid:** Neurological Surgery, Univ Western Ontario 1991; **Fellow:** Skull Base Surgery, Loyola Univ-Stritch Sch Med 1992

Hankinson, Hal L MD [NS] - **Spec Exp:** Brain Tumors; **Hospital:** Presbyterian Hospital - Albuquerque, Albuquerque Regional Med Ctr; **Address:** New Mexico Neurosurgery, 522 Lomas Blvd NE, Albuquerque, NM 87102; **Phone:** 505-247-4253; **Board Cert:** Neurological Surgery 1977; **Med School:** Tulane Univ 1967; **Resid:** Neurological Surgery, UCSF Med Ctr 1975; **Fac Appt:** Clin Prof NS, Univ New Mexico

Harper, Richard L MD [NS] - **Spec Exp:** Spinal Surgery; Brain Tumors & Hemifacial Spasms; **Hospital:** Methodist Hosp - Houston; **Address:** 6560 Fannin St, Ste 1200, Houston, TX 77030; **Phone:** 713-790-1211; **Board Cert:** Neurological Surgery 1983; **Med School:** Baylor Coll Med 1971; **Resid:** Neurological Surgery, Baylor Hosps 1978; **Fac Appt:** Asst Clin Prof NS, Baylor Coll Med

Hassenbusch, Samuel J MD/PhD [NS] - **Spec Exp:** Pain Management; Pain-Cancer; Brain Tumors; Stereotactic Radiosurgery; **Hospital:** UT MD Anderson Cancer Ctr (page 71); **Address:** UT MD Anderson Cancer Ctr, PO Box 301402, Houston, TX 77230-1402; **Phone:** 713-563-8706; **Board Cert:** Neurological Surgery 1992; **Med School:** Johns Hopkins Univ 1978; **Resid:** Surgery, Johns Hopkins Univ 1980; Neurological Surgery, Johns Hopkins Univ 1988; **Fellow:** Research, Keck Fdn-UCSF 1986; **Fac Appt:** Prof NS, Univ Tex, Houston

Jimenez, David MD [NS] - **Spec Exp:** Pediatric Neurosurgery; Craniosynostosis; Endoscopic Strip Craniectomy; Spinal Surgery; **Hospital:** Univ Hlth Sys - Univ Hosp, St Luke's Baptist Hosp; **Address:** Dept of Neurosurgery, 7703 Floyd Curl Drive, MC 7843, San Antonio, TX 78229-3900; **Phone:** 210-567-5625; **Board Cert:** Neurological Surgery 1995; **Med School:** Temple Univ 1985; **Resid:** Neurological Surgery, Temple Univ Hosp 1991; **Fellow:** Pediatric Neurological Surgery, Montefiore Hosp/Einstein Coll Med 1992; **Fac Appt:** Prof NS, Univ Tex, San Antonio

Kline, David G MD [NS] - **Spec Exp:** Peripheral Nerve Disorders; **Hospital:** Ochsner Fdn Hosp; **Address:** Ochsner Clinic, Dept Neurosurgery, 1514 Jefferson Hwy, New Orleans, LA 70121; **Phone:** 504-842-4632; **Board Cert:** Neurological Surgery 1969; **Med School:** Univ Pennsylvania 1960; **Resid:** Surgery, Univ Mich Hosp 1962; Neurological Surgery, Univ Mich Hosp 1967; **Fac Appt:** Prof NS, Louisiana State Univ

Lang Jr, Frederick F MD [NS] - **Spec Exp:** Brain & Spinal Tumors; Neuro-Oncology; **Hospital:** UT MD Anderson Cancer Ctr (page 71); **Address:** Univ Texas MD Anderson Cancer Ctr, Box 301402, Houston, TX 77230-1402; **Phone:** 713-792-2400; **Board Cert:** Neurological Surgery 2000; **Med School:** Yale Univ 1988; **Resid:** Neurological Surgery, NYU Med Ctr 1995; **Fellow:** Neurosurgical Oncology, MD Anderson Cancer Ctr 1996; **Fac Appt:** Prof NS, Univ Tex, Houston

Luerssen, Thomas G MD [NS] - **Spec Exp:** Pediatric Neurosurgery; Brain Injury-Traumatic; **Hospital:** Texas Chldns Hosp - Houston; **Address:** Clinical Care Center, Ste 1230, 6621 Fannin St, Houston, TX 77030; **Phone:** 832-822-3950; **Board Cert:** Neurological Surgery 1985; Pediatric Neurological Surgery 2005; **Med School:** Indiana Univ 1976; **Resid:** Neurological Surgery, Indiana Univ Hosp 1981; **Fellow:** Pediatric Neurological Surgery, Chldns Hosp 1984; **Fac Appt:** Prof NS, Baylor Coll Med

Mapstone, Timothy MD [NS] - **Spec Exp:** Brain Tumors-Adult & Pediatric; Pediatric Neurosurgery; Congenital Anomalies; **Hospital:** OU Med Ctr, Chldns Hosp OU Med Ctr; **Address:** Univ OK Hlth Sci Ctr, Dept Neurosurgery, 1000 N Lincoln Blvd, Ste 400, Oklahoma City, OK 73104; **Phone:** 405-271-4912; **Board Cert:** Neurological Surgery 1985; Pediatric Neurological Surgery 2005; **Med School:** Case West Res Univ 1977; **Resid:** Neurological Surgery, Univ Hosps 1983; **Fellow:** Research, Case West Res; **Fac Appt:** Prof NS, Univ Okla Coll Med

Mickey, Bruce E MD [NS] - **Spec Exp:** Brain Tumors; Skull Base Surgery; **Hospital:** UT Southwestern Med Ctr - Dallas; **Address:** UTSW Med Ctr, Dept Neurosurgery, 5323 Harry Hines Blvd, Dallas, TX 75390-8855; **Phone:** 214-645-2300; **Board Cert:** Neurological Surgery 1987; **Med School:** Univ Tex SW, Dallas 1978; **Resid:** Neurological Surgery, Parkland Meml Hosp 1984; **Fellow:** Research, Righospitalet 1983; **Fac Appt:** Prof NS, Univ Tex SW, Dallas

Papadopoulos, Stephen M MD [NS] - **Spec Exp:** Spinal Surgery; Stereotactic Radiosurgery; **Hospital:** St Joseph's Hosp & Med Ctr - Phoenix; **Address:** Barrow Neurosurg Assocs, 2910 N 3rd Ave, Phoenix, AZ 85013; **Phone:** 602-406-3159; **Board Cert:** Neurological Surgery 1991; **Med School:** Univ Tex, Houston 1978; **Resid:** Neurological Surgery, Univ Mich Med Ctr 1988; **Fellow:** Spinal Surgery, Barrow Neur Inst

Samson, Duke MD [NS] - **Spec Exp:** Vascular Neurosurgery; Cerebrovascular Disease; Arteriovenous Malformations; **Hospital:** UT Southwestern Med Ctr - Dallas, Parkland Meml Hosp - Dallas; **Address:** Univ Tex SW Med Ctr, Dept Neuro Surg, 5323 Harry Hines Blvd, Dallas, TX 75390-8855; **Phone:** 214-648-3529; **Board Cert:** Neurological Surgery 1978; **Med School:** Washington Univ, St Louis 1969; **Resid:** Neurological Surgery, Univ Texas SW Med Ctr 1975; **Fellow:** Neurological Surgery, Ctr Medico-Chirurgical Fech 1973; Neurological Surgery, Univ Zurich 1973; **Fac Appt:** Prof NS, Univ Tex SW, Dallas

Sawaya, Raymond MD [NS] - **Spec Exp:** Brain Tumors; **Hospital:** UT MD Anderson Cancer Ctr (page 71); **Address:** MD Anderson Cancer Ctr, 1515 Holcombe Blvd, Unit 442, Houston, TX 77030; **Phone:** 713-563-8749; **Board Cert:** Neurological Surgery 1985; **Med School:** Lebanon 1974; **Resid:** Neurological Surgery, Univ Cincinnati Med Ctr 1980; Neurological Surgery, Johns Hopkins Med Ctr 1981; **Fellow:** Neuro-Oncology, Natl Inst Hlth 1982; **Fac Appt:** Prof NS, Univ Tex, Houston

Sklar, Frederick H MD [NS] - **Spec Exp:** Pediatric Neurosurgery; Craniofacial Surgery; Hydrocephalus; **Hospital:** Chldns Med Ctr of Dallas, Texas Scottish Rite Hosp for Chldn; **Address:** Center for Pediatric Neurosurgery, 1935 Motor St, Dallas, TX 75235; **Phone:** 214-456-6660; **Board Cert:** Neurological Surgery 1978; Pediatric Neurological Surgery ; **Med School:** Johns Hopkins Univ 1970; **Resid:** Neurological Surgery, Johns Hopkins Hosp 1976; **Fac Appt:** Assoc Clin Prof NS, Univ Tex SW, Dallas

Sonntag, Volker MD [NS] - **Spec Exp:** Spinal Surgery; **Hospital:** St Joseph's Hosp & Med Ctr - Phoenix; **Address:** Barrow Neurosurgery Associates, 2910 N Third Ave, Phoenix, AZ 85013; **Phone:** 602-406-3458; **Board Cert:** Neurological Surgery 1980; **Med School:** Univ Ariz Coll Med 1971; **Resid:** Neurological Surgery, New England Med Ctr 1977; **Fac Appt:** Clin Prof NS, Univ Ariz Coll Med

Neurological Surgery

Spetzler, Robert F MD [NS] - **Spec Exp:** Skull Base Tumors & Surgery; Cerebrovascular Surgery; **Hospital:** St Joseph's Hosp & Med Ctr - Phoenix; **Address:** Barrow Neurosurgical Assocs, 2910 N Third Ave, Phoenix, AZ 85013; **Phone:** 602-406-3489; **Board Cert:** Neurological Surgery 1979; **Med School:** Northwestern Univ 1971; **Resid:** Neurological Surgery, UCSF Med Ctr 1976; **Fac Appt:** Prof S, Univ Ariz Coll Med

Walsh, John W MD/PhD [NS] - **Spec Exp:** Pediatric Neurosurgery; Epilepsy; **Hospital:** Tulane Univ Hosp & Clin; **Address:** 4720 S I-10 Service Rd, New Orleans, LA 70001; **Phone:** 504-988-8000; **Board Cert:** Neurological Surgery 1997; Pediatric Neurological Surgery 1996; **Med School:** UCLA 1966; **Resid:** Neurological Surgery, Peter Bent Brigham Hosp 1974; **Fellow:** Neurological Surgery, Lahey Clin Fdn 1975; **Fac Appt:** Prof NS, Tulane Univ

West Coast and Pacific

Adler Jr, John R MD [NS] - **Spec Exp:** Stereotactic Radiosurgery; Brain Tumors; Acoustic Neuroma; **Hospital:** Stanford Univ Med Ctr; **Address:** Stanford Univ Med Ctr, Dept Neurosurg, 300 Pasteur Drive, rm R 205, Stanford, CA 94305-5327; **Phone:** 650-723-5573; **Board Cert:** Neurological Surgery 1990; **Med School:** Harvard Med Sch 1980; **Resid:** Neurological Surgery, Chldns Hosp 1987; Neurological Surgery, Mass Genl Hosp 1985; **Fellow:** Cerebrovascular Disease, Karolinska Inst 1986; **Fac Appt:** Prof NS, Stanford Univ

Apuzzo, Michael L J MD [NS] - **Spec Exp:** Brain Tumors; Epilepsy/Seizure Disorders; Stereotactic Radiosurgery; **Hospital:** LAC & USC Med Ctr, USC Norris Comp Cancer Ctr; **Address:** 1420 N San Pablo Street, PMBA106, Los Angeles, CA 90033-1029; **Phone:** 323-226-7421; **Board Cert:** Neurological Surgery 1975; **Med School:** Boston Univ 1965; **Resid:** Neurological Surgery, Hartford Hosp; Neurological Surgery, Hartford Hosp 1973; **Fellow:** Neurological Physiology, Yale Univ Hosp; **Fac Appt:** Prof NS, USC Sch Med

Berger, Mitchel S MD [NS] - **Spec Exp:** Brain & Spinal Cord Tumors; Pituitary Tumors; Neuro-Oncology; Pain Management; **Hospital:** UCSF Med Ctr; **Address:** UCSF Med Ctr, Dept Neurosurgery, 505 Parnassus Avenue, M-786, San Francisco, CA 94143-0112; **Phone:** 415-353-3933; **Board Cert:** Neurological Surgery 1991; **Med School:** Univ Miami Sch Med 1979; **Resid:** Neurological Surgery, UCSF Med Ctr 1984; **Fellow:** Neuro-Oncology, UCSF Med Ctr 1985; Pediatric Neurological Surgery, Hosp Sick Chldn 1986; **Fac Appt:** Prof NS, UCSF

Black, Keith L MD [NS] - **Spec Exp:** Brain Tumors; Pituitary Surgery; Trigeminal Neuralgia; **Hospital:** Cedars-Sinai Med Ctr; **Address:** Maxine Dunitz Neurosurgical Inst, 8631 W 3rd St, Ste 800E, Los Angeles, CA 90048; **Phone:** 310-423-7900; **Board Cert:** Neurological Surgery 1990; **Med School:** Univ Mich Med Sch 1981; **Resid:** Neurological Surgery, Univ Michigan Med Ctr 1987; **Fac Appt:** Prof NS, UCLA

Boggan, James E MD [NS] - **Spec Exp:** Skull Base Tumors & Surgery; Pediatric Neurosurgery; **Hospital:** UC Davis Med Ctr; **Address:** Dept Neurological Surgery, 4860 Y St, Ste 3740, Sacramento, CA 95817-2307; **Phone:** 916-734-2371; **Board Cert:** Neurological Surgery 1985; **Med School:** Univ Chicago-Pritzker Sch Med 1976; **Resid:** Neurological Surgery, UCSF Med Ctr 1982; **Fac Appt:** Prof NS, UC Davis

Burchiel, Kim J MD [NS] - **Spec Exp:** Pain Management; Stereotactic Radiosurgery; Epilepsy/Movement Disorders; **Hospital:** OR Hlth & Sci Univ; **Address:** Oregon Hlth & Sci Univ, Dept Neurosurgery, 3303 SW Bond St, MC CH8N, Portland, OR 97239; **Phone:** 503-494-4314; **Board Cert:** Neurological Surgery 1984; **Med School:** UCSD 1976; **Resid:** Neurological Surgery, Univ Wash Med Ctr 1982; **Fac Appt:** Prof NS, Oregon Hlth Sci Univ

Edwards, Michael S MD [NS] - **Spec Exp:** Brain Tumors-Pediatric; Pediatric Neurosurgery; Stereotactic Radiosurgery; **Hospital:** Lucile Packard Chldns Hosp/Stanford Univ Med Ctr; **Address:** Pediatric Neurosurgery, 300 Pasteur Drive, Ste R211, MC 5327, Stanford, CA 94305-5327; **Phone:** 650-497-8775; **Board Cert:** Neurological Surgery 1980; Pediatric Neurological Surgery 2006; **Med School:** Tulane Univ 1970; **Resid:** Neurological Surgery, Oschner Fdn Hosp/Charity Hosp 1977; **Fellow:** Pediatric Neuro-Oncology, UCSF Med Ctr 1978; **Fac Appt:** Prof NS, Stanford Univ

Ellenbogen, Richard MD [NS] - **Spec Exp:** Pediatric Neurosurgery; Chiari's Deformity; Brain Tumors; **Hospital:** Chldns Hosp and Regl Med Ctr - Seattle, Univ Wash Med Ctr; **Address:** 4800 Sand Point Way NE, MS W-7729, Seattle, WA 98105; **Phone:** 206-987-2544; **Board Cert:** Neurological Surgery 1992; Pediatric Neurological Surgery 1998; **Med School:** Brown Univ 1983; **Resid:** Neurological Surgery, Brigham Womens Hosp/Childrens Hosp 1989; **Fac Appt:** Prof NS, Univ Wash

Frazee, John G MD [NS] - **Spec Exp:** Vascular Neurosurgery; Spinal Surgery; Neuro-Endoscopy; **Hospital:** UCLA Med Ctr, VA Med Ctr - W Los Angeles; **Address:** UCLA Med Ctr, Div Neurosurgery, rm 18-211 NPI, Los Angeles, CA 90095-7039; **Phone:** 310-206-1231; **Board Cert:** Neurological Surgery 1984; **Med School:** Univ Rochester 1975; **Resid:** Neurological Surgery, UCLA Med Ctr 1982; **Fac Appt:** Clin Prof NS, UCLA

Giannotta, Steven L MD [NS] - **Spec Exp:** Aneurysm-Cerebral; Skull Base Tumors; Acoustic Neuroma; **Hospital:** USC Univ Hosp - R K Eamer Med Plz, LAC & USC Med Ctr; **Address:** 1520 San Pablo St, Ste 3800, Los Angeles, CA 90033; **Phone:** 323-442-5720; **Board Cert:** Neurological Surgery 1980; **Med School:** Univ Mich Med Sch 1972; **Resid:** Neurological Surgery, Univ Michigan Med Ctr 1978; **Fac Appt:** Prof NS, USC Sch Med

Harsh IV, Griffith MD [NS] - **Spec Exp:** Brain & Spinal Cord Tumors; Skull Base Tumors; Pituitary Tumors; Acoustic Neuroma; **Hospital:** Stanford Univ Med Ctr; **Address:** Stanford Center for Advanced Medicine, 875 Blake Wilbur Drive, MC 5826, Stanford, CA 94305; **Phone:** 650-736-9976; **Board Cert:** Neurological Surgery 1989; **Med School:** Harvard Med Sch 1980; **Resid:** Neurological Surgery, UCSF Med Ctr 1986; **Fellow:** Neuro-Oncology, UCSF Med Ctr 1987; **Fac Appt:** Prof NS, Stanford Univ

Laws Jr, Edward R MD [NS] - **Spec Exp:** Pituitary Surgery; Epilepsy/Seizure Disorders; Brain Tumors; **Hospital:** Stanford Univ Med Ctr, Lucile Packard Chldns Hosp/Stanford Univ Med Ctr; **Address:** Stanford Univ Med Ctr, Dept Neurosurgery, rm CC-2330, MC 5821, Stanford, CA 94305-5821; **Phone:** 650-736-0500; **Board Cert:** Neurological Surgery 1974; **Med School:** Johns Hopkins Univ 1963; **Resid:** Neurological Surgery, Johns Hopkins Hosp 1971; **Fac Appt:** Prof NS, Stanford Univ

Mamelak, Adam N MD [NS] - **Spec Exp:** Brain Tumors; Epilepsy; Spinal Tumors; **Hospital:** Cedars-Sinai Med Ctr, Huntington Memorial Hosp; **Address:** Maxine Dunitz Neurosurgical Institute, 8631 W Third St, Ste 800-East, Los Angeles, CA 90048; **Phone:** 310-423-7900; **Board Cert:** Neurological Surgery 2000; **Med School:** Harvard Med Sch 1990; **Resid:** Neurological Surgery, UCSF Med Ctr 1994; **Fellow:** Epilepsy, UCSF Epilepsy Research Lab 1995

Marshall, Lawrence F MD [NS] - **Spec Exp:** Spinal Surgery; Spinal Cord Surgery; Brain Tumors; Head Injury; **Hospital:** UCSD Med Ctr; **Address:** UCSD Medical Ctr, Dept Neurosurgery, 200 W Arbor Drive, rm 8893, San Diego, CA 92103; **Phone:** 619-543-5540; **Board Cert:** Neurological Surgery 1977; **Med School:** Univ Mich Med Sch 1969; **Resid:** Neurological Surgery, Hosp U Penn 1975; **Fellow:** Neurological Pathology, Glasgow Univ Med Research 1976; **Fac Appt:** Prof NS, UCSD

Neurological Surgery

Martin, Neil A MD [NS] - **Spec Exp:** Vascular Neurosurgery; **Hospital:** UCLA Med Ctr; **Address:** UCLA Med Ctr, Div Neuro Surgery, 10833 LeConte Ave, Box 95-7039, Los Angeles, CA 90095-7039; **Phone:** 310-825-5482; **Board Cert:** Neurological Surgery 1989; **Med School:** Med Coll VA 1978; **Resid:** Neurological Surgery, UCSF Med Ctr 1984; **Fellow:** Neurological Vascular Surgery, Barrow Neuro Inst 1985; **Fac Appt:** Prof NS, UCLA

Mayberg, Marc R MD [NS] - **Spec Exp:** Pituitary Surgery; Stroke/Cerebrovascular Disease; Skull Base Tumors; **Hospital:** Swedish Med Ctr - Seattle; **Address:** Seattle Neuroscience Inst, 550 17th Ave, Ste 500, Seattle, WA 98122; **Phone:** 206-320-2800; **Board Cert:** Neurological Surgery 1988; **Med School:** Mayo Med Sch 1978; **Resid:** Neurological Surgery, Mass Genl Hosp 1984; **Fellow:** Neurological Surgery, Natl Hosp for Nervous Dis 1985

McDermott, Michael W MD [NS] - **Spec Exp:** Brain Tumors; Meningioma; Stereotactic Radiosurgery; Skull Base Tumors; **Hospital:** UCSF Med Ctr; **Address:** UCSF Dept Neurosurgery, 400 Parnassus Ave, rm A808, San Francisco, CA 94143; **Phone:** 415-353-7500; **Board Cert:** Neurological Surgery 2003; **Med School:** Univ Toronto 1982; **Resid:** Neurological Surgery, Univ British Columbia 1988; **Fellow:** Neuro-Oncology, UCSF Med Ctr 1990; **Fac Appt:** Prof NS, UCSF

Ott, Kenneth H MD [NS] - **Spec Exp:** Brain Tumors; Stereotactic Radiosurgery; **Hospital:** Scripps Meml Hosp - La Jolla; **Address:** Neurosurgical Medical Clinic, 501 Washington St, Ste 700, San Diego, CA 92103-2231; **Phone:** 619-297-4481; **Board Cert:** Neurological Surgery 1980; **Med School:** UCSF 1970; **Resid:** Surgery, Mass Genl Hosp 1972; Neurological Surgery, Mass Genl Hosp 1976; **Fac Appt:** Assoc Clin Prof S, UCSD

Pitts, Lawrence H MD [NS] - **Spec Exp:** Acoustic Neuroma; Skull Base Surgery; Spinal Surgery; **Hospital:** UCSF Med Ctr; **Address:** UCSF Dept of Neurosurgery, 400 Parnassus Ave, rm A808, San Francisco, CA 94143; **Phone:** 415-353-7500; **Board Cert:** Neurological Surgery 1978; **Med School:** Case West Res Univ 1969; **Resid:** Neurological Surgery, UCSF Med Ctr 1975; **Fac Appt:** Prof NS, UCSF

Sekhar, Laligam N MD [NS] - **Spec Exp:** Aneurysm-Cerebral; Arteriovenous Malformations; Brain Tumors; Skull Base Tumors; **Hospital:** Harborview Med Ctr, Univ Wash Med Ctr; **Address:** Harborview Med Ctr, UW Med Dept Neurosurg, 325 Ninth Ave, Box 359766, Seattle, WA 98104-2420; **Phone:** 206-744-9300; **Board Cert:** Neurological Surgery 1986; **Med School:** India 1973; **Resid:** Neurology, Univ Cincinnati Med Ctr 1977; Neurology, Univ Pittsburgh Med Ctr 1982; **Fellow:** Skull Base Surgery, Norstadt Krankenhaus 1983; Cerebrovascular Neurosurgery, Univ Zurich Hospital; **Fac Appt:** Prof NS, Univ Wash

Shuer, Lawrence M MD [NS] - **Spec Exp:** Pediatric Neurosurgery; Craniosynostosis; Epilepsy; Chiari's Deformity; **Hospital:** Stanford Univ Med Ctr; **Address:** Stanford Univ Med Ctr, Dept Neurosurgery, 300 Pasteur Drive, rm R229, Stanford, CA 94305; **Phone:** 650-723-5574; **Board Cert:** Neurological Surgery 1986; **Med School:** Univ Mich Med Sch 1978; **Resid:** Neurological Surgery, Stanford Univ 1984; **Fac Appt:** Prof NS, Stanford Univ

Steinberg, Gary K MD/PhD [NS] - **Spec Exp:** Aneurysm-Cerebral; Moya Moya; Arteriovenous Malformations; **Hospital:** Stanford Univ Med Ctr; **Address:** Stanford Univ Hosp, Dept Neurosurg, 300 Pasteur Drive, rm R281, Stanford, CA 94305-5327; **Phone:** 650-723-5575; **Board Cert:** Neurological Surgery 1989; **Med School:** Stanford Univ 1980; **Resid:** Neuropathology, Stanford Univ Med Ctr 1982; Neurological Surgery, Stanford Univ Med Ctr 1987; **Fellow:** Cerebrovascular Neurosurgery, Univ West Ontario 1985; **Fac Appt:** Assoc Prof NS, Stanford Univ

Weiss, Martin H MD [NS] - **Spec Exp:** Brain Tumors; Spinal Cord Tumors; Pituitary Tumors; **Hospital:** USC Univ Hosp - R K Eamer Med Plz; **Address:** LAC-USC Med Ctr, 1200 N State St, Ste 5046, Los Angeles, CA 90033-1029; **Phone:** 323-442-5720; **Board Cert:** Neurological Surgery 1972; **Med School:** Cornell Univ-Weill Med Coll 1963; **Resid:** Surgery, US Army Hosp 1966; Neurological Surgery, Univ Hosp 1970; **Fellow:** Neurological Surgery, NIH-Univ Hosp 1970; **Fac Appt:** Prof NS, USC Sch Med

Yu, John S MD [NS] - **Spec Exp:** Brain Tumors; Spinal Tumors; Clinical Trials; Spinal Surgery; **Hospital:** Cedars-Sinai Med Ctr; **Address:** Cedars Sinai Medical Ctr, 8631 W 3rd St, Ste 800E, Los Angeles, CA 90048; **Phone:** 310-423-7900; **Board Cert:** Neurological Surgery 2002; **Med School:** Harvard Med Sch 1990; **Resid:** Neurological Surgery, Mass General Hosp 1997

Neurological Institute

The Cleveland Clinic Neurological Institute is a fully integrated entity with a disease-specific focus, combining all physicians and other healthcare providers in neurology, neurosurgery, neuroradiology, the behavioral sciences and nursing who treat children and adults with neurological and neurobehavioral disorders. Our staff of more than 100 specialists sees one of the largest and most diverse patient populations in the country. Because of our clinical expertise, academic achievement and innovative research, the Cleveland Clinic Neurological Institute has earned an international reputation for excellence.

Our unique clinical structure allows us to deliver coordinated, comprehensive, multidisciplinary care to our patients through more efficient treatment decision making and consultation for complex cases. Fully integrating specialties along disease lines creates an exciting synergy among Institute physicians who share similar clinical, research and educational interests, to the benefit of patients and physicians alike.

Major advances in the treatment of brain tumors, epilepsy, mood disorders, stroke, movement disorders, pain and spinal disorders are improving quality of life and survival for thousands of patients. For those diseases resistant to available treatments, we believe the innovative model of medicine created with the Neurological Institute will speed research and advances in treatment, resulting in better clinical care and more rapid breakthroughs in the full range of neurological and behavioral disorders.

Centers in the Neurological Institute include: Brain Tumor & Neuro-Oncology Center, Center for Headache & Pain, Center for Neuroimaging, Center for Neurological Restoration, Center for Pediatric Neurology & Neurosurgery, Center for Spine Health, Cerebrovascular Center, Epilepsy Center, Mellen Center for Multiple Sclerosis Treatment & Research, Neuromuscular Center, Psychiatry and Psychology and Sleep Disorders Center

Comprehensive Neurological Care

Cleveland Clinic offers expert diagnostic and treatment options for all neurologic conditions affecting children and adults, including:

- Alzheimer's disease
- ALS (Amyotrophic Lateral Sclerosis)
- Aneurysms
- Arteriovenous Malformations (AVMs)
- Back and Neck Disorders
- Brain and Spine Tumors
- Cerebral Palsy
- Congenital Disorders
- Craniofacial Disorders
- Epilepsy
- Headache
- Hydrocephalus
- Metastatic Tumors
- Movement Disorders
- Neonatal Disorders
- Neurofibromatosis
- Parkinson's Disease
- Peripheral Neuropathies
- Pituitary Disorders
- Psychiatric Disorders
- Skull Base Disorders
- Sleep Disorders
- Stroke

To schedule an appointment or for more information about the Cleveland Clinic Neurological Institute, please call 800.890.2467 or visit www.clevelandclinic.org/neurotopdocs.

Cleveland Clinic Neurological Institute
9500 Euclid Avenue / W14 | Cleveland OH 44195

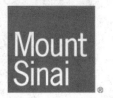

THE MOUNT SINAI MEDICAL CENTER
NEUROSURGERY

One Gustave L. Levy Place (Fifth Avenue and 100th Street)
New York, NY 10029-6574
Physician Referral: 1-800-MD-SINAI (637-4624)
www.mountsinai.org

The Department of Neurosurgery at The Mount Sinai Medical Center was established in 1920, and has gained a distinguished international reputation. Areas of expertise include the skull-base, cerebrovascular, pituitary, acoustic, spinal reconstruction, epilepsy, radiosurgery, stereotactic, primary brain tumor surgery, functional, minimally invasive, and neuroendoscopy. Neurosurgery research at Mount Sinai includes clinical programs, case presentations, and laboratories in the following areas: cerebrovascular, skull-base dissection, spinal cord injury, pituitary endocrinology, cerebral blood flow regulation, gene therapy and brain tumors, and movement disorders.

The Mount Sinai Brain Tumor Program provides comprehensive care to patients with peripheral and central nervous system tumors and with neurological complications of systemic cancer. Our physicians utilize the latest techniques, including computer-assisted image-guided tumor resections and biopsies, advanced skull base approaches, and minimally invasive/endoscopic procedures. The most advanced stereotactic radiosurgery program gives patients a treatment option that does not require open surgery, and gene therapy is an option for selected patients. An interdisciplinary approach includes members of the Departments of Neurology, Radiation Oncology, and Rehabilitation Medicine. Mount Sinai physicians focus not only on survival but also on the quality of the patient's life during and after treatment.

The Mount Sinai Clinical Center for Cranial Base Surgery provides a comprehensive, highly advanced treatment program for lesions of nerve, blood vessel, and brain in the complex structures and remote recesses at the base of the skull. The multidisciplinary Center unites the expertise of surgical specialists in neurosurgery, otolaryngology/head and neck cancer, craniofacial surgery, oral and maxillofacial surgery, and microvascular and reconstructive procedures. Together they have pioneered the development of minimally invasive techniques, including purely endoscopic tumor resection and stereotactic radiosurgery to treat complex skull base lesions. The Center also offers patients the benefit of a wide range of experts in the related fields of neurology, electrophysiology, pathology, radiation oncology, rehabilitation medicine, and medical oncology. Our program is world-renowned for pituitary adenomas, acoustic neuromas, meningiomas, and skull-base lesions.

The Clinical Program for Cerebrovascular Disorders and Stroke at Mount Sinai provides expertise in the evaluation, treatment, and rehabilitation of patients with cerebrovascular diseases. The team evaluates each patient to determine whether vascular lesions can be treated with minimally invasive endovascular techniques from the inside of the blood vessel. Pathologies treated include intracranial aneurysms, arteriovenous malformations of the brain, dura and spinal cord, carotid artery stenosis, intracerebral cerebral hemorrhage, stroke/cerebral infarction, lesions of the skull base, and trigeminal neuralgia.

The Division of Functional and Restorative Neurosurgery utilizes the latest technology to precisely target locations and abnormalities in the brain and spinal cord. Our physicians are focused on the development of minimally invasive neurosurgical techniques that either modulate neural function, replace lost neuronal populations, or halt the neurodegenerative process altogether. Presently, deep brain stimulation (DBS) dominates this field, but many technologies with great potential are on the horizon. Our physicians have been honored by the Dystonia Medical Research Foundation for their pioneering work treating dystonia with DBS. They also use cutting-edge techniques in the treatment of patients with Parkinson's disease, essential tremor, facial nerve disorders, epilepsy and pain.

The Mount Sinai Clinical Program for Stereotactic Neurosurgery has extended the scope of operative tumors by using techniques such as frame-based or frameless stereotaxy, awake and asleep brain mapping, micro-neurosurgery, and endoscopic surgery. Our physicians have been pioneers in computer-assisted techniques since 1993. The development of a precision navigation system and the addition of the Novalis Shaped Beam Surgery system at Mount Sinai have resulted in substantial reductions of wound and neurosurgical morbidity, length of surgery, length of stay, and hospital costs.

The Mount Sinai Center for Spinal Disorders offers comprehensive treatment for all disorders of the spinal column and spinal cord including degenerative disorders (disc herniations, spinal stenosis, spinal instability), trauma, infections, congenital disorders (including scoliosis), and tumors. The neurosurgeons have pioneered endoscopic, minimally invasive surgical approaches to treat disorders of the spine: these approaches have the potential to reduce post-operative pain, speed recovery, shorten hospital stays, reduce disability, and facilitate an early return to work, while providing the same or improved decompression or stabilization.

867

NEUROSURGERY

The Department of Neurosurgery at NYU Medical Center offers the most advanced surgical procedures available anywhere in the world, along with compassionate care and supportive services for patients and their families. In an environment of leading-edge research and medical education, the department's interdisciplinary team of physicians, nurses, and allied health professionals are world-renowned for their highly specialized training and their down-to-earth approach to clinical care. The department also is home to the most sophisticated surgical instrumentation in the region.

Because of the large number of cases referred from all over the world, NYU neurosurgeons have been able to subspecialize in order to develop specific expertise and to provide the best and most up-to-date treatment in a broad range of conditions in adults and children. These include brain, skull base and spinal cord tumors, vascular disorders such as aneurysms and arteriovenous malformations, Parkinson's disease, ruptured disks, degenerative spine disease, epilepsy, peripheral nerve injuries and tumors and many other conditions. Notwithstanding the high technology focus and sophisticated surgical methodology, we firmly believe that quality of our patients' lives is the most important measure of our success.

The Center for the Study and Treatment of Movement Disorders

The Center for Study and Treatment of Movement Disorders provides surgical care for patients with Parkinson's disease and other movement disorders. Its highly focused surgeons implant neuroaugmentative devices ("brain pacemakers") and also have considerable experience in pallidotomy and thalamotomy for those with disabling tremor who may not be candidates for neuroaugmentative surgery. These procedures are performed using the latest computer localization and imaging technology in conjunction with precision electrophysiologic monitoring.

The Gamma Knife

In the recent past, patients with brain abnormalities considered too deep or too delicate to reach with a scalpel had little reason for hope. But with the Gamma Knife, neurosurgeons at NYU Medical Center can now remove deep-seated tumors, vascular malformations, and other sites of dysfunction with outstanding results. Aided by three-dimensional MRI technology that pinpoints the problem area, the neurosurgeon uses the Gamma Knife to destroy tumors with precise doses of radiation. Unlike conventional surgery, this noninvasive procedure is entirely bloodless and woundless, and achieves improved outcomes at lower cost and dramatically reduced recovery time.

Spine Surgery

NYU spinal neurosurgeons stress minimally invasive methods in treating a variety of degenerative spine conditions and in the removal of tumors of the spinal cord and spinal column. Dr. Paul Cooper, Ricciardi Professor of Neurosurgery and Dr Tony Frempong are internationally respected authorities in the management of spinal tumors, spinal reconstruction and stabilization procedures. On-line electrophysiologic monitoring has dramatically improved the neurological postoperative outcome over the past several years. Patients considered to have "inoperable" conditions at other institutions are treated here on a routine basis with excellent postoperative results and a very high level of patient satisfaction..

The Tumor Surgery Program at NYU Medical Center treats patients referred from all over the world. Dr Patrick J Kelly, Ransohoff Professor and Chairman of the Department of Neurosurgery has personally operated on over 6,600 brain tumors and is one of the most experienced brain tumor surgeons in the world. He developed computer-assisted stereotactic volumetric resection, a minimally invasive method for the precision and complete removal of brain tumors with excellent postoperative results. Methods for noninvasive brain mapping using magnetoencephalotomography (MEG), functional MRI and preoperative computer surgical simulations, allow selection of the safest surgical approach that minimizes risk and ensures the best possible clinical outcomes.

With this technology, "Inoperable tumors" become operable tumors at NYU.

689

PENN NEUROSURGERY

Center for Excellence

The Department of Neurosurgery at the University of Pennsylvania provides comprehensive medical and surgical care for people with disorders of the brain, spinal cord and peripheral nervous system. One of the hallmarks of Penn's neurosurgery program is its integration of research and clinical practice, embracing new technologies and seeking the highest quality and best outcomes possible.

The University of Pennsylvania's history of excellence in the research and treatment of neurological diseases dates back to the establishment of the Department of Neurology in 1874. *The Best Doctors in America*® lists more neurologists and neurosurgeons from the Hospital of the University of Pennsylvania than from any other hospital or medical center in the Philadelphia region. In addition, the Hospital of the University of Pennsylvania ranked highest in the region and among the top nationally for medical and surgical treatment of neurological disorders in *U.S.News & World Report*.

Excellence and Expertise

The Penn Gamma Knife® Center at Pennsylvania Hospital offers power, precision and hope to patients suffering from brain tumors and other serious brain disorders. Gamma Knife radiosurgery is noninvasive, effective, and safe, making it the optimal choice for treating a wide variety of conditions including benign or malignant brain tumors, blood vessel malformations,

trigeminal neuralgia (tic douloureux) and tremor. Furthermore, it offers new hope to patients with deep-seated brain lesions once considered inoperable.

The Parkinson's Disease and Movement Disorders Center, recognized by the National Parkinson Foundation as one of its worldwide "Centers of Excellence," was the first and remains one of the only facilities in the area to perform deep brain stimulation for tremor due to Parkinson's disease and movement disorders. The Center for Functional and Restorative Neurosurgery at Pennsylvania Hospital performed more deep brain stimulation procedures in the past year than any other hospital or health system in the United States.

The Brain Tumor Center provides comprehensive evaluation, diagnosis and treatment to patients with brain and spinal tumors and other cancer-related neurological, central nervous system and peripheral nervous system problems. The multidisciplinary approach includes physicians and other health care providers from neurology, neurosurgery, radiation oncology, neuro-oncology, neuropathology, neuroradiology, rehabilitation medicine, neuro-psychiatry and social work.

Programs

- The Brain Tumor Center
- The Center for Brain Injury and Repair
- The Center for Cranial Base Surgery
- Penn Gamma Knife® Center
- The Head Injury Center
- The Interventional Neuro Center
- Neuro Intensive Care
- The Neurosurgery Spine Center
- The Neurovascular Center
- The Parkinson's Disease and Movement Disorders Center
- The Stroke Center

Locations

Hospital of the University of Pennsylvania

Pennsylvania Hospital

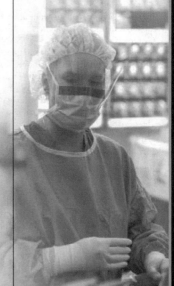

Gamma Knife and Leksell Gamma Knife are U.S. federally registered trademarks of Elekta Instrument S.A., Geneva, Switzerland.

Hospital of the University of Pennsylvania | Penn Presbyterian Medical Center | Pennsylvania Hospital

THE UNIVERSITY OF TEXAS
MD ANDERSON
CANCER CENTER
Making Cancer History®

The University of Texas
M. D. Anderson Cancer Center

1515 Holcombe Blvd.
Houston, Texas 77030-4095
Tel. 713-792-6161
Toll Free 877-MDA-6789
http://www.mdanderson.org

BRAIN AND SPINE CENTER

When faced with a tumor involving the brain, spine or skull base, choosing the right treatment center can make a difference in your outcome. With a team approach to personalized care and neurosurgical innovations not available elsewhere, the Brain and Spine Center offers patients with malignant or benign tumors the most effective treatment and best quality of life.

BrainSUITE

BrainSUITE® is an integrated neurosurgery system that allows for more precise treatment of complicated tumors in sensitive areas of the brain. It is the latest advancement in image-guided surgery, providing views of the tumor site using magnetic resonance imaging (iMRI) obtained during surgery. BrainSUITE's imaging systems provide a highly detailed view of the tumor site, enabling the surgeons to get new images at any time to check their work. This allows them to remove as much tumor as possible while protecting critical areas of the brain.

SKULL BASE PROGRAM

M. D. Anderson is one of the few cancer centers in the country with a specialized program for tumors of the skull base. The Skull Base Tumor Program joins together experts from multiple departments to provide each patient with comprehensive, individualized care – all within the M. D. Anderson setting. Surgeons in the Skull Base Tumor Program use both open and minimally invasive diagnostic and surgical approaches, depending on each patient's unique characteristics.

PROTON THERAPY

M. D. Anderson's Proton Therapy Center opened in May 2006 as the largest and most sophisticated center of its type. Proton therapy allows for the most aggressive cancer therapy possible, deriving its advantage over traditional forms of radiation treatment from its ability to deliver targeted radiation doses to the tumor with remarkable precision. Proton therapy radiation avoids the surrounding tissue, generates fewer side effects, and improves tumor control. It is used to treat cancers brain and skull base, head and neck, and eye.

MORE INFORMATION

For more information or to make an appointment, call 877-MDA-6789, or visit us online at http://www.mdanderson.org.

At M. D. Anderson Cancer Center, our mission is simple – to eliminate cancer. Achieving that goal begins with integrated programs in cancer treatment, clinical trials, education programs and cancer prevention.

We focus exclusively on cancer and have seen cases of every kind. That means you receive expert care no matter what your diagnosis.

Choosing the right partner for cancer care really does make a difference. The fact is, people who choose M. D. Anderson over other hospitals and clinics often have better results. That is how we've been making cancer history for over sixty years.

835

Neurology

A neurologist specializes in the diagnosis and treatment of all types of disease or impaired function of the brain, spinal cord, peripheral nerves, muscles and autonomic nervous system, as well as the blood vessels that relate to these structures. A child neurologist has special skills in the diagnosis and management of neurologic disorders of the neonatal period, infancy, early childhood and adolescence.

Training Required: Four years

Neurology

New England

Amato, Anthony A MD [N] - **Spec Exp:** Peripheral Neuropathy; Neuromuscular Disorders; Muscular Dystrophy; **Hospital:** Brigham & Women's Hosp; **Address:** Brigham & Women's Hosp, Dept Neurology, 75 Francis St, Boston, MA 02115; **Phone:** 617-732-8046; **Board Cert:** Neurology 1991; **Med School:** Univ Cincinnati 1986; **Resid:** Neurology, Wilford Hall USAF Med Ctr 1990; **Fellow:** Neuromuscular Disease, Ohio State Med Ctr 1992; **Fac Appt:** Assoc Prof N, Harvard Med Sch

Armon, Carmel MD [N] - **Spec Exp:** Epilepsy/Seizure Disorders; Amyotrophic Lateral Sclerosis (ALS); **Hospital:** Baystate Med Ctr; **Address:** Baystate Neurology, 759 Chestnut St, Springfield, MA 01199; **Phone:** 413-794-7030; **Board Cert:** Neurology 1990; Clinical Neurophysiology 2002; Vascular Neurology 2005; **Med School:** Israel 1980; **Resid:** Neurology, Mayo Clinic 1988; **Fellow:** Neurology, Mayo Clinic 1989; Clinical Neurophysiology, Duke Univ Med Ctr 1991

Blumenfeld, Hal MD/PhD [N] - **Spec Exp:** Epilepsy/Seizure Disorders; **Hospital:** Yale - New Haven Hosp; **Address:** Yale Dept of Neurology, PO Box 208018, New Haven, CT 06520-8018; **Phone:** 203-785-3865; **Board Cert:** Neurology 1998; **Med School:** Columbia P&S 1992; **Resid:** Neurology, Mass Genl Hosp 1996; **Fellow:** Epilepsy, Yale-New Haven Hosp 1998; **Fac Appt:** Assoc Prof N, Yale Univ

Bromfield, Edward B MD [N] - **Spec Exp:** Epilepsy/Seizure Disorders; Sleep Disorders/Apnea; **Hospital:** Brigham & Women's Hosp; **Address:** Brigham & Women's Hosp, Dept Neurology, Division of Epilepsy and EEG, 75 Francis St, Boston, MA 02115; **Phone:** 617-732-7547; **Board Cert:** Neurology 1989; **Med School:** Harvard Med Sch 1983; **Resid:** Neurology, New York Hosp 1987; **Fellow:** Epilepsy, Natl Inst Hlth/NINDS 1989; **Fac Appt:** Assoc Prof N, Harvard Med Sch

Caplan, Louis Robert MD [N] - **Spec Exp:** Stroke; **Hospital:** Beth Israel Deaconess Med Ctr - Boston; **Address:** Palmer 127 West Campus BIDMC, 330 Brookline Ave, Boston, MA 02215; **Phone:** 617-632-8911; **Board Cert:** Internal Medicine 1969; Neurology 1972; **Med School:** Univ MD Sch Med 1962; **Resid:** Neurology, Boston City Hosp 1969; **Fellow:** Neurology, Harvard 1970; **Fac Appt:** Prof N, Harvard Med Sch

Cole, Andrew J MD [N] - **Spec Exp:** Epilepsy/Seizure Disorders; Rasmussen's Syndrome; **Hospital:** Mass Genl Hosp; **Address:** Mass Genl Hosp-Epilepsy Svc, 55 Fruit St, VBK 830, Boston, MA 02114; **Phone:** 617-726-3311; **Board Cert:** Neurology 1987; **Med School:** Dartmouth Med Sch 1982; **Resid:** Neurology, Neuro Inst-McGill 1986; **Fellow:** Electroencephalography, Neuro Inst-McGill 1987; Neurological Surgery, Johns Hopkins Hosp 1988; **Fac Appt:** Asst Prof N, Harvard Med Sch

Easton, J Donald MD [N] - **Spec Exp:** Stroke; **Hospital:** Rhode Island Hosp; **Address:** 110 Lockwood St, Ste 324, Providence, RI 02903; **Phone:** 401-444-8795; **Board Cert:** Neurology 1971; **Med School:** Univ Wash 1964; **Resid:** Neurology, NY Hosp-Cornell Med Ctr 1968; **Fac Appt:** Prof N, Brown Univ

Feldmann, Edward MD [N] - **Spec Exp:** Cerebrovascular Disease; Stroke; **Hospital:** Rhode Island Hosp; **Address:** 110 Lockwood St, Ste 324, Providence, RI 02903; **Phone:** 401-444-8806; **Board Cert:** Neurology 1988; **Med School:** Harvard Med Sch 1983; **Resid:** Neurology, New York Hosp 1987; **Fellow:** Cerebrovascular Disease, Tufts New Eng Med Ctr 1988; **Fac Appt:** Prof N, Brown Univ

Hafler, David A MD [N] - **Spec Exp:** Multiple Sclerosis; **Hospital:** Brigham & Women's Hosp; **Address:** Harvard Med Sch, 77 Ave Louis Pasteur, NRB 641-D, Boston, MA 02115; **Phone:** 617-525-5330; **Board Cert:** Neurology 1987; **Med School:** Univ Miami Sch Med 1978; **Resid:** Neurology, NY Hosp-Cornell Med Ctr 1982; **Fellow:** Neurological Immunology, Harvard Med Sch 1984; **Fac Appt:** Prof N, Harvard Med Sch

Jobst, Barbara Christine MD [N] - **Spec Exp:** Epilepsy in Pregnancy; Women's Health; **Hospital:** Dartmouth - Hitchcock Med Ctr; **Address:** One Medical Center Drive, Lebanon, NH 03756-1000; **Phone:** 603-650-8309; **Board Cert:** Neurology 2002; **Med School:** Germany 1993; **Resid:** Neurology, Krankenhaus Barmherzigen Bruder 1996; Neurology, Dartmouth-Hitchcock Med Ctr 2000; **Fellow:** Epilepsy, Dartmouth-Hitchcock Med Ctr 2001; **Fac Appt:** Asst Prof N, Dartmouth Med Sch

Kase, Carlos S MD [N] - **Spec Exp:** Stroke; Seizure Disorders; **Hospital:** Boston Med Ctr; **Address:** Boston Univ Sch of Med, 715 Albany St, Neurology C-329, Boston, MA 02118; **Phone:** 617-638-5102; **Board Cert:** Neurology 1980; **Med School:** Chile 1967; **Resid:** Neurology, Mass Genl Hosp 1973; Neurology, Mass Genl Hosp 1978; **Fac Appt:** Prof N, Boston Univ

Kistler, John Philip MD [N] - **Spec Exp:** Stroke; **Hospital:** Mass Genl Hosp; **Address:** Mass Genl Hosp, Stroke Svce, 55 Fruit St VBK Bldg - rm 802, Boston, MA 02114; **Phone:** 617-726-8459; **Board Cert:** Internal Medicine 1970; Neurology 1976; **Med School:** Columbia P&S 1964; **Resid:** Internal Medicine, Columbia Presby Hosp 1968; Neurology, Mass Genl Hosp-Harvard Med Sch 1975; **Fellow:** Cerebrovascular Disease, Mass Genl Hosp 1972; **Fac Appt:** Prof N, Harvard Med Sch

Ropper, Allan MD [N] - **Spec Exp:** Trauma Neurology; Guillain-Barre Syndrome; Neurology-Intensive Care; **Hospital:** St Elizabeth's Med Ctr; **Address:** St Elizabeth Hosp, Dept Neurology, 736 Cambridge St, Boston, MA 02135; **Phone:** 617-789-3300; **Board Cert:** Internal Medicine 1977; Neurology 1980; **Med School:** Cornell Univ-Weill Med Coll 1974; **Resid:** Internal Medicine, UCSF Med Ctr 1976; Neurology, Mass Genl Hosp 1979; **Fac Appt:** Prof N, Tufts Univ

Samuels, Martin Allen MD [N] - **Spec Exp:** Neurologic Aspects of Systemic Disease; **Hospital:** Brigham & Women's Hosp, Mass Genl Hosp; **Address:** Brigham & Women's Hosp, Dept Neurology, 75 Francis St, Neurology ASB-1, rm 158, Boston, MA 02115; **Phone:** 617-732-7432; **Board Cert:** Internal Medicine 1974; Neurology 1978; **Med School:** Univ Cincinnati 1971; **Resid:** Internal Medicine, Boston City Hosp 1975; Neurology, Mass Genl Hosp 1977; **Fellow:** Neurological Pathology, Mass Genl Hosp 1976; **Fac Appt:** Prof N, Harvard Med Sch

Selkoe, Dennis MD [N] - **Spec Exp:** Alzheimer's Disease; **Hospital:** Brigham & Women's Hosp; **Address:** 77 Ave Louis Pasteur HIM 730 Bldg, Boston, MA 02115-5716; **Phone:** 617-525-5200; **Board Cert:** Neurology 1977; **Med School:** Univ VA Sch Med 1969; **Resid:** Neurology, Peter Bent Brigham 1975; **Fellow:** Neurological Biology, Chldns Hosp Med Ctr 1978; **Fac Appt:** Prof N, Harvard Med Sch

Spencer, Susan S MD [N] - **Spec Exp:** Epilepsy/Seizure Disorders; **Hospital:** Yale - New Haven Hosp; **Address:** Yale Univ Sch Med, Dept Neurology, 333 Cedar St, Box 208018, New Haven, CT 06520-8018; **Phone:** 203-785-3865; **Board Cert:** Neurology 1980; Clinical Neurophysiology 1988; **Med School:** Univ Rochester 1974; **Resid:** Neurology, Yale-New Haven Hosp 1978; **Fellow:** Epilepsy, Yale New Haven Hosp 1980; **Fac Appt:** Prof N, Yale Univ

Weiner, Howard L MD [N] - **Spec Exp:** Multiple Sclerosis; Autoimmune Disease; **Hospital:** Brigham & Women's Hosp; **Address:** Harvard Inst Med-Ctr Neuro Disease, 77 Ave Louis Pasteur, Bldg HIM 730, Boston, MA 02115; **Phone:** 617-525-5300; **Board Cert:** Neurology 1978; **Med School:** Univ Colorado 1969; **Resid:** Internal Medicine, Beth Israel 1971; Neurology, Longwood Prog 1974; **Fellow:** Immunology, Univ Colo 1976; **Fac Appt:** Prof N, Harvard Med Sch

Young, Anne MD [N] - **Spec Exp:** Huntington's Disease; Parkinson's Disease; Movement Disorders; **Hospital:** Mass Genl Hosp; **Address:** Mass Genl Hosp, Dept Neurology, 55 Fruit Street, VBK 915, Boston, MA 02114; **Phone:** 617-726-2385; **Board Cert:** Neurology 1981; **Med School:** Johns Hopkins Univ 1973; **Resid:** Neurology, UCSF Med Ctr 1978; **Fac Appt:** Prof N, Harvard Med Sch

Mid Atlantic

Apatoff, Brian R MD/PhD [N] - **Spec Exp:** Multiple Sclerosis; Neuro-Immunology; **Hospital:** NY-Presby Hosp/Weill Cornell (page 66); **Address:** 525 E 68th St, Starr Pavilion, Ste 607, New York, NY 10021; **Phone:** 212-746-4504; **Board Cert:** Neurology 1991; **Med School:** Univ Chicago-Pritzker Sch Med 1984; **Resid:** Neurology, Columbia Presby Med Ctr 1990; **Fellow:** Multiple Sclerosis, Neuro Inst-Columbia Univ 1992; **Fac Appt:** Assoc Prof N, Cornell Univ-Weill Med Coll

Baser, Susan M MD [N] - **Spec Exp:** Parkinson's Disease; Huntington's Disease; Dystonia; Movement Disorders; **Hospital:** Allegheny General Hosp; **Address:** Allegheny Neurology Assocs, 490 E North Ave Prof Bldg - Ste 500, Pittsburgh, PA 15212; **Phone:** 412-359-8860; **Board Cert:** Neurology 1990; **Med School:** Loyola Univ-Stritch Sch Med 1983; **Resid:** Neurology, Univ Pittsburgh 1987; **Fellow:** Neuropharmacology, Natl Inst Hlth 1990; **Fac Appt:** Assoc Prof N, Thomas Jefferson Univ

Bell, Rodney D MD [N] - **Spec Exp:** Stroke; **Hospital:** Thomas Jefferson Univ Hosp; **Address:** Thomas Jefferson University, Dept Neurology, 900 Walnut St, Ste 200, Philadelphia, PA 19107; **Phone:** 215-955-6488; **Board Cert:** Internal Medicine 1975; Neurotology 1981; **Med School:** Oregon Hlth Sci Univ 1971; **Resid:** Internal Medicine, Parkland Meml Hosp 1975; Neurology, Parkland Meml Hosp 1978; **Fac Appt:** Prof N, Thomas Jefferson Univ

Bergey, Gregory K MD [N] - **Spec Exp:** Epilepsy/Seizure Disorders; Epilepsy in Women; Epilepsy in Pregnancy; **Hospital:** Johns Hopkins Hosp - Baltimore (page 61); **Address:** Johns Hopkins Hosp, Neurology, Meyer 2-147, 600 N Wolfe St, Baltimore, MD 21287; **Phone:** 410-955-7338; **Board Cert:** Internal Medicine 1978; Neurology 1984; Clinical Neurophysiology 1997; **Med School:** Univ Pennsylvania 1975; **Resid:** Internal Medicine, Yale-New Haven Hosp 1977; Neurology, Johns Hopkins Hosp 1981; **Fellow:** Neurological Physiology, Natl Inst Health 1983; **Fac Appt:** Prof N, Johns Hopkins Univ

Bressman, Susan MD [N] - **Spec Exp:** Parkinson's Disease; Movement Disorders; Dystonia; **Hospital:** Beth Israel Med Ctr - Petrie Division; **Address:** 10 Union Square East, Ste 2-Q, New York, NY 10003-3314; **Phone:** 212-844-8379; **Board Cert:** Neurology 1983; **Med School:** Columbia P&S 1977; **Resid:** Internal Medicine, New York Hosp 1978; Neurology, Columbia-Presby Med Ctr 1981; **Fellow:** Movement Disorders, Columbia-Presby Med Ctr 1983; **Fac Appt:** Prof N, Albert Einstein Coll Med

Brust, John C M MD [N] - **Spec Exp:** Stroke; Substance Abuse; **Hospital:** Harlem Hosp Ctr, NY-Presby Hosp/Columbia (page 66); **Address:** 506 Lenox Ave, rm 16-101, New York, NY 10037-1802; **Phone:** 212-939-4244; **Board Cert:** Neurology 1971; **Med School:** Columbia P&S 1962; **Resid:** Internal Medicine, Columbia Presby 1966; Neurology, Columbia Presby 1969; **Fac Appt:** Clin Prof N, Columbia P&S

Buchholz, David W MD [N] - **Spec Exp:** Migraine; Restless Legs Syndrome; Headache; **Hospital:** Johns Hopkins Hosp - Baltimore (page 61); **Address:** Johns Hopkins at Green Spring Station, 10753 Falls Rd, Ste 315, Lutherville, MD 21093; **Phone:** 410-583-2830; **Board Cert:** Neurology 1984; **Med School:** Univ Pennsylvania 1979; **Resid:** Neurology, Johns Hopkins Hosp 1983; **Fac Appt:** Assoc Prof N, Johns Hopkins Univ

Caronna, John J MD [N] - **Spec Exp:** Cerebrovascular Disease; **Hospital:** NY-Presby Hosp/Weill Cornell (page 66); **Address:** Dept Neurology, Cornell Univ-Weill Med College, 520 E 70th St, Ste 607, New York, NY 10021; **Phone:** 212-746-2304; **Board Cert:** Neurology 1974; **Med School:** Cornell Univ-Weill Med Coll 1965; **Resid:** Internal Medicine, NY Hosp 1967; Neurology, NY Hosp 1971; **Fellow:** Neurology, NY Hosp 1973; **Fac Appt:** Prof N, Cornell Univ-Weill Med Coll

Charney, Jonathan MD [N] - **Spec Exp:** Headache; Stroke; **Hospital:** Mount Sinai Med Ctr; **Address:** 1111 Park Ave, Ste 1H, New York, NY 10128-1234; **Phone:** 212-831-2886; **Board Cert:** Neurology 1977; **Med School:** NY Med Coll 1969; **Resid:** Neurology, Methodist Hosp-Baylor 1971; Neurology, Columbia-Presby Med Ctr 1973; **Fac Appt:** Asst Prof N, Mount Sinai Sch Med

Cook, Stuart D MD [N] - **Spec Exp:** Multiple Sclerosis; Infectious & Demyelinating Diseases; **Hospital:** UMDNJ-Univ Hosp-Newark; **Address:** 65 Bergen St, rm 1435, Newark, NJ 07101-1709; **Phone:** 973-972-9181; **Board Cert:** Neurology 1970; **Med School:** Univ VT Coll Med 1962; **Resid:** Neurology, Albert Einstein Coll Med 1968; **Fac Appt:** Prof N, UMDNJ-NJ Med Sch, Newark

Cornblath, David R MD [N] - **Spec Exp:** Peripheral Neuropathy; **Hospital:** Johns Hopkins Hosp - Baltimore (page 61); **Address:** 600 N Wolfe St Meyer 6-181A, Baltimore, MD 21287-6965; **Phone:** 410-955-2229; **Board Cert:** Neurology 1982; Clinical Neurophysiology 1994; **Med School:** Case West Res Univ 1977; **Resid:** Neurology, Hosp Univ Penn 1981; **Fellow:** Neurology, Hosp Univ Penn 1982; **Fac Appt:** Prof N, Johns Hopkins Univ

Coyle, Patricia K MD [N] - **Spec Exp:** Multiple Sclerosis; Neuro-Immunology; Lyme Disease; Infections-Neurologic; **Hospital:** Stony Brook Univ Med Ctr; **Address:** SUNY Stony Brook, Dept Neurology, HSC T12-020, Stony Brook, NY 11794-8121; **Phone:** 631-444-2599; **Board Cert:** Neurology 1978; **Med School:** Johns Hopkins Univ 1974; **Resid:** Neurology, Johns Hopkins Hosp 1978; **Fellow:** Neurological Immunology, Johns Hopkins Hosp 1980; **Fac Appt:** Prof N, SUNY Stony Brook

Dalakas, Marinos C MD [N] - **Spec Exp:** Neuromuscular Disorders; **Hospital:** Thomas Jefferson Univ Hosp; **Address:** 900 Walnut St Fl 2, Philadelphia, PA 19107; **Phone:** 212-955-1234; **Board Cert:** Neurology 1980; **Med School:** Greece 1972; **Resid:** Neurology, UMDNJ-Univ Hosp 1977; **Fellow:** Neuromuscular Disease, Natl Inst Hlth 1980

De Angelis, Lisa MD [N] - **Spec Exp:** Neuro-Oncology; **Hospital:** Meml Sloan Kettering Cancer Ctr; **Address:** 1275 York Ave, New York, NY 10021-6007; **Phone:** 212-639-7123; **Board Cert:** Neurology 1986; **Med School:** Columbia P&S 1980; **Resid:** Neurology, Neuro Inst-Presby Hosp 1984; **Fellow:** Neuro-Oncology, Neuro Inst-Presby Hosp 1985; Neuro-Oncology, Meml Sloan-Kettering Cancer Ctr 1986; **Fac Appt:** Prof N, Cornell Univ-Weill Med Coll

DeKosky, Steven T MD [N] - **Spec Exp:** Alzheimer's Disease; **Hospital:** UPMC Presby, Pittsburgh; **Address:** Univ Pittsburgh Physicians, Dept Neurology, 3471 Fifth Ave, Ste 811, Pittsburgh, PA 15213-2593; **Phone:** 412-692-2700; **Board Cert:** Neurology 2004; **Med School:** Univ Fla Coll Med 1974; **Resid:** Internal Medicine, Johns Hopkins Hosp 1975; Neurology, Univ Florida 1978; **Fellow:** Neurological Chemistry, Univ Virginia Hosp 1979; **Fac Appt:** Prof N, Univ Pittsburgh

Devinsky, Orrin MD [N] - **Spec Exp:** Epilepsy; Tuberous Sclerosis; Behavioral Neurology; **Hospital:** NYU Med Ctr (page 67), St Barnabas Med Ctr; **Address:** 403 E 34th St, FL 4, New York, NY 10016-4972; **Phone:** 212-263-8871; **Board Cert:** Neurology 1987; Clinical Neurophysiology 1990; **Med School:** Harvard Med Sch 1982; **Resid:** Neurology, New York Hosp-Cornell Med Ctr 1986; **Fellow:** Epilepsy, Natl Inst Health 1988; **Fac Appt:** Prof N, NYU Sch Med

Dewberry, Robert G MD [N] - **Hospital:** Maryland Genl Hosp; **Address:** Maryland Genl Hosp, Div Neurology, 827 Linden Ave Fl Basement, Baltimore, MD 21201; **Phone:** 410-225-8290; **Board Cert:** Neurology 1992; **Med School:** Univ MD Sch Med 1987; **Resid:** Neurology, Barnes Hospital 1991; **Fellow:** Neurological Muscular Disease, Univ Virginia Hosp 1993

Dichter, Marc A MD [N] - **Spec Exp:** Epilepsy/Seizure Disorders; **Hospital:** Hosp Univ Penn - UPHS (page 72); **Address:** Hosp Univ Pennsylvania, Dept Neurology, 3400 Spruce St 3W Gates Bldg, Philadelphia, PA 19104; **Phone:** 215-349-5166; **Board Cert:** Neurology 1978; **Med School:** NYU Sch Med 1969; **Resid:** Neurology, Beth Israel Hosp/Chldns Hosp/ Brigham Hosp 1975; **Fac Appt:** Prof N, Univ Pennsylvania

Drachman, Daniel B MD [N] - **Spec Exp:** Muscular Dystrophy; Neuromuscular Disorders; Myasthenia Gravis; Amyotrophic Lateral Sclerosis (ALS); **Hospital:** Johns Hopkins Hosp - Baltimore (page 61); **Address:** Johns Hopkins Med Ctr, 600 N Wolfe St, Meyer 5-119, Baltimore, MD 21287-7519; **Phone:** 410-955-5406; **Board Cert:** Neurology 1963; **Med School:** NYU Sch Med 1956; **Resid:** Neurology, Boston City Hosp 1959; Neuropathology, Mallory Inst Path/Boston City Hosp 1960; **Fellow:** Neurology, Harvard Med Sch 1960; **Fac Appt:** Prof N, Johns Hopkins Univ

Dromerick, Alexander MD [N] - **Spec Exp:** Stroke Rehabilitation; **Hospital:** Natl Rehab Hosp, Washington Hosp Ctr; **Address:** NRH-Neuroscience Rsch Ctr, 102 Irving St NW, Washington, DC 20010; **Phone:** 202-877-1000; **Board Cert:** Neurology 1992; **Med School:** Univ MD Sch Med 1986; **Resid:** Neurology, Hosp Univ Penn 1991; **Fellow:** Neurological Rehabilitation, Univ Penn 1992; Neurological Rehabilitation, Cornell-Burke Rehab Ctr 1993

Fahn, Stanley MD [N] - **Spec Exp:** Movement Disorders; Parkinson's Disease; **Hospital:** NY-Presby Hosp/Columbia (page 66); **Address:** 710 W 168th St, Fl 3rd - rm 350, New York, NY 10032; **Phone:** 212-305-5277; **Board Cert:** Neurology 1968; **Med School:** UCSF 1958; **Resid:** Neurology, Neuro Inst-Columbia Presby Hosp 1962; **Fac Appt:** Prof N, Columbia P&S

Feinberg, Todd E MD [N] - **Spec Exp:** Alzheimer's Disease; Stroke Rehabilitation; Brain Injury; **Hospital:** Beth Israel Med Ctr - Petrie Division; **Address:** Beth Israel Med Ctr, Yarmon Neurobehavioral Ctr, First Ave at 16th St, New York, NY 10003; **Phone:** 212-420-4111; **Board Cert:** Psychiatry 1984; Neurology 1987; **Med School:** Mount Sinai Sch Med 1978; **Resid:** Psychiatry, Mount Sinai 1982; Neurology, Mount Sinai 1984; **Fellow:** Behavioral Neurology, Univ Florida 1986; **Fac Appt:** Clin Prof N, Albert Einstein Coll Med

Fink, Matthew E MD [N] - **Spec Exp:** Cerebrovascular Disease; **Hospital:** NY-Presby Hosp/Weill Cornell (page 66); **Address:** NY Cornell Med Ctr Dept Neurology, 525 E 68th St, Ste F106, New York, NY 10021-4870; **Phone:** 212-746-4564; **Board Cert:** Internal Medicine 1980; Vascular Neurology 2005; **Med School:** Univ Pittsburgh 1976; **Resid:** Internal Medicine, Boston Med Ctr 1980; Neurology, Columbia-Presby Hosp 1982; **Fac Appt:** Prof N, Cornell Univ

French, Jacqueline MD [N] - **Spec Exp:** Epilepsy/Seizure Disorders; **Hospital:** Hosp Univ Penn - UPHS (page 72); **Address:** Hosp Univ Penn, Dept Neurology, 3W Gates Bldg, 3400 Spruce St, Philadelphia, PA 19104; **Phone:** 215-349-5166; **Board Cert:** Neurology 1987; **Med School:** Brown Univ 1982; **Resid:** Neurological Surgery, Mount Sinai Hosp 1986; **Fellow:** Epilepsy, Mount Sinai Hosp 1988; Epilepsy, Yale-New Haven Hosp 1989; **Fac Appt:** Prof N, Univ Pennsylvania

Galetta, Steven MD [N] - **Spec Exp:** Neuro-Ophthalmology; Optic Nerve Disorders; Multiple Sclerosis; **Hospital:** Hosp Univ Penn - UPHS (page 72); **Address:** Hosp Univ Penn, Dept Neurology, 3W Gates Bldg, 3400 Spruce St, Philadelphia, PA 19104; **Phone:** 215-662-3381; **Board Cert:** Neurology 1988; **Med School:** Cornell Univ-Weill Med Coll 1983; **Resid:** Neurology, Hosp Univ Penn 1987; **Fellow:** Neurological Ophthalmology, Bascom Palmer Eye Inst 1988; **Fac Appt:** Prof N, Univ Pennsylvania

Gendelman, Seymour MD [N] - **Spec Exp:** Parkinson's Disease; Dementia; Headache; **Hospital:** Mount Sinai Med Ctr; **Address:** 5 E 98th St Fl 7, Box 1139, New York, NY 10029-6501; **Phone:** 212-241-8172; **Board Cert:** Neurology 1971; **Med School:** Geo Wash Univ 1964; **Resid:** Neurology, Mount Sinai Hosp 1968; **Fac Appt:** Clin Prof N, Mount Sinai Sch Med

Gizzi, Martin MD/PhD [N] - **Spec Exp:** Neuro-Ophthalmology; Balance Disorders; Progressive Supranuclear Palsy (PSP); **Hospital:** JFK Med Ctr - Edison, Muhlenberg Regional Med Ctr; **Address:** NJ Neuroscience Insitute, 65 James St, Edison, NJ 08820-3947; **Phone:** 732-321-7010; **Board Cert:** Neurology 1990; **Med School:** Univ Miami Sch Med 1985; **Resid:** Neurology, Mount Sinai Hosp 1989; **Fellow:** Neurological Ophthalmology, Mount Sinai Hosp 1991; **Fac Appt:** Prof N, Seton Hall Univ Sch Grad Med Ed

Glass, Jon MD [N] - **Spec Exp:** Neuro-Oncology; Brain Tumors; Spinal Tumors; **Hospital:** Fox Chase Cancer Ctr (page 59); **Address:** Fox Chase Cancer Ctr, 333 Cottman Ave, Philadelphia, PA 19111; **Phone:** 215-728-3070; **Board Cert:** Neurology 1993; **Med School:** SUNY Downstate 1986; **Resid:** Neurology, Boston Univ 1989; **Fellow:** Neuro-Oncology, Mass Genl Hosp 1991; **Fac Appt:** Asst Prof N, NYU Sch Med

Golbe, Lawrence MD [N] - **Spec Exp:** Parkinson's Disease; Progressive Supranuclear Palsy (PSP); Movement Disorders; **Hospital:** Robert Wood Johnson Univ Hosp - New Brunswick; **Address:** 97 Paterson St, rm 208, New Brunswick, NJ 08901-2160; **Phone:** 732-235-7733; **Board Cert:** Neurology 1984; **Med School:** NYU Sch Med 1978; **Resid:** Internal Medicine, Hahnemann Univ Hosp 1980; Neurology, Bellevue Hosp 1983; **Fac Appt:** Prof N, UMDNJ-RW Johnson Med Sch

Goodgold, Albert MD [N] - **Spec Exp:** Parkinson's Disease; Spinal Cord Disorders; Multiple Sclerosis; Movement Disorders; **Hospital:** NYU Med Ctr (page 67); **Address:** 530 First Ave Fl 5 - Ste 5A, New York, NY 10016; **Phone:** 212-263-7205; **Med School:** Switzerland 1955; **Resid:** Neurology, Bellevue Hosp 1960; **Fac Appt:** Prof N, NYU Sch Med

Griffin, John W MD [N] - **Spec Exp:** Peripheral Neuropathy; Guillain-Barre Syndrome; Diabetic Polyneuropathy; **Hospital:** Johns Hopkins Hosp - Baltimore (page 61); **Address:** 600 N Wolfe St, Meyer 6-113, Baltimore, MD 21287; **Phone:** 410-955-2227; **Board Cert:** Internal Medicine 1974; Neurology 1976; **Med School:** Stanford Univ 1968; **Resid:** Internal Medicine, Johns Hopkins Hosp 1970; Neurology, Johns Hopkins Hosp 1973; **Fac Appt:** Prof N, Johns Hopkins Univ

Hiesiger, Emile MD [N] - **Spec Exp:** Pain Management; Neuro-Oncology; **Hospital:** NYU Med Ctr (page 67), VA Med Ctr - Manhattan; **Address:** 530 1st Ave, Ste 5A, New York, NY 10016-6402; **Phone:** 212-263-6123; **Board Cert:** Neurology 1983; **Med School:** NY Med Coll 1978; **Resid:** Neurology, NYU Med Ctr 1982; **Fellow:** Neurology, Meml Sloan-Kettering Cancer Ctr 1984; **Fac Appt:** Assoc Clin Prof N, NYU Sch Med

Hurtig, Howard MD [N] - **Spec Exp:** Parkinson's Disease; Movement Disorders; **Hospital:** Pennsylvania Hosp (page 72); **Address:** Pennsylvania Hosp Neurological Inst, 330 S 9th St Fl 3, Philadelphia, PA 19107; **Phone:** 215-829-6500; **Board Cert:** Neurology 1976; **Med School:** Tulane Univ 1966; **Resid:** Internal Medicine, New York Hosp 1968; Neurology, Hosp Univ Penn 1973; **Fac Appt:** Prof N, Univ Pennsylvania

Johnson, Kenneth P MD [N] - **Spec Exp:** Multiple Sclerosis; **Hospital:** Univ of MD Med Sys; **Address:** Maryland Ctr for Multiple Sclerosis, 11 S Paca St, Ste 300A, Baltimore, MD 21201-1791; **Phone:** 410-328-5605; **Board Cert:** Neurology 1968; **Med School:** Jefferson Med Coll 1959; **Resid:** Neurology, Buffalo Genl Hosp 1961; Neurology, Univ Hosps 1965; **Fellow:** Neurology, Univ Case West Res 1968; **Fac Appt:** Prof N, Univ MD Sch Med

Jordan, Barry D MD [N] - **Spec Exp:** Brain Injury-Traumatic; Sports Neurology; Alzheimer's Disease; Memory Disorders; **Hospital:** Burke Rehab Hosp; **Address:** Burke Rehabilitation Hosp, 785 Mamaroneck Ave, White Plains, NY 10605; **Phone:** 914-597-2332; **Board Cert:** Neurology 1989; **Med School:** Harvard Med Sch 1981; **Resid:** Neurology, New York Hosp 1986; **Fellow:** Hosp Spec Surgery 1987; UCLA Med Ctr 1998; **Fac Appt:** Assoc Prof N, Cornell Univ-Weill Med Coll

Kolodny, Edwin H MD [N] - **Spec Exp:** Pediatric Neurology; Inherited Disorders of Nervous System; Gaucher Disease; Fabry's Disease; **Hospital:** NYU Med Ctr (page 67), Bellevue Hosp Ctr; **Address:** 403 E 34 St Fl 2, New York, NY 10016-6402; **Phone:** 212-263-8344; **Board Cert:** Neurology 1971; Clinical Genetics 1984; Clinical Biochemical Genetics 1987; **Med School:** NYU Sch Med 1962; **Resid:** Internal Medicine, Bellevue Hosp 1964; Neurology, Mass Genl Hosp 1967; **Fellow:** Neurological Pathology, Mass Genl Hosp 1966; Neurology, Nat Inst Neurol Dis & Stroke 1970; **Fac Appt:** Prof N, NYU Sch Med

Koroshetz, Walter J MD [N] - **Spec Exp:** Stroke; Huntington's Disease; Movement Disorders; **Hospital:** Natl Inst of Hlth - Clin Ctr; **Address:** NIH-NINDS, Bldg 31 - rm 8A52, 31 Center Drive, MS 2540, Bethesda, MD 20892-2540; **Phone:** 301-496-5751; **Board Cert:** Internal Medicine 1982; Neurology 1986; **Med School:** Univ Chicago-Pritzker Sch Med 1979; **Resid:** Internal Medicine, Univ Chicago Med Ctr 1981; Internal Medicine, Mass Genl Hosp 1982; **Fellow:** Neurology, Mass Genl Hosp 1987; Research, Mass Genl Hosp

Krauss, Gregory L MD [N] - **Spec Exp:** Epilepsy/Seizure Disorders; **Hospital:** Johns Hopkins Hosp - Baltimore (page 61); **Address:** Johns Hopkins Hosp, Dept Neurology, 600 N Wolfe St, Meyer 2-147, Baltimore, MD 21287; **Phone:** 410-955-2822; **Board Cert:** Neurology 1990; **Med School:** Oregon Hlth Sci Univ 1985; **Resid:** Neurology, Johns Hopkins Hosp 1989; **Fellow:** Epilepsy, Johns Hopkins Hosp 1991; **Fac Appt:** Assoc Prof N, Johns Hopkins Univ

Krumholz, Allan MD [N] - **Spec Exp:** Epilepsy/Seizure Disorders; **Hospital:** Univ of MD Med Sys; **Address:** Univ Maryland Med System, Dept Neurology, 22 S Greene St, rm N4W46, Baltimore, MD 21201-1544; **Phone:** 410-328-6267; **Board Cert:** Neurology 1977; Clinical Neurophysiology 1996; **Med School:** Ros Franklin Univ/Chicago Med Sch 1970; **Resid:** Internal Medicine, Baltimore City Hosp 1972; Neurology, Johns Hopkins Hosp 1975; **Fellow:** Electroencephalography, Johns Hopkins Hosp 1980; **Fac Appt:** Prof N, Univ MD Sch Med

Kula, Roger W MD [N] - **Spec Exp:** Neuromuscular Disorders; Myasthenia Gravis; Syringomyelia & Spinal Cord Diseases; **Hospital:** N Shore Univ Hosp at Manhasset, Long Island Jewish Med Ctr; **Address:** 865 Northern Blvd, Ste 302, Great Neck, NY 11021; **Phone:** 516-570-4400; **Board Cert:** Internal Medicine 1975; Neurology 1977; **Med School:** Johns Hopkins Univ 1970; **Resid:** Internal Medicine, New York Hosp 1972; Neurology, UCSF Med Ctr 1974; **Fellow:** Neuromuscular Disease, Natl Inst Hlth 1977; **Fac Appt:** Assoc Prof N, SUNY Hlth Sci Ctr

Kuzniecky, Ruben MD [N] - **Spec Exp:** Epilepsy/Seizure Disorders; MRI; **Hospital:** NYU Med Ctr (page 67); **Address:** 403 E 34th St Fl 4, New York, NY 10016; **Phone:** 212-263-8870; **Board Cert:** Neurology 1990; **Med School:** Argentina 1980; **Resid:** Neurology, McGill Univ 1986; **Fellow:** Epilepsy, McGill Univ 1988

Lacomis, David MD [N] - **Spec Exp:** Amyotrophic Lateral Sclerosis (ALS); Muscle Disorders; Myasthenia Gravis; **Hospital:** UPMC Presby, Pittsburgh; **Address:** Dept Neurology -Kaufmann Med Bldg, 3471 Fifth Ave, Ste 810, Pittsburgh, PA 15213; **Phone:** 412-692-4917; **Board Cert:** Neurology 1992; Clinical Neurophysiology 2004; **Med School:** Penn State Univ-Hershey Med Ctr 1987; **Resid:** Neurology, Harvard Affil Hosp 1991; **Fellow:** Neurological Muscular Disease, Univ Massachusetts Med Ctr 1993; **Fac Appt:** Prof N, Univ Pittsburgh

Levine, David N MD [N] - **Spec Exp:** Dementia; Stroke; Spinal Cord Disorders; **Hospital:** NYU Med Ctr (page 67); **Address:** 400 E 34th St, Ste RIRM- 311, New York, NY 10016-4901; **Phone:** 212-263-7744; **Board Cert:** Neurology 1976; **Med School:** Harvard Med Sch 1968; **Resid:** Neurology, Mass Genl Hosp 1974; **Fellow:** Neurology, Mass Genl Hosp 1976; **Fac Appt:** Prof N, NYU Sch Med

Levine, Steven R MD [N] - **Spec Exp:** Stroke; Cerebrovascular Disease; **Hospital:** Mount Sinai Med Ctr; **Address:** Mt Sinai Sch Med, Neurology, Stroke Center, 1 Gustave Levy Pl, Box 1137, New York, NY 10029-6500; **Phone:** 212-241-1970; **Board Cert:** Neurology 1986; Vascular Neurology 2005; **Med School:** Med Coll Wisc 1981; **Resid:** Neurology, Univ Mich Hosps 1985; **Fellow:** Cerebrovascular Disease, Henry Ford Hosp 1987; **Fac Appt:** Prof N, Mount Sinai Sch Med

Liporace, Joyce D MD [N] - **Spec Exp:** Epilepsy in Women; Women's Health; Epilepsy in Pregnancy; **Hospital:** Riddle Meml Hosp; **Address:** Riddle Healthcare 2, 1088 Baltimore Pike, Ste 2205, Media, PA 19063; **Phone:** 610-744-2960; **Board Cert:** Neurological Surgery 1993; Clinical Neurophysiology 1999; **Med School:** Johns Hopkins Univ 1988; **Resid:** Neurology, Hosp U Penn 1992; **Fellow:** Clinical Neurophysiology, Hosp U Penn 1994; **Fac Appt:** Assoc Prof Med, Thomas Jefferson Univ

Neurology

Lipton, Richard MD [N] - **Spec Exp:** Headache; Migraine; Clinical Trials; **Hospital:** Montefiore Med Ctr - Weiler-Einstein Div; **Address:** 1575 Blondell Ave, Ste 225, Bronx, NY 10461-2662; **Phone:** 718-405-8360; **Board Cert:** Neurology 1985; **Med School:** Univ Chicago-Pritzker Sch Med 1980; **Resid:** Neurology, Montefiore Med Ctr 1984; **Fellow:** Neurological Physiology, Montefiore Med Ctr 1985; NeuroEpidemiology, Columbia Univ 1990; **Fac Appt:** Prof N, Albert Einstein Coll Med

Liu, Grant T MD [N] - **Spec Exp:** Pediatric Neuro-Ophthalmology; Neuro-Ophthalmology; **Hospital:** Hosp Univ Penn - UPHS (page 72), Chldns Hosp of Philadelphia, The; **Address:** Hosp Univ Penn, Dept Neurology, 3W Gates Bldg, 3400 Spruce St, Philadelphia, PA 19104; **Phone:** 215-349-8460; **Board Cert:** Neurology 1993; **Med School:** Columbia P&S 1988; **Resid:** Neurology, Harvard-Nolgwood Neurology Program 1992; **Fellow:** Neurological Ophthalmology, Bascom Palmer Eye Inst 1993; **Fac Appt:** Assoc Prof N, Univ Pennsylvania

Logigian, Eric L MD [N] - **Spec Exp:** Neuromuscular Disorders; Electromyography; Lyme Disease; **Hospital:** Univ of Rochester Strong Meml Hosp; **Address:** Univ Rochester, Dept of Neurology, 601 Elmwood Ave, Box 673, Rochester, NY 14642; **Phone:** 585-275-4568; **Board Cert:** Internal Medicine 1981; Neurology 1985; Clinical Neurophysiology 1999; **Med School:** Boston Univ 1978; **Resid:** Internal Medicine, Beth Israel Hosp 1981; Neurology, Mass Genl Hosp 1984; **Fellow:** Clinical Neurophysiology, Mass General Hosp 1985; **Fac Appt:** Prof N, Univ Rochester

Lublin, Fred MD [N] - **Spec Exp:** Multiple Sclerosis; **Hospital:** Mount Sinai Med Ctr; **Address:** Dickinson Ctr for Multiple Sclerosis, 5 E 98th St, Box 1138, New York, NY 10029-6574; **Phone:** 212-241-6854; **Board Cert:** Neurology 1977; **Med School:** Jefferson Med Coll 1972; **Resid:** Neurology, NY Hosp/Cornell Med Ctr 1976; **Fac Appt:** Prof N, Mount Sinai Sch Med

Max, Mitchell B MD [N] - **Spec Exp:** Pain Management; **Hospital:** Natl Inst of Hlth - Clin Ctr; **Address:** National Inst Heath, Fl 3 - rm 3C403, 10 Center Dr, MSC 1258, Bethesda, MD 20892-1258; **Phone:** 301-496-5483; **Board Cert:** Internal Medicine 1978; Neurology 1982; **Med School:** Harvard Med Sch 1974; **Resid:** Internal Medicine, Univ Chicago Hosp 1976; Neurology, New York Hosp- Cornell 1982; **Fellow:** Neurology, Meml Sloan Kettering Cancer Ctr

McArthur, Justin C MD [N] - **Spec Exp:** AIDS/HIV; Multiple Sclerosis; **Hospital:** Johns Hopkins Hosp - Baltimore (page 61); **Address:** Johns Hopkins Hosp, Dept Neurology, 600 N Wolfe St, Meyer 6-109, Baltimore, MD 21287; **Phone:** 410-955-3730; **Board Cert:** Neurology 1986; Internal Medicine 1984; **Med School:** England 1979; **Resid:** Internal Medicine, Johns Hopkins Hosp 1982; Neurology, Johns Hopkins Hosp 1985; **Fac Appt:** Prof N, Johns Hopkins Univ

McDonald, John W MD/PhD [N] - **Spec Exp:** Spinal Cord Injury; Stroke Rehabilitation; **Hospital:** Kennedy Krieger Inst; **Address:** Kennedy Krieger Inst, 707 N Broadway, Ste 518, Baltimore, MD 21205; **Phone:** 443-923-9210; **Med School:** Univ Mich Med Sch 1991; **Resid:** Neurology, Barnes-Jewish Hosp 1995; **Fac Appt:** Assoc Prof N, Johns Hopkins Univ

Mitsumoto, Hiroshi MD [N] - **Spec Exp:** Amyotrophic Lateral Sclerosis (ALS); Neuromuscular Disorders; Clinical Trials; **Hospital:** NY-Presby Hosp/Columbia (page 66); **Address:** Neurological Inst, 710 W 168th St Fl 9 - rm 9001, New York, NY 10032; **Phone:** 212-305-1319; **Board Cert:** Neurology 1978; **Med School:** Japan 1968; **Resid:** Internal Medicine, Toho Univ Hosps 1972; Neurology, Univ Hosps 1976; **Fellow:** Neurological Pathology, Cleveland Clinic 1978; Neuromuscular Disease, Tufts Univ 1981; **Fac Appt:** Prof N, Columbia P&S

Mohr, Jay P MD [N] - **Spec Exp:** Aphasia; Stroke; Aneurysm-Cerebral; **Hospital:** NY-Presby Hosp/Columbia (page 66); **Address:** Neurological Inst-Dept Neurology, 710 W 168 St, rm 615, New York, NY 10032-2603; **Phone:** 212-305-8033; **Board Cert:** Neurology 1971; **Med School:** Univ VA Sch Med 1963; **Resid:** Neurology, Columbia Presby Med Ctr 1966; Neurology, Mass Genl Hosp 1968; **Fellow:** Neurology, Mass Genl Hosp 1969; **Fac Appt:** Clin Prof N, Columbia P&S

Newman, Lawrence C MD [N] - **Spec Exp:** Headache; Pain-Facial; **Hospital:** St Luke's - Roosevelt Hosp Ctr - Roosevelt Div; **Address:** St Luke's-Roosevelt Hosp-Headache Inst, 1000 Tenth Ave, Ste 1C10, New York, NY 10019-1192; **Phone:** 212-523-5869; **Board Cert:** Neurology 2005; **Med School:** Mexico 1983; **Resid:** Internal Medicine, Elmhurst Hosp 1986; Neurology, Montefiore Med Ctr 1989; **Fac Appt:** Assoc Prof N, Albert Einstein Coll Med

Olanow, C Warren MD [N] - **Spec Exp:** Parkinson's Disease; Movement Disorders; **Hospital:** Mount Sinai Med Ctr; **Address:** Dept Neurology, One Gustave L Levy Pl, Box 1137, New York, NY 10029; **Phone:** 212-241-8435; **Med School:** Univ Toronto 1965; **Resid:** Neurology, Toronto Genl Hosp 1968; Neurology, Columbia Presby Hosp 1970; **Fellow:** Neurological Anatomy, Columbia Presby Hosp 1971; **Fac Appt:** Prof N, Mount Sinai Sch Med

Pedley, Timothy A MD [N] - **Spec Exp:** Epilepsy/Seizure Disorders; **Hospital:** NY-Presby Hosp/Columbia (page 66); **Address:** The Neurological Inst, 710 W 168th St, rm 1406, New York, NY 10032; **Phone:** 212-305-6489; **Board Cert:** Neurology 1975; **Med School:** Yale Univ 1969; **Resid:** Neurology, Stanford Univ Hosp 1973; **Fellow:** Clinical Neurophysiology, Stanford Univ Hosp 1975; **Fac Appt:** Prof N, Columbia P&S

Petito, Frank MD [N] - **Spec Exp:** Multiple Sclerosis; Headache; Lyme Disease; **Hospital:** NY-Presby Hosp/Weill Cornell (page 66); **Address:** 525 E 68th St, rm *607, New York, NY 10021-4870; **Phone:** 212-746-2309; **Board Cert:** Neurology 1972; **Med School:** Columbia P&S 1967; **Resid:** Neurology, New York Hosp 1971; **Fac Appt:** Prof N, Cornell Univ-Weill Med Coll

Posner, Jerome MD [N] - **Spec Exp:** Neuro-Oncology; Brain Tumors; **Hospital:** Meml Sloan Kettering Cancer Ctr; **Address:** 1275 York Ave, rm C731, New York, NY 10021-6007; **Phone:** 212-639-7047; **Board Cert:** Neurology 1962; **Med School:** Univ Wash 1955; **Resid:** Neurology, Univ WA Affil Hosp 1959; **Fellow:** Biochemistry, Univ WA Affil Hosp 1963; **Fac Appt:** Prof N, Cornell Univ-Weill Med Coll

Pula, Thaddeus MD [N] - **Spec Exp:** Neurophysiology; Electromyography; **Hospital:** Maryland Genl Hosp; **Address:** Maryland Genl Hosp, Div Neurology, 827 Linden Ave Fl Basement, Baltimore, MD 21201-4606; **Phone:** 410-225-8290; **Board Cert:** Neurology 1981; **Med School:** Univ MD Sch Med 1976; **Resid:** Internal Medicine, Mercy Hosp Med Ctr; **Fellow:** Neurology, Univ Maryland

Reich, Stephen G MD [N] - **Spec Exp:** Movement Disorders; Parkinson's Disease; **Hospital:** Univ of MD Med Sys; **Address:** Univ Maryland Med System, Frenkil Bldg, 16 S Eutaw St Fl 3, Baltimore, MD 21201; **Phone:** 410-328-5858; **Board Cert:** Neurology 1989; **Med School:** Tulane Univ 1983; **Resid:** Neurology, Case West Res Univ Hosp 1987; **Fellow:** Movement Disorders, Johns Hopkins Hosp 1988; **Fac Appt:** Assoc Prof N, Univ MD Sch Med

Relkin, Norman MD/PhD [N] - **Spec Exp:** Alzheimer's Disease; Dementia; Memory Disorders; **Hospital:** NY-Presby Hosp/Columbia (page 66); **Address:** Weill Cornell Memory Disorders Program, 428 E 72nd St, Ste 500, New York, NY 10021; **Phone:** 212-746-2441; **Board Cert:** Neurology 1992; **Med School:** Albert Einstein Coll Med 1987; **Resid:** Neurology, New York Hosp 1991; **Fellow:** Behavioral Neurology, New York Hosp-Cornell 1992; **Fac Appt:** Asst Prof N, Cornell Univ-Weill Med Coll

Rosenfeld, Myrna MD/PhD [N] - **Spec Exp:** Neuro-Oncology; Brain Tumors; **Hospital:** Hosp Univ Penn - UPHS (page 72); **Address:** Hosp Univ Penn, Dept Neurology, 3400 Spruce St, 3W Gates, Philadelphia, PA 19104; **Phone:** 215-746-4707; **Board Cert:** Neurology 1990; **Med School:** Northwestern Univ 1985; **Resid:** Neurology, Northwestern Univ Hosp 1987; Neurology, Univ Hosp Cleveland 1989; **Fellow:** Neuro-Oncology, Meml Sloan Kettering Cancer Ctr; **Fac Appt:** Assoc Prof N, Univ Pennsylvania

Rosenfeld, Steven S MD [N] - **Spec Exp:** Brain Tumors; Gliomas; Neuro-Oncology; **Hospital:** NY-Presby Hosp/Columbia (page 66); **Address:** Neurological Inst of NY-Brain Tumor Ctr, 710 W 168th St, rm 204, New York, NY 10032; **Phone:** 212-305-1718; **Board Cert:** Neurology 1994; **Med School:** Northwestern Univ 1985; **Resid:** Neurology, Duke Univ Med Ctr 1989; **Fellow:** Neuro-Oncology, Duke Univ Med Ctr 1990; **Fac Appt:** Prof N, Columbia P&S

Sage, Jacob MD [N] - **Spec Exp:** Parkinson's Disease; **Hospital:** Robert Wood Johnson Univ Hosp - New Brunswick; **Address:** UMDNJ, Dept Neurology, 97 Paterson St, New Brunswick, NJ 08901-2160; **Phone:** 732-235-7733; **Board Cert:** Neurology 1979; **Med School:** Univ Pittsburgh 1972; **Resid:** Neurology, Univ Pittsburgh Hosps 1978; **Fellow:** Neurological Chemistry, NY Hosp-Cornell 1980; **Fac Appt:** Prof N, UMDNJ-RW Johnson Med Sch

Shoulson, Ira MD [N] - **Spec Exp:** Parkinson's Disease; Movement Disorders; Huntington's Disease; **Hospital:** Univ of Rochester Strong Meml Hosp; **Address:** 1351 Mount Hope Ave, Ste 218, Rochester, NY 14620; **Phone:** 585-275-2585; **Board Cert:** Internal Medicine 1974; Neurology 1980; **Med School:** Univ Rochester 1971; **Resid:** Internal Medicine, Strong Meml Hosp 1973; Neurology, Strong Meml Hosp 1977; **Fellow:** Neurology, Natl Inst Hlth 1975; **Fac Appt:** Prof N, Univ Rochester

Silberstein, Stephen D MD [N] - **Spec Exp:** Headache; Migraine; Pain-Facial; **Hospital:** Thomas Jefferson Univ Hosp; **Address:** Jefferson Headache Center, 111 S 11th St, Ste Gibbon, Philadelphia, PA 19107; **Phone:** 215-955-2243; **Board Cert:** Neurology 1975; **Med School:** Univ Pennsylvania 1967; **Resid:** Internal Medicine, Hosp U Penn 1969; Neurology, Hosp U Penn 1975; **Fac Appt:** Clin Prof N, Temple Univ

Sirdofsky, Michael D MD [N] - **Spec Exp:** Neuromuscular Disorders; Electrodiagnosis; **Hospital:** Georgetown Univ Hosp; **Address:** Pasquerilla Health Care Bldg, Entrance 1 Fl 7, 3800 Resevoir Rd NW, Washington, DC 20007; **Phone:** 202-444-8525; **Board Cert:** Neurology 1981; **Med School:** Georgetown Univ 1976; **Resid:** Neurology, Georgetown Univ Hosp 1980; **Fac Appt:** Assoc Prof N, Georgetown Univ

Sperling, Michael R MD [N] - **Spec Exp:** Epilepsy/Seizure Disorders; **Hospital:** Thomas Jefferson Univ Hosp; **Address:** Thos Jefferson Univ Hosp, Dept Neurology, 900 Walnut St, Ste 200, Philadelphia, PA 19107; **Phone:** 215-955-1222; **Board Cert:** Neurology 1984; Clinical Neurophysiology 1999; **Med School:** Temple Univ 1978; **Resid:** Neurology, Mt Sinai Hosp 1982; **Fellow:** Epilepsy, UCLA Med Ctr 1984; **Fac Appt:** Prof N, Thomas Jefferson Univ

Stern, Matthew MD [N] - **Spec Exp:** Parkinson's Disease; Movement Disorders; Botox Therapy; **Hospital:** Pennsylvania Hosp (page 72); **Address:** Pennsylvania Hosp, Dept Neurology, 330 S 9th St Fl 3, Philadelphia, PA 19107; **Phone:** 215-829-6500; **Board Cert:** Neurology 1983; **Med School:** Duke Univ 1978; **Resid:** Neurology, Hosp Univ Penn 1982; **Fac Appt:** Prof Med, Univ Pennsylvania

Swerdlow, Michael MD [N] - **Spec Exp:** Myasthenia Gravis; Spinal Disorders; Multiple Sclerosis; **Hospital:** Montefiore Med Ctr; **Address:** 3400 Bainbridge Ave, Bronx, NY 10467-2401; **Phone:** 718-920-4178; **Board Cert:** Neurology 1975; **Med School:** Univ Pennsylvania 1967; **Resid:** Internal Medicine, Mount Sinai Hosp 1969; Neurology, Albert Einstein Coll 1972; **Fellow:** Neurology, Natl Inst Hlth 1974; **Fac Appt:** Prof N, Albert Einstein Coll Med

Vas, George A MD [N] - **Spec Exp:** Stroke; Multiple Sclerosis; **Hospital:** SUNY Downstate Med Ctr, Kings County Hosp Ctr; **Address:** 450 Clarkson Ave, Ste A, Brooklyn, NY 11203-2056; **Phone:** 718-270-2502; **Board Cert:** Internal Medicine 1973; Neurology 1977; Clinical Neurophysiology 2002; **Med School:** Univ Pittsburgh 1970; **Resid:** Internal Medicine, New York Hosp 1972; Neurology, New York Hosp 1975; **Fac Appt:** Prof N, SUNY Downstate

Wechsler, Lawrence R MD [N] - **Spec Exp:** Cerebrovascular Disease; Stroke; **Hospital:** UPMC Presby, Pittsburgh, UPMC Shadyside; **Address:** UPMC Stroke Institute, 3471 Fifth Ave, Ste 810, Pittsburgh, PA 15213; **Phone:** 412-692-4920; **Board Cert:** Internal Medicine 1983; Neurology 1984; Clinical Neurophysiology 1994; Vascular Neurology 2005; **Med School:** Univ Pennsylvania 1978; **Resid:** Internal Medicine, Presby-Univ Hosp 1980; Neurology, Mass Genl Hosp 1983; **Fellow:** Clinical Neurophysiology, Mass Genl Hosp 1984; Cerebrovascular Disease, Mass Genl Hosp 1985; **Fac Appt:** Prof N, Univ Pittsburgh

Weinberg, Harold MD [N] - **Spec Exp:** Headache; Spinal Disorders; Neuromuscular Disorders; **Hospital:** NYU Med Ctr (page 67); **Address:** 650 1st Ave Fl 4, New York, NY 10016-3240; **Phone:** 212-213-9339; **Board Cert:** Neurology 1983; **Med School:** Albert Einstein Coll Med 1978; **Resid:** Neurology, Columbia-Presby Med Ctr 1982; **Fellow:** Neuromuscular Disease, Columbia-Presby Med Ctr 1982; **Fac Appt:** Clin Prof N, NYU Sch Med

Weiner, William J MD [N] - **Spec Exp:** Movement Disorders; Parkinson's Disease; Huntington's Disease; **Hospital:** Univ of MD Med Sys; **Address:** Univ Maryland Med System, Dept Neurology, 22 S Greene St, rm N4W46, Baltimore, MD 21201; **Phone:** 410-328-2172; **Board Cert:** Neurology 1975; **Med School:** Univ IL Coll Med 1969; **Resid:** Neurology, Univ Minn 1971; Neurology, Rush-Presby Med Ctr 1973; **Fac Appt:** Prof N, Univ MD Sch Med

Wityk, Robert J MD [N] - **Spec Exp:** Stroke; Cerebrovascular Disease; **Hospital:** Johns Hopkins Hosp - Baltimore (page 61); **Address:** 600 N Wolfe St, Phipps 126-B, Baltimore, MD 21287; **Phone:** 410-955-2228; **Board Cert:** Internal Medicine 1988; Neurology 1992; **Med School:** Case West Res Univ 1985; **Resid:** Internal Medicine, UCSD Med Ctr 1988; Neurology, Mass Genl Hosp 1991; **Fellow:** Cardiovascular Disease, Tufts U-New Eng MC 1992; **Fac Appt:** Assoc Prof N, Johns Hopkins Univ

Zimmerman, Earl A MD [N] - **Spec Exp:** Memory Disorders; Alzheimer's Disease; Dementia; **Hospital:** Albany Med Ctr; **Address:** Albany Med Ctr-Neurology, 43 New Scotland Ave, MC 70, Albany, NY 12208; **Phone:** 518-262-5226; **Board Cert:** Neurology 1970; Internal Medicine 1970; **Med School:** Univ Pennsylvania 1963; **Resid:** Internal Medicine, Presbyterian Hosp 1965; Neurology, Neurological Inst 1968; **Fellow:** Endocrinology, Presbyterian Hosp 1972; **Fac Appt:** Prof N, Albany Med Coll

Neurology

Southeast

Adams, Robert J MD [N] - **Spec Exp:** Stroke; **Hospital:** Med Coll of GA Hosp and Clin; **Address:** Medical Coll of Georgia, Dept Neurology, 1429 Harper St, rm HF1154, Augusta, GA 30912; **Phone:** 706-721-4670; **Board Cert:** Neurology 1987; **Med School:** Univ Ark 1980; **Resid:** Neurology, Med Coll Georgia 1985; **Fac Appt:** Assoc Prof N, Med Coll GA

Berger, Joseph MD [N] - **Spec Exp:** Multiple Sclerosis; AIDS/HIV; Infectious & Demyelinating Diseases; **Hospital:** Univ of Kentucky Chandler Hosp; **Address:** Univ Kentucky, Dept Neurology, Kentucky Clinic, Rm L-445, 740 S Limestone, Lexington, KY 40536; **Phone:** 859-323-5661; **Board Cert:** Neurology 1983; Internal Medicine 1977; **Med School:** Jefferson Med Coll 1974; **Resid:** Internal Medicine, Georgetown Univ Hosp 1977; Neurology, Jackson Meml Hosp 1981; **Fac Appt:** Prof N, Univ KY Coll Med

Bernad, Peter MD [N] - **Spec Exp:** Stroke; Headache; Migraine; Head Injury; **Hospital:** Inova Alexandria Hosp, G Washington Univ Hosp; **Address:** Sherwood Hall Med Ctr, 2616 Sherwood Hall Ln, Ste 201, Alexandria, VA 22306-3154; **Phone:** 703-360-8200; **Board Cert:** Internal Medicine 1979; Neurology 1981; **Med School:** McGill Univ 1974; **Resid:** Internal Medicine, USC Univ Hosp 1976; Neurology, Mass Genl Hosp-Harvard 1979; **Fellow:** Neurological Muscular Disease, Natl Inst Hlth 1981; **Fac Appt:** Assoc Clin Prof N, Geo Wash Univ

Corbett, James MD [N] - **Spec Exp:** Neuro-Ophthalmology; Pseudotumor Cerebri; Neurosarcoidosis; **Hospital:** Univ Hosps & Clins - Jackson; **Address:** Univ Mississippi Med Ctr, Dept Neurology, 2500 N State St, Jackson, MS 39216-4505; **Phone:** 601-984-5501; **Board Cert:** Neurology 2004; **Med School:** Ros Franklin Univ/Chicago Med Sch 1966; **Resid:** Internal Medicine, Rhode Island Hosp 1968; Neurology, Univ Hosp-Case Western Reserve 1971; **Fac Appt:** Prof N, Univ Miss

De Long, Mahlon R MD [N] - **Spec Exp:** Parkinson's Disease; Movement Disorders; **Hospital:** Emory Univ Hosp; **Address:** Emory Clinic, Dept Neurology, 101 Woodruff Cir, Ste 6000, Atlanta, GA 30322; **Phone:** 404-727-3818; **Board Cert:** Neurology 1980; **Med School:** Harvard Med Sch 1966; **Resid:** Neurology, Johns Hopkins Hosp 1976; Internal Medicine, Boston City Hosp 1968; **Fellow:** Neurology, NIMH 1973; **Fac Appt:** Prof N

Dure IV, Leon S MD [N] - **Spec Exp:** Huntington's Disease; Tourette's Syndrome; Movement Disorders; **Hospital:** Univ of Ala Hosp at Birmingham; **Address:** 1600 7th Ave S, Ste 314, Birmingham, AL 35233-0011; **Phone:** 205-939-9100; **Board Cert:** Child Neurology 1991; **Med School:** Baylor Coll Med 1984; **Resid:** Pediatrics, Columbia Presby Hosp 1986; Child Neurology, Texas Chldns Hosp 1989; **Fellow:** Child Neurology, Univ Michigan 1990; **Fac Appt:** Assoc Prof N, Univ Ala

Finkel, Michael MD [N] - **Spec Exp:** Movement Disorders-Lower Limb; ADD/ADHD; Headache in Women; Trauma Neurology; **Hospital:** Physicians Regl Med Ctr; **Address:** Medical Surgical Specialists, 6101 Pine Ridge Rd, Naples, FL 34119; **Phone:** 239-348-4397; **Board Cert:** Neurology 1979; **Med School:** Washington Univ, St Louis 1973; **Resid:** Neurology, Strong Meml Hosp 1977

Glass, Jonathan MD [N] - **Spec Exp:** Neuro-Pathology; Amyotrophic Lateral Sclerosis (ALS); Peripheral Neuropathy; **Hospital:** Emory Univ Hosp, Grady Hlth Sys; **Address:** 1365 Clifton Rd NE, Ste A3100, Atlanta, GA 30322; **Phone:** 404-778-3444; **Board Cert:** Neurology 1990; Clinical Neurophysiology 1996; Neuropathology 1997; **Med School:** Univ VT Coll Med 1985; **Resid:** Neurology, Johns Hopkins Univ 1989; **Fellow:** Neuropathology, Johns Hopkins Univ 1991; **Fac Appt:** Prof N, Emory Univ

Goldstein, Larry B MD [N] - **Spec Exp:** Stroke; Carotid Artery Disease; **Hospital:** Duke Univ Med Ctr, VA Med Ctr - Durham; **Address:** Duke Univ Med Ctr, Box 3651, Durham, NC 27710-0001; **Phone:** 919-684-3801; **Board Cert:** Neurology 1987; Vascular Neurology 2005; **Med School:** Mount Sinai Sch Med 1981; **Resid:** Neurology, Mt Sinai Hosp 1985; **Fellow:** Cerebrovascular Disease, Duke Univ Med Ctr 1986; **Fac Appt:** Prof N, Duke Univ

Gress, Daryl Ray MD [N] - **Spec Exp:** Critical Care; Stroke; **Hospital:** Lynchburg Genl Hosp, Virginia Baptist Hosp; **Address:** 1933 Thomson Drive, Lynchburg, VA 24501; **Phone:** 434-947-3928; **Board Cert:** Neurology 1989; **Med School:** Washington Univ, St Louis 1982; **Resid:** Internal Medicine, Johns Hopkins Hosp 1984; Neurology, Mass Genl Hosp 1987; **Fellow:** Stroke, Mass Genl Hosp 1988

Haley Jr, Elliott Clarke MD [N] - **Spec Exp:** Stroke; **Hospital:** Univ Virginia Med Ctr; **Address:** Univ VA Hlth Sys, Dept Neurology, PO Box 800394, Charlottesville, VA 22908; **Phone:** 434-924-8041; **Board Cert:** Internal Medicine 1978; Neurology 1985; **Med School:** Tulane Univ 1974; **Resid:** Internal Medicine, Univ Va Hosp 1978; Neurology, Univ Va Hosp 1982; **Fellow:** Cerebrovascular Disease, Mass Genl Hosp 1984; **Fac Appt:** Prof N, Univ VA Sch Med

Heilman, Kenneth MD [N] - **Spec Exp:** Behavioral Neurology; Memory Disorders; **Hospital:** Shands Hlthcre at Univ of FL, VA Med Ctr - Gainesville; **Address:** Hlth Ctr Univ Fla Coll Med, Dept Neur, Box 100236, Gainesville, FL 32610-0236; **Phone:** 352-273-5550; **Board Cert:** Neurology 1973; **Med School:** Univ VA Sch Med 1963; **Resid:** Internal Medicine, Bellevue Hosp Ctr 1965; Neurology, Boston City Hosp 1970; **Fac Appt:** Prof N, Univ Fla Coll Med

Hess, David Charles MD [N] - **Spec Exp:** Stroke; Antiphospholipid Syndrome (APS); Autoimmune Cerebrovascular Disease; **Hospital:** Med Coll of GA Hosp and Clin; **Address:** Dept Neurology, 1120 15th St, rm BI-3080, Augusta, GA 30912; **Phone:** 706-721-1691; **Board Cert:** Internal Medicine 1986; Neurology 1990; **Med School:** Univ MD Sch Med 1983; **Resid:** Internal Medicine, Allegheny Genl Hosp 1985; Neurology, Med Coll Ga 1989; **Fellow:** Cerebrovascular Disease, Med Coll Ga 1990; **Fac Appt:** Prof N, Med Coll GA

Hurwitz, Barrie MD [N] - **Spec Exp:** Multiple Sclerosis; Parkinson's Disease; Stroke/Cerebrovascular Disease; **Hospital:** Duke Univ Med Ctr; **Address:** Duke Univ Med Ctr, 122 Baker House, Box 3184, Durham, NC 27710; **Phone:** 919-684-4126; **Board Cert:** Neurology 1979; **Med School:** South Africa 1968; **Resid:** Internal Medicine, Johannesburg Genl Hosp 1973; Neurology, New York Hosp/Sloan Kettering Hosp 1977; **Fellow:** Neurology, New York Hosp-Cornell 1976; **Fac Appt:** Assoc Prof Med, Duke Univ

Kirshner, Howard S MD [N] - **Spec Exp:** Stroke; Aphasia; Neurorehabilitation; Dementia; **Hospital:** Vanderbilt Univ Med Ctr, Vanderbilt Stallworth Rehab Hosp Lp; **Address:** Vanderbilt Univ Med Ctr, Dept Neurology, 2311 Pierce Avve, SGOB-Ste 2306, Nashville, TN 37232-3375; **Phone:** 615-936-1354; **Board Cert:** Neurology 1980; Vascular Neurology 2005; **Med School:** Harvard Med Sch 1972; **Resid:** Neurology, Mass Genl Hosp 1978; **Fellow:** Neurological Science, Natl Inst Hlth 1975; **Fac Appt:** Prof N, Vanderbilt Univ

Kurtzke, Robert MD [N] - **Spec Exp:** Electromyography; Nerve/Muscle Disorders; **Hospital:** Inova Fairfax Hosp, Reston Hosp Ctr; **Address:** Neurology Ctr Fairfax, 3020 Hamaker Ct, Ste 400, Fairfax, VA 22031-2220; **Phone:** 703-876-0800; **Board Cert:** Neurology 1990; Clinical Neurophysiology 2004; **Med School:** Georgetown Univ 1985; **Resid:** Neurology, Neurology Inst-Columbia Presby 1989; **Fellow:** Neurological Muscular Disease, Duke Univ Med Ctr 1990; **Fac Appt:** N, Georgetown Univ

Morgenlander, Joel Charles MD [N] - **Spec Exp:** Nerve/Muscle Disorders; **Hospital:** Duke Univ Med Ctr; **Address:** Duke Univ Med Ctr, Box 3394, Durham, NC 27710; **Phone:** 919-684-6887; **Board Cert:** Neurology 1992; **Med School:** Univ Pittsburgh 1986; **Resid:** Neurology, Duke Univ Med Ctr 1990; **Fellow:** Neurological Muscular Disease, Duke Univ Med Ctr 1991; **Fac Appt:** Assoc Prof N, Duke Univ

Newman, Nancy Jean MD [N] - **Spec Exp:** Neuro-Ophthalmology; **Hospital:** Emory Univ Hosp; **Address:** Emory Eye Center, 1365B Clifton Rd NE, Ste 3600, Atlanta, GA 30322; **Phone:** 404-778-5360; **Board Cert:** Neurology 1989; **Med School:** Harvard Med Sch 1984; **Resid:** Neurology, Mass Genl Hosp 1988; **Fellow:** Neurological Ophthalmology, Mass EE Infirmary 1989; **Fac Appt:** Prof N, Emory Univ

Nolan, Bruce A MD [N] - **Spec Exp:** Sleep Disorders/Apnea; **Hospital:** Jackson Meml Hosp; **Address:** Univ Miami, Dept Neurology, Sleep Disorders Center, 1501 NW 9th Ave, Miami, FL 33136; **Phone:** 305-243-5195; **Board Cert:** Neurology 1974; **Med School:** Wayne State Univ 1966; **Resid:** Neurology, Univ Miami Med Ctr 1970; **Fac Appt:** Assoc Prof N, Univ Miami Sch Med

Oh, Shin Joong MD [N] - **Spec Exp:** Neuromuscular Disorders; Electromyography; **Hospital:** Univ of Ala Hosp at Birmingham; **Address:** Univ AL Hosp, Jefferson Tower, 1720 7th Ave S, Birmingham, AL 35233; **Phone:** 205-934-2121; **Board Cert:** Neurology 1973; Clinical Neurophysiology 2001; **Med School:** Korea 1960; **Resid:** Internal Medicine, Seoul National Univ Hosp 1964; Neurology, Georgetown Univ Hosp 1967; **Fellow:** NeuroEpidemiology, Univ Minnesota Hosps 1968; **Fac Appt:** Prof N, Univ Ala

Patchell, Roy MD [N] - **Spec Exp:** Neuro-Oncology; Brain Tumors; Spinal Tumors; **Hospital:** Univ of Kentucky Chandler Hosp; **Address:** Univ Kentucky Neurosurgery-Chandler Med Ctr, 800 Rose St, MS 105, Lexington, KY 40536; **Phone:** 859-323-5672; **Board Cert:** Neurology 1984; **Med School:** Univ KY Coll Med 1979; **Resid:** Neurology, Johns Hopkins Hosp 1983; **Fellow:** Neuro-Oncology, Meml Sloan-Kettering Canc Ctr 1985; **Fac Appt:** Prof N, Univ KY Coll Med

Phuphanich, Surasak MD [N] - **Spec Exp:** Neuro-Oncology; Brain Tumors; Spinal Tumors; **Hospital:** Emory Univ Hosp; **Address:** Winship Cancer Inst-Emory Univ, 1365 Clifton Rd NE C Bldg Fl 2, Atlanta, GA 30322; **Phone:** 404-778-1900; **Board Cert:** Neurology 1983; **Med School:** Thailand 1975; **Resid:** Neurology, Univ Illinois Med Ctr 1981; **Fellow:** Neuro-Oncology, UCSF Med Ctr 1984; **Fac Appt:** Prof, Emory Univ

Rothrock, John MD [N] - **Spec Exp:** Stroke; Headache; **Hospital:** Univ of Ala Hosp at Birmingham; **Address:** UAB, Dept Neurology, 1813 6th Ave S RWUH Bldg - Ste M226, Birmingham, AL 35249; **Phone:** 205-934-2401; **Board Cert:** Neurology 1984; **Med School:** Univ VA Sch Med 1977; **Resid:** Neurology, Univ Ariz Med Ctr 1981; **Fac Appt:** Prof N, Univ S Ala Coll Med

Sacco, Ralph L MD [N] - **Spec Exp:** Stroke; Stroke Prevention; **Hospital:** Univ of Miami Hosp & Clins/Sylvester Comp Canc Ctr; **Address:** Univ of Miami, Chairman of Neurology, 1120 NW 14th St Fl 8 - Ste 853, Miami, FL 33136; **Phone:** 305-243-7519; **Board Cert:** Neurology 1989; **Med School:** Boston Univ 1983; **Resid:** Neurology, Columbia-Presby Med Ctr 1987; **Fellow:** Cerebrovascular Disease, Columbia-Presby Med Ctr 1989; **Fac Appt:** Prof N, Univ Miami Sch Med

Sadowsky, Carl H MD [N] - **Spec Exp:** Memory Disorders; Alzheimer's Disease; Dementia; **Hospital:** Good Sam Med Ctr - W Palm Beach, Columbia Hosp - W Palm Beach; **Address:** 4631 Congress Ave, Ste 200, West Palm Beach, FL 33407-2234; **Phone:** 561-845-0500 x129; **Board Cert:** Neurology 1977; **Med School:** Cornell Univ 1971; **Resid:** Internal Medicine, Dartmouth-Hitchcock Med Ctr 1973; Neurology, Dartmouth-Hitchcock Med Ctr 1976; **Fac Appt:** Assoc Clin Prof N, Nova SE Univ, Coll Osteo Med

Schatz, Norman J MD [N] - **Spec Exp:** Neuro-Ophthalmology; Multiple Sclerosis & Visual Loss; Vision-Unexplained Loss; **Hospital:** Mount Sinai Med Ctr - Miami, Cleveland Clin - Weston (page 57); **Address:** 4701 N Meridian Ave, Adams Bldg - Ste 500A, Miami Beach, FL 33140; **Phone:** 305-532-2885; **Board Cert:** Neurology 1969; **Med School:** Hahnemann Univ 1961; **Resid:** Neurology, Jefferson Hosp 1965; **Fellow:** Neurological Ophthalmology, Bascom Palmer Eye Inst 1966; **Fac Appt:** Clin Prof N, Univ Pennsylvania

Schold Jr, S Clifford MD [N] - **Spec Exp:** Brain Tumors; Neuro-Oncology; **Hospital:** H Lee Moffitt Cancer Ctr & Research Inst; **Address:** H Lee Moffitt Cancer Ctr, 12902 Magnolia Dr, MCC VP Admin, Tampa, FL 33612; **Phone:** 813-745-7426; **Board Cert:** Neurology 1980; **Med School:** Univ Ariz Coll Med 1973; **Resid:** Neurology, Colorado Med Ctr 1977; **Fellow:** Neuro-Oncology, Sloan-Kettering Cancer Ctr 1978; **Fac Appt:** Prof N, Univ S Fla Coll Med

Sethi, Kapil MD [N] - **Spec Exp:** Parkinson's Disease; Restless Legs Syndrome; Movement Disorders; Botox Therapy; **Hospital:** Med Coll of GA Hosp and Clin; **Address:** Med College Georgia, Dept Neurology, 1429 Harper St, Augusta, GA 30912-0004; **Phone:** 706-721-2798; **Board Cert:** Neurology 1987; **Med School:** India 1976; **Resid:** Neurology, Pgimer 1981; Neurology, Med Coll Georgia 1985; **Fac Appt:** Prof N, Med Coll GA

Valenstein, Edward MD [N] - **Spec Exp:** Neuromuscular Disorders; Multiple Sclerosis; Amyotrophic Lateral Sclerosis (ALS); **Hospital:** Shands Hlthcre at Univ of FL; **Address:** 100 S Newell Drive, Box 100263, Gainesville, FL 32610; **Phone:** 352-265-8408; **Board Cert:** Neurology 1974; Clinical Neurophysiology 1996; **Med School:** Albert Einstein Coll Med 1967; **Resid:** Neurology, Boston City Hosp 1971; **Fac Appt:** Prof N, Univ Fla Coll Med

Watts, Ray L MD [N] - **Spec Exp:** Parkinson's Disease; Movement Disorders; **Hospital:** Univ of Ala Hosp at Birmingham; **Address:** UAB, Dept Neurology, 1720 7th Ave S, Sparks Center, rm 350, Birmingham, AL 35233; **Phone:** 205-934-0683; **Board Cert:** Neurology 1985; **Med School:** Washington Univ, St Louis 1980; **Resid:** Neurology, Mass Genl Hosp 1984; **Fellow:** Electromyography, Mass Genl Hosp 1983; **Fac Appt:** Prof N, Univ Ala

Wooten Jr, George Frederick MD [N] - **Spec Exp:** Movement Disorders; Parkinson's Disease; Tremor; **Hospital:** Univ Virginia Med Ctr; **Address:** Univ VA Hlth Sys, Dept Neuro-McKim Hall, PO Box 800394, Charlottesville, VA 22908; **Phone:** 434-924-8369; **Board Cert:** Neurology 1977; **Med School:** Cornell Univ-Weill Med Coll 1970; **Resid:** Neurology, New York Hosp-Cornell 1977; **Fellow:** Pharmacology, Natl Inst Hlth-NIMH 1974; **Fac Appt:** Prof N, Univ VA Sch Med

Neurology

Midwest

Adams Jr, Harold P MD [N] - **Spec Exp:** Stroke; Cerebrovascular Disease; **Hospital:** Univ Iowa Hosp & Clinics; **Address:** Univ Iowa Hosp, Dept Neurology, 200 Hawkins Drive, rm 2148-RCP, Iowa City, IA 52242; **Phone:** 319-356-4110; **Board Cert:** Neurology 2004; Vascular & Interventional Radiology 2005; **Med School:** Northwestern Univ 1970; **Resid:** Neurology, Univ Iowa Hosp 1974; **Fac Appt:** Prof N, Univ Iowa Coll Med

Ahlskog, J Eric MD/PhD [N] - **Spec Exp:** Parkinson's Disease; Movement Disorders; **Hospital:** Mayo Med Ctr & Clin - Rochester, St Mary's Hosp - Rochester; **Address:** Mayo Clinic, Dept Neur, 200 First St SW, Rochester, MN 55905; **Phone:** 507-538-1038; **Board Cert:** Neurology 1984; **Med School:** Dartmouth Med Sch 1976; **Resid:** Internal Medicine, Univ Chicago Hosps Clins 1978; Neurology, Mayo Grad Sch Med 1981; **Fac Appt:** Prof N, Mayo Med Sch

Alberts, Mark J MD [N] - **Spec Exp:** Stroke/Cerebrovascular Disease; **Hospital:** Northwestern Meml Hosp; **Address:** 675 N St Clair, Galter-Ste 20-100, Chicago, IL 60611; **Phone:** 312-695-7950; **Board Cert:** Neurology 1987; **Med School:** Tufts Univ 1982; **Resid:** Neurology, Duke Univ Med Ctr 1986; **Fellow:** Cerebrovascular Disease, Duke Univ Med Ctr 1987; **Fac Appt:** Prof N, Northwestern Univ

Arnason, Barry G W MD [N] - **Spec Exp:** Multiple Sclerosis; Guillain-Barre Syndrome; Myasthenia Gravis; **Hospital:** Univ of Chicago Hosps; **Address:** 5841 S Maryland Ave, MC 2030, Chicago, IL 60637; **Phone:** 773-702-6222; **Board Cert:** Neurology 1971; **Med School:** Univ Manitoba 1957; **Resid:** Neurology, Mass Genl Hosp 1959; Neurology, Mass Genl Hosp 1962; **Fac Appt:** Prof N, Univ Chicago-Pritzker Sch Med

Bennett, David A MD [N] - **Spec Exp:** Alzheimer's Disease; **Hospital:** Rush Univ Med Ctr; **Address:** Rush Alzheimer's Disease Ctr, 600 S Paulina St, Ste 61028, Chicago, IL 60612; **Phone:** 312-942-4823; **Board Cert:** Neurology 1990; **Med School:** Rush Med Coll 1984; **Resid:** Neurology, Rush-Presby-St Luke's Med Ctr 1989; **Fac Appt:** Assoc Prof N, Rush Med Coll

Broderick, Joseph P MD [N] - **Spec Exp:** Stroke; **Hospital:** Univ Hosp - Cincinnati; **Address:** Univ Cincinnati, Dept Neurology, 231 Bethesda Ave, Ste 3200, Cincinnati, OH 45267-0525; **Phone:** 513-475-8730; **Board Cert:** Neurotology 1988; Vascular Neurology 2005; **Med School:** Univ Cincinnati 1982; **Resid:** Neurology, Mayo Clinic 1986; **Fac Appt:** Clin Prof N, Univ Cincinnati

Brooks, Benjamin R MD [N] - **Spec Exp:** Neuromuscular Disorders; Multiple Sclerosis; Neurotoxicology; **Hospital:** Univ WI Hosp & Clins, VA Hospital, Madison; **Address:** Univ Wisconsin Hosp, Dept Neurology, 600 Highland Ave, rm H6-558, Madison, WI 53792; **Phone:** 608-263-5421; **Board Cert:** Internal Medicine 1974; Neurology 1978; **Med School:** Harvard Med Sch 1970; **Resid:** Neurology, Mass Genl Hosp 1974; Neurology, Natl Inst Neuro Disorders & Stroke-NIH 1976; **Fellow:** Neurovirology, Johns Hopkins Hosp 1978; **Fac Appt:** Prof N, Univ Wisc

Burke, Allan M MD [N] - **Spec Exp:** Cerebrovascular Disease; Neurologic Imaging; **Hospital:** Northwestern Meml Hosp; **Address:** 150 E Huron St, Ste 803, Chicago, IL 60611-2912; **Phone:** 312-944-0063; **Board Cert:** Neurology 1982; Neuroimaging 2002; **Med School:** Columbia P&S 1976; **Resid:** Internal Medicine, NY Hosp 1978; Neurology, Columbia-Presby Med Ctr 1981; **Fellow:** Cerebrovascular Disease, Hosp Univ Penn 1983; **Fac Appt:** Assoc Clin Prof N, Northwestern Univ

Cohen, Jeffrey Alan MD [N] - **Spec Exp:** Multiple Sclerosis; Neuro-Immunology; **Hospital:** Cleveland Clin Fdn (page 57); **Address:** Cleveland Clin - Mellen Ctr, 9500 Euclid Ave, Desk U10, Cleveland, OH 44195; **Phone:** 216-445-8110; **Board Cert:** Neurology 1985; **Med School:** Univ Chicago-Pritzker Sch Med 1980; **Resid:** Neurology, Hosp Univ Penn 1984; **Fellow:** Neurological Immunology, Hosp Univ Penn 1987

Cutrer, F Michael MD [N] - **Spec Exp:** Headache; Pain-Facial; Migraine; **Hospital:** Mayo Med Ctr & Clin - Rochester, Rochester Meth Hosp; **Address:** Mayo Clinic, Dept Neurology, 200 First St NW, Rochester, MN 55905-0001; **Phone:** 507-284-4409; **Board Cert:** Neurology 1993; **Med School:** Univ Miss 1988; **Resid:** Neurology, UCLA Med Ctr 1992; **Fellow:** Neurology, Mass Genl Hosp-Harvard 1994; **Fac Appt:** Asst Prof N, Mayo Med Sch

Elias, Stanton B MD [N] - **Spec Exp:** Multiple Sclerosis; Myasthenia Gravis; **Hospital:** Henry Ford Hosp; **Address:** Henry Ford Hosp, Dept Neurology, 2799 W Grand Blvd, Fl K-11, Detroit, MI 48202-2689; **Phone:** 313-916-7207; **Board Cert:** Neurology 1979; **Med School:** Univ Pittsburgh 1972; **Resid:** Neurology, Duke Univ Med Ctr 1976; **Fellow:** Neurology, Duke Univ Med Ctr 1977

Farlow, Martin MD [N] - **Spec Exp:** Alzheimer's Disease; Neurodegenerative Disorders; Multiple Sclerosis; **Hospital:** Indiana Univ Hosp, Wishard Hlth Srvs; **Address:** Indiana Univ Sch Med, 541 Clinical Drive, rm 291, Indianapolis, IN 46202; **Phone:** 317-274-2291; **Board Cert:** Neurology 1988; **Med School:** Indiana Univ 1979; **Resid:** Neurology, Indiana Univ 1983; **Fac Appt:** Prof N, Indiana Univ

Feldman, Eva L MD/PhD [N] - **Spec Exp:** Neuromuscular Disorders; Amyotrophic Lateral Sclerosis (ALS); Neuropathy; **Hospital:** Univ Michigan Hlth Sys; **Address:** Univ Mich, Dept Neurology, 1500 E Med Ctr Drive, rm 1324 Taubman Ctr, Ann Arbor, MI 48109-0322; **Phone:** 734-936-9020; **Board Cert:** Neurology 1988; **Med School:** Univ Mich Med Sch 1983; **Resid:** Neurology, Johns Hopkins Hosp 1987; **Fellow:** Neuromuscular Disease, Univ Mich Hosps 1988; **Fac Appt:** Prof N, Univ Mich Med Sch

Fox, Jacob H MD [N] - **Spec Exp:** Alzheimer's Disease; Dementia; **Hospital:** Rush Univ Med Ctr; **Address:** Rush Med Ctr, Dept Neurology, 1725 W Harrison St, Ste 1106, Chicago, IL 60612; **Phone:** 312-942-8729; **Board Cert:** Neurology 1974; **Med School:** Univ IL Coll Med 1967; **Resid:** Neurology, Barnes Hosp 1971; **Fac Appt:** Prof N, Rush Med Coll

Furlan, Anthony J MD [N] - **Spec Exp:** Stroke; Thrombolytic Therapy; **Hospital:** Cleveland Clin Fdn (page 57); **Address:** Cleveland Clinic, Dept Neurology, 9500 Euclid Ave, Desk S91, Cleveland, OH 44195-0001; **Phone:** 216-444-5535; **Board Cert:** Neurology 1979; **Med School:** Loyola Univ-Stritch Sch Med 1973; **Resid:** Neurology, Cleveland Clinic 1977; **Fellow:** Cerebrovascular Disease, Mayo Clinic 1978; **Fac Appt:** Assoc Prof N, Ohio State Univ

Gilman, Sid MD [N] - **Spec Exp:** Parkinson's Disease/Movement Disorders; Alzheimer's Disease; Multiple Sclerosis; Epilepsy; **Hospital:** Univ Michigan Hlth Sys; **Address:** Univ Mich, Dept Neurology, 300 N Ingalls 3D15, Ann Arbor, MI 48109-0489; **Phone:** 734-936-1808; **Board Cert:** Neurology 1966; **Med School:** UCLA 1957; **Resid:** Neurology, Boston City Hosp-Harvard 1963; **Fellow:** Neurological Physiology, Boston City Hosp-Harvard 1965; **Fac Appt:** Prof N, Univ Mich Med Sch

Goetz, Christopher MD [N] - **Spec Exp:** Movement Disorders; Parkinson's Disease; Dyskinesias; **Hospital:** Rush Univ Med Ctr; **Address:** 1725 W Harrison St, Ste 755, Chicago, IL 60612-3835; **Phone:** 312-563-2030; **Board Cert:** Neurology 1982; **Med School:** Rush Med Coll 1975; **Resid:** Neurology, Rush-Presby-St Luke's Med Ctr 1976; Neurology, Michael Reese Med Ctr 1977; **Fellow:** Neurology, Rush-Presby-St Luke's Med Ctr 1979; **Fac Appt:** Prof N, Rush Med Coll

Greenberg, Harry S MD [N] - **Spec Exp:** Neuro-Oncology; Brain Tumors; **Hospital:** Univ Michigan Hlth Sys, Vail Valley Med Ctr; **Address:** Taubman Ctr 1914-0316, 1500 E Med Ctr Dr, Ann Arbor, MI 48109-0316; **Phone:** 734-936-9055; **Board Cert:** Neurology 1980; **Med School:** SUNY Upstate Med Univ 1973; **Resid:** Neurology, Stanford Univ Hosp 1977; **Fellow:** Neuro-Oncology, Sloan Kettering Cancer Ctr 1979; **Fac Appt:** Prof N, Univ Mich Med Sch

Hain, Timothy C MD [N] - **Spec Exp:** Neuro-Otology; Balance Disorders; Motion Sickness; **Hospital:** Northwestern Meml Hosp; **Address:** 645 N Michigan Ave, Ste 410, Chicago, IL 60611; **Phone:** 312-274-0197; **Board Cert:** Neurology 1983; **Med School:** Univ IL Coll Med 1978; **Resid:** Neurology, Univ IL 1982; **Fellow:** Neurology, Johns Hopkins Hosp 1984; Psychiatry, Johns Hopkins Hosp 1984; **Fac Appt:** Prof N, Northwestern Univ

Hecox, Kurt E MD [N] - **Spec Exp:** Pediatric Neurology; Epilepsy/Seizure Disorders; Hearing Loss; **Hospital:** Chldns Hosp - Wisconsin; **Address:** Med College Wisconsin, Dept of Neurology, 9000 W Wisconsin Ave, MS CCC540, PO Box 1997, Milwaukee, WI 53226; **Phone:** 414-266-3464; **Board Cert:** Clinical Neurophysiology 1977; **Med School:** UCSD 1971; **Resid:** Neurology, Univ Texas Southwestern Med Ctr 1975; **Fellow:** Pediatric Neurology, Children's Med Ctr/Parkland Hosp 1978; **Fac Appt:** Prof N, Med Coll Wisc

Josephson, David A MD [N] - **Spec Exp:** Electromyography; Epilepsy; Stroke; **Hospital:** St Vincent Hosp & Hlth Svcs - Indianapolis, Comm Hosp N - Indianapolis; **Address:** 8402 Harcourt Rd, Ste 615, Indianapolis, IN 46260; **Phone:** 317-355-1555; **Board Cert:** Neurology 1976; **Med School:** Indiana Univ 1971; **Resid:** Neurology, Univ Mich Med Ctr 1973; Neurology, Indiana Univ Med Ctr 1975; **Fac Appt:** Assoc Clin Prof N, Indiana Univ

Kincaid, John C MD [N] - **Spec Exp:** Neuromuscular Disorders; Electromyography; Pain-Facial; **Hospital:** Indiana Univ Hosp; **Address:** Indiana Univ Hosp, 550 N University Blvd, Ste 1711, Indianapolis, IN 46202; **Phone:** 317-274-0311; **Board Cert:** Neurology 1982; Clinical Neurophysiology 1997; **Med School:** Indiana Univ 1975; **Resid:** Neurology, Indiana Univ 1979; **Fellow:** Electromyography, Mayo Clinic 1980; **Fac Appt:** Prof N, Indiana Univ

Lisak, Robert P MD [N] - **Spec Exp:** Multiple Sclerosis; Myasthenia Gravis; Vasculitis; **Hospital:** Harper Univ Hosp, Detroit Receiving Hospital; **Address:** Wayne State Univ Sch Med, 4201 St Antoine, Hlth Ctr 8D, Detroit, MI 48201; **Phone:** 313-745-4240; **Board Cert:** Neurology 1975; **Med School:** Columbia P&S 1965; **Resid:** Internal Medicine, Bronx Municipal Hosp-Einstein 1969; Neurology, Hosp Univ Penn 1972; **Fac Appt:** Prof N, Wayne State Univ

Logan, William R MD [N] - **Hospital:** St John's Mercy Med Ctr - St Louis; **Address:** St Johns Mercy Med Ctr, Tower B, 621 New Ballas Rd, Ste 5003, St Louis, MO 63141; **Phone:** 314-251-5910; **Board Cert:** Internal Medicine 1981; Neurology 1986; **Med School:** Univ Okla Coll Med 1978; **Resid:** Internal Medicine, Univ MO Hosps 1982; Neurology, Unix Texas Hlth Sci Ctr 1984

Luders, Hans MD/PhD [N] - **Spec Exp:** Epilepsy; **Hospital:** Univ Hosps Case Med Ctr; **Address:** University Hosps-Case Med Ctr, 11100 Euclid Ave, Dept Neurology, Lakeside Bldg - Ste 3200, Cleveland, OH 44195-0001; **Phone:** 216-844-3650; **Board Cert:** Neurology 1985; **Med School:** Chile 1965; **Resid:** Neurology, Neur Inst-Kyushu Univ 1971; **Fellow:** Neurological Physiology, Mayo Grad Sch Med 1975; **Fac Appt:** Prof N, Ohio State Univ

Mahowald, Mark W MD [N] - **Spec Exp:** Sleep Disorders/Apnea; **Hospital:** Hennepin Cnty Med Ctr; **Address:** Minn Regional Sleep Disorders Ctr, 701 Park Ave S, Minneapolis, MN 55415; **Phone:** 612-873-6201; **Board Cert:** Neurology 1976; **Med School:** Univ Minn 1968; **Resid:** Neurology, Fairview Univ Med Ctr 1974; **Fac Appt:** Prof N, Univ Minn

Mendell, Jerry R MD [N] - **Spec Exp:** Neuromuscular Disorders; **Hospital:** Ohio St Univ Med Ctr, Chldn's Hosp - Columbus; **Address:** Columbus Childrens Rsch Inst, 700 Childrens Drive, rm WA-3011, Columbus, OH 43205; **Phone:** 614-722-2203; **Board Cert:** Neurology 1972; **Med School:** Univ Tex SW, Dallas 1966; **Resid:** Neurology, Neurological Inst 1969; Neurology, Natl Inst Hlth 1970; **Fellow:** Neurological Muscular Disease, Natl Inst Hlth 1972; **Fac Appt:** Prof N, Ohio State Univ

Mesulam, Marel MD [N] - **Spec Exp:** Alzheimer's Disease; Tourette's Syndrome; Dementia; **Hospital:** Northwestern Meml Hosp; **Address:** 320 E Superior St, Chicago, IL 60611; **Phone:** 312-908-9339; **Board Cert:** Neurology 1977; **Med School:** Harvard Med Sch 1972; **Resid:** Neurology, Boston City Hosp 1976; **Fac Appt:** Prof N, Northwestern Univ

Mikkelsen, Tommy MD [N] - **Spec Exp:** Brain Tumors; Gliomas; **Hospital:** Henry Ford Hosp, William Beaumont Hosp; **Address:** Henry Ford Hospital, ER 3096, 2799 W Grand Blvd, Detroit, MI 48202; **Phone:** 313-916-8641; **Board Cert:** Neurology 1998; **Med School:** Univ Calgary 1983; **Resid:** Internal Medicine, Calgary General Hosp 1985; Neurology, Montreal Neurological Inst 1988; **Fellow:** Neuro-Oncology, Royal Victoria Hosp 1990; Neuro-Oncology, Ludwig Inst for Cancer Rsch 1992; **Fac Appt:** Assoc Prof N, Case West Res Univ

Mohammad, Yousef M MD [N] - **Spec Exp:** Headache; Migraine; **Hospital:** Ohio St Univ Med Ctr; **Address:** OSU Medical Ctr, Dept Neurology, 1654 Upham Dr, 403 Means, Columbus, OH 43210; **Phone:** 614-293-4974; **Board Cert:** Neurology 2004; **Med School:** Amer Univ Beirut 1989; **Resid:** Neurology, Wayne State Univ Affil Hosps 1996; **Fellow:** Stroke, Emory Univ 1999; **Fac Appt:** Asst Prof N, Ohio State Univ

Montgomery Jr, Erwin B MD [N] - **Spec Exp:** Parkinson's Disease; **Hospital:** Univ WI Hosp & Clins; **Address:** 600 Highland Ave, MS 2425, Madison, WI 53792; **Phone:** 608-263-5430; **Board Cert:** Neurology 1982; **Med School:** SUNY Buffalo 1976; **Resid:** Neurology, Wahington Univ Med Ctr 1980; **Fellow:** Neurological Physiology, Washington Univ Med Ctr 1981; **Fac Appt:** Prof N, Univ Wisc

Morris, John MD [N] - **Spec Exp:** Alzheimer's Disease; **Hospital:** Barnes-Jewish Hosp; **Address:** Memory Diagnostic Ctr, 4488 Forest Park, Ste 160, St Louis, MO 63108-2215; **Phone:** 314-286-1967; **Board Cert:** Internal Medicine 1979; Neurology 1985; **Med School:** Univ Rochester 1974; **Resid:** Internal Medicine, Akron Genl Med Ctr 1979; Neurology, Cleveland Metro Genl Hosp 1982; **Fellow:** Neuropharmacology, Washington Univ 1985; **Fac Appt:** Prof N, Washington Univ, St Louis

Pascuzzi, Robert MD [N] - **Spec Exp:** Neuromuscular Disorders; Amyotrophic Lateral Sclerosis (ALS); Myasthenia Gravis; **Hospital:** Indiana Univ Hosp, Wishard Hlth Srvs; **Address:** Clarian Hlth-Indiana Univ Sch Med, 545 Barnhill Drive, EH 125, Indianapolis, IN 46202; **Phone:** 317-274-4455; **Board Cert:** Neurology 1984; **Med School:** Indiana Univ 1979; **Resid:** Neurology, Univ Va Med Ctr 1983; **Fellow:** Neuromuscular Disease, Univ Va Med Ctr 1985; **Fac Appt:** Prof N, Indiana Univ

Perlmutter, Joel S MD [N] - **Spec Exp:** Parkinson's Disease; Movement Disorders; Huntington's Disease; **Hospital:** Barnes-Jewish Hosp; **Address:** Wash Univ Sch Med, Dept Neurology, 660 S Euclid Ave, Box 8111, St Louis, MO 63110; **Phone:** 314-362-6908; **Board Cert:** Neurology 1985; **Med School:** Univ MO-Columbia Sch Med 1979; **Resid:** Neurology, Barnes Hosp-Wash Univ 1983; **Fellow:** Movement Disorders, Barnes Hosp-Wash Univ 1984; **Fac Appt:** Prof N, Washington Univ, St Louis

Pestronk, Alan MD [N] - **Spec Exp:** Neuromuscular Disorders; Neuropathy; **Hospital:** Barnes-Jewish Hosp; **Address:** Washington Univ Sch Med, Dept Neurology, 660 S Euclid Ave, Box 8111, St Louis, MO 63110; **Phone:** 314-362-6981; **Board Cert:** Neurology 1978; **Med School:** Johns Hopkins Univ 1970; **Resid:** Neurology, Johns Hopkins Hosp 1974; **Fellow:** Neuromuscular Disease, Johns Hopkins Hosp 1977; **Fac Appt:** Prof NPath, Washington Univ, St Louis

Petersen, Ronald C MD/PhD [N] - **Spec Exp:** Alzheimer's Disease; **Hospital:** Mayo Med Ctr & Clin - Rochester; **Address:** Mayo Clinic, Dept Neurology, 200 1st St SW, Rochester, MN 55905; **Phone:** 507-538-1038; **Board Cert:** Neurology 1986; **Med School:** Mayo Med Sch 1980; **Resid:** Neurology, Mayo Clinic 1984; **Fellow:** Behavioral Neurology, Beth Israel Med Ctr 1986; **Fac Appt:** Prof N, Mayo Med Sch

Reder, Anthony T MD [N] - **Spec Exp:** Multiple Sclerosis; Tetanus; Myasthenia Gravis; **Hospital:** Univ of Chicago Hosps; **Address:** Ctr Advanced Medicine, 5758 S Maryland Ave, rm 4D, Chicago, IL 60637-1426; **Phone:** 773-702-6222; **Board Cert:** Neurology 1984; **Med School:** Univ Mich Med Sch 1978; **Resid:** Neurology, Univ Minn Hosps 1982; **Fellow:** Neurological Immunology, Univ Chicago 1984; **Fac Appt:** Assoc Prof N, Univ Chicago-Pritzker Sch Med

Reed, Robert L MD [N] - **Spec Exp:** Multiple Sclerosis; Stroke; **Hospital:** Good Samaritan Hosp - Cincinnati; **Address:** 111 Wellington Pl, Cincinnati, OH 45219; **Phone:** 513-241-2370; **Board Cert:** Neurology 1975; **Med School:** Univ Cincinnati 1966; **Resid:** Internal Medicine, Mayo Grad Sch Med 1970; Neurology, Mayo Grad Sch Med 1973

Rogers, Lisa R DO [N] - **Spec Exp:** Neuro-Oncology; Brain Tumors; Brain Radiation Toxicity; **Hospital:** Univ Michigan Hlth Sys; **Address:** Univ Michigan, Dept Neurology, 1914 Taubman Center, Ann Arbor, MI 48109-0316; **Phone:** 734-615-2994; **Board Cert:** Neurology 1982; **Med School:** Kirksville Coll Osteo Med 1976; **Resid:** Neurology, Cleveland Clinic Fdn 1980; **Fellow:** Neuro-Oncology, Meml-Sloan Kettering Cancer Ctr 1982; **Fac Appt:** Prof N, Univ Mich Med Sch

Roos, Karen MD [N] - **Spec Exp:** Infections-Neurologic; Encephalitis; **Hospital:** Indiana Univ Hosp, Wishard Hlth Srvs; **Address:** Indiana Univ Med Ctr, 550 N University Blvd, rm 4411, Indianapolis, IN 46202-5149; **Phone:** 317-278-6785; **Board Cert:** Neurology 1986; **Med School:** Hahnemann Univ 1981; **Resid:** Neurology, Univ Virginia Med Ctr 1985; **Fac Appt:** Prof N, Indiana Univ

Roos, Raymond MD [N] - **Spec Exp:** Amyotrophic Lateral Sclerosis (ALS); Multiple Sclerosis; Neuromuscular Disorders; **Hospital:** Univ of Chicago Hosps; **Address:** Univ Chicago, Dept Neurology, 5841 S Maryland Ave, MC-2030, Chicago, IL 60637; **Phone:** 773-702-5659; **Board Cert:** Neurology 1976; **Med School:** SUNY Downstate 1968; **Resid:** Neurology, Johns Hopkins Hosp 1974; **Fellow:** Neurology, Natl Inst Neur Dis & Stroke 1971; Neurological Viral Immunology, Johns Hopkins Hosp 1976; **Fac Appt:** Prof N, Univ Chicago-Pritzker Sch Med

Rubin, Susan MD [N] - **Spec Exp:** Multiple Sclerosis in Women; Epilepsy in Pregnancy; Headache in Women; Migraine in Women; **Hospital:** Glenbrook Hosp, Evanston Hosp; **Address:** Glenbrook Hosp, Dept Neurology, 2100 Pfingsten Rd, rm B110, Glenview, IL 60025-1393; **Phone:** 847-657-5875; **Board Cert:** Neurology 1996; **Med School:** Univ IL Coll Med 1988; **Resid:** Neurology, Northwestern Meml Hosp 1993; **Fellow:** Neurology, Northwestern Meml Hosp 1994

Ruff, Robert L MD/PhD [N] - **Spec Exp:** Spinal Cord Injury; Neuro-Rehabilitation; Muscle Disorders; **Hospital:** VA Med Ctr - Cleveland; **Address:** ATTN: Dr. Robert Ruff, Department of Neurology, 10701 East Blvd, Cleveland, OH 44106; **Phone:** 216-791-3800 x5219; **Board Cert:** Neurology 1982; Spinal Cord Injury Medicine 2002; **Med School:** Univ Wash 1976; **Resid:** Neurology, NY-Cornell Hosp 1980; **Fac Appt:** Prof N, Case West Res Univ

Sagar, Stephen M MD [N] - **Spec Exp:** Neuro-Oncology; Brain Tumors; **Hospital:** Univ Hosps Case Med Ctr; **Address:** Univ Hosp Cleveland, Hanna House, 11100 Euclid Ave Fl 5, Cleveland, OH 44106; **Phone:** 216-844-7510; **Board Cert:** Internal Medicine 1976; Neurology 1979; **Med School:** Harvard Med Sch 1972; **Resid:** Internal Medicine, Peter Bent Brigham Hosp 1974; Neurology, Mass Genl Hosp 1977; **Fellow:** Neurology, Chldns Hosp Med Ctr 1979; **Fac Appt:** Prof N, Case West Res Univ

Saper, Joel R MD [N] - **Spec Exp:** Headache; Pain-Chronic after Head Injury; **Hospital:** Chelsea Comm Hosp; **Address:** Michigan Head Pain & Neurological Inst, 3120 Professional Drive, Ann Arbor, MI 48104; **Phone:** 734-677-6000; **Board Cert:** Neurology 1975; Pain Medicine 1996; **Med School:** Univ IL Coll Med 1969; **Resid:** Neurology, Univ Mich Med Ctr 1973; **Fac Appt:** Clin Prof N, Mich State Univ

Schapiro, Randall T MD [N] - **Spec Exp:** Multiple Sclerosis; **Hospital:** Univ Minn Med Ctr, Fairview - Univ Campus; **Address:** Schapiro Center for MS, 4225 Golden Valley Rd, Golden Valley, MN 55422; **Phone:** 763-302-4199; **Board Cert:** Neurology 1976; **Med School:** Univ Minn 1970; **Resid:** Internal Medicine, Wadsworth VA Hosp 1972; Neurology, Univ Minn 1975; **Fac Appt:** Clin Prof N, Univ Minn

Siddique, Teepu MD [N] - **Spec Exp:** Amyotrophic Lateral Sclerosis (ALS); Muscular Dystrophy; Neurogenetics; **Hospital:** Northwestern Meml Hosp; **Address:** Northwestern Univ-Feinberg, Dept Neuro, 303 E Chicago Ave, Tarry Bldg, rm 13-715, Chicago, IL 60611-5935; **Phone:** 312-695-5886; **Board Cert:** Neurology 1980; **Med School:** Pakistan 1973; **Resid:** Neurology, UMDNJ-RW Johnson Med Sch 1979; **Fellow:** Electromyography, Hosp Special Surg-Cornell 1980; Neurological Muscular Disease, Natl Inst Hlth 1981; **Fac Appt:** Prof N, Northwestern Univ

Swanson, Jerry W MD [N] - **Spec Exp:** Headache; **Hospital:** Mayo Med Ctr & Clin - Rochester; **Address:** Mayo Clinic, Dept Neurology, 200 First St SW, Rochester, MN 55905-0001; **Phone:** 507-284-4409; **Board Cert:** Neurology 1984; **Med School:** Northwestern Univ 1977; **Resid:** Neurology, Mayo Clinic 1982; **Fellow:** Electroencephalography, Mayo Clinic; **Fac Appt:** Prof N, Mayo Med Sch

Taylor, Frederick R MD [N] - **Spec Exp:** Headache; Pain-Facial; **Hospital:** Methodist Hosp - Minnesota; **Address:** Park Nicollet Headache Clinic, 6490 Excelsior Blvd, Meadowbrook Bldg, Ste E-500, Minneapolis, MN 55426; **Phone:** 952-993-3432; **Board Cert:** Pediatrics 1982; Neurology 1985; Clinical Neurophysiology 1996; **Med School:** Univ New Mexico 1977; **Resid:** Pediatrics, Univ Wisc Hlth Sci Ctr 1980; Neurology, Univ Wisc Hlth Sci Ctr 1983; **Fellow:** Neurological Physiology, Univ Wisc Hlth Sci Ctr 1984; **Fac Appt:** Assoc Prof N, Univ Minn

Vick, Nicholas A MD [N] - **Spec Exp:** Brain Tumors; Neuro-Oncology; **Hospital:** Evanston Hosp; **Address:** Evanston Hosp, Div Neurology, 2650 Ridge Ave, Evanston, IL 60201; **Phone:** 847-570-2570 x11; **Board Cert:** Neurology 1971; **Med School:** Univ Chicago-Pritzker Sch Med 1965; **Resid:** Neurology, Univ Chicago Hosps 1968; **Fellow:** Neurology, Natl Inst Hlth 1970; **Fac Appt:** Prof N, Northwestern Univ

Vitek, Jerrold Lee MD/PhD [N] - **Spec Exp:** Parkinson's Disease/Movement Disorders; Tremor & Dystonia; **Hospital:** Cleveland Clin Fdn (page 57); **Address:** Cleveland Clinic Fdn, 9500 Euclid Ave, NC30, Cleveland, OH 44195; **Phone:** 216-444-5535; **Board Cert:** Neurology 1992; **Med School:** Univ Minn 1984; **Resid:** Neurology, Johns Hopkins Hosp 1988; **Fac Appt:** Prof N, Cleveland Cl Coll Med/Case West Res

Wiebers, David O MD [N] - **Spec Exp:** Stroke; Aneurysm-Cerebral; **Hospital:** Mayo Med Ctr & Clin - Rochester; **Address:** Mayo Clinic, Dept Neur, 200 First St SW, Rochester, MN 55905-0002; **Phone:** 507-284-9735; **Board Cert:** Neurology 1984; **Med School:** Univ Nebr Coll Med 1975; **Resid:** Neurology, Mayo Clinic 1979; **Fellow:** Cerebrovascular Disease, Mayo Clinic 1980; **Fac Appt:** Prof N, Mayo Med Sch

Windebank, Anthony J MD [N] - **Spec Exp:** Peripheral Neuropathy; Amyotrophic Lateral Sclerosis (ALS); Multiple Sclerosis; **Hospital:** Mayo Med Ctr & Clin - Rochester; **Address:** Mayo Clinic, Dept Neurology, 200 First St SW, Rochester, MN 55905; **Phone:** 507-284-2798; **Board Cert:** Neurology 1982; **Med School:** England 1974; **Resid:** Internal Medicine, Radcliffe Infirm 1977; Neurology, Mayo Clinic 1981; **Fellow:** Neurology, Mayo Clinic 1982; **Fac Appt:** Prof N, Mayo Med Sch

Wright, Robert B MD [N] - **Spec Exp:** Myasthenia Gravis; Migraine; **Hospital:** Rush Univ Med Ctr; **Address:** 1725 W Harrison St, Ste 1118, Chicago, IL 60612-3841; **Phone:** 312-942-5936; **Board Cert:** Neurology 1988; **Med School:** Univ IL Coll Med 1982; **Resid:** Neurology, Rush Presby-St Luke's Med Ctr 1986; **Fellow:** Neuromuscular Disease, Rush Presby-St Luke's Med Ctr 1987; **Fac Appt:** Asst Prof N, Rush Med Coll

Great Plains and Mountains

Barohn, Richard J MD [N] - **Spec Exp:** Peripheral Neuropathy; Myasthenia Gravis; Amyotrophic Lateral Sclerosis (ALS); **Hospital:** Univ of Kansas Hosp; **Address:** Univ Kansas Medical Ctr, Dept Neurology, 3599 Rainbow Blvd, MS 2012, Kansas City, KS 66160; **Phone:** 913-588-6970; **Board Cert:** Neurology 1987; Clinical Neurophysiology 2004; **Med School:** Univ MO-Kansas City 1980; **Resid:** Neurology, Lackland AFB 1985

Bromberg, Mark B MD/PhD [N] - **Spec Exp:** Peripheral Neuropathy; Neuromuscular Disorders; **Hospital:** Univ Utah Hosps and Clins; **Address:** 30 N 1900 East, Ste 3R 210, Salt Lake City, UT 84132; **Phone:** 801-585-6837; **Board Cert:** Neurology 1988; Clinical Neurophysiology 2002; **Med School:** Univ Mich Med Sch 1982; **Resid:** Neurology, Univ Mich Med Ctr 1986; **Fellow:** Electromyography, Univ Mich Med Ctr 1987; **Fac Appt:** Prof N, Univ Utah

Cilo, Mark P MD [N] - **Spec Exp:** Brain Injury; Spinal Cord Injury; **Hospital:** Craig Hosp, Swedish Med Ctr - Englewood; **Address:** 3425 S Clarkson St, Englewood, CO 80113; **Phone:** 303-789-8220; **Board Cert:** Neurology 1979; Spinal Cord Injury Medicine 2003; **Med School:** Mount Sinai Sch Med 1972; **Resid:** Neurology, Mount Sinai Hosp 1976; **Fellow:** Spinal Cord & Brain Injury Rehab, Craig Hosp 1978; **Fac Appt:** Asst Clin Prof Med, Univ Colorado

Filley, Christopher M MD [N] - **Spec Exp:** Leukoencephalopathy; Alzheimer's Disease; Brain Injury-Traumatic; Multiple Sclerosis; **Hospital:** Univ Colorado Hosp, VA Med Ctr; **Address:** Univ CO, Neurology Dept, Behavioral Neurology Section, 4200 E 9th Ave, Ste B183, Denver, CO 80262; **Phone:** 303-315-6461; **Board Cert:** Neurology 1984; **Med School:** Johns Hopkins Univ 1979; **Resid:** Neurology, Univ Colorado Hosp 1983; **Fellow:** Behavioral Neurology, Boston VA Hosp 1984; **Fac Appt:** Prof N, Univ Colorado

Kelts, K Alan MD/PhD [N] - **Spec Exp:** Pediatric Neurology; Sleep Disorders/Apnea; Neuromuscular Disorders; **Hospital:** Rapid City Reg Hosp; **Address:** Black Hills Neurology, 2929 5th St, Ste 240, Rapid City, SD 57701; **Phone:** 605-341-3770; **Board Cert:** Pediatrics 1977; Child Neurology 1978; **Med School:** Univ Rochester 1971; **Resid:** Pediatrics, Chldns & Univ Hosps 1973; Child Neurology, Colorado Med Ctr 1976; **Fellow:** Neurological Muscular Disease, Muscular Dystrophy Assn 1975; **Fac Appt:** Clin Prof N, Univ SD Sch Med

Ringel, Steven MD [N] - **Spec Exp:** Neuromuscular Disorders; **Hospital:** Univ Colorado Hosp; **Address:** Neuromuscular Dept, 4200 E Ninth Ave, Box B 185, Denver, CO 80262; **Phone:** 303-315-7221; **Board Cert:** Neurology 1974; **Med School:** Univ Mich Med Sch 1968; **Resid:** Neurology, Rush-Presby-St Lukes Med Ctr 1972; **Fellow:** Neurology, Natl Inst Neuro Dis-NIH 1976; **Fac Appt:** Prof N, Univ Colorado

Southwest

Ahern, Geoffry L MD/PhD [N] - **Spec Exp:** Behavioral Neurology; Dementia; Alzheimer's Disease; **Hospital:** Univ Med Ctr - Tucson; **Address:** Univ Arizona, Dept Neurology, 1501 N Campbell Ave, Box 245094, Tucson, AZ 85724-5094; **Phone:** 520-694-8888; **Board Cert:** Neurology 1992; **Med School:** Yale Univ 1984; **Resid:** Neurology, Boston Univ Affil Hosps 1988; **Fellow:** Behavioral Neurology, Beth Israel Hosp 1990; **Fac Appt:** Prof N, Univ Ariz Coll Med

Burns, Richard S MD [N] - **Spec Exp:** Movement Disorders; Ataxia; Neurodegenerative Disorders; **Hospital:** St Joseph's Hosp & Med Ctr - Phoenix; **Address:** Barrow Neurological Institute, 500 W Thomas Rd, Ste 300, Phoenix, AZ 85013; **Phone:** 602-406-4931; **Board Cert:** Neurology 1985; **Med School:** Univ Minn 1969; **Resid:** Internal Medicine, Huntington Meml Hosp 1971; Neurology, UC Irvine Med Ctr 1978; **Fellow:** Clinical Pharmacology, Natl Inst Genl Med Sci 1980

Carter, John E MD [N] - **Spec Exp:** Neuro-Ophthalmology; **Hospital:** Univ Hlth Sys - Univ Hosp; **Address:** Univ Tex Hlth Sci Ctr, Div Neurology, 7703 Floyd Curl, rm 5.318T, MC 7883, San Antonio, TX 78229-3900; **Phone:** 210-567-5088; **Board Cert:** Neurology 1978; **Med School:** Univ Ark 1969; **Resid:** Neurology, Boston Univ Med Ctr 1978; Neurological Ophthalmology, Tufts Univ 1979; **Fac Appt:** Assoc Prof N, Univ Tex, San Antonio

Couch Jr, James R MD/PhD [N] - **Spec Exp:** Headache; Stroke; **Hospital:** OU Med Ctr, VA Med Ctr - Oklahoma City; **Address:** 711 S L Young Blvd, Ste 215, Oklahoma City, OK 73104-5021; **Phone:** 405-271-4113; **Board Cert:** Neurology 1974; Clinical Neurophysiology 2002; **Med School:** Baylor Coll Med 1965; **Resid:** Neurology, Washington Univ Med Ctr 1972; **Fellow:** Neuropharmacology, Natl Inst Hlth 1969; **Fac Appt:** Prof N, Univ Okla Coll Med

Coull, Bruce MD [N] - **Spec Exp:** Stroke; Cerebrovascular Disease; **Hospital:** Univ Med Ctr - Tucson; **Address:** 2800 E Ajo Way, Tucson, AZ 85713; **Phone:** 520-874-2700; **Board Cert:** Neurology 1979; Vascular Neurology 2005; **Med School:** Univ Pittsburgh 1972; **Resid:** Neurology, Stanford Univ Med Ctr 1976; **Fac Appt:** Prof N, Univ Ariz Coll Med

Dodick, David MD [N] - **Spec Exp:** Headache; **Hospital:** Mayo Clin Hosp - Scottsdale; **Address:** Mayo Clinic, Dept of Neurology, 13400 E Shea Blvd, Scottsdale, AZ 85259; **Phone:** 480-301-8100; **Board Cert:** Neurology 1996; Vascular Neurology 2005; **Med School:** Dalhousie Univ 1990; **Resid:** Neurology, Mayo Clinic 1994; **Fellow:** Headache, Sunnybrook Hlth Sci Ctr 1996

Ferrendelli, James A MD [N] - **Spec Exp:** Epilepsy/Seizure Disorders; Neuro-Pharmacology; Geriatric Neurology; **Hospital:** Meml Hermann Hosp - Houston; **Address:** UT Houston Sch Med, Dept Neurology, 6431 Fannin St, Ste 7.044, Houston, TX 77030-1501; **Phone:** 713-500-7070; **Board Cert:** Neurology 1973; **Med School:** Univ Colorado 1962; **Resid:** Neurology, Cleveland Metro Genl Hosp 1968; **Fellow:** Neuropharmacology, Washington Univ Med Sch 1971; **Fac Appt:** Prof N, Univ Tex, Houston

Fox, Peter Thornton MD [N] - **Spec Exp:** PET Imaging; **Hospital:** Univ Hlth Sys - Univ Hosp; **Address:** UT Hlth Sci Ctr San Antonio, Rsch Imaging Ctr, 7703 Floyd Curl Drive, MS 6240, San Antonio, TX 78229-3900; **Phone:** 210-567-8150; **Board Cert:** Neurology 1985; **Med School:** Georgetown Univ 1979; **Resid:** Neurology, Washington Univ 1983; **Fellow:** Radiotracer Imaging, Washington Univ 1984; **Fac Appt:** Prof N, Univ Tex, San Antonio

Gilbert, Mark R MD [N] - **Spec Exp:** Brain Tumors; Neuro-Oncology; **Hospital:** UT MD Anderson Cancer Ctr (page 71); **Address:** Univ Tex MD Anderson Cancer Ctr, 1515 Holcombe Blvd, Unit 431, Houston, TX 77030; **Phone:** 713-792-6600; **Board Cert:** Internal Medicine 1985; Neurology 1990; **Med School:** Johns Hopkins Univ 1982; **Resid:** Internal Medicine, Johns Hopkins Hosp 1985; Neurology, Johns Hopkins Hosp 1988; **Fellow:** Neuro-Oncology, Johns Hopkins Hosp 1988; **Fac Appt:** Assoc Prof N, Univ Tex, Houston

Grotta, James MD [N] - **Spec Exp:** Stroke; **Hospital:** Meml Hermann Hosp - Houston; **Address:** UT Houston Med Sch, Dept Neur, 6410 Fannin St, Ste 1014, Houston, TX 77030; **Phone:** 832-325-7080; **Board Cert:** Neurology 1978; **Med School:** Univ VA Sch Med 1971; **Resid:** Neurology, Univ Colorado Hlth Sci Ctr 1977; **Fellow:** Diagnostic Radiology, Mass Genl Hosp 1979; **Fac Appt:** Prof N, Univ Tex, Houston

Hart, Robert G MD [N] - **Spec Exp:** Stroke; **Hospital:** Univ Hlth Sys - Univ Hosp; **Address:** Univ Tex Hlth & Sci Ctr, Dept Neurology, 7703 Floyd Curl, MC 7883, San Antonio, TX 78229-3901; **Phone:** 210-592-0404; **Board Cert:** Neurology 1985; Vascular Neurology 2005; **Med School:** Univ MO-Columbia Sch Med 1977; **Resid:** Neurology, Univ Hosp & Clinic 1981; **Fellow:** Stroke, Oregon Hlth Sci Ctr 1982; **Fac Appt:** Prof N, Univ Tex, San Antonio

Infante, Ernesto MD [N] - **Spec Exp:** Neuromuscular Disorders; Movement Disorders; Headache; **Hospital:** Meml Hermann Hosp - Houston, Park Plaza Hosp; **Address:** 6410 Fannin St, Ste 1014, UT Professional Building Fl 10, Houston, TX 77030; **Phone:** 825-325-7080; **Board Cert:** Neurology 1973; **Med School:** Spain 1964; **Resid:** Neurology, Univ Minn Hosps 1969; **Fellow:** Electromyography, Mayo Clinic 1970; **Fac Appt:** Assoc Clin Prof N, Univ Tex, Houston

Jankovic, Joseph MD [N] - **Spec Exp:** Movement Disorders; Parkinson's Disease; Tourette's Syndrome; **Hospital:** Methodist Hosp - Houston, St Luke's Episcopal Hosp - Houston; **Address:** Parkinson's Dis Ctr & Movement Disorders Clin, 6550 Fannin St, Smith Twr, Ste 1801, Houston, TX 77030; **Phone:** 713-798-5998; **Board Cert:** Neurology 1979; **Med School:** Univ Ariz Coll Med 1973; **Resid:** Neurology, Columbia-Presby Med Ctr 1977; **Fac Appt:** Prof N, Baylor Coll Med

Knoefel, Janice E MD [N] - **Spec Exp:** Geriatric Neurology; Neuro-Rehabilitation; **Hospital:** Univ NM Hlth & Sci Ctr, VA Med Ctr; **Address:** New Mexico VA Hlth Care System, 1501 San Pedro SE, MC 111K, Albuquerque, NM 87108-5153; **Phone:** 505-256-2795; **Board Cert:** Neurology 1983; **Med School:** Ohio State Univ 1977; **Resid:** Internal Medicine, Univ Cincinnati Med Ctr 1979; Neurology, Boston Univ Med Ctr 1982; **Fellow:** Geriatric Medicine, Boston Univ Med Ctr 1983; **Fac Appt:** Prof N, Univ New Mexico

Labiner, David MD [N] - **Spec Exp:** Epilepsy; **Hospital:** Univ Med Ctr - Tucson; **Address:** Dept of Neurology, PO Box 245023, Tuscon, AZ 85724-5023; **Phone:** 520-626-2006; **Board Cert:** Neurology 1992; **Med School:** Med Coll GA 1984; **Resid:** Neurology, Columbia Univ NY Neuro Inst 1988; **Fellow:** Epilepsy, Duke Univ Med Ctr 1989; **Fac Appt:** Prof N, Univ Ariz Coll Med

Levin, Victor A MD [N] - **Spec Exp:** Brain Tumors; Neuro-Oncology; Clinical Trials; **Hospital:** UT MD Anderson Cancer Ctr (page 71); **Address:** 1515 Holcombe Blvd, Unit #431, Houston, TX 77030-4009; **Phone:** 713-792-8297; **Board Cert:** Neurology 1976; **Med School:** Univ Wisc 1966; **Resid:** Neurology, Mass Genl Hosp 1972; **Fac Appt:** Prof Med, Univ Tex, Houston

Nicholl, Jeffrey Scott MD [N] - **Spec Exp:** Seizure Disorders-Emergency Care; Epilepsy; **Hospital:** Tulane Univ Hosp & Clin; **Address:** Tulane Univ Sch Med Dept Neuro TB-52, 1440 Canal St, New Orleans, LA 70112; **Phone:** 504-988-2241; **Board Cert:** Neurology 1999; Psychiatry 1981; Clinical Neurophysiology 2001; Emergency Medicine 2004; **Med School:** Georgetown Univ 1974; **Resid:** Psychiatry, UCLA Neuro Psyc Inst 1979; Neurology, Tulane Univ 1997; **Fellow:** Clinical Neurophysiology, Tulane Univ 1998; Epilepsy, UCLA 2000; **Fac Appt:** Asst Prof N, Tulane Univ

Oommen, Kalarickal MD [N] - **Spec Exp:** Epilepsy; **Hospital:** OU Med Ctr; **Address:** 711 Stanton L Young Blvd, Oklahoma City, OK 73104; **Phone:** 405-271-3635; **Board Cert:** Neurology 1983; **Med School:** India 1973; **Resid:** Psychiatry, AZ Hlth Sci Ctr 1979; Neurology, AZ Hlth Sci Ctr 1982; **Fellow:** Electrocardiography, Med Coll GA 1983; **Fac Appt:** Assoc Prof N, Univ Okla Coll Med

Shapiro, William R MD [N] - **Spec Exp:** Neuro-Oncology; **Hospital:** St Joseph's Hosp & Med Ctr - Phoenix; **Address:** Barrow Neurology Clinics, 500 W Thomas Rd, Ste 300, Phoenix, AZ 85013; **Phone:** 602-406-6262; **Board Cert:** Neurology 1969; **Med School:** UCSF 1961; **Resid:** Internal Medicine, Univ Wash Hosp 1963; Neurology, NY Hosp-Cornell Med Ctr 1966; **Fellow:** Neuro-Oncology, Natl Inst Hlth 1969; **Fac Appt:** Prof N, Univ Ariz Coll Med

Neurology

Sherman, David MD [N] - **Spec Exp:** Cerebrovascular Disease; Stroke; **Hospital:** Univ Hlth Sys - Univ Hosp; **Address:** Univ Tex Hlth Scis Ctr, Div Neur, 7703 Floyd Curl Drive, MC 7883, San Antonio, TX 78229-3900; **Phone:** 210-592-0340; **Board Cert:** Neurology 1976; **Med School:** Univ Okla Coll Med 1967; **Resid:** Internal Medicine, Baylor Affil Hosp 1969; Neurology, UCSD Med Ctr 1974; **Fac Appt:** Prof N, Univ Tex, San Antonio

Suter, Cary MD [N] - **Spec Exp:** Epilepsy; Headache; **Hospital:** Lovelace Medical Center; **Address:** Lovelace Clin Dept of Neurology, 5400 Gibson Blvd SE, Albuquerque, NM 87108; **Phone:** 505-262-7000; **Board Cert:** Neurology 1984; **Med School:** Univ VA Sch Med 1978; **Resid:** Neurology, Univ NM 1982; **Fellow:** Electroencephalography, Mayo Clin 1984

Vollmer, Timothy Lee MD [N] - **Spec Exp:** Multiple Sclerosis; Myasthenia Gravis; Vasculitis of the Nervous System; Stroke; **Hospital:** St Joseph's Hosp & Med Ctr - Phoenix; **Address:** Barrow Neurological Inst, MS Clinic, 500 W Thomas Rd, Ste 300, Phoenix, AZ 85013; **Phone:** 602-406-6209; **Board Cert:** Neurology 1991; **Med School:** Stanford Univ 1983; **Resid:** Neurology, Stanford Univ Hosp 1987; **Fellow:** Neurological Immunology, Stanford Univ Sch Med 1986

Wolinsky, Jerry S MD [N] - **Spec Exp:** Multiple Sclerosis; Clinical Trials; MRI; **Hospital:** Meml Hermann Hosp - Houston; **Address:** Univ Texas Med Sch, 6431 Fannin St, Ste MSB G.150, Houston, TX 77030-1503; **Phone:** 713-500-5010; **Board Cert:** Neurology 1975; **Med School:** Univ IL Coll Med 1969; **Resid:** Neurology, UCSF Med Ctr 1973; **Fellow:** Neuropathology, VA Hosp 1975; **Fac Appt:** Prof N, Univ Tex, Houston

West Coast and Pacific

Adornato, Bruce T MD [N] - **Spec Exp:** Stroke; Neuropathy; Sleep Disorders/Apnea; **Hospital:** Stanford Univ Med Ctr; **Address:** 1101 Welch Rd, Ste C5, Palo Alto, CA 94304-1926; **Phone:** 650-324-4300; **Board Cert:** Internal Medicine 1975; Neurology 1978; **Med School:** UCSD 1972; **Resid:** Internal Medicine, UCSF-Moffitt Hosp 1974; Neurology, UCSF-Moffitt Hosp 1976; **Fellow:** Neurology, Natl Inst Hlth 1978; **Fac Appt:** Clin Prof N, Stanford Univ

Albers, Gregory W MD [N] - **Spec Exp:** Cerebrovascular Disease; Stroke; **Hospital:** Stanford Univ Med Ctr; **Address:** Stanford Univ Med Ctr, Dept Neurology, 300 Pasteur Drive, rm A301, Stanford, CA 94305; **Phone:** 650-723-4448; **Board Cert:** Neurology 1990; **Med School:** UCSD 1984; **Resid:** Neurology, Standford Univ Med Ctr 1988; **Fellow:** Stroke, Standford Univ Med Ctr 1989; **Fac Appt:** Assoc Prof N, Stanford Univ

Aminoff, Michael J MD [N] - **Spec Exp:** Movement Disorders; Parkinson's Disease; **Hospital:** UCSF Med Ctr; **Address:** 505 Parnassus Ave, Fl 3 - rm M348, San Francisco, CA 94143-0216; **Phone:** 415-353-2904; **Board Cert:** Neurology 2004; Clinical Neurophysiology 2000; **Med School:** England 1965; **Resid:** Internal Medicine, Univ London Hosps 1970; Neurology, Middlesex Hosp/Natl Hosp Queen Sq 1972; **Fac Appt:** Prof N, UCSF

Becker, Kyra J MD [N] - **Spec Exp:** Stroke/Cerebrovascular Disease; Neuro-Immunology; Stroke-Young Adults; **Hospital:** Harborview Med Ctr, Univ Wash Med Ctr; **Address:** Harborview Medical Ctr, Dept Neurology, 325 9th Ave, Box 359775, Seattle, WA 98104; **Phone:** 206-731-3251; **Board Cert:** Neurology 1995; **Med School:** Duke Univ 1989; **Resid:** Neurology, Johns Hopkins Hosp 1993; **Fellow:** Critical Care Neurology, Johns Hopkins Hosp 1995; Research, NIH-NINDS 1996; **Fac Appt:** Assoc Prof N, Univ Wash

Bourdette, Dennis MD [N] - **Spec Exp:** Multiple Sclerosis; Guillain-Barre Syndrome; Myasthenia Gravis; **Hospital:** OR Hlth & Sci Univ; **Address:** Oregon Hlth & Sci Univ, Dept Neurology, 3181 SW Sam Jackson Park Rd, MS UHS-42, Portland, OR 97239; **Phone:** 503-494-5759; **Board Cert:** Neurology 1985; **Med School:** UC Davis 1978; **Resid:** Neurology, Oregon Hlth Sci Univ Hosp 1982; **Fellow:** Neurological Immunology, VA Med Ctr 1985; **Fac Appt:** Prof N, Oregon Hlth Sci Univ

Bowen, James MD [N] - **Spec Exp:** Multiple Sclerosis; **Hospital:** Evergreen Hosp Med Ctr; **Address:** Evergreen Multiple Sclerosis Ctr, 12333 NE 130th Ln, Ste 225, Kirkland, WA 98034; **Phone:** 425-899-5350; **Board Cert:** Neurology 1990; **Med School:** Johns Hopkins Univ 1982; **Resid:** Internal Medicine, Univ Washington Med Ctr 1984; Neurology, Univ Washington Med Ctr 1987; **Fac Appt:** Asst Clin Prof N, Univ Wash

Chui, Helena Chang MD [N] - **Spec Exp:** Stroke; Dementia; Alzheimer's Disease; **Hospital:** USC Univ Hosp - R K Eamer Med Plz, Rancho Los Amigos Natl Rehab Ctr; **Address:** Health Care Consultation Center II, 1510 San Pablo St, Ste 618, Los Angeles, CA 90033; **Phone:** 323-442-7591; **Board Cert:** Neurology 1984; **Med School:** Johns Hopkins Univ 1977; **Resid:** Neurology, Univ Iowa Med Ctr 1981; **Fellow:** Behavioral Neurology, Univ Iowa Med Ctr 1979; **Fac Appt:** Prof N, USC Sch Med

Cloughesy, Timothy F MD [N] - **Spec Exp:** Neuro-Oncology; Seizure Disorders; Brain Tumors; **Hospital:** UCLA Med Ctr; **Address:** UCLA Neurological Services, 710 Westwood Plaza, Ste 1-230, Los Angeles, CA 90095; **Phone:** 310-825-5321; **Board Cert:** Neurology 1993; **Med School:** Tulane Univ 1987; **Resid:** Neurology, UCLA Med Ctr 1991; **Fellow:** Neuro-Oncology, Meml Sloan-Kettering Canc Ctr; **Fac Appt:** Clin Prof N, UCLA

Cummings, Jeffrey Lee MD [N] - **Spec Exp:** Neuro-Psychiatry; Alzheimer's Disease; Parkinson's Disease; **Hospital:** UCLA Med Ctr; **Address:** UCLA Med Ctr, Alzheimer's Disease Ctr, 10911 Weyburn Ave, Ste 200, Los Angeles, CA 90095-7226; **Phone:** 310-794-3665; **Board Cert:** Neurology 1979; **Med School:** Univ Wash 1974; **Resid:** Neurology, Boston Univ Sch Med 1978; **Fellow:** Behavioral Neurology and Psychiatry, Boston Univ Sch Med 1979; Neurological Pathology, The Natl Hosp 1980; **Fac Appt:** Assoc Prof N, UCLA

DeGiorgio, Christopher M MD [N] - **Spec Exp:** Epilepsy; Seizure Disorders; Neurocysticercosis; Parasitic Infections; **Hospital:** UCLA Med Ctr; **Address:** UCLA Med Ctr, Dept Neurology, 710 Westwood Plaza, Los Angeles, CA 90095; **Phone:** 310-825-5521; **Board Cert:** Neurology 1987; **Med School:** Loyola Univ-Stritch Sch Med 1981; **Resid:** Neurology, West Los Angeles VA Hosp 1985; **Fellow:** Epilepsy, UCLA Med Ctr 1987; **Fac Appt:** Assoc Prof N, UCLA

Dobkin, Bruce H MD [N] - **Spec Exp:** Stroke; Spinal Cord Injury; Neurologic Rehabilitation; **Hospital:** UCLA Med Ctr; **Address:** UCLA-RNRC, Dept Neuro, 710 Westwood Plaza, Ste 1-129, Los Angeles, CA 90095-1769; **Phone:** 310-794-1195; **Board Cert:** Neurology 1979; **Med School:** Temple Univ 1973; **Resid:** Neurology, UCLA Med Ctr 1977; **Fac Appt:** Prof N, UCLA

Engel, William King MD [N] - **Spec Exp:** Neuromuscular Disorders; **Hospital:** Good Samaritan Hosp - Los Angeles, USC Univ Hosp - R K Eamer Med Plz; **Address:** 637 S Lucas Ave Fl 3, Los Angeles, CA 90017; **Phone:** 213-975-9950; **Board Cert:** Neurology 1962; **Med School:** McGill Univ 1955; **Resid:** Neurology, Natl Inst Hlth 1959; Neurology, Natl Hosp 1960; **Fellow:** Neuromuscular Disease, Natl Inst Hlth 1961; **Fac Appt:** Prof N, USC Sch Med

Neurology

Engstrom, John W MD [N] - **Spec Exp:** Peripheral Nerve Disorders; Neuromuscular Disorders; Spinal Cord Diseases; **Hospital:** UCSF Med Ctr; **Address:** UCSF Med Ctr, Dept Neurology, 500 Parnassus Ave, M798, Box 0114, San Francisco, CA 94143; **Phone:** 415-353-2273; **Board Cert:** Internal Medicine 1984; Neurology 1991; Clinical Neurophysiology 2002; **Med School:** Stanford Univ 1981; **Resid:** Internal Medicine, Johns Hopkins Hosp 1984; Neurology, UCSF Med Ctr 1988; **Fellow:** Neurology, UCSF Med Ctr 1989; **Fac Appt:** Prof N, UCSF

Fisher, Mark MD [N] - **Spec Exp:** Stroke; Cerebrovascular Disease; **Hospital:** UC Irvine Med Ctr; **Address:** UC Irvine Med Ctr, Dept Neurology, 101 The City Drive S Bldg 55 - rm 121, Orange, CA 92868; **Phone:** 714-456-6808; **Board Cert:** Neurology 1981; Vascular Neurology 2005; **Med School:** Univ Cincinnati 1975; **Resid:** Neurology, UCLA-Wadsworth VA Hosp 1980; **Fac Appt:** Prof N, UC Irvine

Fisher, Robert S MD [N] - **Spec Exp:** Epilepsy/Seizure Disorders; **Hospital:** Stanford Univ Med Ctr; **Address:** 300 Pasteur Drive, rm A-343, Stanford, CA 94305-5235; **Phone:** 650-498-3056; **Board Cert:** Neurology 1983; Clinical Neurophysiology 2002; **Med School:** Stanford Univ 1977; **Resid:** Internal Medicine, Stanford Univ 1979; Neurology, Johns Hopkins Hosp 1982

Goodin, Douglas MD [N] - **Spec Exp:** Multiple Sclerosis; **Hospital:** UCSF Med Ctr, VA Med Ctr - San Francisco; **Address:** UCSF MS Ctr, 350 Parnassus Ave, Ste 908, San Francisco, CA 94117; **Phone:** 415-363-4490; **Board Cert:** Neurology 1985; **Med School:** UC Irvine 1978; **Resid:** Neurology, UCSF Med Ctr 1981; **Fac Appt:** Assoc Prof N, UCSF

Graves, Michael C MD [N] - **Spec Exp:** Amyotrophic Lateral Sclerosis (ALS); **Hospital:** UCLA Med Ctr; **Address:** UCLA Neurological Svcs, 300 Medical Plaza, Ste B200, Box 956975, Los Angeles, CA 90095-6975; **Phone:** 310-825-7266; **Board Cert:** Neurology 1977; **Med School:** Stanford Univ 1970; **Resid:** Internal Medicine, UCSD Med Ctr 1972; Neurology, Johns Hopkins Hosp 1975; **Fellow:** Rockefeller Univ Hosp; **Fac Appt:** Assoc Prof N, UCLA

Hauser, Stephen Lawrence MD [N] - **Spec Exp:** Multiple Sclerosis; Epilepsy; **Hospital:** UCSF Med Ctr; **Address:** UCSF MS Ctr, 400 Parnassus Ave Fl 8th, San Francisco, CA 94143-0164; **Phone:** 415-353-2069; **Board Cert:** Internal Medicine 1978; Neurology 1981; **Med School:** Harvard Med Sch 1975; **Resid:** Internal Medicine, NY Presby-Cornell 1977; Neurology, Mass Genl Hosp 1980; **Fellow:** Neurology, Harvard Univ 1980; **Fac Appt:** Prof N, UCSF

Henderson, Victor W MD [N] - **Spec Exp:** Alzheimer's Disease; Dementia; Memory Disorders; **Hospital:** Stanford Univ Med Ctr; **Address:** Stanford Univ Hosp, Dept Neurology, 300 Pasteur Drive, rm A343, Stanford, CA 94305-5235; **Phone:** 650-723-5184; **Board Cert:** Neurology 1981; **Med School:** Johns Hopkins Univ 1976; **Resid:** Internal Medicine, Duke Univ Med Ctr 1977; Neurology, Barnes Hosp- Wash Univ 1980; **Fellow:** Behavioral Neurology, Aphasia Rsch Ctr-Boston Univ 1981; **Fac Appt:** Prof N, Stanford Univ

Langston, J William MD [N] - **Spec Exp:** Parkinson's Disease; Movement Disorders; Tremor; **Hospital:** El Camino Hosp/Camino Hlthcare Sys; **Address:** The Parkinsons Institute, 1170 Morse Ave, Sunnyvale, CA 94089; **Phone:** 408-542-5633; **Board Cert:** Neurology 1986; **Med School:** Univ MO-Columbia Sch Med 1967; **Resid:** Neurology, Stanford Univ 1974; **Fellow:** Neurological Physiology, Stanford Univ

Lutsep, Helmi L MD [N] - **Spec Exp:** Stroke/Cerebrovascular Disease; **Hospital:** OR Hlth & Sci Univ; **Address:** Oregon Stroke Ctr, Oregon HSU, 3181 SW Sam Jackson Park Rd, CR-131, Portland, OR 97239; **Phone:** 503-494-7225; **Board Cert:** Neurology 1994; Vascular Neurology 2005; **Med School:** Mayo Med Sch 1988; **Resid:** Neurology, Mayo Clinic 1992; **Fellow:** Behavioral Neurology, UC Davis Med Ctr 1995; Stroke, Stanford Univ Med Ctr 1996; **Fac Appt:** Assoc Prof N, Oregon Hlth Sci Univ

Morrell, Martha J MD [N] - **Spec Exp:** Epilepsy; Epilepsy in Women; **Hospital:** Stanford Univ Med Ctr; **Address:** 300 Pasteur Drive, rm A-343, MC 5235, Stanford, CA 94305; **Phone:** 650-498-6648; **Board Cert:** Neurology 1989; Clinical Neurophysiology 2003; **Med School:** Stanford Univ 1984; **Resid:** Neurology, Hosp Univ Penn 1988; **Fellow:** Epilepsy, Graduate Hosp-Univ Penn 1990; **Fac Appt:** Prof N, Stanford Univ

Myers, Lawrence W MD [N] - **Spec Exp:** Multiple Sclerosis; Infectious & Demyelinating Diseases; **Hospital:** UCLA Med Ctr; **Address:** UCLA Neurological Services, 300 Medical Plaza, Ste B200, Los Angeles, CA 90095; **Phone:** 310-794-1195; **Board Cert:** Neurology 1975; **Med School:** SUNY Upstate Med Univ 1964; **Resid:** Neurology, UCLA Med Ctr 1971; **Fellow:** Neurology, UCLA Med Ctr 1973; **Fac Appt:** Prof N, UCLA

Nutt Jr, John G MD [N] - **Spec Exp:** Movement Disorders; Parkinson's Disease; **Hospital:** OR Hlth & Sci Univ; **Address:** Oregon Health Science Univ, OP-32, 3181 SW Sam Jackson Park Rd, Portland, OR 97239; **Phone:** 503-494-7230; **Board Cert:** Neurology 1978; **Med School:** Baylor Coll Med 1970; **Resid:** Neurology, Univ Wash Med Ctr 1976; **Fellow:** Pharmacology, Natl Inst Neuro Disorders /Stroke 1978; **Fac Appt:** Prof N, Oregon Hlth Sci Univ

Rosenbaum, Richard B MD [N] - **Spec Exp:** Neuromuscular Disorders; **Hospital:** OR Hlth & Sci Univ; **Address:** Oregon Clinic Neurology Department, 5050 NE Hoyt St, Ste 315, Portland, OR 97213-2975; **Phone:** 503-963-3100; **Board Cert:** Neurology 1979; Internal Medicine 1975; **Med School:** Harvard Med Sch 1971; **Resid:** Internal Medicine, Stanford Med Ctr 1974; Neurology, UCSF Med Ctr 1977; **Fac Appt:** Clin Prof N, Oregon Hlth Sci Univ

Smith, Wade S MD/PhD [N] - **Spec Exp:** Stroke; Pain-Back & Shoulder; **Hospital:** UCSF Med Ctr; **Address:** UCSF, Dept Neurology, 505 Parnassus Ave, Ste M830, Box 0114, San Francisco, CA 94143; **Phone:** 415-353-1489; **Board Cert:** Neurology 1996; **Med School:** Univ Wash 1989; **Resid:** Neurology, UCSF-Moffitt Hosp 1993; **Fellow:** Critical Care Medicine, UCSF-Moffitt Hosp 1994; **Fac Appt:** Asst Clin Prof N, UCSF

Spence, Alexander M MD [N] - **Spec Exp:** Neuro-Oncology; **Hospital:** Univ Wash Med Ctr; **Address:** Univ Wash, Dept Neur, 1959 NE Pacific St, Box 356465, Seattle, WA 98195-0001; **Phone:** 206-543-0252; **Board Cert:** Neurology 1971; **Med School:** Univ Chicago-Pritzker Sch Med 1965; **Resid:** Neurology, Chldns Hosp 1969; Neuropathology, Stanford Univ Med Ctr 1974; **Fac Appt:** Prof N, Univ Wash

Starr, Arnold MD [N] - **Spec Exp:** Auditory Neuropathy; Neurophysiology-Aging; Neurophysiology-Dementia; Hearing Disorders; **Hospital:** UC Irvine Med Ctr; **Address:** Dept Neurology, 1 Medical Plaza Drive, Irvine, CA 92697; **Phone:** 949-824-6088; **Board Cert:** Neurology 1970; Clinical Molecular Genetics 1992; **Med School:** NYU Sch Med 1957; **Resid:** Neurology, Boston City Hosp 1959; **Fellow:** Neurology, Natl Inst Hlth 1962; Clinical Neurophysiology, Inst Neurophysiology 1963; **Fac Appt:** Prof N, UC Irvine

Tanner, Caroline M MD/PhD [N] - **Spec Exp:** Parkinson's Disease; Movement Disorders; Dystonia; **Hospital:** Parkinson's Inst/Movement Disorders Trmt Ctr, The; **Address:** The Parkinson's Institute, 1170 Morse Ave, Sunnyvale, CA 94089; **Phone:** 408-734-2800; **Board Cert:** Neurology 1982; **Med School:** Loyola Univ-Stritch Sch Med 1976; **Resid:** Neurology, Rush-Presby-St Luke's Med Ctr 1980; **Fellow:** Neurological Pharmacology, Rush-Presby-St Luke's Med Ctr 1982

Tetrud, James W MD [N] - **Spec Exp:** Movement Disorders; Parkinson's Disease; Tremor; **Hospital:** Parkinson's Inst/Movement Disorders Trmt Ctr, The; **Address:** The Parkinson's Institute, 1170 Morse Ave, Sunnyvale, CA 94089; **Phone:** 408-734-2800; **Board Cert:** Neurology 1981; **Med School:** NYU Sch Med 1973; **Resid:** Internal Medicine, VetVA Med Ctr-West Los Angeles 1974; Neurology, VA Med Ctr-West Los Angeles 1978

Weiner, Leslie P MD [N] - **Spec Exp:** Multiple Sclerosis; Amyotrophic Lateral Sclerosis (ALS); **Hospital:** USC Univ Hosp - R K Eamer Med Plz, LAC & USC Med Ctr; **Address:** Keck Sch Med, Dept Neurology, 2025 Zonal Ave, RMR - 506, Los Angeles, CA 90089; **Phone:** 323-442-3020; **Board Cert:** Neurology 1969; **Med School:** Univ Cincinnati 1961; **Resid:** Neurology, Baltimore City Hosp 1963; Neurology, Johns Hopkins Hosp 1965; **Fellow:** Neurology, Johns Hopkins Hosp 1969; **Fac Appt:** Prof N, USC Sch Med

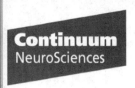

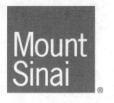

⌐ NewYork-Presbyterian
⌐ The University Hospital of Columbia and Cornell
NewYork-Presbyterian Neuroscience Centers

Affiliated with Columbia University College of Physicians and Surgeons and Weill Medical College of Cornell University

The Neurological Institute of New York at
NewYork-Presbyterian Hospital
Columbia University Medical Center
710 West 168th Street
New York, NY 10032

Weill Cornell Neuroscience Institute at
NewYork-Presbyterian Hospital
Weill Cornell Medical Center
525 East 68th Street
New York, NY 10021

OVERVIEW:

The NewYork-Presbyterian Neuroscience Centers are consistently ranked among the top providers of neurological services in the United States, according to *U.S. News & World Report.* The Centers provide the most innovative, up-to-date treatments to combat the full range of neurological disorders, including:

- Stroke and Cerebrovascular Services – Diagnoses and treatments of Stroke (brain attack), Aneurysms, and Arteriovenous Malformations (AVMs) by leading neurologists, neurosurgeons and interventional neuroradiologists.

- Epilepsy – Comprehensive Epilepsy Centers provide round-the-clock surveillance of adults and children in monitoring unit and functional brain mapping to identify source of a seizure and the most effective treatment.

- Pediatric Neurology/Neurosurgery – Expertise and state-of-the-art care tailored to special needs of children.

- Spinal Disorders – The Spine Center integrates physicians specializing in neurology, neurosurgery, neuroradiology, orthopedics, physiatry (rehabilitative medicine) and anesthesiology/pain management, as well as physical and occupational therapy.

- Neuro-Oncology – Therapeutic interventions include the full spectrum of traditional as well as new and innovative treatments including: surgery, radiation therapy, stereotactic radiosurgery immune therapy and complementary therapies.

- Neuro-Immunology – One of the country's largest Multiple Sclerosis treatment and research programs.

- Neuro-Infectious Diseases – Rapid diagnosis and a wide range of experts.

- Neuromuscular Diseases –Diagnosis and appropriate therapies for improving pain management and quality of life.

- Movement Disorders – Largest regional program offering latest protocols and Deep Brain Stimulation Surgery to reduce/eliminate tremors.

- Memory Disorders – A premier center offering early detection/diagnosis and standard and investigational treatments to help slow or reverse progression of symptoms.

Physician Referral: For physician referral or to learn more about NewYork-Presbyterian Neuroscience Centers call toll free **1-877-NYP-WELL** (1-877-697-9355) or visit our website at **www.nypneuro.org**

HIGHLIGHTS INCLUDE:

- Leading interventional neuroradiology service providing minimally invasive endovascular surgery including carotid stenting, arterial stenosis in the brain and neck, acute stroke, cerebral aneurysms, brain tumors, arteriovenus fistulas and AVMs.

- Participating in NIH-CREST randomized clinical trial evaluating carotid artery stenting as compared to carotid endarterectomy.

- Country's largest program for Parkinson's Disease and other movement disorders; provides deep brain stimulation surgery for controlling Parkinson's.

- Only multidisciplinary academic neurointensive care units in the greater New York area.

- One of 28 specialized Alzheimer's Disease Research Centers sponsored by the National Institute on Aging.

- Intraoperative MRI

NYU Medical Center

550 First Avenue (at 31st Street)
New York, NY 10016
Physician Referral:
(888)7-NYU-MED (888-769-8633)

www.nyumc.org

NEUROLOGY

Dedicated to exceptional patient care, advanced scientific research, and high-quality graduate education, the Department of Neurology at NYU Medical Center evaluates and treats children and adults with a broad spectrum of neurological diseases. Specialty groups within the department deliver integrated care to patients with stroke, cerebrovascular behavioral disorders and dementia, brain tumors, genetic and degenerative diseases, headache and pain syndromes, movement disorders including Parkinson's disease, multiple sclerosis, neuromuscular diseases, and enologic diseases of children. NYU Medical Center is home to the largest multiple sclerosis program in New York.

The clinical mission especially benefits from a 30-bed neurorehabilitation unit, a state-of-the-art neurophysiology laboratory, and a neurogenetics testing facility, each conducted under departmental auspices.

NYU COMPREHENSIVE EPILEPSY CENTER

Among the department's core programs is the NYU Comprehensive Epilepsy Center – the largest epilepsy program in the eastern United States. The center offers testing, evaluation, treatment, drug trials, alternative therapies, and surgical intervention for patients with all forms of epilepsy. Beyond control of seizures, the center aims to improve quality of life by addressing problems of social isolation and helping patients achieve gratification at school, at work, at home, and in their communities.

At present, medications adequately control about 75 percent of those who suffer from recurrent epileptic seizures. But when medications fail to bring these debilitating seizures under control, a patient may be a candidate for surgery.

In the past two decades, enormous strides in understanding, technology, and surgical techniques have made surgery a safe and effective option for patients with intractable seizure disorders. Key to surgical success is functional mapping, which involves testing the brain to make sure it is safe to remove the tissues that are responsible for the seizures. Using a variety of imaging technologies, including MRI, PET, and SPECT, NYU's epileptologists are able to visualize abnormal anatomy and physiology and define a surgical target. Video-EEG recording is the most important test of all for characterizing and localizing seizures.

The most common surgical procedure for epilepsy is temporal lobe

Brain diseases can cause intellectual impairments of profound complexity. The diagnosis and management of the cognitive disabilities accompanying traumatic brain injury or such diseases as stroke, Alzheimer's disease, epilepsy, and systemic illness often require an integrated approach. The Cognitive Neurology Program is an outpatient specialty clinic that serves adults with brain-based memory, perceptual, cognitive, or emotional impairments. Its specialists work closely with other branches of the Department of Neurology, and have close ties with Rusk Institute for Rehabilitation Medicine, where patients receive cognitive rehabilitation and speech therapy.

PHYSICIAN REFERRAL
1-888-7-NYU-MED
(1-888-769-8633)
WWW.NYUMC.ORG

702

PENN NEUROLOGY

Center for Excellence

The University of Pennsylvania's history of excellence in the treatment of neurological diseases dates back to the establishment of the Department of Neurology in 1874. *The Best Doctors in America®* lists more neurologists and neurosurgeons from the Hospital of the University of Pennsylvania than from any other hospital or medical center in the Philadelphia region. In addition, the Hospital of the University of Pennsylvania ranked highest in the region and among the top nationally for medical and surgical treatment of neurological disorders in *U.S.News & World Report.*

Excellence and Expertise

The Parkinson's Disease and Movement Disorders Center is committed to providing exceptional patient care, education, social support services and ongoing research into the causes of Parkinson's disease. Research is an important and ongoing mission of the Parkinson's Disease and Movement Disorders Center, which actively pursues the investigation of the disease as well as exploration of new medications. Five internationally recognized neurologists treat more than 2,000 patients annually. The team also consists of a neurosurgeon, a psychologist, a nurse, a social worker, a physical and occupational therapist and a speech pathologist providing a multidimensional approach to patient care.

The Multiple Sclerosis Center specializes in quality, state-of-the-art care with a personal approach. The comprehensive multidisciplinary team includes neurologists, nurse practitioners and specialists from other disciplines who are available for consultation in the management of genitourinary complications, spasticity and pain. Our program has existed for more than two decades, and basic research to investigate the origin and development of multiple sclerosis has taken place at Penn since 1963.

The Brain Tumor Center provides comprehensive evaluation, diagnosis and treatment to patients with brain and spinal tumors and other cancer-related neurological, central nervous system and peripheral nervous system problems. The multidisciplinary approach includes physicians and other health care providers from neurology, neurosurgery, radiation oncology, neuro-oncology, neuropathology, neuroradiology, rehabilitation medicine, neuro-psychiatry and social work.

Programs

- The Brain Tumor Center
- The Cognitive Neurology Program
- The Center for Brain Injury and Repair
- The Interventional Neuro Center
- The Memory Disorders Clinic
- Multiple Sclerosis Center
- Neuro Intensive Care
- The Neurogenetics Center
- Neuromuscular Disorders Program
- The Neuro-Ophthalmology Service
- The Neuropsychology Service
- The Neurovascular Center
- The Parkinson's Disease and Movement Disorders Center
- The Penn Epilepsy Center
- Penn Center for Sleep Disorders
- Penn Memory Center
- The Stroke Center

Locations

Hospital of the University of Pennsylvania

Pennsylvania Hospital

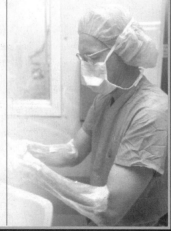

Sponsored Page

Nuclear Medicine

A nuclear medicine specialist employs the properties of radioactive atoms and molecules in the diagnosis and treatment of disease, and in research. Radiation detection and imaging instrument systems are used to detect disease as it changes the function and metabolism of normal cells, tissues and organs. A wide variety of diseases can be found in this way, usually before the structure of the organ involved by the disease can be seen to be abnormal by any other techniques. Early detection of coronary artery disease (including acute heart attack); early cancer detection and evaluation of the effect of tumor treatment; diagnosis of infection and inflammation anywhere in the body; and early detection of blood clot in the lungs, are all possible with these techniques. Unique forms of radioactive molecules can attack and kill cancer cells (e.g., lymphoma, thyroid cancer) or can relieve the severe pain of cancer that has spread to bone.

The nuclear medicine specialist has special knowledge in the biologic effects of radiation exposure, the fundamentals of the physical sciences and the principles and operation of radiation detection and imaging instrumentation systems.

Training required: Three years

Nuclear Medicine

Mid Atlantic

Alavi, Abass MD [NuM] - **Spec Exp:** Brain Tumors; Neurologic Imaging; PET Imaging-Brain; Brain Infections; **Hospital:** Hosp Univ Penn - UPHS (page 72), Chldns Hosp of Philadelphia, The; **Address:** Hosp Univ Penn, Div Nuclear Med, 3400 Spruce St, Donner Bldg rm 110, Philadelphia, PA 19104; **Phone:** 215-662-3014; **Board Cert:** Nuclear Medicine 1973; Internal Medicine 1972; **Med School:** Iran 1964; **Resid:** Internal Medicine, Albert Einstein Med Ctr/Phila VA Hosp 1969; Hematology, Hosp Univ Penn 1970; **Fellow:** Nuclear Medicine, Hosp Univ Penn 1973; **Fac Appt:** Prof Rad, Univ Pennsylvania

Carrasquillo, Jorge A MD [NuM] - **Spec Exp:** Radioimmunotherapy of Cancer; PET Imaging; **Hospital:** Meml Sloan Kettering Cancer Ctr; **Address:** Memorial Sloan Kettering Cancer Ctr, 1275 York Ave, New York, NY 10021; **Phone:** 212-639-2459; **Board Cert:** Internal Medicine 1977; Nuclear Medicine 1982; **Med School:** Univ Puerto Rico 1974; **Resid:** Internal Medicine, Univ Dist Hosp 1977; Nuclear Medicine, Univ Wash Hosp 1982

Freeman, Leonard M MD [NuM] - **Spec Exp:** Nuclear Oncology; Gastrointestinal Disorders; PET Imaging; CT Scan; **Hospital:** Montefiore Med Ctr; **Address:** 111 E 210th St, Bronx, NY 10467-2401; **Phone:** 718-920-6060; **Board Cert:** Diagnostic Radiology 1966; Nuclear Medicine 1972; Nuclear Radiology 1974; **Med School:** Ros Franklin Univ/Chicago Med Sch 1961; **Resid:** Diagnostic Radiology, Bronx Municipal Hosp 1965; **Fac Appt:** Prof NuM, Albert Einstein Coll Med

Goldsmith, Stanley J MD [NuM] - **Spec Exp:** Thyroid Cancer; Neuroendocrine Tumors; PET Imaging; Lymphoma; **Hospital:** NY-Presby Hosp/Weill Cornell (page 66); **Address:** 525 E 68th St Starr Bldg - rm 2-21, New York, NY 10021-9800; **Phone:** 212-746-4588; **Board Cert:** Internal Medicine 1969; Nuclear Medicine 1972; Endocrinology 1972; **Med School:** SUNY Downstate 1962; **Resid:** Internal Medicine, Kings Co Hosp 1967; **Fellow:** Endocrinology, Diabetes & Metabolism, Mt Sinai Hosp 1968; Nuclear Medicine, Bronx VA Hosp 1969; **Fac Appt:** Prof Rad, Cornell Univ-Weill Med Coll

Kramer, Elissa MD [NuM] - **Spec Exp:** Cancer Detection & Staging; Lymphedema Imaging; Radioimmunotherapy of Cancer; **Hospital:** NYU Med Ctr (page 67), Bellevue Hosp Ctr; **Address:** 560 1st Ave, rm HW231, New York, NY 10016-6402; **Phone:** 212-263-7410; **Board Cert:** Nuclear Medicine 1982; Diagnostic Radiology 1982; **Med School:** NYU Sch Med 1977; **Resid:** Diagnostic Radiology, Bellevue Hosp/NYU 1980; **Fellow:** Nuclear Medicine, Bellevue Hosp/NYU 1982; **Fac Appt:** Prof Rad, NYU Sch Med

Larson, Steven M MD [NuM] - **Spec Exp:** Thyroid Cancer; PET Imaging; **Hospital:** Meml Sloan Kettering Cancer Ctr; **Address:** Meml Sloan Kettering Cancer Ctr, Dept Nuclear Medicine, 1275 York Ave, Box 77, New York, NY 10021; **Phone:** 212-639-7373; **Board Cert:** Nuclear Medicine 1972; Internal Medicine 1973; **Med School:** Univ Wash 1965; **Resid:** Internal Medicine, Virginia Mason Hosp 1970; Nuclear Medicine, Natl Inst Hlth 1972; **Fac Appt:** Prof NuM, Cornell Univ-Weill Med Coll

Majd, Massoud MD [NuM] - **Spec Exp:** Pediatric Nuclear Medicine; **Hospital:** Chldns Natl Med Ctr; **Address:** 111 Michigan Ave NW, Washington, DC 20010-2978; **Phone:** 202-884-5088; **Board Cert:** Diagnostic Radiology 1972; Nuclear Medicine 1973; **Med School:** Iran 1960; **Resid:** Diagnostic Radiology, Georgetown Univ Hosp 1965; **Fac Appt:** Prof, Geo Wash Univ

Mountz, James M MD/PhD [NuM] - **Spec Exp:** Neurologic Imaging; Brain Imaging; **Hospital:** UPMC Presby, Pittsburgh; **Address:** UPMC Hlth Sys, Presby Univ Hosp, 200 Lothrop St, PET Facility, rm B 932, Pittsburgh, PA 15213; **Phone:** 412-647-0104; **Board Cert:** Diagnostic Radiology 1985; Nuclear Medicine 1986; **Med School:** Case West Res Univ 1981; **Resid:** Diagnostic Radiology, Univ Michigan Hosps 1985; **Fellow:** Nuclear Medicine, Univ Michigan Hosps 1986; **Fac Appt:** Prof Rad, Univ Pittsburgh

Neumann, Ronald D MD [NuM] - **Hospital:** Natl Inst of Hlth - Clin Ctr; **Address:** NIH Bldg 10, Box 1C-401, 10 Center Dr, MSC 1180, Bethesda, MD 20892-1180; **Phone:** 301-496-6455; **Board Cert:** Nuclear Medicine 1979; **Med School:** Yale Univ 1974; **Resid:** Pathology, Yale-New Haven Hosp 1977; Nuclear Medicine, Yale-New Haven Hosp 1979

Strashun, Arnold M MD [NuM] - **Spec Exp:** Neurologic Imaging; Nuclear Cardiology; Thyroid Disorders; PET Imaging-Brain; **Hospital:** SUNY Downstate Med Ctr, Kings County Hosp Ctr; **Address:** 450 Clarkson Ave Fl 2, Box 1210, Brooklyn, NY 11203; **Phone:** 718-245-3692; **Board Cert:** Internal Medicine 1977; Nuclear Medicine 1979; **Med School:** Baylor Coll Med 1974; **Resid:** Internal Medicine, Baylor Med Ctr 1975; Internal Medicine, Texas Med Ctr 1977; **Fellow:** Nuclear Medicine, VA Med Ctr 1978; Nuclear Medicine, Mount Sinai Hosp 1979; **Fac Appt:** Prof NuM, SUNY Downstate

Strauss, H William MD [NuM] - **Spec Exp:** Cardiac Imaging in Cancer Therapy; Thyroid Disorders; **Hospital:** Meml Sloan Kettering Cancer Ctr; **Address:** Meml Sloan Kettering Cancer Ctr, 1275 York Ave, S-212, Box 77, Nw York, NY 10021; **Phone:** 212-639-7238; **Board Cert:** Nuclear Medicine 1988; **Med School:** SUNY Downstate 1965; **Resid:** Internal Medicine, Downstate Med Ctr 1967; Internal Medicine, Bellevue Hosp 1968; **Fellow:** Nuclear Medicine, Johns Hopkins Hosp 1970; **Fac Appt:** Prof NuM, Cornell Univ-Weill Med Coll

Van Heertum, Ronald L MD [NuM] - **Spec Exp:** PET Imaging; PET Imaging in Alzheimer's Disease; **Hospital:** NY-Presby Hosp/Columbia (page 66); **Address:** NY Presby Hosp, Dept Radiology, 622 W 168th St, Ste HP 3-320, New York, NY 10032; **Phone:** 212-305-7132; **Board Cert:** Diagnostic Radiology 1971; Nuclear Medicine 1973; **Med School:** UMDNJ-NJ Med Sch, Newark 1966; **Resid:** Diagnostic Radiology, St Vincents Hosp 1970; **Fellow:** Diagnostic Radiology, St Vincents Hosp Med Ctr 1971; Nuclear Medicine, SUNY-Upstate Med Ctr 1975; **Fac Appt:** Prof Rad, Columbia P&S

Wahl, Richard L MD [NuM] - **Spec Exp:** Radioimmunotherapy of Cancer; PET Imaging; PET Imaging-Breast; **Hospital:** Johns Hopkins Hosp - Baltimore (page 61); **Address:** Johns Hopkins Hosp, Div Nuclear Medicine, 601 N Caroline St, JHOC-3223, Baltimore, MD 21287; **Phone:** 410-955-7226; **Board Cert:** Diagnostic Radiology 1982; Nuclear Radiology 1983; Nuclear Medicine 1985; **Med School:** Washington Univ, St Louis 1978; **Resid:** Diagnostic Radiology, Mallinckrodt Inst 1982; **Fellow:** Nuclear Radiology, Mallinckrodt Inst 1983; **Fac Appt:** Prof Rad, Johns Hopkins Univ

Southeast

Alazraki, Naomi P MD [NuM] - **Spec Exp:** Nuclear Oncology; **Hospital:** VA Med Ctr - Atlanta, Emory Univ Hosp; **Address:** VA Medical Ctr - Atlanta, 1670 Clairmont Rd, MC 115, Decatur, GA 30033; **Phone:** 404-728-7629; **Board Cert:** Nuclear Medicine 1972; Diagnostic Radiology 1972; **Med School:** Albert Einstein Coll Med 1966; **Resid:** Diagnostic Radiology, Univ Hospital 1971; **Fac Appt:** Prof DR, Emory Univ

Coleman, Ralph E MD [NuM] - **Spec Exp:** PET Imaging; SPECT Imaging; Tumor Imaging; **Hospital:** Duke Univ Med Ctr; **Address:** Duke Univ Med Ctr, Erwin Rd, Box 3949, Durham, NC 27710; **Phone:** 919-684-7244; **Board Cert:** Nuclear Medicine 1974; Internal Medicine 1973; **Med School:** Washington Univ, St Louis 1968; **Resid:** Internal Medicine, Royal Victoria Hosp 1970; **Fellow:** Nuclear Medicine, Mallinckrodt Inst Radiology 1974; **Fac Appt:** Prof DR, Duke Univ

Sandler, Martin P MD [NuM] - **Spec Exp:** Nuclear Endocrinology; Cardiac Imaging; PET Imaging; **Hospital:** Vanderbilt Univ Med Ctr; **Address:** Vanderbilt Univ Med Ctr, O-3300 MCN, 1161 21st Ave S, Nashville, TN 37232-2104; **Phone:** 615-322-0860; **Board Cert:** Nuclear Medicine 1983; **Med School:** South Africa 1972; **Resid:** Internal Medicine, Groote Schur Hosp; **Fellow:** Endocrinology, Diabetes & Metabolism, Vanderbilt Univ Med Ctr 1980; Nuclear Medicine, Vanderbilt Univ Med Ctr 1982; **Fac Appt:** Prof Rad, Vanderbilt Univ

Midwest

Neumann, Donald R MD [NuM] - **Spec Exp:** Nuclear Oncology; Nuclear Cardiology; **Hospital:** Cleveland Clin Fdn (page 57); **Address:** Cleveland Clinic, MFI Dept, 9500 Euclid Ave, MS Gb3, Cleveland, OH 44195; **Phone:** 216-444-2193; **Board Cert:** Diagnostic Radiology 1987; Nuclear Radiology 1990; **Med School:** Wright State Univ 1980; **Resid:** Diagnostic Radiology, Mount Sinai Med Ctr 1987; **Fellow:** Magnetic Resonance Imaging, Mount Sinai Med Ctr 1987

Siegel, Barry A MD [NuM] - **Spec Exp:** Cancer Detection & Staging; PET Imaging; **Hospital:** Barnes-Jewish Hosp, St Louis Chldns Hosp; **Address:** Mallinckrodt Inst of Radiology, 510 S Kingshighway Blvd, St Louis, MO 63110-1016; **Phone:** 314-362-2809; **Board Cert:** Diagnostic Radiology 1977; Nuclear Medicine 1973; Nuclear Radiology 1981; **Med School:** Washington Univ, St Louis 1969; **Resid:** Diagnostic Radiology, Mallinckrodt Inst Radiology 1973; **Fellow:** Nuclear Medicine, Mallinckrodt Inst Radiology 1973; **Fac Appt:** Prof, Washington Univ, St Louis

Silberstein, Edward B MD [NuM] - **Spec Exp:** Thyroid Cancer; Prostate Cancer Pain; Lymphoma; **Hospital:** Univ Hosp - Cincinnati, Jewish Hosp - Kenwood - Cincinnati; **Address:** Univ Hosp, 234 Goodman Ave, G026 Mont Reid Pav, Cincinnati, OH 45219-2364; **Phone:** 513-584-9032; **Board Cert:** Internal Medicine 1980; Nuclear Medicine 1972; Hematology 1972; Medical Oncology 1981; **Med School:** Harvard Med Sch 1962; **Resid:** Internal Medicine, Univ Cincinnati Hosp 1964; Internal Medicine, Univ Hosps-Case Western Reserve 1967; **Fellow:** Hematology, New England Med Ctr 1968; **Fac Appt:** Prof Emeritus Med, Univ Cincinnati

Southwest

Podoloff, Donald MD [NuM] - **Spec Exp:** Prostate Cancer; Breast Cancer; Lymphoma; **Hospital:** UT MD Anderson Cancer Ctr (page 71); **Address:** UT MD Anderson Cancer Ctr, 1515 Holcombe Blvd, Box 57, Houston, TX 77030; **Phone:** 713-745-1160; **Board Cert:** Diagnostic Radiology 1973; Nuclear Medicine 1975; Nuclear Radiology 1975; **Med School:** SUNY Downstate 1964; **Resid:** Internal Medicine, Beth Israel Med Ctr 1968; Diagnostic Radiology, Wilford Hall USAF Med Ctr 1973; **Fac Appt:** Prof Rad, Univ Tex, Houston

West Coast and Pacific

Dae, Michael W MD [NuM] - **Spec Exp:** Nuclear Cardiology; Pediatric Nuclear Medicine; **Hospital:** UCSF Med Ctr; **Address:** UCSF, Dept Radiology, 505 Parnassus Ave, Box 0252, San Francisco, CA 94143-0252; **Phone:** 415-353-1521; **Board Cert:** Pediatrics 1983; Nuclear Medicine 1984; **Med School:** Duke Univ 1976; **Resid:** Pediatrics, Chldns Hosp 1978; **Fellow:** Pediatric Cardiology, UCSF Med Ctr 1982; Nuclear Cardiology, UCSF Med Ctr 1983; **Fac Appt:** Prof, UCSF

Scheff, Alice M MD [NuM] - **Spec Exp:** PET Imaging; Thyroid Disorders; Neurologic Imaging; Cardiac Imaging; **Hospital:** Santa Clara Vly Med Ctr; **Address:** 751 S Bascom Ave, San Jose, CA 95128; **Phone:** 408-885-6970; **Board Cert:** Nuclear Medicine 1982; Nuclear Radiology 1983; **Med School:** Penn State Univ-Hershey Med Ctr 1978; **Resid:** Diagnostic Radiology, Penn State-Hershey Med Ctr 1982; Nuclear Medicine, Penn State-Hershey Med Ctr 1982; **Fellow:** Magnetic Resonance Imaging, Long Beach Meml Med Ctr 1993

Schelbert, Heinrich R MD/PhD [NuM] - **Spec Exp:** Nuclear Cardiology; Coronary Artery Disease; **Hospital:** UCLA Med Ctr; **Address:** B2-085J CHS, Box 95648, Los Angeles, CA 90095-6948; **Phone:** 310-825-3076; **Board Cert:** Nuclear Medicine 1976; **Med School:** Germany 1964; **Resid:** Internal Medicine, Mercy Med Ctr 1968; Cardiovascular Disease, Univ Duesseldorf Sch Med 1972; **Fellow:** Nuclear Medicine, UCSD 1973; Cardiovascular Disease, UCSD 1969

Waxman, Alan D MD [NuM] - **Spec Exp:** PET Imaging-Brain; Thyroid Cancer; Cancer Detection & Staging; **Hospital:** Cedars-Sinai Med Ctr, USC Univ Hosp - R K Eamer Med Plz; **Address:** Cedars-Sinai Med Ctr, Taper Imaging, 8700 Beverly Blvd, rm 1251, Los Angeles, CA 90048-1804; **Phone:** 310-423-2981; **Board Cert:** Nuclear Medicine 1972; **Med School:** USC Sch Med 1963; **Resid:** Nuclear Medicine, Wadsworth VA Hosp 1965; **Fellow:** Internal Medicine, Natl Inst Hlth 1967; **Fac Appt:** Clin Prof DR, USC Sch Med

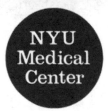

NYU Medical Center

550 First Avenue (at 31st Street)
New York, NY 10016
Physician Referral:
(888)7-NYU-MED (888-769-8633)
www.nyumc.org

NUCLEAR MEDICINE

Nuclear Medicine is an integral part of patient care, offering safe and cost-effective techniques to image the body physiology in order to provide diagnosis, management, treatment, and prevention of disease.

The Division of Nuclear Medicine in the Department of Radiology at NYU Medical Center is an integral component of its world-renowned multidisciplinary care. Offering the latest in technological expertise to medical specialties from pediatrics to cardiology to oncology to psychiatry, nuclear medicine truly cuts across all fields to deliver life-saving diagnoses. There are nearly one hundred different nuclear medicine imaging procedures available, with every major organ system imaged by Positron Emission Tomography (PET) scans.

PET scans are simple imaging studies that allow physicians to view the metabolic function of various organs and tissues in the body. Patients receive a simple injection in the arm of radiolabeled sugar. One hour later patients lie on the imaging table of the scanner while images are taken.

NYU Medical Center houses some of the most advanced radiology equipment in the world, including remote-controlled digital fluoroscopy and advanced digital subtraction angiography with three-dimensional capabilities. There are six high-field, large bore Magnetic Resonance Imaging (MRI) units, an open MRI unit, 10 Computed Tomography (CT) units (seven of which are the latest spiral units) and one of the largest concentration of Single-Photon Emission Computed Tomography (SPECT) gamma cameras in the United States. Over 90% of the reports at Tisch Hospital are dictated directly into the radiology information system using computerized voice recognition technology.

NYU MEDICAL CENTER

The NYU Department of Radiology has a large and distinguished faculty. In a recent year, department members wrote 146 peer-reviewed scientific papers as well as 11 complete texts and 55 chapters for other academic texts. Among the faculty are officers of national and regional scientific and professional societies, members of selective societies, and frequent peer reviewers and editors of professional journals.

PHYSICIAN REFERRAL
(888) 7-NYU-MED
(888-769-8633)
WWW.MYUMC.ORG

Obstetrics & Gynecology

An obstetrician/gynecologist possesses special knowledge, skills and professional capability in the medical and surgical care of the female reproductive system and associated disorders. This physician serves as a consultant to other physicians and as a primary physician for women.

Training Required: Four years *plus* two years in clinical practice before certification is complete.

Obstetrics & Gynecology

New England

Laufer, Marc MD [ObG] - **Spec Exp:** Adolescent Gynecology; Endometriosis; Congenital Anomalies-Gynecologic; Pediatric Gynecology; **Hospital:** Children's Hospital - Boston, Brigham & Women's Hosp; **Address:** Chldns Hosp, Dept of Ped Gynecology, 300 Longwood Ave, Boston, MA 03115; **Phone:** 617-355-5785; **Board Cert:** Obstetrics & Gynecology 2005; **Med School:** Univ Pennsylvania 1986; **Resid:** Obstetrics & Gynecology, Brigham & Womens Hosp/Mass Genl Hosp 1990; **Fellow:** Reproductive Endocrinology, Brigham & Womens Hosp/Chldns Hosp 1992; Gynecology, Chldns Hosp 1992; **Fac Appt:** Assoc Prof ObG, Harvard Med Sch

Noller, Kenneth L MD [ObG] - **Spec Exp:** DES-Exposed Females; Gynecology Only; Cervical Cancer; **Hospital:** Tufts-New England Med Ctr; **Address:** Tufts New England Med Ctr, Box 324, 750 Washington St, Boston, MA 02111; **Phone:** 617-636-2382; **Board Cert:** Obstetrics & Gynecology 1991; **Med School:** Creighton Univ 1970; **Resid:** Obstetrics & Gynecology, Mayo Clinic 1974; **Fac Appt:** Prof ObG, Univ Mass Sch Med

Nour, Nawal M MD [ObG] - **Spec Exp:** Female Genital Cutting (FGC) Education; **Hospital:** Brigham & Women's Hosp; **Address:** Brigham & Women's Hosp, Dept Ob/Gyn, 75 Francis St, Connors Ctr, 3rd Fl, Boston, MA 02115; **Phone:** 617-732-4740; **Board Cert:** Obstetrics & Gynecology 2002; **Med School:** Harvard Med Sch 1994; **Resid:** Obstetrics & Gynecology, Brgham & Women's Hosp 1998

Reilly, Raymond J MD [ObG] - **Spec Exp:** Gynecologic Surgery; **Hospital:** Brigham & Women's Hosp; **Address:** 1 Brookline Pl, Ste 522, Brookline, MA 02445; **Phone:** 617-731-3400; **Board Cert:** Obstetrics & Gynecology 1969; **Med School:** Ireland 1958; **Resid:** Obstetrics & Gynecology, Johns Hopkins Hosp 1964; **Fac Appt:** Assoc Prof ObG, Harvard Med Sch

Mid Atlantic

Amstey, Marvin S MD [ObG] - **Spec Exp:** Infectious Disease; Vulvar Disease/Cancer; **Hospital:** Park Ridge Hosp, Highland Hosp - Rochester; **Address:** 995 Sen Keating Blvd E Bldg - Ste 340, Rochester, NY 14618; **Phone:** 585-368-4455; **Board Cert:** Obstetrics & Gynecology 2003; **Med School:** Duke Univ 1964; **Resid:** Obstetrics & Gynecology, Strong Meml Hosp 1971; **Fellow:** Viral Immunology, Natl Inst Hlth 1967; **Fac Appt:** Prof Emeritus ObG, Univ Rochester

Baxi, Laxmi Vibhakar MD [ObG] - **Spec Exp:** Pregnancy-High Risk; Miscarriage-Recurrent; Multiple Gestation; **Hospital:** NY-Presby Hosp/Columbia (page 66); **Address:** Columbia Presby Med Ctr, Dept OB/GYN, 161 Ft Washington Ave Fl 3 - Ste 408, New York, NY 10032-3713; **Phone:** 212-305-5899; **Board Cert:** Obstetrics & Gynecology 1995; Maternal & Fetal Medicine 1995; **Med School:** India 1963; **Resid:** Obstetrics & Gynecology, King Edward M. Hosp 1969; Obstetrics & Gynecology, St Peter's Med Ctr-Rutgers Univ NJ 1977; **Fellow:** Maternal & Fetal Medicine, Columbia-Presby Med Ctr 1979; **Fac Appt:** Prof ObG, Columbia P&S

Brodman, Michael MD [ObG] - **Spec Exp:** Incontinence-Female; Laparoscopic Surgery; Pelvic Organ Prolapse Repair; Uro-Gynecology; **Hospital:** Mount Sinai Med Ctr; **Address:** Dept of Obstetrics & Gynecology, 5 E 98th St, Box 1170, New York, NY 10029; **Phone:** 212-241-7952; **Board Cert:** Obstetrics & Gynecology 2005; **Med School:** Mount Sinai Sch Med 1982; **Resid:** Obstetrics & Gynecology, Mount Sinai Hosp 1986; **Fellow:** Pelvic Surgery, Mount Sinai Hosp 1987; **Fac Appt:** Assoc Prof ObG, Mount Sinai Sch Med

DeCherney, Alan Hersh MD [ObG] - **Spec Exp:** Infertility-Female; Reproductive Endocrinology; **Hospital:** Natl Inst of Hlth - Clin Ctr; **Address:** NICHD, NIH, Bldg 10, CRC, 1 East, 10 Center Drive, rm 1-3140, MS 1109, Bethesda, MD 20892-5800; **Phone:** 310-770-9667; **Board Cert:** Obstetrics & Gynecology 1989; Reproductive Endocrinology 1979; **Med School:** Temple Univ 1967; **Resid:** Obstetrics & Gynecology, Hosp Univ Penn 1972; **Fac Appt:** Prof ObG, UCLA

Divon, Michael Y MD [ObG] - **Spec Exp:** Maternal & Fetal Medicine; Pregnancy-High Risk; Ultrasound; **Hospital:** Lenox Hill Hosp (page 62); **Address:** 130 E 77th St Fl 2 Black Hall, New York, NY 10021-1851; **Phone:** 212-434-2160; **Board Cert:** Obstetrics & Gynecology 2003; **Med School:** Israel 1979; **Resid:** Obstetrics & Gynecology, Rambam Med Ctr 1983; **Fellow:** Perinatal Medicine, USC Med CTr 1985; Perinatal Medicine, Montefiore Med Ctr 1989; **Fac Appt:** Clin Prof ObG, Albert Einstein Coll Med

Evans, Mark I MD [ObG] - **Spec Exp:** Prenatal Diagnosis; Multiple Gestation; Fetal Therapy; Reproductive Genetics; **Hospital:** Mount Sinai Med Ctr; **Address:** Comprehensive Genetics, 131 E 65th St, New York, NY 10021; **Phone:** 212-744-2590; **Board Cert:** Obstetrics & Gynecology 2005; Clinical Genetics 1984; **Med School:** SUNY Downstate 1978; **Resid:** Obstetrics & Gynecology, Lying-In Hosp 1982; **Fellow:** Clinical Genetics, Natl Inst Hlth 1984; **Fac Appt:** Prof ObG, Mount Sinai Sch Med

Goldstein, Martin MD [ObG] - **Spec Exp:** Incontinence; Laparoscopic Surgery; Uterine Fibroids; Pelvic Organ Prolapse Repair; **Hospital:** Mount Sinai Med Ctr; **Address:** 40 E 84th St, New York, NY 10128-1314; **Phone:** 212-472-6500; **Board Cert:** Obstetrics & Gynecology 1980; **Med School:** SUNY Hlth Sci Ctr 1966; **Resid:** Obstetrics & Gynecology, Mount Sinai Hosp 1971; **Fac Appt:** Assoc Clin Prof ObG, Mount Sinai Sch Med

Lucente, Vincent R MD [ObG] - **Spec Exp:** Uro-Gynecology; Pelvic Floor Reconstruction; Incontinence-Female; **Hospital:** St Luke's Hosp - Bethlehem, Abington Mem Hosp; **Address:** Park Professional Bldg, 2200 W Hamilton St, Ste 111, Allentown, PA 18104; **Phone:** 610-435-9575; **Board Cert:** Obstetrics & Gynecology 2005; **Med School:** SUNY Stony Brook 1985; **Resid:** Obstetrics & Gynecology, N Shore Univ Hosp 1989; **Fellow:** Uro-Gynecology, Methodist Hosp 1990; **Fac Appt:** Clin Prof ObG, Temple Univ

Minkoff, Howard L MD [ObG] - **Spec Exp:** AIDS/HIV in Pregnancy; **Hospital:** Maimonides Med Ctr (page 63); **Address:** Maimonides Med Ctr, Dept Ob-Gyn, 4802 Tenth Ave, Brooklyn, NY 11219; **Phone:** 718-283-7973; **Board Cert:** Obstetrics & Gynecology 1995; Maternal & Fetal Medicine 1995; **Med School:** Penn State Univ-Hershey Med Ctr 1975; **Resid:** Obstetrics & Gynecology, Kings Co Hosp Ctr 1979; Obstetrics & Gynecology, SUNY Hlth Sci Ctr 1981; **Fellow:** Maternal & Fetal Medicine, Kings Co Hosp Ctr 1981; **Fac Appt:** Prof ObG, SUNY Hlth Sci Ctr

Witter, Frank R MD [ObG] - **Spec Exp:** Pregnancy-High Risk; Multiple Gestation; Lupus/SLE in Pregnancy; **Hospital:** Johns Hopkins Hosp - Baltimore (page 61); **Address:** 600 N Wolfe St, Nelson 2170, Baltimore, MD 21287; **Phone:** 410-955-1421; **Board Cert:** Obstetrics & Gynecology 1997; Maternal & Fetal Medicine 1997; **Med School:** Univ Chicago-Pritzker Sch Med 1976; **Resid:** Obstetrics & Gynecology, Johns Hopkins Hosp 1980; **Fellow:** Maternal & Fetal Medicine, Johns Hopkins Hosp 1982; Clinical Pharmacology, Johns Hopkins Hosp 1984; **Fac Appt:** Prof ObG, Johns Hopkins Univ

Young, Bruce MD [ObG] - **Spec Exp:** Infertility; Minimally Invasive Surgery; Twin to Twin Transfusion Syndrome (TTTS); **Hospital:** NYU Med Ctr (page 67); **Address:** 530 1st Ave, HCC-5th Fl, Ste 5G, New York, NY 10016; **Phone:** 212-263-6359; **Board Cert:** Obstetrics & Gynecology 1970; Maternal & Fetal Medicine 1975; **Med School:** NYU Sch Med 1963; **Resid:** Obstetrics & Gynecology, New York Univ Med Ctr 1968; **Fellow:** Reproductive Endocrinology, New York Univ Med Ctr 1968; **Fac Appt:** Prof ObG, NYU Sch Med

Southeast

Duff, W Patrick MD [ObG] - **Spec Exp:** Pregnancy-High Risk; Infectious Disease; Maternal & Fetal Medicine; **Hospital:** Shands Hlthcre at Univ of FL; **Address:** Magnolia Park Women's Health, 3951 NW 48th Terr, Ste 101, Gainesville, FL 32606; **Phone:** 352-265-6200; **Board Cert:** Obstetrics & Gynecology 2003; Maternal & Fetal Medicine 2003; **Med School:** Georgetown Univ 1974; **Resid:** Obstetrics & Gynecology, Walter Reed Med Ctr 1978; **Fellow:** Maternal & Fetal Medicine, UT - San Antonio 1983; **Fac Appt:** Prof ObG, Univ S Fla Coll Med

Filip, Stanley John MD [ObG] - **Spec Exp:** Uterine Fibroids; Menopause Problems; Hysterectomy Alternatives; Endometriosis; **Hospital:** Duke Univ Med Ctr, Durham Regional Hosp; **Address:** 3116 N Duke St, Durham, NC 27704; **Phone:** 919-684-2471; **Board Cert:** Obstetrics & Gynecology 1985; **Med School:** Mount Sinai Sch Med 1979; **Resid:** Obstetrics & Gynecology, Univ Colo Hlth Scis Ctr 1983

Gluck, Paul MD [ObG] - **Spec Exp:** Gynecology; Menopause Problems; Depression in Women; **Hospital:** Baptist Hosp of Miami; **Address:** 8950 N Kendall Drive, Ste 507, Miami, FL 33176-2132; **Phone:** 305-279-3773; **Board Cert:** Obstetrics & Gynecology 2005; **Med School:** NYU Sch Med 1972; **Resid:** Obstetrics & Gynecology, Jackson Meml Hosp 1976; **Fac Appt:** Assoc Clin Prof ObG, Univ Miami Sch Med

Hager, W David MD [ObG] - **Spec Exp:** Gynecologic Infectious Disease; Sexually Transmitted Diseases; **Hospital:** Central Baptist Hosp; **Address:** 1720 Nicholasville Rd, Lexington, KY 40503; **Phone:** 859-278-0363; **Board Cert:** Obstetrics & Gynecology 1993; **Med School:** Univ KY Coll Med 1972; **Resid:** Obstetrics & Gynecology, Univ Kentucky Med Ctr 1976; **Fac Appt:** Prof ObG, Univ KY Coll Med

Kovac, S Robert MD [ObG] - **Spec Exp:** Pelvic Reconstruction; Vaginal Hysterectomy; **Hospital:** Emory Univ Hosp, Grady Hlth Sys; **Address:** Emory Clinic A, Dept Ob/Gyn, 1365 Clifton Rd NE Fl 4, Atlanta, GA 30322; **Phone:** 404-778-3401; **Board Cert:** Obstetrics & Gynecology 1979; **Med School:** Univ MO-Columbia Sch Med 1964; **Resid:** Obstetrics & Gynecology, Barnes JewishHosp 1970; **Fellow:** Reconstructive Pelvic Surgery, Barnes Hosp 1969; **Fac Appt:** Prof ObG, Emory Univ

Lipscomb, Gary H MD [ObG] - **Spec Exp:** Pregnancy-High Risk; Cervical Cancer; Uro-Gynecology; **Hospital:** Regional Med Ctr - Memphis, Baptist Memorial Hospital - Memphis; **Address:** Memphis Medical Ctr, 880 Madison Ave, Ste 3E01, Memphis, TN 38103-3409; **Phone:** 901-448-6632; **Board Cert:** Obstetrics & Gynecology 1997; **Med School:** Univ Tenn Coll Med, Memphis 1981; **Resid:** Obstetrics & Gynecology, Univ Tenn Affil Hosps 1985; **Fac Appt:** Prof ObG, Univ Tenn Coll Med, Memphis

Morgan, Linda S MD [ObG] - **Spec Exp:** Gynecologic Cancer; Women's Health; **Hospital:** Shands Hlthcre at Univ of FL; **Address:** Univ of Florida, PO Box 100294, Dept Ob/Gyn, Gainesville, FL 32610; **Phone:** 352-392-4161; **Board Cert:** Obstetrics & Gynecology 2004; Gynecologic Oncology 2004; **Med School:** Med Coll PA Hahnemann 1975; **Resid:** Obstetrics & Gynecology, Shands Hosp 1979; **Fellow:** Gynecologic Oncology, Mass Genl Hosp 1981; **Fac Appt:** Prof ObG, Univ Fla Coll Med

Sanz, Luis E MD [ObG] - **Spec Exp:** Uro-Gynecology; Hysteroscopic Surgery; Vaginal Reconstructive Surgery; Pelvic Reconstruction; **Hospital:** Virginia Hosp Ctr - Arlington; **Address:** 1625 N George Mason Drive, Ste 475, Arlington, VA 22205; **Phone:** 703-717-4000; **Board Cert:** Obstetrics & Gynecology 1982; **Med School:** Georgetown Univ 1976; **Resid:** Obstetrics & Gynecology, Georgetown Univ Hosp 1980; **Fellow:** Advanced Pelvic Surgery, Georgetown Univ 1982; **Fac Appt:** Prof ObG, Georgetown Univ

Simpson, Joe Leigh MD [ObG] - **Spec Exp:** Prenatal Diagnosis; Ovarian Failure; Infertility/Genetics; **Hospital:** Mount Sinai Med Ctr - Miami; **Address:** Florida International University, University Park HLS 693, 11200 SW H St, Miami, FL 33199; **Phone:** 305-348-0613; **Board Cert:** Obstetrics & Gynecology 2004; Clinical Genetics 1982; **Med School:** Duke Univ 1968; **Resid:** Obstetrics & Gynecology, NY Hosp-Cornell Med Ctr 1973; **Fac Appt:** Prof ObG, Baylor Coll Med

Steege, John F MD [ObG] - **Spec Exp:** Laparoscopic Surgery; Endometriosis; Pain-Pelvic & Perineal; Gynecologic Surgery; **Hospital:** Univ NC Hosps; **Address:** Univ NC-Dept OB/GYN, 7570, Chapel Hill, NC 27599-7570; **Phone:** 919-966-7764; **Board Cert:** Obstetrics & Gynecology 1978; **Med School:** Yale Univ 1972; **Resid:** Obstetrics & Gynecology, Yale - New Haven Hosp 1976; **Fac Appt:** Prof ObG, Univ NC Sch Med

Underwood, Paul MD [ObG] - **Spec Exp:** Pelvic Reconstruction; Women's Health over age 40; **Hospital:** MUSC Med Ctr; **Address:** 1280 Johnnie Dodds Blvd, Ste 200, Mt Pleasant, SC 29464; **Phone:** 843-881-1312; **Board Cert:** Obstetrics & Gynecology 1989; Gynecologic Oncology 1974; **Med School:** Med Univ SC 1959; **Resid:** Obstetrics & Gynecology, Med University SC 1964; **Fellow:** Gynecologic Oncology, MD Anderson Hosp 1967; **Fac Appt:** Prof ObG, Med Univ SC

Midwest

De Lia, Julian E MD [ObG] - **Spec Exp:** Fetal Surgery; Twin to Twin Transfusion Syndrome (TTTS); **Hospital:** Wheaton Franciscan Hlthcare-St Joseph-Milwaukee; **Address:** TTTS Inst, WFHC-St Joseph, 5000 W Chambers St, Milwaukee, WI 53210-1688; **Phone:** 414-447-3535; **Board Cert:** Obstetrics & Gynecology 1993; **Med School:** UMDNJ-NJ Med Sch, Newark 1972; **Resid:** Obstetrics & Gynecology, St Barnabas Med Ctar 1976; **Fac Appt:** Assoc Prof ObG, Med Coll Wisc

DeLancey, John O MD [ObG] - **Spec Exp:** Uro-Gynecology; Incontinence; Pelvic Organ Prolapse Repair; **Hospital:** Univ Michigan Hlth Sys; **Address:** Univ Mich Med Ctr, Dept ObGyn, 1500 E Med Ctr Drive, rm L4100-WH, Ann Arbor, MI 48109-0276; **Phone:** 734-763-6295; **Board Cert:** Obstetrics & Gynecology 1997; **Med School:** Univ Mich Med Sch 1977; **Resid:** Obstetrics & Gynecology, Univ Mich Med Ctr 1981; **Fac Appt:** Prof ObG, Univ Mich Med Sch

Elias, Sherman MD [ObG] - **Spec Exp:** Prenatal Diagnosis; Reproductive Genetics; **Hospital:** Northwestern Meml Hosp; **Address:** Prentice Women's Hosp, 333 E Superior, Ste 490, Chicago, IL 60611-3095; **Phone:** 312-926-6622; **Board Cert:** Obstetrics & Gynecology 1996; Clinical Genetics 2004; **Med School:** Univ KY Coll Med 1972; **Resid:** Obstetrics & Gynecology, Michael Reese Hosp 1973; Obstetrics & Gynecology, Univ Louisville Hosp 1976; **Fellow:** Clinical Genetics, Yale Univ 1975; Clinical Genetics, Northwestern Univ 1978; **Fac Appt:** Prof ObG, Northwestern Univ

Gonik, Bernard MD [ObG] - **Spec Exp:** Maternal & Fetal Medicine; Infectious Disease; Prenatal Diagnosis; **Hospital:** Sinai-Grace Hosp - Detroit; **Address:** 6071 W Outer Drive, Detroit, MI 48235-2624; **Phone:** 313-966-1880; **Board Cert:** Obstetrics & Gynecology 1995; Maternal & Fetal Medicine 1995; **Med School:** Mich State Univ 1978; **Resid:** Obstetrics & Gynecology, Univ Texas Med Sch 1982; **Fellow:** Maternal & Fetal Medicine, Univ Texas Med Sch 1985; **Fac Appt:** Prof ObG, Wayne State Univ

Karram, Mickey M MD [ObG] - **Spec Exp:** Uro-Gynecology; Pelvic Floor Reconstruction; Incontinence-Female; **Hospital:** Good Samaritan Hosp - Cincinnati; **Address:** Good Samaritan Hosp, 375 Dixmyth Ave, Cincinnati, OH 45220; **Phone:** 513-872-2466; **Board Cert:** Obstetrics & Gynecology 1998; **Med School:** Egypt 1982; **Resid:** Obstetrics & Gynecology, Good Samaritan Hosp 1985; **Fellow:** Gynecologic Urology, Harbor Hosp-UCLA 1986; **Fac Appt:** Prof ObG, Univ Cincinnati

Levine, Elliot MD [ObG] - **Spec Exp:** Sexually Transmitted Diseases; Sexual Dysfunction; Vulvar Disease; **Hospital:** Adv Illinois Masonic Med Ctr, Adv Luth Genl Hosp; **Address:** 2825 N Halsted St, Chicago, IL 60657; **Phone:** 773-472-0812; **Board Cert:** Obstetrics & Gynecology 1984; **Med School:** Ros Franklin Univ/Chicago Med Sch 1978; **Resid:** Obstetrics & Gynecology, Illinois Masonic Med Ctr 1982; **Fac Appt:** Asst Prof ObG, Rush Med Coll

Merritt, Diane MD [ObG] - **Spec Exp:** Adolescent Gynecology; Pediatric Gynecology; Endometriosis; **Hospital:** Barnes-Jewish Hosp, St Louis Chldns Hosp; **Address:** Washington University, School of Medicine, 660 S Euclid, St. Louis, MO 63110; **Phone:** 314-362-4211; **Board Cert:** Obstetrics & Gynecology 1984; **Med School:** NYU Sch Med 1975; **Resid:** Surgery, Barnes Hosp-Wash Univ 1977; Obstetrics & Gynecology, Barnes Hosp-Wash Univ 1980; **Fac Appt:** Prof ObG, Washington Univ, St Louis

Muraskas, Erik MD [ObG] - **Spec Exp:** Lupus/SLE in Pregnancy; Heart Disease in Pregnancy; **Hospital:** Loyola Univ Med Ctr; **Address:** 2160 S 1st Ave, Maywood, IL 60153; **Phone:** 708-216-4033; **Board Cert:** Obstetrics & Gynecology 2003; **Med School:** Loyola Univ-Stritch Sch Med 1981; **Resid:** Obstetrics & Gynecology, Loyola Univ-Stritch Sch Med 1985; **Fac Appt:** Assoc Prof ObG, Loyola Univ-Stritch Sch Med

Schreiber, James MD [ObG] - **Spec Exp:** Menstrual Disorders; Infertility; Pregnancy-High Risk; **Hospital:** Barnes-Jewish Hosp; **Address:** 4911 Barnes Hospital Plaza, Box 8064, St Louis, MO 63110; **Phone:** 314-362-4211; **Board Cert:** Obstetrics & Gynecology 1991; Reproductive Endocrinology 1982; **Med School:** Johns Hopkins Univ 1972; **Resid:** Obstetrics & Gynecology, USC-LAC Hosp 1974; Obstetrics & Gynecology, USC-LAC Hosp 1978; **Fellow:** Reproductive Endocrinology, Natl Inst Hlth 1976; **Fac Appt:** Prof ObG, Washington Univ, St Louis

Shulman, Lee MD [ObG] - **Spec Exp:** Prenatal Diagnosis; Breast Cancer Genetics; Ovarian Cancer Genetics; **Hospital:** Northwestern Meml Hosp, Rush Univ Med Ctr; **Address:** Northwestern Univ, Dept Ob/Gyn, 333 E Superior St, Ste 484, Chicago, IL 60611; **Phone:** 312-926-6627; **Board Cert:** Obstetrics & Gynecology 1999; Clinical Genetics 1990; **Med School:** Cornell Univ-Weill Med Coll 1983; **Resid:** Obstetrics & Gynecology, North Shore Univ Hosp 1987; **Fellow:** Reproductive Genetics, Univ Tenn Med Ctr 1989; **Fac Appt:** Prof ObG, Northwestern Univ

Walters, Mark D MD [ObG] - **Spec Exp:** Uro-Gynecology; Vaginal Reconstructive Surgery; Incontinence-Female; Pelvic Organ Proplapse Repair; **Hospital:** Cleveland Clin Fdn (page 57); **Address:** 9500 Euclid Ave, MC A81, Cleveland, OH 44195-0001; **Phone:** 216-445-6586; **Board Cert:** Obstetrics & Gynecology 1996; **Med School:** Ohio State Univ 1980; **Resid:** Obstetrics & Gynecology, New England Med Ctr 1984

Great Plains and Mountains

Bury, Robert MD [ObG] - **Spec Exp:** Infertility; Laser Surgery; Microsurgery; **Hospital:** St. Alexius Med Ctr - Bismarck; **Address:** Mid Dakota Clinic-Center for Women, PO Box 5538, Bismarck, ND 58506; **Phone:** 701-530-6000; **Board Cert:** Obstetrics & Gynecology 1981; **Med School:** Baylor Coll Med 1975; **Resid:** Obstetrics & Gynecology, Baylor Affil Hosp 1979; **Fac Appt:** Clin Prof ObG, Univ ND Sch Med

Southwest

Carr, Bruce MD [ObG] - **Spec Exp:** Infertility-Female; **Hospital:** UT Southwestern Med Ctr - Dallas, Parkland Meml Hosp - Dallas; **Address:** 5323 Harry Hines Blvd, rm U5.104, Dallas, TX 75390-8865; **Phone:** 214-648-8846; **Board Cert:** Obstetrics & Gynecology 2000; Reproductive Endocrinology 2000; **Med School:** Univ Mich Med Sch 1971; **Resid:** Obstetrics & Gynecology, Parkland Meml Hosp 1975; **Fellow:** Reproductive Endocrinology, Univ Texas SW Med Ctr 1980; **Fac Appt:** Prof ObG, Univ Tex SW, Dallas

Faro, Sebastian MD/PhD [ObG] - **Spec Exp:** Infections in Pregnancy; Infectious Disease-Gynecologic; Sexually Transmitted Diseases; **Hospital:** Woman's Hosp TX, The, St Luke's Episcopal Hosp - Houston; **Address:** 7400 Fannin, Ste 840, Houston, TX 77054; **Phone:** 713-799-9091; **Board Cert:** Obstetrics & Gynecology 1991; **Med School:** Creighton Univ 1975; **Resid:** Obstetrics & Gynecology, Creighton Univ 1978; **Fac Appt:** Clin Prof ObG, Univ Tex, Houston

West Coast and Pacific

Eschenbach, David A MD [ObG] - **Spec Exp:** Gynecologic Surgery; Infectious Disease; Vaginal Disorders; **Hospital:** Univ Wash Med Ctr; **Address:** Univ Washington Women's Health Care, 4245 Roosevelt Way NE, Box 354765, Seattle, WA 98105-6920; **Phone:** 206-598-5500; **Board Cert:** Obstetrics & Gynecology 1975; **Med School:** Univ Wisc 1968; **Resid:** Obstetrics & Gynecology, Univ Wash Hosp 1973; **Fellow:** Infectious Disease, Univ Wash Hosp 1974; **Fac Appt:** Prof ObG, Univ Wash

Sweet, Richard L MD [ObG] - **Spec Exp:** Sexually Transmitted Diseases; Infectious Disease-Gynecologic; Women's Health; Infections in Pregnancy; **Hospital:** UC Davis Med Ctr; **Address:** UC Davis Dept of ObGyn, 4860 Y St, Ste 2500, Sacramento, CA 95817; **Phone:** 916-734-6670; **Board Cert:** Obstetrics & Gynecology 1975; **Med School:** Univ Mich Med Sch 1966; **Resid:** Obstetrics & Gynecology, Univ Mich Med Ctr 1973; **Fac Appt:** Prof ObG, UC Davis

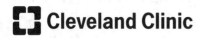
Cleveland Clinic

Obstetrics and Gynecology

Reproductive Endocrinology and Infertility
Our Reproductive Endocrinology and Infertility Program involves close collaboration among male and female infertility specialists, andrologists and embryologists, as well as our colleagues in the Minimally Invasive Surgery Center. Cleveland Clinic reproductive surgeons were among the first to routinely remove advanced endometriosis laparoscopically. Many procedures today are performed with robotic assistance.

Urogynecology and Reconstructive Pelvic Surgery
This Center offers cutting-edge and traditional surgery for urinary incontinence and pelvic organ prolapse, along with medical and behavioral therapy

Center for Female Pelvic Medicine and Reconstructive Surgery
Cleveland Clinic urogynecologists established the Center for Female Pelvic Medicine and Reconstructive Surgery in conjunction with Cleveland Clinic urologists and colorectal surgeons. The sub specialists on this team treat incontinence and prolapse via the abdominal, vaginal and laparoscopic routes.

Maternal-Fetal Medicine/Obstetrics
Cleveland Clinic maternal-fetal medicine specialists provide overall management of complicated pregnancies, beginning with genetic counseling for high-risk patients.

The Fetal Care Center
The Fetal Care Center involves a multidisciplinary team of perinatologists, neonatologists, pediatric surgeons and other specialists. Through collaboration and communication, we provide prenatal diagnosis using state-of-the-art techniques such as high-resolution ultrasound, fetal MRI and fetoscopy. We then apply this information as we develop a management plan for pregnancy, delivery and newborn care.

Menstrual Disorders, Fibroids and Hysteroscopic Services
This Center offers unified and streamlined consultations, workups and treatment for menstrual dysfunction and uterine fibroids in the least invasive manner, so as to preserve a woman's reproductive potential.

Gynecologic Oncology
Our gynecologic oncologists have garnered national and international recognition for expertise in complex reproductive cancers, clinical and basic research, and preventive oncology. Cleveland Clinic gynecologists were among the first to treat early cervical and endometrial cancers laparoscopically. In performing less invasive surgical procedures, we always weigh curative potential against preservation of fertility. We offer oocyte, embryo and ovarian tissue cryopreservation for cancer patients.

Women's Health Center
The Cleveland Clinic Women's Health Center offers a full range of specialized women's health services in one location. We manage menopause, hormone therapy, vulvar disorders, and premenstrual dysthymic disorder and hormonally exacerbated. We offer evaluation and treatment for women with urinary incontinence, osteoporosis or breast concerns. Breast specialists evaluate and treat breast cancer as well as benign breast disease in our center.

To schedule an appointment or for more information about Cleveland Clinic Department of Obstetrics and Gynecology call 800.890.2467 or visit www.clevelandclinic.org/obgyntopdocs

Department of Obstetrics and Gynecology | 9500 Euclid Avenue / W14 | Cleveland OH 44195

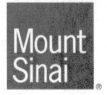

Building on more than a century of leadership in providing healthcare to women, the Department of Obstetrics, Gynecology and Reproductive Science at The Mount Sinai Medical Center offers special expertise in:

• General obstetrics, including genetic counseling, prenatal care, labor and delivery management, and postpartum care. In addition to our talented physicians, other healthcare professionals are integrated into our practice, including genetic counselors, nutritionists, social workers, nurse midwives, childbirth educators, and lactation/breastfeeding specialists.

• High-risk obstetrics, including advanced techniques in prenatal diagnosis and consultations in the management of complicated pregnancies. Our ultrasound unit is recognized for its expertise in fetal anatomy ultrasound assessments. The latest technology, including 4D imaging, is utilized.
Antepartum testing, including amniocentesis, chorionic villus sampling, and fetal blood sampling are all routinely performed at Mount Sinai.

• Reproductive endocrinology and infertility, including diagnosis and treatment of both female and male factor infertility. Treatment options for women include fertility medications, intrauterine insemination, in vitro fertilization, intracytoplasmic sperm injections, and ovum donation.

• General gynecology, including cancer screening, management of abnormal Pap smears, family planning, surgical management of fibroids, endometriosis, and other benign gynecologic conditions. Minimally invasive surgery is offered for many conditions.

• Gynecologic infectious diseases, including the treatment and prevention of sexually transmitted infections and consultations on obstetrical and gynecological infections.

• Gynecologic oncology, including care for women with cancers of the ovary, uterus, cervix, vulva, and vagina.
Minimally invasive surgery for many conditions.

• Urogynecology and reconstructive pelvic surgery, including lower urinary tract disorders.

THE MOUNT SINAI MEDICAL CENTER

Known worldwide for excellence and innovative approaches to prenatal diagnosis and fetal therapy, Mount Sinai's Department of Obstetrics, Gynecology and Reproductive Science has a long tradition of advancing clinical practice through patient-oriented research. Faculty members are pioneering work in diverse areas, including first and second trimester screening for fetal chromosomal abnormalities, vaccines for the prevention of sexually transmitted infections, minimally invasive surgical techniques, and new approaches to the diagnosis and treatment of gender specific cancers.

612

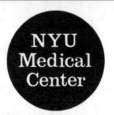

NYU Medical Center

550 First Avenue (at 31st Street)
New York, NY 10016
Physician Referral:
(888)7-NYU-MED (888-769-8633)
www.nyumc.org

WOMEN'S HEALTH

NYU Medical Center supports a comprehensive group of programs and services designed specifically for women's medical needs. Services range from primary care to the most specialized clinical care programs available in the nation. Supported by the most sophisticated research and advanced training at NYU School of Medicine, the Department of Obstetrics and Gynecology at NYU Medical Center offers a unique, abundant blend of high quality therapies and regimens, as well as leading-edge research technologies and methods.

Along with routine gynecological care, many other services are offered including: pelvic ultrasound; aspiration of breast cysts; evaluation of infertility, including the special needs of same-sex couples; colposcopy (a diagnostic evaluation of abnormal pap smears); LEEP (a loop electrosurgical procedure used to diagnose and treat cervical cancer); cryotherapy for vaginal warts; and bone density testing for osteoporosis prevention and treatment.

The Obstetrics program also offers a broad range of services. Among these are prenatal care that gives equal emphasis to the well-being of the mother and of the fetus; fetal monitoring through ultrasound and other techniques; childbirth preparedness and breastfeeding classes; and consultation for high-risk pregnancies, including treatment for women who experience recurrent pregnancy loss.

At NYU Medical Center, the backbone of patient care is the continued research into gynecologic diseases. With world-class faculty leading clinical investigations into disorders that can occur at any stage of a woman's life, doctors at NYU Medical Center are equipped with the latest findings to treat women throughout their lives.

NYU MEDICAL CENTER

Women's Health at
NYU Medical Center

- Obstetrics
- Gynecology
- Maternal-Fetal Medicine
- Gynecologic Oncology
- Reproductive Endocrinology and Infertility
- Reconstructive Pelvic Surgery and Urogynecology
- Endoscopic Pelvic Surgery and Family Planning
- Ultrasound Imaging
- Gynecological Pathology

**PHYSICIAN REFERRAL
(888) 7-NYU-MED
(888-769-8633)
WWW.NYUMC.ORG**

704

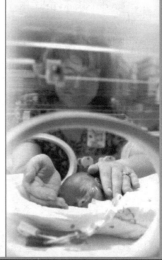

Ophthalmology

An ophthalmologist has the knowledge and professional skills needed to provide comprehensive eye and vision care. Ophthalmologists are medically trained to diagnose, monitor and medically or surgically treat all ocular and visual disorders. This includes problems affecting the eye and its component structures, the eyelids, the orbit and the visual pathways. In so doing, an ophthalmologist prescribes vision services, including glasses and contact lenses.

Training Required: Four years

Ophthalmology

New England

Aiello, Lloyd M MD [Oph] - **Spec Exp:** Diabetic Eye Disease/Retinopathy; **Hospital:** Beth Israel Deaconess Med Ctr - Boston; **Address:** Beetham Eye Inst-Joslin Diabetes Ctr, 1 Joslin Pl, Boston, MA 02215-5397; **Phone:** 617-732-2520; **Board Cert:** Ophthalmology 1966; **Med School:** Boston Univ 1960; **Resid:** Ophthalmology, Mass Eye & Ear Infirm 1964; **Fac Appt:** Assoc Clin Prof Oph, Harvard Med Sch

Duker, Jay S MD [Oph] - **Spec Exp:** Retinal Disorders; Retinal Disorders-Pediatric; Diabetic Eye Disease/Retinopathy; **Hospital:** Tufts-New England Med Ctr; **Address:** New England Eye Ctr, 750 Washington St, Box 450, Boston, MA 02111; **Phone:** 617-636-4600; **Board Cert:** Ophthalmology 1989; **Med School:** Jefferson Med Coll 1984; **Resid:** Ophthalmology, Wills Eye Hosp 1988; **Fellow:** Vitreoretinal Surgery & Disease, Wills Eye Hosp 1990; **Fac Appt:** Assoc Prof Oph, Tufts Univ

Foster, Charles Stephen MD [Oph] - **Spec Exp:** Uveitis; Corneal Disease; Cataract Surgery; **Hospital:** Mass Eye & Ear Infirmary; **Address:** 5 Cambridge Ctr Fl 8, Cambridge, MA 02142; **Phone:** 866-353-6377; **Board Cert:** Ophthalmology 1976; **Med School:** Duke Univ 1969; **Resid:** Ophthalmology, Barnes Hosp 1975; **Fellow:** Cornea, Mass EE Infirm-Harvard 1976; Ocular Immunology, Mass EE Infirm-Harvard 1977; **Fac Appt:** Prof Oph, Harvard Med Sch

Hedges, Thomas R MD [Oph] - **Spec Exp:** Neuro-Ophthalmology; **Hospital:** Tufts-New England Med Ctr; **Address:** New England Med Ctr, 750 Washington St, Box 450, Boston, MA 02111; **Phone:** 617-636-5488; **Board Cert:** Ophthalmology 1980; **Med School:** Tufts Univ 1975; **Resid:** Ophthalmology, Mass EE Infirm 1980; **Fellow:** Neurological Ophthalmology, UCSF Med Ctr 1981; **Fac Appt:** Prof Oph, Tufts Univ

Hunter, David G MD [Oph] - **Spec Exp:** Pediatric Ophthalmology; Eye Muscle Disorders; Strabismus; Cataract-Pediatric; **Hospital:** Children's Hospital - Boston; **Address:** Chlds Hosp Boston, Dept Ophthalmology, 300 Longwood Ave, Fegan 4, Boston, MA 02115; **Phone:** 617-355-6401; **Board Cert:** Ophthalmology 2003; **Med School:** Baylor Coll Med 1987; **Resid:** Ophthalmology, Mass EE Infirm 1991; **Fellow:** Pediatric Ophthalmology, Wilmer Ophthalmic Inst 1992; **Fac Appt:** Assoc Prof Oph, Harvard Med Sch

Kornmehl, Ernest W MD [Oph] - **Spec Exp:** Laser Vision Surgery; Cornea & External Eye Disease; **Hospital:** Mass Eye & Ear Infirmary, Beth Israel Deaconess Med Ctr - Boston; **Address:** Kornmehl Laser Eye Assoc, 44 Washington St, Brookline, MA 02445; **Phone:** 617-232-2090; **Board Cert:** Ophthalmology 1989; **Med School:** SUNY Downstate 1984; **Resid:** Ophthalmology, Yale-New Haven Hosp 1988; **Fellow:** Cornea & Ext Eye Disease, Mass E&E Infirmary 1990; **Fac Appt:** Assoc Clin Prof Oph, Tufts Univ

Miller, Joan W MD [Oph] - **Spec Exp:** Macular Degeneration; Retinal Disorders; **Hospital:** Mass Eye & Ear Infirmary; **Address:** Mass Eye & Ear Infirmary - Ophthalmology, 243 Charles St, Boston, MA 02114; **Phone:** 617-573-3915; **Board Cert:** Ophthalmology 1991; **Med School:** Harvard Med Sch 1985; **Resid:** Ophthalmology, Mass Eye & Ear Infirm 1989; **Fellow:** Retina, Mass Eye & Ear Infirm 1991; **Fac Appt:** Assoc Prof Oph, Harvard Med Sch

Mitchell, Paul Ralph MD [Oph] - **Spec Exp:** Pediatric Ophthalmology; Nystagmus; **Hospital:** CT Chldns Med Ctr, Hartford Hosp; **Address:** 366 Colt Hwy, Route 6, Farmington, CT 06032-2547; **Phone:** 860-409-0449; **Board Cert:** Ophthalmology 1977; **Med School:** Geo Wash Univ 1970; **Resid:** Ophthalmology, Wills Eye Hosp 1976; **Fellow:** Pediatric Ophthalmology, Chldns Hosp MC/Geo Wash 1977; **Fac Appt:** Asst Clin Prof Oph, Univ Conn

Petersen, Robert Allen MD [Oph] - **Spec Exp:** Pediatric Ophthalmology; Retinoblastoma; Retinopathy of Prematurity; **Hospital:** Children's Hospital - Boston, Beth Israel Deaconess Med Ctr - Boston; **Address:** Chldns Hosp, Dept Oph, 300 Longwood Ave, Fegan-4, Boston, MA 02115-5724; **Phone:** 617-355-6401; **Board Cert:** Ophthalmology 1967; **Med School:** Columbia P&S 1959; **Resid:** Internal Medicine, Presby Hosp 1961; Ophthalmology, Mass EE Infirm 1966; **Fellow:** Ophthalmology, Columbia Presby Hosp 1962; Research, Mass EE Infirm 1963; **Fac Appt:** Asst Prof Oph, Harvard Med Sch

Robb, Richard M MD [Oph] - **Spec Exp:** Strabismus; Lacrimal Gland Disorders; Eyelid Problems/Ptosis/Blepharospasm; **Hospital:** Children's Hospital - Boston; **Address:** Chldns Hosp, Dept Ophthalmology, 300 Longwood Ave, Boston, MA 02115; **Phone:** 617-355-6401; **Board Cert:** Ophthalmology 1967; **Med School:** Univ Pennsylvania 1960; **Resid:** Ophthalmology, Mass Eye & Ear Infirm 1965; **Fac Appt:** Assoc Prof Oph, Harvard Med Sch

Rosenthal, Perry MD [Oph] - **Spec Exp:** Corneal Disease; Boston Scleral Lens Prosthesis; **Address:** 464 Hillside Ave, Ste 205, Needham, MA 02494; **Phone:** 781-726-7333; **Board Cert:** Ophthalmology 1965; **Med School:** McGill Univ 1958; **Resid:** Ophthalmology, Mass E&E Infirmary 1963; **Fac Appt:** Asst Clin Prof Oph, Harvard Med Sch

Rubin, Peter A D MD [Oph] - **Spec Exp:** Oculoplastic Surgery; Orbital & Eyelid Tumors/Cancer; Eyelid Cancer & Reconstruction; Eyelid Surgery-Cosmetic & Reconstructive; **Hospital:** Mass Eye & Ear Infirmary; **Address:** Boston Eye Physicians, 44 Washington St, Brookline, MA 02245; **Phone:** 617-232-9600; **Board Cert:** Ophthalmology 1991; **Med School:** Yale Univ 1985; **Resid:** Ophthalmology, Manhattan EET Hosp 1989; **Fellow:** Oculoplastic Surgery, Mass EE Infirm 1990; **Fac Appt:** Assoc Prof Oph, Harvard Med Sch

Tsai, James C MD [Oph] - **Spec Exp:** Glaucoma; **Hospital:** Yale - New Haven Hosp; **Address:** Dept Ophthalmology & Visual Science, 330 Cedar St, PO Box 208061, New Haven, CT 06520-8061; **Phone:** 203-785-2020; **Board Cert:** Ophthalmology 2005; **Med School:** Stanford Univ 1989; **Resid:** Ophthalmology, Doheny Eye Inst/USC 1993; **Fellow:** Glaucoma, Bascom Palmer Eye Inst 1994; Glaucoma, Moorfields Eye Hosp 1995; **Fac Appt:** Assoc Prof Oph, Columbia P&S

Walton, David S MD [Oph] - **Spec Exp:** Glaucoma-Pediatric; Cataract-Pediatric; Neuro-Ophthalmology; **Hospital:** Mass Eye & Ear Infirmary, Mass Genl Hosp; **Address:** 2 Longfellow Pl, Ste 201, Boston, MA 02114; **Phone:** 617-227-3011; **Board Cert:** Ophthalmology 1969; Pediatrics 1983; **Med School:** Duke Univ 1961; **Resid:** Ophthalmology, Mass EE Infirm 1967; **Fellow:** Glaucoma, Mass EE Infirm 1968; **Fac Appt:** Prof Oph, Harvard Med Sch

Ophthalmology

Mid Atlantic

Abramson, David H MD [Oph] - **Spec Exp:** Eye Tumors/Cancer; Orbital Tumors/Cancer; Retinoblastoma; Melanoma-Choroidal (eye); **Hospital:** Meml Sloan Kettering Cancer Ctr; **Address:** 70 E 66th St, New York, NY 10021; **Phone:** 212-744-1700; **Board Cert:** Ophthalmology 1975; **Med School:** Albert Einstein Coll Med 1969; **Resid:** Ophthalmology, Harkness Eye Inst 1974; **Fellow:** Ocular Oncology, Columbia-Presby Med Ctr 1975; **Fac Appt:** Clin Prof Oph, Cornell Univ-Weill Med Coll

Behrens, Myles MD [Oph] - **Spec Exp:** Neuro-Ophthalmology; **Hospital:** NY-Presby Hosp/Columbia (page 66); **Address:** 635 W 165th St, New York, NY 10032-3701; **Phone:** 212-305-5415; **Board Cert:** Ophthalmology 1971; **Med School:** Columbia P&S 1962; **Resid:** Internal Medicine, Columbia Presby Hosp 1964; Ophthalmology, Columbia Presby Hosp 1970; **Fellow:** Neurological Ophthalmology, UCSF Med Ctr 1971; **Fac Appt:** Clin Prof Oph, Columbia P&S

Bressler, Neil M MD [Oph] - **Spec Exp:** Retinal Disorders; **Hospital:** Johns Hopkins Hosp - Baltimore (page 61); **Address:** Wilmer Eye Institute, 550 N Broadway, Ste 115, Baltimore, MD 21205; **Phone:** 410-955-8342; **Board Cert:** Ophthalmology 1987; **Med School:** Johns Hopkins Univ 1982; **Resid:** Internal Medicine, Johns Hopkins Hosp 1983; Ophthalmology, Mass Eye & Ear Infirm 1986; **Fellow:** Retina, Wilmer Inst/Johns Hopkins Hosp 1987; **Fac Appt:** Assoc Prof Oph, Johns Hopkins Univ

Brown, Gary C MD [Oph] - **Spec Exp:** Retinal Disorders; Retinal Vascular Diseases; **Hospital:** Wills Eye Hosp; **Address:** 910 E Willow Grove Ave, Wyndmoor, PA 19038; **Phone:** 215-233-4300; **Board Cert:** Ophthalmology 2003; **Med School:** SUNY Upstate Med Univ 1975; **Resid:** Ophthalmology, Wills Eye Hosp 1979; **Fellow:** Vitreoretinal Disease, Wills Eye Hosp 1981; **Fac Appt:** Prof Oph, Jefferson Med Coll

Brucker, Alexander J MD [Oph] - **Spec Exp:** Retinal Disorders; Retina/Vitreous Surgery; Macular Degeneration; **Hospital:** Penn Presby Med Ctr - UPHS (page 72); **Address:** Univ Penn, Scheie Eye Inst, 51 N 39th St, rm 517, Philadelphia, PA 19104; **Phone:** 215-662-8100; **Board Cert:** Ophthalmology 1977; **Med School:** NY Med Coll 1972; **Resid:** Ophthalmology, Friedenwald Inst 1976; **Fellow:** Retina/Vitreous, Johns Hopkins Hosp 1977; **Fac Appt:** Prof Oph, Univ Pennsylvania

Campochiaro, Peter MD [Oph] - **Spec Exp:** Retina/Vitreous Surgery; **Hospital:** Johns Hopkins Hosp - Baltimore (page 61); **Address:** Wilmer Ophthalmological Inst, 600 N Wolfe St, 719 Maumenee, Baltimore, MD 21287-9277; **Phone:** 410-955-5106; **Board Cert:** Ophthalmology 1983; **Med School:** Johns Hopkins Univ 1978; **Resid:** Ophthalmology, Univ Virginia 1982; **Fellow:** Retina/Vitreous, John Hopkins Univ 1984; **Fac Appt:** Prof Oph, Johns Hopkins Univ

Caputo, Anthony R MD [Oph] - **Spec Exp:** Pediatric Ophthalmology; Strabismus; **Hospital:** Columbus Hosp; **Address:** 556 Eagle Rock Ave, Ste 203, Roseland, NJ 07068-1500; **Phone:** 973-228-3111; **Board Cert:** Ophthalmology 1976; **Med School:** Italy 1969; **Resid:** Ophthalmology, UMDNJ-Univ Hosp 1974; **Fellow:** Ophthalmology, Wills Eye Hosp 1975; **Fac Appt:** Prof Oph, UMDNJ-NJ Med Sch, Newark

Chang, Stanley MD [Oph] - **Spec Exp:** Diabetic Eye Disease/Retinopathy; Macular Disease/Degeneration; Retina/Vitreous Surgery; Retinal Disorders; **Hospital:** NY-Presby Hosp/Columbia (page 66); **Address:** 635 W 165th St, Box 20, New York, NY 10032; **Phone:** 212-305-9535; **Board Cert:** Ophthalmology 1979; **Med School:** Columbia P&S 1974; **Resid:** Ophthalmology, Mass Eye & Ear Infirmary 1978; **Fellow:** Vitreoretinal Surgery, Bascom Palmer Eye Inst 1979; **Fac Appt:** Prof Oph, Columbia P&S

D'Amico, Donald MD [Oph] - **Spec Exp:** Diabetic Eye Disease/Retinopathy; Retinal Detachment; **Hospital:** NY-Presby Hosp/Weill Cornell (page 66); **Address:** Weill Cornell Ophthalmology Associates, 520 E 70th St, Starr Pavilion, Fl 8, New York, NY 10021; **Phone:** 212-746-2860; **Board Cert:** Ophthalmology 1982; **Med School:** Univ IL Coll Med 1977; **Resid:** Ophthalmology, Mass Eye & Ear Infirm 1981; **Fellow:** Vitreoretinal Surgery, Bascom Palmer Eye Inst 1982; **Fac Appt:** Prof Oph, Cornell Univ-Weill Med Coll

Del Priore, Lucian MD/PhD [Oph] - **Spec Exp:** Diabetic Eye Disease/Retinopathy; Macular Degeneration; Retinal Detachment; **Hospital:** NY-Presby Hosp/Columbia (page 66), Manhattan Eye, Ear & Throat Hosp; **Address:** Harkness Eye Inst, 635 W 165th St, New York, NY 10032; **Phone:** 212-305-9535; **Board Cert:** Ophthalmology 1989; **Med School:** Univ Rochester 1982; **Resid:** Ophthalmology, Wilmer Eye Inst/Johns HopkinsHosp 1987; **Fellow:** Glaucoma, Wilmer Eye Inst/Johns Hopkins Hosp 1988; Vitreoretinal Surgery, Wilmer Eye Inst/Johns Hopkins Hosp 1989; **Fac Appt:** Prof Oph, Columbia P&S

Della Rocca, Robert MD [Oph] - **Spec Exp:** Orbital Tumors/Cancer; Eyelid Tumors/Cancer; Thyroid Eye Disease; Oculoplastic Surgery; **Hospital:** New York Eye & Ear Infirm (page 65), Sound Shore Med Ctr - Westchester; **Address:** 310 E 14th St, South Bldg, rm 319, New York, NY 10003; **Phone:** 212-979-4575; **Board Cert:** Ophthalmology 1975; **Med School:** Creighton Univ 1967; **Resid:** Ophthalmology, NY Eye & Ear Infirm 1973; **Fellow:** Oculoplastic Surgery, Albany Med Ctr

Diamond, Gary R MD [Oph] - **Spec Exp:** Pediatric Ophthalmology; Strabismus; Amblyopia; **Hospital:** St Christopher's Hosp for Chldn; **Address:** St. Christopher's Hosp for Chldn, Ophth, Front Street at Erie Ave, Philadelphia, PA 19134-1095; **Phone:** 215-427-8120; **Board Cert:** Ophthalmology 1979; **Med School:** Johns Hopkins Univ 1974; **Resid:** Ophthalmology, Wilmer Inst-Johns Hopkins 1979; **Fellow:** Pediatric Ophthalmology, Chldns Hosp Med Ctr 1979; Pediatric Ophthalmology, Harkness Eye Inst 1979; **Fac Appt:** Prof Oph, Drexel Univ Coll Med

Eagle, Ralph C MD [Oph] - **Spec Exp:** Ophthalmic Pathology; **Hospital:** Wills Eye Hosp; **Address:** Wills Eye Hosp, Dept Pathology, 840 Walnut St, Ste 1410, Philadelphia, PA 19107; **Phone:** 215-928-3280; **Board Cert:** Ophthalmology 1976; **Med School:** Univ Pennsylvania 1970; **Resid:** Ophthalmology, Scheie Eye Inst 1975; **Fellow:** Ophthalmic Pathology, Armed Forces Inst Path 1978; **Fac Appt:** Prof Oph, Jefferson Med Coll

Eggers, Howard M MD [Oph] - **Spec Exp:** Pediatric Ophthalmology; Strabismus; **Hospital:** NY-Presby Hosp/Columbia (page 66); **Address:** 635 W 165th St, Box 21, New York, NY 10032-3724; **Phone:** 212-305-5409; **Board Cert:** Ophthalmology 1978; **Med School:** Columbia P&S 1971; **Resid:** Ophthalmology, Harkness Inst - Presby Hosp 1975; **Fac Appt:** Prof Oph, Columbia P&S

Feldon, Steven E MD [Oph] - **Spec Exp:** Neuro-Ophthalmology; Orbital Surgery; Strabismus; **Hospital:** Univ of Rochester Strong Meml Hosp, Rochester Gen Hosp; **Address:** 601 Elmwood Ave, Box 659, Rochester, NY 14642; **Phone:** 585-275-1126; **Board Cert:** Ophthalmology 1979; **Med School:** Albert Einstein Coll Med 1973; **Resid:** Ophthalmology, Mass Eye & Ear Infirmary 1978; **Fellow:** Ophthalmology, UCSF Med Ctr 1979; **Fac Appt:** Prof Oph, Univ Rochester

Finger, Paul T MD [Oph] - **Spec Exp:** Eye Tumors/Cancer; Orbital Diseases; **Hospital:** New York Eye & Ear Infirm (page 65), NYU Med Ctr (page 67); **Address:** The New York Eye Cancer Ctr, 115 E 61st St, New York, NY 10021-8183; **Phone:** 212-832-8170; **Board Cert:** Ophthalmology 1990; **Med School:** Tulane Univ 1982; **Resid:** Ophthalmology, Manhattan EET Hosp 1986; **Fellow:** Ocular Oncology, N Shore Univ Hosp-Cornell 1987; **Fac Appt:** Clin Prof Oph, NYU Sch Med

Ophthalmology

Flynn, John T MD [Oph] - **Spec Exp:** Pediatric Ophthalmology; Strabismus; Retinopathy of Prematurity; **Hospital:** NY-Presby Hosp/Columbia (page 66); **Address:** Harkness Eye Inst, 635 W 165th St, Flanzer Ste, New York, NY 10032; **Phone:** 212-305-3908; **Board Cert:** Ophthalmology 1967; **Med School:** Northwestern Univ 1956; **Resid:** Ophthalmology, New York Hosp 1964; **Fellow:** Strabismus, Natl Inst Hlth 1965; **Fac Appt:** Prof Oph, Columbia P&S

Fuchs, Wayne MD [Oph] - **Spec Exp:** Diabetic Eye Disease/Retinopathy; Macular Disease/Degeneration; Retina/Vitreous Surgery; Retinal Disorders; **Hospital:** Mount Sinai Med Ctr, Manhattan Eye, Ear & Throat Hosp; **Address:** 121 E 60th St, Ste 5B, New York, NY 10022-1186; **Phone:** 212-319-8205; **Board Cert:** Ophthalmology 1985; **Med School:** Mount Sinai Sch Med 1979; **Resid:** Ophthalmology, Mount Sinai Hosp 1983; **Fellow:** Vitreoretinal Surgery & Disease, New York Hosp/Cornell 1984; **Fac Appt:** Clin Prof Oph, Mount Sinai Sch Med

Gaasterland, Douglas E MD [Oph] - **Spec Exp:** Glaucoma; Laser Surgery; Anterior Segment Surgery; **Hospital:** Georgetown Univ Hosp, G Washington Univ Hosp; **Address:** 2 Wisconsin Cir, Ste 200, Chevy Chase, MD 20815; **Phone:** 301-215-7100; **Board Cert:** Ophthalmology 1971; **Med School:** Johns Hopkins Univ 1965; **Resid:** Ophthalmology, Yale-New Haven Hosp 1970; **Fellow:** Glaucoma, National Eye Inst-NIH 1971; **Fac Appt:** Clin Prof Oph, Geo Wash Univ

Gallin, Pamela F MD [Oph] - **Spec Exp:** Pediatric Ophthalmology; Amblyopia; Strabismus; Tear Duct Problems; **Hospital:** NY-Presby Hosp/Columbia (page 66), Manhattan Eye, Ear & Throat Hosp; **Address:** Columbia Presby Med Ctr, 635 W 165th St, Ste 224, New York, NY 10032-3701; **Phone:** 212-305-5407; **Board Cert:** Ophthalmology 1983; **Med School:** Washington Univ, St Louis 1978; **Resid:** Ophthalmology, Mount Sinai Med Ctr 1982; **Fellow:** Pediatric Ophthalmology, Chldns Natl Med Ctr 1983; Strabismus, Columbia-Presby Med Ctr 1983; **Fac Appt:** Assoc Prof Oph, Columbia P&S

Gentile, Ronald MD [Oph] - **Spec Exp:** Retina/Vitreous Surgery; Diabetic Eye Disease; Macular Degeneration; **Hospital:** New York Eye & Ear Infirm (page 65); **Address:** 2nd Ave at 14th St, South Bldg - Ste 319, New York, NY 10003-4201; **Phone:** 212-979-4120; **Board Cert:** Ophthalmology 1997; **Med School:** SUNY Downstate 1991; **Resid:** Ophthalmology, New York Eye & Ear Infirm 1995; **Fellow:** Vitreoretinal Surgery & Disease, Kresge Eye Inst 1998; **Fac Appt:** Assoc Prof Oph, NY Med Coll

Gibralter, Richard P MD [Oph] - **Spec Exp:** Cataract Surgery; Laser Vision Surgery; Cornea Transplant; Corneal Disease & Surgery; **Hospital:** Manhattan Eye, Ear & Throat Hosp, New York Eye & Ear Infirm (page 65); **Address:** 154 E 71st St, New York, NY 10021-5123; **Phone:** 212-628-2202; **Board Cert:** Ophthalmology 1981; **Med School:** Mount Sinai Sch Med 1976; **Resid:** Ophthalmology, Manhattan EE&T Hosp 1980; **Fellow:** Cornea, Manhattan EE&T Hosp 1981; **Fac Appt:** Asst Prof Oph, NYU Sch Med

Goldberg, Morton MD [Oph] - **Spec Exp:** Macular Disease/Degeneration; Diabetic Eye Disease; Retinal Disorders; **Hospital:** Johns Hopkins Hosp - Baltimore (page 61); **Address:** Johns Hopkins Hosp, 600 N Wolfe St, Woods Bldg 276, Baltimore, MD 21287-9128; **Phone:** 410-955-6846; **Board Cert:** Ophthalmology 1968; **Med School:** Harvard Med Sch 1962; **Resid:** Ophthalmology, Wilmer Ophth Inst 1966; **Fellow:** Ophthalmology, Wilmer Ophth Inst 1967; Research, Johns Hopkins Hosp 1967; **Fac Appt:** Prof Oph, Johns Hopkins Univ

Gorin, Michael B MD [Oph] - **Spec Exp:** Retinal Disorders; Macular Disease/Degeneration; Eye Diseases-Hereditary; **Hospital:** UPMC Presby, Pittsburgh; **Address:** UPMC Eye Center, 203 Lothrop St, Pittsburgh, PA 15213; **Phone:** 412-647-2200; **Board Cert:** Ophthalmology 1987; **Med School:** Univ Pennsylvania 1980; **Resid:** Ophthalmology, Jules Stein Eye Inst/UCLA 1986; **Fellow:** Medical Retina, Moorfields Eye Hosp 1987; **Fac Appt:** Prof Oph, Univ Pittsburgh

Green, William Richard MD [Oph] - **Spec Exp:** Ophthalmic Pathology; Retinal Disorders; **Hospital:** Johns Hopkins Hosp - Baltimore (page 61); **Address:** Johns Hopkins Hosp, Eye Path Lab, 600 N Wolfe St, Maumenee 427, Baltimore, MD 21287; **Phone:** 410-955-3455; **Board Cert:** Ophthalmology 1965; Anatomic Pathology 1970; **Med School:** Univ Louisville Sch Med 1959; **Resid:** Ophthalmology, Wills Eye Hosp 1963; Anatomic Pathology, Temple Univ 1968; **Fellow:** Ophthalmology, Natl Inst Neuro Disease 1965; **Fac Appt:** Prof Oph, Johns Hopkins Univ

Guyton, David Lee MD [Oph] - **Spec Exp:** Strabismus; Pediatric Ophthalmology; **Hospital:** Johns Hopkins Hosp - Baltimore (page 61); **Address:** Johns Hopkins Hosp, 600 N Wolfe, Wilmer 233, Baltimore, MD 21287; **Phone:** 410-955-8314; **Board Cert:** Ophthalmology 1977; **Med School:** Harvard Med Sch 1969; **Resid:** Ophthalmology, Johns Hopkins Hosp 1976; **Fellow:** Pediatric Ophthalmology, Baylor Coll Med 1977; **Fac Appt:** Prof Oph, Johns Hopkins Univ

Hall, Lisabeth MD [Oph] - **Spec Exp:** Pediatric Ophthalmology; Strabismus; Eye Muscle Disorders; Cataract-Pediatric; **Hospital:** New York Eye & Ear Infirm (page 65), Lenox Hill Hosp (page 62); **Address:** 310 E 14th St South Bldg Fl 2, New York, NY 10003-4201; **Phone:** 212-979-4614; **Board Cert:** Ophthalmology 1998; **Med School:** SUNY Stony Brook 1992; **Resid:** Ophthalmology, Manhattan Eye & Ear Infirm 1996; **Fellow:** Pediatric Ophthalmology, Jules Stein Eye Inst 1997; **Fac Appt:** Asst Prof Oph, NY Med Coll

Handa, James T MD [Oph] - **Spec Exp:** Macular Degeneration; Melanoma-Choroidal (eye); Retinoblastoma; **Hospital:** Johns Hopkins Hosp - Baltimore (page 61); **Address:** Johns Hopkins-Wilmer Eye Inst, 1550 Orleans St, rm CRB-144, Baltimore, MD 21287; **Phone:** 410-614-4211; **Board Cert:** Ophthalmology 1991; **Med School:** Univ Pennsylvania 1986; **Resid:** Ophthalmology, Wills Eye Hosp 1990; **Fellow:** Retina/Vitreous, Duke Eye Ctr 1992; Ophthalmic Oncololgy, USC Sch Med 1993; **Fac Appt:** Assoc Prof Oph, Johns Hopkins Univ

Hersh, Peter MD [Oph] - **Spec Exp:** LASIK-Refractive Surgery; Cornea Transplant; Keratoconus; **Hospital:** UMDNJ-Univ Hosp-Newark; **Address:** 300 Frank W Burr Blvd, Teaneck, NJ 07666-6704; **Phone:** 201-883-0505; **Board Cert:** Ophthalmology 1987; **Med School:** Johns Hopkins Univ 1982; **Resid:** Internal Medicine, Lenox Hill Hosp 1983; Ophthalmology, Mass Eye & Ear Infirm 1986; **Fellow:** Cornea & Ext Eye Disease, Mass Eye & Ear Infirm 1987; **Fac Appt:** Prof Oph, UMDNJ-NJ Med Sch, Newark

Iliff, Nicholas Taylor MD [Oph] - **Spec Exp:** Oculoplastic Surgery; Orbital & Eyelid Tumors/Cancer; **Hospital:** Johns Hopkins Hosp - Baltimore (page 61); **Address:** Johns Hopkins Hosp-Wilmer Inst, Maumenee 505, 600 N Wolfe St, Baltimore, MD 21287-9218; **Phone:** 410-955-1112; **Board Cert:** Ophthalmology 1978; **Med School:** Johns Hopkins Univ 1972; **Resid:** Ophthalmology, Johns Hopkins-Wilmer Inst 1977; **Fellow:** Retinal Surgery, Johns Hopkins-Wilmer Inst 1978; Oculoplastic & Reconstructive Surgery, Johns Hopkins-Wilmer Inst 1980; **Fac Appt:** Prof Oph, Johns Hopkins Univ

Ophthalmology

Jaafar, Mohamad S MD [Oph] - **Spec Exp:** Pediatric Ophthalmology; Strabismus-Adult & Pediatric; Glaucoma-Pediatric; **Hospital:** Chldns Natl Med Ctr, G Washington Univ Hosp; **Address:** Childrens Natl Med Ctr, Dept Ophth, 111 Michigan Ave NW, Washington, DC 20010-2970; **Phone:** 202-884-3017; **Board Cert:** Ophthalmology 1997; **Med School:** Amer Univ Beirut 1978; **Resid:** Ophthalmology, Am Univ Beirut Med Ctr 1981; Ophthalmology, Washington Hosp Ctr 1994; **Fellow:** Pediatric Ophthalmology, Chldns Hosp 1982; Pediatric Ophthalmology, Baylor Coll Med 1983; **Fac Appt:** Prof Oph, Geo Wash Univ

Katowitz, James A MD [Oph] - **Spec Exp:** Oculoplastic & Orbital Surgery; Pediatric Ophthalmology; Cornea Plastic Surgery; **Hospital:** Chldns Hosp of Philadelphia, The, Hosp Univ Penn - UPHS (page 72); **Address:** Childrens Hosp, Div Ophthalmology, 34th St & Civic Center Blvd, Wood Bldg Fl 1, Philadelphia, PA 19104; **Phone:** 215-590-2791; **Board Cert:** Ophthalmology 1969; **Med School:** Univ Pennsylvania 1963; **Resid:** Ophthalmology, Hosp Univ Penn 1967; **Fellow:** Oculoplastic Surgery, Queen Victoria Hosp 1968; Oculoplastic Surgery, Moorfield Eye Hosp 1968; **Fac Appt:** Prof Oph, Univ Pennsylvania

Koller, Harold Paul MD [Oph] - **Spec Exp:** Pediatric Ophthalmology; Eye Muscle Surgery; Visual Perception & Learning Disorders; **Hospital:** Wills Eye Hosp, St Christopher's Hosp for Chldn; **Address:** 1650 Huntington Pike, Ste 150, Meadowbrook, PA 19046-8001; **Phone:** 215-947-6660; **Board Cert:** Ophthalmology 1971; **Med School:** Tulane Univ 1964; **Resid:** Ophthalmology, Tulane Hosp Med Ctr 1968; **Fellow:** Pediatric Ophthalmology, Washington Chldn's Hosp 1970; **Fac Appt:** Clin Prof Oph, Thomas Jefferson Univ

Kupersmith, Mark MD [Oph] - **Spec Exp:** Neuro-Ophthalmology; **Hospital:** St Luke's - Roosevelt Hosp Ctr - Roosevelt Div; **Address:** 1000 10th Ave, New York, NY 10009; **Phone:** 212-870-9418; **Board Cert:** Ophthalmology 1981; Neurology 1981; **Med School:** Northwestern Univ 1974; **Resid:** Neurology, NYU Med Ctr 1978; Ophthalmology, NYU Med Ctr 1980; **Fac Appt:** Prof Oph, NYU Sch Med

Liebmann, Jeffrey MD [Oph] - **Spec Exp:** Glaucoma; Cataract Surgery; **Hospital:** New York Eye & Ear Infirm (page 65), Manhattan Eye, Ear & Throat Hosp; **Address:** 121 E 60th St, New York, NY 10022; **Phone:** 212-477-7540 x330; **Board Cert:** Ophthalmology 1989; **Med School:** Boston Univ 1983; **Resid:** Ophthalmology, SUNY Downstate Med Ctr 1987; **Fellow:** Glaucoma, New York EE Infirmary 1988; **Fac Appt:** Clin Prof Oph, NYU Sch Med

Lisman, Richard D MD [Oph] - **Spec Exp:** Oculoplastic Surgery; Eyelid/Tear Duct Reconstruction; Eyelid Surgery-Cosmetic & Reconstructive; Cosmetic Surgery-Eyes; **Hospital:** NYU Med Ctr (page 67), Manhattan Eye, Ear & Throat Hosp; **Address:** 635 Park Ave, New York, NY 10021-6546; **Phone:** 212-585-1405; **Board Cert:** Ophthalmology 1981; **Med School:** NYU Sch Med 1976; **Resid:** Ophthalmology, Manhattan EE Hosp 1980; **Fellow:** Ophthalmic Plastic Surgery, NY Eye & Ear Infirmary 1981; Plastic Surgery, Manhattan EE&T Hosp 1982; **Fac Appt:** Clin Prof Oph, NYU Sch Med

Mackool, Richard J MD [Oph] - **Spec Exp:** Cataract Surgery; LASIK-Refractive Surgery; Lens Implants-Multifocal (Restor); Corneal Disease & Surgery; **Hospital:** New York Eye & Ear Infirm (page 65); **Address:** 31-27 41st St, Astoria, NY 11103; **Phone:** 718-728-3400; **Board Cert:** Ophthalmology 1975; **Med School:** Boston Univ 1968; **Resid:** Ophthalmology, New York EE Infirm 1973; **Fac Appt:** Clin Prof Oph, NYU Sch Med

Magramm, Irene MD [Oph] - **Spec Exp:** Pediatric Ophthalmology; Strabismus; Cataract Surgery; **Hospital:** Manhattan Eye, Ear & Throat Hosp, New York Eye & Ear Infirm (page 65); **Address:** 225 E 64th St, New York, NY 10021; **Phone:** 212-644-5100; **Board Cert:** Ophthalmology 1987; **Med School:** Cornell Univ-Weill Med Coll 1981; **Resid:** Ophthalmology, North Shore Univ Hosp 1985; **Fellow:** Pediatric Ophthalmology, Manhattan EE&T Hosp 1986; **Fac Appt:** Asst Clin Prof Oph, Cornell Univ-Weill Med Coll

Mandel, Eric R MD [Oph] - **Spec Exp:** Laser Vision Surgery; Corneal Disease; PRK-Refractive Surgery; LASIK-Refractive Surgery; **Hospital:** New York Eye & Ear Infirm (page 65), Lenox Hill Hosp (page 62); **Address:** 211 E 70th St, New York, NY 10021-5106; **Phone:** 212-734-0111; **Board Cert:** Ophthalmology 1988; **Med School:** SUNY Stony Brook 1982; **Resid:** Ophthalmology, Lenox Hill Hosp 1986; **Fellow:** Cornea & Ext Eye Disease, Mass EE Infirm 1987

Medow, Norman MD [Oph] - **Spec Exp:** Cataract-Pediatric; Glaucoma-Pediatric; Corneal Disease-Pediatric; **Hospital:** Manhattan Eye, Ear & Throat Hosp, NY-Presby Hosp/Weill Cornell (page 66); **Address:** 225 E 64th St, Ste 6, New York, NY 10021-6690; **Phone:** 212-644-5100; **Board Cert:** Ophthalmology 1975; **Med School:** SUNY Hlth Sci Ctr 1966; **Resid:** Ophthalmology, Manhattan EE&T Hosp 1972; **Fac Appt:** Assoc Clin Prof Oph, Cornell Univ-Weill Med Coll

Miller, Neil MD [Oph] - **Spec Exp:** Neuro-Ophthalmology; Orbital Diseases; Thyroid Eye Disease; **Hospital:** Johns Hopkins Hosp - Baltimore (page 61); **Address:** Johns Hopkins - Wilmer Eye Inst, 600 N Wolfe St, Maumenee - rm 127, Baltimore, MD 21287-0001; **Phone:** 410-955-8679; **Board Cert:** Ophthalmology 1976; **Med School:** Johns Hopkins Univ 1971; **Resid:** Ophthalmology, Johns Hopkins Hosp 1975; **Fellow:** Neurological Ophthalmology, UCSF Med Ctr 1975; **Fac Appt:** Prof Oph, Johns Hopkins Univ

Mills, Monte D MD [Oph] - **Spec Exp:** Pediatric Ophthalmology; Eye Muscle Disorders; Strabismus; **Hospital:** Chldns Hosp of Philadelphia, The; **Address:** Chldns Hosp, Richard D Wood Bldg, 34th St and Civic Center Blvd, Wood Bldg Fl 1, Philadelphia, PA 19104; **Phone:** 215-590-2791; **Board Cert:** Ophthalmology 1993; **Med School:** Baylor Coll Med 1988; **Resid:** Ophthalmology, Mass E&E Infirm 1992; **Fellow:** Pediatric Ophthalmology, Chldns Hosp 1993; **Fac Appt:** Prof Oph, Univ Pennsylvania

Muldoon, Thomas O MD [Oph] - **Spec Exp:** Retina/Vitreous Surgery; Macular Disease/Degeneration; Diabetic Eye Disease/Retinopathy; **Hospital:** New York Eye & Ear Infirm (page 65); **Address:** 310 E 14th St, Ste 402, New York, NY 10003-4201; **Phone:** 212-979-4595; **Board Cert:** Ophthalmology 1971; **Med School:** Univ Rochester 1962; **Resid:** Surgery, St Lukes Hosp 1966; Ophthalmology, New York EE Infirm 1969; **Fellow:** Retinal Surgery, New York EE Infirm 1970; **Fac Appt:** Assoc Clin Prof Oph, NY Med Coll

Odel, Jeffrey G MD [Oph] - **Spec Exp:** Neuro-Ophthalmology; Retinal Disorders; Optic Nerve Disorders; **Hospital:** NY-Presby Hosp/Columbia (page 66); **Address:** 635 W 165th St, rm 316, New York, NY 10032-3701; **Phone:** 212-305-5415; **Board Cert:** Ophthalmology 1981; **Med School:** Univ Rochester 1975; **Resid:** Ophthalmology, Mt Sinai Hosp 1981; **Fellow:** Ophthalmology, Bascom-Palmer Eye Inst 1977; Ophthalmology, Columbia Presby Med Ctr 1982; **Fac Appt:** Assoc Clin Prof Oph, Columbia P&S

Podos, Steven M MD [Oph] - **Spec Exp:** Glaucoma; **Hospital:** Mount Sinai Med Ctr; **Address:** 1465 Madison Ave, New York, NY 10029; **Phone:** 212-241-6752; **Board Cert:** Ophthalmology 1968; **Med School:** Harvard Med Sch 1962; **Resid:** Ophthalmology, Washington Univ-Barnes Hosp 1967; **Fac Appt:** Prof Oph, Mount Sinai Sch Med

Ophthalmology

Quigley, Harry A MD [Oph] - **Spec Exp:** Glaucoma; **Hospital:** Johns Hopkins Hosp - Baltimore (page 61); **Address:** 600 N Wolfe St, Maumenee B-110, Baltimore, MD 21287-9205; **Phone:** 410-955-6052; **Board Cert:** Ophthalmology 1976; **Med School:** Johns Hopkins Univ 1971; **Resid:** Ophthalmology, Wilmer Inst-Johns Hopkins Hosp 1975; **Fellow:** Ophthalmology, Bascom Palmer Eye Inst 1977; **Fac Appt:** Prof Oph, Johns Hopkins Univ

Quinn, Graham E MD [Oph] - **Spec Exp:** Pediatric Ophthalmology; Eye Growth/Development; **Hospital:** Chldns Hosp of Philadelphia, The; **Address:** Chldns Hosp of Philadelphia, Div Ophthalmology, 34th St & Civic Center Blvd, Wood Bldg Fl 1, Philadelphia, PA 19104-4399; **Phone:** 215-590-2791; **Board Cert:** Ophthalmology 1979; **Med School:** Duke Univ 1973; **Resid:** Pathology, Metro Genl Hosp 1975; Ophthalmology, Hosp Univ Penn 1978; **Fellow:** Pediatric Ophthalmology, Childrens Hosp 1979; **Fac Appt:** Prof Oph, Univ Pennsylvania

Raab, Edward L MD [Oph] - **Spec Exp:** Pediatric Ophthalmology; Strabismus-Adult & Pediatric; Glaucoma-Pediatric; **Hospital:** Mount Sinai Med Ctr; **Address:** 5 E 98th St, Fl 7, New York, NY 10029-6501; **Phone:** 212-369-0988; **Board Cert:** Ophthalmology 1966; **Med School:** NYU Sch Med 1958; **Resid:** Ophthalmology, Mount Sinai 1964; **Fellow:** Pediatric Ophthalmology, Chldns Natl Med Ctr 1967; **Fac Appt:** Prof Oph, Mount Sinai Sch Med

Regillo, Carl D MD [Oph] - **Spec Exp:** Retinal Disorders; **Hospital:** Wills Eye Hosp; **Address:** 910 E Willow Grove Ave, Wyndmoor, PA 19038; **Phone:** 215-233-4300; **Board Cert:** Ophthalmology 2004; **Med School:** Harvard Med Sch 1988; **Resid:** Ophthalmology, Wills Eye Hosp 1992; **Fellow:** Retinal Surgery, Wills Eye Hosp 1994; **Fac Appt:** Prof Oph, Jefferson Med Coll

Reynolds, James D MD [Oph] - **Spec Exp:** Pediatric Ophthalmology; Strabismus; Retinopathy of Prematurity; **Hospital:** Women's & Chldn's Hosp of Buffalo, The; **Address:** 3580 Sheridan Drive, Ste 140A, Amherst, NY 14226; **Phone:** 716-834-0113; **Board Cert:** Ophthalmology 1982; **Med School:** SUNY Buffalo 1978; **Resid:** Ophthalmology, Erie CO Med Ctr 1981; **Fellow:** Pediatric Ophthalmology, Pittsburgh EE Hospital 1982; **Fac Appt:** Prof Oph, SUNY Buffalo

Ritch, Robert MD [Oph] - **Spec Exp:** Glaucoma; **Hospital:** New York Eye & Ear Infirm (page 65); **Address:** 310 E 14th St, rm 304S, New York, NY 10003-4201; **Phone:** 212-477-7540; **Board Cert:** Ophthalmology 1977; **Med School:** Albert Einstein Coll Med 1972; **Resid:** Ophthalmology, Mount Sinai Hosp 1976; **Fellow:** Glaucoma, Mount Sinai Hosp 1978; **Fac Appt:** Clin Prof Oph, NY Med Coll

Savino, Peter J MD [Oph] - **Spec Exp:** Neuro-Ophthalmology; **Hospital:** Thomas Jefferson Univ Hosp; **Address:** Wills Eye Hosp, Dept Neuro-Ophthalmology, 840 Walnut St Fl 9 - Ste 930, Philadelphia, PA 19107; **Phone:** 215-928-3130; **Board Cert:** Ophthalmology 1975; **Med School:** Italy 1968; **Resid:** Ophthalmology, Georgetown Med Ctr 1973; **Fellow:** Neurological Ophthalmology, Bascom Palmer Eye Inst 1974; **Fac Appt:** Prof Oph, Thomas Jefferson Univ

Schein, Oliver D MD [Oph] - **Spec Exp:** Cataract Surgery; Corneal Disease & Surgery; **Hospital:** Johns Hopkins Hosp - Baltimore (page 61); **Address:** Johns Hopkins Hosp, 600 N Wolfe St, Wilmer 116, Baltimore, MD 21287; **Phone:** 410-955-7677; **Board Cert:** Internal Medicine 1984; Ophthalmology 1990; **Med School:** Johns Hopkins Univ 1981; **Resid:** Internal Medicine, Johns Hopkins Hosp 1984; Ophthalmology, Mass Eye & Ear Infirm 1987; **Fellow:** Cornea & Ext Eye Disease, Mass Eye & Ear Infirm 1988; **Fac Appt:** Prof Oph, Johns Hopkins Univ

Schiff, William M MD [Oph] - **Spec Exp:** Macular Disease/Degeneration; Diabetic Eye Disease/Retinopathy; Retinal Detachment; **Hospital:** NY-Presby Hosp/Columbia (page 66), St Luke's - Roosevelt Hosp Ctr - Roosevelt Div; **Address:** Columbia Ophthalmic Consultants, 635 W 165th St, New York, NY 10032; **Phone:** 212-305-9535; **Board Cert:** Ophthalmology 2006; **Med School:** NYU Sch Med 1988; **Resid:** Ophthalmology, New York Eye & Ear Infirm 1994; **Fellow:** Retina/Vitreous, NY Hosp-Harkness Eye Inst 1996; **Fac Appt:** Assoc Prof Oph, Columbia P&S

Schuman, Joel S MD [Oph] - **Spec Exp:** Glaucoma; Cataract Surgery; **Hospital:** UPMC Presby, Pittsburgh, UPMC Shadyside; **Address:** Eye & Ear Institute, Ste 816, 203 Lothrop St, Pittsburgh, PA 15213; **Phone:** 412-647-2205; **Board Cert:** Ophthalmology 1990; **Med School:** Mount Sinai Sch Med 1984; **Resid:** Ophthalmology, Med Coll Virginia Hosps 1988; **Fellow:** Glaucoma, Mass EE Infirmary 1990; **Fac Appt:** Prof Oph, Univ Pittsburgh

Sergott, Robert C MD [Oph] - **Spec Exp:** Neuro-Ophthalmology; Optic Nerve Disorders; Glaucoma; Thyroid Eye Disease; **Hospital:** Thomas Jefferson Univ Hosp, Wills Eye Hosp; **Address:** Wills Eye Hosp, Dept Neuro-Opthalmology, 840 Walnut St Fl 9 - Ste 930, Philadelphia, PA 19107; **Phone:** 215-928-3130; **Board Cert:** Ophthalmology 1982; **Med School:** Johns Hopkins Univ 1975; **Resid:** Internal Medicine, Mary Imogene Bassett Hosp 1976; Ophthalmology, Jackson Meml Hosp 1980; **Fellow:** Ophthalmology, Jackson Meml Hosp 1980

Shabto, Uri MD [Oph] - **Spec Exp:** Retinopathy of Prematurity; Macular Disease/Degeneration; Diabetic Eye Disease/Retinopathy; **Hospital:** New York Eye & Ear Infirm (page 65), Beth Israel Med Ctr - Petrie Division; **Address:** 310 E 14th St South Bldg - Ste 419, New York, NY 10003-4201; **Phone:** 212-677-2000; **Board Cert:** Ophthalmology 1991; **Med School:** Harvard Med Sch 1986; **Resid:** Ophthalmology, NY Eye & Ear Infirm 1990; **Fellow:** Vitreoretinal Surgery, Montefiore Hosp 1991; **Fac Appt:** Asst Prof Oph, NYU Sch Med

Shields, Carol L MD [Oph] - **Spec Exp:** Orbital Tumors/Cancer; Melanoma; Retinoblastoma; Pediatric Ophthalmology; **Hospital:** Wills Eye Hosp, Jefferson Hosp - Pittsburgh; **Address:** Wills Eye Hosp, Ocular Oncology Service, 840 Walnut St, Ste 1440, Phildelphia, PA 19107; **Phone:** 215-928-3105; **Board Cert:** Ophthalmology 1989; **Med School:** Univ Pittsburgh 1983; **Resid:** Ophthalmology, Willis Eye Hosp 1988; **Fellow:** Ophthalmic Pathology, Willis Eye Hosp 1988; Ophthalmic Oncololgy, Willis Eye Hosp 1989; **Fac Appt:** Prof Oph, Jefferson Med Coll

Shields, Jerry MD [Oph] - **Spec Exp:** Eye Tumors/Cancer; Pediatric Ophthalmology; Retinoblastoma; **Hospital:** Wills Eye Hosp; **Address:** Wills Eye Hosp, Ocular Oncology Service, 840 Walnut St, Ste 1440, Philadelphia, PA 19107; **Phone:** 215-928-3105; **Board Cert:** Ophthalmology 1972; **Med School:** Univ Mich Med Sch 1964; **Resid:** Ophthalmology, Wills Eye Hosp 1970; **Fellow:** Ophthalmology, Wills Eye Hosp 1972; **Fac Appt:** Prof Oph, Thomas Jefferson Univ

Simon, John W MD [Oph] - **Spec Exp:** Pediatric Ophthalmology; Strabismus; **Hospital:** Albany Med Ctr, St Peter's Hosp - Albany; **Address:** 1220 New Scottland Rd, Ste 202, Slingerlands, NY 12159; **Phone:** 518-533-6502; **Board Cert:** Ophthalmology 1981; **Med School:** Mount Sinai Sch Med 1976; **Resid:** Ophthalmology, Mt Sinai Hosp 1980; **Fellow:** Pediatric Ophthalmology, Wills Eye Hosp 1981; **Fac Appt:** Prof Oph, Albany Med Coll

Stark, Walter J MD [Oph] - **Spec Exp:** Corneal Disease & Transplant; Cataract Surgery; Refractive Surgery; **Hospital:** Johns Hopkins Hosp - Baltimore (page 61); **Address:** Wilmer Eye Institute, 600 N Wolfe St Maumenee Bldg - rm 327, Baltimore, MD 21287-9238; **Phone:** 410-955-5490; **Board Cert:** Ophthalmology 1973; **Med School:** Univ Okla Coll Med 1967; **Resid:** Ophthalmology, Wilmer Inst-Johns Hopkins 1971; **Fac Appt:** Prof Oph, Johns Hopkins Univ

Vander, James F MD [Oph] - **Spec Exp:** Diabetic Eye Disease; Retinal Disorders; Macular Degeneration; **Hospital:** Wills Eye Hosp; **Address:** 910 E Willow Grove Ave, Wyndmoor, PA 19038-7910; **Phone:** 215-233-4300; **Board Cert:** Ophthalmology 1989; **Med School:** Univ Mich Med Sch 1984; **Resid:** Ophthalmology, Univ Michigan Med Ctr 1988; **Fellow:** Retina/Vitreous, Wills Eye Hosp 1990; **Fac Appt:** Prof Oph, Thomas Jefferson Univ

Walsh, Joseph MD [Oph] - **Spec Exp:** Diabetic Eye Disease; Macular Degeneration; Retinal Disorders; **Hospital:** New York Eye & Ear Infirm (page 65), Beth Israel Med Ctr - Petrie Division; **Address:** 310 E 14th St Bldg S Fl 3, New York, NY 10003-4201; **Phone:** 212-979-4500; **Board Cert:** Ophthalmology 2005; **Med School:** Georgetown Univ 1966; **Resid:** Ophthalmology, NY Eye & Ear Infirm 1973; **Fellow:** Retina, Montefiore Hosp Med Ctr 1974; **Fac Appt:** Prof Oph, NY Med Coll

Wang, Frederick MD [Oph] - **Spec Exp:** Pediatric Ophthalmology; Strabismus; Eye Muscle Disorders; **Hospital:** New York Eye & Ear Infirm (page 65), Montefiore Med Ctr; **Address:** 30 E 40th St, Ste 405, New York, NY 10016-1201; **Phone:** 212-684-3980; **Board Cert:** Pediatrics 1978; Ophthalmology 1980; **Med School:** Albert Einstein Coll Med 1972; **Resid:** Pediatrics, Jacobi Med Ctr 1974; Ophthalmology, Albert Einstein 1979; **Fellow:** Pediatric Ophthalmology, Children's Hosp Natl Med Ctr 1980; **Fac Appt:** Clin Prof Oph, Albert Einstein Coll Med

Yannuzzi, Lawrence MD [Oph] - **Spec Exp:** Retina/Vitreous Surgery; Macular Disease/Degeneration; Diabetic Eye Disease; **Hospital:** Manhattan Eye, Ear & Throat Hosp; **Address:** 460 Park Ave Fl 5, New York, NY 10021-4028; **Phone:** 212-861-9797; **Board Cert:** Ophthalmology 1970; **Med School:** Boston Univ 1964; **Resid:** Ophthalmology, Manhattan EE&T Hosp 1968; **Fellow:** Ophthalmology, Manhattan EE&T Hosp 1971; **Fac Appt:** Clin Prof Oph, Columbia P&S

Zaidman, Gerald MD [Oph] - **Spec Exp:** Laser Vision Surgery; Cornea Transplant; Cataract Surgery; **Hospital:** Westchester Med Ctr, Our Lady of Mercy Med Ctr; **Address:** Westchester Med Ctr, Macy Pavilion, Dept Opth, rm 1100, Valhalla, NY 10595; **Phone:** 914-493-1599; **Board Cert:** Ophthalmology 1981; **Med School:** Albert Einstein Coll Med 1975; **Resid:** Ophthalmology, Beth Abraham Hosp 1977; Ophthalmology, Lenox Hill Hosp 1980; **Fellow:** Cornea & Ext Eye Disease, Univ Pittsburgh 1982; **Fac Appt:** Prof Oph, NY Med Coll

Southeast

Aaberg Sr, Thomas M MD [Oph] - **Spec Exp:** Retina/Vitreous Surgery; Diabetic Eye Disease/Retinopathy; Macular Disease/Degeneration; **Hospital:** Emory Univ Hosp, Crawford Long Hosp of Emory Univ; **Address:** Emory University, Dept Ophthalmology, 1365B Clifton Rd NE, rm 4405, Atlanta, GA 30322; **Phone:** 404-778-4182; **Board Cert:** Ophthalmology 1967; **Med School:** Harvard Med Sch 1961; **Resid:** Ophthalmology, Mass EE Infirm 1966; **Fellow:** Vitreoretinal Surgery, Bascom-Palmer Eye Inst 1969; **Fac Appt:** Prof Oph, Emory Univ

Alfonso, Eduardo MD [Oph] - **Spec Exp:** Corneal Disease & Surgery; LASIK-Refractive Surgery; Cataract Surgery; **Hospital:** Bascom Palmer Eye Inst. (page 55), Jackson Meml Hosp; **Address:** Bascom Palmer Eye Institute, 900 NW 17th St, Miami, FL 33136-1119; **Phone:** 305-326-6366; **Board Cert:** Ophthalmology 1985; **Med School:** Yale Univ 1980; **Resid:** Ophthalmology, Bascom Palmer Eye Inst-U Miami 1984; **Fellow:** Cornea, Mass Eye & Ear Hosp 1986; Ophthalmological Pathology, Mass Eye & Ear Hosp 1986; **Fac Appt:** Prof Oph, Univ Miami Sch Med

Anderson, Douglas R MD [Oph] - **Spec Exp:** Glaucoma; **Hospital:** Bascom Palmer Eye Inst. (page 55); **Address:** Bascom Palmer Eye Institute, 900 NW 17th St, Miami, FL 33136-1119; **Phone:** 305-243-2020; **Board Cert:** Ophthalmology 1970; **Med School:** Washington Univ, St Louis 1962; **Resid:** Ophthalmology, UCSF Hosp 1968; **Fellow:** Ophthalmology, Mass Eye & Ear Infirmary 1969; **Fac Appt:** Prof Oph, Univ Miami Sch Med

Buckley, Edward G MD [Oph] - **Spec Exp:** Pediatric Ophthalmology; Strabismus; Cataract-Pediatric; **Hospital:** Duke Univ Med Ctr; **Address:** 2351 Erwin Rd, Durham, NC 27705; **Phone:** 919-684-6084; **Board Cert:** Ophthalmology 1982; **Med School:** Duke Univ 1977; **Resid:** Ophthalmology, Duke Univ Eye Ctr 1981; **Fellow:** Ophthalmology, Bascom Palmer Eye Inst 1983; **Fac Appt:** Prof Oph, Duke Univ

Budenz, Donald L MD [Oph] - **Spec Exp:** Glaucoma; **Hospital:** Bascom Palmer Eye Inst. (page 55); **Address:** Bascom Palmer Eye Inst, 900 NW 17th St, Ste 341, Miami, FL 33136; **Phone:** 305-326-6384; **Board Cert:** Ophthalmology 2003; **Med School:** Harvard Med Sch 1987; **Resid:** Ophthalmology, Scheie Eye Inst 1991; **Fellow:** Glaucoma, Bascom Palmer Eye Inst 1992; **Fac Appt:** Assoc Prof Oph, Univ Miami Sch Med

Capo, Hilda MD [Oph] - **Spec Exp:** Pediatric Ophthalmology; Strabismus; Neuro-Ophthalmology; **Hospital:** Bascom Palmer Eye Inst. (page 55); **Address:** Bascom Palmer Eye Institute, 900 NW 17th St, Miami, FL 33136; **Phone:** 305-326-6555; **Board Cert:** Ophthalmology 1989; **Med School:** Puerto Rico 1982; **Resid:** Ophthalmology, Univ PR Med Sch 1987; **Fellow:** Neurological Ophthalmology, NYU Med Ctr 1989; Pediatric Ophthalmology, Johns Hopkins Hosp 1988; **Fac Appt:** Prof Oph, Univ Miami Sch Med

Culbertson, William MD [Oph] - **Spec Exp:** LASIK-Refractive Surgery; Corneal Disease & Surgery; Cataract Surgery; **Hospital:** Bascom Palmer Eye Inst. (page 55); **Address:** Bascom Palmer Eye Institute, 900 NW 17th St, Miami, FL 33136-1119; **Phone:** 305-326-2020; **Board Cert:** Ophthalmology 1976; **Med School:** Emory Univ 1970; **Resid:** Ophthalmology, Vanderbilt Univ Hosp 1974; **Fellow:** Ophthalmology, Bascom Palmer Eye Inst 1979; **Fac Appt:** Prof Oph, Univ Miami Sch Med

Driebe Jr, William T MD [Oph] - **Spec Exp:** Cornea Transplant; Lens Implants; **Hospital:** Shands Hlthcre at Univ of FL; **Address:** Shands Hlthcare Univ FL, 1600 SW Archer Rd, Box 100284, Gainesville, FL 32610-0284; **Phone:** 352-846-2100; **Board Cert:** Ophthalmology 1984; **Med School:** Univ VA Sch Med 1979; **Resid:** Ophthalmology, Shands Hlthcare Univ FL 1983; **Fellow:** Cornea, Bascom Palmer Eye Inst 1984; **Fac Appt:** Prof Oph, Univ Fla Coll Med

Dutton, Jonathan J MD/PhD [Oph] - **Spec Exp:** Oculoplastic Surgery; Eye Tumors/Cancer; Melanoma-Choroidal (eye); **Hospital:** Univ NC Hosps; **Address:** Univ North Carolina - Dept Ophthalmology, 130 Mason Farm Rd, 5110 Bioinformatics, CB 7040, Chapel Hill, NC 27599; **Phone:** 919-966-5296; **Board Cert:** Ophthalmology 1983; **Med School:** Washington Univ, St Louis 1977; **Resid:** Ophthalmology, Washington Univ Med Ctr 1982; **Fellow:** Oculoplastic Surgery, Univ Iowa Med Ctr 1983; **Fac Appt:** Prof Oph, Univ NC Sch Med

Flynn Jr, Harry W MD [Oph] - **Spec Exp:** Retina/Vitreous Surgery; Diabetic Eye Disease/Retinopathy; **Hospital:** Bascom Palmer Eye Inst. (page 55), Univ of Miami Hosp & Clins/Sylvester Comp Canc Ctr; **Address:** Bascom Palmer Eye Institute, 900 NW 17th St, Miami, FL 33136-1119; **Phone:** 305-326-6118; **Board Cert:** Ophthalmology 1976; **Med School:** Univ VA Sch Med 1971; **Resid:** Ophthalmology, Univ VA Hosp 1975; **Fellow:** Retina, Pacific Med Ctr 1976; **Fac Appt:** Prof Oph, Univ Miami Sch Med

Forster, Richard K MD [Oph] - **Spec Exp:** Cornea Transplant; Cataract Surgery; **Hospital:** Bascom Palmer Eye Inst. (page 55); **Address:** Bascom Palmer Eye Institute, 900 NW 17th St, Miami, FL 33136; **Phone:** 305-243-2020; **Board Cert:** Ophthalmology 1971; **Med School:** Boston Univ 1963; **Resid:** Ophthalmology, Bascom Palmer Eye Inst 1969; **Fellow:** Ophthalmology, Fl Proctor Fdn/UCSF 1969; **Fac Appt:** Prof Oph, Univ Miami Sch Med

Freedman, Sharon MD [Oph] - **Spec Exp:** Pediatric Ophthalmology; Glaucoma-Pediatric; Strabismus-Pediatric; Retinopathy of Prematurity; **Hospital:** Duke Univ Med Ctr; **Address:** Duke Eye Center, DUMC 3082, Durham, NC 27710-0001; **Phone:** 919-684-4584; **Board Cert:** Ophthalmology 1991; **Med School:** Harvard Med Sch 1985; **Resid:** Ophthalmology, Mass Eye & Ear Infirm 1989; **Fellow:** Pediatric Ophthalmology, Childns Hosp 1990; Glaucoma, Duke Eye Ctr 1992; **Fac Appt:** Assoc Prof Oph, Duke Univ

Glaser, Joel MD [Oph] - **Spec Exp:** Neuro-Ophthalmology; Orbital Diseases; **Hospital:** Bascom Palmer Eye Inst. (page 55); **Address:** 801 Arthur Godfrey Rd, Ste 402, Miami Beach, FL 33140-3333; **Phone:** 305-532-2885; **Board Cert:** Ophthalmology 1968; **Med School:** Duke Univ 1963; **Resid:** Ophthalmology, Univ Miami Med Coll 1965; **Fellow:** Neurological Ophthalmology, UCSF Med Ctr 1970; **Fac Appt:** Prof Oph, Univ Miami Sch Med

Gorovoy, Mark S MD [Oph] - **Spec Exp:** LASIK-Refractive Surgery; Corneal Disease & Transplant; Glaucoma; Cataract Surgery; **Hospital:** Southwest Florida Regional Medical Center, Lee Memorial Health Systems; **Address:** 12381 S Cleveland Ave, Ste 300, Fort Myers, FL 33907; **Phone:** 239-939-1444; **Board Cert:** Ophthalmology 1982; **Med School:** Geo Wash Univ 1973; **Resid:** Ophthalmology, George Washington Univ Hosp 1980; **Fellow:** Cornea & Ext Eye Disease, Univ Florida 1982

Grossniklaus, Hans E MD [Oph] - **Spec Exp:** Ophthalmic Pathology; Melanoma-Choroidal (eye); Macular Disease/Degeneration; **Hospital:** Emory Univ Hosp; **Address:** Emory Clinic - LF Montgomery Lab, 1365-B Clifton Rd NE, rm BT428, Atlanta, GA 30322; **Phone:** 404-778-4611; **Board Cert:** Ophthalmology 1985; Anatomic Pathology 1987; **Med School:** Ohio State Univ 1980; **Resid:** Ophthalmology, Case West Res Univ Hosp 1984; Pathology, Case West Res Univ Hosp 1987; **Fellow:** Ophthalmological Pathology, Johns Hopkins Hosp 1985; **Fac Appt:** Prof Oph, Emory Univ

Haik, Barrett MD [Oph] - **Spec Exp:** Eye Tumors/Cancer; **Hospital:** St Jude Children's Research Hosp; **Address:** Univ Tenn Med Group, Ophthamology, 930 Madison Ave, Ste 200, Memphis, TN 38103-3452; **Phone:** 901-448-6650; **Board Cert:** Ophthalmology 1981; **Med School:** Louisiana State Univ 1976; **Resid:** Ophthalmology, Columbia-Presby/Harkness Eye Inst 1980; **Fac Appt:** Prof Oph, Univ Tenn Coll Med, Memphis

Hess, J Bruce MD [Oph] - **Spec Exp:** Pediatric Ophthalmology; Strabismus; **Hospital:** All Children's Hosp, Bayfront Med Ctr; **Address:** 880 6th St S, Ste 350, St Petersburg, FL 33701; **Phone:** 727-767-4393; **Board Cert:** Ophthalmology 1978; **Med School:** Baylor Coll Med 1971; **Resid:** Ophthalmology, Geisinger Med Ctr 1977; **Fellow:** Ophthalmology, Wills Eye Hosp 1978; **Fac Appt:** Assoc Prof Oph, Univ S Fla Coll Med

Holliday, James N MD/PhD [Oph] - **Spec Exp:** Cataract Surgery; Glaucoma; Diabetic Eye Disease; **Hospital:** St Francis Hosp - Memphis, Baptist Memorial Hospital - Memphis; **Address:** 4571 Summer Ave, Memphis, TN 38122; **Phone:** 901-680-0043; **Board Cert:** Ophthalmology 2004; **Med School:** Duke Univ 1987; **Resid:** Ophthalmology, UC Irvine Med Ctr 1992; **Fellow:** Anterior Segment - External Disease, Mayo Clinic 1993

Lambert, Scott R MD [Oph] - **Spec Exp:** Pediatric Ophthalmology; Strabismus; Cataract-Pediatric; **Hospital:** Chldns Hlthcare Atlanta - Egleston, Chldns Hlthcare Atlanta - Scottish Rite; **Address:** Emory Eye Ctr, Dept Ped Opth, 1365 Clifton Rd B Bldg - Ste 4513, Atlanta, GA 30322; **Phone:** 404-778-3431; **Board Cert:** Ophthalmology 1989; **Med School:** Yale Univ 1983; **Resid:** Ophthalmology, UCSF Med Ctr 1987; **Fellow:** Pediatric Ophthalmology, Hosp for Sick Chldn 1988; **Fac Appt:** Prof Oph, Emory Univ

Lee, Paul P MD [Oph] - **Spec Exp:** Glaucoma; **Hospital:** Duke Univ Med Ctr; **Address:** Duke Univ Eye Ctr, Erwin Rd, Wadsworth Bldg, Box 3802, Durham, NC 27710; **Phone:** 919-681-2793; **Board Cert:** Ophthalmology 1991; **Med School:** Univ Mich Med Sch 1986; **Resid:** Ophthalmology, Wilmer Eye Inst/Johns Hopkins 1990; **Fellow:** Glaucoma, Mass EE Infirm 1991; **Fac Appt:** Prof Oph, Duke Univ

McCord, Clinton MD [Oph] - **Spec Exp:** Eyelid Surgery; Oculoplastic Surgery; **Hospital:** Piedmont Hosp; **Address:** 3200 Downwood Cir, Ste 640, Atlanta, GA 30327; **Phone:** 404-351-0051; **Board Cert:** Ophthalmology 1968; **Med School:** Emory Univ 1961; **Resid:** Ophthalmology, Emory Univ Hosp 1965; **Fellow:** Oculoplastic Surgery, Manhattan Eye & Ear Inst 1967; **Fac Appt:** Assoc Clin Prof PlS, Emory Univ

McKeown, Craig A MD [Oph] - **Spec Exp:** Pediatric Ophthalmology; Strabismus-Adult & Pediatric; Eye Muscle Disorders; **Hospital:** Bascom Palmer Eye Inst. (page 55); **Address:** Bascolm Palmer Eye Institute, 900 NW 17th St, Miami, FL 33136; **Phone:** 305-243-2020; **Board Cert:** Ophthalmology 1982; **Med School:** Northwestern Univ 1971; **Resid:** Ophthalmology, Walter Reed Med Ctr 1980; **Fellow:** Pediatric Ophthalmology, Chldns Hosp Natl Med Ctr 1984; Pediatric Ophthalmology, Wilmer Inst-Johns Hospkins 1985; **Fac Appt:** Assoc Prof Oph, Univ Miami Sch Med

Meredith, Travis MD [Oph] - **Spec Exp:** Retina/Vitreous Surgery; Macular Degeneration; Diabetic Eye Disease/Retinopathy; **Hospital:** Univ NC Hosps; **Address:** 5113 Bio Informatics, Box CB#7040, Chapel Hill, NC 27599-7040; **Phone:** 919-966-5509; **Board Cert:** Ophthalmology 1976; **Med School:** Johns Hopkins Univ 1969; **Resid:** Ophthalmology, Wilmer Inst-Johns Hopkins 1971; Ophthalmology, Wilmer Inst-Johns Hopkins 1975; **Fellow:** Vitreoretinal Surgery, Med Coll Wisconsin 1976; **Fac Appt:** Prof Oph, Univ NC Sch Med

Nunery, William R MD [Oph] - **Spec Exp:** Orbital Surgery; Oculoplastic Surgery; Thyroid Eye Disease; **Hospital:** Univ of Louisville Hosp; **Address:** Eye Specialists of Louisville, PSC, 301 E Muhammad Ali Blvd, Louisville, KY 40202; **Phone:** 502-852-7665; **Board Cert:** Ophthalmology 1980; **Med School:** Case West Res Univ 1975; **Resid:** Ophthalmology, Indiana Univ Hosp 1979; **Fellow:** Ophthalmic Plastic Surgery, Emory Univ 1980

Nussbaum, Julian MD [Oph] - **Spec Exp:** Diabetic Eye Disease/Retinopathy; Macular Degeneration; Retinopathy of Prematurity; **Hospital:** Med Coll of GA Hosp and Clin; **Address:** Med Coll Georgia, 1120 15th St Bldg BA 27, Augusta, GA 30912; **Phone:** 706-721-1148; **Board Cert:** Ophthalmology 1981; **Med School:** Univ Miami Sch Med 1976; **Resid:** Internal Medicine, Jackson Memorial Hosp 1977; Ophthalmology, Med Coll Georgia 1980; **Fellow:** Vitreoretinal Surgery, Mass Eye & Ear Infirmary 1982; **Fac Appt:** Prof Oph, Med Coll GA

Ophthalmology

Palmberg, Paul MD/PhD [Oph] - **Spec Exp:** Glaucoma; **Hospital:** Bascom Palmer Eye Inst. (page 55); **Address:** 900 NW 17th St, Miami, FL 33136; **Phone:** 305-326-6386; **Board Cert:** Ophthalmology 1976; **Med School:** Northwestern Univ 1970; **Resid:** Ophthalmology, Washington Univ 1974; Ophthalmology, Barnes Hosp 1977; **Fellow:** Glaucoma, Washington Univ 1976; **Fac Appt:** Prof Oph, Univ Miami Sch Med

Parrish, Richard K MD [Oph] - **Spec Exp:** Glaucoma; Cataract Surgery; Anterior Segment Surgery; **Hospital:** Bascom Palmer Eye Inst. (page 55), Jackson Meml Hosp; **Address:** Bascom Palmer Eye Institute, 900 NW 17th St, Miami, FL 33136; **Phone:** 305-243-2020; **Board Cert:** Ophthalmology 1981; **Med School:** Indiana Univ 1976; **Resid:** Ophthalmology, Wills Eye Hosp 1980; **Fellow:** Glaucoma, Bascom Palmer Eye Inst 1982; **Fac Appt:** Prof Oph, Univ Miami Sch Med

Pollard, Zane F MD [Oph] - **Spec Exp:** Pediatric Ophthalmology; Strabismus; Tear Duct Problems; **Hospital:** Chldns Hlthcare Atlanta - Scottish Rite, Piedmont Hosp; **Address:** 5445 Meridian Mark Rd, Ste 220, Atlanta, GA 30342-4722; **Phone:** 404-255-2419; **Board Cert:** Ophthalmology 1975; **Med School:** Tulane Univ 1966; **Resid:** Surgery, UCSF Med Ctr 1968; Ophthalmology, USC Med Ctr 1973; **Fellow:** Pediatric Ophthalmology, Wills Eye Hosp 1975

Puliafito, Carmen A MD [Oph] - **Spec Exp:** Retinal Disorders; Macular Degeneration; **Hospital:** Bascom Palmer Eye Inst. (page 55); **Address:** 900 NW 17 St, Miami, FL 33136; **Phone:** 305-326-6303; **Board Cert:** Ophthalmology 1983; **Med School:** Harvard Med Sch 1978; **Resid:** Ophthalmology, Mass Eye & Ear Infirm 1982; **Fellow:** Vitreoretinal Surgery, Mass Eye & Ear Infirm 1983; **Fac Appt:** Prof Oph, Univ Miami Sch Med

Rosenfeld, Philip MD [Oph] - **Spec Exp:** Macular Disease/Degeneration; Diabetic Eye Disease/Retinopathy; Retinal Detachment; Retina/Vitreous Surgery; **Hospital:** Bascom Palmer Eye Inst. (page 55); **Address:** Bascom Palmer Eye Institute, 900 NW 17th St, Miami, FL 33136; **Phone:** 305-243-2020; **Board Cert:** Ophthalmology 1997; **Med School:** Johns Hopkins Univ 1988; **Resid:** Ophthalmology, Mass Eye & Ear Infirm 1995; **Fellow:** Retina, Bascom Palmer Eye Inst 1996; **Fac Appt:** Assoc Prof Oph, Univ Fla Coll Med

Sherwood, Mark MD [Oph] - **Spec Exp:** Glaucoma; **Hospital:** Shands Hlthcre at Univ of FL; **Address:** Shands at University of Florida, 1600 SW Archer Rd, Box 100284, Gainesville, FL 32610-0393; **Phone:** 352-392-3451; **Board Cert:** Ophthalmology 1983; **Med School:** England 1976; **Resid:** Ophthalmology, Moorefield's Eye Hosp 1980; **Fellow:** Glaucoma, Wills Eye Hosp 1982; Glaucoma, Moorefield's Eye Hosp 1983; **Fac Appt:** Prof Oph, Univ Fla Coll Med

Sternberg Jr, Paul MD [Oph] - **Spec Exp:** Retina/Vitreous Surgery; Macular Degeneration(Age-Related); Eye Tumors/Cancer; **Hospital:** Vanderbilt Univ Med Ctr, Vanderbilt Children's Hosp; **Address:** Vanderbilt Eye Institute, 8000 Medical Center E, Nashville, TN 37232-8808; **Phone:** 615-936-1453; **Board Cert:** Ophthalmology 1985; **Med School:** Univ Chicago-Pritzker Sch Med 1979; **Resid:** Ophthalmology, Johns Hopkins Hosp 1983; **Fellow:** Vitreoretinal Surgery, Duke Univ Med Ctr 1984; **Fac Appt:** Prof Oph, Vanderbilt Univ

Stulting, R Doyle MD [Oph] - **Spec Exp:** Corneal Disease & Transplant; Laser Vision Surgery; Cataract Surgery; **Hospital:** Emory Univ Hosp; **Address:** The Emory Clinic, Dept Ophthalmology, 1365B Clifton Rd NE, Ste 4500, Atlanta, GA 30322; **Phone:** 404-778-5818; **Board Cert:** Ophthalmology 1982; **Med School:** Duke Univ 1976; **Resid:** Internal Medicine, Barnes Hosp 1978; Ophthalmology, Bascom Palmer Eye Inst 1981; **Fellow:** Cornea, Emory Univ Clinic 1982; **Fac Appt:** Prof Oph, Emory Univ

Tse, David MD [Oph] - **Spec Exp:** Oculoplastic Surgery; Orbital Tumors/Cancer; Lacrimal Gland Disorders; Eyelid Tumors/Cancer; **Hospital:** Bascom Palmer Eye Inst. (page 55), Jackson Meml Hosp; **Address:** Bascom Palmer Eye Inst, 900 NW 17th St, Miami, FL 33136-1119; **Phone:** 305-326-6086; **Board Cert:** Ophthalmology 2002; **Med School:** Univ Miami Sch Med 1976; **Resid:** Ophthalmology, LAC/USC Med Ctr 1981; **Fellow:** Oculoplastic Surgery, Univ Iowa Hosps 1982; **Fac Appt:** Prof Oph, Univ Miami Sch Med

Wang, Ming X MD/PhD [Oph] - **Spec Exp:** Laser Vision Surgery; Anterior Segment Surgery; Corneal Disease; **Hospital:** Saint Thomas Hosp - Nashville; **Address:** 1801 West End Ave, Palmer Plaza, Ste 1150, Nashville, TN 37203; **Phone:** 615-321-8881; **Board Cert:** Ophthalmology 1998; **Med School:** Harvard Med Sch 1991; **Resid:** Ophthalmology, Wills Eye Hosp 1996; **Fellow:** Refractive Surgery, Bascom Palmer Eye Inst 1997; **Fac Appt:** , UC Davis

Waring III, George O MD [Oph] - **Spec Exp:** LASIK-Refractive Surgery; Cataract Surgery; Lens Implants; **Hospital:** Northside Hosp; **Address:** 301 Perimeter Center N, Ste 600, Atlanta, GA 30346; **Phone:** 678-222-5102; **Board Cert:** Ophthalmology 1975; **Med School:** Baylor Coll Med 1967; **Resid:** Ophthalmology, Wills Eye Hosp 1973; **Fellow:** Cornea & Ext Eye Disease, Wills Eye Hosp 1974

Wilson Jr, M Edward MD [Oph] - **Spec Exp:** Cataract-Pediatric; Strabismus-Pediatric; Lens Implants-Pediatric; Pediatric Ophthalmology; **Hospital:** MUSC Chldns Hosp; **Address:** MUSC Storm Eye Inst, 167 Ashley Ave, PO Box 250676, Charleston, SC 29425; **Phone:** 843-792-7622; **Board Cert:** Ophthalmology 1987; **Med School:** Med Univ SC 1980; **Resid:** Ophthalmology, Natl Naval Med Ctr 1986; **Fellow:** Pediatric Ophthalmology, Chldns Hosp - Naval Med Ctr 1987; **Fac Appt:** Prof Oph, Med Univ SC

Midwest

Abrams, Gary W MD [Oph] - **Spec Exp:** Retina/Vitreous Surgery; **Hospital:** Hutzel Hosp - Detroit; **Address:** Kresge Eye Institute, 4717 St Antoine St, Detroit, MI 48201; **Phone:** 313-577-8900; **Board Cert:** Ophthalmology 1977; **Med School:** Univ Okla Coll Med 1968; **Resid:** Ophthalmology, Med Coll Wisc Affil Hosps 1976; **Fellow:** Vitreoretinal Surgery, Bascom Palmer Eye Inst 1978; **Fac Appt:** Prof Oph, Wayne State Univ

Albert, Daniel M MD [Oph] - **Spec Exp:** Eye Tumors/Cancer; Ophthalmic Pathology; **Hospital:** Univ WI Hosp & Clins; **Address:** Dept Ophthalmology/VisualSci, K61412 CSC, 600 Highland Ave, Madison, WI 53792-4673; **Phone:** 608-263-9092; **Board Cert:** Ophthalmology 1969; **Med School:** Univ Pennsylvania 1962; **Resid:** Ophthalmology, Hosp Univ Penn 1966; Neurological Ophthalmology, Natl Inst Hlth 1968; **Fellow:** Pathology, Armed Forces Inst Path 1969; **Fac Appt:** Prof Oph, Univ Wisc

Alward, Wallace MD [Oph] - **Spec Exp:** Glaucoma; **Hospital:** Univ Iowa Hosp & Clinics, VA Med Ctr - Iowa City; **Address:** 200 Hawkins Drive, Iowa City, IA 52242-1009; **Phone:** 319-356-3938; **Board Cert:** Ophthalmology 1987; **Med School:** Ohio State Univ 1976; **Resid:** Ophthalmology, Univ Louisville 1986; **Fellow:** Glaucoma, Univ Miami-Bascom Palmer Eye Inst 1987; **Fac Appt:** Prof Oph, Univ Iowa Coll Med

Appen, Richard E MD [Oph] - **Spec Exp:** Neuro-Ophthalmology; **Hospital:** Univ WI Hosp & Clins; **Address:** Dept Ophth-UNW Hosp, 600 Highland Ave, Madison, WI 53792; **Phone:** 608-263-7171; **Board Cert:** Ophthalmology 1974; **Med School:** Duke Univ 1966; **Resid:** Ophthalmology, Univ Wisconsin & Clinics 1972; **Fellow:** Neurological Ophthalmology, Mass Eye & Ear Infirmary 1973; **Fac Appt:** Prof Oph, Univ Wisc

Ophthalmology

Archer, Steven M MD [Oph] - **Spec Exp:** Pediatric Ophthalmology; **Hospital:** Univ Michigan Hlth Sys; **Address:** Kellogg Eye Center, 1000 Wall St, Ann Arbor, MI 48105-1912; **Phone:** 734-764-7558; **Board Cert:** Ophthalmology 1986; **Med School:** Univ Chicago-Pritzker Sch Med 1978; **Resid:** Ophthalmology, Univ Chicago 1984; **Fellow:** Pediatric Ophthalmology, Indiana Univ 1986; **Fac Appt:** Asst Prof Oph, Univ Mich Med Sch

Azar, Dimitri T MD [Oph] - **Spec Exp:** Cornea Transplant; Cornea & External Eye Disease; Refractive Surgery; **Hospital:** Univ of IL at Chicago Eye & Ear Infirm; **Address:** Univ of Illinois, 1855 West Taylor St, Chicago, IL 60612; **Phone:** 312-996-6590; **Board Cert:** Ophthalmology 1991; **Med School:** Lebanon 1983; **Resid:** Ophthalmology, American Univ Medical Ctr 1986; Ophthalmology, Mass E&E Infirm 1991; **Fellow:** Cornea & Ext Eye Disease, Mass E&E Infirm 1988; Cornea Research, Harvard Med Sch 1991

Baker, John D MD [Oph] - **Spec Exp:** Pediatric Ophthalmology; **Hospital:** Chldns Hosp of Michigan; **Address:** 2355 Monroe Blvd, Dearborn, MI 48124-3009; **Phone:** 313-561-1777; **Board Cert:** Ophthalmology 1974; **Med School:** Wayne State Univ 1967; **Resid:** Ophthalmology, Detroit Genl Hosp 1971; **Fellow:** Pediatric Ophthalmology, Chldns Natl Med Ctr 1972; **Fac Appt:** Clin Prof Oph, Wayne State Univ

Burke, Miles J MD [Oph] - **Spec Exp:** Pediatric Ophthalmology; Eye Muscle Surgery; Amblyopia & Vision Development; **Hospital:** Cincinnati Chldns Hosp Med Ctr, Jewish Hosp - Kenwood - Cincinnati; **Address:** 10475 Montgomery Rd, Ste 4F, Cincinnati, OH 45242-5200; **Phone:** 513-984-4949; **Board Cert:** Ophthalmology 1979; **Med School:** Univ Ariz Coll Med 1974; **Resid:** Ophthalmology, Univ Michigan Med Ctr 1978; **Fellow:** Pediatric Ophthalmology, Wills Eye Hosp 1979

Carter, Keith D MD [Oph] - **Spec Exp:** Oculoplastic & Orbital Surgery; Eyelid Surgery / Blepharoplasty; Botox Therapy; **Hospital:** Univ Iowa Hosp & Clinics; **Address:** Univ Iowa, Dept Ophthalmology, 200 Hawkins Dr, PFP 11136-F, Iowa City, IA 52242; **Phone:** 319-356-2852; **Board Cert:** Ophthalmology 1988; **Med School:** Indiana Univ 1983; **Resid:** Ophthalmology, Univ Michigan Med Ctr 1987; **Fellow:** Oculoplastic Surgery, Univ Iowa 1988; **Fac Appt:** Prof Oph, Univ Iowa Coll Med

Cionni, Robert J MD [Oph] - **Spec Exp:** Cataract Surgery-Lens Implant; **Hospital:** Bethesda North Hosp; **Address:** 1945 Cei Drive, Cincinnati, OH 45242; **Phone:** 513-984-5133; **Board Cert:** Ophthalmology 1991; **Med School:** Univ Cincinnati 1985; **Resid:** Ophthalmology, Univ Louisville Hosp 1987; **Fellow:** Cataract/Lens Implant Surgery, Cincinnati Eye Inst

Del Monte, Monte A MD [Oph] - **Spec Exp:** Pediatric Ophthalmology; Strabismus-Adult; Glaucoma-Pediatric; Cataract-Pediatric; **Hospital:** Univ Michigan Hlth Sys; **Address:** Kellogg Eye Center, 1000 Wall St, Ann Arbor, MI 48105-1912; **Phone:** 734-764-3111; **Board Cert:** Ophthalmology 1982; **Med School:** Johns Hopkins Univ 1974; **Resid:** Pediatrics, Chldns Hosp Med Ctr 1977; Ophthalmology, Wilmer Eye Inst 1981; **Fellow:** Ophthalmology, Wilmer Eye Inst 1978; Pediatric Ophthalmology, Chldns Hosp 1981; **Fac Appt:** Prof Oph, Univ Mich Med Sch

Feder, Robert S MD [Oph] - **Spec Exp:** Corneal Disease; LASIK-Refractive Surgery; Cataract Surgery; **Hospital:** Northwestern Meml Hosp; **Address:** 675 N St Clair St, Fl 15, Chicago, IL 60611-5975; **Phone:** 312-695-8150; **Board Cert:** Ophthalmology 1983; **Med School:** Northwestern Univ 1978; **Resid:** Ophthalmology, Barnes Hosp-Wash Univ 1982; **Fellow:** Cornea & Ext Eye Disease, Univ Iowa 1983; **Fac Appt:** Assoc Prof Oph, Northwestern Univ

France, Thomas D MD [Oph] - **Spec Exp:** Pediatric Ophthalmology; Strabismus-Adult & Pediatric; Amblyopia & Vision Development; **Hospital:** Univ WI Hosp & Clins; **Address:** Univ Station Clinics, Dept Pediatric Ophthalmology, 2880 University Ave, Madison, WI 53705; **Phone:** 608-263-6414; **Board Cert:** Ophthalmology 1971; **Med School:** Northwestern Univ 1962; **Resid:** Ophthalmology, UCSF Med Ctr 1969; **Fellow:** Pediatric Ophthalmology, Chldns Hosp Natl Med Ctr 1970; Pediatric Ophthalmology, Hosp Sick Chldn 1970; **Fac Appt:** Prof Oph, Univ Wisc

Greenwald, Mark MD [Oph] - **Spec Exp:** Pediatric Ophthalmology; **Hospital:** Univ of Chicago Hosps; **Address:** Univ of Chicago, Dept Ophthalmology, 5841 S Maryland Ave, MC 2114, Chicago, IL 60637; **Phone:** 773-834-5685; **Board Cert:** Ophthalmology 1981; **Med School:** Harvard Med Sch 1976; **Resid:** Ophthalmology, Univ Illinois Hosp 1980; **Fellow:** Pediatric Ophthalmology, Children's Hosp 1981; **Fac Appt:** Assoc Prof Oph, Univ Wash

Heuer, Dale K MD [Oph] - **Spec Exp:** Glaucoma; **Hospital:** Froedtert Meml Lutheran Hosp; **Address:** The Eye Institute, 925 N 87th St, Milwaukee, WI 53226; **Phone:** 414-456-2020; **Board Cert:** Ophthalmology 1983; **Med School:** Northwestern Univ 1978; **Resid:** Ophthalmology, Med Coll Wisc Affil Hosp 1982; **Fellow:** Glaucoma, Bascom Palmer Eye Inst 1984; **Fac Appt:** Prof Oph, Med Coll Wisc

Holland, Edward J MD [Oph] - **Spec Exp:** Corneal Disease; Refractive Surgery; Cataract Surgery; **Hospital:** St Elizabeth Med Ctr (South Unit), Bethesda North Hosp; **Address:** 1945 CEI Drive, Cincinnati, OH 45242; **Phone:** 513-984-5133; **Board Cert:** Ophthalmology 1986; **Med School:** Loyola Univ-Stritch Sch Med 1981; **Resid:** Ophthalmology, Univ Minn Med Ctr 1985; **Fellow:** Ophthalmology, Univ Iowa 1986; Ocular Immunology, Natl Eye Inst 1987; **Fac Appt:** Clin Prof Oph, Univ Cincinnati

John, Thomas MD [Oph] - **Spec Exp:** Cornea Transplant & Artificial Cornea; Amniotic Membrane Transplant; Cataract Surgery; Refractive Surgery; **Hospital:** Loyola Univ Med Ctr, Adv S Suburban Hosp; **Address:** 16532 S Oak Park Ave, Ste 201, Tinley Park, IL 60477; **Phone:** 708-429-2223; **Board Cert:** Ophthalmology 1987; **Med School:** India 1977; **Resid:** Ophthalmology, Hosp U Penn 1984; **Fellow:** Cornea & Ext Eye Disease, Univ Rochester Sch Med & Dentistry 1985; Cornea & Ext Eye Disease, Mass Eye & Ear Infirmary 1987; **Fac Appt:** Assoc Clin Prof Oph, Loyola Univ-Stritch Sch Med

Kaufman, Paul L MD [Oph] - **Spec Exp:** Glaucoma; **Hospital:** Univ WI Hosp & Clins; **Address:** Univ Wisconsin Hosp, Dept Ophthalmology, 2870 University Ave, Ste 102, Madison, WI 53705-3611; **Phone:** 608-263-7171; **Board Cert:** Ophthalmology 1976; **Med School:** NYU Sch Med 1967; **Resid:** Ophthalmology, Barnes Hospital 1973; **Fellow:** Ocular Pharmacology, Univ Uppsala 1975; **Fac Appt:** Prof Oph, Univ Wisc

Krachmer, Jay H MD [Oph] - **Spec Exp:** Corneal Disease; **Hospital:** Univ Minn Med Ctr, Fairview - Univ Campus; **Address:** ATTN: Dr. Jay H Krachmer, Dept Ophthalmology, 420 Delaware St SE, MMC 493, Minneapolis, MN 55455; **Phone:** 612-625-4400; **Board Cert:** Ophthalmology 1972; **Med School:** Tulane Univ 1966; **Resid:** Ophthalmology, Univ Hosp 1970; **Fellow:** Cornea, Wills Eye Hosp 1974; **Fac Appt:** Prof Oph, Univ Minn

Krueger, Ronald MD [Oph] - **Spec Exp:** Corneal Disease; Refractive Surgery; **Hospital:** Cleveland Clin Fdn (page 57); **Address:** Cleveland Clinic Fdn - Cole Eye Inst, 9500 Euclid Ave, Desk i32, Cleveland, OH 44195; **Phone:** 216-444-8158; **Board Cert:** Ophthalmology 2003; **Med School:** UMDNJ-NJ Med Sch, Newark 1987; **Resid:** Ophthalmology, Columbia Presby Med Ctr 1991; **Fellow:** Refractive Surgery, Univ Okla Hlth Sci Ctr-McGee Eye Inst; Cornea, USC-Doheny Eye Inst 1993

Ophthalmology

Kushner, Burton J MD [Oph] - **Spec Exp:** Pediatric Ophthalmology; Strabismus-Adult & Pediatric; **Hospital:** Univ WI Hosp & Clins; **Address:** Dept Ophth-UNW Hosp, 600 Highland Ave, Madison, WI 53792; **Phone:** 608-263-7171; **Board Cert:** Ophthalmology 1975; **Med School:** Northwestern Univ 1969; **Resid:** Ophthalmology, Univ Wisc Hosp 1973; **Fellow:** Pediatric Ophthalmology, Bascom Palmer Eye Inst 1974; **Fac Appt:** Prof Oph, Univ Wisc

Lane, Stephen S MD [Oph] - **Spec Exp:** Laser Vision Surgery; Cataract Surgery; **Hospital:** United Hosp; **Address:** Associated Eye Care, 2950 Curve Crest Blvd, Stillwater, MN 55082; **Phone:** 651-275-3000; **Board Cert:** Ophthalmology 1986; **Med School:** Univ Minn 1980; **Resid:** Ophthalmology, MS Hershey Med Ctr 1984; **Fellow:** Cornea & Ext Eye Disease, Univ Minn 1984; **Fac Appt:** Clin Prof Oph, Univ Minn

Lee, Andrew G MD [Oph] - **Spec Exp:** Neuro-Ophthalmology; Optic Nerve Disorders; Optic Nerve Tumors; **Hospital:** Univ Iowa Hosp & Clinics; **Address:** Univ Iowa, Dept Ophthalmology, 200 Hawkins Dr, PFP 11290-E, Iowa City, IA 52242; **Phone:** 319-356-2548; **Board Cert:** Ophthalmology 1995; **Med School:** Univ VA Sch Med 1989; **Resid:** Ophthalmology, Cullen Eye Inst-Baylor 1993; **Fellow:** Neurological Ophthalmology, Wilmer Eye Inst-Johns Hopkins 1994; **Fac Appt:** Prof Oph, Univ Iowa Coll Med

Lewis, Hilel MD [Oph] - **Spec Exp:** Macular Degeneration; Diabetic Eye Disease/Retinopathy; Retinal Disorders; **Hospital:** Cleveland Clin Fdn (page 57); **Address:** Cleveland Clinic, Cole Eye Inst, 9500 Euclid Ave, Desk i30, Cleveland, OH 44195-0001; **Phone:** 216-444-0430; **Board Cert:** Ophthalmology 1990; **Med School:** Mexico 1980; **Resid:** Ophthalmology, Jules Stein Eye Inst-UCLA 1986; **Fellow:** Ocular Pathology, Jules Stein Eye Inst-UCLA 1983; Vitreoretinal Surgery, Med Coll Wisconsin 1987; **Fac Appt:** Prof Oph, Cleveland Cl Coll Med/Case West Res

Lichter, Paul R MD [Oph] - **Spec Exp:** Cataract Surgery; Glaucoma; **Hospital:** Univ Michigan Hlth Sys; **Address:** 1000 Wall St, Ann Arbor, MI 48105; **Phone:** 734-763-5874; **Board Cert:** Ophthalmology 1970; **Med School:** Univ Mich Med Sch 1964; **Resid:** Ophthalmology, Univ Mich Med Ctr 1968; **Fellow:** Ophthalmology, UCSF Med Ctr 1969; **Fac Appt:** Prof Oph, Univ Mich Med Sch

Lindstrom, Richard L MD [Oph] - **Spec Exp:** Corneal Disease; Cataract Surgery; Refractive Surgery; **Hospital:** Abbott - Northwestern Hosp, Phillips Eye Inst; **Address:** 710 E 24th St, Ste 106, Minneapolis, MN 55404; **Phone:** 612-813-3600; **Board Cert:** Ophthalmology 1978; **Med School:** Univ Minn 1972; **Resid:** Ophthalmology, Univ Minn 1979; Ophthalmology, Univ Minn 1980; **Fellow:** Anterior Segment - External Disease, Mary Shields Eye Hosp; Glaucoma, Univ Hosps; **Fac Appt:** Prof Oph, Univ Minn

Lueder, Gregg T MD [Oph] - **Spec Exp:** Retinoblastoma; Eye Tumors-Pediatric; Pediatric Ophthalmology; **Hospital:** St Louis Chldns Hosp; **Address:** St Louis Children's Hospital, One Children's Pl, rm 2S89, St Louis, MO 63110; **Phone:** 314-454-6026; **Board Cert:** Pediatrics 1989; Ophthalmology 2003; **Med School:** Univ Iowa Coll Med 1985; **Resid:** Pediatrics, St Louis Children's Hosp 1988; Ophthalmology, Univ Iowa Med Ctr 1991; **Fellow:** Pediatric Ophthalmology, Hosp for Sick Children 1993; **Fac Appt:** Assoc Prof Oph, Washington Univ, St Louis

Maguire, Leo J MD [Oph] - **Spec Exp:** Cornea Transplant; Refractive Surgery; Boston Scleral Lens Prosthesis; **Hospital:** Mayo Med Ctr & Clin - Rochester; **Address:** Mayo Clinic, Dept Ophthalmology, 200 First St SW, Rochester, MN 55905; **Phone:** 507-284-4152; **Board Cert:** Ophthalmology 1986; **Med School:** Jefferson Med Coll 1980; **Resid:** Ophthalmology, Univ Michigan Med Ctr 1984; **Fellow:** Cornea & Ext Eye Disease, LSU Eye Ctr 1986; **Fac Appt:** Assoc Prof Oph, Mayo Med Sch

Mets, Marilyn MD [Oph] - **Spec Exp:** Pediatric Ophthalmology; Ophthalmic Genetics; Strabismus; Retinal Disorders; **Hospital:** Children's Mem Hosp; **Address:** 2300 Children's Plaza, Box 70, Chicago, IL 60614; **Phone:** 773-880-4346; **Board Cert:** Ophthalmology 2005; **Med School:** Geo Wash Univ 1976; **Resid:** Ophthalmology, Cleveland Clinic Fdn 1980; **Fellow:** Ophthalmology, Natl Chldns Hosp 1981; **Fac Appt:** Prof Oph, Northwestern Univ

Mieler, William F MD [Oph] - **Spec Exp:** Eye Tumors/Cancer; Retina/Vitreous Surgery; Retinoblastoma; **Hospital:** Univ of Chicago Hosps; **Address:** Univ Chicago, Dept Opth & Vis Sci, 5841 S Maryland, rm S-209, MC 211, Chicago, IL 60637; **Phone:** 773-702-3838; **Board Cert:** Ophthalmology 1984; **Med School:** Univ Wisc 1979; **Resid:** Ophthalmology, Bascom-Palmer Eye Inst 1983; **Fellow:** Vitreoretinal Surgery & Disease, Med Ctr Wisconsin Eye Inst 1984; Oculoplastic Surgery, Wills Eye Hosp 1986; **Fac Appt:** Prof Oph, Univ Chicago-Pritzker Sch Med

Nerad, Jeffrey MD [Oph] - **Spec Exp:** Orbital Tumors/Cancer; Eyelid Cancer & Reconstruction; Oculoplastic Surgery; **Hospital:** Univ Iowa Hosp & Clinics; **Address:** Univ Iowa, Dept Ophthalmology, 200 Hawkins Drive, Iowa City, IA 52242; **Phone:** 319-356-2864; **Board Cert:** Ophthalmology 1984; **Med School:** St Louis Univ 1979; **Resid:** Ophthalmology, St Louis Univ Med Ctr 1983; **Fellow:** Oculoplastic & Reconstructive Surgery, Univ Iowa 1984; **Fac Appt:** Prof Oph, Univ Iowa Coll Med

Olitsky, Scott Eric MD [Oph] - **Spec Exp:** Pediatric Ophthalmology; Strabismus; **Hospital:** Chldns Mercy Hosps & Clinics; **Address:** Chldns Mercy Hosp, Dept Oph, 2401 Gillham Rd, Kansas City, MO 64108; **Phone:** 816-234-3046; **Board Cert:** Ophthalmology 1993; **Med School:** Jefferson Med Coll 1988; **Resid:** Ophthalmology, SUNY Buffalo Med Ctr 1992; **Fellow:** Pediatric Ophthalmology, Wills Eye Hosp 1993; **Fac Appt:** Assoc Prof Oph, Univ MO-Kansas City

Osher, Robert H MD [Oph] - **Spec Exp:** Cataract Surgery-Lens Implant; **Address:** 1945 CEI Drive, Cincinnati, OH 45242; **Phone:** 513-984-5133; **Board Cert:** Ophthalmology 1981; **Med School:** Univ Rochester 1976; **Resid:** Ophthalmology, Bascom Palmer Eye Inst 1980; **Fellow:** Ophthalmology, Wills Eye Hosp 1977; Ophthalmology, Bascom Palmer Eye Inst 1981; **Fac Appt:** Prof Oph, Univ Cincinnati

Pepose, Jay MD [Oph] - **Spec Exp:** LASIK-Refractive Surgery; Cataract Surgery; Corneal & External Eye Disease; **Hospital:** Barnes-Jewish Hosp, St John's Mercy Med Ctr - St Louis; **Address:** 1815 Clarkson Rd Chesterfield, MO 63017; **Phone:** 636-728-0111; **Board Cert:** Ophthalmology 1989; **Med School:** UCLA 1982; **Resid:** Ophthalmology, Johns Hopkins Hosp 1987; **Fellow:** Cornea & Ext Eye Disease, Georgetown Univ Med Ctr 1988; **Fac Appt:** Prof Oph, Washington Univ, St Louis

Price, Ronald MD [Oph] - **Spec Exp:** Pediatric Ophthalmology; Strabismus; **Hospital:** MetroHealth Med Ctr, Univ Hosps Case Med Ctr; **Address:** Univ Ophth Assocs, 1611 S Green Rd, Ste 306-C, Cleveland, OH 44121-4128; **Phone:** 216-382-8022; **Board Cert:** Ophthalmology 1971; **Med School:** Columbia P&S 1965; **Resid:** Ophthalmology, Univ Louisville Hosps 1970; **Fellow:** Pediatric Ophthalmology, DC Chldns Hosp 1971; **Fac Appt:** Asst Clin Prof Oph, Case West Res Univ

Putterman, Allen M MD [Oph] - **Spec Exp:** Oculoplastic & Orbital Surgery; Cosmetic Surgery-Face & Eyes; Thyroid Eye Disease; **Hospital:** Michael Reese Hosp & Med Ctr, Univ of IL Med Ctr at Chicago; **Address:** 111 N Wabash Ave, Ste 1722, Chicago, IL 60602-2002; **Phone:** 312-372-2256; **Board Cert:** Ophthalmology 1971; **Med School:** Univ Wisc 1963; **Resid:** Ophthalmology, Michael Reese Hosp 1969; **Fellow:** Oculoplastic Surgery, Manhattan Eye/Ear Infirm 1970; **Fac Appt:** Prof Oph, Univ IL Coll Med

Rogers, Gary L MD [Oph] - **Spec Exp:** Strabismus-Adult & Pediatric; **Hospital:** Chldn's Hosp - Columbus; **Address:** 555 S 18th St, Ste 4C, Columbus, OH 43205; **Phone:** 614-224-6222; **Board Cert:** Ophthalmology 1974; **Med School:** Ohio State Univ 1968; **Resid:** Ophthalmology, Mt Sinai Hosp 1972; **Fellow:** Pediatric Ophthalmology, Chldns Hosp Natl Med Ctr 1974; **Fac Appt:** Clin Prof Oph, Ohio State Univ

Rosenberg, Michael A MD [Oph] - **Spec Exp:** Refractive Surgery; Cataract Surgery; Eye Muscle Surgery; **Hospital:** Northwestern Meml Hosp, Evanston Hosp; **Address:** Northwestern Med Fac Fdn, 675 N St Clair, Ste 15-150, Chicago, IL 60611-5967; **Phone:** 312-695-8150; **Board Cert:** Ophthalmology 1975; **Med School:** Northwestern Univ 1967; **Resid:** Ophthalmology, Bascom Palmer Eye Inst 1973; **Fellow:** Neurological Ophthalmology, UCSF Med Ctr 1974; Refractive Surgery, Univ Monterrey 1998; **Fac Appt:** Assoc Clin Prof Oph, Northwestern Univ

Samuelson, Thomas MD [Oph] - **Spec Exp:** Glaucoma; Cataract Surgery; Anterior Segment Surgery; Refractive Surgery; **Hospital:** Phillips Eye Inst, Regions Hosp - St Paul; **Address:** Minnesota Eye Consultants, 710 E 24th St, Ste 106, Minneapolis, MN 55404-3810; **Phone:** 612-813-3600; **Board Cert:** Ophthalmology 1991; **Med School:** Univ Minn 1985; **Resid:** Ophthalmology, Univ S Fla 1990; **Fellow:** Glaucoma, Wills Eye Hosp 1991; **Fac Appt:** Assoc Clin Prof Oph, Univ Minn

Schachat, Andrew P MD [Oph] - **Spec Exp:** Retina/Vitreous Surgery; Diabetic Eye Disease/Retinopathy; Melanoma-Choroidal (eye); **Hospital:** Cleveland Clin Fdn (page 57); **Address:** The Cleveland Clinic Fdn, Cole Eye Inst, 9500 Euclid Ave, Desk i30, Cleveland, OH 44195; **Phone:** 216-444-0430; **Board Cert:** Ophthalmology 1983; **Med School:** Johns Hopkins Univ 1979; **Resid:** Ophthalmology, Wilmer Inst-John Hopkins Hosp 1982; **Fellow:** Vitreoretinal Surgery & Disease, Wilmer Eye Inst-Johns Hopkins Hosp 1983; **Fac Appt:** Prof Oph

Stone, Edwin MD [Oph] - **Spec Exp:** Retinal Disorders; Eye Diseases-Hereditary; **Hospital:** Univ Iowa Hosp & Clinics; **Address:** Dept Ophthalmology, 200 Hawkins Dr, Pomerantz Bldg, Iowa City, IA 52242; **Phone:** 319-356-2864; **Board Cert:** Ophthalmology 1990; **Med School:** Baylor Coll Med 1985; **Resid:** Ophthalmology, Univ Iowa Hosps 1989; **Fellow:** Retina, Univ Iowa Hosps 1992; **Fac Appt:** Prof Oph, Univ Iowa Coll Med

Summers, C Gail MD [Oph] - **Hospital:** Univ Minn Med Ctr, Fairview - Univ Campus; **Address:** University of Minnesota Medical Ctr, 420 Delaware St SE, MC 493, Minneapolis, MN 55455-0356; **Phone:** 612-625-4400; **Board Cert:** Ophthalmology 1984; **Med School:** Univ Minn 1979; **Resid:** Ophthalmology, Univ Minnesota Med Ctr 1983; **Fellow:** Pediatric Ophthalmology, Unin Minnesota Med Ctr 1984; **Fac Appt:** Prof Oph, Univ Minn

Traboulsi, Elias Iskan MD [Oph] - **Spec Exp:** Pediatric Ophthalmology; Glaucoma-Pediatric; **Hospital:** Cleveland Clin Fdn (page 57); **Address:** Cleveland Clinic Fdn, Cole Eye Inst, 9500 Euclid Ave, Desk i32, Cleveland, OH 44195; **Phone:** 216-444-0430; **Board Cert:** Clinical Genetics 1987; Ophthalmology 1991; **Med School:** Amer Univ Beirut 1982; **Resid:** Ophthalmology, American Univ Beirut Hosp 1985; Ophthalmology, Georgetown Hosp 1989; **Fellow:** Ophthalmology, Johns Hopkins Hosp 1986; Pediatric Ophthalmology, Chldns Hosp Natl Med Ctr 1990; **Fac Appt:** Prof Oph, Ohio State Univ

Trese, Michael T MD [Oph] - **Spec Exp:** Retina/Vitreous Surgery; Retinal Disorders-Pediatric; **Hospital:** William Beaumont Hosp, Chldns Hosp of Michigan; **Address:** 3535 W 13 Mile Rd, Ste 632, Royal Oak, MI 48073-6710; **Phone:** 248-288-2280; **Board Cert:** Ophthalmology 1981; **Med School:** Georgetown Univ 1976; **Resid:** Ophthalmology, J Stein Eye Inst-UCLA 1980; **Fellow:** Retina, Duke Univ Med Ctr 1981; **Fac Appt:** Assoc Clin Prof Oph, Wayne State Univ

Trobe, Jonathan Daniel MD [Oph] - **Spec Exp:** Neuro-Ophthalmology; Optic Nerve Disorders; **Hospital:** Univ Michigan Hlth Sys; **Address:** WK Kellogg Eye Ctr, 1000 Wall St, Ann Arbor, MI 48105-1912; **Phone:** 734-763-5114; **Board Cert:** Ophthalmology 1974; Neurology 1988; **Med School:** Harvard Med Sch 1968; **Resid:** Ophthalmology, Wills Eye Hosp 1972; Neurology, Jackson Meml Hosp/U Miami 1986; **Fellow:** Neurological Ophthalmology, Bascom Palmer Eye Inst 1977; **Fac Appt:** Prof Oph, Univ Mich Med Sch

Tychsen, Lawrence MD [Oph] - **Spec Exp:** Pediatric Ophthalmology; Strabismus; Amblyopia; **Hospital:** St Louis Chldns Hosp, Barnes-Jewish Hosp; **Address:** St Louis Chldns Hosp, 1 Children's Pl, ATTN: Eye Care Ctr, rm 2S89, St Louis, MO 63110; **Phone:** 314-454-6026; **Board Cert:** Ophthalmology 1984; **Med School:** Georgetown Univ 1979; **Resid:** Ophthalmology, Univ Iowa Hosp 1983; **Fellow:** Pediatric Ophthalmology, UCSF Med Ctr 1985; **Fac Appt:** Assoc Prof Oph, Washington Univ, St Louis

Vine, Andrew K MD [Oph] - **Spec Exp:** Melanoma-Choroidal (eye); Retinal Disorders; Macular Degeneration; **Hospital:** Univ Michigan Hlth Sys; **Address:** Univ Michigan-Kellogg Eye Ctr, 1000 Wall St, Ann Arbor, MI 48105; **Phone:** 734-763-5906; **Board Cert:** Ophthalmology 1979; **Med School:** McGill Univ 1972; **Resid:** Ophthalmology, Royal Victoria Hosp 1978; **Fellow:** Pathology, McGill Univ 1975; Retina, UCSF Med Ctr 1980; **Fac Appt:** Prof Oph, Univ Mich Med Sch

Weingeist, Thomas A MD/PhD [Oph] - **Spec Exp:** Retinal Disorders; Eye Tumors/Cancer; **Hospital:** Univ Iowa Hosp & Clinics; **Address:** Univ Iowa, Dept Ophthalmology, 200 Hawkins Drive, Iowa City, IA 52242; **Phone:** 319-356-2864; **Board Cert:** Ophthalmology 1976; **Med School:** Univ Iowa Coll Med 1972; **Resid:** Ophthalmology, Univ Iowa Hosp 1975; **Fellow:** Vitreoretinal Surgery, Univ Iowa 1976; **Fac Appt:** Prof Oph, Univ Iowa Coll Med

Williams, George A MD [Oph] - **Spec Exp:** Retinal Disorders; Macular Degeneration; **Hospital:** William Beaumont Hosp; **Address:** Assoc Retinal Consultants, William Beaumont Bldg, 3535 W 13 Mile Rd, Ste 632, Royal Oak, MI 48073; **Phone:** 248-288-2280; **Board Cert:** Ophthalmology 2005; **Med School:** Northwestern Univ 1978; **Resid:** Ophthalmology, Med Coll Wisconsin 1982; **Fellow:** Retina/Vitreous, Med Coll Wisconsin 1984; **Fac Appt:** Clin Prof Oph, Univ Mich Med Sch

Wilson, Steven E MD [Oph] - **Spec Exp:** PRK-Refractive Surgery; Corneal Disease; **Hospital:** Cleveland Clin Fdn (page 57); **Address:** Cleveland Clinic Fdn - Cole Eye Inst, 9500 Euclid Ave, Ste I32, Cleveland, OH 44195; **Phone:** 216-444-5887; **Board Cert:** Ophthalmology 1990; **Med School:** UCSD 1984; **Resid:** Ophthalmology, Mayo Clinic 1988; **Fellow:** Refractive Surgery, Med Ctr Louisiana-LSU 1990; **Fac Appt:** Prof Oph, Case West Res Univ

Younge, Brian R MD [Oph] - **Spec Exp:** Neuro-Ophthalmology; Temporal Arteritis; Ocular Palsies; **Hospital:** Mayo Med Ctr & Clin - Rochester; **Address:** Mayo Clinic, 200 First St SW, Rochester, MN 55905-0001; **Phone:** 507-284-4567; **Board Cert:** Ophthalmology 1974; **Med School:** Univ Alberta 1965; **Resid:** Ophthalmology, Montreal Genl Hosp 1972; **Fellow:** Neurological Ophthalmology, Mayo Clinic 1974; **Fac Appt:** Prof Oph, Mayo Med Sch

Ophthalmology

Great Plains and Mountains

Anderson, Richard L MD [Oph] - **Spec Exp:** Orbital & Eyelid Tumors/Cancer; Eyelid Problems/Ptosis/Blepharospasm; Cosmetic Surgery-Face & Eyes; **Hospital:** Salt Lake Regional Med Ctr, Intermountain Shriners Hosp; **Address:** 1002 E South Temple, Ste 308, Salt Lake City, UT 84102-1525; **Phone:** 801-363-3355; **Board Cert:** Ophthalmology 1976; **Med School:** Univ Iowa Coll Med 1971; **Resid:** Ophthalmology, Univ Iowa Hosps-Clins 1975; **Fellow:** Oculoplastic & Reconstructive Surgery, Albany Med Ctr 1975; Oculoplastic & Reconstructive Surgery, UCSF Med Ctr 1976; **Fac Appt:** Prof PlS, Univ Utah

Bateman, J Bronwyn MD [Oph] - **Spec Exp:** Pediatric Ophthalmology; Genetic Disorders-Eye; Strabismus; **Hospital:** Chldn's Hosp - Denver, The, Univ Colorado Hosp; **Address:** 1675 N Ursula St, MS F731, Aurora, CO 80045; **Phone:** 720-848-2020; **Board Cert:** Ophthalmology 1979; Clinical Genetics 1982; **Med School:** Columbia P&S 1974; **Resid:** Ophthalmology, UCLA Med Ctr 1978; **Fellow:** Pediatric Ophthalmology, Chldn's Natl Med Ctr 1979; Genetics, Johns Hopkins/Wilmer Inst 1980; **Fac Appt:** Prof Oph, Univ Colorado

Crandall, Alan S MD [Oph] - **Spec Exp:** Glaucoma; Cataract Surgery; **Hospital:** Univ Utah Hosps and Clins; **Address:** Moran Eye Ctr- Univ Utah Hosp, 65 N Medical Way, Salt Lake City, UT 84132; **Phone:** 801-581-2352; **Board Cert:** Ophthalmology 1977; **Med School:** Univ Utah 1973; **Resid:** Ophthalmology, Hosp Univ Penn 1976; **Fellow:** Glaucoma, Scheie Eye Inst; **Fac Appt:** Clin Prof Oph, Univ Utah

Durrie, Daniel MD [Oph] - **Spec Exp:** LASIK-Refractive Surgery; Corneal Disease; **Hospital:** St Luke's Hosp of Kansas City; **Address:** 5520 College Blvd Fl 2 - Ste 201, Overland Park, KS 66211; **Phone:** 913-491-3330; **Board Cert:** Ophthalmology 1979; **Med School:** Univ Nebr Coll Med 1975; **Resid:** Ophthalmology, Univ Nebr Med Coll 1979; **Fellow:** Cornea, Filkins Eye Inst 1980; **Fac Appt:** Asst Clin Prof Oph, Univ Kans

Southwest

Ellis Jr, George S MD [Oph] - **Spec Exp:** Pediatric Ophthalmology; Eye Muscle Disorders; **Hospital:** Children's Hospital - New Orleans, E Jefferson Genl Hosp; **Address:** Children's Hospital, 200 Henry Clay Ave, Ste 3106, New Orleans, LA 70118; **Phone:** 504-896-9426; **Board Cert:** Ophthalmology 1982; **Med School:** Tulane Univ 1977; **Resid:** Ophthalmology, Duke Univ-Eye Ctr 1982; Pediatric Ophthalmology, Hall Eye Clinic 1982; **Fellow:** Pediatric Ophthalmology, Chldns Hosp 1983; **Fac Appt:** Assoc Clin Prof Oph, Tulane Univ

Eustis, Horatio S MD [Oph] - **Spec Exp:** Pediatric Ophthalmology; **Hospital:** Ochsner Fdn Hosp; **Address:** Ochsner Clinic, Dept Oph, 1514 Jefferson Hwy, Fl 10, New Orleans, LA 70121; **Phone:** 504-842-3995; **Board Cert:** Ophthalmology 1985; **Med School:** Louisiana State Univ 1980; **Resid:** Ophthalmology, LSU Eye Ctr 1984; **Fellow:** Pediatric Ophthalmology, Hosp Sick Chldn 1985; Pediatric Ophthalmology, Chldns Hosp; **Fac Appt:** Clin Prof Oph, Louisiana State Univ

Holladay, Jack T MD [Oph] - **Spec Exp:** LASIK-Refractive Surgery; PRK-Refractive Surgery; **Hospital:** Park Plaza Hosp; **Address:** Holladay LASIK Institute, 6802 Mapleridge, Bellaire T Bldg - Ste 200, Houston, TX 77401; **Phone:** 713-668-7337; **Board Cert:** Ophthalmology 1979; **Med School:** Univ Tex, Houston 1974; **Resid:** Ophthalmology, Univ Texas Hlth Sci Ctr 1978; **Fellow:** Ophthalmology, Univ Texas Hlth Sci Ctr 1975; **Fac Appt:** Clin Prof Oph, Baylor Coll Med

Kaufman, Herbert E MD [Oph] - **Spec Exp:** Corneal Disease & Surgery; Laser Vision Surgery; Cataract Surgery; **Hospital:** Med Ctr LA @ New Orleans (Univ Hosp); **Address:** 2820 Napoleon Ave, Ste 750, Baton Rouge, LA 70115; **Phone:** 504-891-1116; **Board Cert:** Ophthalmology 1962; **Med School:** Harvard Med Sch 1956; **Resid:** Ophthalmology, Mass Eye & Ear Infirmary 1962; **Fellow:** Ophthalmology, Natl Inst Hlth 1959; **Fac Appt:** Prof Oph, Louisiana State Univ

Koch, Douglas D MD [Oph] - **Spec Exp:** Cataract Surgery; Refractive Surgery; **Hospital:** Methodist Hosp - Houston; **Address:** 6550 Fannin, Ste 1501, Houston, TX 77030-2704; **Phone:** 713-798-6100; **Board Cert:** Ophthalmology 1982; **Med School:** Harvard Med Sch 1977; **Resid:** Ophthalmology, Baylor Coll Med 1981; **Fellow:** Cornea, Moorfields Eye Hosp 1982; Ophthalmology, Baylor Coll Med 1982; **Fac Appt:** Prof Oph, Baylor Coll Med

Lambert, H Michael MD [Oph] - **Spec Exp:** Retina/Vitreous Surgery; Macular Disease/Degeneration; Diabetic Eye Disease/Retinopathy; **Hospital:** Methodist Hosp - Houston, St Luke's Episcopal Hosp - Houston; **Address:** 2727 Gramercy, Ste 200, Houston, TX 77025-1633; **Phone:** 713-799-9975; **Board Cert:** Ophthalmology 1983; **Med School:** Baylor Coll Med 1977; **Resid:** Ophthalmology, Wilford Hall USAF Med Ctr 1982; **Fellow:** Vitreoretinal Surgery, Duke Univ Eye Ctr 1983; **Fac Appt:** Assoc Clin Prof Oph, Baylor Coll Med

Lewis, Richard Alan MD [Oph] - **Spec Exp:** Eye Diseases-Hereditary; Ophthalmic Genetics; Retinal Disorders; **Hospital:** St Luke's Episcopal Hosp - Houston, Texas Chldns Hosp - Houston; **Address:** Cullen Eye Institute NC-206, Baylor College of Medicine, One Baylor Plaza, Houston, TX 77030; **Phone:** 713-798-6100; **Board Cert:** Ophthalmology 1976; **Med School:** Univ Mich Med Sch 1969; **Resid:** Ophthalmology, Univ Michigan Hospital 1973; **Fellow:** Retina, Univ Michigan Hospital 1974; Macular Disease, Bascom Palmer Eye Inst 1975; **Fac Appt:** Prof Oph, Baylor Coll Med

Mazow, Malcolm L MD [Oph] - **Spec Exp:** Strabismus-Adult; Pediatric Ophthalmology; **Hospital:** Meml Hermann Hosp - Houston; **Address:** 2855 Gramercy St, Houston, TX 77025; **Phone:** 713-668-6828; **Board Cert:** Ophthalmology 1967; **Med School:** Univ Tex Med Br, Galveston 1961; **Resid:** Ophthalmology, Univ Iowa Hosp 1965; **Fellow:** Strabismus, Univ Iowa Hosp 1966; **Fac Appt:** Clin Prof Oph, Univ Tex, Houston

McCulley, James P MD [Oph] - **Spec Exp:** Corneal & External Eye Disease; Laser Vision Surgery; Cataract Surgery; **Hospital:** UT Southwestern Med Ctr - Dallas, Univ Med Ctr - Lubbock; **Address:** Univ Tex SW Med Ctr, Dept Oph, 5323 Harry Hines Blvd, Dallas, TX 75390-9057; **Phone:** 214-648-2020; **Board Cert:** Ophthalmology 1974; **Med School:** Washington Univ, St Louis 1968; **Resid:** Ophthalmology, Mass EE Infirm 1973; **Fellow:** Cornea, Cornea Rsch-Retina Fdn 1974; Cornea, Mass EE Infirm 1974; **Fac Appt:** Prof Oph, Univ Tex SW, Dallas

Miller, Joseph M MD [Oph] - **Spec Exp:** Pediatric Ophthalmology; Strabismus; Amblyopia; **Hospital:** Univ Med Ctr - Tucson; **Address:** Univ Ariz, Dept Ophthalmology & Vision Sci, 655 N Alvernon Way, Ste 108, Tucson, AZ 85711; **Phone:** 520-321-3677; **Board Cert:** Ophthalmology 1991; **Med School:** NE Ohio Univ 1985; **Resid:** Ophthalmology, Yale New Haven Hosp 1990; **Fellow:** Pediatric Ophthalmology, Johns Hopkins Hosp 1991; Refractive Surgery, Univ Arizona Hosp 2001; **Fac Appt:** Prof Oph, Univ Ariz Coll Med

Mims III, James Luther MD [Oph] - **Spec Exp:** Pediatric Ophthalmology; Strabismus-Adult & Pediatric; **Hospital:** Baptist Med Ctr - San Antonio, Methodist Chldns Hosp of South Texas; **Address:** 311 Camden St, Ste 511, San Antonio, TX 78215-2015; **Phone:** 210-225-0084; **Board Cert:** Ophthalmology 1977; **Med School:** Tulane Univ 1968; **Resid:** Ophthalmology, Wills Eye Hosp 1976; **Fellow:** Pediatric Ophthalmology, Wills Eye Hosp 1977; **Fac Appt:** Clin Prof Oph, Univ Tex, San Antonio

Pflugfelder, Stephen C MD [Oph] - **Spec Exp:** Corneal & External Eye Disease; Refractive Surgery; Cataract Surgery; Lens Implants; **Hospital:** Baylor Univ Medical Ctr; **Address:** Cullen Eye Inst-Baylor College of Medicine, 6501 Fannin, Ste NC307, Houston, TX 77030; **Phone:** 713-798-6100; **Board Cert:** Ophthalmology 1987; **Med School:** SUNY Upstate Med Univ 1981; **Resid:** Ophthalmology, Baylor Univ Med Ctr 1985; **Fellow:** Cornea & Ext Eye Disease, Bascom Palmer Eye Inst 1986; **Fac Appt:** Prof Oph, Baylor Coll Med

Piest, Kenneth L MD [Oph] - **Spec Exp:** Eyelid Cancer & Reconstruction; Pediatric Eye Reconstructive Surgery; Orbital Tumors/Cancer; Oculoplastic Surgery; **Hospital:** Metro Methodist Hosp, Baptist Med Ctr - San Antonio; **Address:** Texas Ophthalmic Plastic Surgery, 225 E Sonterra Blvd, Ste 201, San Antonio, TX 78258; **Phone:** 210-494-8859; **Board Cert:** Ophthalmology 1991; **Med School:** Univ IL Coll Med 1984; **Resid:** Ophthalmology, Univ Tex Hlth Scis Ctr 1989; **Fellow:** Ophthalmic Plastic Surgery, Chldns Hosp/Sheie Eye Inst/Univ Penn 1990; Craniofacial Ophthalmic Plastic Surgery, Chldns Hosp/Univ Penn 1991; **Fac Appt:** Assoc Clin Prof Oph, Univ Tex, San Antonio

Richard, James M MD [Oph] - **Spec Exp:** Pediatric Ophthalmology; Eye Muscle Surgery; **Hospital:** Intergris Baptist Med Ctr - OK, Deaconess Hosp - Oklahoma; **Address:** 11013 Hefner Pointe Drive, Oklahoma City, OK 73120-5050; **Phone:** 405-751-2020; **Board Cert:** Ophthalmology 1979; **Med School:** Univ Okla Coll Med 1974; **Resid:** Ophthalmology, Baylor Coll Med 1978; **Fellow:** Pediatric Ophthalmology, Chldns Hosp 1979; Ophthalmology, Johns Hopkins Hosp 1980; **Fac Appt:** Clin Prof Oph, Univ Okla Coll Med

Siatkowski, R Michael MD [Oph] - **Spec Exp:** Pediatric Ophthalmology; Neuro-Ophthalmology; Retinopathy of Prematurity; **Hospital:** OU Med Ctr; **Address:** Dean A Mcgee Eye Institute, 608 Stanton L Young Blvd, Oklahoma City, OK 73104; **Phone:** 405-271-1094; **Board Cert:** Ophthalmology 2003; **Med School:** Jefferson Med Coll 1987; **Resid:** Ophthalmology, St Francis Med Ctr 1991; **Fellow:** Neurological Ophthalmology, Bascom Palmer Eye Inst 1992; Pediatric Ophthalmology, Bascom Palmer Eye Inst 1993; **Fac Appt:** Prof Oph, Univ Okla Coll Med

Soparkar, Charles MD [Oph] - **Spec Exp:** Eye Tumors/Cancer; Orbital & Eyelid Tumors/Cancer; Oculoplastic Surgery; **Hospital:** Methodist Hosp - Houston, Texas Chldns Hosp - Houston; **Address:** Plastic Eye Surg Assocs, 3730 Kirby Drive, Ste 900, Houston, TX 77098; **Phone:** 713-795-0705; **Board Cert:** Ophthalmology 1996; **Med School:** Univ Mass Sch Med 1990; **Resid:** Ophthalmology, Baylor Affil Hosps 1994; **Fellow:** Ophthalmic Oncololgy, Texas Med Ctr 1995

Wallace, R Bruce MD [Oph] - **Spec Exp:** Refractive Surgery; Cataract Surgery; **Hospital:** St Francis Med Ctr; **Address:** 4110 Parliament Drive, Alexandria, LA 71303; **Phone:** 318-448-4488; **Board Cert:** Ophthalmology 1979; **Med School:** Tulane Univ 1974; **Resid:** Ophthalmology, Tulane Univ 1979; **Fac Appt:** Clin Prof Oph, Louisiana State Univ

Wilhelmus, Kirk R MD/PhD [Oph] - **Spec Exp:** Corneal & External Eye Disease; **Hospital:** Methodist Hosp - Houston; **Address:** Cullen Eye Inst, 6550 Fannin St, Smith Tower, Ste 1501, Houston, TX 77030; **Phone:** 713-798-6100; **Board Cert:** Ophthalmology 1981; **Med School:** Vanderbilt Univ 1975; **Resid:** Ophthalmology, Baylor Coll Med 1979; **Fellow:** Cornea & Ext Eye Disease, Moorfields Eye Hosp 1981; **Fac Appt:** Prof Oph, Baylor Coll Med

West Coast and Pacific

Abbott, Richard L MD [Oph] - **Spec Exp:** Refractive Surgery; Cornea & External Eye Disease; **Hospital:** UCSF Med Ctr; **Address:** UCSF, Dept Ophthalmology, 10 Koret Way, K301, San Francisco, CA 94143-0730; **Phone:** 415-502-6265; **Board Cert:** Ophthalmology 1978; **Med School:** Geo Wash Univ 1971; **Resid:** Ophthalmology, Presby-Pacific Med Ctr 1977; **Fellow:** Cornea & Ext Eye Disease, Bascom Palmer Eye Inst 1978; **Fac Appt:** Clin Prof Oph, UCSF

Arnold, Anthony C MD [Oph] - **Spec Exp:** Neuro-Ophthalmology; **Hospital:** UCLA Med Ctr; **Address:** 100 Stein Plaza, Box 957000, Los Angeles, CA 90095-7005; **Phone:** 310-825-4344; **Board Cert:** Ophthalmology 1980; **Med School:** UCLA 1975; **Resid:** Ophthalmology, Jules Stein Eye Inst-UCLA 1979; **Fellow:** Neurological Ophthalmology, Jules Stein Eye Inst-UCLA 1983; **Fac Appt:** Clin Prof Oph, UCLA

Baerveldt, George MD [Oph] - **Spec Exp:** Glaucoma; **Hospital:** UC Irvine Med Ctr; **Address:** UC Irvine Med Ctr, Dept of Ophthalmology, 118 Med Surge I, Irvine, CA 92697-4375; **Phone:** 949-824-2020; **Med School:** South Africa 1967; **Resid:** Ophthalmology, Univ of Witwatersrand 1975; **Fellow:** Neurological Ophthalmology, SUNY Downstate Med Ctr 1975; **Fac Appt:** Prof Oph, UC Irvine

Baylis, Henry I MD [Oph] - **Spec Exp:** Oculoplastic Surgery; **Hospital:** UCLA Med Ctr, Hoag Meml Hosp Presby; **Address:** 1260 15 St, Ste 600, Santa Monica, CA 90404; **Phone:** 310-207-0300; **Board Cert:** Ophthalmology 1969; **Med School:** Univ Mich Med Sch 1960; **Resid:** Ophthalmology, UCLA Med Ctr 1966; **Fellow:** Oculoplastic Surgery, Manhattan EET Hosp 1967; **Fac Appt:** Clin Prof Oph, UCLA

Binder, Perry S MD [Oph] - **Spec Exp:** Refractive Surgery; **Hospital:** Sharp Meml Hosp; **Address:** 8910 Univ Center Lane, Ste 800, San Diego, CA 92122; **Phone:** 858-455-6800; **Board Cert:** Ophthalmology 1975; **Med School:** Northwestern Univ 1969; **Resid:** Ophthalmology, USC Med Ctr 1973; **Fellow:** Cornea, Univ Fla Hosps 1974

Blumenkranz, Mark S MD [Oph] - **Spec Exp:** Retinal Disorders; Macular Degeneration; **Hospital:** Stanford Univ Med Ctr; **Address:** 1225 Crane St, Ste 202, Menlo Park, CA 94025; **Phone:** 650-323-0231; **Board Cert:** Ophthalmology 1980; **Med School:** Brown Univ 1975; **Resid:** Ophthalmology, Stanford Univ Hosp 1979; **Fellow:** Vitreoretinal Surgery, Bascom Palmer Eye Inst 1980; **Fac Appt:** Prof Oph, Stanford Univ

Borchert, Mark S MD [Oph] - **Spec Exp:** Pediatric Ophthalmology; Vision-Unexplained Loss; Optic Nerve Disorders; **Hospital:** Chldns Hosp - Los Angeles (page 56); **Address:** Chldns Hosp, Div Ophthalmology, 4650 Sunset Blvd, MC 88, Los Angeles, CA 90027-6062; **Phone:** 323-669-2344; **Board Cert:** Ophthalmology 1989; **Med School:** Baylor Coll Med 1983; **Resid:** Ophthalmology, LAC-USC Med Ctr 1987; **Fellow:** Neurological Ophthalmology, Mass EE Infirm-Harvard 1988; **Fac Appt:** Assoc Prof Oph, USC Sch Med

Ophthalmology

Boxer Wachler, Brian S MD [Oph] - **Spec Exp:** LASIK-Refractive Surgery; Keratoconus; Corneal Disease & Surgery; **Hospital:** Cedars-Sinai Med Ctr; **Address:** Boxer Wachler Vision Inst, 465 N Roxbury Drive, Ste 902, Los Angeles, CA 90210; **Phone:** 310-860-1900; **Board Cert:** Ophthalmology 1999; **Med School:** Dartmouth Med Sch 1993; **Resid:** Ophthalmology, St Louis Univ Eye Inst 1997; **Fellow:** Refractive Surgery, Univ Kansas Med Ctr 1998

Boxrud, Cynthia Ann MD [Oph] - **Spec Exp:** Oculoplastic Surgery; Eye Tumors/Cancer; Orbital Diseases; **Hospital:** UCLA Med Ctr, St John's Hlth Ctr, Santa Monica; **Address:** 2021 Santa Monica Blvd, Ste 700E, Santa Monica, CA 90404-2208; **Phone:** 310-829-9060; **Board Cert:** Ophthalmology 1997; **Med School:** Case West Res Univ 1986; **Resid:** Ophthalmology, NYU-Bellevue Hosp Ctr 1990; **Fellow:** Ophthalmic Oncololgy, New York Hosp-Cornell Med Ctr 1992; Ophthalmic Plastic Surgery, UCLA - Jules Stein Eye Inst 1993; **Fac Appt:** Asst Prof Oph, UCLA

Caprioli, Joseph MD [Oph] - **Spec Exp:** Glaucoma; Cataract Surgery; **Hospital:** UCLA Med Ctr; **Address:** UCLA-Jules Stein Eye Institute, 100 Stein Plaza, rm 2-273, Los Angeles, CA 90095-7006; **Phone:** 310-794-9442; **Board Cert:** Ophthalmology 1985; **Med School:** SUNY Buffalo 1979; **Resid:** Ophthalmology, Yale-New Haven Hosp. 1983; **Fellow:** Glaucoma, Wills Eye Hosp 1984; **Fac Appt:** Prof Oph, UCLA

Char, Devron H MD [Oph] - **Spec Exp:** Eye Tumors/Cancer; Thyroid Eye Disease; Oculoplastic Surgery; **Hospital:** CA Pacific Med Ctr - Pacific Campus, UCSF Med Ctr; **Address:** 45 Castro St, Ste 309, San Francisco, CA 94114; **Phone:** 415-522-0700; **Board Cert:** Ophthalmology 1978; **Med School:** Univ Minn 1970; **Resid:** Internal Medicine, Mass Genl Hosp 1972; Ophthalmology, UCSF Med Ctr 1977; **Fellow:** Medical Oncology, Natl Cancer Inst 1974; Ophthalmology, UCSF Med Ctr 1978; **Fac Appt:** Prof Oph, Stanford Univ

Choy, Andrew Eng MD [Oph] - **Spec Exp:** Eye Muscle Disorders; Oculoplastic & Orbital Surgery; **Hospital:** Long Beach Meml Med Ctr, Los Alamitos Med Ctr; **Address:** 4100 Long Beach Blvd, Ste 108, Long Beach, CA 90807-2619; **Phone:** 562-426-3925; **Board Cert:** Ophthalmology 1976; **Med School:** USC Sch Med 1969; **Resid:** Neurology, LAC-USC Med Ctr 1971; Ophthalmology, Bellevue Hosp Ctr-NYU 1974; **Fellow:** Strabismus, Columbia-Presby Med Ctr 1975; **Fac Appt:** Assoc Clin Prof Oph, UCLA

Day, Susan H MD [Oph] - **Spec Exp:** Pediatric Ophthalmology; Strabismus; **Hospital:** CA Pacific Med Ctr - Pacific Campus; **Address:** 2340 Clay St, Ste 100, San Francisco, CA 94115; **Phone:** 415-202-1500; **Board Cert:** Ophthalmology 1980; **Med School:** Louisiana State Univ 1975; **Resid:** Ophthalmology, California Pacific Med Ctr 1979; **Fellow:** Pediatric Ophthalmology, Hosp Sick Chldn 1980

De Juan Jr, Eugene MD [Oph] - **Spec Exp:** Retina/Vitreous Surgery; **Hospital:** UCSF Med Ctr; **Address:** 400 Parnassus Ave, San Francisco, CA 94122; **Phone:** 415-353-2800; **Board Cert:** Ophthalmology 1985; **Med School:** Univ S Ala Coll Med 1979; **Resid:** Ophthalmology, Johns Hopkins Hosp 1983; **Fellow:** Vitreoretinal Surgery, Duke Univ Eye Ctr 1984; **Fac Appt:** Prof Oph, UCSF

Demer, Joseph L MD/PhD [Oph] - **Spec Exp:** Pediatric Ophthalmology; Strabismus; Nystagmus; **Hospital:** UCLA Med Ctr; **Address:** Jules Stein Eye Institute, 100 Stein Plaza, MC 700219, Los Angeles, CA 90095-7065; **Phone:** 310-825-5931; **Board Cert:** Ophthalmology 1988; **Med School:** Johns Hopkins Univ 1983; **Resid:** Ophthalmology, Baylor Coll Med 1987; **Fellow:** Pediatric Ophthalmology, Texas Chldns Hosp 1988; **Fac Appt:** Prof Oph, UCLA

Fein, William MD [Oph] - **Spec Exp:** Oculoplastic Surgery; Tear Duct Problems; LASIK-Refractive Surgery; Cosmetic Surgery-Eyes; **Hospital:** Cedars-Sinai Med Ctr; **Address:** 415 N Crescent Drive, Ste 200, Beverly Hills, CA 90210-6812; **Phone:** 310-859-0760; **Board Cert:** Ophthalmology 1969; **Med School:** UC Irvine 1960; **Resid:** Ophthalmology, Los Angeles Co Genl Hosp 1966; **Fellow:** Ophthalmology, Manhattan EET Infirm 1967; **Fac Appt:** Assoc Clin Prof Oph, USC Sch Med

Granet, David Bruce MD [Oph] - **Spec Exp:** Pediatric Ophthalmology; Eye Muscle Disorders; Strabismus; **Hospital:** UCSD Med Ctr, Rady Children's Hosp - San Diego; **Address:** UCSD-Shiley Eye Ctr, 9415 Campus Point Drive, La Jolla, CA 92093; **Phone:** 858-534-2020; **Board Cert:** Ophthalmology 1994; **Med School:** Yale Univ 1987; **Resid:** Ophthalmology, Bellevue Hosp-NYU 1991; **Fellow:** Pediatric Ophthalmology, Chldns Hosp 1993; **Fac Appt:** Assoc Prof Oph, UCSD

Irvine, John A MD [Oph] - **Spec Exp:** Corneal & External Eye Disease; **Hospital:** USC Univ Hosp - R K Eamer Med Plz; **Address:** USC-Doheny Eye Institute, 1450 San Pablo St, Ste 5703, Los Angeles, CA 90033; **Phone:** 323-442-6335; **Board Cert:** Ophthalmology 1989; **Med School:** USC Sch Med 1982; **Resid:** Ophthalmology, Mass EE Infirm/Harvard 1986; **Fellow:** Cornea & Ext Eye Disease, Mass EE Infirm 1987; **Fac Appt:** Prof Oph, USC Sch Med

Isenberg, Sherwin Jay MD [Oph] - **Spec Exp:** Strabismus; Pediatric Ophthalmology; **Hospital:** LAC - Harbor - UCLA Med Ctr, UCLA Med Ctr; **Address:** Jules Stein Eye Institute, 100 Stein Plaza, Los Angeles, CA 90095-7000; **Phone:** 310-825-8840; **Board Cert:** Ophthalmology 1978; **Med School:** UCLA 1973; **Resid:** Ophthalmology, Illinois Ear & Eye Infirm 1977; **Fellow:** Pediatric Ophthalmology, Chldns Hosp Natl Med Ctr 1978; **Fac Appt:** Prof Oph, UCLA

Iwach, Andrew G MD [Oph] - **Spec Exp:** Glaucoma; **Hospital:** UCSF Med Ctr, CA Pacific Med Ctr; **Address:** Glaucoma Ctr of San Francisco, 55 Stevenson St, San Francisco, CA 94105; **Phone:** 415-981-2020; **Board Cert:** Ophthalmology 1991; **Med School:** UCLA 1984; **Resid:** Ophthalmology, Stanford Univ Med Ctr 1988; **Fellow:** Glaucoma, UCSF Med Ctr 1989; **Fac Appt:** Assoc Prof Oph, UCSF

Mahon, Kathleen M K MD [Oph] - **Spec Exp:** Pediatric Ophthalmology; Retinopathy of Prematurity; Eye Muscle Disorders; Glaucoma; **Hospital:** Sunrise Hosp & Med Ctr/Sunrise Chldn's Hosp, Univ Med Ctr - Las Vegas; **Address:** 3201 S Maryland Pkwy, Ste 400, Las Vegas, NV 89109; **Phone:** 702-731-3333; **Board Cert:** Ophthalmology 1980; **Med School:** Univ New Mexico 1975; **Resid:** Ophthalmology, Univ Florida Med Ctr 1979; **Fellow:** Pediatric Ophthalmology, Univ Tex Hlth Sci Ctr 1980; **Fac Appt:** Clin Prof Oph, Univ Nevada

Maloney, Robert K MD [Oph] - **Spec Exp:** Refractive Surgery; LASIK-Refractive Surgery; **Hospital:** UCLA Med Ctr; **Address:** Maloney Vision Inst, 10921 Wilshire Blvd, Ste 900, Los Angeles, CA 90024-4002; **Phone:** 310-208-3937; **Board Cert:** Ophthalmology 1991; **Med School:** UCSF 1985; **Resid:** Ophthalmology, Johns Hopkins Hosp 1989; **Fellow:** Refractive Surgery, Emory Univ Hosp 1991; **Fac Appt:** Clin Prof Oph, UCLA

Manche, Edward E MD [Oph] - **Spec Exp:** LASIK-Refractive Surgery; Corneal Disease & Transplant; PRK-Refractive Surgery; **Hospital:** Stanford Univ Med Ctr; **Address:** 900 Blake Wilbur Dr, rm W3002, Palo Alto, CA 94304-2201; **Phone:** 650-498-7020; **Board Cert:** Ophthalmology 1996; **Med School:** Albert Einstein Coll Med 1990; **Resid:** Ophthalmology, UMDNJ-NJ Med Sch 1994; **Fellow:** Cornea & Ext Eye Disease, Jules Stein Eye Inst-UCLA 1996; **Fac Appt:** Assoc Prof Oph, Stanford Univ

Mannis, Mark MD [Oph] - **Spec Exp:** Cornea Transplant; Refractive Surgery; **Hospital:** UC Davis Med Ctr; **Address:** UC Davis Med Ctr, Dept of Ophthalmology, 4860 Y St, Ste 2400, Sacramento, CA 95817; **Phone:** 916-734-6602; **Board Cert:** Ophthalmology 1980; **Med School:** Univ Fla Coll Med 1975; **Resid:** Ophthalmology, Univ Washington 1979; **Fellow:** Cornea & Ext Eye Disease, Univ IA Hosps & Clins 1980; **Fac Appt:** Prof Oph, UC Davis

Marmor, Michael F MD [Oph] - **Spec Exp:** Retinal Disorders; Retinal Dystrophies; Electroretinograms (ERG); Macular Degeneration; **Hospital:** Stanford Univ Med Ctr; **Address:** California Vitreoretinal Ctr, 1225 Crane St, Ste 202, Menlo Park, CA 94025; **Phone:** 650-323-0231; **Board Cert:** Ophthalmology 1974; **Med School:** Harvard Med Sch 1966; **Resid:** Ophthalmology, Mass EE Infirm 1973; **Fellow:** Neurological Physiology, Natl Inst Mntl Hlth 1970; **Fac Appt:** Prof Oph, Stanford Univ

Masket, Samuel MD [Oph] - **Spec Exp:** Cataract Surgery; Cataract Surgery Revision; **Address:** 2080 Century Park E, Ste 911, Los Angeles, CA 90067; **Phone:** 310-229-1220; **Board Cert:** Ophthalmology 1974; **Med School:** NY Med Coll 1968; **Resid:** Ophthalmology, Metropolitan Hosp Ctr 1972; **Fellow:** Ophthalmology, Columbia Presby Med Ctr 1973; **Fac Appt:** Clin Prof Oph, UCLA

Minckler, Donald S MD [Oph] - **Spec Exp:** Glaucoma; **Hospital:** UC Irvine Med Ctr; **Address:** Gottschalk Medical Plaza-Irvine, 1 Medical Plaza Drive, Irvine, CA 92697; **Phone:** 949-824-2020; **Board Cert:** Ophthalmology 1975; Pathology 1978; **Med School:** Oregon Hlth Sci Univ 1964; **Resid:** Anatomic Pathology, Univ Wash Med Ctr 1970; Ophthalmology, Univ Wash Med Ctr 1973; **Fellow:** Pathology, Armed Forces Inst Path 1975; Glaucoma, Shaffer Assocs-UCSF 1982

Mondino, Bartly John MD [Oph] - **Spec Exp:** Cornea & External Eye Disease; **Hospital:** UCLA Med Ctr; **Address:** 100 Stein Plaza, MC 700619, Los Angeles, CA 90095-7065; **Phone:** 310-825-5053; **Board Cert:** Ophthalmology 1976; **Med School:** Stanford Univ 1971; **Resid:** Ophthalmology, NY Hosp/Cornell Univ 1975; **Fellow:** Cornea & Ext Eye Disease, Univ Pittsburgh Eye & Ear Hosp 1976; **Fac Appt:** Prof Oph, UCLA

Murphree, A Linn MD [Oph] - **Spec Exp:** Pediatric Ophthalmology; Eye Diseases-Hereditary; Retinoblastoma; Orbital Tumors/Cancer; **Hospital:** Chldns Hosp - Los Angeles (page 56), USC Univ Hosp - R K Eamer Med Plz; **Address:** Chldns Hosp, Div Oph, 4650 Sunset Blvd, MS 88, Los Angeles, CA 90027-6016; **Phone:** 323-669-2299; **Board Cert:** Ophthalmology 1978; **Med School:** Baylor Coll Med 1972; **Resid:** Clinical Genetics, Baylor Heed 1973; Ophthalmology, Baylor Coll Med 1976; **Fellow:** Ophthalmology, Wilmer Inst/Johns Hopkins 1977; **Fac Appt:** Prof Oph, USC Sch Med

Nesburn, Anthony B MD [Oph] - **Spec Exp:** Corneal Disease; Laser Vision Surgery; **Hospital:** Cedars-Sinai Med Ctr; **Address:** Cedars-Sinai Med Ctr, 8635 W Third St, Ste 390W, Los Angeles, CA 90048-6101; **Phone:** 310-652-1133; **Board Cert:** Ophthalmology 1969; **Med School:** Harvard Med Sch 1960; **Resid:** Ophthalmology, Mass Eye & Ear Infirm 1968; **Fellow:** Virology, Harvard 1965; **Fac Appt:** Prof Oph, UC Irvine

Palmer, Earl A MD [Oph] - **Spec Exp:** Strabismus; Retinopathy of Prematurity; **Hospital:** OR Hlth & Sci Univ; **Address:** Casey Eye Institute, 3375 SW Terwilliger Blvd, Portland, OR 97239-4197; **Phone:** 503-494-7675; **Board Cert:** Pediatrics 1975; Ophthalmology 1976; **Med School:** Duke Univ 1966; **Resid:** Pediatrics, Univ Colo Med Ctr 1968; Ophthalmology, Oregon Hlth & Sciences Univ 1974; **Fellow:** Pediatric Ophthalmology, Texas Chldns Hosp 1975; **Fac Appt:** Prof Oph, Oregon Hlth Sci Univ

Paul, T Otis MD [Oph] - **Spec Exp:** Pediatric Ophthalmology; Strabismus; **Hospital:** CA Pacific Med Ctr - Pacific Campus, Chldns Hosp - Oakland; **Address:** 2100 Webster St, Ste 214, San Francisco, CA 94115; **Phone:** 415-923-3007; **Board Cert:** Ophthalmology 1974; **Med School:** UCLA 1967; **Resid:** Ophthalmology, Naval Hosp 1972; **Fellow:** Pediatric Ophthalmology, Ca Pacific Med Ctr 1974

Rao, Narsing Adupa MD [Oph] - **Spec Exp:** Uveitis/AIDS; Eye Pathology; **Hospital:** USC Univ Hosp - R K Eamer Med Plz; **Address:** USC Doheny Eye Inst, 1450 San Pablo St, rm DVRZ 211, Los Angeles, CA 90033-4697; **Phone:** 323-442-6645; **Board Cert:** Pathology 1974; Ophthalmology 1977; **Med School:** India 1967; **Resid:** Pathology, Georgetown Hosp 1972; Ophthalmology, Georgetown Hosp 1975; **Fac Appt:** Prof Oph, USC Sch Med

Salz, James J MD [Oph] - **Spec Exp:** LASIK-Refractive Surgery; PRK-Refractive Surgery; Cataract Surgery; **Hospital:** Cedars-Sinai Med Ctr; **Address:** 444 S San Vicente Blvd, Ste 704, Los Angeles, CA 90048-5901; **Phone:** 323-653-3800; **Board Cert:** Ophthalmology 1971; **Med School:** Duke Univ 1965; **Resid:** Ophthalmology, LAC-USC Med Ctr 1969; **Fac Appt:** Clin Prof Oph, USC Sch Med

Seibel, Barry S MD [Oph] - **Spec Exp:** Cataract Surgery; **Hospital:** UCLA Med Ctr; **Address:** 11620 Wilshire Blvd, Ste 711, Los Angeles, CA 90025; **Phone:** 310-273-0323; **Board Cert:** Ophthalmology 1991; **Med School:** Univ Tex, Houston 1985; **Resid:** Ophthalmology, Hollywood Presby Med Ctr 1987; Ophthalmology, USC-Doheny Eye Clin 1989; **Fac Appt:** Asst Clin Prof Oph, UCLA

Seiff, Stuart R MD [Oph] - **Spec Exp:** Oculoplastic Surgery; Orbital Tumors/Cancer; **Hospital:** UCSF Med Ctr, CA Pacific Med Ctr; **Address:** 2100 Webster St, Ste 214, San Francisco, CA 94115; **Phone:** 415-923-3007; **Board Cert:** Ophthalmology 1986; **Med School:** UCSF 1980; **Resid:** Ophthalmology, UCSF Med Ctr 1984; **Fellow:** Ophthalmic Plastic & Reconstructive Surgery, UCLA Med Ctr 1985; Oculoplastic Surgery, Moorfield's Eye Hosp 1986; **Fac Appt:** Prof Oph, UCSF

Serafano, Donald N MD [Oph] - **Spec Exp:** LASIK-Refractive Surgery; Cataract Surgery; Lens Implants; **Hospital:** Los Alamitos Med Ctr, Long Beach Meml Med Ctr; **Address:** 10861 Cherry St, Ste 204, Box 250, Los Alamitos, CA 90720-5403; **Phone:** 562-598-3160; **Board Cert:** Ophthalmology 1978; **Med School:** Wayne State Univ 1971; **Resid:** Ophthalmology, Mayo Clinic 1978; **Fac Appt:** Assoc Clin Prof Oph, USC Sch Med

Smith, Ronald E MD [Oph] - **Spec Exp:** Corneal Disease; Uveitis; **Hospital:** USC Univ Hosp - R K Eamer Med Plz; **Address:** Doheny Eye Clinic, 1450 San Pablo Rd, Ste DEI-5706, Los Angeles, CA 90033; **Phone:** 323-442-6424; **Board Cert:** Ophthalmology 1974; **Med School:** Johns Hopkins Univ 1967; **Resid:** Ophthalmology, Wilmer Oph Inst/Johns Hopkins 1973; **Fellow:** Research, Proctor Fdn/Univ California 1972; **Fac Appt:** Prof Oph, USC Sch Med

Steinert, Roger F MD [Oph] - **Spec Exp:** Refractive Surgery; Cataract Surgery; Cornea Transplant; **Hospital:** UC Irvine Med Ctr; **Address:** Gottschalk Med Plaza, 1 Medical Plaza Drive Fl 2nd, Irvine, CA 92697; **Phone:** 949-824-2020; **Board Cert:** Ophthalmology 1982; **Med School:** Harvard Med Sch 1977; **Resid:** Ophthalmology, Mass EE Infirm 1981; **Fac Appt:** Prof Oph, UC Irvine

Ophthalmology

Stout, John Timothy MD/PhD [Oph] - **Spec Exp:** Retinal Disorders-Pediatric; Retinoblastoma; Retinopathy of Prematurity; **Hospital:** OR Hlth & Sci Univ, Providence St Vincent Med Ctr; **Address:** 3375 SW Terwilliger Blvd, Portland, OR 97239; **Phone:** 503-494-2435; **Board Cert:** Ophthalmology 1999; **Med School:** Baylor Coll Med 1989; **Resid:** Ophthalmology, Doheny Eye Inst 1993; **Fellow:** Ophthalmology, Moorfields Eye Hosp 1994; Retinal Surgery, Doheny Eye Inst 1995; **Fac Appt:** Assoc Prof Oph, Oregon Hlth Sci Univ

Weiss, Avery H MD [Oph] - **Spec Exp:** Pediatric Ophthalmology; Strabismus; Amblyopia; **Hospital:** Chldns Hosp and Regl Med Ctr - Seattle; **Address:** 4800 Sand Point Way NE, MS W-4753, Seattle, WA 98105; **Phone:** 206-987-2177; **Board Cert:** Ophthalmology 1981; **Med School:** Univ Miami Sch Med 1974; **Resid:** Internal Medicine, Barnes Hosp 1976; Ophthalmology, Barnes Hosp 1980; **Fellow:** Research, Barnes Hosp 1977; Pediatric Ophthalmology, Chldns Hosp Natl Med Ctr 1981; **Fac Appt:** Assoc Prof Oph, Univ Wash

Wilson, David Jean MD [Oph] - **Spec Exp:** Eye Tumors/Cancer; Ophthalmic Pathology; **Hospital:** OR Hlth & Sci Univ; **Address:** 3375 SW Terwilliger Blvd, Portland, OR 97239; **Phone:** 503-494-7891; **Board Cert:** Ophthalmology 1986; **Med School:** Baylor Coll Med 1981; **Resid:** Ophthalmology, Univ Oregon 1985; **Fellow:** Ophthalmic Pathology, John Hopkins Hosp 1987; Retina/Vitreous, Mass Eye & Ear Infirm 1988; **Fac Appt:** Prof Oph, Oregon Hlth Sci Univ

Wright, Kenneth W MD [Oph] - **Spec Exp:** Cataract Surgery-Lens Implant; Strabismus-Adult & Pediatric; Pediatric Eye Surgery-Ptosis; Pediatric Ophthalmology; **Hospital:** Cedars-Sinai Med Ctr; **Address:** 520 S San Vincente Blvd, Los Angeles, CA 90048; **Phone:** 310-652-6420; **Board Cert:** Ophthalmology 1983; **Med School:** Boston Univ 1977; **Resid:** Ophthalmology, LAC-USC Med Ctr 1981; **Fellow:** Pediatric Ophthalmology, Johns Hopkins Hosp 1981; Pediatric Ophthalmology, Children's Hosp Natl Med Ctr 1982; **Fac Appt:** Clin Prof Oph, USC Sch Med

Yoshizumi, Marc O MD [Oph] - **Spec Exp:** Retinal Detachment; Diabetic Eye Disease/Retinopathy; Macular Degeneration; **Hospital:** UCLA Med Ctr; **Address:** 200 Stein Plaza Bldg UCLA, Los Angeles, CA 90095-7000; **Phone:** 310-825-4749; **Board Cert:** Ophthalmology 1978; **Med School:** Yale Univ 1970; **Resid:** Internal Medicine, Johns Hopkins Hosp 1972; Ophthalmology, Mass EE Infirm/Harvard 1977; **Fellow:** Neuropathology, Oxford Univ 1971; Retina, Harvard Med Sch 1978; **Fac Appt:** Prof Oph, UCLA

Cleveland Clinic

Cole Eye Institute

Cleveland Clinic Cole Eye Institute is one of the few dedicated, comprehensive eye institutes in the world. We are here to serve the needs of patients and referring physicians for early, accurate diagnosis and excellent, effective patient care. Here, the lines between research and patient care blur. The belief that the two are interdependent and synergistic is the foundation for everything we do. We believe that this approach enhances diagnosis and advances treatment, to the benefit of our patients today and tomorrow.

Our Specialized, Experienced Staff

All of our ophthalmologists have advanced expertise in treating disorders and diseases of a specific part or parts of the eye. This specialized approach offers patients a higher level of care and the assurance that their physicians are experienced in treating even the most unusual eye problems.

- Retina and Vitreous Surgery: Age-related macular degeneration, diabetic retinopathy, inherited retinal diseases and infectious retinopathies.
- Cornea and External Diseases: Diseases of the eye's external surface and cornea, such as inflammatory, infectious and degenerative diseases of the cornea, conjunctiva and lens; corneal tumors; and contact lens-related problems.
- Glaucoma: All forms of this silent thief of sight.
- Neuro-Ophthalmology: Vision problems related to neurologic disorders such as stroke, multiple sclerosis and tumors.
- Oculoplastics and Orbital Surgery: Problems of the orbit and eyelids.
- Ocular Oncology: Primary and metastatic tumors of the eye and eyelids.
- Pediatric Ophthalmology: Strabismus, amblyopia and congenital cataracts.
- Refractive Surgery: Correction of nearsightedness, farsightedness and astigmatism.
- Uveitis: Internal ocular inflammation and infection-related immune system disturbances.

Emergency Services

A Cole Eye Institute ophthalmologist is on-call 24 hours a day for immediate consultation on or treatment of eye emergencies. When necessary, a complete surgical team can be assembled in less than an hour to provide emergency treatment for the most serious cases.

To schedule an appointment or for more information about the Cleveland Clinic Cole Eye Institute call 800.890.2467 or visit www.clevelandclinic.org/eyetopdocs.

Cole Eye Institute | 9500 Euclid Avenue / W14 | Cleveland OH 44195

Why choose Cole Eye Institute?

- Internationally recognized, all subspecialty medical staff.
- Amongst the world's most advanced eye institutes, dedicated to comprehensive and highly specialized ophthalmologic care.
- One of the highest patient volumes in the United States.
- Aggressive research program that bridges the gap between laboratory and patient care and offers access to the latest clinical trials.
- State-of-the-art diagnostic technology and outpatient surgical center.

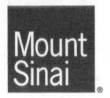

THE MOUNT SINAI MEDICAL CENTER
OPHTHALMOLOGY

One Gustave L. Levy Place (Fifth Avenue and 100th Street)
New York, NY 10029-6574
Physician Referral: 1-800-MD-SINAI (637-4624)
www.mountsinai.org

Specializing in the prevention, diagnosis, and treatment of eye disorders, The Department of Ophthalmology at Mount Sinai offers a variety of sophisticated tests for evaluating patient conditions, including electroretinography, visually evoked potentials, electro-oculography, fundus photography, fluorescein angiography, corneal topography, CT scanning, and MR imaging, as well as new techniques for assessing glaucoma. Ultrasound biomicroscopy (UBM) is a noninvasive method to achieve high-resolution imaging of the inside of the eye. In certain cases of glaucoma (those involving lesions behind the iris or behind a cloudy cornea), it is the only non-invasive way to identify the exact cause of the condition and ascertain optimal treatment. UBM is also an ideal tool to diagnose and manage certain cataract and corneal surgery complications. The pain-free procedure takes about 45 minutes.

Ophthalmology at Mount Sinai features faculty with wide experience in special eye problems and offers comprehensive eye care for the full range of eye disorders, including glaucoma, eye infections, retinal disorders (diabetic retinopathy, macular degeneration, and retinitis pigmentosa), dry eyes (Sjogren's syndrome), allergic reactions to contact lenses, neuro-ophthalmic disorders (double vision and droopy eyelids), corneal and external diseases of the eye, trauma, orbital tumors, and thyroid-related eye problems. We also offer minimally invasive procedures to treat eye disease, including non-laser refractive surgeries, small incision cataract surgery, bladeless laser procedures, and intacs for keratoconus.

Our highly skilled eye surgeons perform corneal transplants, refractive surgery, glaucoma surgery, cataract surgery, ophthalmic plastic surgery, ophthalmic reconstructive surgery, vitreous surgery for complicated retinal detachment, and corneal transplant surgery. We also specialize in the treatment of children with eye conditions.

We feature new imaging methods to assess and follow patients with OCT, HRT II, confocal for corneal problems, glaucoma, and retinal disease. These methods allow for faster, more accurate diagnosis and help determine the best treatment plan for each individual patient.

THE MOUNT SINAI MEDICAL CENTER

Mount Sinai ophthalmologists helped pioneer a new radiofrequency method of correcting farsightedness. Known as Conductive Keratoplasty (CK), the brief procedure is performed in the doctor's office with only topical anesthesia (eye drops). For most farsighted patients—especially those over age 40 whose eyes are naturally aging—the CK procedure eliminates the need for glasses.

623

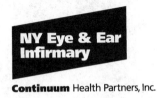

Continuum Health Partners, Inc.

THE NEW YORK EYE AND EAR INFIRMARY
310 East 14th Street
New York, New York 10003
Tel. 212.979.4000   Fax. 212.228.0664
http://www.nyee.edu

PROVIDING EXCEPTIONAL EYE CARE

The Department of Ophthalmology is the region's most comprehensive center for the delivery of primary through tertiary eye care. It is also by far the largest provider of eye care in the metropolitan area—with some 82,000 outpatient visits and 14,000 surgical cases performed each year. More than 250 board-certified ophthalmologists located throughout New York City and its tri-state area comprise the attending Medical Staff.

IN A HIGHLY SPECIALIZED SETTING

As a specialty hospital, the Infirmary is uniquely qualified to handle the most complicated cases. It serves as a nationwide referral center with a commitment to teaching, research, and high-technology based patient care. Computerized ocular imaging equipment includes the new combination of scanning laser ophthalmoscopy with optical coherence tomography, to provide highest resolution in-depth images which detect the smallest defects and assist in the earliest and most accurate diagnosis of diseases such as glaucoma and macular degeneration. Highly experienced staff using state-of-the-art instrumentation have made the Infirmary's 17 operating rooms a national benchmark in efficiency in eye surgery cases.

FOR PATIENTS OF ALL AGES

Staff at the Infirmary are sensitive to the specific needs of patients of all ages. Senior citizens are the vast majority of the Infirmary's 8,000 yearly cataract patients, as well as individuals receiving treatment for age-related macular degeneration. Young children are now 25 percent of the patient population, with conditions such as strabismus, acquired and congenital cataracts, corneal diseases and ocular trauma. For those rare cases of children who have a disease ordinarily associated with age, the Infirmary runs New York's only Pediatric Glaucoma Service. Active adults of all ages utilize the New York Eye Trauma Center and Oculoplastic and Orbital Surgery Services.

Ophthalmology Clinical Services
Ambulatory Care Services
Comprehensive Eye Care
Cornea & Refractive Surgery
Eye Trauma
Glaucoma
Low Vision
Neuro-Ophthalmology
Oculoplastic & Orbital Surgery
Ocular Tumor
Pediatric Ophthalmology & Strabismus
Retinal-Vitreal
Uveitis

Facilities
Ambulatory Surgery Center
Eye Trauma Center
Retina Center

About The New York Eye and Ear Infirmary
Founded in 1820, it is the nation's oldest, continuously operating specialty hospital. More than 10 million people have sought treatment here since its inception.

Physician Referral
1.800.449.HOPE (4673)

Orthopaedic Surgery

An orthopaedic surgeon is trained in the preservation, investigation and restoration of the form and function of the extremities, spine and associated structures by medical, surgical and physical means.

An orthopaedic surgeon is involved with the care of patients whose musculoskeletal problems include congenital deformities, trauma, infections, tumors, metabolic disturbances of the musculoskeletal system, deformities, injuries and degenerative diseases of the spine, hands, feet, knee, hip, shoulder and elbow in children and adults. An orthopaedic surgeon is also concerned with primary and secondary muscular problems and the effects of central or peripheral nervous system lesions of the musculoskeletal system.

Note: *There are many Orthopaedic Surgeons who are trained in Sports Medicine and prefer to be listed under that heading; some trained in Sports Medicine prefer to be listed under Orthopaedics.*

Training Required: Five years (including general surgery training) *plus* two years in clinical practice before final certification is achieved.

Orthopaedic Surgery

New England

Bierbaum, Benjamin MD [OrS] - **Spec Exp:** Hip Replacement; Knee Replacement; **Hospital:** New England Bapt Hosp; **Address:** 830 Boylston St, Ste 106, Chestnut Hill, MA 02467-2502; **Phone:** 617-277-1205; **Board Cert:** Orthopaedic Surgery 1993; **Med School:** Univ Iowa Coll Med 1960; **Resid:** Orthopaedic Surgery, Harvard Affil Hosps 1967; Orthopaedic Surgery, Mass Genl Hosp 1966; **Fellow:** Hip Surgery, Mass Genl Hosp 1968; **Fac Appt:** Clin Prof OrS, Tufts Univ

Browner, Bruce D MD [OrS] - **Spec Exp:** Fractures-Complex; Osteomyelitis; Bone Infections; **Hospital:** Univ of Conn Hlth Ctr, John Dempsey Hosp, Hartford Hosp; **Address:** Med Arts & Rsch Bldg, 4th Fl, 263 Farmington Ave, Farmington, CT 06034-4037; **Phone:** 860-679-6650; **Board Cert:** Orthopaedic Surgery 1997; **Med School:** SUNY Downstate 1973; **Resid:** Orthopaedic Surgery, Albany Med Ctr 1978; **Fellow:** Trauma, Albany Med Ctr 1975; **Fac Appt:** Prof OrS, Univ Conn

Ehrlich, Michael G MD [OrS] - **Spec Exp:** Pediatric Orthopaedic Surgery; **Hospital:** Rhode Island Hosp; **Address:** Rhode Island Hosp, Cooperative Care Bldg, 2 Dudley St, Ste 200, Providence, RI 02905; **Phone:** 401-457-1540; **Board Cert:** Orthopaedic Surgery 1992; **Med School:** Columbia P&S 1963; **Resid:** Orthopaedic Surgery, Bellevue Hosp 1965; Orthopaedic Surgery, Mt Sinai Hosp 1970; **Fac Appt:** Assoc Prof OrS, Harvard Med Sch

Einhorn, Thomas A MD [OrS] - **Spec Exp:** Metabolic Bone Disease; Fractures-Complex; Hip & Knee Replacement; Hip & Knee Reconstruction; **Hospital:** Boston Med Ctr; **Address:** Boston Medical Ctr, Doctors Office Bldg, 720 Harrison Ave, Ste 808, Boston, MA 02118-2393; **Phone:** 617-638-5633; **Board Cert:** Orthopaedic Surgery 1998; **Med School:** Cornell Univ-Weill Med Coll 1976; **Resid:** Orthopaedic Surgery, St Lukes-Roosevelt Hosp 1981; Pediatric Orthopaedic Surgery, Alfred DuPont Inst 1981; **Fellow:** Orthopaedic Surgery, Hosp Special Surgery 1982; **Fac Appt:** Prof OrS, Boston Univ

Friedlaender, Gary E MD [OrS] - **Spec Exp:** Bone & Soft Tissue Tumors; Limb Surgery/Reconstruction; Fractures-Non Union; Bone Tumors-Metastatic; **Hospital:** Yale - New Haven Hosp; **Address:** Yale Univ Sch Med, Dept Orthopedic Surg, 800 Howard Ave YPB Bldg - rm 133, Box 208071, New Haven, CT 06520-8071; **Phone:** 203-737-5656; **Board Cert:** Orthopaedic Surgery 1975; **Med School:** Univ Mich Med Sch 1969; **Resid:** Surgery, Michigan Med Ctr 1971; Orthopaedic Surgery, Yale-New Haven Hosp 1974; **Fellow:** Musculoskeletal Oncology, Mass Genl Hosp 1983; **Fac Appt:** Prof OrS, Yale Univ

Gebhardt, Mark MD [OrS] - **Spec Exp:** Musculoskeletal Tumors; Bone Tumors; **Hospital:** Beth Israel Deaconess Med Ctr - Boston, Children's Hospital - Boston; **Address:** 330 Brookline Ave, Shapiro 2, Boston, MA 02215; **Phone:** 617-667-3940; **Board Cert:** Orthopaedic Surgery 1992; **Med School:** Univ Cincinnati 1975; **Resid:** Surgery, Univ Pittsburg Med Ctr 1977; Orthopaedic Surgery, Harvard 1982; **Fellow:** Pediatric Orthopaedic Surgery, Boston Chldns Hosp 1983; Orthopaedic Oncology, Mass Genl Hosp 1983; **Fac Appt:** Prof OrS, Harvard Med Sch

Jokl, Peter MD [OrS] - **Spec Exp:** Knee Surgery; Sports Medicine; Shoulder Surgery; **Hospital:** Yale - New Haven Hosp; **Address:** Yale Sports Med, Dept Orthopaedics, 800 Howard Ave, New Haven, CT 06519-1369; **Phone:** 203-785-2579; **Board Cert:** Orthopaedic Surgery 1974; **Med School:** Yale Univ 1968; **Resid:** Orthopaedic Surgery, Yale-New Haven Hosp 1972; **Fac Appt:** Prof OrS, Yale Univ

Jupiter, Jesse B MD [OrS] - **Spec Exp:** Upper Extremity Trauma; Hand Surgery; **Hospital:** Mass Genl Hosp, Newton - Wellesley Hosp; **Address:** Yawkey Center, Ste 2100, 55 Fruit St, Boston, MA 02114-2621; **Phone:** 617-726-8530; **Board Cert:** Orthopaedic Surgery 1982; **Med School:** Yale Univ 1972; **Resid:** Surgery, Mass Genl Hosp 1976; Orthopaedic Surgery, Mass Genl Hosp 1979; **Fellow:** Hand Surgery, Univ Louisville 1981; Trauma, AO/ASIF 1980; **Fac Appt:** Prof OrS, Harvard Med Sch

Kasser, James MD [OrS] - **Spec Exp:** Pediatric Orthopaedic Surgery; **Hospital:** Children's Hospital - Boston; **Address:** Chldns Hosp, Dept Ortho Surgery, 300 Longwood Ave, Boston, MA 02115; **Phone:** 617-355-6617; **Board Cert:** Orthopaedic Surgery 1984; **Med School:** Tufts Univ 1976; **Resid:** Orthopaedic Surgery, Tufts Univ 1981; **Fellow:** Pediatric Orthopaedic Surgery, Dupont Inst; **Fac Appt:** Prof OrS, Harvard Med Sch

Kocher, Mininder S MD [OrS] - **Spec Exp:** Pediatric Orthopaedic Surgery; Bone Infections in Children; Limb Lengthening; Pediatric Sports Medicine; **Hospital:** Children's Hospital - Boston; **Address:** Children's Hosp, Dept Orthopaedic Surg, 300 Longwood Ave, Boston, MA 02115; **Phone:** 617-355-6021; **Board Cert:** Orthopaedic Surgery 2002; **Med School:** Duke Univ 1993; **Resid:** Orthopaedic Surgery, Beth Israel Hosp 1999; **Fellow:** Pediatric Orthopaedic Surgery, Chldns Hosp 1999; Sports Medicine, Steadman Hawkins Clin 2000; **Fac Appt:** Asst Prof OrS, Harvard Med Sch

Marsh, James S MD [OrS] - **Spec Exp:** Pediatric Orthopaedic Surgery; **Hospital:** Yale - New Haven Hosp; **Address:** 1200 Boston Post Rd, Ste 201B, Guilford, CT 06437; **Phone:** 203-453-1088; **Board Cert:** Orthopaedic Surgery 2000; **Med School:** Harvard Med Sch 1981; **Resid:** Orthopaedic Surgery, Stanford Univ 1986; **Fellow:** Pediatric Orthopaedic Surgery, Mass Genl Hosp 1987; **Fac Appt:** Assoc Prof OrS, Yale Univ

Ready, John E MD [OrS] - **Spec Exp:** Bone Cancer; Sarcoma-Soft Tissue; Hip & Knee Replacement; Hip & Knee Replacement in Bone Tumors; **Hospital:** Brigham & Women's Hosp, Dana-Farber Cancer Inst; **Address:** Brigham & Women's Hospital, Dept Orthopaedics, 75 Francis St, Boston, MA 02115; **Phone:** 617-732-5368; **Board Cert:** Orthopaedic Surgery 2002; **Med School:** Dalhousie Univ 1982; **Resid:** Orthopaedic Surgery, Dalhousie Univ Hosp 1987; **Fellow:** Orthopaedic Oncology, St Michael's Hosp 1988; Orthopaedic Oncology, Mass Genl Hosp/Childns Hosp 1989

Reilly, Donald T MD [OrS] - **Spec Exp:** Hip & Knee Replacement; **Hospital:** New England Bapt Hosp; **Address:** 125 Parker Hill Ave, Ste 550, Boston, MA 02120; **Phone:** 617-232-6025; **Board Cert:** Orthopaedic Surgery 1984; **Med School:** Case West Res Univ 1975; **Resid:** Orthopaedic Surgery, Harvard Combined Ortho 1981

Scott, Richard David MD [OrS] - **Spec Exp:** Hip Replacement; Knee Replacement; **Hospital:** Brigham & Women's Hosp, New England Bapt Hosp; **Address:** 125 Parker Hill Ave, Boston, MA 02120; **Phone:** 617-738-9151; **Board Cert:** Orthopaedic Surgery 1975; **Med School:** Temple Univ 1968; **Resid:** Orthopaedic Surgery, Mass Genl Hosp 1974; **Fellow:** Orthopaedic Surgery, Mass Genl Hosp 1974; **Fac Appt:** Prof OrS, Harvard Med Sch

Springfield, Dempsey MD [OrS] - **Spec Exp:** Bone Tumors; Soft Tissue Tumors; **Hospital:** Mass Genl Hosp; **Address:** 55 Fruit St, YAW 3700, Boston, MA 02114-2621; **Phone:** 617-724-3700; **Board Cert:** Orthopaedic Surgery 1992; **Med School:** Univ Fla Coll Med 1971; **Resid:** Orthopaedic Surgery, Univ Florida/Shands 1976; **Fellow:** Orthopaedic Surgery, Univ Florida/Shands 1979

Orthopaedic Surgery

Thornhill, Thomas S MD [OrS] - **Spec Exp:** Hip & Knee Replacement; Arthritis; **Hospital:** Brigham & Women's Hosp; **Address:** Brigham & Women's Hosp, Dept Orth Surg, 75 Francis St, Boston, MA 02115; **Phone:** 617-732-5322; **Board Cert:** Internal Medicine 1973; Orthopaedic Surgery 1979; **Med School:** Cornell Univ-Weill Med Coll 1970; **Resid:** Internal Medicine, Peter Brent Brigham Hosp 1972; Orthopaedic Surgery, Harvard Combined Prgm 1978; **Fellow:** Joint Replacement Surgery, Robert Breck Brigham Hosp; **Fac Appt:** Prof OrS, Harvard Med Sch

Weinstein, James DO [OrS] - **Spec Exp:** Pain-Back; Spinal Tumors; **Hospital:** Dartmouth - Hitchcock Med Ctr; **Address:** DHMC, Dept Orthopaedic Surgery, One Medical Ctr Drive, Lebanon, NH 03756; **Phone:** 603-653-3580; **Board Cert:** Orthopaedic Surgery 2002; **Med School:** Chicago Coll Osteo Med 1973; **Resid:** Orthopaedic Surgery, Rush Presby-St Lukes Med Ctr 1983; **Fac Appt:** Prof OrS, Dartmouth Med Sch

Zarins, Bertram MD [OrS] - **Spec Exp:** Knee Injuries/ACL; Arthroscopic Surgery; Shoulder Injuries; **Hospital:** Mass Genl Hosp; **Address:** Mass General Hosp, 175 Cambridge St, Ste 400, Boston, MA 02114; **Phone:** 617-726-3421; **Board Cert:** Orthopaedic Surgery 1994; **Med School:** SUNY Upstate Med Univ 1967; **Resid:** Surgery, Johns Hopkins Hosp 1969; Orthopaedic Surgery, Harvard Ortho Prog 1973; **Fellow:** Sports Medicine, Mass Genl Hosp 1976; **Fac Appt:** Assoc Clin Prof OrS, Harvard Med Sch

Mid Atlantic

Albert, Todd J MD [OrS] - **Spec Exp:** Spinal Surgery; Scoliosis; Spinal Deformity; Spinal Surgery-Cervical; **Hospital:** Thomas Jefferson Univ Hosp; **Address:** Rothman Institute, 925 Chesnut St Fl 5, Philadelphia, PA 19107; **Phone:** 267-339-3500; **Board Cert:** Orthopaedic Surgery 2006; **Med School:** Univ VA Sch Med 1987; **Resid:** Orthopaedic Surgery, Thomas Jefferson Univ Hosp 1992; **Fellow:** Spinal Surgery, Minnesota Spine Ctr 1993; **Fac Appt:** Prof OrS, Thomas Jefferson Univ

Balderston, Richard MD [OrS] - **Spec Exp:** Scoliosis; Spinal Surgery; Spinal Disc Replacement; **Hospital:** Pennsylvania Hosp (page 72); **Address:** 800 Spruce St, 3B Orthopaedics, Philadelphia, PA 19107; **Phone:** 215-829-2222; **Board Cert:** Orthopaedic Surgery 1985; **Med School:** Univ Pennsylvania 1977; **Resid:** Orthopaedic Surgery, Hosp Univ Penn 1982; **Fellow:** Spinal Surgery, Univ Minn Affil Hosp 1983; **Fac Appt:** Clin Prof OrS, Univ Pennsylvania

Baratz, Mark E MD [OrS] - **Spec Exp:** Hand Surgery; Upper Extremity Surgery; Elbow Reconstruction; **Hospital:** Allegheny General Hosp; **Address:** 1307 Federal St Fl 2, Pittsburgh, PA 15212; **Phone:** 412-359-4263; **Board Cert:** Orthopaedic Surgery 2004; Hand Surgery 2004; **Med School:** Univ Pittsburgh 1984; **Resid:** Orthopaedic Surgery, Univ Hlth Ctr 1990; **Fellow:** Orthopaedic Surgery, Univ Hlth Ctr 1987; Hand Surgery, Med Coll Penn 1991; **Fac Appt:** Prof OrS, Drexel Univ Coll Med

Bartolozzi, Arthur R MD [OrS] - **Spec Exp:** Sports Medicine; Arthroscopic Surgery-Knee; **Hospital:** Pennsylvania Hosp (page 72); **Address:** 800 Spruce St Fl 1, Philadelphia, PA 19107; **Phone:** 215-829-2222; **Board Cert:** Orthopaedic Surgery 2000; **Med School:** UCSD 1981; **Resid:** Orthopaedic Surgery, Hosp Univ Penn 1986; **Fellow:** Sports Medicine, UCLA Med Ctr 1987; **Fac Appt:** Assoc Clin Prof OrS, Univ Pennsylvania

Bauman, Phillip MD [OrS] - **Spec Exp:** Foot & Ankle Surgery; Knee Surgery; Dance/Sports Medicine; **Hospital:** St Luke's - Roosevelt Hosp Ctr - Roosevelt Div, NY-Presby Hosp/Columbia (page 66); **Address:** Orthopaedic Assocs of NY, 343 W 58th St, rm 1, New York, NY 10019; **Phone:** 212-765-2260; **Board Cert:** Orthopaedic Surgery 2001; **Med School:** Columbia P&S 1981; **Resid:** Surgery, St Luke's-Roosevelt Hosp Ctr 1983; Orthopaedic Surgery, Columbia-Presby Med Ctr 1987; **Fac Appt:** Asst Prof OrS, Columbia P&S

Benevenia, Joseph MD [OrS] - **Spec Exp:** Limb Sparing Surgery; Bone Cancer; Sarcoma-Soft Tissue; **Hospital:** UMDNJ-Univ Hosp-Newark; **Address:** 140 Bergen St, Ste D-1610, Newark, NJ 07103; **Phone:** 973-972-2153; **Board Cert:** Orthopaedic Surgery 2003; **Med School:** UMDNJ-NJ Med Sch, Newark 1984; **Resid:** Orthopaedic Surgery, UMDNJ-NJ Med Sch Hosp 1988; **Fellow:** Orthopaedic Oncology, Case Western Reserve Univ 1991; **Fac Appt:** Prof OrS, UMDNJ-NJ Med Sch, Newark

Betz, Randal R MD [OrS] - **Spec Exp:** Spinal Cord Injury-Pediatric; Praxis Functional Electrical Stim (FES); **Hospital:** Philadelphia Shriners Hosp; **Address:** Shriners Hospital for Children, 3351 N Broad St, Philadelphia, PA 19140; **Phone:** 215-430-4026; **Board Cert:** Orthopaedic Surgery 1998; Spinal Cord Injury Medicine 1998; **Med School:** Temple Univ 1977; **Resid:** Orthopaedic Surgery, Shriners Hospital 1980; Orthopaedic Surgery, Temple Univ Hospital 1982; **Fellow:** Pediatric Orthopaedic Surgery, DuPont Inst 1983; **Fac Appt:** Prof OrS, Temple Univ

Bigliani, Louis MD [OrS] - **Spec Exp:** Shoulder Surgery; Sports Medicine; Arthroscopic Surgery; **Hospital:** NY-Presby Hosp/Columbia (page 66); **Address:** 622 W 168th St, rm 1130, New York, NY 10032-3720; **Phone:** 212-305-5564; **Board Cert:** Orthopaedic Surgery 1979; **Med School:** Loyola Univ-Stritch Sch Med 1973; **Resid:** Surgery, Roosevelt Hosp 1974; Orthopaedic Surgery, Columbia Presby Med Ctr 1977; **Fac Appt:** Prof OrS, Columbia P&S

Bitan, Fabien D MD [OrS] - **Spec Exp:** Spinal Surgery-Pediatric & Adult; Spinal Disc Replacement; Spinal Deformity & Degeneration; **Hospital:** Lenox Hill Hosp (page 62); **Address:** Phillips Ambulatory Care Ctr, Spine Inst, 130 E 77th St Fl 7, New York, NY 10021; **Phone:** 212-744-8114; **Med School:** France 1981; **Resid:** Orthopaedic Surgery, Hospital Beaujon 1987; Pediatric Orthopaedic Surgery, Hosp des Enfants Malades 1990; **Fellow:** Pediatric Orthopaedic Surgery, Hosp Special Surgery 1997; Spinal Surgery, Beth Israel Med Ctr 1998

Boachie-Adjei, Oheneba MD [OrS] - **Spec Exp:** Spinal Surgery; Scoliosis; **Hospital:** Hosp For Special Surgery (page 60); **Address:** Hospital for Special Surgery, 523 E 72nd St, New York, NY 10021; **Phone:** 212-606-1948; **Board Cert:** Orthopaedic Surgery 2000; **Med School:** Columbia P&S 1980; **Resid:** Surgery, St Vincents Hosp 1982; Orthopaedic Surgery, Hosp Spec Surg 1986; **Fellow:** Orthopaedic Pathology, Hosp Spec Surg 1983; Spinal Surgery, Twin Cities Scoliosis Ctr/Minn Spine Ctr 1987; **Fac Appt:** Assoc Clin Prof S, Cornell Univ-Weill Med Coll

Booth Jr, Robert E MD [OrS] - **Spec Exp:** Knee Replacement; **Hospital:** Pennsylvania Hosp (page 72); **Address:** 800 Spruce St Fl 1, Philadelphia, PA 19107; **Phone:** 215-829-2222; **Board Cert:** Orthopaedic Surgery 1978; **Med School:** Univ Pennsylvania 1971; **Resid:** Surgery, Penn Hosp 1973; Orthopaedic Surgery, Hosp Univ Penn 1977; **Fac Appt:** Clin Prof OrS, Jefferson Med Coll

Bradley, James P MD [OrS] - **Spec Exp:** Sports Medicine; **Hospital:** UPMC St Margaret; **Address:** 200 Delafield Ave, Ste 4010, Pittsburgh, PA 15215; **Phone:** 412-784-5783; **Board Cert:** Orthopaedic Surgery 2001; **Med School:** Georgetown Univ 1982; **Resid:** Surgery, Univ Tennessee 1984; Orthopaedic Surgery, Univ Hlth Ctr 1987; **Fellow:** Sports Medicine, Kerlan-Jobe Ortho Clinic 1988; **Fac Appt:** Assoc Prof OrS, Univ Pittsburgh

Brushart, Thomas M MD [OrS] - **Spec Exp:** Hand Surgery; Peripheral Nerve Surgery; **Hospital:** Johns Hopkins Hosp - Baltimore (page 61); **Address:** 601 N Caroline St, rm 5221, Baltimore, MD 21287-0882; **Phone:** 410-955-9663; **Board Cert:** Orthopaedic Surgery 1985; Hand Surgery 1989; **Med School:** Harvard Med Sch 1978; **Resid:** Orthopaedic Surgery, Harvard Affil Hosps 1981; **Fellow:** Hand Surgery, Curtis Hand Ctr 1983; **Fac Appt:** Prof OrS, Johns Hopkins Univ

Buly, Robert L MD [OrS] - **Spec Exp:** Hip Replacement; Minimally Invasive Surgery; Arthritis; **Hospital:** Hosp For Special Surgery (page 60); **Address:** Hospital for Special Surgery, 535 E 70th St, New York, NY 10021; **Phone:** 212-606-1971; **Board Cert:** Orthopaedic Surgery 2004; **Med School:** Cornell Univ-Weill Med Coll 1985; **Resid:** Orthopaedic Surgery, Hosp for Special Surg 1990; **Fellow:** Hip Surgery, Mueller Fdn 1991; Joint Reconstruction, Case Western Res/ Univ Hosp 1992; **Fac Appt:** Asst Prof OrS, Cornell Univ-Weill Med Coll

Cammisa Jr, Frank P MD [OrS] - **Spec Exp:** Spinal Surgery; Spinal Disc Replacement; Scoliosis; **Hospital:** Hosp For Special Surgery (page 60), NY-Presby Hosp/Weill Cornell (page 66); **Address:** 523 E 72nd St, Fl 3, New York, NY 10021; **Phone:** 212-606-1946; **Board Cert:** Orthopaedic Surgery 2001; **Med School:** Columbia P&S 1982; **Resid:** Surgery, Columbia-Presby Hosp 1983; Orthopaedic Surgery, Hosp for Special Surgery 1987; **Fellow:** Spinal Surgery, Jackson Meml Hosp 1988; **Fac Appt:** Assoc Prof OrS, Cornell Univ-Weill Med Coll

Crossett, Lawrence MD [OrS] - **Spec Exp:** Hip Surgery; Knee Surgery; **Hospital:** UPMC Presby, Pittsburgh, UPMC Shadyside; **Address:** Univ Pittsburgh Physicians, Orthopaedics, 5200 Centre Ave, Ste 415, Pittsburgh, PA 15232; **Phone:** 412-802-4100; **Board Cert:** Orthopaedic Surgery 2000; **Med School:** Temple Univ 1981; **Resid:** Orthopaedic Surgery, Temple Univ Hosp 1986; Orthopaedic Surgery, Shriners Children's Hosp 1984; **Fac Appt:** Asst Prof OrS, Univ Pittsburgh

Davidson, Richard S MD [OrS] - **Spec Exp:** Limb Lengthening (Ilizarov Procedure); Limb Deformities; Foot Deformities; Clubfoot; **Hospital:** Chldns Hosp of Philadelphia, The; **Address:** Children's Hospital, Dept Orthopaedics, 34th St & Civic Ctr Blvd, Wood Center Fl 2, Philadelphia, PA 19104; **Phone:** 215-590-1527; **Board Cert:** Orthopaedic Surgery 1997; **Med School:** NYU Sch Med 1976; **Resid:** Orthopaedic Surgery, Hosp Special Surgery 1981; **Fellow:** Pediatric Orthopaedic Surgery, Hosp Sick Children 1982; **Fac Appt:** Assoc Clin Prof OrS, Univ Pennsylvania

Delahay, John N MD [OrS] - **Spec Exp:** Pediatric Orthopaedic Surgery; Trauma; **Hospital:** Georgetown Univ Hosp; **Address:** 3800 Reservoir Rd NW, PHC Bldg, Ground FL, Washington, DC 20007; **Phone:** 202-444-1438; **Board Cert:** Orthopaedic Surgery 1975; **Med School:** Georgetown Univ 1969; **Resid:** Orthopaedic Surgery, Georgetown Univ Hosp 1974; **Fac Appt:** Prof OrS, Georgetown Univ

Deland, Jonathan T MD [OrS] - **Spec Exp:** Foot & Ankle Surgery; Sports Medicine; Arthritis; **Hospital:** Hosp For Special Surgery (page 60); **Address:** Hosp Spec Surg, Foot & Ankle Service, 535 E 70th St, New York, NY 10021-4099; **Phone:** 212-606-1665; **Board Cert:** Orthopaedic Surgery 2003; **Med School:** Columbia P&S 1980; **Resid:** Orthopaedic Surgery, St Luke's-Rooselvelt Hosp Ctr 1982; Orthopaedic Surgery, Mass Genl Hosp 1987; **Fac Appt:** Asst Prof S, Cornell Univ-Weill Med Coll

Dines, David M MD [OrS] - **Spec Exp:** Shoulder Surgery; Sports Medicine; Shoulder Replacement; **Hospital:** Long Island Jewish Med Ctr, Hosp For Special Surgery (page 60); **Address:** 935 Northern Blvd, Ste 303, Great Neck, NY 11021-5309; **Phone:** 516-482-1037; **Board Cert:** Orthopaedic Surgery 1980; **Med School:** UMDNJ-NJ Med Sch, Newark 1974; **Resid:** Surgery, NY Hosp-Cornell Med Ctr 1976; Orthopaedic Surgery, Hosp Special Surg 1979; **Fac Appt:** Clin Prof OrS, Albert Einstein Coll Med

Donaldson III, William F MD [OrS] - **Spec Exp:** Spinal Surgery; **Hospital:** UPMC Presby, Pittsburgh; **Address:** Univ Pittsburgh Physicians, Orthopaedics, 3471 5th Ave, Ste 1010, Pittsburgh, PA 15213; **Phone:** 412-605-3218; **Board Cert:** Orthopaedic Surgery 1999; **Med School:** Rush Med Coll 1980; **Resid:** Surgery, Rush Presby-St Luke's Med Ctr 1981; Orthopaedic Surgery, Hosp Special Surg 1985; **Fellow:** Spinal Surgery, Hosp Special Surg 1986; **Fac Appt:** Assoc Prof OrS, Univ Pittsburgh

Dormans, John P MD [OrS] - **Spec Exp:** Tumor Surgery-Pediatric; Spinal Surgery-Pediatric; Pediatric Orthopaedic Surgery; **Hospital:** Chldns Hosp of Philadelphia, The; **Address:** Childrens Hosp Philadelphia, 34 St & Civic Center Blvd, Wood Bldg Fl 2-rm 2315, Philadelphia, PA 19104; **Phone:** 215-590-1527; **Board Cert:** Orthopaedic Surgery 2002; **Med School:** Indiana Univ 1983; **Resid:** Orthopaedic Surgery, Michigan State Univ Hosps 1988; **Fellow:** Pediatric Orthopaedic Surgery, Hosp Sick Children 1989; **Fac Appt:** Prof OrS, Univ Pennsylvania

Errico, Thomas MD [OrS] - **Spec Exp:** Spinal Surgery; Spinal Disc Replacement; Scoliosis; **Hospital:** NYU Med Ctr (page 67), Hosp For Joint Diseases (page 68); **Address:** 530 1st Ave, Ste 8U, New York, NY 10016-6402; **Phone:** 212-263-7182; **Board Cert:** Orthopaedic Surgery 1986; **Med School:** UMDNJ-NJ Med Sch, Newark 1978; **Resid:** Orthopaedic Surgery, NYU Med Ctr 1983; **Fellow:** Spinal Surgery, Toronto Genl Hosp 1984; **Fac Appt:** Assoc Clin Prof OrS, NYU Sch Med

Farcy, Jean Pierre MD [OrS] - **Spec Exp:** Spinal Surgery; Spinal Disc Replacement; Sports Medicine; **Hospital:** Hosp For Joint Diseases (page 68); **Address:** 303 2nd Ave, Ste 19, New York, NY 10003; **Phone:** 212-534-7758; **Med School:** France 1967; **Resid:** Orthopaedic Surgery, Univ Marseilles Med Ctr 1967; **Fellow:** Orthopaedic Surgery, Columbia Presby Med Ctr 1983; **Fac Appt:** Assoc Clin Prof OrS, NYU Sch Med

Feldman, David S MD [OrS] - **Spec Exp:** Limb Deformities; Spinal Surgery; Pediatric Orthopaedic Surgery; **Hospital:** Hosp For Joint Diseases (page 68), NYU Med Ctr (page 67); **Address:** 67 Irving Pl Fl 8, New York, NY 10003; **Phone:** 212-533-5310; **Board Cert:** Orthopaedic Surgery 2007; **Med School:** Albert Einstein Coll Med 1988; **Resid:** Orthopaedic Surgery, Hosp for Joint Diseases 1993; **Fellow:** Pediatric Surgery, Hosp For Sick Chldn 1994; **Fac Appt:** Asst Prof OrS, NYU Sch Med

Flatow, Evan MD [OrS] - **Spec Exp:** Rotator Cuff Surgery; Shoulder Injuries; Shoulder Replacement; Shoulder Arthroscopic Surgery; **Hospital:** Mount Sinai Med Ctr; **Address:** 5 E 98th St Fl 9, Box 1188, New York, NY 10029; **Phone:** 212-241-1663; **Board Cert:** Orthopaedic Surgery 2000; **Med School:** Columbia P&S 1981; **Resid:** Surgery, Roosevelt Hosp 1983; Orthopaedic Surgery, Columbia-Presby Med Ctr 1985; **Fellow:** Shoulder Surgery, Columbia-Presby Med Ctr 1987; **Fac Appt:** Prof OrS, Mount Sinai Sch Med

Orthopaedic Surgery

Frassica, Frank J MD [OrS] - **Spec Exp:** Bone Cancer; **Hospital:** Johns Hopkins Hosp - Baltimore (page 61); **Address:** 601 N Caroline St, Ste 5215, Baltimore, MD 21287-0882; **Phone:** 410-955-9300; **Board Cert:** Orthopaedic Surgery 2001; **Med School:** Univ SC Sch Med 1982; **Resid:** Orthopaedic Surgery, Mayo Clinic 1987; **Fellow:** Orthopaedic Oncology, Mayo Clinic 1988; **Fac Appt:** Prof OrS, Johns Hopkins Univ

Fu, Freddie H MD [OrS] - **Spec Exp:** Sports Medicine; Knee Injuries; Shoulder Injuries; **Hospital:** UPMC Presby, Pittsburgh; **Address:** Presbyterian Univ Hospital, Kaufmann Bldg, 3471 5th Ave, Ste 1011, Pittsburgh, PA 15213; **Phone:** 412-605-3265; **Board Cert:** Orthopaedic Surgery 1994; **Med School:** Univ Pittsburgh 1977; **Resid:** Orthopaedic Surgery, Univ Pittsburgh Med Ctr 1982; **Fellow:** Orthopaedic Research, Univ Pittsburgh Med Ctr 1979; **Fac Appt:** Prof OrS, Univ Pittsburgh

Glashow, Jonathan L MD [OrS] - **Spec Exp:** Sports Medicine; Shoulder Surgery; Knee Surgery; Arthroscopic Surgery; **Hospital:** Mount Sinai Med Ctr, Lenox Hill Hosp (page 62); **Address:** 159 E 74th St Fl 1, New York, NY 10021; **Phone:** 212-794-5096; **Board Cert:** Orthopaedic Surgery 2004; **Med School:** Cornell Univ-Weill Med Coll 1984; **Resid:** Orthopaedic Surgery, Lenox Hill Hosp 1989; **Fellow:** Arthroscopic Surgery, S Calif Ortho Inst 1990; Shoulder Surgery, Univ Texas Med Ctr 1990; **Fac Appt:** Assoc Clin Prof OrS, Mount Sinai Sch Med

Grelsamer, Ronald P MD [OrS] - **Spec Exp:** Knee-Patella Problems; Sports Medicine; Knee Reconstruction; Hip Reconstruction; **Hospital:** Mount Sinai Med Ctr; **Address:** Mount Sinai Medical Ctr, Dept Orthopaedics, 5 E 98th St, Box 1188, New York, NY 10029-6574; **Phone:** 212-241-2914; **Board Cert:** Orthopaedic Surgery 2006; **Med School:** Columbia P&S 1979; **Resid:** Orthopaedic Surgery, Columbia Presby Med Ctr 1984; **Fellow:** Hip & Knee Surgery, Columbia Presby Med Ctr 1985; **Fac Appt:** Assoc Prof OrS, Mount Sinai Sch Med

Haas, Steven B MD [OrS] - **Spec Exp:** Knee Surgery; Knee Replacement; Minimally Invasive Surgery; **Hospital:** Hosp For Special Surgery (page 60); **Address:** Hospital for Special Surgery, 535 E 70th St, New York, NY 10021; **Phone:** 212-606-1852; **Board Cert:** Orthopaedic Surgery 2004; **Med School:** Univ Rochester 1985; **Resid:** Orthopaedic Surgery, Hosp Special Surgery 1990; Surgery, Harvard Surg Service 1986; **Fellow:** Knee Surgery, Hosp Special Surgery 1991; **Fac Appt:** Assoc Prof OrS, Cornell Univ-Weill Med Coll

Hamilton, William MD [OrS] - **Spec Exp:** Dance Medicine; Foot & Ankle Surgery; Sports Medicine; **Hospital:** St Luke's - Roosevelt Hosp Ctr - Roosevelt Div; **Address:** 343 W 58th St, New York, NY 10019-1173; **Phone:** 212-765-2260; **Board Cert:** Orthopaedic Surgery 1971; **Med School:** Columbia P&S 1964; **Resid:** Surgery, St Luke's-Roosevelt Hosp Ctr 1966; Orthopaedic Surgery, Columbia-Presby Hosp 1969; **Fellow:** Pediatric Orthopaedic Surgery, Newington Chldrn's Hosp 1970; **Fac Appt:** Clin Prof OrS, Columbia P&S

Hannafin, Jo MD/PhD [OrS] - **Spec Exp:** Sports Medicine-Women; Shoulder Arthroscopic Surgery; Knee Injuries/Ligament Surgery; Ligament Reconstruction; **Hospital:** Hosp For Special Surgery (page 60), NY-Presby Hosp/Weill Cornell (page 66); **Address:** 535 E 70th St, New York, NY 10021-4872; **Phone:** 212-606-1469; **Board Cert:** Orthopaedic Surgery 2005; **Med School:** Albert Einstein Coll Med 1985; **Resid:** Orthopaedic Surgery, Montefiore Hosp Med Ctr 1990; **Fellow:** Sports Medicine, Hosp Special Surg-Cornell 1992; **Fac Appt:** Assoc Prof OrS, Cornell Univ-Weill Med Coll

Hausman, Michael R MD [OrS] - **Spec Exp:** Hand Reconstruction; Elbow Reconstruction; Arthroscopic Surgery; **Hospital:** Mount Sinai Med Ctr; **Address:** 5 E 98th St, Box 1188, New York, NY 10029-6501; **Phone:** 212-241-1658; **Board Cert:** Orthopaedic Surgery 2000; **Med School:** Yale Univ 1979; **Resid:** Surgery, Yale-New Haven Hosp 1981; Orthopaedic Surgery, Yale-New Haven Hosp 1985; **Fellow:** Hand Surgery, Roosevelt Hosp 1987; **Fac Appt:** Assoc Clin Prof OrS, Mount Sinai Sch Med

Healey, John H MD [OrS] - **Spec Exp:** Bone Tumors; Hip & Knee Replacement in Bone Tumors; Prosthetic Reconstruction; Sarcoma-Soft Tissue; **Hospital:** Meml Sloan Kettering Cancer Ctr, Hosp For Special Surgery (page 60); **Address:** 1275 York Ave, Ste A-342, New York, NY 10021-6007; **Phone:** 212-639-7610; **Board Cert:** Orthopaedic Surgery 2005; **Med School:** Univ VT Coll Med 1978; **Resid:** Orthopaedic Surgery, Hosp Special Surg 1983; **Fellow:** Orthopaedic Oncology, Meml Sloan Kettering Cancer Ctr 1984; Orthopaedic Surgery, Hosp Special Surgery 1984; **Fac Appt:** Prof OrS, Cornell Univ-Weill Med Coll

Helfet, David L MD [OrS] - **Spec Exp:** Fractures-Complex; Fractures-Non Union; Trauma; **Hospital:** Hosp For Special Surgery (page 60), NY-Presby Hosp/Weill Cornell (page 66); **Address:** 535 E 70th St, New York, NY 10021; **Phone:** 212-606-1888; **Board Cert:** Orthopaedic Surgery 1984; **Med School:** South Africa 1975; **Resid:** Surgery, Edendale Hosp 1977; Orthopaedic Surgery, Johns Hopkins 1981; **Fellow:** Orthopaedic Surgery, Inselspita Hosp 1981; Orthopaedic Surgery, UCLA Med Ctr 1982; **Fac Appt:** Prof OrS, Cornell Univ-Weill Med Coll

Herzenberg, John E MD [OrS] - **Spec Exp:** Limb Lengthening (Ilizarov Procedure); Limb Deformities; Pediatric Orthopaedic Surgery; Clubfoot; **Hospital:** Sinai Hosp - Baltimore; **Address:** Sinai Hospital, 2401 W Belvedere Ave, Baltimore, MD 21215; **Phone:** 410-601-8700; **Board Cert:** Orthopaedic Surgery 1999; **Med School:** Boston Univ 1979; **Resid:** Orthopaedic Surgery, Duke Univ Med Ctr 1985; **Fellow:** Pediatric Orthopaedic Surgery, Hosp for Sick Children 1986; **Fac Appt:** Prof S, Univ MD Sch Med

Hilibrand, Alan S MD [OrS] - **Spec Exp:** Spinal Surgery; spinal trauma; **Hospital:** Thomas Jefferson Univ Hosp; **Address:** Rothman Institute, 925 Chestnut St, Philadelphia, PA 19107; **Phone:** 267-339-3500; **Board Cert:** Orthopaedic Surgery 1998; **Med School:** Yale Univ 1990; **Resid:** Orthopaedic Surgery, Univ Michigan Hlth System 1996; **Fellow:** Spinal Surgery, Cleveland Spine Inst 1997; **Fac Appt:** Assoc Prof OrS, Thomas Jefferson Univ

Hotchkiss, Robert MD [OrS] - **Spec Exp:** Hand Surgery; Wrist Surgery; Elbow Reconstruction; **Hospital:** Hosp For Special Surgery (page 60), NY-Presby Hosp/Weill Cornell (page 66); **Address:** 535 E 70th St, New York, NY 10021; **Phone:** 212-606-1964; **Board Cert:** Orthopaedic Surgery 2000; Hand Surgery 2000; **Med School:** Johns Hopkins Univ 1980; **Resid:** Surgery, Johns Hopkins Hosp 1982; Orthopaedic Surgery, Johns Hopkins Hosp 1985; **Fellow:** Hand Surgery, Union Meml Hosp 1987; **Fac Appt:** Assoc Prof OrS, Cornell Univ-Weill Med Coll

Hozack, William J MD [OrS] - **Spec Exp:** Hip Surgery; Knee Surgery; Joint Replacement; **Hospital:** Thomas Jefferson Univ Hosp; **Address:** Rothman Institute, 925 Chesnut St Fl 5, Philadelphia, PA 19107; **Phone:** 215-955-3458; **Board Cert:** Orthopaedic Surgery 2000; **Med School:** McGill Univ 1981; **Resid:** Orthopaedic Surgery, Hosp Univ Penn 1986; **Fellow:** Joint Reconstruction, Penn Hosp/Thomas Jefferson Univ 1987; **Fac Appt:** Prof OrS, Jefferson Med Coll

Orthopaedic Surgery

Johnson, Carl A MD [OrS] - **Spec Exp:** Knee Surgery; **Hospital:** Johns Hopkins Hosp - Baltimore (page 61), Johns Hopkins Bayview Med Ctr (page 61); **Address:** Johns Hopkins Univ, Dept Orth Surg, 4940 Eastern Ave, Baltimore, MD 21224; **Phone:** 410-550-0453; **Board Cert:** Orthopaedic Surgery 1983; **Med School:** Johns Hopkins Univ 1976; **Resid:** Surgery, Johns Hopkins Hosp 1978; Orthopaedic Surgery, Johns Hopkins Hosp 1981; **Fac Appt:** Assoc Prof OrS, Johns Hopkins Univ

Kaplan, Frederick S MD [OrS] - **Spec Exp:** Metabolic Bone Disease; Fibrodysplasia Ossificans Progressiv FOP; Progressive Osseous Heteroplasia POH; **Hospital:** Hosp Univ Penn - UPHS (page 72), Thomas Jefferson Univ Hosp; **Address:** U Penn Medical Ctr, Orthopaedic Inst, 3400 Spruce St, 2 Silverstein, MC 4283, Philadelphia, PA 19104; **Phone:** 215-349-8727; **Med School:** Johns Hopkins Univ 1976; **Resid:** Orthopaedic Surgery, Hosp U Penn 1981; **Fellow:** Orthopaedic Research, Hosp U Penn 1982; Musculoskeletal Disorders, Dr Michael Zasloff/U Penn 1991; **Fac Appt:** Prof OrS, Univ Pennsylvania

Keenan, Mary Ann MD [OrS] - **Spec Exp:** Neuro-Orthopaedic Surgery; Arthritis; Deformity Reconstruction; **Hospital:** Hosp Univ Penn - UPHS (page 72), Pennsylvania Hosp (page 72); **Address:** Hosp Univ Penn, Dept Orthopaedic Surg, 3400 Spruce St, 2 Fl- Silverstein, Philadelphia, PA 19104; **Phone:** 215-662-3340; **Board Cert:** Orthopaedic Surgery 1997; **Med School:** Med Coll PA 1976; **Resid:** Orthopaedic Surgery, Albert Einstein Med Ctr 1981; **Fellow:** Arthritis Surgery, Rancho Los Amigos Med Ctr 1981; Neurological Orthopaedic Surgery, Rancho Los Amigos Med Ctr 1982; **Fac Appt:** Prof OrS, Univ Pennsylvania

Kenan, Samuel MD [OrS] - **Spec Exp:** Bone Tumors; Hip Replacement; Knee Replacement; **Hospital:** Hosp For Joint Diseases (page 68), NYU Med Ctr (page 67); **Address:** 317 E 34th St, Ste 903, New York, NY 10016; **Phone:** 212-684-5511; **Med School:** Israel 1976; **Resid:** Orthopaedic Surgery, Hadassah Univ Hosp 1984; **Fellow:** Orthopaedic Pathology, Hosp for Joint Diseases 1987; **Fac Appt:** Prof OrS, NYU Sch Med

Krackow, Kenneth A MD [OrS] - **Spec Exp:** Knee Replacement; Knee Reconstruction; Hip Replacement & Revision; **Hospital:** Buffalo General Hosp; **Address:** Bufffalo Genl Hosp, Dept Orthopaedic Surgery, 100 High St, B276, Buffalo, NY 14203; **Phone:** 716-859-1256; **Board Cert:** Orthopaedic Surgery 1993; **Med School:** Duke Univ 1971; **Resid:** Surgery, Johns Hopkins Hosp 1973; **Fellow:** Orthopaedic Surgery, Johns Hopkins Hosp 1976; **Fac Appt:** Prof OrS, SUNY Buffalo

Lackman, Richard D MD [OrS] - **Spec Exp:** Bone Cancer; Sarcoma; Limb Sparing Surgery; **Hospital:** Hosp Univ Penn - UPHS (page 72), Pennsylvania Hosp (page 72); **Address:** Hosp Univ Penn - Dept Orthopaedic Surg, 3400 Spruce St, 2 Silverstein, Philadelphia, PA 19104; **Phone:** 215-662-3340; **Board Cert:** Orthopaedic Surgery 1985; **Med School:** Univ Pennsylvania 1977; **Resid:** Orthopaedic Surgery, Hosp Univ Penn 1982; **Fellow:** Orthopaedic Oncology, Mayo Clinic 1983; **Fac Appt:** Assoc Prof OrS, Univ Pennsylvania

Lane, Joseph MD [OrS] - **Spec Exp:** Metabolic Bone Disease; Osteoporosis Spinal Fracture; Osteoporosis Spine-Kyphoplasty; Bone Cancer; **Hospital:** Hosp For Special Surgery (page 60), NY-Presby Hosp/Weill Cornell (page 66); **Address:** Hosp for Special Surgery, 535 E 70th St, New York, NY 10021; **Phone:** 212-606-1172; **Board Cert:** Orthopaedic Surgery 1998; **Med School:** Harvard Med Sch 1965; **Resid:** Surgery, Hosp Univ Penn 1967; Orthopaedic Surgery, Hosp Univ Penn 1973; **Fac Appt:** Prof OrS, Cornell Univ-Weill Med Coll

Lauerman, William MD [OrS] - **Spec Exp:** Spinal Deformity-Pediatric & Adult; Spinal Surgery; Pain-Back; Scoliosis; **Hospital:** Georgetown Univ Hosp; **Address:** 3800 Reservoir Rd NW, Spine Surgery Clinic-1 Gorman, Washington, DC 20007; **Phone:** 202-444-8766 x2; **Board Cert:** Orthopaedic Surgery 2001; **Med School:** Georgetown Univ 1982; **Resid:** Orthopaedic Surgery, Georgetown Univ Med Ctr 1987; **Fellow:** Orthopaedic Surgery, Univ Minn-Twin Cities Scoliosis Ctr 1988; **Fac Appt:** Prof OrS, Georgetown Univ

Lehman, Wallace B MD [OrS] - **Spec Exp:** Clubfoot/Foot Deformities in Children; Hip Disorders-Pediatric; Limb Deformities; Blount's Disease; **Hospital:** Hosp For Joint Diseases (page 68), NYU Med Ctr (page 67); **Address:** NYU Hosp Joint Diseases, Dept Ped Orth Surg, 301 E 17th St, Ste 413, New York, NY 10003-3804; **Phone:** 212-598-6403; **Board Cert:** Orthopaedic Surgery 1966; **Med School:** SUNY Hlth Sci Ctr 1958; **Resid:** Orthopaedic Surgery, Hosp Joint Diseases 1963; **Fac Appt:** Prof OrS, NYU Sch Med

Malawer, Martin M MD [OrS] - **Spec Exp:** Bone Tumors; Limb Sparing Surgery; Pediatric Orthopaedic Surgery; Sarcoma; **Hospital:** Washington Hosp Ctr, G Washington Univ Hosp; **Address:** Washington Cancer Institute, 110 Irving St NW, Ste C2173, Washington, DC 20010; **Phone:** 202-877-3970; **Board Cert:** Orthopaedic Surgery 1993; **Med School:** NYU Sch Med 1969; **Resid:** Surgery, Bronx Muni Hosp 1972; Orthopaedic Surgery, Bellevue Hosp Ctr 1975; **Fellow:** Orthopaedic Oncology, Shands Hosp-Univ Florida 1978; **Fac Appt:** Prof OrS, Geo Wash Univ

McAfee, Paul C MD [OrS] - **Spec Exp:** Spinal Surgery; Scoliosis; **Hospital:** St Joseph Med Ctr; **Address:** Scoliosis & Spine Ctr, 7505 Osler Drive, Ste 104, Towson, MD 21204; **Phone:** 410-337-8888; **Board Cert:** Orthopaedic Surgery 1997; **Med School:** SUNY Upstate Med Univ 1979; **Resid:** Orthopaedic Surgery, SUNY Upstate Med Ctr 1984; **Fellow:** Spinal Surgery, Case West Res Univ Hosps 1986; **Fac Appt:** Assoc Prof OrS, Johns Hopkins Univ

McCann, Peter D MD [OrS] - **Spec Exp:** Shoulder Surgery; Elbow Surgery; **Hospital:** Beth Israel Med Ctr - Petrie Division; **Address:** 10 Union Square E, Ste 3M, New York, NY 10003; **Phone:** 212-844-6735; **Board Cert:** Orthopaedic Surgery 1999; **Med School:** Columbia P&S 1980; **Resid:** Surgery, St Vincent's Hosp 1982; Orthopaedic Surgery, Columbia-Presby Med Ctr 1985; **Fellow:** Shoulder Surgery, Columbia-Presby Med Ctr 1986; **Fac Appt:** Assoc Prof OrS, Albert Einstein Coll Med

McFarland, Edward G MD [OrS] - **Spec Exp:** Sports Medicine; **Hospital:** Johns Hopkins Hosp - Baltimore (page 61); **Address:** 10753 Falls Rd, Ste 215, Lutherville, MD 21093; **Phone:** 410-583-2850; **Board Cert:** Orthopaedic Surgery 2001; **Med School:** Univ Louisville Sch Med 1982; **Resid:** Orthopaedic Surgery, Mayo Clinic 1987; **Fellow:** Sports Medicine, Kerlan-Jobe Orthopaedic Group 1989; **Fac Appt:** Assoc Prof OrS, Johns Hopkins Univ

Myerson, Mark MD [OrS] - **Spec Exp:** Foot & Ankle Surgery; **Hospital:** Mercy Medical Center Inc; **Address:** 301 St Paul Pl, Baltimore, MD 21202; **Phone:** 410-659-2800; **Board Cert:** Orthopaedic Surgery 1999; **Med School:** South Africa 1979; **Resid:** Surgery, Sinai Hospital 1981; Orthopaedic Surgery, Johns Hopkins Hosp/Univ MD Hosp 1985; **Fellow:** Foot/Ankle Surgery, Hospital Joint Disease

Neuwirth, Michael MD [OrS] - **Spec Exp:** Scoliosis; Spinal Surgery; **Hospital:** Beth Israel Med Ctr - Petrie Division, Palisades Med Ctr; **Address:** Beth Israel Med Ctr - Spine Institute, 10 Union Square E, Ste 5P, New York, NY 10003-3314; **Phone:** 212-844-8692; **Board Cert:** Orthopaedic Surgery 1980; **Med School:** SUNY Hlth Sci Ctr 1974; **Resid:** Orthopaedic Surgery, Hosp for Joint Diseases 1978; **Fellow:** Spinal Surgery, Rush-Presbyterian Med Ctr 1979; **Fac Appt:** Assoc Clin Prof OrS, NYU Sch Med

Orthopaedic Surgery

Nicholas, Stephen J MD [OrS] - **Spec Exp:** Sports Medicine; Shoulder & Knee Surgery; Arthroscopic Surgery; **Hospital:** Lenox Hill Hosp (page 62); **Address:** 130 E 77th St, New York, NY 10021-1803; **Phone:** 212-737-3301; **Board Cert:** Orthopaedic Surgery 2005; **Med School:** NY Med Coll 1986; **Resid:** Orthopaedic Surgery, Hosp for Special Surgery 1991; **Fellow:** Sports Medicine, Lenox Hill Hosp 1992

O'Keefe, Regis J MD/PhD [OrS] - **Spec Exp:** Bone & Soft Tissue Tumors; Reconstructive Surgery; **Hospital:** Univ of Rochester Strong Meml Hosp, Highland Hosp - Rochester; **Address:** Univ Rochester, Dept Orthopaedic Surgery, 601 Elmwood Ave, Box 665, Rochester, NY 14642; **Phone:** 585-275-3100; **Board Cert:** Orthopaedic Surgery 1996; **Med School:** Harvard Med Sch 1985; **Resid:** Surgery, New Eng Deaconess Hosp/Harvard 1986; Orthopaedic Surgery, Univ Rochester 1992; **Fellow:** Orthopaedic Oncology, Mass Genl Hosp 1993; **Fac Appt:** Prof S, Univ Rochester

O'Leary, Patrick MD [OrS] - **Spec Exp:** Spinal Surgery; **Hospital:** Hosp For Special Surgery (page 60); **Address:** 1015 Madison Ave Fl 4, New York, NY 10021; **Phone:** 212-249-8100; **Board Cert:** Orthopaedic Surgery 1983; **Med School:** Ireland 1968; **Resid:** Surgery, Roosevelt Hosp. 1972; Orthopaedic Surgery, Hosp Spec Surg-Cornell 1975; **Fellow:** Spinal Surgery, Univ Toronto Genl Ortho Hosp 1976; **Fac Appt:** Assoc Clin Prof OrS, Cornell Univ-Weill Med Coll

Paley, Dror MD [OrS] - **Spec Exp:** Limb Lengthening (Ilizarov Procedure); Limb Deformities; Pediatric Orthopaedic Surgery; **Hospital:** Sinai Hosp - Baltimore, Univ of MD Med Sys; **Address:** Rubin Institute for Advanced Ortho, 2401 W Belvedere Ave, Baltimore, MD 21215; **Phone:** 410-601-4200; **Board Cert:** Orthopaedic Surgery 2000; **Med School:** Univ Toronto 1979; **Resid:** Orthopaedic Surgery, Univ Toronto Hosp 1985; **Fellow:** Hand Surgery, SunnyBrook Hosp 1986; Pediatric Orthopaedic Surgery, Hosp for Sick Children 1987; **Fac Appt:** Assoc Prof S, Univ MD Sch Med

Palmer, Andrew MD [OrS] - **Spec Exp:** Hand Surgery; **Hospital:** Univ. Hosp.- SUNY Upstate, Crouse Hosp; **Address:** 550 Harrison St, Ste 128, Syracuse, NY 13202-3096; **Phone:** 315-464-8624; **Board Cert:** Orthopaedic Surgery 1978; **Med School:** SUNY Upstate Med Univ 1972; **Resid:** Orthopaedic Surgery, Univ Mich Med Ctr 1976; **Fellow:** Hand Surgery, Mayo Clinic 1977; **Fac Appt:** Prof OrS, SUNY Upstate Med Univ

Pellicci, Paul MD [OrS] - **Spec Exp:** Hip Replacement-Young Adults; Hip Resurfacing; Knee Replacement; **Hospital:** Hosp For Special Surgery (page 60), NY-Presby Hosp/Weill Cornell (page 66); **Address:** 535 E 70th St, New York, NY 10021-4872; **Phone:** 212-606-1010; **Board Cert:** Orthopaedic Surgery 1982; **Med School:** Cornell Univ-Weill Med Coll 1975; **Resid:** Surgery, New York Hosp 1976; Orthopaedic Surgery, Hosp for Special Surgery 1980; **Fellow:** Joint Replacement Surgery, Brigham & Womens Hosp 1981; **Fac Appt:** Prof OrS, Cornell Univ-Weill Med Coll

Ramsey, Matthew L MD [OrS] - **Spec Exp:** Shoulder Surgery; Elbow Surgery; Sports Medicine; **Hospital:** Penn Presby Med Ctr - UPHS (page 72), Hosp Univ Penn - UPHS (page 72); **Address:** Penn Presby Med Ctr, Dept Ortho Surg, 51 N 39th St, 1 Cupp Bldg Fl 1, Philadelphia, PA 19104; **Phone:** 215-662-3340; **Board Cert:** Orthopaedic Surgery 1998; **Med School:** SUNY Hlth Sci Ctr 1990; **Resid:** Orthopaedic Surgery, Thomas Jefferson Univ Hosp 1996; **Fellow:** Shoulder Surgery, Hosp Univ Penn 1996; **Fac Appt:** Assoc Prof OrS, Univ Pennsylvania

Ranawat, Chitranjan MD [OrS] - **Spec Exp:** Hip Replacement; Knee Replacement; **Hospital:** Lenox Hill Hosp (page 62), Hosp For Special Surgery (page 60); **Address:** 130 E 77th St, FL 11, New York, NY 10021-1851; **Phone:** 212-434-4700; **Board Cert:** Orthopaedic Surgery 1969; **Med School:** India 1958; **Resid:** Surgery, MY Hosp 1963; Orthopaedic Surgery, Albany Med Ctr 1965; **Fellow:** Orthopaedic Surgery, Hosp Special Surg 1969; **Fac Appt:** Prof OrS, Cornell Univ-Weill Med Coll

Rechtine, Glenn MD [OrS] - **Spec Exp:** Spinal Surgery; **Hospital:** Univ of Rochester Strong Meml Hosp; **Address:** Strong Meml Hosp, Dept Orthopaedics, 601 Elmwood Ave, Box 665, Rochester, NY 14618; **Phone:** 585-275-2225; **Board Cert:** Orthopaedic Surgery 1982; **Med School:** Univ S Fla Coll Med 1975; **Resid:** Orthopaedic Surgery, Naval Regional Med Ctr 1980; **Fellow:** Spinal Surgery, Case West Res Univ 1981; **Fac Appt:** Prof OrS, Univ Rochester

Rokito, Andrew MD [OrS] - **Spec Exp:** Shoulder & Elbow Surgery; Knee Surgery; Arthroscopic Surgery; Sports Medicine; **Hospital:** Hosp For Joint Diseases (page 68), NYU Med Ctr (page 67); **Address:** 301 E 17th St, Ste 1402, New York, NY 10003; **Phone:** 212-598-6008; **Board Cert:** Orthopaedic Surgery 2005; **Med School:** Boston Univ 1988; **Resid:** Orthopaedic Surgery, Hosp Joint Diseases 1993; **Fellow:** Sports Medicine, Kerlan-Jobe Ortho Clin 1994; **Fac Appt:** Asst Prof OrS, NYU Sch Med

Rosier, Randy MD/PhD [OrS] - **Spec Exp:** Bone Disorders-Metabolic; **Hospital:** Univ of Rochester Strong Meml Hosp; **Address:** Univ Rochester, Dept Orthopaedic Surgery, 601 Elmwood Ave, Box 665, Rochester, NY 14642; **Phone:** 585-275-3100; **Board Cert:** Orthopaedic Surgery 1998; **Med School:** Univ Rochester 1978; **Resid:** Orthopaedic Surgery, Univ Iowa Hosp 1984; **Fellow:** Univ Iowa Hosp 1983; **Fac Appt:** Prof OrS, Univ Rochester

Rothman, Richard MD [OrS] - **Spec Exp:** Hip Replacement; Knee Replacement; **Hospital:** Thomas Jefferson Univ Hosp; **Address:** Rothman Institute, 925 Chestnut St Fl 5, Philadelphia, PA 19107; **Phone:** 267-339-3500; **Board Cert:** Orthopaedic Surgery 1970; **Med School:** Univ Pennsylvania 1962; **Resid:** Orthopaedic Surgery, Jefferson Hosp 1968; **Fac Appt:** Prof OrS, Jefferson Med Coll

Roye, David MD [OrS] - **Spec Exp:** Pediatric Orthopaedic Surgery; Scoliosis; Hip Disorders-Pediatric; **Hospital:** NY-Presby Hosp/Columbia (page 66), Greenwich Hosp; **Address:** Morgan Stanley Chlds Hosp NewYork-Presby, 3959 Broadway, 8 North, New York, NY 10032-1559; **Phone:** 212-305-5475; **Board Cert:** Orthopaedic Surgery 1981; **Med School:** Columbia P&S 1975; **Resid:** Orthopaedic Surgery, Columbia-Presby Med Ctr 1979; **Fellow:** Orthopaedic Surgery, Hosp for Sick Chldn 1980; **Fac Appt:** Prof OrS, Columbia P&S

Rozbruch, S Robert MD [OrS] - **Spec Exp:** Limb Lengthening; Limb Deformities; Bone Disorders; Fractures-Complex; **Hospital:** Hosp For Special Surgery (page 60), NY-Presby Hosp/Weill Cornell (page 66); **Address:** 535 E 70th St, New York, NY 10021; **Phone:** 212-606-1415; **Board Cert:** Orthopaedic Surgery 1998; **Med School:** Cornell Univ-Weill Med Coll 1990; **Resid:** Orthopaedic Surgery, Hosp Special Surgery 1995; **Fellow:** Trauma, Univ Bern Hosp 1997; Limb Lengthening, Intl Ctr Limb Length/Univ MD 1999; **Fac Appt:** Asst Prof OrS, Cornell Univ-Weill Med Coll

Salvati, Eduardo A MD [OrS] - **Spec Exp:** Hip Surgery; Hip & Knee Replacement; **Hospital:** Hosp For Special Surgery (page 60); **Address:** Hosp for Spec Surg, 535 E 70th Street, New York, NY 10021; **Phone:** 212-606-1472; **Board Cert:** Orthopaedic Surgery 1972; **Med School:** Argentina 1963; **Resid:** Orthopaedic Surgery, Univ Florence Ortho Clinic 1965; Orthopaedic Surgery, Hosp Buenos Aires 1969; **Fellow:** Hip Surgery, Hosp For Spec Surg 1972; **Fac Appt:** Clin Prof OrS, Cornell Univ-Weill Med Coll

Orthopaedic Surgery

Sandhu, Harvinder S MD [OrS] - Spec Exp: Minimally Invasive Surgery; Spinal Disc Replacement; Spinal Surgery; **Hospital:** Hosp For Special Surgery (page 60), NY-Presby Hosp/Weill Cornell (page 66); **Address:** 535 E 70th St, New York, NY 10021; **Phone:** 212-606-1798; **Board Cert:** Orthopaedic Surgery 2007; **Med School:** Northwestern Univ 1987; **Resid:** Orthopaedic Surgery, Univ Hosp-SUNY Hlth Sci Ctr 1992; **Fellow:** Spinal Surgery, UCLA Med Ctr 1993; **Fac Appt:** Assoc Prof OrS, Cornell Univ-Weill Med Coll

Scott, W Norman MD [OrS] - Spec Exp: Knee Injuries; Knee Replacement; Sports Medicine; **Hospital:** Lenox Hill Hosp (page 62), Franklin Hosp Med Ctr; **Address:** 210 E 64th St, New York, NY 10021-7471; **Phone:** 212-434-4301; **Board Cert:** Orthopaedic Surgery 1978; **Med School:** Cornell Univ-Weill Med Coll 1972; **Resid:** Surgery, St Luke's-Roosevelt Hosp Ctr 1974; Orthopaedic Surgery, Hosp Special Surg 1977; **Fac Appt:** Clin Prof OrS, Cornell Univ-Weill Med Coll

Sculco, Thomas P MD [OrS] - Spec Exp: Hip Replacement; Knee Replacement; Minimally Invasive Surgery; Joint Replacement; **Hospital:** Hosp For Special Surgery (page 60); **Address:** 535 E 70th St, Ste 238, New York, NY 10021-4872; **Phone:** 212-606-1475; **Board Cert:** Orthopaedic Surgery 1976; **Med School:** Columbia P&S 1969; **Resid:** Surgery, Roosevelt Hosp 1971; Orthopaedic Surgery, Hosp For Special Surgery 1974; **Fellow:** Orthopaedic Surgery, The London Hosp 1975

Sherman, Orrin MD [OrS] - Spec Exp: Knee Injuries/ACL; Shoulder Surgery; Sports Medicine; Arthroscopic Surgery; **Hospital:** NYU Med Ctr (page 67), Hosp For Joint Diseases (page 68); **Address:** 530 1st Ave, Ste 8U, New York, NY 10016-6402; **Phone:** 212-263-8961; **Board Cert:** Orthopaedic Surgery 1997; **Med School:** Geo Wash Univ 1978; **Resid:** Orthopaedic Surgery, NYU Med Ctr 1983; **Fellow:** Sports Medicine, So Cal Orthopedic Inst 1984; **Fac Appt:** Assoc Prof OrS, NYU Sch Med

Spivak, Jeffrey M MD [OrS] - Spec Exp: Spinal Surgery; Scoliosis; Sports Medicine Back Injuries; **Hospital:** Hosp For Joint Diseases (page 68), NYU Med Ctr (page 67); **Address:** Hospital for Joint Diseases, Spine Ctr, 301 E 17th St, Ste 400, New York, NY 10003-3804; **Phone:** 212-598-6696; **Board Cert:** Orthopaedic Surgery 2006; **Med School:** Cornell Univ-Weill Med Coll 1986; **Resid:** Orthopaedic Surgery, Hosp for Joint Diseases 1992; **Fellow:** Spinal Surgery, Thomas Jefferson Univ Hosp 1993; **Fac Appt:** Asst Prof OrS, NYU Sch Med

Sponseller, Paul D MD [OrS] - Spec Exp: Cerebral Palsy; Scoliosis; Pediatric Orthopaedic Surgery; **Hospital:** Johns Hopkins Hosp - Baltimore (page 61); **Address:** 601 N Caroline St, Ste 5212, Baltimore, MD 21287-0882; **Phone:** 410-955-3136; **Board Cert:** Orthopaedic Surgery 2000; **Med School:** Univ Mich Med Sch 1980; **Resid:** Orthopaedic Surgery, Univ Wisc Hosp 1985; **Fellow:** Pediatric Orthopaedic Surgery, Chldns Hosp-Harvard 1986; **Fac Appt:** Prof OrS, Johns Hopkins Univ

Strongwater, Allan MD [OrS] - Spec Exp: Pediatric Orthopaedic Surgery; Cerebral Palsy; Deformity Reconstruction; **Hospital:** Hosp For Joint Diseases (page 68), NYU Med Ctr (page 67); **Address:** 301 E 17th St, New York, NY 10003; **Phone:** 212-598-6190; **Board Cert:** Orthopaedic Surgery 1997; **Med School:** Rush Med Coll 1978; **Resid:** Orthopaedic Surgery, Yale-New Haven Hosp 1983; Pediatric Orthopaedic Surgery, Hosp Joint Diseases 1984; **Fac Appt:** Clin Prof OrS, NYU Sch Med

Stuchin, Steven MD [OrS] - **Spec Exp:** Hand Surgery; Arthritis; Hip & Knee Replacement; **Hospital:** Hosp For Joint Diseases (page 68), Lenox Hill Hosp (page 62); **Address:** 301 E 17th St, Ste 1402, New York, NY 10003-3804; **Phone:** 212-598-6708; **Board Cert:** Orthopaedic Surgery 1984; **Med School:** Columbia P&S 1976; **Resid:** Surgery, Roosevelt Hosp 1978; Orthopaedic Surgery, Hosp For Special Surg 1981; **Fellow:** Hand Surgery, Thomas Jefferson Univ Hosp 1982; **Fac Appt:** Assoc Prof OrS, NYU Sch Med

Tischler, Henry MD [OrS] - **Spec Exp:** Hip Replacement & Revision; Knee Replacement & Revision; Hip Reconstruction; **Hospital:** New York Methodist Hosp, St Vincent Cath Med Ctrs - Manhattan; **Address:** Brooklyn Spine & Arthritis Ctr, 263 7th Ave, Ste 2B, Brooklyn, NY 11215; **Phone:** 718-246-8700; **Board Cert:** Orthopaedic Surgery 2006; **Med School:** SUNY Downstate 1985; **Resid:** Orthopaedic Surgery, SUNY Downstate Med Ctr 1990; **Fellow:** Orthopaedic Surgery, Tampa Gen Hosp/Fla Osteo Inst 1991; **Fac Appt:** Asst Prof OrS, SUNY Hlth Sci Ctr

Vaccaro, Alexander R MD [OrS] - **Spec Exp:** Spinal Surgery; spinal trauma; Spinal Cord Injury; **Hospital:** Thomas Jefferson Univ Hosp; **Address:** Rothman Institute, 925 Chestnut St Fl 5, Philadelphia, PA 19107; **Phone:** 267-339-3500; **Board Cert:** Orthopaedic Surgery 2006; **Med School:** Georgetown Univ 1989; **Resid:** Orthopaedic Surgery, Thos Jefferson Univ Hosp 1994; **Fellow:** Spinal Surgery, UCSD Med Ctr 1995; **Fac Appt:** Prof OrS, Thomas Jefferson Univ

Wapner, Keith L MD [OrS] - **Spec Exp:** Foot & Ankle Surgery; Tendon Surgery; Arthritis; **Hospital:** Pennsylvania Hosp (page 72); **Address:** The Farm Journal Bldg Fl 5, 230 W Washington Square, Philadelphia, PA 19106-3500; **Phone:** 215-829-3668; **Board Cert:** Orthopaedic Surgery 1999; **Med School:** Temple Univ 1980; **Resid:** Surgery, Hosp Univ Penn 1981; Orthopaedic Surgery, Hosp Univ Penn 1985; **Fellow:** Joint Reconstruction, Ohio St Univ Med Ctr 1986; Foot/Ankle Surgery, UCSF Med Ctr 1987; **Fac Appt:** Clin Prof OrS, Univ Pennsylvania

Warren, Russell MD [OrS] - **Spec Exp:** Knee Injuries/Ligament Surgery; Shoulder Reconstruction; Shoulder Replacement; Sports Medicine; **Hospital:** Hosp For Special Surgery (page 60), NY-Presby Hosp/Weill Cornell (page 66); **Address:** 535 E 70th St, New York, NY 10021-4892; **Phone:** 212-606-1178; **Board Cert:** Orthopaedic Surgery 1974; **Med School:** SUNY Upstate Med Univ 1966; **Resid:** Surgery, St Lukes Hosp 1968; Orthopaedic Surgery, Hosp For Special Surgery 1973; **Fellow:** Shoulder Surgery, Columbia-Presby Med Ctr 1977; **Fac Appt:** Prof OrS, Cornell Univ-Weill Med Coll

Wickiewicz, Thomas L MD [OrS] - **Spec Exp:** Shoulder Surgery; Sports Medicine; Knee Surgery; **Hospital:** Hosp For Special Surgery (page 60), NY-Presby Hosp/Weill Cornell (page 66); **Address:** 535 E 70th St, New York, NY 10021; **Phone:** 212-606-1450; **Board Cert:** Orthopaedic Surgery 1984; **Med School:** UMDNJ-NJ Med Sch, Newark 1976; **Resid:** Orthopaedic Surgery, Hosp for Special Surg 1981; **Fellow:** Sports Medicine, UCLA Med Ctr 1982; **Fac Appt:** Clin Prof OrS, Cornell Univ-Weill Med Coll

Wiesel, Sam W MD [OrS] - **Spec Exp:** Spinal Surgery; **Hospital:** Georgetown Univ Hosp; **Address:** 3800 Reservoir Rd NW, PHC Bldg Fl Ground, Washington, DC 20007-2113; **Phone:** 202-444-8766 x2; **Board Cert:** Orthopaedic Surgery 1977; **Med School:** Univ Pennsylvania 1971; **Resid:** Orthopaedic Surgery, Hosp Univ Penn 1976; **Fellow:** Orthopaedic Surgery, Hosp Univ Penn 1973; **Fac Appt:** Prof OrS, Georgetown Univ

Orthopaedic Surgery

Williams, Gerald MD [OrS] - **Spec Exp:** Shoulder Arthroscopic Surgery; Shoulder Reconstruction; Shoulder Cartilage Implant; Shoulder Replacement; **Hospital:** Methodist Hosp, Thomas Jefferson Univ Hosp; **Address:** Rothman Institute, 925 Chestnut St, Philadelphia, PA 19107; **Phone:** 267-339-3500; **Board Cert:** Orthopaedic Surgery 2003; **Med School:** Temple Univ 1984; **Resid:** Orthopaedic Surgery, Univ Texas San Antonio Afill Hosp 1989; **Fellow:** Shoulder Surgery, Univ Texas San Antonio 1990; **Fac Appt:** Prof OrS, Thomas Jefferson Univ

Zuckerman, Joseph MD [OrS] - **Spec Exp:** Shoulder Surgery; Hip Replacement; Knee Replacement; Joint Replacement; **Hospital:** Hosp For Joint Diseases (page 68), NYU Med Ctr (page 67); **Address:** Hosp for Joint Diseases, Dept Ortho Surg, 301 E 17th St Fl 14 - Ste 1402, New York, NY 10003; **Phone:** 212-598-6674; **Board Cert:** Orthopaedic Surgery 2004; **Med School:** Med Coll Wisc 1978; **Resid:** Orthopaedic Surgery, Univ WA Med Ctr 1983; **Fellow:** Arthritis Surgery, Brigham & Womans Hosp 1984; Shoulder Surgery, Mayo Clinic 1984; **Fac Appt:** Prof OrS, NYU Sch Med

Southeast

Beaty, James H MD [OrS] - **Spec Exp:** Pediatric Orthopaedic Surgery; Clubfoot; Fractures-Pediatric; **Hospital:** Le Bonheur Chldns Med Ctr, Baptist Memorial Hospital - Memphis; **Address:** Campbell Clinic, 1211 Union Ave, Ste 500, Memphis, TN 38104; **Phone:** 901-759-3125; **Board Cert:** Orthopaedic Surgery 2007; **Med School:** Univ Tenn Coll Med, Memphis 1976; **Resid:** Surgery, Baptist Meml Hosp 1979; Orthopaedic Surgery, Campbell Clin Fdn 1981; **Fellow:** Pediatric Orthopaedic Surgery, Alfred I Dupont Inst 1982; **Fac Appt:** Prof OrS, Univ Tenn Coll Med, Memphis

Boden, Scott D MD [OrS] - **Spec Exp:** Spinal Disorders; Spinal Surgery; Spinal Disc Replacement; Microdiscectomy; **Hospital:** Emory Univ Hosp; **Address:** 59 Executive Park S, Ste 3000, Atlanta, GA 30329; **Phone:** 404-778-7143; **Board Cert:** Orthopaedic Surgery 2005; **Med School:** Univ Pennsylvania 1986; **Resid:** Orthopaedic Surgery, George Washington Univ Hosp 1991; **Fellow:** Spinal Surgery, Case Western Res Univ Hosp 1992; **Fac Appt:** Prof OrS, Emory Univ

Cuckler, John MD [OrS] - **Spec Exp:** Hip Replacement; Knee Replacement; **Hospital:** Univ of Ala Hosp at Birmingham; **Address:** UAB Div Orthopedics, FOT 930, 510 20th St S, Birmingham, AL 35294; **Phone:** 205-975-2663; **Board Cert:** Orthopaedic Surgery 1999; **Med School:** NYU Sch Med 1975; **Resid:** Orthopaedic Surgery, Hosp Univ Penn 1980; **Fac Appt:** Prof OrS, Univ Ala

Curl, Walton W MD [OrS] - **Spec Exp:** Sports Medicine; **Hospital:** Wake Forest Univ Baptist Med Ctr (page 73); **Address:** Wake Forest Med Ctr, Comp Rehab, 131 Miller St, Winston-Salem, NC 27103; **Phone:** 336-716-8091; **Board Cert:** Orthopaedic Surgery 1980; **Med School:** Duke Univ 1974; **Resid:** Orthopaedic Surgery, Letterman Army Med Ctr 1978; **Fellow:** Sports Medicine, Keller Army Hosp 1979; **Fac Appt:** Prof OrS, Wake Forest Univ

Eismont, Frank MD [OrS] - **Spec Exp:** Spinal Surgery; **Hospital:** Jackson Meml Hosp; **Address:** Univ Miami Sch Med, Dept Orth Surg, PO Box 016960, D-27, Miami, FL 33101; **Phone:** 305-243-3000; **Board Cert:** Orthopaedic Surgery 1994; **Med School:** Univ Rochester 1973; **Resid:** Orthopaedic Surgery, Case Western Res Univ Hosp 1978; **Fellow:** Spinal Surgery, Case Western Res Univ Hosp 1979; Spinal Surgery, PA Hosp 1980; **Fac Appt:** Prof OrS, Univ Miami Sch Med

Garrett, William MD [OrS] - **Spec Exp:** Sports Medicine; Shoulder & Knee Surgery; Shoulder & Knee Reconstruction; **Hospital:** Duke Univ Med Ctr; **Address:** Duke Univ Med Ctr, Box 3338, Durham, NC 27710; **Phone:** 919-684-5678; **Board Cert:** Orthopaedic Surgery 1985; **Med School:** Duke Univ 1976; **Resid:** Orthopaedic Surgery, Duke Univ Med Ctr 1982; **Fac Appt:** Prof OrS, Duke Univ

Goldner, Richard MD [OrS] - **Spec Exp:** Upper Extremity Surgery; Hand Surgery; **Hospital:** Duke Univ Med Ctr; **Address:** DUMC, Box 2093, Durham, NC 27710; **Phone:** 919-613-7797; **Board Cert:** Orthopaedic Surgery 1982; Hand Surgery 2000; **Med School:** Duke Univ 1974; **Resid:** Orthopaedic Surgery, Univ Virginia 1980; Surgery, Duke Univ Med Ctr 1976; **Fellow:** Hand Surgery, Duke Univ Med Ctr 1981; **Fac Appt:** Assoc Prof OrS, Duke Univ

Johnson, Darren L MD [OrS] - **Spec Exp:** Knee Injuries; Sports Medicine; **Hospital:** Univ of Kentucky Chandler Hosp; **Address:** Univ Kentucky, Dept Orthopaedic Surgery, 740 S Limestone, Ste K-401, Lexington, KY 40536-0284; **Phone:** 859-257-4969; **Board Cert:** Orthopaedic Surgery 2006; **Med School:** UCLA 1987; **Resid:** Orthopaedic Surgery, LAC-USC Med Ctr 1992; **Fellow:** Sports Medicine, Univ Pittsburgh 1993; **Fac Appt:** Assoc Prof OrS, Univ KY Coll Med

Karas, Spero G MD [OrS] - **Spec Exp:** Sports Medicine; Shoulder Reconstruction; Elbow Reconstruction; Knee Reconstruction; **Hospital:** Emory Univ Hosp; **Address:** Emory Healthcare Sports Medicine, 59 Executive Park Drive S, Ste 1000, Atlanta, GA 30329; **Phone:** 404-778-3350; **Board Cert:** Orthopaedic Surgery 2002; **Med School:** Indiana Univ 1993; **Resid:** Orthopaedic Surgery, Duke Univ Med Ctr 1999; **Fellow:** Orthopaedic Surgery, Steadman Hawkins Clinic 2000; **Fac Appt:** Assoc Prof OrS, Emory Univ

Kneisl, Jeffrey S MD [OrS] - **Spec Exp:** Bone Cancer; Musculoskeletal Tumors; **Hospital:** Carolinas Med Ctr; **Address:** Carolinas Med Ctr, 1001 Blythe Blvd, Ste 602, Charlotte, NC 28203; **Phone:** 704-355-5982; **Board Cert:** Orthopaedic Surgery 2000; **Med School:** Northwestern Univ 1980; **Resid:** Orthopaedic Surgery, Northwestern Univ 1987; **Fellow:** Orthopaedic Oncology, Univ Chicago 1990

Laurencin, Cato T MD/PhD [OrS] - **Spec Exp:** Shoulder & Knee Surgery; Sports Medicine; **Hospital:** Univ Virginia Med Ctr; **Address:** University Virginia Medical Ctr, PO Box 800159, Charlottesville, VA 22908; **Phone:** 434-243-0250; **Board Cert:** Orthopaedic Surgery 2004; **Med School:** Harvard Med Sch 1987; **Resid:** Orthopaedic Surgery, Harvard Combined Program 1993; **Fellow:** Sports Medicine & Shoulder Surgery, New York Hosp-Cornell Med Ctr 1994; **Fac Appt:** Clin Prof OrS, Univ VA Sch Med

Nunley, James MD [OrS] - **Spec Exp:** Arthritis; Ankle Replacement & Revision; Foot & Ankle Surgery; Hand & Wrist Surgery; **Hospital:** Duke Univ Med Ctr; **Address:** Duke Univ Med Ctr, Box 2093, Durham, NC 27710-0001; **Phone:** 919-613-7797; **Board Cert:** Orthopaedic Surgery 1981; **Med School:** Tulane Univ 1973; **Resid:** Orthopaedic Surgery, Duke Univ Med Ctr 1979; **Fellow:** Hand Surgery, Duke Univ Med Ctr 1980; **Fac Appt:** Prof OrS, Duke Univ

Pettrone, Frank A MD [OrS] - **Spec Exp:** Sports Medicine; Shoulder & Knee Surgery; **Hospital:** Virginia Hosp Ctr - Arlington; **Address:** 1635 N George Mason Drive, Ste 310, Arlington, VA 22205-3616; **Phone:** 703-525-6100; **Board Cert:** Orthopaedic Surgery 1975; **Med School:** Georgetown Univ 1969; **Resid:** Orthopaedic Surgery, Georgetown Hosp 1974; **Fac Appt:** Clin Prof OrS, Georgetown Univ

Orthopaedic Surgery

Poehling, Gary G MD [OrS] - **Spec Exp:** Hand Surgery; Arthroscopic Surgery; Sports Medicine; **Hospital:** Wake Forest Univ Baptist Med Ctr (page 73); **Address:** 131 Miller St, Winston Salem, NC 27103; **Phone:** 336-716-8091; **Board Cert:** Orthopaedic Surgery 1977; **Med School:** Marquette Sch Med 1968; **Resid:** Surgery, Duke Univ Med Ctr 1970; Orthopaedic Surgery, Duke Univ Med Ctr 1976; **Fac Appt:** Prof OrS, Wake Forest Univ

Richardson, William J MD [OrS] - **Spec Exp:** Spinal Surgery; Spinal Deformity & Trauma; Spinal Disc Replacement; **Hospital:** Duke Univ Med Ctr; **Address:** DUMC, Box 2093, Durham, NC 27710; **Phone:** 919-613-7797; **Board Cert:** Orthopaedic Surgery 2000; **Med School:** Eastern VA Med Sch 1979; **Resid:** Orthopaedic Surgery, Duke Univ Med Ctr 1986; **Fellow:** Spinal Surgery, Totonto General Hosp 1987

Scarborough, Mark MD [OrS] - **Spec Exp:** Bone Tumors; Sarcoma; **Hospital:** Shands Hlthcre at Univ of FL; **Address:** Shands Healthcare Univ FL, 3450 Hull Rd, Gainesville, FL 32611; **Phone:** 352-273-7000; **Board Cert:** Orthopaedic Surgery 2003; **Med School:** Univ Fla Coll Med 1985; **Resid:** Orthopaedic Surgery, Univ Texas Med Ctr 1990; **Fellow:** Orthopaedic Surgery, Mass Genl Hosp 1991; **Fac Appt:** Prof OrS, Univ Fla Coll Med

Schwartz, Herbert S MD [OrS] - **Spec Exp:** Bone Tumors-Metastatic; Bone Tumors; Pelvic Surgery-Complex; **Hospital:** Vanderbilt Univ Med Ctr, Baptist Hosp - Nashville; **Address:** Vanderbilt Med Ctr Ortho Institute, South Tower, rm 4200, Medical Ctr East, Nashville, TN 37232-8774; **Phone:** 615-343-8612; **Board Cert:** Orthopaedic Surgery 1992; **Med School:** Univ Chicago-Pritzker Sch Med 1981; **Resid:** Orthopaedic Surgery, Univ Chicago Hosps 1986; **Fellow:** Orthopaedic Oncology, Mayo Clinic 1987; **Fac Appt:** Prof OrS, Vanderbilt Univ

Scully, Sean P MD [OrS] - **Spec Exp:** Bone Cancer; Sarcoma; Musculoskeletal Tumors; Knee Replacement & Revision; **Hospital:** Cedars Med Ctr - Miami; **Address:** Cedars Medical Ctr, East Bldg, 1400 NW 12th Ave Fl 4, Miami, FL 33136; **Phone:** 305-325-4683; **Board Cert:** Orthopaedic Surgery 1995; **Med School:** Univ Rochester 1980; **Resid:** Orthopaedic Surgery, Duke Univ Med Ctr 1985; **Fellow:** Orthopaedic Oncology, Mass General Hosp 1987; Research, Natl Inst Health 1988; **Fac Appt:** Prof OrS, Univ Miami Sch Med

Spengler, Dan M MD [OrS] - **Spec Exp:** Spinal Surgery; **Hospital:** Vanderbilt Univ Med Ctr, Saint Thomas Hosp - Nashville; **Address:** Vanderbilt Univ-Med Ctr North, 1161 21st Ave S, rm D4221, Nashville, TN 37232-2550; **Phone:** 615-343-6364; **Board Cert:** Orthopaedic Surgery 1988; **Med School:** Univ Mich Med Sch 1966; **Resid:** Orthopaedic Surgery, Univ Mich Med Ctr 1973; **Fellow:** Orthopaedic Surgery, Case West Res Hosps 1974; **Fac Appt:** Prof OrS, Vanderbilt Univ

Spindler, Kurt P MD [OrS] - **Spec Exp:** Sports Medicine; Arthroscopic Surgery; **Hospital:** Vanderbilt Univ Med Ctr; **Address:** Vanderbilt Orthopaedic Inst, Medical Center E, S Tower, Ste 4200, Nashville, TN 37232-8774; **Phone:** 615-322-7878; **Board Cert:** Orthopaedic Surgery 2004; **Med School:** Univ Pennsylvania 1985; **Resid:** Orthopaedic Surgery, Hosp Univ Penn 1990; **Fellow:** Sports Medicine, Cleveland Clinic Fdn 1991; **Fac Appt:** Prof OrS, Vanderbilt Univ

Taft, Timothy MD [OrS] - **Spec Exp:** Sports Medicine; Knee Injuries/ACL; Shoulder Surgery; **Hospital:** Univ NC Hosps; **Address:** UNC Orthopaedics, CB # 7055, Chapel Hill, NC 27599-7055; **Phone:** 919-962-6637; **Board Cert:** Orthopaedic Surgery 1976; **Med School:** Univ MO-Columbia Sch Med 1969; **Resid:** Orthopaedic Surgery, UNC Hosps 1974; Orthopaedic Surgery, N Carolina Ortho Hosp 1972; **Fac Appt:** Prof OrS, Univ NC Sch Med

Uribe, John MD [OrS] - **Spec Exp:** Shoulder & Elbow Surgery; Arthroscopic Surgery; Sports Medicine; **Hospital:** Doctors' Hosp, Jackson Meml Hosp; **Address:** 1150 Campo Sano Ave, Ste 200, Coral Gables, FL 33146-6960; **Phone:** 305-669-3320; **Board Cert:** Orthopaedic Surgery 1982; **Med School:** Univ NC Sch Med 1976; **Resid:** Orthopaedic Surgery, Jackson Memorial Hosp 1981; **Fellow:** Sports Medicine, Hughston Sports Med Hosp 1985; **Fac Appt:** Assoc Prof OrS, Univ Miami Sch Med

Ward, William G MD [OrS] - **Spec Exp:** Bone Tumors; Soft Tissue Tumors; Reconstructive Surgery; **Hospital:** Wake Forest Univ Baptist Med Ctr (page 73), Forsyth Med Ctr; **Address:** Wake Forest Med Ctr, Comprehensive Rehab, 131 Miller St, Winston Salem, NC 77103; **Phone:** 336-716-8200; **Board Cert:** Orthopaedic Surgery 2004; **Med School:** Duke Univ 1975; **Resid:** Surgery, Duke Univ Med Ctr 1985; Orthopaedic Surgery, Duke Univ Med Ctr 1989; **Fellow:** Sports Medicine, Cleveland Clinic 1990; Orthopaedic Oncology, UCLA Med Ctr 1991; **Fac Appt:** Prof OrS, Wake Forest Univ

Webb, Lawrence MD [OrS] - **Spec Exp:** Trauma; Pelvic & Acetabular Fractures; Fractures-Complex & Non Union; **Hospital:** Wake Forest Univ Baptist Med Ctr (page 73); **Address:** Wake Forest Med Ctr, Medical Center Blvd, Winston Salem, NC 27157-1070; **Phone:** 336-716-3606; **Board Cert:** Orthopaedic Surgery 2005; **Med School:** Temple Univ 1978; **Resid:** Orthopaedic Surgery, Bowman Gray Affil Hosp 1983; **Fellow:** Trauma, Harborview Med Ctr 1984; **Fac Appt:** Prof OrS, Wake Forest Univ

Weiner, Richard L MD [OrS] - **Spec Exp:** Knee Surgery; Shoulder Surgery; Hip Surgery; **Hospital:** St Mary's Med Ctr - W Palm Bch, Palm Beach Gardens Med Ctr; **Address:** 733 US Highway 1, North Palm Beach, FL 33408-4508; **Phone:** 561-840-1090; **Board Cert:** Orthopaedic Surgery 2004; **Med School:** Univ Pennsylvania 1986; **Resid:** Orthopaedic Surgery, UMDNJ-Univ Hosp 1991

Midwest

Bach Jr, Bernard R MD [OrS] - **Spec Exp:** Sports Medicine; Knee Surgery; Knee Injuries/ACL; **Hospital:** Rush Univ Med Ctr; **Address:** 1725 W Harrison St, Ste 1063, Chicago, IL 60612; **Phone:** 312-243-4244; **Board Cert:** Orthopaedic Surgery 2000; **Med School:** Univ Cincinnati 1979; **Resid:** Surgery, New Eng Deaconess Hosp 1981; Orthopaedic Surgery, Mass Genl Hosp 1985; **Fellow:** Sports Medicine, Hosp Special Surg 1986; **Fac Appt:** Prof OrS, Rush Med Coll

Bergfeld, John A MD [OrS] - **Spec Exp:** Sports Medicine; Knee Ligament Reconstruction; Cartilage Damage; Musculoskeletal Disorders; **Hospital:** Cleveland Clin Fdn (page 57); **Address:** The Cleveland Clinic, 9500 Euclid Ave, A41, Cleveland, OH 44195-5027; **Phone:** 216-444-2618; **Board Cert:** Orthopaedic Surgery 1972; **Med School:** Temple Univ 1964; **Resid:** Surgery, Cleveland Clinic 1966; Orthopaedic Surgery, Cleveland Clinic 1970

Biermann, J Sybil MD [OrS] - **Spec Exp:** Sarcoma; Bone Cancer; Multiple Myeloma; Limb Sparing Surgery; **Hospital:** Univ Michigan Hlth Sys; **Address:** Univ Michigan Cancer Ctr, 1500 E Medical Ctr Drive, 7304 CCGC, Ann Arbor, MI 48109-0948; **Phone:** 734-647-8902; **Board Cert:** Orthopaedic Surgery 2004; **Med School:** Stanford Univ 1987; **Resid:** Orthopaedic Surgery, Univ Iowa Hosp 1992; **Fellow:** Orthopaedic Oncology, Univ Chicago Hosps 1993; **Fac Appt:** Assoc Prof OrS, Univ Mich Med Sch

Blaha, John David MD [OrS] - **Spec Exp:** Hip & Knee Replacement; **Hospital:** Univ Michigan Hlth Sys; **Address:** Univ Michigan, Dept Orthopaedic Surg, 1500 E Medical Ctr Dr, 2912 Taubman, Ann Arbor, MI 48109; **Phone:** 734-647-9961; **Board Cert:** Orthopaedic Surgery 1979; **Med School:** Univ Mich Med Sch 1973; **Resid:** Surgery, Univ Mich Hosp 1975; Orthopaedic Surgery, Univ Mich Hosp 1978; **Fellow:** Joint Replacement Surgery, Univ London 1980; **Fac Appt:** Prof OrS, Univ Mich Med Sch

Bohlman, Henry H MD [OrS] - **Spec Exp:** Spinal Surgery-Cervical; **Hospital:** Univ Hosps Case Med Ctr; **Address:** Univ Hosps of Cleveland, Dept Ortho Surg, 11100 Euclid Ave, Cleveland, OH 44106-1736; **Phone:** 216-844-1025; **Board Cert:** Orthopaedic Surgery 1972; **Med School:** Univ MD Sch Med 1964; **Resid:** Surgery, Univ Hosp 1966; Orthopaedic Surgery, Johns Hopkins Hosp 1970; **Fellow:** Spinal Surgery, Johns Hopkins Hosp 1968; **Fac Appt:** Prof OrS, Case West Res Univ

Bridwell, Keith MD [OrS] - **Spec Exp:** Spinal Deformity; Scoliosis; Spinal Surgery; **Hospital:** Barnes-Jewish Hosp, St Louis Chldns Hosp; **Address:** 1 Barnes Jewish Hosp Plaza, Ste 11300, West Pav, Dept Ortho Surg, Campus Box 8233, St. Louis, MO 63110; **Phone:** 314-747-2500; **Board Cert:** Orthopaedic Surgery 1985; **Med School:** Washington Univ, St Louis 1977; **Resid:** Orthopaedic Surgery, Barnes Hosp-Wash Univ 1981; **Fellow:** Spinal Surgery, Rush Presby-St Lukes Med Ctr; **Fac Appt:** Prof OrS, Washington Univ, St Louis

Buckwalter, Joseph MD [OrS] - **Spec Exp:** Bone Cancer; Bone Tumors-Metastatic; Fractures-Complex; **Hospital:** Univ Iowa Hosp & Clinics; **Address:** Univ Iowa Hosps, Orthopaedics, 200 Hawkins Drive, Iowa City, IA 52242; **Phone:** 319-356-2595; **Board Cert:** Orthopaedic Surgery 1991; **Med School:** Univ Iowa Coll Med 1974; **Resid:** Orthopaedic Surgery, Iowa Hosp 1979; **Fac Appt:** Prof OrS, Univ Iowa Coll Med

Callaghan, John J MD [OrS] - **Spec Exp:** Hip & Knee Replacement; Sports Medicine; **Hospital:** Univ Iowa Hosp & Clinics; **Address:** Univ Iowa, Dept Orthopaedics, 200 Hawkins Drive, Iowa City, IA 52242; **Phone:** 319-356-3110; **Board Cert:** Orthopaedic Surgery 2000; **Med School:** Loyola Univ-Stritch Sch Med 1978; **Resid:** Orthopaedic Surgery, Univ Iowa Hosp 1983; **Fellow:** Orthopaedic Surgery, Hosp Special Surg 1984; **Fac Appt:** Prof OrS, Univ Iowa Coll Med

Cofield, Robert H MD [OrS] - **Spec Exp:** Shoulder Surgery; Rotator Cuff Surgery; Shoulder Injuries; **Hospital:** Mayo Med Ctr & Clin - Rochester; **Address:** Mayo Clinic, Dept Ortho Surg, 200 First St SW, Rochester, MN 55905-0001; **Phone:** 507-284-9219; **Board Cert:** Orthopaedic Surgery 2004; **Med School:** Univ KY Coll Med 1969; **Resid:** Surgery, Charity Hosp - Tulane Div 1971; Orthopaedic Surgery, Mayo Clinic 1975; **Fac Appt:** Prof S, Mayo Med Sch

Ebraheim, Nabil A MD [OrS] - **Spec Exp:** Trauma; Fractures-Complex; **Hospital:** Univ of Toledo Med Ctr; **Address:** Univ of Toledo Med Ctr, Orthopaedics, 3065 Arlington Ave, MS 1094, Toledo, OH 43614; **Phone:** 419-383-4020; **Board Cert:** Orthopaedic Surgery 2007; **Med School:** Egypt 1975; **Resid:** Orthopaedic Surgery, St Clare's Hosp 1980; Orthopaedic Surgery, SUNY-Downstate Med Ctr 1983; **Fellow:** Trauma, Univ Maryland Hosps 1984; **Fac Appt:** Prof OrS, Med Coll OH

Galante, Jorge O MD [OrS] - **Spec Exp:** Hip Replacement; Knee Replacement; **Hospital:** Rush Univ Med Ctr; **Address:** 1725 W Harrison St, Ste 1063, Chicago, IL 60612-3841; **Phone:** 312-432-2344; **Board Cert:** Orthopaedic Surgery 1968; **Med School:** Argentina 1958; **Resid:** Orthopaedic Surgery, Michael Reese Hosp 1961; Orthopaedic Surgery, Univ Illinois Hosps 1964; **Fellow:** Orthopaedic Surgery, Univ Goteborg 1967; **Fac Appt:** Prof OrS, Rush Med Coll

Goitz, Henry MD [OrS] - **Spec Exp:** Sports Medicine; Arthroscopic Surgery; **Hospital:** Henry Ford Hosp; **Address:** Henry Ford Hosp, Ctr for Athletic Med, 6525 2nd Ave, Detroit, MI 48202; **Phone:** 313-972-4066; **Board Cert:** Orthopaedic Surgery 2005; **Med School:** UMDNJ-Rutgers Med Sch 1985; **Resid:** Surgery, Univ Virginia 1987; Orthopaedic Surgery, Univ Virginia 1991; **Fellow:** Sports Medicine & Hand Surgery, Univ Virginia 1992; Sports Medicine, American Sports Med Inst 1993

Goldberg, Victor M MD [OrS] - **Spec Exp:** Hip & Knee Replacement; Arthritis; **Hospital:** Univ Hosps Case Med Ctr; **Address:** Univ Hosps of Cleveland, Dept Ortho Surg, 11100 Euclid Ave, Cleveland, OH 44106; **Phone:** 216-844-3044; **Board Cert:** Orthopaedic Surgery 1992; **Med School:** SUNY Downstate 1964; **Resid:** Surgery, Univ Hosp 1966; Orthopaedic Surgery, Hosp Special Surg 1971; **Fac Appt:** Prof OrS, Case West Res Univ

Goldstein, Wayne MD [OrS] - **Spec Exp:** Hip Replacement; Knee Replacement; **Hospital:** Adv Luth Genl Hosp; **Address:** 9000 Waukegan Rd, Ste 200, Morton Grove, IL 60053; **Phone:** 847-375-3000; **Board Cert:** Orthopaedic Surgery 1997; **Med School:** Univ IL Coll Med 1978; **Resid:** Orthopaedic Surgery, Univ Ilinois Med Ctr 1983; **Fellow:** Brigham & Women's Hosp-Harvard 1984; **Fac Appt:** Assoc Clin Prof OrS, Univ Chicago-Pritzker Sch Med

Graf, Ben K MD [OrS] - **Spec Exp:** Sports Medicine; **Hospital:** Univ WI Hosp & Clins; **Address:** 600 Highland Ave, rm K4-735, Madison, WI 53792-3228; **Phone:** 608-263-8850; **Board Cert:** Orthopaedic Surgery 1998; **Med School:** Univ Wisc 1979; **Resid:** Orthopaedic Surgery, Univ Wisc Hosps 1984; **Fellow:** Sports Medicine, Long Beach Meml Hosp 1985; **Fac Appt:** Assoc Prof S, Univ Wisc

Grant, Richard E MD [OrS] - **Spec Exp:** Hip & Knee Replacement; Spinal Surgery-Low Back; Sickle Cell Disease-Hip Surgery; **Hospital:** Univ Hosps Case Med Ctr; **Address:** Univ Hosps Cleveland, Dept Ortho Surgery, 11100 Euclid Ave, Cleveland, OH 44106; **Phone:** 216-844-1118; **Board Cert:** Orthopaedic Surgery 2007; **Med School:** Howard Univ 1976; **Resid:** Orthopaedic Surgery, Wilford Hall Med Ctr-Lackland 1984; **Fellow:** Joint Arthroplasty, Ohio State Univ Hosp; Spinal Cord Injury Medicine, St Lukes/Baylor Univ; **Fac Appt:** Prof OrS, Howard Univ

Hensinger, Robert MD [OrS] - **Spec Exp:** Pediatric Orthopaedic Surgery; Spinal Surgery-Pediatric; **Hospital:** Univ Michigan Hlth Sys; **Address:** Univ Michigan Med Ctr, Dept Ortho Surg, 2912 Taubman Ctr, 1500 E Medical Ctr Dr, Ann Arbor, MI 48109-0328; **Phone:** 734-936-5780; **Board Cert:** Orthopaedic Surgery 2007; **Med School:** Univ Mich Med Sch 1964; **Resid:** Orthopaedic Surgery, Univ Michigan 1966; Orthopaedic Surgery, Univ Michigan 1971; **Fellow:** Pediatric Orthopaedic Surgery, Al DuPont Inst 1972; **Fac Appt:** Prof OrS, Univ Mich Med Sch

Iannotti, Joseph MD/PhD [OrS] - **Spec Exp:** Shoulder Surgery; **Hospital:** Cleveland Clin Fdn (page 57); **Address:** 9500 Euclid Ave/Desk A41, Cleveland, OH 44195-5027; **Phone:** 216-445-5151; **Board Cert:** Orthopaedic Surgery 2006; **Med School:** Northwestern Univ 1979; **Resid:** Orthopaedic Surgery, Hosp Univ Penn 1984; **Fellow:** Orthopaedic Surgery, Hosp Univ Penn 1985; **Fac Appt:** Prof OrS, Cleveland Cl Coll Med/Case West Res

Orthopaedic Surgery

Joyce, Michael J MD [OrS] - **Spec Exp:** Bone & Soft Tissue Tumors; Fractures-Complex & Non Union; Musculoskeletal Tissue Banking; Pelvic & Acetabular Fractures; **Hospital:** Cleveland Clin Fdn (page 57); **Address:** Cleveland Clinic, Dept Orthopaedic Surgery, 9500 Euclid Ave, Desk A41, Cleveland, OH 44195; **Phone:** 216-444-4282; **Board Cert:** Orthopaedic Surgery 1985; **Med School:** Univ Louisville Sch Med 1976; **Resid:** Surgery, Johns Hopkins Hosp 1978; Orthopaedic Surgery, Harvard Combined Program 1981; **Fellow:** Orthopaedic Oncology, Mass General Hosp 1982; Trauma, Univ Toronto-Sunnybrook Hosp 1983; **Fac Appt:** Assoc Clin Prof OrS, Case West Res Univ

Lenke, Lawrence G MD [OrS] - **Spec Exp:** Spinal Surgery; Spinal Deformity; Scoliosis; **Hospital:** Barnes-Jewish Hosp; **Address:** Washington Univ Sch Med, 1 Barnes Hospital Plaza, Ste 11300, West Pavilion, St Louis, MO 63110; **Phone:** 314-747-2500; **Board Cert:** Orthopaedic Surgery 1994; **Med School:** Northwestern Univ 1986; **Resid:** Orthopaedic Surgery, Barnes-Jewish Hosp 1990; **Fellow:** Spinal Surgery, Barnes-Jewish Hosp 1992; **Fac Appt:** Prof OrS, Washington Univ, St Louis

Lock, Terrence Ralph MD [OrS] - **Spec Exp:** Sports Medicine; Arthroscopic Surgery; Shoulder & Knee Reconstruction; **Hospital:** Henry Ford Hosp, Bon Secours Cottage Hosp; **Address:** 6525 2nd Ave, Detroit, MI 48202; **Phone:** 313-972-4085; **Board Cert:** Orthopaedic Surgery 2002; **Med School:** Wayne State Univ 1983; **Resid:** Orthopaedic Surgery, Wayne St Univ Sch Med 1988; **Fellow:** Sports Medicine, Mass Genl Hosp 1989

Manoli II, Arthur MD [OrS] - **Spec Exp:** Foot & Ankle Surgery; Reconstructive Surgery; **Hospital:** St Joseph Mercy Oakland Hosp; **Address:** 44555 Woodward Ave, Ste 105, Pontiac, MI 48341; **Phone:** 248-858-6773; **Board Cert:** Orthopaedic Surgery 2005; **Med School:** Univ Mich Med Sch 1970; **Resid:** Surgery, Oakwood Hosp 1972; Orthopaedic Surgery, Wayne St Univ Affil Hosps 1975; **Fellow:** Ankle and Foot Surgery, Univ Wash/Vanderbilt Univ 1990

Martell, John M MD [OrS] - **Spec Exp:** Hip Replacement; Knee Replacement; Knee Surgery; **Hospital:** Univ of Chicago Hosps; **Address:** 5841 S Maryland Ave, MC 3079, Chicago, IL 60637-1463; **Phone:** 773-702-7297; **Board Cert:** Orthopaedic Surgery 2002; **Med School:** Univ Chicago-Pritzker Sch Med 1983; **Resid:** Orthopaedic Surgery, Univ Chicago Hosps 1988; **Fellow:** Joint Replacement Surgery, Rush Presby-St Luke's Med Ctr 1989; **Fac Appt:** Assoc Prof OrS, Univ Chicago-Pritzker Sch Med

McDonald, Douglas J MD [OrS] - **Spec Exp:** Bone Tumors; Ewing's Sarcoma; Reconstructive Surgery; **Hospital:** Barnes-Jewish Hosp; **Address:** Ctr Advanced Med, Orthopaedic Surg Ctr, 4921 Parkview Pl Fl 6 - Ste A, Box 8605, St Louis, MO 63110; **Phone:** 314-747-2500; **Board Cert:** Orthopaedic Surgery 2001; **Med School:** Univ Minn 1982; **Resid:** Orthopaedic Surgery, Mayo Clinic 1987; **Fellow:** Orthopaedic Oncology, Mayo Clinic 1988; **Fac Appt:** Prof OrS, Washington Univ, St Louis

Muschler, George F MD [OrS] - **Spec Exp:** Hip Replacement; Knee Replacement; Fractures-Non Union; Fractures-Complex; **Hospital:** Cleveland Clin Fdn (page 57); **Address:** Cleveland Clinic, Dept Orthopaedic Surg, 9500 Euclid Ave, Desk A41, Cleveland, OH 44195-0001; **Phone:** 216-444-5338; **Board Cert:** Orthopaedic Surgery 2001; **Med School:** Northwestern Univ 1981; **Resid:** Orthopaedic Surgery, Univ Texas SW Med Ctr 1986; **Fellow:** Metabolic Bone Research, Hosp Special Surgery 1988; Musculoskeletal Oncology, Meml Sloan Kettering Cancer Ctr 1988; **Fac Appt:** Prof OrS, Cleveland Cl Coll Med/Case West Res

Nuber, Gordon MD [OrS] - **Spec Exp:** Shoulder Reconstruction; Cartilage Damage; Elbow Surgery; **Hospital:** Northwestern Meml Hosp; **Address:** Northwestern Orthopaedic Institute, 680 N Lakeshore Dr, Ste 1028, Chicago, IL 60611-4451; **Phone:** 312-664-6848; **Board Cert:** Orthopaedic Surgery 2004; **Med School:** Wayne State Univ 1978; **Resid:** Orthopaedic Surgery, Northwestern Meml Hosp 1983; **Fellow:** Sports Medicine, Natl Hlth Inst 1984; **Fac Appt:** Clin Prof OrS, Northwestern Univ

Pinzur, Michael S MD [OrS] - **Spec Exp:** Diabetes-Amputation; Foot & Ankle Surgery; Amputation Surgery; **Hospital:** Loyola Univ Med Ctr; **Address:** Loyola Univ Med Ctr, Dept Orth Surg, 2160 S 1st Ave, Maywood, IL 60153-3304; **Phone:** 708-216-4993; **Board Cert:** Orthopaedic Surgery 1980; **Med School:** Rush Med Coll 1974; **Resid:** Orthopaedic Surgery, Northwest Meml Hosp 1979; **Fac Appt:** Prof OrS, Loyola Univ-Stritch Sch Med

Polly, David W MD [OrS] - **Spec Exp:** Spinal Surgery; Amputation Surgery; Scoliosis; **Hospital:** Univ Minn Med Ctr, Fairview - Univ Campus; **Address:** Univ Minnesota, Orthopaedic Dept, 2450 Riverside Ave S, rm 200, Minneapolis, MN 55454; **Phone:** 612-273-9400; **Board Cert:** Orthopaedic Surgery 1994; **Med School:** Uniformed Srvs Univ, Bethesda 1985; **Resid:** Orthopaedic Surgery, Walter Reed Army Med Ctr 1991; **Fellow:** Spinal Surgery, Univ Minn 1992

Riew, K Daniel MD [OrS] - **Spec Exp:** Spinal Surgery-Cervical; Minimally Invasive Spinal Surgery; Spinal Microsurgery; **Hospital:** Barnes-Jewish Hosp; **Address:** Ctr for Advanced Med-Spine Ctr, 4921 Parkview Pl, CAM Bldg Fl 12 - Ste A, St. Louis, MO 63110; **Phone:** 314-747-2500; **Board Cert:** Internal Medicine 1987; Orthopaedic Surgery 1997; **Med School:** Case West Res Univ 1984; **Resid:** Internal Medicine, NY Hosp-Cornell Med Ctr 1987; Orthopaedic Surgery, George Wash Univ Med Ctr 1994; **Fellow:** Spinal Surgery, Case West Res Univ 1995; **Fac Appt:** Prof OrS, Washington Univ, St Louis

Rosenberg, Aaron G MD [OrS] - **Spec Exp:** Hip & Knee Replacement; Hip & Knee Reconstruction; **Hospital:** Rush Univ Med Ctr; **Address:** 1725 W Harrison St, Ste 1063, Chicago, IL 60612-3828; **Phone:** 312-432-2340; **Board Cert:** Orthopaedic Surgery 1997; **Med School:** Albany Med Coll 1978; **Resid:** Orthopaedic Surgery, Rush Presby-St Lukes Med Ctr 1983; **Fellow:** Arthritis Surgery, Mass Genl Hosp 1984; **Fac Appt:** Prof OrS, Rush Med Coll

Schafer, Michael F MD [OrS] - **Spec Exp:** Sports Medicine; Spinal Surgery; Scoliosis; **Hospital:** Northwestern Meml Hosp, Children's Mem Hosp; **Address:** 675 N St Clair, Ste 17-100, Chicago, IL 60611-5968; **Phone:** 312-695-6800; **Board Cert:** Orthopaedic Surgery 1983; **Med School:** Univ Iowa Coll Med 1967; **Resid:** Orthopaedic Surgery, Northwestern Univ Hosp 1972; **Fellow:** Spinal Surgery, Natl Fdn Traveling Fellowship 1973; **Fac Appt:** Prof OrS, Northwestern Univ

Shelbourne, K Donald MD [OrS] - **Spec Exp:** Knee Surgery; Arthroscopic Surgery; Knee Rehabilitation (Non-Surgical); **Hospital:** Methodist Hosp - Indianapolis; **Address:** 1815 N Capitol Ave, Ste 600, Indianapolis, IN 46202-1288; **Phone:** 317-924-8636; **Board Cert:** Orthopaedic Surgery 1984; **Med School:** Indiana Univ 1976; **Resid:** Orthopaedic Surgery, Indiana Univ Hosp 1981; **Fellow:** Sports Medicine, Univ Wisconsin 1982; **Fac Appt:** Assoc Clin Prof OrS, Indiana Univ

Orthopaedic Surgery

Simon, Michael MD [OrS] - **Spec Exp:** Bone Tumors; Soft Tissue Tumors; Pediatric Orthopaedic Cancers; **Hospital:** Univ of Chicago Hosps; **Address:** 5841 S Maryland Ave, MC 3079, Univ of Chicago, Chicago, IL 60637; **Phone:** 773-702-6144; **Board Cert:** Orthopaedic Surgery 1992; **Med School:** Univ Mich Med Sch 1967; **Resid:** Surgery, Univ Mich Med Ctr 1969; Orthopaedic Surgery, Univ Mich Med Ctr 1974; **Fellow:** Orthopaedic Oncology, Univ Fla 1975; **Fac Appt:** Prof S, Univ Chicago-Pritzker Sch Med

Stulberg, S David MD [OrS] - **Spec Exp:** Hip & Knee Replacement; Arthritis; Shoulder Surgery; **Hospital:** Northwestern Meml Hosp; **Address:** 680 N Lake Shore Drive, Ste 1028, Chicago, IL 60611; **Phone:** 312-664-6848; **Board Cert:** Orthopaedic Surgery 1977; **Med School:** Univ Mich Med Sch 1969; **Resid:** Orthopaedic Surgery, Mass General Hosp 1974; **Fellow:** Research, Hosp Sick Chldn 1976; **Fac Appt:** Prof OrS, Northwestern Univ

Swiontkowski, Marc F MD [OrS] - **Spec Exp:** Osteomyelitis; Fractures-Non Union; Trauma; Bone Infections; **Hospital:** Univ Minn Med Ctr, Fairview - Univ Campus; **Address:** Univ Minnesota, Orthopaedic Dept, 2450 Riverside Ave S, rm 200, Minneapolis, MN 55454; **Phone:** 612-273-9400; **Board Cert:** Orthopaedic Surgery 2004; **Med School:** USC Sch Med 1979; **Resid:** Orthopaedic Surgery, Univ Washington Med Ctr 1984; **Fac Appt:** Prof OrS, Univ Minn

Weinstein, Stuart L MD [OrS] - **Spec Exp:** Scoliosis; Hip Disorders & Dysplasia; Hip Disorders-Pediatric; Spinal Deformity; **Hospital:** Univ Iowa Hosp & Clinics; **Address:** Univ Iowa, Dept Orthopaedics, 200 Hawkins Drive, Iowa City, IA 52242-1009; **Phone:** 319-356-1872; **Board Cert:** Orthopaedic Surgery 1995; **Med School:** Univ Iowa Coll Med 1972; **Resid:** Orthopaedic Surgery, Univ Iowa Hosps 1976; **Fac Appt:** Prof OrS, Univ Iowa Coll Med

Wixson, Richard L MD [OrS] - **Spec Exp:** Hip & Knee Replacement; **Hospital:** Northwestern Meml Hosp; **Address:** 676 N St Clair, Ste 450, Chicago, IL 60611; **Phone:** 312-943-7850; **Board Cert:** Orthopaedic Surgery 1979; **Med School:** Univ Wisc 1972; **Resid:** Orthopaedic Surgery, Henry Ford Hosp 1977; Orthopaedic Surgery, New Eng Baptist Hosp 1979; **Fellow:** Orthopaedic Surgery, Mass Genl Hosp 1978; **Fac Appt:** Clin Prof OrS, Northwestern Univ

Yamaguchi, Ken MD [OrS] - **Spec Exp:** Shoulder Surgery; Elbow Surgery; Rotator Cuff Surgery; **Hospital:** Barnes-Jewish Hosp; **Address:** One Barnes Hosp Plaza, Dept Orthopaedic Surg, 11300 West Pavilion, St Louis, MO 63110-1036; **Phone:** 314-747-2534; **Board Cert:** Orthopaedic Surgery 1997; **Med School:** Geo Wash Univ 1989; **Resid:** Orthopaedic Surgery, George Wash Univ Med Ctr 1994; **Fellow:** Shoulder Surgery, Columbia Presby Med Ctr 1995; **Fac Appt:** Prof OrS, Washington Univ, St Louis

Zdeblick, Thomas MD [OrS] - **Spec Exp:** Spinal Surgery; **Hospital:** Univ WI Hosp & Clins; **Address:** 600 Highland Ave, rm K4-739 CSC, Madison, WI 53792-7375; **Phone:** 608-265-3207; **Board Cert:** Orthopaedic Surgery 2002; **Med School:** Tufts Univ 1982; **Resid:** Orthopaedic Surgery, Case West Res Univ 1988; **Fellow:** Spinal Surgery, Johns Hopkins Univ 1989; **Fac Appt:** Prof OrS, Univ Wisc

Great Plains and Mountains

Coughlin, Michael MD [OrS] - **Spec Exp:** Foot & Ankle Surgery; **Hospital:** St Alphonsus Regl Med Ctr; **Address:** 901 N Curtis Rd, Ste 503, Boise, ID 83706; **Phone:** 208-377-1000; **Board Cert:** Orthopaedic Surgery 1980; **Med School:** Oregon Hlth Sci Univ 1974; **Resid:** Orthopaedic Surgery, UCSF Med Ctr 1978; **Fellow:** Foot/Ankle Surgery, Samuel Merritt Hosp 1979; **Fac Appt:** Clin Prof OrS, Oregon Hlth Sci Univ

Dunn, Harold K MD [OrS] - **Spec Exp:** Hip Reconstruction; Knee Reconstruction; **Hospital:** Univ Utah Hosps and Clins; **Address:** Univ Utah, Orthopaedic Ctr, 590 Wakara Way, Salt Lake City, UT 84108; **Phone:** 801-587-5428; **Board Cert:** Orthopaedic Surgery 1983; **Med School:** Baylor Coll Med 1963; **Resid:** Orthopaedic Surgery, Univ New Mexico Affil Hosp 1967; Orthopaedic Surgery, Baylor Coll Med 1969; **Fac Appt:** Prof OrS, Univ Utah

Garvin, Kevin L MD [OrS] - **Spec Exp:** Hip Surgery; Knee Surgery; Joint Replacement; **Hospital:** Nebraska Med Ctr; **Address:** Orthopaedic Clinic, 989265 Nebraska Medical Ctr Fl 2, Omaha, NE 68198-9265; **Phone:** 402-559-8000; **Board Cert:** Orthopaedic Surgery 2001; **Med School:** Med Coll Wisc 1982; **Resid:** Orthopaedic Surgery, Univ Hosp of Arizona 1987; **Fellow:** Hip Surgery, Hosp for Special Surgery 1988; **Fac Appt:** Prof OrS, Univ Nebr Coll Med

Millett, Peter J MD [OrS] - **Spec Exp:** Shoulder Surgery; Sports Medicine; Arthroscopic Surgery; **Hospital:** Vail Valley Med Ctr; **Address:** Steadman-Hawkins Clinic, 181 W Meadow Drive, Ste 400, Vail, CO 81657; **Phone:** 970-476-1100; **Board Cert:** Orthopaedic Surgery 2003; **Med School:** Dartmouth Med Sch 1995; **Resid:** Orthopaedic Surgery, Hosp Special Surgery 2000; **Fellow:** Sports Medicine, Steadman Hawkins Clinic 2001

Randall, R Lor MD [OrS] - **Spec Exp:** Bone Tumors; Sarcoma-Soft Tissue; Pediatric Orthopaedic Surgery; **Hospital:** Univ Utah Hosps and Clins, Primary Children's Med Ctr; **Address:** Ped Ortho Surg, Primary Chlds Med Ctr, 100 N Medical Drive, Ste 4550, SLC, UT 84113, Salt Lake City, UT 84113; **Phone:** 801-662-5600; **Board Cert:** Orthopaedic Surgery 2001; **Med School:** Yale Univ 1992; **Resid:** Orthopaedic Surgery, UCSF Med Ctr 1997; **Fellow:** Musculoskeletal Oncology, Univ WA Med Ctr 1998; **Fac Appt:** Assoc Prof OrS, Univ Utah

Rosenberg, Thomas D MD [OrS] - **Spec Exp:** Knee Surgery; Sports Medicine; **Hospital:** Ortho Spec Hosp, The (TOSH); **Address:** 1820 Sidewinder Drive, Park City, UT 84060; **Phone:** 435-655-6600; **Board Cert:** Orthopaedic Surgery 1979; **Med School:** Univ Utah 1973; **Resid:** Orthopaedic Surgery, Univ Utah Affil Hosps 1977; **Fellow:** Sports Medicine, Univ Wisconsin Hosp 1978

Saltzman, Charles L MD [OrS] - **Spec Exp:** Foot & Ankle Surgery; **Hospital:** Univ Utah Hosps and Clins; **Address:** Univ Utah, Dept Orthopaedic Surgery, 590 Wakara Way, Salt Lake City, UT 84108; **Phone:** 801-587-5404; **Board Cert:** Orthopaedic Surgery 2004; **Med School:** Univ NC Sch Med 1985; **Resid:** Orthopaedic Surgery, Univ Michigan Med Ctr; **Fellow:** Orthopaedic Surgery, Mayo Clinic; **Fac Appt:** Prof OrS, Univ Utah

Steadman, J Richard MD [OrS] - **Spec Exp:** Knee-Microfracture Surgery; Sports Medicine; **Hospital:** Vail Valley Med Ctr; **Address:** Steadman-Hawkins Sports Medicine Clinic, 181 W Meadow Drive, Ste 400, Vail, CO 81657; **Phone:** 970-476-1100; **Board Cert:** Orthopaedic Surgery 1972; **Med School:** Univ Tex SW, Dallas 1963; **Resid:** Orthopaedic Surgery, Charity Hosp 1966; Orthopaedic Surgery, Louisiana St Univ Hosp 1967

Wiedel, Jerome D MD [OrS] - **Spec Exp:** Hip/Knee Replacement; Reconstructive Surgery; **Hospital:** Univ Colorado Hosp; **Address:** 1635 N Ursula St, Ste 4100, PO Box 6510, MS F722, Aurora, CO 80045; **Phone:** 720-848-1900; **Board Cert:** Orthopaedic Surgery 1993; **Med School:** Univ Nebr Coll Med 1964; **Resid:** Orthopaedic Surgery, Univ Colorado Med Ctr 1971; **Fellow:** Reconstructive Surgery, Robert Jones-A Hunt Ortho Hosp 1972; **Fac Appt:** Prof OrS, Univ Colorado

Orthopaedic Surgery

Wilkins, Ross M MD [OrS] - **Spec Exp:** Bone Cancer; **Hospital:** Presby - St Luke's Med Ctr, Porter Adventist Hosp; **Address:** 1601 E 19th Ave, Ste 3300, Denver, CO 80218; **Phone:** 303-837-0072; **Board Cert:** Orthopaedic Surgery 2006; **Med School:** Wayne State Univ 1978; **Resid:** Orthopaedic Surgery, Univ Colorado Med Ctr 1983; **Fellow:** Orthopaedic Oncology, Mayo Clinic 1984

Southwest

Aronson, James MD [OrS] - **Spec Exp:** Limb Lengthening (Ilizarov Procedure); Hip Disorders & Dysplasia; Clubfoot; Limb Deformities; **Hospital:** Arkansas Chldns Hosp; **Address:** Arkansas Chldns Hosp, Dept Orthopaedics, 800 Marshall St, Slot 839, Little Rock, AR 72202; **Phone:** 501-364-1468; **Board Cert:** Orthopaedic Surgery 1997; **Med School:** Univ Pittsburgh 1975; **Resid:** Surgery, Maine Med Ctr 1977; Orthopaedic Surgery, Duke Univ Med Ctr 1982; **Fellow:** Pediatric Orthopaedic Surgery, Alfred I DuPont Inst 1983; **Fac Appt:** Prof OrS, Univ Ark

Brodsky, James W MD [OrS] - **Spec Exp:** Foot & Ankle Surgery; **Hospital:** Baylor Univ Medical Ctr; **Address:** 411 N Washington Ave, Ste 7000, Dallas, TX 75246-1777; **Phone:** 214-823-7090; **Board Cert:** Orthopaedic Surgery 1998; **Med School:** Case West Res Univ 1979; **Resid:** Orthopaedic Surgery, Bellevue Hosp Ctr/NYU 1981; Orthopaedic Surgery, Baylor Coll Med 1984; **Fellow:** Foot/Ankle Surgery, Rancho Los Amigos/USC/LAC Hosp 1985; **Fac Appt:** Clin Prof OrS, Univ Tex SW, Dallas

Bucholz, Robert MD [OrS] - **Spec Exp:** Trauma; **Hospital:** Parkland Meml Hosp - Dallas, UT Southwestern Med Ctr - Dallas; **Address:** Univ Tex SW Med Sch, Dept Ortho Surg, 5323 Harry Hines Blvd, Dallas, TX 75390-8882; **Phone:** 214-648-3068; **Board Cert:** Orthopaedic Surgery 1994; **Med School:** Yale Univ 1973; **Resid:** Orthopaedic Surgery, Yale-New Haven Hosp 1977; **Fac Appt:** Prof OrS, Univ Tex SW, Dallas

Cooper, Daniel E MD [OrS] - **Spec Exp:** Sports Medicine; Knee Surgery; **Hospital:** Baylor Univ Medical Ctr, Mary Shiels Hosp; **Address:** The Carrell Clinic, 9301 N Central Expwy Ave, Ste 400, Dallas, TX 75231; **Phone:** 214-220-2468; **Board Cert:** Orthopaedic Surgery 2002; **Med School:** Univ Tex SW, Dallas 1984; **Resid:** Orthopaedic Surgery, Univ Texas Health Scis Ctr 1989; **Fellow:** Sports Medicine, Hospital for Special Surgery 1990

Dabezies, Eugene MD [OrS] - **Spec Exp:** Hand Surgery; Trauma; **Hospital:** Univ Med Ctr - Lubbock; **Address:** 3502 9th St, Medical Office Plaza, Ste 450, Lubbock, TX 79415; **Phone:** 806-743-4263; **Board Cert:** Orthopaedic Surgery 1992; **Med School:** Tulane Univ 1960; **Resid:** Orthopaedic Surgery, Charity Hosp 1965; **Fellow:** Hand Surgery, Rancho Los Amigos Natl Rehab Ctr; **Fac Appt:** Prof OrS, Texas Tech Univ

Gugenheim Jr, Joseph J MD [OrS] - **Spec Exp:** Limb Lengthening (Ilizarov Procedure); Limb Deformities; **Hospital:** Texas Ortho Hosp; **Address:** Foundren Orthopaedic Group, 7401 S Main St, Houston, TX 77030; **Phone:** 713-799-2300; **Board Cert:** Orthopaedic Surgery 1978; **Med School:** Northwestern Univ 1972; **Resid:** Orthopaedic Surgery, Baylor Univ Hosp 1976; **Fellow:** Pediatric Orthopaedic Surgery, Boston Chldns Hosp 1977; **Fac Appt:** Assoc Prof S, Baylor Coll Med

Hochschuler, Stephen H MD [OrS] - **Spec Exp:** Spinal Surgery; **Hospital:** Presby Hosp - Plano; **Address:** Texas Back Institute, 6020 W Parker Rd, Ste 200, Plano, TX 75093-7916; **Phone:** 972-608-5000; **Board Cert:** Orthopaedic Surgery 1978; **Med School:** Harvard Med Sch 1968; **Resid:** Surgery, Boston City Hosp 1971; Orthopaedic Surgery, Univ Texas SW Med Ctr 1976

Mabrey, Jay D MD [OrS] - **Spec Exp:** Knee Replacement & Revision; Hip Replacement & Revision; Arthroscopic Surgery-Hip; **Hospital:** Baylor Univ Medical Ctr; **Address:** Baylor Univ Med Ctr, Dept Orthopaedics, 3500 Gaston Ave Bldg Hob Fl 6, Dallas, TX 75246-9990; **Phone:** 214-820-3434; **Board Cert:** Orthopaedic Surgery 2000; **Med School:** Cornell Univ-Weill Med Coll 1981; **Resid:** Orthopaedic Surgery, Duke Univ MC 1987; Surgery, Duke Univ MC 1983; **Fellow:** Joint Replacement Surgery, Hosp Special Surg 1991; **Fac Appt:** Clin Prof OrS, Univ Tex SW, Dallas

Paulos, Leon MD [OrS] - **Spec Exp:** Sports Medicine; Shoulder & Knee Surgery; **Hospital:** St Luke's Episcopal Hosp - Houston; **Address:** 6620 Main, Ste 1325, Houston, TX 77030; **Phone:** 713-986-6010; **Board Cert:** Orthopaedic Surgery 1980; **Med School:** Univ Utah 1973; **Resid:** Orthopaedic Surgery, Univ Utah Sch Med 1978; **Fellow:** Sports Medicine, Atlanta Sports Med Fdn 1978; Sports Medicine, Univ Hosp 1979

Simmons Jr, James W MD [OrS] - **Spec Exp:** Spinal Surgery; **Hospital:** Methodist Spec & Transpl Hosp; **Address:** 12770 Cimarron Path, Ste 132, San Antonio, TX 78249; **Phone:** 210-614-3900; **Board Cert:** Orthopaedic Surgery 1969; **Med School:** Univ Miss 1962; **Resid:** Orthopaedic Surgery, Martin AMC 1964; Orthopaedic Surgery, Brooke Genl Hosp 1967; **Fac Appt:** Clin Prof OrS, Univ Tex Med Br, Galveston

Souryal, Tarek O MD [OrS] - **Spec Exp:** Sports Medicine; Knee Injuries/ACL; **Hospital:** Presby Hosp of Dallas; **Address:** 6901 Snider Plaza, Ste 200, Dallas, TX 75205; **Phone:** 214-369-7733; **Board Cert:** Orthopaedic Surgery 2001; **Med School:** Univ Tex, San Antonio 1982; **Resid:** Orthopaedic Surgery, UTSW Med Ctr 1987; **Fellow:** Sports Medicine, Sports Med Clin N Tex 1987; Sports Medicine, Hughston Ortho Clinic 1988; **Fac Appt:** Clin Prof OrS, Univ Tex SW, Dallas

Trick, Lorence Wain MD [OrS] - **Spec Exp:** Hip Replacement; Knee Replacement; **Hospital:** SW TX Meth Hosp, Nix Med Ctr; **Address:** 4647 Medical Drive, San Antonio, TX 78229; **Phone:** 210-567-0924; **Board Cert:** Orthopaedic Surgery 1973; **Med School:** Geo Wash Univ 1967; **Resid:** Orthopaedic Surgery, Wilford Hall USAF Med Ctr 1972; **Fellow:** Orthopaedic Surgery, New Eng Baptist Med Ctr; **Fac Appt:** Clin Prof OrS, Univ Tex, San Antonio

Wirth, Michael A MD [OrS] - **Spec Exp:** Shoulder Surgery; Joint Replacement; **Hospital:** Univ Hlth Sys - Univ Hosp; **Address:** Univ Tex Hlth Sci Ctr, Dept Orth, 7703 Floyd Curl Drive, MC 7774, San Antonio, TX 78229-3900; **Phone:** 210-567-5135; **Board Cert:** Orthopaedic Surgery 2004; **Med School:** Oregon Hlth Sci Univ 1985; **Resid:** Orthopaedic Surgery, Univ Texas Hlth Sci Ctr 1990; **Fellow:** Shoulder Surgery, Charles Rockwood Jr MD 1991; **Fac Appt:** Prof OrS, Univ Tex, San Antonio

West Coast and Pacific

Anderson, Lesley J MD [OrS] - **Spec Exp:** Knee Injuries/ACL; Knee Cartilage/Meniscus Transplants; Cartilage Damage; Shoulder Surgery; **Hospital:** CA Pacific Med Ctr; **Address:** 2100 Webster St, Ste 309, San Francisco, CA 94115-2376; **Phone:** 415-923-3029; **Board Cert:** Orthopaedic Surgery 2007; **Med School:** Penn State Univ-Hershey Med Ctr 1976; **Resid:** Orthopaedic Surgery, UCLA Med Ctr 1983; **Fellow:** Sports Medicine/Knee Surgery, Blazina Ortho Clinic 1984; **Fac Appt:** Asst Clin Prof OrS, UCSF

Orthopaedic Surgery

Bradford, David S MD [OrS] - **Spec Exp:** Scoliosis; Spinal Deformity; Spinal Surgery; **Hospital:** UCSF Med Ctr; **Address:** 500 Parnassus Ave Fl 3, Box 0728, San Francisco, CA 94143-0728; **Phone:** 415-353-2808; **Board Cert:** Orthopaedic Surgery 1988; **Med School:** Univ Pennsylvania 1962; **Resid:** Orthopaedic Surgery, Columbia-Presbyterian Med Ctr 1968; **Fellow:** Orthopaedic Surgery, Columbia-Presbyterian Med Ctr 1969; **Fac Appt:** Prof OrS, UCSF

Cannon Jr, W Dilworth MD [OrS] - **Spec Exp:** Sports Medicine; Knee Surgery; **Hospital:** UCSF Med Ctr; **Address:** 1701 Divisadero St, Ste 240, San Francisco, CA 94115-1351; **Phone:** 415-353-7566; **Board Cert:** Orthopaedic Surgery 1972; **Med School:** Columbia P&S 1963; **Resid:** Surgery, St Vincents Hosp 1965; Orthopaedic Surgery, NY Ortho Hosp 1970; **Fellow:** Orthopaedic Surgery, Royal Natl Ortho Hosp 1971; **Fac Appt:** Clin Prof OrS, UCSF

Carragee, Eugene J MD [OrS] - **Spec Exp:** Spinal Surgery; Spinal Disc Replacement; **Hospital:** Stanford Univ Med Ctr; **Address:** Stanford Univ Hospital, Orthopaedics/Spine Ctr, 300 Pasteur Drive, rm R171, Stanford, CA 94304; **Phone:** 650-725-5905; **Board Cert:** Orthopaedic Surgery 2005; **Med School:** Stanford Univ 1982; **Resid:** Internal Medicine, Stanford Univ Hosp 1984; Orthopaedic Surgery, Stanford Univ Hosp 1988; **Fac Appt:** Prof OrS, Stanford Univ

Chambers, Richard Byron MD [OrS] - **Spec Exp:** Diabetes-Amputation; **Hospital:** Rancho Los Amigos Natl Rehab Ctr; **Address:** 7601 E Imperial Hwy, rm HB-145, Downey, CA 90242; **Phone:** 562-401-7225; **Board Cert:** Orthopaedic Surgery 1977; **Med School:** Columbia P&S 1971; **Resid:** Surgery, NY Hosp; Orthopaedic Surgery, Hosp Special Surg

Conrad, Ernest U MD [OrS] - **Spec Exp:** Pediatric Orthopaedic Surgery; Bone Tumors; Sarcoma; **Hospital:** Chldns Hosp and Regl Med Ctr - Seattle, Univ Wash Med Ctr; **Address:** Children's Hosp & Regional Med Ctr, 4800 Sand Point Way, MS B6553, Seattle, WA 98105; **Phone:** 206-987-5096; **Board Cert:** Orthopaedic Surgery 1999; **Med School:** Univ VA Sch Med 1979; **Resid:** Orthopaedic Surgery, Hosp for Special Surgery 1984; **Fellow:** Orthopaedic Oncology, Univ Fla Coll Med 1985; Pediatric Orthopaedic Surgery, Hosp for Sick Chldn 1986; **Fac Appt:** Prof OrS, Univ Wash

Copp, Steven N MD [OrS] - **Spec Exp:** Foot & Ankle Surgery; Hip & Knee Replacement; **Hospital:** Scripps Green Hosp; **Address:** Scripps Clinic, Dept Orthopedic Surgery, 10666 N Torrey Pines Rd, La Jolla, CA 92037; **Phone:** 858-554-8519; **Board Cert:** Orthopaedic Surgery 2002; **Med School:** UCSD 1983; **Resid:** Orthopaedic Surgery, UCSD Med Ctr 1988

Delamarter, Rick B MD [OrS] - **Spec Exp:** Spinal Surgery; Minimally Invasive Spinal Surgery; Spinal Disc Replacement; **Hospital:** St John's Hlth Ctr, Santa Monica; **Address:** Spine Inst at Saint John's Health Ctr, 1301 20th St, Ste 400, Santa Monica, CA 90404; **Phone:** 310-828-7757; **Board Cert:** Orthopaedic Surgery 2000; **Med School:** Oregon Hlth Sci Univ 1981; **Resid:** Orthopaedic Surgery, UCLA Med Ctr 1986; **Fac Appt:** Assoc Prof S, UCLA

Dillingham, Michael F MD [OrS] - **Hospital:** Stanford Univ Med Ctr; **Address:** 500 Arguello St, Ste 100, Redwood City, CA 94063; **Phone:** 650-851-4900; **Board Cert:** Orthopaedic Surgery 1977; Physical Medicine & Rehabilitation 1979; **Med School:** Stanford Univ 1971; **Resid:** Orthopaedic Surgery, Standford Univ Med Ctr 1975; Physical Medicine & Rehabilitation, Santa Clara Valley Med Ctr 1977; **Fellow:** Spinal Surgery, Santa Clara Valley Med Ctr 1976; **Fac Appt:** Clin Prof OrS, Stanford Univ

Dorr, Lawrence Douglas MD [OrS] - **Spec Exp:** Hip & Knee Replacement; **Hospital:** Centinela Freeman Reg Med Ctr-Centinela; **Address:** The Arthritis Institute, 501 E Hardy St, Ste 300, Inglewood, CA 90301-4058; **Phone:** 310-695-4800; **Board Cert:** Orthopaedic Surgery 1978; **Med School:** Univ Iowa Coll Med 1967; **Resid:** Orthopaedic Surgery, LAC-USC Med Ctr 1976; **Fellow:** Joint Replacement Surgery, Hosp Special Surg 1977; **Fac Appt:** Prof OrS, USC Sch Med

Eckardt, Jeffrey J MD [OrS] - **Spec Exp:** Bone Tumors; Soft Tissue Tumors; Limb Sparing Surgery; **Hospital:** Santa Monica - UCLA Med Ctr, UCLA Med Ctr; **Address:** UCLA Med Ctr, Dept Ortho Surg/Oncology, 1250 16th St Tower # 745, Santa Monica, CA 90404; **Phone:** 310-319-3816; **Board Cert:** Orthopaedic Surgery 1981; **Med School:** Cornell Univ-Weill Med Coll 1971; **Resid:** Orthopaedic Surgery, UCLA Med Ctr 1979; **Fellow:** Orthopaedic Oncology, Mayo Clinic 1980; **Fac Appt:** Prof OrS, UCLA

Finerman, Gerald MD [OrS] - **Spec Exp:** Sports Medicine; Hip & Knee Replacement; **Hospital:** UCLA Med Ctr, Santa Monica - UCLA Med Ctr; **Address:** UCLA Med Ctr, Dep Orthopaedic Surgery, 10833 Le Conte Ave, rm 76-131, Los Angeles, CA 90095; **Phone:** 310-825-6019; **Board Cert:** Orthopaedic Surgery 1971; **Med School:** Johns Hopkins Univ 1962; **Resid:** Surgery, Johns Hopkins Hosp 1964; Orthopaedic Surgery, Johns Hopkins Hosp 1969; **Fac Appt:** Prof OrS, UCLA

Garfin, Steven R MD [OrS] - **Spec Exp:** Spinal Surgery; **Hospital:** UCSD Med Ctr; **Address:** UCSD, Dept Orthopedic Surgery, 4150 Regents Park Row, La Jolla, CA 92037; **Phone:** 858-657-8200; **Board Cert:** Orthopaedic Surgery 1982; **Med School:** Univ Minn 1972; **Resid:** Orthopaedic Surgery, UCSD Med Ctr 1979; **Fellow:** Spinal Surgery, Pennsylvania Hosp 1981; **Fac Appt:** Prof OrS, UCSD

Goodman, Stuart B MD/PhD [OrS] - **Spec Exp:** Arthritis; Joint Replacement; Reconstructive Surgery; **Hospital:** Stanford Univ Med Ctr, Lucile Packard Chldns Hosp/Stanford Univ Med Ctr; **Address:** Stanford Univ, Div Ortho Surgery, 300 Pasteur, rm R-I05, Stanford, CA 94305-2200; **Phone:** 650-723-7072; **Board Cert:** Orthopaedic Surgery 1998; **Med School:** Univ Toronto 1978; **Resid:** Orthopaedic Surgery, Univ Toronto 1984; **Fellow:** Orthopaedic Surgery, Univ Toronto 1985; **Fac Appt:** Prof OrS, Stanford Univ

Hansen, Sigvard MD [OrS] - **Spec Exp:** Ankle Replacement & Revision; Deformity Reconstruction; Neuromuscular Disorders; **Hospital:** Harborview Med Ctr, Univ Wash Med Ctr; **Address:** Foot & Ankle Institute, 325 9th Ave, Box 359799, Seattle, WA 98104; **Phone:** 206-731-4830; **Board Cert:** Orthopaedic Surgery 1993; **Med School:** Univ Wash 1961; **Resid:** Orthopaedic Surgery, Univ Washington Affil Hosps 1969; **Fellow:** Orthopaedic Surgery, Sheffield Chldrns Hosp 1970; **Fac Appt:** Prof OrS, Univ Wash

Lowenberg, David W MD [OrS] - **Spec Exp:** Osteomyelitis; Limb Lengthening (Ilizarov Procedure); Fractures-Complex & Non Union; Bone Infections; **Hospital:** CA Pacific Med Ctr; **Address:** Dept of Orthopaedic Surgery, 2100 Webster St, Ste 117, San Francisco, CA 94115; **Phone:** 415-600-3835; **Board Cert:** Orthopaedic Surgery 2003; **Med School:** UCLA 1985; **Resid:** Orthopaedic Surgery, UCSF Med Ctr 1990; **Fac Appt:** Assoc Prof OrS, UCSF

Luck Jr, James V MD [OrS] - **Spec Exp:** Hemophilia Related Disease; Hip & Knee Replacement; Musculoskeletal Tumors; **Hospital:** Santa Monica - UCLA Med Ctr; **Address:** 2400 S Flower St, Fl 3, Los Angeles, CA 90007-2660; **Phone:** 213-749-8255; **Board Cert:** Orthopaedic Surgery 2000; **Med School:** USC Sch Med 1967; **Resid:** Orthopaedic Surgery, Orthopaedic Hosp 1973; **Fellow:** Orthopaedic Oncology, Orthopaedic Hosp 1974; Reconstructive Surgery, Rancho Los Amigos 1974; **Fac Appt:** Prof OrS, UCLA

Matsen, Frederick MD [OrS] - **Spec Exp:** Shoulder Replacement; Elbow Replacement; Rotator Cuff Surgery; **Hospital:** Univ Wash Med Ctr; **Address:** Bone & Joint Ctr, UWMC-Roosevelt, 4245 Roosevelt Way NE, Box 354740, Seattle, WA 98105; **Phone:** 206-598-4288; **Board Cert:** Orthopaedic Surgery 1978; **Med School:** Baylor Coll Med 1968; **Resid:** Orthopaedic Surgery, Univ Washington Med Ctr 1974; **Fac Appt:** Prof OrS, Univ Wash

O'Donnell, Richard John MD [OrS] - **Spec Exp:** Bone Cancer; Sarcoma-Soft Tissue; Pediatric Orthopaedic Cancers; **Hospital:** UCSF Med Ctr; **Address:** 1600 Divisadero St Fl 4th, San Francisco, CA 94115; **Phone:** 415-885-3800; **Board Cert:** Orthopaedic Surgery 1999; **Med School:** Harvard Med Sch 1989; **Resid:** Orthopaedic Surgery, Mass Genl Hosp 1995; **Fellow:** Musculoskeletal Oncology, Univ WA Med Ctr 1996; **Fac Appt:** Assoc Prof OrS, UCSF

Patzakis, Michael J MD [OrS] - **Spec Exp:** Osteomyelitis; Fractures-Non Union; Joint Infections; **Hospital:** USC Univ Hosp - R K Eamer Med Plz; **Address:** 1200 N State St GNH3900, Los Angeles, CA 90033-1029; **Phone:** 323-226-7201; **Board Cert:** Orthopaedic Surgery 1983; **Med School:** Ohio State Univ 1963; **Resid:** Orthopaedic Surgery, LAC-USC Med Ctr 1968; **Fellow:** Rheumatology, Univ CO Med Ctr 1969; **Fac Appt:** Prof OrS, USC Sch Med

Peterson, Davis C MD [OrS] - **Spec Exp:** Spinal Surgery; Scoliosis; Trauma; **Hospital:** Providence Alaska Med Ctr, Alaska Regl Hosp; **Address:** 3260 Providence Drive, Ste 200, Anchorage, AK 99508-4603; **Phone:** 907-563-3145; **Board Cert:** Orthopaedic Surgery 1999; **Med School:** Baylor Coll Med 1980; **Resid:** Orthopaedic Surgery, Madigan Army Med Ctr 1986; **Fellow:** Spinal Surgery, St Luke's Med Ctr 1990

Sangeorzan, Bruce J MD [OrS] - **Spec Exp:** Foot & Ankle Surgery; Trauma; **Hospital:** Harborview Med Ctr, Univ Wash Med Ctr; **Address:** 325 9th Ave, Box 359798, Seattle, WA 98104-2499; **Phone:** 206-731-4830; **Board Cert:** Orthopaedic Surgery 2000; **Med School:** Wayne State Univ 1981; **Resid:** Orthopaedic Surgery, Wayne State Univ 1986; **Fellow:** Univ Wash 1987; Foot/Ankle Surgery, Univ Wash 1987; **Fac Appt:** Prof OrS, Univ Wash

Schmalzried, Thomas P MD [OrS] - **Spec Exp:** Hip Replacement; **Hospital:** Orthopaedic Hosp; **Address:** 2400 S Flower St, Los Angeles, CA 90007; **Phone:** 213-742-1075; **Board Cert:** Orthopaedic Surgery 2004; **Med School:** UCLA 1984; **Resid:** Orthopaedic Surgery, UCLA Med Ctr 1990; **Fellow:** Orthopaedic Surgery, UCLA Med Ctr 1987; Hip Surgery, Mass Genl Hosp/Harvard 1991; **Fac Appt:** Asst Prof OrS, UCLA

Schurman, David J MD [OrS] - **Spec Exp:** Hip & Knee Replacement; Sports Medicine; Bone Infections; **Hospital:** Stanford Univ Med Ctr; **Address:** 300 Pasteur Drive, Ste R144, Stanford, CA 94305-5341; **Phone:** 650-723-7608; **Board Cert:** Orthopaedic Surgery 1994; **Med School:** Columbia P&S 1965; **Resid:** Surgery, Mount Sinai Hosp 1967; Orthopaedic Surgery, UCLA Med Ctr 1972; **Fellow:** Arthritis Surgery, UCLA Med Ctr 1973; **Fac Appt:** Prof OrS, Stanford Univ

Singer, Daniel I MD [OrS] - **Spec Exp:** Hand Surgery; Bone Cancer; Hand & Upper Extremity Tumors; **Hospital:** Queen's Med Ctr - Honolulu, Kapiolani Med Ctr @ Pali Momi; **Address:** Queen's Physicians' Office Blg 1, 1380 Lusitana St, Ste 615, Honolulu, HI 96813-2442; **Phone:** 808-521-8109; **Board Cert:** Orthopaedic Surgery 2000; Hand Surgery 2000; **Med School:** Boston Univ 1979; **Resid:** Surgery, Univ Conn Hlth Ctr 1981; Orthopaedic Surgery, Univ Hawaii 1984; **Fellow:** Hand Surgery, Thomas Jefferson Univ Med Ctr 1985; Microvascular Surgery, St Vincent's Hosp 1985; **Fac Appt:** Assoc Prof OrS, Univ Hawaii JA Burns Sch Med

Thalgott, John S MD [OrS] - **Spec Exp:** Spinal Surgery; **Hospital:** Valley Hosp Med Ctr, Sunrise Hosp & Med Ctr/Sunrise Chldn's Hosp; **Address:** 600 S Rancho Drive, Ste 107, Las Vegas, NV 89106; **Phone:** 702-878-8370; **Board Cert:** Orthopaedic Surgery 2000; **Med School:** Washington Univ, St Louis 1979; **Resid:** Orthopaedic Surgery, Barnes Hosp-Wash Univ Med Ctr 1981; Orthopaedic Surgery, LAC/USC Med Ctr 1985; **Fellow:** Spinal Surgery, St Charles Genl Hosp

Tolo, Vernon T MD [OrS] - **Spec Exp:** Pediatric Orthopaedic Surgery; Spinal Deformity-Pediatric; Skeletal Dysplasia; **Hospital:** Chldns Hosp - Los Angeles (page 56), USC Univ Hosp - R K Eamer Med Plz; **Address:** Chldns Hosp LA, 4650 W Sunset Blvd, MS 69, Los Angeles, CA 90027-6062; **Phone:** 323-669-4658; **Board Cert:** Orthopaedic Surgery 1977; **Med School:** Johns Hopkins Univ 1968; **Resid:** Orthopaedic Surgery, Johns Hopkins Hosp 1975; **Fellow:** Pediatric Orthopaedic Surgery, Hosp Sick Chldn 1976; **Fac Appt:** Prof OrS, USC Sch Med

Vail, Thomas Parker MD [OrS] - **Spec Exp:** Hip & Knee Replacement; Hip Resurfacing; Arthritis; Osteonecrosis; **Hospital:** UCSF Med Ctr; **Address:** UCSF Med Center, Box 0728, MU326W, 500 Parnassus Ave, San Francisco, CA 94143; **Phone:** 415-502-7335; **Board Cert:** Orthopaedic Surgery 1994; **Med School:** Loyola Univ-Stritch Sch Med 1985; **Resid:** Thoracic Surgery, Duke Univ Med Ctr 1987; Orthopaedic Surgery, Duke Univ Med Ctr 1991; **Fellow:** Reconstructive Surgery, North Amer/Euro Trav Prgm 1992; **Fac Appt:** Prof OrS, UCSF

Watkins III, Robert G MD [OrS] - **Spec Exp:** Spinal Surgery; Spinal Disc Replacement; **Address:** 13160 Mindanao Way, Ste 325, Marina Del Rey, CA 90292; **Phone:** 310-361-6202; **Board Cert:** Orthopaedic Surgery 1982; **Med School:** Univ Tenn Coll Med, Memphis 1969; **Resid:** Orthopaedic Surgery, LAC-USC Med Ctr 1978; **Fellow:** Spinal Surgery, Jones-Hunt Orth Hosp 1979; **Fac Appt:** Assoc Prof OrS, USC Sch Med

Yoo, Jung MD [OrS] - **Spec Exp:** Spinal Surgery; **Hospital:** OR Hlth & Sci Univ; **Address:** 3181 SW Sam Jackson Park Rd, MC OP-31, Portland, OR 97239; **Phone:** 503-494-6406; **Board Cert:** Orthopaedic Surgery 2004; **Med School:** Univ Chicago-Pritzker Sch Med 1984; **Resid:** Orthopaedic Surgery, Case Western Reserve Univ 1990; **Fellow:** Orthopaedic Surgery, SUNY Hlth Sci Ctr 1991; **Fac Appt:** Prof OrS, Oregon Hlth Sci Univ

Childrens Hospital Los Angeles

4650 Sunset Boulevard
Los Angeles, California 90027
www.ChildrensHospitalLA.org

ChildrensHospitalLosAngeles

International Leader in Pediatrics

Childrens Hospital Los Angeles is acknowledged throughout the United States and around the world for its leadership in pediatric and adolescent health. It is able to offer the very best in multidisciplinary care, with 85 pediatric subspecialties and dozens of special services for children and families. Its physicians are recognized as leaders. Its treatments set the standard of care. Its research is recognized worldwide.

The Heart Institute

The Heart Institute is known throughout the world as a leader in the treatment of pediatric heart disease, offering the most advanced diagnostic and treatment modalities available in cardiology, cardio thoracic surgery, cardio thoracic transplantation and intensive care, as well as innovation in cardiac research. Physicians provide comprehensive care to 8,000 children each year – fetus through adolescent – who have congenital or acquired heart and lung disorders. For information contact (323) 669-4148.

Center for Endocrinology, Diabetes and Metabolism

The Center for Endocrinology, Diabetes and Metabolism is at the forefront of patient care, basic and clinical research in diabetes, obesity, growth, bone metabolism and endocrinology. More than 2,000 children and adolescents with Type 1 and Type 2 diabetes are under the care of its pediatric diabetes specialists, certified diabetes educators and nutritionists – one of the largest programs of its kind in America. For information contact (323) 669-4604.

Childrens Center for Cancer and Blood Diseases

The Childrens Center for Cancer and Blood Diseases is the nation's largest pediatric hematology/oncology program. Physician- scientists integrate their laboratory experience with their clinical expertise in an approach to medical problem-solving that enables them to move effectively from "Bench to Bedside." Breakthroughs in the treatment of childhood cancer, many pioneered at Childrens Hospital Los Angeles, offer children, teenagers and young adults the most advanced treatment available anywhere. For information contact (323) 669-2121.

Childrens Orthopaedic Center

The Childrens Orthopaedic Center is one of the nation's most comprehensive programs dedicated to pediatric musculoskeletal care, education and research. Its Scoliosis and Spine Disorders Program, one of the largest in the country, is the only one of its kind in Los Angeles County devoted exclusively to the pediatric population. Its state-of-the-art Motion Analysis Laboratory is designed to analyze muscle activity and joint movements in children who have difficulty walking, such as those with cerebral palsy, spina bifida and congenital leg conditions. For information contact (323) 669-2142.

602

Cleveland Clinic

Orthopaedic Surgery

The Cleveland Clinic Department of Orthopaedic Surgery has a long history of excellence and innovation in treating musculoskeletal injuries and diseases. For the past several years, *U.S.News & World Report* has consistently ranked the Department of Orthopaedic Surgery among the nation's top five orthopaedic programs.

Foot & Ankle Center – All specialists and surgeons in the Cleveland Clinic Foot and Ankle Center have extensive training in the diagnosis and care of foot and ankle disorders. Our staff of orthopaedic surgeons, podiatrists, nurse clinicians, certified pedorthists and technicians deliver state-of-the-art care exclusively for the foot and ankle.

Joint Replacement – Cleveland Clinic Section of Adult Reconstruction treats osteoarthritis and rheumatoid arthritis of the hip and knee joints, fractures of these joints, and performs joint replacement and revision surgery. At the frontier of surgical developments, our experienced surgeons offer the most advanced implants and minimally invasive techniques to restore patient mobility.

Pediatrics – The Section of Pediatric Orthopaedic Surgery handles more than 11,000 outpatient visits each year. Our physicians offer expertise in the management of all musculoskeletal conditions, including treatment of spinal deformity, hip dysplasia, clubfoot, leg lengthening and limb deformity correction, fractures and growth plate injuries, neuromuscular disorders and sports injuries.

Spine Institute – Cleveland Clinic Spine Institute (CCSI) diagnoses and treats more than 13,000 patients annually. The institute brings together the expertise of specialists in neurosurgery, orthopaedic surgery and non-surgical spine care. CCSI integrates the functions of research, clinical practice, and education.

Research and Education

Established in 2001, the Cleveland Clinic Orthopaedic Research Center (ORC) is a unique collaboration that taps into the synergy between Orthopaedic Surgery and Biomedical Engineering. The Center's mission is to advance the health and treatment of people with disorders of the musculoskeletal system through basic and applied scientific investigation, and to train future leaders in musculoskeletal care, research and education. Recent developments, such as harvesting bone marrow cells to generate new bone tissue, help to advance patient care.

Trauma – Cleveland Clinic has been a leader in the treatment of fracture non-union and in the development of methods to improve outcomes through advanced bone-grafting techniques. Innovative procedures offered are the Ilizarov/Taylor Spatial Frame techniques and the use of fresh frozen osteochondral allografts for traumatic defects in and around the knee.

Tumor – One of the largest multi-disciplinary musculoskeletal tumor centers, we have expertise in treating bone and soft tissue sarcomas and performing limb salvage.

To schedule an appointment or for more information about the Cleveland Clinic Department of Orthopaedic Surgery call 800.890.2467 or visit www.clevelandclinic.org/orthotopdocs.

Department of Orthopaedic Surgery | 9500 Euclid Avenue / W14 | Cleveland OH 44195

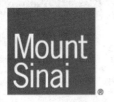

THE MOUNT SINAI MEDICAL CENTER
ORTHOPAEDICS

One Gustave L. Levy Place (Fifth Avenue and 100th Street)
New York, NY 10029-6574
Physician Referral: 1-800-MD-SINAI (637-4624)
www.mountsinai.org

In addition to offering depth and breadth of expertise, The **Leni and Peter W. May Department of Orthopaedics** is known for personalized care. The faculty and staff invest the time to get to know their patients as individuals, ensuring that they receive direct care from subspecialty-trained orthopedists. The faculty share expertise in surgery of the foot and ankle, knee, hip, hand, elbow, shoulder, and spine; total joint replacement (knee, hip, foot and ankle, and shoulder); microvascular surgery; cancer surgery; and minimally invasive surgery. Taking a whole-patient approach to care, they work in close collaboration with specialists in geriatrics, neurology, oncology, pathology, and rehabilitation medicine.

INVESTIGATION AND INNOVATION

Recent years have seen successive refinements in the techniques of orthopedic surgery at Mount Sinai, including the design and composition of the prostheses used in joint replacements that has lead to improved postoperative function. Faculty members have also been instrumental in the design and perfection of hip and shoulder prosthesis. Additionally, Mount Sinai has broadened the applications of arthroscopic surgery—the fiberoptic technology that first heralded the arrival of minimally invasive surgery.

Mount Sinai orthopedic scientists are also known for their studies of "wear and tear" diseases of the skeletal system. Researchers are currently investigating bone wear at the microscopic level, rotator cuff degeneration, factors that predict hip fractures, the effects of microgravity on aging of bones and tissue, how joints of the foot degenerate, methods of determining bone strength, and how genetic alterations change the skeleton's function.

USE OF CUTTING-EDGE TECHNOLOGY

Mount Sinai uses 3-D imaging technology during many of its total knee and total hip replacement surgeries. This allows the surgeon to see multiple views of the anatomy, provides a more exact placement of implants, and lets the surgeon review the joint's range of motion with the implant installed in its final position.

THE MOUNT SINAI MEDICAL CENTER

Today at Mount Sinai, arthroscopy is used to repair not only the knee, but virtually every joint. Converting what used to be major open surgery to outpatient procedures, this has dramatically shortened rehabilitation and return-to-work times. Even more significantly, it has allowed many more patients to get help for painful, function-limiting conditions. That is the case for many elderly or frail patients who would be physically unable to undergo major surgery. The fact that such procedures are now more widely accessible is enhancing the quality of life for many patients and allowing them to lead more active lives.

624

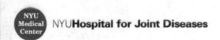

550 First Avenue (at 31st Street)
New York, NY 10016
Physician Referral:
(888)7-NYU-MED (888-769-8633
www.nyumc.org

301 East 17th Street (at 2nd Ave.)
New York, NY 10003
Physician Referral:
(888) HJD-D OCS (888-453-3627)
www.nyuhjd.org

ORTHOPAEDIC SERVICES

Leaders in the treatment of adult and children's bone and joint disorders.

The NYU Hospital for Joint Diseases Department of Orthopaedic Surgery offers the following services and treatments:

General Orthopaedics	Arthritis and Joint Replacement Center
The Spine Center	Arthroscopic Surgery
Pediatric Orthopaedics	Bone Tumors/Orthopaedic Oncology
Foot and Ankle Surgery	Hand Surgery
Limb Lengthening and Bone Growth	Occupational and Industrial Orthopaedic Care
Sports Medicine	Shoulder and Elbow Service
Center for Neuromuscular and Developmental Disorders	The Harkness Center for Dance Injuries
Orthopaedic Urgent Care Center	

NYU Hospital for Joint Diseases provides care at NYU Tisch Hospital, NYU Hospital for Joint Diseases, Manhattan VA, Jamaica Hospital, and Bellevue Hospital Center, where more than 15,000 surgical procedures are performed each year. The orthopaedic faculty maintains offices in all five boroughs as well as in Rockland County and New Jersey.

NYUHJD Orthopaedic Programs and Services

More than 12,000 surgical procedures are performed at the NYU Hospital for Joint Diseases annually. Among our programs and services, we offer the following:

The Joint Replacement Center of NYC: Patients have access to physicians and surgeons highly specialized in treating degenerative joint conditions. Utilizing state-of-the-art techniques, the Center's surgeons are renowned for their expertise in knee, hip and shoulder replacements, complex joint revisions, as well as minimally invasive surgeries. Our center is one of the most active in the world, performing over 2,500 joint replacements annually.

The Spine Center: Provides comprehensive treatment of adult and pediatric spine disorders including lower back pain, neck pain, scoliosis, osteoporosis and the most complex spine problems. We perform minimally invasive spinal fusions that reduce incision size and lead to a speedier recovery. Our Spine Center is distinguished as one of the first in the country to successfully perform artificial disc implantation. We perform over 1,300 spinal procedures each year.

Pediatric Orthopaedic Service: Our skilled specialists provide orthopaedic care for children of all ages with the full spectrum of clinical conditions including neuromuscular diseases such as cerebral palsy, spina bifida and muscular dystrophies and congenital conditions such a clubfoot, hip dysplasia, and limb deformities. Our interdisciplinary approach teams orthopaedic surgeons with pediatric specialists to provide the most up-to-date continuity of care.

Diabetes Foot and Ankle Center: Our main goal is the prevention of foot problems and their recurrence. We offer patients an interdisciplinary team of dedicated medical professionals to provide the most advanced

705

PENN ORTHOPAEDICS

Penn Orthopaedics, a leader in treating patients with musculoskeletal injuries and disorders from the most common to the most complex, provides comprehensive, quality care that ranks among the very best in the nation. Our multidisciplinary team of surgeons and staff use the latest technology and techniques to get people – grandparents and professional athletes alike – back in motion.

Programs

Penn Orthopaedics offers specialized services and programs to treat a wide range of orthopaedic problems, including:
• Foot and ankle
• Hand
• Hip and knee replacements
• Neuro-orthopaedics
• Orthopaedic oncology
• Shoulder and elbow
• Spine
• Sports medicine

Leadership

As recognized clinical leaders, our doctors offer state-of-the-art treatment options, including:

• Advanced minimally invasive joint replacement procedures, such as one and two-incision hip replacements, and surgical navigation, which improves accuracy in hip and knee replacements
• Upper extremity services dedicated to the treatment of shoulder, elbow, wrist and hand disorders

• Treatment for malignant and benign tumors of the bone and soft tissue
• Neuro-orthopaedic procedures to restore range of motion for patients with permanent disabilities following stroke, head injury or cerebral palsy.

Our physicians serve on the boards of the nation's premiere orthopaedic organizations and publish articles in many of the leading orthopaedic journals in the world.

Also a noted research group, Penn Orthopaedics is helping to create the next generation of orthopaedic care, in areas including tissue engineering, tendon healing and biomechanics of the shoulder and spine. Additionally, we are one of the most prominent recipients of orthopaedic grants from the National Institutes of Health.

Expertise

Penn Orthopaedics is consistently recognized as a national leader in outstanding care. Many of our surgeons are listed among the *Best Doctors in America*, and a number of our physicians are listed annually in *Philadelphia* magazine's "Top Docs" issue.

Locations

Hospital of the
University of Pennsylvania

Penn Presbyterian Medical Center

Pennsylvania Hospital

Penn Sports Medicine Center *at Weightman Hall*

Penn Medicine at Cherry Hill

Penn Medicine at Radnor

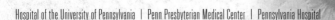

Hospital of the University of Pennsylvania | Penn Presbyterian Medical Center | Pennsylvania Hospital

Wake Forest University Baptist
M E D I C A L   C E N T E R ®

Orthopaedics

Medical Center Boulevard • Winston-Salem, NC 27157 • 336-716-2011
Health On-Call® (Patient access) 1-800-446-2255
PAL® (Physician-to-physician calls) 1-800-277-7654
www.wfubmc.edu

Wake Forest University Baptist Medical Center offers comprehensive programs in all facets of bone and joint care including innovative therapies that are setting the standards for orthopaedics, bone and joint replacement and sports medicine. Surgeons here are pioneers in the use of botox® injections for treating spasticity disorders.

PROGRAM HIGHLIGHTS

The **Wake Forest Institute for Tissue Engineering** is leading the way in the use of patients' own cells to develop tissues and organs in the laboratory. Multiple projects underway that would benefit patients with orthopaedic injuries include the development of ligament and meniscus replacements, technologies to improve nerve regeneration and methods of bone regeneration.

The **Orthopaedic Oncology Program** offers a comprehensive team of specialists who provide the most advanced diagnostic technologies and treatment modalities available for patients with benign or malignant bone and soft tissue tumors. The program utilizes limb-sparing techniques and offers expertise in limb salvage and reconstruction.

The **Comprehensive Joint Replacement Program** employs the most advanced technologies and surgical techniques for hip and knee replacements and specialized after-surgery care. The Program is one of only a few in North Carolina to offer hip resurfacing, an alternative to hip replacement for patients who want to remain active after surgery.

The **Upper Extremity Program** offers nationally and internationally recognized experts utilizing minimally invasive arthroscopy procedures for the shoulder, elbow and wrist to treat degenerative conditions as well as traumatic injuries such as rotator cuff tears. The program has multiple specialists who provide joint replacements of all joints in the arm, particularly the shoulder, wrist, elbow and hand. The Hand Therapy Center, one of the first in North Carolina, offers integrated physician and therapy teams specially trained in the care and management of upper extremity disorders.

Pediatric Orthopaedic Services offers experts with specialty training in acquired and congenital disorders of children, and nerve disorders as simple as carpal tunnel procedures and as complex as nerve reconstruction involving the brachial plexus, incorporating a multidisciplinary approach with neurologists, therapists and rehabilitation specialists. The Pediatric Physical and Occupational Therapy Center boasts a specialty-trained dedicated staff.

The **Sports Medicine Program** is comprised of a network of the region's most qualified physicians and therapists working collaboratively to provide the most comprehensive, evidence-based approach to treatment of sports related injuries. The team utilizes an individualized approach to treating athletes and persons whose physical abilities have been limited by injury, degenerative disease or aging.

It is the only center in the state to use "motion monitor" technology in a clinical setting. This sophisticated system allows therapists to analyze motion – such as running, pitching or a golf swing - on a computer, allowing the therapist to look at the body as an interconnected system and to develop more comprehensive treatment and performance enhancement programs.

Wake Forest Baptist has 13 digital operating rooms for orthopaedic surgeries – more than any other center in the United States. This technology enables physicians to capture procedures on video and still images so the patient can be followed appropriately.

KNOWLEDGE MAKES ALL THE DIFFERENCE.

Otolaryngology

An otolaryngologist-head and neck surgeon provides comprehensive medical and surgical care for patients with diseases and disorders that affect the ears, nose, throat, the respiratory and upper alimentary systems and related structures of the head and neck.

An otolaryngologist diagnoses and provides medical and/or surgical therapy or prevention of diseases, allergies, neoplasms, deformities, disorders and/or injuries of the ears, nose, sinuses, throat, respiratory and upper alimentary systems, face, jaws and the other head and neck systems. Head and neck oncology, facial plastic and reconstructive surgery and the treatment of disorders of hearing and voice are fundamental areas of expertise.

Training Required: Five years

Certification in the following subspecialty requires additional training and examination.

Plastic Surgery within the Head and Neck: An otolaryngologist with additional training in plastic and reconstructive procedures within the head, face, neck and associated structures, including cutaneous head and neck oncology and reconstruction, management of maxillofacial trauma, soft tissue repair and neural surgery.

(continued on the next page)

Facial Plastic and Reconstructive Surgery is not a recognized ABMS subspecialty. However this designation has been included because the certification process is meaningful and rigorous. It is awarded to those doctors who hold a current ABMS certification in Otolaryngology, but those board certified in Plastic Surgery, Ophthalmology, or Dermatology are also eligible. Certification requires a post-graduate fellowship in Facial Plastic and Reconstructive Surgery followed by a written examination.

This field is diverse and involves a wide age range of patients, from the newborn to the aged. While both cosmetic and reconstructive surgeries are practiced, there are many additional procedures which interface with them.

Otolaryngology

New England

Deschler, Daniel G MD [Oto] - **Spec Exp:** Head & Neck Cancer; Head & Neck Reconstruction; Salivary Gland Tumors & Surgery; **Hospital:** Mass Eye & Ear Infirmary; **Address:** Mass Eye & Ear Infirmary, Head & Neck Surgery, 243 Charles St, Boston, MA 02114; **Phone:** 617-573-4100; **Board Cert:** Otolaryngology 1996; **Med School:** Harvard Med Sch 1990; **Resid:** Otolaryngology, UCSF Med Ctr 1995; **Fellow:** Facial Plastic & Reconstructive Surgery, Hahneman U Med Ctr 1996; **Fac Appt:** Assoc Prof Oto, Harvard Med Sch

Gliklich, Richard E MD [Oto] - **Spec Exp:** Cosmetic Surgery-Face & Neck; Rhinoplasty; Skin Laser Surgery-Resurfacing; **Hospital:** Mass Eye & Ear Infirmary; **Address:** Mass Eye & Ear Infirmary, 243 Charles St Fl 9, Boston, MA 02114; **Phone:** 617-573-4105; **Board Cert:** Otolaryngology 1994; Facial Plastic & Reconstructive Surgery 1996; **Med School:** Harvard Med Sch 1988; **Resid:** Otolaryngology, Mass E&E Infirmary 1993; **Fellow:** Otolaryngology, Mass E&E Infirmary 1994; **Fac Appt:** Assoc Prof Oto, Harvard Med Sch

Grundfast, Kenneth MD [Oto] - **Spec Exp:** Hearing Loss; Pediatric Otolaryngology; **Hospital:** Boston Med Ctr; **Address:** Boston Medical Center, 830 Harrison Ave, Ste 1400, Boston, MA 02119; **Phone:** 617-638-8124; **Board Cert:** Otolaryngology 1977; **Med School:** SUNY Upstate Med Univ 1969; **Resid:** Surgery, Sibley Meml Hosp 1974; Otolaryngology, Boston-Affil Hosps 1977; **Fellow:** Pediatric Otolaryngology, Chldns Hosp 1978; **Fac Appt:** Prof Oto, Boston Univ

Kveton, John MD [Oto] - **Spec Exp:** Ear Disorders; Cochlear Implants; Acoustic Neuroma; **Hospital:** Yale - New Haven Hosp, Hosp of St Raphael; **Address:** 46 Prince St, Ste 601, New Haven, CT 06519-1634; **Phone:** 203-752-1726; **Board Cert:** Otolaryngology 1982; Neurotology 2004; **Med School:** St Louis Univ 1978; **Resid:** Otolaryngology, Yale-New Haven Hosp 1982; **Fellow:** Neurotology, The Otology Group 1983; **Fac Appt:** Clin Prof Oto, Yale Univ

McKenna, Michael J MD [Oto] - **Spec Exp:** Skull Base Surgery; Otology; Neuro-Otology; **Hospital:** Mass Eye & Ear Infirmary; **Address:** Massachusetts Eye & Ear Infirmary, 243 Charles St, Boston, MA 02114-3002; **Phone:** 617-573-3672; **Board Cert:** Otolaryngology 1988; Neurotology 2004; **Med School:** USC Sch Med 1982; **Resid:** Otolaryngology, Mass Eye & Ear Infirm 1988; **Fellow:** Neurotology, Otologic Med Group 1989; **Fac Appt:** Prof Oto, Harvard Med Sch

Metson, Ralph MD [Oto] - **Spec Exp:** Sinus Disorders/Surgery; Facial Plastic Surgery; **Hospital:** Mass Eye & Ear Infirmary; **Address:** Zero Emerson Pl, Ste 2D, Boston, MA 02114; **Phone:** 617-227-4366; **Board Cert:** Otolaryngology 1985; **Med School:** UCSD 1979; **Resid:** Otolaryngology, UCLA Med Ctr 1985; **Fac Appt:** Assoc Clin Prof Oto, Harvard Med Sch

Nadol, Joseph B MD [Oto] - **Spec Exp:** Ear Disorders/Surgery; Hearing Disorders; Cochlear Implants; **Hospital:** Mass Eye & Ear Infirmary; **Address:** Mass Eye & Ear Infirmary, 243 Charles St, Boston, MA 02114-3096; **Phone:** 617-573-3632; **Board Cert:** Otolaryngology 1975; Neurotology 2005; **Med School:** Johns Hopkins Univ 1970; **Resid:** Surgery, Beth Israel Hosp 1972; Otolaryngology, Mass Eye & Ear Infirmary 1975; **Fac Appt:** Prof Oto, Harvard Med Sch

Otolaryngology

Poe, Dennis MD [Oto] - **Spec Exp:** Cochlear Implants; Neuro-Otology; Ear Disorders/Surgery; **Hospital:** Children's Hospital - Boston; **Address:** Chldns Hosp, Dept Otolaryngology, 300 Longwood Ave, LO-367, Boston, MA 02115-5724; **Phone:** 617-355-3794; **Board Cert:** Otolaryngology 1987; Neurotology 2004; **Med School:** SUNY Upstate Med Univ 1982; **Resid:** Surgery, Univ Mass Med Ctr 1983; Otolaryngology, Univ Chicago Hosps 1987; **Fellow:** Otology & Neurotology, Otology Group 1988; **Fac Appt:** Assoc Prof Oto, Harvard Med Sch

Randolph, Gregory W MD [Oto] - **Spec Exp:** Thyroid Disorders; Thyroid Cancer; Parathyroid Disease; **Hospital:** Mass Eye & Ear Infirmary; **Address:** Mass Eye & Ear Infirmary, 243 Charles St Fl 2, Boston, MA 02114; **Phone:** 617-573-4115; **Board Cert:** Otolaryngology 1993; **Med School:** Cornell Univ-Weill Med Coll 1987; **Resid:** Otolaryngology, Mass E&E Infirmary 1992; **Fellow:** Thyroid Oncology, Mass E&E Infirmary 1993; **Fac Appt:** Asst Prof Oto, Harvard Med Sch

Rauch, Steven D MD [Oto] - **Spec Exp:** Hearing & Balance Disorders; Meniere's Disease; Neuro-Otology; **Hospital:** Mass Eye & Ear Infirmary; **Address:** Mass Eye & Ear Infirmary, Dept Otolary, 243 Charles St, Boston, MA 02114; **Phone:** 617-573-3644; **Board Cert:** Otolaryngology 1984; **Med School:** Univ Cincinnati 1979; **Resid:** Surgery, U Mass Med Ctr 1981; Otolaryngology, Mass E&E Infirmary 1984; **Fac Appt:** Assoc Prof Oto, Harvard Med Sch

Sasaki, Clarence T MD [Oto] - **Spec Exp:** Head & Neck Cancer; Skull Base Surgery; Voice Disorders; Swallowing Disorders; **Hospital:** Yale - New Haven Hosp, Hosp of St Raphael; **Address:** Yale Sch Med, Dept Otolaryngology, 333 Cedar St, Box 208041, New Haven, CT 06520-8041; **Phone:** 203-785-2592; **Board Cert:** Otolaryngology 1973; **Med School:** Yale Univ 1966; **Resid:** Surgery, Mary Hitchcock Hosp 1968; Otolaryngology, Yale-New Haven Hosp 1973; **Fellow:** Head and Neck Surgery, Univ of Milan 1978; Skull Base Surgery, Univ Zurich 1982; **Fac Appt:** Prof Oto, Yale Univ

Vining, Eugenia MD [Oto] - **Spec Exp:** Sinus Disorders/Surgery; **Hospital:** Yale - New Haven Hosp, Hosp of St Raphael; **Address:** 46 Prince St, Ste 601, New Haven, CT 06519; **Phone:** 203-752-1726; **Board Cert:** Otolaryngology 1993; **Med School:** Yale Univ 1987; **Resid:** Otolaryngology, Yale-New Haven Hosp 1991; Otolaryngology, Yale-New Haven Hosp 1992; **Fellow:** Sinus Surgery, Univ Penn Med Ctr 1993

Zeitels, Steven MD [Oto] - **Spec Exp:** Laryngeal Disorders; Voice Disorders; Head & Neck Surgery; **Hospital:** Mass Genl Hosp; **Address:** Mass Genl Hospital, 1 Bowdoin Square Fl 11, Boston, MA 02114; **Phone:** 617-726-1444; **Board Cert:** Otolaryngology 1988; **Med School:** Boston Univ 1982; **Resid:** Surgery, Univ Hosp-Boston City Hosp 1983; Otolaryngology, Boston Univ-Tufts Univ 1987; **Fellow:** Head and Neck Surgery, Boston VA Med Ctr-Boston Univ 1988; **Fac Appt:** Assoc Prof Oto, Harvard Med Sch

Mid Atlantic

Abramson, Allan MD [Oto] - **Spec Exp:** Head & Neck Cancer & Surgery; Laryngeal Cancer; Hearing Disorders; **Hospital:** Long Island Jewish Med Ctr; **Address:** LIJ Med Ctr, Dept Otolaryngology, 270-05 76th Ave, Ste 1120, New Hyde Park, NY 11040; **Phone:** 516-470-7555; **Board Cert:** Otolaryngology 1972; **Med School:** SUNY Downstate 1967; **Resid:** Surgery, LI Jewish-Hillside Med Ctr 1969; Otolaryngology, Mount Sinai Med Ctr 1972; **Fac Appt:** Prof Oto, Albert Einstein Coll Med

Arriaga, Moises Alberto MD [Oto] - **Spec Exp:** Hearing Loss; Acoustic Neuroma; Balance Disorders; Otology & Neurotology; **Hospital:** Allegheny General Hosp, Mercy Hosp - Pittsburgh; **Address:** 420 E North Ave, Ste 402, Pittsburgh, PA 15212; **Phone:** 412-359-6690; **Board Cert:** Otolaryngology 1990; Neurotology 2004; **Med School:** Brown Univ 1985; **Resid:** Otolaryngology, Univ Pittsburgh Med Ctr 1990; **Fellow:** Neurotology, House Ear Clinic 1991; **Fac Appt:** Assoc Clin Prof Oto, Univ Pittsburgh

Aviv, Jonathan MD [Oto] - **Spec Exp:** Voice Disorders; Swallowing Disorders; Vocal Cord Disorders; Endoscopy; **Hospital:** NY-Presby Hosp/Columbia (page 66); **Address:** 16 E 60th St, Ste 470, New York, NY 10022-1002; **Phone:** 212-326-8475; **Board Cert:** Otolaryngology 1990; **Med School:** Columbia P&S 1985; **Resid:** Surgery, Mount Sinai Med Ctr 1987; Otolaryngology, Mount Sinai Med Ctr 1990; **Fellow:** Otolaryngology, Mount Sinai Med Ctr 1991; **Fac Appt:** Prof Oto, Columbia P&S

Blitzer, Andrew MD/DDS [Oto] - **Spec Exp:** Voice Disorders; Swallowing Disorders; Nasal & Sinus Surgery; Botox Therapy; **Hospital:** St Luke's - Roosevelt Hosp Ctr - Roosevelt Div, NY-Presby Hosp/Columbia (page 66); **Address:** 425 W 59th St Fl 10, New York, NY 10019-1104; **Phone:** 212-262-9500; **Board Cert:** Otolaryngology 1977; **Med School:** Mount Sinai Sch Med 1973; **Resid:** Surgery, Beth Israel Med Ctr 1974; Otolaryngology, Mount Sinai Hosp 1977; **Fac Appt:** Clin Prof Oto, Columbia P&S

Bolger, William E MD [Oto] - **Spec Exp:** Nasal & Sinus Surgery; Encephalocele; **Hospital:** Suburban Hosp - Bethesda; **Address:** Suburban ENT Associates, 6420 Rockledge Drive, Ste 4200, Bethesda, MD 20817; **Phone:** 301-896-6840; **Board Cert:** Otolaryngology 1992; **Med School:** Uniformed Srvs Univ, Bethesda 1986; **Resid:** Otolaryngology, Willford Hall USAF Med Ctr 1991; **Fellow:** Sinus Surgery, Univ Penn Med Ctr 1992; **Fac Appt:** Prof Oto, Uniformed Srvs Univ, Bethesda

Carrau, Ricardo L MD [Oto] - **Spec Exp:** Skull Base Tumors & Surgery; Nasal & Sinus Cancer & Surgery; Swallowing Disorders; **Hospital:** UPMC Presby, Pittsburgh; **Address:** Eye & Ear Institute, 200 Lothrop St, Ste 500, Pittsburgh, PA 15213; **Phone:** 412-647-2100; **Board Cert:** Otolaryngology 1987; **Med School:** Univ Puerto Rico 1981; **Resid:** Surgery, University Hosp 1984; Head and Neck Surgery, University Hosp 1987; **Fellow:** Head and Neck Oncology, Univ Pittsburgh Med Ctr 1990; **Fac Appt:** Assoc Prof Oto, Univ Pittsburgh

Chalian, Ara A MD [Oto] - **Spec Exp:** Head & Neck Cancer; Head & Neck Reconstruction; Thyroid Cancer; Reconstructive Plastic Surgery; **Hospital:** Hosp Univ Penn - UPHS (page 72); **Address:** Hosp U Penn, Dept Otolaryngology, 3400 Spruce St, Silverstein Bldg, Philadelphia, PA 19104; **Phone:** 215-349-5559; **Board Cert:** Otolaryngology 1994; **Med School:** Indiana Univ 1988; **Resid:** Surgery, Indiana Univ Hosp 1990; Otolaryngology, Indiana Univ Hosp 1993; **Fellow:** Molecular Biology, Hosp U Penn 1994; Head and Neck Surgery, Hosp U Penn 1995; **Fac Appt:** Assoc Prof Oto, Univ Pennsylvania

Close, Lanny G MD [Oto] - **Spec Exp:** Skull Base Surgery; Head & Neck Cancer; Sinus Disorders/Surgery; Endoscopic Sinus Surgery; **Hospital:** NY-Presby Hosp/Columbia (page 66); **Address:** 16 E 60th St, Ste 470, New York, NY 10022; **Phone:** 212-326-8475; **Board Cert:** Otolaryngology 1977; **Med School:** Baylor Coll Med 1972; **Resid:** Surgery, Johns Hopkins Hosp 1974; Otolaryngology, Baylor Affil Hosps 1977; **Fellow:** Head and Neck Surgery, MD Anderson Cancer Ctr 1979; **Fac Appt:** Prof Oto, Columbia P&S

Costantino, Peter D MD [Oto] - **Spec Exp:** Skull Base Tumors; Head & Neck Cancer; Craniofacial Surgery/Reconstruction; **Hospital:** St Luke's - Roosevelt Hosp Ctr - Roosevelt Div, NY-Presby Hosp/Columbia (page 66); **Address:** 1000 W 10th Ave, Ste 5G-80, New York, NY 10019-1104; **Phone:** 212-523-6756; **Board Cert:** Otolaryngology 1990; Facial Plastic & Reconstructive Surgery 2000; **Med School:** Northwestern Univ 1984; **Resid:** Surgery, Northwestern Meml Hosp 1986; Otolaryngology, Northwestern Meml Hosp 1989; **Fellow:** Head and Neck Surgery, Northwestern Meml Hosp 1990; Skull Base Surgery, Univ Pittsburgh 1991; **Fac Appt:** Prof Oto, Columbia P&S

Cummings, Charles MD [Oto] - **Spec Exp:** Head & Neck Cancer & Surgery; Laryngeal Disorders; Laryngeal Cancer; **Hospital:** Johns Hopkins Hosp - Baltimore (page 61); **Address:** Johns Hopkins Outpt Ctr, Otolaryngology, 601 N Caroline St Fl 6, Baltimore, MD 21287; **Phone:** 410-955-7400; **Board Cert:** Otolaryngology 1968; **Med School:** Univ VA Sch Med 1961; **Resid:** Surgery, Univ Virginia Hosp 1965; Otolaryngology, Mass Genl Hosp 1968; **Fac Appt:** Prof Oto, Johns Hopkins Univ

Davidson, Bruce J MD [Oto] - **Spec Exp:** Head & Neck Cancer; Thyroid Disorders; **Hospital:** Georgetown Univ Hosp; **Address:** Georgetown Univ Med Ctr, Dept Oto, 3800 Reservoir Rd NW, 1st fl Gorman, Washington, DC 20007; **Phone:** 202-444-8186; **Board Cert:** Otolaryngology 1993; **Med School:** W VA Univ 1987; **Resid:** Otolaryngology, Georgetown Univ Med Ctr 1992; **Fellow:** Otolaryngology, Memorial Sloan-Kettering Cancer Ctr 1994; **Fac Appt:** Asst Prof Oto, Georgetown Univ

Edelstein, David R MD [Oto] - **Spec Exp:** Nasal & Sinus Disorders; Endoscopic Sinus Surgery; Sleep Disorders/Apnea; **Hospital:** Manhattan Eye, Ear & Throat Hosp, Lenox Hill Hosp (page 62); **Address:** 1421 3rd Ave Fl 4, New York, NY 10028; **Phone:** 212-452-1500; **Board Cert:** Otolaryngology 1985; **Med School:** Boston Univ 1980; **Resid:** Otolaryngology, Mount Sinai Hosp 1984; **Fac Appt:** Clin Prof Oto, Cornell Univ-Weill Med Coll

Fried, Marvin P MD [Oto] - **Spec Exp:** Endoscopic Sinus Surgery; Laryngeal & Voice Disorders; Head & Neck Tumors; **Hospital:** Montefiore Med Ctr, Montefiore Med Ctr - Weiler-Einstein Div; **Address:** 3400 Bainbridge Ave Fl 3, Bronx, NY 10467; **Phone:** 718-920-4646; **Board Cert:** Otolaryngology 1975; **Med School:** Tufts Univ 1969; **Resid:** Surgery, Jewish Hosp 1971; Otolaryngology, Barnes Hosp 1975; **Fellow:** Stroke, Washington Univ 1976; **Fac Appt:** Prof Oto, Albert Einstein Coll Med

Genden, Eric M MD [Oto] - **Spec Exp:** Head & Neck Cancer & Surgery; Head & Neck Reconstruction; Airway Reconstruction; Thyroid & Parathyroid Cancer & Surgery; **Hospital:** Mount Sinai Med Ctr; **Address:** Mt Sinai Sch Med Dept Otolar, 1 Gustave L. Levy Pl, Box 1191, New York, NY 10029; **Phone:** 212-241-9410; **Board Cert:** Otolaryngology 1999; Facial Plastic & Reconstructive Surgery 2000; **Med School:** Mount Sinai Sch Med 1992; **Resid:** Otolaryngology, Barnes Jewish Hosp 1998; **Fellow:** Head and Neck Surgery, Mount Sinai Med Ctr 1999; **Fac Appt:** Assoc Prof Oto, Mount Sinai Sch Med

Gold, Scott MD [Oto] - **Spec Exp:** Endoscopic Sinus Surgery; Sinus Disorders/Surgery; **Hospital:** Beth Israel Med Ctr - Petrie Division, Mount Sinai Med Ctr; **Address:** 36A E 36th St, Ste 200, New York, NY 10016-3401; **Phone:** 212-889-8575; **Board Cert:** Otolaryngology 1983; **Med School:** Mount Sinai Sch Med 1979; **Resid:** Otolaryngology, Mount Sinai Med Ctr 1983; **Fac Appt:** Asst Clin Prof Oto, Mount Sinai Sch Med

Har-El, Gady MD [Oto] - **Spec Exp:** Head & Neck Cancer; Sinus Disorders/Surgery; Thyroid & Parathyroid Surgery; Skull Base Surgery; **Hospital:** Lenox Hill Hosp (page 62), Manhattan Eye Ear and Throat Hosp; **Address:** 186 E 76th St, Floor 2, New York, NY 10021; **Phone:** 212-434-2323; **Board Cert:** Otolaryngology 1992; **Med School:** Israel 1982; **Resid:** Otolaryngology, SUNY Downstate Med Ctr 1991; **Fac Appt:** Prof Oto, SUNY Hlth Sci Ctr

Hicks Jr, Wesley L MD/DDS [Oto] - **Spec Exp:** Head & Neck Cancer & Surgery; Reconstructive Surgery; **Hospital:** Roswell Park Cancer Inst; **Address:** Roswell Park Cancer Inst, Head & Neck Surg, Elm & Carlton Sts, Buffalo, NY 14263; **Phone:** 716-845-3158; **Board Cert:** Otolaryngology 1993; **Med School:** SUNY Buffalo 1984; **Resid:** Otolaryngology, Manhattan Eye Ear & Throat Hosp 1988; Otolaryngology, New York Hosp/Meml Sloan Kettering Cancer Ctr 1989; **Fellow:** Head and Neck Surgery, Stanford Univ Med Ctr 1990; **Fac Appt:** Assoc Prof Oto, SUNY Buffalo

Hirsch, Barry MD [Oto] - **Spec Exp:** Hearing Loss; Ear Infections; Ear Tumors; Skull Base Tumors; **Hospital:** UPMC Presby, Pittsburgh; **Address:** 200 Lothrop St, Ste 500, Ear Nose Throat Inst, Dept Otolaryngology, Pittsburgh, PA 15213; **Phone:** 412-647-2100; **Board Cert:** Otolaryngology 1982; Neurotology 2005; **Med School:** Univ Pennsylvania 1977; **Resid:** Otolaryngology, Univ Pittsburgh Med Ctr 1982; **Fellow:** Neurotology, Univ Pittsburgh 1985; Neurotology, Univ Zurich 1986; **Fac Appt:** Prof Oto, Univ Pittsburgh

Hurst, Michael K MD/DDS [Oto] - **Spec Exp:** Nasal Allergy; Sleep Disorders/Apnea; Thyroid Surgery; **Hospital:** WV Univ Hosp - Ruby Memorial, Monongalia Genl Hosp; **Address:** 1188 Pineview Drive, Morgantown, WV 26505; **Phone:** 304-599-3959; **Board Cert:** Otolaryngology 1994; **Med School:** Marshall Univ 1988; **Resid:** Otolaryngology, Univ West Virginia Hosps 1993; **Fac Appt:** Assoc Prof Oto, W VA Univ

Johnson, Jonas T MD [Oto] - **Spec Exp:** Head & Neck Surgery; Head & Neck Cancer; Sleep Disorders/Apnea/Snoring; **Hospital:** UPMC Presby, Pittsburgh, Magee-Womens Hosp - UPMC; **Address:** Univ Physicians UPMC, Eye & Ear Inst, 200 Lothrop St, Ste 300, Pittsburgh, PA 15213; **Phone:** 412-647-2100; **Board Cert:** Otolaryngology 1977; **Med School:** SUNY Upstate Med Univ 1972; **Resid:** Surgery, Med Coll Virginia Hosps 1974; Otolaryngology, SUNY-Univ Hosp 1977; **Fac Appt:** Prof Oto, Univ Pittsburgh

Josephson, Jordan S MD [Oto] - **Spec Exp:** Endoscopic Sinus Surgery; Sinus Surgery; Nasal & Sinus Disorders; Sleep Apnea; **Hospital:** Manhattan Eye, Ear & Throat Hosp, Lenox Hill Hosp (page 62); **Address:** 111 E 77th St, New York, NY 10021-1802; **Phone:** 212-717-1773; **Board Cert:** Otolaryngology 1988; **Med School:** SUNY Downstate 1983; **Resid:** Otolaryngology, LI Jewish Med Ctr 1988; **Fellow:** Sinus Surgery, Johns Hopkins Hosp 1989

Keane, William M MD [Oto] - **Spec Exp:** Head & Neck Cancer & Surgery; Thyroid Cancer; Sinus Disorders/Surgery; **Hospital:** Thomas Jefferson Univ Hosp; **Address:** Thomas Jefferson Hosp, 925 Chestnut St Fl 6, Philadelphia, PA 19107; **Phone:** 215-955-6760; **Board Cert:** Otolaryngology 1978; **Med School:** Harvard Med Sch 1970; **Resid:** Surgery, Strong Meml Hosp 1972; Otolaryngology, Univ Penn Hosp 1977; **Fac Appt:** Prof Oto, Thomas Jefferson Univ

Otolaryngology

Kennedy, David W MD [Oto] - **Spec Exp:** Sinus Disorders/Surgery; Skull Base Tumors & Surgery; Endoscopic Sinus Surgery; Minimally Invasive Transnasal Surgery; **Hospital:** Hosp Univ Penn - UPHS (page 72), Pennsylvania Hosp (page 72); **Address:** Hosp Univ Penn, Dept Oto/Head & Neck Surg, 3400 Spruce St Ravdin Bldg Fl 5, Philadelphia, PA 19104; **Phone:** 215-662-6971; **Board Cert:** Otolaryngology 1978; **Med School:** Ireland 1972; **Resid:** Surgery, Johns Hopkins Hosp 1974; Otolaryngology, Johns Hopkins Hosp 1978; **Fac Appt:** Prof Oto, Univ Pennsylvania

Koch, Wayne Martin MD [Oto] - **Spec Exp:** Head & Neck Cancer; Sinus Tumors; **Hospital:** Johns Hopkins Hosp - Baltimore (page 61); **Address:** Johns Hopkins Hosp, Dept Otolaryngology, 601 N Caroline St, rm 6221, Baltimore, MD 21287; **Phone:** 410-955-4906; **Board Cert:** Otolaryngology 1987; **Med School:** Univ Pittsburgh 1982; **Resid:** Otolaryngology, Tufts-Boston Univ Hosps 1987; **Fellow:** Surgical Oncology, Johns Hopkins Hosp 1989; **Fac Appt:** Assoc Prof Oto, Johns Hopkins Univ

Koufman, Jamie A MD [Oto] - **Spec Exp:** Voice Disorders; Laryngeal Disorders; **Hospital:** New York Eye & Ear Infirm (page 65); **Address:** NY Eye & Ear Infirmary, 9 W 67th St, New York, NY 10023; **Phone:** 212-884-8277; **Board Cert:** Otolaryngology 1978; **Med School:** Boston Univ 1973; **Resid:** Surgery, Hartford Hosp 1975; Otolaryngology, Boston Univ Med Ctr 1978

Kraus, Dennis MD [Oto] - **Spec Exp:** Head & Neck Cancer; Skull Base Tumors; Thyroid & Parathyroid Surgery; **Hospital:** Meml Sloan Kettering Cancer Ctr; **Address:** Memorial Sloan Kettering Cancer Ctr, 1275 York Ave, Box 285, New York, NY 10021-6007; **Phone:** 212-639-5621; **Board Cert:** Otolaryngology 1990; **Med School:** Univ Rochester 1985; **Resid:** Surgery, Cleveland Clinic Hosp 1987; Otolaryngology, Cleveland Clinic Hosp 1990; **Fellow:** Head and Neck Surgery, Meml Sloan Kettering Cancer Ctr 1991; **Fac Appt:** Prof Oto, Cornell Univ-Weill Med Coll

Krespi, Yosef MD [Oto] - **Spec Exp:** Nasal & Sinus Cancer & Surgery; Sleep Disorders/Apnea; Head & Neck Cancer & Surgery; Laser Surgery; **Hospital:** St Luke's - Roosevelt Hosp Ctr - Roosevelt Div; **Address:** 425 W 59th St Fl 10, New York, NY 10019-1128; **Phone:** 212-262-4444; **Board Cert:** Otolaryngology 1981; **Med School:** Israel 1973; **Resid:** Surgery, Mount Sinai Hosp 1976; Otolaryngology, Mount Sinai Hosp 1980; **Fellow:** Surgery, Northwestern Meml Hosp 1981; **Fac Appt:** Clin Prof Oto, Columbia P&S

Lawson, William MD [Oto] - **Spec Exp:** Sinus Disorders/Surgery; Cosmetic Surgery-Face; Head & Neck Cancer; Skull Base Surgery; **Hospital:** Mount Sinai Med Ctr; **Address:** 5 E 98th St Fl 8, Box 1191, New York, NY 10029-6501; **Phone:** 212-241-9410; **Board Cert:** Otolaryngology 1974; **Med School:** NYU Sch Med 1965; **Resid:** Surgery, Bronx VA Hosp 1967; Otolaryngology, Mount Sinai Hosp 1973; **Fellow:** Otolaryngology, Mount Sinai Hosp 1970; **Fac Appt:** Prof Oto, Mount Sinai Sch Med

Linstrom, Christopher MD [Oto] - **Spec Exp:** Cochlear Implants; Acoustic Neuroma; Encephalocele; Cholesteatoma; **Hospital:** New York Eye & Ear Infirm (page 65), St Vincent Cath Med Ctrs - Manhattan; **Address:** NY Eye & Ear Infirmary, Dept Otolaryngology, 310 E 14th St Fl 6, New York, NY 10003-4201; **Phone:** 212-979-4200; **Board Cert:** Otolaryngology 1987; **Med School:** McGill Univ 1982; **Resid:** Surgery, Geo Wash Med Ctr 1984; Otolaryngology, New York Hosp 1987; **Fellow:** Otology & Neurotology, Michigan Ear Inst 1989; **Fac Appt:** Assoc Prof Oto, NY Med Coll

Minor, Lloyd B MD [Oto] - **Spec Exp:** Balance Disorders; Neuro-Otology; Meniere's Disease; **Hospital:** Johns Hopkins Hosp - Baltimore (page 61); **Address:** 601 N Caroline St, rm 6210, Baltimore, MD 21287; **Phone:** 410-955-1080; **Board Cert:** Otolaryngology 1993; Neurotology 2004; **Med School:** Brown Univ 1982; **Resid:** Otolaryngology, Univ Chicago Hosps 1992; **Fellow:** Otolaryngology, Ear Foundation/Baptist Hosp 1993; **Fac Appt:** Prof Oto, Johns Hopkins Univ

Moscatello, Augustine L MD [Oto] - **Spec Exp:** Nasal & Sinus Disorders; Head & Neck Surgery; **Hospital:** Westchester Med Ctr; **Address:** 1055 Sawmill River Rd, Ste 101, Ardsley, NY 10502; **Phone:** 914-693-7636; **Board Cert:** Otolaryngology 1987; **Med School:** Mount Sinai Sch Med 1982; **Resid:** Surgery, Mount Sinai Hosp 1987; Otolaryngology, Mount Sinai Hosp 1987; **Fac Appt:** Assoc Prof Oto, NY Med Coll

Myers, Eugene MD [Oto] - **Spec Exp:** Head & Neck Surgery; Parotid Gland Tumors; Paragangliomas; **Hospital:** UPMC Montefiore, Western Penn Hosp; **Address:** UPMC Health System, Dept Otolaryngology, 200 Lothrop St, EEI Inst Fl 3 - Ste 300, Pittsburgh, PA 15213-2546; **Phone:** 412-647-2111; **Board Cert:** Otolaryngology 1966; **Med School:** Temple Univ 1960; **Resid:** Surgery, VA Hosp 1962; Otolaryngology, Mass EE Infirm 1965; **Fellow:** Otolaryngology, Harvard Med Sch 1965; Head and Neck Surgery, St Vincent's Hosp 1968; **Fac Appt:** Prof Oto, Univ Pittsburgh

Niparko, John MD [Oto] - **Spec Exp:** Ear Disorders/Surgery; Neuro-Otology; **Hospital:** Johns Hopkins Hosp - Baltimore (page 61); **Address:** Johns Hopkins Hosp, Dept Otolaryngology, 601 N Caroline St, rm 6223, Baltimore, MD 21287-0910; **Phone:** 410-955-2689; **Board Cert:** Otolaryngology 1986; Neurotology 2004; **Med School:** Univ Mich Med Sch 1980; **Resid:** Surgery, William Beaumont Hosp 1982; Otolaryngology, Univ Michigan Hosp 1986; **Fellow:** Otolaryngology, Univ Michigan Hosp; **Fac Appt:** Prof Oto, Johns Hopkins Univ

O'Malley Jr, Bert W MD [Oto] - **Spec Exp:** Head & Neck Cancer; Sinus Tumors; Skull Base Tumors; **Hospital:** Hosp Univ Penn - UPHS (page 72); **Address:** Hosp Univ Penn, Dept Oto, 3400 Spruce St, 5 Ravdin, Philadelphia, PA 19104; **Phone:** 215-615-4325; **Board Cert:** Otolaryngology 1995; **Med School:** Univ Tex SW, Dallas 1988; **Resid:** Surgery, UTSW Med Ctr/Parkland Meml Hosp 1989; Otolaryngology, Baylor Coll Med 1993; **Fellow:** Head and Neck Oncology, Univ Pittsburgh 1994; Skull Base Surgery, Univ Pittsburgh 1995; **Fac Appt:** Prof Oto, Univ Pennsylvania

Papel, Ira D MD [Oto] - **Spec Exp:** Rhinoplasty; Cosmetic Surgery-Face; Reconstructive Surgery-Face; Skin Cancer/Facial Reconstruction; **Hospital:** Greater Baltimore Med Ctr, Johns Hopkins Hosp - Baltimore (page 61); **Address:** 1838 Greene Tree Rd, Ste 370, Baltimore, MD 21208; **Phone:** 410-486-3400; **Board Cert:** Otolaryngology 1986; Facial Plastic & Reconstructive Surgery 1991; **Med School:** Boston Univ 1981; **Resid:** Otolaryngology, Johns Hopkins Hosp 1986; **Fellow:** Facial Plastic Surgery, UCSF Med Ctr 1987; **Fac Appt:** Assoc Prof Oto, Johns Hopkins Univ

Parisier, Simon C MD [Oto] - **Spec Exp:** Cochlear Implants; Hearing Loss; Ear Infections; **Hospital:** New York Eye & Ear Infirm (page 65), Beth Israel Med Ctr - Petrie Division; **Address:** NY Eye & Ear Infirmary - Otolaryngology, 310 E 14th St, 6th Fl - Window 5, New York, NY 10003-4297; **Phone:** 212-979-4542; **Board Cert:** Otolaryngology 1967; **Med School:** Boston Univ 1961; **Resid:** Otolaryngology, Mount Sinai Hosp 1966; **Fac Appt:** Prof Oto, NY Med Coll

Pastorek, Norman MD [Oto] - **Spec Exp:** Cosmetic Surgery-Face & Eyes; Rhinoplasty; Eyelid Surgery; **Hospital:** NY-Presby Hosp/Weill Cornell (page 66), Manhattan Eye, Ear & Throat Hosp; **Address:** 12 E 88th St, New York, NY 10128-0535; **Phone:** 212-987-4700; **Board Cert:** Otolaryngology 1970; Facial Plastic & Reconstructive Surgery 1991; **Med School:** Univ IL Coll Med 1964; **Resid:** Surgery, Hines VA Hosp 1967; Otolaryngology, Univ Illinois Med Ctr 1969; **Fac Appt:** Clin Prof Oto, Cornell Univ-Weill Med Coll

Persky, Mark S MD [Oto] - **Spec Exp:** Head & Neck Cancer; Skull Base Tumors; Thyroid Cancer; **Hospital:** Beth Israel Med Ctr - Petrie Division; **Address:** 10 Union Square East, Ste 4J, New York, NY 10003; **Phone:** 212-844-8648; **Board Cert:** Otolaryngology 1976; **Med School:** SUNY Upstate Med Univ 1972; **Resid:** Otolaryngology, Bellevue Hosp 1976; **Fellow:** Head and Neck Surgery, Beth Israel Med Ctr 1977; **Fac Appt:** Clin Prof Oto, Albert Einstein Coll Med

Picken, Catherine A MD [Oto] - **Spec Exp:** Head & Neck Reconstruction; Thyroid Disorders; Sinus Disorders/Surgery; **Hospital:** Georgetown Univ Hosp; **Address:** 2021 K St, Ste 206, Washington, DC 20006; **Phone:** 202-785-5000; **Board Cert:** Otolaryngology 1989; **Med School:** Northwestern Univ 1979; **Resid:** Surgery, Natl Heart Lung Blood Inst 1983; Otolaryngology, Georgetown Univ Hosp 1989; **Fac Appt:** Assoc Prof Oto, Georgetown Univ

Quatela, Vito C MD [Oto] - **Spec Exp:** Facial Plastic Surgery; Rhinoplasty; **Hospital:** Univ of Rochester Strong Meml Hosp, Rochester Gen Hosp; **Address:** 973 East Ave, Ste 100, Rochester, NY 14607; **Phone:** 585-244-1000; **Board Cert:** Otolaryngology 1985; Facial Plastic & Reconstructive Surgery 1991; **Med School:** Northwestern Univ 1979; **Resid:** Surgery, Med Ctr Hosp Vermont 1981; Otolaryngology, Northwestern Univ Hosp 1985; **Fellow:** Facial Plastic Surgery, Tulane Univ 1986; Facial Plastic Surgery, Oregon Hlth Science Univ 1987; **Fac Appt:** Assoc Clin Prof Oto, Univ Rochester

Rosen, Clark A MD [Oto] - **Spec Exp:** Voice Disorders; **Hospital:** UPMC Presby, Pittsburgh; **Address:** 200 Lothrop St, Ste 500, Pittsburgh, PA 15213; **Phone:** 412-647-7464; **Board Cert:** Otolaryngology 1995; **Med School:** Rush Med Coll 1989; **Resid:** Otolaryngology, Oregon Hlth Sci Univ 1994; **Fellow:** Otolaryngology, Univ Tenn Med Ctr 1995; **Fac Appt:** Assoc Prof Oto, Univ Pittsburgh

Sataloff, Robert T MD [Oto] - **Spec Exp:** Neuro-Otology; Voice Disorders; **Hospital:** Thomas Jefferson Univ Hosp; **Address:** 1721 Pine Street, Philadelphia, PA 19103-6701; **Phone:** 215-545-3322; **Board Cert:** Otolaryngology 1980; **Med School:** Jefferson Med Coll 1975; **Resid:** Otolaryngology, Univ Mich Hosp 1980; **Fellow:** Neurotology, Univ Mich Hosp 1981; **Fac Appt:** Prof Oto, Drexel Univ Coll Med

Schaefer, Steven D MD [Oto] - **Spec Exp:** Sinus Disorders/Surgery; Head & Neck Surgery; Endoscopic Surgery; **Hospital:** New York Eye & Ear Infirm (page 65), Beth Israel Med Ctr - Petrie Division; **Address:** NY Eye & Ear Infirm, Dept Otolaryngology, 310 E 14th St, New York, NY 10003-4201; **Phone:** 212-979-4200; **Board Cert:** Otolaryngology 1978; **Med School:** UC Irvine 1972; **Resid:** Surgery, UCLA Med Ctr 1974; Otolaryngology, Stanford Med Ctr 1977; **Fac Appt:** Prof Oto, NY Med Coll

Schley, W Shain MD [Oto] - **Spec Exp:** Nasal & Sinus Disorders; Throat Disorders; Voice Disorders; **Hospital:** NY-Presby Hosp/Weill Cornell (page 66); **Address:** 449 E 68th St Fl 2 - Ste DS 10, New York, NY 10021-6310; **Phone:** 212-746-2223; **Board Cert:** Otolaryngology 1973; **Med School:** Emory Univ 1966; **Resid:** Surgery, St Luke's-Roosevelt Hosp Ctr 1968; Otolaryngology, New York Hosp 1973; **Fac Appt:** Assoc Clin Prof Oto, Cornell Univ-Weill Med Coll

Setzen, Michael MD [Oto] - **Spec Exp:** Nasal & Sinus Surgery; Rhinoplasty; Sleep Disorders/Apnea; Snoring/Sleep Apnea; **Hospital:** N Shore Univ Hosp at Manhasset, St Francis Hosp - The Heart Ctr (page 70); **Address:** 333 E Shore Rd, Ste 102, Manhasset, NY 11030-2900; **Phone:** 516-482-8778; **Board Cert:** Otolaryngology 1982; **Med School:** South Africa 1974; **Resid:** Surgery, Cleveland Clinic Fdn 1978; Otolaryngology, Barnes Jewish Hosp 1982; **Fac Appt:** Assoc Clin Prof Oto, NYU Sch Med

Shapshay, Stanley M MD [Oto] - **Spec Exp:** Laryngeal Cancer; Vocal Cord Disorders; **Hospital:** Albany Med Ctr; **Address:** University Ear, Nose & Throat Ctr, 35 Hackett Blvd, Albany, NY 12208; **Phone:** 518-262-5575; **Board Cert:** Otolaryngology 1975; **Med School:** Med Coll VA 1968; **Resid:** Surgery, New England Med Ctr 1971; Otolaryngology, Boston Med Ctr 1975; **Fellow:** Surgery, Serafimer Hosp/Karolinska Med Sch 1972

Snyderman, Carl H MD [Oto] - **Spec Exp:** Skull Base Tumors & Surgery; Sinus Tumors; Head & Neck Cancer; Endoscopic Surgery; **Hospital:** UPMC Presby, Pittsburgh; **Address:** Eye Ear Inst, Dept of Otolaryngology, 200 Lothrop St, Ste 500, Pittsburgh, PA 15213; **Phone:** 412-647-2100; **Board Cert:** Otolaryngology 1987; **Med School:** Univ Chicago-Pritzker Sch Med 1982; **Resid:** Otolaryngology, Eye-Ear Hosp/Univ Pittsburgh 1987; **Fellow:** Skull Base Surgery, Eye-Ear Hosp/Univ Pittsburgh 1988; **Fac Appt:** Prof Oto, Univ Pittsburgh

Stewart, Michael G MD [Oto] - **Spec Exp:** Nasal & Sinus Disorders; Sleep Disorders/Apnea; Head & Neck Trauma; **Hospital:** NY-Presby Hosp/Weill Cornell (page 66); **Address:** Weill Cornell Physicians, 1305 York Ave Fl 5th, New York, NY 10011; **Phone:** 646-962-6673; **Board Cert:** Otolaryngology 1995; **Med School:** Johns Hopkins Univ 1988; **Resid:** Otolaryngology, Baylor Coll Med 1993; **Fac Appt:** Prof Oto, Cornell Univ-Weill Med Coll

Strome, Scott MD [Oto] - **Spec Exp:** Microvascular Surgery; Head & Neck Cancer; **Hospital:** Univ of MD Med Sys; **Address:** 16 S Eutaw St, Ste 500, Baltimore, MD 21201; **Phone:** 410-328-6467; **Board Cert:** Otolaryngology 1998; **Med School:** Harvard Med Sch 1991; **Resid:** Otolaryngology, Univ Michigan 1997; **Fellow:** Head and Neck Surgery, Allegheny Genl Hosp/Med Coll PA 1998; Microvascular Surgery, Allegheny Genl Hosp/Med Coll PA 1998; **Fac Appt:** Prof Oto, Univ MD Sch Med

Urken, Mark MD [Oto] - **Spec Exp:** Head & Neck Cancer & Surgery; Head & Neck Cancer Reconstruction; Thyroid & Parathyroid Cancer & Surgery; Salivary Gland Tumors & Surgery; **Hospital:** Beth Israel Med Ctr - Petrie Division; **Address:** Inst for Head, Neck & Thyroid Cancer, 10 Union Square E, Ste 5B, New York, NY 10003-3314; **Phone:** 212-844-8775; **Board Cert:** Otolaryngology 1986; **Med School:** Univ VA Sch Med 1981; **Resid:** Otolaryngology, Mount Sinai Hosp 1986; **Fellow:** Microvascular Surgery, Mercy Hosp 1987; **Fac Appt:** Prof Oto, Albert Einstein Coll Med

Waner, Milton MD [Oto] - **Spec Exp:** Pediatric Facial Plastic Surgery; Hemangiomas; Vascular Malformations; **Hospital:** St Luke's - Roosevelt Hosp Ctr - St Luke's Hosp, Beth Israel Med Ctr - Petrie Division; **Address:** 1725 York Ave, Ste 2E, New York, NY 10128; **Phone:** 212-987-0979; **Med School:** South Africa 1977; **Resid:** Surgery, Univ of Witwatersrand 1980; Otolaryngology, Univ of Witwatersrand 1984; **Fellow:** Otolaryngology, Univ Cincinnatti Med Ctr 1985

Weinstein, Gregory MD [Oto] - **Spec Exp:** Head & Neck Cancer; Laryngeal Cancer; **Hospital:** Hosp Univ Penn - UPHS (page 72); **Address:** Hosp Univ Penn, Dept Otolaryngology, 3400 Spruce St, 5 Ravdin, Philadelphia, PA 19104; **Phone:** 215-349-5390; **Board Cert:** Otolaryngology 1990; **Med School:** NY Med Coll 1985; **Resid:** Otolaryngology, Univ Iowa Hosp 1990; **Fellow:** Head and Neck Oncology, UC Davis Med Ctr 1991; **Fac Appt:** Assoc Prof Oto, Univ Pennsylvania

Otolaryngology

Woo, Peak MD [Oto] - **Spec Exp:** Voice Disorders; Laryngeal Disorders; Laryngeal Cancer; **Hospital:** Mount Sinai Med Ctr; **Address:** 5 E 98th St Fl 1, Box 1653, New York, NY 10029-6501; **Phone:** 212-241-9425; **Board Cert:** Otolaryngology 1983; **Med School:** Boston Univ 1978; **Resid:** Otolaryngology, Boston Univ Med Ctr 1983; **Fac Appt:** Prof Oto, Mount Sinai Sch Med

Zalzal, George MD [Oto] - **Spec Exp:** Airway Disorders; Laryngeal & Tracheal Disorders; Ear Disorders/Surgery; **Hospital:** Chldns Natl Med Ctr; **Address:** Childrens Natl Med Ctr, Dept Otolaryngology, 111 Michigan Ave NW, Washington, DC 20010; **Phone:** 202-884-2159; **Board Cert:** Otolaryngology 1996; **Med School:** Lebanon 1979; **Resid:** Otolaryngology, American Univ Hosp 1983; **Fellow:** Pediatric Otolaryngology, Univ Cincinnati 1985; **Fac Appt:** Prof Ped, Geo Wash Univ

Southeast

Balkany, Thomas Jay MD [Oto] - **Spec Exp:** Ear Disorders/Surgery; Neuro-Otology; Cochlear Implants; Hearing Loss; **Hospital:** Bascom Palmer Eye Inst. (page 55), Jackson Meml Hosp; **Address:** PO Box 016960, Miami, FL 33101; **Phone:** 305-585-7129; **Board Cert:** Otolaryngology 1977; **Med School:** Univ Miami Sch Med 1972; **Resid:** Surgery, St Joseph Hosp 1974; Otolaryngology, Colo Med Ctr 1977; **Fellow:** Otology & Neurotology, House Ear Inst; **Fac Appt:** Clin Prof Oto, Univ Miami Sch Med

Becker, Ferdinand F MD [Oto] - **Spec Exp:** Cosmetic Surgery-Face; **Hospital:** Indian River Mem Hosp; **Address:** 5070 N A1A, Ste A, Vero Beach, FL 32963-1229; **Phone:** 772-234-3700; **Board Cert:** Otolaryngology 1972; **Med School:** Tulane Univ 1965; **Resid:** Surgery, Charity Hosp 1969; Otolaryngology, Charity Hosp 1972; **Fac Appt:** Asst Clin Prof Oto, Univ Fla Coll Med

Bumpous, Jeffrey MD [Oto] - **Spec Exp:** Head & Neck Cancer; Head & Neck Reconstruction; Thyroid & Parathyroid Cancer & Surgery; **Hospital:** Univ of Louisville Hosp, Norton Hosp; **Address:** 601 S Floyd St, Ste 700, Louisville, KY 40202-1845; **Phone:** 502-583-8303; **Board Cert:** Otolaryngology 1994; **Med School:** Univ Louisville Sch Med 1989; **Resid:** Otolaryngology, Univ Louisville Hosp 1993; **Fellow:** Head and Neck Surgery, Univ Pittsburgh 1994; **Fac Appt:** Prof Oto, Univ Louisville Sch Med

Burkey, Brian MD [Oto] - **Spec Exp:** Parotid Gland Tumors; Head & Neck Cancer; Reconstructive Microvascular Surgery; **Hospital:** Vanderbilt Univ Med Ctr, Saint Thomas Hosp - Nashville; **Address:** Vanderbilt Univ, Dept Otolaryngology, 1215 21st Ave South, 7209 MCE-South Tower, Nashville, TN 37232-0014; **Phone:** 615-322-6180; **Board Cert:** Otolaryngology 1992; **Med School:** Univ VA Sch Med 1986; **Resid:** Otolaryngology, Univ Mich Med Ctr 1991; **Fellow:** Microsurgery, Ohio State Univ 1991; **Fac Appt:** Assoc Prof Oto, Vanderbilt Univ

Cassisi, Nicholas J MD [Oto] - **Spec Exp:** Head & Neck Cancer; Voice Disorders; **Hospital:** Shands Hlthcre at Univ of FL; **Address:** Shands Healthcare at Univ FL, 1600 SW Archer Rd, Box 100383, Gainesville, FL 32610; **Phone:** 352-265-8989; **Board Cert:** Otolaryngology 1971; **Med School:** Univ Miami Sch Med 1965; **Resid:** Surgery, Jackson Memorial Hosp 1967; Otolaryngology, Barnes Hosp - Washington U 1971; **Fac Appt:** Prof Oto, Univ Fla Coll Med

Day, Terrence A MD [Oto] - **Spec Exp:** Head & Neck Cancer; Reconstructive Microvascular Surgery; Skull Base Surgery; Facial Plastic & Reconstructive Surgery; **Hospital:** MUSC Med Ctr; **Address:** MUSC, Dept Otolaryngology, 135 Rutledge Ave, Ste 1130, Box 250550, Charleston, SC 29425; **Phone:** 843-792-0719; **Board Cert:** Otolaryngology 1996; **Med School:** Univ Okla Coll Med 1989; **Resid:** Otolaryngology, LSU Med Ctr 1995; **Fellow:** Head & Neck Surgical Oncology, UC Davis Med Ctr 1996; Maxillofacial Surgery, Univ Hosp; **Fac Appt:** Assoc Prof Oto, Med Univ SC

Farmer, Joseph MD [Oto] - **Spec Exp:** Ear Disorders; Hearing Disorders; Balance Disorders; **Hospital:** Duke Univ Med Ctr; **Address:** 1559 Stead-Blue Zone, South Hospital, Durham, NC 27710; **Phone:** 919-684-6968; **Board Cert:** Otolaryngology 1971; **Med School:** Duke Univ 1962; **Resid:** Surgical Oncology, Natl Cancer Inst 1967; Otolaryngology, Duke Univ Med Ctr 1970; **Fellow:** Thoracic Surgery, Duke Univ Med Ctr 1964; **Fac Appt:** Prof Oto, Duke Univ

Farrior, Edward MD [Oto] - **Spec Exp:** Rhinoplasty; Ear Reshaping (Otoplasty); Facial Plastic Surgery; **Hospital:** Tampa Genl Hosp; **Address:** 2908 W Azeele St, Tampa, FL 33609-3109; **Phone:** 813-875-3223; **Board Cert:** Otolaryngology 1987; Facial Plastic & Reconstructive Surgery 1992; **Med School:** Univ VA Sch Med 1982; **Resid:** Otolaryngology, Univ Mich Hosps 1987; **Fellow:** Facial Plastic & Reconstructive Surgery, Tampa Genl Hosp 1988; **Fac Appt:** Assoc Clin Prof S, Univ S Fla Coll Med

Farrior, Joseph Brown MD [Oto] - **Spec Exp:** Otosclerosis/Stapedectomy; Hearing Loss; Meniere's Disease; Otology; **Hospital:** St Joseph's Hosp - Tampa, Tampa Genl Hosp; **Address:** 2727 Martin Luther King Blvd, Tampa, FL 33607; **Phone:** 800-342-3277; **Board Cert:** Otolaryngology 1981; **Med School:** Emory Univ 1975; **Resid:** Surgery, Johns Hopkins Hosp 1977; Otolaryngology, Johns Hopkins Hosp 1981; **Fellow:** Otolaryngology, Farrior Clin/St Josephs Hosp 1980; **Fac Appt:** Assoc Clin Prof Oto, Univ S Fla Coll Med

Goodwin, W Jarrard Jarrard MD [Oto] - **Spec Exp:** Head & Neck Cancer; **Hospital:** Univ of Miami Hosp & Clins/Sylvester Comp Canc Ctr, Jackson Meml Hosp; **Address:** Dept Otolaryngology, 1475 NW 12th Ave, Ste 4037, Miami, FL 33136-1015; **Phone:** 305-243-4387; **Board Cert:** Otolaryngology 1978; **Med School:** Albany Med Coll 1972; **Resid:** Surgery, Univ Miami/Jackson Hosp Meml Hosp 1973; Otolaryngology, Univ Miami/Jackson Hosp 1977; **Fellow:** Head & Neck Surgical Oncology, MD Anderson Hosp 1980; **Fac Appt:** Prof Oto, Univ Miami Sch Med

Gross, Charles W MD [Oto] - **Spec Exp:** Sinus Disorders/Surgery; Pediatric Otolaryngology; **Hospital:** Univ Virginia Med Ctr; **Address:** UVA Health System, PO Box 800713, Charlottesville, VA 22908-0713; **Phone:** 434-924-5934; **Board Cert:** Otolaryngology 1967; **Med School:** Univ VA Sch Med 1961; **Resid:** Surgery, Beckley Meml Hosp 1963; Otolaryngology, Mass EE Infirm 1966; **Fac Appt:** Prof Oto, Univ VA Sch Med

Kuhn, Frederick MD [Oto] - **Spec Exp:** Endoscopic Sinus Surgery; Allergic Fungal Sinusitis; Rhinoplasty Revision; **Hospital:** Meml Hlth Univ Med Ctr - Savannah, St Joseph's-Candler Hosp; **Address:** Georgia Nasal & Sinus Inst, 4750 Waters Ave, Ste 112, Savannah, GA 31404; **Phone:** 912-355-1070; **Board Cert:** Otolaryngology 1972; **Med School:** Univ Okla Coll Med 1966; **Resid:** Surgery, Univ Oklahoma Hosp 1967; Surgery, St Lukes Hosp 1968; **Fellow:** Otolaryngology, Barnes Hosp/Wash Univ 1972

Otolaryngology

Lambert, Paul R MD [Oto] - **Spec Exp:** Neuro-Otology; Acoustic Neuroma; **Hospital:** MUSC Med Ctr; **Address:** MUSC, Dept Otolaryngology, 135 Rutledge Ave, Box 250550, Charleston, SC 29425; **Phone:** 843-792-3531; **Board Cert:** Otolaryngology 1981; Neurotology 2004; **Med School:** Duke Univ 1976; **Resid:** Surgery, UCLA Med Ctr 1978; Otolaryngology, UCLA Med Ctr 1981; **Fellow:** Neurotology, Otologic Med Group 1982; **Fac Appt:** Prof Oto, Med Univ SC

Lanza, Donald MD [Oto] - **Spec Exp:** Skull Base Tumors; Sinus Disorders/Surgery; Rhinitis; Graves' Disease-Eye Surgery; **Hospital:** St Anthony's Hosp - St Petersburg, All Children's Hosp; **Address:** 900 Carillon Pkwy, Ste 200, St. Petersburg, FL 33716-1108; **Phone:** 727-573-0074; **Board Cert:** Otolaryngology 1990; **Med School:** SUNY Hlth Sci Ctr 1985; **Resid:** Surgery, Albany Med Ctr 1987; Otolaryngology, Albany Med Ctr 1990; **Fellow:** Rhinology, Johns Hopkins Univ 1990; Rhinology, Univ Penn 1991

Levine, Paul A MD [Oto] - **Spec Exp:** Head & Neck Cancer; Head & Neck Reconstruction; Skull Base Tumors; **Hospital:** Univ Virginia Med Ctr; **Address:** UVA Hlth Systems, Dept Otolaryngology, PO Box 800713, Charlottesville, VA 22908; **Phone:** 434-924-5593; **Board Cert:** Otolaryngology 1978; **Med School:** Albany Med Coll 1973; **Resid:** Otolaryngology, Yale-New Haven Hosp 1977; **Fellow:** Head and Neck Surgery, Stanford Med Ctr 1978; **Fac Appt:** Prof Oto, Univ VA Sch Med

Mangat, Devinder S MD [Oto] - **Spec Exp:** Cosmetic & Reconstructive Surgery-Face; **Hospital:** St Elizabeth Med Ctr (South Unit); **Address:** 133 Barnwood Drive, Edgewood, KY 41017; **Phone:** 859-331-9600; **Board Cert:** Otolaryngology 1978; Facial Plastic & Reconstructive Surgery 1991; **Med School:** Univ KY Coll Med 1973; **Resid:** Surgery, Univ Ky Med Ctr 1975; Otolaryngology, Univ Okla Hlth Scis Ctr 1978; **Fellow:** Facial Plastic Surgery, McCullough Clinic 1979; **Fac Appt:** Assoc Prof Oto, Univ Cincinnati

Mattox, Douglas MD [Oto] - **Spec Exp:** Neuro-Otology; Ear Tumors; Skull Base Surgery; **Hospital:** Emory Univ Hosp, Chldns Hlthcare Atlanta - Scottish Rite; **Address:** Emory Univ Hospital, Dept Otolaryngology, 1365-A Clifton Rd NE, Atlanta, GA 30322; **Phone:** 404-778-3381; **Board Cert:** Otolaryngology 1977; Neurotology 2004; **Med School:** Yale Univ 1973; **Resid:** Otolaryngology, Stanford Univ Hosp 1977; **Fellow:** Neurotology, Ugo Fisch, MD 1985; **Fac Appt:** Prof Oto, Emory Univ

Netterville, James MD [Oto] - **Spec Exp:** Head & Neck Surgery; Head & Neck Cancer; Vocal Cord Disorders; Skull Base Tumors; **Hospital:** Vanderbilt Univ Med Ctr, Vanderbilt Children's Hosp; **Address:** Vanderbilt Univ Med Ctr, Dept Oto, 7209 Med Ctr East, South Twr, 1215 21st Ave S, Nashville, TN 37232-8605; **Phone:** 615-343-8840; **Board Cert:** Otolaryngology 1985; **Med School:** Univ Tenn Coll Med, Memphis 1980; **Resid:** Surgery, Methodist Hosp 1982; Otolaryngology, Univ Tenn 1985; **Fellow:** Surgical Oncology, Univ Iowa 1986; **Fac Appt:** Prof Oto, Vanderbilt Univ

Osguthorpe, John D MD [Oto] - **Spec Exp:** Head & Neck Cancer; Thyroid & Parathyroid Cancer & Surgery; Nasal & Sinus Disorders; Salivary Gland Tumors & Surgery; **Hospital:** MUSC Med Ctr; **Address:** MUSC Med Ctr-Dept Otolaryngology, 135 Rutledge Ave, Ste 1130, Box 250550, Charleston, SC 29425; **Phone:** 843-792-3533; **Board Cert:** Otolaryngology 1978; **Med School:** Univ Utah 1973; **Resid:** Surgery, UCLA 1975; Otolaryngology, UCLA 1978; **Fellow:** Skull Base Surgery, Univ Zurich 1989; **Fac Appt:** Prof Oto, Med Univ SC

Peters, Glenn E MD [Oto] - **Spec Exp:** Head & Neck Cancer & Surgery; Skull Base Surgery; Thyroid & Parathyroid Cancer & Surgery; **Hospital:** Univ of Ala Hosp at Birmingham; **Address:** UAB Med Ctr, Div of Head & Neck Surgery, 1530 3rd Ave S, BDB 563 Ave S, Birmingham, AL 35294-0012; **Phone:** 205-934-9777; **Board Cert:** Otolaryngology 1985; **Med School:** Louisiana State Univ 1980; **Resid:** Surgery, Bapt Med Ctr 1982; Otolaryngology, Univ Alabama Hosp 1984; **Fellow:** Head & Neck Surgical Oncology, Johns Hopkins Hosp 1987; **Fac Appt:** Prof S, Univ Ala

Pillsbury, Harold C MD [Oto] - **Spec Exp:** Cochlear Implants; Neuro-Otology; Ear Disorders/Surgery; **Hospital:** Univ NC Hosps; **Address:** 130 Mason Farm Rd, 1115 Bioinformatics Bldg, Box CB 7070, Chapel Hill, NC 27599-7070; **Phone:** 919-966-8926; **Board Cert:** Otolaryngology 1978; Neurotology 2004; **Med School:** Geo Wash Univ 1972; **Resid:** Surgery, Univ NC Hosp 1973; Otolaryngology, NC Meml Hosp 1976; **Fac Appt:** Prof Oto, Univ NC Sch Med

Pitman, Karen MD [Oto] - **Spec Exp:** Head & Neck Cancer & Surgery; Swallowing Disorders; Thyroid & Parathyroid Cancer & Surgery; Sentinel Node Surgery; **Hospital:** Univ Hosps & Clins - Jackson; **Address:** Univ Mississippi Med Ctr, 2500 N State St, Jackson, MS 39216; **Phone:** 601-984-5160; **Board Cert:** Otolaryngology 1995; **Med School:** Uniformed Srvs Univ, Bethesda 1987; **Resid:** Otolaryngology, Naval Med Ctr 1994; **Fellow:** Head and Neck Oncology, Univ Pittsburgh 1996; **Fac Appt:** Assoc Prof Oto, Univ Miss

Poole, Michael D MD/PhD [Oto] - **Spec Exp:** Pediatric Otolaryngology; Ear & Sinus Infections; Sleep Disorders/Apnea; **Hospital:** Meml Hlth Univ Med Ctr - Savannah, St Joseph's-Candler Hosp; **Address:** Georgia Ear Institute, 4700 Waters Ave, Savannah, GA 31404; **Phone:** 912-350-5000; **Board Cert:** Otolaryngology 1986; **Med School:** Univ NC Sch Med 1981; **Resid:** Otolaryngology, NC Meml Hosp 1986; **Fac Appt:** Prof Oto, Mercer Univ Sch Med

Postma, Gregory N MD [Oto] - **Spec Exp:** Voice Disorders; **Hospital:** Med Coll of GA Hosp and Clin; **Address:** Med Coll Georgia, Voice & Swallowing Center, 1120 15th St, BP-4109, Augusta, GA 30912; **Phone:** 706-721-6100; **Board Cert:** Otolaryngology 1994; **Med School:** Hahnemann Univ 1984; **Resid:** Otolaryngology, Oakland Naval Hosp 1992; Otolaryngology, Univ N Carolina Hosps 1993; **Fellow:** Otolaryngology, Vanderbilt Univ 1996

Sillers, Michael MD [Oto] - **Spec Exp:** Nasal & Sinus Disorders; Sinus Disorders/Surgery; **Hospital:** St Vincent's Hosp - Birmingham, Brookwood Med Ctr; **Address:** Alabama Nasal & Sinus Ctr, 7191 Cahaba Valley Rd, Ste 301, Birmingham, AL 35242; **Phone:** 205-980-2091; **Board Cert:** Otolaryngology 1994; **Med School:** Univ Ala 1988; **Resid:** Otolaryngology, Univ Alabama Hosp 1993; **Fellow:** Sinus Surgery, Med Coll Georgia 1994; **Fac Appt:** Asst Prof S, Univ Ala

Silverstein, Herbert MD [Oto] - **Spec Exp:** Ear Disorders/Surgery; Meniere's Disease; **Hospital:** Sarasota Meml Hosp; **Address:** 1901 Floyd St, Silverstein Inst, Sarasota, FL 34239; **Phone:** 941-366-9222; **Board Cert:** Otolaryngology 1967; **Med School:** Temple Univ 1961; **Resid:** Surgery, Hosp Univ Penn 1963; Otolaryngology, Mass EE Infirm 1966; **Fac Appt:** Clin Prof S, Univ S Fla Coll Med

Stringer, Scott P MD [Oto] - **Spec Exp:** Nasal & Sinus Disorders; Head & Neck Cancer; Thyroid & Parathyroid Cancer & Surgery; **Hospital:** Univ Hosps & Clins - Jackson; **Address:** Univ Mississippi Med Ctr, Dept Otolaryngology, 2500 N State St, Jackson, MS 39216-4505; **Phone:** 601-984-5160; **Board Cert:** Otolaryngology 1987; **Med School:** Univ Tex SW, Dallas 1982; **Resid:** Surgery, Univ Tex SW Med Ctr 1984; Otolaryngology, Univ Tex SW Med Ctr 1988; **Fac Appt:** Prof Oto, Univ Miss

Otolaryngology

Terris, David J MD [Oto] - **Spec Exp:** Head & Neck Cancer; Sleep Disorders/Apnea; Sinus Disorders; **Hospital:** Med Coll of GA Hosp and Clin; **Address:** MCG Health System-Dept of Otolaryngology, 1120 15th St, rm BP4134, Augusta, GA 30912; **Phone:** 706-721-4400; **Board Cert:** Otolaryngology 1994; **Med School:** Duke Univ 1988; **Resid:** Surgery, Stanford Univ Med Ctr 1989; Otolaryngology, Stanford Univ Med Ctr 1993; **Fellow:** Head and Neck Surgery, Stanford Univ Med Ctr 1994; **Fac Appt:** Prof Oto, Med Coll GA

Tucci, Debara Lyn MD [Oto] - **Spec Exp:** Skull Base Surgery; Middle Ear Disorders; Otology; **Hospital:** Duke Univ Med Ctr; **Address:** 1559 Stead-Blue Zone, South Hospital, Durham, NC 27710; **Phone:** 919-684-6968; **Board Cert:** Otolaryngology 1990; **Med School:** Univ VA Sch Med 1985; **Resid:** Otolaryngology, Univ Va Hlth Sci Ctr 1990; **Fellow:** Otology & Neurotology, Univ Mich Med Ctr 1992; **Fac Appt:** Assoc Prof S, Duke Univ

Valentino, Joseph MD [Oto] - **Spec Exp:** Head & Neck Cancer; Reconstructive Microvascular Surgery; Thyroid Cancer; **Hospital:** Univ of Kentucky Chandler Hosp; **Address:** 740 S Limestone St, rm B-317, Lexington, KY 40536-0284; **Phone:** 859-257-5405; **Board Cert:** Otolaryngology 1993; **Med School:** UMDNJ-RW Johnson Med Sch 1987; **Resid:** Otolaryngology, Univ Minn 1992; **Fellow:** Otolaryngology, Univ Iowa Coll Med 1993; **Fac Appt:** Assoc Prof Oto, Univ KY Coll Med

Wazen, Jack J MD [Oto] - **Spec Exp:** Skull Base Surgery; Meniere's Disease; Acoustic Neuroma; **Hospital:** Sarasota Meml Hosp; **Address:** 1901 Floyd St, Silverstein Inst, Sarasota, FL 34239; **Phone:** 941-366-9222; **Board Cert:** Otolaryngology 1983; **Med School:** Lebanon 1978; **Resid:** Surgery, St Lukes Hosp 1980; Otolaryngology, Columbia Presby Hosp 1983; **Fellow:** Neurotology, Ear Rsch Fdn 1984; **Fac Appt:** Assoc Clin Prof Oto, Columbia P&S

Weissler, Mark Christian MD [Oto] - **Spec Exp:** Head & Neck Cancer; Laryngeal & Tracheal Disorders; Voice Disorders; **Hospital:** Univ NC Hosps; **Address:** G0412 Neurosciences Hosp UNC, CB 7070, Chapel Hill, NC 27599-7070; **Phone:** 919-843-3796; **Board Cert:** Otolaryngology 1985; **Med School:** Boston Univ 1980; **Resid:** Surgery, Mass Genl Hosp 1982; Otolaryngology, Mass Eye & Ear Infirm 1985; **Fellow:** Head and Neck Oncology, Univ Cincinnati 1986; **Fac Appt:** Prof Oto, Univ NC Sch Med

Midwest

Arts, H Alexander MD [Oto] - **Spec Exp:** Skull Base Tumors & Surgery; Neuro-Otology; Hearing Loss; Cochlear Implants; **Hospital:** Univ Michigan Hlth Sys; **Address:** Univ Michigan Health Systems, Dept Otolaryngology, 1500 E Medical Ctr Dr, 1904 Taubman Ctr, Ann Arbor, MI 48109; **Phone:** 734-936-8006; **Board Cert:** Otolaryngology 1992; Neurotology 2004; **Med School:** Baylor Coll Med 1983; **Resid:** Surgery, Univ Washington Med Ctr 1985; Otolaryngology, Univ Washington Med Ctr 1990; **Fellow:** Neurotology, Univ Virginia 1991; **Fac Appt:** Prof Oto, Univ Mich Med Sch

Baim, Howard MD [Oto] - **Spec Exp:** Head & Neck Surgery; Sleep Disorders/Apnea; Sinus Disorders; **Hospital:** Adv Illinois Masonic Med Ctr, Highland Park Hosp; **Address:** 2532 N Lincoln Ave, Chicago, IL 60614-2468; **Phone:** 773-883-1177; **Board Cert:** Otolaryngology 1978; **Med School:** Univ IL Coll Med 1973; **Resid:** Surgery, Illinois Met Grp Hosps 1975; Otolaryngology, Illinois EE Infirmary 1978; **Fac Appt:** Asst Clin Prof Oto, Univ IL Coll Med

Baker, Shan Ray MD [Oto] - **Spec Exp:** Cosmetic Surgery-Face & Neck; Reconstructive Surgery; **Hospital:** Univ Michigan Hlth Sys; **Address:** Ctr Facial & Cosmetic Surgery, 19900 Haggerty Rd, Ste 103, Livonia, MI 48152-1054; **Phone:** 734-432-7634; **Board Cert:** Otolaryngology 1977; Facial Plastic & Reconstructive Surgery 1990; **Med School:** Univ Iowa Coll Med 1971; **Resid:** Surgery, UCSD Med Ctr 1973; Otolaryngology, Univ Iowa Hosps 1977; **Fac Appt:** Prof Oto, Univ Mich Med Sch

Bastian, Robert W MD [Oto] - **Spec Exp:** Voice Disorders; Swallowing Disorders; Laryngeal Disorders; **Hospital:** Adv Good Samaritan Hosp; **Address:** Bastian Voice Inst, 3010 Highland Parkway, Ste 550, Downers Grove, IL 60515-5500; **Phone:** 630-724-1100; **Board Cert:** Otolaryngology 1983; **Med School:** Washington Univ, St Louis 1978; **Resid:** Surgery, Barnes Hosp 1979; Otolaryngology, Barnes Hosp 1983; **Fellow:** Otolaryngology, Hosp Foch 1983

Beatty, Charles W MD [Oto] - **Spec Exp:** Otology & Neuro-Otology; Acoustic Neuroma; Meniere's Disease; **Hospital:** Mayo Med Ctr & Clin - Rochester; **Address:** Mayo Clinic, Dept Otolaryngology, 200 1st St SW Fl W5, Rochester, MN 55905; **Phone:** 507-284-8532; **Board Cert:** Otolaryngology 1982; **Med School:** Univ Iowa Coll Med 1977; **Resid:** Otolaryngology, Mayo Clinic 1982; **Fac Appt:** Prof Oto, Mayo Med Sch

Benninger, Michael S MD [Oto] - **Spec Exp:** Voice Disorders; Nasal & Sinus Disorders; Sinus Disorders/Surgery; **Hospital:** Henry Ford Hosp; **Address:** 2799 W Grand Blvd, rm k807, Detroit, MI 48202; **Phone:** 313-916-3275; **Board Cert:** Otolaryngology 1988; **Med School:** Case West Res Univ 1983; **Resid:** Surgery, Cleveland Clin Fdn 1985; Otolaryngology, Cleveland Clin Fdn 1988

Bojrab, Dennis I MD [Oto] - **Spec Exp:** Otology & Neuro-Otology; Facial Nerve Disorders; Skull Base Tumors; **Hospital:** Providence Hosp - Southfield, William Beaumont Hosp; **Address:** Michigan Ear Inst, 30055 Northwestern Hwy, Ste 101, Farmington Hills, MI 48334; **Phone:** 248-865-4444; **Board Cert:** Otolaryngology 1985; **Med School:** Indiana Univ 1979; **Resid:** Surgery, Butterworth Hosp 1981; Otolaryngology, Univ Indiana Sch Med 1984; **Fellow:** Skull Base Surgery, Vanderbilt Univ Med Ctr 1985; **Fac Appt:** Prof Oto, Wayne State Univ

Bradford, Carol MD [Oto] - **Spec Exp:** Head & Neck Cancer; Melanoma-Head & Neck; Skin Cancer-Head & Neck; **Hospital:** Univ Michigan Hlth Sys; **Address:** A A Taubman Health Care Ctr, 1500 E Medical Center Drive, rm 1904-TC, Ann Arbor, MI 48109-0312; **Phone:** 734-936-8050; **Board Cert:** Otolaryngology 1993; **Med School:** Univ Mich Med Sch 1986; **Resid:** Otolaryngology, Univ Michigan Med Ctr 1992; **Fellow:** Head and Neck Surgery, Univ Michigan Med Ctr 1988; **Fac Appt:** Prof Oto, Univ Mich Med Sch

Branham, Gregory H MD [Oto] - **Spec Exp:** Cosmetic & Reconstructive Surgery-Face; Nasal Surgery; Botox Therapy; Skin Laser Surgery-Resurfacing; **Hospital:** Washington Univ Med Ctr, Barnes-Jewish Hosp; **Address:** 605 Old Ballas Rd, Ste 100, Saint Louis, MO 63141; **Phone:** 314-432-7760; **Board Cert:** Otolaryngology 1989; Facial Plastic & Reconstructive Surgery 1993; **Med School:** Washington Univ, St Louis 1983; **Resid:** Otolaryngology, St Louis Univ Hosp 1989; **Fellow:** Facial Plastic & Reconstructive Surgery, Washington Univ 1990; **Fac Appt:** Assoc Prof Oto, St Louis Univ

Caldarelli, David D MD [Oto] - **Spec Exp:** Laryngeal & Vocal Cord Surgery; Sinus Disorders/Surgery; Ear Disorders/Surgery; Meniere's Disease; **Hospital:** Rush Univ Med Ctr; **Address:** 1725 W Harrison St, rm 308, Chicago, IL 60612; **Phone:** 312-733-4341; **Board Cert:** Otolaryngology 1970; **Med School:** Univ IL Coll Med 1965; **Resid:** Surgery, Presby-St Lukes Hosp 1967; Otolaryngology, Univ Illinois Eye/Ear Infirm 1970; **Fac Appt:** Prof Oto, Rush Med Coll

Otolaryngology

Christiansen, Thomas A MD [Oto] - **Hospital:** Abbott - Northwestern Hosp, Univ Minn Med Ctr, Fairview - Univ Campus; **Address:** 2211 Park Ave S, Minneapolis, MN 55404; **Phone:** 612-871-1144; **Board Cert:** Otolaryngology 1973; **Med School:** Univ IL Coll Med 1968; **Resid:** Otolaryngology, Univ of MN Hosp 1974; **Fac Appt:** Asst Clin Prof Oto, Univ Minn

Corey, Jacquelynne P MD [Oto] - **Spec Exp:** Nasal & Sinus Disorders; Allergy; Voice Disorders; **Hospital:** Univ of Chicago Hosps; **Address:** Univ Chicago Hosps-Otolaryngology, 5841 S Maryland Ave, Chicago, IL 60637; **Phone:** 773-702-1865; **Board Cert:** Otolaryngology 1985; **Med School:** Univ IL Coll Med 1979; **Resid:** Otolaryngology, Rush Presby-St Lukes Med Ctr 1984; **Fac Appt:** Assoc Prof Oto, Univ Chicago-Pritzker Sch Med

Driscoll, Colin L W MD [Oto] - **Spec Exp:** Acoustic Neuroma; Cochlear Implants; Meniere's Disease; Cholesteatoma; **Hospital:** Mayo Med Ctr & Clin - Rochester; **Address:** Mayo Clinic, Dept Otolaryngology, 200 1st St SW, W5, Rochester, MN 55905-0001; **Phone:** 507-284-4065; **Board Cert:** Otolaryngology 1998; **Med School:** Univ New Mexico 1992; **Resid:** Otolaryngology, Mayo Clinic 1997; **Fellow:** Neurotology, UCSF Med Ctr 1998; Skull Base Surgery, UCSF Med Ctr 1999; **Fac Appt:** Assoc Prof Oto, Mayo Med Sch

Ford, Charles N MD [Oto] - **Spec Exp:** Voice Disorders; Laryngeal Disorders; **Hospital:** Univ WI Hosp & Clins; **Address:** Univ of WI Hosp & Clinics, 600 Highland Avenue-K4-714, Madison, WI 53792-3284; **Phone:** 608-263-0192; **Board Cert:** Otolaryngology 1971; **Med School:** Univ Louisville Sch Med 1965; **Resid:** Otolaryngology, Henry Ford Hosp 1970; **Fac Appt:** Prof Oto, Univ Wisc

Friedman, Michael MD [Oto] - **Spec Exp:** Sleep Disorders/Apnea/Snoring; Thyroid & Parathyroid Surgery; Sinus Disorders/Surgery; **Hospital:** Adv Illinois Masonic Med Ctr, Rush Univ Med Ctr; **Address:** 30 N Michigan St, Ste 1107, Chicago, IL 60602-3747; **Phone:** 312-236-3642; **Board Cert:** Otolaryngology 1977; **Med School:** Univ IL Coll Med 1972; **Resid:** Surgery, Illinois Masonic Hosp 1974; Otolaryngology, Univ Illinois Med Ctr 1977; **Fac Appt:** Prof Oto, Rush Med Coll

Funk, Gerry F MD [Oto] - **Spec Exp:** Head & Neck Cancer; Head & Neck Reconstruction; Head & Neck Trauma; **Hospital:** Univ Iowa Hosp & Clinics; **Address:** UIHC, Dept Otolaryngology, 200 Hawkins Drive, Iowa City, IA 52242-1009; **Phone:** 319-356-2165; **Board Cert:** Otolaryngology 1992; **Med School:** Univ Chicago-Pritzker Sch Med 1986; **Resid:** Surgery, LAC-USC Med Ctr 1987; Otolaryngology, LAC-USC Med Ctr 1991; **Fellow:** Head and Neck Surgery, Univ Iowa Hosp 1992; **Fac Appt:** Prof Oto, Univ Iowa Coll Med

Gantz, Bruce MD [Oto] - **Spec Exp:** Cochlear Implants; Neuro-Otology; Skull Base Surgery; **Hospital:** Univ Iowa Hosp & Clinics; **Address:** Univ Hosp & Clins, Dept Otolaryngology, 200 Hawkins Drive, rm 21201PFP, Iowa City, IA 52242-1078; **Phone:** 319-356-2173; **Board Cert:** Otolaryngology 1980; Neurotology 2004; **Med School:** Univ Iowa Coll Med 1974; **Resid:** Otolaryngology, Univ Iowa Hosps 1980; **Fellow:** Neurotology, Univ Zurich 1982; **Fac Appt:** Prof Oto, Univ Iowa Coll Med

Gluckman, Jack L MD [Oto] - **Spec Exp:** Head & Neck Cancer; Head & Neck Surgery; **Hospital:** Univ Hosp - Cincinnati, Good Samaritan Hosp - Cincinnati; **Address:** Univ Cincinnati Medical Center, Head & Neck Surgery MSB 6505, 231 Albert B Sabin Way, Box 670528, Cincinnati, OH 45267-0528; **Phone:** 513-558-0017; **Board Cert:** Otolaryngology 1990; **Med School:** South Africa 1967; **Resid:** Surgery, St James Hosp 1971; Otolaryngology, Groote Schuur Hosp 1974; **Fellow:** Otolaryngology, Univ Cincinnati Med Ctr 1979; **Fac Appt:** Prof Oto, Univ Cincinnati

Goebel, Joel Alan MD [Oto] - **Spec Exp:** Dizziness; Hearing Disorders; Otology & Neurotology; **Hospital:** Barnes-Jewish Hosp, St Louis Chldns Hosp; **Address:** Barnes Jewish Hosp South, 660 S Euclid, Box 8115, St Louis, MO 63110; **Phone:** 314-362-7509; **Board Cert:** Otolaryngology 1985; **Med School:** Washington Univ, St Louis 1980; **Resid:** Otolaryngology, Barnes Hosp/Wash Univ 1985; **Fac Appt:** Prof Oto, Washington Univ, St Louis

Haughey, Bruce MD [Oto] - **Spec Exp:** Reconstructive Surgery-Face; Head & Neck Cancer; Head & Neck Reconstruction; **Hospital:** Barnes-Jewish Hosp; **Address:** Barnes Jewish Hosp South, 660 S Euclid Ave, Box 8115, St Louis, MO 63110; **Phone:** 314-362-7509; **Board Cert:** Otolaryngology 1984; **Med School:** New Zealand 1976; **Resid:** Surgery, Univ Auckland 1980; Otolaryngology, Univ Iowa Med Ctr 1984; **Fac Appt:** Prof Oto, Washington Univ, St Louis

Hilger, Peter A MD [Oto] - **Spec Exp:** Head & Neck Surgery; Facial Plastic Surgery; **Hospital:** Regions Hosp - St Paul, Fairview Southdale Hosp; **Address:** Centennial Lakes Med Bldg, 7373 France Ave S, Ste 410, Edina, MN 55435; **Phone:** 952-844-0404; **Board Cert:** Otolaryngology 1979; **Med School:** Univ Minn 1974; **Resid:** Surgery, Univ Minn Hosp 1975; Otolaryngology, Univ Minn Hosp 1979; **Fellow:** Plastic Surgery, Mass Eye & Ear Infirm 1980; **Fac Appt:** Asst Prof Oto, Univ Minn

Jones, Paul John MD [Oto] - **Spec Exp:** Pediatric Otolaryngology; **Hospital:** Rush Univ Med Ctr; **Address:** 1725 W Harrison St, Ste 938, Chicago, IL 60612; **Phone:** 312-942-2175; **Board Cert:** Otolaryngology 1989; **Med School:** Rush Med Coll 1983; **Resid:** Otolaryngology, Rush Presby St Lukes Med Ctr 1988; **Fac Appt:** Asst Prof Oto, Rush Med Coll

Kartush, Jack MD [Oto] - **Spec Exp:** Ear Disorders/Surgery; Balance Disorders; **Hospital:** Providence Hosp - Southfield; **Address:** Michigan Ear Inst, 30055 Northwestern Hwy, Ste 101, Farmington Hills, MI 48334; **Phone:** 248-865-4444; **Board Cert:** Otolaryngology 1984; **Med School:** Univ Mich Med Sch 1978; **Resid:** Otolaryngology, Univ Mich Med Ctr 1984; **Fellow:** Neurotology, Univ Mich Med Ctr 1985; **Fac Appt:** Assoc Clin Prof Oto, Wayne State Univ

Kern, Robert MD [Oto] - **Spec Exp:** Head & Neck Cancer; Sinus Disorders/Surgery; Rhinoplasty; **Hospital:** Northwestern Meml Hosp, Stroger Hosp of Cook Co; **Address:** 675 N St Clair St, Ste 15-200, Chicago, IL 60611; **Phone:** 312-695-8182; **Board Cert:** Otolaryngology 1990; **Med School:** Jefferson Med Coll 1985; **Resid:** Otolaryngology, Wayne State Affil Hosp 1990; **Fellow:** Research, Natl Inst Hlth 1991; **Fac Appt:** Prof Oto, Northwestern Univ

Lavertu, Pierre MD [Oto] - **Spec Exp:** Thyroid Cancer; Head & Neck Cancer; Skull Base Tumors; **Hospital:** Univ Hosps Case Med Ctr; **Address:** Univ Hosps, Dept Oto-Head & Neck Surg, 11100 Euclid Ave, Cleveland, OH 44106-5045; **Phone:** 216-844-4773; **Board Cert:** Otolaryngology 1981; **Med School:** Univ Montreal 1976; **Resid:** Otolaryngology, Univ Montreal Med Ctr 1981; **Fellow:** Head and Neck Surgery, Univ Montreal Med Ctr 1982; Head and Neck Surgery, Cleveland Clinic 1983; **Fac Appt:** Prof Oto, Case West Res Univ

Leonetti, John P MD [Oto] - **Spec Exp:** Skull Base Tumors & Surgery; Acoustic Neuroma; Neuro-Otology; **Hospital:** Loyola Univ Med Ctr; **Address:** Loyola University Medical Ctr, Dept Otolaryngology, 2160 S First Ave Bldg 105 - rm 1870, Maywood, IL 60153; **Phone:** 708-216-4804; **Board Cert:** Otolaryngology 1987; **Med School:** Loyola Univ-Stritch Sch Med 1982; **Resid:** Otolaryngology, Loyola Univ Med Ctr 1987; Research, House Ear Inst; **Fellow:** Neurotology, Barnes Hosp 1988; **Fac Appt:** Prof Oto, Loyola Univ-Stritch Sch Med

Marentette, Lawrence MD [Oto] - **Spec Exp:** Skull Base Tumors & Surgery; Facial Plastic & Reconstructive Surgery; **Hospital:** Univ Michigan Hlth Sys; **Address:** Univ Michigan Health Systems, Dept Oto, 1500 E Med Ctr Drive, 1904 Taubman Ctr, Ann Arbor, MI 48109; **Phone:** 734-936-8051; **Board Cert:** Otolaryngology 1981; Facial Plastic & Reconstructive Surgery 1995; **Med School:** Wayne State Univ 1976; **Resid:** Otolaryngology, Wayne State Univ 1980; **Fellow:** Maxillofacial Surgery, Univ of Zurich 1985; **Fac Appt:** Prof Oto, Univ Mich Med Sch

Miyamoto, Richard T MD [Oto] - **Spec Exp:** Neuro-Otology; Acoustic Neuroma; Middle Ear Disorders; Cochlear Implants; **Hospital:** Indiana Univ Hosp, Riley Hosp for Children; **Address:** 702 Barnhill Drive, rm 0860, Indianapolis, IN 46202-5128; **Phone:** 317-274-3556; **Board Cert:** Otolaryngology 1975; Neurotology 2004; **Med School:** Univ Mich Med Sch 1970; **Resid:** Surgery, Butterworth Hosp 1972; Otolaryngology, Indiana Univ Hosps 1975; **Fellow:** Otology & Neurotology, Otologic Med Grp 1978; **Fac Appt:** Prof Oto, Indiana Univ

Naclerio, Robert MD [Oto] - **Spec Exp:** Head & Neck Surgery; Pediatric Otolaryngology; Sinus Disorders/Surgery; **Hospital:** Univ of Chicago Hosps; **Address:** Univ Chicago Hosps, 5841 S Maryland Ave, MC 1035, Chicago, IL 60637; **Phone:** 773-702-0080; **Board Cert:** Otolaryngology 1983; **Med School:** Baylor Coll Med 1976; **Resid:** Surgery, Johns Hopkins Hosp 1978; Otolaryngology, Baylor Coll Med 1980; **Fellow:** Clinical Immunology, Johns Hopkins Hosp 1982; **Fac Appt:** Prof Oto, Univ Chicago-Pritzker Sch Med

Olsen, Kerry D MD [Oto] - **Spec Exp:** Head & Neck Cancer & Surgery; Esthesioneuroblastoma; Salivary Gland Tumors & Surgery; Skull Base Tumors; **Hospital:** Mayo Med Ctr & Clin - Rochester; **Address:** Mayo Clinic, Dept Otolaryngology, 200 1st St SW, Rochester, MN 55905-0001; **Phone:** 507-284-3542; **Board Cert:** Otolaryngology 1981; **Med School:** Mayo Med Sch 1976; **Resid:** Otolaryngology, Mayo Clinic 1981; **Fac Appt:** Prof Oto, Mayo Med Sch

Paparella, Michael MD [Oto] - **Spec Exp:** Hearing Disorders; Neuro-Otology; Meniere's Disease; **Hospital:** Univ Minn Med Ctr, Fairview - Riverside Campus; **Address:** Paparella Ear, Head & Neck Institute, 701 25th Ave S, Ste 200, Minneapolis, MN 55454-1443; **Phone:** 612-339-2836; **Board Cert:** Otolaryngology 1963; **Med School:** Univ Mich Med Sch 1957; **Resid:** Otolaryngology, Henry Ford Hosp 1961; **Fac Appt:** Clin Prof Oto, Univ Minn

Pelzer, Harold J MD/DDS [Oto] - **Spec Exp:** Head & Neck Cancer; Swallowing Disorders; **Hospital:** Northwestern Meml Hosp; **Address:** 675 N St Clair, Ste 15-200, Chicago, IL 60611; **Phone:** 312-695-8182; **Board Cert:** Otolaryngology 1985; **Med School:** Northwestern Univ 1979; **Resid:** Surgery, Northwestern Meml Hosp 1983; **Fellow:** Head and Neck Surgery, Northwestern Meml Hosp 1985; **Fac Appt:** Assoc Prof Oto, Northwestern Univ

Pensak, Myles MD [Oto] - **Spec Exp:** Skull Base Tumors; Facial Paralysis; Hearing & Balance Disorders; **Hospital:** Univ Hosp - Cincinnati, Good Samaritan Hosp - Cincinnati; **Address:** Univ Medical Arts Building, 222 Piedmont Ave, Ste 5200, Cincinnati, OH 45219; **Phone:** 513-475-8400; **Board Cert:** Otolaryngology 1983; Neurotology 2004; **Med School:** NY Med Coll 1978; **Resid:** Surgery, Upstate Med Ctr 1980; Otolaryngology, Yale Univ 1983; **Fellow:** Otology & Neurotology, The Otology Group 1984; **Fac Appt:** Prof Oto, Univ Cincinnati

Petruzzelli, Guy MD/PhD [Oto] - **Spec Exp:** Head & Neck Cancer & Surgery; Skull Base Tumors; Thyroid Cancer; **Hospital:** Loyola Univ Med Ctr; **Address:** Loyola Univ Med Ctr, 2160 S 1st Ave, Bldg 105 - rm 1870, Maywood, IL 60153; **Phone:** 708-216-9183; **Board Cert:** Otolaryngology 1993; **Med School:** Rush Med Coll 1987; **Resid:** Otolaryngology, Univ Pittsburgh Med Ctr 1992; **Fellow:** Head and Neck Oncology, Univ Pittsburgh Med Ctr 1993; Skull Base Surgery, Univ Pittsburgh Ctr Cranial Base Surg; **Fac Appt:** Prof Oto, Loyola Univ-Stritch Sch Med

Piccirillo, Jay MD [Oto] - **Spec Exp:** Sleep Disorders/Apnea; Sinus Disorders/Surgery; **Hospital:** Barnes-Jewish Hosp; **Address:** Wash Univ Sch Med, Dept ENT, 660 S Euclid Ave, Box 8115, St Louis, MO 63110; **Phone:** 314-362-7509; **Board Cert:** Otolaryngology 1990; **Med School:** Univ VT Coll Med 1985; **Resid:** Otolaryngology, Albany Med Ctr 1990; **Fellow:** Yale Univ 1992; **Fac Appt:** Asst Prof Oto, Washington Univ, St Louis

Schuller, David MD [Oto] - **Spec Exp:** Head & Neck Cancer; Head & Neck Surgery; **Hospital:** Arthur G James Cancer Hosp & Research Inst, Ohio St Univ Med Ctr; **Address:** 300 W 10th Ave, rm 518, Columbus, OH 43210; **Phone:** 614-293-8074; **Board Cert:** Otolaryngology 1975; **Med School:** Ohio State Univ 1970; **Resid:** Otolaryngology, Ohio State Univ Affil Hosps 1975; Surgery, Univ Hosps 1973; **Fellow:** Head and Neck Surgery, Pack Med Fdn 1973; Head and Neck Oncology, Univ Iowa 1976; **Fac Appt:** Prof Oto, Ohio State Univ

Siegel, Gordon J MD [Oto] - **Spec Exp:** Head & Neck Cancer; Nasal & Sinus Disorders; Cosmetic Surgery-Face; **Hospital:** Northwestern Meml Hosp; **Address:** 3 E Huron St Fl 1, Chicago, IL 60611-2705; **Phone:** 312-988-7777; **Board Cert:** Otolaryngology 1984; **Med School:** Ros Franklin Univ/Chicago Med Sch 1978; **Resid:** Otolaryngology, Northwestern Univ 1982; **Fac Appt:** Asst Clin Prof Oto, Northwestern Univ

Stankiewicz, James MD [Oto] - **Spec Exp:** Endoscopic Sinus Surgery; Rhinosinusitis; Nasal & Sinus Disorders; **Hospital:** Loyola Univ Med Ctr; **Address:** Loyola Univ Med Ctr, Dept Oto, 2160 S First Ave, Maywood, IL 60153-5590; **Phone:** 708-216-8563; **Board Cert:** Otolaryngology 1978; **Med School:** Univ Chicago-Pritzker Sch Med 1974; **Resid:** Otolaryngology, Univ Chicago Hosp 1978; **Fac Appt:** Prof Oto, Loyola Univ-Stritch Sch Med

Strome, Marshall MD [Oto] - **Spec Exp:** Sleep Disorders/Apnea; Voice Disorders; Head & Neck Cancer; **Hospital:** Cleveland Clin Fdn (page 57); **Address:** Cleveland Clinic Fdn, 9500 Euclid Ave, Ste A71, Cleveland, OH 44195; **Phone:** 216-444-6686; **Board Cert:** Otolaryngology 1970; **Med School:** Univ Mich Med Sch 1964; **Resid:** Surgery, Harper Hosp 1966; Otolaryngology, Univ Michigan Hosp 1970; **Fac Appt:** Prof Oto, Cleveland Cl Coll Med/Case West Res

Szachowicz II, Edward H MD [Oto] - **Spec Exp:** Cosmetic Surgery-Face; Rhinoplasty; **Hospital:** Abbott - Northwestern Hosp; **Address:** Centennial Lakes Med Bldg, 7373 France Ave S, Ste 508, Edina, MN 55435-4538; **Phone:** 952-835-5665; **Board Cert:** Otolaryngology 1984; **Med School:** Univ IL Coll Med 1979; **Resid:** Surgery, Fairview Univ Med Ctr 1980; Otolaryngology, Fairview Univ Med Ctr 1984; **Fellow:** Facial Plastic Surgery, Fairview Univ Med Ctr 1986; **Fac Appt:** Asst Clin Prof Oto, Univ Minn

Otolaryngology

Teknos, Theodoros N MD [Oto] - **Spec Exp:** Head & Neck Cancer; Thyroid Cancer; Facial Plastic & Reconstructive Surgery; Reconstructive Microvascular Surgery; **Hospital:** Univ Michigan Hlth Sys; **Address:** Univ Mich Med Ctr, TC 1904, 1500 E Med Ctr Drive, Ann Arbor, MI 48109; **Phone:** 734-936-3172; **Board Cert:** Otolaryngology 1997; **Med School:** Harvard Med Sch 1991; **Resid:** Otolaryngology, Mass Eye & Ear Hosp 1996; **Fellow:** Head and Neck Surgery, Vanderbilt Univ Med Ctr 1997; **Fac Appt:** Assoc Prof Oto, Univ Mich Med Sch

Telian, Steven A MD [Oto] - **Spec Exp:** Cochlear Implants; Ear Disorders/Surgery; Acoustic Neuroma; **Hospital:** Univ Michigan Hlth Sys; **Address:** Univ Mich Med Ctr, Dept Oto-HNS, 1500 E Med Ctr Dr, Taubman Ctr, rm 1904, Ann Arbor, MI 48109-0312; **Phone:** 734-936-8006; **Board Cert:** Otolaryngology 1985; **Med School:** Univ Pennsylvania 1980; **Resid:** Otolaryngology, Hosp Univ Penn 1985; **Fellow:** Neurotology, Univ Mich Med Ctr 1986; **Fac Appt:** Prof Oto, Univ Mich Med Sch

Toriumi, Dean MD [Oto] - **Spec Exp:** Rhinoplasty; Cosmetic Surgery-Face; Reconstructive Plastic Surgery; **Hospital:** Univ of IL Med Ctr at Chicago; **Address:** 60 E Delaware Ave Fl 14 - Ste 1460, Chicago, IL 60611; **Phone:** 312-255-8812; **Board Cert:** Otolaryngology 1988; **Med School:** Rush Med Coll 1981; **Resid:** Surgery, Univ Illinois Med Ctr 1985; Otolaryngology, Northwestern Univ Med Sch 1987; **Fellow:** Facial Plastic Surgery, Tulane Med Sch 1988; Facial Plastic Surgery, Virginia Mason Med Ctr 1989; **Fac Appt:** Assoc Prof Oto, Univ IL Coll Med

Wackym, Phillip MD [Oto] - **Spec Exp:** Cochlear Implants; Acoustic Neuroma; Head & Neck Surgery; **Hospital:** Froedtert Meml Lutheran Hosp, Chldns Hosp - Wisconsin; **Address:** Med Coll Wisconsin, Dept Otolaryngology, 9200 W Wisconsin Ave, Milwaukee, WI 53226; **Phone:** 414-805-3666; **Board Cert:** Otolaryngology 1992; **Med School:** Vanderbilt Univ 1985; **Resid:** Neurological Surgery, UCLA Med Ctr 1987; Head and Neck Surgery, UCLA Med Ctr 1991; **Fellow:** Otology & Neurotology, Univ Iowa 1992; Neurological Science, UCLA Med Ctr 1995; **Fac Appt:** Prof Oto, Med Coll Wisc

Wiet, Richard J MD [Oto] - **Spec Exp:** Acoustic Neuroma; Hearing Loss; Otosclerosis/Stapedectomy; **Hospital:** Hinsdale Hosp, Northwestern Meml Hosp; **Address:** 950 N York Rd, Ste 102, Hinsdale, IL 60521; **Phone:** 630-789-3110; **Board Cert:** Otolaryngology 1976; Neurotology 2004; **Med School:** Loyola Univ-Stritch Sch Med 1971; **Resid:** Otolaryngology, Cincinnati Med Ctr 1976; **Fellow:** Neurotology, Univ Zurich/Ear Fdn 1979; **Fac Appt:** Clin Prof Oto, Northwestern Univ

Wilson, Keith M MD [Oto] - **Spec Exp:** Head & Neck Cancer & Surgery; Voice Disorders; **Hospital:** Univ Hosp - Cincinnati; **Address:** Univ Cincinnati Medical Ctr, 222 Piedmont Ave, Ste 5200, Cincinnati, OH 45219; **Phone:** 513-475-8351; **Board Cert:** Otolaryngology 1992; **Med School:** Cornell Univ-Weill Med Coll 1986; **Resid:** Otolaryngology, St Louis Univ Med Ctr 1991; **Fellow:** Head & Neck Surgical Oncology, Ohio State Med Ctr 1992; **Fac Appt:** Assoc Prof Oto, Univ Cincinnati

Wolf, Gregory T MD [Oto] - **Spec Exp:** Head & Neck Cancer; Laryngeal Cancer; **Hospital:** Univ Michigan Hlth Sys; **Address:** Univ Mich Med Ctr, Dept Oto-HNS, 1500 E Med Ctr, Taubman Ctr, rm 1904, Ann Arbor, MI 48109-0312; **Phone:** 734-936-8029; **Board Cert:** Otolaryngology 1978; **Med School:** Univ Mich Med Sch 1973; **Resid:** Surgery, Georgetown Univ Hosp 1975; Otolaryngology, SUNY Upstate Med Ctr 1978; **Fac Appt:** Prof Oto, Univ Mich Med Sch

Woodson, B Tucker MD [Oto] - **Spec Exp:** Sleep Disorders/Apnea; **Hospital:** Froedtert Meml Lutheran Hosp, Chldns Hosp - Wisconsin; **Address:** 9200 W Wisconsin Ave, Froedtert West ENT Clinic, Milwaukee, WI 53226-3522; **Phone:** 414-805-7667; **Board Cert:** Otolaryngology 1988; **Med School:** Univ MO-Columbia Sch Med 1983; **Resid:** Surgery, Henry Ford Hosp 1984; Otolaryngology, Henry Ford Hosp 1988; **Fac Appt:** Assoc Prof Oto, Med Coll Wisc

Woodson, Gayle Ellen MD [Oto] - **Spec Exp:** Voice Disorders; Swallowing Disorders; **Hospital:** St John's Hosp - Springfield, Memorial Med Ctr - Springfield; **Address:** SIU Sch Med, Div Oto - Head & Neck Surg, PO Box 19662, Springfield, IL 62794; **Phone:** 217-545-6099; **Board Cert:** Otolaryngology 1981; **Med School:** Baylor Coll Med 1976; **Resid:** Surgery, Johns Hopkins Hosp 1978; Otolaryngology, Baylor Coll Med 1981; **Fellow:** Laryngology, Inst Laryngology and Otology 1982; **Fac Appt:** Prof Oto, Southern IL Univ

Young, Nancy MD [Oto] - **Spec Exp:** Cochlear Implants; Cholesteatoma; Hearing Loss; Baha Implant; **Hospital:** Children's Mem Hosp, Glenbrook Hosp; **Address:** Children's Memorial, Div Otolaryngology, 2300 Children's Plaza, Box 265, Chicago, IL 60614; **Phone:** 800-543-7362; **Board Cert:** Otolaryngology 1987; **Med School:** NYU Sch Med 1982; **Resid:** Surgery, Montefiore Med Ctr 1984; Otolaryngology, Northwestern Univ Hosp 1987; **Fellow:** Neurotology, Hinsdale Hosp 1988; **Fac Appt:** Assoc Prof Oto, Northwestern Univ

Great Plains and Mountains

Bentz, Brandon G MD [Oto] - **Spec Exp:** Head & Neck Cancer & Surgery; Skull Base Tumors; **Hospital:** Univ Utah Hosps and Clins; **Address:** Univ Utah Hospitals, Dept Otolaryngology, 50 N Medical Drive, rm 3C120, Salt Lake City, UT 84132; **Phone:** 801-581-7515; **Board Cert:** Otolaryngology 2001; **Med School:** Northwestern Univ 1993; **Resid:** Otolaryngology, Northwestern Univ Med Ctr 1997; **Fellow:** Head & Neck Surgical Oncology, Meml Sloan Kettering Cancer Ctr 1999; **Fac Appt:** Asst Prof Oto, Univ Utah

Chowdhury, Khalid MD [Oto] - **Spec Exp:** Skull Base Tumors & Surgery; Craniofacial Surgery; Cosmetic Surgery-Face; **Hospital:** Presby - St Luke's Med Ctr, Chldn's Hosp - Denver, The; **Address:** Center for Craniofacial Surgery, 1601 E 19th Ave, Ste 3000, Denver, CO 80218; **Phone:** 303-839-5155; **Board Cert:** Otolaryngology 1990; Facial Plastic & Reconstructive Surgery 1995; **Med School:** Univ Saskatchewan 1982; **Resid:** Surgery, Univ Saskatchewan Hosp 1985; Otolaryngology, McGill Univ Hosps 1989; **Fellow:** Craniofacial Surgery, Univ Bern Hosp 1990; Facial Plastic & Reconstructive Surgery, Univ Bern Hosp 1990; **Fac Appt:** Assoc Prof Oto, Univ Colorado

Denenberg, Steven M MD [Oto] - **Spec Exp:** Cosmetic Surgery-Face; Rhinoplasty; **Hospital:** Nebraska Meth Hosp, Nebraska Med Ctr; **Address:** 7640 Pacific St, Omaha, NE 68114-5421; **Phone:** 402-391-7640; **Board Cert:** Otolaryngology 1984; Facial Plastic & Reconstructive Surgery 1992; **Med School:** Univ Nebr Coll Med 1980; **Resid:** Otolaryngology, Stanford Univ Med Ctr 1984; **Fellow:** Facial Plastic Surgery, McCollough Ctr 1985; **Fac Appt:** Asst Clin Prof Oto, Univ Nebr Coll Med

Jenkins, Herman A MD [Oto] - **Spec Exp:** Ear Disorders/Surgery; Neuro-Otology; Acoustic Neuroma; **Hospital:** Univ Colorado Hosp, Chldn's Hosp - Denver, The; **Address:** Univ Colorado Hosp, Dept Otolaryngology, PO Box 6510, MS F737, Aurora, CO 80045; **Phone:** 720-848-2820; **Board Cert:** Otolaryngology 1977; Neurotology 2004; **Med School:** Vanderbilt Univ 1970; **Resid:** Surgery, UCLA Med Ctr 1972; Otolaryngology, UCLA Med Ctr 1977; **Fellow:** Neurotology, Univ Hosp 1980; **Fac Appt:** Prof Oto, Univ Colorado

Otolaryngology

Leopold, Donald Arthur MD [Oto] - **Spec Exp:** Olfactory Disorders; Sinus Disorders/Surgery; **Hospital:** Nebraska Med Ctr; **Address:** Univ Nebr, Dept Oto-Head & Neck Surg, 981225 Nebraska Med Ctr, Omaha, NE 68198-1225; **Phone:** 402-559-8007; **Board Cert:** Otolaryngology 1978; Facial Plastic & Reconstructive Surgery 1991; **Med School:** Ohio State Univ 1973; **Resid:** Surgery, St Luke's Med Ctr 1974; Otolaryngology, Univ Iowa 1978; **Fac Appt:** Prof Oto, Univ Nebr Coll Med

Southwest

Alford, Bobby R MD [Oto] - **Spec Exp:** Neurovestibular Disease; Thyroid Surgery; Head & Neck Surgery; Hearing & Balance Disorders; **Hospital:** Methodist Hosp - Houston; **Address:** Baylor Coll Med, Neurosensory Ctr, One Baylor Plaza, Ste NA-102, Houston, TX 77030; **Phone:** 713-798-3200; **Board Cert:** Otolaryngology 1962; **Med School:** Baylor Coll Med 1956; **Resid:** Otolaryngology, Baylor Coll Med 1960; **Fellow:** Otology, Univ Tex Med Branch 1961; Neurological Physiology, Johns Hopkins Med Sch 1962; **Fac Appt:** Prof Oto, Baylor Coll Med

Clayman, Gary Lee MD/DMD [Oto] - **Spec Exp:** Thyroid Cancer & Surgery; Salivary Gland Tumors & Surgery; Head & Neck Cancer; **Hospital:** UT MD Anderson Cancer Ctr (page 71); **Address:** Univ TX/MD Anderson Cancer Center, 1515 Holcombe Blvd, Box 441, Houston, TX 77030-4009; **Phone:** 713-792-8837; **Board Cert:** Otolaryngology 1992; **Med School:** NE Ohio Univ 1986; **Resid:** Surgery, Hennepin Co Med Ctr 1987; Otolaryngology, Univ Minn 1991; **Fellow:** Head and Neck Surgery, MD Anderson Cancer Ctr 1993; **Fac Appt:** Prof Oto, Univ Tex, Houston

Coker, Newton J MD [Oto] - **Spec Exp:** Acoustic Neuroma; Cochlear Implants; Skull Base Tumors; **Hospital:** Methodist Hosp - Houston, Texas Chldns Hosp - Houston; **Address:** Baylor Coll Medicine, One Baylor Plaza, MS NA-102, Houston, TX 77030; **Phone:** 713-798-3200; **Board Cert:** Otolaryngology 1981; Neurotology 2004; **Med School:** Med Coll GA 1976; **Resid:** Surgery, Med Coll Georgia 1978; Otolaryngology, Med Coll Georgia 1981; **Fellow:** Otology & Neurotology, University Hosp 1982; **Fac Appt:** Prof Oto, Baylor Coll Med

Daspit, C Phillip MD [Oto] - **Spec Exp:** Hearing & Balance Disorders; Skull Base Tumors & Surgery; Cochlear Implants; **Hospital:** St Joseph's Hosp & Med Ctr - Phoenix; **Address:** 222 W Thomas Rd, Ste 114, Phoenix, AZ 85013; **Phone:** 602-279-5444; **Board Cert:** Otolaryngology 1977; **Med School:** Louisiana State Univ 1968; **Resid:** Surgery, UCSF Med Ctr 1973; Otolaryngology, Ft Miley VA Hosp 1977; **Fellow:** Otology & Neurotology, House Ear Inst 1978; Skull Base Surgery, House Ear Inst 1978; **Fac Appt:** Clin Prof S, Univ Ariz Coll Med

Donovan, Donald T MD [Oto] - **Spec Exp:** Head & Neck Cancer; Voice Disorders; Thyroid Disorders; **Hospital:** Methodist Hosp - Houston, St Luke's Episcopal Hosp - Houston; **Address:** 6550 Fannin St, Ste 1727, Houston, TX 77030; **Phone:** 713-798-3380; **Board Cert:** Otolaryngology 1981; **Med School:** Baylor Coll Med 1976; **Resid:** Surgery, Baylor Affil Hosps 1978; Otolaryngology, Baylor Affil Hosps 1981; **Fellow:** Head and Neck Surgery, Columbia-Presby Med Ctr 1982; **Fac Appt:** Prof Oto, Baylor Coll Med

Gianoli, Gerard MD [Oto] - **Spec Exp:** Dizziness; Hearing Loss; Ear Disorders; **Hospital:** North Oaks Med Ctr; **Address:** 17050 Medical Center Drive, Ste 315, The Ear & Balance Institute, Baton Rouge, LA 70816-3249; **Phone:** 225-293-6973; **Board Cert:** Otolaryngology 1993; Neurotology 2004; **Med School:** Tulane Univ 1986; **Resid:** Pediatrics, Tulane Univ 1988; Otolaryngology, Tulane Univ 1992; **Fellow:** Otology & Neurotology, Michigan Ear Inst; **Fac Appt:** Assoc Clin Prof Oto, Tulane Univ

Hanna, Ehab YN MD [Oto] - **Spec Exp:** Skull Base Tumors & Surgery; Head & Neck Cancer & Surgery; **Hospital:** UT MD Anderson Cancer Ctr (page 71); **Address:** Univ Tex MD Anderson Cancer Ctr, 1515 Holcolmbe Blvd, Unit 441, Houston, TX 77030; **Phone:** 713-745-1815; **Board Cert:** Otolaryngology 1994; **Med School:** Egypt 1982; **Resid:** Otolaryngology, Cleveland Clinic 1989; Otolaryngology, Cleveland Clinic 1993; **Fellow:** Otolaryngology, Univ Pittsburgh Med Ctr 1994; **Fac Appt:** Asst Prof Oto, Univ Tex, Houston

Hayden, Richard E MD [Oto] - **Spec Exp:** Head & Neck Surgery; Facial Plastic & Reconstructive Surgery; Microvascular Surgery; **Hospital:** Mayo Clin Hosp - Scottsdale; **Address:** Mayo Clinic, Dept Otolaryngology, 5777 E Mayo Blvd, Phoenix, AZ 85054; **Phone:** 480-342-2629; **Board Cert:** Otolaryngology 1978; **Med School:** McGill Univ 1974; **Resid:** Otolaryngology, Univ Toronto 1978; **Fellow:** Head and Neck Oncology, MD Anderson Hosp 1979; Radiation Oncology, Princess Margaret Hosp 1980; **Fac Appt:** Prof Oto, Mayo Med Sch

Johnson Jr, Calvin M MD [Oto] - **Spec Exp:** Ear Disorders/Surgery; Nasal Surgery; Cosmetic Surgery-Face; **Address:** Hedgewood Surgical Ctr, 2427 St Charles Ave, New Orleans, LA 70130; **Phone:** 504-895-7642; **Board Cert:** Otolaryngology 1974; **Med School:** Tulane Univ 1967; **Resid:** Surgery, Tulane Univ Sch Med 1971; Otolaryngology, Tulane Univ Sch Med 1974; **Fellow:** Facial Plastic Surgery, Amer Academy Facial Plastic & Recon Surg 1975

Macias, John D MD [Oto] - **Spec Exp:** Otology; Neuro-Otology; Cochlear Implants; **Hospital:** Banner Good Samaritan Regl Med Ctr - Phoenix, Phoenix Children's Hosp; **Address:** 1515 N 9th St, Ste B, Phoenix, AZ 85006-2523; **Phone:** 602-257-4228; **Board Cert:** Otolaryngology 1994; Neurotology 2005; **Med School:** Stanford Univ 1988; **Resid:** Otolaryngology, Univ Iowa Hosps & Clins 1993; **Fellow:** Otology, Ear Fdn/Otology Grp 1994

Medina, Jesus MD [Oto] - **Spec Exp:** Head & Neck Cancer; **Hospital:** OU Med Ctr; **Address:** Univ OK Hlth Sci Ctr, Dept Oto-WP 1290, PO Box 26901, Oklahoma City, OK 73190; **Phone:** 405-271-8047; **Board Cert:** Otolaryngology 1980; **Med School:** Peru 1974; **Resid:** Surgery, Wayne St Univ Affil Hosp 1977; Otolaryngology, Wayne St Univ Affil Hosp 1980; **Fellow:** Head and Neck Surgery, Univ Tex Sys Cancer Ctrs 1981; **Fac Appt:** Prof Oto, Univ Okla Coll Med

Myers, Jeffrey N MD/PhD [Oto] - **Spec Exp:** Head & Neck Cancer; Melanoma-Head & Neck; Tongue Cancer; **Hospital:** UT MD Anderson Cancer Ctr (page 71); **Address:** Univ Texas MD Anderson Cancer Ctr, 1515 Holcombe Blvd, Box 441, Houston, TX 77030; **Phone:** 713-745-2667; **Board Cert:** Otolaryngology 1997; **Med School:** Univ Pennsylvania 1991; **Resid:** Otolaryngology, Univ Pittsburgh Med Ctr 1996; **Fellow:** Head & Neck Surgical Oncology, MD Anderson Cancer Ctr 1997; **Fac Appt:** Assoc Prof Oto, Univ Tex, Houston

Nuss, Daniel W MD [Oto] - **Spec Exp:** Head & Neck Cancer; Skull Base Tumors & Surgery; **Hospital:** Our Lady of the Lake Regl Med Ctr; **Address:** LSU Sch Med, Dept Otolaryngology, 533 Bolivar St Fl 5, New Orleans, LA 70112; **Phone:** 225-765-1475; **Board Cert:** Otolaryngology 1987; **Med School:** Louisiana State Univ 1981; **Resid:** Surgery, Charity Hosp 1983; Otolaryngology, LSU Med Ctr 1987; **Fellow:** Surgical Oncology, MD Anderson Hosp & Tumor Inst 1984; Head and Neck Surgery, Ctr Cranial Base Surg-Univ Pittsbur 1991; **Fac Appt:** Prof Oto, Louisiana State Univ

Otolaryngology

Otto, Randal A MD [Oto] - **Spec Exp:** Head & Neck Cancer; Thyroid & Parathyroid Cancer & Surgery; Sinus Disorders/Surgery; **Hospital:** Univ Hlth Sys - Univ Hosp, Audie L Murphy Meml Vets Hosp; **Address:** 7703 Floyd Curl Drive, MS 7777, San Antonio, TX 78229-3900; **Phone:** 210-358-0490; **Board Cert:** Otolaryngology 1987; **Med School:** Univ MO-Columbia Sch Med 1981; **Resid:** Pathology, Queens Med Ctr 1982; Otolaryngology, Univ Missouri 1987; **Fac Appt:** Prof Oto, Univ Tex, San Antonio

Suen, James Y MD [Oto] - **Spec Exp:** Head & Neck Cancer; Vascular Lesions-Head & Neck; Laryngeal Disorders; **Hospital:** UAMS Med Ctr, Arkansas Chldns Hosp; **Address:** Univ Hosp Arkansas Med Scis, 4301 W Markham St, Slot 543, Little Rock, AR 72205; **Phone:** 501-686-8224; **Board Cert:** Otolaryngology 1973; **Med School:** Univ Ark 1966; **Resid:** Surgery, Univ Arkansas Med Ctr 1970; Otolaryngology, Univ Arkansas Med Ctr 1973; **Fellow:** Head and Neck Surgery, MD Anderson Cancer Ctr-Tumor Inst 1974; **Fac Appt:** Prof Oto, Univ Ark

Weber, Randal S MD [Oto] - **Spec Exp:** Skin Cancer; Thyroid & Parathyroid Cancer & Surgery; Salivary Gland Tumors & Surgery; Head & Neck Cancer; **Hospital:** UT MD Anderson Cancer Ctr (page 71); **Address:** 1515 Holcombe Blvd, Unit 441, Houston, TX 77030-4009; **Phone:** 713-745-0497; **Board Cert:** Otolaryngology 1985; **Med School:** Univ Tenn Coll Med, Memphis 1976; **Resid:** Surgery, Baylor Coll Med 1982; Otolaryngology, Baylor Coll Med 1985; **Fellow:** Head and Neck Surgery, MD Anderson Cancer Ctr 1986; **Fac Appt:** Prof Oto, Univ Tex, Houston

West Coast and Pacific

Berke, Gerald S MD [Oto] - **Spec Exp:** Head & Neck Surgery; Head & Neck Cancer; Voice Disorders; **Hospital:** UCLA Med Ctr; **Address:** 200 UCLA Med Plaza, Ste 550, Los Angeles, CA 90095; **Phone:** 310-825-5179; **Board Cert:** Otolaryngology 1984; **Med School:** USC Sch Med 1978; **Resid:** Otolaryngology, LAC-USC Med Ctr 1979; **Fellow:** Head and Neck Surgery, UCLA Med Ctr 1984; **Fac Appt:** Prof Oto, UCLA

Brackmann, Derald E MD [Oto] - **Spec Exp:** Ear Disorders/Surgery; Facial Nerve Disorders; Acoustic Neuroma; **Hospital:** St Vincent's Med Ctr - Los Angeles, USC Univ Hosp - R K Eamer Med Plz; **Address:** House Clinic, 2100 W 3rd St, Fl 1st, Los Angeles, CA 90057-1902; **Phone:** 213-483-9930; **Board Cert:** Otolaryngology 1971; Neurotology 2005; **Med School:** Univ IL Coll Med 1962; **Resid:** Otolaryngology, LAC/USC Med Ctr 1970; **Fellow:** Otology & Neurotology, House Ear Clinic 1971; **Fac Appt:** Clin Prof Oto, USC-Keck School of Medicine

Courey, Mark S MD [Oto] - **Spec Exp:** Laryngeal Disorders; Swallowing Disorders; Laryngeal Cancer; **Hospital:** UCSF - Mt Zion Med Ctr, UCSF Med Ctr; **Address:** UCSF Voice & Swallowing Ctr, 2330 Post St Fl 5, San Francisco, CA 94115; **Phone:** 415-885-7700; **Board Cert:** Otolaryngology 1993; **Med School:** SUNY Buffalo 1987; **Resid:** Otolaryngology, SUNY-Buffalo Med Ctr 1992; **Fellow:** Laryngology, Vanderbilt Univ 1993; **Fac Appt:** Prof Oto, UCSF

De la Cruz, Antonio MD [Oto] - **Spec Exp:** Otosclerosis/Stapedectomy; Skull Base Surgery; Otology; **Hospital:** St Vincent's Med Ctr - Los Angeles, Torrance Memorial Med Ctr; **Address:** 2100 W 3rd St Fl 1, Los Angeles, CA 90057; **Phone:** 213-483-9930; **Board Cert:** Otolaryngology 1973; **Med School:** Costa Rica 1967; **Resid:** Surgery, Univ Miami Med Ctr 1970; Otolaryngology, Univ Miami Med Ctr 1973; **Fellow:** Otology & Neurotology, House Ear Clinic 1974; **Fac Appt:** Clin Prof Oto, USC Sch Med

Donald, Paul MD [Oto] - **Spec Exp:** Skull Base Tumors & Surgery; Head & Neck Cancer; **Hospital:** UC Davis Med Ctr; **Address:** 2521 Stockton Blvd, rm 7200, Sacramento, CA 95817; **Phone:** 916-734-2832; **Board Cert:** Otolaryngology 1973; **Med School:** Univ British Columbia Fac Med 1964; **Resid:** Surgery, St Pauls Hosp 1969; Otolaryngology, Univ Iowa Hosp 1973; **Fac Appt:** Prof Oto, UC Davis

Eisele, David W MD [Oto] - **Spec Exp:** Salivary Gland Tumors & Surgery; Head & Neck Cancer; Thyroid Cancer; **Hospital:** UCSF Med Ctr; **Address:** UCSF, Dept Head & Neck Surgery, 400 Parnassus Ave, Ste A 730, San Francisco, CA 94143-0342; **Phone:** 415-502-0498; **Board Cert:** Otolaryngology 1988; **Med School:** Cornell Univ-Weill Med Coll 1982; **Resid:** Surgery, Univ Wash Med Ctr 1984; Otolaryngology, Univ Wash Med Ctr 1988; **Fac Appt:** Prof Oto, UCSF

Fee Jr, Willard E MD [Oto] - **Spec Exp:** Head & Neck Cancer; Parotid Gland Tumors; Thyroid Cancer; **Hospital:** Stanford Univ Med Ctr; **Address:** Stanford Cancer Ctr, 875 Lake Wilber Dr, CC-2227, Stanford, CA 94305-5826; **Phone:** 650-725-6500; **Board Cert:** Otolaryngology 1974; **Med School:** Univ Colorado 1969; **Resid:** Surgery, Wadsworth VA Hosp 1971; Otolaryngology, UCLA Med Ctr 1974; **Fac Appt:** Prof Oto, Stanford Univ

Harris, Jeffrey P MD/PhD [Oto] - **Spec Exp:** Neuro-Otology; Hearing & Balance Disorders; Skull Base Surgery; **Hospital:** UCSD Med Ctr, VA San Diego Hlthcre Sys; **Address:** UCSD Med Ctr, 200 W Arbor Drive, San Diego, CA 92103-8895; **Phone:** 619-543-7896; **Board Cert:** Otolaryngology 1974; Neurotology 2004; **Med School:** Univ Pennsylvania 1974; **Resid:** Otolaryngology, Mass EE Infirmary 1979; **Fellow:** Neurological Surgery, Univ Zurich Med Ctr 1983; **Fac Appt:** Prof S, UCSD

Jackler, Robert K MD [Oto] - **Spec Exp:** Neuro-Otology; Skull Base Surgery; Ear Tumors; **Hospital:** Stanford Univ Med Ctr; **Address:** Stanford Univ Med Ctr, Dept Head & Neck Surg, 801 Welch Rd, Stanford, CA 94305-5739; **Phone:** 650-725-6500; **Board Cert:** Otolaryngology 1984; Neurotology 2004; **Med School:** Boston Univ 1979; **Resid:** Otolaryngology, UCSF Med Ctr 1984; **Fellow:** Otolaryngology, Oto Med Grp 1985; **Fac Appt:** Prof Oto, Stanford Univ

Kamer, Frank M MD [Oto] - **Spec Exp:** Rhinoplasty; Cosmetic Surgery-Face; **Hospital:** Cedars-Sinai Med Ctr, UCLA Med Ctr; **Address:** Cedars-Sinai Med Ctr, Lasky Clinic, 201 S Lasky Drive, Beverly Hills, CA 90212-3647; **Phone:** 310-556-8155; **Board Cert:** Otolaryngology 1971; **Med School:** Albert Einstein Coll Med 1963; **Resid:** Surgery, LI Jewish Hosp 1965; Otolaryngology, Mt Sinai Hosp 1970; **Fac Appt:** Prof Oto, UCLA

Keller, Gregory S MD [Oto] - **Spec Exp:** Cosmetic Surgery-Face; **Hospital:** Santa Barbara Cottage Hosp, UCLA Med Ctr; **Address:** 221 E Pueblo St, Ste A, Santa Barbara, CA 93105; **Phone:** 805-687-6408; **Board Cert:** Otolaryngology 1976; **Med School:** Univ IL Coll Med 1971; **Resid:** Surgery, Cottage Hosp 1973; Otolaryngology, Univ Illinois 1976; **Fac Appt:** Assoc Clin Prof S, UCLA

Larrabee Jr, Wayne F MD [Oto] - **Spec Exp:** Cosmetic Surgery-Face; Eyelid Surgery; Rhinoplasty; Nasal Surgery; **Hospital:** Swedish Med Ctr - Seattle, Univ Wash Med Ctr; **Address:** Facial Plastic Surgery Ctr, 600 Broadway Ste 280, Seattle, WA 98122-5371; **Phone:** 206-386-3550; **Board Cert:** Otolaryngology 1979; Facial Plastic & Reconstructive Surgery 1991; **Med School:** Tulane Univ 1971; **Resid:** Surgery, Charity Hosp 1976; Otolaryngology, Tulane Univ Med Ctr 1979; **Fac Appt:** Clin Prof Oto, Univ Wash

Otolaryngology

McMenomey, Sean O MD [Oto] - **Spec Exp:** Otology & Neuro-Otology; Skull Base Tumors & Surgery; Head & Neck Surgery; Stereotactic Radiosurgery; **Hospital:** OR Hlth & Sci Univ, Providence St Vincent Med Ctr; **Address:** Oregon Hlth & Sci Univ, Dept Otolaryngology, 3181 SW Sam Jackson Park Rd, MC PV-01, Portland, OR 97239; **Phone:** 503-494-8135; **Board Cert:** Otolaryngology 1993; **Med School:** St Louis Univ 1987; **Resid:** Otolaryngology, Oregon Health Sci Ctr 1992; **Fellow:** Otology & Neurotology, Baptist Hosp 1993; **Fac Appt:** Assoc Prof Oto, Oregon Hlth Sci Univ

Powell, Nelson B MD/DDS [Oto] - **Spec Exp:** Sleep Disorders/Apnea; Maxillofacial Surgery; **Hospital:** Stanford Univ Med Ctr; **Address:** 750 Welch Rd, Ste 317, Palo Alto, CA 94304; **Phone:** 650-328-0511; **Board Cert:** Otolaryngology 1984; **Med School:** Univ Wash 1979; **Resid:** Surgery, Stanford Univ Hosp & Clinics 1980; Otolaryngology, Stanford Univ Hosp 1983; **Fac Appt:** Clin Prof S, Stanford Univ

Rice, Dale MD [Oto] - **Spec Exp:** Head & Neck Cancer; Sinus Disorders/Surgery; **Hospital:** USC Univ Hosp - R K Eamer Med Plz; **Address:** USC Keck Sch Med, 1200 N State St, Box 795, Los Angeles, CA 90033-1029; **Phone:** 323-442-5790; **Board Cert:** Otolaryngology 1976; **Med School:** Univ Mich Med Sch 1968; **Resid:** Surgery, Univ Mich Med Ctr 1976; Otolaryngology, Univ Mich Med Ctr 1976; **Fac Appt:** Prof Oto, USC Sch Med

Senders, Craig W MD [Oto] - **Spec Exp:** Pediatric Otolaryngology; Cleft Palate/Lip; Endoscopic Sinus Surgery; Sleep Disorders/Apnea; **Hospital:** UC Davis Med Ctr; **Address:** UC Davis, Dept Oto-Head & Neck Surg, 2521 Stockton Blvd, Ste 7200, Sacramento, CA 95817; **Phone:** 916-734-5400; **Board Cert:** Otolaryngology 1984; **Med School:** Oregon Hlth Sci Univ 1979; **Resid:** Otolaryngology, Univ Iowa Hosps & Clins 1983; **Fellow:** Maxillofacial Surgery, Univ Iowa Hosps & Clins 1984; **Fac Appt:** Prof Oto, UC Davis

Sinha, Uttam K MD [Oto] - **Spec Exp:** Head & Neck Cancer; Voice Disorders; **Hospital:** USC Univ Hosp - R K Eamer Med Plz, House Ear Inst; **Address:** 1200 N State St, rm 4136, Los Angeles, CA 90033; **Phone:** 323-226-7315; **Board Cert:** Otolaryngology 1998; **Med School:** India 1985; **Resid:** Otolaryngology, LAC-USC Med Ctr 1995; **Fellow:** Mount Sinai Med Sch 1988; LAC-USC Med Ctr 1990; **Fac Appt:** Asst Prof Oto, USC Sch Med

Wax, Mark K MD [Oto] - **Spec Exp:** Facial Nerve Disorders; Skull Base Tumors & Surgery; Facial Plastic & Reconstructive Surgery; **Hospital:** OR Hlth & Sci Univ; **Address:** Oregon Hlth Scis Univ-Dept Otolaryngology, 3181 SW Sam Jackson Park Rd, Ste PV-01, Portland, OR 97201; **Phone:** 503-494-5355; **Board Cert:** Otolaryngology 1985; Facial Plastic & Reconstructive Surgery 1987; **Med School:** Univ Toronto 1980; **Resid:** Otolaryngology, Univ Toronto 1985; Surgery, Cedars-Sinai Med Ctr 1983; **Fellow:** Head and Neck Surgery, St Michaels Hosp 1991; **Fac Appt:** Prof Oto, Oregon Hlth Sci Univ

Weisman, Robert A MD [Oto] - **Spec Exp:** Head & Neck Cancer; Clinical Trials; Thyroid & Parathyroid Cancer & Surgery; Head & Neck Cancer Reconstruction; **Hospital:** UCSD Med Ctr; **Address:** Moores-UCSD Cancer Center, 3855 Health Sciences Drive, MC 0987, La Jolla, CA 92093-0987; **Phone:** 858-822-6197; **Board Cert:** Otolaryngology 1978; **Med School:** Washington Univ, St Louis 1973; **Resid:** Head and Neck Surgery, UCLA Med Ctr 1978; **Fac Appt:** Prof S, UCSD

Weymuller, Ernest MD [Oto] - **Spec Exp:** Head & Neck Cancer; Sinus Disorders/Surgery; **Hospital:** Univ Wash Med Ctr; **Address:** 1959 NE Pacific St, Box 356161, Seattle, WA 98195-6161; **Phone:** 206-598-4022; **Board Cert:** Otolaryngology 1973; **Med School:** Harvard Med Sch 1966; **Resid:** Surgery, Vanderbilt Univ Hosp 1968; Otolaryngology, Mass Eye and Ear Infirm 1973; **Fac Appt:** Prof Oto, Univ Wash

Cleveland Clinic

Head and Neck Institute

The specialists at the Cleveland Clinic Head and Neck Institute have been recognized nationally and internationally as leaders in this multidisciplinary field. The Institute is composed of specialists with extensive training in all areas, including:

Audiology: Audiologists provide the non-medical management of hearing disorders including comprehensive audiologic evaluation and treatment through the use of assistive listening devices, hearing aids, Baha Hearing Systems, and cochlear implants.

Facial Aesthetic and Reconstructive Surgery: Surgeons perform a broad range of procedures, from office-based treatments including Botox and Restylane injections to operative procedures ranging from rhinoplasty and facelifts to major facial reconstructive surgery.

Head and Neck Surgery: Evaluation and treatment of both benign and malignant head and neck tumors. Patients are seen in a team fashion by surgeons, radiation therapists and oncologists to facilitate optimal treatment.

Laryngotracheal Reconstruction: Laryngeal airway obstruction, esophageal reflux, tracheal aspiration, and voice preservation and rehabilitation and removal of upper and lower respiratory foreign bodies.

Nasal and Sinus Disorders: Treatment of a wide variety of sinonasal conditions, including rhinosinusitis, nasal polyps, fungal sinusitis, septal deviation, nasal obstruction and inhalant allergies. Minimally invasive, computer-aided, endoscopic techniques for revision sinus surgery, CSF leaks and neoplasms of the nose, sinuses and skull base.

Otology-Neurotology: Care of all forms of otologic disorders, including middle and posterior cranial fossa surgery for cerebellopontine and skull base tumors. Immune-mediated inner ear disease (deafness), Meniere's disease and cochlear implantation are also handled here.

Pediatric Otolaryngology: Treatment of all forms of pediatric otolaryngologic disorders, with support from Cleveland Clinic Children's Hospital, a pediatric intensive care unit, and numerous other pediatric specialists on staff.

Speech-Language Pathology: Comprehensive evaluation and treatment for all speech, language, voice, cognitive and swallowing disorders. Services are provided to pediatric through geriatric patient populations via an interdisciplinary medical care model.

Vestibular and Balance Disorders: Diagnosis and vestibular rehabilitation from dizziness, disequilibrium.

To schedule an appointment or for more information about the Cleveland Clinic Head and Neck Institute call 800.890.2467 or visit www.clevelandclinic.org/headandnecktopdocs.

Head and Neck Institute | 9500 Euclid Avenue / W14 | Cleveland OH 44195

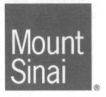

THE MOUNT SINAI MEDICAL CENTER
OTOLARYNGOLOGY – EAR, NOSE, AND THROAT

One Gustave L. Levy Place (Fifth Avenue and 100th Street)
New York, NY 10029-6574
Physician Referral: 1-800-MD-SINAI (637-4624)
www.mountsinai.org

One of the oldest and most respected departments in the nation, Mount Sinai's Department of Otolaryngology is consistently ranked among the top in the nation and in 2006, *US News & World Report* ranked the department #19 in the nation. All physicians are board-certified specialists dedicated to healing disorders of the ear, nose, throat, head, and neck, including the following:

Robotic Surgery - The Department is spearheading the use of robotic surgery to treat head and neck cancers. The DaVinci Surgical System®, a cutting edge technology, magnifies the surgical field and gives surgeons greater visualization, dexterity, and precision during an operation, resulting in less invasive surgical techniques and reduced scarring while improving outcomes.

Endoscopic Surgery – This technique enables surgeons to remove tumors of the voice box, skull base, and neck without external incisions. Many patients are discharged the same day instead of being admitted for an inpatient stay.

Cranial Base Surgery – Surgeons at Mount Sinai have developed techniques to endoscopically remove skull-base tumors through the nose, leaving no visible sign of surgery. Interdisciplinary teams provide expertise in the diagnosis and treatment of tumors, vascular lesions, and trauma at the base of the brain.

Thyroid and Parathyroid Surgery – Minimally invasive thyroidectomy and parathyroidectomy can be performed through a one-inch incision. We believe that a team approach involving an experienced surgeon, a dedicated endocrinologist, and a team of physicians trained in nuclear medicine is of critical importance for the treatment of thyroid cancers.

Audiology – All aspects of audiology are covered at Mount Sinai, including the performance and interpretation of audiograms, brainstem evoked potentials, otoacoustic emission testing, neonatal hearing screening, and evaluations for assisted listening devices.

Facial Plastic and Cosmetic Surgery – Our reconstructive facial surgeons and specialists in facial cosmetic surgery use state-of-the-art endoscopic techniques.

Head and Neck Reconstructive Surgery – The Department has some of the most experienced reconstructive surgeons in the world, specializing in microvascular free tissue transfer.

Hearing, Facial Nerve, and Balance Disorders – Multidisciplinary teams provide treatment for a broad range of adult and pediatric neuro-otologic and otologic disorders.

Maxillofacial Prosthodontics – Complete services to restore speech and chewing abilities and minimize cosmetic defects, are offered.

Nasal and Sinus Surgery – Renowned rhinologists treat all inflammatory and infectious diseases of the nose and sinuses.

Oral and Maxillofacial Surgery – All treatment options are provided for patients with congenital, acquired, or traumatic problems of the oral cavity, jaws, and associated structures.

Additionally, The Grabscheid Voice Center offers the highest level of medical care for the professional voice, along with a profound understanding of the special medical, psychological, and professional needs of singers, actors, and lecturers.

THE MOUNT SINAI MEDICAL CENTER

Mount Sinai's Multidisciplinary Head and Neck Cancer Team has gained national recognition for its expertise and innovation in the management of head, neck, and skull-base cancer. Mount Sinai has a nationally recognized team of experts in minimally invasive and endoscopic head and neck surgery. The team is comprised of a group of surgeons and oncologists focused on the curative treatment for head and neck malignancies. The expert team works to cure tumors of the oral cavity, jaw, and larynx and preserve each patient's quality of life. Speech and swallowing rehabilitation therapists work with patients to help them fully recover. Mount Sinai is on the cutting edge of head and neck cancer therapy, reconstruction, and rehabilitation.

615

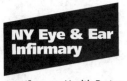

NY Eye & Ear Infirmary

Continuum Health Partners, Inc.

THE NEW YORK EYE AND EAR INFIRMARY

310 East 14th Street
New York, New York 10003
Tel. 212.979.4000   Fax. 212.228.0664
http://www.nyee.edu

PROVIDING EXCEPTIONAL CARE OF THE EAR, NOSE, THROAT, AND HEAD & NECK

Established in 1820 the Department of Otolaryngology/Head & Neck Surgery is the first training program in this specialty in the Western Hemisphere. Over nearly two centuries the department has evolved to be an international referral center for the medical and surgical treatment of diseases of the ear, nose, and throat.

OUTSTANDING SERVICES:

Facial Plastic Surgery: In-office or ambulatory procedures utilizing computer imaging, new techniques and materials produce outstanding results with minimal incisions, rapid recovery and a natural, youthful appearance.

Head & Neck Oncology: A multi-disciplinary team including board-certified surgeons, medical & radiation oncologists, nutritionists and rehabilitation specialists insure rapid recovery from complex, life-saving surgical procedures and return to daily activities.

Thyroid Center: A comprehensive program to streamline the diagnosis and treatment of thyroid diseases and cancers. A highly skilled team of surgeons, endocrinologists and radiologists manage the patient's care.

Voice & Swallowing Institute: Combining the expertise of physicians, speech pathologists and a voice physiologist to diagnose and treat voice problems – not only for performing artists but also for teachers, stockbrokers, receptionists, salespeople – anyone for whom voice is an important part of life.

Ear Institute (Otology – Neuro-otology): Specializing in the care of chronic ear disease including hearing loss, cochlear implantation, dizziness, tinnitus, intra cranial tumors and facial nerve disorders. Our advanced otologic and vestibular diagnostic labs assist physicians in treatment.

Pediatric Otolaryngology: Treating children has long been a priority at the Infirmary. Pediatric care ranges from middle ear infection, tonsil and adenoid disease, and neck masses to complex sinus and airway diseases.

Rhinology and Sinus Surgery: Internationally known specialists utilize minimally invasive techniques to treat disorders from sinusitis to intra cranial tumors

Otolaryngology Clinical Services

Facial Plastic & Reconstructive Surgery
Head & Neck Oncology
Thyroid Center
General Otolaryngology
Laryngology
Swallowing Disorders
Voice & Vocal Dynamics
Otology & Neuro-otology
Cochlear Implantation
Pediatric Otolaryngology
Rhinology & Sinus Surgery

Facilities

Ambulatory Care Services
Faculty Practice
Teaching Practice
Hearing Aid Dispensary
Vestibular Rehabilitation

About The New York Eye and Ear Infirmary

The Infirmary is the nation's oldest, continuously operating specialty hospital and one of the most experienced in terms of the number of patients it treats and complexity of its cases. Each year the otolaryngology department performs more than 6,000 surgeries and sees more than 60,000 visits from outpatients

Physician Referral
1.800.449.HOPE (4673)

NYU Medical Center

550 First Avenue (at 31st Street)
New York, NY 10016
Physician Referral:
(888)7-NYU-MED (888-769-8633)
www.nyumc.org

OTOLARYNGOLOGY (EAR, NOSE AND THROAT)

Treating the full spectrum of ear, nose, throat, head and neck disorders, the Department of Otolaryngology at NYU Medical Center (www.med.nyu/ent) provides state-of-the-art patient care and research through the following programs:

Cochlear Implants – the first center in the U.S. to use a multichannel cochlear implant in a profoundly deaf adult, in 1984. Since then we have implanted more than 1700 adults and children from the age of 6 months to 85 years.

Sinus and Nasal Disorders – comprehensive diagnosis and minimally invasive treatment of sinus and nasal disorders

Facial Plastic Surgery – plastic and reconstructive surgery for a variety of problems, including nasal obstruction, facial trauma, defects left after removing skin and other facial cancers, facial paralysis and spasm, congenital malformations.

Head and Neck Surgery – state of the art treatment for benign and cancerous diseases of the nasopharynx, larynx, tongue, mouth, mandible, neck and face.

Sleep Apnea – repairing the collapse of soft tissue that leads to snoring and sleep apnea (a dangerous condition in which snorers stop breathing repeatedly during the night, taxing the heart and leaving the snorer unrested)

Skull Base Surgery – minimally invasive and advanced surgical approaches to the tumors of the anterior and posterior skull base such as acoustic neuroma, esthesioneuroblastoma, NF2, chordoma, chondrosarcoma, encephalocele.

Swallowing Disorders – the only center of its kind in New York City, providing comprehensive diagnosis, treatment and therapy for swallowing disorders

Voice Center – state-of-the-art biofeedback and therapy to rectify problems in speech

Advanced Otologic Medicine & Surgery – treating patients with disorders of the ear and conditions that affect hearing, balance and facial nerve function

The cochlear implant program at NYU Cochlear Implant Center is one of the nation's finest. Since it set the standard in 1984 by implanting a profoundly deaf adult, the Center has been the site of numerous studies and research trials that will continue to improve the technologies available. www.med.nyu.edu/cochlear

Adults and children travel from all over the world to get their cochlear implant at NYU Medical Center.

Physician Referral
(888) 7-NYU-MED
(888-769-8633)
www.med.nyu.edu

687

Sponsored Page

Pain Medicine

subspecialty of Anesthesiology, Neurology, and in Physical Medicine and Rehabilitation or Psychiatry

Some physicians who have their primary board certification in anesthesiology, neurology, physical medicine and rehabilitation, or psychiatry have completed additional training and passed an examination in the subspecialty called pain management. These doctors provide a high level of care, either as a primary physician or consultant, for patients experiencing problems with acute, chronic and/or cancer pain in both hospital and ambulatory settings.

For more information about the main specialties of these physicians, see **Anesthesiology, Neurology, Physical Medicine** and **Rehabilitation** or **Psychiatry** section(s).

Training Required: Number of years required for primary specialty *plus* additional training and examination

Pain Medicine

New England

Abrahm, Janet L MD [PM] - **Spec Exp:** Palliative Care; Pain-Cancer; **Hospital:** Dana-Farber Cancer Inst; **Address:** Dana-Farber Cancer Institute, 44 Binney St, Shields-Warren 420, Boston, MA 02115; **Phone:** 617-632-6464; **Board Cert:** Internal Medicine 1976; Medical Oncology 1981; Hematology 1978; **Med School:** UCSF 1973; **Resid:** Internal Medicine, Mass Genl Hosp 1975; Internal Medicine, Moffitt Hosp-UCSF 1977; **Fellow:** Hematology, Mass Genl Hosp 1976; Hematology & Oncology, Hosp Univ Penn 1980; **Fac Appt:** Assoc Prof Med, Harvard Med Sch

Berde, Charles Benjamin MD/PhD [PM] - **Spec Exp:** Pain Management-Pediatric; Critical Care; **Hospital:** Children's Hospital - Boston, Spaulding Rehab Hosp; **Address:** Chldns Hosp, Dept Anes, 300 Longwood Ave, Bader 3, Boston, MA 02115; **Phone:** 617-355-6995; **Board Cert:** Pediatrics 1988; Anesthesiology 1988; Pain Medicine 2004; **Med School:** Stanford Univ 1980; **Resid:** Pediatrics, Chldns Hosp 1983; Anesthesiology, Mass Genl Hosp 1985; **Fellow:** Pediatric Anesthesiology, Chldns Hosp 1985; **Fac Appt:** Prof Ped, Harvard Med Sch

Carr, Daniel B MD [PM] - **Spec Exp:** Pain-Neuropathic; Pain-Chronic; Headache; **Hospital:** Tufts-New England Med Ctr, St Elizabeth's Med Ctr; **Address:** New England Med Ctr, Dept Anesthesia, Box NEMC298, 750 Washington St, Boston, MA 02111; **Phone:** 617-636-9710; **Board Cert:** Internal Medicine 1979; Endocrinology 1981; Anesthesiology 2001; Pain Medicine 2004; **Med School:** Columbia P&S 1976; **Resid:** Internal Medicine, Columbia-Presby Med Ctr 1979; Anesthesiology, Mass Genl Hosp 1986; **Fellow:** Endocrinology, Mass Genl Hosp 1981; **Fac Appt:** Prof Anes, Tufts Univ

Loder, Elizabeth W MD [PM] - **Spec Exp:** Headache; Migraine; **Hospital:** Brigham & Women's Hosp, Faulkner Hosp; **Address:** 1153 Centre St, Ste 4970, Boston, MA 02130; **Phone:** 617-983-7580; **Board Cert:** Internal Medicine 2000; **Med School:** Univ ND Sch Med 1985; **Resid:** Internal Medicine, Faulkner Hosp 1989; **Fellow:** Pain Medicine, Graham Headache Ctr 1990; **Fac Appt:** Asst Prof Med, Harvard Med Sch

Mid Atlantic

De Leon-Casasola, Oscar MD [PM] - **Spec Exp:** Pain-Acute; Pain-Chronic; Pain-Cancer; **Hospital:** Roswell Park Cancer Inst; **Address:** Roswell Park Cancer Inst, Anesthesia/Pain Med, Elm & Carlton Sts, Buffalo, NY 14263; **Phone:** 716-845-4595; **Board Cert:** Anesthesiology 1991; Critical Care Medicine 1993; Pain Medicine 2005; **Med School:** Guatemala 1982; **Resid:** Surgery, SUNY-Downstate Med Ctr 1986; Anesthesiology, Univ Buffalo 1989; **Fac Appt:** Prof Anes, SUNY Buffalo

Dubois, Michel MD [PM] - **Spec Exp:** Pain-Back & Neck; Pain-Neuropathic; **Hospital:** NYU Med Ctr (page 67), Bellevue Hosp Ctr; **Address:** 317 E 34th St, Ste 902, New York, NY 10016-4974; **Phone:** 212-201-1004; **Board Cert:** Anesthesiology 1985; Pain Medicine 2004; **Med School:** France 1974; **Resid:** Anesthesiology, Georgetown Univ Hosp 1980; London Hosp 1976; **Fellow:** Pain Medicine, Georgetown Univ Hosp 1983; **Fac Appt:** Prof Anes, NYU Sch Med

Foley, Kathleen M MD [PM] - **Spec Exp:** Palliative Care; Pain-Cancer; **Hospital:** Meml Sloan Kettering Cancer Ctr; **Address:** Meml Sloan Kettering Cancer Ctr, Pain Care, 1275 York Ave, Box 52, New York, NY 10021-6007; **Phone:** 212-639-7050; **Board Cert:** Neurology 1977; **Med School:** Cornell Univ-Weill Med Coll 1969; **Resid:** Neurology, New York Hosp 1974; **Fellow:** Clinical Genetics, New York Hosp 1971; **Fac Appt:** Prof N, Cornell Univ-Weill Med Coll

Jain, Subhash MD [PM] - **Spec Exp:** Pain-Cancer; Pain-Pelvic; Reflex Sympathetic Dystrophy (RSD); Pain-Neuropathic; **Hospital:** Beth Israel Med Ctr - Petrie Division; **Address:** 360 S 72nd St, Ste C, New York, NY 10021; **Phone:** 212-439-6100; **Board Cert:** Anesthesiology 1994; Pain Medicine 1998; **Med School:** India 1968; **Resid:** Surgery, St Vincent Med Ctr 1977; Anesthesiology, New York Hosp 1979; **Fellow:** Pain Medicine, New York Hosp/Meml Sloan Kettering Cancer Ctr 1980; **Fac Appt:** Assoc Prof Anes, Cornell Univ-Weill Med Coll

Kreitzer, Joel MD [PM] - **Spec Exp:** Pain-Back; Pain-Cancer; Pain-Neuropathic; **Hospital:** Mount Sinai Med Ctr, Mount Sinai Hosp of Queens (page 64); **Address:** Upper East Side Pain Medicine, 1540 York Ave, New York, NY 10028; **Phone:** 212-288-2180; **Board Cert:** Anesthesiology 1990; Pain Medicine 2003; **Med School:** Albert Einstein Coll Med 1985; **Resid:** Anesthesiology, Mount Sinai Hosp 1989; **Fellow:** Pain Medicine, Mount Sinai Hosp 1989; **Fac Appt:** Assoc Clin Prof Anes, Mount Sinai Sch Med

Lema, Mark J MD/PhD [PM] - **Spec Exp:** Pain-Cancer; Pain-Acute; Pain-Neuropathic; **Hospital:** Roswell Park Cancer Inst; **Address:** Roswell Park Cancer Inst, Dept Pain Medicine, Elm & Carlton St, Buffalo, NY 14263-0001; **Phone:** 716-845-3240; **Board Cert:** Anesthesiology 1987; Pain Medicine 2004; **Med School:** SUNY Downstate 1982; **Resid:** Anesthesiology, Brigham & Women's Hosp 1984; **Fellow:** Physiology, SUNY Buffalo Genl Hosp 1978; **Fac Appt:** Prof Anes, SUNY Buffalo

Ngeow, Jeffrey MD [PM] - **Spec Exp:** Pain-Musculoskeletal-Spine & Neck; Acupuncture; Reflex Sympathetic Dystrophy (RSD); Pain-Neuropathic; **Hospital:** Hosp For Special Surgery (page 60); **Address:** 535 E 70th St, New York, NY 10021-4872; **Phone:** 212-606-1059; **Board Cert:** Anesthesiology 1980; Pain Medicine 2005; **Med School:** England 1971; **Resid:** Anesthesiology, Peter Bent Brigham Hosp 1977; **Fellow:** Pain Medicine, Tufts New England Med Ctr 1978; **Fac Appt:** Assoc Clin Prof Anes, Cornell Univ-Weill Med Coll

Portenoy, Russell MD [PM] - **Spec Exp:** Pain-Cancer; Palliative Care; **Hospital:** Beth Israel Med Ctr - Petrie Division; **Address:** Beth Israel Med Ctr, Dept Pain Medicine/Palliative Care, First Ave at 16th St, New York, NY 10003; **Phone:** 212-844-1403; **Board Cert:** Neurology 1985; **Med School:** Univ MD Sch Med 1980; **Resid:** Neurology, Albert Einstein 1984; **Fellow:** Pain Medicine, Meml Sloan-Kettering Cancer Ctr 1985; **Fac Appt:** Prof N, Albert Einstein Coll Med

Raja, Srinivasa MD [PM] - **Spec Exp:** Pain-Neuropathic; Herpetic Neuralgia (Shingles); Reflex Sympathetic Dystrophy (RSD); **Hospital:** Johns Hopkins Hosp - Baltimore (page 61); **Address:** 600 N Wolfe St Bldg Osler Fl 2 - rm 292, Baltimore, MD 21287; **Phone:** 410-955-1822; **Board Cert:** Anesthesiology 1982; Pain Medicine 1993; **Med School:** India 1974; **Resid:** Anesthesiology, Univ Washington Med Ctr 1979; **Fellow:** Pain Medicine, Univ Virginia Hosp 1981; **Fac Appt:** Prof Anes, Johns Hopkins Univ

Pain Medicine

Sarno, John E MD [PM] - **Spec Exp:** Pain-Mind/Body Disorder; **Hospital:** NYU Med Ctr (page 67); **Address:** Rusk Institute, Ground Floor, 400 E 34th St, rm 30, New York, NY 10016-4901; **Phone:** 212-263-6035; **Board Cert:** Physical Medicine & Rehabilitation 1965; **Med School:** Columbia P&S 1950; **Resid:** Physical Medicine & Rehabilitation, NYU Med Ctr 1952; Pediatrics, Babies Hosp/Columbia-Presby Med Ctr 1961; **Fellow:** Physical Medicine & Rehabilitation, NYU Med Ctr 1963; **Fac Appt:** Clin Prof PMR, NYU Sch Med

Staats, Peter MD [PM] - **Spec Exp:** Pain-Cancer; Pain-Back; **Hospital:** Riverview Med Ctr (page 59), CentraState Med Ctr; **Address:** Metzger Staats Pain Mgmt, LLC, 160 Avenue at the Commons, Ste 1, Shrewsbury, NJ 07702; **Phone:** 732-380-0200; **Board Cert:** Anesthesiology 1994; Pain Medicine 2005; **Med School:** Univ Mich Med Sch 1989; **Resid:** Anesthesiology, Johns Hopkins Hosp 1993; **Fellow:** Pain Medicine, Johns Hopkins Hosp 1994

Weinberger, Michael L MD [PM] - **Spec Exp:** Pain-Cancer; Pain-Back; **Hospital:** NY-Presby Hosp/Columbia (page 66); **Address:** 630 W 168th St, PH5, rm 500, New York, NY 10032-3720; **Phone:** 212-305-7114; **Board Cert:** Internal Medicine 1986; Anesthesiology 1990; Pain Medicine 2004; Hospice & Palliative Medicine 2006; **Med School:** Columbia P&S 1983; **Resid:** Internal Medicine, St Vincent's Hosp 1986; Anesthesiology, Columbia-Presby Med Ctr 1989; **Fellow:** Pain Medicine, Meml Sloan Kettering Cancer Ctr 1990; **Fac Appt:** Assoc Prof Anes, Columbia P&S

Southeast

Anghelescu, Doralina L MD [PM] - **Spec Exp:** Pain Management-Pediatric; Pain-Cancer; **Hospital:** St Jude Children's Research Hosp; **Address:** St Jude Chldn's Rsch Hosp, Anesthesiology, 332 N Lauderdale, rm B3035, MS 130, Memphis, TN 38105; **Phone:** 901-495-4034; **Board Cert:** Anesthesiology 1998; Pain Medicine 2001; **Med School:** Romania 1985; **Resid:** Anesthesiology, Univ NMex Hosp 1997; **Fellow:** Pain Medicine, Chldns Natl Med Ctr 1998; Pain Medicine, Univ NMex Hosp 1999

Baumann, Patricia L MD [PM] - **Hospital:** Crawford Long Hosp of Emory Univ, Emory Univ Hosp; **Address:** 550 Peachtree St Fl 7 - Ste 7085, Atlanta, GA 30308; **Phone:** 404-686-2410; **Board Cert:** Anesthesiology 1993; Pain Medicine 2005; **Med School:** Emory Univ 1988; **Resid:** Anesthesiology, Emory Univ Med Ctr 1992; **Fac Appt:** Asst Prof Anes, Emory Univ

Berger, Jerry J MD [PM] - **Spec Exp:** Herpetic Neuralgia (Shingles); Complex Regional Pain Syndrome-CRPS; **Hospital:** Shands Hlthcre at Univ of FL; **Address:** Shands at Univ Florida, 1600 SW Archer Rd, Box 100254, Gainesville, FL 32610; **Phone:** 352-265-0077; **Board Cert:** Anesthesiology 1981; Pain Medicine 1993; **Med School:** Duke Univ 1977; **Resid:** Anesthesiology, Shands-Univ Florida 1980; **Fellow:** Pain Medicine, Shands-Univ Florida 1981; **Fac Appt:** Asst Prof Anes, Univ Fla Coll Med

Payne, Richard MD [PM] - **Spec Exp:** Palliative Care; Pain-Neuropathic; **Hospital:** Duke Univ Med Ctr; **Address:** Duke Inst on Care at the End of Life, Box 90968, Durham, NC 27705; **Phone:** 919-660-3553; **Board Cert:** Neurology 1984; **Med School:** Harvard Med Sch 1977; **Resid:** Internal Medicine, Peter Bent Brigham Hosp 1979; Neurology, New York Hosp 1982; **Fellow:** Neuro-Oncology, Meml Sloan Kettering Cancer Ctr 1984

Rauck, Richard L MD [PM] - **Spec Exp:** Pain-Cancer; Spinal Cord Stimulation; Complex Regional Pain Syndrome-CRPS; **Hospital:** Forsyth Med Ctr, Wake Forest Univ Baptist Med Ctr (page 73); **Address:** Carolinas Pain Institute, 145 Kimel Park Drive, Ste 330, Winston Salem, NC 27103; **Phone:** 336-765-6181; **Board Cert:** Anesthesiology 1987; Pain Medicine 2005; **Med School:** Bowman Gray 1982; **Resid:** Anesthesiology, Univ Cincinnati Hosp 1985; **Fellow:** Pain Medicine, Univ Cincinnati Hosp 1986; **Fac Appt:** Assoc Prof Anes, Wake Forest Univ

Midwest

Abram, Stephen E MD [PM] - **Hospital:** Froedtert Meml Lutheran Hosp; **Address:** Med Coll Wisconsin-Pain Mgmt Ctr, Tosa Ctr Fl 1st, 1155 N Mayfair Rd, Wauwatosa, WI 53226; **Phone:** 414-456-7600; **Board Cert:** Anesthesiology 2001; Pain Medicine 2004; **Med School:** Jefferson Med Coll 1970; **Resid:** Anesthesiology, Mary Hitchcock Meml Hosp 1973; **Fac Appt:** Prof Anes, Med Coll Wisc

Benzon, Honorio T MD [PM] - **Spec Exp:** Pain-Back; Complex Regional Pain Syndrome-CRPS; Pain-Neuropathic; Pain-Cancer; **Hospital:** Northwestern Meml Hosp; **Address:** 675 N Saint Clair St Fl 20, Ste 20-100, Chicago, IL 60611-3015; **Phone:** 312-695-2500; **Board Cert:** Anesthesiology 1995; Pain Medicine 2004; **Med School:** Philippines 1971; **Resid:** Anesthesiology, Univ Cincinnati Med Ctr 1975; Anesthesiology, Northwestern Meml Hosp 1976; **Fellow:** Research, Brigham & Womens Hosp 1986; **Fac Appt:** Prof Anes, Northwestern Univ

Covington, Edward C MD [PM] - **Spec Exp:** Pain-Chronic; **Hospital:** Cleveland Clin Fdn (page 57); **Address:** Cleveland Clinic, Desk C21, 9500 Euclid Ave, Cleveland, OH 44195; **Phone:** 216-444-5964; **Board Cert:** Psychiatry 1978; Addiction Psychiatry 1998; Pain Medicine 2001; **Med School:** Univ Tenn Coll Med, Memphis 1970; **Resid:** Psychiatry, Mayo Clinic 1975

Green, Carmen R MD [PM] - **Spec Exp:** Racial/Ethnic Disparities in Pain Care; **Hospital:** Univ Michigan Hlth Sys; **Address:** Univ Hosp, Acute Pain Management Svc, 1500 E Med Ctr Drive, rm 1H247, Ann Arbor, MI 48109-0048; **Phone:** 734-936-4240; **Board Cert:** Anesthesiology 1996; Pain Medicine 1998; **Med School:** Mich State Univ 1987; **Resid:** Anesthesiology, Univ Mich Med Ctr 1989; **Fellow:** Pain Medicine, Univ Mich Med Ctr 1992; **Fac Appt:** Asst Prof Anes, Univ Mich Med Sch

Harden, R Norman MD [PM] - **Spec Exp:** Pain-Back; Reflex Sympathetic Dystrophy (RSD); Fibromyalgia; Headache; **Hospital:** Rehab Inst - Chicago; **Address:** 1030 N Clark St, Ste 320, Chicago, IL 60610; **Phone:** 312-238-7800; **Med School:** Med Coll GA 1984; **Resid:** Neurology, Univ South Carolina Med Ctr 1985; **Fellow:** Pain Medicine, Rehab Inst - Georgia 1989; **Fac Appt:** Asst Prof PMR, Northwestern Univ

Huntoon, Marc MD [PM] - **Spec Exp:** Pain-Cancer; Pain-after Spinal Intervention; Palliative Care; **Hospital:** Mayo Med Ctr & Clin - Rochester; **Address:** Mayo Clinic - Pain Medicine, 200 First St SW, Rochester, MN 55905; **Phone:** 507-266-9240; **Board Cert:** Anesthesiology 2003; Pain Medicine 2004; **Med School:** Wayne State Univ 1985; **Resid:** Anesthesiology, Naval Hosp Med Ctr 1991; **Fellow:** Pain Medicine, Naval Hosp Med Ctr 1992

Robbins, Lawrence D MD [PM] - **Spec Exp:** Headache; Migraine; Psychopharmacology; **Hospital:** Highland Park Hosp, Evanston Hosp; **Address:** 1535 Lake Cook Rd, Ste 506, Northbrook, IL 60062-1451; **Phone:** 847-480-9399; **Board Cert:** Pain Medicine 1995; **Med School:** Univ IL Coll Med 1981; **Resid:** Neurology, Univ Illinois 1985; **Fellow:** Pain Medicine, Diamond Headache Clinic 1986; **Fac Appt:** Asst Prof N, Rush Med Coll

Pain Medicine

Rosenquist, Richard W MD [PM] - **Spec Exp:** Complex Regional Pain Syndrome-CRPS; Pain-Back; Headache/Facial Pain; **Hospital:** Univ Iowa Hosp & Clinics, VA Med Ctr - Iowa City; **Address:** Center Pain Medicine-Dept Anesthesia, 200 Hawkins Drive, Iowa City, IA 52242; **Phone:** 319-356-2320; **Board Cert:** Anesthesiology 1988; Pain Medicine 2004; **Med School:** Northwestern Univ 1984; **Resid:** Anesthesiology, Northwestern Univ Med Ctr 1987; **Fellow:** Anesthesiology & Pain Management, Emory Univ 1988; **Fac Appt:** Prof Anes, Univ Iowa Coll Med

Swarm, Robert A MD [PM] - **Spec Exp:** Pain-Acute; Pain-Chronic; Pain-Cancer; **Hospital:** Barnes-Jewish Hosp; **Address:** Ctr for Advanced Med-Pain Mngmt Ctr, 4921 Parkview Pl, Ste 10A, MS 90-35-706, St Louis, MO 63110; **Phone:** 314-362-8820; **Board Cert:** Anesthesiology 1990; Pain Medicine 2004; **Med School:** Washington Univ, St Louis 1983; **Resid:** Surgery, Barnes Hosp 1986; Anesthesiology, Barnes Hosp 1989; **Fellow:** Pain Medicine, Univ Sydney; **Fac Appt:** Assoc Prof Anes, Washington Univ, St Louis

Weisman, Steven Jay MD [PM] - **Spec Exp:** Pain Management-Pediatric; Palliative Care-Pediatric; Reflex Sympathetic Dystrophy (RSD); **Hospital:** Chldns Hosp - Wisconsin; **Address:** Chldns Hosp Wisconsin, 9000 W Wisconsin Ave, MS 792, Milwaukee, WI 53226-3518; **Phone:** 414-266-2775; **Board Cert:** Pediatrics 1982; Pediatric Hematology-Oncology 1984; Anesthesiology 1996; **Med School:** Albert Einstein Coll Med 1978; **Resid:** Pediatrics, Chldns Hosp 1981; Anesthesiology, Univ Conn Hlth Ctr 1994; **Fellow:** Pediatric Hematology-Oncology, Indiana Univ Sch Med 1984; **Fac Appt:** Prof Anes, Med Coll Wisc

Great Plains and Mountains

Fine, Perry G MD [PM] - **Spec Exp:** Pain-Cancer; Palliative Care; Pain-Chronic; **Hospital:** Univ Utah Hosps and Clins; **Address:** 546 S Chipeta Way, Ste 200, Salt Lake City, UT 84108; **Phone:** 801-581-7246; **Board Cert:** Anesthesiology 1985; Pain Medicine 2004; **Med School:** Med Coll VA 1981; **Resid:** Anesthesiology, Univ Utah Hlth Sci Ctr 1984; **Fellow:** Pain Medicine, Univ Toronto 1985; **Fac Appt:** Prof Anes, Univ Utah

Waldman, Steven D MD [PM] - **Spec Exp:** Pain-Neuropathic; **Hospital:** Doctors Hosp; **Address:** The Headache & Pain Ctr, 4801 College Blvd, Leawood, KS 66211; **Phone:** 913-491-6451; **Board Cert:** Anesthesiology 1983; Pain Medicine 2004; **Med School:** Univ MO-Kansas City 1977; **Resid:** Anesthesiology, Mayo Clinic 1980; **Fac Appt:** Clin Prof Anes, Univ MO-Kansas City

Southwest

Burton, Allen W MD [PM] - **Spec Exp:** Pain-Cancer; Palliative Care; **Hospital:** UT MD Anderson Cancer Ctr (page 71); **Address:** MD Anderson Cancer Ctr, Dept Anesth, 1400 Holcombe Blvd, Unit 409, Houston, TX 77030; **Phone:** 713-745-7246; **Board Cert:** Anesthesiology 1996; Pain Medicine 1998; **Med School:** Baylor Coll Med 1991; **Resid:** Anesthesiology, Brigham & Women's Hosp 1995; **Fellow:** Pain Medicine, U Texas Med Branch Hosp 1998; **Fac Appt:** Assoc Prof Anes, Univ Tex Med Br, Galveston

Driver, Larry C MD [PM] - **Spec Exp:** Pain-Cancer; Palliative Care; **Hospital:** UT MD Anderson Cancer Ctr (page 71); **Address:** MD Andeson Cancer Ctr, Dept Pain Medicine, 1400 Holcombe Blvd, Unit 409, Houston, TX 77030; **Phone:** 713-745-7246; **Board Cert:** Anesthesiology 1992; Pain Medicine 2002; **Med School:** Univ Tex, San Antonio 1980; **Resid:** Anesthesiology, Univ Colorado Hlth Sci Ctr 1984; **Fellow:** Pain Medicine, MD Anderson Cancer Ctr 1999; **Fac Appt:** Assoc Prof Anes, Univ Tex, Houston

Racz, Gabor MD [PM] - **Spec Exp:** Pain-after Spinal Intervention; Reflex Sympathetic Dystrophy (RSD); Pain-Back, Head & Neck; Headache/Facial Pain; **Hospital:** Univ Med Ctr - Lubbock; **Address:** 3601 4th St, rm 1C282, Lubbock, TX 79430-0002; **Phone:** 806-743-3112; **Board Cert:** Anesthesiology 1993; Pain Medicine 1993; **Med School:** England 1962; **Resid:** Anesthesiology, SUNY Upstate Med Ctr 1969; **Fac Appt:** Prof Anes, Texas Tech Univ

Ramamurthy, Somayaji MD [PM] - **Spec Exp:** Pain-Back; Pain-Chronic; **Hospital:** Univ Hlth Sys - Univ Hosp; **Address:** Univ Tex Hlth Sci Ctr, Dept Anes, 7703 Floyd Curl Drive, MC 783, San Antonio, TX 78229-3900; **Phone:** 210-567-4543; **Board Cert:** Anesthesiology 1972; Pain Medicine 2003; **Med School:** India 1965; **Resid:** Anesthesiology, Cook Co Hosp 1970; **Fac Appt:** Prof Anes, Univ Tex, San Antonio

Rogers, James N MD [PM] - **Spec Exp:** Pain-Chronic; Pain-Acute; **Hospital:** Univ Hlth Sys - Univ Hosp; **Address:** Univ Texas Hlth Sci Ctr, Dept Anes, 7703 Floyd Curl Drive, MC 783, San Antonio, TX 78229-3900; **Phone:** 210-567-4543; **Board Cert:** Anesthesiology 1993; Pain Medicine 1994; **Med School:** Univ Ariz Coll Med 1987; **Resid:** Anesthesiology, Bexar Co Hosp 1991; **Fellow:** Pain Medicine, Bexar Co Hosp 1992; **Fac Appt:** Prof Anes, Univ Tex, San Antonio

Walsh, Nicolas MD [PM] - **Spec Exp:** Pain-Back; Trauma Rehabilitation; Post Polio Syndrome (PPS); **Hospital:** Univ Hlth Sys - Univ Hosp, Audie L Murphy Meml Vets Hosp; **Address:** Univ Tex Hlth Sci Ctr, Rehab Med (7798), 7703 Floyd Curl Drive, San Antonio, TX 78229-3901; **Phone:** 210-567-5350; **Board Cert:** Physical Medicine & Rehabilitation 1983; Pain Medicine 2000; **Med School:** Univ Colorado 1979; **Resid:** Physical Medicine & Rehabilitation, Univ Tex Hlth Sci Ctr 1982; **Fac Appt:** Prof PMR, Univ Tex, San Antonio

West Coast and Pacific

Anderson, Corrie MD [PM] - **Spec Exp:** Pain Management-Pediatric; **Hospital:** Chldns Hosp and Regl Med Ctr - Seattle, Univ Wash Med Ctr; **Address:** Chldns Hosp & Regl Med Ctr, Dept Anesth, 4800 Sands Point Way NE, rm W9825, Seattle, WA 98105; **Phone:** 206-987-2704; **Board Cert:** Anesthesiology 1994; **Med School:** Stanford Univ 1982; **Resid:** Pediatrics, Childrens Hosp 1985; Anesthesiology, Brigham & Womens Hosp 1987; **Fellow:** Pediatric Anesthesiology, Childrens Hosp 1988; **Fac Appt:** Prof Anes, Univ Wash

Du Pen, Stuart L MD [PM] - **Spec Exp:** Pain-Cancer; Pain-Chronic; **Hospital:** Overlake Hosp Med Ctr, Harrison Meml Hosp; **Address:** 1135 116th Ave NE, Ste 110, Bellevue, WA 98004; **Phone:** 425-289-3140; **Board Cert:** Anesthesiology 1972; Pain Medicine 1993; **Med School:** St Louis Univ 1967; **Resid:** Anesthesiology, Virginia Mason Med Ctr 1971; **Fac Appt:** Assoc Clin Prof Anes, Univ Wash

Ferrante, F Michael MD [PM] - **Spec Exp:** Pain-Back & Neck; Reflex Sympathetic Dystrophy (RSD); Botox for Pain; Pain-Neuropathic; **Hospital:** Santa Monica - UCLA Med Ctr, UCLA Med Ctr; **Address:** UCLA Pain Program, 1245 16th St, Ste 225, Santa Monica, CA 90404; **Phone:** 310-319-2241; **Board Cert:** Internal Medicine 1985; Anesthesiology 1987; Pain Medicine 2004; **Med School:** NY Med Coll 1980; **Resid:** Internal Medicine, Emory Univ Affil Hosp 1983; Anesthesiology, Emory Univ Affil Hosp 1986; **Fellow:** Infectious Disease, Barnes Hosp-Wash Univ 1984; Pain Medicine, Brigham & Women's Hosp 1987; **Fac Appt:** Prof Anes, UCLA

Fishman, Scott M MD [PM] - **Spec Exp:** Pain-Cancer; Pain-Chronic; Psychiatry in Pain Management; **Hospital:** UC Davis Med Ctr; **Address:** UC Davis Med Ctr, Pain Management Clinic, 4860 Y St, Ste 2700, Sacramento, CA 95817; **Phone:** 916-734-7246; **Board Cert:** Internal Medicine 1994; Psychiatry 1998; **Med School:** Univ Mass Sch Med 1990; **Resid:** Internal Medicine, Greenwich Hosp 1993; Psychiatry, Mass Genl Hosp 1996; **Fellow:** Pain Medicine, Mass Genl Hosp 1995; **Fac Appt:** Assoc Prof Anes, UC Davis

Fitzgibbon, Dermot R MD [PM] - **Spec Exp:** Pain-Cancer; **Hospital:** Univ Wash Med Ctr; **Address:** Univ Wash Med Ctr, Dept Anesthesiology, 1959 NE Pacific St, Box 356540, Seattle, WA 98195; **Phone:** 206-598-4260; **Board Cert:** Anesthesiology 1996; Pain Medicine 1998; **Med School:** Ireland 1983; **Resid:** Anesthesiology, St Vincent's Hosp 1992; Anesthesiology, Univ Washington Med Ctr 1995; **Fellow:** Pain Medicine, Univ Wash-Pain Mngmt Clinic 1994; **Fac Appt:** Assoc Prof Anes, Univ Wash

Prager, Joshua Philip MD [PM] - **Spec Exp:** Complex Regional Pain Syndrome-CRPS; **Hospital:** UCLA Med Ctr; **Address:** 100 UCLA Med Plaza, Ste 760, Los Angeles, CA 90095; **Phone:** 310-264-7246 x100; **Board Cert:** Internal Medicine 1984; Anesthesiology 1987; Pain Medicine 2004; **Med School:** Stanford Univ 1981; **Resid:** Internal Medicine, UCLA Med Ctr 1984; Anesthesiology, Mass Genl Hosp 1986; **Fac Appt:** Asst Clin Prof Anes, UCLA

Ready, L Brian MD [PM] - **Spec Exp:** Pain-Cancer; **Hospital:** Tacoma Genl Hosp; **Address:** 1901 S Union Ave, Ste A244, Tacoma, WA 98405; **Phone:** 253-459-6509; **Med School:** Canada 1967; **Resid:** Anesthesiology, Univ Washington Med Ctr 1975

Rosner, Howard L MD [PM] - **Spec Exp:** Pain-after Spinal Intervention; Pain-Cancer; Pain-Back; **Hospital:** Cedars-Sinai Med Ctr; **Address:** 444 S San Vincente Blvd, Ste 1101, Cedars-Sinai Med Ctr,Mark Goodson Bldg, Los Angeles, CA 90048; **Phone:** 310-423-9612; **Board Cert:** Anesthesiology 1989; Pain Medicine 2004; **Med School:** Univ Miami Sch Med 1980; **Resid:** Anesthesiology, Mass Genl Hosp 1983; **Fellow:** Pain Medicine, Columbia-Presby Med Ctr

Rowbotham, Michael C MD [PM] - **Spec Exp:** Reflex Sympathetic Dystrophy (RSD); Pain-Nerve Injury; Herpetic Neuralgia (Shingles); **Hospital:** UCSF - Mt Zion Med Ctr; **Address:** 1701 Divisadero St, Ste 480, San Francisco, CA 94115; **Phone:** 415-885-7246; **Board Cert:** Neurology 1989; **Med School:** UCSF 1979; **Resid:** Neurology, Boston Univ 1986; Neurology, UCSF 1987; **Fellow:** Neurological Pharmacology, UCSF 1980; Pain Medicine, UCSF 1989; **Fac Appt:** Assoc Prof N, UCSF

Slatkin, Neal E MD [PM] - **Spec Exp:** Pain-Cancer; Palliative Care; **Hospital:** City of Hope Natl Med Ctr & Beckman Rsch; **Address:** City of Hope Supportive Care NW Bldg, 1500 E Duarte Rd, rm 1218, Duarte, CA 91010; **Phone:** 626-256-4673 x63991; **Board Cert:** Neurology 1982; Pain Medicine 2000; **Med School:** SUNY Stony Brook 1976; **Resid:** Neurology, Bellevue Hosp Ctr-NYU 1978; Neurology, Med Coll Va 1981; **Fellow:** Neurology, Med Coll Va 1982; Neuro-Oncology, Meml Sloan-Kettering Cancer Ctr 1984; **Fac Appt:** Asst Clin Prof Med, USC-Keck School of Medicine

Wallace, Mark S MD [PM] - **Spec Exp:** Pain-Chronic; Pain-Cancer; Palliative Care; **Hospital:** UCSD Med Ctr; **Address:** 9300 Campus Point Drive, MC 7651, La Jolla, CA 92037; **Phone:** 858-657-6035; **Board Cert:** Anesthesiology 1992; Pain Medicine 2005; **Med School:** Creighton Univ 1987; **Resid:** Anesthesiology, Univ Maryland Hosp 1991; **Fellow:** Pain Medicine, UCSD Med Ctr 1994; **Fac Appt:** Assoc Prof Anes, UCSD

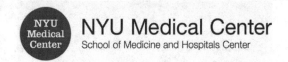

NYU Medical Center
School of Medicine and Hospitals Center

NYU Medical Center
550 First Avenue (at 31st Street)
New York, NY 10016
Physician Referral:
(888) 7-NYU-MED (888-769-8633)
www.nyumc.org

The International Center for the Study and Treatment of Pain at NYU

We have recently changed our name to The International Center for the Study and Treatment of Pain at NYU to reflect our reputation as a comprehensive, state-of-the-art, multidisciplinary, patient-centered care facility. We are an international center serving corporate business and individuals from all over the world. At this Center, clinicians and scientists gather to advance scientific knowledge by stimulating multispecialty cooperative projects involving basic and clinical sciences related to acute and chronic pain mechanisms, pain prevention, rehabilitation and clinical care to promote novel modality and analgesic development.

The International Center for the Study & Treatment of Pain at NYU was awarded the American Pain Society's 2007 Clinical Center of Excellence Award to honor programs that exemplify the provision of outstanding, multidisciplinary clinical care to patients. This prestigious award was given to only six programs across the country and our award presents the only award in NYC.

For more information, please contact us:

International Center for the Study and Treatment of Pain
NYU Medical Center
317 East 34th Street, Suite 902
New York, NY 10016
Tel: 212-263-7316
Fax: 212-685-5365
www.nyumc.org

> **Mission**
>
> The core mission of The International Center for the Study & Treatment of Pain at NYU is to preserve, improve and comfort human life. This mission will be achieved through the provision of superior clinical care, academic excellence, and innovative research.

Pathology

A pathologist deals with the causes and nature of disease and contributes to diagnosis, prognosis and treatment through knowledge gained by the laboratory application of the biologic, chemical and physical sciences.

A pathologist uses information gathered from the microscopic examination of tissue specimens, cells and body fluids, and from clinical laboratory tests on body fluids and secretions for the diagnosis, exclusion and monitoring of disease.

Training Required: Five to seven years

Certification in the following subspecialty requires additional training and examination.

Dermatopathology: A dermatopathologist has the expertise to diagnose and monitor diseases of the skin including infectious, immunologic, degenerative and neoplastic diseases. This entails the examination and interpretation of specially prepared tissue sections, cellular scrapings and smears of skin lesions by means of routine and special (electron and flourescent) microscopes.

Pathology

New England

Bhan, Atul Kumar MD [Path] - **Spec Exp:** Immunopathology; Liver Pathology; Liver Cancer; **Hospital:** Mass Genl Hosp; **Address:** Mass Genl Hosp, Dept Path, 55 Fruit St, Warren 501, Boston, MA 02114-2620; **Phone:** 617-726-2588; **Board Cert:** Anatomic Pathology 1976; Immunopathology 1985; **Med School:** India 1965; **Resid:** Pathology, Boston Univ Hosp 1971; Pathology, Chldns Univ Hosp 1974; **Fac Appt:** Prof Path, Harvard Med Sch

Connolly, James Leo MD [Path] - **Spec Exp:** Breast Pathology; Breast Cancer; **Hospital:** Beth Israel Deaconess Med Ctr - Boston; **Address:** BIDMC, Dept Path, 330 Brookline Ave, rm ES 112, Boston, MA 02215-5400; **Phone:** 617-667-4344; **Board Cert:** Anatomic Pathology 1980; **Med School:** Vanderbilt Univ 1974; **Resid:** Anatomic Pathology, Beth Israel Hosp 1978; **Fac Appt:** Prof Path, Harvard Med Sch

DeLellis, Ronald A MD [Path] - **Spec Exp:** Thyroid Cancer; Endocrine Pathology; **Hospital:** Rhode Island Hosp, Miriam Hosp; **Address:** Rhode Island Hospital, Dept Pathology, 593 Eddy St, Providence, RI 02903-4923; **Phone:** 401-444-5154; **Board Cert:** Anatomic Pathology 1997; **Med School:** Tufts Univ 1966; **Resid:** Anatomic Pathology, Natl Inst Hlth 1971; **Fellow:** Pathology, Univ Hosp 1973; **Fac Appt:** Prof Path, Brown Univ

Fletcher, Christopher MD [Path] - **Spec Exp:** Soft Tissue Tumors; Sarcoma; Surgical Pathology; **Hospital:** Brigham & Women's Hosp, Dana-Farber Cancer Inst; **Address:** Brigham & Women's Hospital, Dept Pathology, 75 Francis St, Boston, MA 02115-6110; **Phone:** 617-732-8558; **Med School:** England 1981; **Resid:** Pathology, St Thomas Hosp 1985; **Fellow:** Pathology, St Thomas Hosp 1986; **Fac Appt:** Prof Path, Harvard Med Sch

Harris, Nancy L MD [Path] - **Spec Exp:** Lymphoma; Hematopathology; **Hospital:** Mass Genl Hosp; **Address:** Mass Genl Hosp, Dept Path, 55 Fruit St, Warren 211, Boston, MA 02114; **Phone:** 617-726-5155; **Board Cert:** Anatomic Pathology 1978; Clinical Pathology 1978; **Med School:** Stanford Univ 1970; **Resid:** Pathology, Beth Israel Hosp 1978; **Fellow:** Immunopathology, Mass Genl Hosp 1980; **Fac Appt:** Prof Path, Harvard Med Sch

Mark, Eugene J MD [Path] - **Spec Exp:** Lung Pathology; Cardiac Pathology; Forensic Pathology; **Hospital:** Mass Genl Hosp; **Address:** Mass Genl Hosp, Dept Path, 55 Fruit St, Warren 246, Boston, MA 02114; **Phone:** 617-726-8891; **Board Cert:** Anatomic & Clinical Pathology 1973; Dermatopathology 1975; **Med School:** Harvard Med Sch 1967; **Resid:** Pathology, Mass Genl Hosp 1972; **Fellow:** Pathology, Kantons Hospital 1966; **Fac Appt:** Prof Path, Harvard Med Sch

Odze, Robert D MD [Path] - **Spec Exp:** Gastrointestinal Pathology; Liver Pathology; **Hospital:** Brigham & Women's Hosp; **Address:** Brigham & Women's Hosp, Dept Pathology, 75 Francis St, Boston, MA 02115; **Phone:** 617-732-7549; **Board Cert:** Anatomic Pathology 1990; **Med School:** McGill Univ 1984; **Resid:** Surgery, McGill Univ 1987; Pathology, McGill Univ 1990; **Fellow:** Gastrointestinal Pathology, New England Deaconess Med Ctr 1991; **Fac Appt:** Assoc Prof Path, Harvard Med Sch

Rennke, Helmut G MD [Path] - **Spec Exp:** Kidney Pathology; **Hospital:** Brigham & Women's Hosp; **Address:** Brigham & Womens Hosp, Dept Pathology, 75 Francis St Emory Bldg, Boston, MA 02115; **Phone:** 617-732-6518; **Board Cert:** Anatomic Pathology 1980; **Med School:** Chile 1971; **Resid:** Pathology, Boston City Hosp 1974; Pathology, Peter Bent Brigham Hosp 1977; **Fac Appt:** Prof Path, Harvard Med Sch

Schnitt, Stuart J MD [Path] - **Spec Exp:** Breast Pathology; Breast Cancer; **Hospital:** Beth Israel Deaconess Med Ctr - Boston; **Address:** Beth Israel Deaconess Med Ctr, Dept Pathology, 330 Brookline Ave, rm ES 112, Boston, MA 02215-5400; **Phone:** 617-667-4344; **Board Cert:** Anatomic & Clinical Pathology 1983; **Med School:** Albany Med Coll 1979; **Resid:** Anatomic Pathology, Beth Israel Deaconess Med Ctr; **Fellow:** Surgical Pathology, Beth Israel Deaconess Med Ctr; **Fac Appt:** Assoc Prof Path, Harvard Med Sch

Young, Robert H MD [Path] - **Spec Exp:** Ovarian Cancer; Breast Cancer; **Hospital:** Mass Genl Hosp; **Address:** Mass Genl Hosp, Dept Pathology, 55 Fruit St, Warren 215, Boston, MA 02114; **Phone:** 617-726-8892; **Board Cert:** Anatomic Pathology 1980; **Med School:** Ireland 1974; **Resid:** Pathology, Mass Genl Hosp 1979; Pathology, Dublin Univ 1977; **Fac Appt:** Prof Path, Harvard Med Sch

Mid Atlantic

Brooks, John S MD [Path] - **Spec Exp:** Tumor Diagnosis; Sarcoma; Bone & Soft Tissue Pathology; **Hospital:** Pennsylvania Hosp (page 72), Hosp Univ Penn - UPHS (page 72); **Address:** Pennsylvania Hospital, Preston 6 FL, 800 Spruce St, Philadelphia, PA 19107; **Phone:** 215-829-3541; **Board Cert:** Anatomic Pathology 1978; Immunopathology 1983; **Med School:** Thomas Jefferson Univ 1974; **Resid:** Pathology, osp U Penn 1978; **Fellow:** Immunopathology, Hosp U Penn 1978; **Fac Appt:** Prof Path, Univ Pennsylvania

Burger, Peter MD [Path] - **Spec Exp:** Brain Tumors; Neuro-Pathology; **Hospital:** Johns Hopkins Hosp - Baltimore (page 61); **Address:** Johns Hopkins Hosp-Division Pathology, 600 N Wolfe St, rm 710, Baltimore, MD 21287; **Phone:** 410-955-8378; **Board Cert:** Anatomic Pathology 1976; Neuropathology 1976; **Med School:** Northwestern Univ 1966; **Resid:** Anatomic Pathology, Duke Univ Med Ctr 1973; **Fellow:** Neuropathology, Duke Univ Med Ctr 1973

Demetris, A Jake MD [Path] - **Spec Exp:** Transplant Pathology; Liver Pathology; **Hospital:** UPMC Presby, Pittsburgh; **Address:** UPMC - Montefiore, 3459 5th Ave, rm E741, Pittsburgh, PA 15213; **Phone:** 412-647-2067; **Board Cert:** Anatomic & Clinical Pathology 1987; **Med School:** Univ Pittsburgh 1982; **Resid:** Anatomic & Clinical Pathology, Univ Pittsburgh Med Ctr 1986; **Fac Appt:** Prof Path, Univ Pittsburgh

Dorfman, Howard D MD [Path] - **Spec Exp:** Bone Tumors; Soft Tissue Tumors; Joint Pathology; **Hospital:** Montefiore Med Ctr, Montefiore Med Ctr - Weiler-Einstein Div; **Address:** Montefiore-Orthopaedic Pathology Div, 111 E 210th St, Bronx, NY 10467-2401; **Phone:** 718-920-5622; **Board Cert:** Anatomic Pathology 1958; **Med School:** SUNY Downstate 1951; **Resid:** Pathology, Mt Sinai Hosp 1953; Surgical Pathology, Columbia-Presby Med Ctr 1958; **Fellow:** Pathology, Mt Sinai Med Ctr 1954; **Fac Appt:** Prof Path, Albert Einstein Coll Med

Ehya, Hormoz MD [Path] - **Spec Exp:** Cytopathology; Breast Pathology; Lung Pathology; **Hospital:** Fox Chase Cancer Ctr (page 59); **Address:** Fox Chase Cancer Center, 333 Cottman Ave, rm C427, Philadelphia, PA 19111-2497; **Phone:** 215-728-5389; **Board Cert:** Anatomic Pathology 1979; Cytopathology 1989; **Med School:** Iran 1974; **Resid:** Pathology, Univ Miss Med Ctr 1979; **Fellow:** Cytopathology, Meml Sloan-Kettering Cancer Ctr 1980

Pathology

Epstein, Jonathan MD [Path] - **Spec Exp:** Bladder Cancer; Urologic Cancer; Prostate Cancer; Urologic Pathology; **Hospital:** Johns Hopkins Hosp - Baltimore (page 61); **Address:** 401 N Broadway, Weinberg 2242, Baltimore, MD 21231; **Phone:** 410-955-5043; **Board Cert:** Anatomic Pathology 1986; **Med School:** Boston Univ 1981; **Resid:** Pathology, Johns Hopkins Hosp 1985; **Fellow:** Pathology, Meml Sloan Kettering Cancer Ctr 1984; **Fac Appt:** Prof Path, Johns Hopkins Univ

Gupta, Prabodh K MD [Path] - **Spec Exp:** Lung Pathology; Cervical Cancer; Fine Needle Aspiration Biopsy; **Hospital:** Hosp Univ Penn - UPHS (page 72); **Address:** Hosp Univ Penn - Cytopathology, 3400 Spruce St, 6 Founders, Philadelphia, PA 19104; **Phone:** 215-662-3238; **Board Cert:** Anatomic Pathology 1975; Cytopathology 1989; **Med School:** India 1965; **Resid:** Pathology, All India Inst Med Scis 1967; **Fellow:** Pathology, Mass Genl Hosp 1968; Johns Hopkins Hosp 1969; **Fac Appt:** Prof Path, Univ Pennsylvania

Hruban, Ralph H MD [Path] - **Spec Exp:** Gastrointestinal Pathology; Pancreatic Cancer; **Hospital:** Johns Hopkins Hosp - Baltimore (page 61); **Address:** Johns Hopkins Hosp, Dept Pathology, 401 N Broadway Bldg Weinberg - rm 2242, Baltimore, MD 21231; **Phone:** 410-955-9132; **Board Cert:** Anatomic Pathology 1990; **Med School:** Johns Hopkins Univ 1985; **Resid:** Pathology, Johns Hopkins Hosp 1990; **Fellow:** Meml Sloan Kettering Cancer Ctr 1989; **Fac Appt:** Prof Path, Johns Hopkins Univ

Jaffe, Elaine S MD [Path] - **Spec Exp:** Lymphoma; Hematopathology; **Hospital:** Natl Inst of Hlth - Clin Ctr; **Address:** NIH/NCI - Lab Pathology, 10 Center Drive Bldg 10 - rm 2N202, Bethesda, MD 20892; **Phone:** 301-496-0183; **Board Cert:** Anatomic Pathology 1974; **Med School:** Univ Pennsylvania 1969; **Resid:** Pathology, Clinical Ctr/NIH 1972; **Fellow:** Hematopathology, Natl Cancer Inst 1974; **Fac Appt:** Clin Prof Path, Geo Wash Univ

Kahn, Leonard B MD [Path] - **Spec Exp:** Bone Pathology; Head & Neck Pathology; Soft Tissue Tumors; **Hospital:** Long Island Jewish Med Ctr, N Shore Univ Hosp at Manhasset; **Address:** 270-05 76th Ave, rm B67, New Hyde Park, NY 11040-1433; **Phone:** 718-470-7491; **Board Cert:** Anatomic Pathology 1980; **Med School:** South Africa 1960; **Resid:** Pathology, Univ Cape Town 1966; **Fellow:** Pathology, Washington Univ Sch Med 1969; **Fac Appt:** Prof Path, Albert Einstein Coll Med

Katzenstein, Anna-Luise A MD [Path] - **Spec Exp:** Lung Cancer; Pulmonary Pathology; Interstitial Lung Disease; **Hospital:** Univ. Hosp.- SUNY Upstate, Crouse Hosp; **Address:** SUNY Upstate Medical Univ, 766 Irving Ave, Weiskotten, rm 2106, Syracuse, NY 13210; **Phone:** 315-464-7125; **Board Cert:** Anatomic Pathology 1976; **Med School:** Johns Hopkins Univ 1971; **Resid:** Pathology, Univ Hospital 1975; **Fellow:** Surgical Pathology, Barnes Hosp-Wash Univ 1976; **Fac Appt:** Prof Path, SUNY Upstate Med Univ

Knowles, Daniel MD [Path] - **Spec Exp:** Lymph Node Pathology; Bone Marrow Pathology; Lymphoma; **Hospital:** NY-Presby Hosp/Weill Cornell (page 66); **Address:** Cornell-Weill Med Coll- Dept Pathology, 1300 York Ave, rm C302, New York, NY 10021; **Phone:** 212-746-6464; **Board Cert:** Anatomic Pathology 1978; Immunopathology 1984; **Med School:** Univ Chicago-Pritzker Sch Med 1973; **Resid:** Anatomic Pathology, Columbia-Presby Med Ctr 1975; **Fellow:** Immunopathology, Rockefeller Univ 1977; **Fac Appt:** Prof Path, Cornell Univ-Weill Med Coll

Kurman, Robert J MD [Path] - **Spec Exp:** Gynecologic Pathology; Ovarian Cancer; Uterine Cancer; **Hospital:** Johns Hopkins Hosp - Baltimore (page 61); **Address:** Johns Hopkins Hosp, Dept Pathology, 401 N Broadway, Weinberg-2242, Baltimore, MD 21231; **Phone:** 410-955-0471; **Board Cert:** Anatomic Pathology 1972; Obstetrics & Gynecology 1980; **Med School:** SUNY Upstate Med Univ 1968; **Resid:** Pathology, Peter Bent Brigham Hosp/Mass Genl Hosp 1977; Obstetrics & Gynecology, LAC Hosp/USC 1978; **Fellow:** Obstetrics & Gynecology, Harvard Univ 1973; **Fac Appt:** Prof Path, Johns Hopkins Univ

Li Volsi, Virginia A MD [Path] - **Spec Exp:** Endocrine Cancers; Thyroid Cancer; Gynecologic Cancer; **Hospital:** Hosp Univ Penn - UPHS (page 72); **Address:** Hosp Univ Penn - Pathology, 3400 Spruce St 6 Founders Bldg - Ste 6030, Philadelphia, PA 19104; **Phone:** 215-662-6545; **Board Cert:** Anatomic Pathology 1974; **Med School:** Columbia P&S 1969; **Resid:** Anatomic Pathology, Presbyterian Hosp 1974; **Fac Appt:** Prof Path, Univ Pennsylvania

McCormick, Steven MD [Path] - **Spec Exp:** Ophthalmic Pathology; Head & Neck Pathology; Fine Needle Aspiration Biopsy; **Hospital:** New York Eye & Ear Infirm (page 65); **Address:** 310 E 14th St, New York, NY 10003; **Phone:** 212-979-4156; **Board Cert:** Anatomic Pathology 1988; **Med School:** W VA Univ 1984; **Resid:** Anatomic Pathology, West Va Univ Hosp 1988; **Fellow:** Ophthalmic Pathology, West Va Univ Hosp 1988; **Fac Appt:** Assoc Prof Path, NY Med Coll

McNutt, N Scott MD [Path] - **Spec Exp:** Dermatopathology; **Address:** Rockefeller Univ, Krueger Laboratory, 1230 York Ave, New York, NY 10021; **Phone:** 212-327-8086; **Board Cert:** Anatomic Pathology 1973; Dermatopathology 1979; **Med School:** Harvard Med Sch 1966; **Resid:** Pathology, Mass Genl Hosp 1970; **Fellow:** Pathology, Mass Genl Hosp 1972

Mies, Carolyn MD [Path] - **Spec Exp:** Breast Cancer; **Hospital:** Hosp Univ Penn - UPHS (page 72); **Address:** Hosp Univ Penn - Surgical Pathology, 3400 Spruce St, Founders 6, Philadelphia, PA 19104; **Phone:** 215-662-6503; **Board Cert:** Anatomic Pathology 1980; **Med School:** Rush Med Coll 1980; **Resid:** Pathology, Tufts-New England Med Ctr 1982; Pathology, New England Deaconess Hosp 1984; **Fellow:** Surgical Pathology, Meml Sloan Kettering Cancer Ctr 1986; **Fac Appt:** Assoc Prof Path, Univ Pennsylvania

Montgomery, Elizabeth A MD [Path] - **Spec Exp:** Barrett's Esophagus; Esophageal Cancer; Gastrointestinal Pathology; **Hospital:** Johns Hopkins Hosp - Baltimore (page 61); **Address:** Johns Hopkins Univ, Dept Pathology, 401 N Broadway Weinberg Bldg - rm 2242, Baltimore, MD 21231; **Phone:** 410-614-2308; **Board Cert:** Anatomic Pathology 1988; Cytopathology 1994; **Med School:** Geo Wash Univ 1984; **Resid:** Pathology, Walter Reed AMC 1988; **Fac Appt:** Assoc Prof Path, Johns Hopkins Univ

Orenstein, Jan M MD/PhD [Path] - **Spec Exp:** Prostate Cancer; Tumor Banking; AIDS/HIV; **Hospital:** G Washington Univ Hosp; **Address:** Geo Wash Univ Med Ctr Dept Path, 502 Ross Hall, 2300 Eye St NW, Washington, DC 20037; **Phone:** 202-994-2943; **Board Cert:** Anatomic Pathology 1977; **Med School:** SUNY Downstate 1971; **Resid:** Pathology, Presby Hosp 1973; Pathology, Natl Cancer Inst 1977; **Fac Appt:** Prof Path, Geo Wash Univ

Patchefsky, Arthur S MD [Path] - **Spec Exp:** Breast Cancer; Pulmonary Pathology; Sarcoma; **Hospital:** Fox Chase Cancer Ctr (page 59); **Address:** Fox Chase Cancer Center, 7701 Burholme Ave, rm C4333, Philadelphia, PA 19111; **Phone:** 215-728-5390; **Board Cert:** Anatomic Pathology 1969; **Med School:** Hahnemann Univ 1963; **Resid:** Pathology, John Hopkins Hosp 1966; Pathology, Hosp U Penn 1967; **Fellow:** Pathology, Meml Sloan Kettering Cancer Ctr 1968; **Fac Appt:** Prof Path, Thomas Jefferson Univ

Rosen, Paul P MD [Path] - **Spec Exp:** Breast Pathology; Breast Cancer; **Hospital:** NY-Presby Hosp/Weill Cornell (page 66); **Address:** New York Presbyterian, Dept Pathology, 525 E 68th St, Starr 1031, New York, NY 10021-4870; **Phone:** 212-746-6482; **Board Cert:** Anatomic & Clinical Pathology 1969; Pathology 1998; **Med School:** Columbia P&S 1964; **Resid:** Pathology, Presby Hosp 1966; Pathology, VA Hosp 1968; **Fellow:** Pathology, Meml Hosp Cancer Ctr 1970; **Fac Appt:** Prof Path, Cornell Univ-Weill Med Coll

Rosenblum, Marc MD [Path] - **Spec Exp:** Neuropathology; Cytopathology; **Hospital:** Meml Sloan Kettering Cancer Ctr; **Address:** Dept Pathology, 1275 York Ave, New York, NY 10021; **Phone:** 212-639-8410; **Board Cert:** Anatomic Pathology 1984; Pathology 1998; Neuropathology 1988; **Med School:** Univ Miami Sch Med 1979; **Resid:** Anatomic Pathology, Mount Sinai Med Ctr 1984; **Fellow:** Pathology, Meml Sloan-Kettering Cancer Ctr 1985; Neurological Pathology, Bellevue-NYU Med Ctr 1987; **Fac Appt:** Prof Path, Cornell Univ

Ross, Jeffrey S MD [Path] - **Spec Exp:** Urologic Cancer; Prostate Cancer; Breast Cancer; **Hospital:** Albany Med Ctr; **Address:** Albany Med Coll, Dept Path, 47 New Scotland Ave, MC 8, Albany, NY 12208; **Phone:** 518-262-5471; **Board Cert:** Anatomic & Clinical Pathology 1974; **Med School:** SUNY Buffalo 1970; **Resid:** Pathology, Mass Genl Hosp 1974; **Fellow:** Pathology, Harvard Med Sch 1974; **Fac Appt:** Prof Path, Albany Med Coll

Sanchez, Miguel A MD [Path] - **Spec Exp:** Breast Cancer; Thyroid Cancer; **Hospital:** Englewood Hosp & Med Ctr; **Address:** Englewood Hosp & Med Ctr, Dept Pathology, 350 Engle St, Englewood, NJ 07631-1898; **Phone:** 201-894-3423; **Board Cert:** Anatomic Pathology 1975; Clinical Pathology 1979; Cytopathology 1991; **Med School:** Spain 1969; **Resid:** Pathology, Englewood Hosp 1972; Pathology, Temple Univ 1973; **Fellow:** Pathology, Meml Sloan Kettering Cancer Ctr 1974; **Fac Appt:** Assoc Prof Path, Mount Sinai Sch Med

Schiller, Alan L MD [Path] - **Spec Exp:** Bone & Joint Pathology; Soft Tissue Pathology; Bone Tumors; **Hospital:** Mount Sinai Med Ctr; **Address:** Mt Sinai Sch Med, Dept Pathology, 1 Gustave Levy Pl, Box 1194, New York, NY 10029-6500; **Phone:** 212-241-8014; **Board Cert:** Anatomic Pathology 1973; **Med School:** Ros Franklin Univ/Chicago Med Sch 1967; **Resid:** Pathology, Mass Genl Hosp 1972; **Fac Appt:** Prof Path, Mount Sinai Sch Med

Schlaepfer, William W MD [Path] - **Spec Exp:** Neurofilament Metabolism; Neuro-Pathology; **Hospital:** Hosp Univ Penn - UPHS (page 72); **Address:** 609 Stellar Chance Lab, 422 Curie Blvd, Philadelphia, PA 19104-6100; **Phone:** 215-662-7372; **Board Cert:** Anatomic Pathology 1964; Neuropathology 1964; **Med School:** Yale Univ 1958; **Resid:** Pathology, Grace-New Haven Comm Hosp 1961; **Fac Appt:** Prof Path, Univ Pennsylvania

Silverberg, Steven G MD [Path] - **Spec Exp:** Gynecologic Pathology; Breast Pathology; Urologic Pathology; Endocrine Pathology; **Hospital:** Univ of MD Med Sys; **Address:** Univ Maryland Med Ctr, Dept Pathology, 22 S Greene St, Baltimore, MD 21201; **Phone:** 410-328-5072; **Board Cert:** Anatomic Pathology 1969; **Med School:** Johns Hopkins Univ 1962; **Resid:** Pathology, Yale-New Haven Hosp 1965; **Fellow:** Surgical Pathology, Meml Sloan Kettering Cancer Ctr 1966; **Fac Appt:** Prof Path, Univ MD Sch Med

Swerdlow, Steven H MD [Path] - **Spec Exp:** Lymphoma; Hematopathology; Transplant Pathology; **Hospital:** UPMC Presby, Pittsburgh; **Address:** UPMC-Presby Hosp, Div Hematopathology, 200 Lothrop St, rm C606, Pittsburgh, PA 15213-2536; **Phone:** 412-647-5191; **Board Cert:** Anatomic Pathology 2005; Clinical Pathology 2005; **Med School:** Harvard Med Sch 1975; **Resid:** Pathology, Beth Israel Hosp 1979; **Fellow:** Hematopathology, Vanderbilt Univ 1981; Hematopathology, St Bartholmew's Hosp 1983; **Fac Appt:** Prof Path, Univ Pittsburgh

Tomaszewski, John E MD [Path] - **Spec Exp:** Kidney Pathology; Immunopathology; Kidney Pathology; Uterine Cancer; **Hospital:** Hosp Univ Penn - UPHS (page 72); **Address:** Hosp Univ Penn, Dept Pathology & Lab Med, 3400 Spruce St, 6 Founders Bldg, Ste 6042, Philadelphia, PA 19104; **Phone:** 215-662-6852; **Board Cert:** Anatomic Pathology 1982; Immunopathology 1983; **Med School:** Univ Pennsylvania 1977; **Resid:** Pathology, Hosp Univ Penn 1982; **Fellow:** Surgical Pathology, Hosp Univ Penn 1983; **Fac Appt:** Prof Path, Univ Pennsylvania

Tornos, Carmen MD [Path] - **Spec Exp:** Gynecologic Cancer; Breast Cancer; Ovarian Cancer; **Hospital:** Stony Brook Univ Med Ctr; **Address:** Stony Brook Univ Hosp, Dept Pathology, Level 2, rm 766, Stony Brook, NY 11794-7025; **Phone:** 631-444-2222; **Board Cert:** Anatomic & Clinical Pathology 1997; **Med School:** Spain 1977; **Resid:** Hematology, Ciudad Sanitaria Valle de Hebron 1982; Anatomic & Clinical Pathology, Univ Texas HSC 1989; **Fellow:** Surgical Pathology, MD Anderson Cancer Ctr 1990; **Fac Appt:** Prof Path, SUNY Stony Brook

Travis, William MD [Path] - **Spec Exp:** Pulmonary Pathology; Lung Cancer; Interstitial Lung Disease; **Hospital:** Meml Sloan Kettering Cancer Ctr; **Address:** Meml Sloan-Kettering Canc Ctr, Dept Path, 1275 York Ave, New York, NY 10021; **Phone:** 212-639-5905; **Board Cert:** Anatomic & Clinical Pathology 1985; **Med School:** Univ Fla Coll Med 1981; **Resid:** Anatomic Pathology, New England Deaconess Hosp 1983; Clinical Pathology, Mayo Clinic 1985; **Fellow:** Surgical Pathology, Mayo Clinic 1986

Yousem, Samuel A MD [Path] - **Spec Exp:** Pulmonary Pathology; Transplant-Lung (Pathology); Lung Cancer; **Hospital:** UPMC Presby, Pittsburgh; **Address:** Dept Pathology, A-610, Presbyterian Campus, 200 Lothrop St, Pittsburgh, PA 15213; **Phone:** 412-647-6193; **Board Cert:** Anatomic Pathology 1985; Cytopathology 1997; **Med School:** Univ MD Sch Med 1981; **Resid:** Pathology, Stanford Univ Med Ctr 1983; **Fellow:** Surgical Pathology, Stanford Univ Med Ctr 1984; **Fac Appt:** Prof Path, Univ Pittsburgh

Southeast

Banks, Peter MD [Path] - **Spec Exp:** Hematopathology; Lymphoma; **Hospital:** Carolinas Med Ctr; **Address:** Dept Pathology, 1000 Blythe Blvd, 4th Fl Lab, Charlotte, NC 28232; **Phone:** 704-355-2251; **Board Cert:** Anatomic Pathology 1997; **Med School:** Harvard Med Sch 1971; **Resid:** Pathology, National Cancer Inst 1974; Pathology, Duke Univ Med Ctr 1975; **Fellow:** Surgical Pathology, Univ Minn Med Ctr 1976; **Fac Appt:** Prof Path, Univ NC Sch Med

Bostwick, David MD [Path] - **Spec Exp:** Urologic Pathology; Prostate Cancer; Bladder Cancer; **Address:** 4355 Innslake Drive, Glen Allen, VA 23060; **Phone:** 804-967-9225; **Board Cert:** Anatomic Pathology 1985; **Med School:** Univ MD Sch Med 1979; **Resid:** Pathology, Stanford Univ Med Ctr 1981; **Fellow:** Surgical Pathology, Stanford Univ Med Ctr 1984

Braylan, Raul MD [Path] - **Spec Exp:** Hematopathology; Leukemia; Lymphoma; **Hospital:** Shands Hlthcre at Univ of FL; **Address:** Univ Florida, Dept Hematopathology, PO Box 100275, Gainesville, FL 32610; **Phone:** 352-392-3477; **Board Cert:** Anatomic Pathology 1972; **Med School:** Argentina 1960; **Resid:** Anatomic Pathology, Mt Sinai Hosp 1965; Anatomic Pathology, Einstein Affil Hosps 1967; **Fellow:** Anatomic Pathology, Meml Sloan Kettering Cancer Hosp 1968; Hematopathology, Univ Chicago Hosps 1973; **Fac Appt:** Prof Path, Univ Fla Coll Med

Chesney, Carolyn M MD [Path] - **Spec Exp:** Hematopathology; Bleeding/Coagulation Disorders; **Hospital:** Univ of Tennesee Mem Hosp; **Address:** Dept of Pathology-Coag Lab, 6019 Walnut Grove, Memphis, TN 38120; **Phone:** 901-226-5650; **Board Cert:** Internal Medicine 1972; Hematology 1999; **Med School:** Vanderbilt Univ 1968; **Resid:** Internal Medicine, Vanderbilt Univ Hosp 1970; **Fellow:** Internal Medicine, Mass Genl Hosp 1972; **Fac Appt:** Prof Med, Univ Tenn Coll Med, Memphis

Crawford, James M MD/PhD [Path] - **Spec Exp:** Liver Pathology; Gastrointestinal Pathology; Gastrointestinal Cancer; **Hospital:** Shands Hlthcre at Univ of FL; **Address:** Univ Florida, Dept Pathology, 1600 SW Archer Rd, rm M649, Box 100275, Gainesville, FL 32610-0275; **Phone:** 352-392-3741; **Board Cert:** Anatomic Pathology 1987; **Med School:** Duke Univ 1982; **Resid:** Pathology, Brigham & Women's Hosp 1984; **Fellow:** Gastrointestinal Pathology, Brigham & Women's Hosp 1987; **Fac Appt:** Prof Path, Univ Fla Coll Med

Masood, Shahla MD [Path] - **Spec Exp:** Breast Cancer; Breast Pathology; **Hospital:** Shands Jacksonville; **Address:** Univ of Florida, Dept Pathology, 655 W 8th St, Jacksonville, FL 32209-6511; **Phone:** 904-244-4387; **Board Cert:** Anatomic & Clinical Pathology 1998; Cytopathology 1990; **Med School:** Iran 1973; **Resid:** Anatomic Pathology, University Hosp 1977; **Fac Appt:** Prof Path, Univ Fla Coll Med

McCurley, Thomas L MD [Path] - **Spec Exp:** Hematopathology; Immunopathology; **Hospital:** Vanderbilt Univ Med Ctr, VA Med Ctr - Nashville; **Address:** Vanderbilt Univ Hosp, Dept Pathology, 21st & Garland Ave, Nashville, TN 37232; **Phone:** 615-343-9167; **Board Cert:** Anatomic & Clinical Pathology 1981; Immunopathology 1986; Hematology 1999; **Med School:** Vanderbilt Univ 1974; **Resid:** Internal Medicine, UCSF Med Ctr 1976; Pathology, Vanderbilt Univ Med Ctr 1981; **Fellow:** Hematopathology, Vanderbilt Univ Med Ctr 1984; **Fac Appt:** Assoc Prof Path, Vanderbilt Univ

Mills, Stacey E MD [Path] - **Spec Exp:** Breast Pathology; Ear, Nose & Throat Cancer; Surgical Pathology; **Hospital:** Univ Virginia Med Ctr; **Address:** Univ VA Hlth System, Dept Pathology, PO Box 800214, Charlottesville, VA 22908-0214; **Phone:** 434-982-4406; **Board Cert:** Anatomic Pathology 1999; **Med School:** Univ VA Sch Med 1977; **Resid:** Pathology, Univ Virginia Med Ctr 1980; **Fellow:** Pathology, Univ Virginia 1981; **Fac Appt:** Prof Path, Univ VA Sch Med

Norenberg, Michael D MD [Path] - **Spec Exp:** Liver Pathology; Parkinson's Disease; **Hospital:** Jackson Meml Hosp; **Address:** Jackson Meml Hosp, Dept Pathology, 1611 NW 12th Ave Holtz Ctr, rm 2142, Miami, FL 33136; **Phone:** 305-585-7017; **Board Cert:** Anatomic Pathology 1972; Neuropathology 1974; **Med School:** Univ Rochester 1965; **Resid:** Pathology, Strong Meml Hosp 1970; **Fellow:** Neuropathology, Strong Meml Hosp 1972; **Fac Appt:** Prof Path, Univ Miami Sch Med

Page, David L MD [Path] - **Spec Exp:** Breast Cancer; **Hospital:** Vanderbilt Univ Med Ctr; **Address:** Vanderbilt Univ, MCN, 1161 21st Ave S, rm C 3309, Nashville, TN 37232-2561; **Phone:** 615-322-3759; **Board Cert:** Anatomic Pathology 1972; Dermatopathology 1974; **Med School:** Johns Hopkins Univ 1966; **Resid:** Pathology, Mass Genl Hosp 1969; Pathology, Johns Hopkins Hosp 1972; **Fac Appt:** Prof Path, Vanderbilt Univ

Petito, Carol MD [Path] - **Spec Exp:** Neuro-Pathology; **Hospital:** Jackson Meml Hosp; **Address:** Univ Miami Sch Med, Dept Pathology (R-5), 1550 NW 10th Ave, PAP Bldg - Fl 4, rm 417, Miami, FL 33136; **Phone:** 305-243-3584; **Board Cert:** Anatomic Pathology 1973; Neuropathology 1973; **Med School:** Columbia P&S 1967; **Resid:** Pathology, NY Hosp-Cornell Med Ctr 1970; Neuropathology, Armed Forces Inst; **Fac Appt:** Prof Path, Univ Miami Sch Med

Sewell, C Whitaker MD [Path] - **Spec Exp:** Breast Pathology; Surgical Pathology; **Hospital:** Emory Univ Hosp; **Address:** Emory Univ Hosp, Dept Pathology, 1364 Clifton Rd NE, rm H185, Atlanta, GA 30322; **Phone:** 404-712-7003; **Board Cert:** Anatomic Pathology 1974; Clinical Pathology 1974; **Med School:** Emory Univ 1969; **Resid:** Pathology, Emory Univ Hosp 1974; **Fac Appt:** Prof Path, Emory Univ

Weiss, Sharon MD [Path] - **Spec Exp:** Soft Tissue Pathology; Surgical Pathology; Sarcoma; **Hospital:** Emory Univ Hosp, Crawford Long Hosp of Emory Univ; **Address:** Emory Univ Hosp, Dept Path, 1364 Clifton Rd NE, rm H180, Atlanta, GA 30322; **Phone:** 404-712-0708; **Board Cert:** Anatomic Pathology 1974; **Med School:** Johns Hopkins Univ 1971; **Resid:** Pathology, Johns Hopkins Hosp 1975; **Fac Appt:** Prof Path, Emory Univ

Midwest

Allred, D Craig MD [Path] - **Spec Exp:** Breast Cancer; Breast Pathology; Breast Cancer Risk Assessment; **Hospital:** Barnes-Jewish Hosp; **Address:** Washington Univ Sch Med, Path & Immunology, 660 S Euclid Ave, Box 8118, St Louis, MO 63110; **Phone:** 314-362-6313; **Board Cert:** Anatomic Pathology 1984; **Med School:** Univ Utah 1979; **Resid:** Anatomic Pathology, Univ Conn Hlth Ctr 1983; **Fellow:** Immunopathology, Univ Conn Hlth Ctr 1982; **Fac Appt:** Prof Path, Baylor Coll Med

Appelman, Henry MD [Path] - **Spec Exp:** Gastrointestinal Pathology; Liver Pathology; **Hospital:** Univ Michigan Hlth Sys; **Address:** Univ Michigan, Dept of Pathology, 1500 E Medical Center Drive, Ann Arbor, MI 48109-0054; **Phone:** 734-936-6770; **Board Cert:** Anatomic & Clinical Pathology 1966; **Med School:** Univ Mich Med Sch 1961; **Resid:** Pathology, Univ Mich Med Ctr 1966; **Fac Appt:** Prof Path, Univ Mich Med Sch

Balla, Andre K MD/PhD [Path] - **Spec Exp:** Prostate Cancer; Gynecologic Pathology; Tumor Banking; **Hospital:** Univ of IL Med Ctr at Chicago; **Address:** Univ IL at Chicago, Dept Path, 840 S Wood St, rm 130, MC 847, Chicago, IL 60612; **Phone:** 312-996-3879; **Board Cert:** Anatomic & Clinical Pathology 1988; **Med School:** Brazil 1972; **Resid:** Pathology, Hahnemann Univ Hosp 1988; **Fellow:** Clinical Immunology, Scripps Clin Rsch Fdn 1981; **Fac Appt:** Prof Path, Univ IL Coll Med

Cohen, Michael B MD [Path] - **Spec Exp:** Urologic Cancer; Cytopathology; **Hospital:** Univ Iowa Hosp & Clinics, VA Med Ctr - Iowa City; **Address:** Univ Iowa - Dept Pathology, 200 Hawkins Drive, C670GH, Iowa City, IA 52242; **Phone:** 319-384-9609; **Board Cert:** Anatomic Pathology 1998; Cytopathology 1996; **Med School:** Albany Med Coll 1982; **Resid:** Pathology, UCSF Hosps & Clinics 1986; **Fellow:** Cytopathology, UCSF Hosps & Clinics 1987; **Fac Appt:** Prof Path, Univ Iowa Coll Med

Pathology

Gambetti, Pierluigi MD [Path] - **Spec Exp:** Neuro-Pathology; Neurodegenerative Disorders; Creutzfeldt-Jakob Disease (CJD); **Hospital:** Univ Hosps Case Med Ctr; **Address:** Case Western Reserve Univ, Inst Path, 2085 Adelbert Rd, rm 419, Cleveland, OH 44106; **Phone:** 216-368-0587; **Board Cert:** Neuropathology 1981; **Med School:** Italy 1960; **Resid:** Neurology, Univ Bologna Med Ctr 1963; **Fellow:** Neurological Pathology, Institut Bunge 1965; Neurological Pathology, Hosp Univ Penn 1968; **Fac Appt:** Prof Path, Case West Res Univ

Goldblum, John R MD [Path] - **Spec Exp:** Soft Tissue Pathology; Esophageal Cancer; Gastrointestinal Pathology; Sarcoma; **Hospital:** Cleveland Clin Fdn (page 57); **Address:** Cleveland Clinic, Anatomic Pathology L25, 9500 Euclid Ave, Cleveland, OH 44195; **Phone:** 216-444-8238; **Board Cert:** Anatomic Pathology 1993; **Med School:** Univ Mich Med Sch 1989; **Resid:** Anatomic Pathology, Univ Michigan Hosps 1993; **Fac Appt:** Prof Path, Cleveland Cl Coll Med/Case West Res

Greenson, Joel K MD [Path] - **Spec Exp:** Liver Cancer; Gastrointestinal Pathology; Liver Pathology; **Hospital:** Univ Michigan Hlth Sys; **Address:** Univ Michigan Hospitals, Dept Pathology, 1500 E Medical Center Drive, rm 2G332, Ann arbor, MI 48109-0054; **Phone:** 734-936-6776; **Board Cert:** Anatomic & Clinical Pathology 1988; **Med School:** Univ Mich Med Sch 1984; **Resid:** Pathology, Cedars-Sinai Med Ctr 1988; **Fellow:** Gastrointestinal Pathology, Johns Hopkins Hosp 1990; **Fac Appt:** Prof Path, Univ Mich Med Sch

Kurtin, Paul J MD [Path] - **Spec Exp:** Lymph Node Pathology; Bone Marrow Pathology; Lymphoma; **Hospital:** Mayo Med Ctr & Clin - Rochester; **Address:** Mayo Clinic - Dept Pathology, 200 First St SW, Hilton 1156A, Rochester, MN 55905; **Phone:** 507-284-4939; **Board Cert:** Anatomic & Clinical Pathology 1983; Hematology 1988; **Med School:** Mcd Coll Wisc 1979; **Resid:** Anatomic & Clinical Pathology, Vanderbilt Univ mED cTR 1983; **Fellow:** Hematopathology, Brigham & Women's Hosp 1984; Surgical Pathology, Brigham & Women's Hosp 1986; **Fac Appt:** Prof Path, Mayo Med Sch

Mitros, Frank A MD [Path] - **Spec Exp:** Liver Pathology; Gastrointestinal Pathology; Surgical Pathology; **Hospital:** Univ Iowa Hosp & Clinics; **Address:** Univ Iowa Hosp & Clins, Dept Pathology, 200 Hawkins Dr, 5244B RCP, Iowa City, IA 52242; **Phone:** 319-356-1760; **Board Cert:** Anatomic Pathology 1979; **Med School:** UMDNJ-NJ Med Sch, Newark 1969; **Resid:** Pathology, Univ Chicago Hosps 1976; **Fac Appt:** Prof Path, Univ Iowa Coll Med

Myers, Jeffrey L MD [Path] - **Spec Exp:** Lung Cancer; Lung Pathology; **Hospital:** Univ Michigan Hlth Sys; **Address:** Univ Michigan, 2G332 UH, 1500 E Medical Ctr Drive, Ann Arbor, MI 48109; **Phone:** 734-936-1888; **Board Cert:** Anatomic Pathology 1986; **Med School:** Washington Univ, St Louis 1981; **Resid:** Anatomic Pathology, Barnes Jewish Hosp 1984; **Fellow:** Surgical Pathology, U Alabama Med Ctr 1985; **Fac Appt:** Prof Path, Univ Mich Med Sch

Petras, Robert E MD [Path] - **Spec Exp:** Gastrointestinal Pathology; **Address:** Ameripath GI Institute, 7730 First Pl, Ste A, Oakwood Village, OH 44146; **Phone:** 440-703-2100; **Board Cert:** Anatomic & Clinical Pathology 2004; **Med School:** Ohio State Univ 1978; **Resid:** Anatomic & Clinical Pathology, Cleveland Clinic 1982; **Fellow:** Gastrointestinal Pathology, St Marks Hosp; **Fac Appt:** Assoc Prof Path, NE Ohio Univ

Scheithauer, Bernd MD [Path] - **Spec Exp:** Brain Tumors; Pituitary Tumors; Neuro-Pathology; Pituitary Disorders; **Hospital:** Mayo Med Ctr & Clin - Rochester, St Mary's Hosp - Rochester; **Address:** Mayo Clinic, Dept Pathology, 200 First St SW, Rochester, MN 55905; **Phone:** 507-284-8350; **Board Cert:** Anatomic Pathology 1979; Neuropathology 1979; **Med School:** Loma Linda Univ 1973; **Resid:** Anatomic Pathology, Stanford Univ Med Ctr 1976; Neuropathology, Stanford Univ Med Ctr 1978; **Fac Appt:** Prof Path, Mayo Med Sch

Suster, Saul M MD [Path] - **Spec Exp:** Lung Cancer; Mediastinal Tumors; Surgical Pathology; **Hospital:** Ohio St Univ Med Ctr; **Address:** Ohio State Univ Med Ctr, E-411 Doan Hall, 410 W 10th Ave, Columbus, OH 43210-1240; **Phone:** 614-293-7625; **Board Cert:** Anatomic & Clinical Pathology 1988; **Med School:** Ecuador 1976; **Resid:** Anatomic Pathology, Tel Aviv Univ Med Ctr 1984; Anatomic & Clinical Pathology, Mt Sinai Med Ctr 1988; **Fellow:** Surgical Pathology, Yale-New Haven Hosp 1990; **Fac Appt:** Prof Path, Ohio State Univ

Ulbright, Thomas M MD [Path] - **Spec Exp:** Testicular Cancer; Gynecologic Pathology; **Hospital:** Indiana Univ Hosp; **Address:** Clarion Pathology Laboratory, 350 W 11th St, rm 4014, Indianapolis, IN 46202; **Phone:** 317-491-6498; **Board Cert:** Anatomic Pathology 1980; **Med School:** Washington Univ, St Louis 1975; **Resid:** Pathology, Barnes Jewish Hosp 1978; Surgical Pathology, Barnes Jewish Hosp 1979; **Fellow:** Gynecologic Pathology, St Johns Mercy Med Ctr 1980; **Fac Appt:** Prof Path, Indiana Univ

Great Plains and Mountains

De Masters, Bette K MD [Path] - **Spec Exp:** Neuro-Pathology; Brain Tumors; **Hospital:** Univ Colorado Hosp, Chldn's Hosp - Denver, The; **Address:** Univ Colo Hlth Sci Ctr, Dept Path, Box 6511, MS 8104, Denver, CO 80262; **Phone:** 303-724-3704; **Board Cert:** Anatomic & Clinical Pathology 1982; Neuropathology 1985; **Med School:** Univ Wisc 1977; **Resid:** Internal Medicine, Presby Hosp 1979; Pathology, Univ Colo Med Sch 1982; **Fellow:** Neurological Pathology, Univ Colo/Univ Kansas 1984; **Fac Appt:** Prof Path, Univ Colorado

Rodgers III, George M MD/PhD [Path] - **Spec Exp:** Hematopathology; Anemia-Cancer Related; **Hospital:** Univ Utah Hosps and Clins; **Address:** Univ Utah Med Ctr - Div Hematology, 30 N 1900 E, rm 4C416, Salt Lake City, UT 84132; **Phone:** 801-585-3229; **Board Cert:** Internal Medicine 1979; Hematology 1982; **Med School:** Tulane Univ 1976; **Resid:** Internal Medicine, Baylor Affil Hosps 1979; **Fellow:** Hematology, UCSF Med Ctr 1982; **Fac Appt:** Prof Med, Univ Utah

Thor, Ann D MD [Path] - **Spec Exp:** Breast Cancer; Gynecologic Cancer; **Hospital:** Univ Colorado Hosp; **Address:** Univ Colorado Hlth Sci Ctr, Dept Pathology, Box 6511, MS 8104, Aurora, CO 80045-0508; **Phone:** 303-724-3704; **Board Cert:** Anatomic Pathology 1987; Cytopathology 1989; **Med School:** Vanderbilt Univ 1981; **Resid:** Pathology, Vanderbilt Univ 1983; **Fellow:** Immunopathology, Natl Cancer Inst 1986; Gynecologic Pathology, Mass Genl Hosp 1990; **Fac Appt:** Prof Path, Univ Colorado

Weisenburger, Dennis MD [Path] - **Spec Exp:** Hematopathology; Lymphoma; **Hospital:** Nebraska Med Ctr; **Address:** Univ Nebraska Med Ctr, Dept Pathology, 983135 Nebraska Medical Center, Omaha, NE 68198-3135; **Phone:** 402-559-7688; **Board Cert:** Anatomic & Clinical Pathology 1979; **Med School:** Univ Minn 1974; **Resid:** Anatomic Pathology, Univ Iowa Hosps 1978; **Fellow:** Hematopathology, City of Hope Natl Med Ctr 1980; **Fac Appt:** Prof Path, Univ Nebr Coll Med

Southwest

Bruner, Janet M MD [Path] - **Spec Exp:** Brain Tumors; Neuro-Pathology; **Hospital:** UT MD Anderson Cancer Ctr (page 71); **Address:** MD Anderson Cancer Ctr, 1515 Holcombe Blvd, Ste 85, Houston, TX 77030; **Phone:** 713-792-6127; **Board Cert:** Anatomic Pathology 1997; Neuropathology 1984; **Med School:** Med Coll OH 1979; **Resid:** Anatomic & Clinical Pathology, Med Coll Ohio Hosp 1982; **Fellow:** Neurological Pathology, Baylor Coll Med 1984

Pathology

Cagle, Philip MD [Path] - **Spec Exp:** Pulmonary Pathology; Lung Cancer; Mesothelioma; **Hospital:** Methodist Hosp - Houston; **Address:** Methodist Hospital, Dept Pathology, 6565 Fannin St, Ste 227, Houston, TX 77030; **Phone:** 713-441-6478; **Board Cert:** Anatomic & Clinical Pathology 1985; **Med School:** Univ Tenn Coll Med, Memphis 1981; **Fac Appt:** Prof Path, Baylor Coll Med

Colby, Thomas V MD [Path] - **Spec Exp:** Pulmonary Pathology; Surgical Pathology; Lung Cancer; **Hospital:** Mayo Clin Hosp - Scottsdale; **Address:** Mayo Clinic, Dept Path, 13400 E Shea Blvd, Scottsdale, AZ 85259; **Phone:** 480-301-8021; **Board Cert:** Anatomic Pathology 1978; **Med School:** Univ Mich Med Sch 1974; **Resid:** Anatomic Pathology, Stanford Univ Hosp 1978; **Fellow:** Surgical Pathology, Stanford Univ Hosp; **Fac Appt:** Prof Path, Mayo Med Sch

Foucar, M Kathryn MD [Path] - **Spec Exp:** Leukemia; Lymph Node Pathology; Bone Marrow Pathology; **Hospital:** Univ NM Hlth & Sci Ctr; **Address:** TriCore Reference Lab, Hematopathology, 1001 Woodward Pl NE, Albuquerque, NM 87102; **Phone:** 505-938-8457; **Board Cert:** Anatomic & Clinical Pathology 1978; **Med School:** Ohio State Univ 1974; **Resid:** Anatomic Pathology, Univ NM Health & Sci Ctr 1976; Anatomic Pathology, Univ Minn Med Ctr 1978; **Fellow:** Surgical Pathology, Univ Minn Med Ctr 1979; **Fac Appt:** Prof Path, Univ New Mexico

Grogan, Thomas M MD [Path] - **Spec Exp:** Immunopathology; Lymphoma; **Hospital:** Univ Med Ctr - Tucson; **Address:** Univ Med Ctr, Dept Pathology, 1501 N Campbell Ave, rm 5212, Tucson, AZ 85724; **Phone:** 520-626-7477; **Board Cert:** Anatomic Pathology 1976; **Med School:** Geo Wash Univ 1971; **Resid:** Pathology, Letterman Army Med Ctr 1976; **Fellow:** Immunopathology, Stanford Univ Sch Med 1979; **Fac Appt:** Prof Path, Univ Ariz Coll Med

Hamilton, Stanley R MD [Path] - **Spec Exp:** Surgical Pathology; Gastrointestinal Pathology; Liver Pathology; **Hospital:** UT MD Anderson Cancer Ctr (page 71); **Address:** Univ Texas MD Anderson Cancer Ctr, 1515 Holcombe Blvd, Unit 85, Houston, TX 77030-4009; **Phone:** 713-792-2040; **Board Cert:** Anatomic & Clinical Pathology 1978; **Med School:** Indiana Univ 1973; **Resid:** Pathology, Johns Hopkins Hosp 1978; **Fellow:** St Marks Hosp 1979; **Fac Appt:** Prof Path, Univ Tex, Houston

Kinney, Marsha C MD [Path] - **Spec Exp:** Hematopathology; Lymphoma; Leukemia; **Hospital:** Univ Hlth Sys - Univ Hosp; **Address:** Univ Tex Hlth & Sci Ctr, Dept Path, 7703 Floyd Curl Drive, MC 775, San Antonio, TX 78229-3900; **Phone:** 210-567-4098; **Board Cert:** Anatomic & Clinical Pathology 1985; Hematology 1998; **Med School:** Univ Tex SW, Dallas 1981; **Resid:** Pathology, Vanderbilt Univ Med Ctr 1985; **Fellow:** Hematopathology, Vanderbilt Univ Med Ctr 1988; **Fac Appt:** Prof Path, Univ Tex, San Antonio

Leslie, Kevin O MD [Path] - **Spec Exp:** Pulmonary Pathology; Lung Cancer; Surgical Pathology; **Hospital:** Mayo Clin Hosp - Scottsdale; **Address:** Mayo Clinic, Scottsdale, 13400 E Shea Blvd, Scottsdale, AZ 85259; **Phone:** 480-301-8021; **Board Cert:** Anatomic & Clinical Pathology 1982; **Med School:** Albert Einstein Coll Med 1976; **Resid:** Anatomic & Clinical Pathology, Univ Colorado Health Sci Ctr 1982; **Fellow:** Surgical Pathology, Stanford Univ Med Ctr 1983; **Fac Appt:** Prof Path, Mayo Med Sch

Moran, Cesar A MD [Path] - **Spec Exp:** Lung Cancer; Mediastinal Tumors; Mesothelioma; **Hospital:** UT MD Anderson Cancer Ctr (page 71); **Address:** MD Anderson Cancer Ctr, Dept Pathology, 1515 Holcombe Blvd, rm G1-3738, Houston, TX 77030; **Phone:** 713-792-8134; **Board Cert:** Anatomic Pathology 1992; **Med School:** Guatemala 1981; **Resid:** Anatomic Pathology, Mt Sinai Med Ctr 1988; **Fellow:** Surgical Pathology, Yale-New Haven Med Ctr 1989; **Fac Appt:** Prof Path, Univ Tex, Houston

Prieto, Victor G MD/PhD [Path] - **Spec Exp:** Dermatopathology; Melanoma; Skin Cancer; **Hospital:** UT MD Anderson Cancer Ctr (page 71); **Address:** MD Anderson Cancer Ctr, Dept Pathology, 1515 Holcombe Blvd, Box 85, Houston, TX 77030; **Phone:** 713-792-0918; **Board Cert:** Anatomic Pathology 1995; Dermatopathology 1997; **Med School:** Spain 1986; **Resid:** Pathology, New York Hosp-Cornell Med Ctr 1993; **Fellow:** Pathology, Meml Sloan Kettering Cancer Ctr 1995; Dermatopathology, New York Hosp-Cornell Med Ctr 1996; **Fac Appt:** Prof Path, Univ Tex, Houston

Rashid, Asif MD/PhD [Path] - **Spec Exp:** Gastrointestinal Pathology; Liver Pathology; **Hospital:** UT MD Anderson Cancer Ctr (page 71); **Address:** MD Anderson Cancer Ctr, Dept Pathology, 1515 Holcombe Blvd, Box 85, Houston, TX 77030; **Phone:** 713-745-1101; **Board Cert:** Anatomic Pathology 1994; **Med School:** Pakistan 1984; **Resid:** Anatomic Pathology, Mass Gnrl Hosp 1993; **Fellow:** Anatomic Pathology, Mass Gnrl Hosp 1994; Anatomic Pathology, Johns Hopkins Med Inst 1996

Roberts, William C MD [Path] - **Spec Exp:** Preventive Cardiology; Cardiac Pathology; **Hospital:** Baylor Univ Medical Ctr; **Address:** Baylor Univ Med Ctr, Heart & Vascular Inst, 3500 Gaston Ave, Dallas, TX 75246-2017; **Phone:** 214-820-7911; **Board Cert:** Anatomic Pathology 1965; **Med School:** Emory Univ 1958; **Resid:** Anatomic Pathology, Natl Heart Inst-NIH 1962; Internal Medicine, Johns Hopkins Hosp 1963; **Fellow:** Cardiovascular Disease, Natl Heart Inst-NIH 1964

Silva, Elvio G MD [Path] - **Spec Exp:** Gynecologic Pathology; Gynecologic Cancer; **Hospital:** UT MD Anderson Cancer Ctr (page 71), Cedars-Sinai Med Ctr; **Address:** MD Anderson Cancer Ctr, Dept Pathology, 1515 Holcombe Blvd, Box 85, Houston, TX 77030; **Phone:** 713-792-3154; **Board Cert:** Anatomic Pathology 1997; **Med School:** Argentina 1969; **Resid:** Pathology, National Univ Med Ctr 1975; Anatomic Pathology, Univ Toronto 1978; **Fellow:** Surgical Pathology, MD Anderson Cancer Ctr 1979; **Fac Appt:** Prof Path

Walker, David H MD [Path] - **Spec Exp:** Infections-Emerging; Tropical Diseases; Biodefense; **Hospital:** UTMB - John Sealy Hospital, Houston Shriners Hosp; **Address:** UT Med Br Galveston, Dept Path, 301 University Blvd, Galveston, TX 77555-0609; **Phone:** 409-772-3989; **Board Cert:** Anatomic & Clinical Pathology 1974; **Med School:** Vanderbilt Univ 1969; **Resid:** Anatomic & Clinical Pathology, Peter Bent Brigham Hosp 1973; **Fellow:** Pathology, Harvard 1973; **Fac Appt:** Prof Path, Univ Tex Med Br, Galveston

Wheeler, Thomas M MD [Path] - **Spec Exp:** Thyroid Disorders; Thyroid Cancer; **Hospital:** Ben Taub General Hosp; **Address:** Baylor Coll Med, Dept Pathology, One Baylor Plaza, rm T203, Houston, TX 77030; **Phone:** 713-798-4664; **Board Cert:** Anatomic & Clinical Pathology 1999; Cytopathology 1990; **Med School:** Baylor Coll Med 1977; **Resid:** Pathology, Baylor Coll Med 1981; **Fac Appt:** Prof Path, Baylor Coll Med

West Coast and Pacific

Arber, Daniel A MD [Path] - **Spec Exp:** Bone Marrow Pathology; Lymph Node Pathology; Spleen Pathology; **Hospital:** Stanford Univ Med Ctr, Lucile Packard Chldns Hosp/Stanford Univ Med Ctr; **Address:** Clinic Laboratories, Stanford Univ Med Ctr, 300 Pasteur Drive, rm H1507, MC 5627, Stanford, CA 94305; **Phone:** 650-725-5604; **Board Cert:** Anatomic & Clinical Pathology 1991; Hematology 1993; **Med School:** Univ Tex, San Antonio 1986; **Resid:** Anatomic & Clinical Pathology, Scott & White Meml Hosp 1991; **Fellow:** Hematopathology, City of Hope Natl Med Ctr 1993; **Fac Appt:** Prof Path, Stanford Univ

Pathology

Bollen, Andrew W MD [Path] - **Spec Exp:** Neuro-Pathology; Brain Tumors; Brain Infections; **Hospital:** UCSF Med Ctr, CA Pacific Med Ctr - Pacific Campus; **Address:** Dept Pathology/Neuropathology, 505 Parnassus Ave, M551, Box 0102, San Francisco, CA 94143-0511; **Phone:** 415-476-5236; **Board Cert:** Clinical Pathology 1993; Anatomic Pathology 1992; Neuropathology 1992; **Med School:** UCSD 1985; **Resid:** Anatomic Pathology, UCSF Med Ctr 1991; **Fellow:** Neuropathology, UCSF Med Ctr 1989; **Fac Appt:** Prof Path, UCSF

Chandrasoma, Parakrama T MD [Path] - **Spec Exp:** Gastrointestinal Pathology; Gastrointestinal Cancer; Neuro-Pathology; **Hospital:** LAC & USC Med Ctr; **Address:** LAC-USC Med Ctr, Dept Path, 1200 N State St, rm 16-905, Los Angeles, CA 90033; **Phone:** 323-226-4600; **Board Cert:** Anatomic Pathology 1982; **Med School:** Sri Lanka 1971; **Resid:** Anatomic Pathology, Univ Sri Lanka 1978; Anatomic Pathology, LAC-USC Med Ctr 1982; **Fac Appt:** Prof Path, USC Sch Med

Cochran, Alistair J MD [Path] - **Spec Exp:** Melanoma; Dermatopathology; **Hospital:** UCLA Med Ctr; **Address:** UCLA Med Ctr, Dept Path & Med, 10833 Le Conte Ave, rm 13145CHS, MC 173216, Los Angeles, CA 90095-1713; **Phone:** 310-825-2743; **Med School:** Scotland 1966; **Resid:** Dermatopathology, Western Infirmary 1968; **Fellow:** Immunology, Karolinska Inst 1970; **Fac Appt:** Prof Path, UCLA

Cote, Richard J MD [Path] - **Spec Exp:** Lymph Node Pathology; Bladder Cancer; Breast Cancer; **Hospital:** USC Norris Comp Cancer Ctr, USC Univ Hosp - R K Eamer Med Plz; **Address:** 1441 Eastlake Ave, rm 2424, Los Angeles, CA 90033; **Phone:** 323-865-0212; **Board Cert:** Anatomic Pathology 1987; **Med School:** Univ Chicago-Pritzker Sch Med 1980; **Resid:** Pathology, New York Hosp-Cornell 1987; **Fellow:** Pathology, Meml Sloan-Kettering Cancer Ctr 1990; **Fac Appt:** Prof Path, USC-Keck School of Medicine

Dubeau, Louis MD/PhD [Path] - **Spec Exp:** Ovarian Cancer; Breast Cancer; **Hospital:** USC Norris Comp Cancer Ctr; **Address:** USC Norris Cancer Ctr, Dept Pathology, 1441 Eastlake Ave, rm 7320, Los Angeles, CA 90033-1048; **Phone:** 323-865-0720; **Board Cert:** Anatomic Pathology 1984; **Med School:** McGill Univ 1979; **Resid:** Anatomic Pathology, McGill Univ Med Ctr 1984; **Fac Appt:** Prof Path, USC Sch Med

Ferrell, Linda MD [Path] - **Spec Exp:** Liver Pathology; **Hospital:** UCSF Med Ctr; **Address:** UCSF Med Ctr, Dept Pathology, 505 Parnassus Ave, rm M590, San Francisco, CA 94143-0102; **Phone:** 415-353-1090; **Board Cert:** Anatomic Pathology 1982; **Med School:** Univ Kans 1977; **Resid:** Anatomic Pathology, UCSF Med Ctr 1981; Anatomic Pathology, Univ Kansas Med Ctr 1979; **Fac Appt:** Prof Path, UCSF

Fishbein, Michael C MD [Path] - **Spec Exp:** Cardiovascular Pathology; Pulmonary Pathology; **Hospital:** UCLA Med Ctr; **Address:** 10833 Le Conte Ave, Los Angeles, CA 90095-1732; **Phone:** 310-825-9731; **Board Cert:** Anatomic & Clinical Pathology 1975; **Med School:** Univ IL Coll Med 1971; **Resid:** Anatomic & Clinical Pathology, UCLA-Harbor General Hosp 1975; **Fellow:** Pathology, Heart Lung Inst-NIH 1975; **Fac Appt:** Prof Path, UCLA

Govindarajan, Sugantha MD [Path] - **Spec Exp:** Liver Pathology; **Hospital:** Rancho Los Amigos Natl Rehab Ctr; **Address:** Rancho Los Amigos Natl Rehab Ctr, Pathology, 7601 E Imperial Hwy, Bldg JPI - rm B170, Downey, CA 90242; **Phone:** 562-401-8996; **Board Cert:** Anatomic Pathology 1976; **Med School:** India 1969; **Resid:** Pathology, St Lukes Hosp 1976; **Fellow:** Pathology, Cleveland Clinic 1977; **Fac Appt:** Prof Path, USC Sch Med

Hammar, Samuel P MD [Path] - **Spec Exp:** Lung Cancer; Pulmonary Pathology; **Hospital:** Harrison Meml Hosp; **Address:** Diagnostic Specialties Laboratory, 700 Lebo Blvd, Bremerton, WA 98310; **Phone:** 360-479-7707; **Board Cert:** Anatomic & Clinical Pathology 1975; **Med School:** Univ Wash 1970

Hendrickson, Michael MD [Path] - **Spec Exp:** Gynecologic Cancer; Gynecologic Pathology; **Hospital:** Stanford Univ Med Ctr; **Address:** Stanford Univ Med Ctr, Surg Path Lab, 300 Pasteur Drive, rm L230, MC 5324, Stanford, CA 94305; **Phone:** 650-725-5169; **Board Cert:** Anatomic Pathology 1975; **Med School:** Stanford Univ 1971; **Resid:** Anatomic Pathology, Stanford Univ Med Sch 1974; **Fac Appt:** Prof Path, Stanford Univ

Kanel, Gary Craig MD [Path] - **Spec Exp:** Liver Disease; **Hospital:** USC Univ Hosp - R K Eamer Med Plz; **Address:** USC Univ Hosp, Dept Pathology, 1500 San Pablo St, Los Angeles, CA 90033; **Phone:** 323-226-8591; **Board Cert:** Anatomic & Clinical Pathology 1979; **Med School:** Tufts Univ 1974; **Resid:** Pathology, Tufts-New England Med Ctr 1976; Pathology, Univ Chicago Hosp 1977; **Fellow:** Pathology, Tufts-New England Med Ctr 1979; **Fac Appt:** Prof Path, USC Sch Med

Kempson, Richard MD [Path] - **Spec Exp:** Breast Pathology; Gynecologic Pathology; **Hospital:** Stanford Univ Med Ctr; **Address:** 300 Pasteur Drive, Ste H2110, Stanford, CA 94305-5243; **Phone:** 650-723-7211; **Board Cert:** Anatomic Pathology 1963; **Med School:** Tulane Univ 1955; **Resid:** Surgical Pathology, Barnes Hosp 1963; **Fellow:** Anatomic Pathology, Tulane Univ Med Ctr 1962; **Fac Appt:** Prof Path, Stanford Univ

Koss, Michael N MD [Path] - **Spec Exp:** Pulmonary Pathology; Lung Cancer; Mediastinal Tumors; **Hospital:** USC Norris Comp Cancer Ctr, USC Univ Hosp - R K Eamer Med Plz; **Address:** Hoffman Medical Research Bldg, rm 209, 2011 Zonal Ave, Los Angeles, CA 90033; **Phone:** 323-226-6507; **Board Cert:** Anatomic Pathology 1979; **Med School:** Stanford Univ 1970; **Resid:** Pathology, Columbia Presby Med Ctr 1974; **Fellow:** Renal Pathology, Columbia Presby Med Ctr 1975; Pulmonary Pathology, Armed Forces Inst Path 1978; **Fac Appt:** Prof Path, USC Sch Med

Le Boit, Philip E MD [Path] - **Spec Exp:** Cutaneous Lymphoma; Skin Cancer; Dermatopathology; **Hospital:** UCSF Med Ctr; **Address:** UCSF - Dermatopathology Section, 1701 Divisadero St, Ste 350, San Francisco, CA 94115; **Phone:** 415-353-7546; **Board Cert:** Anatomic Pathology 1983; Clinical Pathology 1986; Dermatopathology 1983; **Med School:** Albany Med Coll 1979; **Resid:** Anatomic Pathology, UCSF Med Ctr 1981; Clinical Pathology, Mt Sinai Hosp 1982; **Fellow:** Dermatopathology, New York Hosp-Cornell Med Ctr 1983; **Fac Appt:** Prof Path, UCSF

Nathwani, Bharat N MD [Path] - **Spec Exp:** Hematopathology; Leukemia; Lymphoma; **Hospital:** LAC & USC Med Ctr; **Address:** LAC & USC Med Ctr, Dept Pathology, 1200 N State St, rm 2422, Los Angeles, CA 90033-4526; **Phone:** 323-226-7064; **Board Cert:** Anatomic Pathology 1977; **Med School:** India 1969; **Resid:** Pathology, JJ Group-Grant Med Ctr 1972; Pathology, Rush-Presby-St Lukes Med Ctr 1974; **Fellow:** Hematopathology, City Hope Natl Med Ctr 1975; **Fac Appt:** Prof Path, USC Sch Med

Sibley, Richard K MD [Path] - **Spec Exp:** Kidney Pathology; Breast Pathology; Liver Pathology; **Hospital:** Stanford Univ Med Ctr; **Address:** Stanford Univ Med Ctr, Dept Pathology, 300 Pasteur Drive, rm H2110, MC 5243, Stanford, CA 94305; **Phone:** 650-723-7211; **Board Cert:** Anatomic Pathology 1975; **Med School:** Univ Tex SW, Dallas 1971; **Resid:** Anatomic Pathology, Univ Chicago Hosps 1974; **Fellow:** Stanford Univ Med Ctr 1975; **Fac Appt:** Prof Path, Stanford Univ

True, Lawrence D MD [Path] - **Spec Exp:** Urologic Pathology; Prostate Cancer; Bladder Cancer; **Hospital:** Univ Wash Med Ctr; **Address:** Univ Wash Med Ctr, Dept Anatomic Path, 1959 NE Pacific St, rm BB220, Box 356100, Seattle, WA 98195-6100; **Phone:** 206-598-6400; **Board Cert:** Anatomic Pathology 1981; **Med School:** Tulane Univ 1971; **Resid:** Pathology, Univ Colo Hlth Sci Ctr 1980; **Fac Appt:** Prof Path, Univ Wash

Warnke, Roger A MD [Path] - **Spec Exp:** Lymphoma; Hematopathology; **Hospital:** Stanford Univ Med Ctr; **Address:** Stanford Univ, Dept Pathology, 300 Pasteur Drive, Ste L235, Stanford, CA 94305; **Phone:** 650-725-5167; **Board Cert:** Anatomic Pathology 1975; **Med School:** Washington Univ, St Louis 1971; **Resid:** Pathology, Stanford Univ Med Ctr 1973; **Fellow:** Surgical Pathology, Stanford Univ Med Ctr 1975; Immunology, Stanford Univ Med Ctr 1976; **Fac Appt:** Prof Path, Stanford Univ

Weiss, Lawrence M MD [Path] - **Spec Exp:** Lymphoma; Hematopathology; Adrenal Pathology; **Hospital:** City of Hope Natl Med Ctr & Beckman Rsch; **Address:** City of Hope Natl Med Ctr, Div Pathology, 1500 E Duarte Rd, Duarte, CA 91010-0269; **Phone:** 626-359-8111 x62456; **Board Cert:** Anatomic Pathology 1985; **Med School:** Univ MD Sch Med 1981; **Resid:** Pathology, Brigham & Women's Hosp 1983; **Fellow:** Pathology, Stanford Univ Hosp 1984

Wilczynski, Sharon P MD/PhD [Path] - **Spec Exp:** Gynecologic Cancer; Breast Cancer; Ovarian Cancer; Clinical Trials; **Hospital:** City of Hope Natl Med Ctr & Beckman Rsch; **Address:** City Hope Natl Med Ctr-Dept of Pathology, 1500 E Duarte Blvd, Duarte, CA 91010; **Phone:** 626-256-4673 x62456; **Board Cert:** Anatomic & Clinical Pathology 1985; Cytopathology 1991; **Med School:** Med Coll PA Hahnemann 1981; **Resid:** Pathology, Hosp Univ Penn 1983; Anatomic & Clinical Pathology, Long Beach Meml Hosp 1985; **Fac Appt:** Prof Path, USC-Keck School of Medicine

Pediatrics

A pediatrician is concerned with the physical, emotional and social health of children from birth to young adulthood. Care encompasses a broad spectrum of health services ranging from preventive healthcare to the diagnosis and treatment of acute and chronic diseases.

A pediatrician deals with biological, social and environmental influences on the developing child, and with the impact of disease and dysfunction on development.

Training Required: Three years

Pediatric Allergy and Immunology: An allergist-immunologist is trained in evaluation, physical and laboratory diagnosis and management of disorders involving the immune system. Selected examples of such conditions include asthma, anaphylaxis, rhinitis, eczema and adverse reactions to drugs, foods and insect stings as well as immune deficiency diseases (both acquired and congenital), defects in host defense and problems related to autoimmune disease, organ transplantation or malignancies of the immune system. As our understanding of the immune system develops, the scope of this specialty is widening.

Training Required: Prior certification in pediatrics *plus* two years in allergy/immunology. (Training programs are available at some medical centers to provide individuals with expertise in both allergy/immunology and pediatric pulmonology. Such individuals are candidates for dual certification.)

(continued on next page)

Certification in one of the following subspecialties requires additional training and examination.

Pediatric Cardiology: A pediatric cardiologist provides comprehensive care to patients with cardiovascular problems. This specialist is skilled in selecting, performing and evaluating the structural and functional assessment of the heart and blood vessels and the clinical evaluation of cardiovascular disease.

Pediatric Critical Care Medicine: A pediatrician who cares for children who are victims of life threatening disorders such as severe accidents, shock and diabetic acidosis.

Pediatric Endocrinology: A pediatrician who provides expert care to infants, children and adolescents who have diseases that result from an abnormality in the endocrine glands (glands which secrete hormones). These diseases include diabetes mellitus, growth failure, unusual size for age, early or late pubertal development, birth defects, the genital anomalies and disorders of the thyroid, the adrenal and pituitary glands.

Pediatric Gastroenterology: A pediatrician who specializes in the diagnosis and treatment of diseases of the digestive systems of infants, children and adolescents. This specialist treats conditions such as abdominal pain, ulcers, diarrhea, cancer and jaundice and performs complex diagnostic and therapeutic procedures using lighted scopes to see internal organs.

Pediatric Hematology-Oncology: A pediatrician trained in the combination of pediatrics, hematology and oncology to recognize and manage pediatric blood disorders and cancerous diseases.

Pediatric Infectious Diseases: A pediatrician trained to care for children in the diagnosis, treatment and prevention of infectious diseases. This specialist can apply specific knowledge to effect a better outcome for pediatric infections with complicated courses, underlying diseases that predispose to unusual or severe infections, unclear diagnoses, uncommon diseases and complex or investigational treatments.

Pediatric Nephrology: A pediatrician who deals with the normal and abnormal development and maturation of the kidney and urinary tract, the mechanisms by which the kidney can be damaged, the evaluation and treatment of renal diseases, fluid and electrolyte abnormalities, hypertension and renal replacement therapy.

Pediatric Otolaryngology: A pediatric otolaryngologist has special expertise in the management of infants and children with disorders that include congenital and acquired conditions involving the aerodigestive tract, nose and paranasal sinuses, the ear and other areas of the head and neck. The pediatric otolaryngologist has special skills in the diagnosis, treatment and management of childhood disorders of voice, speech, language and hearing.

Pediatric Pulmonology: A pediatrician dedicated to the prevention and treatment of all respiratory diseases affecting infants, children and young adults. This specialist is knowledgeable about the growth and development of the lung, assessment of respiratory function in infants and children and experienced in a variety of invasive and noninvasive diagnostic techniques.

Pediatric Rheumatology: A pediatrician who treats diseases of joints, muscle, bones and tendons. A pediatric rheumatologist diagnoses and treats arthritis, back pain, muscle strains, common athletic injuries and "collagen" diseases.

Pediatric Surgery: A surgeon with expertise in the management of surgical conditions in premature and newborn infants, children and adolescents.

Pediatrics

New England

Palfrey, Judith S MD [Ped] - **Spec Exp:** Special Health Care Needs (CSHCN); Developmental Disorders; **Hospital:** Children's Hospital - Boston; **Address:** Children's Hospital Wolbach Bldg, 300 Longwood Ave, rm 220, Boston, MA 02115; **Phone:** 617-355-6714; **Board Cert:** Pediatrics 1976; Developmental-Behavioral Pediatrics 2002; **Med School:** Columbia P&S 1971; **Resid:** Pediatrics, Albert Einstein Coll Med 1974; **Fac Appt:** Prof Ped, Harvard Med Sch

Rappaport, Leonard MD [Ped] - **Spec Exp:** Developmental & Behavioral Disorders; **Hospital:** Children's Hospital - Boston, Brigham & Women's Hosp; **Address:** 319 Longwood Ave Fl 4, Boston, MA 02115-5710; **Phone:** 617-277-7320; **Board Cert:** Pediatrics 1983; Developmental-Behavioral Pediatrics 2002; **Med School:** Yale Univ 1977; **Resid:** Pediatrics, Chldns Hosp 1980; **Fellow:** Developmental-Behavioral Pediatrics, Chldns Hosp 1982; **Fac Appt:** Assoc Prof Ped, Harvard Med Sch

Sallan, Stephen MD [Ped] - **Spec Exp:** Pediatric Cancers; Leukemia; **Hospital:** Children's Hospital - Boston; **Address:** Dana Farber Cancer Inst, Dept Ped Oncology, 44 Binney St, Ste 1642, Boston, MA 02115; **Phone:** 617-632-3316; **Board Cert:** Pediatrics 1972; **Med School:** Wayne State Univ 1967; **Resid:** Pediatrics, Chldns Hosp 1969; Pediatrics, Hosp Sick Chldn 1970; **Fellow:** Pediatric Oncology, Chldns Hosp Med Ctr 1975; **Fac Appt:** Prof Ped, Harvard Med Sch

Shaywitz, Sally E MD [Ped] - **Spec Exp:** Learning Disorders; Dyslexia; **Hospital:** Yale - New Haven Hosp; **Address:** Yale Univ Sch Med, Dept Peds, 333 Cedar St, rm LMP-3089, New Haven, CT 06520; **Phone:** 203-785-4641; **Board Cert:** Pediatrics 1971; **Med School:** Albert Einstein Coll Med 1966; **Resid:** Pediatrics, Albert Einstein Coll Med 1970; **Fellow:** Pediatrics, Bronx Muni Hosp Ctr 1968; Behavioral Pediatrics, Albert Einstein Coll Med 1970; **Fac Appt:** Prof Ped, Yale Univ

Mid Atlantic

Berlin Jr, Cheston M MD [Ped] - **Spec Exp:** Phenylketonuria (PKU); Tourette's Syndrome; **Hospital:** Penn State Milton S Hershey Med Ctr; **Address:** Penn State Univ Coll Med, Pediatrics, PO Box 850, Hershey, PA 17033; **Phone:** 717-531-8006; **Board Cert:** Pediatrics 1982; **Med School:** Harvard Med Sch 1962; **Resid:** Pediatrics, Children's Hosp 1967; **Fac Appt:** Prof Ped, Penn State Univ-Hershey Med Ctr

Burgess, David B MD [Ped] - **Spec Exp:** Developmental & Behavioral Disorders; ADD/ADHD; Autism; **Hospital:** Chldns Hosp of Philadelphia, The; **Address:** Children's Hosp Philadelphia, Specialty Care Ctr, 4009 Black Horse Pike, Mays Landing, NJ 08330; **Phone:** 609-677-7895; **Board Cert:** Pediatrics 1978; Developmental-Behavioral Pediatrics 2004; **Med School:** Univ Wisc 1973; **Resid:** Pediatrics, Charity Hosp 1977; **Fellow:** Child Development, JFK Child Dev Ctr, Univ Colorado 1980; **Fac Appt:** Assoc Clin Prof Ped, Univ Pennsylvania

Cohen, Herbert J MD [Ped] - **Spec Exp:** Developmental & Behavioral Disorders; Developmental Delay; **Hospital:** Montefiore Med Ctr; **Address:** Children's Evaluation Rehab Ctr, 1410 Pelham Pkwy S, Ste 237, Bronx, NY 10461-1116; **Phone:** 718-430-8522; **Board Cert:** Pediatrics 1964; **Med School:** SUNY Hlth Sci Ctr 1959; **Resid:** Pediatrics, New York Hosp 1962; **Fellow:** Developmental-Behavioral Pediatrics, Albert Einstein 1966; **Fac Appt:** Prof Ped, Albert Einstein Coll Med

Cohen, William I MD [Ped] - **Spec Exp:** Developmental & Behavioral Disorders; Down Syndrome; Hypnosis; Family Therapy; **Hospital:** Chldns Hosp of Pittsburgh - UPMC; **Address:** Children's Hosp Pittsburgh, Pediatrics, Child Development Unit, 3705 Fifth Ave, Pittsburgh, PA 15213; **Phone:** 412-692-5560; **Board Cert:** Pediatrics 1979; Developmental-Behavioral Pediatrics 2002; **Med School:** SUNY Buffalo 1975; **Resid:** Pediatrics, Children's Hosp 1978; **Fellow:** Developmental-Behavioral Pediatrics, Children's Hosp 1980; **Fac Appt:** Prof Ped, Univ Pittsburgh

Hofkosh, Dena MD [Ped] - **Spec Exp:** Developmental & Behavioral Disorders; Developmental Disorders-Infants; **Hospital:** Chldns Hosp of Pittsburgh - UPMC; **Address:** Childrens Hosp of Pittsburgh, Pediatrics, Child Development Unit, 3705 Fifth Ave, Pittsburgh, PA 15213; **Phone:** 412-692-6541; **Board Cert:** Pediatrics 1984; Neurodevelopmental Disabilities 2001; **Med School:** NYU Sch Med 1979; **Resid:** Pediatrics, Univ Pittsburgh Med Ctr 1982; **Fellow:** Ambulatory Pediatrics, Univ Pittsburgh Med Ctr 1984; **Fac Appt:** Prof Ped, Univ Pittsburgh

Ludwig, Stephen MD [Ped] - **Spec Exp:** Child Abuse; Emergency Medicine; **Hospital:** Chldns Hosp of Philadelphia, The; **Address:** Childrens Hosp of Philadelphia, 34th St and Civic Center Blvd, rm 9557, Philadelphia, PA 19104; **Phone:** 215-590-2162; **Board Cert:** Pediatrics 1992; Pediatric Emergency Medicine 2000; **Med School:** Temple Univ 1971; **Resid:** Pediatrics, Chldns Hosp Natl Med Ctr 1974; **Fac Appt:** Prof Ped, Univ Pennsylvania

Oeffinger, Kevin MD [Ped] - **Spec Exp:** Cancer Survivors-Late Effects of Therapy; **Hospital:** Meml Sloan Kettering Cancer Ctr; **Address:** 1275 York Ave, New York, NY 10021; **Phone:** 212-639-8469; **Board Cert:** Family Medicine 2000; **Med School:** Univ Tex, San Antonio 1984; **Resid:** Family Medicine, Baylor Coll Med 1985; **Fellow:** Family Medicine, Fam Practice Faculty Dev Ctr 1999; Natl Cancer Inst 2000

Offit, Paul A MD [Ped] - **Spec Exp:** Infectious Disease; Vaccines; **Hospital:** Chldns Hosp of Philadelphia, The; **Address:** Children's Hospital of Philadelphia, Abramson Bldg, 34th St & Civic Center Blvd, Ste 1202D, Philadelphia, PA 19104; **Phone:** 215-590-2017; **Board Cert:** Pediatrics 1982; **Med School:** Univ MD Sch Med 1977; **Resid:** Pediatrics, Children's Hosp 1980; **Fac Appt:** Assoc Clin Prof Ped, Univ Pennsylvania

Pasquariello Jr, Patrick S MD [Ped] - **Spec Exp:** Chronic Fatigue Syndrome; Failure to Thrive; Spina Bifida; **Hospital:** Chldns Hosp of Philadelphia, The; **Address:** Chldns Hosp, Diagnostic Ctr, 3400 Civic Center Blvd, Wood Bldg - rm 3335, Philadelphia, PA 19104; **Phone:** 215-590-4020; **Board Cert:** Pediatrics 1963; **Med School:** Jefferson Med Coll 1956; **Resid:** Pediatrics, Chldns Hosp 1963; **Fac Appt:** Prof Ped, Univ Pennsylvania

Vining, Eileen P MD [Ped] - **Spec Exp:** Pediatric Neurology; Epilepsy; Rasmussen's Syndrome; **Hospital:** Johns Hopkins Hosp - Baltimore (page 61); **Address:** Johns Hopkins Hospital, 600 N Wolfe St Meyer Bldg - rm 2-147, Baltimore, MD 21287; **Phone:** 410-955-9100; **Board Cert:** Pediatrics 1977; **Med School:** Johns Hopkins Univ 1972; **Resid:** Pediatrics, Children's Hosp 1974; **Fellow:** Developmental-Behavioral Pediatrics, JFK Inst/Johns Hopkins Hosp 1976; **Fac Appt:** Assoc Prof Ped, Johns Hopkins Univ

Southeast

Levine, Melvin D MD [Ped] - **Spec Exp:** Learning Disorders; Developmental Disorders; **Hospital:** Univ NC Hosps; **Address:** Ctr for Study of Development & Learning, 1450 Raleigh Rd, Ste 100, Chapel Hill, NC 27517; **Phone:** 919-966-1020; **Board Cert:** Pediatrics 1971; **Med School:** Harvard Med Sch 1966; **Resid:** Pediatrics, Chldns Hosp 1969; **Fac Appt:** Prof Ped, Univ NC Sch Med

Pediatrics

Midwest

Berman, Brian MD [Ped] - **Spec Exp:** Sickle Cell Disease; Thrombotic Disorders; Hemophilia; **Hospital:** Rainbow Babies & Chldns Hosp; **Address:** Rainbow Babies & Chldn's Hosp, 11100 Euclid Ave, MS MTH6019, Cleveland, OH 44106-6019; **Phone:** 216-844-3752; **Board Cert:** Pediatrics 1989; Pediatric Hematology-Oncology 1989; **Med School:** Temple Univ 1975; **Resid:** Pediatrics, St Chris Hosp for Chldn 1978; **Fellow:** Pediatric Hematology-Oncology, Yale-New Haven Hosp 1980; **Fac Appt:** Prof Ped, Case West Res Univ

Bull, Marilyn J MD [Ped] - **Spec Exp:** Developmental Disorders; Down Syndrome; Birth Defects; **Hospital:** Riley Hosp for Children; **Address:** 702 Barnhill Drive, rm 1601, Indianapolis, IN 46202; **Phone:** 317-274-4846; **Board Cert:** Pediatrics 1973; Clinical Genetics 1982; Neurodevelopmental Disabilities 2001; **Med School:** Univ Mich Med Sch 1968; **Resid:** Pediatrics, Children's Meml Hosp 1972; **Fellow:** Genetics, Boston Floating Hosp 1973; **Fac Appt:** Prof Ped, Indiana Univ

Fost, Norman C MD [Ped] - **Spec Exp:** Ethics; **Hospital:** Univ WI Hosp & Clins; **Address:** Univ Wisconsin Chldns Hosp, 600 Highland Ave, Madison, WI 53792-4108; **Phone:** 608-265-6050; **Board Cert:** Pediatrics 1970; **Med School:** Yale Univ 1964; **Resid:** Pediatrics, Johns Hopkins Hosp 1971; **Fellow:** Pediatrics, Harvard Sch Public Hlth 1973; **Fac Appt:** Prof Ped, Univ Wisc

Jacob, Molly MD [Ped] - **Spec Exp:** Asthma; ADD/ADHD; Nutrition; **Hospital:** Children's Mem Hosp, Adv Illinois Masonic Med Ctr; **Address:** 3000 N Halstead Ave, Ste 825, Chicago, IL 60657; **Phone:** 773-528-3403; **Board Cert:** Pediatrics 1980; **Med School:** India 1968; **Resid:** Pediatrics, Ill Masonic Med Ctr 1979; **Fellow:** Ambulatory Pediatrics, Ill Masonic Med Ctr 1979; **Fac Appt:** Asst Clin Prof Ped, Univ IL Coll Med

Lantos, John MD [Ped] - **Spec Exp:** Chronic Disease; Palliative Care; Ethics; **Hospital:** La Rabida Chlds Hosp, Univ of Chicago Hosps; **Address:** 5841 S Maryland Ave, MC 6082, Chicago, IL 60637; **Phone:** 773-702-6602; **Board Cert:** Pediatrics 1986; **Med School:** Univ Pittsburgh 1981; **Resid:** Pediatrics, Chldns Natl Med Ctr 1984; **Fellow:** Clinical Ethics, Univ Chicago; **Fac Appt:** Prof Ped, Univ Chicago-Pritzker Sch Med

Mendelsohn, Janis MD [Ped] - **Hospital:** Univ of Chicago Hosps; **Address:** 5841 S Maryland Ave, MC 1057, Chicago, IL 60637; **Phone:** 773-702-6169; **Board Cert:** Pediatrics 1973; **Med School:** Univ Tenn Coll Med, Memphis 1967; **Resid:** Pediatrics, Chldns Meml Hosp 1971; **Fac Appt:** Assoc Clin Prof Ped, Univ Chicago-Pritzker Sch Med

West Coast and Pacific

Berkowitz, Carol D MD [Ped] - **Spec Exp:** Behavioral Pediatrics; Child Abuse; **Hospital:** LAC - Harbor - UCLA Med Ctr; **Address:** LAC-Harbor-UCLA Med Ctr, 1000 W Carson St, Box 437, Torrance, CA 90509-2910; **Phone:** 310-222-3091; **Board Cert:** Pediatrics 2000; Pediatric Emergency Medicine 2006; **Med School:** Columbia P&S 1969; **Resid:** Pediatrics, Roosevelt Hosp 1972; **Fac Appt:** Clin Prof Ped, UCLA

Feldman, Kenneth W MD [Ped] - **Spec Exp:** Child Abuse; **Hospital:** Chldns Hosp and Regl Med Ctr - Seattle; **Address:** Odessa Brown Chldns Clin, 2101 E Yesler Way, Ste 100, Seattle, WA 98122; **Phone:** 206-987-7225; **Board Cert:** Pediatrics 1975; **Med School:** Univ Wisc 1970; **Resid:** Pediatrics, Chldns Regl Med Ctr 1974; **Fac Appt:** Clin Prof Ped, Univ Wash

Jones Jr, Kenneth Lyons MD [Ped] - **Spec Exp:** Genetic Disorders; Dysmorphology; **Hospital:** UCSD Med Ctr; **Address:** 200 W Arbor Drive, MC 8446, San Diego, CA 92123-8446; **Phone:** 619-543-2040; **Board Cert:** Pediatrics 1971; **Med School:** Hahnemann Univ 1966; **Resid:** Pediatrics, Chldns Ortho Hosp 1969; **Fac Appt:** Prof Ped, UCSD

Miller, Carol A MD [Ped] - **Spec Exp:** Neonatal Critical Care; **Hospital:** UCSF Med Ctr; **Address:** UCSF Med Ctr, Dept Primary Peds, 400 Parnassus Ave Fl 2, San Francisco, CA 94143; **Phone:** 415-353-2000; **Board Cert:** Pediatrics 1981; **Med School:** Stanford Univ 1975; **Resid:** Pediatrics, Mt Zion Hosp 1977; **Fellow:** Neonatology, Mt Zion Hosp 1979; **Fac Appt:** Clin Prof Ped, UCSF

Pantell, Robert H MD [Ped] - **Spec Exp:** Fevers in Infants; **Hospital:** UCSF Med Ctr; **Address:** UCSF Med Ctr, Dept Primary Peds, 400 Parnassus Ave Fl 2, San Francisco, CA 94143; **Phone:** 415-353-2000; **Board Cert:** Pediatrics 1974; **Med School:** Boston Univ 1969; **Resid:** Pediatrics, NC Meml Hosp 1972; **Fellow:** Pediatrics, Stanford Univ Hosp 1977; **Fac Appt:** Prof Ped, UCSF

Zeltzer, Lonnie K MD [Ped] - **Spec Exp:** Pain Management; Adolescent Health; Complementary Medicine; **Hospital:** Mattel Chldns Hosp at UCLA; **Address:** UCLA Pediatric Pain Program, 10833 Le Conte Ave, #22-464 MDCC, Los Angeles, CA 90095-1752; **Phone:** 310-825-0731; **Board Cert:** Pediatrics 1976; **Med School:** Univ Cincinnati 1970; **Resid:** Pediatrics, Univ Ariz Hosp 1973; **Fellow:** Adolescent Medicine, Chldns Hosp 1976; **Fac Appt:** Prof Ped, UCLA

Pediatric Allergy & Immunology

New England

Klein, Robert B MD [PA&I] - **Spec Exp:** Asthma; **Hospital:** Rhode Island Hosp; **Address:** Rhode Island Hosp, Dept of Pediatrics, 593 Eddy St, Providence, RI 02903; **Phone:** 401-444-8639; **Board Cert:** Pediatrics 1976; Allergy & Immunology 1977; **Med School:** Switzerland 1971; **Resid:** Pediatrics, Dartmouth/Hitchcock Med Ctr 1974; **Fellow:** Allergy & Immunology, UCLA 1976; **Fac Appt:** Prof Ped, Brown Univ

Mid Atlantic

Kamani, Naynesh R MD [PA&I] - **Spec Exp:** Stem Cell Transplant; Immunotherapy; Bone Marrow Transplant; **Hospital:** Chldns Natl Med Ctr; **Address:** Chldns Natl Med Ctr, Div Hematology, 111 Michigan Ave NW, Washington, DC 20010; **Phone:** 202-884-2800; **Board Cert:** Pediatrics 1983; Pediatric Allergy & Immunology 1983; **Med School:** Ethiopia 1975; **Resid:** Pediatrics, Downstate Med Ctr-Kings Co Hosp 1981; **Fellow:** Pediatric Allergy & Immunology, Children's Hosp 1983; **Fac Appt:** Prof Ped, Geo Wash Univ

Sampson, Hugh MD [PA&I] - **Spec Exp:** Food Allergy; Anaphylaxis; Eczema; **Hospital:** Mount Sinai Med Ctr; **Address:** Mt Sinai Sch Med, Dept Peds, 1 Gustave Levy Pl, Box 1198, New York, NY 10029-6500; **Phone:** 212-241-5548; **Board Cert:** Pediatrics 1980; Allergy & Immunology 1981; **Med School:** SUNY Buffalo 1975; **Resid:** Pediatrics, Chldns Meml Hosp 1979; **Fellow:** Allergy & Immunology, Duke Univ Med Ctr 1980; **Fac Appt:** Prof Ped, Mount Sinai Sch Med

Pediatric Allergy & Immunology

Schuberth, Kenneth Charles MD [PA&I] - Spec Exp: Allergy; **Hospital:** Johns Hopkins Hosp - Baltimore (page 61), Greater Baltimore Med Ctr; **Address:** 10807 Falls Rd, Ste 200, Lutherville, MD 21093; **Phone:** 410-321-9393; **Board Cert:** Pediatrics 1979; Allergy & Immunology 1983; **Med School:** Johns Hopkins Univ 1973; **Resid:** Pediatrics, Johns Hopkins Hosp 1978; **Fellow:** Allergy & Immunology, Johns Hopkins Hosp 1980; **Fac Appt:** Assoc Prof Ped, Johns Hopkins Univ

Skoner, David Peter MD [PA&I] - Spec Exp: Asthma & Allergy; Rhinitis; **Hospital:** Allegheny General Hosp; **Address:** Allegheny Genl Hosp, Div Asthma Allergy & Immunology, 320 E North Ave, Fl 7 - South Tower, Pittsburgh, PA 15212; **Phone:** 412-359-6640; **Board Cert:** Pediatrics 1985; Allergy & Immunology 1985; **Med School:** Temple Univ 1980; **Resid:** Pediatrics, Chldns Hosp Med Ctr 1983; **Fellow:** Allergy & Immunology, Chldns Hosp 1985; **Fac Appt:** Prof Ped, Drexel Univ Coll Med

Sly, R Michael MD [PA&I] - Spec Exp: Asthma; Allergy; Atopic Dermatitis; **Hospital:** Chldns Natl Med Ctr; **Address:** Children's Natl Med Ctr, Dept Allergy & Immunology, 111 Michigan Ave NW, Washington, DC 20010-2970; **Phone:** 202-884-2610; **Board Cert:** Pediatrics 1980; Allergy & Immunology 1987; **Med School:** Washington Univ, St Louis 1960; **Resid:** Pediatrics, St Louis Chldns Hosp 1962; Pediatrics, Univ Kentucky Med Ctr 1963; **Fellow:** Pediatric Allergy & Immunology, UCLA Med Ctr 1967; **Fac Appt:** Prof Ped, Geo Wash Univ

Wood, Robert Alan MD [PA&I] - Spec Exp: Food Allergy; Asthma; **Hospital:** Johns Hopkins Hosp - Baltimore (page 61); **Address:** 600 N Wolfe St, CMSC-1102, Baltimore, MD 21287; **Phone:** 410-955-5883; **Board Cert:** Pediatrics 1987; Allergy & Immunology 1997; **Med School:** Univ Rochester 1982; **Resid:** Pediatrics, Johns Hopkins Hosp 1985; **Fellow:** Allergy & Immunology, Johns Hopkins Hosp 1988; **Fac Appt:** Prof Ped, Johns Hopkins Univ

Southeast

Buckley, Rebecca Hatcher MD [PA&I] - Spec Exp: Immune Deficiency; Allergy; Eczema; **Hospital:** Duke Univ Med Ctr; **Address:** Duke Univ Sch Medicine, Box 2898, Durham, NC 27710-2898; **Phone:** 919-684-2922; **Board Cert:** Pediatrics 1963; Allergy & Immunology 1977; Clinical & Laboratory Immunology 1986; **Med School:** Univ NC Sch Med 1958; **Resid:** Pediatrics, Duke Univ Med Ctr 1961; **Fellow:** Pediatric Allergy & Immunology, Duke Univ Med Ctr 1963; Immunology, Duke Univ Med Ctr 1965; **Fac Appt:** Prof Ped, Duke Univ

Kelly, Cynthia S MD [PA&I] - Spec Exp: Asthma; Rhinitis; Sinusitis; **Hospital:** Chldns Hosp of King's Daughters; **Address:** Chlds Hosp of The Kings Daughters, 601 Childrens Lane, Norfolk, VA 23507; **Phone:** 757-668-8255; **Board Cert:** Pediatrics 2004; Allergy & Immunology 1997; **Med School:** Wayne State Univ 1985; **Resid:** Pediatrics, Univ Mich 1987; **Fellow:** Allergy & Immunology, UCLA 1988; Pediatric Infectious Disease, Vanderbilt Univ 1989; **Fac Appt:** Assoc Prof Ped, Eastern VA Med Sch

Ownby, Dennis R MD [PA&I] - Spec Exp: Food Allergy; Anaphylaxis; **Hospital:** Med Coll of GA Hosp and Clin; **Address:** Allergy & Immunology, 1120 15th St Bldg BG - rm 1019, Augusta, GA 30912-0004; **Phone:** 706-721-2390; **Board Cert:** Pediatrics 1977; Pediatric Allergy & Immunology 1993; Clinical & Laboratory Immunology 1986; **Med School:** Med Coll OH 1972; **Resid:** Pediatrics, Duke Med Ctr 1974; **Fellow:** Pediatric Allergy & Immunology, Duke Med Ctr 1977; **Fac Appt:** Prof Ped, Med Coll GA

Midwest

Blum, Paul MD [PA&I] - **Spec Exp:** Asthma; **Hospital:** Univ Minn Med Ctr, Fairview - Univ Campus; **Address:** 3955 Parklawn Ave, Ste 210, Edina, MN 55435; **Phone:** 952-831-4454; **Board Cert:** Pediatrics 1973; Allergy & Immunology 1981; **Med School:** Univ Minn 1968; **Resid:** Pediatrics, Univ Minnesota Hosp 1971; **Fellow:** Allergy & Immunology, UCLA Med Ctr 1980; **Fac Appt:** Asst Clin Prof Ped, Univ Minn

Lemanske Jr, Robert F MD [PA&I] - **Spec Exp:** Asthma; Allergy; Immune Deficiency; **Hospital:** Univ WI Hosp & Clins; **Address:** 600 Highland Ave, rm K4/916 CSC, Madison, WI 53792; **Phone:** 608-265-2206; **Board Cert:** Pediatrics 1980; Allergy & Immunology 1981; **Med School:** Univ Wisc 1975; **Resid:** Pediatrics, Univ Wisc Hosp 1978; **Fellow:** Allergy & Immunology, Univ Wisc Hosp 1980; Allergy & Immunology, Natl Inst Health 1983; **Fac Appt:** Prof Ped, Univ Wisc

Pongracic, Jacqueline MD [PA&I] - **Spec Exp:** Latex Allergy; Asthma; Food Allergy; **Hospital:** Children's Mem Hosp, Northwestern Meml Hosp; **Address:** 2300 Children's Plaza, Box 60, Chicago, IL 60614; **Phone:** 773-327-3710; **Board Cert:** Internal Medicine 1988; Allergy & Immunology 2001; **Med School:** Northwestern Univ 1985; **Resid:** Internal Medicine, North Shore Univ Hosp 1988; **Fellow:** Allergy & Immunology, Johns Hopkins Hosp 1991; **Fac Appt:** Asst Prof Ped, Northwestern Univ

Strunk, Robert MD [PA&I] - **Spec Exp:** Asthma; **Hospital:** St Louis Chldns Hosp; **Address:** One Children's Place, Dept Pediatrics, Box 8116-NWT, St Louis, MO 63110; **Phone:** 314-454-2694; **Board Cert:** Pediatrics 1974; Allergy & Immunology 1987; **Med School:** Northwestern Univ 1968; **Resid:** Pediatrics, Cincinnati Chldns Hosp 1970; **Fellow:** Pediatric Allergy & Immunology, Boston Chldns Hosp 1974; **Fac Appt:** Prof Ped, Washington Univ, St Louis

Wolf, Raoul MD [PA&I] - **Spec Exp:** Asthma; Allergy; Immune Deficiency; **Hospital:** Univ of Chicago Hosps, La Rabida Chlds Hosp; **Address:** La Rabida Chldns Hosp, Dept A&I, E 65th St at Lake Michigan, Chicago, IL 60649; **Phone:** 773-753-8637; **Board Cert:** Pediatrics 1980; Allergy & Immunology 1983; **Med School:** South Africa 1969; **Resid:** Pediatrics, Baragwanath Hosp 1973; Pediatrics, Transvaal Meml Hosp Chldn 1976; **Fellow:** Allergy & Immunology, Chldns Hosp Med Ctr 1979; **Fac Appt:** Prof Ped, Univ Chicago-Pritzker Sch Med

Great Plains and Mountains

Bock, S Allan MD [PA&I] - **Spec Exp:** Asthma up to age 50; Allergy up to age 50; Food Allergy; **Hospital:** Boulder Community Hospital, Natl Jewish Med & Rsch Ctr; **Address:** Boulder Asthma & Allergy Clinics, 3950 Broadway, Boulder, CO 80304; **Phone:** 303-444-5991; **Board Cert:** Pediatrics 1977; Allergy & Immunology 1977; **Med School:** Univ MD Sch Med 1972; **Resid:** Pediatrics, Colo Med Ctr/Natl Jewish Med Ctr 1974; **Fellow:** Allergy & Immunology, Colo Med Ctr/Natl Jewish Med Ctr 1976; **Fac Appt:** Clin Prof Ped, Univ Colorado

Gelfand, Erwin MD [PA&I] - **Spec Exp:** Immune Deficiency; Asthma; Allergy-Pediatric & Adult; **Hospital:** Natl Jewish Med & Rsch Ctr, Chldn's Hosp - Denver, The; **Address:** National Jewish Med & Research Ctr, 1400 Jackson St, Denver, CO 80206; **Phone:** 303-398-1196; **Board Cert:** Pediatrics 1972; **Med School:** McGill Univ 1966; **Resid:** Pediatrics, Montreal Children's Hosp 1968; Pediatrics, Children's Hosp Med Ctr 1969; **Fellow:** Immunology, Children's Hosp Med Ctr 1971; **Fac Appt:** Prof Ped, Univ Colorado

Pediatric Allergy & Immunology

Leung, Donald MD/PhD [PA&I] - **Spec Exp:** Atopic Dermatitis; Asthma; **Hospital:** Natl Jewish Med & Rsch Ctr, Chldn's Hosp - Denver, The; **Address:** 1400 Jackson St, Bldg K - Ste 926I, Denver, CO 80206; **Phone:** 303-398-1379; **Board Cert:** Pediatrics 1982; Allergy & Immunology 1983; Clinical & Laboratory Immunology 1990; **Med School:** Univ Chicago-Pritzker Sch Med 1977; **Resid:** Pediatrics, Childrens Hosp 1979; **Fellow:** Allergy & Immunology, Childrens Hosp 1981; **Fac Appt:** Prof Ped, Univ Colorado

Southwest

Bahna, Sami L MD [PA&I] - **Spec Exp:** Food Allergy; Asthma; Eczema; **Hospital:** Louisiana State Univ Hosp; **Address:** LSU Hlth Scis Ctr, Dept Pediatrics, 1501 Kings Hwy, Shreveport, LA 71103; **Phone:** 318-675-7625; **Board Cert:** Pediatrics 1980; Allergy & Immunology 1981; **Med School:** Egypt 1964; **Resid:** Pediatrics, Univ Maryland Hosp 1975; **Fellow:** Allergy & Immunology, Harbor-UCLA Med Ctr 1978; **Fac Appt:** Prof Ped, Louisiana State Univ

Shearer, William T MD [PA&I] - **Spec Exp:** AIDS/HIV; Immune Deficiency; **Hospital:** Texas Chldns Hosp - Houston; **Address:** Tex Chldns Hosp, Div A&I, 6621 Fannin, St Fl 3, MC FC 330.01, Houston, TX 77030-2399; **Phone:** 832-824-1319; **Board Cert:** Pediatrics 1986; Allergy & Immunology 1989; Clinical & Laboratory Immunology 1986; **Med School:** Washington Univ, St Louis 1970; **Resid:** Pediatrics, Chldns Hosp-Wash Univ 1972; **Fellow:** Allergy & Immunology, Barnes Hosp-Wash Univ 1974; **Fac Appt:** Prof Ped, Baylor Coll Med

West Coast and Pacific

Church, Joseph A MD [PA&I] - **Spec Exp:** AIDS/HIV; Immune Deficiency; **Hospital:** Chldns Hosp - Los Angeles (page 56); **Address:** Immunology and Allergy, Children Hosp LA, 4650 W Sunset Blvd, MS 75, Los Angeles, CA 90027; **Phone:** 323-669-2501; **Board Cert:** Pediatrics 1977; Allergy & Immunology 1977; **Med School:** UMDNJ-NJ Med Sch, Newark 1972; **Resid:** Pediatrics, Chldns Hosp/Natl Med Ctr 1974; **Fellow:** Allergy & Immunology, Georgetown Med Ctr 1976; **Fac Appt:** Prof Ped, USC Sch Med

Cowan, Morton J MD [PA&I] - **Spec Exp:** Immunodeficiency Disorders; Stem Cell Transplant-Fetal; Bone Marrow Transplant; **Hospital:** UCSF Med Ctr; **Address:** UCSF Med Ctr, Peds BMT Program, 505 Parnassus Ave, rm R679, San Francisco, CA 94143-1278; **Phone:** 415-476-2188; **Board Cert:** Pediatrics 1981; Allergy & Immunology 1983; **Med School:** Univ Pennsylvania 1970; **Resid:** Surgery, Duke Univ Med Ctr 1972; Pediatrics, UCSF Med Ctr 1977; **Fellow:** Research, Natl Inst Hlth 1975; Immunology, UCSF Med Ctr; **Fac Appt:** Prof Ped, UCSF

Epstein, Stuart Zane MD [PA&I] - **Spec Exp:** Asthma & Allergy; Food Allergy; **Hospital:** Cedars-Sinai Med Ctr; **Address:** 9735 Wilshire Blvd, Ste 121, Beverly Hills, CA 90212-2101; **Phone:** 310-274-6853; **Board Cert:** Pediatrics 1998; Allergy & Immunology 1999; **Med School:** Univ IL Coll Med 1978; **Resid:** Pediatrics, Cedars Sinai Med Ctr 1980; **Fellow:** Pediatrics, UC Irvine 1981; Pediatrics, USC Med Ctr 1982; **Fac Appt:** Assoc Clin Prof Ped, UCLA

Fanous, Yvonne F MD [PA&I] - **Spec Exp:** Asthma & Allergy; Cystic Fibrosis; Immune Deficiency; **Hospital:** Loma Linda Univ Med Ctr; **Address:** 11370 Anderson St, Ste B-100, Loma Linda, CA 92354; **Phone:** 909-558-2388; **Board Cert:** Pediatrics 1983; Allergy & Immunology 1985; **Med School:** Egypt 1973; **Resid:** Pediatrics, Texas Tech Univ Hosp 1980; Pediatrics, Loma Linda Univ 1981; **Fellow:** Allergy & Immunology, UC Irvine 1983; **Fac Appt:** Assoc Prof A&I, Loma Linda Univ

Stiehm, E Richard MD [PA&I] - **Spec Exp:** Immune Deficiency; Allergy; Pediatric Rheumatology; **Hospital:** UCLA Med Ctr; **Address:** UCLA Children's Hosp, 22-387 MDCC, 10833 Le Conte Ave, Los Angeles, CA 90095-3075; **Phone:** 310-825-6481; **Board Cert:** Pediatrics 1964; Allergy & Immunology 1974; **Med School:** Univ Wisc 1957; **Resid:** Pediatrics, Babies Hosp 1963; **Fellow:** Allergy & Immunology, Univ Wisc 1959; Allergy & Immunology, UCSF 1965; **Fac Appt:** Prof Ped, UCLA

Wara, Diane W MD [PA&I] - **Spec Exp:** AIDS/HIV; Immune Deficiency; **Hospital:** UCSF Med Ctr; **Address:** 505 Parnassus Ave, Box 0107, San Francisco, CA 94143; **Phone:** 415-476-2865; **Board Cert:** Pediatrics 1974; Allergy & Immunology 1975; **Med School:** UC Irvine 1969; **Resid:** Pediatrics, UCSF Med Ctr 1972; **Fellow:** Immunology, UCSF Med Ctr 1975; **Fac Appt:** Prof Ped, UCSF

Pediatric Cardiology

New England

Lock, James E MD [PCd] - **Spec Exp:** Interventional Cardiology; Angioplasty-Pulmonary Artery; Cardiac Catheterization; **Hospital:** Children's Hospital - Boston; **Address:** Chldns Hosp, Dept Cardiology, 300 Longwood Ave, Farley 2, Boston, MA 02115-5724; **Phone:** 617-355-7313; **Board Cert:** Pediatrics 1978; Pediatric Cardiology 1981; **Med School:** Stanford Univ 1973; **Resid:** Pediatrics, Univ Minn Hosp 1975; Pediatric Cardiology, Univ Minn Hosp 1977; **Fellow:** Cardiovascular Disease, Hosp Sick Chldn 1979; **Fac Appt:** Prof Ped, Harvard Med Sch

Newburger, Jane MD [PCd] - **Spec Exp:** Kawasaki Disease; Cholesterol/Lipid Disorders; Congenital Heart Disease; **Hospital:** Children's Hospital - Boston, Brigham & Women's Hosp; **Address:** Chldns Hosp, Dept Ped Cardiology, 300 Longwood Ave, Farley Bldg Fl 2, Boston, MA 02115-5724; **Phone:** 617-355-5427; **Board Cert:** Pediatrics 1979; Pediatric Cardiology 1983; **Med School:** Harvard Med Sch 1974; **Resid:** Pediatrics, Chldns Hosp Med Ctr 1976; **Fellow:** Pediatric Cardiology, Chldns Hosp Med Ctr 1979; **Fac Appt:** Prof Ped, Harvard Med Sch

Walsh, Edward Patrick MD [PCd] - **Spec Exp:** Cardiac Electrophysiology; Arrhythmias; **Hospital:** Children's Hospital - Boston; **Address:** Chldns Hosp, Dept Cardiology, 300 Longwood Ave, Bader 2, Boston, MA 02115; **Phone:** 617-355-6328; **Board Cert:** Pediatrics 1985; Pediatric Cardiology 1985; **Med School:** Univ Pennsylvania 1979; **Resid:** Pediatrics, Chldns Hosp 1982; **Fellow:** Pediatric Cardiology, Chldns Hosp 1985; **Fac Appt:** Assoc Prof Ped, Harvard Med Sch

Mid Atlantic

Beerman, Lee MD [PCd] - **Spec Exp:** Congenital Heart Disease-Adult & Child; Arrhythmias; **Hospital:** Chldns Hosp of Pittsburgh - UPMC; **Address:** Chldns Hosp-Heart Ctr, 3705 5th Ave, Fl 2 - rm 2820, Pittsburgh, PA 15213-2524; **Phone:** 412-692-5540; **Board Cert:** Pediatrics 1979; Pediatric Cardiology 1979; **Med School:** Univ Pittsburgh 1974; **Resid:** Pediatrics, Chldns Hosp 1977; **Fellow:** Pediatric Cardiology, Chldns Hosp 1979; **Fac Appt:** Prof Ped, Univ Pittsburgh

Pediatric Cardiology

Biancaniello, Thomas MD [PCd] - **Spec Exp:** Congenital Heart Disease; Fetal Echocardiography; Interventional Cardiology; Cardiac Catheterization; **Hospital:** Stony Brook Univ Med Ctr; **Address:** Stony Brook Univ Hosp, Dept Pediatrics, 100 Nicholls Rd, Stony Brook, NY 11794-0001; **Phone:** 631-444-5437; **Board Cert:** Pediatrics 1979; Pediatric Cardiology 1981; **Med School:** NY Med Coll 1975; **Resid:** Pediatrics, North Shore Univ Hosp 1977; **Fellow:** Pediatric Cardiology, Cincinnati Chldns Hosp 1980; **Fac Appt:** Prof Ped, SUNY Stony Brook

Bierman, Fredrick MD [PCd] - **Spec Exp:** Fetal Echocardiography; Kawasaki Disease; Congenital Heart Disease; **Hospital:** Schneider Chldn's Hosp; **Address:** Chldns Heart Ctr, Schneider Chldns Hosp, 269-01 76th Ave, rm 139, New Hyde Park, NY 11040; **Phone:** 718-470-7350; **Board Cert:** Pediatrics 1978; Pediatric Cardiology 1981; **Med School:** SUNY Downstate 1973; **Resid:** Pediatrics, Mount Sinai Med Ctr 1976; **Fellow:** Pediatric Cardiology, Harvard Chldns Hosp 1979; **Fac Appt:** Prof Ped, Albert Einstein Coll Med

Brenner, Joel I MD [PCd] - **Spec Exp:** Congenital Heart Disease; **Hospital:** Johns Hopkins Hosp - Baltimore (page 61), Greater Baltimore Med Ctr; **Address:** Johns Hopkins Hosp, Pediatric Cardiology, 600 N Wolfe St, Brady 522, Baltimore, MD 21287; **Phone:** 410-955-5987; **Board Cert:** Pediatrics 1975; Pediatric Cardiology 1977; **Med School:** NY Med Coll 1970; **Resid:** Pediatrics, New York Hosp 1972; **Fellow:** Pediatric Cardiology, Yale-New Haven Hosp 1974; **Fac Appt:** Assoc Prof Ped, Johns Hopkins Univ

Cooper, Rubin MD [PCd] - **Spec Exp:** Congenital Heart Disease; Rheumatic Heart Disease; Kawasaki Disease; **Hospital:** NYPresby-Morgan Stanley Children's Hosp, NY Hosp Queens; **Address:** 525 E 68th St, Ste F695B, New York, NY 10021; **Phone:** 212-746-3561; **Board Cert:** Pediatrics 1976; Pediatric Cardiology 1979; **Med School:** NY Med Coll 1971; **Resid:** Pediatrics, Strong Meml Hosp 1973; **Fellow:** Pediatric Cardiology, Strong Meml Hosp 1975; **Fac Appt:** Prof Ped, Cornell Univ-Weill Med Coll

Gewitz, Michael MD [PCd] - **Spec Exp:** Neonatal Cardiology; Kawasaki Disease; Echocardiography; Heart Failure; **Hospital:** Westchester Med Ctr, Vassar Bros Med Ctr; **Address:** Maria Fareri Chldns Hosp/NY Med Coll, Rte 100, Munger Pavillion, Ste 618, Valhalla, NY 10595; **Phone:** 914-594-4370; **Board Cert:** Pediatrics 1979; Pediatric Cardiology 1981; **Med School:** Hahnemann Univ 1974; **Resid:** Pediatrics, Chldns Hosp 1976; Pediatrics, Hosp Sick Chldn 1977; **Fellow:** Pediatric Cardiology, Yale-New Haven Hosp 1979; **Fac Appt:** Prof Ped, NY Med Coll

Hellenbrand, William E MD [PCd] - **Spec Exp:** Interventional Cardiology; **Hospital:** NYPresby-Morgan Stanley Children's Hosp, Robert Wood Johnson Univ Hosp - New Brunswick; **Address:** Morgan Stanley Chlds Hosp of NY-Presby, 3959 Broadway Fl 2N - Ste 255, New York, NY 10032; **Phone:** 212-305-6069; **Board Cert:** Pediatrics 1975; Pediatric Cardiology 1977; **Med School:** SUNY Downstate 1970; **Resid:** Pediatrics, Yale-New Haven Hosp 1972; **Fellow:** Pediatric Cardiology, Yale-New Haven Hosp 1976; **Fac Appt:** Prof Ped, Columbia P&S

Parness, Ira A MD [PCd] - **Spec Exp:** Echocardiography; Congenital Heart Disease; Fetal Echocardiography; **Hospital:** Mount Sinai Med Ctr; **Address:** 1 Gustave Levy Pl, Box 1201, New York, NY 10029-6500; **Phone:** 212-241-8662; **Board Cert:** Pediatrics 1984; Pediatric Cardiology 1985; **Med School:** SUNY Downstate 1979; **Resid:** Pediatrics, Brookdale Hosp 1982; **Fellow:** Pediatric Cardiology, Children's Hosp 1985; **Fac Appt:** Assoc Prof Ped, Mount Sinai Sch Med

Radtke, Wolfgang MD [PCd] - **Spec Exp:** Interventional Cardiology; Cardiac Catheterization; Congenital Heart Disease-Adult & Child; **Hospital:** Alfred I duPont Hosp for Children; **Address:** Nemours Cardiac Ctr, 1600 Rockland Rd, Wilmington, DE 19803; **Phone:** 302-651-6600; **Board Cert:** Pediatrics 2002; **Med School:** Germany 1980; **Resid:** Pediatrics, Kiel Univ Chldns Hosp; **Fellow:** Pediatric Cardiology, Chldns Hosp; **Fac Appt:** Prof Ped, Jefferson Med Coll

Velvis, Harm MD [PCd] - **Spec Exp:** Cardiac Catheterization; Congenital Heart Disease; Heart Disease in Down Syndrome; **Hospital:** Albany Med Ctr, St Peter's Hosp - Albany; **Address:** Pediatric Cardiology, Albany Med Ctr, 319 S Manning Blvd, Ste 203, Albany, NY 12208-1743; **Phone:** 518-489-3292; **Board Cert:** Pediatric Cardiology 2002; **Med School:** Netherlands 1980; **Resid:** Pediatrics, Albany Med Ctr 1987; **Fellow:** Pediatric Cardiology, UCSF Med Ctr 1990; **Fac Appt:** Assoc Clin Prof Ped, Albany Med Coll

Walsh, Christine A MD [PCd] - **Spec Exp:** Arrhythmias; Congenital Heart Disease; Syncope; **Hospital:** Montefiore Med Ctr, Montefiore Med Ctr - Weiler-Einstein Div; **Address:** 3415 Bainbridge Ave, Bronx, NY 10467-2401; **Phone:** 718-741-2310; **Board Cert:** Pediatrics 1978; Pediatric Cardiology 1983; Pediatric Critical Care Medicine 2003; **Med School:** Yale Univ 1973; **Resid:** Pediatrics, Columbia-Presby Med Ctr 1976; **Fellow:** Pediatric Cardiology, Columbia-Presby Med Ctr 1980; **Fac Appt:** Prof Ped, Albert Einstein Coll Med

Weinberg, Paul M MD [PCd] - **Spec Exp:** Cardiac Pathology; Cardiac MRI; **Hospital:** Chldns Hosp of Philadelphia, The; **Address:** Chldns Hosp, Div Cardiology, 34th St & Civic Ctr Blvd, Philadelphia, PA 19104; **Phone:** 215-590-3274; **Board Cert:** Pediatrics 1974; Pediatric Cardiology 1975; **Med School:** Jefferson Med Coll 1969; **Resid:** Pediatrics, Chldns Hosp 1971; Cardiology & Pathology, Chldns Hosp Med Ctr 1977; **Fellow:** Pediatric Cardiology, Chldns Hosp 1973; **Fac Appt:** Prof Ped, Univ Pennsylvania

Southeast

Boucek, Mark M MD [PCd] - **Spec Exp:** Transplant Medicine-Heart; Cardiac Catheterization; Heart Failure; Interventional Cardiology; **Hospital:** Joe Di Maggio Chldns Hosp; **Address:** J Dimaggio Chldns Hosp, Dept Ped Cardiology, 1150 N 35th Ave, Hollywood, FL 33021; **Phone:** 954-985-6939; **Board Cert:** Pediatrics 1982; Pediatric Cardiology 1983; **Med School:** Univ Miami Sch Med 1977; **Resid:** Pediatrics, Vanderbilt Univ Hosp 1979; **Fellow:** Pediatric Cardiology, Univ Utah Hlth Sci Ctr 1981; **Fac Appt:** Clin Prof Ped, Univ Hlth Sci, Coll Osteo Med

Bricker, John Timothy MD [PCd] - **Spec Exp:** Transplant Medicine-Heart; Congenital Heart Disease-Adult; **Hospital:** Univ of Kentucky Chandler Hosp; **Address:** Chairman, Department of Pediatrics, 740 S Limestone Ave, rm J-406, Lexington, KY 40536-0284; **Phone:** 859-323-5481 x297; **Board Cert:** Pediatrics 1981; Pediatric Cardiology 1997; **Med School:** Ohio State Univ 1976; **Resid:** Pediatrics, Tex Chldns Hosp 1980; **Fellow:** Pediatric Cardiology, Tex Chldns Hosp 1983; **Fac Appt:** Prof Ped, Univ KY Coll Med

Colvin, Edward V MD [PCd] - **Spec Exp:** Congenital Heart Disease-Adult & Child; Fetal Echocardiography; Transplant Medicine-Heart; **Hospital:** Univ of Ala Hosp at Birmingham, Children's Hospital - Birmingham; **Address:** Hillman Bldg 320, 620 20th St S, Birmingham, AL 35233; **Phone:** 205-934-3460; **Board Cert:** Pediatrics 1982; Pediatric Cardiology 1985; **Med School:** Univ Ala 1977; **Resid:** Pediatrics, Chldns Hosp 1980; **Fellow:** Pediatric Cardiology, Baylor Coll Med 1983; **Fac Appt:** Prof Ped, Univ Ala

Pediatric Cardiology

Epstein, Michael L MD [PCd] - **Spec Exp:** Congenital Heart Disease; **Hospital:** All Children's Hosp; **Address:** All Children's Hospital, VP Med Affairs, 801 Sixth St S, St Petersburg, FL 33701; **Phone:** 727-767-6900; **Board Cert:** Pediatrics 1976; Pediatric Cardiology 1981; **Med School:** Univ Tex Med Br, Galveston 1971; **Resid:** Pediatrics, Univ Ariz Hlth Sci Ctr 1974; **Fellow:** Pediatric Cardiology, Univ Minn Hosp 1979; **Fac Appt:** Prof Ped, Wayne State Univ

Fish, Frank A MD [PCd] - **Spec Exp:** Arrhythmias-Pediatric & Adult; Congenital Heart Disease; Pacemakers; **Hospital:** Vanderbilt Univ Med Ctr, Vanderbilt Children's Hosp; **Address:** Vanderbilt Chldns Hosp, Div Peds Cardiology, 2200 Children's Way, Ste 5230, Nashville, TN 37232; **Phone:** 615-322-7447; **Board Cert:** Pediatrics 1987; Pediatric Cardiology 1999; **Med School:** Indiana Univ 1983; **Resid:** Pediatrics, Indiana Univ Hosp 1986; **Fellow:** Pediatric Cardiology, Vanderbilt Univ Med Ctr 1989; Pediatric Cardiology, Chldns Meml Hosp 1990; **Fac Appt:** Assoc Prof Ped, Vanderbilt Univ

Fricker, Frederick Jay MD [PCd] - **Spec Exp:** Transplant Medicine-Heart; **Hospital:** Shands Hlthcre at Univ of FL; **Address:** Shands Hlthcre, Div Pediatric Cardiology, 1600 SW Archer Rd, Box 100296, Gainesville, FL 32610-0296; **Phone:** 352-273-7770; **Board Cert:** Pediatrics 1975; Pediatric Cardiology 1981; **Med School:** Loyola Univ-Stritch Sch Med 1970; **Resid:** Pediatrics, Children's Hosp 1973; **Fellow:** Pediatric Cardiology, Children's Hosp 1977; **Fac Appt:** Prof Ped, Univ Fla Coll Med

Moskowitz, William B MD [PCd] - **Spec Exp:** Cardiac Catheterization; Transplant Medicine-Heart; **Hospital:** Med Coll of VA Hosp; **Address:** Childrens Heart Ctr, Med Coll Virginia, 1200 E Broad St, PO Box 980543, Richmond, VA 23298; **Phone:** 804-828-9143; **Board Cert:** Pediatrics 1983; Pediatric Cardiology 1985; **Med School:** Univ S Fla Coll Med 1978; **Resid:** Pediatrics, Childrens Hosp 1981; **Fellow:** Pediatric Cardiology, Childrens Hosp 1984; **Fac Appt:** Prof Ped, Med Coll VA

Tamer, Dolores MD [PCd] - **Spec Exp:** Kawasaki Disease; **Hospital:** Jackson Meml Hosp, Univ of Miami Hosp & Clins/Sylvester Comp Canc Ctr; **Address:** Univ Miami, Dept Peds, PO Box 016960 (R-76), Miami, FL 33101-6960; **Phone:** 305-585-6683; **Board Cert:** Pediatrics 1966; Pediatric Cardiology 1967; **Med School:** SUNY Buffalo 1961; **Resid:** Pediatrics, Chldns Hosp 1963; Pediatrics, Chldns Hosp 1964; **Fellow:** Pediatrics, Chldns Hosp 1965; **Fac Appt:** Prof Ped, Univ Miami Sch Med

Wolff, Grace S MD [PCd] - **Spec Exp:** Arrhythmias; Cardiac Electrophysiology; Syncope; **Hospital:** Jackson Meml Hosp; **Address:** 1475 NW 12th Ave, Miami, FL 33101; **Phone:** 305-585-6683; **Board Cert:** Pediatrics 1990; Pediatric Cardiology 1990; **Med School:** Med Coll Wisc 1965; **Resid:** Pediatrics, Colum-Presby Med Ctr 1969; **Fellow:** Pediatric Cardiology, Children's Hosp 1971; **Fac Appt:** Prof Ped, Univ Miami Sch Med

Young, Ming-Lon MD [PCd] - **Spec Exp:** Cardiac Electrophysiology; Arrhythmias; **Hospital:** Jackson Meml Hosp, Univ of Miami Hosp & Clins/Sylvester Comp Canc Ctr; **Address:** Univ Miami, Dept Peds, PO Box 016960 (R-76), Miami, FL 33101-6960; **Phone:** 305-585-6683; **Board Cert:** Pediatric Cardiology 1985; Pediatrics 1985; **Med School:** Taiwan 1976; **Resid:** Preventive Medicine, Johns Hopkins Hosp 1979; Pediatrics, St Agnes Hosp 1981; **Fellow:** Pediatric Cardiology, Univ Miami Hosps 1985; **Fac Appt:** Prof Ped, Univ Miami Sch Med

Zahn, Evan M MD [PCd] - **Spec Exp:** Interventional Cardiology; Ventricular Septal Defect (Amplatzer R); Congenital Heart Disease; **Hospital:** Miami Children's Hosp, Baptist Hosp of Miami; **Address:** 3100 SW 62nd Ave Fl 2, Miami, FL 33155-4045; **Phone:** 305-666-6511 x4285; **Board Cert:** Pediatric Cardiology 2000; Pediatrics 1989; **Med School:** NY Med Coll 1986; **Resid:** Pediatrics, Univ Colorado Hosp 1989; **Fellow:** Interventional Cardiology, Hosp for Sick Children 1992

Midwest

Ackerman, Michael J MD [PCd] - **Spec Exp:** Long QT Interval Syndrome; Sudden Infant Death Syndrome (SIDS); Hypertrophic Cardiomyopathy (HCM); **Hospital:** Mayo Med Ctr & Clin - Rochester; **Address:** Mayo Clinic, 200 First St SW, Rochester, MN 55905; **Phone:** 507-284-0101; **Board Cert:** Pediatrics 1998; **Med School:** Mayo Med Sch 1995; **Resid:** Pediatric & Adolescent Medicine, Mayo Clinic 1998; **Fellow:** Pediatric Cardiology, Mayo Clinic 2000; **Fac Appt:** Assoc Prof Ped, Mayo Med Sch

Agarwala, Brojendra MD [PCd] - **Spec Exp:** Congenital Heart Disease; **Hospital:** Univ of Chicago Hosps; **Address:** 5839 S Maryland Ave, rm C-104, MC 4051, Chicago, IL 60637; **Phone:** 773-702-6172; **Board Cert:** Pediatrics 1970; Pediatric Cardiology 1978; **Med School:** India 1965; **Resid:** Pediatrics, St Vincent Hosp Med Ctr 1969; **Fellow:** Pediatric Cardiology, NYU Med Ctr 1972; **Fac Appt:** Prof Ped, Univ Chicago-Pritzker Sch Med

Artman, Michael MD [PCd] - **Spec Exp:** Congenital Heart Disease; Heart Failure; Cardiac Electrophysiology; **Hospital:** Univ Iowa Hosp & Clinics; **Address:** Univ Iowa Hosp & Clinics, Peds 2636 JCP, 200 Hawkins Drive, Iowa City, IA 52242; **Phone:** 319-356-0469; **Board Cert:** Pediatrics 1983; Pediatric Cardiology 1985; **Med School:** Tulane Univ 1978; **Resid:** Pediatrics, Vanderbilt Univ Hosp 1981; **Fellow:** Pediatric Cardiology, Vanderbilt Univ Hosp 1983; **Fac Appt:** Prof Ped, Univ Iowa Coll Med

Beekman III, Robert H MD [PCd] - **Spec Exp:** Interventional Cardiology; Cardiac Catheterization; **Hospital:** Cincinnati Chldns Hosp Med Ctr; **Address:** Cincinnati Chldns Hosp Med Ctr, Div Cardiology, 3333 Burnet Ave, MC 2003, Cincinnati, OH 45229-3026; **Phone:** 513-636-7072; **Board Cert:** Pediatrics 1981; Pediatric Cardiology 1983; **Med School:** Duke Univ 1976; **Resid:** Pediatrics, UCLA Med Ctr 1979; **Fellow:** Pediatric Cardiology, Univ Mich Hosp 1982; **Fac Appt:** Prof Ped, Univ Cincinnati

Caldwell, Randall MD [PCd] - **Spec Exp:** Transplant Medicine-Heart; Echocardiography; **Hospital:** Riley Hosp for Children, Clarian Hlth Ptrs; **Address:** 702 Barnhill Drive, RR-127, Indianapolis, IN 46202-5128; **Phone:** 317-274-8906; **Board Cert:** Pediatrics 1976; Pediatric Cardiology 1978; **Med School:** Indiana Univ 1971; **Resid:** Pediatrics, Indiana Med Ctr 1975; **Fellow:** Pediatric Cardiology, Indiana Med Ctr 1978; **Fac Appt:** Prof Ped, Indiana Univ

Cetta Jr, Frank MD [PCd] - **Spec Exp:** Congenital Heart Disease-Adult; Congenital Heart Disease; **Hospital:** Mayo Med Ctr & Clin - Rochester; **Address:** Mayo Clinic, Gonda 6-138 NW, 200 First St SW, Rochester, MN 55905; **Phone:** 507-266-0676; **Board Cert:** Pediatrics 2000; Pediatric Cardiology 2003; **Med School:** Loyola Univ-Stritch Sch Med 1987; **Resid:** Internal Medicine, Loyola Medical Ctr 1991; Pediatrics, Loyola Medical Ctr 1991; **Fac Appt:** Assoc Prof Ped, Mayo Med Sch

Dick, Macdonald MD [PCd] - **Spec Exp:** Cardiac Electrophysiology; **Hospital:** Mott Chldns Hosp; **Address:** C.S. Motts Chldns Hosp, Dept Ped Cardio, 1500 E Med Ctr Drive, rm L1242, Box 0204, Ann Arbor, MI 48109; **Phone:** 734-936-7418; **Board Cert:** Pediatrics 1989; Pediatric Cardiology 1989; **Med School:** Univ VA Sch Med 1967; **Resid:** Pediatrics, Univ Va Hosp 1971; **Fellow:** Pediatric Cardiology, Chldns Hosp Med Ctr 1974; **Fac Appt:** Prof Ped, Univ Mich Med Sch

Driscoll, David J MD [PCd] - **Spec Exp:** Exercise Physiology; Klippel-Trenaunay Syndrome; Cardiomyopathy; **Hospital:** Mayo Med Ctr & Clin - Rochester; **Address:** Mayo Clinic - Pediatric Cardiology, 200 1st St SW, Rochester, MN 55905-0001; **Phone:** 507-284-3297; **Board Cert:** Pediatrics 1976; Pediatric Cardiology 1999; **Med School:** Marquette Sch Med 1970; **Resid:** Pediatrics, Milwaukee Chldns Hosp 1972; Pediatrics, Milwaukee Chldns Hosp 1975; **Fellow:** Pediatric Cardiology, Baylor Coll Med 1978; **Fac Appt:** Prof Ped, Mayo Med Sch

Hijazi, Ziyad M MD [PCd] - **Spec Exp:** Interventional Cardiology; Congenital Heart Disease; Coarctation of the Aorta; **Hospital:** Univ of Chicago Hosps; **Address:** Univ Chicago Chldns Hosp, Congenital Heart Ctr, 5839 S Maryland Ave, rm C104, MC 4051, Chicago, IL 60637; **Phone:** 773-702-6172; **Board Cert:** Pediatrics 2000; Pediatric Cardiology 2000; **Med School:** Jordan 1982; **Resid:** Pediatrics, Yale-New Haven Hosp 1988; **Fellow:** Pediatric Cardiology, Yale-New Haven Hosp 1991; **Fac Appt:** Prof Ped, Univ Chicago-Pritzker Sch Med

Latson, Larry A MD [PCd] - **Spec Exp:** Congenital Heart Disease; Interventional Cardiology; **Hospital:** Cleveland Clin Fdn (page 57); **Address:** Cleveland Clinic Fdn, Ped Cardiology, 9500 Euclid Ave, Desk M41, Cleveland, OH 44195; **Phone:** 216-445-6532; **Board Cert:** Pediatrics 1981; Pediatric Cardiology 1983; Pediatric Critical Care Medicine 2003; **Med School:** Baylor Coll Med 1976; **Resid:** Pediatrics, Baylor Coll Med 1978; **Fellow:** Pediatric Cardiology, Baylor Coll Med 1981; **Fac Appt:** Prof Ped, Case West Res Univ

O'Laughlin, Martin P MD [PCd] - **Spec Exp:** Cardiac Catheterization; Congenital Heart Disease-Adult & Child; Interventional Cardiology; **Hospital:** Chldns Mercy Hosps & Clinics, St Luke's Hosp of Kansas City; **Address:** 4400 Broadway, Ste 400, Kansas City, MO 64111; **Phone:** 816-931-5440; **Board Cert:** Pediatrics 1985; Pediatric Cardiology 2003; **Med School:** Columbia P&S 1980; **Resid:** Pediatrics, Baylor Coll Med 1984; **Fellow:** Pediatric Cardiology, Texas Chldns Hosp/Baylor 1987

Porter, Co-burn Joseph MD [PCd] - **Spec Exp:** Arrhythmias; Arrhythmias-Fetal; Transplant Medicine-Heart; **Hospital:** St Mary's Hosp - Rochester; **Address:** Mayo Med Ctr, Dept Ped Cardiology, 200 First St SW, Rochester, MN 55905-0001; **Phone:** 507-284-3297; **Board Cert:** Pediatrics 1977; Pediatric Cardiology 1983; **Med School:** Creighton Univ 1972; **Resid:** Pediatrics, Univ Colo Hlth Sci Ctr 1975; **Fellow:** Pediatric Cardiology, Baylor Coll Med 1977; Pediatric Cardiology, Baylor Coll Med 1981; **Fac Appt:** Prof Ped, Mayo Med Sch

Rocchini, Albert P MD [PCd] - **Spec Exp:** Congenital Heart Disease; Interventional Cardiology; Hypertension in Obesity; **Hospital:** Univ Michigan Hlth Sys; **Address:** Mott Chldns Hosp, Dept Ped Cardiology, 1500 E Med Ctr Drive, rm L1242, Box 0204, Ann Arbor, MI 48109-0204; **Phone:** 734-936-8993; **Board Cert:** Pediatrics 1989; Pediatric Cardiology 1989; **Med School:** Univ Pittsburgh 1972; **Resid:** Pediatrics, Univ Minn 1974; **Fellow:** Pediatric Cardiology, Chldns Hosp 1977; **Fac Appt:** Prof Ped, Univ Mich Med Sch

Rosenthal, Amnon MD [PCd] - **Spec Exp:** Congenital Heart Disease; Congenital Heart Disease-Young Adult; **Hospital:** Univ Michigan Hlth Sys; **Address:** Univ Mich-Mott Children's Hosp, 1500 E Medical Ctr, rm L1242 Women's, Box 0204, Ann Arbor, MI 48109-0204; **Phone:** 734-764-5176; **Board Cert:** Pediatrics 1986; Pediatric Cardiology 1986; **Med School:** Albany Med Coll 1959; **Resid:** Pediatrics, Boston Chldns Hosp 1962; **Fellow:** Cardiovascular Disease, Boston Chldns Hosp 1968; **Fac Appt:** Prof Ped, Univ Mich Med Sch

Sodt, Peter C MD [PCd] - **Spec Exp:** Congenital Heart Disease; Arrhythmias; Pacemakers; **Hospital:** Children's Mem Hosp, St Alexius Med Ctr; **Address:** 1555 N Barrington Rd, Ste 430, Hoffman Estates, IL 60194; **Phone:** 847-884-1212; **Board Cert:** Pediatrics 1986; Pediatric Cardiology 2002; **Med School:** Northwestern Univ 1980; **Resid:** Pediatrics, Oregon Hlth Scis Univ 1984; **Fellow:** Pediatric Cardiology, Univ Chicago 1986; **Fac Appt:** Assoc Clin Prof Ped, Northwestern Univ

Great Plains and Mountains

Minich, Lois LuAnn MD [PCd] - **Spec Exp:** Echocardiography; **Hospital:** Primary Children's Med Ctr; **Address:** Primary Chlds Med Ctr, Dept Ped Cardiology, 100 N Medical, Ste 1500, Salt Lake City, UT 84113; **Phone:** 801-662-5400; **Board Cert:** Pediatrics 2000; Pediatric Cardiology 2000; **Med School:** W VA Univ 1986; **Resid:** Pediatrics, Fletcher Allen Health Care 1989; **Fellow:** Pediatric Cardiology, Univ Michigan Hosps 1992

Southwest

Dreyer, William J MD [PCd] - **Spec Exp:** Congenital Heart Disease; Transplant Medicine-Heart; Cardiomyopathy; **Hospital:** Texas Chldns Hosp - Houston; **Address:** Texas Chldns Hosp, 6621 Fannin St, MS 19345C, Houston, TX 77030; **Phone:** 832-826-5659; **Board Cert:** Pediatrics 1987; Pediatric Cardiology 2006; **Med School:** Univ Fla Coll Med 1981; **Resid:** Pediatrics, UCSF Med Ctr 1984; **Fellow:** Pediatric Cardiology, Baylor Coll Med 1988; **Fac Appt:** Assoc Prof Ped, Baylor Coll Med

Friedman, Richard Alan MD [PCd] - **Spec Exp:** Cardiac Electrophysiology; **Hospital:** Texas Chldns Hosp - Houston; **Address:** Texas Children's Hospital, 6621 Fannin St, MC 19345-C, Houston, TX 77030-2303; **Phone:** 832-826-5600; **Board Cert:** Pediatrics 1986; Pediatric Cardiology 2003; **Med School:** Univ Pittsburgh 1980; **Resid:** Pediatrics, Baylor Affil Hosps 1983; **Fellow:** Pediatric Cardiology, Baylor Affil Hosps 1985; **Fac Appt:** Assoc Prof Ped, Baylor Coll Med

Gillette, Paul C MD [PCd] - **Spec Exp:** Arrhythmias; **Hospital:** Cook Chldns Med Ctr, Harris Methodist Hosp - Fort Worth; **Address:** Pediatric Cardiology, 901 7th Ave, Ste 310, Fort Worth, TX 76104; **Phone:** 682-885-2140; **Board Cert:** Pediatrics 1974; Pediatric Cardiology 1975; **Med School:** Med Univ SC 1969; **Resid:** Pediatrics, Baylor Coll Med 1972; **Fellow:** Pediatric Cardiology, Baylor Coll Med 1974

Mahony, Lynn MD [PCd] - **Spec Exp:** Congenital Heart Disease; Marfan's Syndrome; Congestive Heart Failure; **Hospital:** Chldns Med Ctr of Dallas; **Address:** 1935 Motor St, Dallas, TX 75235; **Phone:** 214-456-2333; **Board Cert:** Pediatrics 1979; Pediatric Cardiology 1997; **Med School:** Stanford Univ 1975; **Resid:** Pediatrics, Stanford Univ 1978; **Fellow:** Pediatric Cardiology, UCSF Med Ctr 1981; **Fac Appt:** Assoc Prof Ped, Univ Tex SW, Dallas

Pediatric Cardiology

Moodie, Douglas MD [PCd] - **Spec Exp:** Marfan's Syndrome; Congenital Heart Disease-Adult & Child; **Hospital:** Ochsner Fdn Hosp; **Address:** Ochsner Chldns Heart Inst, 1315 Jefferson Hwy, New Orleans, LA 70121; **Phone:** 504-842-4827; **Board Cert:** Pediatrics 1977; Pediatric Cardiology 1977; **Med School:** Med Coll Wisc 1972; **Resid:** Pediatrics, Mayo Clinic 1974; **Fellow:** Pediatric Cardiology, Mayo Clinic 1977

Rogers Jr, James H MD [PCd] - **Spec Exp:** Congenital Heart Disease; **Hospital:** Christus Santa Rosa Children's Hosp, Univ Hlth Sys - Univ Hosp; **Address:** Childrens Heart Network, 1901 Babcock Rd, Ste 301, San Antonio, TX 78229; **Phone:** 210-341-7722; **Board Cert:** Pediatrics 1976; Pediatric Cardiology 1977; **Med School:** Med Coll GA 1971; **Resid:** Pediatrics, Wilford Hall USAF Med Ctr 1974; **Fellow:** Pediatric Cardiology, Med Coll Georgia 1976; **Fac Appt:** Clin Prof Ped, Univ Tex, San Antonio

West Coast and Pacific

Bernstein, Daniel MD [PCd] - **Spec Exp:** Transplant Medicine-Heart; Cardiomyopathy; **Hospital:** Lucile Packard Chldns Hosp/Stanford Univ Med Ctr, Stanford Univ Med Ctr; **Address:** Lucile Packard Chldns Hosp, Div Ped Card, 750 Welch Rd, Ste 305, Palo Alto, CA 94304-1510; **Phone:** 650-723-7913; **Board Cert:** Pediatrics 1984; Pediatric Cardiology 1985; **Med School:** NYU Sch Med 1978; **Resid:** Pediatrics, Montefiore Hosp-Einstein 1982; **Fellow:** Pediatric Cardiology, UCSF 1986; **Fac Appt:** Prof Ped, Stanford Univ

Boucek Jr, Robert J MD [PCd] - **Spec Exp:** Congenital Heart Disease; Cardiomyopathy; Transplant Medicine-Heart; **Hospital:** Chldns Hosp and Regl Med Ctr - Seattle; **Address:** 4800 Sand Point Way NE, MS G0035, Seattle, WA 98105; **Phone:** 206-987-2015; **Board Cert:** Pediatrics 1974; Pediatric Cardiology 1977; **Med School:** Tulane Univ 1969; **Resid:** Pediatrics, Duke Univ Med Ctr 1971; **Fellow:** Ambulatory Pediatrics, US Naval Hosp 1973; Pediatric Cardiology, Vanderbilt Med Ctr 1976; **Fac Appt:** Prof Ped, Univ Wash

Hohn, Arno R MD [PCd] - **Spec Exp:** Hypertension; Preventive Cardiology; **Hospital:** Chldns Hosp - Los Angeles (page 56), LAC & USC Med Ctr; **Address:** Chldns Hosp, Div Cardiology, 4650 Sunset Blvd, MS 34, Los Angeles, CA 90027; **Phone:** 323-669-2535; **Board Cert:** Pediatrics 1986; Pediatric Cardiology 1986; **Med School:** NY Med Coll 1956; **Resid:** Pediatrics, Chldns Hosp 1958; Pediatrics, Chldns Hosp 1962; **Fellow:** Pediatric Cardiology, Chldns Hosp 1963; **Fac Appt:** Prof Ped, USC Sch Med

Perry, Stanton Bruce MD [PCd] - **Spec Exp:** Interventional Cardiology; **Hospital:** Lucile Packard Chldns Hosp/Stanford Univ Med Ctr; **Address:** L Packard Chldns Hosp, Ped Cardiology, 750 Welch Rd, Ste 305, Palo Alto, CA 94304; **Phone:** 650-723-7913; **Board Cert:** Pediatrics 1986; Pediatric Cardiology 1988; **Med School:** Iceland 1978; **Resid:** Pediatrics, St Louis Chldns Hosp 1983; **Fellow:** Pediatric Cardiology, Chldns Hosp 1984; **Fac Appt:** Assoc Prof Ped, Stanford Univ

Takahashi, Masato MD [PCd] - **Spec Exp:** Kawasaki Disease; Cardiac Catheterization; Congenital Heart Disease-Adult; **Hospital:** Chldns Hosp - Los Angeles (page 56), USC Univ Hosp - R K Eamer Med Plz; **Address:** Chldns Hosp-LA, Div Cardiology, 4650 Sunset Blvd, MS 34, Los Angeles, CA 90027-6062; **Phone:** 323-669-4634; **Board Cert:** Pediatrics 1966; Pediatric Cardiology 1992; **Med School:** Indiana Univ 1960; **Resid:** Pediatrics, Ind Med Ctr 1963; **Fellow:** Pediatric Cardiology, UCLA Med Ctr 1967; **Fac Appt:** Prof Ped, USC Sch Med

Teitel, David F MD [PCd] - **Hospital:** UCSF Med Ctr; **Address:** UCSF, Dept Ped Cardiology, 400 Parnassus Ave, rm A2962, Box 0379, San Francisco, CA 94143-0379; **Phone:** 415-353-2008; **Board Cert:** Pediatrics 1980; Pediatric Cardiology 1983; **Med School:** Univ Toronto 1975; **Resid:** Pediatrics, Childrens Hosp 1980; **Fellow:** Pediatric Cardiology, UCSF Med Ctr 1982; **Fac Appt:** Prof Ped, UCSF

Pediatric Critical Care Medicine

New England

Fleisher, Gary R MD [PCCM] - **Spec Exp:** Infectious Disease; Trauma; **Hospital:** Children's Hospital - Boston; **Address:** Chldns Hosp, Dept Med, 300 Longwood Ave, Hunnewell 350, Boston, MA 02115-5724; **Phone:** 617-355-5022; **Board Cert:** Emergency Medicine 2001; Pediatrics 1992; Pediatric Emergency Medicine 2007; Pediatric Infectious Disease 1999; **Med School:** Jefferson Med Coll 1973; **Resid:** Pediatrics, Chldns Hosp 1976; Pediatrics, Chldns Hosp 1977; **Fellow:** Infectious Disease, Chldns Hosp 1979; **Fac Appt:** Prof Ped, Harvard Med Sch

Mid Atlantic

Fuhrman, Bradley P MD [PCCM] - **Hospital:** Women's & Chldn's Hosp of Buffalo, The; **Address:** Chldns Hosp Buffalo, Dept Ped Critical Care, 219 Bryant St, Buffalo, NY 14222-2006; **Phone:** 716-878-7442; **Board Cert:** Pediatrics 1992; Pediatric Critical Care Medicine 2003; Neonatal-Perinatal Medicine 1979; Pediatric Cardiology 1979; **Med School:** NYU Sch Med 1971; **Resid:** Pediatrics, Univ Minnesota Med Ctr 1973; **Fellow:** Pediatric Cardiology, Univ Minnesota 1974; Neonatal-Perinatal Medicine, Univ Minnesota 1979; **Fac Appt:** Prof Ped, SUNY Buffalo

Nichols, David Gregory MD [PCCM] - **Spec Exp:** Respiratory Failure; Mechanical Ventilation; **Hospital:** Johns Hopkins Hosp - Baltimore (page 61); **Address:** Johns Hopkins Hosp - Pediatric CCM, 733 N Broadway, Ste 115, Baltimore, MD 21205; **Phone:** 410-955-8401; **Board Cert:** Pediatrics 1982; Anesthesiology 1984; Pediatric Critical Care Medicine 2003; **Med School:** Mount Sinai Sch Med 1977; **Resid:** Pediatrics, Childrens Hosp 1980; Anesthesiology, Hosp Univ Penn 1983; **Fellow:** Critical Care Anesthesiology, Childrens Hosp 1983; **Fac Appt:** Prof Ped, Johns Hopkins Univ

Thompson, Ann Ellen MD [PCCM] - **Spec Exp:** Mechanical Ventilation; Critical Care; Respiratory Failure; **Hospital:** Chldns Hosp of Pittsburgh - UPMC; **Address:** Chldns Hosp, Dept Ped Crit Care, 3705 Fifth Ave Bldg Main Tower - rm 6840, Pittsburgh, PA 15213-2584; **Phone:** 412-692-5164; **Board Cert:** Anesthesiology 1980; Pediatrics 1992; Pediatric Critical Care Medicine 2003; **Med School:** Tufts Univ 1974; **Resid:** Pediatrics, Chldns Hosp 1977; Anesthesiology, Hosp Univ Penn 1980; **Fellow:** Pediatric Critical Care Medicine, Chldns Hosp 1979; **Fac Appt:** Prof Ped, Univ Pittsburgh

Midwest

Sarnaik, Ashok P MD [PCCM] - **Spec Exp:** Critical Care; Perinatal Medicine; **Hospital:** Chldns Hosp of Michigan; **Address:** Chldns Hosp, Div Crit Care Med, 3901 Beaubien St, Detroit, MI 48201-2119; **Phone:** 313-745-5629; **Board Cert:** Pediatrics 1975; Neonatal-Perinatal Medicine 1979; Pediatric Critical Care Medicine 2003; **Med School:** India 1969; **Resid:** Pediatrics, JJ Hosp-Bombay Univ 1971; Pediatrics, Chldns Hosp Mich 1974; **Fellow:** Neonatal-Perinatal Medicine, Chldns Hosp Mich 1975; **Fac Appt:** Prof Ped, Wayne State Univ

Pediatric Critical Care Medicine

Great Plains and Mountains

Dean, Jonathan M MD [PCCM] - **Hospital:** Primary Children's Med Ctr; **Address:** Primary Chlds Med Ctr, Pediatric ICU, 100 N Medical Drive, Salt Lake City, UT 84113; **Phone:** 801-587-7572; **Board Cert:** Pediatrics 1981; Pediatric Critical Care Medicine 2003; **Med School:** Northwestern Univ 1977; **Resid:** Pediatrics, Children's Hosp 1981; **Fellow:** Pediatric Critical Care Medicine, Johns Hopkins Hosp 1983; **Fac Appt:** Prof Ped, Univ Utah

Southwest

Anand, Kanwaljeet Singh MD/PhD [PCCM] - **Spec Exp:** Pain Management; Critical Care; **Hospital:** Arkansas Chldns Hosp; **Address:** Arkansas Chldns Hosp, Div CCM, 800 Marshall St, Sturg-slot 512-12, Little Rock, AR 72202-3591; **Phone:** 501-364-3568; **Board Cert:** Pediatric Critical Care Medicine 2004; **Med School:** India 1981; **Resid:** Pediatrics, Chldns Hosp 1991; Neonatal-Perinatal Medicine, John Radcliffe Hosp 1985; **Fellow:** Pediatric Critical Care Medicine, Mass Genl Hosp 1993; **Fac Appt:** Prof Ped, Univ Ark

Perez Fontan, J Julio MD [PCCM] - **Spec Exp:** Respiratory Failure; **Hospital:** UT Southwestern Med Ctr - Dallas; **Address:** UT SW Med Ctr, Dept Peds, 5323 Harry Hines Blvd, Dallas, TX 75390-9063; **Phone:** 214-648-3563; **Board Cert:** Pediatrics 1987; Pediatric Critical Care Medicine 2003; **Med School:** Spain 1977; **Resid:** Pediatrics, Chldns Hosp/Univ Barcelona 1981; **Fellow:** Critical Care Medicine, UCSF Med Ctr 1984; **Fac Appt:** Prof Ped, Univ Tex SW, Dallas

Schwarz, Adam J MD [PCCM] - **Hospital:** Phoenix Children's Hosp; **Address:** Phoenix Children's Hosp, Critical Care, 1919 E Thomas Rd, Ste 1891, Phoenix, AZ 85016; **Phone:** 602-546-1784; **Board Cert:** Pediatrics 2001; Pediatric Critical Care Medicine 2004; **Med School:** Stanford Univ 1990; **Resid:** Pediatrics, Stanford Med Ctr 1993; **Fellow:** Pediatric Critical Care Medicine, Harbor-UCLA Med Ctr 1996; **Fac Appt:** Assoc Clin Prof Ped

Taylor, Richard P MD [PCCM] - **Hospital:** Univ Hlth Sys - Univ Hosp; **Address:** Univ Texas HSC, Dept Ped Critical Care, 7703 Floyd Curl Drive, San Antonio, TX 78229; **Phone:** 210-567-5314; **Board Cert:** Internal Medicine 1988; Pediatrics 1989; Pediatric Critical Care Medicine 2004; **Med School:** Univ Tex Med Br, Galveston 1984; **Resid:** Internal Medicine, St Joseph Mercy Hosp 1988; Pediatrics, UNiv Michigan Med Ctr 1988; **Fellow:** Pediatric Critical Care Medicine, Univ Michigan Med Ctr 1995; **Fac Appt:** Assoc Prof Ped

Thomas, James A MD [PCCM] - **Hospital:** Chldns Med Ctr of Dallas; **Address:** Children's Medical Ctr of Dallas, PICU, 1935 Motor St, Dallas, TX 75235; **Phone:** 214-456-5095; **Board Cert:** Pediatrics 2000; Pediatric Critical Care Medicine 2004; **Med School:** Stanford Univ 1989; **Resid:** Pediatrics, Children's Hosp 1992; **Fellow:** Pediatric Critical Care Medicine, U Texas SW Med Ctr 1996

West Coast and Pacific

Brill, Judith Eileen MD [PCCM] - **Hospital:** Mattel Chldns Hosp at UCLA; **Address:** UCLA, Dept Peds-Div Crit Care, 10833 Le Conte Ave, rm 12-494 MDCC, Los Angeles, CA 90095-1752; **Phone:** 310-825-9124; **Board Cert:** Pediatrics 1982; Anesthesiology 1986; Pediatric Critical Care Medicine 2003; **Med School:** Harvard Med Sch 1977; **Resid:** Pediatrics, Chldns Hosp Med Ctr 1979; Pediatrics, UCLA Med Ctr 1981; **Fellow:** Anesthesiology, Mass Genl Hosp 1982; **Fac Appt:** Prof Med, UCLA

Zimmerman, Jerry John MD [PCCM] - **Spec Exp:** Inflammation in Critical Illness; Sepsis; Septic Shock; **Hospital:** Chldns Hosp and Regl Med Ctr - Seattle, Harborview Med Ctr; **Address:** Children's Hosp & Regl Med Ctr, 4800 Sandpoint Way NE, rm W9813, Seattle, WA 98105-0371; **Phone:** 206-987-2170; **Board Cert:** Pediatrics 1992; Pediatric Critical Care Medicine 2003; **Med School:** Univ Wisc 1979; **Resid:** Pediatrics, Univ Wisconsin Hosp 1982; **Fellow:** Pediatric Critical Care Medicine, Childrens Natl Med Ctr 1984; **Fac Appt:** Prof Ped, Univ Wash

Pediatric Endocrinology

New England

Casella, Samuel Joseph MD [PEn] - **Spec Exp:** Thyroid Disorders; Growth/Development Disorders; **Hospital:** Dartmouth - Hitchcock Med Ctr; **Address:** Darthmouth-Hitchcock Med Ctr, Ped Endocrinology, One Medical Center Drive, Lebanon, NH 03756; **Phone:** 603-653-9877; **Board Cert:** Pediatrics 1985; Pediatric Endocrinology 1986; **Med School:** SUNY Upstate Med Univ 1981; **Resid:** Pediatrics, Upstate Med Ctr 1984; **Fellow:** Pediatric Endocrinology, NC Meml Hosp-Univ NC 1986; **Fac Appt:** Assoc Prof Ped, Johns Hopkins Univ

Levitsky, Lynne Lipton MD [PEn] - **Spec Exp:** Diabetes; Growth/Development Disorders; Cushing's Syndrome; **Hospital:** Mass Genl Hosp; **Address:** Mass Genl Hosp, Ped Endo, 55 Fruit St, YAW-6800, Boston, MA 02114-2696; **Phone:** 617-726-2909; **Board Cert:** Pediatrics 1971; Pediatric Endocrinology 1978; **Med School:** Yale Univ 1966; **Resid:** Pediatrics, Children's Hosp 1968; **Fellow:** Pediatric Endocrinology, Univ Maryland Hosp 1970; **Fac Appt:** Assoc Prof Ped, Harvard Med Sch

Ludwig, David S MD/PhD [PEn] - **Spec Exp:** Obesity; Nutrition; **Hospital:** Children's Hospital - Boston; **Address:** Chldns Hosp, Div Endocrinology, 333 Longwood Ave Fl 6 - rm 624, Boston, MA 02115; **Phone:** 617-355-7476; **Board Cert:** Pediatric Endocrinology 2003; **Med School:** Stanford Univ 1990; **Resid:** Pediatrics, Chldns Hosp 1993; **Fellow:** Pediatric Endocrinology, Chldns Hosp 1995; **Fac Appt:** Asst Prof Ped, Harvard Med Sch

Tamborlane, William V MD [PEn] - **Spec Exp:** Diabetes; **Hospital:** Yale - New Haven Hosp; **Address:** Yale Pediatric Endocrinology, 333 Cedar St, rm 3091-LMP, New Haven, CT 06510-3289; **Phone:** 203-764-6747; **Board Cert:** Pediatrics 1978; Pediatric Endocrinology 1986; **Med School:** Georgetown Univ 1972; **Resid:** Pediatrics, Georgetown Univ Hosp 1975; **Fellow:** Pediatric Endocrinology, Yale-NewHaven Hosp 1977; **Fac Appt:** Prof Ped, Yale Univ

Mid Atlantic

Arslanian, Silva MD [PEn] - **Spec Exp:** Diabetes; Obesity; **Hospital:** Chldns Hosp of Pittsburgh - UPMC; **Address:** Chldns Hosp Pittsburgh, Div Endocrinology, 3705 5th Ave, DeSoto Wing, rm 4A 400-11, Pittsburgh, PA 15213; **Phone:** 412-692-6565; **Board Cert:** Pediatrics 1983; Pediatric Endocrinology 1983; **Med School:** Lebanon 1978; **Resid:** Pediatrics, American Univ Hosp 1980; **Fellow:** Pediatric Endocrinology, Chldns Hosp 1983; **Fac Appt:** Prof Ped, Univ Pittsburgh

Becker, Dorothy J MD [PEn] - **Spec Exp:** Diabetes; **Hospital:** Chldns Hosp of Pittsburgh - UPMC; **Address:** Children's Hosp Pittsburgh, Div Endocrinology, 3705 5th Ave, 4A-400 DeSoto, Pittsburgh, PA 15213; **Phone:** 412-692-5172; **Board Cert:** Pediatrics 1978; Pediatric Endocrinology 1978; **Med School:** South Africa 1964; **Resid:** Pediatrics, Univ Capetown 1972; Endocrinology, Diabetes & Metabolism, Univ Capetown 1974; **Fellow:** Pediatric Endocrinology, Univ Pittsburgh 1976; **Fac Appt:** Prof Ped, Univ Pittsburgh

Pediatric Endocrinology

Moshang Jr, Thomas MD [PEn] - **Spec Exp:** Growth/Development Disorders; **Hospital:** Chldns Hosp of Philadelphia, The; **Address:** Chldns Hosp of Philaelphia, Div Endocrinology, 34th St and Civic Center Blvd, rm 8416, Philadelphia, PA 19104; **Phone:** 215-590-3174; **Board Cert:** Pediatrics 1967; Pediatric Endocrinology 1978; **Med School:** Univ MD Sch Med 1962; **Resid:** Pediatrics, Chldns Hosp 1965; **Fellow:** Pediatric Endocrinology, Chldns Hosp 1970; **Fac Appt:** Prof Ped, Univ Pennsylvania

New, Maria I MD [PEn] - **Spec Exp:** Adrenal Disorders; **Hospital:** Mount Sinai Med Ctr; **Address:** Mount Sinai Medical Ctr, 1 Gustave L Levy Pl, Box 1198, New York, NY 10029; **Phone:** 212-241-8210; **Board Cert:** Pediatrics 1960; **Med School:** Univ Pennsylvania 1954; **Resid:** Pediatrics, New York Hosp 1957; **Fellow:** Pediatric Endocrinology, New York Hosp 1958; Endocrinology, Diabetes & Metabolism, New York Hosp 1964; **Fac Appt:** Prof Ped, Cornell Univ-Weill Med Coll

Oberfield, Sharon E MD [PEn] - **Spec Exp:** Adrenal Disorders; Neuroendocrine Growth Disorders; Growth Disorders; **Hospital:** NYPresby-Morgan Stanley Children's Hosp; **Address:** 630 W 168th St PH East Bldg - Ste 522, New York, NY 10032; **Phone:** 212-305-6559; **Board Cert:** Pediatrics 1979; Pediatric Endocrinology 2000; **Med School:** Cornell Univ-Weill Med Coll 1974; **Resid:** Pediatrics, NY Hosp-Cornell 1976; **Fellow:** Pediatric Endocrinology, NY Hosp-Cornell 1979; **Fac Appt:** Prof Ped, Columbia P&S

Plotnick, Leslie Parker MD [PEn] - **Spec Exp:** Diabetes; Growth Disorders; **Hospital:** Johns Hopkins Hosp - Baltimore (page 61); **Address:** Johns Hopkins Hospital, Dept Pediatric Endocrinology, Baltimore, MD 21287; **Phone:** 410-955-6463; **Board Cert:** Pediatrics 1975; Pediatric Endocrinology 1978; **Med School:** Univ MD Sch Med 1970; **Resid:** Pediatrics, Johns Hopkins Hosp 1972; **Fellow:** Pediatric Endocrinology, Johns Hopkins Hosp 1974; **Fac Appt:** Prof Ped, Johns Hopkins Univ

Sklar, Charles A MD [PEn] - **Spec Exp:** Cancer Survivors-Late Effects of Therapy; Growth Disorders in Childhood Cancer; Pituitary Disorders; **Hospital:** Meml Sloan Kettering Cancer Ctr; **Address:** 1275 York Ave, Box 151, New York, NY 10021; **Phone:** 212-639-8138; **Board Cert:** Pediatrics 1979; Pediatric Endocrinology 1980; **Med School:** USC Sch Med 1974; **Resid:** Pediatrics, Childrens Hosp 1976; **Fellow:** Pediatric Endocrinology, UCSF Med Ctr 1979; **Fac Appt:** Assoc Prof Ped, Cornell Univ-Weill Med Coll

Sperling, Mark A MD [PEn] - **Spec Exp:** Diabetes; Growth/Development Disorders; Hypoglycemia; **Hospital:** Chldns Hosp of Pittsburgh - UPMC, UPMC Presby, Pittsburgh; **Address:** Chldns Hosp Pittsburgh, Endocrinology, 3705 Fifth Ave, DeSot Bldg, Fl 4A - Ste 400, Pittsburgh, PA 15213-2524; **Phone:** 412-692-5172; **Board Cert:** Pediatrics 1986; Pediatric Endocrinology 1986; **Med School:** Australia 1962; **Resid:** Internal Medicine, Prince Henry Hosp 1964; Pediatrics, Royal Chldns Hosp 1968; **Fellow:** Pediatric Endocrinology, Chldns Hosp 1970; **Fac Appt:** Prof Ped, Univ Pittsburgh

Stanley, Charles MD [PEn] - **Spec Exp:** Hyperinsulinism-Congenital; Hypoglycemia; **Hospital:** Chldns Hosp of Philadelphia, The; **Address:** Chldns Hosp, Div Endocrinology, 34th St & Civic Ctr Blvd, rm 8416, Philadelphia, PA 19104; **Phone:** 215-590-3174; **Board Cert:** Pediatrics 1976; Pediatric Endocrinology 1978; **Med School:** Univ VA Sch Med 1970; **Resid:** Pediatrics, Chldns Hosp 1972; **Fellow:** Pediatric Endocrinology, Chldns Hosp 1976; **Fac Appt:** Prof Ped, Univ Pennsylvania

Southeast

Diamond, Frank MD [PEn] - **Spec Exp:** Growth Disorders; Obesity; Calcium Disorders in Newborn; **Hospital:** All Children's Hosp, Tampa Genl Hosp; **Address:** 801 6th St, St Petersburg, FL 33701; **Phone:** 727-767-4237; **Board Cert:** Pediatrics 1979; Pediatric Endocrinology 1980; **Med School:** Penn State Univ-Hershey Med Ctr 1974; **Resid:** Pediatrics, Chldns Hosp-Univ Alabama 1976; **Fellow:** Pediatric Endocrinology, Chldns Hosp-Univ Penn 1978; **Fac Appt:** Prof Ped, Univ S Fla Coll Med

Freemark, Michael S MD [PEn] - **Spec Exp:** Thyroid Disorders; Neuroendocrine Growth Disorders; Diabetes; **Hospital:** Duke Univ Med Ctr, Durham Regional Hosp; **Address:** Duke Univ Med Ctr, Erwin Rd, Bell Bldg, rm 305, Box 3080, Durham, NC 27710-0001; **Phone:** 919-684-8350; **Board Cert:** Pediatrics 1980; Pediatric Endocrinology 1984; **Med School:** Duke Univ 1976; **Resid:** Pediatrics, Duke Univ Med Ctr 1979; **Fellow:** Pediatric Endocrinology, Duke Univ Med Ctr 1984; Pediatric Endocrinology, Hospital Necker Enfants Malades 1993; **Fac Appt:** Prof Ped, Duke Univ

Friedman, Nancy E MD [PEn] - **Spec Exp:** Calcium Disorders; Bone Disorders-Metabolic; Growth/Development Disorders; Cancer Survivors-Late Effects of Therapy; **Hospital:** Duke Univ Med Ctr; **Address:** Duke Consultative Services, 3713 Benson Drive, Ste 202, Durham, NC 27609; **Phone:** 919-684-3772; **Board Cert:** Pediatrics 1979; Pediatric Endocrinology 2003; **Med School:** Med Coll VA 1975; **Resid:** Pediatrics, Childrens Hosp Med Ctr 1977; Pediatrics, Childrens Meml Hosp 1978; **Fellow:** Endocrinology, Diabetes & Metabolism, Michael Reese Hosp 1980; **Fac Appt:** Asst Clin Prof Ped, Duke Univ

Key Jr, L Lyndon MD [PEn] - **Spec Exp:** Osteopetrosis; Osteoporosis-Juvenile; **Hospital:** MUSC Med Ctr; **Address:** MUSC Med Ctr, Dept Pediatrics, 135 Rutledge Ave, Box 250561, Charleston, SC 29425; **Phone:** 843-792-6807; **Board Cert:** Pediatrics 1983; Pediatric Endocrinology 1983; **Med School:** Univ NC Sch Med 1977; **Resid:** Pediatrics, Duke Univ Med Ctr 1980; **Fellow:** Endocrinology, Chldns Hosp 1983; **Fac Appt:** Prof Ped, Med Univ SC

Meacham, Lillian R MD [PEn] - **Spec Exp:** Growth Disorders in Childhood Cancer; Cancer Survivors-Late Effects of Therapy; **Hospital:** Emory Univ Hosp; **Address:** Emory Childrens Ctr, 2015 Uppergate Drive, Altanta, GA 30322; **Phone:** 404-727-5753; **Board Cert:** Pediatrics 2006; Pediatric Endocrinology 2006; **Med School:** Emory Univ 1984; **Resid:** Pediatrics, Emory Univ Hosp 1987; **Fellow:** Pediatric Endocrinology, Emory Univ Hosp 1990; **Fac Appt:** Assoc Prof Ped, Emory Univ

Schwartz, Robert P MD [PEn] - **Hospital:** Wake Forest Univ Baptist Med Ctr (page 73); **Address:** Wake Forest Univ Sch Med-Dept Pediatrics, Med Ctr Blvd, Winston-Salem, NC 27157-0001; **Phone:** 336-716-3199; **Board Cert:** Pediatrics 1994; Pediatric Endocrinology 2002; **Med School:** Univ Fla Coll Med 1968; **Resid:** Pediatrics, Charlotte Meml Hosp 1970; Pediatrics, Duke Univ Med Ctr 1971; **Fellow:** Pediatric Endocrinology, Duke Univ Med Ctr 1971; Pediatric Endocrinology, Duke Univ Med Ctr 1974; **Fac Appt:** Prof Ped, Wake Forest Univ

Silverstein, Janet H MD [PEn] - **Spec Exp:** Diabetes; Growth/Development Disorders; **Hospital:** Shands Hlthcre at Univ of FL, Shands at Alachua Gen Hosp; **Address:** Univ Florida - Shands Hlthcare, 1600 SW Archer Rd, Box 100296, Gainesville, FL 32610-3003; **Phone:** 352-334-1390; **Board Cert:** Pediatrics 1975; Pediatric Endocrinology 2004; **Med School:** Univ Pennsylvania 1970; **Resid:** Pediatrics, Chldns Hosp 1972; Pediatrics, Chldns Hosp 1975; **Fellow:** Pediatric Endocrinology, Duke Univ Med Ctr 1977; **Fac Appt:** Prof Ped, Univ Fla Coll Med

Pediatric Endocrinology

Midwest

Allen, David Bruce MD [PEn] - **Spec Exp:** Growth Disorders; Pubertal Disorders; **Hospital:** Univ WI Hosp & Clins; **Address:** 600 Highland Ave, H4/448 CSC-Pediatrics, Madison, WI 53792; **Phone:** 608-263-5835; **Board Cert:** Pediatrics 1986; Pediatric Endocrinology 2004; **Med School:** Duke Univ 1980; **Resid:** Pediatrics, Univ Wisc Hosp 1985; **Fellow:** Pediatric Endocrinology, Univ Wisc Hosp 1988; **Fac Appt:** Prof Ped, Univ Wisc

Eugster, Erica MD [PEn] - **Spec Exp:** Pubertal Disorders; Turner Syndrome; **Hospital:** Riley Hosp for Children; **Address:** Riley Chldns Hosp, 702 Barnhill Drive, rm 5960, Indianapolis, IN 46202; **Phone:** 317-274-3889; **Board Cert:** Pediatrics 2002; Pediatric Endocrinology 2005; **Med School:** Med Coll PA 1990; **Resid:** Pediatrics, Marshfield Clin-St Josephs Hosp 1994; **Fellow:** Pediatric Endocrinology, Univ Minn Hosp 1994; **Fac Appt:** Prof Ped, Indiana Univ

Gutai, James MD [PEn] - **Hospital:** Chldns Hosp of Michigan, Marquette Genl Hosp; **Address:** Morris J Hood Comp Diabetes Ctr, 4201 St Antoine St, Univ Hlth Ctr, Ste 9A-6, Detroit, MI 48201; **Phone:** 313-577-0133; **Board Cert:** Pediatrics 1977; Pediatric Endocrinology 1980; **Med School:** Temple Univ 1970; **Resid:** Pediatrics, Johns Hopkins Hosp 1976; **Fellow:** Pediatric Endocrinology, Johns Hopkins Hosp 1976; **Fac Appt:** Prof Ped, Wayne State Univ

Levy, Richard Alshuler MD [PEn] - **Spec Exp:** Growth Disorders; Pituitary Disorders; Thyroid Disorders; **Hospital:** Rush - Copley Med Ctr, Ingalls Meml Hosp; **Address:** 1725 W Harrison St, Ste 328, Chicago, IL 60612-3863; **Phone:** 312-942-8989; **Board Cert:** Internal Medicine 1976; Pediatrics 1983; Endocrinology 1985; Pediatric Endocrinology 1986; **Med School:** Louisiana State Univ 1971; **Resid:** Internal Medicine, Univ Mass Med Ctr 1977; Pediatrics, Beth Israel Hosp 1978; **Fellow:** Endocrinology, Diabetes & Metabolism, Barnes Hosp/Washington Univ 1982; **Fac Appt:** Asst Prof Ped, Rush Med Coll

Maurer, William MD [PEn] - **Spec Exp:** Growth Disorders; Thyroid Disorders; Diabetes; **Hospital:** OSF Saint Francis Med Ctr; **Address:** 320 E Armstrong Ave, Peoria, IL 61603; **Phone:** 309-624-9680; **Board Cert:** Pediatrics 1971; Pediatric Endocrinology 1978; **Med School:** Ohio State Univ 1966; **Resid:** Pediatrics, Columbus Chldns Hosp 1968; **Fellow:** Pediatric Endocrinology, Columbus Chldns Hosp 1970; Pediatric Endocrinology, Duke Univ Med Ctr 1975; **Fac Appt:** Asst Clin Prof Ped, Univ IL Coll Med at Peoria

Menon, Ram K MD [PEn] - **Spec Exp:** Growth/Development Disorders; Diabetes; **Hospital:** Univ Michigan Hlth Sys; **Address:** Univ Mich Med Ctr, D1205 Med Prof Bldg, 1500 E Medical Ctr Drive, Box 0718, Ann Arbor, MI 48109; **Phone:** 734-764-5175; **Board Cert:** Pediatrics 2002; Pediatric Endocrinology 2003; **Med School:** India 1979; **Resid:** Pediatrics, All India Inst of Medical Science 1984; **Fellow:** Pediatric Endocrinology, Children's Hosp 1989; **Fac Appt:** Assoc Prof Ped, Univ Mich Med Sch

Rogers, Douglas G MD [PEn] - **Spec Exp:** Diabetes; Growth/Development Disorders; Thyroid Disorders; **Hospital:** Cleveland Clin Fdn (page 57); **Address:** Div Pediatric Endocrinology, 9500 Euclid Ave, Box A120, Cleveland, OH 44195-0001; **Phone:** 216-445-8048; **Board Cert:** Pediatrics 1984; Pediatric Endocrinology 1986; **Med School:** Ros Franklin Univ/Chicago Med Sch 1978; **Resid:** Pediatrics, Cardinal Glennon Chldns Hosp 1981; **Fellow:** Endocrinology, Diabetes & Metabolism, St Louis Chldns Hosp 1985

Rosenfield, Robert L MD [PEn] - **Spec Exp:** Polycystic Ovarian Syndrome; Pubertal Disorders; Menstrual Disorders; **Hospital:** Univ of Chicago Hosps; **Address:** 5841 S Maryland Ave, MC 5053, Chicago, IL 60637-1463; **Phone:** 773-702-6169; **Board Cert:** Pediatrics 1986; Pediatric Endocrinology 1986; **Med School:** Northwestern Univ 1960; **Resid:** Pediatrics, Chldns Hosp 1963; **Fellow:** Pediatric Endocrinology, Chldns Hosp 1968; **Fac Appt:** Prof Ped, Univ Chicago-Pritzker Sch Med

White, Neil H MD [PEn] - **Spec Exp:** Diabetes; Hypoglycemia; **Hospital:** St Louis Chldns Hosp; **Address:** Washington University School of Medicine, 660 S Euclid Ave, Box 8208, St Louis, MO 63110-1010; **Phone:** 314-454-6051; **Board Cert:** Pediatrics 1981; Pediatric Endocrinology 1983; **Med School:** Albert Einstein Coll Med 1975; **Resid:** Pediatrics, St Louis Chldns Hosp 1977; **Fellow:** Endocrinology, Diabetes & Metabolism, Washington Univ 1979; **Fac Appt:** Prof Ped, Washington Univ, St Louis

Zimmerman, Donald MD [PEn] - **Spec Exp:** Growth Disorders in Childhood Cancer; Thyroid Cancer; Thyroid Disorders; Growth/Development Disorders; **Hospital:** Children's Mem Hosp; **Address:** Children's Memorial Hosp, 2300 Children's Plaza, Box 54, Chicago, IL 60614; **Phone:** 773-327-7740; **Board Cert:** Internal Medicine 1977; Endocrinology 1979; Pediatrics 1983; Pediatric Endocrinology 1983; **Med School:** Univ IL Coll Med 1974; **Resid:** Internal Medicine, Johns Hopkins Hosp 1977; Pediatrics, Mayo Grad Sch Med 1981; **Fellow:** Endocrinology, Diabetes & Metabolism, Mayo Grad Sch Med 1980; **Fac Appt:** Prof Ped, Northwestern Univ

Great Plains and Mountains

Foster, Carol M MD [PEn] - **Spec Exp:** Diabetes; Growth/Development Disorders; Pubertal Disorders; **Hospital:** Primary Children's Med Ctr, Univ Utah Hosps and Clins; **Address:** Utah Diabetes Ctr, 615 Arapeen Drive, Ste 100, Salt Lake City, UT 84108; **Phone:** 801-581-7761; **Board Cert:** Pediatrics 1983; Pediatric Endocrinology 1983; **Med School:** Washington Univ, St Louis 1978; **Resid:** Pediatrics, Univ Utah Hlth Scis Ctr 1981; **Fellow:** Pediatric Endocrinology, Natl Inst Hlth 1984; **Fac Appt:** Prof Med, Univ Utah

Kappy, Michael S MD/PhD [PEn] - **Spec Exp:** Growth/Development Disorders; Thyroid Disorders; Pubertal Disorders; **Hospital:** Chldn's Hosp - Denver, The; **Address:** Childrens Hosp, Dept Ped Endocrinology, 1056 E 19th Ave, Box B265, Denver, CO 80218; **Phone:** 303-861-6061; **Board Cert:** Pediatrics 1973; Pediatric Endocrinology 1980; **Med School:** Univ Wisc 1967; **Resid:** Pediatrics, Univ Colorado Med Ctr 1972; **Fellow:** Pediatric Endocrinology, Johns Hopkins Hosp 1980; **Fac Appt:** Prof Ped, Univ Colorado

Klingensmith, Georgeanna MD [PEn] - **Spec Exp:** Diabetes; **Hospital:** Chldn's Hosp - Denver, The; **Address:** Barbara Davis Ctr for Childhood Diabetes, MS B140, PO Box 6511, Aurora, CO 80045-0511; **Phone:** 303-724-2323; **Board Cert:** Pediatrics 1976; Pediatric Endocrinology 2000; **Med School:** Duke Univ 1971; **Resid:** Pediatrics, Childrens Hosp 1973; **Fellow:** Pediatric Endocrinology, Johns Hopkins Hosp 1976; Pediatric Endocrinology, Childrens Hosp 1974; **Fac Appt:** Prof Ped, Univ Colorado

Southwest

Kirkland III, John L MD [PEn] - **Spec Exp:** Growth/Development Disorders; Thyroid Disorders; **Hospital:** Texas Chldns Hosp - Houston; **Address:** Texas Chldns Hosp, Endo Clinic, 6621 Fannin St, Houston, TX 77030; **Phone:** 832-822-3670; **Board Cert:** Pediatrics 1973; Pediatric Endocrinology 1978; **Med School:** Univ NC Sch Med 1968; **Resid:** Pediatrics, Baylor 1970; Pediatrics, Guys Hosp 1970; **Fellow:** Pediatric Endocrinology, Baylor 1973; Molecular Endocrinology, Univ of Texas 1978; **Fac Appt:** Prof Ped, Baylor Coll Med

Pediatric Endocrinology

West Coast and Pacific

Geffner, Mitchell Eugene MD [PEn] - **Spec Exp:** Growth Disorders; Pubertal Disorders; Thyroid Disorders; **Hospital:** Chldns Hosp - Los Angeles (page 56); **Address:** Chlds Hosp LA, Div Endocrinology, 4650 Sunset Blvd, MS 61, Los Angeles, CA 90027; **Phone:** 323-669-7032; **Board Cert:** Pediatrics 1980; Pediatric Endocrinology 1983; **Med School:** Albert Einstein Coll Med 1975; **Resid:** Pediatrics, LAC-USC Med Ctr 1979; **Fellow:** Pediatric Endocrinology, UCLA Med Ctr 1982; **Fac Appt:** Prof Ped, USC Sch Med

Kaufman, Francine R MD [PEn] - **Spec Exp:** Diabetes; Growth/Development Disorders; **Hospital:** Chldns Hosp - Los Angeles (page 56), USC Univ Hosp - R K Eamer Med Plz; **Address:** Chldns Hosp, Div Endocrinology, 4650 W Sunset Blvd, MS 61, Los Angeles, CA 90027; **Phone:** 323-669-4606; **Board Cert:** Pediatrics 1980; Pediatric Endocrinology 1983; **Med School:** Ros Franklin Univ/Chicago Med Sch 1976; **Resid:** Pediatrics, Children's Hosp 1978; **Fellow:** Pediatric Endocrinology, Children's Hosp 1980; **Fac Appt:** Prof Ped, USC Sch Med

Wilson, Darrell M MD [PEn] - **Spec Exp:** Diabetes; Growth Disorders; **Hospital:** Stanford Univ Med Ctr; **Address:** Stanford Univ Med Ctr - Pediatrics, 300 Pasteur Rd, Ste G-313, MC 520, Stanford, CA 94305-5208; **Phone:** 650-723-5791; **Board Cert:** Pediatrics 1982; Pediatric Endocrinology 2003; **Med School:** UCSD 1977; **Resid:** Pediatrics, Stanford Univ Med Ctr 1980; **Fellow:** Endocrinology, Diabetes & Metabolism, Stanford Univ Med Ctr 1984; **Fac Appt:** Prof Ped, Stanford Univ

Pediatric Gastroenterology

New England

Kleinman, Ronald E MD [PGe] - **Spec Exp:** Transplant Medicine-Liver; Nutrition; **Hospital:** Mass Genl Hosp, N Shore Children's Hosp; **Address:** Mass Genl Hosp, Div Ped GI/Nutrition, 55 Fruit St, VBK 107, Boston, MA 02114; **Phone:** 617-726-8705; **Board Cert:** Pediatrics 1992; Pediatric Gastroenterology 2005; **Med School:** NY Med Coll 1972; **Resid:** Pediatrics, Albert Einstein Coll Med 1977; **Fellow:** Pediatric Gastroenterology, Mass Genl Hosp 1980; **Fac Appt:** Prof Ped, Harvard Med Sch

Mid Atlantic

Baker Jr, Robert D MD/PhD [PGe] - **Spec Exp:** Gastroesophageal Reflux Disease (GERD); Cystic Fibrosis; Nutrition; **Hospital:** Women's & Chldn's Hosp of Buffalo, The; **Address:** Children's Hospital, Div Gastroenterology, 219 Bryant St, Buffalo, NY 14222-2006; **Phone:** 716-878-7793; **Board Cert:** Pediatrics 1978; Pediatric Gastroenterology 2005; **Med School:** Temple Univ 1972; **Resid:** Pediatrics, Buffalo Chldns Hosp 1975; **Fellow:** Gastroenterology, Mass Genl Hosp/Chldns Hosp Med Ctr 1983; Nutritional Biochemistry, MIT 1984; **Fac Appt:** Prof Ped, SUNY Buffalo

Baker, Susan S MD/PhD [PGe] - **Spec Exp:** Nutrition; Obesity; Liver Disease; **Hospital:** Women's & Chldn's Hosp of Buffalo, The; **Address:** Childrens Hospital, Dept Pediatrics, 219 Bryant St, Buffalo, NY 14201-2099; **Phone:** 716-878-7793; **Board Cert:** Pediatrics 1978; Pediatric Gastroenterology 2004; **Med School:** Temple Univ 1972; **Resid:** Pediatrics, Buffalo Chldns Hosp 1975; **Fellow:** Nutrition, MIT 1981; Gastroenterology, Mass Genl Hosp 1984; **Fac Appt:** Prof Ped, SUNY Buffalo

Baldassano, Robert N MD [PGe] - **Spec Exp:** Inflammatory Bowel Disease; Ulcerative Colitis; Crohn's Disease; **Hospital:** Chldns Hosp of Philadelphia, The; **Address:** Chldns Hosp of Philadelphia, GI/Nutrition, 324 S 34th St, Philadelphia, PA 19104-4399; **Phone:** 215-590-3630; **Board Cert:** Pediatrics 1989; Pediatric Gastroenterology 2000; **Med School:** SUNY Downstate 1984; **Resid:** Pediatrics, Childrens Hosp 1988; **Fellow:** Pediatric Gastroenterology, Childrens Hosp 1991; **Fac Appt:** Assoc Prof Ped, Univ Pennsylvania

Benkov, Keith J MD [PGe] - **Spec Exp:** Inflammatory Bowel Disease/Crohn's; Liver Disease; Celiac Disease; **Hospital:** Mount Sinai Med Ctr, Englewood Hosp & Med Ctr; **Address:** 5 E 98th St, Box 1656, New York, NY 10029; **Phone:** 212-241-5415; **Board Cert:** Pediatrics 1984; Pediatric Gastroenterology 1998; **Med School:** Mount Sinai Sch Med 1979; **Resid:** Pediatrics, Mount Sinai Hosp 1982; **Fellow:** Pediatric Gastroenterology, Mount Sinai Hosp 1984; **Fac Appt:** Assoc Prof Ped, Mount Sinai Sch Med

Fasano, Alessio MD [PGe] - **Spec Exp:** Celiac Disease; Diarrheal Diseases; Nutrition; **Hospital:** Univ of MD Med Sys; **Address:** 20 Penn St, rm 351, Baltimore, MD 21201; **Phone:** 410-706-5501; **Med School:** Italy ; **Resid:** Pediatrics, Univ Naples; **Fellow:** Univ Naples; **Fac Appt:** Prof Ped, Univ MD Sch Med

Hillemeier, A Craig MD [PGe] - **Spec Exp:** Gastroesophageal Reflux Disease (GERD); Inflammatory Bowel Disease/Crohn's; **Hospital:** Penn State Milton S Hershey Med Ctr, Penn State Chldns Hosp; **Address:** Hershey Med Ctr, Dept Ped, 500 University Drive, MC H085, Hershey, PA 17033-0850; **Phone:** 717-531-6700; **Board Cert:** Pediatrics 1981; Pediatric Gastroenterology 1998; **Med School:** Loyola Univ-Stritch Sch Med 1976; **Resid:** Pediatrics, Loyola Univ Stritch 1978; **Fellow:** Pediatric Gastroenterology, Yale New Haven Med Ctr 1982; **Fac Appt:** Prof Ped, Penn State Univ-Hershey Med Ctr

Levy, Joseph MD [PGe] - **Spec Exp:** Celiac Disease; Irritable Bowel Syndrome; Gastroesophageal Reflux Disease (GERD); Nutrition in Autism; **Hospital:** NYU Med Ctr (page 67); **Address:** 160 E 32nd St, Fl 2, New York, NY 10016; **Phone:** 212-263-5407; **Board Cert:** Pediatrics 1979; Pediatric Gastroenterology 1990; **Med School:** Israel 1973; **Resid:** Pediatrics, Beth Israel Med Ctr 1977; **Fellow:** Research, Columbia-Presby Med Ctr 1975; Pediatric Gastroenterology, Columbia-Presby Med Ctr 1979; **Fac Appt:** Prof Ped, Columbia P&S

Newman, Leonard MD [PGe] - **Spec Exp:** Inflammatory Bowel Disease; Celiac Disease; **Hospital:** Westchester Med Ctr, Our Lady of Mercy Med Ctr; **Address:** NY Med College, Dept Ped, Munger Pavillion - rm 123, Valhalla, NY 10595; **Phone:** 914-594-4610; **Board Cert:** Pediatrics 1975; Pediatric Gastroenterology 1990; **Med School:** NY Med Coll 1970; **Resid:** Pediatrics, UCSD Med Ctr 1972; Pediatrics, NY Med Coll 1973; **Fellow:** Gastroenterology, Bronx Lebanon Hosp/Einstein 1974; **Fac Appt:** Prof Ped, NY Med Coll

Oliva-Hemker, Maria M MD [PGe] - **Spec Exp:** Inflammatory Bowel Disease/Crohn's; Ulcerative Colitis; Malabsorption Syndrome; **Hospital:** Johns Hopkins Hosp - Baltimore (page 61); **Address:** Johns Hopkins Hosp, Ped GI & Nutrition, 600 N Wolfe St, Brady 320, Baltimore, MD 21287-2631; **Phone:** 410-955-8765; **Board Cert:** Pediatrics 2000; Pediatric Gastroenterology 2000; **Med School:** Johns Hopkins Univ 1986; **Resid:** Pediatrics, Johns Hopkins Hosp 1989; **Fellow:** Gastroenterology, Johns Hopkins Hosp 1992; **Fac Appt:** Assoc Prof Ped, Johns Hopkins Univ

Piccoli, David A MD [PGe] - **Spec Exp:** Liver Disease; Inflammatory Bowel Disease; **Hospital:** Chldns Hosp of Philadelphia, The; **Address:** Chlds Hosp of Philadelphia, Div Gastroenterology/Nutrition, 34th St and Civic Ctr Blvd, Ste 9S20C, Philadelphia, PA 19104; **Phone:** 215-590-1678; **Board Cert:** Pediatrics 1984; Pediatric Gastroenterology 2005; **Med School:** Harvard Med Sch 1979; **Resid:** Pediatrics, Chldns Hosp Med Ctr 1983; **Fellow:** Gastroenterology, Chldns Hosp 1986; **Fac Appt:** Prof Ped, Univ Pennsylvania

Pediatric Gastroenterology

Schwarz, Kathleen B MD [PGe] - **Spec Exp:** Hepatitis B & C; Transplant Medicine-Liver; Liver Disease; **Hospital:** Johns Hopkins Hosp - Baltimore (page 61); **Address:** Johns Hopkins Pediatric GI, 600 N Wolfe St, Brady 320, Baltimore, MD 21287-0005; **Phone:** 410-955-8769; **Board Cert:** Pediatrics 1977; Pediatric Gastroenterology 2005; **Med School:** Washington Univ, St Louis 1972; **Resid:** Pediatrics, St Louis Chldns Hosp 1974; **Fellow:** Pediatric Gastroenterology, St Louis Chldns Hosp 1976; **Fac Appt:** Prof Ped, Johns Hopkins Univ

Schwarz, Steven M MD [PGe] - **Spec Exp:** Gastroesophageal Reflux Disease (GERD); Nutrition; Endoscopy; **Hospital:** Long Island Coll Hosp, Beth Israel Med Ctr - Petrie Division; **Address:** LI Coll Hosp - Dept of Pediatrics, 339 Hicks St, Brooklyn, NY 11201-5514; **Phone:** 718-780-1146; **Board Cert:** Pediatrics 1979; Pediatric Gastroenterology 1998; **Med School:** Columbia P&S 1974; **Resid:** Pediatrics, Columbia-Presby Med Ctr 1977; **Fellow:** Pediatric Gastroenterology, Stanford Univ Med Ctr 1978; Pediatric Gastroenterology, Columbia-Presby Med Ctr 1980; **Fac Appt:** Prof Ped, SUNY Downstate

Spivak, William MD [PGe] - **Spec Exp:** Inflammatory Bowel Disease/Crohn's; Ulcerative Colitis; Gastroesophageal Reflux Disease (GERD); **Hospital:** Lenox Hill Hosp (page 62); **Address:** 177 E 87th St, Ste 305, New York, NY 10128; **Phone:** 212-369-7700; **Board Cert:** Pediatrics 1981; Pediatric Gastroenterology 2005; **Med School:** Albert Einstein Coll Med 1976; **Resid:** Pediatrics, Jacobi Med Ctr 1979; **Fellow:** Gastroenterology, Childrens Hosp 1982; Research, Brigham & Womens Hosp 1982; **Fac Appt:** Clin Prof Ped, Cornell Univ-Weill Med Coll

Squires, Robert H MD [PGe] - **Spec Exp:** Liver Disease; **Hospital:** Chldns Hosp of Pittsburgh - UPMC; **Address:** Children's Hosp Pittsburgh, Gastroenterology, 3705 Fifth Ave, Pittsburgh, PA 15213; **Phone:** 412-692-5180; **Board Cert:** Pediatrics 1981; Pediatric Gastroenterology 2005; **Med School:** Univ Tex Med Br, Galveston 1977; **Resid:** Pediatrics, Children's Hosp 1979; **Fellow:** Pediatric Gastroenterology, Children's Hosp 1982; **Fac Appt:** Prof Ped, Univ Pittsburgh

Suchy, Frederick J MD [PGe] - **Spec Exp:** Hepatitis; Liver Disease; **Hospital:** Mount Sinai Med Ctr; **Address:** Mount Sinai Medical Ctr, 1 Gustave Levy Pl, Box 1198, New York, NY 10029; **Phone:** 212-241-6933; **Board Cert:** Pediatrics 1982; Pediatric Gastroenterology 2004; **Med School:** Univ Cincinnati 1974; **Resid:** Pediatrics, Chidren's Hosp Med Ctr 1978; **Fellow:** Pediatric Gastroenterology, Chidren's Hosp Med Ctr 1981; **Fac Appt:** Prof Ped, Mount Sinai Sch Med

Treem, William R MD [PGe] - **Spec Exp:** Liver Disease; Inflammatory Bowel Disease; Celiac Disease; **Hospital:** SUNY Downstate Med Ctr, Long Island Coll Hosp; **Address:** SUNY Downstate Med Ctr, Dept Peds, 445 Lennox Rd, Box 49, Brooklyn, NY 11203; **Phone:** 718-270-4714; **Board Cert:** Pediatrics 1982; Pediatric Gastroenterology 2005; **Med School:** Stanford Univ 1977; **Resid:** Pediatrics, Children's Hosp 1980; **Fellow:** Pediatric Gastroenterology, Univ Penn Hosp 1985; **Fac Appt:** Prof Ped, SUNY Downstate

Southeast

Hill, Ivor D MD [PGe] - **Spec Exp:** Celiac Disease; Inflammatory Bowel Disease; Diarrheal Diseases; **Hospital:** Wake Forest Univ Baptist Med Ctr (page 73); **Address:** Wake Forest Univ Sch Med, Div Ped Gastro, Medical Center Blvd, Winston Salem, NC 27157; **Phone:** 336-716-3009; **Board Cert:** Pediatrics 2000; Pediatric Gastroenterology 2003; **Med School:** South Africa 1972; **Resid:** Pediatrics, Addington Hosp 1976; Pediatrics, Red Cross Chldns Hosp 1977; **Fellow:** Pediatric Gastroenterology, Red Cross Chlds Hosp 1980; **Fac Appt:** Prof Ped, Wake Forest Univ

Novak, Donald A MD [PGe] - **Spec Exp:** Liver Disease; **Hospital:** Shands Hlthcre at Univ of FL; **Address:** Shands @ Univ Florida, Div Ped Gastro, 1600 SW Archer Rd, Box 100296, Gainesville, FL 32610-0296; **Phone:** 352-392-6410; **Board Cert:** Pediatrics 1987; Pediatric Gastroenterology 1990; **Med School:** Univ S Fla Coll Med 1981; **Resid:** Pediatrics, Univ South Fla 1984; **Fellow:** Pediatric Gastroenterology, Childrens Hosp 1987; **Fac Appt:** Prof Ped, Univ Fla Coll Med

Thompson, John F MD [PGe] - **Spec Exp:** Inflammatory Bowel Disease/Crohn's; Short Bowel Syndrome; Transplant Medicine-Intestine; **Hospital:** Jackson Meml Hosp, Baptist Hosp of Miami; **Address:** Jackson Meml Hospital, Dept Pediatrics, Div GI & Nutrition, 1601 NW 12th Ave, rm 3005A, MC D820, Miami, FL 33136; **Phone:** 305-243-6426; **Board Cert:** Pediatrics 1983; Pediatric Gastroenterology 2005; **Med School:** Loyola Univ-Stritch Sch Med 1977; **Resid:** Pediatrics, Wylers Chldns Hosp-Univ Chicago 1980; **Fellow:** Pediatric Gastroenterology, Babies Hosp-Columbia Univ 1985; **Fac Appt:** Prof Ped, Univ Miami Sch Med

Ulshen, Martin H MD [PGe] - **Spec Exp:** Intestinal Disorders; Liver Disease; Inflammatory Bowel Disease; **Hospital:** Duke Univ Med Ctr; **Address:** Duke Univ Med Ctr, Box 3009, Durham, NC 27710; **Phone:** 919-684-5068; **Board Cert:** Pediatrics 1993; Pediatric Gastroenterology 2005; **Med School:** Univ Rochester 1969; **Resid:** Pediatrics, Univ North Carolina Hosps 1970; Pediatrics, Univ Colorado 1974; **Fellow:** Pediatric Gastroenterology, Univ Colorado 1975; Pediatric Gastroenterology, Chldns Hosp 1977; **Fac Appt:** Prof Ped, Duke Univ

Midwest

Berman, James MD [PGe] - **Spec Exp:** Inflammatory Bowel Disease/Crohn's; Nutrition; Ulcerative Colitis; **Hospital:** Loyola Univ Med Ctr, Adv Luth Genl Hosp; **Address:** Loyola Univ Med Ctr, Dept Ped Gastro, 2160 S 1st Ave Bldg 105 - rm 3346, Maywood, IL 60153-3304; **Phone:** 708-327-9073; **Board Cert:** Pediatrics 1986; Pediatric Gastroenterology 2005; **Med School:** Univ Pittsburgh 1981; **Resid:** Pediatrics, Chldns Hosp 1984; **Fellow:** Pediatric Gastroenterology, Mass Genl Hosp/Chldns Hosp 1987; **Fac Appt:** Asst Prof Ped, Loyola Univ-Stritch Sch Med

Cohen, Mitchell B MD [PGe] - **Spec Exp:** Inflammatory Bowel Disease; Diarrheal Diseases; Celiac Disease; **Hospital:** Cincinnati Chldns Hosp Med Ctr; **Address:** Chldns Hosp Med Ctr, Div Gastroenterology, 3333 Burnet Ave, rm 4210, MS 2010, Cincinnati, OH 45229-3026; **Phone:** 513-636-4415; **Board Cert:** Pediatrics 1981; Pediatric Gastroenterology 2005; **Med School:** Mount Sinai Sch Med 1977; **Resid:** Pediatrics, Johns Hopkins Hosp 1980; **Fellow:** Pediatric Gastroenterology, Chldns Hosp Med Ctr 1986; **Fac Appt:** Prof Ped, Univ Cincinnati

El-Youssef, Mounif MD [PGe] - **Spec Exp:** Liver Disease; **Hospital:** Mayo Med Ctr & Clin - Rochester; **Address:** Mayo Clinic, Div Ped Gastroenterology, 200 First St SW, Rochester, MN 55905; **Phone:** 507-284-2141; **Board Cert:** Pediatrics 1998; Pediatric Gastroenterology 1998; **Med School:** Belgium 1982; **Resid:** Pediatrics, Cleveland Clinic 1987; **Fellow:** Pediatric Gastroenterology, Harvard Med Sch 1990

Gunasekaran, T S MD [PGe] - **Spec Exp:** Gastroesophageal Reflux Disease (GERD); Esophageal Disorders; Inflammatory Bowel Disease; Pain-Abdominal Recurrent; **Hospital:** Adv Luth Genl Hosp, Loyola Univ Med Ctr; **Address:** Lutheran Genl Chldns Hosp, Dept Ped GI, 1675 Dempster St, Park Ridge, IL 60068; **Phone:** 847-723-7700; **Board Cert:** Pediatrics 2000; Pediatric Gastroenterology 2000; **Med School:** India 1977; **Resid:** Pediatrics 1982; Pediatrics 1987; **Fellow:** Pediatric Gastroenterology, BC Childrens Hosp 1992; **Fac Appt:** Assoc Clin Prof Ped, Loyola Univ-Stritch Sch Med

Pediatric Gastroenterology

Kirschner, Barbara S MD [PGe] - **Spec Exp:** Ulcerative Colitis; Pain-Abdominal Recurrent; Inflammatory Bowel Disease/Crohn's; **Hospital:** Univ of Chicago Hosps; **Address:** Univ Chicago Comer Childrens Hosp, 5839 S Maryland Ave, Ste C-474, MC 4085, Chicago, IL 60637; **Phone:** 773-702-6418; **Board Cert:** Pediatrics 1972; Pediatric Gastroenterology 2004; **Med School:** Med Coll PA Hahnemann 1967; **Resid:** Pediatrics, Univ Chicago Hosps 1970; **Fellow:** Pediatric Gastroenterology, Univ Chicago 1977; **Fac Appt:** Prof Ped, Univ Chicago-Pritzker Sch Med

Molleston, Jean P MD [PGe] - **Spec Exp:** Liver Disease; Inflammatory Bowel Disease/Crohn's; Intestinal Disorders; **Hospital:** Riley Hosp for Children; **Address:** Indiana Univ-Riley Chldns Hosp, Div Ped Gastroenterology, 702 Barnhill Drive, rm ROC 4210, Indianapolis, IN 46202-5225; **Phone:** 317-274-3774; **Board Cert:** Pediatric Gastroenterology 2003; **Med School:** Washington Univ, St Louis 1986; **Resid:** Pediatrics, Chldns Hosp 1988; **Fellow:** Pediatric Gastroenterology, Washington Univ Med Ctr 1991; **Fac Appt:** Assoc Clin Prof Ped, Indiana Univ

Rothbaum, Robert J MD [PGe] - **Spec Exp:** Inflammatory Bowel Disease; **Hospital:** St Louis Chldns Hosp, Barnes-Jewish Hosp; **Address:** 1 Children's Pl, Ste 11E10, St Louis, MO 63110; **Phone:** 314-454-6173; **Board Cert:** Pediatrics 1981; Pediatric Gastroenterology 2004; **Med School:** Univ Chicago-Pritzker Sch Med 1976; **Resid:** Pediatrics, St Louis Chldns Hosp 1978; **Fellow:** Ambulatory Pediatrics, St Louis Chldns Hosp 1979; Pediatric Gastroenterology, Chldns Hosp Med Ctr 1982; **Fac Appt:** Prof Ped, Washington Univ, St Louis

Rudolph, Colin D MD [PGe] - **Spec Exp:** Feeding Disorders; Nutrition; Gastrointestinal Motility Disorders; Gastrointestinal Functional Disorders; **Hospital:** Chldns Hosp - Wisconsin; **Address:** Children's Hospital of Wisconsin, 9000 W Wisconsin Ave, Ste 604, Milwaukee, WI 53226; **Phone:** 414-266-3690; **Board Cert:** Pediatrics 1987; Pediatric Gastroenterology 2005; **Med School:** Case West Res Univ 1982; **Resid:** Pediatrics, Children's Hosp 1984; **Fellow:** Pediatric Gastroenterology, UCSF Med Ctr 1986; **Fac Appt:** Assoc Prof Ped, Univ Wisc

Whitington, Peter F MD [PGe] - **Spec Exp:** Transplant Medicine-Liver; Liver Disease; **Hospital:** Children's Mem Hosp; **Address:** Chldns Meml Hosp, Div Ped Gastro, 2300 Children's Plaza, Box 57, Chicago, IL 60614; **Phone:** 773-880-4643; **Board Cert:** Pediatrics 1977; Pediatric Gastroenterology 2005; **Med School:** Univ Tenn Coll Med, Memphis 1971; **Resid:** Pediatrics, Univ Tenn Hosp 1975; **Fellow:** Gastroenterology, Johns Hopkins Hosp 1977; Gastroenterology, Univ Wisconsin 1978; **Fac Appt:** Prof Ped, Northwestern Univ

Wyllie, Robert MD [PGe] - **Spec Exp:** Inflammatory Bowel Disease/Crohn's; Esophageal Disorders; **Hospital:** Cleveland Clin Fdn (page 57); **Address:** Cleveland Clinic, Dept Peds Gastro, 9500 Euclid Ave, Desk A111, Cleveland, OH 44195; **Phone:** 216-444-2237; **Board Cert:** Pediatrics 1982; Pediatric Gastroenterology 1997; **Med School:** Indiana Univ 1976; **Resid:** Pediatrics, Indiana Univ Med Ctr 1979; **Fellow:** Pediatric Gastroenterology, Indiana Univ Med Ctr 1980

Great Plains and Mountains

Hoffenberg, Edward J MD [PGe] - **Spec Exp:** Inflammatory Bowel Disease/Crohn's; Celiac Disease; **Hospital:** Chldn's Hosp - Denver, The, Univ Colorado Hosp; **Address:** Chldns Hosp, Div Gastroenterology, 1056 E 19th Ave, Box 290, Denver, CO 80218; **Phone:** 303-861-6669; **Board Cert:** Pediatrics 1989; Pediatric Gastroenterology 2000; **Med School:** Case West Res Univ ; **Resid:** Pediatrics, Rainbow Babies & Chldns Hosp; **Fellow:** Pediatric Gastroenterology, Chldns Hosp; **Fac Appt:** Assoc Prof Ped, Univ Colorado

Krebs, Nancy F MD [PGe] - **Spec Exp:** Obesity; Nutrition; **Hospital:** Chldn's Hosp - Denver, The; **Address:** Children's Hospital, Health Ctr, 1056 E 19th Ave Fl 1, Denver, CO 80218; **Phone:** 303-837-2571; **Board Cert:** Pediatrics 1999; Pediatric Gastroenterology 2003; **Med School:** Univ Colorado 1987; **Resid:** Pediatrics, Univ Colorado Health Sci Ctr 1990; **Fellow:** Pediatric Gastroenterology, Univ Colorado Health Sci Ctr 1992; Nutrition, Univ Colorado Health Sci Ctr 1993; **Fac Appt:** Prof Ped, Univ Colorado

Vanderhoof, Jon Arvid MD [PGe] - **Spec Exp:** Nutrition; Short Bowel Syndrome; Probiotics; **Hospital:** Nebraska Med Ctr, Children's Hosp - Omaha; **Address:** Univ Nebraska Med Ctr, 985160 Nebraska Med Ctr, Omaha, NE 68198-5160; **Phone:** 402-559-2412; **Board Cert:** Pediatrics 1993; Pediatric Gastroenterology 1998; **Med School:** Univ Nebr Coll Med 1972; **Resid:** Pediatrics, Univ Nebr Coll Med 1974; **Fellow:** Pediatric Gastroenterology, UCLA Med Ctr 1976; **Fac Appt:** Prof Ped, Univ Nebr Coll Med

Southwest

Klish, William John MD [PGe] - **Hospital:** Texas Chldns Hosp - Houston; **Address:** 6701 Fannin St, MC CCC 1010, Houston, TX 77030-2303; **Phone:** 832-822-3131; **Board Cert:** Pediatrics 1992; Pediatric Gastroenterology 1998; **Med School:** Univ Wisc 1967; **Resid:** Pediatrics, Baylor Coll Med 1972; **Fellow:** Nutrition, Baylor Coll Med 1974; **Fac Appt:** Prof Ped, Baylor Coll Med

Rhoads, J Marc MD [PGe] - **Spec Exp:** Diarrheal Diseases; Inflammatory Bowel Disease; Intestinal Disorders; **Hospital:** Meml Hermann Hosp - Houston; **Address:** Univ Texas Hlth Sci Ctr, Dept Pediatrics-Gastroenterology, 6431 Fannin, MSB 3.137, Houston, TX 77030; **Phone:** 832-325-6516; **Board Cert:** Pediatrics 1986; Pediatric Gastroenterology 2005; **Med School:** Johns Hopkins Univ 1980; **Resid:** Pediatrics, UCLA Med Ctr 1983; **Fellow:** Pediatric Gastroenterology, Hosp for Sick Children 1986; **Fac Appt:** Prof Ped, Univ Tex, Houston

West Coast and Pacific

Christie, Dennis L MD [PGe] - **Hospital:** Chldns Hosp and Regl Med Ctr - Seattle; **Address:** Chldns Hosp Med Ctr, Div Gastroenterology, 4800 Sand Point Way NE, Box A-5950, Seattle, WA 98105-3901; **Phone:** 206-987-2521; **Board Cert:** Pediatrics 1992; Pediatric Gastroenterology 2005; **Med School:** Northwestern Univ 1968; **Resid:** Pediatrics, Univ Wash Med Ctr 1971; **Fellow:** Pediatric Gastroenterology, UCLA Ctr Hlth Sci 1976; **Fac Appt:** Prof Ped, Univ Wash

Heyman, Melvin Bernard MD [PGe] - **Spec Exp:** Inflammatory Bowel Disease/Crohn's; Short Bowel Syndrome; Gastroesophageal Reflux Disease (GERD); **Hospital:** UCSF Med Ctr; **Address:** UCSF, Dept Ped Gastroenterology, 500 Parnassus Ave, Box 0136, San Francisco, CA 94143-0136; **Phone:** 415-476-5892; **Board Cert:** Pediatrics 1981; Pediatric Gastroenterology 2005; **Med School:** UCLA 1976; **Resid:** Pediatrics, LAC-USC Med Ctr 1979; **Fellow:** Gastroenterology, UCLA Med Ctr 1981; Nutrition, Human Nutrition Res Ctr 1990; **Fac Appt:** Prof Ped, UCSF

McDiarmid, Suzanne V MD [PGe] - **Spec Exp:** Transplant Medicine-Liver; Transplant Medicine-Intestine; Transplant Immunology; **Hospital:** UCLA Med Ctr; **Address:** UCLA Med Ctr, 200 Medical Plaza, Ste 265, Los Angeles, CA 90095; **Phone:** 310-206-6134; **Board Cert:** Pediatrics 1984; Pediatric Gastroenterology 2000; **Med School:** New Zealand 1976; **Resid:** Pediatrics, UCLA Med Center 1980; **Fac Appt:** Prof Ped, UCLA

Pediatric Gastroenterology

Sinatra, Frank R MD [PGe] - **Spec Exp:** Liver Disease; **Hospital:** Women & Children's Hosp - LA, Chldns Hosp - Los Angeles (page 56); **Address:** Women's & Children's Hospital, 1240 N Mission Rd, rm L902, Los Angeles, CA 90033; **Phone:** 323-226-3691; **Board Cert:** Pediatrics 1992; Pediatric Gastroenterology 2005; **Med School:** USC Sch Med 1971; **Resid:** Pediatrics, Children's Hosp 1974; **Fellow:** Gastroenterology, Stanford Univ Med Ctr 1976; **Fac Appt:** Prof Ped, USC Sch Med

Pediatric Hematology-Oncology

New England

Fisher, David E MD/PhD [PHO] - **Spec Exp:** Melanoma; **Hospital:** Dana-Farber Cancer Inst; **Address:** Dana-Faber Cancer Inst, Dana 630, 44 Binney St, Boston, MA 02115; **Phone:** 617-632-4916; **Board Cert:** Internal Medicine 1989; Medical Oncology 1991; **Med School:** Cornell Univ-Weill Med Coll 1985; **Resid:** Internal Medicine, Mass Genl Hosp 1988; **Fellow:** Pediatric Hematology-Oncology, Dana-Faber CAncer Inst 1992; **Fac Appt:** Prof Ped, Harvard Med Sch

Grier, Holcombe E MD [PHO] - **Spec Exp:** Bone Cancer; Ewing's Sarcoma; **Hospital:** Dana-Farber Cancer Inst, Children's Hospital - Boston; **Address:** Dana Farber Cancer Inst, 44 Binney St, G350, Boston, MA 02115; **Phone:** 617-632-3971; **Board Cert:** Pediatrics 1983; Internal Medicine 1980; Pediatric Hematology-Oncology 1998; **Med School:** Univ Pennsylvania 1976; **Resid:** Pediatrics, NC Meml Hosp 1980; Internal Medicine, NC Meml Hosp 1980; **Fellow:** Pediatric Oncology, Dana Farber Children's Hosp 1984; **Fac Appt:** Assoc Prof Ped, Harvard Med Sch

Israel, Mark A MD [PHO] - **Spec Exp:** Neuro-Oncology; Brain Tumors; Neuroblastoma; **Hospital:** Dartmouth - Hitchcock Med Ctr; **Address:** Norris Cotton Cancer Ctr, One Medical Center Drive, Lebanon, NH 03756; **Phone:** 603-653-3611; **Board Cert:** Pediatrics 1982; **Med School:** Albert Einstein Coll Med 1973; **Resid:** Pediatrics, Chldns Hosp Med Ctr 1975; **Fellow:** Pediatric Hematology-Oncology, Natl Cancer Inst 1981; **Fac Appt:** Prof Ped, Dartmouth Med Sch

Kieran, Mark MD/PhD [PHO] - **Spec Exp:** Brain Tumors; **Hospital:** Children's Hospital - Boston, Dana-Farber Cancer Inst; **Address:** Dana Farber Cancer Inst, 44 Binney St, Shields Warren Ste 331, Boston, MA 02115; **Phone:** 617-632-2680; **Board Cert:** Pediatrics 2000; Pediatric Hematology-Oncology 1996; **Med School:** Canada 1986; **Resid:** Pediatrics, Montreal Chldns Hosp 1992; **Fellow:** Pediatric Hematology-Oncology, Chldns Hosp 1995; **Fac Appt:** Asst Prof Ped, Harvard Med Sch

Schwartz, Cindy Lee MD [PHO] - **Spec Exp:** Hodgkin's Disease; Bone Cancer; Cancer Survivors-Late Effects of Therapy; **Hospital:** Rhode Island Hosp; **Address:** RI Hospital, Dept Ped-Div Ped Hem/Onc, 593 Eddy St, MPS, rm 117, Providence, RI 02903-4923; **Phone:** 401-444-5171; **Board Cert:** Pediatrics 1985; Pediatric Hematology-Oncology 2002; **Med School:** Brown Univ 1979; **Resid:** Pediatrics, Johns Hopkins Hosp 1982; **Fellow:** Pediatric Hematology-Oncology, Johns Hopkins Hosp 1985; **Fac Appt:** Prof Med, Brown Univ

Weinstein, Howard J MD [PHO] - **Spec Exp:** Bone Marrow Transplant; Leukemia; Lymphoma; **Hospital:** Mass Genl Hosp; **Address:** 55 Fruit St, Yawkey 8B-8893, Boston, MA 02114-2622; **Phone:** 617-724-3315; **Board Cert:** Pediatrics 1977; **Med School:** Univ MD Sch Med 1972; **Resid:** Pediatrics, Mass Genl Hosp 1974; **Fellow:** Pediatric Hematology-Oncology, Dana Farber Cancer Inst/Chldns Hosp 1977; **Fac Appt:** Prof Ped, Harvard Med Sch

Mid Atlantic

Adamson, Peter C MD [PHO] - **Spec Exp:** Drug Development; Clinical Trials; Rhabdomyosarcoma; Pediatric Cancers; **Hospital:** Chldns Hosp of Philadelphia, The; **Address:** Chldns Hosp of Philadelphia, 34th St & Civic Ctr Blvd Abramson Bldg, Philadelphia, PA 19104; **Phone:** 215-590-2299; **Board Cert:** Pediatrics 1988; Pediatric Hematology-Oncology 2005; **Med School:** Cornell Univ-Weill Med Coll 1984; **Resid:** Pediatrics, Children's Hosp 1987; **Fellow:** Pediatric Hematology-Oncology, Natl Cancer Inst 1990; **Fac Appt:** Assoc Prof Pharm, Univ Pennsylvania

Arceci, Robert J MD/PhD [PHO] - **Spec Exp:** Leukemia; Histiocytoma; Bone Marrow Transplant; **Hospital:** Johns Hopkins Hosp - Baltimore (page 61); **Address:** Kimmel Cancer Ctr, Bunting-Blaustein Bldg, 1650 Orleans St, CRB 2M51, Baltimore, MD 21231-1000; **Phone:** 410-502-7519; **Board Cert:** Pediatrics 1987; Pediatric Hematology-Oncology 2005; **Med School:** Univ Rochester 1981; **Resid:** Pediatrics, Chldns Hosp 1983; **Fellow:** Pediatric Hematology-Oncology, Chldns Hosp/Dana Farber Cancer Ctr 1986; **Fac Appt:** Prof Ped, Johns Hopkins Univ

Brecher, Martin L MD [PHO] - **Spec Exp:** Brain Tumors; Lymphoma; Hodgkin's Disease; Leukemia; **Hospital:** Roswell Park Cancer Inst, Women's & Chldn's Hosp of Buffalo, The; **Address:** Roswell Park Cancer Inst, Dept Pediatrics, Elm & Carlton Sts, Buffalo, NY 14263; **Phone:** 716-845-2333; **Board Cert:** Pediatrics 1977; Pediatric Hematology-Oncology 1978; **Med School:** SUNY Buffalo 1972; **Resid:** Pediatrics, Buffalo Chldns Hosp 1975; **Fellow:** Hematology & Oncology, Buffalo Chldns Hosp/Roswell Park Cancer Inst 1977; **Fac Appt:** Prof Ped, SUNY Buffalo

Brodeur, Garrett MD [PHO] - **Spec Exp:** Neuroblastoma; **Hospital:** Chldns Hosp of Philadelphia, The; **Address:** Chldns Hosp Philadelphia, 34th St & Civic Ctr Blvd Abramson Bldg, Philadelphia, PA 19104; **Phone:** 215-590-2817; **Board Cert:** Pediatrics 1980; Pediatric Hematology-Oncology 1980; **Med School:** Washington Univ, St Louis 1975; **Resid:** Pediatrics, St Louis Childrens Hosp 1977; **Fellow:** Pediatric Hematology-Oncology, St Jude Childrens Rsch Hosp 1979; **Fac Appt:** Prof Ped, Univ Pennsylvania

Bussel, James MD [PHO] - **Spec Exp:** Autoimmune Disease; Bleeding/Coagulation Disorders; **Hospital:** NY-Presby Hosp/Weill Cornell (page 66), Lenox Hill Hosp (page 62); **Address:** 525 E 68th St, rm P-695, New York, NY 10021; **Phone:** 212-746-3474; **Board Cert:** Pediatrics 1979; Pediatric Hematology-Oncology 1981; **Med School:** Columbia P&S 1975; **Resid:** Pediatrics, Chldns Hosp 1978; **Fellow:** Pediatric Hematology-Oncology, NY Hosp 1981; **Fac Appt:** Prof Ped, Cornell Univ-Weill Med Coll

Cairo, Mitchell S MD [PHO] - **Spec Exp:** Bone Marrow Transplant; Leukemia; Lymphoma; **Hospital:** NYPresby-Morgan Stanley Children's Hosp; **Address:** Babies/Chldns Hosp-Presby Med Ctr, 3959 Broadway, CHONY-11, Central-1114, New York, NY 10032; **Phone:** 212-305-8316; **Board Cert:** Pediatrics 1980; Pediatric Hematology-Oncology 1982; **Med School:** UCSF 1976; **Resid:** Pediatrics, UCLA Med Ctr 1978; **Fellow:** Pediatric Hematology-Oncology, Indiana Univ Med Ctr 1981; **Fac Appt:** Prof Ped, Columbia P&S

Carroll, William L MD [PHO] - **Spec Exp:** Pediatric Cancers; Leukemia; **Hospital:** NYU Med Ctr (page 67); **Address:** NYU Med Ctr, Div Ped Hem/Onc, 160 E 32nd St Fl 2, New York, NY 10016; **Phone:** 212-263-9947; **Board Cert:** Pediatrics 1984; Pediatric Hematology-Oncology 1987; **Med School:** UC Irvine 1978; **Resid:** Pediatrics, Chldns Hosp Med Ctr 1981; **Fellow:** Pediatric Hematology-Oncology, Stanford Univ 1987; **Fac Appt:** Prof Ped, NYU Sch Med

Chen, Allen R MD/PhD [PHO] - **Spec Exp:** Bone Marrow Transplant; Hodgkin's Disease; Immunotherapy; Graft vs Host Disease; **Hospital:** Johns Hopkins Hosp - Baltimore (page 61); **Address:** Johns Hopkins Hosp, Div Peds Oncology, 1650 Orleans St, CRB 2M53, Baltimore, MD 21231; **Phone:** 410-955-7385; **Board Cert:** Pediatrics 2002; **Med School:** Duke Univ 1986; **Resid:** Pediatrics, Chldns Hosp Med Ctr 1989; **Fellow:** Pediatric Hematology-Oncology, Fred Hutchinson Canc Ctr 1993; Bone Marrow Transplant, Fred Hutchinson Canc Ctr 1994; **Fac Appt:** Assoc Prof Ped, Johns Hopkins Univ

Civin, Curt Ingraham MD [PHO] - **Spec Exp:** Pediatric Cancers; Leukemia; Bone Marrow Transplant; **Hospital:** Johns Hopkins Hosp - Baltimore (page 61); **Address:** 1650 Orleans St, rm CRB-2M44, Baltimore, MD 21231-1000; **Phone:** 410-955-8816; **Board Cert:** Pediatrics 1979; Pediatric Hematology-Oncology 1980; **Med School:** Harvard Med Sch 1974; **Resid:** Pediatrics, Chldns Hosp 1976; **Fellow:** Pediatric Hematology-Oncology, Natl Cancer Inst 1979; **Fac Appt:** Prof Ped, Johns Hopkins Univ

Garvin, James MD/PhD [PHO] - **Spec Exp:** Bone Marrow Transplant; Brain Tumors; Pediatric Cancers; **Hospital:** NYPresby-Morgan Stanley Children's Hosp, St Joseph's Regl Med Ctr - Paterson; **Address:** 161 Fort Washington Ave Fl 7 - rm 708, New York, NY 10032; **Phone:** 212-305-8685; **Board Cert:** Pediatrics 1982; Pediatric Hematology-Oncology 1984; **Med School:** Jefferson Med Coll 1976; **Resid:** Pediatrics, Chldns Hosp 1978; Pediatrics, Middlesex Hosp 1979; **Fellow:** Pediatric Hematology-Oncology, Dana Farber Cancer Inst/Childrens Hosp 1982; **Fac Appt:** Clin Prof Ped, Columbia P&S

Giardina, Patricia MD [PHO] - **Spec Exp:** Thalassemia; **Hospital:** NY-Presby Hosp/Weill Cornell (page 66); **Address:** 525 E 68th St, rm P 695, New York, NY 10021; **Phone:** 212-746-3400; **Board Cert:** Pediatrics 1974; Pediatric Hematology-Oncology 1974; **Med School:** NY Med Coll 1968; **Resid:** Pediatrics, Lenox Hill Hosp; Pediatrics, NY Hosp-Cornell Med Ctr

Green, Daniel M MD [PHO] - **Spec Exp:** Wilms' Tumor; Fertility in Cancer Survivors; Cancer Survivors-Late Effects of Therapy; **Hospital:** Roswell Park Cancer Inst, Women's & Chldn's Hosp of Buffalo, The; **Address:** Roswell Park Cancer Inst, Dept Pediatrics, Elm & Carlton Sts, Buffalo, NY 14263; **Phone:** 716-845-2334; **Board Cert:** Pediatrics 1986; Pediatric Hematology-Oncology 1997; **Med School:** St Louis Univ 1973; **Resid:** Pediatrics, Boston City Hosp 1975; **Fellow:** Pediatric Hematology-Oncology, Chldn's Hosp Med Ctr 1978; **Fac Appt:** Prof Ped, SUNY Buffalo

Helman, Lee Jay MD [PHO] - **Spec Exp:** Solid Tumors; **Hospital:** Natl Inst of Hlth - Clin Ctr; **Address:** National Cancer Inst, NIH, 31 Center Drive, rm 3A11, Bethesda, MD 20892-2440; **Phone:** 301-496-4257; **Board Cert:** Internal Medicine 1983; Medical Oncology 1985; **Med School:** Univ MD Sch Med 1980; **Resid:** Internal Medicine, Barnes Hosp 1983; **Fellow:** Oncology, Natl Inst Hlth 1986

Kamen, Barton A MD/PhD [PHO] - **Spec Exp:** Drug Development; Leukemia; **Hospital:** Robert Wood Johnson Univ Hosp - New Brunswick; **Address:** Cancer Inst of New Jersey, 195 Little Albany St, rm 3507, New Brunswick, NJ 08903; **Phone:** 732-235-8864; **Board Cert:** Pediatrics 1981; Pediatric Hematology-Oncology 1987; **Med School:** Case West Res Univ 1976; **Resid:** Pediatrics, Yale-New Haven Hosp 1978; **Fellow:** Pediatric Hematology-Oncology, Yale-New Haven Hosp 1980; **Fac Appt:** Prof Ped, UMDNJ-RW Johnson Med Sch

Kushner, Brian H MD [PHO] - **Spec Exp:** Neuroblastoma; Bone Marrow Transplant; Immunotherapy; **Hospital:** Meml Sloan Kettering Cancer Ctr; **Address:** 1275 York Ave, rm H1113, New York, NY 10021-6007; **Phone:** 212-639-6793; **Board Cert:** Pediatrics 1983; Pediatric Hematology-Oncology 1987; **Med School:** Johns Hopkins Univ 1976; **Resid:** Pediatrics, Columbia-Presby Med Ctr 1978; Pediatrics, New York Hosp 1979; **Fellow:** Pediatric Hematology-Oncology, Boston Chldns Hosp 1980; Pediatric Hematology-Oncology, Meml Sloan Kettering Cancer Ctr 1986; **Fac Appt:** Prof Ped, Cornell Univ-Weill Med Coll

Lange, Beverly MD [PHO] - **Spec Exp:** Leukemia; Brain & Spinal Cord Tumors; **Hospital:** Chldns Hosp of Philadelphia, The; **Address:** Chldns Hosp Philadelphia, Div of Oncol, 34th St & Civic Ctr Blvd Abramson Bldg, Philadelphia, PA 19104; **Phone:** 215-590-2249; **Board Cert:** Pediatrics 1976; Pediatric Hematology-Oncology 1997; **Med School:** Temple Univ 1971; **Resid:** Pediatrics, Philadelphia Genl Hosp 1973; **Fellow:** Pediatric Oncology, Chldns Hosp; **Fac Appt:** Prof Ped, Univ Pennsylvania

Lanzkowsky, Philip MD [PHO] - **Spec Exp:** Solid Tumors; Leukemia; **Hospital:** Schneider Chldn's Hosp, N Shore Univ Hosp at Manhasset; **Address:** 269-01 76th Ave, Ste CH102, New Hyde Park, NY 11040-1434; **Phone:** 718-470-3460; **Board Cert:** Pediatrics 1966; Pediatric Hematology-Oncology 1974; **Med School:** South Africa 1954; **Resid:** Pediatrics, Red Cross War Meml Chldns Hosp 1960; Pediatrics, St Mary's Hosp 1961; **Fellow:** Pediatric Hematology-Oncology, Duke Univ Med Ctr 1962; Pediatric Hematology-Oncology, Univ UT Hosp 1963; **Fac Appt:** Prof Ped, Albert Einstein Coll Med

Lipton, Jeffrey M MD/PhD [PHO] - **Spec Exp:** Bone Marrow Failure Disorders; Stem Cell Transplant; Bone Marrow Transplant; **Hospital:** Schneider Chldn's Hosp; **Address:** Div Hem-Onc & Stem Cell Transplant, 269-01 76th Ave, rm 255, MC-07670, New Hyde Park, NY 11040-1433; **Phone:** 718-470-3460; **Board Cert:** Pediatrics 1981; **Med School:** St Louis Univ 1975; **Resid:** Pediatrics, Boston Chldns Hosp 1977; **Fellow:** Pediatric Hematology-Oncology, Boston Chldns Hosp/Dana Farber Cancer Inst 1979; **Fac Appt:** Prof Ped, Albert Einstein Coll Med

Meek, Rita S MD [PHO] - **Hospital:** Alfred I duPont Hosp for Children, Christiana Care Hlth Svs; **Address:** Dupont Hosp for Children, Div Hem-Onc, 1600 Rockland Rd, Wilmington, DE 19899; **Phone:** 302-651-5500; **Board Cert:** Pediatrics 1979; Pediatric Hematology-Oncology 1980; **Med School:** Geo Wash Univ 1974; **Resid:** Pediatrics, Childns Hosp Natl Med Ctr 1977; **Fellow:** Pediatric Hematology-Oncology, Chldns Hosp Natl Med Ctr 1979; **Fac Appt:** Assoc Clin Prof Ped, Jefferson Med Coll

Meyers, Paul MD [PHO] - **Spec Exp:** Pediatric Cancers; Bone Tumors; Sarcoma; **Hospital:** Meml Sloan Kettering Cancer Ctr, NY-Presby Hosp/Weill Cornell (page 66); **Address:** 1275 York Ave, Box 471, New York, NY 10021-6007; **Phone:** 212-639-5952; **Board Cert:** Pediatrics 1978; Pediatric Hematology-Oncology 1978; **Med School:** Mount Sinai Sch Med 1973; **Resid:** Pediatrics, Mt Sinai Hosp 1976; **Fellow:** Pediatric Hematology-Oncology, New York Hosp-Cornell 1979; **Fac Appt:** Prof Ped, Cornell Univ-Weill Med Coll

O'Reilly, Richard MD [PHO] - **Spec Exp:** Bone Marrow Transplant; **Hospital:** Meml Sloan Kettering Cancer Ctr, NY-Presby Hosp/Weill Cornell (page 66); **Address:** 1275 York Ave, rm H1409, New York, NY 10021; **Phone:** 212-639-5957; **Board Cert:** Pediatrics 1974; **Med School:** Univ Rochester 1968; **Resid:** Pediatrics, Chldrns Hosp 1972; **Fellow:** Infectious Disease, Chldrns Hosp 1973; **Fac Appt:** Prof Ped, Cornell Univ-Weill Med Coll

Parker, Robert MD [PHO] - **Spec Exp:** Pediatric Cancers; Bleeding/Coagulation Disorders; Platelet Disorders; Lymphoma; **Hospital:** Stony Brook Univ Med Ctr; **Address:** Stony Brook Univ Hosp, Dept Peds, HSC T-11, Rm 029, Stony Brook, NY 11794-8111; **Phone:** 631-444-7720; **Board Cert:** Pediatrics 1983; Pediatric Hematology-Oncology 1984; **Med School:** Brown Univ 1976; **Resid:** Internal Medicine, Roger Williams Med Ctr 1977; Pediatrics, Rhode Island Hosp 1979; **Fellow:** Pediatric Hematology-Oncology, Natl Cancer Inst 1981; Hematology, Natl Cancer Inst 1984; **Fac Appt:** Prof Ped, SUNY Stony Brook

Rausen, Aaron R MD [PHO] - **Spec Exp:** Leukemia & Lymphoma; Bone Tumors; Retinoblastoma; **Hospital:** NYU Med Ctr (page 67), Lenox Hill Hosp (page 62); **Address:** NYU Medical Ctr, 160 E 32nd St Fl 2, New York, NY 10016; **Phone:** 212-263-7144; **Board Cert:** Pediatrics 1960; Pediatric Hematology-Oncology 1974; **Med School:** SUNY Downstate 1954; **Resid:** Pediatrics, Bellevue Hosp 1956; Pediatrics, Mount Sinai 1959; **Fellow:** Hematology, Chldns Hosp 1961; **Fac Appt:** Prof Ped, NYU Sch Med

Reaman, Gregory MD [PHO] - **Spec Exp:** Leukemia; Lymphoma; Cancer Survivors-Late Effects of Therapy; **Hospital:** Chldns Natl Med Ctr; **Address:** Childrens National Med Ctr, 111 Michigan Ave NW, Washington, DC 20010-2916; **Phone:** 202-884-2800; **Board Cert:** Pediatrics 1978; Pediatric Hematology-Oncology 1978; **Med School:** Loyola Univ-Stritch Sch Med 1973; **Resid:** Hematology, Montreal Chldns Hosp 1975; Pediatrics, Montreal Chldns Hosp 1976; **Fellow:** Pediatric Oncology, Natl Cancer Inst 1979; **Fac Appt:** Prof Ped, Geo Wash Univ

Rheingold, Susan R MD [PHO] - **Spec Exp:** Leukemia; Clinical Trials; Complementary Medicine; **Hospital:** Chldns Hosp of Philadelphia, The; **Address:** Chldns Hosp Phila - Div Oncology, 34th & Civic Ctr Blvd, Philadelphia, PA 19104; **Phone:** 215-590-3025; **Board Cert:** Pediatrics 2003; Pediatric Hematology-Oncology 2000; **Med School:** Univ Pennsylvania 1992; **Resid:** Pediatrics, Johns Hopkins Hosp 1995; **Fellow:** Pediatric Hematology-Oncology, Chldns Hosp 1999; **Fac Appt:** Asst Prof Ped, Univ Pennsylvania

Ritchey, Arthur MD [PHO] - **Spec Exp:** Leukemia; Bleeding/Coagulation Disorders; **Hospital:** Chldns Hosp of Pittsburgh - UPMC; **Address:** Chldns Hosp, Div Hematology/Oncology, 3705 Fifth Ave, Desoto Wing 4B, Ste 385, Pittsburgh, PA 15213; **Phone:** 412-692-5055; **Board Cert:** Pediatrics 1977; Pediatric Hematology-Oncology 2000; **Med School:** Univ Cincinnati 1972; **Resid:** Pediatrics, Johns Hopkins Hosp 1975; **Fellow:** Pediatric Hematology-Oncology, Yale-New Haven Hosp 1980; **Fac Appt:** Prof Ped, Univ Pittsburgh

Steinherz, Peter G MD [PHO] - **Spec Exp:** Leukemia & Lymphoma; Pediatric Cancers; Wilms' Tumor; **Hospital:** Meml Sloan Kettering Cancer Ctr, NY-Presby Hosp/Weill Cornell (page 66); **Address:** Memorial Sloan Kettering Cancer Ctr, 1275 York Ave, Box 411, New York, NY 10021; **Phone:** 212-639-7951; **Board Cert:** Pediatrics 1973; Pediatric Hematology-Oncology 1978; **Med School:** Albert Einstein Coll Med 1968; **Resid:** Pediatrics, New York Hosp-Cornell 1971; **Fellow:** Pediatric Hematology-Oncology, New York Hosp-Cornell 1975; **Fac Appt:** Prof Ped, Cornell Univ-Weill Med Coll

Weiner, Michael MD [PHO] - **Spec Exp:** Hodgkin's Disease; Lymphoma; Leukemia; **Hospital:** NY-Presby Hosp/Columbia (page 66), St Joseph's Regl Med Ctr - Paterson; **Address:** 161 Fort Washington Ave, Irving Pavilion-FL 7, New York, NY 10032-3710; **Phone:** 212-305-9770; **Board Cert:** Pediatrics 1980; Pediatric Hematology-Oncology 1980; **Med School:** SUNY Hlth Sci Ctr 1972; **Resid:** Pediatrics, Montefiore Med Ctr 1974; **Fellow:** Pediatric Hematology-Oncology, NYU Med Ctr 1976; Pediatric Hematology-Oncology, Johns Hopkins Hosp 1977; **Fac Appt:** Prof Ped, Columbia P&S

Southeast

Falletta, John MD [PHO] - **Spec Exp:** Hematologic Malignancies; **Hospital:** Duke Univ Med Ctr; **Address:** Duke Univ Med Ctr, 2424 Erwin Rd, Durham, NC 27710; **Phone:** 919-668-5111; **Board Cert:** Pediatrics 1972; Pediatric Hematology-Oncology 1974; **Med School:** Univ Kans 1966; **Resid:** Pediatrics, Texas Childrens Hosp 1971; **Fellow:** Pediatric Hematology-Oncology, Baylor Coll Med 1973; **Fac Appt:** Prof Ped, Duke Univ

Friedman, Henry S MD [PHO] - **Spec Exp:** Neuro-Oncology; Brain & Spinal Cord Tumors; **Hospital:** Duke Univ Med Ctr; **Address:** Brain Tumor Ctr-Duke Univ, Baker House, DUMC, rm 047, Box 3624, Durham, NC 27710; **Phone:** 919-684-5301; **Board Cert:** Pediatrics 1982; Pediatric Hematology-Oncology 1982; **Med School:** SUNY Upstate Med Univ 1977; **Resid:** Pediatrics, SUNY Upstate Med Ctr 1980; **Fellow:** Pediatric Hematology-Oncology, Duke Univ Med Ctr 1983; **Fac Appt:** Prof Ped, Duke Univ

Graham-Pole, John R MD [PHO] - **Spec Exp:** Bone Marrow Transplant; Palliative Care; Arts in the Healing Process; **Hospital:** Shands Hlthcre at Univ of FL; **Address:** Shands Hosp, Dept Ped Hem-Onc, 1600 SW Archer Rd, rm M401, Gainesville, FL 32610-0296; **Phone:** 352-392-5633; **Board Cert:** Pediatrics 1983; Pediatric Hematology-Oncology 1987; **Med School:** England 1966; **Resid:** Pediatrics, Hosp Sick Chldn 1968; Pediatrics, Royal Hosp Sick Chldn 1970; **Fellow:** Pediatric Hematology-Oncology, Royal Hosp Sick Chldn 1971; **Fac Appt:** Prof Ped, Univ Fla Coll Med

Keller Jr, Frank G MD [PHO] - **Spec Exp:** Leukemia; Hodgkin's Disease; **Hospital:** Emory Univ Hosp; **Address:** Emory Healthcare Pediatrics Dept, 2105 Uppergate Drive NE Fl 4, Atlanta, GA 30322; **Phone:** 404-727-5740; **Board Cert:** Pediatric Hematology-Oncology 2002; **Med School:** Univ NC Sch Med 1986; **Resid:** Pediatrics, Vanderbilt Univ Med Ctr 1990; **Fellow:** Pediatric Hematology-Oncology, Duke Univ Med Ctr 1993; **Fac Appt:** Assoc Prof Ped, Emory Univ

Kuttesch, John F MD [PHO] - **Spec Exp:** Brain Tumors; Brain Tumors-Recurrent; **Hospital:** Vanderbilt Children's Hosp; **Address:** Vanderbilt Univ Med Ctr, 2220 Pierce Ave, Rm 397 PRB, Nashville, TN 37232-6310; **Phone:** 615-936-1762; **Board Cert:** Pediatrics 2000; Pediatric Hematology-Oncology 2000; **Med School:** Univ Tex, Houston 1985; **Resid:** Pediatrics, Vanderbilt Univ Med Ctr 1988; **Fellow:** Pediatric Hematology-Oncology, St Judes Chldns Hosp 1992; **Fac Appt:** Assoc Prof Ped, Vanderbilt Univ

Olson, Thomas A MD [PHO] - **Spec Exp:** Platelet Disorders; Sarcoma; Brain Tumors; **Hospital:** Emory Univ Hosp; **Address:** 3 W AFLAC Outpatient Ctr, 1405 Clifton Rd NE, Atlanta, GA 30322; **Phone:** 404-785-1200; **Board Cert:** Pediatrics 1982; Pediatric Hematology-Oncology 1984; **Med School:** Loyola Univ-Stritch Sch Med 1978; **Resid:** Pediatrics, Walter Reed AMC 1981; **Fellow:** Pediatric Hematology-Oncology, Walter Reed AMC 1983; **Fac Appt:** Assoc Prof Ped, Emory Univ

Pui, Ching Hon MD [PHO] - **Spec Exp:** Leukemia; Lymphoma; **Hospital:** St Jude Children's Research Hosp; **Address:** St Jude Chldns Rsch Hosp, 332 N Lauderdale St, Memphis, TN 38105; **Phone:** 901-495-3335; **Board Cert:** Pediatrics 1980; Pediatric Hematology-Oncology 1982; **Med School:** Taiwan 1976; **Resid:** Pediatrics, St Jude Chldns Rsch Hosp 1979; **Fellow:** Hematology & Oncology, St Jude Chldns Rsch Hosp 1981; **Fac Appt:** Prof Ped, Univ Tenn Coll Med, Memphis

Pediatric Hematology-Oncology

Rosoff, Phillip M MD [PHO] - **Spec Exp:** Cancer Survivors-Late Effects of Therapy; Down Syndrome; Leukemia; **Hospital:** Duke Univ Med Ctr; **Address:** Duke Univ Med Ctr, Box 2916, Durham, NC 27710-0001; **Phone:** 919-684-3401; **Board Cert:** Pediatrics 1984; Pediatric Hematology-Oncology 2002; **Med School:** Case West Res Univ 1978; **Resid:** Pediatrics, Chldns Hosp 1980; **Fellow:** Pediatric Hematology-Oncology, Chldns Hosp/Dana Farber Cancer Inst 1984; **Fac Appt:** Assoc Prof Ped, Duke Univ

Toledano, Stuart R MD [PHO] - **Spec Exp:** Leukemia; Solid Tumors; Retinoblastoma; **Hospital:** Jackson Meml Hosp; **Address:** Univ Miami, Dept Peds-Div Ped Hem/Onc, (R-131) P.O. Box 016960, Miami, FL 33101; **Phone:** 305-585-5635; **Board Cert:** Pediatrics 1986; Pediatric Hematology-Oncology 1986; **Med School:** SUNY Buffalo 1972; **Resid:** Pediatrics, Montefiore Med Ctr 1975; **Fellow:** Pediatric Hematology-Oncology, Montefiore Med Ctr 1975; Pediatric Oncology, Childrens Hosp 1979; **Fac Appt:** Prof Ped, Univ Miami Sch Med

Wang, Winfred C MD [PHO] - **Spec Exp:** Sickle Cell Disease; Bone Marrow Failure Disorders; Anemia-Aplastic; **Hospital:** St Jude Children's Research Hosp, Le Bonheur Chldns Med Ctr; **Address:** St Jude Chldn Rsch Hosp, 332 N Lauderdale St, rm S4041, Memphis, TN 38105-2729; **Phone:** 901-495-3497; **Board Cert:** Pediatrics 1972; Pediatric Hematology-Oncology 1974; **Med School:** Univ Chicago-Pritzker Sch Med 1967; **Resid:** Pediatrics, Montefiore Med Ctr 1969; Pediatrics, Kauikeolani Chldn's Hosp 1970; **Fellow:** Pediatric Hematology-Oncology, UCSF 1975; **Fac Appt:** Prof Ped, Univ Tenn Coll Med, Memphis

Midwest

Boxer, Laurence MD [PHO] - **Spec Exp:** Congenital Neutropenia-Severe; Anemias & Red Cell Disorders; Thrombotic Disorders; Anemia-Aplastic; **Hospital:** Univ Michigan Hlth Sys; **Address:** Univ Michigan, L-2110 Womens Hosp, 1500 E Medical Ctr Dr, Box 0238, Ann Arbor, MI 48109-0238; **Phone:** 734-764-7127; **Board Cert:** Pediatrics 1971; Pediatric Hematology-Oncology 1974; **Med School:** Stanford Univ 1966; **Resid:** Pediatrics, Yale-New Haven Hosp 1968; Pediatrics, Stanford Univ Hosp 1969; **Fellow:** Hematology, Childrens Hosp-Harvard 1974; **Fac Appt:** Prof Ped, Univ Mich Med Sch

Castle, Valerie MD [PHO] - **Spec Exp:** Neuroblastoma; Bleeding/Coagulation Disorders; Cancer Survivors-Late Effects of Therapy; **Hospital:** Univ Michigan Hlth Sys; **Address:** Univ Mich Comp Cancer Ctr & Geriatric Ctr, 1500 E Med Ctr Drive, Desk B1-358, Ann Arbor, MI 48109-0911; **Phone:** 734-936-9814; **Board Cert:** Pediatrics 2000; Pediatric Hematology-Oncology 1998; **Med School:** McMaster Univ 1983; **Resid:** Pediatrics, McMaster Univ Med Ctr 1986; **Fellow:** Pediatric Hematology-Oncology, Univ Mich Hosps 1989; **Fac Appt:** Prof Ped, Univ Mich Med Sch

Cohn, Susan L MD [PHO] - **Spec Exp:** Neuroblastoma; **Hospital:** Children's Mem Hosp, Evanston Hosp; **Address:** Children's Memorial Hosp, 2300 Children's Plaza, Box 30, Chicago, IL 60614; **Phone:** 773-880-4562; **Board Cert:** Pediatrics 1985; Pediatric Hematology-Oncology 1987; **Med School:** Univ IL Coll Med 1980; **Resid:** Pediatrics, Michael Reese Hosp 1984; **Fellow:** Hematology & Oncology, Children's Memorial Hosp 1985; **Fac Appt:** Prof Ped, Northwestern Univ

Davies, Stella M MD/PhD [PHO] - **Spec Exp:** Leukemia; Bone Marrow Transplant; Stem Cell Transplant; **Hospital:** Cincinnati Chldns Hosp Med Ctr; **Address:** Cincinnati Chldns Hosp Med Ctr, 3333 Burnet Ave, MLC 7015, Cincinnati, OH 45229-3039; **Phone:** 513-636-2469; **Med School:** England 1981; **Resid:** Pediatrics, Univ Newcastle Med Ctr 1985; **Fellow:** Pediatric Hematology-Oncology, Univ Minn Med Ctr 1993; **Fac Appt:** Prof Ped, Univ Cincinnati

DeBaun, Michael R MD [PHO] - **Spec Exp:** Sickle Cell Disease; **Hospital:** St Louis Chldns Hosp; **Address:** St Louis Children's Hospital, One Children's Pl Fl 9S, St Louis, MO 63110; **Phone:** 314-454-6018; **Board Cert:** Pediatrics 2001; Pediatric Hematology-Oncology 2002; **Med School:** Stanford Univ 1987; **Resid:** Pediatrics, St Louis Children's Hosp 1990; **Fellow:** Pediatric Hematology-Oncology, St Louis Children's Hosp 1993; **Fac Appt:** Assoc Prof Ped, Washington Univ, St Louis

Fallon, Robert J MD/PhD [PHO] - **Spec Exp:** Lymphoma; Hodgkin's Disease; Stem Cell Transplant; **Hospital:** Riley Hosp for Children; **Address:** Riley Childrens Hospital, 702 Barnhill Drive, rm Riley 4340, Indianapolis, IN 46202; **Phone:** 317-274-8784; **Board Cert:** Internal Medicine 1983; Medical Oncology 1985; **Med School:** NYU Sch Med 1980; **Resid:** Internal Medicine, Brigham & Womens Hosp 1983; **Fellow:** Hematology & Oncology, Brigham & Womens Hosp/Dana Farber Cancer Inst 1985; **Fac Appt:** Prof Ped, Indiana Univ

Ferrara, James MD [PHO] - **Spec Exp:** Bone Marrow Transplant; Graft vs Host Disease; Inflammatory Cytokines; **Hospital:** Univ Michigan Hlth Sys; **Address:** Univ Michigan Comprehensive Cancer Ctr, 1500 E Medical Center Drive, Ste 6308, Ann Arbor, MI 48109-0942; **Phone:** 734-615-1340; **Board Cert:** Pediatrics 2004; **Med School:** Georgetown Univ 1980; **Resid:** Pediatrics, Children's Hosp 1982; **Fellow:** Pediatric Hematology-Oncology, Children's Hosp 1985; **Fac Appt:** Prof Ped, Univ Mich Med Sch

Hayani, Ammar MD [PHO] - **Spec Exp:** Leukemia; Solid Tumors; **Hospital:** Adv Christ Med Ctr, Central DuPage Hosp; **Address:** Hope Children's Hospital, 4440 W 95th St, Oak Lawn, IL 60453-2600; **Phone:** 708-684-4094; **Board Cert:** Pediatrics 1989; Pediatric Hematology-Oncology 2005; **Med School:** Syria 1982; **Resid:** Pediatrics, Louisiana State Univ 1987; **Fellow:** Pediatric Hematology-Oncology, Baylor Coll Med 1991

Hayashi, Robert J MD [PHO] - **Spec Exp:** Bone Marrow Transplant; Cancer Survivors-Late Effects of Therapy; Leukemia; **Hospital:** St Louis Chldns Hosp; **Address:** St Louis Chldns Hosp, Div Ped Hem Onc, One Children's Pl Fl 9S, Box 8116, St Louis, MO 63110; **Phone:** 314-454-6018; **Board Cert:** Pediatrics 2000; Pediatric Hematology-Oncology 2000; **Med School:** Washington Univ, St Louis 1986; **Resid:** Pediatrics, St Louis Children's Hosp 1989; **Fellow:** Pediatric Hematology-Oncology, Johns Hopkins Hosp 1992; **Fac Appt:** Asst Prof Ped, Washington Univ, St Louis

Hilden, Joanne M MD [PHO] - **Spec Exp:** Brain Tumors; Leukemia & Lymphoma; Bone Tumors; Soft Tissue Tumors; **Hospital:** St Vincent Hosp & Hlth Svcs - Indianapolis; **Address:** 8402 Harcourt Rd, Ste 603, Indianapolis, IN 46260; **Phone:** 317-338-3466; **Board Cert:** Pediatrics 2006; Pediatric Hematology-Oncology 2002; **Med School:** Univ Minn 1988; **Resid:** Pediatrics, Univ Minn Med Ctr 1991; **Fellow:** Pediatric Hematology-Oncology, Univ Minn Med Ctr 1994; **Fac Appt:** Assoc Prof Ped, Indiana Univ

Hord, Jeffrey D MD [PHO] - **Spec Exp:** Hematologic Malignancies; Bone Marrow Failure Disorders; Sickle Cell Disease; **Hospital:** Children's Hosp & Med Ctr-Akron; **Address:** Akron Childrens Hosp, Hematology/Oncology, One Perkins Square, Akron, OH 44308; **Phone:** 330-543-8580; **Board Cert:** Pediatrics 2000; Pediatric Hematology-Oncology 2004; **Med School:** Univ KY Coll Med 1989; **Resid:** Pediatrics, Childrens Hosp 1992; **Fellow:** Pediatric Hematology-Oncology, Vanderbilt Univ Med Ctr 1995; **Fac Appt:** Assoc Prof Ped, NE Ohio Univ

Lusher, Jeanne M MD [PHO] - **Hospital:** Chldns Hosp of Michigan; **Address:** Children's Hospital Michigan, Div Hem/Onc, 3901 Beaubien Blvd, Detroit, MI 48201; **Phone:** 313-745-5515; **Board Cert:** Pediatrics 1986; Pediatric Hematology-Oncology 1986; **Med School:** Univ Cincinnati 1960; **Resid:** Pediatrics, Charity Hosp/Tulane Univ 1963; **Fellow:** Hematology & Oncology, Charity Hosp/Tulane Univ 1965; Hematology & Oncology, Saint Louis Children's Hosp 1966; **Fac Appt:** Prof Ped, Wayne State Univ

Nachman, James MD [PHO] - **Spec Exp:** Leukemia & Lymphoma; Bone Tumors; Hodgkin's Disease; **Hospital:** Univ of Chicago Hosps; **Address:** Univ Chicago Hosps, 5841 S Maryland Ave, rm C-429, MC 406, Chicago, IL 60637; **Phone:** 773-702-6808; **Board Cert:** Pediatrics 1979; Pediatric Hematology-Oncology 1980; **Med School:** Johns Hopkins Univ 1974; **Resid:** Pediatrics, Chldns Meml Hosp 1977; Pediatrics, Fell-Wylers Chldns Hosp 1980; **Fellow:** Pediatric Hematology-Oncology, Chldns Meml Hosp 1979; **Fac Appt:** Prof Ped, Univ Chicago-Pritzker Sch Med

Neglia, Joseph MD [PHO] - **Spec Exp:** Cancer Survivors-Late Effects of Therapy; **Hospital:** Univ Minn Med Ctr, Fairview - Univ Campus; **Address:** Univ Minnesota-Div Ped Hem/Oncology, 420 Delaware St SE, MMC 484, Minneapolis, MN 55455; **Phone:** 612-626-2778; **Board Cert:** Pediatrics 1986; Pediatric Hematology-Oncology 1987; **Med School:** Loma Linda Univ 1981; **Resid:** Pediatrics, Baylor Coll Med 1984; **Fellow:** Pediatric Hematology-Oncology, Univ Minn Hosp 1987; **Fac Appt:** Prof Ped, Univ Minn

Peters, Charles MD [PHO] - **Spec Exp:** Bone Marrow Transplant; Metabolic Storage Diseases; Gaucher Disease; **Hospital:** Chldns Mercy Hosps & Clinics; **Address:** 2401 Gillham Rd, Kansas City, MO 64108; **Phone:** 816-234-3265; **Board Cert:** Pediatric Hematology-Oncology 2002; **Med School:** St Louis Univ 1983; **Resid:** Pediatrics, Johns Hopkins Hosp 1986; **Fellow:** Pediatric Hematology-Oncology, Univ Mich Hosp 1989

Puccetti, Diane MD [PHO] - **Spec Exp:** Brain Tumors; Neuro-Oncology; Cancer Survivors-Late Effects of Therapy; **Hospital:** Univ WI Hosp & Clins; **Address:** Univ Wisconsin Childrens Hosp, 600 Highland Ave, MC 4116, Madison, WI 53792; **Phone:** 608-263-6420; **Board Cert:** Pediatrics 1989; Pediatric Hematology-Oncology 1998; **Med School:** Med Coll OH 1985; **Resid:** Pediatrics, UC-Irvine Med Ctr 1986; Pediatrics, Med Coll Ohio 1988; **Fellow:** Pediatric Hematology-Oncology, Riley Hosp Chldn 1991; **Fac Appt:** Assoc Clin Prof Ped, Univ Wisc

Salvi, Sharad MD [PHO] - **Spec Exp:** Leukemia; Bleeding/Coagulation Disorders; Anemia; **Hospital:** Adv Christ Med Ctr, Central DuPage Hosp; **Address:** Hope Chldns Hosp, 4440 W 95th St, Oak Lawn, IL 60453; **Phone:** 708-684-4094; **Board Cert:** Pediatrics 1982; Pediatric Hematology-Oncology 1982; **Med School:** India 1974; **Resid:** Pediatrics, Lincoln Meml Hosp 1979; **Fellow:** Pediatric Hematology-Oncology, Chldns Hosp/Roswell Park Meml Cancer Inst 1981

Shapiro, Amy D MD [PHO] - **Spec Exp:** Hemophilia; **Hospital:** St Vincent Hosp & Hlth Svcs - Indianapolis; **Address:** Indiana Hemophilia & Thrombosis Ctr, 8402 Harcourt Rd, Ste 500, Indianapolis, IN 46260; **Phone:** 317-871-0000; **Board Cert:** Pediatrics 1986; Pediatric Hematology-Oncology 1987; **Med School:** NYU Sch Med 1980; **Resid:** Pediatrics, Univ Colo Hlth Sci Ctr 1982; **Fellow:** Pediatric Hematology-Oncology, Univ Colo Hlth Sci Ctr 1983

Sondel, Paul M MD [PHO] - **Spec Exp:** Immunotherapy; Stem Cell Transplant; Pediatric Cancers; **Hospital:** Univ WI Hosp & Clins; **Address:** Univ Wisconsin Childrens Hosp, 600 Highland Ave, K4-448 Clin Sci Ctr, Madison, WI 53792-4672; **Phone:** 608-263-6200; **Board Cert:** Pediatrics 1981; **Med School:** Harvard Med Sch 1977; **Resid:** Pediatrics, Univ Wisconsin Hosp 1980; **Fellow:** Research, Sidney Farber Cancer Inst/Harvard 1975; **Fac Appt:** Prof Ped, Univ Wisc

Valentino, Leonard A MD [PHO] - **Spec Exp:** Bleeding/Coagulation Disorders; Thrombotic Disorders; Hemophilia; **Hospital:** Rush Univ Med Ctr, Rush - Copley Med Ctr; **Address:** Rush Univ Med Ctr, 1725 W Harrison St, Chicago, IL 60612-3828; **Phone:** 312-942-5983; **Board Cert:** Pediatrics 2000; Pediatric Hematology-Oncology 1998; **Med School:** Creighton Univ 1984; **Resid:** Pediatrics, Univ Illinios Med Ctr 1987; **Fellow:** Pediatric Hematology-Oncology, UCLA Med Ctr 1990; **Fac Appt:** Assoc Prof Ped, Rush Med Coll

Yaddanapudi, Ravindranath MD [PHO] - **Spec Exp:** Leukemia; **Hospital:** Chldns Hosp of Michigan; **Address:** Children's Hospital Michigan, Div Hem/Onc, 3901 Beaubien Blvd, Detroit, MI 48201; **Phone:** 313-745-5515; **Board Cert:** Pediatrics 1970; Pediatric Hematology-Oncology 1974; **Med School:** India 1964; **Resid:** Pathology, Western Penn Hosp 1967; Pediatrics, Children's Hosp 1969; **Fellow:** Pediatric Hematology-Oncology, Children's Hosp Michigan 1971; **Fac Appt:** Prof Ped, Wayne State Univ

Great Plains and Mountains

Coccia, Peter MD [PHO] - **Spec Exp:** Bone Marrow Transplant; Leukemia & Lymphoma; Solid Tumors; **Hospital:** Nebraska Med Ctr, Children's Hosp - Omaha; **Address:** Univ Nebr Med Ctr, Dept Pediatrics, 982168 Nebraska Med Ctr, Omaha, NE 68198-2168; **Phone:** 402-559-7257; **Board Cert:** Clinical Pathology 1972; Hematology 1975; Pediatrics 1976; Pediatric Hematology-Oncology 1976; **Med School:** SUNY Upstate Med Univ 1968; **Resid:** Pathology, Upstate Med Ctr 1970; Pediatrics, Univ Minn 1973; **Fellow:** Pediatric Hematology-Oncology, Univ Minn 1974; **Fac Appt:** Prof Ped, Univ Nebr Coll Med

Manco-Johnson, Marilyn MD [PHO] - **Spec Exp:** Hemophilia; Thrombotic Disorders; **Hospital:** Chldn's Hosp - Denver, The, Univ Colorado Hosp; **Address:** Univ Colorado, Hemophilia Ctr, Box 6507, MS F416, Aurora, CO 80045-0507; **Phone:** 303-724-0365; **Board Cert:** Pediatrics 1979; Pediatric Hematology-Oncology 1980; **Med School:** Jefferson Med Coll 1974; **Resid:** Pediatrics, Univ Colorado Affil Hosps 1977; **Fellow:** Pediatric Hematology-Oncology, Chldn's Hosp/Colorado Med Ctr 1981; **Fac Appt:** Prof Ped, Univ Colorado

Odom, Lorrie F MD [PHO] - **Spec Exp:** Leukemia; Solid Tumors; Cancer Survivors-Late Effects of Therapy; **Hospital:** Presby - St Luke's Med Ctr, Chldn's Hosp - Denver, The; **Address:** Rocky Mountain Ped Hem Onc, 1601 E 19th Ave, Box 6600, Denver, CO 80218; **Phone:** 303-832-2344; **Board Cert:** Pediatrics 1974; Pediatric Hematology-Oncology 1976; **Med School:** Univ Colorado 1969; **Resid:** Pediatrics, Childrens Hosp 1972; **Fellow:** Pediatric Hematology-Oncology, Dana-Farber Cancer Inst 1974; Pediatric Hematology-Oncology, Univ Colorado Med Ctr 1975; **Fac Appt:** Clin Prof Ped, Univ Colorado

Southwest

Abella, Esteban MD [PHO] - **Spec Exp:** Leukemia; Anemia-Aplastic; Neuroblastoma; Bone Marrow Transplant; **Hospital:** Banner Desert Med Ctr, St Joseph's Hosp & Med Ctr - Phoenix; **Address:** 1432 S Dobson, Ste 107, Mesa, AZ 85202; **Phone:** 480-833-1123; **Board Cert:** Pediatrics 1998; Pediatric Hematology-Oncology 2002; **Med School:** Dominican Republic 1985; **Resid:** Pediatrics, Chldns Hosp Michigan 1988; **Fellow:** Pediatric Hematology-Oncology, Chldns Hosp Michigan/Wayne St Univ 1991

Pediatric Hematology-Oncology

Baranko, Paul MD [PHO] - **Spec Exp:** Leukemia; Kidney Cancer; Wilms' Tumor; **Hospital:** Phoenix Children's Hosp; **Address:** Phoenix Children's Hosp, 1919 E Thomas Rd, Phoenix, AZ 85016; **Phone:** 602-546-0920; **Board Cert:** Pediatrics 1986; Pediatric Hematology-Oncology 1986; **Med School:** Indiana Univ 1965; **Resid:** Pediatrics, Indiana Med Ctr 1967; Pediatrics, St Josephs Hosp 1968; **Fellow:** Pediatric Hematology-Oncology, Los Angeles Chldns Hosp 1971; **Fac Appt:** Clin Prof Ped, Univ Ariz Coll Med

Berg, Stacey MD [PHO] - **Hospital:** Texas Chldns Hosp - Houston; **Address:** Texas Chldns Cancer Ctr, Ped Hem-Onc, 6621 Fannin St, MC 3-3320, Houston, TX 77030; **Phone:** 832-824-4588; **Board Cert:** Pediatrics 2007; Pediatric Hematology-Oncology 2007; **Med School:** Univ Pittsburgh 1985; **Resid:** Pediatrics, Chldns Hosp 1988; **Fellow:** Pediatric Hematology-Oncology, Natl Inst Hlth 1991

Buchanan, George R MD [PHO] - **Spec Exp:** Sickle Cell Disease; Thrombotic Disorders; Hemophilia; Leukemia; **Hospital:** Chldns Med Ctr of Dallas; **Address:** Univ Texas SW Med Ctr, Peds Hem Onc, 5323 Harry Hines Blvd, MC 9063, Dallas, TX 75390-9063; **Phone:** 214-456-2382; **Board Cert:** Pediatrics 1975; Pediatric Hematology-Oncology 2000; **Med School:** Univ Chicago-Pritzker Sch Med 1970; **Resid:** Pediatrics, Chldn's Meml Hosp 1973; **Fellow:** Hematology & Oncology, Chldn's Meml Hosp 1975; **Fac Appt:** Prof Ped, Univ Tex SW, Dallas

Graham, Michael L MD [PHO] - **Spec Exp:** Bone Marrow Transplant; Leukemia; Stem Cell Transplant; **Hospital:** Univ Med Ctr - Tucson; **Address:** Univ Arizona Hlth Science Ctr, 1501 N Campbell Ave, rm 4341, Box 245073, Tucson, AZ 85724-5073; **Phone:** 520-626-6527; **Board Cert:** Pediatrics 1980; Pediatric Hematology-Oncology 1984; **Med School:** Brown Univ 1975; **Resid:** Pediatrics, Johns Hopkins Hosp 1978; Pediatric Hematology-Oncology, Johns Hopkins Hosp 1980; **Fellow:** Medical Oncology, Yale-New Haven Hosp 1982; **Fac Appt:** Assoc Prof Ped, Univ Ariz Coll Med

Hoots, William K MD [PHO] - **Spec Exp:** Hemophilia; **Hospital:** UT MD Anderson Cancer Ctr (page 71); **Address:** Gulf States, Hemophilia & Thrombophilia Ctr, 6655 Travis, Ste 400 HMC, Houston, TX 77030; **Phone:** 713-500-8360; **Board Cert:** Pediatrics 1980; Pediatric Hematology-Oncology 1980; **Med School:** Univ NC Sch Med 1975; **Resid:** Pediatrics, Chldns Med Ctr 1978; **Fellow:** Pediatric Hematology-Oncology, Univ NC Med Ctr 1980; **Fac Appt:** Prof Ped, Univ Tex, Houston

Murphy, Sharon B MD [PHO] - **Spec Exp:** Lymphoma, Non-Hodgkin's; Leukemia; **Hospital:** Univ Hlth Sys - Univ Hosp; **Address:** UTHSCSA - Children's Cancer Research Inst, 8403 Floyd Curl Drive, MS 7784, San Antonio, TX 78229-3900; **Phone:** 210-562-9000; **Board Cert:** Pediatrics 1990; Pediatric Hematology-Oncology 1990; **Med School:** Harvard Med Sch 1969; **Resid:** Pediatrics, Univ Colorado Med Ctr 1971; **Fellow:** Pediatric Hematology-Oncology, Chldns Hosp 1973; **Fac Appt:** Prof Ped, Univ Tex, San Antonio

Scher, Charles D MD [PHO] - **Spec Exp:** Sickle Cell Disease; Leukemia; **Hospital:** Tulane Univ Hosp & Clin; **Address:** Tulane Univ Hosp, Dept Pediatrics, 1430 Tulane Ave, Box SL-37, New Orleans, LA 70112; **Phone:** 504-988-5412; **Board Cert:** Pediatrics 1972; **Med School:** Univ Pennsylvania 1965; **Resid:** Pediatrics, Bronx Muni Hosp Ctr 1967; Pediatrics, Chldns Hosp Med Ctr 1972; **Fellow:** Pediatric Hematology-Oncology, Chldns Hosp Med Ctr 1974; **Fac Appt:** Prof Ped, Tulane Univ

Wall, Donna A MD [PHO] - **Spec Exp:** Bone Marrow & Stem Cell Transplant; Immunotherapy; **Hospital:** Methodist Chldns Hosp of South Texas, Christus Santa Rosa Children's Hosp; **Address:** Texas Transplant Inst, 7711 Louis Pasteur, Ste 708, San Antonio, TX 78229; **Phone:** 210-575-7268; **Board Cert:** Pediatrics 1986; Pediatric Hematology-Oncology 1987; **Med School:** Canada 1981; **Resid:** Pediatrics, NY Presby-Columbia Med Ctr 1983; Pediatrics, New England Med Ctr 1985; **Fellow:** Pediatric Hematology-Oncology, Dana Farber Cancer Inst 1986

West Coast and Pacific

Andrews, Robert G MD [PHO] - **Spec Exp:** Bone Marrow Transplant; Leukemia; Lymphoma; **Hospital:** Chldns Hosp and Regl Med Ctr - Seattle; **Address:** Fred Hutchinson Cancer Research Ctr, D2-373, 1100 Fairview Ave N, Seattle, WA 98109-1024; **Phone:** 206-288-1024; **Board Cert:** Pediatrics 1984; Pediatric Hematology-Oncology 1984; **Med School:** Univ Minn 1976; **Resid:** Pediatrics, New England Med Ctr 1979; **Fellow:** Pediatric Hematology-Oncology, Children's Hosp Med Ctr 1983; **Fac Appt:** Assoc Prof Ped, Univ Wash

Geyer, J Russell MD [PHO] - **Spec Exp:** Brain Tumors; **Hospital:** Chldns Hosp and Regl Med Ctr - Seattle, Providence Alaska Med Ctr; **Address:** Chldns Hosp & Reg Med Ctr - Div Hem/Onc, 4800 Sands Point Way NE, MS B-6553, Seattle, WA 98105; **Phone:** 206-987-2106; **Board Cert:** Pediatrics 1983; Pediatric Hematology-Oncology 1987; **Med School:** Wayne State Univ 1977; **Resid:** Pediatrics, Chldns Hosp Michigan 1980; **Fellow:** Pediatric Hematology-Oncology, Univ Michigan Med Ctr 1981; **Fac Appt:** Prof Ped, Univ Wash

Glader, Bertil MD [PHO] - **Spec Exp:** Genetic Blood Disorders; Hemophilia; **Hospital:** Lucile Packard Chldns Hosp/Stanford Univ Med Ctr; **Address:** 1000 Welch Rd, Ste 300, Palo Alto, CA 94305; **Phone:** 650-497-8953; **Board Cert:** Pediatrics 1982; Pediatric Hematology-Oncology 2005; Hematology 1983; **Med School:** Northwestern Univ 1968; **Resid:** Pediatrics, Chldns Hosp Med Ctr 1973; **Fellow:** Hematology, Chldns Hosp Med Ctr 1975; **Fac Appt:** Prof Ped, Stanford Univ

Horn, Biljana N MD [PHO] - **Spec Exp:** Bone Marrow Transplant; Brain Tumors; Stem Cell Transplant; Immunotherapy; **Hospital:** UCSF Med Ctr; **Address:** UCSF Med Ctr, Pediatric BMT Program, 505 Parnassus Ave, rm M-659, San Francisco, CA 94143; **Phone:** 415-476-2188; **Board Cert:** Pediatrics 2005; Pediatric Hematology-Oncology 2004; **Med School:** Croatia 1983; **Resid:** Pediatrics, Rainbow Babies & Chldns Hosp 1991; **Fellow:** Pediatric Hematology-Oncology, Natl Cancer Inst 1994; Pediatric Neuro-Oncology, UCSF 1998; **Fac Appt:** Assoc Prof Ped, UCSF

Kadota, Richard P MD [PHO] - **Spec Exp:** Bone Marrow Transplant; Brain Tumors; Clinical Trials; **Hospital:** Rady Children's Hosp - San Diego; **Address:** Children's Hospital San Diego, 3020 Children's Way, MC 5035, San Diego, CA 92123; **Phone:** 858-966-5811; **Board Cert:** Pediatrics 1984; Pediatric Hematology-Oncology 1984; **Med School:** Northwestern Univ 1979; **Resid:** Pediatrics, Mayo Clinic 1983; **Fellow:** Pediatric Hematology-Oncology, Mayo Clinic 1985; **Fac Appt:** Clin Prof Ped, UCSD

Link, Michael P MD [PHO] - **Spec Exp:** Stem Cell Transplant; **Hospital:** Lucile Packard Chldns Hosp/Stanford Univ Med Ctr, Stanford Univ Med Ctr; **Address:** 1000 Welch Rd, Ste 300, Palo Alto, CA 94304; **Phone:** 650-723-5535; **Board Cert:** Pediatrics 1979; Pediatric Hematology-Oncology 1980; **Med School:** Stanford Univ 1974; **Resid:** Pediatrics, Chldns Hosp Med Ctr 1976; **Fellow:** Hematology & Oncology, Dana Farber Cancer Inst 1979; **Fac Appt:** Prof Ped, Stanford Univ

Pediatric Hematology-Oncology

Matthay, Katherine K MD [PHO] - **Spec Exp:** Neuroblastoma; Bone Marrow & Stem Cell Transplant; **Hospital:** UCSF Med Ctr; **Address:** UCSF, Dept Ped Onc, 505 Parnassus Ave, Box 0106, San Francisco, CA 94143; **Phone:** 415-476-0603; **Board Cert:** Pediatrics 1979; Pediatric Hematology-Oncology 1980; **Med School:** Univ Pennsylvania 1973; **Resid:** Pediatrics, Univ Colorado 1976; **Fellow:** Pediatric Hematology-Oncology, UCSF 1979; **Fac Appt:** Prof Ped, UCSF

Nicholson, Henry Stacy MD [PHO] - **Spec Exp:** Brain Tumors; Cancer Survivors-Late Effects of Therapy; **Hospital:** Doernbecher Chldns Hosp/OHSU, OR Hlth & Sci Univ; **Address:** OR Hlth Scis Univ, 709 SW Gaines Rd, Portland, OR 97239; **Phone:** 503-494-4265; **Board Cert:** Pediatrics 2000; Pediatric Hematology-Oncology 2000; **Med School:** Med Coll GA 1985; **Resid:** Pediatrics, Chldns National Med Ctr 1988; **Fellow:** Pediatric Hematology-Oncology, Chldns National Med Ctr 1991; **Fac Appt:** Prof Ped, Oregon Hlth Sci Univ

Rosenthal, Joseph MD [PHO] - **Spec Exp:** Bone Marrow Transplant; Clinical Trials; **Hospital:** City of Hope Natl Med Ctr & Beckman Rsch; **Address:** City of Hope Med Ctr, 1500 E Duarte Rd, Duarte, CA 91010; **Phone:** 626-256-4673 x68442; **Board Cert:** Pediatrics 2003; Pediatric Hematology-Oncology 2004; **Med School:** Israel 1984; **Resid:** Pediatrics, Soroka MC 1988; Pediatrics, Chldrn Hosp 1995; **Fellow:** Pediatric Hematology-Oncology, Univ Colorado 1991; Pediatric Hematology-Oncology, Chldrn Hosp 1994; **Fac Appt:** Assoc Prof Ped, USC-Keck School of Medicine

Sakamoto, Kathleen M MD [PHO] - **Spec Exp:** Fanconi's Anemia; **Hospital:** Chldns Hosp - Los Angeles (page 56); **Address:** Mattel Chldns Hosp UCLA, Div Hem-Onc, 10833 Le Conte Ave, Los Angeles, CA 90095-1752; **Phone:** 310-825-6708; **Board Cert:** Pediatrics 2000; Pediatric Hematology-Oncology 2000; **Med School:** Univ Cincinnati 1985; **Resid:** Pediatrics, Children's Hosp 1988; **Fellow:** Pediatric Hematology-Oncology, Children's Hosp 1991; **Fac Appt:** Prof Ped, UCLA

Siegel, Stuart E MD [PHO] - **Spec Exp:** Leukemia; Infections in Cancer Patients; Psychiatry in Childhood Cancer; Solid Tumors; **Hospital:** Chldns Hosp - Los Angeles (page 56), Ventura Cnty Med Ctr; **Address:** Children's Hospital, 4650 Sunset Blvd, MS 54, Los Angeles, CA 90027-6062; **Phone:** 323-669-2205; **Board Cert:** Pediatrics 1973; Pediatric Hematology-Oncology 1976; **Med School:** Boston Univ 1967; **Resid:** Pediatrics, Univ Minnesota Hosps 1969; **Fellow:** Pediatric Hematology-Oncology, Natl Cancer Inst 1972; **Fac Appt:** Prof Ped, USC Sch Med

Wilkinson, Robert W MD [PHO] - **Hospital:** Kapiolani Med Ctr for Women & Chldn; **Address:** Kapiolani Med Ctr for Women & Children, 1319 Punahou St, Ste 1050, Honolulu, HI 96826; **Phone:** 808-942-8144; **Board Cert:** Pediatrics 1986; Pediatric Hematology-Oncology 1986; **Med School:** Tulane Univ 1967; **Resid:** Pediatrics, Los Angeles Co-USC Med Ctr 1971; **Fellow:** Pediatric Hematology-Oncology, Los Angeles Co-USC Med Ctr 1972; **Fac Appt:** Assoc Prof Ped, Univ Hawaii JA Burns Sch Med

Pediatric Infectious Disease

New England

Andiman, Warren A MD [PInf] - **Spec Exp:** AIDS/HIV; Viral Infections; **Hospital:** Yale - New Haven Hosp; **Address:** 333 Cedar St, rm 418 LSOG, Box 208064, New Haven, CT 06520-8064; **Phone:** 203-785-4730; **Board Cert:** Pediatrics 1975; **Med School:** Albert Einstein Coll Med 1969; **Resid:** Pediatrics, Babies Hosp-Columbia Presby 1971; **Fellow:** Pediatric Infectious Disease, Yale Univ Sch Med 1973; **Fac Appt:** Prof Ped, Yale Univ

Baltimore, Robert MD [PInf] - **Spec Exp:** Neonatal Infections; Hospital Acquired Infections; **Hospital:** Yale - New Haven Hosp; **Address:** Yale Univ Sch Med, Dept Pediatrics, 333 Cedar St, Box 208064, New Haven, CT 06520-8064; **Phone:** 203-785-4655; **Board Cert:** Pediatrics 1975; Pediatric Infectious Disease 2002; **Med School:** SUNY Buffalo 1968; **Resid:** Pediatrics, Univ Chicago Hosps 1971; **Fellow:** Infectious Disease, Boston City Hosp-Harvard 1976; **Fac Appt:** Prof Ped, Yale Univ

Durbin Jr, William Applebee MD [PInf] - **Hospital:** UMass Meml - Univ Campus; **Address:** 55 Lake Ave N, Worcester, MA 01655; **Phone:** 508-856-2650; **Board Cert:** Pediatrics 1978; Pediatric Infectious Disease 2002; **Med School:** Columbia P&S 1972; **Resid:** Pediatrics, Boston Chlns Hosp 1977; **Fellow:** Infectious Disease, Boston Chldns Hosp/Beth Israel 1979; **Fac Appt:** Prof Ped, Univ Mass Sch Med

Jenson, Hal B MD [PInf] - **Spec Exp:** Viral Infections; Tumor Virology; Vaccines; **Hospital:** Baystate Med Ctr; **Address:** 759 Chestnut St, Springfield, MA 01199; **Phone:** 419-794-5588; **Board Cert:** Pediatrics 1985; Pediatric Infectious Disease 2002; **Med School:** Geo Wash Univ 1979; **Resid:** Pediatrics, Rainbow Babies-Chldns Hosp. 1983; **Fellow:** Pediatric Infectious Disease, Yale Univ Sch Med 1985; **Fac Appt:** Prof Ped, Tufts Univ

Shapiro, Eugene D MD [PInf] - **Spec Exp:** Lyme Disease; Vaccines; **Hospital:** Yale - New Haven Hosp; **Address:** Chldns Hosp at Yale New Haven, 333 Cedar St, Box 208064, New Haven, CT 06520-8064; **Phone:** 203-688-4518; **Board Cert:** Pediatrics 1980; Pediatric Infectious Disease 2002; **Med School:** UCSF 1976; **Resid:** Pediatrics, Chldns Hosp 1979; **Fellow:** Pediatric Infectious Disease, Chldns Hosp 1981; Research, Yale Univ 1983; **Fac Appt:** Prof Ped, Yale Univ

Mid Atlantic

Borkowsky, William MD [PInf] - **Spec Exp:** AIDS/HIV; **Hospital:** NYU Med Ctr (page 67), Bellevue Hosp Ctr; **Address:** 550 1st Ave, Dept Pediatrics, New York, NY 10016; **Phone:** 212-263-6513; **Board Cert:** Pediatrics 1979; Infectious Disease 1979; **Med School:** NYU Sch Med 1979; **Resid:** Pediatrics, Bellevue Hosp Ctr 1975; **Fellow:** Infectious Disease, Bellevue Hosp Ctr-NYU 1978; **Fac Appt:** Prof Ped, NYU Sch Med

Krilov, Leonard MD [PInf] - **Spec Exp:** Infections-Respiratory; Infections in Int'l Adopted Children; Chronic Fatigue Syndrome; Lyme Disease; **Hospital:** Winthrop - Univ Hosp; **Address:** 120 Mineola Blvd, Ste 210, Mineola, NY 11501; **Phone:** 516-663-9570; **Board Cert:** Pediatrics 2001; Pediatric Infectious Disease 2001; **Med School:** Columbia P&S 1978; **Resid:** Pediatrics, Johns Hopkins Hosp 1981; **Fellow:** Pediatric Infectious Disease, Chldns Hosp 1984; **Fac Appt:** Prof Ped, SUNY Stony Brook

Long, Sarah S MD [PInf] - **Spec Exp:** Whooping Cough; Vaccines; Antibiotic Resistance; **Hospital:** St Christopher's Hosp for Chldn; **Address:** St Christopher's Hosp for Children, Erie Ave at Front St, Ste 1112, Philadelphia, PA 19134; **Phone:** 215-427-5201; **Board Cert:** Pediatrics 2002; Pediatric Infectious Disease 2002; **Med School:** Jefferson Med Coll 1970; **Resid:** Pediatrics, St Christophers Hosp Chldn 1973; **Fellow:** Pediatric Infectious Disease, Temple Univ Sch Med 1975; **Fac Appt:** Prof Ped, Drexel Univ Coll Med

Munoz, Jose Luis MD [PInf] - **Spec Exp:** Lyme Disease; Immune Deficiency; AIDS/HIV; **Hospital:** Westchester Med Ctr; **Address:** Ped Infectious Disease, 19 Bradhurst Ave, Hawthorne, NY 10532; **Phone:** 914-493-8333; **Board Cert:** Pediatrics 1989; Pediatric Infectious Disease 2002; **Med School:** Yale Univ 1978; **Resid:** Pediatrics, Yale New Haven Hosp 1981; **Fellow:** Pediatric Infectious Disease, Univ Rochester 1984; **Fac Appt:** Assoc Prof Ped, NY Med Coll

Pediatric Infectious Disease

Saiman, Lisa MD [PInf] - **Spec Exp:** Cystic Fibrosis Infection; Fungal Infections; Hospital Acquired Infections; Tuberculosis; **Hospital:** NYPresby-Morgan Stanley Children's Hosp; **Address:** 650 W 168th St Fl PH1 W - rm 470, New York, NY 10032; **Phone:** 212-305-9446; **Board Cert:** Pediatrics 1987; Pediatric Infectious Disease 2002; **Med School:** Albert Einstein Coll Med 1983; **Resid:** Pediatrics, Babies Hosp/NY Presbyterian 1986; **Fellow:** Infectious Disease, Babies Hosp/NY Prebyterian 1989; **Fac Appt:** Assoc Clin Prof Ped, Columbia P&S

Singh, Nalini MD [PInf] - **Hospital:** Chldns Natl Med Ctr; **Address:** Chldns National Med Ctr, Div Inf Disease, 111 Michigan Ave NW, Ste 3.5 West Wing, rm 100, Washington, DC 20010; **Phone:** 202-884-5051; **Board Cert:** Pediatrics 1982; Pediatric Infectious Disease 2005; **Med School:** India 1973; **Resid:** Pediatrics, U Mass Med Ctr 1979; **Fellow:** Infectious Disease, Natl Inst Hlth 1982; **Fac Appt:** Assoc Prof Ped, Geo Wash Univ

Southeast

Clements III, Dennis A MD/PhD [PInf] - **Hospital:** Duke Univ Med Ctr; **Address:** Duke Univ Med Center, Box 2802, Durham, NC 27710; **Phone:** 919-681-4080; **Board Cert:** Pediatrics 1978; Pediatric Infectious Disease 2004; **Med School:** Univ Rochester 1973; **Resid:** Pediatrics, Duke Univ Med Ctr 1976; **Fellow:** Pediatric Infectious Disease, Duke Univ Med Ctr 1988; **Fac Appt:** Assoc Prof Ped, Duke Univ

Edwards, Kathryn M MD [PInf] - **Spec Exp:** Vaccines; Clinical Trials; **Hospital:** Vanderbilt Univ Med Ctr; **Address:** Vanderbilt Univ, Peds Infectious Disease, 1161 21st Ave S, CCC-5323, Med Ctr N, Nashville, TN 37232-2581; **Phone:** 615-322-8792; **Board Cert:** Pediatrics 1978; Pediatric Infectious Disease 2005; **Med School:** Univ Iowa Coll Med 1973; **Resid:** Pediatrics, Childrens Meml Hosp 1976; **Fellow:** Pediatric Infectious Disease, Childrens Meml Hosp 1980; **Fac Appt:** Prof Ped, Vanderbilt Univ

Emmanuel, Patricia MD [PInf] - **Spec Exp:** Infections in Immunocompromised Patients; AIDS/HIV; Congenital Infections; **Hospital:** Tampa Genl Hosp, All Children's Hosp; **Address:** 17 Davis Blvd, Ste 313, Tampa, FL 33606; **Phone:** 813-259-8800; **Board Cert:** Pediatrics 2004; Pediatric Infectious Disease 2002; **Med School:** Univ Fla Coll Med 1986; **Resid:** Pediatrics, Univ So Fla 1989; **Fellow:** Infectious Disease, Univ So Fla 1993; **Fac Appt:** Assoc Prof Ped, Univ S Fla Coll Med

Givner, Laurence Bruce MD [PInf] - **Spec Exp:** Streptococcal Infections; Rocky Mountain Spotted Fever; **Hospital:** Wake Forest Univ Baptist Med Ctr (page 73), Brenner Chldrn's Hosp; **Address:** Wake Forest Univ Sch Med, Dept Ped, Medical Center Blvd, Winston Salem, NC 27157-0001; **Phone:** 336-716-6568; **Board Cert:** Pediatrics 1984; Pediatric Infectious Disease 2001; **Med School:** Univ MD Sch Med 1978; **Resid:** Pediatrics, Univ Maryland 1982; **Fellow:** Infectious Disease, Baylor Coll Med 1984; **Fac Appt:** Prof Ped, Wake Forest Univ

Ingram, David MD [PInf] - **Hospital:** WakeMed New Bern; **Address:** WakeMed - Andrews Ctr, 3024 New Bern Ave, Raleigh, NC 27610; **Phone:** 919-350-2800; **Board Cert:** Pediatrics 1980; Pediatric Infectious Disease 1994; **Med School:** Yale Univ 1967; **Resid:** Pediatrics, Yale-New Haven Hosp 1971; **Fellow:** Pediatric Infectious Disease, Chldns Hosp Med Ctr 1973; **Fac Appt:** Prof Ped, Univ NC Sch Med

McKinney Jr, Ross E MD [PInf] - **Spec Exp:** Infections in Immunocompromised Patients; **Hospital:** Duke Univ Med Ctr; **Address:** Duke Univ Med Ctr, Box 3461, Durham, NC 27710; **Phone:** 919-684-6335; **Board Cert:** Pediatrics 1983; Pediatric Infectious Disease 2002; **Med School:** Univ Rochester 1979; **Resid:** Pediatrics, Duke Univ Med Ctr 1985; **Fellow:** Pediatric Infectious Disease, Duke Univ Med Ctr 1982; **Fac Appt:** Assoc Prof Ped, Duke Univ

Mitchell, Charles D MD [PInf] - **Spec Exp:** AIDS/HIV; Viral Infections; **Hospital:** Jackson Meml Hosp; **Address:** Miller Sch Med, Div Infectious Disease, PO Box 016960, Miami, FL 33101; **Phone:** 305-243-2700; **Board Cert:** Pediatric Infectious Disease 2002; Pediatrics 1986; **Med School:** Univ Tex Med Br, Galveston 1977; **Resid:** Pediatrics, Univ Minn Hosp 1981; **Fellow:** Pediatric Infectious Disease, Univ Minn Hosp 1984; **Fac Appt:** Asst Prof Ped, Univ Miami Sch Med

Scott, Gwendolyn MD [PInf] - **Spec Exp:** AIDS/HIV; **Hospital:** Jackson Meml Hosp, Univ of Miami Hosp & Clins/Sylvester Comp Canc Ctr; **Address:** Univ Miami, Dept Peds-Div Inf Dis/Immun, PO Box 016960 (D4-4), Miami, FL 33101; **Phone:** 305-243-6676; **Board Cert:** Pediatrics 1978; Pediatric Infectious Disease 2002; **Med School:** UCSF 1972; **Resid:** Pediatrics, San Francisco Genl Hosp 1973; Pediatrics, Univ Maryland Hosp 1975; **Fellow:** Pediatric Infectious Disease, Univ Miami 1978; **Fac Appt:** Prof Ped, Univ Miami Sch Med

Midwest

Kleiman, Martin B MD [PInf] - **Spec Exp:** Histoplasmosis; Blastomycosis; Meningitis; AIDS/HIV; **Hospital:** Riley Hosp for Children; **Address:** 702 Barnhill Drive, Ste ROC4380, Indianapolis, IN 46202; **Phone:** 317-274-7260; **Board Cert:** Pediatrics 1973; Pediatric Infectious Disease 2002; **Med School:** SUNY Upstate Med Univ 1968; **Resid:** Pediatrics, Upstate Med Ctr 1971; **Fellow:** Infectious Disease, Johns Hopkins Hosp 1976; **Fac Appt:** Prof Ped, Indiana Univ

Shulman, Stanford MD [PInf] - **Spec Exp:** Kawasaki Disease; Streptococcal Infections; **Hospital:** Children's Mem Hosp, Northwestern Meml Hosp; **Address:** Children's Meml Hosp, 2300 Children's Plaza, Box 20, Chicago, IL 60614-3318; **Phone:** 773-880-4187; **Board Cert:** Pediatrics 1972; Pediatric Infectious Disease 2002; **Med School:** Univ Chicago-Pritzker Sch Med 1967; **Resid:** Pediatrics, Univ Chicago Hosps 1970; **Fellow:** Infectious Disease, Shands Hosp-Univ Florida 1973; **Fac Appt:** Prof Ped, Northwestern Univ

Wald, Ellen MD [PInf] - **Spec Exp:** Urinary Tract Infections; Infections-Respiratory; Meningitis; **Hospital:** Univ WI Hosp & Clins; **Address:** Univ Wisconsin Chldns Hosp, 600 Highland Ave, Box 4108, Madison, WI 57392; **Phone:** 608-263-8558; **Board Cert:** Pediatrics 1973; Pediatric Infectious Disease 2002; **Med School:** SUNY Downstate 1968; **Resid:** Pediatrics, Kings Co Hosp 1971; **Fellow:** Infectious Disease, Univ Maryland Hosp 1973; **Fac Appt:** Prof Ped, Univ Wisc

Southwest

Baker, Carol J MD [PInf] - **Spec Exp:** Streptococcal Infections; Neonatal Infections; Vaccines; **Hospital:** Texas Chldns Hosp - Houston, Ben Taub General Hosp; **Address:** Baylor Coll Med, Dept Peds, One Baylor Plaza, rm 302 A, MC BTM320, Houston, TX 77030; **Phone:** 713-798-4790; **Board Cert:** Pediatrics 1973; Pediatric Infectious Disease 2002; **Med School:** Baylor Coll Med 1968; **Resid:** Pediatrics, Baylor Coll Med 1971; **Fellow:** Pediatric Infectious Disease, Baylor Coll Med 1973; Infectious Disease, Boston City Hosp/Harvard Med Sch 1974; **Fac Appt:** Prof Ped, Baylor Coll Med

Pediatric Infectious Disease

Jacobs, Richard F MD [PInf] - **Spec Exp:** Tuberculosis; Viral Infections; Drug Discovery & Development; **Hospital:** Arkansas Chldns Hosp, UAMS Med Ctr; **Address:** 800 Marshall St, Slot 512-11, Little Rock, AR 72202-3591; **Phone:** 501-364-1416; **Board Cert:** Pediatrics 1982; Pediatric Infectious Disease 2002; **Med School:** Univ Ark 1977; **Resid:** Pediatrics, Ark Chldns Hosp 1980; **Fellow:** Infectious Disease, Univ Washington 1982; **Fac Appt:** Prof Ped, Univ Ark

Kaplan, Sheldon MD [PInf] - **Spec Exp:** Pneumococcal Infections; Meningitis; **Hospital:** Texas Chldns Hosp - Houston; **Address:** Texas Chldns Hosp, Div Infectious Disease, 6621 Fannin St, MC 3-2371, Houston, TX 77030; **Phone:** 832-824-4330; **Board Cert:** Pediatrics 1978; Pediatric Infectious Disease 2002; **Med School:** Univ MO-Columbia Sch Med 1973; **Resid:** Pediatrics, St Louis Chldns Hosp 1975; **Fellow:** Pediatric Infectious Disease, St Louis Chldns Hosp 1977; **Fac Appt:** Prof Ped, Baylor Coll Med

Kline, Mark MD [PInf] - **Spec Exp:** AIDS/HIV; **Hospital:** Texas Chldns Hosp - Houston; **Address:** Texas Children's Hosp, 6621 Fannin St, MC CCC1210, Houston, TX 77030; **Phone:** 832-822-1038; **Board Cert:** Pediatrics 1987; Pediatric Infectious Disease 2002; **Med School:** Baylor Coll Med 1981; **Resid:** Pediatrics, Baylor Coll Med 1985; **Fellow:** Pediatric Infectious Disease, Baylor Coll Med 1987; **Fac Appt:** Prof Ped, Baylor Coll Med

McCracken Jr, George H MD [PInf] - **Spec Exp:** Meningitis; Antibiotic Resistance; **Hospital:** UT Southwestern Med Ctr - Dallas; **Address:** Univ Texas SW Med Ctr, Dept Peds, 5323 Harry Hines Blvd, Ste F3-202, MC 9063, Dallas, TX 75390-9063; **Phone:** 214-456-6500; **Board Cert:** Pediatrics 1967; Pediatric Infectious Disease 2002; **Med School:** Cornell Univ-Weill Med Coll 1962; **Resid:** Pediatrics, NY-Cornell Med Ctr 1965; Pediatrics, Univ Texas SW Med Ctr 1966

West Coast and Pacific

Bradley, John S MD [PInf] - **Spec Exp:** Meningitis; Brain Infections; **Hospital:** Rady Children's Hosp - San Diego; **Address:** 3020 Children's Way, MC 5041, San Diego, CA 92123; **Phone:** 858-966-7785; **Board Cert:** Pediatrics 1981; Pediatric Infectious Disease 2002; **Med School:** UC Davis 1976; **Resid:** Pediatrics, UC Davis Med Ctr 1980; **Fellow:** Pediatric Infectious Disease, Stanford Univ Hosp; **Fac Appt:** Assoc Clin Prof Ped, UCSD

Bryson, Yvonne J MD [PInf] - **Spec Exp:** AIDS/HIV; Herpes Simplex; **Hospital:** UCLA Med Ctr; **Address:** 10833 Le Conte Ave, MDCC, rm 22-442, Los Angeles, CA 90095-1752; **Phone:** 310-825-5235; **Board Cert:** Pediatrics 1976; **Med School:** Univ Tex SW, Dallas 1970; **Resid:** Pediatrics, UCSD Med Ctr 1974; **Fellow:** Infectious Disease, UCSD Med Ctr 1976; **Fac Appt:** Prof Ped, UCLA

Cherry, James D MD [PInf] - **Spec Exp:** Vaccines; Infections-Respiratory; Viral Infections; **Hospital:** Mattel Chldns Hosp at UCLA, UCLA Med Ctr; **Address:** David Geffen Sch Med at UCLA, Dept Ped, 10833 Le Conte Ave, rm 22-442, Los Angeles, CA 90095-1752; **Phone:** 310-825-5226; **Board Cert:** Pediatrics 1962; Pediatric Infectious Disease 2002; **Med School:** Univ VT Coll Med 1957; **Resid:** Pediatrics, Boston City Hosp 1959; Pediatrics, Kings Co Hosp 1960; **Fellow:** Infectious Disease, Boston City Hosp 1962; Epidemiology, London Sch Hygiene & Trop Med 1983; **Fac Appt:** Prof Ped, UCLA

Mason, Wilbert Henry MD [PInf] - **Spec Exp:** Kawasaki Disease; **Hospital:** Chldns Hosp - Los Angeles (page 56), USC Univ Hosp - R K Eamer Med Plz; **Address:** Chldns Hosp, Div Inf Dis, 4650 Sunset Blvd, MS 51, Los Angeles, CA 90027-6062; **Phone:** 323-669-2509; **Board Cert:** Pediatrics 1975; Pediatric Infectious Disease 2002; **Med School:** UC Irvine 1970; **Resid:** Pediatrics, Chldns Hosp 1973; **Fellow:** Infectious Disease, Chldns Hosp 1974; **Fac Appt:** Assoc Clin Prof Ped, USC Sch Med

Petru, Ann MD [PInf] - **Spec Exp:** AIDS/HIV; **Hospital:** Chldns Hosp - Oakland; **Address:** Childrens Hosp, Div Infectious Disease, 747 52nd St, Oakland, CA 94609; **Phone:** 510-428-3336; **Board Cert:** Pediatrics 1983; Pediatric Infectious Disease 2002; **Med School:** UCSF 1978; **Resid:** Pediatrics, Chldns Hosp Med Ctr 1982; **Fellow:** Pediatric Infectious Disease, Chldns Hosp Med Ctr 1983; **Fac Appt:** Asst Clin Prof Med, UCSF

Pediatric Nephrology

New England

Friedman, Aaron MD [PNep] - **Spec Exp:** Hypertension; Transplant Medicine-Kidney; Growth Disorders; **Hospital:** Rhode Island Hosp; **Address:** RIH Dept of Pediatrics, 593 Eddy St, Hasbro 125, Providence, RI 02903; **Phone:** 401-444-5648; **Board Cert:** Pediatrics 1979; Pediatric Nephrology 2003; **Med School:** SUNY Upstate Med Univ 1974; **Resid:** Pediatrics, Univ Wisconsin 1976; **Fellow:** Pediatric Nephrology, Univ Wisconsin 1980; **Fac Appt:** Prof Ped, Univ Wisc

Harmon, William E MD [PNep] - **Hospital:** Children's Hospital - Boston; **Address:** Chldns Hosp, Div Nephrology, 300 Longwood Ave, Hunnewell 319, Boston, MA 02115; **Phone:** 617-355-6129; **Board Cert:** Pediatrics 1976; **Med School:** Case West Res Univ 1971; **Resid:** Pediatrics, Chldns Hosp Med Ctr 1976; **Fellow:** Pediatric Nephrology, Chldns Hosp Med Ctr 1979; **Fac Appt:** Assoc Prof Ped, Harvard Med Sch

Mid Atlantic

Dabbagh, Shermine MD [PNep] - **Spec Exp:** Kidney Disease; Kidney Failure-Chronic; Transplant Medicine-Kidney; **Hospital:** Alfred I duPont Hosp for Children; **Address:** Dupont Hosp for Children, Div Nephrology, 1600 Rockland Rd, PO Box 269, Wilmington, DE 19899; **Phone:** 302-651-4426; **Board Cert:** Pediatrics 1985; Pediatric Nephrology 1985; **Med School:** Lebanon 1979; **Resid:** Pediatrics, Univ Virginia Hosp 1981; **Fellow:** Pediatric Nephrology, Univ Wisconsin 1984

Fivush, Barbara A MD [PNep] - **Spec Exp:** Transplant Medicine-Kidney; **Hospital:** Johns Hopkins Hosp - Baltimore (page 61); **Address:** Johns Hopkins Hosp-Div. Nephrology, 200 N Wolfe St, rm 3055, Baltimore, MD 21287; **Phone:** 410-955-2467; **Board Cert:** Pediatrics 1984; Pediatric Nephrology 2003; **Med School:** Boston Univ 1978; **Resid:** Pediatrics, Johns Hopkins Hosp 1981; **Fellow:** Pediatric Nephrology, Johns Hopkins Hosp 1983; Pediatric Nephrology, Childns Hosp Natl Med Ctr 1984; **Fac Appt:** Assoc Prof Ped, Johns Hopkins Univ

Kaplan, Bernard S MD [PNep] - **Spec Exp:** Hemolytic Uremic Syndrome; Polycystic Kidney Disease; **Hospital:** Chldns Hosp of Philadelphia, The; **Address:** Chldns Hosp of Philadelphia, Div Nephrology, 34 St & Civic Ctr Blvd, rm 2143, Philadelphia, PA 19104; **Phone:** 215-590-2449; **Board Cert:** Pediatrics 1972; Pediatric Nephrology 1974; **Med School:** South Africa 1964; **Resid:** Pediatrics, Baragwanath Hosp, Transvaal Meml Hosp 1970; Nephrology, Royal Victoria Hosp 1973; **Fellow:** Nephrology, Montreal Chldns Hosp 1972; **Fac Appt:** Prof Ped, Univ Pennsylvania

Mendley, Susan MD [PNep] - **Spec Exp:** Transplant Medicine-Kidney; Hypertension; Dialysis Care; **Hospital:** Univ of MD Med Sys; **Address:** Univ Maryland Med System, 22 S Greene St, Pediatric Nephrol N5W67, Baltimore, MD 21201; **Phone:** 410-328-5303; **Board Cert:** Internal Medicine 1988; Nephrology 2000; **Med School:** Boston Univ 1984; **Resid:** Internal Medicine, Univ Chicago Hosps 1987; **Fellow:** Nephrology, Univ Chicago 1990; Pediatric Nephrology, Chldns Meml Hosp/Northwestern Univ 1991; **Fac Appt:** Asst Prof Ped, Univ MD Sch Med

Pediatric Nephrology

Nash, Martin MD [PNep] - **Spec Exp:** Nephrotic Syndrome; Kidney Failure; Urinary Abnormalities; **Hospital:** NYPresby-Morgan Stanley Children's Hosp; **Address:** Morgan Stanley Chlds Hosp of NY-Presby, 3959 Broadway, rm 701, New York, NY 10032-1559; **Phone:** 212-305-5825; **Board Cert:** Pediatrics 1969; Nephrology 1974; **Med School:** Duke Univ 1964; **Resid:** Internal Medicine, Georgetown Univ Hosp 1965; Pediatrics, Columbia-Presby Med Ctr 1967; **Fellow:** Pediatric Nephrology, Montefiore Med Ctr 1971; **Fac Appt:** Clin Prof Ped, Columbia P&S

Roskes, Saul David MD [PNep] - **Hospital:** Johns Hopkins Hosp - Baltimore (page 61); **Address:** 10807 Falls Rd, Ste 200, Lutherville, MD 21093; **Phone:** 410-321-9393; **Board Cert:** Pediatrics 1970; Pediatric Nephrology 1976; **Med School:** Johns Hopkins Univ 1963; **Resid:** Pediatrics, Bronx Muni Hosp Ctr 1965; Pediatrics, Johns Hopkins Hosp 1968; **Fac Appt:** Assoc Prof Ped, Johns Hopkins Univ

Southeast

Chandar, Jayanthi MD [PNep] - **Spec Exp:** Kidney Disease; Transplant Medicine-Kidney; Renal Replacement Therapy; **Hospital:** Jackson Meml Hosp; **Address:** Univ Miami, Dept Peds-Div Nephrology, PO Box 016960 (M-714), Miami, FL 33163; **Phone:** 305-585-6726; **Board Cert:** Pediatric Nephrology 2003; Pediatrics 2004; **Med School:** India 1983; **Resid:** Pediatrics, Jackson Memorial Hosp 1987; **Fellow:** Pediatric Nephrology, Jackson Memorial Hosp; **Fac Appt:** Assoc Prof Ped, Univ Miami Sch Med

Fennell III, Robert S MD [PNep] - **Spec Exp:** Transplant Medicine-Kidney; Kidney Failure-Chronic; **Hospital:** Shands Hlthcre at Univ of FL; **Address:** Shands Healthcare at Univ Florida, 1600 SW Archer Rd, Box 100296, Gainesville, FL 32610-0296; **Phone:** 352-392-4434; **Board Cert:** Pediatrics 1974; Pediatric Nephrology 2000; **Med School:** Univ Fla Coll Med 1964; **Resid:** Pediatrics, Shands Teaching Hosp 1971; **Fellow:** Pediatric Nephrology, Shands Teaching Hosp 1973; **Fac Appt:** Prof Ped, Univ Fla Coll Med

Garin, Eduardo Humberto MD [PNep] - **Hospital:** Shands Hlthcre at Univ of FL; **Address:** Shands Healthcare, Dept Ped Nephrology, 1600 SW Archer Rd, rm HD214, Box 100296, Gainesville, FL 32610; **Phone:** 352-392-4434; **Board Cert:** Pediatrics 1976; Pediatric Nephrology 1976; **Med School:** Chile 1970; **Resid:** Pediatrics, Univ Hosp and Clinics 1973; **Fellow:** Pediatric Nephrology, Shands Hosp Univ FL 1975; **Fac Appt:** Prof Ped, Univ S Fla Coll Med

Neiberger, Richard E MD/PhD [PNep] - **Spec Exp:** Kidney Disease-Genetic; **Hospital:** Shands Hlthcre at Univ of FL; **Address:** Univ Florida College of Medicine, Div Pediatric Nephrology, 1600 SW Archer Rd, Gainesville, FL 32610; **Phone:** 352-392-4434; **Board Cert:** Pediatrics 1999; Nephrology 1999; **Med School:** Univ Louisville Sch Med 1982; **Resid:** Pediatrics, Montefiore Med Ctr 1985; **Fellow:** Pediatric Nephrology, Montefiore Med Ctr 1988; **Fac Appt:** Assoc Prof Ped, Univ Fla Coll Med

Wyatt, Robert J MD [PNep] - **Spec Exp:** Kidney Disease-Autoimmune; Berger's Disease (IgA Nephropathy); **Hospital:** Le Bonheur Chldns Med Ctr; **Address:** Univ Tennessee, Dept Peds, 777 Washington Ave, Ste P110, Memphis, TN 38105; **Phone:** 901-448-2070; **Board Cert:** Pediatrics 1978; Pediatric Nephrology 1979; **Med School:** Med Coll GA 1973; **Resid:** Pediatrics, Kentucky Med Ctr 1976; **Fellow:** Pediatric Nephrology, Cincinnati Chldns Hosp 1979; **Fac Appt:** Prof Ped, Univ Tenn Coll Med, Memphis

Zilleruelo, Gaston E MD [PNep] - **Spec Exp:** Transplant Medicine-Kidney; Nephrotic Syndrome; Congenital Anomalies-Genitourinary; **Hospital:** Jackson Meml Hosp, Broward General Med Ctr; **Address:** Univ Miami, Dept Peds-Div Nephrology, PO Box 016960 (M-714), Miami, FL 33136; **Phone:** 305-585-6726; **Board Cert:** Pediatrics 1979; Pediatric Nephrology 1991; **Med School:** Chile 1969; **Resid:** Pediatrics, L Calvo-Mackenna Chldns Hosp 1972; Pediatrics, Jackson Meml Hosp 1977; **Fellow:** Pediatric Nephrology, Jackson Meml Hosp 1979; **Fac Appt:** Prof Ped, Univ Miami Sch Med

Midwest

Andreoli, Sharon MD [PNep] - **Spec Exp:** Kidney Disease; Hypertension; **Hospital:** Riley Hosp for Children, Indiana Univ Hosp; **Address:** 699 West Drive, rm 213, Indianapolis, IN 46202; **Phone:** 317-278-0854; **Board Cert:** Pediatrics 1983; Pediatric Nephrology 1985; **Med School:** Indiana Univ 1978; **Resid:** Pediatrics, James W Riley Hosp 1981; **Fellow:** Pediatric Nephrology, Univ Minnesota 1981; Pediatric Nephrology, James W Riley Hosp/Indiana Univ 1984; **Fac Appt:** Prof Ped, Indiana Univ

Avner, Ellis D MD [PNep] - **Spec Exp:** Polycystic Kidney Disease; Kidney Disease-Genetic; **Hospital:** Chldns Hosp - Wisconsin; **Address:** Medical Coll Wisconsin, 999 92nd Ave, Milwaukee, WI 53226; **Phone:** 414-337-7702; **Board Cert:** Pediatrics 1980; Pediatric Nephrology 1982; **Med School:** Univ Pennsylvania 1975; **Resid:** Pediatrics, Chldns Hosp Med Ctr 1978; **Fellow:** Pediatric Nephrology, Chldns Hosp Med Ctr 1980; **Fac Appt:** Prof Ped, Med Coll Wisc

Bunchman, Timothy E MD [PNep] - **Spec Exp:** Lupus/SLE; **Hospital:** DeVos Children's Hosp; **Address:** DeVos Ped Nephrology/Transplant, 221 Michigan Ave NE, MC 083, Grand Rapids, MI 49503; **Phone:** 616-391-3788; **Board Cert:** Pediatrics 1986; Pediatric Nephrology 2003; **Med School:** Loyola Univ-Stritch Sch Med 1981; **Resid:** Internal Medicine & Pediatrics, St Louis Univ 1982; Pediatrics, St Louis Univ 1984; **Fellow:** Pediatric Nephrology, Mayo Clinic 1986; Pediatric Nephrology, Univ Minn 1987; **Fac Appt:** Prof Ped, Univ Mich Med Sch

Cohn, Richard MD [PNep] - **Spec Exp:** Transplant Medicine-Kidney; Nephrotic Syndrome; Kidney Disease-Chronic; **Hospital:** Children's Mem Hosp; **Address:** Childrens Meml Hosp, 2300 Children's Plaza, MC-37, Chicago, IL 60614-3394; **Phone:** 773-327-3930; **Board Cert:** Pediatrics 1978; Pediatric Nephrology 1979; **Med School:** Albert Einstein Coll Med 1972; **Resid:** Pediatrics, Johns Hopkins Hosp 1975; **Fellow:** Pediatric Nephrology, Univ Minn 1978; **Fac Appt:** Prof Ped, Northwestern Univ

Davis, Ira D MD [PNep] - **Spec Exp:** Kidney Failure-Chronic; Transplant Medicine-Kidney; **Hospital:** Rainbow Babies & Chldns Hosp; **Address:** Rainbow Babies & Chldns Hosp, Div Pediatric Nephrology, 11100 Euclid Ave, Ste 787, Cleveland, OH 44106; **Phone:** 216-844-1389; **Board Cert:** Pediatrics 1999; Pediatric Nephrology 1999; **Med School:** Univ Minn 1980; **Resid:** Pediatrics, Univ Hosps-Case West Res 1987; **Fellow:** Pediatric Nephrology, Univ Minn Hosps 1990; **Fac Appt:** Assoc Prof Ped, Case West Res Univ

Kashtan, Clifford MD [PNep] - **Spec Exp:** Transplant Medicine-Kidney; Kidney Disease-Genetic; **Hospital:** Univ Minn Med Ctr, Fairview - Univ Campus; **Address:** Univ Minn, Dept Peds, 420 Delaware St SEd, MMC 491, Minneapolis, MN 55455; **Phone:** 612-626-2922; **Board Cert:** Pediatrics 1983; Pediatric Nephrology 2003; **Med School:** Wayne State Univ 1978; **Resid:** Pediatrics, Boston City Hosp 1981; **Fellow:** Pediatric Nephrology, Mass Genl Hosp 1984; Pediatric Nephrology, Univ Minnesota Hosp 1987; **Fac Appt:** Prof Ped, Univ Minn

Pediatric Nephrology

Langman, Craig MD [PNep] - **Spec Exp:** Kidney Stones; Osteoporosis-Juvenile; Oxalosis; **Hospital:** Children's Mem Hosp, Evanston Hosp; **Address:** Children's Meml Hosp, 2300 N Children's Plaza, Box 37, Chicago, IL 60614-3394; **Phone:** 773-327-3930; **Board Cert:** Pediatrics 1982; Pediatric Nephrology 1982; **Med School:** Hahnemann Univ 1977; **Resid:** Pediatrics, Chldns Hosp 1979; **Fellow:** Pediatric Nephrology, Chldns Hosp 1981; **Fac Appt:** Prof Ped, Northwestern Univ

Nevins, Thomas E MD [PNep] - **Spec Exp:** Kidney Failure-Chronic; Transplant Medicine-Kidney; Hypertension; **Hospital:** Univ Minn Med Ctr, Fairview - Univ Campus; **Address:** Fairview Univ Med Ctr, Dept Peds, 420 Delaware St SE, MMC-491, Minneapolis, MN 55455-0374; **Phone:** 612-626-2922; **Board Cert:** Pediatrics 1975; Pediatric Nephrology 1992; **Med School:** Washington Univ, St Louis 1969; **Resid:** Pediatrics, Univ Minnesota Hosps 1972; **Fellow:** Nephrology, Univ Minnesota Hosps 1978; **Fac Appt:** Prof Ped, Univ Minn

Warady, Bradley MD [PNep] - **Spec Exp:** Dialysis-Peritoneal; Transplant Medicine-Kidney; Kidney Disease-Chronic; **Hospital:** Chldns Mercy Hosps & Clinics; **Address:** Chldns Mercy Hosps & Clins, Dept Ped Nephrology, 2401 Gillham Rd, Kansas City, MO 64108; **Phone:** 816-234-3010; **Board Cert:** Pediatrics 1984; Pediatric Nephrology 1985; **Med School:** Univ IL Coll Med 1979; **Resid:** Pediatrics, Chldns Mercy Hosp 1982; **Fellow:** Pediatric Nephrology, Colorado Univ Med Ctr 1984

West Coast and Pacific

Alexander, Steven R MD [PNep] - **Spec Exp:** Kidney Failure; Transplant Medicine-Kidney; Nephrotic Syndrome; **Hospital:** Lucile Packard Chldns Hosp/Stanford Univ Med Ctr; **Address:** Stanford Univ Med Ctr, Dept Peds, 300 Pasteur Drive, rm G306, Stanford, CA 94305-5208; **Phone:** 650-723-7903; **Board Cert:** Pediatrics 1986; Pediatric Nephrology 1986; **Med School:** Baylor Coll Med 1971; **Resid:** Pediatrics, Baylor Affil Hosps 1976; **Fellow:** Pediatric Nephrology, Baylor Affil Hosps 1978; **Fac Appt:** Prof Ped, Stanford Univ

Ettenger, Robert B MD [PNep] - **Spec Exp:** Transplant Medicine-Kidney; Hypertension in Children; Urinary Tract Infections; Kidney Disease; **Hospital:** UCLA Med Ctr, Mattel Chldns Hosp at UCLA; **Address:** Mattel Chldns Hosp, Dept Ped Nephrology, 10833 Le Conte Ave, Box 951752, Los Angeles, CA 90095; **Phone:** 310-206-6987; **Board Cert:** Pediatrics 1986; Pediatric Nephrology 1986; **Med School:** Univ Pennsylvania 1968; **Resid:** Pediatrics, St Christophers Hosp Chldn 1971; **Fellow:** Pediatric Nephrology, Chldns Hosp 1975; **Fac Appt:** Prof Ped, UCLA

Flynn, Joseph T MD [PNep] - **Spec Exp:** Hypertension; Dialysis Care; **Hospital:** Chldns Hosp and Regl Med Ctr - Seattle; **Address:** Children's Hospital, Ped Nephrology, PO Box 5371, Seattle, WA 98105; **Phone:** 206-987-2524; **Board Cert:** Pediatrics 2001; Pediatric Nephrology 2001; **Med School:** SUNY Upstate Med Univ 1987; **Resid:** Pediatrics, St Christophers Hosp 1990; **Fellow:** Pediatric Nephrology, St Christophers Hosp 1993; **Fac Appt:** Prof Ped, Univ Wash

Jordan, Stanley C MD [PNep] - **Spec Exp:** Transplant Medicine-Kidney; **Hospital:** Cedars-Sinai Med Ctr; **Address:** Cedars Sinai Med Ctr, Div Ped Nephrology, 8635 W 3rd St, Ste 590W, Los Angeles, CA 90048; **Phone:** 310-423-2624; **Board Cert:** Pediatrics 1978; Pediatric Nephrology 1979; Clinical & Laboratory Immunology 1988; **Med School:** Univ NC Sch Med 1973; **Resid:** Pediatrics, UCLA Med Ctr 1976; Pediatric Nephrology, UCLA Med Ctr 1977; **Fellow:** Renal Immunology, Scripps Clinic 1978; Dialysis & Tranplantation, Chldns Hosp 1980; **Fac Appt:** Prof Ped, UCLA

McDonald, Ruth A MD [PNep] - **Spec Exp:** Transplant Medicine-Kidney; Kidney Disease; **Hospital:** Chldns Hosp and Regl Med Ctr - Seattle; **Address:** 4800 Sand Point Way NE, MS M1-5, Seattle, WA 98105; **Phone:** 206-987-2524; **Board Cert:** Pediatric Nephrology 2005; **Med School:** Univ Minn 1987; **Resid:** Pediatrics, Chldns Hosp & Med Ctr 1990; **Fellow:** Pediatric Nephrology, Chldns Hosp & Med Ctr 1993; **Fac Appt:** Assoc Prof Ped, Univ Wash

Stapleton, F Bruder MD [PNep] - **Spec Exp:** Kidney Stones; Uric Acid Disorders; **Hospital:** Chldns Hosp and Regl Med Ctr - Seattle; **Address:** 4800 Sand Point Way NE, MS T0112, Seattle, WA 98105-3901; **Phone:** 206-987-2150; **Board Cert:** Pediatrics 1989; Pediatric Nephrology 1997; **Med School:** Univ Kans 1972; **Resid:** Pediatrics, Univ Washington Med Ctr 1974; **Fellow:** Pediatric Nephrology, Univ Kansas Med Ctr 1977; **Fac Appt:** Prof Ped, Univ Wash

Watkins, Sandra MD [PNep] - **Spec Exp:** Kidney Failure-Chronic; Hemolytic Uremic Syndrome; **Hospital:** Chldns Hosp and Regl Med Ctr - Seattle; **Address:** 4800 Sand Point Way NE, MS M1-5, Seattle, WA 98105; **Phone:** 206-987-2524; **Board Cert:** Pediatrics 1987; Pediatric Nephrology 1988; **Med School:** Univ Tex, Houston 1981; **Resid:** Pediatrics, Univ Wash Chldns Hosp 1984; **Fellow:** Nephrology, Univ Wash Sch Med 1986; **Fac Appt:** Prof Ped, Univ Wash

Pediatric Otolaryngology

New England

Cunningham, Michael MD [PO] - **Spec Exp:** Head & Neck Tumors; Sinus Disorders; Hemangiomas; **Hospital:** Mass Eye & Ear Infirmary, Mass Genl Hosp; **Address:** Mass Eye & Ear Infirmary, 243 Charles St, Boston, MA 02114; **Phone:** 617-573-4250; **Board Cert:** Otolaryngology 1988; **Med School:** Univ Rochester 1981; **Resid:** Pediatrics, Mass General Hosp 1983; Otolaryngology, U Pittsburgh Eye & Ear Hosp 1988; **Fellow:** Pediatric Otolaryngology, Mass Eye & Ear Infirm 1989; **Fac Appt:** Assoc Prof Oto, Harvard Med Sch

Eavey, Roland D MD [PO] - **Spec Exp:** Ear Reconstruction/Microtia; Ear Disorders/Surgery; **Hospital:** Mass Eye & Ear Infirmary; **Address:** Mass Eye & Ear Infirmary, 243 Charles St, Boston, MA 02114-3002; **Phone:** 617-573-3190; **Board Cert:** Pediatrics 1982; Otolaryngology 1981; **Med School:** Univ Pennsylvania 1975; **Resid:** Pediatrics, Chldns Hosp 1977; Surgery, Kaiser Hosp 1978; **Fellow:** Otolaryngology, Mass EE Infirm 1981; **Fac Appt:** Assoc Prof Oto, Harvard Med Sch

Healy, Gerald MD [PO] - **Hospital:** Children's Hospital - Boston; **Address:** Chldns Hosp, Dept Otolaryngology, 300 Longwood Ave, LO-367, Boston, MA 02115; **Phone:** 617-355-5064; **Board Cert:** Otolaryngology 1972; **Med School:** Boston Univ 1967; **Resid:** Surgery, Boston Univ Hosps 1969; Otolaryngology, Boston Univ Hosps 1972; **Fac Appt:** Prof Oto, Harvard Med Sch

McGill, Trevor MD [PO] - **Spec Exp:** Head & Neck Tumors; Cholesteatoma; Lymphatic Malformations-Head & Neck; Hemangiomas; **Hospital:** Children's Hospital - Boston; **Address:** Childrens Hosp, Dept Otolaryngology, 333 Longwood Ave, Boston, MA 02115; **Phone:** 617-355-6460; **Board Cert:** Otolaryngology 1988; **Med School:** Ireland 1967; **Resid:** Otolaryngology, Royal Natl Throat Nose & Ear Hosp 1974; **Fellow:** Otolaryngology, Mass Eye & Ear Infirmary 1976; **Fac Appt:** Prof Oto, Harvard Med Sch

Pediatric Otolaryngology

Mid Atlantic

April, Max M MD [PO] - **Spec Exp:** Sinus Disorders; Neck Masses; Laryngeal Disorders; **Hospital:** NY-Presby Hosp/Weill Cornell (page 66), Long Island Jewish Med Ctr; **Address:** Weill-Cornell Medical Ctr, Dept Otolaryngology, 1305 York Ave Fl 5, New York, NY 10021; **Phone:** 646-962-2225; **Board Cert:** Otolaryngology 1990; **Med School:** Boston Univ 1985; **Resid:** Otolaryngology, Boston Univ Med Ctr 1990; **Fellow:** Pediatric Otolaryngology, Johns Hopkins Hosp 1991

Bluestone, Charles D MD [PO] - **Spec Exp:** Otology; Sinusitis; **Hospital:** Chldns Hosp of Pittsburgh - UPMC; **Address:** Chldn Hosp, Dept Otolaryngology, 3705 5th Ave, Pittsburgh, PA 15213-2524; **Phone:** 412-692-5902; **Board Cert:** Otolaryngology 1963; **Med School:** Univ Pittsburgh 1958; **Resid:** Otolaryngology, Eye and Ear Infirmary 1962; **Fac Appt:** Prof Oto, Univ Pittsburgh

Dolitsky, Jay MD [PO] - **Spec Exp:** Ear Infections; Neck Masses; **Hospital:** New York Eye & Ear Infirm (page 65), St Vincent Cath Med Ctrs - Manhattan; **Address:** 404 Park Ave S Fl 12, New York, NY 10016; **Phone:** 212-679-3499; **Board Cert:** Otolaryngology 1990; **Med School:** SUNY Downstate 1981; **Resid:** Otolaryngology, Manhattan EE 1990; **Fellow:** Pediatric Otolaryngology, Children's Hosp 1992; **Fac Appt:** Assoc Prof Oto, NY Med Coll

Goldsmith, Ari J MD [PO] - **Spec Exp:** Voice Disorders; Airway Disorders; Hearing Loss; Sleep Apnea; **Hospital:** Schneider Chldn's Hosp; **Address:** 212-45 26th Ave, Ste 1, Bayside, NY 11360; **Phone:** 718-631-8899; **Board Cert:** Otolaryngology 1994; **Med School:** Albert Einstein Coll Med 1988; **Resid:** Otolaryngology, LI Jewish Hosp 1993; **Fellow:** Pediatric Otolaryngology, Children's Hospital 1994; **Fac Appt:** Assoc Prof Oto, SUNY Hlth Sci Ctr

Haddad Jr, Joseph MD [PO] - **Spec Exp:** Ear Infections; Sinus Disorders; Cleft Palate/Lip; **Hospital:** NYPresby-Morgan Stanley Children's Hosp; **Address:** Morgan Stanley Chldns Hosp of NY-Presby, 3959 Broadway, Ste 501N, New York, NY 10032-1559; **Phone:** 212-305-8933; **Board Cert:** Otolaryngology 1988; **Med School:** NYU Sch Med 1983; **Resid:** Surgery, Columbia-Presby Hosp 1985; Otolaryngology, Columbia-Presby Hosp 1988; **Fellow:** Pediatric Otolaryngology, Childrens Hosp 1990; **Fac Appt:** Clin Prof Oto, Columbia P&S

Jones, Jacqueline MD [PO] - **Spec Exp:** Sinus Disorders/Surgery; **Hospital:** NY-Presby Hosp/Weill Cornell (page 66), Lenox Hill Hosp (page 62); **Address:** 1175 Park Ave, Ste 1A, New York, NY 10128; **Phone:** 212-996-2559; **Board Cert:** Otolaryngology 1989; **Med School:** Cornell Univ-Weill Med Coll 1984; **Resid:** Otolaryngology, Hosp Univ Penn 1989; **Fellow:** Pediatric Otolaryngology, Chldns Hosp 1990; **Fac Appt:** Assoc Prof Oto, Cornell Univ-Weill Med Coll

Potsic, William P MD [PO] - **Spec Exp:** Ear Disorders/Surgery; Ear Tumors; Hearing Disorders; **Hospital:** Chldns Hosp of Philadelphia, The; **Address:** Childrens Hosp of Philadelphia, 34 St & Civic Center Blvd, Wood Bldg, Fl 1, Philadelphia, PA 19104; **Phone:** 215-590-3440; **Board Cert:** Otolaryngology 1974; **Med School:** Emory Univ 1969; **Resid:** Otolaryngology, Univ Chicago Hosps 1974; **Fac Appt:** Prof Oto, Univ Pennsylvania

Rosenfeld, Richard M MD [PO] - **Spec Exp:** Sinus Disorders/Surgery; Head & Neck Surgery; Cochlear Implants; Ear Disorders/Surgery; **Hospital:** Long Island Coll Hosp, SUNY Downstate Med Ctr; **Address:** Univ Otolaryngologists, 134 Atlantic Ave, Brooklyn, NY 11201; **Phone:** 718-780-1498; **Board Cert:** Otolaryngology 1989; **Med School:** SUNY Buffalo 1984; **Resid:** Otolaryngology, Mount Sinai Med Ctr 1989; **Fellow:** Pediatric Otolaryngology, Chldn's Hosp 1991; **Fac Appt:** Prof Oto, SUNY Downstate

Tunkel, David E MD [PO] - **Spec Exp:** Laryngeal Disorders; Otology; Head & Neck Surgery; **Hospital:** Johns Hopkins Hosp - Baltimore (page 61); **Address:** 601 N Caroline St, rm 6161, Baltimore, MD 21287; **Phone:** 410-955-1559; **Board Cert:** Otolaryngology 1990; **Med School:** Johns Hopkins Univ 1984; **Resid:** Surgery, Johns Hopkins Hosp 1986; Otolaryngology, Johns Hopkins Hosp 1990; **Fellow:** Pediatric Otolaryngology, Childrens Natl Med Ctr 1991; **Fac Appt:** Assoc Prof Oto, Johns Hopkins Univ

Ward, Robert MD [PO] - **Spec Exp:** Airway Disorders; Sinus Disorders/Surgery; Choanal Atresia; **Hospital:** NY-Presby Hosp/Weill Cornell (page 66), Manhattan Eye, Ear & Throat Hosp; **Address:** 1305 York Ave Fl 5, New York, NY 10021; **Phone:** 646-962-2224; **Board Cert:** Otolaryngology 1986; **Med School:** Cornell Univ-Weill Med Coll 1981; **Resid:** Surgery, New York Hosp 1983; Otolaryngology, New York Hosp 1986; **Fellow:** Pediatric Otolaryngology, Chldns Hosp 1986; **Fac Appt:** Assoc Clin Prof Oto, Cornell Univ-Weill Med Coll

Southeast

Darrow, David H MD/DDS [PO] - **Spec Exp:** Airway Disorders; Sinus Disorders; Otology; Neck Masses; **Hospital:** Chldns Hosp of King's Daughters; **Address:** Chldns Hosp of Kings Daughters, Div Otolaryngology, 601 Childrens Lane, Norfolk, VA 23507; **Phone:** 757-668-9327; **Board Cert:** Otolaryngology 1994; **Med School:** Duke Univ 1987; **Resid:** Otolaryngology, UCSD Med Ctr 1993; **Fellow:** Pediatric Otolaryngology, Chldns Meml Hosp 1994; **Fac Appt:** Assoc Prof Oto, Eastern VA Med Sch

Drake, Amelia MD [PO] - **Spec Exp:** Head & Neck Surgery; **Hospital:** Univ NC Hosps; **Address:** 130 Mason Farm Rd, 1115 Bio Informatics Bldg, Box 7070, Chapel Hill, NC 27599; **Phone:** 919-966-8926; **Board Cert:** Otolaryngology 1987; **Med School:** Univ NC Sch Med 1981; **Resid:** Otolaryngology, Univ Michigan Hosps 1986

Jahrsdoerfer, Robert A MD [PO] - **Spec Exp:** Hearing Loss; Aural Atresia Repair; Neuro-Otology; **Hospital:** Univ Virginia Med Ctr; **Address:** UVA Health System, Dept Otolaryngology, PO Box 800713, Charlottesville, VA 22908-0713; **Phone:** 434-982-1885; **Board Cert:** Otolaryngology 1966; **Med School:** Univ VA Sch Med 1961; **Resid:** Surgery, Stamford Hosp 1963; Otolaryngology, Yale-New Haven Hosp 1966; **Fac Appt:** Prof Oto, Univ VA Sch Med

Orobello Jr, Peter W MD [PO] - ; **Address:** 801 6th St S, Ste 7535, St Petersburg, FL 33701; **Phone:** 727-767-4305; **Board Cert:** Otolaryngology 1988; **Med School:** Univ Cincinnati 1983; **Resid:** Surgery, Univ Cincinnati Med Ctr 1984; Otolaryngology, Univ Cincinnati Med Ctr 1988; **Fellow:** Pediatric Otolaryngology, Johns Hopkins Hosp 1989; **Fac Appt:** Asst Clin Prof Ped, Univ S Fla Coll Med

Midwest

Arnold, James E MD [PO] - **Spec Exp:** Airway Disorders; Otology; Ear Tumors; **Hospital:** Rainbow Babies & Chldns Hosp, Univ Hosps Case Med Ctr; **Address:** University Hosp Cleveland, Lakeside Bldg, 11100 Euclid Ave Fl 4, Cleveland, OH 44106-2602; **Phone:** 216-844-5031; **Board Cert:** Otolaryngology 1982; **Med School:** Univ Tex, San Antonio 1977; **Resid:** Otolaryngology, Fitzsimons Army Med Ctr 1982; **Fellow:** Pediatric Otolaryngology, Childrens Hosp 1987; **Fac Appt:** Prof Oto, Case West Res Univ

Pediatric Otolaryngology

Belenky, Walter MD [PO] - **Spec Exp:** Cochlear Implants; Airway Disorders; **Hospital:** Chldns Hosp of Michigan; **Address:** Chldns Hosp, Dept Ped Oto, 3901 Beaubien Fl 3, Detroit, MI 48201; **Phone:** 313-745-9048; **Board Cert:** Otolaryngology 1970; **Med School:** Univ Mich Med Sch 1963; **Resid:** Surgery, William Beaumont Hosps 1965; Otolaryngology, Wayne Affil Hosp 1968

Cotton, Robin MD [PO] - **Spec Exp:** Tracheal Surgery; Head & Neck Surgery; Sinusitis; **Hospital:** Cincinnati Chldns Hosp Med Ctr; **Address:** Cincinnati Chldns Hosp, 3333 Burnet Ave, ML 2018, Cincinnati, OH 45229-3039; **Phone:** 513-636-4355; **Board Cert:** Otolaryngology 1972; **Med School:** England 1965; **Resid:** Otolaryngology, Univ Birmingham 1968; Otolaryngology, Univ Toronto Med Ctr 1972; **Fellow:** Head and Neck Surgery, Univ Cincinnati Med Ctr 1973; **Fac Appt:** Prof Oto, Univ Cincinnati

Holinger, Lauren D MD [PO] - **Spec Exp:** Airway Disorders; Swallowing Disorders; Cough-Chronic; **Hospital:** Children's Mem Hosp; **Address:** Chldns Meml Hosp, Dept Otolaryngology, 2300 N Childrens Plaza, Box 25, Chicago, IL 60614-3394; **Phone:** 773-880-4457; **Board Cert:** Otolaryngology 1975; **Med School:** Ros Franklin Univ/Chicago Med Sch 1971; **Resid:** Surgery, Univ Colorado Affil Hosp 1972; Otolaryngology, Univ Colorado Affil Hosp 1975; **Fellow:** Pediatric Otolaryngology, Chldns Meml Hosp 1976; **Fac Appt:** Prof Oto, Northwestern Univ

Katz, Robert L MD [PO] - **Spec Exp:** Ear Infections; Sinus Disorders/Surgery; Hearing Loss; **Hospital:** Cleveland Clin Fdn (page 57); **Address:** 29800 Bainbridge Rd, Solon, OH 44139-2202; **Phone:** 440-519-6950; **Board Cert:** Otolaryngology 1968; **Med School:** Case West Res Univ 1963; **Resid:** Surgery, Mount Sinai Hosp 1965; Otolaryngology, Mass EE Infirm/Chldns Hosp 1968; **Fac Appt:** Clin Prof Oto, Case West Res Univ

Miller, Robert P MD [PO] - **Spec Exp:** Ear Disorders/Surgery; Airway Disorders; Sinus Disorders; **Hospital:** Adv Luth Genl Hosp, Children's Mem Hosp; **Address:** 8780 W Golf Rd, Ste 200, Niles, IL 60714; **Phone:** 847-674-5585; **Board Cert:** Otolaryngology 1978; **Med School:** Loyola Univ-Stritch Sch Med 1974; **Resid:** Otolaryngology, Univ Illinois Hosps 1978; **Fellow:** Pediatric Otolaryngology, Chldns Hosp Med Ctr 1987; **Fac Appt:** Asst Clin Prof Oto, Univ IL Coll Med

Myer III, Charles M MD [PO] - **Spec Exp:** Airway Disorders; Head & Neck Tumors; Neck Masses; **Hospital:** Cincinnati Chldns Hosp Med Ctr; **Address:** Cincinnati Chldns Hosp, Dept Oto, 3333 Burnet Ave Bldg C Fl 3 - Ste 375, Cincinnati, OH 45229; **Phone:** 513-636-4355; **Board Cert:** Otolaryngology 1984; **Med School:** Univ Ala 1978; **Resid:** Otolaryngology, Univ Cincinnati 1984; **Fellow:** Otolaryngology, Chldns Hosp 1985; **Fac Appt:** Prof Oto, Univ Cincinnati

Great Plains and Mountains

Chan, Kenny H MD [PO] - **Spec Exp:** Ear Infections; Sinusitis; **Hospital:** Chldn's Hosp - Denver, The, Porter Adventist Hosp; **Address:** Chldns Hosp, Dept Otolaryngology, 1056 E 19th Ave, Box B455, Denver, CO 80218; **Phone:** 303-764-8501; **Board Cert:** Otolaryngology 1984; **Med School:** Loma Linda Univ 1977; **Resid:** Surgery, Oregon Hlth Sci Univ 1978; Otolaryngology, Loma Linda Univ Hosp 1983; **Fellow:** Pediatric Otolaryngology, Chldns Hosp 1987; **Fac Appt:** Prof Oto, Univ Colorado

Lusk, Rodney P MD [PO] - **Spec Exp:** Cochlear Implants; Sinus Disorders/Surgery; Sleep Disorders/Apnea; **Hospital:** Boys Town Natl Rsch Hosp, Children's Hosp - Omaha; **Address:** Boystown National Research Hosp, 555 N 30th St, Omaha, NE 68131; **Phone:** 402-498-6502; **Board Cert:** Otolaryngology 1982; **Med School:** Univ MO-Columbia Sch Med 1977; **Resid:** Head and Neck Surgery, Univ Iowa Hosp & Clinics 1982; **Fellow:** Pediatric Otolaryngology, Chldns Hosp 1983

Southwest

Bower, Charles MD [PO] - **Spec Exp:** Airway Disorders; Sleep Disorders/Apnea; Sinus Disorders/Surgery; **Hospital:** Arkansas Chldns Hosp, UAMS Med Ctr; **Address:** Arkansas Chldns Hosp, Dept Ped Oto, 800 Marshall St, Slot 836, Little Rock, AR 72202-3510; **Phone:** 501-364-1047; **Board Cert:** Otolaryngology 1990; **Med School:** Univ Ark 1985; **Resid:** Otolaryngology, Univ Ark Med Ctr 1991; **Fellow:** Pediatric Otolaryngology, Chldns Hosp 1992; **Fac Appt:** Assoc Prof Oto, Univ Ark

Duncan III, Newton O MD [PO] - **Spec Exp:** Sinus Disorders; Airway Disorders; Head & Neck Surgery; **Hospital:** Texas Chldns Hosp - Houston, Methodist Hosp - Houston; **Address:** Childrens Ear Nose & Throat, 6550 Fannin St, Ste 2001, Houston, TX 77030-2709; **Phone:** 713-796-2001; **Board Cert:** Otolaryngology 1986; **Med School:** Baylor Coll Med 1978; **Resid:** Surgery, Baylor Coll Med 1983; Otolaryngology, Baylor Coll Med 1986; **Fellow:** Pediatric Otolaryngology, Univ Wash 1991; Pediatric Otolaryngology, Royal Alexandra Hosp Chld 1992; **Fac Appt:** Asst Clin Prof Oto, Baylor Coll Med

Friedman, Ellen M MD [PO] - **Spec Exp:** Airway Disorders; Lymphatic Malformations-Head & Neck; **Hospital:** Texas Chldns Hosp - Houston; **Address:** 67010 Fannin, Ste 540, MC CC6102, Houston, TX 77030; **Phone:** 832-822-3250; **Board Cert:** Otolaryngology 1981; **Med School:** Albert Einstein Coll Med 1975; **Resid:** Surgery, Montefiore Hosp 1976; Otolaryngology, Washington Hosp Ctr 1979; **Fellow:** Pediatric Otolaryngology, Boston Chldns Hosp; **Fac Appt:** Prof Oto, Baylor Coll Med

West Coast and Pacific

Crockett, Dennis M MD [PO] - **Spec Exp:** Head & Neck Cancer; Airway Disorders; **Hospital:** Chldns Hosp - Los Angeles (page 56), USC Univ Hosp - R K Eamer Med Plz; **Address:** USC Health Consultation Ctr #2, 1450 San Pablo St, Ste 4600, Los Angeles, CA 90033; **Phone:** 323-442-5790; **Board Cert:** Otolaryngology 1985; **Med School:** USC Sch Med 1979; **Resid:** Otolaryngology, LAC-USC Med Ctr 1984; **Fellow:** Pediatrics, Boston Chldns Hosp 1985; **Fac Appt:** Assoc Prof Oto, USC Sch Med

Geller, Kenneth Allen MD [PO] - **Spec Exp:** Airway Disorders; Sinus Disorders/Surgery; Head & Neck Cancer; **Hospital:** Chldns Hosp - Los Angeles (page 56), Huntington Memorial Hosp; **Address:** Chldns Hosp, Div Otolaryngology, 4650 Sunset Blvd, MS 58, Los Angeles, CA 90027; **Phone:** 323-669-2145; **Board Cert:** Otolaryngology 1978; **Med School:** USC Sch Med 1972; **Resid:** Surgery, Wadsworth VA Hosp 1975; Otolaryngology, UCLA Hlth Scis Ctr 1978; **Fellow:** Pediatric Otolaryngology, Chldns Hosp 1979; **Fac Appt:** Assoc Clin Prof Oto, USC Sch Med

Pediatric Otolaryngology

Inglis, Andrew MD [PO] - **Spec Exp:** Airway Disorders; Voice Disorders; **Hospital:** Chldns Hosp and Regl Med Ctr - Seattle; **Address:** Children's Hospital & Medical Ctr, 4800 Sand Point Way NE, MS W7729, Seattle, WA 98105-0371; **Phone:** 206-987-2105; **Board Cert:** Otolaryngology 1987; **Med School:** Med Coll PA Hahnemann 1981; **Resid:** Surgery, Virginia Mason Hosp 1983; Otolaryngology, Univ Washington Hosps 1987; **Fellow:** Pediatric Otolaryngology, Royal Alexandria Hosp Chldn 1987; **Fac Appt:** Assoc Prof Oto, Univ Wash

Richardson, Mark A MD [PO] - **Spec Exp:** Sinus Disorders; Airway Disorders; Lymphatic Malformations-Head & Neck; **Hospital:** Doernbecher Chldns Hosp/OHSU, Providence St Vincent Med Ctr; **Address:** Dept Oto/HNS, 3181 SW Sam Jackson Park Rd, PV-01, Portland, OR 97239; **Phone:** 503-494-5350; **Board Cert:** Otolaryngology 1979; **Med School:** Med Univ SC 1975; **Resid:** Otolaryngology, Med Univ Hosp 1979; **Fellow:** Pediatric Otolaryngology, Chldns Hosp Med Ctr 1980; **Fac Appt:** Prof Oto, Oregon Hlth Sci Univ

Rosbe, Kristina MD [PO] - **Spec Exp:** Airway Disorders; Sinus Surgery-Pediatric; Cochlear Implants; Neck Masses; **Hospital:** UCSF Med Ctr; **Address:** UCSF Med Ctr, Dept Otolaryngology, 400 Parnassus Ave, Box 0342, San Francisco, CA 94143-0342; **Phone:** 415-353-2757; **Board Cert:** Orthopaedic Surgery 1999; **Med School:** Dartmouth Med Sch 1993; **Resid:** Surgery, Univ N Carolina Hosps 1994; Otolaryngology, Univ N Carolina Hosps 1998; **Fellow:** Pediatric Otolaryngology, Chldns Hosp 2000; **Fac Appt:** Assoc Prof Ped, UCSF

Pediatric Pulmonology

New England

Lapey, Allen MD [PPul] - **Spec Exp:** Cystic Fibrosis; Asthma; Food Allergy; **Hospital:** Mass Genl Hosp; **Address:** 15 Parkman St, POB 101, Boston, MA 02114; **Phone:** 617-726-8707; **Board Cert:** Pediatrics 1972; Allergy & Immunology 1978; Pediatric Pulmonology 2003; **Med School:** Univ Rochester 1966; **Resid:** Pediatrics, Chldns Hosp 1968; **Fellow:** Pediatric Pulmonology, Mass Genl Hosp 1972; Allergy & Immunology, Mass Genl Hosp 1972; **Fac Appt:** Asst Clin Prof Ped, Harvard Med Sch

Mid Atlantic

Borowitz, Drucy S MD [PPul] - **Spec Exp:** Cystic Fibrosis; **Hospital:** Women's & Chldn's Hosp of Buffalo, The; **Address:** Women & Children's Hospital, 219 Bryant St, Buffalo, NY 14222; **Phone:** 716-878-7524; **Board Cert:** Pediatrics 1984; Pediatric Gastroenterology 2006; **Med School:** Cornell Univ-Weill Med Coll 1979; **Resid:** Pediatrics, UCSF Med Ctr 1982; **Fellow:** Nutrition, UCSF Med Ctr 1983

Dozor, Allen J MD [PPul] - **Spec Exp:** Asthma; Cystic Fibrosis; **Hospital:** Westchester Med Ctr; **Address:** NY Med College, Munger Pavilion, Pediatric Pulmonology, Ste 106, Valhalla, NY 10595-1600; **Phone:** 914-493-7585; **Board Cert:** Pediatrics 1981; Pediatric Pulmonology 2003; **Med School:** Penn State Univ-Hershey Med Ctr 1977; **Resid:** Pediatrics, St Vincent's Hosp & Med Ctr 1980; **Fellow:** Pediatric Pulmonology, Chldns Hosp 1982; **Fac Appt:** Prof Ped, NY Med Coll

Kattan, Meyer MD [PPul] - **Spec Exp:** Asthma; Cystic Fibrosis; **Hospital:** Mount Sinai Med Ctr, Englewood Hosp & Med Ctr; **Address:** Mount Sinai Medical Ctr, One Gustave L Levy Pl, Box 1202B, New York, NY 10029; **Phone:** 212-241-7788; **Board Cert:** Pediatrics 1980; Pediatric Pulmonology 2003; **Med School:** McGill Univ 1973; **Resid:** Pediatrics, Chldns Hosp 1975; Pediatrics, Hosp for Sick Children 1976; **Fellow:** Pulmonary Disease, Hosp for Sick Children 1978; **Fac Appt:** Prof Ped, Mount Sinai Sch Med

Loughlin, Gerald M MD [PPul] - **Spec Exp:** Sleep Disorders/Apnea; Swallowing Disorders; Asthma & Chronic Lung Disease; Breathing Disorders; **Hospital:** NY-Presby Hosp/Weill Cornell (page 66); **Address:** Cornell Med Coll, Dept Peds, 525 E 68th St, rm M-622, New York, NY 10021-4870; **Phone:** 212-746-4111; **Board Cert:** Pediatrics 1993; Pediatric Pulmonology 2003; **Med School:** Univ Rochester 1973; **Resid:** Pediatrics, Univ Ariz Med Ctr 1973; **Fellow:** Pediatric Pulmonology, Univ Ariz Med Ctr 1977; **Fac Appt:** Prof Ped, Cornell Univ-Weill Med Coll

Marcus, Carole L MD [PPul] - **Spec Exp:** Sleep Disorders/Apnea; **Hospital:** Chldns Hosp of Philadelphia, The; **Address:** Chldns Hosp of Philadelphia, Wood Bldg 5FL, 34th St & Civic Ctr Blvd, Philadelphia, PA 19104; **Phone:** 215-590-3749; **Board Cert:** Pediatrics 2000; Pediatric Pulmonology 2000; **Med School:** South Africa 1982; **Resid:** Pediatrics, LIJ/SUNY Brooklyn Med Ctr 1986; **Fellow:** Pediatric Pulmonology, Chldns Hosp 1991; **Fac Appt:** Assoc Prof Ped, Univ Pennsylvania

Quittell, Lynne MD [PPul] - **Spec Exp:** Cystic Fibrosis; Asthma; **Hospital:** NYPresby-Morgan Stanley Children's Hosp; **Address:** Morgan Stanley Chlds Hosp of NY-Presby, 3959 Broadway Fl 7, New York, NY 10032-1551; **Phone:** 212-305-5122; **Board Cert:** Pediatrics 1986; Pediatric Pulmonology 2004; **Med School:** Israel 1981; **Resid:** Pediatrics, Schneider Chldns Hosp 1984; **Fellow:** Pediatric Pulmonology, St Christopher's Hosp 1988; **Fac Appt:** Assoc Prof Ped, Columbia P&S

Zeitlin, Pamela L MD [PPul] - **Spec Exp:** Cystic Fibrosis; **Hospital:** Johns Hopkins Hosp - Baltimore (page 61), Mt Washington Ped Hosp; **Address:** 200 N Wolfe St, Baltimore, MD 21287; **Phone:** 410-955-2035; **Board Cert:** Pediatrics 1988; Pediatric Pulmonology 2000; **Med School:** Yale Univ 1983; **Resid:** Pediatrics, Johns Hopkins Hosp 1986; **Fellow:** Pediatric Pulmonology, Johns Hopkins Hosp 1989; **Fac Appt:** Prof Ped, Johns Hopkins Univ

Southeast

Murphy, Thomas M MD [PPul] - **Spec Exp:** Cystic Fibrosis; Asthma; Pneumonia; **Hospital:** Duke Univ Med Ctr; **Address:** Duke Univ Med Ctr, Box 2994, Durham, NC 27710; **Phone:** 919-684-3364; **Board Cert:** Internal Medicine 1976; Pediatrics 2003; Pediatric Pulmonology 2004; **Med School:** Univ Rochester 1973; **Resid:** Internal Medicine, Georgetown Univ Hosp 1976; **Fellow:** Pediatric Pulmonology, Georgetown Univ Hosp 1978; **Fac Appt:** Assoc Prof Ped, Duke Univ

Sallent, Jorge MD [PPul] - **Spec Exp:** Chronic Lung Disease of Infancy; Asthma & Chronic Lung Disease; Lung Injuries - RSV Related; **Hospital:** St Mary's Med Ctr - W Palm Bch, Palms - West Hosp; **Address:** Pediatric Respiratory Ctr, 500 US Highway 1, Lake Park, FL 33403-3598; **Phone:** 561-863-0105; **Board Cert:** Pediatrics 1984; Pediatric Pulmonology 2003; **Med School:** Dominican Republic 1978; **Resid:** Pediatrics, Orlando Regional Med Ctr 1983; **Fellow:** Pediatric Pulmonology, Univ Florida 1986; **Fac Appt:** Asst Prof Ped, Univ Fla Coll Med

Sherman, James MD [PPul] - **Spec Exp:** Asthma; Airway Disorders; Cough-Chronic; **Hospital:** Carilion Roanoke Meml Hosp; **Address:** 102 Highland Ave, Ste 203, Roanoke, VA 24013; **Phone:** 540-985-9835; **Board Cert:** Pediatrics 1981; Pediatric Pulmonology 2003; **Med School:** Univ S Fla Coll Med 1975; **Resid:** Pediatrics, SUNY Upstate Med Ctr 1977; Pediatrics, Tampa Genl Hosp- Univ So Florida 1978; **Fellow:** Pediatric Pulmonology, Rainbow Babies & Children's Hosp 1981; **Fac Appt:** Prof Ped, Univ Fla Coll Med

Pediatric Pulmonology

Midwest

Davis, Pamela B MD [PPul] - **Spec Exp:** Cystic Fibrosis; **Hospital:** Rainbow Babies & Chldns Hosp; **Address:** Case West Reserve Univ, Biomed Rsch Bldg, 10900 Euclid Ave Fl 8, MS 4948, Cleveland, OH 44106-4948; **Phone:** 216-368-4370; **Board Cert:** Internal Medicine 1976; Pulmonary Disease 1980; Pediatrics 2004; Pediatric Pulmonology 2000; **Med School:** Duke Univ 1974; **Resid:** Internal Medicine, Duke Univ Med Ctr 1975; **Fellow:** Pulmonary Disease, Natl Inst Hlth 1979; **Fac Appt:** Prof Ped, Case West Res Univ

Kemp, James S MD [PPul] - **Spec Exp:** Sudden Infant Death Syndrome (SIDS); Breathing Disorders; **Hospital:** Cardinal Glennon Mem Children's Hosp; **Address:** Cardinal Glennon Chldns Hosp, Dept Ped Pulm, 1465 S Grand Blvd, St Louis, MO 63104; **Phone:** 314-268-6439; **Board Cert:** Pediatrics 1981; Pediatric Pulmonology 2000; **Med School:** Creighton Univ 1976; **Resid:** Pediatrics, Cardinal Glennon Chldns Hosp 1978; Pediatrics, Baylor Univ 1979; **Fellow:** Pediatric Pulmonology, Texas Chldns Hosp 1988; **Fac Appt:** Assoc Prof Ped, St Louis Univ

Kim, Young-Jee MD [PPul] - **Spec Exp:** Asthma; Chest Wall Deformities-Pediatric; Rare Lung Disease-Pediatric; **Hospital:** Riley Hosp for Children; **Address:** Riley Chldns Hosp - Dept Ped Pulm, 702 Barnhill Rd, ROC-rm 4270, Indianapolis, IN 46202-5128; **Phone:** 317-274-7208; **Board Cert:** Pediatric Pulmonology 2006; **Med School:** South Korea 1986; **Resid:** Pediatrics, Duke Univ Med Ctr 1995; **Fellow:** Pediatric Pulmonology, Yale Univ Med Sch 1991; Pediatric Pulmonology, Riley Hosp Chldn 1998; **Fac Appt:** Assoc Prof Ped, Indiana Univ

Konstan, Michael W MD [PPul] - **Spec Exp:** Cystic Fibrosis; **Hospital:** Rainbow Babies & Chldns Hosp; **Address:** Rainbow Babies & Chldns Hosp, Div Ped Pulmonology, 11100 Euclid Ave, rm 3001, MS 6006, Cleveland, OH 44106-2624; **Phone:** 216-844-1997; **Board Cert:** Pediatrics 1986; Pediatric Pulmonology 2004; **Med School:** Case West Res Univ 1982; **Resid:** Pediatrics, Children's Hosp 1985; **Fellow:** Pediatric Pulmonology, Rainbow Babies & Chldns Hosp 1988; **Fac Appt:** Prof Ped, Case West Res Univ

Kurachek, Stephen Charles MD [PPul] - **Spec Exp:** Critical Care; Asthma; **Hospital:** Chldns Hosp and Clinics - Minneapolis; **Address:** 2545 Chicago Ave S, Ste 617, Minneapolis, MN 55404; **Phone:** 612-863-3226; **Board Cert:** Pediatrics 1985; Pediatric Pulmonology 2004; Pediatric Critical Care Medicine 2003; **Med School:** Univ Miami Sch Med 1978; **Resid:** Pediatrics, Univ Hosp 1981; **Fellow:** Pulmonary Disease, Boston Chldns Hosp 1984; **Fac Appt:** Asst Clin Prof Ped, Univ Minn

Stern, Robert C MD [PPul] - **Spec Exp:** Cystic Fibrosis; Lung Disease; **Hospital:** Rainbow Babies & Chldns Hosp; **Address:** Div Ped Pulmonary Disease, 11100 Euclid Ave, Cleveland, OH 44106-1736; **Phone:** 216-844-3267; **Board Cert:** Pediatrics 1968; Pediatric Pulmonology 2002; **Med School:** Albert Einstein Coll Med 1963; **Resid:** Pediatrics, Univ Hosp 1965; Pediatrics, Bronx Muni Hosp Ctr 1966; **Fellow:** Pediatric Pulmonology, Univ Hosp; **Fac Appt:** Prof Ped, Case West Res Univ

Great Plains and Mountains

Accurso, Frank J MD [PPul] - **Spec Exp:** Cystic Fibrosis; **Hospital:** Chldn's Hosp - Denver, The; **Address:** Childrens Hosp, 1056 E 19th Ave, Box B-395, Denver, CO 80218; **Phone:** 303-837-2522; **Board Cert:** Pediatrics 1980; Pediatric Pulmonology 2003; **Med School:** Albert Einstein Coll Med 1974; **Resid:** Pediatrics, Univ Colo Hlth Sci Ctr 1977; **Fellow:** Pulmonary Disease, Univ Colo Hlth Sci Ctr 1980; **Fac Appt:** Prof Ped, Univ Colorado

Larsen, Gary MD [PPul] - **Hospital:** Natl Jewish Med & Rsch Ctr; **Address:** Natl Jewish Med & Rsrch Ctr, 1400 Jackson St, rm J303, Denver, CO 80206-2761; **Phone:** 303-398-1617; **Board Cert:** Pediatrics 1976; Pediatric Pulmonology 2003; **Med School:** Columbia P&S 1971; **Resid:** Pediatrics, Univ Colorado Med Ctr 1974; **Fellow:** Pediatric Pulmonology, Univ Colorado Med Ctr 1978; **Fac Appt:** Prof Ped, Univ Colorado

Southwest

Fan, Leland Lane MD [PPul] - **Spec Exp:** Interstitial Lung Disease; **Hospital:** Texas Chldns Hosp - Houston; **Address:** 6701 Fannin St, MC CCC 1040.01, Houston, TX 77030; **Phone:** 832-822-3300; **Board Cert:** Pediatrics 1978; Pediatric Pulmonology 2002; Pediatric Critical Care Medicine 2003; **Med School:** Baylor Coll Med 1973; **Resid:** Pediatrics, UCSF Med Ctr 1975; Pediatrics, Univ Colo Hlth Sci Ctr 1976; **Fellow:** Pediatric Pulmonary & Critical Care, Univ Colo Hlth Sci Ctr 1978; **Fac Appt:** Prof Ped, Baylor Coll Med

Morgan, Wayne J MD [PPul] - **Spec Exp:** Cystic Fibrosis; Asthma; **Hospital:** Univ Med Ctr - Tucson, Tucson Med Ctr; **Address:** Univ Arizona Hlth Sci Ctr, Div Pediatric Pulmonology, 1501 N Campbell Ave, Box 245073, Tucson, AZ 85724; **Phone:** 520-626-7780; **Board Cert:** Pediatrics 1982; Pediatric Pulmonology 2003; **Med School:** McGill Univ 1976; **Resid:** Pediatrics, Montreal Chldns Hosp 1980; **Fellow:** Pediatric Pulmonology, Univ Ariz Hlth Sci 1982; **Fac Appt:** Prof Ped, Univ Ariz Coll Med

Warren, Robert H MD [PPul] - **Spec Exp:** Muscular Dystrophy; Pulmonary Rehabilitation; **Hospital:** Arkansas Chldns Hosp; **Address:** Arkansas Chldns Hosp, Pulmonary Med, 800 Marshall St, Slot 512-17, Little Rock, AR 72202; **Phone:** 501-364-1006; **Board Cert:** Pediatrics 1973; Pediatric Pulmonology 2003; **Med School:** Univ Ark 1967; **Resid:** Pediatrics, LSU Med Ctr 1971; **Fellow:** Pediatric Pulmonology, Tulane Univ Sch Med; **Fac Appt:** Assoc Prof Ped, Univ Ark

West Coast and Pacific

Keens, Thomas G MD [PPul] - **Spec Exp:** Sudden Infant Death Syndrome (SIDS); Breathing Disorders; **Hospital:** Chldns Hosp - Los Angeles (page 56); **Address:** Chldns Hosp, Div Pulmonology, 4650 W Sunset Blvd, Box 83, Los Angeles, CA 90027-6062; **Phone:** 323-669-2101; **Board Cert:** Pediatrics 1978; Neonatal-Perinatal Medicine 1983; Pediatric Pulmonology 2003; **Med School:** UCSD 1972; **Resid:** Pediatrics, Chldns Hosp 1975; **Fellow:** Pediatric Pulmonology, Hosp Sick Chldn 1977; **Fac Appt:** Prof Ped, USC Sch Med

Platzker, Arnold CG MD [PPul] - **Spec Exp:** Asthma; Chronic Lung Disease; Cystic Fibrosis; **Hospital:** Chldns Hosp - Los Angeles (page 56), Mattel Chldns Hosp at UCLA; **Address:** Chldns Hosp, Div Ped Pulmonology, 4650 Sunset Blvd, Box 83, Los Angeles, CA 90027-6062; **Phone:** 323-669-2101; **Board Cert:** Pediatrics 1967; Neonatal-Perinatal Medicine 1975; Pediatric Pulmonology 2002; **Med School:** Tufts Univ 1962; **Resid:** Pediatrics, City Hosp 1964; Pediatrics, Stanford Univ Med Ctr 1966; **Fellow:** Pediatric Pulmonology, UCSF Med Ctr 1971; Neonatal-Perinatal Medicine, UCSF Med Ctr 1971; **Fac Appt:** Prof Ped, USC Sch Med

Ramsey, Bonnie W MD [PPul] - **Spec Exp:** Cystic Fibrosis; **Hospital:** Chldns Hosp and Regl Med Ctr - Seattle; **Address:** Chldns Hosp & Regl Med Ctr, 1100 Olive Way, Ste 500, MS MPW 5-4, Seattle, WA 98101; **Phone:** 206-987-5725; **Board Cert:** Pediatrics 1981; Pediatric Pulmonology 2006; **Med School:** Harvard Med Sch 1976; **Resid:** Pediatrics, Chldns Hosp 1978; Pediatrics, Chldns Hosp 1979; **Fellow:** Pediatric Critical Care Medicine, Chldns Hosp 1981; **Fac Appt:** Prof Ped, Univ Wash

Pediatric Pulmonology

Redding, Gregory MD [PPul] - **Spec Exp:** Asthma; Chest Wall Deformities-Pediatric; Intersitial Lung Disease; **Hospital:** Chldns Hosp and Regl Med Ctr - Seattle; **Address:** Pulmonary Div, Chlds Hosp & Regl Med Ctr, 4800 Sand Point Way NE, MS G-0038, Seattle, WA 98105; **Phone:** 206-987-2174; **Board Cert:** Pediatrics 1993; Pediatric Pulmonology 2003; **Med School:** Stanford Univ 1974; **Resid:** Pediatrics, Harbor-UCLA Affil Hosps 1977; **Fellow:** Pediatric Pulmonology, Univ Colo Affil Hosps 1980; **Fac Appt:** Prof Ped, Univ Wash

Pediatric Rheumatology

New England

McCarthy, Paul L MD [PRhu] - **Spec Exp:** Lupus/SLE; Juvenile Arthritis; Dermatomyositis; Vasculitis; **Hospital:** Yale - New Haven Hosp; **Address:** Yale Schl Med, 333 Cedar St, Box 208064, New Haven, CT 06520-3206; **Phone:** 203-688-2475; **Board Cert:** Pediatrics 1974; Pediatric Rheumatology 2007; **Med School:** Georgetown Univ 1969; **Resid:** Pediatrics, Chldns Hosp 1972; **Fellow:** Pediatrics, Chldns Hosp 1974; **Fac Appt:** Prof Ped, Yale Univ

Mid Atlantic

Finkel, Terri H MD [PRhu] - **Spec Exp:** Juvenile Arthritis; Lupus/SLE; Vasculitis; **Hospital:** Chldns Hosp of Philadelphia, The; **Address:** Chldns Hosp of Philadelphia, Div Rheum, 34th St & Civic Ctr Blvd, Chldns Seashore House, rm 236, Philadelphia, PA 19104; **Phone:** 215-590-2547; **Board Cert:** Pediatrics 1988; Pediatric Rheumatology 2002; **Med School:** Stanford Univ 1982; **Resid:** Pediatrics, Univ Colorado Med Ctr 1985; **Fellow:** Pediatric Rheumatology, Natl Jewish Med Ctr 1990; **Fac Appt:** Assoc Prof Ped

Haines, Kathleen A MD [PRhu] - **Spec Exp:** Juvenile Arthritis; Lupus/SLE; Immune Deficiency; **Hospital:** Hackensack Univ Med Ctr, NYU Med Ctr (page 67); **Address:** Hackensack Univ Med Ctr, Don Imus Ped Ctr, 30 Prospect Ave Fl 3, Hackensack, NJ 07601; **Phone:** 201-996-5306; **Board Cert:** Pediatrics 1980; Allergy & Immunology 1981; Pediatric Rheumatology 2007; **Med School:** Albert Einstein Coll Med 1975; **Resid:** Pediatrics, New York Hosp 1977; **Fellow:** Allergy & Immunology, New York Hosp 1980; Rheumatology, NYU Med Sch 1982; **Fac Appt:** Assoc Prof Ped, UMDNJ-NJ Med Sch, Newark

Ilowite, Norman T MD [PRhu] - **Spec Exp:** Juvenile Arthritis; Lyme Disease; Lupus/SLE; **Hospital:** Montefiore Med Ctr; **Address:** Montefiore Children's Hosp, Rheumatology, 3415 Bainbridge Ave, Bronx, NY 10467; **Phone:** 718-741-2456; **Board Cert:** Pediatrics 1985; Clinical & Laboratory Immunology 1990; Pediatric Rheumatology 2000; **Med School:** SUNY Downstate 1979; **Resid:** Pediatrics, Chldns Hosp Natl Med Ctr 1982; **Fellow:** Pediatric Rheumatology, Univ WA Med Ctr 1984; **Fac Appt:** Prof Ped, Albert Einstein Coll Med

Lehman, Thomas MD [PRhu] - **Spec Exp:** Arthritis; Scleroderma; Lupus/SLE; Rheumatoid Arthritis; **Hospital:** Hosp For Special Surgery (page 60), NY-Presby Hosp/Weill Cornell (page 66); **Address:** 535 E 70th St, New York, NY 10021-4872; **Phone:** 212-606-1151; **Board Cert:** Pediatrics 1979; Pediatric Rheumatology 2007; **Med School:** Jefferson Med Coll 1974; **Resid:** Pediatrics, Chldns Hosp 1976; Pediatrics, UCSF Med Ctr 1977; **Fellow:** Pediatric Rheumatology, Chldns Hosp 1979; Rheumatology, Natl Inst Hlth 1983; **Fac Appt:** Prof Ped, Cornell Univ-Weill Med Coll

Sherry, David D MD [PRhu] - **Spec Exp:** Pain-Musculoskeletal; Reflex Sympathetic Dystrophy (RSD); Juvenile Arthritis; Lupus/SLE; **Hospital:** Chldns Hosp of Philadelphia, The; **Address:** Chldns Hosp of Phildelphia, Div Rheum, 34th St & Civic Ctr Blvd, rm 236, Chldns Seashore House, Philadelphia, PA 19104; **Phone:** 215-590-2547; **Board Cert:** Pediatrics 1981; Pediatric Rheumatology 2000; **Med School:** Texas Tech Univ 1977; **Resid:** Pediatrics, Duke Univ Med Ctr 1980; **Fellow:** Pediatric Rheumatology, Univ British Columbia 1982; **Fac Appt:** Prof Ped, Univ Pennsylvania

Sills, Edward M MD [PRhu] - **Spec Exp:** Juvenile Arthritis; Lupus/SLE; Dermatomyositis; **Hospital:** Johns Hopkins Hosp - Baltimore (page 61); **Address:** Johns Hopkins Hosp, 200 N Wolfe St, Ste 2-127, Baltimore, MD 21205; **Phone:** 410-955-6145; **Board Cert:** Pediatrics 1968; Pediatric Rheumatology 2000; **Med School:** NYU Sch Med 1963; **Resid:** Pediatrics, Bronx Muni Hosp 1967; **Fac Appt:** Assoc Prof Ped, Johns Hopkins Univ

Southeast

Schanberg, Laura E MD [PRhu] - **Spec Exp:** Rheumatic Diseases of Childhood; Fibromyalgia; **Hospital:** Duke Univ Med Ctr; **Address:** Duke Univ Med Ctr, Box 3212, Durham, NC 27710; **Phone:** 919-684-6575; **Board Cert:** Pediatrics 2000; Pediatric Rheumatology 2000; **Med School:** Duke Univ 1984; **Resid:** Pediatrics, Duke Univ Med Ctr 1987; **Fellow:** Pediatric Rheumatology, Duke Univ Med Ctr 1991; **Fac Appt:** Asst Prof Ped, Duke Univ

Sleasman, John W MD [PRhu] - **Spec Exp:** Infectious Disease; Immunodeficiency Disorders; **Hospital:** All Children's Hosp; **Address:** All Childrens Hosp, Div Ped Immun/Rheumatology, 801 6th St, Box 9350, St Petersburg, FL 33701; **Phone:** 727-553-1257; **Board Cert:** Pediatrics 1988; Diagnostic Lab Immunology 1990; **Med School:** Univ Tenn Coll Med, Memphis 1981; **Resid:** Pediatrics, Shands Hosp 1984; **Fellow:** Pediatric Infectious Disease, Shands Hosp 1987; Immunology, Dana Farber Cancer Inst 1988

Midwest

Passo, Murray H MD [PRhu] - **Hospital:** Cincinnati Chldns Hosp Med Ctr; **Address:** Chldns Hosp Med Ctr, Dept Ped Rheum, 3333 Burnet Ave, ML4010, Cincinnati, OH 45229-3039; **Phone:** 513-636-4676; **Board Cert:** Pediatrics 1979; Pediatric Rheumatology 2000; **Med School:** Indiana Univ 1974; **Resid:** Pediatrics, Riley Chldns Hosp 1977; **Fellow:** Rheumatology, Ind Univ Hosps 1979

Wagner-Weiner, Linda MD [PRhu] - **Spec Exp:** Lupus/SLE; Juvenile Arthritis; Vasculitis; **Hospital:** La Rabida Chlds Hosp, Univ of Chicago Hosps; **Address:** La Rabida Chldns Hosp, East 65th Street at Lake Michigan, Chicago, IL 60649; **Phone:** 773-753-8644; **Board Cert:** Pediatrics 1984; Pediatric Rheumatology 2000; **Med School:** Rush Med Coll 1979; **Resid:** Pediatrics, Univ Chicago Hosps 1982; **Fellow:** Pediatric Rheumatology, Univ Chicago/La Rabida Chldns Hosp 1984; **Fac Appt:** Asst Prof Ped, Univ Chicago-Pritzker Sch Med

Southwest

Myones, Barry Lee MD [PRhu] - **Spec Exp:** Vasculitis; Kawasaki Disease; Dermatomyositis; Scleroderma; **Hospital:** Texas Chldns Hosp - Houston; **Address:** Tex Chldns Hosp, Ped Rheum Ctr, 6701 Fannin St Fl 11, Houston, TX 77030; **Phone:** 832-824-3830; **Board Cert:** Pediatrics 1983; Pediatric Rheumatology 2000; **Med School:** Albany Med Coll 1977; **Resid:** Pediatrics, Duke Univ Med Ctr 1980; **Fellow:** Pediatric Rheumatology, Chldns Hosp-Stanford 1983; Rheumatology, Univ N Carolina 1988; **Fac Appt:** Assoc Clin Prof Ped, Baylor Coll Med

Pediatric Rheumatology

Warren, Robert Wells MD [PRhu] - **Spec Exp:** Juvenile Arthritis; Lupus/SLE; **Hospital:** Texas Chldns Hosp - Houston; **Address:** Tex Chldns Hosp, Ped Rheumatology Ctr, 6701 Fannin Fl 11, Houston, TX 77030-2303; **Phone:** 832-824-3830; **Board Cert:** Pediatrics 1983; Allergy & Immunology 1983; Pediatric Rheumatology 2000; **Med School:** Washington Univ, St Louis 1978; **Resid:** Pediatrics, Duke Univ Med Ctr 1980; **Fellow:** Rheumatology, Duke Univ Med Ctr 1983; **Fac Appt:** Assoc Prof Ped, Baylor Coll Med

Wilking, Andrew MD [PRhu] - **Spec Exp:** Arthritis; Lupus/SLE; Dermatomyositis; **Hospital:** Texas Chldns Hosp - Houston; **Address:** Tex Chldns Hosp, Ped Rheum Ctr, 6701 Fannin St Fl 11, Houston, TX 77030; **Phone:** 832-824-3830; **Board Cert:** Pediatrics 1985; **Med School:** Columbia P&S 1978; **Resid:** Pediatrics, Babies Hosp 1981; **Fellow:** Pediatric Rheumatology, Tex Chldns Hosp 1983; **Fac Appt:** Assoc Prof Ped, Baylor Coll Med

West Coast and Pacific

Bernstein, Bram Henry MD [PRhu] - **Spec Exp:** Juvenile Arthritis; Lupus/SLE; Vasculitis; **Hospital:** Chldns Hosp - Los Angeles (page 56), Miller Children's Hosp; **Address:** Chldns Hosp, MS 60, 4650 W Sunset Blvd, Los Angeles, CA 90027-6062; **Phone:** 323-669-2119; **Board Cert:** Pediatrics 1969; Pediatric Rheumatology 2000; **Med School:** McGill Univ 1964; **Resid:** Pediatrics, Chldns Hosp 1967; Rheumatology, Chldns Hosp 1968; **Fellow:** Rheumatology, Vancouver Genl Hosp 1970; **Fac Appt:** Clin Prof Ped, Univ SC Sch Med

Emery, Helen M MD [PRhu] - **Spec Exp:** Rheumatic Diseases of Childhood; **Hospital:** Chldns Hosp and Regl Med Ctr - Seattle, Univ Wash Med Ctr; **Address:** Chldns Hosp & Regl Med Ctr, Ped Rheum, 4800 Sand Point Way NE, MS M1-8, Seattle, WA 98105; **Phone:** 206-987-2057; **Board Cert:** Pediatrics 1992; Pediatric Rheumatology 2000; **Med School:** Australia 1971; **Resid:** Pediatrics, Chldns Orth Hosp-Univ Wash 1975; **Fellow:** Pediatric Rheumatology, Chldns Orth Hosp-Univ Wash 1977; **Fac Appt:** Prof Ped, Univ Wash

Sandborg, Christy MD [PRhu] - **Spec Exp:** Lupus/SLE; **Hospital:** Stanford Univ Med Ctr; **Address:** 300 Pasteur Drive, Stanford, CA 94305; **Phone:** 650-736-7642; **Board Cert:** Pediatrics 1984; Pediatric Rheumatology 2000; **Med School:** UCLA 1977; **Resid:** Pediatrics, Chldns Hosp 1979; **Fellow:** Pediatric Rheumatology, Chldns Hosp 1981; **Fac Appt:** Prof Ped, Stanford Univ

Pediatric Surgery

New England

Jennings, Russell W MD [PS] - **Spec Exp:** Fetal Surgery; Pediatric Cardiac Surgery; Robotic Surgery; **Hospital:** Children's Hospital - Boston, Brigham & Women's Hosp; **Address:** Chldns Hosp, Fegan 3, 300 Longwood Ave, Boston, MA 02115; **Phone:** 617-355-3038; **Board Cert:** Surgery 1995; Pediatric Surgery 1998; **Med School:** UCSF 1986; **Resid:** Surgery, UCSF Med Ctr 1991; **Fellow:** Fetal Surgery, Fetal Trmt Ctr/UCSF Med Ctr 1994; Pediatric Surgery, Chldns Hosp 1996; **Fac Appt:** Asst Prof S, Harvard Med Sch

Latchaw, Laurie MD [PS] - **Spec Exp:** Thoracic Surgery; Cancer Surgery; Lung Disease in Newborns; Neonatal Surgery; **Hospital:** Dartmouth - Hitchcock Med Ctr; **Address:** Dartmouth-Hitchcock Med Ctr, Dept Ped Surg, One Medical Center Drive, Lebanon, NH 03756; **Phone:** 603-653-9883; **Board Cert:** Surgery 2001; Pediatric Surgery 2003; **Med School:** Rush Med Coll 1976; **Resid:** Surgery, Univ Texas 1981; **Fellow:** Pediatric Surgery, Montreal Chldns Hosp 1983; **Fac Appt:** Assoc Prof S, Dartmouth Med Sch

Mayer Jr, John E MD [PS] - **Spec Exp:** Pediatric Cardiothoracic Surgery; **Hospital:** Children's Hospital - Boston; **Address:** Chldns Hosp, Dept Cardiac Surg, 300 Longwood Ave, Bader 273, Boston, MA 02115; **Phone:** 617-355-8258; **Board Cert:** Thoracic Surgery 2001; **Med School:** Yale Univ 1972; **Resid:** Surgery, Univ Minn Med Ctr 1979; **Fellow:** Cardiothoracic Surgery, Univ Minn Med Ctr 1981; **Fac Appt:** Prof S, Harvard Med Sch

Moss, R Lawrence MD [PS] - **Spec Exp:** Congenital Anomalies; Cancer Surgery; Minimally Invasive Surgery; **Hospital:** Yale - New Haven Hosp; **Address:** Dept Surgery-Ped Surgery, PO Box 208062, New Haven, CT 06520-8062; **Phone:** 203-785-2701; **Board Cert:** Surgery 1999; Pediatric Surgery 1996; Surgical Critical Care 2000; **Med School:** UCSD 1986; **Resid:** Surgery, Virginia Mason Med Ctr 1991; Surgical Critical Care, Chldns Mem Hosp 1992; **Fellow:** Pediatric Surgery, Chldns Mem Hosp 1994; **Fac Appt:** Prof S, Yale Univ

Tracy Jr, Thomas F MD [PS] - **Spec Exp:** Thoracic Surgery; Endoscopic Surgery; Fetal Surgery; Hirschprung's Disease; **Hospital:** Rhode Island Hosp; **Address:** 2 Dudley St, Ste 180, Providence, RI 02905; **Phone:** 401-421-1939; **Board Cert:** Surgery 1996; Pediatric Surgery 2006; **Med School:** Israel 1981; **Resid:** Surgery, Med Coll Virginia 1986; **Fellow:** Pediatric Surgery, Columbia Presby Med Ctr 1988; **Fac Appt:** Prof S, Brown Univ

Vacanti, Joseph P MD [PS] - **Spec Exp:** Transplant-Liver; **Hospital:** Mass Genl Hosp; **Address:** Mass General Hospital Warren Bldg, 55 Fruit St, rm 1157, Boston, MA 02114-2696; **Phone:** 617-724-1725; **Board Cert:** Pediatric Surgery 1997; **Med School:** Univ Nebr Coll Med 1974; **Resid:** Surgery, Mass Genl Hosp 1980; Pediatric Surgery, Children's Hosp 1983; **Fac Appt:** Prof S, Harvard Med Sch

Mid Atlantic

Adzick, N Scott MD [PS] - **Spec Exp:** Fetal Surgery; Twin to Twin Transfusion Syndrome (TTTS); Neonatal Surgery; **Hospital:** Chldns Hosp of Philadelphia, The; **Address:** St 5113 Wood Bldg, Chldns Hosp-Philadelphia, 34th St & Civic Ctr Blvd, Philadelphia, PA 19104-4399; **Phone:** 215-590-2727; **Board Cert:** Surgery 1997; Surgical Critical Care 1991; Pediatric Surgery 1999; **Med School:** Harvard Med Sch 1979; **Resid:** Surgery, Mass Genl Hosp 1986; Pediatric Surgery, Chldns Hosp 1988; **Fellow:** Research, UCSF Med Ctr 1985; **Fac Appt:** Prof S, Univ Pennsylvania

Alexander, Frederick MD [PS] - **Spec Exp:** Transplant-Bowel; Solid Tumors; Congenital Anomalies-Gastrointestinal; **Hospital:** Hackensack Univ Med Ctr; **Address:** Joseph M Sanzari Chldns Hosp-HUMC, 30 Prospect Ave, Ste PC331, Hackensack, NJ 07601; **Phone:** 201-996-2921; **Board Cert:** Pediatric Surgery 1999; **Med School:** Columbia P&S 1976; **Resid:** Surgery, Brigham-Womens Hosp 1984; **Fellow:** Pediatric Surgery, Chldns Hosp 1986; **Fac Appt:** Clin Prof S

Barksdale Jr, Edward M MD [PS] - **Spec Exp:** Gastrointestinal Surgery; Nutrition in Bowel Disorders; Neuroblastoma; Minimally Invasive Surgery; **Hospital:** Chldns Hosp of Pittsburgh - UPMC, Allegheny General Hosp; **Address:** Childrens Hosp Pittsburgh, 3705 Fifth Ave, rm 4A-485, Pittsburgh, PA 15213; **Phone:** 412-692-8735; **Board Cert:** Surgery 2002; Pediatric Surgery 2003; **Med School:** Harvard Med Sch 1984; **Resid:** Surgery, Mass Genl Hosp 1992; **Fellow:** Surgical Research, Mass Genl Hosp 1989; Pediatric Surgery, Childrens Hosp 1994; **Fac Appt:** Assoc Prof S, Univ Pittsburgh

Colombani, Paul M MD [PS] - **Spec Exp:** Thoracic Surgery; Transplant-Kidney; Transplant-Liver; Cancer Surgery; **Hospital:** Johns Hopkins Hosp - Baltimore (page 61); **Address:** 600 N Wolfe St Harvey 319 Bldg, Baltimore, MD 21287; **Phone:** 410-955-2717; **Board Cert:** Surgery 2003; Pediatric Surgery 2003; **Med School:** Univ KY Coll Med 1976; **Resid:** Surgery, Geo Wash Univ Hosp 1981; **Fellow:** Pediatric Surgery, Johns Hopkins Hosp 1983; **Fac Appt:** Prof S, Johns Hopkins Univ

Dolgin, Stephen MD [PS] - **Spec Exp:** Neonatal Surgery; Ulcerative Colitis; Laparoscopy & Thoracostomy; Inflammatory Bowel Disease/Crohn's; **Hospital:** Schneider Chldn's Hosp, N Shore Univ Hosp at Manhasset; **Address:** Schneider Children's Hosp, Pediatric Surgery, 269-10 76th Ave, New Hyde Park, NY 11040; **Phone:** 718-470-3636; **Board Cert:** Surgery 2000; Pediatric Surgery 2003; Surgical Critical Care 2000; **Med School:** NYU Sch Med 1977; **Resid:** Surgery, Peter Bent Brigham Hosp 1982; Pediatric Surgery, Chldns Meml Hosp 1984; **Fac Appt:** Prof S, Albert Einstein Coll Med

Eichelberger, Martin R MD [PS] - **Spec Exp:** Trauma; **Hospital:** Chldns Natl Med Ctr; **Address:** Childrens National Med Ctr, 111 Michigan Ave NW, Washington, DC 20010; **Phone:** 202-884-2151; **Board Cert:** Surgery 1979; Pediatric Surgery 2003; **Med School:** Hahnemann Univ 1971; **Resid:** Surgery, Case-Western Res Hosp 1978; **Fellow:** Pediatric Surgery, Childrens Hosp 1980; **Fac Appt:** Prof S, Geo Wash Univ

Flake, Alan W MD [PS] - **Spec Exp:** Fetal Surgery; Stem Cell Transplant-Fetal; Neonatal Surgery; **Hospital:** Chldns Hosp of Philadelphia, The; **Address:** Children's Hosp, Dept Surgery, 34th St & Civic Center Blvd, Abramson 1116, Philadelphia, PA 19104; **Phone:** 215-590-3671; **Board Cert:** Surgery 2000; Pediatric Surgery 1999; **Med School:** Univ Ark 1981; **Resid:** Surgery, UCSF Med Ctr 1988; **Fellow:** Pediatric Surgery, Chldns Hosp Med Ctr 1990; **Fac Appt:** Prof S, Univ Pennsylvania

Ginsburg, Howard B MD [PS] - **Spec Exp:** Neonatal Surgery; Tumor Surgery; Pediatric Urology; Gastrointestinal Surgery; **Hospital:** NYU Med Ctr (page 67), Bellevue Hosp Ctr; **Address:** NYU Medical Ctr, Div Pediatric Surgery, 530 1st Ave, Ste 10W, New York, NY 10016-6402; **Phone:** 212-263-7391; **Board Cert:** Surgery 1978; Pediatric Surgery 2001; **Med School:** Univ Cincinnati 1972; **Resid:** Surgery, NYU-Bellvue Hosp 1977; Pediatric Surgery, Columbia-Presby Med Ctr 1979; **Fellow:** Pediatric Surgery, Mass Genl Hosp 1980; **Fac Appt:** Assoc Prof S, NYU Sch Med

Gittes, George K MD [PS] - **Spec Exp:** Gastrointestinal Surgery; **Hospital:** Chldns Hosp of Pittsburgh - UPMC; **Address:** Childrens Hosp Pittsburgh, Dept Surgery, 3705 Fifth Ave, Ste 4A-485, Pittsburgh, PA 15213; **Phone:** 412-692-7280; **Board Cert:** Surgery 2003; Pediatric Surgery 1998; **Med School:** Harvard Med Sch 1987; **Resid:** Surgery, UCSF Med Ctr 1994; **Fellow:** Pediatric Surgery, Childrens Mercy Hosp 1995; **Fac Appt:** Prof S, Univ Pittsburgh

Glick, Philip L MD [PS] - **Spec Exp:** Robotic Surgery; Neonatal Surgery; Pediatric Cancers; Chest Wall Deformities; **Hospital:** Women's & Chldn's Hosp of Buffalo, The, Roswell Park Cancer Inst; **Address:** Children's Hosp Buffalo, Dept Pediatric Surgery, 219 Bryant St, Buffalo, NY 14222-2006; **Phone:** 716-878-7449; **Board Cert:** Surgery 1996; Pediatric Surgery 1997; Surgical Critical Care 1999; **Med School:** UCSF 1979; **Resid:** Surgery, UCSF Med Ctr 1985; **Fellow:** Fetal Surgery, UCSF Med Ctr 1984; Pediatric Surgery, Chldn's Hosp Med Ctr 1988; **Fac Appt:** Prof S, SUNY Buffalo

La Quaglia, Michael MD [PS] - **Spec Exp:** Cancer Surgery; Neuroblastoma; Liver Tumors; Colon & Rectal Cancer; **Hospital:** Meml Sloan Kettering Cancer Ctr, NY-Presby Hosp/Weill Cornell (page 66); **Address:** 1275 York Ave, Box 325, New York, NY 10021-6007; **Phone:** 212-639-7002; **Board Cert:** Surgery 2003; Pediatric Surgery 1997; **Med School:** UMDNJ-NJ Med Sch, Newark 1976; **Resid:** Surgery, Mass Genl Hosp 1983; **Fellow:** Cardiothoracic Surgery, Broadgreen Ctr 1984; Pediatric Surgery, Chldns Hosp 1985; **Fac Appt:** Prof S, Cornell Univ-Weill Med Coll

Quaegebeur, Jan M MD [PS] - **Spec Exp:** Arterial Switch; Heart Valve Surgery; Congenital Heart Surgery; **Hospital:** NYPresby-Morgan Stanley Children's Hosp; **Address:** Morgan Stanley Chlds Hosp of NY-Presby, 3959 Broadway, Ste 276, New York, NY 10032; **Phone:** 212-305-5975; **Med School:** Belgium 1969; **Resid:** Surgery, St Michel Clinic 1973; **Fellow:** Thoracic Surgery, Baylor Coll Med 1974; Thoracic Surgery, Univ Hosp 1978; **Fac Appt:** Prof S, Columbia P&S

Schwartz, Marshall Z MD [PS] - **Spec Exp:** Gastrointestinal Surgery; Neonatal Surgery; Transplant-Kidney; **Hospital:** St Christopher's Hosp for Chldn, Thomas Jefferson Univ Hosp; **Address:** St Christopher's Hosp for Chldn, Dept of Surgery, Erie at Front St, Ste 2204, Philadelphia, PA 19134; **Phone:** 215-427-5446; **Board Cert:** Surgery 1998; Pediatric Surgery 1999; **Med School:** Univ Minn 1970; **Resid:** Surgery, Univ Minnesota Hosp 1972; Pediatric Surgery, Chldns Hosp Med Ctr - Harvard Med Sch 1974; **Fellow:** Surgery, Univ Minnesota Hosp 1975; **Fac Appt:** Prof S, Jefferson Med Coll

Shlasko, Edward MD [PS] - **Spec Exp:** Laparoscopic Surgery; Robotic Surgery; **Hospital:** Maimonides Med Ctr (page 63), Mount Sinai Med Ctr; **Address:** Dept Ped Surg, 921 49th St, Brooklyn, NY 11219-2923; **Phone:** 718-283-7384; **Board Cert:** Surgery 1999; Pediatric Surgery 2001; **Med School:** Columbia P&S 1985; **Resid:** Surgery, Mount Sinai Hosp 1991; **Fellow:** Surgical Oncology, NIH-NCI Surg Branch 1989; Pediatric Surgery, SUNY Hlth Sci Ctr 1993; **Fac Appt:** Assoc Prof S, Mount Sinai Sch Med

Spray, Thomas L MD [PS] - **Spec Exp:** Cardiac Surgery-Adult & Pediatric; Transplant-Heart & Lung; Neonatal & Infant Cardiac Surgery; **Hospital:** Chldns Hosp of Philadelphia, The, Hosp Univ Penn - UPHS (page 72); **Address:** Children's Hosp of Philadelphia, Surgery, 34th St & Civic Center Blvd, Ste 8527, Philadelphia, PA 19104; **Phone:** 215-590-2708; **Board Cert:** Thoracic Surgery 1993; **Med School:** Duke Univ 1973; **Resid:** Surgery, Duke Univ Med Ctr 1975; Cardiothoracic Surgery, Duke Univ Med Ctr 1983; **Fac Appt:** Prof S, Univ Pennsylvania

Stolar, Charles J H MD [PS] - **Spec Exp:** Pediatric Cancers; Neonatal Surgery; Diaphragmatic hernia; **Hospital:** NYPresby-Morgan Stanley Children's Hosp; **Address:** Morgan Stanley Chldns Hosp NY-Presby, 3959 Broadway, Fl 2 - rm 215 North, New York, NY 10032; **Phone:** 212-342-8586; **Board Cert:** Surgery 2001; Pediatric Surgery 1996; **Med School:** Georgetown Univ 1974; **Resid:** Surgery, Univ Illinois Hosp 1980; **Fellow:** Pediatric Surgery, Chldns Hosp Natl Med Ctr 1982; **Fac Appt:** Prof S, Columbia P&S

Velcek, Francisca MD [PS] - **Spec Exp:** Anorectal Malformations; Pediatric Gynecology; Neonatal Surgery; Hernia; **Hospital:** Lenox Hill Hosp (page 62), Long Island Coll Hosp; **Address:** 965 5th Ave, New York, NY 10021; **Phone:** 212-744-9396; **Board Cert:** Surgery 1974; Pediatric Surgery 1997; **Med School:** Philippines 1966; **Resid:** Surgery, St Clares Hosp 1971; Pediatric Surgery, SUNY Downstate Med Ctr 1975; **Fellow:** Pediatric Surgery, SUNY Downstate Med Ctr 1973; **Fac Appt:** Prof S, SUNY Hlth Sci Ctr

Pediatric Surgery

Weber, Thomas K MD [PS] - **Hospital:** Albany Med Ctr; **Address:** Albany Medical Ctr, 47 New Scotland Ave, MC 61, Albany, NY 12208; **Phone:** 518-262-5831; **Board Cert:** Surgery 2005; **Med School:** Ohio State Univ 1971; **Resid:** Surgery, Univ MI Hosp & Hlth Ctr 1977; **Fellow:** Pediatric Surgery, Chldns Natl Med Ctr 1979; **Fac Appt:** Prof S, Albany Med Coll

Southeast

Bond, Sheldon J MD [PS] - **Spec Exp:** Pediatric Cancers; Fetal Surgery; Trauma; **Hospital:** Kosair Chldn's Hosp; **Address:** University Pediatric Surgery Assocs, 234 E Gray St, Ste 766, Louisville, KY 40202; **Phone:** 502-583-7337; **Board Cert:** Surgery 1998; Pediatric Surgery 1999; Surgical Critical Care 2001; **Med School:** Med Coll Wisc 1983; **Resid:** Surgery, Univ Louisville Med Ctr 1989; **Fellow:** Fetal Surgery, UCSF Med Ctr; Pediatric Surgery, Chldns Natl Med Ctr 1991; **Fac Appt:** Prof S, Univ Louisville Sch Med

Davidoff, Andrew M MD [PS] - **Spec Exp:** Neuroblastoma; Cancer Surgery; **Hospital:** St Jude Children's Research Hosp, Le Bonheur Chldns Med Ctr; **Address:** St Jude Chldns Rsch Hosp, Dept Surg, 332 N Lauderdale St, Memphis, TN 38105; **Phone:** 901-495-4060; **Board Cert:** Surgery 1995; Pediatric Surgery 1998; **Med School:** Univ Pennsylvania 1987; **Resid:** Surgery, Duke Med Ctr 1994; **Fellow:** Pediatric Surgery, Chldns Hosp 1996; **Fac Appt:** Assoc Prof S, Univ Tenn Coll Med, Memphis

Drucker, David E MD [PS] - **Spec Exp:** Thoracic Surgery; Cancer Surgery; Gastrointestinal Surgery; **Hospital:** Meml Regl Hosp - Hollywood; **Address:** 1150 N 35th Ave, Ste 555, Hollywood, FL 33021-5431; **Phone:** 954-981-0072; **Board Cert:** Surgery 1997; Pediatric Surgery 1999; Surgical Critical Care 2001; **Med School:** Brown Univ 1982; **Resid:** Surgery, Med Coll Virginia Hosps 1988; **Fellow:** Pediatric Surgery, Chldns Hosp 1990

Fallat, Mary E MD [PS] - **Spec Exp:** Trauma; Burn Care; **Hospital:** Kosair Chldn's Hosp, Univ of Louisville Hosp; **Address:** University Pediatric Surgery Assocs, 234 E Gray St, Ste 766, Louisville, KY 40202; **Phone:** 502-583-7337; **Board Cert:** Surgery 1995; Pediatric Surgery 1997; **Med School:** SUNY Upstate Med Univ 1979; **Resid:** Surgery, Univ Louisville Med Ctr 1985; **Fellow:** Research, Mass Genl Hosp 1983; Pediatric Surgery, Chldns Natl Med Ctr 1987; **Fac Appt:** Prof S, Univ Louisville Sch Med

Georgeson, Keith E MD [PS] - **Spec Exp:** Hirschsprung's Disease; Minimally Invasive Surgery; Gastroesophageal Reflux Disease (GERD); **Hospital:** Children's Hospital - Birmingham; **Address:** Chlds Hosp of Alabama, Dept Ped Surgery, 1600 7th Ave S, Ste ACC300, Birmingham, AL 35233-1711; **Phone:** 205-939-9688; **Board Cert:** Surgery 2000; Pediatric Surgery 1995; **Med School:** Loma Linda Univ 1969; **Resid:** Surgery, Loma Linda Univ Med Ctr 1973; Pediatric Surgery, Chldn's Hosp Mich 1975; **Fac Appt:** Prof S, Univ Ala

Nakayama, Don Ken MD [PS] - **Spec Exp:** Neonatal Surgery; Minimally Invasive Surgery; **Hospital:** New Hanover Reg Med Ctr; **Address:** 2131 S 17th St, PO Box 9025, Wilmington, NC 28402; **Phone:** 910-343-7001; **Board Cert:** Pediatric Surgery 1995; Surgery 2003; **Med School:** UCSF 1978; **Resid:** Surgery, UCSF Hosps 1984; **Fellow:** Pediatric Surgery, Childrens Hosp 1986; **Fac Appt:** Prof S, Univ NC Sch Med

Nuss, Donald MD [PS] - **Spec Exp:** Chest Wall Deformities; Minimally Invasive Surgery; **Hospital:** Chldns Hosp of King's Daughters; **Address:** Chldns Surg Specialty Grp, 601 Childrens Ln, Ste Pectus, Norfolk, VA 23507; **Phone:** 757-668-7703; **Board Cert:** Surgery 1973; Pediatric Surgery 1997; **Med School:** South Africa 1963; **Resid:** Surgery, Mayo Clinic 1971; Pediatric Surgery, Red Cross Chldns Hosp 1973; **Fac Appt:** Prof S, Eastern VA Med Sch

Paidas, Charles N MD [PS] - **Spec Exp:** Pediatric Cancers; Chest Wall Deformities; Pediatric Transplant Surgery; Hernia; **Hospital:** Tampa Genl Hosp, Univ of S FL - Tampa; **Address:** Tampa Genl Hosp, Div Ped Surgery, 2 Columbia Drive, rm 6441, Tampa, FL 33606; **Phone:** 813-259-0929; **Board Cert:** Surgery 1999; Pediatric Surgery 2001; Surgical Critical Care 2002; **Med School:** NY Med Coll 1981; **Resid:** Surgery, NY Med Coll Affil Hosps 1987; **Fellow:** Pediatric Surgery, Johns Hopkins Hosp 1991; **Fac Appt:** Prof S, Univ S Fla Coll Med

Rice, Henry MD [PS] - **Spec Exp:** Neonatal Surgery; Cancer Surgery; **Hospital:** Duke Univ Med Ctr; **Address:** Duke Univ Med Ctr, Dept Ped Surg, Box 3815, Durham, NC 27710; **Phone:** 919-681-5077; **Board Cert:** Surgery 1997; Pediatric Surgery 2000; **Med School:** Yale Univ 1988; **Resid:** Surgery, Univ Wash Affil Hosps 1996; **Fellow:** Pediatric Surgery, Chldns Hosp of Buffalo 1998; **Fac Appt:** Assoc Prof S, Duke Univ

Ricketts, Richard R MD [PS] - **Spec Exp:** Neonatal Surgery; Cancer Surgery; Gastrointestinal Surgery; **Hospital:** Chldns Hlthcare Atlanta - Egleston; **Address:** 1975 Century Blvd, Ste 6, Atlanta, GA 30345; **Phone:** 404-982-9938; **Board Cert:** Surgery 2004; Pediatric Surgery 2001; **Med School:** Northwestern Univ 1973; **Resid:** Surgery, LAC-USC Med Ctr 1978; **Fellow:** Pediatric Surgery, Chldns Meml Hosp 1980; **Fac Appt:** Prof S, Emory Univ

Rodgers, Bradley Moreland MD [PS] - **Spec Exp:** Thoracic Surgery; Neonatal Surgery; Minimally Invasive Surgery; **Hospital:** Univ Virginia Med Ctr; **Address:** U VA Chldns Hosp, Dept Surgery, PO Box 800709, Charlottesville, VA 22908; **Phone:** 434-924-2673; **Board Cert:** Surgery 1997; Pediatric Surgery 2005; Thoracic Surgery 1975; **Med School:** Johns Hopkins Univ 1966; **Resid:** Surgery, Duke Univ Med Ctr 1968; Cardiothoracic Surgery, Duke Univ Med Ctr 1973; **Fellow:** Pediatric Surgery, Chldns Hosp 1974; **Fac Appt:** Prof S, Univ VA Sch Med

Shochat, Stephen J MD [PS] - **Spec Exp:** Cancer Surgery; Chest Wall Deformities; **Hospital:** St Jude Children's Research Hosp; **Address:** St Jude Childrens Research Hosp, Dept Surgery, 332 N Lauderdale St, Memphis, TN 38105; **Phone:** 901-495-2911; **Board Cert:** Surgery 1969; Thoracic Surgery 1975; Pediatric Surgery 2005; **Med School:** Med Coll VA 1963; **Resid:** Surgery, Barnes Hosp 1964; Pediatric Surgery, Boston Children's Hosp 1968; **Fellow:** Thoracic Surgery, George Washington Univ Med Ctr 1974; **Fac Appt:** Prof S, Univ Tenn Coll Med, Memphis

Stylianos, Steven MD [PS] - **Spec Exp:** Trauma; Neonatal Surgery; Chest Wall Deformities; **Hospital:** Miami Children's Hosp; **Address:** Miami Childrens Hosp, 3200 SW 60th Court, Ste 201, Miami, FL 33155; **Phone:** 305-662-8320; **Board Cert:** Surgery 2002; Pediatric Surgery 2003; **Med School:** NYU Sch Med 1983; **Resid:** Surgery, Columbia-Presby Med Ctr 1988; Pediatric Surgery, Chldns Hosp 1992; **Fellow:** Pediatric Trauma, New England Med Ctr 1990; **Fac Appt:** Assoc Prof S, Univ Miami Sch Med

Weinberger, Malvin MD [PS] - **Spec Exp:** Neonatal Surgery; Trauma; Cancer Surgery; **Hospital:** Miami Children's Hosp, Baptist Hosp of Miami; **Address:** 3200 SW 60th Ct, Ste 201, Miami, FL 33155-4070; **Phone:** 305-662-8320; **Board Cert:** Surgery 1970; Pediatric Surgery 1995; **Med School:** Temple Univ 1962; **Resid:** Surgery, Temple Univ Hosp 1969; Pediatric Surgery, Chldns Hosp/Ohio St Univ Hosp 1971; **Fac Appt:** Assoc Clin Prof S, Univ Miami Sch Med

Midwest

Aiken, John Judson MD [PS] - **Spec Exp:** Tumor Surgery; Chest Wall Deformities; Hernia; **Hospital:** Chldns Hosp - Wisconsin; **Address:** 999 N 92nd St, Ste C-320, Milwaukee, WI 53226; **Phone:** 414-266-6550; **Board Cert:** Surgery 2004; Pediatric Surgery 2000; **Med School:** Univ Cincinnati 1984; **Resid:** Surgery, Mass Genl Hosp 1991; **Fellow:** Pediatric Surgery, Chldns Hosp; **Fac Appt:** Assoc Prof S, Med Coll Wisc

Bove, Edward MD [PS] - **Spec Exp:** Pediatric Cardiothoracic Surgery; Hypoplastic Left Heart Syndrome; Congenital Heart Surgery; **Hospital:** Univ Michigan Hlth Sys; **Address:** C.S. Mott Chldns Hosp, Dept Surg, 1500 E Med Ctr Drive, rm F7830, Box 0223, Ann Arbor, MI 48109-0223; **Phone:** 734-936-4980; **Board Cert:** Thoracic Surgery 1998; **Med School:** Albany Med Coll 1972; **Resid:** Surgery, Univ Mich Med Ctr 1976; Thoracic Surgery, Univ Mich Med Ctr 1979; **Fellow:** Pediatric Cardiac Surgery, Hosp Sick Chldn 1980; **Fac Appt:** Prof S, Univ Mich Med Sch

Crombleholme, Timothy M MD [PS] - **Spec Exp:** Fetal Surgery; Twin to Twin Transfusion Syndrome (TTTS); **Hospital:** Cincinnati Chldns Hosp Med Ctr, Univ Hosp - Cincinnati; **Address:** Fetal Care Center of Cincinnati, 3333 Burnet Ave, MC 2023, Cincinnati, OH 45229; **Phone:** 513-636-9608; **Board Cert:** Surgery 2003; Pediatric Surgery 1994; **Med School:** Tufts Univ 1984; **Resid:** Surgery, UCSF Med Ctr 1991; **Fellow:** Pediatric Surgery, Tufts-New England Med Ctr 1993; **Fac Appt:** Prof S, Univ Cincinnati

Duncan, Brian W MD [PS] - **Spec Exp:** Pediatric Cardiac Surgery; Neonatal & Infant Cardiac Surgery; Transplant-Heart-Pediatric; **Hospital:** Cleveland Clin Fdn (page 57); **Address:** Cleveland Clinic, Children's Hospital, 9500 Euclid Ave, Desk M41, Cleveland, OH 44195; **Phone:** 216-444-9365; **Board Cert:** Surgery 2004; Thoracic Surgery 1997; **Med School:** Indiana Univ 1985; **Resid:** Surgery, Mass General Hosp 1992; Thoracic Surgery, Mass General Hosp 1995; **Fellow:** Surgical Research, UCSF Med Ctr; **Fac Appt:** Prof S, Cleveland Cl Coll Med/Case West Res

Ehrlich, Peter F MD [PS] - **Spec Exp:** Pediatric Cancers; Wilms' Tumor; Thyroid Cancer; **Hospital:** Mott Chldns Hosp, Mich State Univ-Hurley Med Ctr; **Address:** Mott Children's Hospital, 1500 E Medical Center Drive, rm F3970, Ann Arbor, MI 48109-0245; **Phone:** 734-764-4151; **Board Cert:** Surgery 1997; Pediatric Surgery 2000; **Med School:** Canada 1989; **Resid:** Surgery, Univ Toronto Med Ctr 1996; **Fellow:** Pediatric Surgery, Children's Natl Med Ctr 1998; **Fac Appt:** Assoc Clin Prof S, Univ Mich Med Sch

Grosfeld, Jay L MD [PS] - **Spec Exp:** Cancer Surgery; Neonatal Surgery; **Hospital:** Riley Hosp for Children; **Address:** 702 Barnhill Drive, Ste 2500, Indianapolis, IN 46202-5200; **Phone:** 317-274-5716; **Board Cert:** Surgery 1989; Pediatric Surgery 2000; **Med School:** NYU Sch Med 1961; **Resid:** Surgery, Bellevue-NYU Hosp 1966; Pediatric Surgery, Ohio State Univ 1970; **Fellow:** Surgical Oncology, Chldns Hosp 1970; **Fac Appt:** Prof S, Indiana Univ

Holterman, Mark J MD [PS] - **Spec Exp:** Minimally Invasive Surgery; Neonatal Surgery; Transplant-Liver; Transplant-Bowel; **Hospital:** Univ of IL Med Ctr at Chicago; **Address:** Univ of Illinos, Pediatric Surgery, 840 S Wood St, Ste 416, MC 95, Chicago, IL 60612; **Phone:** 312-413-7707; **Board Cert:** Surgery 2001; Pediatric Surgery 1998; **Med School:** Univ VA Sch Med 1985; **Resid:** Surgery, Univ Virginia Hosp 1993; **Fellow:** Pediatric Surgery, Childrens Hosp & Med Ctr 1993; **Fac Appt:** Assoc Prof S, Univ IL Coll Med

Ilbawi, Michel MD [PS] - **Spec Exp:** Cardiac Surgery; Congenital Anomalies; Cardiovascular Surgery; **Hospital:** Adv Christ Med Ctr, Adv Luth Genl Hosp; **Address:** Hope Chldns Hosp at Adv Christ Med Ctr, 4440 W 95th St, Oak Lawn, IL 60453; **Phone:** 708-684-3029; **Board Cert:** Thoracic Surgery 1998; **Med School:** Lebanon 1971; **Resid:** Surgery, American Univ Hosp 1975; Thoracic Surgery, Univ Hosps 1977; **Fellow:** Thoracic Surgery, Chldns Meml Hosp 1978; **Fac Appt:** Clin Prof S, Univ IL Coll Med

Lobe, Thom E MD [PS] - **Spec Exp:** Minimally Invasive Surgery; Robotic Surgery; Pediatric Urology; **Hospital:** Iowa Methodist Med Ctr; **Address:** Blank Children's Hospital, 1212 Pleasant St, Ste 300, Des Moines, IA 50309; **Phone:** 515-241-6000; **Board Cert:** Surgery 1989; Pediatric Surgery 1989; **Med School:** Univ MD Sch Med 1975; **Resid:** Surgery, Ohio State Univ Med Ctr 1979; Pediatric Surgery, Childrens Hosp 1981

Mavroudis, Constantine MD [PS] - **Spec Exp:** Congenital Heart Disease; Transplant-Heart & Lung; Coronary Artery Surgery; **Hospital:** Children's Mem Hosp; **Address:** 2300 Childrens Plaza , Box 22, Chicago, IL 60614-3318; **Phone:** 773-880-4378; **Board Cert:** Surgery 2000; Thoracic Surgery 2000; **Med School:** Univ VA Sch Med 1973; **Resid:** Surgery, UCSF Med Ctr 1979; **Fellow:** Surgery, UCSF Med Ctr 1977; **Fac Appt:** Prof S, Northwestern Univ

Oldham, Keith T MD [PS] - **Spec Exp:** Neonatal Surgery; Thoracic Surgery; Gastrointestinal Surgery; **Hospital:** Chldns Hosp - Wisconsin; **Address:** 999 N 92nd St, Ste 320, Milwaukee, WI 53226; **Phone:** 414-266-6550; **Board Cert:** Surgery 2000; Pediatric Surgery 1991; Surgical Critical Care 1995; **Med School:** Med Coll VA 1976; **Resid:** Surgery, Univ Wash Med Ctr 1981; **Fellow:** Pediatric Surgery, Univ Cincinnati Chldns Hosp 1983; **Fac Appt:** Prof S, Med Coll Wisc

Pena, Alberto MD [PS] - **Spec Exp:** Imperforate Anus; Anorectal Malformations; Colon & Rectal Surgery; **Hospital:** Cincinnati Chldns Hosp Med Ctr; **Address:** Cincinnati Chlds Hosp Med Ctr, 3333 Burnet Ave, ML 2023, Cincinnati, OH 45229; **Phone:** 513-636-3238; **Med School:** Mexico 1962; **Resid:** Surgery, Military Hosp 1966; **Fellow:** Pediatric Surgery, Childrens Hosp 1971; Cardiovascular Surgery, Childrens Hosp 1969

Reynolds, Marleta MD [PS] - **Spec Exp:** Critical Care; Trauma; Congenital Anomalies; **Hospital:** Children's Mem Hosp; **Address:** Chldns Meml Hosp, Dept Ped Surg, 2300 Children's Plaza, Box 63, Chicago, IL 60614; **Phone:** 773-880-4292; **Board Cert:** Surgery 1991; Thoracic Surgery 1995; Pediatric Surgery 1993; **Med School:** Tulane Univ 1976; **Resid:** Surgery, Tulane Univ Affil Hosp 1981; Pediatric Surgery, Chldns Meml Hosp 1983; **Fellow:** Cardiothoracic Surgery, Northwestern Univ 1985; **Fac Appt:** Asst Prof S, Northwestern Univ

Sato, Thomas T MD [PS] - **Spec Exp:** Neonatal Surgery; Congenital Anomalies; Laparoscopy & Thoracostomy; **Hospital:** Chldns Hosp - Wisconsin; **Address:** 999 N 92nd St, Ste C320, Milwaukee, WI 53226; **Phone:** 414-266-6550; **Board Cert:** Surgery 2007; Pediatric Surgery 1998; **Med School:** USC Sch Med 1988; **Resid:** Surgery, Univ Wash Med Ctr 1995; **Fellow:** Surgery, Harborview Med Ctr 1993; Pediatric Surgery, Chldns Natl Med Ctr 1997; **Fac Appt:** Assoc Prof S, Med Coll Wisc

Pediatric Surgery

Sheldon, Curtis MD [PS] - **Spec Exp:** Pediatric Urology; Genitourinary Reconstruction; Transplant-Kidney-Pediatric; **Hospital:** Cincinnati Chldns Hosp Med Ctr; **Address:** Childrens Hosp, Div Pediatric Urology, 3333 Burnet Ave, MC 5037, Cincinnati, OH 45229; **Phone:** 513-636-4975; **Board Cert:** Surgery 1993; Urology 1982; Pediatric Surgery 1997; **Med School:** UCSD 1976; **Resid:** Urology, Univ Minnesota Affil Hosp 1981; Surgery, Univ Minnesota Affil Hosp 1983; **Fellow:** Pediatric Surgery, Chldns Hosp Med Ctr 1985; Pediatric Urology, Hosp for Sick Chldn 1986; **Fac Appt:** Prof S, Univ Cincinnati

Warner, Brad MD [PS] - **Spec Exp:** Gastrointestinal Surgery; Neonatal Surgery; Cancer Surgery; **Hospital:** Cincinnati Chldns Hosp Med Ctr; **Address:** Cincinnati Chlds Hosp, Div Ped Surg, 3333 Burnet Ave, MLC 2023, Cincinnati, OH 45229; **Phone:** 513-636-4371; **Board Cert:** Surgery 1998; Pediatric Surgery 2001; **Med School:** Univ MO-Kansas City 1982; **Resid:** Surgery, Univ Cincinnati Med Ctr 1989; **Fellow:** Pediatric Surgery, Chldns Hosp Med Ctr 1991; **Fac Appt:** Prof S, Univ Cincinnati

Great Plains and Mountains

Karrer, Frederick M MD [PS] - **Spec Exp:** Liver Surgery; Transplant-Liver; Critical Care; **Hospital:** Chldn's Hosp - Denver, The, Denver Health Med Ctr; **Address:** Children's Hospital, Dept Surgery, 1950 Ogden St, B323, Denver, CO 80218-1022; **Phone:** 303-861-6571; **Board Cert:** Surgery 1996; Pediatric Surgery 1997; Surgical Critical Care 1998; **Med School:** Univ Nebr Coll Med 1979; **Resid:** Surgery, Univ Ariz Med Ctr 1984; Pediatric Surgery, Children's Meml Hosp 1988; **Fellow:** Transplant Surgery, Univ Pittsburgh 1986; **Fac Appt:** Prof S, Univ Colorado

Meyers, Rebecka L MD [PS] - **Spec Exp:** Transplant-Liver; Tumor Surgery-Pediatric; Biliary Surgery; Pancreatic Surgery; **Hospital:** Univ Utah Hosps and Clins; **Address:** Primary Chlds Med Ctr, Dept Ped Surg, 100 N Medical Drive, Ste 2600, Salt Lake City, UT 84113; **Phone:** 801-588-3350; **Board Cert:** Surgery 2003; Pediatric Surgery 1996; **Med School:** Oregon Hlth Sci Univ 1985; **Resid:** Surgery, UCSF 1990; **Fellow:** Research, Cardio Rsch Inst-UCSF 1992; Pediatric Surgery, St Christopher's Hosp for Chldn 1994; **Fac Appt:** Assoc Prof S, Univ Utah

Ziegler, Moritz M MD [PS] - **Spec Exp:** Hirschsprung's Disease; Gastrointestinal Surgery; Neuroblastoma; Tumor Surgery-Pediatric; **Hospital:** Chldn's Hosp - Denver, The; **Address:** Chldns Hosp, Dept Surgery, 1056 E 19th Ave, Box 323, Denver, CO 80218; **Phone:** 303-861-6524; **Board Cert:** Surgery 1975; Pediatric Surgery 1995; **Med School:** Univ Mich Med Sch 1968; **Resid:** Surgery, Univ Penn Hosp 1975; Pediatric Surgery, Chldns Hosp 1977; **Fellow:** Surgical Oncology, Amer Oncologic Hosp 1975; **Fac Appt:** Prof S, Univ Colorado

Southwest

Arensman, Robert MD [PS] - **Spec Exp:** Congenital Anomalies; **Hospital:** Ochsner Fdn Hosp, Tulane Univ Hosp & Clin; **Address:** 1514 Jefferson Hwy, New Orleans, LA 70121; **Phone:** 504-842-3907; **Board Cert:** Surgery 1979; Pediatric Surgery 1989; **Med School:** Univ IL Coll Med 1969; **Resid:** Surgery, Univ Illinois Med Ctr 1972; Surgery, Univ Illinois Med Ctr 1976; **Fellow:** Pediatric Surgery, Chldns Natl Med Ctr 1978

Foglia, Robert P MD [PS] - **Spec Exp:** Congenital Anomalies; Burn Care; **Hospital:** Chldns Med Ctr of Dallas; **Address:** 1935 Motor St, Dallas, TX 75235; **Phone:** 214-456-6040; **Board Cert:** Surgery 2002; Pediatric Surgery 1995; Surgical Critical Care 1993; **Med School:** Georgetown Univ 1974; **Resid:** Surgery, UCLA Med Ctr 1981; **Fellow:** Pediatric Surgery, Chldns Hosp Natl Med Ctr 1983; **Fac Appt:** Prof S, Univ Tex SW, Dallas

Jackson, Richard J MD [PS] - **Spec Exp:** Cancer Surgery; Neonatal Surgery; Robotic Surgery; **Hospital:** Arkansas Chldns Hosp; **Address:** Arkansas Chldns Hosp - Ped Surgery, 800 Marshall St, MS 837, Little Rock, AR 72202; **Phone:** 501-364-1446; **Board Cert:** Surgery 1997; Pediatric Surgery 2001; Surgical Critical Care 1998; **Med School:** W VA Univ 1983; **Resid:** Surgery, W Va Univ Hosps 1988; Pediatric Surgery, Chldns Hosp 1989; **Fellow:** Pediatric Critical Care Medicine, Chldns Hosp-Univ Pittsburgh 1990; Pediatric Surgery, Chldns Hosp-Univ Pittsburgh 1992; **Fac Appt:** Assoc Prof S, Univ Ark

Nuchtern, Jed MD [PS] - **Spec Exp:** Thoracic Surgery; Cancer Surgery; Laparoscopic Surgery; **Hospital:** Texas Chldns Hosp - Houston, Ben Taub General Hosp; **Address:** Texas Children's Hosp, 6621 Fannin St, MC CC650, Houston, TX 77030; **Phone:** 832-822-3135; **Board Cert:** Surgery 2003; Surgical Critical Care 2002; Pediatric Surgery 1998; **Med School:** Harvard Med Sch 1985; **Resid:** Surgery, Univ Washington 1992; Pediatric Surgery, Baylor Coll Med 1995; **Fellow:** Cellular Molecular Biology, Natl Inst Hlth 1990; **Fac Appt:** Assoc Prof S, Baylor Coll Med

West Coast and Pacific

Albanese, Craig MD [PS] - **Spec Exp:** Fetal Surgery; Laparoscopic Surgery; Twin to Twin Transfusion Syndrome (TTTS); **Hospital:** Lucile Packard Chldns Hosp/Stanford Univ Med Ctr; **Address:** 780 Welch Rd, Ste 206, MC 5733, Palo Alto, CA 94304; **Phone:** 650-723-6439; **Board Cert:** Surgery 2000; Pediatric Surgery 2003; **Med School:** SUNY Hlth Sci Ctr 1986; **Resid:** Surgery, Mt Sinai Med Ctr 1991; **Fellow:** Pediatric Surgery, Chldns Hosp 1994; **Fac Appt:** Prof S, Stanford Univ

Atkinson, James B MD [PS] - **Spec Exp:** Laparoscopic Surgery; Cancer Surgery; Colorectal Anomalies; **Hospital:** UCLA Med Ctr, Northridge Hosp Med Ctr - Roscoe Campus; **Address:** 10833 LeConte Ave, Box 709818, Los Angeles, CA 90095; **Phone:** 310-206-2429; **Board Cert:** Surgery 2001; Pediatric Surgery 2003; **Med School:** Wake Forest Univ 1976; **Resid:** Surgery, UCLA Med Ctr 1981; **Fellow:** Pediatric Surgery, Chldns Hosp 1983; **Fac Appt:** Prof S, UCLA

Ford, Henri R MD [PS] - **Spec Exp:** Minimally Invasive Surgery; Trauma; **Hospital:** Chldns Hosp - Los Angeles (page 56); **Address:** 4650 Sunset Blvd, MS 100, Los Angeles, CA 90027; **Phone:** 323-669-2104; **Board Cert:** Surgery 2002; Pediatric Surgery 2005; **Med School:** Harvard Med Sch 1984; **Resid:** Surgery, New York Hosp 1991; **Fellow:** Pediatric Surgery, Chldns Hosp Pittsburgh 1995

Harrison, Michael R MD [PS] - **Spec Exp:** Fetal Surgery; Twin to Twin Transfusion Syndrome (TTTS); Spina Bifida; **Hospital:** UCSF Med Ctr, CA Pacific Med Ctr - Pacific Campus; **Address:** 533 Parnassus Ave, Ste U149, Box 0570, San Francisco, CA 94143-0570; **Phone:** 415-476-2538; **Board Cert:** Pediatric Surgery 1999; **Med School:** Harvard Med Sch 1969; **Resid:** Surgery, Mass Genl Hosp 1971; Surgery, Mass Genl Hosp 1975; **Fellow:** Pediatric Surgery, Rikshospitalet 1976; Pediatric Surgery, Chldns Hosp 1978; **Fac Appt:** Prof S, UCSF

Hilfiker, Mary L MD/PhD [PS] - **Hospital:** UCSD Med Ctr; **Address:** 8010 Frost St, Ste 414, San Diego, CA 92123; **Phone:** 858-966-7711; **Board Cert:** Surgery 2004; Pediatric Surgery 2000; **Med School:** Wright State Univ 1988; **Resid:** Surgery, U New Mexico Med Ctr 1993; **Fellow:** Pelvic Surgery, SUNY-Children's Hosp 1995; **Fac Appt:** Assoc Clin Prof S, UCSD

Pediatric Surgery

Krummel, Thomas M MD [PS] - **Spec Exp:** Minimally Invasive Surgery; Robotic Surgery; Fetal Surgery; **Hospital:** Lucile Packard Chldns Hosp/Stanford Univ Med Ctr, Stanford Univ Med Ctr; **Address:** Dept Surgery, 701B Welch Rd, Ste 225, MC 5784, Stanford, CA 94305-5784; **Phone:** 650-498-4292; **Board Cert:** Surgery 2004; Pediatric Surgery 1997; **Med School:** Univ Wisc 1977; **Resid:** Surgery, Med Coll Va Hosp 1983; Pediatric Surgery, Chldns Hosp 1985; **Fellow:** Surgery, Med Coll Va Hosp 1980; Fetal Surgery, UCSF Med Ctr; **Fac Appt:** Prof S, Stanford Univ

Sawin, Robert S MD [PS] - **Spec Exp:** Pediatric Cancers; Thoracic Surgery; Neonatal Surgery-Gastrointestinal; **Hospital:** Chldns Hosp and Regl Med Ctr - Seattle; **Address:** Chldns Hosp & Regl Med Ctr, PO Box 5371, MS W7724, Seattle, WA 98105; **Phone:** 206-987-2039; **Board Cert:** Surgery 1998; Surgical Critical Care 2001; Pediatric Surgery 1999; **Med School:** Univ Pittsburgh 1982; **Resid:** Surgery, Brigham Women's Hosp 1987; **Fellow:** Pediatric Surgery, Chldns Hosp 1989; **Fac Appt:** Prof S, Univ Wash

Stein, James E MD [PS] - **Hospital:** Chldns Hosp - Los Angeles (page 56); **Address:** Children's Hospital of LA, 4650 Sunset Blvd, MS 100, Los Angeles, CA 90027; **Phone:** 323-669-2491; **Board Cert:** Surgery 2004; Pediatric Surgery 2005; **Med School:** Tufts Univ 1986; **Resid:** Surgery, Tufts New England Med Ctr 1993; Research, Boston Chldn's Hosp 1991; **Fellow:** Pediatric Surgery, Royal Chldns Hosp 1994; Pediatric Surgery, Babies Hosp/Columbia Presby 1996; **Fac Appt:** Assoc Prof S, USC Sch Med

Bascom Palmer
EYE INSTITUTE

University of Miami
Miller School of Medicine
www.bascompalmer.org
(800) 329-7000

Miami
900 NW 17th Street
Miami, FL 33136
(305) 326-6000
(800) 329-7000

Naples
311 9th Street North
Naples, FL 34102
(239) 659-3937

Plantation
1000 South Pine Island Road
Plantation, FL 33324
(239) 659-3937

Palm Beach Gardens
7101 Fairway Drive
Palm Beach Gardens, FL 33418
(561) 515-1500

INTERNATIONALLY ACCLAIMED

Bascom Palmer Eye Institute is committed to the protection and preservation of the treasured gift of sight. The Institute's full-time faculty of internationally-respected physicians and scientists are skilled in every ophthalmic subspecialty. Bascom Palmer Eye Institute, which serves as the Department of Ophthalmology for the University of Miami Miller School of Medicine in Miami, Florida, is recognized as one of the world's finest and most progressive centers for ophthalmic care, research and education.

BASCOM PALMER EYE INSTITUTE EARNS TOP RATINGS

Bascom Palmer Eye Institute continues to be rated as one of the nation's best ophthalmic hospitals by board-certified ophthalmologists from across the United States. In 2004, 2005 and 2006 Bascom Palmer was named the #1 eye hospital in the United States by *U.S.News & World Report*. Bascom Palmer has also received the #1 ranking for its Clinical (Patient Care) and Residency programs by *Ophthalmology Times*, which annually ranks the top ophthalmology programs in the United States.

PEDIATRIC OPHTHALMOLOGISTS DIAGNOSE AND TREAT CHILDHOOD EYE DISEASE AND DISORDERS

Bascom Palmer Eye Institute is one of only a few centers giving special attention to the diverse ophthalmic needs of children from infancy through adolescence- a critical time when clear vision plays an important role in mental, physical, and social development. As a major referral center serving the southeastern United States, the Caribbean and South America, the Institute treats approximately 7,000 children annually in its William and Norma Horvitz Children's Clinic, an outstanding ophthalmic facility designed specifically for pediatric care. Our spacious outpatient clinic is specifically designed to meet the unique ophthalmic and social needs of children with visual deficiencies as well as adults and children with strabismus. The clinic's diagnostic and treatment services encompass the common eye disorders of childhood, such as amblyopia and strabismus, as well as rare disorders affecting infants and children. With the support of the extensive resources of the entire Bascom Palmer Eye Institute, The Horvitz Clinic specializes in the blinding and visually-impairing diseases of childhood including congenital cataracts, congenital glaucoma, retinopathy of prematurity, detached retinas, ocular infections, hereditary disorders and tumors.

Childrens Hospital Los Angeles

4650 Sunset Boulevard
Los Angeles, California 90027
www.ChildrensHospitalLA.org

ChildrensHospitalLosAngeles

International Leader in Pediatrics

Childrens Hospital Los Angeles is acknowledged throughout the United States and around the world for its leadership in pediatric and adolescent health. It is able to offer the very best in multidisciplinary care, with 85 pediatric subspecialties and dozens of special services for children and families. Its physicians are recognized as leaders. Its treatments set the standard of care. Its research is recognized worldwide.

The Heart Institute

The Heart Institute is known throughout the world as a leader in the treatment of pediatric heart disease, offering the most advanced diagnostic and treatment modalities available in cardiology, cardio thoracic surgery, cardio thoracic transplantation and intensive care, as well as innovation in cardiac research. Physicians provide comprehensive care to 8,000 children each year – fetus through adolescent – who have congenital or acquired heart and lung disorders. For information contact (323) 669-4148.

Center for Endocrinology, Diabetes and Metabolism

The Center for Endocrinology, Diabetes and Metabolism is at the forefront of patient care, basic and clinical research in diabetes, obesity, growth, bone metabolism and endocrinology. More than 2,000 children and adolescents with Type 1 and Type 2 diabetes are under the care of its pediatric diabetes specialists, certified diabetes educators and nutritionists – one of the largest programs of its kind in America. For information contact (323) 669-4604.

Childrens Center for Cancer and Blood Diseases

The Childrens Center for Cancer and Blood Diseases is the nation's largest pediatric hematology/oncology program. Physician- scientists integrate their laboratory experience with their clinical expertise in an approach to medical problem-solving that enables them to move effectively from "Bench to Bedside." Breakthroughs in the treatment of childhood cancer, many pioneered at Childrens Hospital Los Angeles, offer children, teenagers and young adults the most advanced treatment available anywhere. For information contact (323) 669-2121.

Childrens Orthopaedic Center

The Childrens Orthopaedic Center is one of the nation's most comprehensive programs dedicated to pediatric musculoskeletal care, education and research. Its Scoliosis and Spine Disorders Program, one of the largest in the country, is the only one of its kind in Los Angeles County devoted exclusively to the pediatric population. Its state-of-the-art Motion Analysis Laboratory is designed to analyze muscle activity and joint movements in children who have difficulty walking, such as those with cerebral palsy, spina bifida and congenital leg conditions. For information contact (323) 669-2142.

602

Cleveland Clinic

Children's Hospital

Cleveland Clinic Children's Hospital is ranked among the top pediatric hospitals in the United States, with more that 50 pediatricians recognized as "Best Doctors in America." Cleveland Clinic Children's Hospital specialists are nationally recognized for sophisticated diagnosis and innovative care of complex or chronic medical conditions affecting infants, children and adolescents as well as nationally funded research initiatives that are leading to advanced treatments for young patients.

- Our Center for Pediatric and Congenital Heart Disease is known for groundbreaking catheter and surgical treatments.
- As part of Cleveland Clinic's Neurological Institute, our pediatric epilepsy specialists offer highly specialized diagnosis and surgery for different seizure disorders.
- Our pediatric digestive disease specialists utilize breakthrough technology to diagnose and treat gastrointestinal problems.
- Children's Hospital oncologists are national leaders in the treatment of childhood leukemia and other cancers
- A comprehensive Fetal Care Center with maternal-fetal medicine specialists to diagnose fetal problems and treat them in the womb or immediately after birth.

In addition, Cleveland Clinic Children's Hospital has the only comprehensive pediatric transplant center in Northern Ohio, offering heart, lung, liver and kidney transplantation and follow-up.

Our Pediatric ICU offers outstanding outcomes, saving many more young lives than similar centers, largely due to the 24-hour presence of seasoned critical care specialists. Our Pediatric Critical Care Transport Service transferred over 1,000 patients to our Children's Hospital from more than 13 states in 2006.

Our expertise in specialty pediatrics extends into the realm of long-term care for developmental, behavioral and rehabilitation needs. The Cleveland Clinic Children's Hospital for Rehabilitation, Shaker Campus, serves pediatric patients with chronic or complex medical conditions as one of just a handful of freestanding accredited pediatric rehabilitation hospitals in the country, and the only one in Ohio.

To schedule an appointment or for more information about the Cleveland Clinic Children's Hospital call 800.890.2467 or visit www.clevelandclinic.org/childrenstopdocs.

Children's Hospital | 9500 Euclid Avenue / W14 | Cleveland OH 44195

Cleveland Clinic Children's Hospital

More than 150 Cleveland Clinic pediatricians and pediatric specialists offer advanced specialty and subspecialty care and rehabilitation for acute illnesses and injuries, as well as chronic and disabling conditions, in our Children's Hospital. Children with serious or complex medical problems such as congenital heart disease, cancer, epilepsy and digestive disorders are treated at our Main Campus. Our Shaker Campus is home to the Cleveland Clinic Children's Hospital for Rehabilitation and developmental, behavioral, therapeutic and rehabilitation programs that promote functional independence in children.

Sponsored Page

NewYork-Presbyterian

⌐ The University Hospital of Columbia and Cornell

✤ Morgan Stanley
⚘ Children's Hospital
⁄ of NewYork-Presbyterian
Columbia University Medical Center

3959 Broadway, New York, NY 10032

Komansky Center
for Children's Health
⌐ NewYork-Presbyterian Hospital
⌐ Weill Cornell Medical Center

525 East 68th Street, New York, NY 10021

Sponsorship: Voluntary Not-for-Profit

Beds: 387

Accreditation: Joint Commission on Accreditation of Healthcare Organizations (JCAHO)

OVERVIEW:

NewYork-Presbyterian brings together the outstanding pediatric services and resources of the Morgan Stanley Children's Hospital and the Komansky Center for Children's Health to create one of the largest, most comprehensive children's hospital in the world.

With more than 1,000 pediatricians and medical and surgical subspecialists on staff, and teams of specially trained pediatric health professionals, NewYork-Presbyterian provides the highest level of care from infancy to adolescence. The Hospital's expertise in addressing simple and complex medical conditions and the psychological and emotional issues that accompany them is unparalleled. The Hospital offers:

- Adolescent Medicine
- Allergy
- Anesthesiology and Pain Management
- Cardiology
- Child Development and Behavioral Medicine
- Critical Care
- Dermatology
- Diabetes and Endocrinology
- Gastroenterology
- Genetics
- Hematology
- Infectious Disease
- Neonatal-Perinatal Medicine
- Nephrology
- Neurology
- Neurosurgery
- Oncology
- Primary Care
- Psychiatry and Mental Health
- Rheumatology
- Laboratory and Radiology Diagnostic Services
- Pediatric Emergency Care in emergency medicine, burn and trauma
- Surgical Services in cardiac, dental, oral and maxillofacial, general neurosurgery, ophthalmology, orthopedics, otolaryngology, plastic surgery, transplantation and urology

Physician Referral: For a physician referral or for information, call **1-800-245-KIDS** (1-800-245-5437) or visit our website at **www.childrensnyp.org**

CHILDREN'S HOSPITAL HIGHLIGHTS INCLUDE:

- One of the country's largest and most successful pediatric cardiology and cardiac surgery programs.

- Only provider in the region to offer three major transplant surgeries – heart, liver and kidney.

- One of three Level 1-designated Pediatric Trauma Centers in New York State and only one in New York City.

- Nationally recognized pediatric oncologists. Bone marrow transplantation program is one of the largest in the nation.

- Sophisticated neonatal intensive care that sets standards nationwide.

- Referral center and regional resource for hospitals needing expertise of our pediatric intensive care units. Seriously ill children can be transferred to NewYork-Presbyterian through the Pediatric Critical Care Transport Program.

NYU Medical Center

550 First Avenue (at 31st Street)
New York, NY 10016
Physician Referral:
(888)7-NYU-MED (888-769-8633)
www.nyumc.org

NYU CHILDREN'S HEALTH

NYU Medical Center's Children's Health Team is comprised of some of the best clinical specialists in the country. Among the programs they offer are:

Apnea/SIDS Program —identifying and treating of infants with apnea and infants who are are at increased risk for SIDS

Center for Child and Adolescent Sports Medicine – developmentally sensitive and comprehensive evaluation and treatment of sports-related injuries in children

NYU- Hospital for Joint Diseases Center for Children – holistic outpatient treatment of children and adolescents with a wide range of orthopaedic and neurological conditions

Child Study Center – advancing the field of mental health for children and adolescents through evidence-based practice, science, and education

Cochlear Implant Program – restoring hearing to profoundly deaf children

Craniofacial Program – treating facial deformities discovered at birth
Epilepsy Program – state-of-the-art evaluation and multidisciplinary treatment of children with epilepsy

Familial Dysautonomia Program – the only center in the U.S. providing care to individuals affected with this genetic disorder

Hassenfeld Children's Center – comprehensive outpatient care for children with cancer and blood disorders

Headache Center – thorough diagnosis and evaluation to help pediatric patients manage frequency and severity of chronic headaches

Hemangiomas and Vascular Malformation Program – multidisciplinary care for children with hemangiomas and vascular malformations

Orthopaedic Immediate Care Center at the Hospital for Joint Diseases– evaluation and treatment of urgent pediatric and adult orthopaedic problems, such as fractures

Pediatric Rehabilitation Service – multi-disciplinary pediatric rehabilitation for a variety of congenital and acquired disabilities on an inpatient and outpatient basis

Preschool and Early Intervention Program – individualized educational and early intervention services for children under five

Stem Cell Transplant Program – Using stem cell transplant to treat brain and other solid tumors, under the auspices of the Hassenfeld Children's Center, which was the site of much of the original stem cell harvest and transplantation research.

NYU MEDICAL CENTER

Children's Services at NYU Medical Center provides comprehensive, family-centered care for children with all types of conditions. Specialized care for children are provided in the following areas:

- Adolescent Medicine
- Allergy
- Anesthesia
- Cardiology
- Cardio-Vascular Surgery
- Critical Care
- Dermatology
- Developmental Pediatrics
- Dysautonomia
- Emergency Medicine
- Endocrinology
- Epilepsy
- Gastroenterology
- Genetics
- Hematology
- Infectious Diseases
- Neonatology
- Nephrology
- Neurology
- Neurosurgery
- Oncology
- Ophthamology
- Orthopaedics
- Otolaryngology
- Pediatrics
- Plastic Surgery/Cranial Facial
- Psychiatry
- Pulmonology
- Radiology
- Rehabilitation Medicine
- Rheumatology
- Surgery
- Urology

706

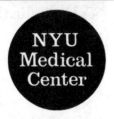

NYU Medical Center

550 First Avenue (at 31st Street)
New York, NY 10016
Physician Referral:
(888)7-NYU-MED (888-769-8633)
www.nyumc.org

PEDIATRIC ALLERGY AND IMMUNOLOGY

NYU Medical Center's Children's Health Team is comprised of some of the best clinical specialists in the country. Among the programs they offer are:

Apnea/SIDS Program –identifying and treating of infants with apnea and infants who are are at increased risk for SIDS.

Center for Child and Adolescent Sports Medicine – developmentally sensitive and comprehensive evaluation and treatment of sports-related injuries in children.

NYU- Hospital for Joint Diseases Center for Children – holistic outpatient treatment of children and adolescents with a wide range of orthopaedic and neurological conditions.

Child Study Center – advancing the field of mental health for children and adolescents through evidence-based practice, science, and education.

Cochlear Implant Program – restoring hearing to profoundly deaf children.

Craniofacial Program – treating facial deformities discovered at birth.

Epilepsy Program – state-of-the-art evaluation and multidisciplinary treatment of children with epilepsy.

Familial Dysautonomia Program – the only center in the U.S. providing care to individuals affected with this genetic disorder.

Hassenfeld Children's Center – comprehensive outpatient care for children with cancer and blood disorders.

Headache Center – thorough diagnosis and evaluation to help pediatric patients manage frequency and severity of chronic headaches.

Hemangiomas and Vascular Malformation Program – multidisciplinary care for children with hemangiomas and vascular malformations.

Orthopaedic Immediate Care Center at the Hospital for Joint Diseases Orthopaedic Institute – evaluation and treatment of urgent pediatric and adult orthopaedic problems, such as fractures.

Pediatric Rehabilitation Service – multi-disciplinary pediatric rehabilitation for a variety of congenital and acquired disabilities on an inpatient and outpatient basis.

Preschool and Early Intervention Program – individualized educational and early intervention services for children under five.

Stem Cell Transplant Program – Using stem cell transplant to treat brain and other solid tumors, under the auspices of the Hassenfeld Children's Center, which was the site of much of the original stem cell harvest and transplantation research.

707

NYU MEDICAL CENTER

NYU Children's Health provides family-centered care for pediatric allergy problems within the setting of a world-class academic medical center. Our allergy specialists work side-by-side with physicians from many other medical specialties and have ready access to their expertise, to optimize your child's treatment. Together, these teams will work with you to determine the therapy or combination of therapies that is right for you and your child.

NYU Medical Center also enjoys a strong history in pediatric immunology. Perhaps its most important achievement is the discovery of a vaccine for rubella. But that is by no means its only achievement. With a superb clinical faculty and staff that is highly committed to basic science and clinical research, NYU Medical Center continues to conduct research that positively and directly impacts on children's health.

Physician Referral
(866) CHILD-NYU
(866-244-5369)
www.nyuchildrens.org

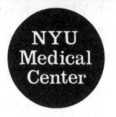

NYU Medical Center

550 First Avenue (at 31st Street)
New York, NY 10016
Physician Referral:
(888)7-NYU-MED (888-769-8633)
www.nyumc.org

PEDIATRIC CARDIOLOGY

NYU's Pediatric Cardiology Program is motivated by an academic approach to patient care. A leader for more than three decades, the Pediatric Cardiology Program remains at the forefront of innovation in both research and clinical care. It is also an outstanding training ground for future pediatricians dedicated to the heart health of children.

There is a long list of recent advances that are benefiting infants, children, and young adults with a wide range of heart problems. First, a growing emphasis on minimally invasive surgical techniques allows for quicker recoveries and shorter hospital stays. Various clinical sub-disciplines further support the Pediatric Cardiology Program, including:

Cardiothoracic Surgery – corrective procedures for all types of congenital and acquired heart disease.

Pediatric Cardiac Critical Care – intensive care for children with heart disease, provided capably and compassionately by a staff of pediatric cardiologists, neonatologists, cardiac anesthesiologists, respiratory therapists, and pediatric intensive care nurses.

Pediatric Non-Invasive Cardiac Imaging – the use of echocardiography and magnetic resonance imaging (MRI) to diagnose and monitor a wide range of cardiac abnormalities.

Pediatric Cardiac Electrophysiology – a wide array of diagnostic and therapeutic services, including arrhythmia detection and pacemaker placement.

Pediatric Interventional Cardiac Catheterization – the treatment of serious heart conditions in a nonsurgical setting, sometimes used in combination with open-heart surgery.

Pediatric Cardiopulmonary Exercise Laboratory – assesses the cardiorespiratory response of exercise in children as young as three and four years old. The Lab features some of the most sophisticated equipment in the region for measuring oxygen consumption, cardiac output, and lung capacity.

NYU MEDICAL CENTER

At NYU, a child's heart health is a family affair.

The Pediatric Cardiology staff at NYU is vigilant in helping children stay in contact with their parents during a stay at the Medical Center.

Whenever possible, parents are welcome to stay overnight in their child's room on the pediatric floor. Social workers and child life experts are always on hand to give families the information and support they need to cope with their child's disease during and after their hospital stay.

**Physician Referral
(866) CHILD-NYU
(866-244-5369)
www.nyuchildrens.org**

708

NYU Medical Center

550 First Avenue (at 31st Street)
New York, NY 10016
Physician Referral:
(888)7-NYU-MED (888-769-8633)
www.nyumc.org

PEDIATRIC CRITICAL CARE

When children experience medical problems, they deserve the most compassionate, state-of-the-art medical care possible. Yet, pediatric patients have needs, medical and emotional, that are unique and different from those of adults. To better meet these needs, Tisch Hospital at NYU Medical Center has recently completed a major expansion and improvement of its Pediatric Intensive Care Unit (PICU).

In most hospitals, pediatric patients recover in specialized areas annexed to the adult units for their particular ailment. For example, children recovering from neurosurgery would have awakened in a pediatric section of the neurosurgery unit to find a crowded and noisy recovery room that did not cater to their unique physical and emotional needs. At NYU, they recover in an environment developed especially for them, with a multidisciplinary staff assembled just for them.

The PICU at NYU Medical Center has the added advantage of being a real resource to referring physicians, providing them with the technology, expertise and time-saving procedures that can help them save lives.

At NYU Medical Center, parents are viewed as integral members of the healthcare team because each child's recovery is strongly influenced by continued family involvement. In recognition of this, each room has a rollaway sofa or chair so one parent can spend the night in close proximity to the child for the duration of their stay. In addition, there is a special family room that was created to give families a quiet place to gather together. Of course, the PICU staff also strives to keep children in contact with their parents and to keep parents informed throughout their child's stay.

NYU MEDICAL CENTER

Understanding that healthcare concerns and pediatric emergencies may occur at any time, the PICU staff is available around the clock to provide a second opinion, consult on a specific case, or help expedite a patients' admission. Social services are also available, and there is an on-site pharmacy within the unit.

The new PICU has been equipped with state-of-the-art monitors, dialysis machines, ventilators, and an isolation room. Special capabilities are available to monitor patients who have had surgery for epilepsy.

For children who stay in the PICU for more than a week, physician and occupational therapists will help develop a postdischarge rehabilitation plan. In addition, PICU patients are assigned a social worker, when necessary, to provide referrals for home care and other services.

709

GASTROENTEROLOGY

The mission of the Division of Gastroenterology at NYU Medical Center is excellence in the delivery of patient care, research, and education in diseases of the gastrointestinal tract. Its physicians bring with them a rich body of knowledge in the diagnosis and management of inflammatory bowel disease, peptic ulcer disease, esophageal disorders, gastrointestinal cancer, and liver, biliary, and pancreatic diseases. Their multidisciplinary approach insures the greatest possible patient care at NYU's three acclaimed, academically integrated teaching hospitals: Tisch Hospital (New York University Hospital), Bellevue Hospitals Center, and the New York Harbor Health Care System (Manhattan Veterans Hospital).

Members of the Division of Gastroenterology are nationally recognized leaders who are involved in numerous studies in the field of gastroenterology and hepatology, including clinical research in liver diseases (especially hepatitis C), endoscopy, colon cancer screening, acute and chronic GI bleeding, and Helicobacter pylori.

Always at the forefront of new technologies, NYU's gastroenterologists work side-by-side with radiologists to perform virtual colonoscopies, a new minimally invasive technique for finding early-stage cancers in the colon.

Virtual colonoscopy is a new screening test in which a radiologist uses a CAT (Computer Assisted Tomography) scanner and sophisticated image processing computers to actually recreate and evaluate the inner surface of the colon. The CAT scanner provides the x-ray images; the image-processing computers create the 3-D display for the final interpretation by the referring gastroenterologist. The study gives a complete evaluation of the entire surface of the colon and can be performed quickly, with little discomfort and extremely accurate readings.

NYU MEDICAL CENTER

The colon and the rectum are the final sections of the large intestine. In the United States, approximately 150,000 people are diagnosed with colorectal cancer every year and of these, approximately 55,000 will die of the disease. Cancer of the colon is the second leading cause of cancer death in the United States. Most experts agree that it is preventable, and NYU is on the cutting edge of 21st century research into quicker, safer, and more accurate diagnosis and treatment, with its advanced video colonoscopy and noninvasive radiologic techniques.

**Physician Referral
(888) 7-NYU-MED
(888-769-8633)
www.nyumc.org**

696

PEDIATRIC HEMATOLOGY PROGRAM

For decades, children with chronic blood diseases have come to NYU Medical Center's Pediatric Hematology Program for comprehensive medical care, including a full range of psychosocial support services to meet every need. Members of the program's expert staff are guided by a patient- and family-centered approach to care, with all the advantages of a leading academic medical center at their fingertips.

The Program addresses the needs of patients with red blood cell disorders, including a variety of anemias and thalassemias – problems of hemoglobin metabolism – as well as vascular problems and malformations, coagulation disorders, and numerous other hemostatic abnormalities.

Patients requiring hospitalization are treated on the pediatric floor of Tisch Hospital, where they benefit from its advanced diagnostic and therapeutic expertise and the support of all pediatric subspecialties. Families are actively encouraged to become knowledgeable about their children's disease and its management. Our multidisciplinary team works closely with the patient's primary care physician to coordinate both medical and psychosocial care.

PSYCHOSOCIAL SERVICES

To help children and families cope with their disease and to prevent later psychological trauma, our behavioral health professionals are committed to a holistic approach to patient care. Among the services we provide are art therapy, relaxation training, play therapy, psychiatric evaluation, neuropsychological assessment, individual and group counseling, and patient education.

THE PEDIATRIC SPECIAL HEMATOLOGY LABORATORY

As a service to clinicians, the Pediatric Special Hematology Laboratory provides comprehensive hemostasis and red cell testing. Tests have been adapted so that small quantities of blood can be drawn from pediatric patients. The Laboratory's repertoire of test procedures is routinely upgraded to incorporate the latest developments in the field. It strives to provide fast, precise test information that leads to effective treatments while maintaining rigorous quality control standards.

711

NYU
Medical
Center

NYU Medical Center

550 First Avenue (at 31st Street)
New York, NY 10016
Physician Referral:
(888)7-NYU-MED (888-769-8633)
www.nyumc.org

PEDIATRIC INFECTIOUS DISEASES

PEDIATRIC INFECTIOUS DISEASES CLINIC

One major provider of health care services for mothers and children with HIV infection in Manhattan is the Pediatric Infectious Diseases (PID) Family Clinic at Bellevue Hospital, which follows over 300 families, including more than 120 children who are HIV-positive. Initiated in 1982 with the aid of private philanthropy and now funded in large part by federal support, this program has made major contributions to the understanding of the transmission of HIV from mothers to children and has contributed to their improved care and longevity.

The PID multidisciplinary health care team maintains a close relationship with patients and follows them closely, providing the majority of medical and psychosocial care for HIV-infected children on an outpatient basis. Thus far, the team has proved successful, as indicated by the average daily census of less than one HIV-infected child.

ADOLESCENT HIV CLINIC

The Bellevue Adolescent Clinic provides free, confidential HIV testing, pre- and post-test counseling, complete medical evaluations, comprehensive medical care, and referral to clinical trials for HIV-positive teens. NYU Medical Center was recently designated a Reaching for Excellence in Adolescent Care and Health (REACH) site, an NIH/HRSA-funded project. REACH's primary goal is to increase understanding of the natural history of HIV in teens.

DAY HOSPITAL PROGRAM

In addition to the outpatient program, children requiring intravenous infusions during the course of their illness are seen in the Pediatric AIDS Day Hospital. Candidates for infusion include patients receiving intravenous gammaglobulin or those with vomiting, diarrhea and/or decreased oral intake who would benefit from intravenous hydration. While these children do not routinely require hospitalization, they do require 4-6 hour periods of observation with adequate nursing and physician supervision. The Pediatric AIDS Day Hospital provides the medical, nursing, psychological, and social support services these patients require, maintaining an organized and efficient delivery of care, as well as providing a facility in which innovative treatments can be developed and implemented. Pediatric patients can also use the new Day Hospital for non-acute care outside of regular clinic hours.

NYU MEDICAL CENTER

Medical services are provided for the children by Pediatric Infectious Disease attendings, post-doctoral fellows, a pediatrician, with a dermatologist and a pedodontist available on call. Psychologists provide developmental testing. Medical care for parents is provided in the same clinic by adult infectious diseases specialists and an obstetrician/ gynecologist, who see parents while their children are being seen. In addition to nursing, staff also include public health advisors who screen mothers for risk factors, counsel, and initiate testing, as well as provide follow-up for mothers in prenatal care; a counselor who makes home visits, provides emotional support, and aids in the follow-up effort; and a full range of clinical social work and child life services.

Since 1988, the Division has been funded as an AIDS clinical trials unit by the National Institutes of Health, one of thirty units in the United States named to study the effectiveness and safety of medications used to treat HIV disease.

The Division has an interest in a variety of infections, including:

- Human Immunodeficiency Virus (HIV) infection
- Cytomegalovirus infection
- Tuberculosis
- Pneumocystis Carinii infection
- Measles virus infection
- Hepatitis B and C infections
- Pneumococcal infections

712

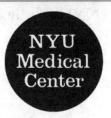

NYU Medical Center

550 First Avenue (at 31st Street)
New York, NY 10016
Physician Referral:
(888)7-NYU-MED (888-769-8633)
www.nyumc.org

PEDIATRIC NEPHROLOGY

The kidneys are a vital organ system in the body, and taking care of a child's kidneys and renal tract is of great importance to his or her growth into adulthood. In addition to clearing the blood of metabolic waste products, the kidneys perform vital support services to other systems. They help bone marrow produce red blood cells, and they are critical in producing the active form of Vitamin D that helps a child's bones grow strong.

NYU Medical Center prides itself in its ability to provide full, comprehensive care to pediatric patients with renal disease. Its physicians provide an expert, nondiscriminatory approach to treatment, regardless of a patient's age, race, sex, or insurance coverage. Furthermore, through the AT&T Language Line Services, the pediatric nephrology team is able to communicate with any patient, tearing down the often-frustrating language barrier. It also has several staff members that speak fluent Spanish.

Along with the diagnosis and treatment of these conditions, NYU Medical Center is dedicated to taking care of children with acute and chronic renal failure, and has an active program for treating children with end stage renal disease with dialysis and renal transplantation. Services offered include diagnostic evaluation, ongoing treatment, renal biopsy, hemodialysis, and peritoneal dialysis. And thanks to a desire to be on the forefront of technology, NYU Medical Center has for over a decade led the charge towards living donor transplantation and minimally invasive procedures.

NYU offers living donor kidney transplantation to patients with end stage renal failure, and thanks to new surgical techniques including minimally invasive kidney extraction, family members and other donors to donate a kidney to a loved one in need has become easier. Hospitalization lasts 1-2 days, and most donors return to normal activity in around one or two weeks, which means a faster return to daily activites after the surgery.

713

NYU Medical Center

550 First Avenue (at 31st Street)
New York, NY 10016
Physician Referral:
(888)7-NYU-MED (888-769-8633)
www.nyumc.org

PEDIATRIC PULMONOLOGY

On the forefront of technology, NYU pediatric lung care specialists utilize minimally invasive techniques, providing complete pediatric general surgical and thoracic services for infants, children and adolescents. This includes surgery for congenital and acquired problems, surgery in premature infants, tumor surgery, surgery on the lungs, esophageal surgery and repair of chest wall deformities. With over a decade of experience in using minimally invasive techniques to treat these problems and state-of-the-art instruments and techniques, the team of pediatricians can perform these procedures with minimal discomfort, little scarring, and limited hospitalization. Consultation requests for conditions prenatally diagnosed are welcome.

Because NYU Medical Center is committed to comprehensive care through an interdisciplinary approach, its pediatric lung specialists are able to join forces with other centers, departments, and divisions within the medical center. Pulmonary care at the NYU Infant Apnea/SIDS Program of Neonatology, within the Department Pediatrics, for example, is specially designed and dedicated to the identification and treatment of infants with apnea and infants who are at an increased risk for sudden infant death syndrome (SIDS). The program consists of physicians and nurses specially trained in this area, and it provides testing and treatment for apnea and identification of high risk infants. Physicians and nurses also supply extensive education to the surrounding community and around-the-clock support to families of high risk infants.

NYU MEDICAL CENTER

The Infant Apnea program is only one of many pediatric pulmonary services offered. Among other areas of comprehensive diagnostic and therapeutic care for children with a wide range of respiratory conditions and disorders includes the following:

• Asthma

• Airway abnormalities

• Bronchopulmonary Dysplasia (BPD)

• Lung diseases in children with developmental delay and orthopedic conditions

• Gastroesophageal Reflux Disease (GERD)

• Neuromuscular diseases

• Apnea and sleep disorders

• Sinus problems

**Physician Referral
(866) CHILD-NYU
(866-244-5369)
www.nyuchildrens.org**

714

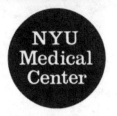

NYU Medical Center

550 First Avenue (at 31st Street)
New York, NY 10016
Physician Referral:
(888)7-NYU-MED (888-769-8633)
www.nyumc.org

PEDIATRIC RHEUMATOLOGY

CAUSES OF ARTHRITIS IN CHILDREN

Arthritis is the term used to describe inflammation and swelling of the tissues in a joint. Perhaps surprisingly, viruses are the most common cause of arthritis in children. This type of arthritis is usually temporary and passes quickly without permanent damage. However, a bacterial joint infection is a more urgent matter. Called septic arthritis, this painful condition requires urgent care to prevent the spread of infection and the possibility of permanent damage to the joint. At its first sign, NYU's expert medical staff are quick to take steps to fight the infection at its source. Normally, septic arthritis is completely cured with antibiotics.

JUVENILE IDIOPATHIC ARTHRITIS

An umbrella term for several different patterns of arthritis in children, Juvenile Idiopathic Arthritis (JIA) refers to arthritic disorders caused by an autoimmune reaction. Autoimmune disease occurs when the body begins to attack its own tissues as if they were foreign substances. NYU's pediatric rheumatologists are expert in diagnosing and treating at least seven different types of JIA. These are diagnosed by putting together a total picture that includes the age of the child and the presence of associated arthritis in the family. The physician also considers which joints have been tender and swollen and for how long, and which laboratory tests are abnormal.

Although JIA is not curable at present, rheumatologists have learned that aggressive, early treatment with methotrexate and injections of corticosteroids into the joints can usually prevent significant damage. The increased use of methotrexate in combination with newly discovered biologic agents, such as Etanercept and Infliximab, gives even greater reason for optimism. Juvenile arthritis, once a crippler of children, is fast becoming a highly manageable disease.

NYU MEDICAL CENTER

Rheumatic disease in children can differ in origin from the same condition in adults, and there are differences in how they are treated. NYU Medical Center houses a program in Pediatric Rheumatology that is uniquely tailored to the needs of young patients with inflammatory and noninflammatory disorders of the muscle, connective tissue, blood vessels, and skin. At NYU, children's physical and psychological development are important contributing factors in the total treatment equation.

NYU's outstanding specialists give children the compassionate care they need – easing their painful symptoms and helping them manage their disease over the long term.

**Physician Referral
(866) CHILD-NYU
(866-244-5369)
www.nyuchildrens.org**

715

PEDIATRIC SURGERY

When it comes to surgery, children are not just smaller versions of adults. NYU Medical Center provides comprehensive pediatric surgical care that starts even before the child is admitted and may continue long after patient discharge. In addition to its top-quality surgeons and surgical nurses, the Medical Center offers a wide array of Child Life Services to help children and their families become familiar with the hospital environment and allay fears that often accompany a hospital stay.

SURGICAL EXPERTISE

Besides general surgical services, NYU is renowned for its achievements in the full spectrum of pediatric surgical specialties, including transplant, neurosurgery, thoracic surgery, cancer surgery, abdominal surgery, and reconstructive surgery, among others. With more than a decade of experience using minimally invasive techniques to treat a broad range of medical problems, NYU surgeons strive to cut pain and scarring down to size and keep children as safe and comfortable as humanly possible. Shorter hospital stays and faster recovery – both benefits associated with minimally invasive surgery – mean that children can return home and resume their lives far sooner than in the recent past.

CHILD LIFE SERVICES

The pediatric unit at Tisch Hospital is home to a Child Life Program that focuses on creating a supportive environment for children undergoing surgery. The Program comprises many small services that add up to a total approach to caring for the whole child and supporting families in the process. Just a few examples of these services are:

• *Pre-Admission Orientation and Information* – Informational packets are available for families through pre-admission testing and doctors' offices. Parents and their children are also encouraged to attend an orientation session with a member of the Child Life staff.
• *Therapeutic Play* – To help children face the challenges they may encounter during their hospital stay, therapists use arts and crafts, music, horticulture, games, and cooking.
• *Pediatric Library and Computer Center* – A great variety of children's books, videos, and audiotapes are available in the pediatric library, which also houses two computers with Internet access.
• *Teen Esteem Workshop Series* – In cooperation with the Social Work Department, this workshop series was developed to address the special needs of teenagers who are living with chronic or life-threatening illnesses.

NYU MEDICAL CENTER

Warmth, contact, and caring make all the difference in the world when a youngster is recovering from surgery. At every point, Child Life staff and volunteers reach out to each child in many different ways. Too sick to visit the playroom? A volunteer will make an individual bedside visit to make sure the young patient's needs are being met. Just a little bit lonely? Foster grandparents are on hand to comfort, console, and entertain children whose parents may be unable to be present during the day. And since everyone knows happiness is a warm puppy, a group of specially trained dogs and their owners volunteer regularly for special visits with eligible children.

Physician Referral
(866) CHILD-NYU
(866-244-5369)
www.nyuchildrens.org

716

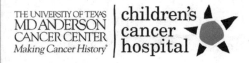

**Children's Cancer Center at
The University of Texas
M. D. Anderson Cancer Center**

1515 Holcombe Blvd.
Houston, Texas 77030-4095
Tel. 713-792-6161 Toll Free 877-MDA-6789
www.mdanderson.org/children

THE CHILDRENS CANCER HOSPITAL AT
M. D. ANDERSON CANCER CENTER

At M. D. Anderson, hope is real. We've helped thousands of children survive cancer with the best possible outcomes and quality of life. Unlike most children's hospitals, we do only one thing — treat cancer. Every patient benefits from our extensive knowledge of both common and rare tumors, as well as a strong research program that works to find new pediatric treatments.

At the Children's Cancer Hospital, kids rule — not cancer. At M. D. Anderson, we treat the whole child, not just the cancer. Each patient has a team of specialists to address medical, psychological and developmental issues related to cancer or its treatments. Counseling and support groups help both you and your child overcome fears and concerns. Our in-house classroom allows them to keep up with schoolwork. Even after treatment is finished, follow-up programs will monitor and manage any long-term side effects.

PROTON THERAPY

M. D. Anderson's Proton Therapy Center opened in May 2006 as the largest and most sophisticated center of its type. Proton therapy radiation is one of the most advanced technologies available for treating children's cancer. It allows for the most aggressive cancer therapy possible, while keeping the harm to growing bodies and side effects to a minimum.

MORE INFORMATION

For more information or to make an appointment, call 877-MDA-6789, or visit us online at http://www.mdanderson.org/children.

At M. D. Anderson Cancer Center, our mission is simple – to eliminate cancer. Achieving that goal begins with integrated programs in cancer treatment, clinical trials, education programs and cancer prevention.

We focus exclusively on cancer and have seen cases of every kind. That means you receive expert care no matter what your diagnosis.

Choosing the right partner for cancer care really does make a difference. The fact is, people who choose M. D. Anderson over other hospitals and clinics often have better results. That is how we've been making cancer history for over sixty years.

Wake Forest University Baptist
MEDICAL CENTER ®

Medical Center Boulevard • Winston-Salem, NC 27157
336-716-2011
Health On-Call® (Patient access) 1-800-446-2255
Physician Inquiries (PAL®) 1-800-277-7654
www.brennerchildrens.org

Brenner Children's
Hospital & Health Services

AN OPTIMAL PLACE FOR HEALING

Building on its tradition of excellence, Brenner Children's Hospital is housed in a state-of-the-art, 160-bed pediatric facility — an innovative environment designed to meet the complex needs of young patients and their families. Brenner Children's holistic care approach, outstanding facility, medical excellence and depth of pediatric subspecialty expertise – including western North Carolina's only Level IV nursery — have made it the resource for children's health in this region.

FAMILY-CENTERED

The pediatric tower exemplifies the gold standard for quality care and comfort, with spacious private rooms that encourage parents to room-in, a rooftop garden and play area, soothing quiet areas and interactive play centers. A Ronald McDonald Family Room –one of the first in the world—offers parents a comfortable place for respite and refreshment.

HOLISTIC CARE

Brenner Children's Hospital reflects a "whole child" philosophy. Every effort is made to meet emotional, spiritual and social needs as children receive expert medical care. Child Life specialists help patients and families cope with issues of hospitalization and illness.

COMMITTED TO CHILDREN'S HEALTH

Staffed by Wake Forest University School of Medicine faculty, Brenner Children's Hospital is committed to children's health research. Examples include the National Institutes of Health (NIH) Pediatric Heart Network. Brenner Children's Hospital joins other children's hospitals in the nation conducting clinical trials on patients with heart defects.

To make an appointment or find a specialist at Brenner Children's Hospital, call Health On-Call® at 1-800-446-2255.

PEDIATRIC EXPERTISE

- Brenner Children's Hospital is western North Carolina's only full service pediatric facility. More than 85 pediatric specialists and subspecialists provide expert care for critically ill children from N.C., W.V., TN, VA and S.C.

- Brenner Children's Hospital offers children highly specialized, minimally invasive procedures often not available elsewhere in the Southeast, such as outpatient heart surgery for patent ductus arteriosus. Pediatric specialists manage every aspect of care.

- Brenner Children's neonatal intensive care nursery (the region's only Level IV nursery) participates in research to find new therapies and treatments.

- Brenner Children's houses the area's only pediatric Emergency Department, where children receive emergency care designed specifically for them.

- The Wake Forest Baptist ECMO (heart/lung) unit is one of only a few centers in the U.S. that supports newborns and children.

- Brenner Children's is one of eight centers in the United States participating in the National Institutes of Health (NIH) Pediatric Heart Network, which searches for the best ways to care for patients with heart defects.

- Our pediatric oncologists and nurses participate in a national Children's Oncology Group, a group of national researchers who evaluate current therapies used in treating children with cancer. This ensures that our children have access to the best cancer treatments available.

KNOWLEDGE MAKES ALL THE DIFFERENCE.

Sponsored Page

Physical Medicine & Rehabilitation

Physical medicine and rehabilitation, also referred to as rehabilitation medicine, is the medical specialty concerned with diagnosing, evaluating and treating patients with physical disabilities. These disabilities may arise from conditions affecting the musculoskeletal system such as neck and back pain, sports injuries, or other painful conditions affecting the limbs, for example carpal tunnel syndrome. Alternatively, the disabilities may result from neurological trauma or disease such as spinal cord injury, head injury or stroke.

A physician certified in physical medicine and rehabilitation is often called a physiatrist. The primary goal of the physiatrist is to achieve maximal restoration of physical, psychological, social and vocational function through comprehensive rehabilitation. Pain management is often an important part of the role of the physiatrist. For diagnosis and evaluation, a physiatrist may include the techniques of electromyography to supplement the standard history, physical, X-ray and laboratory examinations. The physiatrist has expertise in the appropriate use of therapeutic exercise, prosthetics (artificial limbs), orthotics and mechanical and electrical devices.

Training Required: Four years *plus* one year clinical practice.

Certification in the following subspecialty requires additional training and examination.

Spinal Cord Injury Medicine: A physician who addresses the prevention, diagnosis, treatment and management of traumatic spinal cord injury and non-traumatic etiologies of spinal cord dysfunction by working in an interdisciplinary manner. Care is provided to patients of all ages on a lifelong basis and covers related medical, physical, psychological and vocational disabilities and complications.

Physical Medicine & Rehabilitation

New England

Frontera, Walter R MD/PhD [PMR] - **Spec Exp:** Sports Medicine; Musculoskeletal Disorders; **Hospital:** Spaulding Rehab Hosp, Mass Genl Hosp; **Address:** Spaulding Rehab Hosp-Physical Med Rehab, 125 Nashua St, Boston, MA 02114; **Phone:** 617-573-7180; **Board Cert:** Physical Medicine & Rehabilitation 1985; **Med School:** Univ Puerto Rico 1979; **Resid:** Physical Medicine & Rehabilitation, Univ Hosp/Univ Puerto Rico 1983; **Fac Appt:** Assoc Prof PMR, Harvard Med Sch

Silver, Julie K MD [PMR] - **Spec Exp:** Polio Rehabilitation; **Hospital:** Spaulding Rehab Hosp; **Address:** Spaulding Rehabilitation Outpatient Ctr, 570 Worcester Rd, Framingham, MA 01702; **Phone:** 508-872-2200; **Board Cert:** Physical Medicine & Rehabilitation 2006; **Med School:** Georgetown Univ 1991; **Resid:** Physical Medicine & Rehabilitation, Natl Rehab Hosp 1995; **Fac Appt:** Asst Prof PMR, Harvard Med Sch

Mid Atlantic

Ahn, Jung Hwan MD [PMR] - **Spec Exp:** Spinal Cord Injury; Stroke Rehabilitation; Neurologic Rehabilitation; **Hospital:** NYU Med Ctr (page 67); **Address:** 400 E 34th St, rm 421, New York, NY 10016-4901; **Phone:** 212-263-6122; **Board Cert:** Physical Medicine & Rehabilitation 1980; Spinal Cord Injury Medicine 1998; **Med School:** South Korea 1970; **Resid:** Obstetrics & Gynecology, Elmhurst City Hosp - Mt Sinai 1976; Physical Medicine & Rehabilitation, NYU Med Ctr 1979; **Fellow:** Spinal Cord Injury Medicine, NYU Med Ctr 1980; **Fac Appt:** Clin Prof PMR, NYU Sch Med

Aseff, John N MD [PMR] - **Spec Exp:** Electrodiagnosis; Pain-Soft Tissue; **Hospital:** Natl Rehab Hosp, Washington Hosp Ctr; **Address:** National Rehabilitation Hosp, 102 Irving St NW, Washington, DC 20010; **Phone:** 202-877-1916; **Board Cert:** Physical Medicine & Rehabilitation 1978; **Med School:** Ohio State Univ 1973; **Resid:** Surgery, Univ Hosps Cleveland 1975; Physical Medicine & Rehabilitation, Ohio State Univ Hosps 1977; **Fac Appt:** Assoc Clin Prof PMR, Georgetown Univ

Bach, John MD [PMR] - **Spec Exp:** Mechanical Ventilation; Spinal Cord Injury; Neuromuscular Disorders; **Hospital:** UMDNJ-Univ Hosp-Newark; **Address:** 150 Bergen St, Ste B403, Newark, NJ 07103; **Phone:** 973-972-7195; **Board Cert:** Physical Medicine & Rehabilitation 1986; **Med School:** UMDNJ-NJ Med Sch, Newark 1976; **Resid:** Physical Medicine & Rehabilitation, NYU Med Ctr 1980; **Fellow:** Neurological Muscular Disease, Univ Hosp 1983; **Fac Appt:** Prof PMR, UMDNJ-NJ Med Sch, Newark

Ballard, Pamela H MD [PMR] - **Spec Exp:** Spinal Cord Injury; Spasticity Management; Neuromuscular Disorders; **Hospital:** Natl Rehab Hosp; **Address:** 102 Irving St NW, Ste 2164, Washington, DC 20010; **Phone:** 202-877-1621; **Board Cert:** Physical Medicine & Rehabilitation 1991; Spinal Cord Injury Medicine 1999; **Med School:** Howard Univ 1986; **Resid:** Physical Medicine & Rehabilitation, Sinai Hosp 1990

Braddom, Randall L MD [PMR] - **Spec Exp:** Electromyography; Pain-Neck; Pain-Low Back; Musculoskeletal Disorders; **Hospital:** Riverview Med Ctr (page 59); **Address:** Orthopaedic, Sports Medicine & Rehab Ctr, 80 Oak Hill Rd, rm 368, Red Bank, NJ 07701; **Phone:** 732-741-2313; **Board Cert:** Physical Medicine & Rehabilitation 1974; **Med School:** Ohio State Univ 1968; **Resid:** Physical Medicine & Rehabilitation, Ohio State Univ Hosp 1973; **Fac Appt:** Clin Prof PMR, UMDNJ-NJ Med Sch, Newark

De Lateur, Barbara J MD [PMR] - **Spec Exp:** Frailty Syndrome; **Hospital:** Johns Hopkins Bayview Med Ctr (page 61); **Address:** Johns Hopkins Bayview Med Ctr, Rehab, AA Bldg Fl 01 - rm 1661, Baltimore, MD 21224; **Phone:** 410-550-5299; **Board Cert:** Physical Medicine & Rehabilitation 1970; **Med School:** Univ Wash 1963; **Resid:** Physical Medicine & Rehabilitation, Univ Wash Hosp 1968; **Fac Appt:** Prof PMR, Johns Hopkins Univ

Esquenazi, Alberto M MD [PMR] - **Spec Exp:** Amputee Rehabilitation; Mobility Evaluation & Treatment; Polio Rehabilitation; **Hospital:** MossRehab Hosp; **Address:** Moss Rehab Hosp, 60 E Township Line Rd, Philadelphia, PA 19027; **Phone:** 215-663-6676; **Board Cert:** Physical Medicine & Rehabilitation 1986; **Med School:** Mexico 1981; **Resid:** Physical Medicine & Rehabilitation, Temple Univ 1985; **Fellow:** Gait and Prosthetics, Moss Rehab Hosp 1986; **Fac Appt:** Prof PMR, Jefferson Med Coll

Evans, Sarah Helen MD [PMR] - **Spec Exp:** Pediatric Rehabilitation Medicine; **Hospital:** Chldns Natl Med Ctr; **Address:** Children's National Medical Ctr, Pediatric Rehabilitation, 111 Michigan Ave NW, Washington, DC 20010; **Phone:** 202-884-3094; **Board Cert:** Physical Medicine & Rehabilitation 1992; Pediatrics 2002; Pediatric Rehabilitation Medicine 2003; **Med School:** Univ MD Sch Med 1984; **Resid:** Pediatrics, Univ Colorado Hlth Sci Ctr 1987; **Fellow:** Physical Medicine & Rehabilitation, Univ Colorado Hlth Sci Ctr 1988; Pediatric Rehabilitation Medicine, Children's Hosp 1989; **Fac Appt:** Assoc Prof PMR, Univ Colorado

Feinberg, Joseph Hunt MD [PMR] - **Spec Exp:** Peripheral Nerve Disorders; Spinal Rehabilitation; Electrodiagnosis; Sports Medicine; **Hospital:** Hosp For Special Surgery (page 60), Kessler Inst for Rehab - W Orange; **Address:** 535 E 70th St, New York, NY 10021-4872; **Phone:** 212-606-1568; **Board Cert:** Physical Medicine & Rehabilitation 1991; **Med School:** Albany Med Coll 1983; **Resid:** Surgery, Mt Sinai Hosp 1985; Physical Medicine & Rehabilitation, Rusk Inst Rehab 1990; **Fellow:** Orthopaedic Pathology, Hosp Spec Surg 1986; Orthopaedic Biomechanics, Univ Iowa Hosp & Clins 1987; **Fac Appt:** Assoc Prof PMR, Cornell Univ-Weill Med Coll

Fried, Guy W MD [PMR] - **Spec Exp:** Brain Injury Rehabilitation; Spinal Cord Injury; Neutogenic Bladder; **Hospital:** Magee Rehab Hosp; **Address:** Magee Hospital, 1513 Race St, Philadelphia, PA 19102-1177; **Phone:** 215-587-3394; **Board Cert:** Physical Medicine & Rehabilitation 1990; Spinal Cord Injury Medicine 1999; Pain Medicine 2000; **Med School:** Yale Univ 1985; **Resid:** Physical Medicine & Rehabilitation, Thom Jefferson Univ Hosp 1989; **Fac Appt:** Asst Prof PMR, Thomas Jefferson Univ

Kirshblum, Steven C MD [PMR] - **Spec Exp:** Spinal Cord Injury; **Hospital:** Kessler Inst for Rehab - W Orange, St Barnabas Med Ctr; **Address:** 1199 Pleasant Valley Way, West Orange, NJ 07052-1424; **Phone:** 973-731-3600 x2258; **Board Cert:** Physical Medicine & Rehabilitation 1991; Spinal Cord Injury Medicine 1998; **Med School:** Ros Franklin Univ/Chicago Med Sch 1986; **Resid:** Physical Medicine & Rehabilitation, Mount Sinai Med Ctr 1990; **Fac Appt:** Prof PMR, UMDNJ-NJ Med Sch, Newark

Lutz, Gregory MD [PMR] - **Spec Exp:** Spinal Rehabilitation; Sports Medicine; Pain-Low Back; **Hospital:** Hosp For Special Surgery (page 60), Univ Med Ctr - Princeton; **Address:** 535 E 70th St, New York, NY 10021-4898; **Phone:** 212-606-1648; **Board Cert:** Physical Medicine & Rehabilitation 2003; **Med School:** Georgetown Univ 1988; **Resid:** Physical Medicine & Rehabilitation, Mayo Clinic 1992; **Fellow:** Sports Medicine, Hosp For Spec Surg 1993; **Fac Appt:** Assoc Prof PMR, Cornell Univ-Weill Med Coll

Physical Medicine & Rehabilitation

Ma, Dong M MD [PMR] - **Spec Exp:** Electromyography; Musculoskeletal Disorders; **Hospital:** Rusk Inst of Rehab Med (page 69), NYU Med Ctr (page 67); **Address:** 400 E 34th St, rm 211, New York, NY 10016; **Phone:** 212-263-6338; **Board Cert:** Physical Medicine & Rehabilitation 1979; **Med School:** South Korea 1968; **Resid:** Physical Medicine & Rehabilitation, NYU Med Ctr 1975; **Fellow:** Physical Medicine & Rehabilitation, NYU Med Ctr 1977; **Fac Appt:** Clin Prof PMR, NYU Sch Med

Marino, Ralph J MD [PMR] - **Spec Exp:** Spinal Cord Injury; **Hospital:** Thomas Jefferson Univ Hosp; **Address:** 132 S 10th St, 375 Main Bldg, Philadelphia, PA 19107; **Phone:** 215-955-1200; **Board Cert:** Physical Medicine & Rehabilitation 1988; Spinal Cord Injury Medicine 2000; **Med School:** Jefferson Med Coll 1982; **Resid:** Physical Medicine & Rehabilitation, Thos Jefferson Univ Hosp 1987; **Fac Appt:** Assoc Prof PMR, Jefferson Med Coll

Mayer, Nathaniel MD [PMR] - **Spec Exp:** Motor Control Analysis; Spasticity Management; Brain Injury Rehabilitation; **Hospital:** MossRehab Hosp; **Address:** Moss Rehab Hosp, Drucker Brain Injury Ctr, 60 E Township Line Rd, Elkins Park, PA 19027; **Phone:** 215-663-6681; **Board Cert:** Physical Medicine & Rehabilitation 1976; **Med School:** Albert Einstein Coll Med 1968; **Resid:** Physical Medicine & Rehabilitation, Temple Univ Hosp 1973; **Fac Appt:** Prof PMR, Temple Univ

Munin, Michael C MD [PMR] - **Spec Exp:** Spasticity Management; Amputee Rehabilitation; Hip Surgery Rehabilitation; Electrodiagnosis; **Hospital:** UPMC Presby, Pittsburgh, UPMC Inst Rehab & Rsch; **Address:** Univ Pittsburgh Physicians, 3471 Fifth Ave, Kaufman Bldg Ste 1103, Pittsburgh, PA 15213; **Phone:** 412-692-4400; **Board Cert:** Physical Medicine & Rehabilitation 1993; **Med School:** Jefferson Med Coll 1988; **Resid:** Physical Medicine & Rehabilitation, Thomas Jefferson Univ Hosp 1992; **Fac Appt:** Assoc Prof PMR, Univ Pittsburgh

Myers, Stanley J MD [PMR] - **Spec Exp:** Muscular Dystrophy; Stroke Rehabilitation; Neuromuscular Disorders; **Hospital:** NY-Presby Hosp/Weill Cornell (page 66); **Address:** Columbia Presby Rehab Associates, 180 Fort Washington Ave, HP Ste 199, PH50B, New York, NY 10032-3710; **Phone:** 212-305-3535; **Board Cert:** Physical Medicine & Rehabilitation 1971; **Med School:** SUNY Downstate 1961; **Resid:** Internal Medicine, Maimonides Medical Ctr 1964; Physical Medicine & Rehabilitation, Columbia-Presby Hosp 1969; **Fellow:** Neurological Muscular Disease, Maimonides Medical Ctr 1965; **Fac Appt:** Prof PMR, Columbia P&S

Ragnarsson, Kristjan T MD [PMR] - **Spec Exp:** Spinal Cord Injury; Brain Injury Rehabilitation; Pain-Back & Neck; **Hospital:** Mount Sinai Med Ctr; **Address:** 5 E 98th St, New York, NY 10029-6501; **Phone:** 212-659-9370; **Board Cert:** Physical Medicine & Rehabilitation 1976; **Med School:** Iceland 1969; **Resid:** Physical Medicine & Rehabilitation, NYU Med Ctr 1974; **Fellow:** Spinal Cord & Brain Injury Rehab, NYU Med Ctr 1975; **Fac Appt:** Prof PMR, Mount Sinai Sch Med

Slipman, Curtis W MD [PMR] - **Spec Exp:** Spinal Rehabilitation; Pain Management; **Hospital:** Hosp Univ Penn - UPHS (page 72); **Address:** Hosp Univ Penn, Dept Rehab Med, 3400 Spruce St White Bldg Fl Ground, Philadelphia, PA 19104; **Phone:** 215-662-3259; **Board Cert:** Physical Medicine & Rehabilitation 1987; **Med School:** Baylor Coll Med 1983; **Resid:** Physical Medicine & Rehabilitation, Columbia-Presby Med Ctr 1986; **Fac Appt:** Assoc Prof PMR, Univ Pennsylvania

Stubblefield, Michael MD [PMR] - **Spec Exp:** Cancer Rehabilitation; Pain-Cancer; Spasticity Management; Electrodiagnosis; **Hospital:** Meml Sloan Kettering Cancer Ctr; **Address:** Meml Sloan Kettering Cancer Ctr, 1275 York Ave, Box 349, New York, NY 10021; **Phone:** 212-639-7834; **Board Cert:** Internal Medicine 2001; Physical Medicine & Rehabilitation 2002; **Med School:** Columbia P&S 1996; **Resid:** Internal Medicine, Columbia Presby Med Ctr 2001; Physical Medicine & Rehabilitation, Columbia Presby Med Ctr 2001

Zafonte, Ross DO [PMR] - **Spec Exp:** Brain Injury Rehabilitation; Spinal Cord Injury; **Hospital:** UPMC Presby, Pittsburgh, UPMC Inst Rehab & Rsch; **Address:** Lillian Kaufman Bldg, 3471 Fifth Ave, Ste 201, Pittsburgh, PA 15213-3221; **Phone:** 412-648-6979; **Board Cert:** Physical Medicine & Rehabilitation 1990; **Med School:** Nova SE Univ, Coll Osteo Med 1985; **Resid:** Physical Medicine & Rehabilitation, Mt Sinai Med Ctr 1989; **Fac Appt:** Clin Prof PMR, Univ Pittsburgh

Southeast

Brown-Jackson, Amie L MD [PMR] - **Spec Exp:** Spinal Cord Injury; **Hospital:** Univ of Ala Hosp at Birmingham, Children's Hospital - Birmingham; **Address:** Univ Alabama-Spine Rehab Ctr, 619 19th St S, Ste 190, Birmingham, AL 35249; **Phone:** 205-934-4131; **Board Cert:** Physical Medicine & Rehabilitation 1990; **Med School:** Univ Ala 1984; **Resid:** Physical Medicine & Rehabilitation, Univ Alabama Med Ctr 1987; **Fac Appt:** Prof PMR, Univ Ala

Cardenas, Diana D MD [PMR] - **Spec Exp:** Spinal Cord Injury; Spina Bifida; **Hospital:** Univ of Miami Hosp & Clins/Sylvester Comp Canc Ctr, Jackson Meml Hosp; **Address:** Univ Miami, Dept Rehab Medicine, PO Box 016960 (D461), Miami, FL 33101; **Phone:** 305-243-9516; **Board Cert:** Physical Medicine & Rehabilitation 1977; **Med School:** Univ Tex SW, Dallas 1973; **Resid:** Physical Medicine & Rehabilitation, Univ Wash Affil Hosps 1976; **Fac Appt:** Prof PMR, Univ Miami Sch Med

Creamer, Michael DO [PMR] - **Spec Exp:** Spinal Cord Injury; Pain Management; Electrodiagnosis; **Hospital:** Orlando Regl Med Ctr, Florida Hosp - Orlando; **Address:** 100 W Gore St, Ste 203, Orlando, FL 32806-1041; **Phone:** 407-649-8707; **Board Cert:** Physical Medicine & Rehabilitation 1992; Spinal Cord Injury Medicine 1998; Pain Medicine 2000; **Med School:** Chicago Coll Osteo Med 1987; **Resid:** Physical Medicine & Rehabilitation, Rehab Inst Chicago 1991; **Fac Appt:** Asst Prof Med, Univ Fla Coll Med

Diamond, Paul T MD [PMR] - **Spec Exp:** Neurorehabilitation; Geriatric Rehabilitation; **Hospital:** Univ Virginia Med Ctr; **Address:** Univ of Virginia Hlth Sci Ctr, Dept Rehabilitation, 545 Ray C Hunt Drive, Ste 240, Charlottesville, VA 22903; **Phone:** 434-243-5622; **Board Cert:** Internal Medicine 1989; Physical Medicine & Rehabilitation 2003; **Med School:** Univ VA Sch Med 1986; **Resid:** Internal Medicine, Johns Hospkins Bayview Hosp 1989; Physical Medicine & Rehabilitation, Sinai/Johns Hopkins Hosp 1992; **Fac Appt:** Assoc Prof PMR, Univ VA Sch Med

Gater Jr, David R MD/PhD [PMR] - **Spec Exp:** Spinal Cord Injury; Exercise Physiology; Electrodiagnosis; **Hospital:** Hunter Holmes McGuire VA Med Ctr, VCU Med Ctr; **Address:** 1201 E Broadrock Blvd, Richmond, VA 23249; **Phone:** 804-675-5000 x5455; **Board Cert:** Physical Medicine & Rehabilitation 1997; Spinal Cord Injury Medicine 1999; Electrodiagnostic Medicine 1998; **Med School:** Univ Ariz Coll Med 1992; **Resid:** Physical Medicine & Rehabilitation, UC Davis Med Ctr 1994; **Fac Appt:** Prof PMR, Va Commonwealth Univ

Physical Medicine & Rehabilitation

Kerrigan, D Casey MD [PMR] - **Spec Exp:** Gait Disorders; **Hospital:** Univ Virginia Med Ctr; **Address:** Univ Va, Dept Physical Med Rehab, 545 Ray C Hunt Drive, Ste 240, Charlottesville, VA 22908-1004; **Phone:** 434-243-0378; **Board Cert:** Physical Medicine & Rehabilitation 1992; **Med School:** Harvard Med Sch 1987; **Resid:** Physical Medicine & Rehabilitation, UCLA Med Ctr 1991; **Fac Appt:** Prof PMR, Univ VA Sch Med

Lipkin, David L MD [PMR] - **Spec Exp:** Geriatric Rehabilitation; Pain-Back; Rheumatology; **Hospital:** Mount Sinai Med Ctr - Miami; **Address:** PO Box 630127, Miami, FL 33163-0127; **Phone:** 305-672-1256; **Board Cert:** Physical Medicine & Rehabilitation 1971; **Med School:** Belgium 1964; **Resid:** Pediatrics, Jersey City Med Ctr 1966; Physical Medicine & Rehabilitation, Bronx Muni Hosp 1969; **Fellow:** Research, Natl Inst Hlth-Einstein Coll Med 1969; **Fac Appt:** Assoc Clin Prof PMR, Univ Miami Sch Med

Nelson, Maureen R MD [PMR] - **Spec Exp:** Pediatric Rehabilitation Medicine; Brachial Plexus Palsy; Electrodiagnosis; **Hospital:** Carolinas Med Ctr; **Address:** Carolinas Rehab, Dept PM&R, 1100 Blythe Blvd, Charlotte, NC 28203; **Phone:** 704-355-4330; **Board Cert:** Physical Medicine & Rehabilitation 1990; Pediatric Rehabilitation Medicine 2003; **Med School:** Univ IL Coll Med 1985; **Resid:** Physical Medicine & Rehabilitation, Univ Tex Hlth Scis Ctr 1989; **Fellow:** Pediatric Rehabilitation Medicine, Alfred I Dupont Inst 1990; **Fac Appt:** Assoc Clin Prof PMR, Univ NC Sch Med

Midwest

Chen, David MD [PMR] - **Spec Exp:** Spinal Cord Injury; **Hospital:** Rehab Inst - Chicago; **Address:** 345 E Superior St, Ste 1146, Chicago, IL 60611; **Phone:** 312-238-0764; **Board Cert:** Physical Medicine & Rehabilitation 1992; Spinal Cord Injury Medicine 1998; **Med School:** Univ IL Coll Med 1987; **Resid:** Physical Medicine & Rehabilitation, Northwestern Med Sch 1991; **Fac Appt:** Asst Prof PMR, Northwestern Univ

Clairmont, Albert MD [PMR] - **Spec Exp:** Spasticity Management; Electrodiagnosis; **Hospital:** Ohio St Univ Med Ctr; **Address:** Dodd Hall - Davis Center, 480 Medical Center Drive, Columbus, OH 43210; **Phone:** 614-293-4837; **Board Cert:** Physical Medicine & Rehabilitation 1985; Pediatrics 1985; **Med School:** Jamaica 1974; **Resid:** Pediatrics, Columbus Chldns Hosp 1981; Physical Medicine & Rehabilitation, Ohio St Univ Hosps 1983; **Fac Appt:** Assoc Clin Prof PMR, Ohio State Univ

Colachis III, Samuel C MD [PMR] - **Spec Exp:** Spinal Cord Injury; Electrodiagnosis; **Hospital:** Ohio St Univ Med Ctr; **Address:** Dodd Hall - Davis Center, 480 Medical Center Drive, Columbus, OH 43210; **Phone:** 614-293-4837; **Board Cert:** Physical Medicine & Rehabilitation 1988; Spinal Cord Injury Medicine 2003; **Med School:** USC Sch Med 1984; **Resid:** Physical Medicine & Rehabilitation, Ohio State Univ Hosps 1987; **Fellow:** Electrodiagnosis, Ohio State Univ Hosps 1988; **Fac Appt:** Assoc Prof PMR, Ohio State Univ

Dillingham, Timothy R MD [PMR] - **Spec Exp:** Electrodiagnosis; Electromyography; Amputee Rehabilitation; **Hospital:** Froedtert Meml Lutheran Hosp; **Address:** Froedtert Memorial Hospital, 9200 W Wisconsin Ave, rm 2183, Milwaukee, WI 53226; **Phone:** 414-805-7343; **Board Cert:** Physical Medicine & Rehabilitation 1991; **Med School:** Univ Wash 1986; **Resid:** Physical Medicine & Rehabilitation, Univ Wash Affil Hosps 1990; **Fac Appt:** Prof PMR, Med Coll Wisc

Frost, Frederick S MD [PMR] - **Spec Exp:** Spinal Cord Injury; Stroke Rehabilitation; Geriatric Rehabilitation; **Hospital:** Cleveland Clin Fdn (page 57); **Address:** Cleveland Clinic Fdn, 9500 Euclid Ave, MC C21, Cleveland, OH 44195; **Phone:** 216-445-2006; **Board Cert:** Physical Medicine & Rehabilitation 1988; Spinal Cord Injury Medicine 1998; **Med School:** Northwestern Univ 1983; **Resid:** Physical Medicine & Rehabilitation, Northwestern Meml Hosp 1987; **Fellow:** Spinal Cord Injury Medicine, Rehab Inst Chicago; **Fac Appt:** Asst Prof PMR, Cleveland Cl Coll Med/Case West Res

Gittler, Michelle MD [PMR] - **Spec Exp:** Spinal Cord Injury; Amputee Rehabilitation; **Hospital:** Schwab Rehab Hosp, Univ of Chicago Hosps; **Address:** 1401 S California Blvd, Chicago, IL 60608; **Phone:** 773-522-5853; **Board Cert:** Physical Medicine & Rehabilitation 2003; Spinal Cord Injury Medicine 1998; **Med School:** Univ IL Coll Med 1988; **Resid:** Physical Medicine & Rehabilitation, Rehab Inst Chicago 1992; **Fac Appt:** Assoc Clin Prof S, Univ Chicago-Pritzker Sch Med

Haig, Andrew MD [PMR] - **Spec Exp:** International Rehabilitation; Pain-Back & Neck; Electrodiagnosis; **Hospital:** Univ Michigan Hlth Sys, VA Med Ctr - Ann Arbor; **Address:** Univ Michigan Spine Program, 325 E Eisenhower, Burlington Bldg - Ste 100, Ann Artbor, MI 48108-3346; **Phone:** 734-763-4300; **Board Cert:** Physical Medicine & Rehabilitation 1987; Pain Medicine 2002; **Med School:** Med Coll Wisc 1983; **Resid:** Physical Medicine & Rehabilitation, Northwestern Univ 1986; **Fac Appt:** Assoc Prof PMR, Univ Mich Med Sch

Kuiken, Todd A MD/PhD [PMR] - **Spec Exp:** Amputee Rehabilitation; Prosthesis Control; Gait Disorders; **Hospital:** Rehab Inst - Chicago; **Address:** Rehab Inst of Chicago, 345 E Superior St, rm 1309, Chicago, IL 60611; **Phone:** 312-238-8072; **Board Cert:** Physical Medicine & Rehabilitation 2006; **Med School:** Northwestern Univ 1990; **Resid:** Physical Medicine & Rehabilitation, Rehab Inst Chicago 1995; **Fac Appt:** Assoc Prof PMR, Northwestern Univ

La Ban, Myron M MD [PMR] - **Spec Exp:** Pain-Back; Electromyography; **Hospital:** William Beaumont Hosp; **Address:** 3535 W Thirteen Mile Rd, Ste 437, Royal Oak, MI 48073; **Phone:** 248-288-2237; **Board Cert:** Physical Medicine & Rehabilitation 1967; **Med School:** Univ Mich Med Sch 1961; **Resid:** Physical Medicine & Rehabilitation, Univ Ohio Hosps 1965; **Fac Appt:** Clin Prof PMR, Ohio State Univ

Leonard Jr, James A MD [PMR] - **Spec Exp:** Amputee Rehabilitation; Electrodiagnosis; **Hospital:** Univ Michigan Hlth Sys; **Address:** Univ Michigan, Dept Physical Med & Rehab, 325 E Eisenhower Pkwy, Ste 100, Ann Arbor, MI 48108; **Phone:** 734-936-7175; **Board Cert:** Physical Medicine & Rehabilitation 1977; **Med School:** Univ Mich Med Sch 1972; **Resid:** Physical Medicine & Rehabilitation, Univ Mich Med Ctr 1975; **Fac Appt:** Clin Prof PMR, Univ Mich Med Sch

Mysiw, W Jerry MD [PMR] - **Spec Exp:** Brain Injury Rehabilitation; **Hospital:** Ohio St Univ Med Ctr; **Address:** Dodd Hall - Davis Center, 480 Medical Center Drive, Columbus, OH 43210-1245; **Phone:** 614-293-4837; **Board Cert:** Physical Medicine & Rehabilitation 1985; **Med School:** Ohio State Univ 1981; **Resid:** Physical Medicine & Rehabilitation, Ohio State Univ Med Ctr 1984; **Fac Appt:** Assoc Prof PMR, Ohio State Univ

Nobunaga, Austin MD [PMR] - **Spec Exp:** Spinal Cord Injury; Electrodiagnosis; **Hospital:** Univ Hosp - Cincinnati; **Address:** Univ Cincinnati Coll Med, Dept PM&R, 151 W Galbraith Rd, South Pavillion, Cincinnati, OH 45216; **Phone:** 513-948-2707; **Board Cert:** Physical Medicine & Rehabilitation 1990; Spinal Cord Injury Medicine 1999; **Med School:** Univ Mich Med Sch 1985; **Resid:** Physical Medicine & Rehabilitation, Rehab Inst Chicago 1989

Press, Joel MD [PMR] - **Spec Exp:** Sports Medicine; Pain-Back; Musculoskeletal Injuries; **Hospital:** Rehab Inst - Chicago, Northwestern Meml Hosp; **Address:** Ctr for Spine, Sports & Occup Rehab, 1030 N Clark St, Ste 500, Chicago, IL 60610; **Phone:** 312-238-7767; **Board Cert:** Physical Medicine & Rehabilitation 1988; **Med School:** Univ IL Coll Med 1984; **Resid:** Physical Medicine & Rehabilitation, Northwestern Meml Hosp 1988; **Fac Appt:** Assoc Clin Prof PMR, Northwestern Univ

Roth, Elliot MD [PMR] - **Spec Exp:** Stroke Rehabilitation; Neurologic Rehabilitation; Geriatric Rehabilitation; **Hospital:** Rehab Inst - Chicago, Northwestern Meml Hosp; **Address:** Rehab Inst Chicago, 345 E Superior St, rm 0-821, Chicago, IL 60611-2654; **Phone:** 312-238-4637; **Board Cert:** Physical Medicine & Rehabilitation 1987; **Med School:** Northwestern Univ 1982; **Resid:** Physical Medicine & Rehabilitation, Northwestern Univ 1985; **Fellow:** Physical Medicine & Rehabilitation, Rehab Inst Chicago 1986; **Fac Appt:** Prof PMR, Northwestern Univ

Sisung, Charles MD [PMR] - **Spec Exp:** Rheumatic Diseases of Childhood; Trauma Rehabilitation; Burn Care; **Hospital:** Rehab Inst - Chicago; **Address:** 345 E Superior St, rm 1158, Chicago, IL 60611; **Phone:** 312-238-1246; **Board Cert:** Pediatrics 2004; Physical Medicine & Rehabilitation 1991; Pediatric Rehabilitation Medicine 2003; **Med School:** Univ Mich Med Sch 1981; **Resid:** Pediatrics, Mott Chldns Hosp/Univ Mich 1984; Physical Medicine & Rehabilitation, Schwab Rehab Hosp 1989; **Fellow:** Pediatric Rheumatology, Univ Chicago Hosps 1991; **Fac Appt:** Asst Prof PMR, Northwestern Univ

Sliwa, James A DO [PMR] - **Spec Exp:** Polio Rehabilitation; Multiple Sclerosis; Pain-Back; **Hospital:** Rehab Inst - Chicago; **Address:** Rehab Inst Chicago, 345 E Superior St, rm 1108, Chicago, IL 60611-3015; **Phone:** 312-238-4093; **Board Cert:** Physical Medicine & Rehabilitation 2005; **Med School:** Chicago Coll Osteo Med 1980; **Resid:** Physical Medicine & Rehabilitation, Rehab Inst 1984; **Fac Appt:** Prof PMR, Northwestern Univ

Smith, Joanne MD [PMR] - **Spec Exp:** Pain-Pelvic; Pain-Back; **Hospital:** Rehab Inst - Chicago, Northwestern Meml Hosp; **Address:** Rehab Inst of Chicago, 345 E Superior St, Ste 1507, Chicago, IL 60611; **Phone:** 312-238-0815; **Board Cert:** Physical Medicine & Rehabilitation 2003; **Med School:** Mich State Univ 1988; **Resid:** Physical Medicine & Rehabilitation, Northwestern Univ 1992; **Fac Appt:** Asst Prof PMR, Northwestern Univ

Volshteyn, Oksana MD [PMR] - **Spec Exp:** Spinal Cord Injury; **Hospital:** Rehab Inst St. Louis, Barnes-Jewish Hosp; **Address:** 4444 Forest Park, Campus Box 8518, St Louis, MO 63108; **Phone:** 314-658-3887; **Board Cert:** Physical Medicine & Rehabilitation 1986; Spinal Cord Injury Medicine 1999; **Med School:** Russia 1976; **Resid:** Physical Medicine & Rehabilitation, Barnes Jewish Hosp 1985; **Fac Appt:** Assoc Prof N, Washington Univ, St Louis

Great Plains and Mountains

Lammertse, Daniel MD [PMR] - **Spec Exp:** Spinal Cord Injury; **Hospital:** Craig Hosp; **Address:** CNS Med Grp, 3425 S Clarkson St, Engelwood, CO 80113; **Phone:** 303-789-8220; **Board Cert:** Physical Medicine & Rehabilitation 1980; Spinal Cord Injury Medicine 1998; **Med School:** Ohio State Univ 1976; **Resid:** Physical Medicine & Rehabilitation, Ohio State Univ Hosp 1979; **Fac Appt:** Assoc Clin Prof PMR, Univ Colorado

Mason, Kristin MD [PMR] - **Spec Exp:** Neurologic Rehabilitation; Electrodiagnosis; Musculoskeletal Injuries; **Hospital:** Swedish Med Ctr - Englewood; **Address:** Rehabilitation Assocs of Colorado, 8515 Pearl St, Ste 100, Thornton, CO 80229; **Phone:** 303-286-2888; **Board Cert:** Physical Medicine & Rehabilitation 2003; **Med School:** Baylor Coll Med 1988; **Resid:** Physical Medicine & Rehabilitation, Rehab Inst Chicago 1992

Matthews, Dennis J MD [PMR] - **Spec Exp:** Brain Injury Rehabilitation; Neuromuscular Disorders; Cerebral Palsy; **Hospital:** Chldn's Hosp - Denver, The; **Address:** Chldns Hosp, Dept Rehabilitation, 1056 E 19th Ave Ave, Box 285, Denver, CO 80218-1007; **Phone:** 303-861-6633; **Board Cert:** Physical Medicine & Rehabilitation 1979; Pediatric Rehabilitation Medicine 2003; **Med School:** Univ Colorado 1975; **Resid:** Physical Medicine & Rehabilitation, Univ Minnesota Hosps 1978; **Fellow:** Research, Univ Minnesota Hosps 1978; **Fac Appt:** Assoc Prof PMR, Univ Colorado

Southwest

Barber, Douglas Byron MD [PMR] - **Spec Exp:** Spinal Cord Injury; **Hospital:** Audie L Murphy Meml Vets Hosp; **Address:** Univ Hlth Sci Ctr, Dept of Rehab Med, 7703 Floyd Curl Drive, MC 7798, San Antonio, TX 78229-3900; **Phone:** 210-567-5353; **Board Cert:** Physical Medicine & Rehabilitation 1992; Spinal Cord Injury Medicine 1999; **Med School:** Univ Tex, Houston 1987; **Resid:** Physical Medicine & Rehabilitation, Univ TX Hlth Scis Ctr 1991; **Fac Appt:** Assoc Prof PMR, Univ Tex, San Antonio

Donovan, William Henry MD [PMR] - **Spec Exp:** Spinal Cord Injury; Amputee Rehabilitation; **Hospital:** TIRR; **Address:** 1333 Moursund St, Ste E-103, Houston, TX 77030-3405; **Phone:** 713-797-5912; **Board Cert:** Physical Medicine & Rehabilitation 1975; **Med School:** Albany Med Coll 1966; **Resid:** Internal Medicine, Marquette Univ 1968; Physical Medicine & Rehabilitation, Univ Wash 1972; **Fac Appt:** Prof PMR, Univ Tex, Houston

Dumitru, Daniel MD/PhD [PMR] - **Spec Exp:** Electrodiagnosis; **Address:** Univ Tex Hlth Sci Ctr, Dept Rehab Med, 7703 Floyd Curl Drive, San Antonio, TX 78229-3900; **Phone:** 210-567-5347; **Board Cert:** Physical Medicine & Rehabilitation 1984; **Med School:** Univ Cincinnati 1980; **Resid:** Physical Medicine & Rehabilitation, VA Hosp/Univ Hosp 1983; **Fac Appt:** Prof PMR, Univ Tex, San Antonio

Francisco, Gerard E MD [PMR] - **Spec Exp:** Spasticity Management; Brain Injury Rehabilitation; Stroke Rehabilitation; **Hospital:** TIRR; **Address:** The Inst Rehab & Rsch, 1333 Moursund St, Houston, TX 77030-3405; **Phone:** 713-797-5246; **Board Cert:** Physical Medicine & Rehabilitation 1995; **Med School:** Philippines 1989; **Resid:** Physical Medicine & Rehabilitation, UMDNJ-Univ Hosp 1994; **Fellow:** Physical Medicine & Rehabilitation, Baylor Coll Med 1995; **Fac Appt:** Assoc Clin Prof PMR, Univ Tex, Houston

Ivanhoe, Cindy MD [PMR] - **Spec Exp:** Brain Injury Rehabilitation; **Hospital:** TIRR; **Address:** 1333 Moursund St, Ste D-110, Houston, TX 77030-3405; **Phone:** 713-942-7300; **Board Cert:** Physical Medicine & Rehabilitation 1993; **Med School:** Mexico 1984; **Resid:** Physical Medicine & Rehabilitation, Univ Ill Coll Med 1992; **Fellow:** Brain Injury, Baylor Coll Med 1993; **Fac Appt:** Asst Prof PMR, Baylor Coll Med

Kevorkian, Charles G MD [PMR] - **Spec Exp:** Stroke Rehabilitation; Neuromuscular Disorders; Electrodiagnosis; **Hospital:** St Luke's Episcopal Hosp - Houston; **Address:** Baylor Coll Med, Dept PMR, 6624 Fannin St, Ste 2330, Houston, TX 77030-2335; **Phone:** 713-798-4061; **Board Cert:** Physical Medicine & Rehabilitation 1980; **Med School:** Australia 1972; **Resid:** Physical Medicine & Rehabilitation, Prince Henry Hosp 1976; Physical Medicine & Rehabilitation, Mayo Clinic 1979; **Fac Appt:** Assoc Prof PMR, Baylor Coll Med

Physical Medicine & Rehabilitation

King, John Chandler MD [PMR] - **Spec Exp:** Stroke Rehabilitation; Electrodiagnosis; Pain-Chronic; **Hospital:** Univ Hlth Sys - Univ Hosp, Audie L Murphy Meml Vets Hosp; **Address:** Univ Tex Hlth Sci Ctr, Dept Rehab Med, 7703 Floyd Curl Drive, MC 7798, San Antonio, TX 78229-3900; **Phone:** 210-567-5345; **Board Cert:** Physical Medicine & Rehabilitation 1987; Spinal Cord Injury Medicine 2000; **Med School:** Oral Roberts Sch Med 1983; **Resid:** Physical Medicine & Rehabilitation, Baylor Coll Med 1986; **Fac Appt:** Prof PMR, Univ Tex, San Antonio

West Coast and Pacific

Herring, Stanley A MD [PMR] - **Spec Exp:** Sports Medicine; Pain-Back; Spinal Rehabilitation; **Hospital:** Harborview Med Ctr; **Address:** 325 9th Ave, Box 359721, Seattle, WA 98104; **Phone:** 206-744-0401; **Board Cert:** Physical Medicine & Rehabilitation 1983; **Med School:** Univ Tex SW, Dallas 1979; **Resid:** Physical Medicine & Rehabilitation, Univ Washington 1982; **Fac Appt:** Clin Prof PMR, Univ Wash

Jaffe, Kenneth M MD [PMR] - **Spec Exp:** Brain Injury; Spinal Cord Injury; Limb Deficiency-Arthrogryposis; **Hospital:** Chldns Hosp and Regl Med Ctr - Seattle; **Address:** 4800 Sand Point Way NE, Seattle, WA 98105; **Phone:** 206-987-2114; **Board Cert:** Pediatrics 1980; Physical Medicine & Rehabilitation 1982; **Med School:** Harvard Med Sch 1975; **Resid:** Pediatrics, Univ Wash-Chldns Hosp 1980; Physical Medicine & Rehabilitation, Univ Wash Affil Hosp 1982; **Fac Appt:** Prof PMR, Univ Wash

Kraft, George Howard MD [PMR] - **Spec Exp:** Multiple Sclerosis; Spinal Cord Injury; Electrodiagnosis; **Hospital:** Univ Wash Med Ctr; **Address:** 1959 NE Pacific St, Box 356490, Seattle, WA 98195; **Phone:** 206-598-3344; **Board Cert:** Physical Medicine & Rehabilitation 1969; Spinal Cord Injury Medicine 1998; **Med School:** Ohio State Univ 1963; **Resid:** Physical Medicine & Rehabilitation, UCSF-Moffitt Hosp 1965; Physical Medicine & Rehabilitation, Ohio State Univ Med Ctr 1967; **Fac Appt:** Prof PMR, Univ Wash

Massagli, Teresa Luisa MD [PMR] - **Spec Exp:** Spinal Cord Injury-Pediatric; Brain Injury Rehabiliation-Pediatric; **Hospital:** Chldns Hosp and Regl Med Ctr - Seattle; **Address:** Chldns Hosp & Regl Med Ctr, PO Box 5371, MS W6847, Seattle, WA 98105-3916; **Phone:** 206-987-2180; **Board Cert:** Pediatrics 1987; Physical Medicine & Rehabilitation 1989; Spinal Cord Injury Medicine 1998; **Med School:** Yale Univ 1982; **Resid:** Pediatrics, Yale-New Haven Hosp 1985; **Fellow:** Physical Medicine & Rehabilitation, Univ Washington 1988; **Fac Appt:** Prof PMR, Univ Wash

Robinson, Lawrence R MD [PMR] - **Spec Exp:** Electrodiagnosis; Electromyography; Botox Therapy; **Hospital:** Harborview Med Ctr, Univ Wash Med Ctr; **Address:** Clinical Affairs, Box 356380, University of Washington, Seattle, WA 98195-6380; **Phone:** 206-543-6232; **Board Cert:** Physical Medicine & Rehabilitation 1987; **Med School:** Baylor Coll Med 1982; **Resid:** Physical Medicine & Rehabilitation, Northwestern Meml Hosp 1985; **Fac Appt:** Prof PMR, Univ Wash

Saal, Jeffrey A MD [PMR] - **Spec Exp:** Pain-Lower Back (IDET procedure); Spinal Rehabilitation; Sports Medicine; **Hospital:** Stanford Univ Med Ctr; **Address:** 500 Arguello St, Ste 100, Redwood City, CA 94063; **Phone:** 650-851-4900; **Board Cert:** Internal Medicine 1978; Physical Medicine & Rehabilitation 1982; **Med School:** Tulane Univ 1975; **Resid:** Internal Medicine, VA Med Ctr 1978; Physical Medicine & Rehabilitation, Stanford Univ Affil Hosps 1981; **Fac Appt:** Assoc Clin Prof PMR, UC Irvine

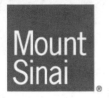

THE MOUNT SINAI MEDICAL CENTER
REHABILITATION MEDICINE

One Gustave L. Levy Place (Fifth Avenue and 100th Street)
New York, NY 10029-6574
Physician Referral: 1-800-MD-SINAI (637-4624)
www.mountsinai.org

The Department of Rehabilitation Medicine at The Mount Sinai Medical Center is a center of excellence in the delivery of complete care for people with disabilities. A wide range of comprehensive patient care services are available for individuals with spinal cord injuries, brain injuries, and a variety of neuromuscular, musculosketetal, and chronic conditions. We are CARF-accredited for our inpatient spinal cord and brain injury programs, the only such accredited programs in New York State, as well as for our comprehensive rehabilitation medicine program.

Our Team-Oriented Approach is pivotal to successful rehabilitation. The interdisciplinary team approach at Mount Sinai takes advantage of each discipline's expertise to provide quality coordinated care. Our experienced professionals evaluate each patient and meet regularly to develop and implement individualized treatment plans in partnership with patients and their families. Our goal is to make each individual with a disability maximally self-sufficient and mobile and able to return to community life.

The Mount Sinai Rehabilitation Center team is led by Kristjan T. Ragnarsson, MD, whose leadership and innovative approach to patient care has had a major impact in the field of Rehabilitation Medicine. The Center includes physicians, primary rehab nurses, nurse practitioners, and professional staff in physical therapy, occupational therapy, speech therapy, nutrition, social work, psychology, therapeutic recreation, and vocational counseling. Special rehabilitation medicine programs include the following:

• **The Spinal Cord Injury (SCI) Rehabilitation Program** provides comprehensive care to individuals with spinal cord injuries. This includes a full range of innovative medical and rehabilitation services. For example, our "Do It" program is a unique outpatient program that facilitates community integration.

• **The Brain Injury (BI) Rehabilitation Program** provides comprehensive care to individuals with brain injuries. It is well recognized that the treatment of individuals with cognitive and behavioral challenges is critical to community integration. Our program contains specialists uniquely qualified to meet these challenges.

• **Sports Therapy Center** is a comprehensive outpatient physical and occupational therapy facility offering individualized treatments for individuals with a variety of musculoskeletal conditions. It is conveniently located in midtown Manhattan.

THE MOUNT SINAI MEDICAL CENTER

Department of Rehabilitation Medicine

• Consistently ranked among the top rehabilitation centers in *U.S. News & World Report*

• One of the 14 designated programs by the National Institute on Disability and Rehabilitation Research (NIDRR) as a Model of System Care for Spinal Cord Injury.

• The *only* Research and Training Center for Traumatic Brain Intervention

• The only Model System for Spinal Cord Injury in New York State

• One of only a few programs in the country designated by NIDRR as a Model Systems of Care in Spinal Cord Injury, Traumatic Brain Injury and as a Research and Training Center.

• One of 16 programs designated by the National Institute on Disability and Rehabilitation Research (NIDRR) as a Model System of Care for Traumatic Brain Injury.

• The Only Medical System for Traumatic Brain Injury in New York State.

618

Sponsored Page

Plastic Surgery

A plastic surgeon deals with the repair, reconstruction or replacement of physical defects of form or function involving the skin, musculoskeletal system, craniomaxillofacial structures, hand, extremities, breast and trunk and external genitalia. He/she uses aesthetic surgical principles not only to improve undesirable qualities of normal structures (commonly called "cosmetic surgery") but in all reconstructive procedures as well.

A plastic surgeon possesses special knowledge and skill in the design and surgery of grafts, flaps, free tissue transfer and replantation. Competence in the management of complex wounds, the use of implantable materials, and in tumor surgery is required.

Training Required: Five to seven years

Certification in one of the following subspecialties requires additional training and examination.

Plastic Surgery within the Head and Neck: A plastic surgeon with additional training in plastic and reconstructive procedures within the head, face, neck and associated structures, including cutaneous head and neck oncology and reconstruction, management of maxillofacial trauma, soft tissue repair and neural surgery.

The field is diverse and involves a wide age range of patients, from the newborn to the aged. While both cosmetic and reconstructive surgery are practiced, there are many additional procedures which interface with them.

Surgery of the Hand (see Hand Surgery)

Plastic Surgery

New England

Ariyan, Stephan MD [PlS] - **Spec Exp:** Melanoma; **Hospital:** Yale - New Haven Hosp; **Address:** New Haven Hospital, 60 Temple St, Ste 7C, New Haven, CT 06510-2716; **Phone:** 203-786-3000; **Board Cert:** Plastic Surgery 1978; **Med School:** NY Med Coll 1966; **Resid:** Surgery, Yale-New Haven Hosp 1975; Plastic Surgery, Yale-New Haven Hosp 1976; **Fellow:** Surgical Oncology, Yale-New Haven Hosp 1971; **Fac Appt:** Clin Prof S, Yale Univ

Collins, Eva Dale MD [PlS] - **Spec Exp:** Breast Cancer; Breast Reconstruction; **Hospital:** Dartmouth - Hitchcock Med Ctr; **Address:** Darthmouth-Hitchcock Med Ctr, Div Plas Surgery, One Medical Center Drive, Lebanon, NH 03756; **Phone:** 603-650-5148; **Board Cert:** Plastic Surgery 1997; **Med School:** Emory Univ 1989; **Resid:** Plastic Surgery, Washington Univ Med Ctr 1994; **Fellow:** Microsurgery, Washington Univ Med Ctr 1995; **Fac Appt:** Assoc Prof S, Dartmouth Med Sch

Constantian, Mark B MD [PlS] - **Spec Exp:** Rhinoplasty; Rhinoplasty Revision; Nasal Reconstruction; **Hospital:** St Joseph Hosp, Southern NH Med Ctr; **Address:** 19 Tyler St, Ste 302, Nashua, NH 03060-2951; **Phone:** 603-880-7700; **Board Cert:** Plastic Surgery 1979; **Med School:** Univ VA Sch Med 1972; **Resid:** Surgery, Boston Univ Med Ctr 1976; **Fellow:** Plastic Reconstructive Surgery, Medical Coll VA 1978

Eriksson, Elof MD/PhD [PlS] - **Spec Exp:** Abdominoplasty; Cosmetic Surgery-Breast; Skin Laser Surgery; **Hospital:** Brigham & Women's Hosp; **Address:** Brigham & Women's Hosp, Div Plas Surg, 75 Francis St, Boston, MA 02115; **Phone:** 617-732-5093; **Board Cert:** Plastic Surgery 1980; **Med School:** Sweden 1969; **Resid:** Surgery, Chicago Affil Hosps 1977; **Fellow:** Plastic Surgery, Med Coll Va 1979; **Fac Appt:** Prof PlS, Harvard Med Sch

Feldman, Joel MD [PlS] - **Spec Exp:** Cosmetic Surgery-Face; Burns-Reconstructive Plastic Surgery; **Hospital:** Mount Auburn Hosp, Mass Genl Hosp; **Address:** 300 Mt Auburn St, Ste 304, Cambridge, MA 02138; **Phone:** 617-661-5998; **Board Cert:** Surgery 1975; Plastic Surgery 1977; **Med School:** Harvard Med Sch 1969; **Resid:** Surgery, Mass Genl Hosp 1974; Plastic Surgery, Johns Hopkins Hosp 1976; **Fac Appt:** Assoc Clin Prof PlS, Harvard Med Sch

Gallico, G Gregory MD [PlS] - **Hospital:** Mass Genl Hosp; **Address:** 170 Commonwealth Ave, Boston, MA 02116; **Phone:** 617-267-5553; **Board Cert:** Plastic Surgery 1982; **Med School:** Harvard Med Sch 1973; **Resid:** Surgery, Mass Genl Hosp 1980; Plastic Surgery, Mass Genl Hosp 1981; **Fellow:** Immunology, Oxford Univ Med Sch 1977; **Fac Appt:** Assoc Clin Prof S, Harvard Med Sch

May Jr, James W MD [PlS] - **Spec Exp:** Cosmetic Surgery; Breast Reconstruction; Hand Surgery; **Hospital:** Mass Genl Hosp; **Address:** Mass Genl Hosp, 15 Parkman St, WACC 453, Boston, MA 02114; **Phone:** 617-726-8220; **Board Cert:** Surgery 1975; Plastic Surgery 1977; **Med School:** Northwestern Univ 1969; **Resid:** Plastic Surgery, Mass Genl Hosp 1975; **Fellow:** Hand Surgery, Univ Louisville 1975; **Fac Appt:** Prof S, Harvard Med Sch

Meara, John MD/DMD [PIS] - **Spec Exp:** Cleft Palate/Lip; Craniofacial Surgery-Pediatric; **Hospital:** Children's Hospital - Boston; **Address:** Department of Plastic Surgery, 300 Longwood Ave, Hunnewell 158, Boston, MA 02115; **Phone:** 617-355-4401; **Board Cert:** Plastic Surgery 2001; Otolaryngology 1998; **Med School:** Univ Mich Med Sch 1990; **Resid:** Plastic Surgery, Brigham & Womens & The Chldns Hosps 1999; Otolaryngology, Mass Eye & Ear Infirmary 1997; **Fellow:** Craniofacial Surgery, Royal Chldns Hosp 2000; **Fac Appt:** Assoc Prof PlS, Harvard Med Sch

Mulliken, John B MD [PIS] - **Spec Exp:** Pediatric Plastic Surgery; Cleft Palate/Lip; Vascular Malformations; **Hospital:** Children's Hospital - Boston; **Address:** Chldns Hosp, Div Plas Surg, 300 Longwood Ave, Hunnewell-1, Boston, MA 02115-5724; **Phone:** 617-355-7686; **Board Cert:** Surgery 1972; Plastic Surgery 1975; **Med School:** Columbia P&S 1964; **Resid:** Surgery, Mass Genl Hosp 1970; Plastic Surgery, Johns Hopkins Hosp 1974; **Fac Appt:** Prof S, Harvard Med Sch

Orgill, Dennis MD [PIS] - **Spec Exp:** Wound Healing/Care; Burns-Reconstructive Plastic Surgery; **Hospital:** Brigham & Women's Hosp; **Address:** Brigham & Women's Hosp, Dept Plas Surg, 75 Francis St, Boston, MA 02115; **Phone:** 617-732-5456; **Board Cert:** Surgery 2000; Plastic Surgery 1994; **Med School:** Harvard Med Sch 1985; **Resid:** Surgery, Brigham & Women's Hosp 1990; **Fellow:** Plastic Surgery, Brigham & Women's Hosp 1992; **Fac Appt:** Assoc Prof S, Harvard Med Sch

Stadelmann, Wayne K MD [PIS] - **Spec Exp:** Melanoma-Head & Neck; Breast Reconstruction; Breast Augmentation; **Hospital:** Concord Hospital, Elliot Hosp; **Address:** 248 Pleasant St, Ste 201, Concord, NH 03301; **Phone:** 603-224-5200; **Board Cert:** Plastic Surgery 1999; **Med School:** Univ Chicago-Pritzker Sch Med 1990; **Resid:** Surgery, Univ Chicago Hosps 1994; Plastic Surgery, Univ S Florida/H Lee Moffit Cancer Ctr 1997

Stahl, Richard S MD [PIS] - **Spec Exp:** Breast Reconstruction; Chest Wall Tumors; Chest Wall Reconstruction; Abdominal Wall Reconstruction; **Hospital:** Yale - New Haven Hosp, Hosp of St Raphael; **Address:** 5 Durham Rd, Guilford, CT 06437; **Phone:** 203-458-4440; **Board Cert:** Surgery 2001; Plastic Surgery 1984; **Med School:** Vanderbilt Univ 1976; **Resid:** Surgery, Yale New Haven Hosp 1981; Plastic Surgery, Emory Univ Med Ctr 1983; **Fac Appt:** Clin Prof S, Yale Univ

Sullivan, Patrick K MD [PIS] - **Spec Exp:** Cosmetic Surgery-Face; Cosmetic Surgery-Breast; Rhinoplasty; **Hospital:** Rhode Island Hosp; **Address:** 235 Plain St, Ste 502, Providence, RI 02905; **Phone:** 401-831-8300; **Board Cert:** Otolaryngology 1985; Plastic Surgery 1989; **Med School:** Mayo Med Sch 1979; **Resid:** Otolaryngology, Univ Colo Hlth Scis Ctr 1984; Plastic Surgery, Rhode Island Hosp 1986; **Fellow:** Craniofacial Surgery, Dr Paul Tessier & Dr Hugo Obwegeser 1987; **Fac Appt:** Assoc Prof PlS, Brown Univ

Mid Atlantic

Aston, Sherrell MD [PIS] - **Spec Exp:** Cosmetic Surgery-Face; Rhinoplasty; Cosmetic Surgery-Breast; Liposuction & Body Contouring; **Hospital:** Manhattan Eye, Ear & Throat Hosp, NYU Med Ctr (page 67); **Address:** 728 Park Ave, New York, NY 10021; **Phone:** 212-249-6000; **Board Cert:** Surgery 1974; Plastic Surgery 1978; **Med School:** Univ VA Sch Med 1968; **Resid:** Surgery, UCLA Med Ctr 1973; Plastic Surgery, New York Univ 1975; **Fellow:** Surgery, Johns Hopkins Hosp 1970; **Fac Appt:** Prof PlS, NYU Sch Med

Plastic Surgery

Attinger, Christopher E MD [PlS] - **Spec Exp:** Limb Surgery/ Reconstruction; Diabetic Leg/Foot; Wound Healing/Care; Lower Limb Reconstruction; **Hospital:** Georgetown Univ Hosp; **Address:** Georgetown Univ Hosp - The Limb Center, 3800 Resorvoir Rd, 1 Main West, Washington, DC 20007; **Phone:** 202-444-5462; **Board Cert:** Plastic Surgery 1992; **Med School:** Yale Univ 1981; **Resid:** Surgery, Brigham & Women's Hosp 1986; Plastic Surgery, NYU Med Ctr 1989; **Fellow:** Vascular Surgery, Brigham & Women's Hosp 1987; Hand Surgery, NYU Med Ctr 1990; **Fac Appt:** Prof PlS, Georgetown Univ

Baker, Daniel MD [PlS] - **Spec Exp:** Cosmetic Surgery-Face; Reconstructive Surgery-Face; Rhinoplasty; **Hospital:** Manhattan Eye, Ear & Throat Hosp; **Address:** 65 E 66th St, New York, NY 10021; **Phone:** 212-734-9695; **Board Cert:** Plastic Surgery 1978; **Med School:** Columbia P&S 1968; **Resid:** Surgery, UCSF Med Ctr 1975; Plastic Surgery, NYU Med Ctr 1977; **Fellow:** Head and Neck Surgery, NYU Med Ctr/St Vincents Hosp 1978; **Fac Appt:** Assoc Prof PlS, NYU Sch Med

Bartlett, Scott P MD [PlS] - **Spec Exp:** Craniofacial Surgery/Reconstruction; Pediatric Plastic Surgery; Facial Plastic & Reconstructive Surgery; **Hospital:** Hosp Univ Penn - UPHS (page 72), Chldns Hosp of Philadelphia, The; **Address:** Hosp Univ Penn, 3400 Spruce St, Philadelphia, PA 19104-4227; **Phone:** 215-662-2096; **Board Cert:** Plastic Surgery 1987; **Med School:** Washington Univ, St Louis 1975; **Resid:** Surgery, Mass Genl Hosp 1983; Plastic Surgery, Mass Genl Hosp 1985; **Fellow:** Craniofacial Surgery, Hosp Univ Penn 1986; **Fac Appt:** Prof PlS, Univ Pennsylvania

Boyajian, Michael J MD [PlS] - **Spec Exp:** Pediatric Plastic Surgery; **Hospital:** Chldns Natl Med Ctr; **Address:** Chldns Natl Med Ctr, 111 Michigan Ave NW, Ste 4W-100, Washington, DC 20010-2978; **Phone:** 202-884-2150; **Board Cert:** Plastic Surgery 1984; **Med School:** NYU Sch Med 1976; **Resid:** Surgery, Univ Colo Med Ctr 1979; Surgery, Univ Cincinnati Hosp 1981; **Fellow:** Plastic Surgery, Brigham & Women's Hosp 1983; Craniofacial Surgery, Chldns Hosp 1983; **Fac Appt:** Asst Prof PlS, Geo Wash Univ

Bucky, Louis P MD [PlS] - **Spec Exp:** Cosmetic Surgery-Face; Botox Therapy; Cosmetic Surgery-Breast; Liposuction & Body Contouring; **Hospital:** Pennsylvania Hosp (page 72), Hosp Univ Penn - UPHS (page 72); **Address:** 230 W Washington Square, Ste 101, Philadelphia, PA 19106; **Phone:** 215-829-6320; **Board Cert:** Plastic Surgery 1997; **Med School:** Harvard Med Sch 1986; **Resid:** Surgery, Mass Genl Hosp 1992; Plastic Surgery, Mass Genl Hosp 1994; **Fellow:** Microsurgery, Meml Sloan Kettering Cancer Ctr 1995; Craniofacial Surgery, Miami Chldns Hosp 1996; **Fac Appt:** Assoc Prof S, Univ Pennsylvania

Chiu, David T.W. MD [PlS] - **Spec Exp:** Hand & Microvascular Surgery; Cosmetic Surgery-Face; Peripheral Nerve Surgery; **Hospital:** NYU Med Ctr (page 67), Lenox Hill Hosp (page 62); **Address:** 900 Park Ave, New York, NY 10021-0231; **Phone:** 212-879-8880; **Board Cert:** Plastic Surgery 1982; Hand Surgery 2000; **Med School:** Columbia P&S 1973; **Resid:** Surgery, Barnes Jewish Hosp 1977; Plastic Surgery, Columbia-Presby Med Ctr 1979; **Fellow:** Hand Surgery, NYU Med Ctr 1980; **Fac Appt:** Prof S, NYU Sch Med

Cordeiro, Peter G MD [PlS] - **Spec Exp:** Reconstructive Surgery; Breast Reconstruction; Facial Plastic & Reconstructive Surgery; **Hospital:** Meml Sloan Kettering Cancer Ctr, Manhattan Eye, Ear & Throat Hosp; **Address:** Meml Sloan Kettering Cancer Ctr, 1275 York Ave, rm C1193, New York, NY 10021-6007; **Phone:** 212-639-2521; **Board Cert:** Surgery 1998; Plastic Surgery 1994; **Med School:** Harvard Med Sch 1983; **Resid:** Surgery, New Eng Deaconess Hosp-Harvard 1989; Plastic Surgery, NYU Med Ctr 1991; **Fellow:** Microsurgery, Meml Sloan-Kettering Cancer Ctr. 1992; Craniofacial Surgery, Univ Miami 1992; **Fac Appt:** Prof S, Cornell Univ-Weill Med Coll

Cutting, Court MD [PlS] - **Spec Exp:** Cleft Palate/Lip; Reconstructive Plastic Surgery; Rhinoplasty; Craniofacial Surgery/Reconstruction; **Hospital:** NYU Med Ctr (page 67); **Address:** 333 E 34th St, Ste 1K, New York, NY 10016-6481; **Phone:** 212-447-6229; **Board Cert:** Otolaryngology 1980; Plastic Surgery 1986; **Med School:** Univ Chicago-Pritzker Sch Med 1975; **Resid:** Otolaryngology, Univ Iowa Hosps 1980; Plastic Surgery, NYU Med Ctr 1983; **Fellow:** Craniofacial Surgery, NYU Med Ctr 1984; **Fac Appt:** Prof PlS, NYU Sch Med

Dagum, Alexander B MD [PlS] - **Spec Exp:** Reconstructive Plastic Surgery; Microvascular Surgery; Hand Surgery; **Hospital:** Stony Brook Univ Med Ctr; **Address:** SUNY Health Science Ctr, T19-060, Box 8191, Stony Brook, NY 11794-8191; **Phone:** 631-444-8210; **Board Cert:** Plastic Surgery 2003; Hand Surgery 2004; **Med School:** Canada 1987; **Resid:** Surgery, Univ Ottawa Civic Hosp 1988; Plastic Surgery, Univ Toronto Med Ctr 1993; **Fellow:** Microsurgery, Univ Toronto Med Ctr 1984; Hand Surgery, Stony Brook Univ Hosp 1995; **Fac Appt:** Assoc Prof S, SUNY Stony Brook

Deleyiannis, Frederic W B MD [PlS] - **Spec Exp:** Head & Neck Reconstruction; Maxillofacial Surgery; Craniofacial Surgery; Pediatric Plastic Surgery; **Hospital:** UPMC Presby, Pittsburgh, Chldns Hosp of Pittsburgh - UPMC; **Address:** Falk Medical Bldg, 3601 Fifth Ave, Ste 6B, Pittsburgh, PA 15213; **Phone:** 412-648-9670; **Board Cert:** Otolaryngology 2000; Plastic Surgery 2003; **Med School:** Yale Univ 1992; **Resid:** Otolaryngology, Univ Washington Med Ctr 1999; Plastic Surgery, Univ Pittsburgh Med Ctr 2003; **Fellow:** Head and Neck Surgery, Univ Oviedo Med Ctr 2000; Reconstructive Microsurgery, Univ Pittsburgh Med Ctr 2000; **Fac Appt:** Asst Prof PlS, Univ Pittsburgh

Dufresne, Craig R MD [PlS] - **Spec Exp:** Craniofacial Surgery; Cosmetic Surgery; **Hospital:** Inova Fairfax Hosp; **Address:** 5530 Wisconsin Ave, Ste 1235, Chevy Chase, MD 20815; **Phone:** 301-654-9151; **Board Cert:** Plastic Surgery 1986; **Med School:** Columbia P&S 1977; **Resid:** Surgery, Johns Hopkins Hosp 1982; Plastic Surgery, NYU Med Ctr 1984; **Fellow:** Craniofacial Surgery, NYU Med Ctr 1985; **Fac Appt:** Clin Prof PlS, Georgetown Univ

Gold, Alan MD [PlS] - **Spec Exp:** Cosmetic Surgery; Cosmetic Surgery-Face & Eyes; Nasal Surgery; **Hospital:** N Shore Univ Hosp at Manhasset, N Shore Univ Hosp at Glen Cove; **Address:** 833 Northern Blvd, Ste 240, Great Neck, NY 11021-5308; **Phone:** 516-498-2800; **Board Cert:** Plastic Surgery 1979; **Med School:** SUNY Downstate 1971; **Resid:** Surgery, N Shore Univ Hosp 1975; Plastic Surgery, Kings County-Suny Med Ctr 1978; **Fellow:** Hand Surgery, Nassau County Med Ctr 1976; **Fac Appt:** Assoc Clin Prof S, Cornell Univ-Weill Med Coll

Hidalgo, David MD [PlS] - **Spec Exp:** Cosmetic Surgery-Face; Cosmetic Surgery-Breast; Rhinoplasty; Reconstructive Surgery; **Hospital:** Manhattan Eye, Ear & Throat Hosp, NY-Presby Hosp/Weill Cornell (page 66); **Address:** 655 Park Ave Fl 1, New York, NY 10021-5937; **Phone:** 212-517-9777; **Board Cert:** Plastic Surgery 1987; **Med School:** Georgetown Univ 1978; **Resid:** Surgery, NYU Med Ctr 1983; Plastic Surgery, NYU Med Ctr 1985; **Fellow:** Microsurgery, NYU Med Ctr 1986; **Fac Appt:** Clin Prof S, Cornell Univ-Weill Med Coll

Hoffman, Lloyd MD [PlS] - **Spec Exp:** Cosmetic Surgery-Face; Liposuction; Breast Reconstruction; **Hospital:** NY-Presby Hosp/Columbia (page 66), Lenox Hill Hosp (page 62); **Address:** 12 E 68th St, New York, NY 10021; **Phone:** 212-861-1640; **Board Cert:** Plastic Surgery 1989; **Med School:** Northwestern Univ 1978; **Resid:** Surgery, New York Hosp 1983; Plastic Surgery, NYU Med Ctr 1986; **Fellow:** Hand Surgery, NYU Med Ctr 1987; **Fac Appt:** Assoc Prof PlS, Cornell Univ-Weill Med Coll

Hurwitz, Dennis J MD [PlS] - **Spec Exp:** Body Contouring; Cosmetic Surgery-Face; Rhinoplasty; **Hospital:** Magee-Womens Hosp - UPMC, Chldns Hosp of Pittsburgh - UPMC; **Address:** 3109 Forbes Ave, Ste 500, Pittsburgh, PA 15213; **Phone:** 412-802-6100; **Board Cert:** Plastic Surgery 2005; **Med School:** Univ MD Sch Med 1970; **Resid:** Surgery, Dartmouth Med Ctr 1975; Plastic Surgery, Univ Pittsburgh Med Ctr 1977; **Fellow:** Craniofacial Surgery 1977; **Fac Appt:** Prof S, Univ Pittsburgh

Imber, Gerald MD [PlS] - **Spec Exp:** Cosmetic Surgery-Face; Eyelid Surgery; **Hospital:** NY-Presby Hosp/Weill Cornell (page 66); **Address:** 1009 5th Ave, Lower Level, New York, NY 10028; **Phone:** 212-472-1800; **Board Cert:** Plastic Surgery 1976; **Med School:** SUNY Downstate 1966; **Resid:** Surgery, LI Jewish Med Ctr 1972; Plastic Surgery, NY Hosp 1974; **Fac Appt:** Asst Clin Prof S, Cornell Univ-Weill Med Coll

Klatsky, Stanley A MD [PlS] - **Spec Exp:** Cosmetic Surgery-Face; Cosmetic Surgery-Breast; Liposuction & Body Contouring; **Hospital:** Johns Hopkins Hosp - Baltimore (page 61), Northwest Hosp Ctr; **Address:** 1304 Bellona Ave, Lutherville, MD 21093; **Phone:** 410-616-3000; **Board Cert:** Plastic Surgery 1970; **Med School:** Univ MD Sch Med 1962; **Resid:** Surgery, Sinai Hosp 1966; Plastic Surgery, Columbia-Presby Med Ctr 1968; **Fac Appt:** Assoc Prof S, Johns Hopkins Univ

Leipziger, Lyle S MD [PlS] - **Spec Exp:** Cosmetic Surgery-Face & Eyes; Cosmetic Surgery-Breast; Breast Reconstruction; Liposuction & Body Contouring; **Hospital:** N Shore Univ Hosp at Manhasset, Long Island Jewish Med Ctr; **Address:** 825 Northern Blvd Fl 3, Great Neck, NY 11021; **Phone:** 516-465-8787; **Board Cert:** Plastic Surgery 1994; **Med School:** Cornell Univ-Weill Med Coll 1985; **Resid:** Plastic Surgery, New York Hosp 1990; **Fellow:** Craniofacial Surgery, Johns Hopkins Hosp 1991; **Fac Appt:** Asst Prof S, Albert Einstein Coll Med

Little, John W MD [PlS] - **Spec Exp:** Cosmetic Surgery-Face; **Hospital:** Georgetown Univ Hosp; **Address:** 1145 19th St NW, Ste 802, Washington, DC 20036; **Phone:** 202-467-6700; **Board Cert:** Surgery 1975; Plastic Surgery 1977; **Med School:** Harvard Med Sch 1969; **Resid:** Surgery, Case Western Reserve Affil Hosps 1974; Plastic Surgery, Case Western Reserve Affil Hosps 1975; **Fellow:** Plastic Surgery, Jackson Meml Hosp 1977; **Fac Appt:** Clin Prof PlS, Georgetown Univ

Manders, Ernest K MD [PlS] - **Spec Exp:** Facial Nerve Disorders; **Hospital:** UPMC Presby, Pittsburgh, Magee-Womens Hosp - UPMC; **Address:** 3550 Terrace St, Ste 668, Scaife Hall, Div Plastic Surgery, Pittsburgh, PA 15261; **Phone:** 412-648-8100; **Board Cert:** Surgery 1998; Plastic Surgery 1982; **Med School:** Harvard Med Sch 1972; **Resid:** Surgery, Univ Michigan Med Ctr 1979; Plastic Surgery, Univ Michigan Med Ctr 1981; **Fellow:** Viral Oncology, Natl Insts of Allergy-Infectious Disease 1975; **Fac Appt:** Prof S, Univ Pittsburgh

Manson, Paul MD [PlS] - **Spec Exp:** Cosmetic Surgery; Facial Trauma/Fractures; Skin Cancer; **Hospital:** Johns Hopkins Hosp - Baltimore (page 61), Univ of MD Med Sys; **Address:** 601 N Caroline St, McElderry-8152F, Baltimore, MD 21287; **Phone:** 410-955-9470; **Board Cert:** Plastic Surgery 1979; **Med School:** Northwestern Univ 1968; **Resid:** Surgery, New Eng Deaconess Hosp 1971; Plastic Surgery, Johns Hopkins Hosp 1978; **Fellow:** Surgery, Lahey Clinic 1974; **Fac Appt:** Prof PlS, Johns Hopkins Univ

Matarasso, Alan MD [PlS] - **Spec Exp:** Cosmetic Surgery-Face & Eyes; Rhinoplasty; Liposuction & Body Contouring; Abdominoplasty; **Hospital:** Manhattan Eye, Ear & Throat Hosp, New York Eye & Ear Infirm (page 65); **Address:** 1009 Park Ave, New York, NY 10028-0936; **Phone:** 212-249-7500; **Board Cert:** Plastic Surgery 1986; **Med School:** Univ Miami Sch Med 1979; **Resid:** Surgery, Montefiore Med Ctr 1983; Plastic Surgery, Montefiore Med Ctr 1985; **Fellow:** Plastic Surgery, Manhattan EET Hosp/NYU 1985; **Fac Appt:** Clin Prof PlS, Albert Einstein Coll Med

McCarthy, Joseph G MD [PlS] - **Spec Exp:** Craniofacial Surgery-Pediatric; Reconstructive Surgery-Face; Cosmetic Surgery-Face; **Hospital:** NYU Med Ctr (page 67), Manhattan Eye, Ear & Throat Hosp; **Address:** 722 Park Ave, New York, NY 10021-4954; **Phone:** 212-628-4420; **Board Cert:** Surgery 1972; Plastic Surgery 1974; **Med School:** Columbia P&S 1964; **Resid:** Surgery, Columbia-Presby Med Ctr 1971; Plastic Surgery, NYU Med Ctr 1973; **Fac Appt:** Prof S, NYU Sch Med

Napoli, Joseph A MD/DDS [PlS] - **Spec Exp:** Cleft Palate/Lip; Maxillofacial Surgery; Craniofacial Surgery-Pediatric; **Hospital:** Alfred I duPont Hosp for Children; **Address:** Al duPont Hosp for Children, 1600 Rockland Rd, Wilmington, DE 19803; **Phone:** 302-651-4200; **Board Cert:** Plastic Surgery 2004; **Med School:** Columbia P&S 1987; **Resid:** Oral & Maxillofacial Surgery, Columbia-Presby Med Ctr 1985; Plastic Reconstructive Surgery, Dartmouth-Hitchcock Med Ctr 2001; **Fellow:** Craniofacial Surgery, Royal Chldns Hosp 2002; Pediatric Plastic Surgery, Royal Chldns Hosp 2002

Noone, R Barrett MD [PlS] - **Spec Exp:** Breast Reconstruction; Cosmetic Surgery; **Hospital:** Bryn Mawr Hosp, Lankenau Hosp; **Address:** 888 Glenbrook Ave, Bryn Mawr, PA 19010-2506; **Phone:** 610-527-4833; **Board Cert:** Surgery 1972; Plastic Surgery 1974; **Med School:** Univ Pennsylvania 1965; **Resid:** Surgery, Hosp Univ Penn 1971; Plastic Surgery, Hosp Univ Penn 1973; **Fac Appt:** Clin Prof S, Univ Pennsylvania

Pitman, Gerald H MD [PlS] - **Spec Exp:** Cosmetic Surgery-Face; Liposuction; Abdominoplasty; **Hospital:** Manhattan Eye, Ear & Throat Hosp, NYU Med Ctr (page 67); **Address:** 170 E 73rd St, New York, NY 10021-4352; **Phone:** 212-517-2600; **Board Cert:** Plastic Surgery 1978; **Med School:** Univ Pennsylvania 1968; **Resid:** Surgery, Columbia-Presby Hosp 1975; Plastic Surgery, NYU Med Ctr 1977; **Fellow:** Microsurgery, NYU Med Ctr 1981; **Fac Appt:** Clin Prof PlS, NYU Sch Med

Posnick, Jeffrey C MD/DMD [PlS] - **Spec Exp:** Cosmetic Surgery-Face; Craniofacial Surgery/Reconstruction; Maxillofacial Surgery; **Hospital:** Georgetown Univ Hosp; **Address:** 5530 Wisconsin Ave, Ste 1250, Chevy Chase, MD 20815; **Phone:** 301-986-9475; **Board Cert:** Plastic Surgery 1988; **Med School:** Vanderbilt Univ 1979; **Resid:** Surgery, Mass Genl Hosp 1983; Plastic Surgery, Eastern Virginia Med Sch 1986; **Fellow:** Craniofacial Surgery, Hosp Univ Penn/Chldns Hosp 1983; **Fac Appt:** Clin Prof PlS, Georgetown Univ

Ramirez, Oscar M MD [PlS] - **Spec Exp:** Cosmetic Surgery-Face; Facial Implants (Endoscopic); Breast Reduction; **Hospital:** Greater Baltimore Med Ctr; **Address:** 2219 York Rd, Ste 100, Timonium, MD 21093; **Phone:** 410-560-7090; **Board Cert:** Plastic Surgery 1985; **Med School:** Peru 1976; **Resid:** Surgery, Franklin Sq Hosp 1982; Plastic Surgery, Univ Pittsburgh Affil Hosps 1984; **Fellow:** Craniofacial Surgery, Manuel Gea Gonzalez Hosp 1984; **Fac Appt:** Asst Clin Prof S, Johns Hopkins Univ

Serletti, Joseph M MD [PlS] - **Spec Exp:** Breast Reconstruction; Reconstructive Surgery; Cosmetic Surgery; **Hospital:** Hosp Univ Penn - UPHS (page 72); **Address:** Hosp Univ Penn, 3400 Spruce St, 10 Penn Tower, Philadelphia, PA 19104; **Phone:** 215-662-3743; **Board Cert:** Plastic Surgery 2003; **Med School:** Univ Rochester 1982; **Resid:** Surgery, U Rochester Med Ctr 1986; Plastic Surgery, U Rochester Med Ctr 1988; **Fellow:** Reconstructive Surgery, Johns Hopkins Hosp 1990; **Fac Appt:** Prof PlS, Univ Pennsylvania

Seyfer, Alan MD [PlS] - **Spec Exp:** Chest Wall Reconstruction; Cleft Palate/Lip; Hand Surgery; **Hospital:** W Reed Army Med Ctr; **Address:** USUHS-School of Medicine, 4301 Jones Bridge Rd, Bethesda, MD 20814; **Phone:** 301-295-0441; **Board Cert:** Hand Surgery 1999; Plastic Surgery 1982; **Med School:** Louisiana State Univ 1973; **Resid:** Surgery, Fitzsimons AMC 1978; Plastic Surgery, Walter Reed AMC 1981; **Fellow:** Hand Surgery, Duke Univ Med Ctr 1980; **Fac Appt:** Prof S, Uniformed Srvs Univ, Bethesda

Siebert, John W MD [PlS] - **Spec Exp:** Facial Plastic & Reconstructive Surgery; Microsurgery; Cosmetic Surgery-Face; **Hospital:** NYU Med Ctr (page 67), Manhattan Eye, Ear & Throat Hosp; **Address:** 50 E 71 St, New York, NY 10021; **Phone:** 212-737-8300; **Board Cert:** Plastic Surgery 1991; **Med School:** Univ Wisc 1981; **Resid:** Surgery, Mass Genl Hosp 1986; Plastic Surgery, NYU Med Ctr 1988; **Fellow:** Microsurgery, NYU Med Ctr 1989; **Fac Appt:** Assoc Prof S, NYU Sch Med

Slezak, Sheri MD [PlS] - **Spec Exp:** Breast Reconstruction; **Hospital:** Univ of MD Med Sys; **Address:** Univ Maryland, Dept Plastic Surgery, 22 S Greene St, rm S8D12, Baltimore, MD 21201; **Phone:** 410-328-2360; **Board Cert:** Plastic Surgery 1991; **Med School:** Harvard Med Sch 1980; **Resid:** Surgery, Columbia-Presby Med Ctr 1985; Plastic Surgery, Johns Hopkins Hosp 1989; **Fac Appt:** Assoc Prof PlS, Univ MD Sch Med

Spear, Scott L MD [PlS] - **Spec Exp:** Breast Reconstruction; Cosmetic Surgery-Face; **Hospital:** Georgetown Univ Hosp; **Address:** Georgetown Univ Hosp, Div Plastic Surg, 3800 Reservoir Rd NW, 1 PHC, Washington, DC 20007; **Phone:** 202-444-8612; **Board Cert:** Plastic Surgery 1981; **Med School:** Univ Chicago-Pritzker Sch Med 1972; **Resid:** Surgery, Beth Israel Hosp 1978; Plastic Surgery, Univ Miami Hosps 1980; **Fellow:** Plastic Surgery, Hosp St Louis 1981; **Fac Appt:** Prof PlS, Georgetown Univ

Spence, Robert J MD [PlS] - **Spec Exp:** Burns-Reconstructive Plastic Surgery; Scleroderma; Tissue Banking; **Hospital:** Johns Hopkins Bayview Med Ctr (page 61), Johns Hopkins Hosp - Baltimore (page 61); **Address:** 4940 Eastern Ave, Baltimore, MD 21224-2780; **Phone:** 410-550-0411; **Board Cert:** Plastic Surgery 1981; **Med School:** Johns Hopkins Univ 1972; **Resid:** Surgery, Johns Hopkins Hops 1974; Surgery, Hershey Med Ctr 1978; **Fellow:** Plastic Surgery, Johns Hopkins Hosp 1980; **Fac Appt:** Assoc Prof S, Johns Hopkins Univ

Spinelli, Henry M MD [PlS] - **Spec Exp:** Cosmetic Surgery; Craniofacial Surgery/Reconstruction; Oculoplastic & Orbital Surgery; **Hospital:** NY-Presby Hosp/Weill Cornell (page 66), Manhattan Eye, Ear & Throat Hosp; **Address:** 875 Fifth Ave, New York, NY 10021-4952; **Phone:** 212-570-6235; **Board Cert:** Ophthalmology 1987; Plastic Surgery 1993; **Med School:** NYU Sch Med 1981; **Resid:** Ophthalmology, Manhattan EET Hosp 1985; Plastic Reconstructive Surgery, NYU-Bellevue Hosp 1990; **Fellow:** Craniofacial Surgery, NYU Med Ctr 1991; **Fac Appt:** Clin Prof S, Cornell Univ-Weill Med Coll

Staffenberg, David A MD [PlS] - **Spec Exp:** Craniofacial Surgery/Reconstruction; Pediatric Plastic Surgery; Facial Plastic & Reconstructive Surgery; Cosmetic Surgery-Face; **Hospital:** Montefiore Med Ctr; **Address:** 3353 Bainbridge Ave, Bronx, NY 10467; **Phone:** 718-920-4462; **Board Cert:** Plastic Surgery 1999; **Med School:** NY Med Coll 1989; **Resid:** Surgery, Maimonides Med Ctr 1995; Plastic Surgery, Emory Univ Med Ctr 1997; **Fellow:** Craniofacial Surgery, UCLA Med Ctr 1998; **Fac Appt:** Assoc Prof PlS, Albert Einstein Coll Med

Sultan, Mark MD [PlS] - **Spec Exp:** Breast Reconstruction; Cosmetic Surgery-Breast; Cosmetic Surgery-Face; **Hospital:** St Luke's - Roosevelt Hosp Ctr - Roosevelt Div, Beth Israel Med Ctr - Petrie Division; **Address:** 1100 Park Ave, New York, NY 10128; **Phone:** 212-360-0700; **Board Cert:** Plastic Surgery 1992; **Med School:** Columbia P&S 1982; **Resid:** Surgery, Columbia-Presby Hosp 1987; Plastic Surgery, Columbia-Presby Hosp 1990; **Fellow:** Head and Neck Surgery, Emory Univ Hosp 1989; **Fac Appt:** Assoc Prof S, Columbia P&S

Tabbal, Nicolas MD [PlS] - **Spec Exp:** Rhinoplasty; Cosmetic Surgery-Face; Eyelid Surgery; **Hospital:** Manhattan Eye, Ear & Throat Hosp; **Address:** 521 Park Ave, New York, NY 10021-8140; **Phone:** 212-644-5800; **Board Cert:** Plastic Surgery 1980; **Med School:** Lebanon 1972; **Resid:** Surgery, Am Univ Med Ctr 1976; Plastic Surgery, Akron City Hosp 1979; **Fellow:** Surgery, Upstate Med Ctr 1977; Reconstructive Microsurgery, NYU Med Ctr 1980

Thorne, Charles MD [PlS] - **Spec Exp:** Cosmetic Surgery-Face & Breast; Ear Reconstruction/Microtia; Craniofacial Surgery; **Hospital:** NYU Med Ctr (page 67), Manhattan Eye, Ear & Throat Hosp; **Address:** 812 Park Ave, New York, NY 10021-2759; **Phone:** 212-794-0044; **Board Cert:** Plastic Surgery 1991; **Med School:** UCLA 1981; **Resid:** Surgery, Mass Genl Hosp 1986; Plastic Surgery, NYU Med Ctr 1988; **Fellow:** Craniofacial Surgery, NYU Med Ctr 1989; **Fac Appt:** Assoc Prof PlS, NYU Sch Med

Vander Kolk, Craig Alan MD [PlS] - **Spec Exp:** Cosmetic Surgery; Cleft Palate/Lip; Craniofacial Surgery/Reconstruction; **Hospital:** Johns Hopkins Hosp - Baltimore (page 61); **Address:** Johns Hopkins Outpatient Ctr, 601 N Caroline St Fl 8, Baltimore, MD 21287; **Phone:** 410-955-6897; **Board Cert:** Plastic Surgery 1989; **Med School:** Univ Mich Med Sch 1980; **Resid:** Surgery, Univ Mich Med Ctr 1983; Plastic Surgery, Univ Mich Med Ctr 1986; **Fellow:** Hand Surgery, St Vincents Hosp 1985; Craniofacial Surgery, Chldns Hosp 1987; **Fac Appt:** Assoc Prof PlS, Johns Hopkins Univ

Whitaker, Linton A MD [PlS] - **Spec Exp:** Cosmetic Surgery-Face; Craniofacial Surgery/Reconstruction; Facial Tumors; Eyelid Surgery; **Hospital:** Hosp Univ Penn - UPHS (page 72), Chldns Hosp of Philadelphia, The; **Address:** Hosp Univ Penn -10 Penn Tower, 3400 Spruce St, Philadelphia, PA 19104; **Phone:** 215-662-2048; **Board Cert:** Surgery 1970; Plastic Surgery 1978; **Med School:** Tulane Univ 1962; **Resid:** Surgery, Dartmouth Affl Hosp 1969; Plastic Surgery, Hosp Univ Penn 1971; **Fac Appt:** Prof PlS, Univ Pennsylvania

Zide, Barry M MD/DMD [PlS] - **Spec Exp:** Facial Surgery-Chin; Hemangiomas; Facial Reconstruction-Cancer; Craniofacial Surgery-Pediatric; **Hospital:** NYU Med Ctr (page 67), Lenox Hill Hosp (page 62); **Address:** 420 E 55th St, Ste 1D, New York, NY 10022-5140; **Phone:** 212-421-2424; **Board Cert:** Plastic Surgery 1981; **Med School:** Tufts Univ 1973; **Resid:** Surgery, Stanford Med Ctr 1976; Plastic Surgery, U NC Hosp 1978; **Fellow:** Head and Neck Oncology, Roswell Park Cancer Inst 1979; Craniofacial Surgery, NYU Med Ctr 1980; **Fac Appt:** Prof PlS, NYU Sch Med

Southeast

Allen, Robert J MD [PlS] - **Spec Exp:** Breast Reconstruction; **Hospital:** E Cooper Reg Med Ctr, Ochsner Baptist Med Ctr; **Address:** 125 Doughty St, Ste 480, Charleston, SC 29403; **Phone:** 888-890-3437; **Board Cert:** Plastic Surgery 1985; **Med School:** Med Univ SC 1976; **Resid:** Surgery, LSU Med Ctr 1982; Plastic Surgery, LSU Med Ctr 1981; **Fellow:** Microsurgery, NYU Med Ctr 1983; **Fac Appt:** Assoc Clin Prof PlS, Louisiana State Univ

Argenta, Louis Charles MD [PlS] - **Spec Exp:** Pediatric Plastic Surgery; Craniofacial Surgery; Wound Healing/Care; **Hospital:** Wake Forest Univ Baptist Med Ctr (page 73); **Address:** WFU Bapt Med Ctr, Dept Plastic Surg, Medical Center Blvd, Winston Salem, NC 27157-1075; **Phone:** 336-716-4171; **Board Cert:** Plastic Surgery 1982; **Med School:** Univ Mich Med Sch 1969; **Resid:** Surgery, Univ Mich Hosp 1977; Plastic Surgery, Univ Mich Hosp 1979; **Fellow:** Craniofacial Surgery, Hosp Foch 1982; **Fac Appt:** Prof PlS, Wake Forest Univ

Plastic Surgery

Beasley, Michael MD [PlS] - **Spec Exp:** Breast Reconstruction & Augmentation; Liposuction; Body Contouring; **Hospital:** Presby Hosp - Charlotte; **Address:** 2215 Randolph Rd, Charlotte, NC 28207-1523; **Phone:** 704-372-6846; **Board Cert:** Plastic Surgery 1989; **Med School:** Univ NC Sch Med 1980; **Resid:** Surgery, NC Meml Hosp 1985; Plastic Surgery, Emory Univ Hosp 1987; **Fellow:** Plastic Surgery, St. Joseph Hospital 1987; **Fac Appt:** Assoc Clin Prof PlS, Univ NC Sch Med

Bermant, Michael A MD [PlS] - **Spec Exp:** Gynecomastia & Cosmetic Breast Surgery; Rhinoplasty & Ear Reshaping (Otoplasty); Liposuction & Body Contouring; Body Contouring after Weight Loss; **Hospital:** CJW Med Ctr; **Address:** 11601 Ironbridge Rd, Ste 201, Chester, VA 23831; **Phone:** 804-748-7737; **Board Cert:** Plastic Surgery 1991; **Med School:** Northwestern Univ 1978; **Resid:** Surgery, St Vincents Hosp 1982; Plastic Surgery, St Louis Univ Med Ctr 1984; **Fellow:** Microsurgery, NYU Med Ctr 1985

Carraway, James Howard MD [PlS] - **Spec Exp:** Oculoplastic Surgery; Cosmetic Surgery-Face; Eyelid Surgery; **Hospital:** Sentara Leigh Hosp; **Address:** 5589 Greenwich Rd, Ste 100, Virginia Beach, VA 23462; **Phone:** 757-557-0300; **Board Cert:** Surgery 1972; Plastic Surgery 1974; **Med School:** Univ VA Sch Med 1962; **Resid:** Surgery, Norfolk Med Ctr 1970; Plastic Surgery, Eastern VA Med Ctr 1973; **Fellow:** Plastic Surgery, Glasgow Royal Infirmary 1970; **Fac Appt:** Prof PlS, Eastern VA Med Sch

Cruse, C Wayne MD [PlS] - **Spec Exp:** Burns-Reconstructive Plastic Surgery; **Hospital:** Tampa Genl Hosp; **Address:** 12902 Magnolia Dr, Ste 4035, Tampa, FL 33612; **Phone:** 813-972-8414; **Board Cert:** Plastic Surgery 1981; **Med School:** Univ Louisville Sch Med 1972; **Resid:** Surgery, Univ S Fla Hosp 1977; Plastic Surgery, Univ KY Hosp-Chandler Med Ctr 1979; **Fac Appt:** Prof S, Univ S Fla Coll Med

Fix, R Jobe MD [PlS] - **Spec Exp:** Breast Reconstruction; Hand Surgery; Microsurgery; **Hospital:** Univ of Ala Hosp at Birmingham, Children's Hospital - Birmingham; **Address:** Univ of Alabama Hosp, Div Plastic Surg, 510 S 20th St, FOT-Ste 1102, Birmingham, AL 35294; **Phone:** 205-934-3358; **Board Cert:** Surgery 1997; Hand Surgery 2001; Plastic Surgery 1991; **Med School:** Univ Nebr Coll Med 1982; **Resid:** Surgery, Valley Med Ctr 1987; Plastic Surgery, Univ Ala Hosp 1989; **Fac Appt:** Prof PlS, Univ Ala

Georgiade, Gregory MD [PlS] - **Spec Exp:** Breast Reconstruction; Cleft Palate/Lip; **Hospital:** Duke Univ Med Ctr; **Address:** Duke Univ Med Ctr, Box 3960, Durham, NC 27710; **Phone:** 919-684-3039; **Board Cert:** Plastic Surgery 1981; Surgery 1990; **Med School:** Duke Univ 1973; **Resid:** Surgery, Duke Univ Med Ctr 1978; Plastic Surgery, Duke Univ Med Ctr 1980; **Fac Appt:** Prof S, Duke Univ

Gregory, Richard O MD [PlS] - **Spec Exp:** Skin Laser Surgery; Cosmetic Surgery-Face; Facial Rejuvenation; **Hospital:** Florida Hosp Celebration Hlth; **Address:** 400 Celebration Pl, Ste A320, Celebration, FL 34747; **Phone:** 407-303-4250; **Board Cert:** Plastic Surgery 1981; **Med School:** Indiana Univ 1971; **Resid:** Surgery, Duke Univ Med Ctr 1977; Plastic Surgery, Duke Univ Med Ctr 1979; **Fellow:** Hand Surgery, Univ Louisville Hlth Sci Ctr 1979; **Fac Appt:** Assoc Clin Prof PlS, Univ S Fla Coll Med

Grotting, James MD [PlS] - **Spec Exp:** Cosmetic Surgery-Face & Body; Cosmetic Surgery-Breast; Breast Reconstruction; **Hospital:** Healthsouth Med Ctr - Birmingham; **Address:** One Inverness Center Pkwy, Ste 100, Birmingham, AL 35242-4865; **Phone:** 205-930-1600; **Board Cert:** Plastic Surgery 1986; **Med School:** Univ Minn 1978; **Resid:** Surgery, Univ Wash Affil Hosp 1983; Plastic Surgery, UCSF Med Ctr 1985; **Fac Appt:** Clin Prof PlS, Univ Ala

Hagan, Kevin Francis MD [PlS] - **Spec Exp:** Reconstructive Surgery; Breast Surgery; Cosmetic Surgery; **Hospital:** Vanderbilt Univ Med Ctr; **Address:** Vanderbilt Univ Med Ctr, Dept Plastic Surg, D-4207 Med Ctr N, Nashville, TN 37232; **Phone:** 615-936-3574; **Board Cert:** Plastic Surgery 1983; **Med School:** Johns Hopkins Univ 1974; **Resid:** Surgery, Med Coll VA Hosps 1979; Plastic Surgery, UCSF Med Ctr 1982; **Fellow:** Microsurgery, Dr Harry Buncke Med Clinic 1980; **Fac Appt:** Assoc Prof PlS, Vanderbilt Univ

Hester Jr, T Roderick MD [PlS] - **Spec Exp:** Cosmetic Surgery-Face; Breast Reconstruction; **Hospital:** Emory Univ Hosp; **Address:** 3200 Downwood Cir, Ste 6340, Atlanta, GA 30327-1624; **Phone:** 404-351-0051; **Board Cert:** Plastic Surgery 1980; Surgery 1973; **Med School:** Emory Univ 1967; **Resid:** Surgery, Emory Affil Hosps 1972; Plastic Reconstructive Surgery, Emory Affil Hosps 1978

Hunstad, Joseph P MD [PlS] - **Spec Exp:** Cosmetic Surgery-Face & Body; Cosmetic Dermatology; **Hospital:** Carolinas Med Ctr-Univ; **Address:** 8605 Cliff Cameron Drive, Ste 100, Charlotte, NC 28269; **Phone:** 704-549-0500; **Board Cert:** Plastic Surgery 1989; **Med School:** Mich State Univ 1981; **Resid:** Surgery, Butterworth Hosp 1984; Plastic Surgery, Grand Rapids Area Med Ed Ct 1986; **Fellow:** Reconstructive Microsurgery, MECOM MicSurg Inst 1987

Kelly, Kevin J MD/DDS [PlS] - **Spec Exp:** Craniofacial Surgery; Cosmetic Surgery; Maxillofacial Surgery; **Hospital:** Vanderbilt Univ Med Ctr; **Address:** Vanderbilt Univ Med Ctr, Dept Plastic Surgery, 1161 21st Ave S, rm D4207, Nashville, TN 37232-2345; **Phone:** 615-322-2350; **Board Cert:** Plastic Surgery 1991; **Med School:** SUNY Downstate 1982; **Resid:** Surgery, Albany Med Ctr 1986; Plastic Surgery, Albany Med Ctr 1988; **Fellow:** Craniofacial Surgery, Johns Hopkins Med Ctr 1989; **Fac Appt:** Assoc Prof PlS, Vanderbilt Univ

Levin, L Scott MD [PlS] - **Spec Exp:** Toe-to-Hand Transfer; Reconstructive Microvascular Surgery; Microsurgery; **Hospital:** Duke Univ Med Ctr; **Address:** Duke Univ Med Ctr, Baker Bldg - rm 134, Box 3945, Durham, NC 27710; **Phone:** 919-613-7797; **Board Cert:** Orthopaedic Surgery 2004; Hand Surgery 2004; Plastic Surgery 1993; **Med School:** Temple Univ 1982; **Resid:** Orthopaedic Surgery, Duke Univ Med Ctr 1988; Plastic Surgery, Duke Univ Med Ctr 1989; **Fac Appt:** Prof S, Duke Univ

Mast, Bruce A MD [PlS] - **Spec Exp:** Breast Reconstruction & Augmentation; Body Contouring; Cosmetic Surgery-Face; Wound Healing/Care; **Hospital:** North Florida Regl Med Ctr, Shands at Alachua Gen Hosp; **Address:** 4340 Newberry Rd, Ste 301, Gainesville, FL 32607; **Phone:** 352-372-9414; **Board Cert:** Surgery 1995; Plastic Surgery 1998; **Med School:** UMDNJ-RW Johnson Med Sch 1987; **Resid:** Surgery, Med Coll Virginia 1993; Plastic Surgery, Univ Pittsburgh 1995; **Fac Appt:** Asst Clin Prof PlS, Univ Fla Coll Med

Matthews, David MD [PlS] - **Spec Exp:** Craniofacial Surgery/Reconstruction; **Hospital:** Carolinas Med Ctr, Presby Hosp - Charlotte; **Address:** 1719 South Blvd, Ste B, Charlotte, NC 28203-2747; **Phone:** 704-375-2955; **Board Cert:** Plastic Surgery 1983; **Med School:** Univ Cincinnati 1974; **Resid:** Surgery, Hosp Univ Penn 1980; Plastic Surgery, Hosp Univ Penn 1982; **Fellow:** Craniofacial Surgery, Royal Melbourne Hosp; **Fac Appt:** Clin Prof PlS, Univ NC Sch Med

Maxwell, G Patrick MD [PlS] - **Spec Exp:** Breast Reconstruction; **Hospital:** Baptist Hosp - Nashville, Centennial Med Ctr; **Address:** 2021 Church St, Ste 310, Baptist Medical Plaza Two, Nashville, TN 37203; **Phone:** 615-284-8200; **Board Cert:** Plastic Surgery 1981; **Med School:** Vanderbilt Univ 1972; **Resid:** Surgery, Johns Hopkins Hosp 1976; Plastic Surgery, Johns Hopkins Hosp 1979; **Fellow:** Microsurgery, Davies Med Ctr 1975; **Fac Appt:** Asst Clin Prof PlS, Vanderbilt Univ

Plastic Surgery

McCraw, John MD [PlS] - **Spec Exp:** Breast Reconstruction; **Hospital:** Univ Hosps & Clins - Jackson; **Address:** Univ Mississippi Med Ctr, Div Plastic Surg, 2500 N State St, Jackson, MS 39216; **Phone:** 601-815-1343; **Board Cert:** Surgery 1972; Plastic Surgery 1974; **Med School:** Univ MO-Columbia Sch Med 1966; **Resid:** Orthopaedic Surgery, Duke U Med Ctr 1969; Surgery, Univ Florida Med Ctr 1972; **Fellow:** Plastic Surgery, Univ Florida Med Ctr 1973; **Fac Appt:** Prof PlS, Univ Miss

Molnar, Joseph MD/PhD [PlS] - **Spec Exp:** Burns-Reconstructive Plastic Surgery; Reconstructive Microvascular Surgery; Hand Surgery; **Hospital:** Wake Forest Univ Baptist Med Ctr (page 73); **Address:** Wake Forest Univ Sch Med, Dept Plastic Surg, Medical Ctr Blvd, Winston-Salem, NC 27157-1075; **Phone:** 336-716-0432; **Board Cert:** Plastic Surgery 2005; Hand Surgery 2000; **Med School:** Ohio State Univ 1977; **Resid:** Surgery, Univ Wash Med Ctr 1989; Plastic Surgery, Med Coll VA 1992; **Fellow:** Trauma, Mass General Hosp 1985; Hand Surgery, Med Coll Wisc 1994; **Fac Appt:** Asst Prof PlS, Wake Forest Univ

Morgan, Raymond F MD [PlS] - **Spec Exp:** Cosmetic Surgery; Laser Surgery; Hand Surgery; **Hospital:** Univ Virginia Med Ctr; **Address:** Univ VA Hlth Sys, Dept Plas Surg, PO Box 800376, Charlottesville, VA 22908; **Phone:** 434-924-2413; **Board Cert:** Plastic Surgery 1983; Hand Surgery 2005; **Med School:** W VA Univ 1976; **Resid:** Surgery, Johns Hopkins Hosp 1980; Plastic Surgery, Johns Hopkins Hosp 1982; **Fellow:** Hand Surgery, Union Meml Hosp; **Fac Appt:** Prof PlS, Univ VA Sch Med

Nahai, Foad MD [PlS] - **Spec Exp:** Cosmetic Surgery-Breast; Cosmetic Surgery-Face; Liposuction; **Hospital:** Piedmont Hosp, St Joseph's Hosp - Atlanta; **Address:** 3200 Downwood Circle, Ste 640, Atlanta, GA 30327; **Phone:** 404-351-0051; **Board Cert:** Plastic Surgery 1980; **Med School:** England 1969; **Resid:** Surgery, Johns Hopkins Affil Hosps 1972; Surgery, Emory Univ Affil Hosps 1975; **Fellow:** Plastic Surgery, Emory Univ Affil Hosps 1978

Smith Jr, David J MD [PlS] - **Spec Exp:** Breast Reconstruction; Burns-Reconstructive Plastic Surgery; **Hospital:** Univ of S FL - Tampa; **Address:** Univ South Florida, Div Plastic Surg, 4 Columbia Drive, Ste 650, Tampa, FL 33606; **Phone:** 813-259-0929; **Board Cert:** Plastic Surgery 1981; **Med School:** Indiana Univ 1973; **Resid:** Plastic Surgery, Ind Univ 1980; Surgery, Emory Univ-Grady Hosp 1978; **Fellow:** Hand Surgery, Univ Louisville 1979; **Fac Appt:** Prof S, Univ S Fla Coll Med

Stuzin, James M MD [PlS] - **Spec Exp:** Cosmetic Surgery-Face; Eyelid Surgery; Skin Laser Surgery-Resurfacing; **Hospital:** Mercy Hosp - Miami; **Address:** 3225 Aviation Ave, Ste 100-200, Coconut Grove, FL 33133; **Phone:** 305-854-8828; **Board Cert:** Plastic Surgery 1989; **Med School:** Univ Fla Coll Med 1978; **Resid:** Surgery, Univ Wash Affil Hosp 1983; Plastic Surgery, NYU Med Ctr 1986; **Fellow:** Craniofacial Surgery, UCLA Med Ctr 1987

Tobin, Gordon R MD [PlS] - **Spec Exp:** Reconstructive Plastic Surgery; Transplant-Hand; Cosmetic Surgery; **Hospital:** Univ of Louisville Hosp, Jewish Hosp HlthCre Svcs Inc; **Address:** 601 S Floyd St, Ste 700, Louisville, KY 40202; **Phone:** 502-583-8303; **Board Cert:** Plastic Surgery 1978; **Med School:** UCSF 1969; **Resid:** Surgery, Univ Ariz Affil Hosps 1975; Plastic Surgery, Univ Ariz Affil Hosps 1976; **Fellow:** Pediatric Plastic Surgery, Univ Miami 1973; Cosmetic Plastic Surgery, Univ Miami 1973; **Fac Appt:** Prof PlS, Univ Louisville Sch Med

Vasconez, Luis O MD [PlS] - **Spec Exp:** Cosmetic Surgery-Face; Breast Reconstruction; **Hospital:** Univ of Ala Hosp at Birmingham; **Address:** 510 20th St S, FOT 1102, Birmingham, AL 35294-3411; **Phone:** 205-934-3245; **Board Cert:** Surgery 1970; Plastic Surgery 1971; **Med School:** Washington Univ, St Louis 1962; **Resid:** Surgery, Strong Meml Hosp 1970; Plastic Surgery, Shands Hosp-Univ FL 1969; **Fac Appt:** Prof S, Univ Ala

Wolfe, S Anthony MD [PlS] - **Spec Exp:** Craniofacial Surgery/Reconstruction; Maxillofacial Surgery; Cosmetic Surgery; **Hospital:** South Miami Hosp, Miami Children's Hosp; **Address:** 6280 Sunset Drive, Ste 400, Miami, FL 33143; **Phone:** 305-662-4111; **Board Cert:** Surgery 1973; Plastic Surgery 1978; **Med School:** Harvard Med Sch 1965; **Resid:** Surgery, Peter Bent Brigham Hosp 1972; Plastic Surgery, Jackson Meml Hosp 1974; **Fac Appt:** Assoc Clin Prof PlS, Univ Miami Sch Med

Midwest

Bauer, Bruce MD [PlS] - **Spec Exp:** Cleft Palate/Lip; Vascular Birthmarks; Ear Reconstruction/Microtia; Pigmented Lesions; **Hospital:** Children's Mem Hosp, Evanston NW Hlthcare; **Address:** Chldns Meml Hosp, 2300 Childrens Plaza, Box 93, Chicago, IL 60614; **Phone:** 773-327-2440; **Board Cert:** Plastic Surgery 1980; **Med School:** Northwestern Univ 1974; **Resid:** Surgery, Northwestern Meml Hosp 1977; Plastic Surgery, Northwestern Meml Hosp 1979; **Fac Appt:** Prof S, Northwestern Univ

Bentz, Michael L MD [PlS] - **Spec Exp:** Pediatric Plastic Surgery; Facial Deformities/Reconstruction; Hand Surgery; Hand Reconstruction; **Hospital:** Univ WI Hosp & Clins, Meriter Hosp; **Address:** Univ Wisconsin Hosp, 600 Highland Ave, CSC, rm G5-361, Madison, WI 53792-3236; **Phone:** 608-263-1367; **Board Cert:** Surgery 1998; Plastic Surgery 1994; Hand Surgery 1994; **Med School:** Temple Univ 1984; **Resid:** Surgery, Temple Univ Hosp 1989; Plastic Surgery, Univ Pittsburgh Med Ctr 1992; **Fellow:** Research, Univ Pittsburgh 1990; **Fac Appt:** Prof S, Univ Wisc

Billmire, David A MD [PlS] - **Spec Exp:** Cleft Palate/Lip; Reconstructive Plastic Surgery; **Hospital:** Cincinnati Chldns Hosp Med Ctr, Univ Hosp - Cincinnati; **Address:** 3333 Burnet Ave, MC 2020, Cincinnati, OH 45229; **Phone:** 513-636-7181; **Board Cert:** Plastic Surgery 1985; **Med School:** Ohio State Univ 1975; **Resid:** Surgery, Univ Hosp 1982; Plastic Surgery, Univ Hosp 1984; **Fellow:** Craniofacial Surgery, Texas Craniofacial Fdn; **Fac Appt:** Assoc Clin Prof S, Univ Cincinnati

Brandt, Keith MD [PlS] - **Spec Exp:** Breast Reconstruction; Reconstructive Surgery; Microsurgery; Hand & Wrist Surgery; **Hospital:** Barnes-Jewish Hosp, St Louis Chldns Hosp; **Address:** 660 S Euclid, Box 8238, St Louis, MO 63110-1010; **Phone:** 314-747-0541; **Board Cert:** Surgery 1999; Plastic Surgery 2003; Hand Surgery 2005; **Med School:** Univ Tex, Houston 1983; **Resid:** Surgery, Univ Nebraska Med Ctr 1989; Plastic Surgery, Univ Tennessee 1991; **Fellow:** Hand Surgery, Wash Univ 1992; Microsurgery, Wash Univ 1993; **Fac Appt:** Prof S, Washington Univ, St Louis

Buchman, Steven R MD [PlS] - **Spec Exp:** Pediatric Plastic Surgery; Craniofacial Surgery-Pediatric; Craniofacial Surgery; **Hospital:** Mott Chldns Hosp, Univ Michigan Hlth Sys; **Address:** Mott Children's Hospital, 1500 E Med Ctr Drive, rm 7859, Ann Arbor, MI 48109; **Phone:** 734-763-8063; **Board Cert:** Plastic Surgery 2005; **Med School:** Univ VA Sch Med 1985; **Resid:** Surgery, Hosp U Penn 1990; Plastic Surgery, Hosp U Penn 1992; **Fellow:** Craniofacial Surgery, UCLA Med Ctr 1993; **Fac Appt:** Prof PlS, Univ Mich Med Sch

Canady, John MD [PlS] - **Spec Exp:** Cleft Palate/Lip; Craniofacial Surgery; Pediatric Plastic Surgery; **Hospital:** Univ Iowa Hosp & Clinics; **Address:** Univ Iowa Hosp, Dept Plastic Surg & Otolaryngology, 200 Hawkins Drive, rm 21262 PFP, Iowa City, IA 52240; **Phone:** 319-356-2168; **Board Cert:** Otolaryngology 1988; Plastic Surgery 1992; **Med School:** Univ Iowa Coll Med 1983; **Resid:** Otolaryngology, Univ Iowa Hosp 1988; Plastic Surgery, Univ Kansas Med Ctr 1990; **Fac Appt:** Prof PlS, Univ Iowa Coll Med

Coleman, John J MD [PlS] - **Spec Exp:** Cancer Reconstruction; Breast Reconstruction; Head & Neck Surgery; **Hospital:** Indiana Univ Hosp; **Address:** 545 Barnhill Dr, Emerson Hall, Ste 232, Indianapolis, IN 46202-5120; **Phone:** 317-274-8106; **Board Cert:** Surgery 1998; Plastic Surgery 1981; **Med School:** Harvard Med Sch 1973; **Resid:** Surgery, Emory Univ Affil Hosp 1978; Plastic Surgery, Emory Univ Affil Hosp 1979; **Fellow:** Surgical Oncology, Univ Maryland Med Ctr; **Fac Appt:** Prof S, Indiana Univ

Hammond, Dennis MD [PlS] - **Spec Exp:** Breast Surgery; Breast Reduction; **Hospital:** Spectrum Hlth Blodgett Campus; **Address:** 4070 Lake Drive SE, Ste 202, Grand Rapids, MI 49546; **Phone:** 616-464-4420; **Board Cert:** Plastic Surgery 1994; **Med School:** Univ Mich Med Sch 1985; **Resid:** Plastic Surgery, Grand Rapids Med Edu & Res Ctr 1990; **Fellow:** Plastic Surgery, Baptist Hosp 1991; Hand & Microvascular Surgery, Med Coll Wisconsin 1992

Kane, Alex A MD [PlS] - **Spec Exp:** Pediatric Plastic Surgery; Craniofacial Surgery; Cleft Palate/Lip; **Hospital:** St Louis Chldns Hosp, Barnes-Jewish Hosp; **Address:** St Louis Children's Hospital, One Children's Pl, Ste 11 West 7, St Louis, MO 63110; **Phone:** 314-454-4894; **Board Cert:** Plastic Surgery 2001; **Med School:** Dartmouth Med Sch 1991; **Resid:** Surgery, Barnes Jewish Hosp 1994; Plastic Surgery, Barnes Jewish Hosp 1998; **Fellow:** Craniofacial Surgery, Chang-Gung Meml Hosp 1999; Craniofacial Imaging, Natl Lab for Diagnostic Research 1999; **Fac Appt:** Asst Prof S, Washington Univ, St Louis

Kuzon Jr, William M MD/PhD [PlS] - **Spec Exp:** Facial Paralysis Reconstruction; Abdominal Wall Reconstruction; Gender Reassignment Surgery; **Hospital:** Univ Michigan Hlth Sys; **Address:** Univ Michigan, Dept Surgery, Taubman Ctr, 1500 E Medical Center Drive, rm 2130, Ann Arbor, MI 48109-0340; **Phone:** 734-936-5890; **Board Cert:** Plastic Surgery 1994; **Med School:** Univ Rochester 1981; **Resid:** Plastic Surgery, Univ Toronto Med Ctr 1990; **Fellow:** Microvascular Surgery, Univ Toronto Med Ctr 1991; Hand & Microvascular Surgery, Univ Pittsburgh Med Ctr 1992; **Fac Appt:** Prof PlS, Univ Mich Med Sch

MacKinnon, Susan E MD [PlS] - **Spec Exp:** Microsurgery; Nerve Surgery & Transplantation; Hand Surgery; Reconstructive Surgery; **Hospital:** Barnes-Jewish Hosp; **Address:** University of Washington, Sch Med, Dr. MacKinnon, 660 S Euclid Ave, Box 8238, St Louis, MO 63110; **Phone:** 314-362-4586; **Med School:** Canada 1975; **Resid:** Surgery, Queens Univ-Kingston 1978; Plastic Surgery, Univ Toronto Med Ctr 1980; **Fellow:** Neurological Surgery, Univ Toronto Med Ctr 1981; Hand Surgery, Union Meml Hosp 1982; **Fac Appt:** Prof S, Washington Univ, St Louis

Marsh, Jeffrey L MD [PlS] - **Spec Exp:** Cleft Palate/Lip; Craniofacial Surgery/Reconstruction; Pediatric Plastic Surgery; **Hospital:** St John's Mercy Med Ctr - St Louis; **Address:** 621 S New Ballas Rd, Ste 260A, St Louis, MO 63141; **Phone:** 314-251-4772; **Board Cert:** Plastic Surgery 1979; **Med School:** Johns Hopkins Univ 1970; **Resid:** Surgery, UCLA Med Ctr 1975; Plastic Surgery, Univ Va Hosp 1977; **Fellow:** Craniofacial Surgery, Cannisburn Hosp; Craniofacial Surgery, Clinic Belvedere Hosp; **Fac Appt:** Clin Prof PlS, St Louis Univ

Mustoe, Thomas A MD [PlS] - **Spec Exp:** Cosmetic Surgery-Face; Cosmetic Surgery-Breast; Rhinoplasty; **Hospital:** Northwestern Meml Hosp, Evanston Hosp; **Address:** NW Med Faculty Fdn-Plastic Surgery, 675 North St Clair St Fl 19 - Ste 250, Chicago, IL 60611-5975; **Phone:** 312-695-6022; **Board Cert:** Otolaryngology 1983; Plastic Surgery 1987; **Med School:** Harvard Med Sch 1978; **Resid:** Surgery, Brigham & Womens Hosp 1980; Otolaryngology, Mass Eye & Ear Infirmary 1983; **Fellow:** Plastic Surgery, Brigham & Womens Hosp 1985; **Fac Appt:** Prof S, Northwestern Univ

Polley, John W MD [PlS] - **Spec Exp:** Craniofacial Surgery; Cosmetic Surgery; Pediatric Plastic Surgery; Maxillofacial Surgery; **Hospital:** Rush Univ Med Ctr; **Address:** Rush U Med Ctr, Plastic Surgery, 1725 W Harrison St, Ste 425, Professional Bldg, Chicago, IL 60612-3841; **Phone:** 312-563-3000; **Board Cert:** Plastic Surgery 1992; **Med School:** Northwestern Univ 1983; **Resid:** Surgery, Mich State Univ 1986; Plastic Surgery, Mich State Univ 1988; **Fellow:** Craniofacial Surgery, Chang Gung Meml Hosp 1989; Hosp for Sick Chldn 1990; **Fac Appt:** Prof PlS, Rush Med Coll

Puckett, Charles L MD [PlS] - **Spec Exp:** Cosmetic & Reconstructive Surgery; Breast Surgery; **Hospital:** Univ of Missouri Hosp & Clins, Columbia Regional Hosp; **Address:** 1 Hospital Drive, Ste M349, Columbia, MO 65212-5276; **Phone:** 573-882-2275; **Board Cert:** Surgery 1972; Plastic Surgery 1977; **Med School:** Wake Forest Univ 1966; **Resid:** Surgery, Duke Univ Med Ctr 1971; Plastic Surgery, Duke Univ Med Ctr 1976; **Fac Appt:** Prof S, Univ MO-Columbia Sch Med

Rees, Riley S MD [PlS] - **Spec Exp:** Wound Healing/Care; Melanoma; **Hospital:** Univ Michigan Hlth Sys, VA Med Ctr - Ann Arbor; **Address:** University of Michigan, 2130 Taubman Ctr, 1500 E Medical Center Drive, Box 0340, Ann Arbor, MI 48109-0340; **Phone:** 734-615-3435; **Board Cert:** Plastic Surgery 1981; **Med School:** Univ Utah 1972; **Resid:** Surgery, LSU Med Ctr 1978; Plastic Surgery, Vanderbilt Univ Med Ctr 1980; **Fac Appt:** Prof S, Univ Mich Med Sch

Sanger, James MD [PlS] - **Spec Exp:** Reconstructive Surgery; Hand Surgery; Microsurgery; **Hospital:** Froedtert Meml Lutheran Hosp, Chldns Hosp - Wisconsin; **Address:** Med Coll Wisc, Dept Plastic Surg, 8700 Watertown Plank Rd, Milwaukee, WI 53226; **Phone:** 414-805-5451; **Board Cert:** Plastic Surgery 1982; Hand Surgery 1999; **Med School:** Univ Wisc 1974; **Resid:** Surgery, LAC-Harbor UCLA Med Ctr 1979; Plastic Surgery, Med Coll Wisc Affil Hosps 1981; **Fellow:** Hand Surgery, Med Coll Wisc Affil Hosps 1982; **Fac Appt:** Prof PlS, Med Coll Wisc

Siemionow, Maria MD/PhD [PlS] - **Spec Exp:** Microsurgery; Peripheral Nerve Surgery; Reconstructive Plastic Surgery; Transplant Surgery; **Hospital:** Cleveland Clin Fdn (page 57); **Address:** Cleveland Clin Fdn, 9500 Euclid Ave, MC A60, Cleveland, OH 44195; **Phone:** 216-445-2405; **Med School:** Poland 1974; **Resid:** Surgery, Inst Orth & Rehab Med; **Fellow:** Plastic Surgery, Univ Hosp; Microsurgery, Univ Louisville Hosp

Sood, Rajiv MD [PlS] - **Spec Exp:** Burns-Reconstructive Plastic Surgery; Pediatric Hand Surgery; **Hospital:** Wishard Hlth Srvs, Riley Hosp for Children; **Address:** Indiana Univ School Med, Plastic Surgery, 1001 W 10th St Fl D-4, Indianapolis, IN 46202; **Phone:** 317-278-1022; **Board Cert:** Plastic Surgery 1994; Hand Surgery 2006; **Med School:** Albany Med Coll 1984; **Resid:** Surgery, Temple Univ Hosp 1989; **Fellow:** Plastic Surgery, Cleveland Clinic Fdn 1991; Hand Surgery, Union Meml Hosp 1992; **Fac Appt:** Prof S, Indiana Univ

Vogt, Peter MD [PlS] - **Spec Exp:** Cosmetic Surgery; **Hospital:** Mercy Hosp - Coon Rapids, Unity Hosp - Fridley; **Address:** 319 Barry Ave S, Ste 300, Wayzata, MN 55391; **Phone:** 952-473-1111; **Board Cert:** Plastic Surgery 1974; **Med School:** Canada 1965; **Resid:** Surgery, Montreal Genl Hosp 1970; Plastic Surgery, Winnipeg Hlth Scis Ctr 1973

Walton Jr, Robert Lee MD [PlS] - **Spec Exp:** Cosmetic Surgery-Face; Nasal Reconstruction; Breast Reconstruction; **Hospital:** Univ of Chicago Hosps, Resurrection Hlth Care St Joseph Hosp; **Address:** 60 E Delaware, Ste 1430, Chicago, IL 60611; **Phone:** 312-337-7795; **Board Cert:** Plastic Surgery 1980; **Med School:** Univ Kans 1972; **Resid:** Surgery, Johns Hopkins Hosp 1974; Plastic Surgery, Yale-New Haven Hosp 1978; **Fellow:** Hand Surgery, Hartford Hosp 1978; **Fac Appt:** Prof PlS, Univ Chicago-Pritzker Sch Med

Plastic Surgery

Wilkins, Edwin G MD [PlS] - **Spec Exp:** Breast Reconstruction; Lower Limb Reconstruction; Microsurgery; **Hospital:** Univ Michigan Hlth Sys; **Address:** Univ Mich, Div Plastic Surg, 1500 E Med Ctr Drive, rm 2130 Taubman Ctr, Ann Arbor, MI 48109-0340; **Phone:** 734-998-6022; **Board Cert:** Plastic Surgery 1991; **Med School:** Wake Forest Univ 1981; **Resid:** Surgery, Charlotte Meml Hosp 1986; Plastic Surgery, Vanderbilt Univ Med Ctr 1988; **Fellow:** Reconstructive Microsurgery, Univ Louisville Sch Med 1989; **Fac Appt:** Assoc Prof PlS, Univ Mich Med Sch

Yetman, Randall John MD [PlS] - **Spec Exp:** Breast Reconstruction; Melanoma; **Hospital:** Cleveland Clin Fdn (page 57); **Address:** 9500 Euclid Ave, Desk A60, Cleveland, OH 44195; **Phone:** 216-444-6908; **Board Cert:** Plastic Surgery 1984; **Med School:** Univ Miami Sch Med 1975; **Resid:** Surgery, Montefiore Med Ctr 1979; Plastic Surgery, NY Cornell Med Ctr 1981; **Fellow:** Plastic Surgery, Cleveland Clin Fdn 1982

Young, Vernon Leroy MD [PlS] - **Spec Exp:** Breast Augmentation; Skin Laser Surgery-Resurfacing; Body Contouring after Weight Loss; **Hospital:** Barnes-Jewish West County Hosp; **Address:** 969 N Mason Rd, Ste 170, St Louis, MO 63141; **Phone:** 314-628-8200; **Board Cert:** Plastic Surgery 1981; **Med School:** Univ KY Coll Med 1970; **Resid:** Surgery, Univ KY Med Ctr 1977; Plastic Surgery, Barnes Hosp-Wash Univ 1979; **Fac Appt:** Prof S, Washington Univ, St Louis

Zins, James MD [PlS] - **Spec Exp:** Cosmetic Surgery-Face; Maxillofacial Surgery; Craniofacial Surgery; **Hospital:** Cleveland Clin Fdn (page 57); **Address:** Department of Plastic Surgery, 9500 Euclid Ave, Desk A-60, Cleveland, OH 44195; **Phone:** 216-444-6901; **Board Cert:** Plastic Surgery 1985; **Med School:** Univ Pennsylvania 1974; **Resid:** Surgery, Hosp Univ Penn 1980; Plastic Surgery, Hosp Univ Penn 1982; **Fellow:** Craniofacial Surgery, Hosp Univ Penn 1978; Maxillofacial Surgery, Hosp Sick Chldn 1983

Great Plains and Mountains

Grossman, John A MD [PlS] - **Spec Exp:** Cosmetic Surgery; **Hospital:** Rose Med Ctr, Cedars-Sinai Med Ctr; **Address:** 4600 Hale Pkwy, Ste 100, Denver, CO 80220; **Phone:** 303-320-5566; **Board Cert:** Surgery 1974; Plastic Surgery 1976; **Med School:** Cornell Univ-Weill Med Coll 1967; **Resid:** Surgery, Boston City Hosp 1973; Plastic Surgery, Univ Colo Hlth Scis Ctr 1975; **Fellow:** Surgery, Harvard Med Sch 1973

Ketch, Lawrence L MD [PlS] - **Spec Exp:** Pediatric Plastic Surgery; Craniofacial Surgery; Cleft Palate/Lip; **Hospital:** Univ Colorado Hosp, Chldn's Hosp - Denver, The; **Address:** 1056 E 19th Ave, Box B467, Denver, CO 80218; **Phone:** 303-861-6409; **Board Cert:** Plastic Surgery 1982; Hand Surgery 1992; **Med School:** Univ Colorado 1974; **Resid:** Surgery, Univ Colo Affil Hosp 1979; **Fellow:** Plastic Surgery, Univ Miami 1981; **Fac Appt:** Prof S, Univ Colorado

Knize, David Maurice MD [PlS] - **Spec Exp:** Cosmetic Surgery-Face; Liposuction; Breast Augmentation; **Hospital:** Swedish Med Ctr - Englewood, Centura Porter Adventist Hosp; **Address:** 3701 S Clarkson St, Englewood, CO 80113; **Phone:** 303-761-9990; **Board Cert:** Surgery 1971; Plastic Surgery 1975; **Med School:** Univ Tex SW, Dallas 1963; **Resid:** Surgery, Univ Colo Med Ctr 1969; Plastic Surgery, NYU Med Ctr 1974; **Fac Appt:** Assoc Clin Prof PlS, Univ Colorado

Southwest

Barone, Constance M MD [PlS] - **Spec Exp:** Craniofacial Surgery; Craniosynostosis; Cosmetic Surgery; **Hospital:** Univ Hlth Sys - Univ Hosp, Christus Santa Rosa Children's Hosp; **Address:** Div Plastic Surg, 7703 Floyd Curl Drive, MC 7844, San Antonio, TX 78229-3900; **Phone:** 210-257-1883; **Board Cert:** Plastic Surgery 1991; **Med School:** Mount Sinai Sch Med 1982; **Resid:** Surgery, Temple Univ Hosp 1987; Plastic Surgery, NYU Med Ctr 1989; **Fellow:** Craniofacial Surgery, Montefiore/Einstein Coll Med 1992; **Fac Appt:** Prof PlS, Univ Tex, San Antonio

Barton Jr, Fritz MD [PlS] - **Spec Exp:** Cosmetic Surgery-Face; Liposuction & Body Contouring; **Hospital:** Baylor Univ Medical Ctr; **Address:** Dallas Plastic Surgery Institute, 411 N Washington Ave, Ste 6000, LB13, Dallas, TX 75246; **Phone:** 214-821-9355; **Board Cert:** Surgery 1975; Plastic Surgery 1977; **Med School:** Univ Tex SW, Dallas 1967; **Resid:** Surgery, Parkland Meml Hosp 1974; NYU Med Ctr 1976; **Fac Appt:** Prof PlS, Univ Tex SW, Dallas

Beals, Stephen P MD [PlS] - **Spec Exp:** Craniofacial Surgery; Pediatric Plastic Surgery; Cosmetic Surgery-Face; **Hospital:** St Joseph's Hosp & Med Ctr - Phoenix, Phoenix Children's Hosp; **Address:** 500 W Thomas Rd, Ste 960, Phoenix, AZ 85013-4223; **Phone:** 602-266-9066; **Board Cert:** Plastic Surgery 1986; **Med School:** Wayne State Univ 1978; **Resid:** Surgery, William Beaumont Hospital 1983; Plastic Surgery, Phoenix Plastic Surgery Inst 1985; **Fellow:** Craniofacial Surgery, Hospital for Sick Children 1985; **Fac Appt:** Asst Prof PlS, Mayo Med Sch

Burns, Alton J MD [PlS] - **Spec Exp:** Cosmetic Surgery; Skin Laser Surgery; Vascular Birthmarks; **Hospital:** Baylor Univ Medical Ctr, Chldns Med Ctr of Dallas; **Address:** 411 N Washington St, Ste 6000, Dallas, TX 75246; **Phone:** 214-823-1978; **Board Cert:** Plastic Surgery 1990; **Med School:** Univ Tex SW, Dallas 1981; **Resid:** Surgery, Univ Utah Hosp 1986; Plastic Surgery, Univ Tex SW Med Ctr 1988; **Fellow:** Vascular Anomalies, Chldns Hosp 1988; **Fac Appt:** Asst Prof PlS, Univ Tex SW, Dallas

Byrd, H Stephenson MD [PlS] - **Spec Exp:** Cosmetic Surgery-Face; Craniofacial Surgery; Pediatric Plastic Surgery; **Hospital:** Baylor Univ Medical Ctr; **Address:** 411 N Washington Ave, Ste 6000, Dallas, TX 75246-1713; **Phone:** 214-821-9662; **Board Cert:** Plastic Surgery 1980; **Med School:** Univ Tex Med Br, Galveston 1972; **Resid:** Surgery, Univ Utah Med Ctr 1977; Plastic Surgery, Dallas Co Hosp-Parkland Meml 1979; **Fac Appt:** Clin Prof PlS, Univ Tex SW, Dallas

Colon, Gustavo MD [PlS] - **Spec Exp:** Cosmetic Surgery; **Hospital:** E Jefferson Genl Hosp; **Address:** 4224 Houma Blvd, Ste 120, Metairie, LA 70006; **Phone:** 504-888-4297; **Board Cert:** Plastic Surgery 1978; **Med School:** Univ MD Sch Med 1964; **Resid:** Surgery, US Public Hlth Svc Hosp 1969; Plastic Surgery, Tulane Affil Prog 1971; **Fac Appt:** Prof S, Tulane Univ

Friedland, Jack A MD [PlS] - **Spec Exp:** Cleft Palate/Lip; Cosmetic Surgery-Face & Body; Cosmetic Surgery-Breast; Eyelid Surgery; **Hospital:** St Joseph's Hosp & Med Ctr - Phoenix, Scottsdale Hlthcare - Shea; **Address:** 101 E Coronado Rd, Phoenix, AZ 85004; **Phone:** 480-905-1700; **Board Cert:** Surgery 1971; Plastic Surgery 1975; **Med School:** Northwestern Univ 1965; **Resid:** Surgery, NYU Med Ctr & Bellevue Hosp-NYU 1970; Plastic Reconstructive Surgery, NYU Medical Ctr 1974; **Fac Appt:** Assoc Prof PlS, Mayo Med Sch

Gunter, Jack MD [PlS] - **Spec Exp:** Rhinoplasty; Rhinoplasty Revision; **Hospital:** Presby Hosp of Dallas; **Address:** 8144 Walnut Hill Lane, Ste 170, Dallas, TX 75231-4218; **Phone:** 214-369-8123; **Board Cert:** Otolaryngology 1969; Plastic Surgery 1981; **Med School:** Univ Okla Coll Med 1963; **Resid:** Surgery, Univ Ark Med Ctr 1965; Otolaryngology, Tulane Univ Hosp 1968; **Fellow:** Mercy Hosp 1969; Plastic Surgery, Univ Mich Hosp 1980; **Fac Appt:** Clin Prof PlS, Univ Tex SW, Dallas

Hamra, Sameer T MD [PlS] - **Spec Exp:** Cosmetic Surgery-Face; Rhinoplasty; **Hospital:** Mary Shiels Hosp; **Address:** 2731 Lemmon Ave E, Ste 306, Dallas, TX 75204; **Phone:** 214-754-9001; **Board Cert:** Surgery 1970; Plastic Surgery 1977; **Med School:** Univ Okla Coll Med 1963; **Resid:** Plastic Surgery, NYU Med Ctr 1973; Surgery, Univ Okla 1968; **Fellow:** Surgery, Univ Lausanne 1966; **Fac Appt:** Asst Clin Prof S, Univ Tex SW, Dallas

Kelly, John M MD [PlS] - **Spec Exp:** Cosmetic Surgery-Face; Breast Surgery; Liposuction; **Hospital:** Intergris Baptist Med Ctr - OK; **Address:** 3301 NW 63rd St, Oklahoma City, OK 73116-3705; **Phone:** 405-842-9732; **Board Cert:** Surgery 1970; Plastic Surgery 1978; **Med School:** Univ Ark 1963; **Resid:** Surgery, Univ Virginia Hosp 1969; Plastic Surgery, Johns Hopkins Hosp 1971; **Fac Appt:** Clin Prof S, Univ Okla Coll Med

Meltzer, Toby R MD [PlS] - **Spec Exp:** Gender Reassignment Surgery; Penile Inversion Technique; Breast Augmentation; **Hospital:** Scottsdale Hlthcare - Osborn; **Address:** 7025 N Scottsdale Rd, Ste 302, Scottsdale, AZ 85253; **Phone:** 866-876-6329; **Board Cert:** Plastic Surgery 1992; **Med School:** Louisiana State Univ 1983; **Resid:** Surgery, Charity Hosp Louisiana 1988; Plastic Surgery, Univ Michigan Med Ctr 1990; **Fellow:** Burn Surgery, Wayne State Univ 1987; **Fac Appt:** Asst Clin Prof S, Univ Ariz Coll Med

Menick, Frederick J MD [PlS] - **Spec Exp:** Reconstructive Surgery-Face; Breast Reconstruction; Cancer Reconstruction; Cosmetic Surgery; **Hospital:** St Joseph's Hosp - Tucson; **Address:** 1102 N Eldorado Pl, Tucson, AZ 85712; **Phone:** 520-881-4525; **Board Cert:** Plastic Surgery 1983; **Med School:** Yale Univ 1970; **Resid:** Surgery, Stanford Med Ctr; Surgery, Univ Ariz Med Ctr 1979; **Fellow:** Plastic Surgery, Queen Victoria Hosp/UC Irvine 1982; **Fac Appt:** Assoc Clin Prof S, Univ Ariz Coll Med

Nath, Rahul Kumar MD [PlS] - **Spec Exp:** Brachial Plexus Palsy; Peripheral Nerve Surgery; **Hospital:** Meml Hermann Hosp - Houston, Methodist Hosp - Houston; **Address:** Texas Nerve & Paralysis Inst, 2201 W Holcombe Blvd, Ste 225, Houston, TX 77030; **Phone:** 713-592-9900; **Board Cert:** Plastic Surgery 1998; **Med School:** Northwestern Univ 1988; **Resid:** Surgery, Northwestern Med Ctr 1991; Plastic Surgery, Washington Univ 1994; **Fellow:** Washington Univ 1996

Robb, Geoffrey L MD [PlS] - **Spec Exp:** Breast Reconstruction; Head & Neck Cancer Reconstruction; Facial Plastic & Reconstructive Surgery; **Hospital:** UT MD Anderson Cancer Ctr (page 71), St Luke's Episcopal Hosp - Houston; **Address:** 1515 Holcombe Blvd, Unit 443, Houston, TX 77030; **Phone:** 713-794-1247; **Board Cert:** Otolaryngology 1979; Plastic Surgery 1986; **Med School:** Univ Miami Sch Med 1974; **Resid:** Otolaryngology, Naval Reg Med Ctr 1979; Plastic Surgery, Univ Pittsburgh 1985; **Fellow:** Microvascular Surgery, Univ Pittsburgh; **Fac Appt:** Prof PlS, Univ Tex, Houston

Rohrich, Rod J MD [PlS] - **Spec Exp:** Nasal Surgery; Rhinoplasty; Breast Reconstruction; Wound Healing/Care; **Hospital:** UT Southwestern Med Ctr - Dallas, Baylor Univ Medical Ctr; **Address:** Univ Tex SW Med Ctr, Plastic Surgery, 5323 Harry Hines Blvd, Dallas, TX 75390-9132; **Phone:** 214-648-3119; **Board Cert:** Plastic Surgery 1987; Hand Surgery 1990; **Med School:** Baylor Coll Med 1979; **Resid:** Plastic Surgery, Univ Mich Hosp 1985; Plastic Surgery, Radcliffe Infirm/Oxford 1983; **Fellow:** Hand Surgery, Mass Genl Hosp-Harvard 1987; **Fac Appt:** Prof PlS, Univ Tex SW, Dallas

Schusterman, Mark A MD [PlS] - **Spec Exp:** Breast Reconstruction; Cancer Reconstruction; Cosmetic Surgery-Face & Breast; **Hospital:** St Luke's Episcopal Hosp - Houston, Park Plaza Hosp; **Address:** 6624 Fannin St, Ste 1420, Houston, TX 77030; **Phone:** 713-794-0368; **Board Cert:** Plastic Surgery 1989; **Med School:** Univ Louisville Sch Med 1980; **Resid:** Surgery, Univ Hosp 1985; Pediatric Surgery, Univ Pittsburgh Med Ctr 1987; **Fellow:** Microsurgery, Univ Pittsburgh Med Ctr 1988; **Fac Appt:** Clin Prof PlS, Baylor Coll Med

Stal, Samuel MD [PlS] - **Spec Exp:** Pediatric Plastic Surgery; Craniofacial Surgery; Cleft Palate/Lip; Maxillofacial Surgery; **Hospital:** Texas Chldns Hosp - Houston; **Address:** Texas Children's Hosp, 6621 Fannin St, MC CCC 620.10, Houston, TX 77030; **Phone:** 832-822-3180; **Board Cert:** Otolaryngology 1981; Plastic Surgery 1982; **Med School:** Loyola Univ-Stritch Sch Med 1974; **Resid:** Otolaryngology, Univ Chicago Hosps 1979; Plastic Surgery, Baylor College Med 1981; **Fellow:** Craniofacial Surgery, Enfant Malade Hosp 1982; **Fac Appt:** Prof Oto, Baylor Coll Med

Tebbetts, John B MD [PlS] - **Spec Exp:** Breast Augmentation; Rhinoplasty; Liposuction; **Hospital:** Mary Shiels Hosp, Baylor Univ Medical Ctr; **Address:** 2801 Lemmon Ave W, Ste 300, Dallas, TX 75204-2398; **Phone:** 214-220-2712; **Board Cert:** Surgery 1978; Plastic Surgery 1980; **Med School:** Univ Tex Med Br, Galveston 1972; **Resid:** Surgery, Univ Utah Med Ctr 1977; Plastic Surgery, Dallas Co Hospital-Parkland Meml Hosp 1979; **Fac Appt:** Asst Clin Prof PlS, Univ Tex SW, Dallas

Yuen, James C MD [PlS] - **Spec Exp:** Hand Reconstruction; Breast Reconstruction; Head & Neck Cancer Reconstruction; Chest Wall Reconstruction; **Hospital:** UAMS Med Ctr; **Address:** Univ Aransas for Med Scis, Plastic Surgery, 4301 W Markham, Ste 720, Little Rock, AR 72212; **Phone:** 501-686-8711; **Board Cert:** Surgery 1991; Plastic Surgery 1995; **Med School:** Med Coll VA 1985; **Resid:** Surgery, W Virginia Med Ctr 1990; Plastic Reconstructive Surgery, Duke Univ Med Ctr 1993; **Fellow:** Hand & Microvascular Surgery, Kleinert Inst of Hand & Microsurgery 1991; **Fac Appt:** Assoc Prof S, Univ Ark

West Coast and Pacific

Alter, Gary J MD [PlS] - **Spec Exp:** Genitourinary Reconstruction; Gender Reassignment Surgery; **Hospital:** Cedars-Sinai Med Ctr, UCLA Med Ctr; **Address:** 416 N Bedford Drive, Ste 400, Beverly Hills, CA 90210-4318; **Phone:** 310-275-5566; **Board Cert:** Plastic Surgery 1997; Urology 1981; **Med School:** UCLA 1973; **Resid:** Urology, Baylor Med Ctr 1979; Plastic Surgery, Mayo Clinic 1992; **Fellow:** Genitourinary Surgery, Eastern Va Med Sch 1992; **Fac Appt:** Clin Prof PlS, UCLA

Andersen, James S MD [PlS] - **Spec Exp:** Cancer Reconstruction; Breast Reconstruction; Head & Neck Reconstruction; **Hospital:** City of Hope Natl Med Ctr & Beckman Rsch; **Address:** City of Hope National Cancer Ctr, Div Plastic Surgery, 1500 E Duarte Rd, Duarte, CA 91010; **Phone:** 626-301-8278; **Board Cert:** Plastic Surgery 1994; **Med School:** Jefferson Med Coll 1983; **Resid:** Surgery, Hosp U Penn 1989; Plastic Surgery, Hosp U Penn 1991; **Fellow:** Microsurgery, USC Med Ctr 1992; **Fac Appt:** Assoc Clin Prof S, USC Sch Med

Brent, Burton D MD [PlS] - **Spec Exp:** Ear Reconstruction/Microtia; **Hospital:** El Camino Hosp/Camino Hlthcare Sys; **Address:** 2995 Woodside Rd, Ste 300, Woodside, CA 94062-2401; **Phone:** 650-851-5300; **Board Cert:** Plastic Surgery 1974; **Med School:** Ros Franklin Univ/Chicago Med Sch 1963; **Resid:** Surgery, University Hosp 1970; Plastic Surgery, Loyola Univ Med Ctr 1973; **Fellow:** Plastic Surgery, Canniesburn Hosp; **Fac Appt:** Assoc Clin Prof PlS, Stanford Univ

Brink, Robert Ross MD [PlS] - **Spec Exp:** Cosmetic Surgery; **Hospital:** Mills - Peninsula Hlth Svcs; **Address:** 66 Bovet Rd, Ste 101, San Mateo, CA 94402-3126; **Phone:** 650-570-6066; **Board Cert:** Plastic Surgery 1980; **Med School:** Univ Mich Med Sch 1970; **Resid:** Surgery, UC Davis Med Ctr 1977; Plastic Surgery, UCSF Med Ctr 1979

Carstens, Michael H MD [PlS] - **Spec Exp:** Pediatric Plastic Surgery; Cleft Palate/Lip; Vascular Birthmarks; Ear Reconstruction/Microtia; **Hospital:** Cardinal Glennon Mem Children's Hosp; **Address:** 3635 Vista Ave Fl 3, Plastic Surgery, St Louis, CA 63110; **Phone:** 314-268-4010; **Board Cert:** Plastic Surgery 1996; **Med School:** Stanford Univ 1981; **Resid:** Surgery, Boston Univ Med Ctr 1987; **Fellow:** Plastic Reconstructive Surgery, Univ Pittsburgh 1989; Craniofacial Surgery, Univ Pittsburgh 1990; **Fac Appt:** Prof PlS, Univ MO-Columbia Sch Med

Cohen, Steven R MD [PlS] - **Spec Exp:** Craniofacial Surgery-Pediatric; Craniofacial Surgery/Reconstruction; **Hospital:** Rady Children's Hosp - San Diego, UCSD Med Ctr; **Address:** 8899 Univ Center Ln, Ste 350, San Diego, CA 92122; **Phone:** 858-453-7224; **Board Cert:** Plastic Surgery 1992; **Med School:** Geo Wash Univ 1980; **Resid:** Surgery, Columbia-Presby Med Ctr 1982; Surgery, Dartmouth-Hitchcock Med Ctr 1987; **Fellow:** Plastic Surgery, Hosp Univ Penn 1989; Craniofacial Surgery, UCLA Med Ctr 1990

Daniel, Rollin K MD [PlS] - **Spec Exp:** Cosmetic Surgery-Face; Rhinoplasty; **Hospital:** Hoag Meml Hosp Presby; **Address:** 1441 Avocado Ave, Ste 308, Newport Beach, CA 92660; **Phone:** 949-721-0494; **Board Cert:** Plastic Surgery 1977; **Med School:** Columbia P&S 1972; **Resid:** Plastic Surgery, McGill Univ Affil Hosps 1975; Hand Surgery, Univ Louisville Hosp 1976; **Fellow:** Craniofacial Surgery, Toronto Genl Hosp

Fisher, Garth MD [PlS] - **Spec Exp:** Cosmetic Surgery-Face; Cosmetic Surgery-Breast; Rhinoplasty; **Hospital:** St John's Hlth Ctr, Santa Monica; **Address:** 120 S Spalding Drive, Ste 222, Beverly Hills, CA 90212; **Phone:** 310-273-5995; **Board Cert:** Plastic Surgery 1993; **Med School:** Univ Miss 1984; **Resid:** Surgery, UC Irvine Medical Ctr 1989; Plastic Surgery, UC Irvine Medical Ctr 1991

Flowers, Robert MD [PlS] - **Spec Exp:** Coronal Canthopexy; **Hospital:** Queen's Med Ctr - Honolulu; **Address:** 677 Ala Moana Blvd, Ste 1011, Honolulu, HI 96813; **Phone:** 808-521-1999; **Board Cert:** Plastic Surgery 1971; **Med School:** Univ Ala 1960; **Resid:** Surgery, Cleveland Clinic 1966; Plastic Surgery, Cleveland Clinic 1968; **Fac Appt:** Asst Clin Prof S, Univ Hawaii JA Burns Sch Med

Fodor, Peter B MD [PlS] - **Spec Exp:** Cosmetic Surgery; Liposuction & Body Contouring; **Hospital:** Olympia Med Ctr, Century City Hosp; **Address:** 2080 Century Park E, Ste 710, Century City, CA 90067; **Phone:** 310-203-9818; **Board Cert:** Plastic Surgery 1977; **Med School:** Univ Wisc 1966; **Resid:** Surgery, Columbia-Presby Med Ctr 1968; Plastic Surgery, St Luke's Hosp 1976; **Fac Appt:** Assoc Clin Prof S, UCLA

Garner, Warren L MD [PlS] - **Spec Exp:** Burns-Reconstructive Plastic Surgery; Wound Healing/Care; Skin Healing; **Hospital:** LAC & USC Med Ctr, USC Univ Hosp - R K Eamer Med Plz; **Address:** 1450 San Pablo St, Ste 2000, Los Angeles, CA 90033; **Phone:** 323-442-6470; **Board Cert:** Surgical Critical Care 2001; Plastic Surgery 1991; **Med School:** Univ Kans 1978; **Resid:** Surgery, Ohio State Univ Hosp 1985; Plastic Surgery, Wash Univ Hosp 1989; **Fellow:** Critical Care Medicine, Ohio State Univ Hosp 1986; **Fac Appt:** Assoc Prof S, USC Sch Med

Gruss, Joseph MD [PlS] - **Spec Exp:** Maxillofacial & Craniofacial Surgery; Facial Trauma/Fractures; Cleft Palate/Lip; Pediatric Plastic Surgery; **Hospital:** Chldns Hosp and Regl Med Ctr - Seattle, Harborview Med Ctr; **Address:** Childrens Hosp & Regional Med Ctr, 4800 Sand Point Way NE, Box 5371, Seattle, WA 98105-3901; **Phone:** 206-987-2039; **Med School:** South Africa 1969; **Resid:** Plastic Surgery, Toronto Western Hosp 1976; Plastic Surgery, Hosp for Sick Children 1976; **Fellow:** Surgical Oncology, Princess Margaret Hosp 1977; Head and Neck Surgery, Princess Margaret Hosp 1977; **Fac Appt:** Prof PlS, Univ Wash

Hardesty, Robert MD [PlS] - **Spec Exp:** Cosmetic Surgery-Face & Body; Cosmetic & Reconstructive Surgery; Body Contouring; Cosmetic Surgery-Breast; **Hospital:** Riverside Comm Hosp, Loma Linda Univ Med Ctr; **Address:** 4646 Brockton Ave, Ste 302, Riverside, CA 92506; **Phone:** 951-686-7600; **Board Cert:** Surgery 1984; Plastic Surgery 1989; **Med School:** Loma Linda Univ 1978; **Resid:** Surgery, Loma Linda Univ Med Ctr 1983; Plastic Surgery, Univ Pittsburgh 1986; **Fellow:** Pediatric Plastic Surgery, Washington Univ Chldns Hosp 1987; **Fac Appt:** Clin Prof PlS, Loma Linda Univ

Hoefflin, Steven M MD [PlS] - **Spec Exp:** Cosmetic Surgery-Face; Reconstructive Surgery; **Hospital:** St John's Hlth Ctr, Santa Monica; **Address:** 1530 Arizona Ave, Santa Monica, CA 90404-1234; **Phone:** 310-451-4733; **Board Cert:** Plastic Surgery 1978; **Med School:** UCLA 1972; **Resid:** Surgery, UCLA Med Ctr 1974; Plastic Surgery, UCLA Med Ctr 1977; **Fac Appt:** Assoc Clin Prof PlS, UCLA

Horowitz, Jed H MD [PlS] - **Spec Exp:** Cosmetic Surgery-Breast; Cosmetic Surgery-Face; **Hospital:** Hoag Meml Hosp Presby, Orange Coast Memorial Med Ctr; **Address:** 7677 Center Ave, Ste 401, Huntington Beach, CA 92647-3098; **Phone:** 714-902-1100; **Board Cert:** Plastic Surgery 1986; **Med School:** SUNY Buffalo 1977; **Resid:** Surgery, Grady Meml Hosp/Emory Univ 1983; **Fellow:** Plastic Surgery, Univ Virginia 1985; **Fac Appt:** Asst Clin Prof PlS, USC Sch Med

Jewell, Mark L MD [PlS] - **Spec Exp:** Liposuction & Body Contouring; Cosmetic Surgery-Face; Breast Reconstruction; Cosmetic Surgery-Breast; **Address:** 630 E 13th Ave, Eugene, OR 97401; **Phone:** 541-683-3234; **Board Cert:** Plastic Surgery 1981; **Med School:** Univ Kans 1973; **Resid:** Surgery, LAC-Harbor Med Ctr 1976; Plastic Surgery, Erlanger Hosp 1979; **Fellow:** Burn Surgery, LAC-USC Med Ctr 1977; **Fac Appt:** Asst Clin Prof PlS, Oregon Hlth Sci Univ

Kawamoto Jr, Henry K MD [PlS] - **Spec Exp:** Cosmetic Surgery; Craniofacial Surgery; Maxillofacial Surgery; **Hospital:** UCLA Med Ctr, St John's Hlth Ctr, Santa Monica; **Address:** 1301 20th St, Ste 460, Santa Monica, CA 90404; **Phone:** 310-829-0391; **Board Cert:** Surgery 1972; Plastic Surgery 1976; **Med School:** USC Sch Med 1964; **Resid:** Surgery, Columbia-Presby Med Ctr 1971; Plastic Surgery, NYU Med Ctr 1973; **Fellow:** Craniofacial Surgery, Dr Paul Tessier 1974; **Fac Appt:** Clin Prof PlS, UCLA

Plastic Surgery

Koplin, Lawrence M MD [PlS] - **Spec Exp:** Cosmetic Surgery-Face; **Hospital:** Cedars-Sinai Med Ctr; **Address:** 465 N Roxbury Drive, Ste 800, Beverly Hills, CA 90210; **Phone:** 310-277-3223; **Board Cert:** Plastic Surgery 1985; **Med School:** Baylor Coll Med 1976; **Resid:** Surgery, Kaiser Fdn Hosp 1981; Plastic Surgery, St Joseph Hosp 1983

Leaf, Norman MD [PlS] - **Spec Exp:** Cosmetic Surgery-Face; Cosmetic Surgery-Breast; **Hospital:** Cedars-Sinai Med Ctr, UCLA Med Ctr; **Address:** 436 N Bedford, Ste 103, Beverly Hills, CA 90210-4310; **Phone:** 310-274-8001; **Board Cert:** Surgery 1973; Plastic Surgery 1974; **Med School:** Univ Chicago-Pritzker Sch Med 1966; **Resid:** Surgery, Univ Chicago Hosps 1972; Plastic Surgery, Univ Chicago Hosps 1973; **Fellow:** Research, Univ Chicago Hosp-US Pub Hlth Svc-NIH 1969; **Fac Appt:** Asst Clin Prof PlS, UCLA

Lesavoy, Malcolm A MD [PlS] - **Spec Exp:** Reconstructive Surgery; Cosmetic Surgery; Hand Surgery; **Hospital:** UCLA Med Ctr; **Address:** 16311 Ventura Blvd, Ste 550, Encino, CA 91436-4314; **Phone:** 818-986-8270; **Board Cert:** Plastic Surgery 1977; **Med School:** Ros Franklin Univ/Chicago Med Sch 1969; **Resid:** Surgery, Univ Chicago Hosps 1974; Plastic Surgery, Univ Miami Hosp/Clinics 1976; **Fac Appt:** Clin Prof PlS, UCLA

Markowitz, Bernard Lloyd MD [PlS] - **Spec Exp:** Cosmetic Surgery-Face; Craniofacial Surgery/Reconstruction; **Hospital:** UCLA Med Ctr, Cedars-Sinai Med Ctr; **Address:** 9675 Brighton Way, Ste 350, Beverly Hills, CA 90210; **Phone:** 310-205-5557; **Board Cert:** Plastic Surgery 1989; **Med School:** NYU Sch Med 1979; **Resid:** Surgery, NYU Med Ctr 1984; Plastic Surgery, NYU Med Ctr 1986; **Fellow:** Maxillofacial Surgery, Johns Hopkins Hosp 1987; Microvascular Surgery, Johns Hopkins Hosp 1987; **Fac Appt:** Clin Prof PlS, UCLA

Marten, Timothy James MD [PlS] - **Spec Exp:** Cosmetic Surgery-Face; Facial Rejuvenation; **Hospital:** CA Pacific Med Ctr, St Mary's Med Ctr - San Fran; **Address:** Marten Clinic of Plastic Surgery, 450 Sutter St, Ste 2222, San Francisco, CA 94108-4207; **Phone:** 415-677-9937; **Board Cert:** Plastic Surgery 1993; **Med School:** UC Davis 1982; **Resid:** Surgery, Kaiser Fdn Hosp 1987; Plastic Surgery, Univ Illinois Chicago Hosp 1989; **Fellow:** Cosmetic Plastic Surgery, Connell Aesthetic Network 1990; Cosmetic Plastic Surgery, Baker, Gordon, & Stuzin

Miller, Timothy A MD [PlS] - **Spec Exp:** Cosmetic Surgery-Face; Eyelid Cancer & Reconstruction; Skin Cancer; Nasal Reconstruction; **Hospital:** UCLA Med Ctr; **Address:** UCLA Med Ctr, Div Plastic Surg, 200 UCLA Med Plaza, Ste 465, Los Angeles, CA 90095-8344; **Phone:** 310-825-5644; **Board Cert:** Surgery 1971; Plastic Surgery 1973; **Med School:** UCLA 1963; **Resid:** Surgery, Johns Hopkins Hosp; Thoracic Surgery, UCLA Med Ctr 1969; **Fellow:** Plastic Surgery, Univ Pittsburgh 1971; **Fac Appt:** Prof S, UCLA

Nichter, Larry S MD [PlS] - **Spec Exp:** Breast Reconstruction & Augmentation; Cosmetic Surgery-Face; Liposuction & Body Contouring; Hand Surgery; **Hospital:** Hoag Meml Hosp Presby, Orange Coast Memorial Med Ctr; **Address:** 7677 Center Ave, Ste 401, Huntingdon Beach, CA 92647-3098; **Phone:** 714-902-1100; **Board Cert:** Plastic Surgery 1986; **Med School:** Boston Univ 1978; **Resid:** Surgery, UCLA Medical Ctr 1982; Plastic Surgery, Univ Virginia Med Ctr 1985; **Fellow:** Hand & Microvascular Surgery, Univ Virginia 1983; Craniofacial Surgery, Univ Virginia 1985; **Fac Appt:** Clin Prof PlS, Univ SC Sch Med

Paul, Malcolm D MD [PlS] - **Spec Exp:** Cosmetic Surgery-Face; Cosmetic Surgery-Breast; Liposuction & Body Contouring; **Hospital:** Hoag Meml Hosp Presby; **Address:** 1401 Avocado Ave, Ste 810, Newport Beach, CA 92660-8708; **Phone:** 949-760-5047; **Board Cert:** Plastic Surgery 1976; **Med School:** Univ MD Sch Med 1969; **Resid:** Surgery, Geo Wash Med Ctr 1973; Plastic Surgery, Geo Wash Med Ctr 1975; **Fac Appt:** Clin Prof S, UC Irvine

Rand, Richard Pierce MD [PlS] - **Spec Exp:** Cosmetic Surgery-Face; Cosmetic Surgery-Breast; Abdominoplasty; **Hospital:** Overlake Hosp Med Ctr; **Address:** 1135 116th Ave NE, Ste 630, Bellevue, WA 98004-4623; **Phone:** 425-688-8828; **Board Cert:** Surgery 1998; Plastic Surgery 1991; **Med School:** Univ Mich Med Sch 1981; **Resid:** Surgery, Tufts-New England Med Ctr 1986; Plastic Surgery, Emory Univ Hosp 1989; **Fellow:** Craniofacial Surgery, Univ Miami 1989; **Fac Appt:** Assoc Prof S, Univ Wash

Reinisch, John F MD [PlS] - **Spec Exp:** Ear Reconstruction/Mocrotia; Cleft Palate/Lip; Craniofacial Surgery/Reconstruction; **Hospital:** Chldns Hosp - Los Angeles (page 56); **Address:** 4650 Sunset Blvd, MS 96, Los Angeles, CA 90027; **Phone:** 323-669-4544; **Board Cert:** Plastic Surgery 1980; **Med School:** Harvard Med Sch 1970; **Resid:** Surgery, Univ Mich Med Ctr 1975; Plastic Surgery, Univ Virginia Hosp 1978; **Fac Appt:** Prof S, USC Sch Med

Ristow, Brunno MD [PlS] - **Spec Exp:** Cosmetic Surgery-Face; Facial Plastic & Reconstructive Surgery; Rhinoplasty; Nasal Reconstruction; **Hospital:** CA Pacific Med Ctr - Pacific Campus; **Address:** 2100 Webster St, Ste 501, San Francisco, CA 94115-2381; **Phone:** 415-202-1507; **Board Cert:** Plastic Surgery 1975; **Med School:** Brazil 1966; **Resid:** Surgery, NY Hosp-Cornell Med Ctr 1971; Plastic Surgery, NYU Med Ctr 1973; **Fellow:** Plastic Surgery, NYU Med Ctr 1968

Romano, James John MD [PlS] - **Spec Exp:** Cosmetic Surgery; Cosmetic Surgery-Breast; Rhinoplasty; **Hospital:** Seton Med Ctr, CA Pacific Med Ctr - CA Campus; **Address:** 126 Post St, Ste 618, San Francisco, CA 94108; **Phone:** 415-981-3911; **Board Cert:** Plastic Surgery 1990; **Med School:** Eastern VA Med Sch 1980; **Resid:** Surgery, Georgetown Univ Hosp 1985; Plastic Surgery, Johns Hopkins Hosp 1988; **Fac Appt:** Asst Prof PlS, USC Sch Med

Rosenberg, Howard L MD [PlS] - **Spec Exp:** Cosmetic Surgery-Breast; Cosmetic Surgery-Face; Liposuction; **Hospital:** El Camino Hosp/Camino Hlthcare Sys; **Address:** 2204 Grant Rd, Ste 201, Mountain View, CA 94040; **Phone:** 650-961-2652; **Board Cert:** Surgery 1975; Plastic Surgery 1977; **Med School:** Johns Hopkins Univ 1969; **Resid:** Surgery, UCLA Med Ctr 1974; Plastic Surgery, Stanford Univ Med Ctr 1976; **Fac Appt:** Asst Clin Prof PlS, Stanford Univ

Sherman, Randolph MD [PlS] - **Spec Exp:** Facial Paralysis; Breast Reconstruction; Limb Surgery/Reconstruction; **Hospital:** USC Univ Hosp - R K Eamer Med Plz, Cedars-Sinai Med Ctr; **Address:** 1450 San Pablo St, Ste 2000, Los Angeles, CA 90033; **Phone:** 323-442-6482; **Board Cert:** Surgery 2004; Plastic Surgery 1986; Hand Surgery 2000; **Med School:** Univ MO-Columbia Sch Med 1977; **Resid:** Surgery, UCSF Hosps 1981; Surgery, State Univ of New York 1983; **Fellow:** Plastic Surgery, USC Med Ctr 1985; **Fac Appt:** Prof S, USC Sch Med

Singer, Robert MD [PlS] - **Spec Exp:** Cosmetic Surgery-Face; Cosmetic Surgery-Breast; Liposuction & Body Contouring; **Hospital:** Scripps Meml Hosp - La Jolla; **Address:** 9834 Genesee Ave, Ste 100, La Jolla, CA 92037-1214; **Phone:** 858-455-0290; **Board Cert:** Plastic Surgery 1977; **Med School:** SUNY Buffalo 1967; **Resid:** Surgery, Stanford Med Ctr 1969; Plastic Surgery, Vanderbilt Univ Hosp 1976; **Fellow:** Neurological Surgery, Rigs Hosp-Kommunes Hosp 1976

Stevenson, Thomas R MD [PlS] - **Spec Exp:** Breast Reconstruction; Cosmetic Surgery-Face; Cosmetic Surgery-Breast; **Hospital:** UC Davis Med Ctr, Sutter Gen Hosp; **Address:** 3301 C St, Ste 1100, Sacramento, CA 95816; **Phone:** 916-734-4323; **Board Cert:** Plastic Surgery 1983; Hand Surgery 1994; Surgery 2003; **Med School:** Univ Kans 1972; **Resid:** Surgery, Univ Virginia Hosp 1978; Plastic Surgery, Emory Univ Hosp 1982; **Fac Appt:** Prof PlS, UC Davis

Wells, James H MD [PlS] - **Spec Exp:** Cleft Palate/Lip; Breast Surgery; **Hospital:** Long Beach Meml Med Ctr; **Address:** 2880 Atlantic Ave, Ste 290, Long Beach, CA 90806; **Phone:** 562-595-6543; **Board Cert:** Plastic Surgery 1978; **Med School:** Univ Tex Med Br, Galveston 1966; **Resid:** Surgery, Ochsner Fdn Hosp 1971; Plastic Surgery, Univ Virginia Hosp 1975

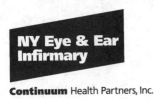

Continuum Health Partners, Inc.

THE NEW YORK EYE AND EAR INFIRMARY

310 East 14th Street
New York, New York 10003
Tel. 212.979.4000   Fax. 212.228.0664
http://www.nyee.edu

PROVIDING EXCEPTIONAL CARE

The Department of Plastic & Reconstructive Surgery is one of the region's most comprehensive centers for surgery which restores the body and spirit. More than 1,500 procedures a year are performed here, and 50 of the most noted board-certified plastic surgeons located throughout New York City and tri-state area comprise the attending medical staff.

IN A HIGHLY SPECIALIZED SETTING

As a specialty hospital, the Infirmary is uniquely qualified to handle the most complicated cases. It serves as a nationwide referral center with a commitment to teaching, research, and high-technology based patient care. Highly experienced staff using state-of-the-art instrumentation have made the Infirmary's 17 operating rooms a national benchmark in efficiency. In addition, private premium patient accommodations are available to assure that the hospital experience is as comfortable and convenient as possible.

FOR PATIENTS OF ALL AGES

Clinical innovations are improving people's lives. A unique procedure to transfer tissue is performed by microvascular surgeons to repair or reattach missing digits and thumbs. Infirmary surgeons perform miracles on children born with cleft lip and palate malformation. Those seeking elective cosmetic surgery are offered an array of options including endoscopic face lifts, a refinement of the facial plastic operation that uses straw-like telescopic instrument inserted through small incisions to smooth wrinkles from "beneath" the skin; no-incision eyelid plasty; and liposuction for reshaping body contours.

**Plastic Surgery
Clinical Services**

Facial plasty

Eyelid plastic operations

Nasal plastic operations

Breast augmentation
Breast reduction procedures
and suspension

Liposuction

Abdominoplasty

Facial resurfacing and
dermabrasion

Botox

**About
The New York Eye
and Ear Infirmary**

Founded in 1820, it is the nation's oldest, continuously operating specialty hospital Throughout its history, the Infirmary has led clinical advances and research in vision, hearing, speech and restoration of the physical appearance.

**Physician Referral
1.800.449.HOPE (4673)**

Preventive & Occupational Medicine

A preventive medicine specialist focuses on the health of individuals and defined populations in order to protect, promote and maintain health and well-being, and to prevent disease, disability and premature death. A preventive medicine physician may be a specialist in general preventive medicine, public health, occupational medicine, or aerospace medicine. This specialist works with large population groups as well as with individual patients to promote health and understand the risks of disease, injury, disability, and death, seeking to modify and eliminate these risks.

Training Required: Three years

Occupational Medicine

New England

Cullen, Mark R MD [OM] - **Spec Exp:** Mesothelioma; **Hospital:** Yale - New Haven Hosp; **Address:** 135 College St, Ste 392, New Haven, CT 06510; **Phone:** 203-785-6434; **Board Cert:** Internal Medicine 1979; Occupational Medicine 1986; **Med School:** Yale Univ 1976; **Resid:** Internal Medicine, Yale-New Haven Hosp 1980; **Fac Appt:** Prof Med, Yale Univ

Mid Atlantic

Brandt-Rauf, Paul W MD [OM] - **Spec Exp:** Occupational Medicine; Environmental Medicine; **Address:** Columbia Univ Sch Public Hlth, Dept Env Hlth Sci, 60 Haven Ave, Ste B1 - rm 106, New York, NY 10032-2604; **Phone:** 212-305-3464; **Board Cert:** Internal Medicine 1984; Occupational Medicine 1986; **Med School:** Columbia P&S 1979; **Resid:** Pathology, Columbia Presby Hosp 1981; Internal Medicine, Georgetown Univ Hosp 1983; **Fellow:** Occupational Medicine, Columbia Presby Hosp 1984; **Fac Appt:** Prof OM, Columbia P&S

Gochfeld, Michael MD/PhD [OM] - **Spec Exp:** Environmental Medicine; Chemical Exposure; Mercury Toxic Exposure; **Hospital:** Robert Wood Johnson Univ Hosp - New Brunswick; **Address:** Enviro & Occupational Health - EOHSI, 170 Frelinghuysen Rd, Ste 200, Piscataway, NJ 08854; **Phone:** 732-445-0123 x627; **Board Cert:** Occupational Medicine 1983; **Med School:** Albert Einstein Coll Med 1965; **Resid:** Behavioral Medicine, Rockefeller Univ 1977; **Fac Appt:** Prof OM, UMDNJ-RW Johnson Med Sch

Landrigan, Philip MD [OM] - **Spec Exp:** Environmental Health in Children; **Hospital:** Mount Sinai Med Ctr; **Address:** Dept of Comm & Prev Med, One Gustave Levy Pl, Box 1057, New York, NY 10029-6500; **Phone:** 212-241-6173; **Board Cert:** Pediatrics 1973; Public Health & Genl Preventive Med 1979; Occupational Medicine 1983; **Med School:** Harvard Med Sch 1967; **Resid:** Internal Medicine, Metro Genl Hosp 1968; Pediatrics, Chldns Hosp 1970; **Fellow:** Epidemiology, Ctrs for Disease Control 1973; Occupational Medicine, Univ London 1977; **Fac Appt:** Prof Ped, Mount Sinai Sch Med

West Coast and Pacific

Harber, Philip I MD [OM] - **Spec Exp:** Occupational Medicine; Environmental Medicine; **Hospital:** UCLA Med Ctr; **Address:** UCLA Med Ctr, Dept Occupational Med, 10880 Wilshire Blvd, Ste 1800, Los Angeles, CA 90024; **Phone:** 310-794-8144; **Board Cert:** Internal Medicine 1979; Pulmonary Disease 1980; Occupational Medicine 1982; **Med School:** Univ Pennsylvania 1972; **Resid:** Internal Medicine, Georgetown Univ Med Ctr 1978; Occupational Medicine, Johns Hopkins Hosp 1980; **Fellow:** Pulmonary Disease, Johns Hopkins Hosp 1980; **Fac Appt:** Assoc Prof Med, UCLA

Preventive Medicine

Mid Atlantic

Cahill, John MD [PrM] - **Spec Exp:** Tropical Diseases; International Health; Disaster Relief Medicine; **Hospital:** St Luke's - Roosevelt Hosp Ctr - Roosevelt Div, St Luke's - Roosevelt Hosp Ctr - St Luke's Hosp; **Address:** 425 W 59th St, Ste 8A, New York, NY 10019; **Phone:** 212-492-5500; **Board Cert:** Emergency Medicine 2001; **Med School:** Mount Sinai Sch Med 1996; **Resid:** Emergency Medicine, Rhode Island Hosp 1997; Emergency Medicine, Rhode Island Hosp 2000; **Fellow:** Tropical Medicine, Royal Coll Surgeons 1998; **Fac Appt:** Asst Clin Prof Med, Columbia P&S

Hoffman, Robert S MD [PrM] - **Spec Exp:** Poison Control; Bioterrorism Preparedness; **Hospital:** NYU Med Ctr (page 67), Bellevue Hosp Ctr; **Address:** NY Poison Control Ctr, 455 1st Ave, rm 123, New York, NY 10016; **Phone:** 212-340-4494; **Board Cert:** Internal Medicine 1987; Emergency Medicine 2005; Medical Toxicology 1999; **Med School:** NYU Sch Med 1984; **Resid:** Internal Medicine, NYU Med Ctr 1987; **Fellow:** Medical Toxicology, NYU Med Ctr 1989; **Fac Appt:** Asst Clin Prof EM, NYU Sch Med

Lane, Dorothy S MD [PrM] - **Spec Exp:** Women's Health; Cancer Prevention; Health Promotion & Disease Prevention; **Hospital:** Stony Brook Univ Med Ctr; **Address:** Stony Brook Univ Sch Med, HSC L2, rm 142, Stony Brook, NY 11794-8437; **Phone:** 631-444-2094; **Board Cert:** Public Health & Genl Preventive Med 1970; Family Medicine 2000; **Med School:** Columbia P&S 1965; **Resid:** Public Health & Genl Preventive Med, NY Health Dept 1968; **Fac Appt:** Prof PrM, SUNY Stony Brook

Pearson, Thomas A MD/PhD [PrM] - **Spec Exp:** Preventive Cardiology; Cholesterol/Lipid Disorders; **Hospital:** Univ of Rochester Strong Meml Hosp; **Address:** Cardiac Rehabilitation, 2400 S Clinton Ave H Bldg - Ste 130, Rochester, NY 14618; **Phone:** 585-341-7100; **Board Cert:** Internal Medicine 1983; Preventive Medicine 1986; **Med School:** Johns Hopkins Univ 1976; **Resid:** Preventive Medicine, Johns Hopkins Hosp 1979; Internal Medicine, Johns Hopkins Hosp 1980; **Fellow:** Cardiovascular Disease, Johns Hopkins Hosp 1983; **Fac Appt:** Prof PrM, Univ Rochester

Weiss, Stanley H MD [PrM] - **Spec Exp:** Cancer Epidemiology & Control; AIDS Related Infections; Bioterrorism Preparedness; Infections in Cancer Patients; **Hospital:** UMDNJ-Univ Hosp-Newark; **Address:** NJ Medical School, 30 Bergen St, ADMC, Ste 1614, Newark, NJ 07107-3000; **Phone:** 973-972-7716; **Board Cert:** Internal Medicine 1981; Medical Oncology 1985; **Med School:** Harvard Med Sch 1978; **Resid:** Internal Medicine, Montefiore Med Ctr 1981; **Fellow:** Medical Oncology, National Cancer Inst 1985; Epidemiology, National Cancer Inst 1987; **Fac Appt:** Prof PrM, UMDNJ-NJ Med Sch, Newark

Southeast

Frank, Erica MD [PrM] - **Spec Exp:** Women Physicians; Physicians' Health; Cholesterol/Lipid Disorders; **Hospital:** Emory Univ Hosp; **Address:** Emory Univ, Dept Fam/ Preventive Medicine, 1365 Clifton Rd NE, Atlanta, GA 30322; **Phone:** 404-616-5603; **Board Cert:** Public Health & Genl Preventive Med 1992; **Med School:** Mercer Univ Sch Med 1988; **Resid:** Preventive Medicine, Yale-New Haven Medical Ctr 1990; **Fellow:** Research, Stanford Medical Ctr 1993; **Fac Appt:** Assoc Prof PrM, Emory Univ

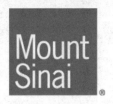

THE MOUNT SINAI MEDICAL CENTER
OCCUPATIONAL AND ENVIRONMENTAL MEDICINE

One Gustave L. Levy Place (Fifth Avenue and 100th Street)
New York, NY 10029-6574
Physician Referral: 1-800-MD-SINAI (637-4624)
www.mountsinai.org

A REPUTATION FOR EXCELLENCE

The Irving J. Selikoff Clinical Center for Occupational and Environmental Medicine is an internationally respected diagnostic and treatment center. The mission of the Center is to prevent occupational disease in the workplace and reduce morbidity and mortality associated with work. To achieve this goal, we utilize a preventive medicine model that includes three integrated components:

• *Clinical Care* – These services include the diagnosis, treatment, and management of occupational diseases and work-related musculoskeletal disorders for current and retired workers. We offer disability assessment and rehabilitation services to facilitate safe return to work and appropriate accommodations. Our social work services include counseling regarding the financial, social, and psychological aspects of occupational disease.

• *Disease Prevention Services* – These services include educating patients, health care providers, workers, unions, employers, and communities on the signs and symptoms of occupational disease. Comprehensive industrial hygiene and ergonomic services are available to evaluate exposures and recommend effective preventive measures. Technical assistance and consultation services are provided for employers, unions, and public health agencies.

• *Surveillance* and *Data Management* – We study the pattern and prevalence of occupational disease and identify new associations between workplace exposure and disease.

To promote disease prevention, the Center treats each newly identified case of occupational disease as a potential sentinel health event, that is, as a signal that there may be other similar cases of disease in the patient's co-workers. This approach, coupled with our efforts to reduce workplace hazards, places the Center's impact well beyond individual patient evaluations. To help achieve our goal of improving public health by preventing occupational and environmental disease, we work closely with labor unions, employers, government and service organizations, health care providers, and community organizations.

The Clinical Center has satellite sites in Westchester County and Queens, where staff physicians see patients several days a week. Some of the services available at the Irving J. Selikoff Center for Occupational and Environmental Medicine include:

• Assistance in evaluating specific workplace environments and suggesting ways of eliminating dangerous conditions
• Educational programs for employers, government agencies, unions, and workers on workplace health issues
• Aid in getting worker compensation and other available legal benefits
• Social work services to help with the social, psychological, and financial problems caused by work-related health problems
• Epidemiologic services

Pediatric Environmental Health Specialty Unit
We provide consultation and medical care for children with toxic environmental exposures and with diseases of suspected environmental origin. This unit serves New York, New Jersey, Puerto Rico, and the Virgin Islands.

World Trade Center Medical Monitoring and Treatment Program
This federally-funded program is available to workers and volunteers who participated in the rescue, recovery, and clean-up efforts following the 9/11 attacks. Services include:
• Medical evaluations for possible WTC-related health conditions
• Treatment at no cost for WTC workers covered under federally-funded program
• Mental health services
• Social work services to assist with Workers' Compensation and related benefits
• Patient education regarding WTC-related and other occupational health concerns

613

Psychiatry

A psychiatrist specializes in the prevention, diagnosis and treatment of mental, addictive and emotional disorders such as schizophrenia and other psychotic disorders, mood disorders, anxiety disorders, substance-related disorders, sexual and gender identity disorders and adjustment disorders. The psychiatrist is able to understand the biologic, psychologic and social components of illness, and therefore is uniquely prepared to treat the whole person. A psychiatrist is qualified to order diagnostic laboratory tests and to prescribe medications, evaluate and treat psychologic and interpersonal problems and to intervene with families who are coping with stress, crises and other problems in living.

Training Required: Four years

Certification in one of the following subspecialties requires additional training and examination.

Addiction Psychiatry: A psychiatrist who focuses on the evaluation and treatment of individuals with alcohol, drug, or other substance-related disorders and of individuals with the dual diagnosis of substance-related and other psychiatric disorders.

Child and Adolescent Psychiatry: A psychiatrist with additional training in the diagnosis and treatment of developmental, behavioral, emotional and mental disorders of childhood and adolescence.

Geriatric Psychiatry: A psychiatrist with expertise in the prevention, evaluation, diagnosis and treatment of mental and emotional disorders in the elderly. The geriatric psychiatrist seeks to improve the psychiatric care of the elderly both in health and in disease.

Psychiatry

New England

Baldessarini, Ross MD [Psyc] - **Spec Exp:** Bipolar/Mood Disorders; Schizophrenia; Psychotic Disorders; **Hospital:** McLean Hosp, Mass Genl Hosp; **Address:** McLean Hosp, Mailman Rsch Ctr, 115 Mill St, Belmont, MA 02478; **Phone:** 617-855-3203; **Board Cert:** Psychiatry 1972; **Med School:** Johns Hopkins Univ 1963; **Resid:** Psychiatry, Johns Hopkins Hosp 1969; **Fellow:** Psychiatry, Natl Inst Mntl Hlth 1966; **Fac Appt:** Prof Psyc, Harvard Med Sch

Block, Susan D MD [Psyc] - **Spec Exp:** Psychiatry in Cancer; **Hospital:** Dana-Farber Cancer Inst; **Address:** Dana Farber Cancer Inst, 44 Binney St, Ste SW411, Boston, MA 02115; **Phone:** 617-632-6181; **Board Cert:** Psychiatry 1984; **Med School:** Case West Res Univ 1977; **Resid:** Internal Medicine, Beth Israel Hosp 1980; Psychiatry, Beth Israel Hosp 1982; **Fac Appt:** Assoc Prof Psyc, Harvard Med Sch

Bowers Jr, Malcolm B MD [Psyc] - **Spec Exp:** Schizophrenia-Consultation; Depression-Consultation; **Hospital:** Yale - New Haven Hosp; **Address:** Yale Univ - Dept Psychiatry, 300 George St, Ste 901, New Haven, CT 06511; **Phone:** 203-785-2121; **Board Cert:** Psychiatry 1970; **Med School:** Washington Univ, St Louis 1958; **Resid:** Psychiatry, Yale-New Haven Hosp 1965; **Fellow:** Psychiatry, Yale-New Haven Hosp 1964; **Fac Appt:** Prof Psyc, Yale Univ

Cohen, Bruce M MD [Psyc] - **Spec Exp:** Psychopharmacology; **Hospital:** McLean Hosp; **Address:** 115 Mill St, Belmont, MA 02478; **Phone:** 617-855-3227; **Board Cert:** Psychiatry 1979; **Med School:** Case West Res Univ 1975; **Resid:** Psychiatry, McLean Hospital 1978; **Fac Appt:** Prof Psyc, Harvard Med Sch

Friedman, Matthew J MD/PhD [Psyc] - **Spec Exp:** Post Traumatic Stress Disorder; Psychopharmacology; Anxiety & Mood Disorders; **Hospital:** VA Aff Med Ctr - White River Junction, Dartmouth - Hitchcock Med Ctr; **Address:** National Center for PTSD, VA Medical Ctr, 215 N Main St, White River Junction, VT 05009; **Phone:** 802-296-5132; **Board Cert:** Psychiatry 1976; **Med School:** Univ KY Coll Med 1976; **Resid:** Psychiatry, Mass Genl Hosp 1972; Psychiatry, Dartmouth Hitchcock Med Ctr 1973; **Fac Appt:** Prof Psyc, Dartmouth Med Sch

Goff, Donald C MD [Psyc] - **Spec Exp:** Schizophrenia; Psychopharmacology; **Hospital:** Mass Genl Hosp; **Address:** Erich Lindemann Mental Health Ctr, Freedom Trail Clinic, 25 Staniford St, Boston, MA 02114; **Phone:** 617-912-7800; **Board Cert:** Psychiatry 1986; **Med School:** UCLA 1980; **Resid:** Psychiatry, Mass Genl Hosp 1984; **Fellow:** Psychopharmacology, Tufts New Engl Med Ctr 1985; **Fac Appt:** Assoc Prof Psyc, Harvard Med Sch

Herman, John B MD [Psyc] - **Spec Exp:** Depression; Anxiety Disorders; **Hospital:** Mass Genl Hosp; **Address:** Mass Genl Hosp, Dept Psychiatry, 55 Fruit St, Bulfinch 351, Boston, MA 02114-3139; **Phone:** 617-726-2993; **Board Cert:** Psychiatry 1987; **Med School:** Univ Wisc 1980; **Resid:** Psychiatry, Mass Genl Hosp 1984; **Fac Appt:** Asst Prof Psyc, Harvard Med Sch

Jenike, Michael Andrew MD [Psyc] - **Spec Exp:** Obsessive-Compulsive Disorder; Geriatric Psychiatry; **Hospital:** Mass Genl Hosp; **Address:** Obsessive Compulsive Disorders Unit, 185 Cambridge St, Ste 2200, Boston, MA 02114; **Phone:** 617-726-6766; **Board Cert:** Psychiatry 1984; **Med School:** Univ Okla Coll Med 1978; **Resid:** Psychiatry, Mass Genl Hosp 1982; **Fellow:** Psychiatry, Harvard Med Sch; Psychiatry, Mass Genl Hosp; **Fac Appt:** Prof Psyc, Harvard Med Sch

McGlashan, Thomas MD [Psyc] - **Spec Exp:** Schizophrenia-Early Detection/Treatment; Personality Disorders; **Hospital:** Connecticut Mental Hlth Ctr, Yale - New Haven Hosp; **Address:** Yale Univ Sch Med, Dept Psychiatry, 301 Cedar St, New Haven, CT 06519; **Phone:** 203-737-2077; **Board Cert:** Psychiatry 1973; **Med School:** Univ Pennsylvania 1967; **Resid:** Psychiatry, Mass Mental Hlth Ctr 1971; **Fac Appt:** Prof Psyc, Yale Univ

Phillips, Katharine MD [Psyc] - **Spec Exp:** Body Dysmorphic Disorder (BDD); Eating Disorders; **Hospital:** Butler Hosp; **Address:** Butler Hosp, Dept Psychiatry, 345 Blackstone Blvd, Providence, RI 02906; **Phone:** 401-455-6490; **Board Cert:** Psychiatry 1992; **Med School:** Dartmouth Med Sch 1987; **Resid:** Psychiatry, McLean Hosp 1991; **Fac Appt:** Prof Psyc, Brown Univ

Pitman, Roger Keith MD [Psyc] - **Spec Exp:** Post Traumatic Stress Disorder; **Hospital:** Mass Genl Hosp; **Address:** Mass Genl Hosp, Rm 2616, Bldg 149, 13th St, Charlestown, MA 02129; **Phone:** 617-726-5333; **Board Cert:** Psychiatry 1975; Forensic Psychiatry 2004; **Med School:** Univ VT Coll Med 1969; **Resid:** Psychiatry, Tufts-New England Med Ctr/VA Med Ctr 1973; **Fellow:** Behavioral Neurology, Beth Israel Hosp/Harvard; **Fac Appt:** Prof Psyc, Harvard Med Sch

Pope Jr, Harrison G MD [Psyc] - **Spec Exp:** Addiction/Substance Abuse; Psychopharmacology; **Hospital:** McLean Hosp; **Address:** McLean Hosp, Dept Psychiatry, 115 Mill St, Belmont, MA 02478; **Phone:** 617-855-2911; **Board Cert:** Psychiatry 1980; **Med School:** Harvard Med Sch 1974; **Resid:** Psychiatry, McLean Hosp 1977; **Fac Appt:** Prof Psyc, Harvard Med Sch

Price, Lawrence H MD [Psyc] - **Spec Exp:** Mood Disorders; Anxiety Disorders; Depression; **Hospital:** Butler Hosp; **Address:** Butler Hospital, Dept Psychiatry, 345 Blackstone Blvd, Providence, RI 02906; **Phone:** 401-455-6533; **Board Cert:** Psychiatry 1983; **Med School:** Univ Mich Med Sch 1978; **Resid:** Psychiatry, Yale-New Haven Hosp 1982; **Fellow:** Psychiatry, Yale-New Haven Hosp 1983; **Fac Appt:** Prof Psyc, Brown Univ

Rasmussen, Steven A MD [Psyc] - **Spec Exp:** Obsessive-Compulsive Disorder; **Hospital:** Butler Hosp; **Address:** Butler Hosp, 345 Blackstone Blvd, Providence, RI 02906; **Phone:** 401-455-6209; **Board Cert:** Psychiatry 1983; **Med School:** Brown Univ 1977; **Resid:** Psychiatry, Yale Univ 1981; **Fac Appt:** Assoc Prof Psyc, Brown Univ

Rosenbaum, Jerrold F MD [Psyc] - **Spec Exp:** Anxiety & Mood Disorders; **Hospital:** Mass Genl Hosp; **Address:** 55 Fruit St, Bulfinch 351, Boston, MA 02114; **Phone:** 617-726-3482; **Board Cert:** Psychiatry 1978; **Med School:** Yale Univ 1973; **Resid:** Psychiatry, Mass Genl Hosp 1977; **Fac Appt:** Prof Psyc, Harvard Med Sch

Salzman, Carl MD [Psyc] - **Spec Exp:** Psychopharmacology; Geriatric Psychiatry; Psychotherapy; **Hospital:** MA Mental Hlth Ctr, Beth Israel Deaconess Med Ctr - Boston; **Address:** Havard Medical School, Dept Psychiatry, 25 Shattuck St, Boston, MA 02115; **Phone:** 617-998-5006; **Board Cert:** Psychiatry 1970; **Med School:** SUNY Upstate Med Univ 1963; **Resid:** Psychiatry, Mass Mental Hlth Ctr 1967; Psychiatry, Natl Inst Mental Hlth 1969; **Fac Appt:** Prof Psyc, Harvard Med Sch

Shapiro, Edward R MD [Psyc] - **Spec Exp:** Psychoanalysis; **Hospital:** Austen Riggs Ctr; **Address:** Austen Riggs Ctr, 25 Main St, PO Box 962, Stockbridge, MA 01262; **Phone:** 413-298-5511; **Board Cert:** Psychiatry 1974; **Med School:** Harvard Med Sch 1968; **Resid:** Psychiatry, Mass Mental Hlth Ctr 1972; **Fellow:** Natl Inst Mental Hlth 1974; **Fac Appt:** Assoc Clin Prof Psyc, Harvard Med Sch

Psychiatry

van der Kolk, Bessel MD [Psyc] - **Spec Exp:** Post Traumatic Stress Disorder; Child Abuse; **Hospital:** Boston Med Ctr, Arbour Hospital - Boston; **Address:** 16 Braddock Park, Boston, MA 02116-5804; **Phone:** 617-247-1720; **Board Cert:** Psychiatry 1976; **Med School:** Univ Chicago-Pritzker Sch Med 1970; **Resid:** Psychiatry, Harvard Med Sch 1974; **Fac Appt:** Prof Psyc, Boston Univ

Yonkers, Kimberly A MD [Psyc] - **Spec Exp:** Anxiety & Mood Disorders; Premenstrual Dysphoric Disorder; **Hospital:** Yale - New Haven Hosp; **Address:** 142 Temple St, Ste 301, New Haven, CT 06510; **Phone:** 203-764-6621; **Board Cert:** Psychiatry 1991; **Med School:** Columbia P&S 1986; **Resid:** Psychiatry, McLean Hosp 1990; **Fellow:** Psychiatry, McLean Hosp 1992; **Fac Appt:** Assoc Prof Psyc, Yale Univ

Mid Atlantic

Akhtar, Salman MD [Psyc] - **Spec Exp:** Psychoanalysis; **Hospital:** Thomas Jefferson Univ Hosp; **Address:** Jefferson Medical College, 833 Chestnut St, Ste 210, Philadelphia, PA 19107; **Phone:** 215-955-2547; **Board Cert:** Psychiatry 1977; **Med School:** India 1968; **Resid:** Psychiatry, UMDNJ Med Ctr 1974; Psychiatry, Univ Virginia Med Ctr 1976; **Fellow:** Psychoanalysis, Philadelphia Psych Inst 1986

Alexopoulos, George MD [Psyc] - **Spec Exp:** Geriatric Psychiatry; Depression; Psychopharmacology; **Hospital:** NY-Presby Hosp/Weill Cornell (page 66); **Address:** 21 Bloomingdale Rd, White Plains, NY 10605; **Phone:** 914-997-5767; **Board Cert:** Psychiatry 1978; Geriatric Psychiatry 2001; **Med School:** Greece 1970; **Resid:** Psychiatry, UMDNJ Univ Hosp 1976; Psychiatry, NY Presby Hosp-Westch Div 1977; **Fellow:** Biological Psychiatry, NY Hosp-Cornell Med Ctr 1978; **Fac Appt:** Prof Psyc, Cornell Univ-Weill Med Coll

Appelbaum, Paul S MD [Psyc] - **Spec Exp:** Forensic Psychiatry; Depression; Anxiety & Mood Disorders; **Hospital:** NY-Presby Hosp/Columbia (page 66); **Address:** NY State Psychiatric Inst, 1051 Riverside Drive, rm 6706, Box 122, New York, NY 10032; **Phone:** 212-543-4184; **Board Cert:** Psychiatry 1981; Forensic Psychiatry 2004; **Med School:** Harvard Med Sch 1976; **Resid:** Psychiatry, Mass Mental Health Ctr 1980; **Fac Appt:** Prof Psyc, Columbia P&S

Basch, Samuel MD [Psyc] - **Spec Exp:** Psychiatry in Cancer; Psychiatry in Physical Illness; Psychopharmacology; Psychoanalysis; **Hospital:** Mount Sinai Med Ctr; **Address:** 10 E 85th St, Ste 1B, New York, NY 10028-0412; **Phone:** 212-427-0344; **Board Cert:** Psychiatry 1970; **Med School:** Hahnemann Univ 1961; **Resid:** Psychiatry, Mount Sinai Hosp 1965; **Fellow:** Psychoanalysis, Columbia Presby Hosp 1976; **Fac Appt:** Clin Prof Psyc, Mount Sinai Sch Med

Blumenfield, Michael MD [Psyc] - **Spec Exp:** Psychopharmacology; Psychosomatic Disorders; Disaster Psychiatry; Liaison Psychiatry; **Hospital:** Westchester Med Ctr, White Plains Hosp Ctr; **Address:** 16 Donellan Rd, Scarsdale, NY 10583-2008; **Phone:** 914-472-5035; **Board Cert:** Psychiatry 1970; Psychosomatic Medicine 2005; **Med School:** SUNY Downstate 1964; **Resid:** Psychiatry, Kings County Hosp 1968; **Fellow:** Psychosomatic Medicine, Kings County Hosp 1971; **Fac Appt:** Prof Psyc, NY Med Coll

Boronow, John Joseph MD [Psyc] - **Spec Exp:** Psychotic Disorders; Schizophrenia; **Hospital:** Sheppard Pratt Hlth Sys; **Address:** 6501 N Charles St, rm TJ-113, Towson, MD 21284; **Phone:** 410-938-4306; **Board Cert:** Psychiatry 1983; **Med School:** Yale Univ 1977; **Resid:** Psychiatry, New York Hosp 1981; **Fellow:** Psychopharmacology, Natl Inst Mntl Hlth 1983; **Fac Appt:** Assoc Clin Prof Psyc, Univ MD Sch Med

Brandt, Harry A MD [Psyc] - **Spec Exp:** Eating Disorders; **Hospital:** St Joseph Med Ctr, Sheppard Pratt Hlth Sys; **Address:** Ctr Eating Disorders, 6535 N Charles St, Ste 300, Baltimore, MD 21204; **Phone:** 410-938-5252; **Board Cert:** Psychiatry 1989; **Med School:** Univ MD Sch Med 1983; **Resid:** Psychiatry, Univ Maryland Hosp 1986; **Fellow:** Biological Psychiatry, Natl Inst Mental Hlth 1988; **Fac Appt:** Assoc Clin Prof Psyc, Univ MD Sch Med

Breitbart, William MD [Psyc] - **Spec Exp:** Psychiatry in Cancer; AIDS Related Cancers; Pain-Cancer; Palliative Care; **Hospital:** Meml Sloan Kettering Cancer Ctr; **Address:** Meml Sloan Kettering Cancer Center, 641 Lexington Ave Fl 7, New York, NY 10021; **Phone:** 646-888-0020; **Board Cert:** Internal Medicine 1982; Psychiatry 1986; Psychosomatic Medicine 2005; **Med School:** Albert Einstein Coll Med 1978; **Resid:** Internal Medicine, Bronx Muni Hosp Ctr 1982; Psychiatry, Bronx Muni Hosp Ctr 1984; **Fellow:** Psychiatric Oncology, Meml Sloan Kettering Cancer Ctr 1986; **Fac Appt:** Prof Psyc, Cornell Univ-Weill Med Coll

Brodkin, Edward S MD [Psyc] - **Spec Exp:** Autism; Learning Disorders (Social); Asperger's Syndrome; **Hospital:** Hosp Univ Penn - UPHS (page 72); **Address:** Univ Penn Sch Med, Translational Rsch Lab, 125 S 31st St, rm 2220, Philadelphia, PA 19104-3403; **Phone:** 215-573-1159; **Board Cert:** Psychiatry 2006; **Med School:** Harvard Med Sch 1992; **Resid:** Psychiatry, Yale-New Haven Hosp 1996; **Fellow:** Neurological Biology, Yale Univ Sch Med 1998; Genetics, Princeton Univ 2002; **Fac Appt:** Asst Prof Psyc, Univ Pennsylvania

Bronheim, Harold MD [Psyc] - **Spec Exp:** Psychiatry in Body Image Awareness; Relationship Problems; Psychiatry in Physical Illness/Depressed; Liaison Psychiatry; **Hospital:** Mount Sinai Med Ctr; **Address:** 1155 Park Ave, New York, NY 10128-1209; **Phone:** 212-996-5777; **Board Cert:** Psychiatry 1985; Internal Medicine 1986; Psychosomatic Medicine 2005; **Med School:** SUNY Hlth Sci Ctr 1980; **Resid:** Psychiatry, Mount Sinai Hosp 1984; **Fellow:** Internal Medicine, Beth Israel Hosp 1985; **Fac Appt:** Clin Prof Psyc, Mount Sinai Sch Med

Cohen, Mitchell J MD [Psyc] - **Spec Exp:** Pain-Chronic; Psychiatry in Physical Illness; Anxiety Disorders; **Hospital:** Thomas Jefferson Univ Hosp; **Address:** 833 Chestnut St E, Ste 210B, Philadelphia, PA 19107; **Phone:** 215-955-6592; **Board Cert:** Psychiatry 1989; Pain Medicine 2002; **Med School:** Med Coll PA 1984; **Resid:** Psychiatry, Johns Hopkins Hosp 1988; **Fac Appt:** Prof Psyc, Thomas Jefferson Univ

DePaulo Jr, J Raymond MD [Psyc] - **Spec Exp:** Bipolar/Mood Disorders; Depression; **Hospital:** Johns Hopkins Hosp - Baltimore (page 61); **Address:** Johns Hopkins Hosp, Dept Psychiatry, 600 N Wolfe St, Meyer 4-113, Baltimore, MD 21287-7413; **Phone:** 410-955-3130; **Board Cert:** Psychiatry 1977; **Med School:** Johns Hopkins Univ 1972; **Resid:** Psychiatry, Johns Hopkins Hosp 1977; **Fac Appt:** Prof Psyc, Johns Hopkins Univ

Doghramji, Karl MD [Psyc] - **Spec Exp:** Sleep Disorders/Apnea; Narcolepsy; **Hospital:** Thomas Jefferson Univ Hosp; **Address:** 1015 Walnut St, Curtis Bldg Fl 3 - rm 319, Philadelphia, PA 19107; **Phone:** 215-955-6175; **Board Cert:** Psychiatry 1986; **Med School:** Thomas Jefferson Univ 1980; **Resid:** Psychiatry, Thomas Jefferson Univ Hosp 1984; **Fellow:** Sleep Medicine, Montefiore Med Ctr; **Fac Appt:** Prof Psyc, Thomas Jefferson Univ

Eaton Jr, James S MD [Psyc] - **Spec Exp:** Anxiety Disorders; Sexual Orientation Issues; Depression; Diagnostic Second Opinions; **Hospital:** Georgetown Univ Hosp, G Washington Univ Hosp; **Address:** 4214 50th St NW, Washington, DC 20016; **Phone:** 202-333-5796; **Board Cert:** Psychiatry 1976; **Med School:** Tulane Univ 1962; **Resid:** Internal Medicine, Tulane Univ Med Ctr 1966; Psychiatry, Tulane Univ Med Ctr 1968; **Fellow:** Psychoanalysis, Tulane Univ Med Ctr 1973; **Fac Appt:** Clin Prof Psyc, Georgetown Univ

Psychiatry

Eth, Spencer MD [Psyc] - **Spec Exp:** Forensic Psychiatry; Post Traumatic Stress Disorder; **Hospital:** St Vincent Cath Med Ctrs - Manhattan; **Address:** 144 W 12th St, rm 174, New York, NY 10011-8202; **Phone:** 212-604-8196; **Board Cert:** Child & Adolescent Psychiatry 1982; Geriatric Psychiatry 2000; Forensic Psychiatry 2005; Addiction Psychiatry 1998; **Med School:** UCLA 1976; **Resid:** Psychiatry, NY Cornell Med Ctr 1979; **Fellow:** Child & Adolescent Psychiatry, Cedars -Sinai Med Ctr 1981; **Fac Appt:** Prof Psyc, NY Med Coll

First, Michael B MD [Psyc] - **Spec Exp:** Psychotherapy; Psychopharmacology; Forensic Psychiatry; **Hospital:** NY-Presby Hosp/Columbia (page 66); **Address:** NY State Psychiatric Inst, Unit 60, 1051 Riverside Drive, New York, NY 10032; **Phone:** 212-543-5531; **Board Cert:** Psychiatry 1989; **Med School:** Univ Pittsburgh 1983; **Resid:** Psychiatry, NY State Psych Inst 1987; **Fellow:** Psychiatric Research, NY State Psych Inst 1988; **Fac Appt:** Clin Prof Psyc, Columbia P&S

Ganguli, Rohan MD [Psyc] - **Spec Exp:** Schizophrenia; **Hospital:** Western Psych Inst & Clin - UPMC; **Address:** Western Psyc Inst & Clinic, 3811 O'Hara St, Pittsburgh, PA 15213; **Phone:** 412-246-5006; **Board Cert:** Psychiatry 1980; **Med School:** India 1973; **Resid:** Psychiatry, Memorial Univ 1978; Psychiatry, Univ Pittsburgh Med Ctr 1978; **Fac Appt:** Prof Psyc, Univ Pittsburgh

Halmi, Katherine MD [Psyc] - **Spec Exp:** Eating Disorders; **Hospital:** NY-Presby Hosp/Weill Cornell (page 66); **Address:** NY Presby Hosp - Westchester Div, 21 Bloomingdale Rd, White Plains, NY 10605; **Phone:** 914-997-5875; **Board Cert:** Pediatrics 1970; Psychiatry 1977; **Med School:** Univ Iowa Coll Med 1965; **Resid:** Pediatrics, Univ Iowa Hosp 1968; Psychiatry, Univ Iowa Hosp 1972; **Fellow:** Child Development, Univ Iowa Hosp 1969; **Fac Appt:** Prof Psyc, Cornell Univ-Weill Med Coll

Hollander, Eric MD [Psyc] - **Spec Exp:** Obsessive-Compulsive Disorder; Anxiety Disorders; Autism; **Hospital:** Mount Sinai Med Ctr; **Address:** 300 Central Park West, Ste 1C, New York, NY 10024-1513; **Phone:** 212-873-4051; **Board Cert:** Psychiatry 1987; **Med School:** SUNY Hlth Sci Ctr 1982; **Resid:** Internal Medicine, Mount Sinai Hosp 1983; Psychiatry, Mount Sinai Hosp 1986; **Fellow:** Psychiatry, Columbia-Presby Med Ctr 1988; **Fac Appt:** Prof Psyc, Mount Sinai Sch Med

Kavey, Neil B MD [Psyc] - **Spec Exp:** Narcolepsy; Sleep Disorders/Apnea; **Hospital:** NY-Presby Hosp/Columbia (page 66); **Address:** Columbia Presby Med Ctr, Sleep Disorders Ctr, 161 Ft Washington Ave Fl 3 - rm 346, New York, NY 10032; **Phone:** 212-305-1860; **Board Cert:** Psychiatry 1976; Sleep Medicine 2003; **Med School:** Columbia P&S 1969; **Resid:** Psychiatry, Columbia Presby Med Ctr 1973; **Fac Appt:** Clin Prof Psyc, Columbia P&S

Klagsbrun, Samuel C MD [Psyc] - **Spec Exp:** Psychiatry in Cancer; Psychiatry in Terminal Illness; **Hospital:** Four Winds Hosp; **Address:** Four Winds Hospital, 800 Cross River Rd, Katonah, NY 10536; **Phone:** 914-763-8151; **Board Cert:** Psychiatry 1977; **Med School:** Ros Franklin Univ/Chicago Med Sch 1962; **Resid:** Psychiatry, Yale-New Haven Hosp 1966; **Fac Appt:** Clin Prof Psyc, Albert Einstein Coll Med

Kunkel, Elisabeth J MD [Psyc] - **Spec Exp:** Psychiatry in Cancer; Psychiatry in Physical Illness; **Hospital:** Thomas Jefferson Univ Hosp; **Address:** Thomas Jefferson Univ, 1020 Samson St, Thompson Bldg, Ste 1652, Philadelphia, PA 19107; **Phone:** 215-955-9545; **Board Cert:** Psychiatry 1989; Geriatric Psychiatry 1994; Addiction Psychiatry 1998; Psychosomatic Medicine 2005; **Med School:** McGill Univ 1983; **Resid:** Psychiatry, NYU Med Ctr 1987; **Fellow:** Liaison Psychiatry, Meml Sloan Kettering Cancer Ctr 1989; **Fac Appt:** Prof Psyc, Jefferson Med Coll

Kupfer, David J MD [Psyc] - **Spec Exp:** Bipolar/Mood Disorders; Sleep Disorders/Apnea; **Hospital:** Western Psych Inst & Clin - UPMC; **Address:** Western Psychiatric Inst & Clinic, 3811 O'Hara St, Pittsburgh, PA 15213-2593; **Phone:** 412-246-6777; **Board Cert:** Psychiatry 1978; **Med School:** Yale Univ 1965; **Resid:** Psychiatry, Yale-New Haven Hosp 1970; Psychiatry, Natl Inst Mental Hlth 1969; **Fellow:** Psychiatry, Yale-New Haven Hosp 1967; **Fac Appt:** Prof Psyc, Univ Pittsburgh

Lawson, William B MD [Psyc] - **Spec Exp:** Bipolar/Mood Disorders; Addiction/Substance Abuse; Dual Diagnosis; **Hospital:** Howard Univ Hosp; **Address:** Howard Univ Hosp, Dept Psychiatry, 2041 Georgia Ave NW, Ste 5B01, Washington, DC 20060; **Phone:** 202-865-6611; **Board Cert:** Psychiatry 1984; Addiction Psychiatry 1994; **Med School:** Univ Chicago-Pritzker Sch Med 1978; **Resid:** Psychiatry, Stanford Univ Med Ctr 1981; Psychiatry, Natl Inst Mental Hlth 1982; **Fellow:** Neuropsychiatry, Natl Inst Mental Hlth 1984; **Fac Appt:** Prof Psyc, Howard Univ

Loewenstein, Richard MD [Psyc] - **Spec Exp:** Trauma Psychiatry; Dissociative Disorders; Child Abuse; **Hospital:** Sheppard Pratt Hlth Sys; **Address:** 6501 N Charles St, Ste A305, Box 6815, Baltimore, MD 21204; **Phone:** 410-938-5070; **Board Cert:** Psychiatry 1980; **Med School:** Yale Univ 1975; **Resid:** Psychiatry, Yale Affil Hosps 1979; **Fellow:** Psychiatry, NIH,NIMH-Biol Psych Br 1982; **Fac Appt:** Assoc Clin Prof Psyc, Univ MD Sch Med

Manevitz, Alan MD [Psyc] - **Spec Exp:** Marital/Family/Sex Therapy; Fibromyalgia Syndrome (FMS); Post Traumatic Stress Disorder; ADD/ADHD; **Hospital:** NY-Presby Hosp/Weill Cornell (page 66), Lenox Hill Hosp (page 62); **Address:** 60 Sutton Place South, Ste 1CN, New York, NY 10022; **Phone:** 212-751-5072; **Board Cert:** Psychiatry 1987; **Med School:** Columbia P&S 1980; **Resid:** Psychiatry, New York Hosp 1984; **Fellow:** Psychopharmacology, New York Hosp 1985; **Fac Appt:** Assoc Clin Prof Psyc, Cornell Univ-Weill Med Coll

Marin, Deborah B MD [Psyc] - **Spec Exp:** Alzheimer's Disease; **Hospital:** Mount Sinai Med Ctr; **Address:** Mount Sinai Hospital, One Gustave L Levy Pl, Box 1068, New York, NY 10029; **Phone:** 212-241-7139; **Board Cert:** Psychiatry 1990; **Med School:** Mount Sinai Sch Med 1984; **Resid:** Psychiatry, Mount Sinai Hosp 1988; **Fellow:** Psychiatry, New York Hosp-Cornell Med Ctr 1991; **Fac Appt:** Prof Psyc, Mount Sinai Sch Med

McCann, Merle C MD [Psyc] - **Hospital:** Sheppard Pratt Hlth Sys; **Address:** Sheppard & Enoch Pratt Hosp, 6501 N Charles St,, rm PJ-111, Baltimore, MD 21204; **Phone:** 410-938-3000; **Board Cert:** Psychiatry 1986; **Med School:** Med Coll VA 1981; **Resid:** Psychiatry, Geo Wash Univ Hosp 1985; **Fac Appt:** Asst Clin Prof Psyc, Univ MD Sch Med

McHugh, Paul MD [Psyc] - **Spec Exp:** Neuro-Psychiatry; Huntington's Disease; **Hospital:** Johns Hopkins Hosp - Baltimore (page 61); **Address:** Johns Hopkins Hosp - Psychiatry, 600 N Wolfe St, Meyer-127, Baltimore, MD 21287; **Phone:** 410-502-3150; **Board Cert:** Neurology 1967; Psychiatry 1968; **Med School:** Harvard Med Sch 1956; **Resid:** Neurology, Mass Genl Hosp 1960; Psychiatry, Maudsley Hosp 1961; **Fac Appt:** Prof Psyc, Johns Hopkins Univ

Roose, Steven MD [Psyc] - **Spec Exp:** Depression in the Elderly; **Hospital:** NY-Presby Hosp/Columbia (page 66); **Address:** NY State Psychiatric Institute, 1051 Riverside Drive, New York, NY 10032; **Phone:** 212-831-8644; **Board Cert:** Psychiatry 1979; **Med School:** Mount Sinai Sch Med 1974; **Resid:** Psychiatry, NY Psychiatric Inst 1978; **Fellow:** Research, Columbia-Presby Med Ctr 1981; **Fac Appt:** Clin Prof Psyc, Columbia P&S

Rosse, Richard B MD [Psyc] - **Hospital:** VA Med Ctr - Washington; **Address:** DC VA Medical Center, 50 Irving St NW, Mental Health Dept, rm 3A154, MC 116A, Washington, DC 20422-0001; **Phone:** 202-745-8156; **Board Cert:** Psychiatry 1986; **Med School:** Univ MD Sch Med 1980; **Resid:** Psychiatry, Georgetown Univ Med Ctr 1984; **Fac Appt:** Assoc Prof Psyc, Georgetown Univ

Sadock, Virginia MD [Psyc] - **Spec Exp:** Psychotherapy; Sexual Dysfunction; Anxiety & Depression; Marital/Family/Sex Therapy; **Hospital:** NYU Med Ctr (page 67); **Address:** 4 E 89th St, Ste 1E, New York, NY 10128; **Phone:** 212-427-0885; **Board Cert:** Psychiatry 1975; **Med School:** NY Med Coll 1970; **Resid:** Psychiatry, Metropolitan Hosp 1973; **Fac Appt:** Clin Prof Psyc, NYU Sch Med

Samberg, Eslee MD [Psyc] - **Spec Exp:** Psychoanalysis; **Hospital:** NY-Presby Hosp/Weill Cornell (page 66); **Address:** 2211 Broadway, Ste 1H, New York, NY 10024-6263; **Phone:** 212-874-7725; **Board Cert:** Psychiatry 1983; **Med School:** Cornell Univ-Weill Med Coll 1978; **Resid:** Psychiatry, NY Hosp-Cornell Med Ctr 1982; **Fac Appt:** Assoc Clin Prof Psyc, Cornell Univ-Weill Med Coll

Shear, M Katherine MD [Psyc] - **Spec Exp:** Panic Disorder; Anxiety Disorders; Bereavement/Traumatic Grief; Phobias; **Address:** 1255 Amsterdam Ave, New York, NY 10027; **Phone:** 412-897-7449; **Board Cert:** Internal Medicine 1975; Psychiatry 1981; **Med School:** Tufts Univ 1972; **Resid:** Internal Medicine, Mt Sinai Hosp 1976; Psychiatry, Payne Whitney Clin 1979; **Fellow:** Psychosomatic Medicine, Montefiore Hosp 1980; **Fac Appt:** Prof Psyc, Colombia

Simon, Robert I MD [Psyc] - **Spec Exp:** Forensic Psychiatry; **Hospital:** Suburban Hosp - Bethesda, Sibley Mem Hosp; **Address:** 8008 Horseshoe Ln, Potomac, MD 20854; **Phone:** 301-983-1270; **Board Cert:** Psychiatry 1969; Forensic Psychiatry 1994; **Med School:** Tufts Univ 1960; **Resid:** Psychiatry, Jackson Meml Hosp 1966; **Fac Appt:** Prof Psyc, Georgetown Univ

Stone, Michael H MD [Psyc] - **Spec Exp:** Personality Disorders; Psychoanalysis; Forensic Psychiatry; **Address:** 225 Central Park West, Ste 114, New York, NY 10024-6027; **Phone:** 212-758-2000; **Board Cert:** Psychiatry 1971; **Med School:** Cornell Univ-Weill Med Coll 1958; **Resid:** Internal Medicine, Bellevue Hosp 1961; Psychiatry, NYS Psych Inst 1966; **Fellow:** Hematology, Meml Sloan Kettering Cancer Ctr 1962; Medical Oncology, Meml Sloan Kettering Cancer Ctr 1963; **Fac Appt:** Clin Prof Psyc, Columbia P&S

Sussman, Norman MD [Psyc] - **Spec Exp:** Psychopharmacology; Anxiety & Mood Disorders; Bipolar/Mood Disorders; **Hospital:** NYU Med Ctr (page 67); **Address:** 150 E 58th St, Fl 27, New York, NY 10155; **Phone:** 212-588-9722; **Board Cert:** Psychiatry 1980; **Med School:** NY Med Coll 1975; **Resid:** Psychiatry, Metropolitan Hosp Ctr 1977; Psychiatry, Westchester Co Med Ctr 1978; **Fac Appt:** Clin Prof Psyc, NYU Sch Med

Thase, Michael E MD [Psyc] - **Spec Exp:** Anxiety & Mood Disorders; Psychopharmacology; Depression; **Hospital:** Western Psych Inst & Clin - UPMC; **Address:** Western Psych Inst & Clinic, 3811 O'Hara St, Pittsburgh, PA 15213; **Phone:** 412-246-5290; **Board Cert:** Psychiatry 1984; **Med School:** Ohio State Univ 1979; **Resid:** Psychiatry, Western Psych Inst 1983; **Fellow:** Research, Univ Pittsburgh Sch Med 1984; **Fac Appt:** Prof Psyc, Univ Pittsburgh

Uhde, Thomas W MD [Psyc] - **Spec Exp:** Anxiety & Mood Disorders; Depression; **Hospital:** Penn State Milton S Hershey Med Ctr; **Address:** Penn State Univ Coll Med, Dept Psychiatry, PO Box 850, MC H073, Hershey, PA 17033; **Phone:** 717-531-8515; **Board Cert:** Psychiatry 1984; **Med School:** Univ Louisville Sch Med 1975; **Resid:** Psychiatry, Yale-New Haven Hosp 1979; **Fellow:** Psychiatry, Natl Inst Mental Hlth 1981; **Fac Appt:** Prof Psyc, Penn State Univ-Hershey Med Ctr

Wait, Susan B MD [Psyc] - **Spec Exp:** Post Traumatic Stress Disorder; Dissociative Disorders; Anxiety & Mood Disorders; Dialectical Behavioral Therapy; **Hospital:** Sheppard Pratt Hlth Sys; **Address:** Sheppard Pratt Hlth System, 6501 N Charles St, Baltimore, MD 21285; **Phone:** 410-938-5076; **Board Cert:** Psychiatry 1993; **Med School:** Med Coll PA Hahnemann 1987; **Resid:** Psychiatry, Sheppard Pratt Hosp 1991; **Fac Appt:** Assoc Clin Prof Psyc, Univ MD Sch Med

Walsh, B Timothy MD [Psyc] - **Spec Exp:** Eating Disorders; **Hospital:** NY State Psychiatric Inst, NY-Presby Hosp/Columbia (page 66); **Address:** NY State Psychiatric Inst-Unit 98, 1051 Riverside Dr, New York, NY 10032-2695; **Phone:** 212-543-5316; **Board Cert:** Psychiatry 1978; **Med School:** Harvard Med Sch 1972; **Resid:** Internal Medicine, Dartmouth Affil Hosps 1973; Psychiatry, Bronx Muni Hosp Ctr 1977; **Fac Appt:** Prof Psyc, Columbia P&S

Southeast

Blazer II, Dan G MD/PhD [Psyc] - **Spec Exp:** Geriatric Psychiatry; Mood Disorders; **Hospital:** Duke Univ Med Ctr; **Address:** Duke Univ Med Ctr, Dept Psychiatary, 3521 Hospital S, Box 3003, Durham, NC 27710-3003; **Phone:** 919-684-4128; **Board Cert:** Psychiatry 1977; Geriatric Psychiatry 2000; **Med School:** Univ Tenn Coll Med, Memphis 1969; **Resid:** Psychiatry, Duke Univ Med Ctr 1975; **Fellow:** Liaison Psychiatry, Montefiore Hosp 1976; **Fac Appt:** Prof Psyc, Duke Univ

Canterbury II, Randolph J MD [Psyc] - **Spec Exp:** Panic Disorder; Depression; Substance Abuse; **Hospital:** Univ Virginia Med Ctr; **Address:** U Virginia Health Science Ctr, Box 800623, Charlottesville, VA 22908; **Phone:** 434-243-5719; **Board Cert:** Internal Medicine 1983; Psychiatry 1985; Psychosomatic Medicine 2005; **Med School:** W VA Univ 1979; **Resid:** Internal Medicine, Univ Va Hosp 1983; Psychiatry, Univ Va Hosp 1985; **Fac Appt:** Prof Psyc, Univ VA Sch Med

Dell, Diana L MD [Psyc] - **Spec Exp:** Postpartum Depression (PPD); Menstrual Disorders (PMS); Pregnancy & Mental Health Issues; Women's Health-Mental & Reproductive; **Hospital:** Duke Univ Med Ctr; **Address:** Duke University Medical Ctr, Box 3263, Durham, NC 27710; **Phone:** 919-668-2570; **Board Cert:** Psychiatry 2001; Obstetrics & Gynecology 1998; **Med School:** Louisiana State Univ 1982; **Resid:** Obstetrics & Gynecology, Charity Hosp 1986; Psychiatry, Univ N Carolina Hosps 1998; **Fellow:** Psychosomatic Medicine, Univ Toronto 1999; **Fac Appt:** Asst Prof Psyc, Duke Univ

Eisdorfer, Carl MD/PhD [Psyc] - **Spec Exp:** Aging and Dementia; Alzheimer's Disease; Depression; **Hospital:** Jackson Meml Hosp, Mount Sinai Med Ctr - Miami; **Address:** Mental Hlth Hosp Ctr, 1695 NW Ninth Ave, rm 3204, Miami, FL 33136-1024; **Phone:** 305-355-9040; **Board Cert:** Psychiatry 1974; **Med School:** Duke Univ 1964; **Resid:** Psychiatry, Duke Univ Med Ctr 1967; **Fac Appt:** Prof Psyc, Univ Miami Sch Med

Giustra Jr, Lawrence J MD [Psyc] - **Spec Exp:** Depression; Mood Disorders; Suicide; **Hospital:** Emory Univ Hosp; **Address:** 1970 Cliff Valley Way NE, Ste 202, Atlanta, GA 30329; **Phone:** 404-325-2139; **Board Cert:** Psychiatry 1982; **Med School:** Johns Hopkins Univ 1976; **Resid:** Psychiatry, Mass General Hosp 1980; **Fac Appt:** Asst Prof Psyc, Emory Univ

Kendler, Kenneth S MD [Psyc] - **Spec Exp:** Schizophrenia; Mood Disorders; **Hospital:** Med Coll of VA Hosp; **Address:** Med Coll VA, Dept Psyc, PO Box 980126, Richmond, VA 23298-0126; **Phone:** 804-828-8590; **Board Cert:** Psychiatry 1981; **Med School:** Stanford Univ 1976; **Resid:** Psychiatry, Yale-New Haven Hosp 1980; **Fac Appt:** Prof Psyc, Med Coll VA

Klapheke, Martin M MD [Psyc] - **Spec Exp:** Transplantation Psychiatry; Psychoanalysis; **Hospital:** Univ of Louisville Hosp; **Address:** 2010 Cherokee Pkwy, Ste 3, Louisville, KY 40204; **Phone:** 502-456-1770; **Board Cert:** Psychiatry 1985; **Med School:** Univ KY Coll Med 1979; **Resid:** Psychiatry, Mayo Grad Sch Med 1982; **Fellow:** Child & Adolescent Psychiatry, Mayo Grad Sch Med 1984; Psychoanalysis, Topeka Inst Psychoanalysis 1994; **Fac Appt:** Clin Prof Psyc, Univ Louisville Sch Med

Levy, Steven T MD [Psyc] - **Spec Exp:** Depression; Anxiety & Mood Disorders; Bipolar/Mood Disorders; **Hospital:** Emory Univ Hosp; **Address:** Emory Univ Psychoanalytic Inst, 2004 Ridgewood Rd, Ste 300, Atlanta, GA 30322; **Phone:** 404-727-0397; **Board Cert:** Psychiatry 1976; **Med School:** Duke Univ 1969; **Resid:** Psychiatry, Yale-New Haven Hosp 1973; **Fac Appt:** Prof Psyc, Emory Univ

McCall, William V MD [Psyc] - **Spec Exp:** Sleep Disorders; Electroconvulsive Therapy (ECT); Depression; **Hospital:** Wake Forest Univ Baptist Med Ctr (page 73); **Address:** Wake Forest U Sch of Med, Dept Psychiatry, Medical Center Blvd, WInston-Salem, NC 27157; **Phone:** 336-716-2911; **Board Cert:** Psychiatry 1990; Geriatric Psychiatry 2005; **Med School:** Duke Univ 1984; **Resid:** Psychiatry, Duke Univ Med Ctr 1987; **Fellow:** Sleep Medicine, Duke Univ Med Ctr 1988; **Fac Appt:** Prof Psyc, Wake Forest Univ

Powers, Pauline MD [Psyc] - **Spec Exp:** Eating Disorders; **Hospital:** Tampa Genl Hosp; **Address:** University S Fla, Dept Psychiatry, 3515 E Fletcher Ave, Tampa, FL 33613-4706; **Phone:** 813-974-2926; **Board Cert:** Psychiatry 1977; **Med School:** Univ Iowa Coll Med 1971; **Resid:** Psychiatry, Univ Iowa Med Ctr 1974; Psychiatry, Univ Calif-Davis Med Ctr 1975; **Fac Appt:** Prof Psyc, Univ S Fla Coll Med

Ray, Albert MD [Psyc] - **Spec Exp:** Pain Management; Stress Management; Headache; **Hospital:** Baptist Hosp of Miami; **Address:** 8603 S Dixie Hwy, Ste 401, Miami, FL 33143; **Phone:** 305-595-4681; **Board Cert:** Psychiatry 1976; Pain Medicine 1999; **Med School:** UMDNJ-NJ Med Sch, Newark 1970; **Resid:** Psychiatry, Monmouth Med Center 1973; **Fac Appt:** Assoc Clin Prof Psyc, Univ Miami Sch Med

Weiner, Richard D MD/PhD [Psyc] - **Spec Exp:** Bipolar/Mood Disorders; Electroconvulsive Therapy (ECT); Depression; Schizophrenia; **Hospital:** Duke Univ Med Ctr, VA Med Ctr - Durham; **Address:** Duke Univ Medical Ctr, Dept Psychiatry, Box 3309, Durham, NC 27710; **Phone:** 919-681-8742; **Board Cert:** Psychiatry 1979; Clinical Neurophysiology 2003; **Med School:** Duke Univ 1973; **Resid:** Psychiatry, Duke Univ Med Ctr 1976; **Fellow:** Electroencephalography, Duke Univ Med Ctr 1977; **Fac Appt:** Prof Psyc, Duke Univ

Weisler, Richard H MD [Psyc] - **Spec Exp:** Depression; Bipolar/Mood Disorders; **Hospital:** Duke Univ Med Ctr; **Address:** 700 Spring Forest Rd, Ste 125, Raleigh, NC 27609; **Phone:** 919-872-5900; **Board Cert:** Psychiatry 1982; **Med School:** Univ NC Sch Med 1977; **Resid:** Psychiatry, Duke Univ Med Ctr 1982; **Fac Appt:** Assoc Prof Psyc, Duke Univ

Midwest

Andersen, Arnold MD [Psyc] - **Spec Exp:** Eating Disorders; **Hospital:** Univ Iowa Hosp & Clinics; **Address:** Univ Iowa, Dept Psychiatry, 200 Hawkins Drive, rm 2880-JPP, Iowa City, IA 52242; **Phone:** 319-356-1354; **Board Cert:** Psychiatry 1980; **Med School:** Cornell Univ-Weill Med Coll 1968; **Resid:** Psychiatry, New York Hosp 1970; Psychiatry, Johns Hopkins Hosp 1976; **Fellow:** Psychiatry, Natl Inst Mental Hlth 1975; **Fac Appt:** Prof Psyc, Univ Iowa Coll Med

Calabrese, Joseph R MD [Psyc] - **Spec Exp:** Bipolar/Mood Disorders; Mood Disorders from Substance Abuse; Depression; **Hospital:** Univ Hosps Case Med Ctr; **Address:** Case Western Reserve Univ, 11400 Euclid Ave, rm 200, Cleveland, OH 44106; **Phone:** 216-844-2865; **Board Cert:** Psychiatry 1989; **Med School:** Ohio State Univ 1980; **Resid:** Psychiatry, Cleveland Clinic 1984; **Fellow:** Biological Psychiatry, Natl Inst Mental Hlth 1986; **Fac Appt:** Prof Psyc, Case West Res Univ

Cloninger, C Robert MD [Psyc] - **Spec Exp:** Personality Disorders; **Hospital:** Barnes-Jewish Hosp; **Address:** Wash Univ Sch Med, Dept Psyc, 660 S Euclid Ave, Box 8134, St Louis, MO 63110; **Phone:** 314-362-7005; **Board Cert:** Psychiatry 1975; **Med School:** Washington Univ, St Louis 1970; **Resid:** Psychiatry, Barnes Hosp 1973; Psychiatry, Renard Hosp-Wash Univ 1973; **Fac Appt:** Prof Psyc, Washington Univ, St Louis

Crow, Scott J MD [Psyc] - **Spec Exp:** Eating Disorders; Obesity; **Hospital:** Univ Minn Med Ctr, Fairview - Univ Campus; **Address:** Univ Minn, Dept Psychiatry, 2450 Riverside Ave, F282/2A West, Minneapolis, MN 55454; **Phone:** 612-273-9807; **Board Cert:** Psychiatry 1994; Geriatric Psychiatry 1995; **Med School:** Univ Minn 1988; **Resid:** Psychiatry, Univ Minn 1992; **Fellow:** Psychiatry, Univ Minn 1992; **Fac Appt:** Prof Psyc, Univ Minn

Greden, John MD [Psyc] - **Spec Exp:** Anxiety & Mood Disorders; Depression; **Hospital:** Univ Michigan Hlth Sys; **Address:** Univ Mich, Dept Psyc, 4250 Plymouth Rd, Ann Arbor, MI 48109; **Phone:** 734-763-9629; **Board Cert:** Psychiatry 1975; **Med School:** Univ Minn 1967; **Resid:** Psychiatry, Univ Minn Med Ctr 1969; Psychiatry, Walter Reed AMC 1972; **Fac Appt:** Prof Psyc, Univ Mich Med Sch

Janicak, Philip G MD [Psyc] - **Spec Exp:** Psychopharmacology; Mood Disorders; Psychotic Disorders; **Hospital:** Rush Univ Med Ctr; **Address:** Rush Univ Med Ctr, Dept Psych, 1720 W Polk St, M Field Bldg, rm 107, Chicago, IL 60612-4328; **Phone:** 312-942-7287; **Board Cert:** Psychiatry 1978; **Med School:** Loyola Univ-Stritch Sch Med 1973; **Resid:** Psychiatry, McGaw Hosp/Loyola Med Ctr 1976; **Fac Appt:** Prof Psyc, Rush Med Coll

Levine, Stephen B MD [Psyc] - **Spec Exp:** Sexual Dysfunction; Relationship Problems; Sexual Identity Issues; **Hospital:** Univ Hosps Case Med Ctr; **Address:** 23230 Chagrin Blvd, Ste 350, Beachwood, OH 44122-5446; **Phone:** 216-831-2900; **Board Cert:** Psychiatry 1976; **Med School:** Case West Res Univ 1967; **Resid:** Psychiatry, Univ Hosps Cleveland 1973; **Fac Appt:** Clin Prof Psyc, Case West Res Univ

Locala, Joseph MD [Psyc] - **Spec Exp:** Psychiatry in Transplant Patients; Mood Disorders; Anxiety Disorders; **Hospital:** Cleveland Clin Fdn (page 57); **Address:** Cleveland Clinic, 11100 Euclid Ave, Hanna Pavillion, Cleveland, OH 44106; **Phone:** 216-844-3414; **Board Cert:** Psychiatry 1996; **Med School:** Temple Univ 1989; **Resid:** Psychiatry, Medical Ctr Hosp 1993; **Fellow:** Cleveland Clinic 1994

McCallum, Kimberli E MD [Psyc] - **Spec Exp:** Eating Disorders; **Hospital:** St Luke's Hosp - Chesterfield, MO; **Address:** McCallum Place, 100 S Brentwood Blvd, Ste 350, Clayton, MO 63105; **Phone:** 314-863-7700; **Board Cert:** Psychiatry 1993; Child & Adolescent Psychiatry 1994; **Med School:** Yale Univ 1986; **Resid:** Psychiatry, UCLA Neuropsyc Inst 1991; **Fellow:** Child Psychiatry, Washington Univ 1993; **Fac Appt:** Assoc Clin Prof Psyc, Washington Univ, St Louis

Nurnberger Jr, John J MD/PhD [Psyc] - **Spec Exp:** Depression; Mood Disorders; **Hospital:** Indiana Univ Hosp; **Address:** Institute Psychiatric Research-IUMC, 791 Union Dr, Indianapolis, IN 46202-2873; **Phone:** 317-278-4344; **Board Cert:** Psychiatry 1981; **Med School:** Indiana Univ 1975; **Resid:** Psychiatry, Columbia-Presby Med Ctr 1978; **Fac Appt:** Prof Psyc, Indiana Univ

Renshaw, Domeena MD [Psyc] - **Spec Exp:** Sexual Dysfunction; Sexual Problems in Children; **Hospital:** Loyola Univ Med Ctr; **Address:** Loyola Univ Hosp, Dept Psychiatry, 2160 S 1st Ave, Maywood, IL 60153; **Phone:** 708-216-3752; **Board Cert:** Psychiatry 1972; **Med School:** South Africa 1960; **Resid:** Pediatrics, Chldns Hosp/Harvard 1963; Psychiatry, Loyola Univ Med Ctr 1968; **Fac Appt:** Prof Psyc, Loyola Univ-Stritch Sch Med

Strakowski, Stephen M MD [Psyc] - **Spec Exp:** Bipolar/Mood Disorders; Psychotic Disorders; Dual Diagnosis; Addiction/Substance Abuse; **Hospital:** Univ Hosp - Cincinnati; **Address:** Univ Cincinnati Coll Med, Dept Psychiatry, 231 Albert Sabin Way, Cincinnati, OH 45267-0559; **Phone:** 513-558-2958; **Board Cert:** Psychiatry 1993; **Med School:** Vanderbilt Univ 1988; **Resid:** Psychiatry, McLean Hosp-Harvard Med Sch 1992; **Fac Appt:** Prof Psyc, Univ Cincinnati

Wooten, Virgil D MD [Psyc] - **Spec Exp:** Sleep Disorders; **Hospital:** Bethesda North Hosp, Good Samaritan Hosp - Cincinnati; **Address:** Bethesda Sleep Ctr, 10475 Montgomery Rd, Ste 1D, Concinnati, OH 45242; **Phone:** 513-745-1690; **Board Cert:** Psychiatry 1985; **Med School:** Univ Ark 1980; **Resid:** Psychiatry, Univ Hosp-VA Hosp 1984; **Fellow:** Sleep Medicine, Univ Hosp 1985

Zorumski, Charles F MD [Psyc] - **Spec Exp:** Neuro-Psychiatry; Psychopharmacology; **Hospital:** Barnes-Jewish Hosp; **Address:** 660 S Euclid Ave, Box CB8134, St Louis, MO 63110-1010; **Phone:** 314-747-2680; **Board Cert:** Psychiatry 1984; **Med School:** St Louis Univ 1978; **Resid:** Psychiatry, Barnes-Jewish Hosp 1982; **Fac Appt:** Prof Psyc, Washington Univ, St Louis

Great Plains and Mountains

Freedman, Robert MD [Psyc] - **Spec Exp:** Schizophrenia; **Hospital:** Univ Colorado Hosp; **Address:** Univ Colorado, Dept Psychiatry, 4200 E 9th Ave, Box C249-32, Denver, CO 80262; **Phone:** 303-315-8403; **Board Cert:** Psychiatry 1980; **Med School:** Harvard Med Sch 1972; **Resid:** Psychiatry, Univ Chicago Hosps & Clins 1978; **Fellow:** Neuropharmacology, NIMH-Neuropharm Lab / St Elizabeth's Hosp; **Fac Appt:** Prof Psyc, Univ Colorado

Greiner, Carl B MD [Psyc] - **Spec Exp:** Psychiatry in Cancer; Psychiatry in Physical Illness; Palliative Care; Post Traumatic Stress Disorder; **Hospital:** Nebraska Med Ctr; **Address:** Dept of Psychiatry, 2626 St Mary's Ave, Omaha, NE 68105; **Phone:** 402-354-6360; **Board Cert:** Psychiatry 1984; Forensic Psychiatry 1999; **Med School:** Univ Cincinnati 1978; **Resid:** Psychiatry, Univ Cincinnati Med Ctr 1982; **Fac Appt:** Prof Psyc, Univ Nebr Coll Med

Mitchell, James E MD [Psyc] - **Spec Exp:** Eating Disorders; **Hospital:** MeritCare Hosp; **Address:** NeuroPsychiatric Research Inst, 120 S 8th St, 2nd Fl, Fargo, ND 58103; **Phone:** 701-293-1335; **Board Cert:** Psychiatry 1979; **Med School:** Northwestern Univ 1972; **Resid:** Psychiatry, Fairview-Univ Med Ctr 1976; **Fac Appt:** Prof Psyc, Univ ND Sch Med

Weiner, Kenneth L MD [Psyc] - **Spec Exp:** Eating Disorders; **Hospital:** Denver Health Med Ctr; **Address:** Eating Disorder Ctr of Denver, 950 S Cherry St, Ste 1010, Denver, CO 80246; **Phone:** 303-771-0861; **Board Cert:** Psychiatry 1983; **Med School:** Tufts Univ 1977; **Resid:** Psychiatry, Univ Colorado Hlth Sci Ctr 1981; **Fac Appt:** Asst Clin Prof Psyc, Univ Colorado

Wilson, Daniel R MD/PhD [Psyc] - **Spec Exp:** Psychopharmacology; Forensic Psychiatry; **Hospital:** Creighton Univ Med Ctr; **Address:** 3528 Dodge St, Omaha, NE 68131; **Phone:** 402-345-8828; **Board Cert:** Psychiatry 1989; Forensic Psychiatry 1998; **Med School:** Univ Iowa Coll Med 1983; **Resid:** Psychiatry, McLean Hosp 1987; **Fellow:** Geriatric Psychiatry, McLean Hosp 1987; Genetics, Cambridge Univ 1993; **Fac Appt:** Prof Psyc, Creighton Univ

Southwest

Avery, Eric N MD [Psyc] - **Spec Exp:** Depression; Dementia; Arts in the Healing Process; AIDS/HIV Liaison Psychiatry; **Hospital:** UT Med Br Hosp at Galveston; **Address:** Univ Texas Medical Branch, Dept Psychiatry, 301 University Blvd, Route 186, Galveston, TX 77555; **Phone:** 409-747-5784; **Board Cert:** Psychiatry 2003; **Med School:** Univ Tex Med Br, Galveston 1974; **Resid:** Psychiatry, NY State Psych Inst 1978; **Fellow:** Liaison Psychiatry for AIDS/HIV, NY State Psych Inst 1994; **Fac Appt:** Asst Prof Psyc, Univ Tex Med Br, Galveston

Bowden, Charles MD [Psyc] - **Spec Exp:** Bipolar/Mood Disorders; **Hospital:** Univ Hlth Sys - Univ Hosp; **Address:** Univ Tex Hlth Sci Ctr, Dept Psychiatry, 7703 Floyd Curl Drive, MC 7792, San Antonio, TX 78229-3900; **Phone:** 210-567-5555; **Board Cert:** Psychiatry 1970; **Med School:** Baylor Coll Med 1964; **Resid:** Psychiatry, NY State Psyc Inst/Columbia-Presby Med Ctr 1968; **Fac Appt:** Prof Psyc, Univ Tex, San Antonio

Davidson, Joyce Eileen MD [Psyc] - **Spec Exp:** Obsessive-Compulsive Disorder; Bipolar/Mood Disorders; Schizophrenia; **Hospital:** Menninger Clinic; **Address:** 2801 Gessner Drive, Houston, TX 77080; **Phone:** 713-275-5419; **Board Cert:** Psychiatry 1988; **Med School:** Univ MO-Kansas City 1979; **Resid:** Psychiatry, Karl Menninger Sch Psyc 1982; **Fellow:** Child & Adolescent Psychiatry, Karl Menninger Sch Psyc 1984

Gabbard, Glen O MD [Psyc] - **Spec Exp:** Personality Disorders-Borderline; Cognitive Psychotherapy; Psychoanalysis; **Hospital:** Baylor Univ Medical Ctr; **Address:** 6655 Travis, Ste 500, Houston, TX 77030; **Phone:** 713-798-6397; **Board Cert:** Psychiatry 1979; **Med School:** Rush Med Coll 1975; **Resid:** Psychiatry, Menninger Sch Psyc 1978; **Fellow:** Psychoanalysis, Topeka Inst Psychoanalysis 1984; **Fac Appt:** Clin Prof Psyc, Univ Kans

Gelenberg, Alan MD [Psyc] - **Spec Exp:** Psychopharmacology; Mood Disorders; Depression; **Hospital:** Univ Med Ctr - Tucson; **Address:** Univ Arizona, Dept Psychiatry, 1501 N Campbell Ave, Tucson, AZ 85724-5002; **Phone:** 520-626-6586; **Board Cert:** Psychiatry 1975; **Med School:** Univ Pennsylvania 1969; **Resid:** Psychiatry, Mass General Hosp 1973; **Fac Appt:** Prof Psyc, Univ Ariz Coll Med

Haque, Waheedul MD [Psyc] - **Spec Exp:** Depression; Panic Disorder; **Hospital:** UT Med Br Hosp at Galveston; **Address:** Univ Texas Med Branch, Dept Psychiatry, 301 University Blvd, Route 0190, Galveston, TX 77555; **Phone:** 409-747-9722; **Board Cert:** Psychiatry 1970; **Med School:** India 1962; **Resid:** Psychiatry, Barnes Jewish Med Ctr 1969; **Fac Appt:** Prof Psyc, Univ Tex Med Br, Galveston

Hirschfeld, Robert M A MD [Psyc] - **Spec Exp:** Bipolar/Mood Disorders; **Hospital:** UT Med Br Hosp at Galveston; **Address:** 301 University Blvd, 1.302 Rebecca Sealy Hosp, Galveston, TX 77555-0188; **Phone:** 409-747-9791; **Board Cert:** Psychiatry 1975; **Med School:** Univ Mich Med Sch 1968; **Resid:** Psychiatry, Stanford Med Ctr 1972; **Fac Appt:** Prof Psyc, Univ Tex Med Br, Galveston

Mohl, Paul C MD [Psyc] - **Spec Exp:** Psychopharmacology; Psychotherapy; **Hospital:** UT Southwestern Med Ctr - Dallas; **Address:** 5323 Harry Hines Blvd, Dallas, TX 75390-9070; **Phone:** 214-648-7312; **Board Cert:** Psychiatry 1977; **Med School:** Duke Univ 1971; **Resid:** Psychiatry, Duke Univ Hosp 1974; **Fac Appt:** Prof Psyc, Univ Tex SW, Dallas

Trivedi, Madhukar H MD [Psyc] - **Spec Exp:** Depression; Mood Disorders; **Hospital:** UT Southwestern Med Ctr - Dallas, Parkland Meml Hosp - Dallas; **Address:** Univ of Texas Southwestern Med Ctr, 5959 Harry Hines Blvd, Bldg I, Dallas, TX 75235; **Phone:** 214-648-0188; **Board Cert:** Psychiatry 1994; **Med School:** India 1980; **Resid:** Psychiatry, Univ General Hosp 1985; Psychiatry, Henry Ford Hosp 1990; **Fellow:** Brain Imaging, U Texas SW Med Ctr 1992; **Fac Appt:** Prof Psyc, Univ Tex SW, Dallas

Weiner, Myron MD [Psyc] - **Spec Exp:** Psychiatry-Geriatric; Alzheimer's Disease; **Hospital:** UT Southwestern Med Ctr - Dallas; **Address:** Univ Texas SW Med Ctr, 5323 Harry Hines Blvd, Dallas, TX 75390-9129; **Phone:** 214-648-9353; **Board Cert:** Psychiatry 1966; Geriatric Psychiatry 2001; **Med School:** Tulane Univ 1957; **Resid:** Psychiatry, Parkland Hosp 1963; **Fellow:** Geriatric Psychiatry, Mt Sinai Med Ctr 1985; **Fac Appt:** Prof Psyc, Univ Tex SW, Dallas

Yager, Joel MD [Psyc] - **Spec Exp:** Eating Disorders; Depression; **Hospital:** Univ NM Hlth & Sci Ctr; **Address:** Univ NM Sch Med, Dept Psyc/MSC09 5030, 1 University of New Mexico, Albuquerque, NM 87131-0001; **Phone:** 505-272-5416; **Board Cert:** Psychiatry 1971; **Med School:** Albert Einstein Coll Med 1965; **Resid:** Psychiatry, Bronx Muni Hosp Ctr 1969; **Fac Appt:** Prof Psyc, Univ New Mexico

West Coast and Pacific

Burt, Vivien Kleinman MD/PhD [Psyc] - **Spec Exp:** Women's Health-Mental Health; Impulse-Control Disorders; **Hospital:** UCLA Neuropsychiatric Hosp, VA Med Ctr - W Los Angeles; **Address:** 300 Medical Plaza, Ste 2337, Los Angeles, CA 90095; **Phone:** 310-562-4942; **Board Cert:** Psychiatry 1990; **Med School:** McGill Univ 1984; **Resid:** Psychiatry, UCLA-Neurpsyc Inst 1988; **Fac Appt:** Assoc Prof Psyc, UCLA

Bystritsky, Alexander MD/PhD [Psyc] - **Spec Exp:** Obsessive-Compulsive Disorder; Anxiety Disorders; Psychopharmacology; **Hospital:** UCLA Neuropsychiatric Hosp; **Address:** 300 UCLA Med Plaza, Ste 2200, Box 956968, Los Angeles, CA 90095-6968; **Phone:** 310-206-5133; **Board Cert:** Psychiatry 1988; **Med School:** Russia 1977; **Resid:** Psychiatry, NYU Med Ctr 1985; **Fellow:** Psychiatry, UCLA 1987; **Fac Appt:** Prof Psyc, UCLA

Eisendrath, Stuart J MD [Psyc] - **Spec Exp:** Depression; Munchausen Syndrome; Cognitive Psychotherapy; **Hospital:** UCSF Med Ctr; **Address:** UCSF Med Ctr, 401 Parnassus Ave, MC-0984, San Francisco, CA 94143-0984; **Phone:** 415-476-7868; **Board Cert:** Psychiatry 1980; **Med School:** Med Coll Wisc 1974; **Resid:** Psychiatry, Langley Porter NPI 1978; **Fellow:** Liaison Psychiatry, Langley Porter NPI 1979; **Fac Appt:** Prof Psyc, UCSF

Fann, Jesse R MD [Psyc] - **Spec Exp:** Psychiatry in Physical Illness; Psychiatry in Neurological Disorders; Psychiatry in Cancer; **Hospital:** Univ Wash Med Ctr, Harborview Med Ctr; **Address:** Univ Washington Med Ctr, Psychiatry-Box 356560, 1959 NE Pacific St, Seattle, WA 98195-0001; **Phone:** 206-685-3925; **Board Cert:** Psychiatry 2005; **Med School:** Northwestern Univ 1989; **Resid:** Psychiatry, Univ Washington Med Ctr 1993; **Fellow:** Liaison Psychiatry, Univ Washington Med Ctr 1995; **Fac Appt:** Asst Prof Psyc, Univ Wash

Friedman, Barry MD [Psyc] - **Spec Exp:** Psychopharmacology; Psychoanalysis; **Address:** 435 N Bedford Dr, Ste 112, Beverly Hills, CA 90210; **Phone:** 310-274-4372; **Board Cert:** Psychiatry 1974; **Med School:** UCSF 1965; **Resid:** Psychiatry, UCLA Med Ctr 1971; **Fellow:** Psychoanalysis, Los Angeles Psychoanalytic Inst 1992; **Fac Appt:** Assoc Clin Prof Psyc, UCLA

Gitlin, Michael Jay MD [Psyc] - **Spec Exp:** Mood Disorders; **Hospital:** UCLA Neuropsychiatric Hosp; **Address:** UCLA NPI-Mood Disorders Clinic, 300 Medical Plaza, Ste 2200, Los Angeles, CA 90095-6968; **Phone:** 310-206-3654; **Board Cert:** Psychiatry 1981; **Med School:** Univ Pennsylvania 1975; **Resid:** Psychiatry, UCLA Med Ctr 1979; **Fac Appt:** Prof Psyc, UCLA

Guilleminault, Christian MD [Psyc] - **Spec Exp:** Sleep Disorders/Apnea; **Hospital:** Stanford Univ Med Ctr; **Address:** 401 Quarry Rd, Ste 3301A, Stanford, CA 94305; **Phone:** 650-723-6601; **Med School:** France 1968; **Fac Appt:** Prof Psyc, Stanford Univ

Keepers, George MD [Psyc] - **Spec Exp:** Neuro-Psychiatry; ADD/ADHD; **Hospital:** OR Hlth & Sci Univ; **Address:** 3181 SW Sam Jackson Park Rd, MC UHN80, Portland, OR 97239; **Phone:** 503-494-8144; **Board Cert:** Psychiatry 1984; **Med School:** Baylor Coll Med 1977; **Resid:** Psychiatry, Oregon Hlth Sci Univ 1981; **Fac Appt:** Prof Psyc, Oregon Hlth Sci Univ

Koran, Lorrin Michael MD [Psyc] - **Spec Exp:** Depression; Obsessive-Compulsive Disorder; Compulsive Shopping/Buying; **Hospital:** Stanford Univ Med Ctr; **Address:** Stanford Med Ctr, Dept Psychiatry, 401 Quarry Rd, rm 2363, Stanford, CA 94305; **Phone:** 650-723-2423; **Board Cert:** Psychiatry 1973; **Med School:** Harvard Med Sch 1966; **Resid:** Psychiatry, Stanford Univ Hosp 1970; **Fac Appt:** Prof Psyc, Stanford Univ

Leuchter, Andrew Francis MD [Psyc] - **Spec Exp:** Depression; **Hospital:** UCLA Neuropsychiatric Hosp; **Address:** 10833 Le Conte Ave, rm 37-452, Los Angeles, CA 90095; **Phone:** 310-825-0207; **Board Cert:** Psychiatry 1986; Geriatric Psychiatry 2001; **Med School:** Baylor Coll Med 1980; **Resid:** Psychiatry, UCLA-Neuro Psyc Inst & Hosp 1984; **Fellow:** Geriatric Psychiatry, UCLA Med Ctr 1986; **Fac Appt:** Prof Psyc, UCLA

Liberman, Robert Paul MD [Psyc] - **Spec Exp:** Schizophrenia; Psychotic Disorders; Psychiatric Rehabilitation; **Hospital:** UCLA Neuropsychiatric Hosp; **Address:** UCLA Neuropsychiatric Institute, 760 Westwood Plaza, Los Angeles, CA 90095; **Phone:** 310-206-1616; **Board Cert:** Psychiatry 1969; **Med School:** Johns Hopkins Univ 1963; **Resid:** Psychiatry, Mass Mntl Hlth Ctr 1967; **Fellow:** Pharmacology, UCSF Med Ctr 1961; Research, Harvard Med Sch 1968; **Fac Appt:** Prof Psyc, UCLA

Marder, Stephen Robert MD [Psyc] - **Spec Exp:** Schizophrenia; Psychopharmacology; **Hospital:** VA Med Ctr - W Los Angeles, UCLA Med Ctr; **Address:** West Los Angeles VA - Gr LA Hlth Svcs, 11301 Wilshire Blvd, Bldg MIRECC 210A, Los Angeles, CA 90073; **Phone:** 310-268-3647; **Board Cert:** Psychiatry 1977; **Med School:** SUNY Buffalo 1971; **Resid:** Psychiatry, LAC-USC Med Ctr 1975; **Fac Appt:** Prof Psyc, UCLA

Marmar, Charles MD [Psyc] - **Spec Exp:** Post Traumatic Stress Disorder; Bereavement/Traumatic Grief; **Hospital:** VA Med Ctr - San Francisco; **Address:** 4150 Clement St Bldg 8 - rm 320-1, Mental Hlth Svc 116A, San Francisco, CA 94941; **Phone:** 415-221-4810 x3436; **Board Cert:** Psychiatry 1982; **Med School:** Univ Manitoba 1970; **Resid:** Psychiatry, Univ Toronto Hosp 1976; **Fellow:** Anxiety Disorder, Langley Porter Inst-UCSF 1978; **Fac Appt:** Prof Psyc, UCSF

Nelson, J Craig MD [Psyc] - **Spec Exp:** Geriatric Psychiatry; Psychopharmacology; Mood Disorders; **Hospital:** UCSF Med Ctr; **Address:** UCSF-Langley Porter Psychiatric Inst, 401 Parnassus Ave, Box 0984, San Francisco, CA 94143-0984; **Phone:** 415-476-7500; **Board Cert:** Psychiatry 1974; Geriatric Psychiatry 2002; **Med School:** Univ Wisc 1968; **Resid:** Psychiatry, Yale-New Haven Hosp 1970; Psychiatry, Yale-New Haven Hosp 1974; **Fac Appt:** Prof Psyc, UCSF

Neppe, Vernon M MD/PhD [Psyc] - **Spec Exp:** Neuro-Psychiatry; Psychopharmacology; Forensic Psychiatry; Behavioral Disorders; **Hospital:** Northwest Hosp, Overlake Hosp Med Ctr; **Address:** Pacific Neuropsychiatric Inst, 10330 Meridian Ave N, Ste 380, Seattle, WA 98133-9463; **Phone:** 206-527-6289; **Board Cert:** Psychiatry 1988; Forensic Psychiatry 1994; Geriatric Psychiatry 2001; **Med School:** South Africa 1973; **Resid:** Neurology, Univ Witwatersrand 1979; Psychiatry, Univ Witwatersrand 1980; **Fellow:** Psychopharmacology, NY Hosp/Cornell Med Ctr 1983; Neuropsychiatry, NY Hosp/Cornell Med Ctr 1983

Norman, Kim Peter MD [Psyc] - **Spec Exp:** Eating Disorders/Obesity; Personality Disorders; Dual Diagnosis; **Hospital:** UCSF Med Ctr; **Address:** UCSF-Langley Porter Psyc Inst, 401 Parnassus Ave, rm 250, Box A-221, San Francisco, CA 94143; **Phone:** 415-476-7402; **Board Cert:** Psychiatry 1983; **Med School:** Albert Einstein Coll Med 1977; **Resid:** Psychiatry, Langley Porter Psyc Inst 1981; **Fac Appt:** Clin Prof Psyc, UCSF

Pi, Edmond Hsin-Tung MD [Psyc] - **Spec Exp:** Psychopharmacology; Cross-Cultural Psychiatry; Anxiety Disorders; **Hospital:** LAC & USC Med Ctr; **Address:** LAC USC Healthcare Network, 1200 N State St, rm 10-621, Los Angeles, CA 90033; **Phone:** 323-226-7975; **Board Cert:** Psychiatry 1980; **Med School:** South Korea 1972; **Resid:** Psychiatry, SUNY-Stony Brook Affil Hosp 1977; Psychiatry, Univ Kentucky Hosp-Chandler Med Ctr 1978; **Fac Appt:** Prof Psyc, USC Sch Med

Pynoos, Robert Sidney MD [Psyc] - **Spec Exp:** Post Traumatic Stress Disorder; **Hospital:** UCLA Neuropsychiatric Hosp; **Address:** Natl Ctr for Child Traumatic Stress-UCLA, 11150 W Olympic Blvd, Ste 650, Los Angeles, CA 90064; **Phone:** 310-235-2633; **Board Cert:** Psychiatry 1980; **Med School:** Columbia P&S 1972; **Resid:** Pediatrics, Mt Sinai Hosp; Psychiatry, NY Presby-Cornell Med Ctr; **Fac Appt:** Prof Psyc, UCLA

Raskind, Murray MD [Psyc] - **Spec Exp:** Geriatric Psychiatry; Alzheimer's Disease; Post Traumatic Stress Disorder; **Hospital:** VA Puget Sound Hlth Care Sys, Univ Wash Med Ctr; **Address:** VA Puget Sound Health Care System, Mental Hlth Svc 116, 1660 S Columbia Way, Seattle, WA 98108; **Phone:** 206-768-5375; **Board Cert:** Psychiatry 1976; Geriatric Psychiatry 2001; **Med School:** Columbia P&S 1968; **Resid:** Internal Medicine, Harlem Hosp Ctr 1970; Psychiatry, Univ Wash Affil Hosps 1973; **Fac Appt:** Prof Psyc, Univ Wash

Reus, Victor I MD [Psyc] - **Spec Exp:** Psychopharmacology; Bipolar/Mood Disorders; Behavioral Disorders; **Hospital:** UCSF Med Ctr; **Address:** 401 Parnassus Ave, San Francisco, CA 94143-0984; **Phone:** 415-476-7478; **Board Cert:** Psychiatry 1977; Geriatric Psychiatry 2000; **Med School:** Univ MD Sch Med 1973; **Resid:** Psychiatry, Univ Wisc Med Ctr 1976; **Fellow:** Biological Psychiatry, Natl Inst Mntl Hlth 1978; **Fac Appt:** Prof Psyc, UCSF

Roy-Byrne, Peter MD [Psyc] - **Spec Exp:** Anxiety & Mood Disorders; Panic Disorder; Bipolar/Mood Disorders; Post Traumatic Stress Disorder; **Hospital:** Harborview Med Ctr, Univ Wash Med Ctr; **Address:** 325 9th Ave, Box 359911, Seattle, WA 98104; **Phone:** 206-341-4200; **Board Cert:** Psychiatry 1983; **Med School:** Tufts Univ 1978; **Resid:** Psychiatry, UCLA Neuropsych Inst 1982; **Fellow:** Biological Psychiatry, Natl Inst Hlth - NIMH 1984; **Fac Appt:** Prof Psyc, Univ Wash

Schatzberg, Alan F MD [Psyc] - **Spec Exp:** Anxiety & Mood Disorders; Psychopharmacology; **Hospital:** Stanford Univ Med Ctr; **Address:** Stanford Univ, Dept Psychiatry, 401 Quarry Rd, Ste 3301A, Stanford, CA 94305-5717; **Phone:** 650-723-6811; **Board Cert:** Psychiatry 1975; **Med School:** NYU Sch Med 1968; **Resid:** Psychiatry, Mass Mental Hlth Ctr 1972; **Fellow:** Psychiatry, Mass Mental Hlth Ctr/Harvard 1972; **Fac Appt:** Prof Psyc, Stanford Univ

Spiegel, David MD [Psyc] - **Spec Exp:** Hypnosis; Psychiatry in Cancer; Post Traumatic Stress Disorder; **Hospital:** Stanford Univ Med Ctr; **Address:** Stanford Univ Sch Medicine, Dept Psychiatry & Behavioral Sciences, 401 Quarry Rd, rm 2325, Stanford, CA 94305-5718; **Phone:** 650-723-6421; **Board Cert:** Psychiatry 1976; **Med School:** Harvard Med Sch 1971; **Resid:** Psychiatry, Mass Mental Hlth Ctr 1974; Psychiatry, Cambridge Hosp-Harvard Med Sch 1974; **Fellow:** Community Psychiatry, Harvard Med Sch 1974; **Fac Appt:** Prof Psyc, Stanford Univ

Stein, Murray Brent MD [Psyc] - **Spec Exp:** Anxiety Disorders; Panic Disorder; Post Traumatic Stress Disorder; **Hospital:** UCSD Med Ctr, VA San Diego Hlthcre Sys; **Address:** UCSD Dept Psychiatry, 8950 Villa La Jolla Drive, Ste B218, La Jolla, CA 92037; **Phone:** 858-534-6400; **Board Cert:** Psychiatry 1989; **Med School:** Univ Manitoba 1983; **Resid:** Psychiatry, Univ Toronto Hosp 1986; Psychiatry, Natl Inst Mental Hlth-NIH 1987; **Fellow:** Anxiety Disorder, Natl Inst Mental Hlth-NIH 1990; **Fac Appt:** Prof Psyc, UCSD

Strouse, Thomas B MD [Psyc] - **Spec Exp:** Psychiatry in Cancer; Pain-Cancer; Psychiatry in Physical Illness; Psychopharmacology; **Hospital:** Cedars-Sinai Med Ctr, UCLA Med Ctr; **Address:** Cedars-Sinai Outpatient Cancer Ctr, 8700 Beverly Blvd, Ste C2000, Los Angeles, CA 90048-1804; **Phone:** 310-423-0637; **Board Cert:** Psychiatry 1993; Pain Medicine 2000; **Med School:** Case West Res Univ 1987; **Resid:** Psychiatry, UCLA Med Ctr 1991; **Fac Appt:** Assoc Clin Prof Psyc, UCLA

Sullivan, Mark MD/PhD [Psyc] - **Spec Exp:** Psychiatry in Heart Disease Patients; Pain-Chronic; Psychiatry in Terminal Illness; **Hospital:** Univ Wash Med Ctr; **Address:** Univ Washington, Dept Psych, 1959 NE Pacific St, Box 356560, Seattle, WA 98195; **Phone:** 206-543-3925; **Board Cert:** Psychiatry 1991; **Med School:** Vanderbilt Univ 1984; **Resid:** Psychiatry, Univ Washington Med Ctr 1988; **Fac Appt:** Assoc Prof Psyc, Univ Wash

Weinstock, Robert MD [Psyc] - **Spec Exp:** Adolescent Psychiatry; Addiction/Substance Abuse; **Hospital:** Cedars-Sinai Med Ctr; **Address:** 1823 Sawtelle Blvd, Los Angeles, CA 90025; **Phone:** 310-477-9933; **Board Cert:** Psychiatry 1975; Forensic Psychiatry 2004; Addiction Psychiatry 1996; **Med School:** NYU Sch Med 1966; **Resid:** Psychiatry, McLean Hosp 1970; Child & Adolescent Psychiatry, McLean Hosp 1972; **Fellow:** Psychiatric Research, Boston Univ 1974; **Fac Appt:** Clin Prof Psyc, UCLA

Zerbe, Kathryn J MD [Psyc] - **Spec Exp:** Eating Disorders; Women's Health-Mental Health; Psychoanalysis; **Hospital:** OR Hlth & Sci Univ; **Address:** 3181 SW Sam Jackson Park Rd, MC OP02, Portland, OR 97201-3098; **Phone:** 503-494-1009; **Board Cert:** Psychiatry 1984; **Med School:** Temple Univ 1978; **Resid:** Psychiatry, Menninger Clin 1982; Psychoanalysis, Topeka Inst for Psychoanalysis 1992; **Fac Appt:** Prof Psyc, Oregon Hlth Sci Univ

Zisook, Sidney MD [Psyc] - **Spec Exp:** Bereavement/Traumatic Grief; Depression; Suicide; **Hospital:** VA San Diego Hlthcre Sys, UCSD Med Ctr; **Address:** UCSD, Dept Psychiatry, 9500 Gilman Drive, MS 9116A, La Jolla, CA 92093; **Phone:** 858-534-4040; **Board Cert:** Psychiatry 1975; **Med School:** Loyola Univ-Stritch Sch Med 1969; **Resid:** Psychiatry, Mass Genl Hosp 1973; **Fellow:** Psychiatry, Harvard 1973; **Fac Appt:** Prof Psyc, UCSD

Addiction Psychiatry

New England

Schottenfeld, Richard MD [AdP] - **Spec Exp:** Drug Abuse; Alcohol Abuse; **Hospital:** Yale - New Haven Hosp; **Address:** Connecticut Mental Health Ctr, 34 Park St, rm S-204, New Haven, CT 06519; **Phone:** 203-974-7349; **Board Cert:** Psychiatry 1984; **Med School:** Yale Univ 1976; **Resid:** Psychiatry, Yale Psych Inst 1982; **Fellow:** Epidemiology, Yale Univ 1984; **Fac Appt:** Assoc Prof Psyc, Yale Univ

Ziedonis, Douglas M MD [AdP] - **Spec Exp:** Nicotine Dependence; **Hospital:** UMass Memorial Med Ctr; **Address:** U Mass Medical School, Dept Psychiatry, 55 Lake Ave N, Worcester, MA 01655; **Phone:** 508-856-3066; **Board Cert:** Psychiatry 1994; Addiction Psychiatry 2006; **Med School:** Penn State Univ-Hershey Med Ctr 1985; **Resid:** Psychiatry, UCLA Med Ctr 1989; **Fellow:** Addiction Psychiatry, UCLA Med Ctr 1990; **Fac Appt:** Prof Psyc, Univ Mass Sch Med

Mid Atlantic

Frances, Richard J MD [AdP] - **Spec Exp:** Alcohol Abuse; Substance Abuse; Forensic Psychiatry; **Hospital:** Silver Hill Hosp, NYU Med Ctr (page 67); **Address:** 510 E 86th St, Ste 1D, New York, NY 10028; **Phone:** 212-861-0570; **Board Cert:** Psychiatry 1976; Addiction Psychiatry 2002; **Med School:** NYU Sch Med 1971; **Resid:** Psychiatry, Bronx Meml Hosp 1974; **Fellow:** Psychoanalysis, NY Psychanal Inst 1978; **Fac Appt:** Clin Prof Psyc, NYU Sch Med

Galanter, Marc MD [AdP] - **Spec Exp:** Alcohol Abuse; Drug Abuse; **Hospital:** NYU Med Ctr (page 67); **Address:** 285 Central Park West, New York, NY 10024-3006; **Phone:** 212-877-4093; **Board Cert:** Psychiatry 1974; Addiction Psychiatry 2002; **Med School:** Albert Einstein Coll Med 1967; **Resid:** Psychiatry, Bronx Muni Hosp-Einstein 1971; **Fac Appt:** Prof Psyc, NYU Sch Med

Kampman, Kyle M MD [AdP] - **Spec Exp:** Addiction/Substance Abuse; Cocaine Addiction; Opiate Addiction; **Hospital:** Hosp Univ Penn - UPHS (page 72); **Address:** Univ Penn Treatment Rsch Ctr, 3900 Chesnut St, Philadelphia, PA 19104; **Phone:** 215-222-3815; **Board Cert:** Psychiatry 2004; Addiction Psychiatry 2006; **Med School:** Tulane Univ 1985; **Resid:** Psychiatry, Univ Penn 1993; **Fellow:** Substance Abuse, Univ Penn 1994; **Fac Appt:** Assoc Prof Psyc, Univ Pennsylvania

Kleber, Herbert MD [AdP] - **Spec Exp:** Opiate Addiction; Cocaine Addiction; Drug Abuse; **Hospital:** NY-Presby Hosp/Columbia (page 66), NY State Psychiatric Inst; **Address:** 1051 Riverside Dr, New York, NY 10032-1007; **Phone:** 212-543-5570; **Med School:** Jefferson Med Coll 1960; **Resid:** Psychiatry, Yale-New Haven Hosp 1964; **Fac Appt:** Prof Psyc, Columbia P&S

Strain, Eric C MD [AdP] - **Spec Exp:** Addiction/Substance Abuse; Dual Diagnosis; Opiate Addiction; **Hospital:** Johns Hopkins Bayview Med Ctr (page 61); **Address:** 4940 Eastern Ave, Baltimore, MD 21224; **Phone:** 410-550-0016; **Board Cert:** Psychiatry 1989; Addiction Psychiatry 2002; **Med School:** Ohio State Univ 1984; **Resid:** Psychiatry, Johns Hopkins Hosp 1988; **Fellow:** Addiction Psychiatry, Johns Hopkins Hosp 1990; **Fac Appt:** Prof Psyc, Johns Hopkins Univ

Southeast

Anton, Raymond F MD [AdP] - **Spec Exp:** Alcohol Abuse; Clinical Trials; **Hospital:** MUSC Med Ctr; **Address:** MUSC Dept Psychiatry, 67 President St, PO Box 250861, Charleston, SC 29425; **Phone:** 843-792-1226; **Board Cert:** Psychiatry 1982; Addiction Psychiatry 1997; **Med School:** UMDNJ-Rutgers Med Sch 1976; **Resid:** Psychiatry, Yale-New Haven Hosp/CT Mental Health Ctr 1980; **Fac Appt:** Prof Psyc, Med Univ SC

Brady, Kathleen T MD/PhD [AdP] - **Spec Exp:** Addiction/Substance Abuse; **Hospital:** MUSC Med Ctr; **Address:** MUSC Inst of Psychiatry, 67 President St, Box 250861, Charleston, SC 29425; **Phone:** 843-792-9888; **Board Cert:** Psychiatry 1992; Addiction Psychiatry 2002; **Med School:** Med Univ SC 1985; **Resid:** Psychiatry, Med Univ SC 1989; **Fellow:** Addiction Psychiatry, Med Univ SC 1989; **Fac Appt:** Prof Psyc, Med Univ SC

McCance-Katz, Elinore F MD/PhD [AdP] - **Spec Exp:** Addiction/Substance Abuse; Psychopharmacology; **Hospital:** Med Coll of VA Hosp; **Address:** Med Coll Va, Dept Psychiatry, 1200 E Broad St, Box 980109, Richmond, VA 23298-0109; **Phone:** 804-828-5351; **Board Cert:** Psychiatry 1993; Addiction Psychiatry 2002; **Med School:** Univ Conn 1987; **Resid:** Psychiatry, Inst of Living 1990; Psychiatry, Yale Univ Sch Med 1991; **Fellow:** Neuropsychopharmacology, Yale Univ Sch Med 1991; **Fac Appt:** Prof Psyc, Med Coll VA

Midwest

Miller, Sheldon I MD [AdP] - **Spec Exp:** Addiction/Substance Abuse; **Hospital:** Northwestern Meml Hosp; **Address:** 40 Timberline Drive, Lemont, IL 60439; **Phone:** 630-257-9600; **Board Cert:** Psychiatry 1972; **Med School:** Tufts Univ 1964; **Resid:** Psychiatry, Univ Hosps 1968; **Fac Appt:** Prof Psyc, Northwestern Univ

Great Plains and Mountains

Crowley, Thomas J MD [AdP] - **Spec Exp:** Addiction/Substance Abuse; Conduct Disorder; **Hospital:** Univ Colorado Hosp; **Address:** 4200 E 9th Ave, Box C268-35, Denver, CO 80262; **Phone:** 303-315-7573; **Board Cert:** Psychiatry 1971; **Med School:** Univ Minn 1962; **Resid:** Psychiatry, Univ Minnesota Hosp 1966; **Fac Appt:** Prof Psyc, Univ Colorado

Howell, Elizabeth F MD [AdP] - **Spec Exp:** Opiate Addiction; Alcohol Abuse; Addiction/Substance Abuse; Pain Management; **Hospital:** Univ Utah Hosps and Clins; **Address:** Univ Utah Neuropsychiatric Inst, 501 Chipeta Way, Salt Lake City, UT 84108; **Phone:** 801-585-1575; **Board Cert:** Psychiatry 1985; Addiction Psychiatry 2003; **Med School:** Med Univ SC 1980; **Resid:** Psychiatry, Med Univ South Carolina 1984; **Fellow:** Psychiatric Research, Med Univ South Carolina 1985; **Fac Appt:** Assoc Clin Prof Psyc, Univ Utah

Child & Adolescent Psychiatry

Southwest

Kosten, Thomas MD [AdP] - **Spec Exp:** Cocaine Addiction; Alcohol Abuse; Psychopharmacology; Opiate Addiction; **Hospital:** VA Med Ctr N TX Hlth Sys, UT MD Anderson Cancer Ctr (page 71); **Address:** Michael DeBakey VA Medical Ctr, 2002 Holcombe Blvd, Research - Building 110, Houston, TX 77030; **Phone:** 713-794-7032; **Board Cert:** Psychiatry 1984; Addiction Psychiatry 2002; **Med School:** Cornell Univ-Weill Med Coll 1977; **Resid:** Psychiatry, Yale-New Haven Hosp 1981; **Fellow:** Epidemiology, Yale-New Haven Hosp 1983; **Fac Appt:** Prof Psyc, Baylor Coll Med

West Coast and Pacific

Schuckit, Marc A MD [AdP] - **Spec Exp:** Alcohol Abuse; Psychopharmacology; **Hospital:** VA San Diego Hlthcre Sys; **Address:** VA San Diego Healthcare System, Dept Psychiatry (116A), 3350 La Jolla Village Drive, San Diego, CA 92161-2002; **Phone:** 858-552-8585 x7978; **Board Cert:** Psychiatry 1974; **Med School:** Washington Univ, St Louis 1968; **Resid:** Psychiatry, Washington Univ 1971; Psychiatry, UC San Diego 1972; **Fac Appt:** Prof Psyc, UCSD

Walker, R Dale MD [AdP] - **Spec Exp:** Alcohol Abuse; Drug Abuse; Substance Abuse; **Hospital:** OR Hlth & Sci Univ; **Address:** 840 SW Gaines Rd, MC GH156, Portland, OR 97239; **Phone:** 503-494-3703; **Board Cert:** Psychiatry 1982; Addiction Psychiatry 1993; **Med School:** Univ Okla Coll Med 1972; **Resid:** Psychiatry, Univ Oklahoma Med Ctr 1973; Psychiatry, UCSD Med Ctr 1977; **Fellow:** Public Health & Genl Preventive Med, Andriga Stampur; **Fac Appt:** Prof Psyc, Oregon Hlth Sci Univ

Child & Adolescent Psychiatry

New England

Biederman, Joseph MD [ChAP] - **Spec Exp:** ADD/ADHD; Anxiety & Mood Disorders; Psychopharmacology; **Hospital:** Mass Genl Hosp; **Address:** 55 Fruit St Yawkey Bldg - rm 6900, Boston, MA 02114; **Phone:** 617-726-1743; **Board Cert:** Psychiatry 1983; Child & Adolescent Psychiatry 1984; **Med School:** Brazil 1971; **Resid:** Psychiatry, Hadassah Univ Hosp 1977; Child & Adolescent Psychiatry, Harvard Chldns Hosp 1979; **Fellow:** Psychiatry, Mass Genl Hosp 1981; **Fac Appt:** Prof Psyc, Harvard Med Sch

Coyle, Joseph MD [ChAP] - **Spec Exp:** Neuro-Psychiatry; Psychiatric Genetics; Mental Retardation; **Hospital:** McLean Hosp; **Address:** McLean Hospital, 115 Mill St, Belmont, MA 02478-1048; **Phone:** 617-855-2101; **Board Cert:** Psychiatry 1980; **Med School:** Johns Hopkins Univ 1969; **Resid:** Psychiatry, Johns Hopkins Hosp 1976; **Fellow:** Psychopharmacology, NIMH 1973; **Fac Appt:** Prof Psyc, Harvard Med Sch

Fritz, Gregory K MD [ChAP] - **Spec Exp:** Asthma; Psychosomatic Disorders; **Hospital:** Rhode Island Hosp; **Address:** RI Hosp, Child & Family Psychiatry, 1 Hoppin St Fl 2, Providence, RI 02903; **Phone:** 401-444-7573; **Board Cert:** Psychiatry 1977; Child & Adolescent Psychiatry 1978; **Med School:** Tufts Univ 1971; **Resid:** Psychiatry, San Mateo Co Hosp 1974; Child & Adolescent Psychiatry, Stanford Univ Med Ctr 1977; **Fac Appt:** Prof Psyc, Brown Univ

Herzog, David B MD [ChAP] - **Spec Exp:** Eating Disorders; Somatic Disorders-Adolescent; **Hospital:** Mass Genl Hosp; **Address:** 2 Longfellow Place, Ste 200, Boston, MA 02114; **Phone:** 617-724-0799; **Board Cert:** Pediatrics 1980; Psychiatry 1982; Child & Adolescent Psychiatry 1986; **Med School:** Mexico 1973; **Resid:** Pediatrics, Univ Wisc 1975; Pediatrics, Boston City Hosp 1976; **Fellow:** Child & Adolescent Psychiatry, Chldns Hosp 1978; Psychiatry, Mass Genl Hosp 1980; **Fac Appt:** Prof Psyc, Harvard Med Sch

Hudziak, James MD [ChAP] - **Spec Exp:** ADD/ADHD; Obsessive-Compulsive Disorder; Psychopharmacology; **Hospital:** FAHC - Med Ctr Campus; **Address:** Univ Vermont Med Sch, Dept Psychiatry, 1 S Prospect Dr, MCHS-Arnold 6-UHC Campus, Burlington, VT 05401; **Phone:** 802-847-4560; **Board Cert:** Psychiatry 2005; Child & Adolescent Psychiatry 2005; **Med School:** Univ Minn 1988; **Resid:** Child & Adolescent Psychiatry, St Louis Chldns Hosp 1991; **Fac Appt:** Assoc Prof Psyc, Univ VT Coll Med

King, Robert A MD [ChAP] - **Spec Exp:** Tourette's Syndrome; Obsessive-Compulsive Disorder; Psychoanalysis; **Hospital:** Yale - New Haven Hosp; **Address:** 230 S Frontage Rd, Box 207900, New Haven, CT 06519-1124; **Phone:** 203-785-5880; **Board Cert:** Psychiatry 1974; Child & Adolescent Psychiatry 1981; **Med School:** Harvard Med Sch 1968; **Resid:** Pediatrics, Chldns Hosp 1969; Psychiatry, Mass Mental Hlth Ctr 1971; **Fellow:** Child Psychiatry, Chldns Hosp 1972; Child Psychiatry, Chldns Hosp Natl Med Ctr 1974; **Fac Appt:** Prof Psyc, Yale Univ

Leckman, James F MD [ChAP] - **Spec Exp:** Tourette's Syndrome; Obsessive-Compulsive Disorder; Autism; **Hospital:** Yale - New Haven Hosp; **Address:** Yale Child Study Ctr, 230 S Frontage Rd, Box 207900, New Haven, CT 06520; **Phone:** 203-785-7971; **Board Cert:** Psychiatry 1980; Child & Adolescent Psychiatry 1982; **Med School:** Univ New Mexico 1973; **Resid:** Psychiatry, Yale Univ 1979; Child & Adolescent Psychiatry, Yale Chld Stdy Ctr 1980; **Fellow:** Psychiatry, Natl Inst Mental Hlth 1976; **Fac Appt:** Prof Psyc, Yale Univ

Leonard, Henrietta MD [ChAP] - **Spec Exp:** Neuro-Psychiatry; Anxiety Disorders; Obsessive-Compulsive Disorder; **Hospital:** Rhode Island Hosp; **Address:** RI Hosp, Child & Family Psyc, 593 Eddy St, Providence, RI 02903; **Phone:** 401-444-3762; **Board Cert:** Psychiatry 1987; Child & Adolescent Psychiatry 1988; **Med School:** Geo Wash Univ 1982; **Resid:** Psychiatry, Geo Wash Univ Med Ctr 1985; **Fellow:** Child & Adolescent Psychiatry, Chldns Hosp 1987; **Fac Appt:** Prof Psyc, Brown Univ

Spencer, Thomas MD [ChAP] - **Spec Exp:** ADD/ADHD; **Hospital:** Mass Genl Hosp; **Address:** Mass General Hospital, 55 Fruit St, Ste YAW 6900, Boston, MA 02114; **Phone:** 617-726-1731; **Board Cert:** Psychiatry 1984; Child & Adolescent Psychiatry 1993; **Med School:** Univ Wisc 1978; **Resid:** Psychiatry, New England Med Ctr 1984; **Fellow:** Child & Adolescent Psychiatry, Mass General Hosp 1992; **Fac Appt:** Assoc Prof Psyc, Harvard Med Sch

Volkmar, Fred R MD [ChAP] - **Spec Exp:** Autism; Asperger's Syndrome; Developmental Disorders; Mental Retardation; **Hospital:** Yale - New Haven Hosp; **Address:** Yale Child Study Ctr, 230 S Frontage Rd, Box 207900, New Haven, CT 06519-1124; **Phone:** 203-785-2510; **Board Cert:** Psychiatry 1981; Child & Adolescent Psychiatry 1988; **Med School:** Stanford Univ 1976; **Resid:** Psychiatry, Stanford Univ 1980; Child & Adolescent Psychiatry, Yale Univ Child Study Ctr 1982; **Fac Appt:** Prof Psyc, Yale Univ

Child & Adolescent Psychiatry

Wilens, Timothy MD [ChAP] - **Spec Exp:** ADD/ADHD; Bipolar/Mood Disorders; Addiction/Substance Abuse; **Hospital:** Mass Genl Hosp; **Address:** Mass Genl Hosp, Dept Psyc, 55 Fruit St Yawkey Bldg - Ste 6A, Boston, MA 02114; **Phone:** 617-724-5600; **Board Cert:** Psychiatry 1990; Child & Adolescent Psychiatry 1991; Addiction Psychiatry 1994; **Med School:** Univ Mich Med Sch 1985; **Resid:** Internal Medicine, Henry Ford Hosp 1986; Psychiatry, Mass Genl Hosp 1988; **Fellow:** Child & Adolescent Psychiatry, Mass Genl Hosp 1990; **Fac Appt:** Assoc Prof Psyc, Harvard Med Sch

Mid Atlantic

Abright, Arthur R MD [ChAP] - **Spec Exp:** Bipolar/Mood Disorders; ADD/ADHD; Post Traumatic Stress Disorder; Autism; **Hospital:** St Vincent Cath Med Ctrs - Manhattan; **Address:** 144 W 12th St, New York, NY 10011-8202; **Phone:** 212-604-8213; **Board Cert:** Psychiatry 1978; Child & Adolescent Psychiatry 1981; **Med School:** Univ Tex SW, Dallas 1973; **Resid:** Psychiatry, St Vincent's Hosp 1974; Psychiatry, NY Hosp-Cornell Med Ctr 1977; **Fellow:** Child & Adolescent Psychiatry, NY Hosp-Cornell Med Ctr 1979; **Fac Appt:** Clin Prof Psyc, NY Med Coll

Bird, Hector MD [ChAP] - **Spec Exp:** ADD/ADHD; Anxiety & Depression; Personality Disorders; **Hospital:** NY-Presby Hosp/Columbia (page 66); **Address:** 145 Central Park West, Ste 1CC, New York, NY 10023-2004; **Phone:** 212-874-5311; **Board Cert:** Psychiatry 1975; Child & Adolescent Psychiatry 1977; **Med School:** Yale Univ 1965; **Resid:** Psychiatry, NY State Psych Inst 1971; Child & Adolescent Psychiatry, NY State Psych Inst 1972; **Fellow:** Psychoanalysis, WA White Institute 1977; **Fac Appt:** Prof Psyc, Columbia P&S

Bogrov, Michael MD [ChAP] - **Spec Exp:** ADD/ADHD; Mood Disorders; **Hospital:** Sheppard Pratt Hlth Sys, Johns Hopkins Hosp - Baltimore (page 61); **Address:** 6501 N Charles St, P.O. Box 6815, Towson, MD 21204-6815; **Phone:** 410-938-4913; **Board Cert:** Psychiatry 1993; Child & Adolescent Psychiatry 1994; **Med School:** Emory Univ 1987; **Resid:** Psychiatry, Univ Maryland 1990; Child & Adolescent Psychiatry, Johns Hopkins Hosp 1992; **Fac Appt:** Asst Prof Psyc, Johns Hopkins Univ

Brent, David A MD [ChAP] - **Spec Exp:** Suicide; **Hospital:** UPMC Presby, Pittsburgh; **Address:** Western Psych Inst & Clinic, 3811 O'Hara St, Ste 315 BFT, Pittsburgh, PA 15213-2593; **Phone:** 412-246-5596; **Board Cert:** Pediatrics 1981; Psychiatry 1982; Child & Adolescent Psychiatry 1983; **Med School:** Jefferson Med Coll 1974; **Resid:** Psychiatry, Western Psych Inst 1982; **Fellow:** Psychiatry, Univ Colorado Med Ctr 1976; **Fac Appt:** Prof Psyc, Univ Pittsburgh

Coffey, Barbara J MD [ChAP] - **Spec Exp:** Tourette's Syndrome; ADD/ADHD; Obsessive-Compulsive Disorder; **Hospital:** NYU Med Ctr (page 67); **Address:** NYU Child Study Ctr, 577 1st Ave, New York, NY 10016; **Phone:** 212-263-3926; **Board Cert:** Psychiatry 1981; Child & Adolescent Psychiatry 1986; **Med School:** Tufts Univ 1975; **Resid:** Psychiatry, Boston Univ 1978; Child & Adolescent Psychiatry, Tufts Univ 1980; **Fac Appt:** Assoc Prof Psyc, NYU Sch Med

Egan, James Harold MD [ChAP] - **Spec Exp:** Psychopharmacology; Psychotherapy; Behavioral Disorders; Mood Disorders; **Hospital:** Brook Lane Hlth Services; **Address:** Brook Lane Health Services, 13218 Brook Lane Dr, PO Box 1945, Hagerstown, MD 21742; **Phone:** 301-733-0330; **Board Cert:** Psychiatry 1973; Child & Adolescent Psychiatry 1975; **Med School:** Columbia P&S 1964; **Resid:** Psychiatry, St Vincents Hosp 1969; Child & Adolescent Psychiatry, St Lukes Hosp 1971; **Fac Appt:** Clin Prof Ped, Geo Wash Univ

Foley, Carmel MD [ChAP] - **Spec Exp:** Mood Disorders; **Hospital:** Schneider Chldn's Hosp; **Address:** Schneider Chldns Hosp, 269-01 76th Ave Fl 4, New Hyde Park, NY 11040; **Phone:** 718-470-3550; **Board Cert:** Psychiatry 1979; Child & Adolescent Psychiatry 1981; Addiction Psychiatry 1997; Forensic Psychiatry 1999; **Med School:** Ireland 1972; **Resid:** Psychiatry, St Patrick's Hosp 1976; Psychiatry, Lafayette Clinic 1977; **Fellow:** Child & Adolescent Psychiatry, Lafayette Clinic 1979; **Fac Appt:** Assoc Prof Psyc, Albert Einstein Coll Med

Fornari, Victor MD [ChAP] - **Spec Exp:** Eating Disorders; Trauma Psychiatry; **Hospital:** N Shore Univ Hosp at Manhasset, Long Island Jewish Med Ctr; **Address:** N Shore Univ Hosp, Dept Psychiatry, 400 Community Drive, Manhasset, NY 11030-3815; **Phone:** 516-562-3051; **Board Cert:** Psychiatry 1984; Child & Adolescent Psychiatry 1985; **Med School:** SUNY Downstate 1979; **Resid:** Psychiatry, Hosp Univ Penn 1982; **Fellow:** Child & Adolescent Psychiatry, LIJ Med Ctr 1984; **Fac Appt:** Assoc Prof Psyc, NYU Sch Med

Greenspan, Stanley MD [ChAP] - **Spec Exp:** Autism; Infant/Toddler Psychiatry; **Hospital:** G Washington Univ Hosp; **Address:** 7201 Glenbrook Rd, Bethesda, MD 20814; **Phone:** 301-657-2348; **Board Cert:** Psychiatry 1972; **Med School:** Yale Univ 1966; **Resid:** Psychiatry, Columbia-Presby Psych Inst 1969; **Fellow:** Child & Adolescent Psychiatry, Childrens Hosp Natl Med Ctr 1971; **Fac Appt:** Clin Prof Psyc, Geo Wash Univ

Hertzig, Margaret MD [ChAP] - **Spec Exp:** Developmental Disorders; ADD/ADHD; **Hospital:** NY-Presby Hosp/Weill Cornell (page 66); **Address:** 525 E 68th St, Box 140, New York, NY 10021; **Phone:** 212-746-5712; **Board Cert:** Psychiatry 1968; Child & Adolescent Psychiatry 1975; **Med School:** NYU Sch Med 1960; **Resid:** Pediatrics, Jewish Hosp 1962; Psychiatry, Bellevue Psych Hosp 1964; **Fellow:** Psychiatric Research, NYU Sch Med 1966; **Fac Appt:** Prof Psyc, Cornell Univ-Weill Med Coll

Kestenbaum, Clarice J MD [ChAP] - **Spec Exp:** Anxiety Disorders; Psychodynamic Psychotherapy; **Hospital:** NY-Presby Hosp/Columbia (page 66); **Address:** 15 W 81st St, New York, NY 10032; **Phone:** 212-873-1020; **Board Cert:** Psychiatry 1971; Child & Adolescent Psychiatry 1975; **Med School:** UCLA 1960; **Resid:** Psychiatry, Columbia Presby Med Ctr 1963; Child & Adolescent Psychiatry, Columbia Presby Med Ctr 1965; **Fac Appt:** Clin Prof Psyc, Columbia P&S

Koplewicz, Harold MD [ChAP] - **Spec Exp:** Anxiety Disorders; Psychopharmacology; **Hospital:** NYU Med Ctr (page 67), Bellevue Hosp Ctr; **Address:** NYU Child Study Center, 577 First Ave, Ste 221A, New York, NY 10016; **Phone:** 212-263-6205; **Board Cert:** Psychiatry 1983; Child & Adolescent Psychiatry 1984; **Med School:** Albert Einstein Coll Med 1978; **Resid:** Psychiatry, New York Hosp-Westchester Div 1981; Child & Adolescent Psychiatry, NY State Psyc Inst 1983; **Fellow:** Psychiatric Research, NY State Psyc Inst 1985; **Fac Appt:** Prof Psyc, NYU Sch Med

Pomeroy, John C MD [ChAP] - **Spec Exp:** Autism; Mental Retardation; Developmental Disorders; **Hospital:** Stony Brook Univ Med Ctr; **Address:** The Cody Center for Autism, 5 Medical Drive, Port Jefferson Stn, NY 11776; **Phone:** 631-632-3070; **Board Cert:** Psychiatry 1984; Child & Adolescent Psychiatry 1988; **Med School:** England 1973; **Resid:** Psychiatry, St.Mary's Hosp 1979; **Fellow:** Child & Adolescent Psychiatry, Univ Iowa Hosps 1981; **Fac Appt:** Assoc Prof Psyc, SUNY Stony Brook

Pruitt, David B MD [ChAP] - **Hospital:** Univ of MD Med Sys; **Address:** Univ Maryland, Div Child & Adolescent Psychiatry, 701 S Pratt St, Ste 429, Baltimore, MD 21201; **Phone:** 410-328-3522; **Board Cert:** Psychiatry 1979; Child & Adolescent Psychiatry 1981; **Med School:** Univ Tex, Houston 1974; **Resid:** Psychiatry, Hosp Univ Penn 1978; Child & Adolescent Psychiatry, Child Guidance Ctr 1979; **Fac Appt:** Prof Psyc, Univ MD Sch Med

Rapoport, Judith MD [ChAP] - **Spec Exp:** Schizophrenia; Obsessive-Compulsive Disorder; **Hospital:** Natl Inst of Hlth - Clin Ctr; **Address:** NIMH-Child Psychiatry Bldg 10, 10 Center Dr, MSC 1600, rm 3N202, Bethesda, MD 20892-1600; **Phone:** 301-496-6081; **Board Cert:** Psychiatry 1969; Child & Adolescent Psychiatry 1969; **Med School:** Harvard Med Sch 1959; **Resid:** Psychiatry, Mass Mental Hlth Ctr 1961; Psychiatry, St Elizabeth Hosp 1962; **Fellow:** Karolinska Inst 1964; Child & Adolescent Psychiatry, Childns Hosp 1966

Riddle, Mark A MD [ChAP] - **Spec Exp:** Psychopharmacology; Anxiety Disorders; Mood Disorders; **Hospital:** Johns Hopkins Hosp - Baltimore (page 61), Mt Washington Ped Hosp; **Address:** 600 N Wolfe St, CMSC-346, Baltimore, MD 21287-3325; **Phone:** 410-955-2320; **Board Cert:** Psychiatry 1982; Child & Adolescent Psychiatry 1986; **Med School:** Indiana Univ 1977; **Resid:** Psychiatry, Yale-New Haven Hosp 1981; **Fellow:** Child & Adolescent Psychiatry, Yale Child Study Ctr 1983; **Fac Appt:** Prof Psyc, Johns Hopkins Univ

Rostain, Anthony L MD [ChAP] - **Spec Exp:** ADD/ADHD; Autism; Tourette's Syndrome; Asperger's Syndrome; **Hospital:** Chldns Hosp of Philadelphia, The, Penn Presby Med Ctr - UPHS (page 72); **Address:** Hosp U Penn, Dept Psychiatry, 3535 Market St Fl 2, Philadelphia, PA 19104; **Phone:** 215-746-7210; **Board Cert:** Pediatrics 1985; Psychiatry 1988; Child & Adolescent Psychiatry 1989; **Med School:** NYU Sch Med 1980; **Resid:** Pediatrics, Children's Hosp 1983; Psychiatry, Hosp U Penn 1987; **Fellow:** Child Psychiatry, Philadelphia Child Guidance Clin 1988; **Fac Appt:** Assoc Prof Psyc, Univ Pennsylvania

Ryan, Neal D MD [ChAP] - **Spec Exp:** Mood Disorders; Depression; **Hospital:** Western Psych Inst & Clin - UPMC; **Address:** Western Psyc Inst & Clinic, 3811 O'Hara St, TDH - rm 720E, Pittsburgh, PA 15213-2593; **Phone:** 412-246-5316; **Board Cert:** Psychiatry 1983; Child & Adolescent Psychiatry 1987; **Med School:** Yale Univ 1978; **Resid:** Psychiatry, NY State Psych Inst 1982; **Fellow:** Psychiatric Research, Columbia Univ 1984; **Fac Appt:** Prof Psyc, Univ Pittsburgh

Turecki, Stanley K MD [ChAP] - **Spec Exp:** Temperamentally Difficult Child; ADD/ADHD; Parenting Issues; **Hospital:** Lenox Hill Hosp (page 62), Beth Israel Med Ctr - Petrie Division; **Address:** 136 E 64th St, Ste 1B, New York, NY 10021-2137; **Phone:** 212-355-2535; **Board Cert:** Psychiatry 1978; Child & Adolescent Psychiatry 1981; **Med School:** South Africa 1961; **Resid:** Psychiatry, Tara Hospital 1969; Child & Adolescent Psychiatry, Mt Sinai Hosp 1971

Walkup, John MD [ChAP] - **Spec Exp:** Anxiety Disorders; **Hospital:** Johns Hopkins Hosp - Baltimore (page 61); **Address:** Johns Hopkins Hosp, Dept Child Psyc, 600 N Wolfe St, CMSC 314, Baltimore, MD 21287; **Phone:** 410-955-5823 x1; **Board Cert:** Psychiatry 1987; Child & Adolescent Psychiatry 1992; **Med School:** Univ Minn 1982; **Resid:** Psychiatry, Yale Univ Med Sch 1985; Child & Adolescent Psychiatry, Yale Chld Study Ctr 1988; **Fac Appt:** Asst Prof Psyc, Johns Hopkins Univ

Southeast

Deas, Deborah V MD [ChAP] - **Spec Exp:** Addiction/Substance Abuse; Dual Diagnosis; Substance Abuse in ADHD Patients; **Hospital:** MUSC Med Ctr; **Address:** MUSC, Ctr for Drug & Alcohol Programs, 67 President St, Charleston, SC 29425; **Phone:** 843-792-5214; **Board Cert:** Psychiatry 2005; Addiction Psychiatry 1997; **Med School:** Med Univ SC 1989; **Resid:** Psychiatry, MUSC Med Ctr 1992; **Fellow:** Child & Adolescent Psychiatry, MUSC Med Ctr 1994; Addiction Psychiatry, MUSC/Natl Inst Alcohol Abuse & Alcoholism 1994; **Fac Appt:** Prof Psyc, Med Univ SC

Heston, Jerry D MD [ChAP] - **Hospital:** Le Bonheur Chldns Med Ctr, St Jude Children's Research Hosp; **Address:** Child & Adolescent Psychiatric Assocs, 1135 Cully Rd, Ste 100, Cordova, TN 38106; **Phone:** 901-752-1980; **Board Cert:** Psychiatry 1988; Pediatrics 2004; Child & Adolescent Psychiatry 1989; **Med School:** Univ S Fla Coll Med 1981; **Resid:** Pediatrics, LeBonheur Chldns Hosp 1984; Psychiatry, Univ Tennessee 1986; **Fellow:** Child & Adolescent Psychiatry, Univ Tennessee 1988

March, John MD [ChAP] - **Spec Exp:** Anxiety Disorders; Obsessive-Compulsive Disorder; **Hospital:** Duke Univ Med Ctr; **Address:** Duke Univ Med Ctr- Box 3527, 718 Rutherford St, Durham, NC 27710; **Phone:** 919-416-2404; **Board Cert:** Psychiatry 1992; Child & Adolescent Psychiatry 1992; **Med School:** UCLA 1978; **Resid:** Family Medicine, Santa Monica Hosp Med Ctr 1981; Psychiatry, Univ Wisconsin Hosp 1988; **Fellow:** Child & Adolescent Psychiatry, Univ Wisconsin Hosp 1990; **Fac Appt:** Prof Psyc, Duke Univ

Sexson, Sandra G B MD [ChAP] - **Spec Exp:** Psychiatry in Transplant Patients; Death & Dying; **Hospital:** Med Coll of GA Hosp and Clin; **Address:** Medical College Georgia, Div Child/Adolescent Psych, 1515 Pope Ave, Augusta, GA 30912; **Phone:** 706-721-6699; **Board Cert:** Psychiatry 1980; Child & Adolescent Psychiatry 1981; **Med School:** Univ Miss 1971; **Resid:** Psychiatry, Tex Hlth Sci Ctr 1974; Child & Adolescent Psychiatry, Washington Univ 1978; **Fellow:** Child & Adolescent Psychiatry, Washington Univ 1978; **Fac Appt:** Prof Psyc, Med Coll GA

Wright, Harry MD [ChAP] - **Spec Exp:** Infant/Toddler Psychiatry; Autism & Developmental Disorders; Anxiety Disorders; **Hospital:** William S Hall Psyc Inst, Richland Mem Hosp; **Address:** 3555 Harden St, Ste 104, Columbia, SC 29203-6894; **Phone:** 803-434-4250; **Board Cert:** Psychiatry 1982; Child & Adolescent Psychiatry 1984; **Med School:** Univ Pennsylvania 1976; **Resid:** Psychiatry, William S Hall Psyc Inst 1979; **Fellow:** Child & Adolescent Psychiatry, William S Hall Psyc Inst-Univ South Carolina 1981; **Fac Appt:** Prof Psyc, Univ SC Sch Med

Midwest

Alessi, Norman E MD [ChAP] - **Spec Exp:** Mood Disorders; Telepsychiatry; Psychopharmacology; **Hospital:** Univ Michigan Hlth Sys; **Address:** 825 Victors Way, Ste 310, Ann Arbor, MI 48108-2830; **Phone:** 734-222-6222; **Board Cert:** Psychiatry 1982; Child & Adolescent Psychiatry 1985; **Med School:** Emory Univ 1976; **Resid:** Psychiatry, Univ Mich Med Ctr 1980; Child & Adolescent Psychiatry, Univ Mich Med Ctr 1981; **Fellow:** Child & Adolescent Psychiatry, Univ Mich Med Ctr 1983; **Fac Appt:** Prof Emeritus Psyc, Univ Mich Med Sch

Boxer, Gary MD [ChAP] - **Spec Exp:** ADD/ADHD; Parenting Issues; Mood Disorders; **Hospital:** St Louis Chldns Hosp; **Address:** St Louis Chldns Hosp, Dept Psychiatry, 24 S Kingshighway Blvd, St Louis, MO 63108; **Phone:** 314-286-1740; **Board Cert:** Psychiatry 1986; Child & Adolescent Psychiatry 1988; **Med School:** Univ Colorado 1980; **Resid:** Psychiatry, Univ Michigan Med Ctr 1983; **Fellow:** Child Psychiatry, Univ Colorado 1985; **Fac Appt:** Assoc Prof Psyc

Child & Adolescent Psychiatry

Campo, John V MD [ChAP] - **Spec Exp:** Psychosomatic Disorders; Psychiatry in Physical Illness; **Hospital:** Chldn's Hosp - Columbus, Ohio St Univ Med Ctr; **Address:** Columbus Chldn's Hosp, 700 Childrens Drive, Timken Hall H2K, Columbus, OH 43205; **Phone:** 614-722-2291; **Board Cert:** Pediatrics 1986; Psychiatry 1989; Child & Adolescent Psychiatry 1993; **Med School:** Univ Pennsylvania 1982; **Resid:** Pediatrics, Childrens Hosp 1985; Psychiatry, West Psych Inst Clin 1989

Dulcan, Mina K MD [ChAP] - **Spec Exp:** ADD/ADHD; **Hospital:** Children's Mem Hosp; **Address:** Chldns Meml Hosp, Dept Psyc, 2300 Children's Plaza, Box 10, Chicago, IL 60614; **Phone:** 773-880-4811; **Board Cert:** Psychiatry 1978; Child & Adolescent Psychiatry 1979; **Med School:** Penn State Univ-Hershey Med Ctr 1974; **Resid:** Psychiatry, Western Psych Inst/Clinic 1977; Child & Adolescent Psychiatry, Western Psych Inst/Clinic 1978; **Fac Appt:** Prof Psyc, Northwestern Univ

Leventhal, Bennett MD [ChAP] - **Spec Exp:** Autism; ADD/ADHD; Psychopharmacology; **Hospital:** Univ of IL Med Ctr at Chicago; **Address:** Univ Illinois, Dept Psychiatry, 1747 W Roosevelt Rd, MC 747, Chicago, IL 60608; **Phone:** 312-355-3026; **Board Cert:** Psychiatry 1979; Child & Adolescent Psychiatry 1980; **Med School:** Louisiana State Univ 1974; **Resid:** Psychiatry, Duke Univ Med Ctr 1978; **Fellow:** Child & Adolescent Psychiatry, Duke Univ Med Ctr 1977; **Fac Appt:** Prof Psyc, Univ IL Coll Med

Luby, Joan L MD [ChAP] - **Spec Exp:** Mood Disorders in Preschool Children; Autism; **Hospital:** Barnes-Jewish Hosp; **Address:** Wash Univ Sch Med, Dept Psychiatry, 660 S Euclid Ave, Box 8134, St Louis, MO 63110; **Phone:** 314-286-2730; **Board Cert:** Psychiatry 1993; Child & Adolescent Psychiatry 1993; **Med School:** Wayne State Univ 1985; **Resid:** Psychiatry, Stanford Univ Sch Med 1988; **Fellow:** Child & Adolescent Psychiatry, Stanford Univ Sch Med 1990; **Fac Appt:** Assoc Prof Psyc, Washington Univ, St Louis

McDougle, Christopher J MD [ChAP] - **Spec Exp:** Autism & Developmental Disorders; Obsessive-Compulsive Disorder; Tourette's Syndrome; **Hospital:** Riley Hosp for Children, Methodist Hosp - Indianapolis; **Address:** 1111 W 10th St, Psychiatry Bldg - rm A-305, Indianapolis, IN 46202-4800; **Phone:** 317-274-8162; **Board Cert:** Psychiatry 1992; Child & Adolescent Psychiatry 2006; **Med School:** Indiana Univ 1986; **Resid:** Psychiatry, Yale Univ 1990; **Fellow:** Child & Adolescent Psychiatry, Yale Child Study Ctr 1995; **Fac Appt:** Prof Psyc, Indiana Univ

Slomowitz, Marcia MD [ChAP] - **Spec Exp:** ADD/ADHD; Bipolar/Mood Disorders; Depression; **Hospital:** Northwestern Meml Hosp; **Address:** 333 N Michigan Ave, Ste 1125, Chicago, IL 60601; **Phone:** 312-726-1083; **Board Cert:** Psychiatry 1982; Child & Adolescent Psychiatry 1983; **Med School:** Univ Wisc 1977; **Resid:** Psychiatry, Univ Cincinnati 1980; **Fellow:** Child & Adolescent Psychiatry, Univ Cincinnati 1982; **Fac Appt:** Asst Prof Psyc, Northwestern Univ

Todd, Richard D MD/PhD [ChAP] - **Spec Exp:** ADD/ADHD; Mood Disorders; Autism; **Hospital:** St Louis Chldns Hosp; **Address:** St Louis Chldns Hosp, Dept Psychiatry, 24 S Kingshighway Blvd, St Louis, MO 63108; **Phone:** 314-286-1740; **Board Cert:** Psychiatry 1988; Child & Adolescent Psychiatry 1989; **Med School:** Univ Tex, San Antonio 1981; **Resid:** Psychiatry, Stanford Univ Med Ctr 1984; **Fellow:** Child Psychiatry, Wash Univ 1986; **Fac Appt:** Prof Psyc, Washington Univ, St Louis

Great Plains and Mountains

Sokol, Mae Sandra MD [ChAP] - **Spec Exp:** Eating Disorders; Obesity; Compulsive Exercise; **Hospital:** Creighton Univ Med Ctr, Children's Hosp - Omaha; **Address:** Creighton Univ School of Medicine, 3528 Dodge St, Omaha, NE 68131; **Phone:** 402-345-7100; **Board Cert:** Psychiatry 1986; Child & Adolescent Psychiatry 1987; **Med School:** Belgium 1980; **Resid:** Psychiatry, Bellevue Hosp-NYU Med Ctr 1984; **Fellow:** Child & Adolescent Psychiatry, Bellevue Hosp-NYU Med Ctr 1986; **Fac Appt:** Assoc Prof Psyc, Creighton Univ

Southwest

Bleiberg, Efrain MD [ChAP] - **Spec Exp:** Trauma Psychiatry; Personality Disorders; **Hospital:** Menninger Clinic; **Address:** Menninger Hosp & Clinic, 2801 Gessner Drive, Box 809045, Houston, TX 77280-9045; **Phone:** 713-275-5213; **Board Cert:** Psychiatry 1985; Child & Adolescent Psychiatry 1986; **Med School:** Mexico 1976; **Resid:** Psychiatry, Menninger Fdn 1980; **Fellow:** Child & Adolescent Psychiatry, Menninger Fdn 1981

Emslie, Graham J MD [ChAP] - **Spec Exp:** Depression; **Hospital:** Chldns Med Ctr of Dallas; **Address:** UT SW Med Ctr at Dallas, 5323 Harry Hines Blvd, Dallas, TX 75390-8589; **Phone:** 214-456-5921; **Board Cert:** Psychiatry 1981; **Med School:** Scotland 1974; **Resid:** Psychiatry, Univ Rochester 1978; Child & Adolescent Psychiatry, Stanford Med Ctr 1981; **Fac Appt:** Prof Psyc, Univ Tex SW, Dallas

Sargent III, A John MD [ChAP] - **Spec Exp:** Eating Disorders; Suicide; Family Therapy; Trauma Psychiatry; **Hospital:** Ben Taub General Hosp, Texas Chldns Hosp - Houston; **Address:** Baylor Coll Med, Dept Psychiatry, One Baylor Plaza, Houston, TX 77030-3411; **Phone:** 713-798-7889; **Board Cert:** Pediatrics 1979; Psychiatry 1988; Child & Adolescent Psychiatry 1989; **Med School:** Univ Rochester 1973; **Resid:** Pediatrics, Univ Wisc Hosp 1977; Child & Adolescent Psychiatry, Phila Child Guidance Ctr 1980; **Fellow:** Ambulatory Pediatrics, Univ Wisc Hosp 1976; **Fac Appt:** Prof Psyc, Baylor Coll Med

Zeanah Jr, Charles H MD [ChAP] - **Spec Exp:** Attachment Disorders; Abuse/Neglect; Adoption-International; **Hospital:** Tulane Univ Hosp & Clin; **Address:** Tulane Univ Sch Med, Dept Psych & Neurology, 1440 Canal St, TB-52, New Orleans, LA 70112-2715; **Phone:** 504-988-5402; **Board Cert:** Psychiatry 1983; Child & Adolescent Psychiatry 1983; **Med School:** Tulane Univ 1977; **Resid:** Psychiatry, Duke Univ Med Ctr 1980; Child & Adolescent Psychiatry, Stanford Univ Med Ctr 1982; **Fellow:** Research, Stanford Univ Med ctr 1984; **Fac Appt:** Prof Psyc, Tulane Univ

West Coast and Pacific

King, Bryan H MD [ChAP] - **Spec Exp:** Mental Retardation; Autism; Self-Injurious Behavior (SIB); **Hospital:** Chldns Hosp and Regl Med Ctr - Seattle; **Address:** Chldns Hosp & Regl Med Ctr, Dept Psych, 4800 Sand Point Way NE, MS W3636, Seattle, WA 98105; **Phone:** 206-987-2760; **Board Cert:** Psychiatry 1991; Child & Adolescent Psychiatry 2004; **Med School:** Med Coll Wisc 1983; **Resid:** Psychiatry, UCLA Neuropsych Inst 1987; **Fellow:** Child & Adolescent Psychiatry, UCLA Neuropsych Inst 1990; **Fac Appt:** Prof Psyc, Univ Wash

McCracken, James Thomas MD [ChAP] - **Spec Exp:** Obsessive-Compulsive Disorder; Tourette's Syndrome; **Hospital:** UCLA Neuropsychiatric Hosp; **Address:** UCLA Neuropsyc Hosp, 760 Westwood Plaza, Ste 48-270, Los Angeles, CA 90027; **Phone:** 310-825-0470; **Board Cert:** Psychiatry 1986; Child & Adolescent Psychiatry 1988; **Med School:** Baylor Coll Med 1980; **Resid:** Psychiatry, Duke Univ Med Ctr 1984; **Fellow:** Child & Adolescent Psychiatry, UCLA Neuropsych Inst 1985; **Fac Appt:** Prof Psyc, UCLA

McKelvey, Robert S MD [ChAP] - **Spec Exp:** Suicide; Depression; Cross-Cultural Psychiatry; **Hospital:** Doernbecher Chldns Hosp/OHSU; **Address:** Oregon Hlth Sci Univ, 3181 SW Sam Jackson Park Rd, MC DC7P, Portland, OR 97239; **Phone:** 503-418-5775; **Board Cert:** Psychiatry 1980; Child & Adolescent Psychiatry 1982; **Med School:** Dartmouth Med Sch 1974; **Resid:** Psychiatry, Cambridge Hosp 1977; Child & Adolescent Psychiatry, McLean Hosp 1979; **Fac Appt:** Prof Psyc, Oregon Hlth Sci Univ

Ponton, Lynn Elisabeth MD [ChAP] - **Spec Exp:** Behavioral Disorders; Eating Disorders; **Hospital:** UCSF Med Ctr; **Address:** 201 Edgewood Ave, San Francisco, CA 94117; **Phone:** 415-664-3039; **Board Cert:** Psychiatry 1985; Child & Adolescent Psychiatry 1985; **Med School:** Univ Wisc 1978; **Resid:** Psychiatry, Hosp Univ Penn 1980; Psychiatry, UCSF Med Ctr 1981; **Fellow:** Child & Adolescent Psychiatry, UCSF Med Ctr 1983; **Fac Appt:** Prof Psyc, UCSF

Russell, Andrew T MD [ChAP] - **Spec Exp:** ADD/ADHD; Schizophrenia; Developmental Disorders; **Hospital:** UCLA Neuropsychiatric Hosp; **Address:** Neuropsych Inst - UCLA, 760 Westwood Plaza, Los Angeles, CA 90024; **Phone:** 310-825-0389; **Board Cert:** Psychiatry 1980; Child & Adolescent Psychiatry 1988; **Med School:** Univ Colorado 1970; **Resid:** Psychiatry, UCLA Med Ctr 1973; **Fellow:** Child & Adolescent Psychiatry, UCLA Med Ctr 1977; **Fac Appt:** Prof Psyc, UCLA

Steiner, Hans MD [ChAP] - **Spec Exp:** Aggression Disorders; Eating Disorders; Trauma Psychiatry; **Hospital:** Stanford Univ Med Ctr; **Address:** Division Child Psych & Child Devlp, 401 Quarry Rd, Ste MC 5719, Stanford, CA 94305-5719; **Phone:** 650-723-5511; **Board Cert:** Psychiatry 1979; Child & Adolescent Psychiatry 1981; **Med School:** Austria 1972; **Resid:** Psychiatry, SUNY Syracuse Med Ctr 1976; **Fellow:** Child & Adolescent Psychiatry, Univ Mich Hosps 1978; **Fac Appt:** Prof Psyc, Stanford Univ

Terr, Lenore Cagen MD [ChAP] - **Spec Exp:** Trauma Psychiatry; Forensic Psychiatry; Psychotherapy; **Hospital:** UCSF Med Ctr; **Address:** 450 Sutter St, Ste 2534, San Francisco, CA 94108-4204; **Phone:** 415-433-7800; **Board Cert:** Psychiatry 1968; Child & Adolescent Psychiatry 1969; **Med School:** Univ Mich Med Sch 1961; **Resid:** Psychiatry, Univ Mich Med Ctr 1964; **Fellow:** Child & Adolescent Psychiatry, Univ Mich 1966; **Fac Appt:** Clin Prof Psyc, UCSF

Geriatric Psychiatry

Mid Atlantic

Greenwald, Blaine MD [GerPsy] - **Spec Exp:** Depression; Dementia; **Hospital:** Long Island Jewish Med Ctr, N Shore Univ Hosp at Forest Hills; **Address:** 75-59 263rd St, Div Geriatric Psychiatry, Glen Oaks, NY 11004; **Phone:** 718-470-8159; **Board Cert:** Psychiatry 1983; Geriatric Psychiatry 2001; **Med School:** NY Med Coll 1978; **Resid:** Psychiatry, Mount Sinai Hosp 1982; **Fellow:** Geriatric Psychiatry, Mount Sinai Hosp/Bronx VA Hosp 1983; **Fac Appt:** Assoc Prof Psyc, Albert Einstein Coll Med

Kennedy, Gary MD [GerPsy] - **Spec Exp:** Alzheimer's Disease; Dementia; Depression; **Hospital:** Montefiore Med Ctr; **Address:** Dept Psyc & Behav Science, 446 E 86th St, rm 11C, New York, NY 10028; **Phone:** 718-920-4236; **Board Cert:** Psychiatry 1980; Geriatric Psychiatry 2000; Psychosomatic Medicine 2005; **Med School:** Univ Tex, San Antonio 1975; **Resid:** Psychiatry, VA Hosp-Univ Texas 1979; **Fellow:** Geriatric Psychiatry, Montefiore Hosp 1984; **Fac Appt:** Prof Psyc, Albert Einstein Coll Med

Klement, Maria MD [GerPsy] - **Spec Exp:** Dementia; **Hospital:** Sheppard Pratt Hlth Sys; **Address:** 6501 N Charles St, Central Gibson Bldg, rm 109, Baltimore, MD 21285; **Phone:** 410-938-5000; **Board Cert:** Psychiatry 1972; **Med School:** Med Coll PA Hahnemann 1959; **Resid:** Psychiatry, Philadelphia Genl Hosp 1962; Psychiatry, Sheppard Pratt Hosp 1963

Lyketsos, Constantine G MD [GerPsy] - **Spec Exp:** Alzheimer's Disease; Neuro-Psychiatry; Depression; **Hospital:** Johns Hopkins Hosp - Baltimore (page 61), Johns Hopkins Bayview Med Ctr (page 61); **Address:** Johns Hopkins Hosp, 550 N Broadway, Ste 308, Baltimore, MD 21205; **Phone:** 410-550-0062; **Board Cert:** Psychiatry 1994; Geriatric Psychiatry 1995; Psychosomatic Medicine 2005; **Med School:** Washington Univ, St Louis 1988; **Resid:** Psychiatry, Johns Hopkins Hosp 1992; **Fellow:** Neuropsychiatry, Johns Hopkins Hosp 1994; **Fac Appt:** Prof Psyc, Johns Hopkins Univ

Reisberg, Barry MD [GerPsy] - **Spec Exp:** Alzheimer's Disease; Dementia; Depression; **Hospital:** NYU Med Ctr (page 67); **Address:** Aging & Dementia Rsch Ctr - NYU, 550 First Ave, THN 316, New York, NY 10016; **Phone:** 212-263-8550; **Board Cert:** Psychiatry 1976; Geriatric Psychiatry 2000; **Med School:** NY Med Coll 1972; **Resid:** Psychiatry, Metropolitan Hosp 1975; **Fellow:** Psychiatric Research, Univ London 1975; **Fac Appt:** Prof Psyc, NYU Sch Med

Rosen, Jules MD [GerPsy] - **Spec Exp:** Alzheimer's Disease; Dementia; **Hospital:** Western Psych Inst & Clin - UPMC, UPMC Presby, Pittsburgh; **Address:** Western Psych Inst & Clin, 3811 O'Hara St, Pittsburgh, PA 15213; **Phone:** 412-246-5900; **Board Cert:** Psychiatry 1984; Geriatric Psychiatry 2003; **Med School:** Univ Cincinnati 1978; **Resid:** Psychiatry, Univ Mich Med Ctr 1982; **Fac Appt:** Prof Psyc, Univ Pittsburgh

Rovner, Barry W MD [GerPsy] - **Spec Exp:** Alzheimer's Disease; Behavioral Problems & Dementia; Depression; **Hospital:** Thomas Jefferson Univ Hosp; **Address:** Jefferson Hospital for Neuroscience, 900 Walnut St Fl 4, Philadelphia, PA 19107; **Phone:** 215-503-1254; **Board Cert:** Psychiatry 1985; Geriatric Psychiatry 2000; **Med School:** Jefferson Med Coll 1980; **Resid:** Psychiatry, Johns Hopkins Hosp 1984; **Fac Appt:** Assoc Prof Psyc, Jefferson Med Coll

Streim, Joel E MD [GerPsy] - **Spec Exp:** Psychiatry in Chronic Medical Illness; Psychiatric Barriers to Physical Rehab; Alzheimer's Disease; **Hospital:** Hosp Univ Penn - UPHS (page 72), VA Med Ctr; **Address:** Univ Penn, Dept Geriatric Psychiatry, 3535 Market St Fl 3, Philadelphia, PA 19104; **Phone:** 215-615-3086; **Board Cert:** Psychiatry 1988; Geriatric Psychiatry 2000; **Med School:** Univ Rochester 1978; **Resid:** Psychiatry, Univ Wisconsin 1985; **Fellow:** Liaison Psychiatry, Univ Rochester/Strong Mem 1981; Geriatric Psychiatry, VA Med Ctr 1988; **Fac Appt:** Prof Psyc, Univ Pennsylvania

Geriatric Psychiatry

Southeast

Holroyd, Suzanne MD [GerPsy] - **Spec Exp:** Dementia; Psychoses-Late Onset; Mood Disorders; **Hospital:** Univ Virginia Med Ctr; **Address:** Univ of Virginia Health Sys, Dept Psych, Box 800623, Chalottesville, VA 22908; **Phone:** 434-924-2241; **Board Cert:** Psychiatry 1992; Geriatric Psychiatry 2004; **Med School:** Univ VA Sch Med 1986; **Resid:** Psychiatry, Johns Hopkins Hosp 1990; **Fellow:** Geriatric Psychiatry, Johns Hopkins Hosp 1991; **Fac Appt:** Prof Psyc, Univ VA Sch Med

Stein, Elliott M MD [GerPsy] - **Spec Exp:** Anxiety & Depression; Memory Disorders; Dementia; Stress Management; **Hospital:** Mount Sinai Med Ctr - Miami; **Address:** Mount Sinai Med Ctr, 4300 Alton Rd, Warner Bldg, Ste 360, Miami Beach, FL 33140; **Phone:** 305-534-3636; **Board Cert:** Psychiatry 1979; Geriatric Psychiatry 2001; **Med School:** Univ Miami Sch Med 1973; **Resid:** Psychiatry, Herrick Meml Hosp 1976; **Fac Appt:** Assoc Clin Prof Psyc, Univ Miami Sch Med

Tune, Larry MD [GerPsy] - **Spec Exp:** Alzheimer's Disease; Dementia; Psychopharmacology; Psychoses-Late Onset; **Hospital:** Wesley Woods Ger Hosp; **Address:** Wesley Woods Health Ctr, Dept Psychiatry, 1841 Clifton Rd NE, Atlanta, GA 30329; **Phone:** 404-728-4969; **Board Cert:** Psychiatry 1991; Geriatric Psychiatry 2004; **Med School:** Univ VA Sch Med 1975; **Resid:** Psychiatry, Johns Hopkins Hosp 1979; Neurology, Johns Hopkins Hosp 1983; **Fellow:** Psychopharmacology, Johns Hopkins Univ 1981; **Fac Appt:** Prof Psyc, Emory Univ

Midwest

Grossberg, George MD [GerPsy] - **Spec Exp:** Alzheimer's Disease; Depression; Behavioral Problems & Dementia; **Hospital:** St Louis Univ Hosp; **Address:** St Louis Univ Sch Med, Dept Psychiatry, 1221 S Grand Blvd, St Louis, MO 63104; **Phone:** 314-577-8721; **Board Cert:** Psychiatry 1982; Geriatric Psychiatry 2001; **Med School:** St Louis Univ 1975; **Resid:** Psychiatry, St Louis Univ Med Ctr 1979; **Fac Appt:** Prof Psyc, St Louis Univ

Luchins, Daniel MD [GerPsy] - **Spec Exp:** Dementia; Mental Retardation; **Hospital:** Univ of Chicago Hosps; **Address:** Univ Chicago, Dept Psychiatry, 5841 S Maryland Ave, MC 3077, Chicago, IL 60637-1463; **Phone:** 773-702-9716; **Board Cert:** Psychiatry 1978; Geriatric Psychiatry 2001; **Med School:** McGill Univ 1973; **Resid:** Psychiatry, Douglas Hosp 1976; Psychiatry, St Marys Hosp 1977; **Fellow:** Psychiatry, Allan Meml Inst 1977; **Fac Appt:** Assoc Prof Psyc, Univ Chicago-Pritzker Sch Med

Mellow, Alan M MD/PhD [GerPsy] - **Spec Exp:** Dementia; Depression; **Hospital:** Univ Michigan Hlth Sys; **Address:** Univ Mich, Dept Geriatric Psyc, 1500 E Med Ctr Drive, rm 1127, Box 0920, Ann Arbor, MI 48109; **Phone:** 734-222-4350; **Board Cert:** Psychiatry 1988; Geriatric Psychiatry 1991; **Med School:** Northwestern Univ 1981; **Resid:** Internal Medicine, Univ Chicago Hosp 1982; Psychiatry, McLean Hosp-Harvard 1985; **Fellow:** Psychiatry, Natl Inst Mental Hlth 1988; **Fac Appt:** Prof Psyc, Univ Mich Med Sch

Great Plains and Mountains

Burke, William J MD [GerPsy] - **Spec Exp:** Depression; Dementia; Alzheimer's Disease; Panic Disorder; **Hospital:** Nebraska Med Ctr; **Address:** Nebraska Medical Ctr, Dept Psychiatry, 985580 Nebraska Medical Ctr, Omaha, NE 68198-5580; **Phone:** 402-354-6591; **Board Cert:** Psychiatry 1986; Geriatric Psychiatry 2001; **Med School:** Univ Nebr Coll Med 1980; **Resid:** Internal Medicine, Univ Nebraska Med Ctr 1981; Psychiatry, Wash Univ Barnes Hosp 1984; **Fac Appt:** Prof Psyc, Univ Nebr Coll Med

West Coast and Pacific

Borson, Soo MD [GerPsy] - **Spec Exp:** Alzheimer's Disease; Psychiatry in Physical Illness; Dementia; Memory Disorders; **Hospital:** Univ Wash Med Ctr; **Address:** 4225 Roosevelt Way NE, Box 354694, Seattle, WA 98105-6008; **Phone:** 206-598-7792; **Board Cert:** Psychiatry 1985; Geriatric Psychiatry 2000; **Med School:** Stanford Univ 1969; **Resid:** Psychiatry, Univ Wash 1979; **Fellow:** Geriatric Psychiatry, Univ Wash 1981; **Fac Appt:** Prof Psyc, Univ Wash

Kramer, Barry Alan MD [GerPsy] - **Spec Exp:** Electroconvulsive Therapy (ECT); Depression; **Hospital:** Cedars-Sinai Med Ctr, Kaiser Permanente LA Med Ctr; **Address:** Cedars-Sinai Medical Ctr, 8730 Alden Drive, rm C-306, Los Angeles, CA 90048; **Phone:** 310-423-4014; **Board Cert:** Psychiatry 1978; Geriatric Psychiatry 2001; **Med School:** Hahnemann Univ 1974; **Resid:** Psychiatry, Montefiore Hosp & Med Ctr 1977; **Fellow:** Geriatric Psychiatry, UCLA-USC Long Term Gero Ctr 1986

Small, Gary W MD [GerPsy] - **Spec Exp:** Dementia; Alzheimer's Disease; Memory Disorders; **Hospital:** UCLA Med Ctr; **Address:** UCLA, Neuropsych Inst, 760 Westwood Plaza, 88-201 NPI, Los Angeles, CA 90024-1759; **Phone:** 310-825-0291; **Board Cert:** Psychiatry 1983; Geriatric Psychiatry 2001; **Med School:** USC Sch Med 1977; **Resid:** Psychiatry, Mass Genl Hosp 1981; **Fellow:** Psychiatry, UCLA Med Ctr 1983; **Fac Appt:** Prof Psyc, UCLA

Veith, Richard MD [GerPsy] - **Spec Exp:** Depression in Cardiovascular Disease; **Hospital:** Univ Wash Med Ctr; **Address:** Univ Washington Health Sciences Ctr, BB 1644, Box 356560, Seattle, WA 98195; **Phone:** 206-543-3752; **Board Cert:** Psychiatry 1979; Geriatric Psychiatry 2000; **Med School:** Univ Wash 1973; **Resid:** Psychiatry, Univ Wash Med Ctr 1977; **Fac Appt:** Prof Psyc, Univ Wash

Cleveland Clinic

Psychiatry and Psychology

The Cleveland Clinic Department of Psychiatry and Psychology offers the full range of mental health and behavioral services for children, adolescents and adults. Our highly trained staff, offering expert clinical evaluation and treatment, includes psychiatrists, psychologists, clinical nurse specialists, social workers, counselors and therapists.

In addition to evaluating and treating patients, our staff educates trainees, professionals and the public on the latest developments in psychiatry and the behavioral sciences.

We are ranked among the top 20 psychiatric programs in the country, according to *U.S.News and World Report's* survey of America's Best Hospitals.

The Department of Psychiatry and Psychology includes:
- Adult Psychiatry
- Child and Adolescent Psychiatry
- Chemical Dependency
- Chronic Pain Management
- General Psychology
- Neuropsychology
- Psychosomatic Medicine
- Psychiatric Occupational Therapy

Our staff treats a wide range of symptoms and problems involving personal or family crises. Among the types of problems for which children and adults seek our professional help:
- Mood and Anxiety Disorders
- Attention Deficit Disorder
- Eating Disorders
- Sleeping Problems
- Disruptive Behavior
- Schizophrenia
- Chronic Pain
- Substance Abuse
- Stress
- Work/Life/Family Problems

Our staff provides individualized assessments, medication management and counseling for individuals, couples, groups and families. The department offers care through outpatient, urgent care and routine visits, as well as inpatient treatment programs.

The department is part of the Cleveland Clinic Neurological Institute, a fully integrated entity with a disease-specific focus, combining all physicians and other healthcare providers in neurology, neurosurgery, neuroradiology, the behavioral sciences and nursing who treat children and adults with neurological and neurobehavioral disorders. Our staff of more than 100 specialists sees one of the largest and most diverse patient populations in the country. Because of our clinical expertise, academic achievement and innovative research, the Cleveland Clinic Neurological Institute has earned an international reputation for excellence.

Our staff also serves as consultants for patients admitted to Cleveland Clinic medical and surgical units, and are key team members in the treatment of many conditions including epilepsy, movement disorders, organ transplantation, morbid obesity, chronic pain, headaches and cancer. Through the Psychiatric Neuromodulation Center we offer both traditional and novel treatments to patients with psychiatric disorders resistant to common therapies.

To schedule an appointment or for more information about the Cleveland Clinic Department of Psychiatry and Psychology call 800.890.2467 or visit www.clevelandclinic.org/psychtopdocs.

Department of Psychiatry and Psychology | 9500 Euclid Avenue / W14 | Cleveland OH 44195

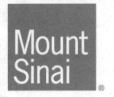

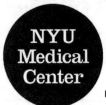

**NEW YORK UNIVERSITY
CHILD STUDY CENTER**

NYU Child Study Center

577 First Avenue
New York, NY 10016
212 263 6622
www.AboutOurKids.org

CHILD AND ADOLESCENT PSYCHIATRY

The New York University Child Study Center is dedicated to increasing the awareness of child and adolescent psychiatric disorders and improving the research necessary to advance the prevention, identification, and treatment of these disorders on a national scale. Last year, the Child Study Center was named the Department of Child and Adolescent Psychiatry within the NYU School of Medicine, making it only the second independent department of child and adolescent psychiatry in the country.

The NYU Child Study Center is built around nine research-driven Institutes focused on key mental health problems facing children and adolescents. The Child Study Center's premiere clinicians implement the knowledge gained from research, resulting in care that incorporates the most up-to-date information about the causes, symptoms, and treatments of mental disorders. The treatment options include Cognitive-Behavioral Therapy, behavioral therapy, family and couples therapy, parent training, group sessions, and medication. School consultation and academic remediation are also available. Specialized programs include:

- ADHD and Behavior Disorders Service
- Anxiety and Mood Disorders Service
- Asperger Syndrome Service – including a Lab for Advanced Learning and Teaching
- Autism Spectrum Disorders Service
- Early Childhood Service
- Eating Disorders Service
- Family Divorce Support Service
- Family Studies Program
- Learning and Academic Achievement Service
- Pediatric Weight Management Program
- Psychopharmacology Service
- Psychiatry and The Law Service
- Tourette's and Movement Disorders Service
- Trauma and Bereavement Service

A key goal of the NYU Child Study Center is to increase the body of scientific knowledge of child and adolescent mental illness. Since its founding in 1997, the Child Study Center has published over 400 articles in peer-reviewed journals and its faculty has made thousands of presentations at national and international scientific meetings.

Education and Training at NYU Child Study Center

The Education and Training component of the NYU Child Study Center is committed to a tripartite goal: to excel in clinical service delivery, the training of child and adolescent psychiatrists and psychologists, and the pursuit of meaningful research. Moreover, we aim to educate thoughtful and productive practitioners who will be innovative leaders and help to shepherd the field of child and adolescent psychiatry well into the 21st Century.

The NYU Child Study Center offers the following training programs:

- Graduate Residency Program in Child and Adolescent Psychiatry
- Psychology Externs
- Summer Program for Kids
- Post-Doctoral Fellows
- Psychology Interns
- Research Training

For more information or to apply to a training program, visit www.AboutOurKids.org/education/apply or call Dr. Jess Shatkin at 212 263 4769.

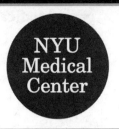

550 First Avenue (at 31st Street)
New York, NY 10016
Physician Referral: (888) 7-NYU-MED
(888-769-8633) www.nyumedicalcenter.org

BEHAVIORAL HEALTH

TREATING MENTAL ILLNESS AND EMOTIONAL DISORDERS

The Behavioral Health Program at NYU Medical Center offers the most up-to-date, scientifically validated treatments available for a wide range of disorders, including: stress/anxiety, schizophrenia, depression, shyness, insomnia, low self-esteem, women's issues, sexual difficulties, panic attacks and phobias, manic-depression, obsessions and compulsions, and attention deficit/hyperactivity disorder.

The Program serves its patients through a variety of approaches, including career counseling, assertiveness training, marital/couples counseling, and individual, group, or family therapy.

BEHAVIORAL HEALTH AT NYU COMPRISES THREE COMPONENTS:

• A 22 bed inpatient unit services an adult population including a Young Adult Program. The service combines comprehensive diagnostic assessment and treatment including psychopharma-cology, neuropsychology, psychotherapies, and electroconvulsive therapy. A multidisciplinary team approach provides a continuum of behavioral and therapeutic modalities.

• The Outpatient Psychiatry Program provides treatment to adults suffering from a broad range of mental disorders including anxiety, depression, bipolar disorder, schizoaffective disorder, schizophrenia, insomnia, adult attention-deficit hyperactivity disorder (ADHD), and personality disorders. Treatment options include individual psychotherapy, medication, or the combination.

• The Program in Human Sexuality provides a comprehensive and in-depth examination of a full range of sexual disorders, such as erectile disorder, premature ejaculation, male orgasmic disorder, female orgasmic and arousal disorders, vaginisumus, dyspareunia, lack of desire, the unconsummated marriage and sexual incompatibility between partners. Developed over the years to include the most recent advances in the field, the Program ensures that couples and individuals who seek treatment receive individualized care appropriate to their condition.

PEACE OF MIND

At NYU Medical Center, scientific innovation goes hand in hand with patient care. Our physician-scientists continue to lead the way in the burgeoning field of psychopharmacology. With the rapid pace of scientific discovery at NYU, people with mood disorders and their families stand to reap the benefits of medical research sooner rather than later. A number of clinical studies are currently under way to test new treatments for depression and bipolar disorder, with potentially lifealtering results for the millions who suffer from these debilitating mental illnesses.

PSYCHIATRY

In close collaboration with the NYU School of Medicine, which has one of the largest and most distinguished psychiatry faculties in the United States, the NYU Medical Center Department of Psychiatry offers these special services:

The Inpatient Unit is an academic service which combines comprehensive diagnostic assessment and treatment including psychopharmacology, neuropsychology, psychotherapies, and electroconvulsive therapy (ECT). For more information please call 212-263-5567.

Behavioral Health Program is the outpatient psychiatric service including licensed psychiatrists, psychologists and social workers. It offers a variety of the most up-to-date and scientifically validated treatments including psychotherapy, medication management or a combination. For more information, please call 212-263-7419.

NYU MEDICAL CENTER

NYU Medical Center is a national training center for mental health professionals, offering a fully-accredited graduate program whose goal is to train and prepare the next generation of mental health professionals to meet the demands of a complex and expanding field and to translate research into advanced clinical care and effective treatments.

Committed to patient care, research, and training, the Department of Psychiatry at NYU Medical Center is home to some of the nation's most respected clinical psychiatrists and psychologists, with specialties in psychoanalysis, psychopharmacology, behavioral therapy, child psychiatry, geriatric psychiatry, neuropsychiatry, and positron emission tomography.

**Physician Referral
(888) 7-NYU-MED
(888-769-8633)
www.nyumc.org**

718

Pulmonary Disease

a subspecialty of Internal Medicine

An internist who treats diseases of the lungs and airways. The pulmonologist diagnoses and treats cancer, pneumonia, pleurisy, asthma, occupational diseases, bronchitis, sleep disorders, emphysema and other complex disorders of the lungs.

Training Required: Three years in internal medicine *plus* additional training and examination for certification in pulmonary disease.

Pulmonary Disease

New England

Beamis, John MD [Pul] - **Spec Exp:** Interventional Pulmonology; Bronchoscopy; **Hospital:** Lahey Clin; **Address:** Lahey Clinic, 41 Mall Rd, Burlington, MA 01805; **Phone:** 781-744-3240; **Board Cert:** Internal Medicine 1974; Pulmonary Disease 1978; Critical Care Medicine 1999; **Med School:** Univ VT Coll Med 1970; **Resid:** Internal Medicine, New Eng Deacones Hosp 1973; **Fellow:** Pulmonary Disease, New Eng Deacones Hosp 1974; Pulmonary Disease, Naval Hosp 1977; **Fac Appt:** Assoc Prof Med, Tufts Univ

Braman, Sidney MD [Pul] - **Spec Exp:** Asthma; Chronic Obstructive Lung Disease (COPD); **Hospital:** Rhode Island Hosp; **Address:** Rhode Island Hosp, Div Pulmonology, 593 Eddy St, Providence, RI 02903; **Phone:** 401-444-3567; **Board Cert:** Internal Medicine 1971; Pulmonary Disease 1972; **Med School:** Temple Univ 1967; **Resid:** Internal Medicine, Philadelphia Genl Hosp 1969; **Fellow:** Pulmonary Disease, Hosp Univ Penn 1970; Pulmonary Disease, Walter Reed AMC 1971; **Fac Appt:** Prof Med, Brown Univ

Celli, Bartolome MD [Pul] - **Spec Exp:** Chronic Obstructive Lung Disease (COPD); Mechanical Ventilation; Respiratory Failure; **Hospital:** St Elizabeth's Med Ctr; **Address:** St Elizabeth's Med Ctr, Dept Pulmonary Disease, 736 Cambridge St, Boston, MA 02135; **Phone:** 617-789-2545; **Board Cert:** Internal Medicine 1975; Pulmonary Disease 1978; **Med School:** Venezuela 1971; **Resid:** Internal Medicine, St Vincent Hosp 1973; Internal Medicine, Boston City Hosp 1976; **Fellow:** Pulmonary Disease, Boston Univ Med Ctr 1977; **Fac Appt:** Prof Med, Tufts Univ

Christiani, David MD [Pul] - **Spec Exp:** Occupational Lung Disease; **Hospital:** Mass Genl Hosp, MA Respiratory Hosp; **Address:** Mass Genl Hosp, Pulm Assocs, 55 Fruit St Cox 201B Bldg, Boston, MA 02114; **Phone:** 617-726-1721; **Board Cert:** Internal Medicine 1979; Occupational Medicine 1984; Pulmonary Disease 1988; **Med School:** Tufts Univ 1976; **Resid:** Internal Medicine, Boston City Hosp 1979; Occupational Medicine, Harvard Sch Public Health 1981; **Fellow:** Pulmonary Disease, Mass Genl Hosp 1987; **Fac Appt:** Prof Med, Harvard Med Sch

Elias, Jack A MD [Pul] - **Spec Exp:** Asthma; Emphysema; Chronic Obstructive Lung Disease (COPD); **Hospital:** Yale - New Haven Hosp; **Address:** Yale Sch Med, Pulmonary Section, 300 Cedar St, S441-TAC, New Haven, CT 06520-8057; **Phone:** 203-785-4163; **Board Cert:** Internal Medicine 1979; Allergy & Immunology 1981; Pulmonary Disease 1982; **Med School:** Univ Pennsylvania 1976; **Resid:** Internal Medicine, Tufts-New England Med Ctr 1978; Internal Medicine, Hosp Univ Penn 1979; **Fellow:** Allergy & Immunology, Hosp Univ Penn 1982; Pulmonary Disease, Hosp Univ Penn 1982; **Fac Appt:** Prof Med, Yale Univ

Ernst, Armin MD [Pul] - **Spec Exp:** Interventional Pulmonology; Tracheal Stenosis; Airway Disorders; **Hospital:** Beth Israel Deaconess Med Ctr - Boston, Children's Hospital - Boston; **Address:** Beth Israel Deaconess Med Ctr, 330 Brookline Ave, Boston, MA 02215; **Phone:** 617-632-8252; **Board Cert:** Internal Medicine 2003; Pulmonary Disease 1996; Critical Care Medicine 1997; **Med School:** Germany 1988; **Resid:** Internal Medicine, Thoraxklinik-Univ Heidelberg; Internal Medicine, Univ Tex Hlth Sci Ctr 1993; **Fellow:** Pulmonary Critical Care Medicine, Deaconess Med Ctr/Brigham & Women's 1996; Interventional Pulmonology, Thoraxklinik-Univ Heidelberg; **Fac Appt:** Assoc Prof Med, Harvard Med Sch

Fanta, Christopher MD [Pul] - **Spec Exp:** Asthma; Chronic Obstructive Lung Disease (COPD); Bronchiectasis; **Hospital:** Brigham & Women's Hosp, Faulkner Hosp; **Address:** 75 Francis St, Boston, MA 02115; **Phone:** 617-732-6770; **Board Cert:** Internal Medicine 1978; Pulmonary Disease 1980; **Med School:** Harvard Med Sch 1975; **Resid:** Internal Medicine, Peter Bent Brigham Hosp 1978; **Fellow:** Pulmonary Disease, Peter Bent Brigham Hosp 1980; **Fac Appt:** Assoc Prof Med, Harvard Med Sch

Friedman, Lloyd Neal MD [Pul] - **Spec Exp:** Tuberculosis; Critical Care; **Hospital:** Milford Hosp, Yale - New Haven Hosp; **Address:** Milford Hospital, 300 Seaside Ave, Milford, CT 06460; **Phone:** 203-876-4288; **Board Cert:** Internal Medicine 1983; Pulmonary Disease 1988; Critical Care Medicine 1999; **Med School:** Yale Univ 1979; **Resid:** Internal Medicine, Beth Israel Med Ctr 1980; Internal Medicine, Oregon Hlth Scis Univ 1983; **Fellow:** Pulmonary Intensive Care, Yale-New Haven Hosp 1988; **Fac Appt:** Clin Prof Med, Yale Univ

Irwin, Richard S MD [Pul] - **Spec Exp:** Cough; Asthma; Chronic Obstructive Lung Disease (COPD); **Hospital:** UMass Meml - Meml Campus; **Address:** 55 Lake Ave N, Worcester, MA 01655-0002; **Phone:** 508-856-1919; **Board Cert:** Internal Medicine 1972; Pulmonary Disease 1974; Critical Care Medicine 1997; **Med School:** Tufts Univ 1968; **Resid:** Internal Medicine, Tufts-New England Med Ctr 1970; **Fellow:** Pulmonary Disease, Columbia-Presby Hosp 1972; **Fac Appt:** Prof Med, Univ Mass Sch Med

Mahler, Donald A MD [Pul] - **Spec Exp:** Chronic Obstructive Lung Disease (COPD); Asthma; Breathing Disorders; **Hospital:** Dartmouth - Hitchcock Med Ctr; **Address:** Dartmouth-Hitchcock Med Ctr, Div Pulmonary Med, One Medical Center Drive, Lebanon, NH 03756-0001; **Phone:** 603-650-5533; **Board Cert:** Internal Medicine 1978; Pulmonary Disease 1980; **Med School:** Loyola Univ-Stritch Sch Med 1972; **Resid:** Internal Medicine, Dartmouth-Hitchcock Med Ctr 1977; **Fellow:** Pulmonary Disease, Yale-New Haven Hosp 1980; **Fac Appt:** Prof Med, Dartmouth Med Sch

Matthay, Richard MD [Pul] - **Spec Exp:** Lung Cancer; Lupus/SLE; Autoimmune Disease; Chronic Obstructive Lung Disease (COPD); **Hospital:** Yale - New Haven Hosp; **Address:** 333 Cedar St, rm 105-LCI, Box 208057, New Haven, CT 06520-3206; **Phone:** 203-785-4198; **Board Cert:** Internal Medicine 1973; Pulmonary Disease 1976; Critical Care Medicine 1997; **Med School:** Tufts Univ 1970; **Resid:** Internal Medicine, Univ Colorado Med Ctr 1973; **Fellow:** Pulmonary Critical Care Medicine, Univ Colorado Med Ctr 1975; **Fac Appt:** Prof Med, Yale Univ

Metersky, Mark L MD [Pul] - **Spec Exp:** Pulmonary Infections; Asthma; Pulmonary Hypertension; **Hospital:** Univ of Conn Hlth Ctr, John Dempsey Hosp; **Address:** Univ Conn Hlth Ctr, 263 Farmington Ave, Farmington, CT 06030-1321; **Phone:** 860-679-3343; **Board Cert:** Internal Medicine 1988; Pulmonary Disease 2003; Critical Care Medicine 2003; **Med School:** NYU Sch Med 1985; **Resid:** Internal Medicine, Boston City Hosp 1988; **Fellow:** Pulmonary Critical Care Medicine, UCSD Med Ctr 1992; **Fac Appt:** Assoc Prof Med, Univ Conn

Millman, Richard P MD [Pul] - **Spec Exp:** Sleep Disorders/Apnea; **Hospital:** Rhode Island Hosp; **Address:** RI Hosp, Div Pulm, Crit Care & Sleep Med, 593 Eddy St, APC 701, Providence, RI 02903-4923; **Phone:** 401-444-2670; **Board Cert:** Internal Medicine 1979; Pulmonary Disease 1982; Critical Care Medicine 1999; **Med School:** Univ Pennsylvania 1976; **Resid:** Internal Medicine, Univ Mich Hosp 1979; **Fellow:** Pulmonary Disease, Univ Penn Med Ctr 1981; **Fac Appt:** Prof Med, Brown Univ

Pulmonary Disease

Nardell, Edward MD [Pul] - **Spec Exp:** Tuberculosis; **Hospital:** Brigham & Women's Hosp; **Address:** Center for Health and Human Rights, 651 Huntington Ave, Boston, MA 02120; **Phone:** 617-432-6937; **Board Cert:** Internal Medicine 1975; Pulmonary Disease 1982; **Med School:** Hahnemann Univ 1972; **Resid:** Internal Medicine, Hahnemann Univ Hosp 1975; **Fellow:** Pulmonary Disease, Mass Genl Hosp 1977; **Fac Appt:** Assoc Prof Med, Harvard Med Sch

Parsons, Polly E MD [Pul] - **Spec Exp:** Critical Care; **Hospital:** FAHC - UHC Campus; **Address:** Fletcher Allen Health Care, 111 Colchester Ave, Patrick 311, Burlington, VT 05401; **Phone:** 802-847-6177; **Board Cert:** Internal Medicine 1981; Pulmonary Disease 1986; Critical Care Medicine 1989; **Med School:** Univ Ariz Coll Med 1978; **Resid:** Internal Medicine, Univ Colorado Hosp 1981; **Fellow:** Pulmonary Disease, Univ Colorado Hosp 1985; **Fac Appt:** Prof Med, Univ VT Coll Med

Redlich, Carrie MD [Pul] - **Spec Exp:** Occupational Lung Disease; **Hospital:** Yale - New Haven Hosp; **Address:** Yale Occupational & Environmental Med, 135 College St Fl 3 - Ste 392, New Haven, CT 06510; **Phone:** 203-785-4197; **Board Cert:** Internal Medicine 1986; Pulmonary Disease 2002; Occupational Medicine 1990; **Med School:** Yale Univ 1982; **Resid:** Internal Medicine, Yale-New Haven Hosp 1986; Occupational Medicine, Yale-New Haven Hosp 1987; **Fellow:** Pulmonary Disease, Univ Washington 1989; **Fac Appt:** Assoc Prof Med, Yale Univ

Reilly Jr, John Joseph MD [Pul] - **Spec Exp:** Transplant Medicine-Lung; Emphysema; Chronic Obstructive Lung Disease (COPD); **Hospital:** Brigham & Women's Hosp; **Address:** 75 Francis St, Clinics 3, Boston, MA 02115; **Phone:** 617-732-7599; **Board Cert:** Internal Medicine 1984; Pulmonary Disease 1986; Critical Care Medicine 1997; **Med School:** Harvard Med Sch 1981; **Resid:** Internal Medicine, Brigham & Women's Hosp 1984; **Fellow:** Pulmonary Disease, Brigham & Women's Hosp 1987; **Fac Appt:** Assoc Prof Med, Harvard Med Sch

Rochester, Carolyn MD [Pul] - **Spec Exp:** Chronic Obstructive Lung Disease (COPD); **Hospital:** VA Conn Hlthcre Sys, Yale - New Haven Hosp; **Address:** Yale Univ Sch Med, Pulm & Crit Care Sect, 300 Cedar St, Box 208057, New Haven, CT 06520-8057; **Phone:** 203-785-3207; **Board Cert:** Internal Medicine 1986; Pulmonary Disease 2002; **Med School:** Columbia P&S 1983; **Resid:** Internal Medicine, Columbia Presby Med Ctr 1986; **Fellow:** Pulmonary Disease, Colombia Presby Med Ctr 1988; **Fac Appt:** Asst Prof Med, Yale Univ

White, David P MD [Pul] - **Spec Exp:** Sleep Disorders/Apnea; **Hospital:** Brigham & Women's Hosp; **Address:** Sleep Disorders Program, 75 Francis St, Boston, MA 02115; **Phone:** 617-732-5778; **Board Cert:** Internal Medicine 1978; Pulmonary Disease 1982; Critical Care Medicine 1997; **Med School:** Emory Univ 1975; **Resid:** Internal Medicine, Univ Colo Med Ctr 1978; **Fellow:** Pulmonary Disease, Univ Colo Med Ctr 1982; **Fac Appt:** Assoc Prof Med, Harvard Med Sch

Mid Atlantic

Arcasoy, Selim M MD [Pul] - **Spec Exp:** Transplant Medicine-Lung; Chronic Obstructive Lung Disease (COPD); Interstitial Lung Disease; **Hospital:** NY-Presby Hosp/Columbia (page 66); **Address:** Ctr for Advanced Lung Dis/Transp, 622 W 168th St, PH, Fl 14E - rm 104, New York, NY 10032-3720; **Phone:** 212-305-6589; **Board Cert:** Internal Medicine 2003; Pulmonary Disease 1996; Critical Care Medicine 1997; **Med School:** Turkey 1990; **Resid:** Internal Medicine, SUNY Downstate Med Ctr 1994; **Fellow:** Pulmonary Critical Care Medicine, Univ Pittsburgh Med Ctr 1998; **Fac Appt:** Assoc Prof Med, Columbia P&S

Bascom, Rebecca MD [Pul] - **Spec Exp:** Environmental Diseases; Chemical Exposure; **Hospital:** Penn State Milton S Hershey Med Ctr; **Address:** Hershey Med Ctr, PO Box 850, MC HO41, Hershey, PA 17033-0850; **Phone:** 717-531-6525; **Board Cert:** Internal Medicine 1982; Occupational Medicine 1987; Pulmonary Disease 1988; Critical Care Medicine 1998; **Med School:** Oregon Hlth Sci Univ 1979; **Resid:** Internal Medicine, Johns Hopkins Univ 1982; Occupational Medicine, Johns Hopkins Univ 1985; **Fellow:** Pulmonary Disease, Johns Hopkins Univ 1985; **Fac Appt:** Prof Med, Penn State Univ-Hershey Med Ctr

Greenberg, Harly MD [Pul] - **Spec Exp:** Sleep Disorders/Apnea; Lung Disease; Critical Care; **Hospital:** Long Island Jewish Med Ctr, N Shore Univ Hosp at Manhasset; **Address:** North Shore LIJ Sleep Disorders Ctr, 410 Lakeville Rd, Ste 105, New Hyde Park, NY 11040; **Phone:** 516-465-3899; **Board Cert:** Internal Medicine 1985; Pulmonary Disease 1988; **Med School:** NYU Sch Med 1982; **Resid:** Internal Medicine, North Shore Univ Hosp 1985; **Fellow:** Pulmonary Disease, NYU-Bellevue Hosp Ctr 1987; **Fac Appt:** Assoc Prof Med, Albert Einstein Coll Med

Hansen-Flaschen, John MD [Pul] - **Spec Exp:** Interstitial Lung Disease; Diagnostic Problems; Chronic Obstructive Lung Disease (COPD); **Hospital:** Hosp Univ Penn - UPHS (page 72); **Address:** Hosp Univ Penn, Div Pulm, Allergy and Crit Care, 3400 Spruce St Radvin Bldg Fl 3 - Ste F, Philadelphia, PA 19104; **Phone:** 215-662-3202; **Board Cert:** Pulmonary Disease 1982; Critical Care Medicine 1988; Internal Medicine 1979; **Med School:** NYU Sch Med 1976; **Resid:** Internal Medicine, Hosp Univ Penn 1979; **Fellow:** Pulmonary Disease, Hosp Univ Penn 1981; Critical Care Medicine, Hosp Univ Penn 1982; **Fac Appt:** Prof Med, Univ Pennsylvania

Kamholz, Stephan MD [Pul] - **Spec Exp:** Critical Care; Tuberculosis; Transplant Medicine-Lung; **Hospital:** N Shore Univ Hosp at Manhasset, Long Island Jewish Med Ctr; **Address:** 300 Community Drive, Dept Medicine, 4DSU, Manhasset, NY 11030; **Phone:** 516-562-4310; **Board Cert:** Internal Medicine 1987; Pulmonary Disease 1978; Critical Care Medicine 1997; **Med School:** NY Med Coll 1972; **Resid:** Internal Medicine, Montefiore Hosp Med Ctr 1975; **Fellow:** Pulmonary Disease, Montefiore Hosp Med Ctr 1977; **Fac Appt:** Prof Med, NYU Sch Med

Libby, Daniel MD [Pul] - **Spec Exp:** Asthma; Lung Cancer; Interstitial Lung Disease; **Hospital:** NY-Presby Hosp/Weill Cornell (page 66); **Address:** 635 Madison Ave, 11th Fl, New York, NY 10021; **Phone:** 212-628-6611; **Board Cert:** Internal Medicine 1977; Pulmonary Disease 1980; **Med School:** Baylor Coll Med 1974; **Resid:** Internal Medicine, New York Hosp 1977; **Fellow:** Pulmonary Disease, New York Hosp 1979; **Fac Appt:** Clin Prof Med, Cornell Univ-Weill Med Coll

Nash, Thomas MD [Pul] - **Spec Exp:** Asthma; Cough; Pneumonia; **Hospital:** NY-Presby Hosp/Weill Cornell (page 66); **Address:** 310 E 72nd St, New York, NY 10021-4726; **Phone:** 212-734-6612; **Board Cert:** Internal Medicine 1981; Infectious Disease 1984; Pulmonary Disease 1988; **Med School:** NYU Sch Med 1978; **Resid:** Internal Medicine, New York Hosp-Cornell 1981; **Fellow:** Infectious Disease, New York Hosp-Cornell 1985; Pulmonary Disease, Meml Sloan Kettering Cancer Ctr 1985; **Fac Appt:** Assoc Clin Prof Med, NYU Sch Med

Niederman, Michael MD [Pul] - **Spec Exp:** Infections-Respiratory; Emphysema; Respiratory Failure; Pneumonia; **Hospital:** Winthrop - Univ Hosp; **Address:** 222 Station Plaza N, Ste 400, Mineola, NY 11501-3893; **Phone:** 516-663-2834; **Board Cert:** Internal Medicine 1980; Pulmonary Disease 1983; Critical Care Medicine 1997; **Med School:** Boston Univ 1977; **Resid:** Internal Medicine, Northwestern Univ Med Ctr 1980; **Fellow:** Pulmonary Disease, Yale-New Haven Hosp 1983; **Fac Appt:** Prof Med, SUNY Stony Brook

Pulmonary Disease

Pack, Allan MD/PhD [Pul] - **Spec Exp:** Sleep Disorders/Apnea; **Hospital:** Hosp Univ Penn - UPHS (page 72); **Address:** Penn Sleep Center, 3624 Market St, Ste 201, Philadelphia, PA 19104; **Phone:** 215-615-3669; **Med School:** Scotland 1967; **Resid:** Internal Medicine, Univ Glasgow Med Ctr 1972; **Fellow:** Pulmonary Disease, Univ Glasgow Med Ctr 1975; **Fac Appt:** Prof Med, Univ Pennsylvania

Palevsky, Harold I MD [Pul] - **Spec Exp:** Pulmonary Hypertension; Pulmonary Vascular Disease; Thromboembolic Disorders; **Hospital:** Penn Presby Med Ctr - UPHS (page 72), Hosp Univ Penn - UPHS (page 72); **Address:** Penn Presbyterian Medical Ctr, 39th & Market Sts, PHI Bldg-Fl 1 Rear, Philadelphia, PA 19104; **Phone:** 215-662-8717; **Board Cert:** Internal Medicine 2007; Pulmonary Disease 2007; Critical Care Medicine 2007; **Med School:** Med Coll VA 1978; **Resid:** Internal Medicine, Hosp Univ Penn 1981; **Fellow:** Pulmonary Critical Care Medicine, Hosp Univ Penn 1984; **Fac Appt:** Prof Med, Univ Pennsylvania

Reichman, Lee B MD [Pul] - **Spec Exp:** Tuberculosis; Mycobacterial Infections; **Hospital:** UMDNJ-Univ Hosp-Newark; **Address:** 225 Warren St, Box 1709, Newark, NJ 07103-3535; **Phone:** 973-972-3270; **Board Cert:** Internal Medicine 1972; Pulmonary Disease 1972; **Med School:** NYU Sch Med 1964; **Resid:** Internal Medicine, Bellevue Hosp 1965; Internal Medicine, Harlem Hosp 1969; **Fellow:** Pulmonary Disease, Harlem Hosp-Columbia P&S 1970; **Fac Appt:** Prof Med, UMDNJ-NJ Med Sch, Newark

Rogers, Robert M MD [Pul] - **Spec Exp:** Pulmonary Alveolar Proteinosis; Emphysema; Chronic Obstructive Lung Disease (COPD); Asthma; **Hospital:** UPMC Presby, Pittsburgh; **Address:** Univ Pittsburgh - Div Pulmonary Medicine, 3459 5th Ave, rm NW628, Box MUH, Pittsburgh, PA 15213; **Phone:** 412-692-2210; **Board Cert:** Internal Medicine 1967; Pulmonary Disease 1969; **Med School:** Univ Pennsylvania 1960; **Resid:** Internal Medicine, Univ Hosps Cleveland 1963; Pulmonary Disease, Case West Res 1964; **Fellow:** Pulmonary Disease, Univ Penn 1965; Physiology, Univ Penn 1968; **Fac Appt:** Prof Med, Univ Pittsburgh

Rossman, Milton D MD [Pul] - **Spec Exp:** Beryllium-induced Lung Disease; Sarcoidosis; Interstitial Lung Disease; **Hospital:** Hosp Univ Penn - UPHS (page 72); **Address:** Hosp of Univ Penn, 3400 Spruce St, 834W Gates Bldg, Philadelphia, PA 19104-4283; **Phone:** 215-662-6413; **Board Cert:** Internal Medicine 1975; Pulmonary Disease 1978; **Med School:** Jefferson Med Coll 1970; **Resid:** Internal Medicine, Univ Hosps 1975; **Fellow:** Pulmonary Disease, Hosp Univ Penn 1977; **Fac Appt:** Prof Med, Univ Pennsylvania

Schluger, Neil MD [Pul] - **Spec Exp:** Tuberculosis; Pulmonary Infections; Chronic Obstructive Lung Disease (COPD); **Hospital:** NY-Presby Hosp/Columbia (page 66); **Address:** Div Pulm, Allergy & Crit Care Med, 630 W 168th St, PH-8 East, Rm 101, New York, NY 10032; **Phone:** 212-305-9817; **Board Cert:** Internal Medicine 1988; Pulmonary Disease 2003; **Med School:** Univ Pennsylvania 1985; **Resid:** Internal Medicine, St Lukes Hosp 1989; **Fellow:** Pulmonary Critical Care Medicine, NY Hosp-Cornell 1992; **Fac Appt:** Assoc Prof Med, Columbia P&S

Schwab, Richard MD [Pul] - **Spec Exp:** Sleep Disorders/Apnea; **Hospital:** Hosp Univ Penn - UPHS (page 72); **Address:** Penn Sleep Center, 3624 Market St Fl 2 - Ste 201, Philadelphia, PA 19104; **Phone:** 215-662-7772; **Board Cert:** Internal Medicine 1986; Pulmonary Disease 2000; Critical Care Medicine 2000; **Med School:** Univ Pennsylvania 1983; **Resid:** Internal Medicine, Hosp Univ Penn 1986; **Fellow:** Pulmonary Critical Care Medicine, Hosp Univ Penn 1991; **Fac Appt:** Asst Prof Med, Univ Pennsylvania

Steiger, David MD [Pul] - **Spec Exp:** Rheumatologic Diseases of the Lung; Asthma; Pulmonary Embolism; Critical Care; **Hospital:** Hosp For Joint Diseases (page 68), NYU Med Ctr (page 67); **Address:** 305 2nd Ave, Ste 16, New York, NY 10003; **Phone:** 212-598-6091; **Board Cert:** Internal Medicine 1987; Pulmonary Disease 2002; Critical Care Medicine 2005; **Med School:** England 1981; **Resid:** Internal Medicine, St Thomas's Hosp 1984; Internal Medicine, St Lukes Hosp 1989; **Fellow:** Pulmonary Disease, UCSF Med Ctr 1994; **Fac Appt:** Asst Prof Med, NYU Sch Med

Steinberg, Harry MD [Pul] - **Spec Exp:** Asthma; Emphysema; Lung Cancer; **Hospital:** Long Island Jewish Med Ctr, N Shore Univ Hosp at Manhasset; **Address:** LI Jewish Med Ctr, Dept Med, 270-05 76th Ave, New Hyde Park, NY 11040-1433; **Phone:** 718-465-5400; **Med School:** Temple Univ 1966; **Resid:** Internal Medicine, LI Jewish Med Ctr 1969; Pulmonary Critical Care Medicine, LI Jewish Med Ctr 1970; **Fellow:** Pulmonary Disease, Hosp U Penn 1974; **Fac Appt:** Clin Prof Med, Albert Einstein Coll Med

Stover-Pepe, Diane E MD [Pul] - **Spec Exp:** Interstitial Lung Disease; Pulmonary Infections; Pulmonary Disease/Immunocompromised; **Hospital:** Meml Sloan Kettering Cancer Ctr; **Address:** 1275 York Ave, rm H819, New York, NY 10021; **Phone:** 212-639-8380; **Board Cert:** Internal Medicine 1975; Pulmonary Disease 1978; **Med School:** Albert Einstein Coll Med 1970; **Resid:** Internal Medicine, Harlem Hosp Ctr 1972; Internal Medicine, NY Hosp-Cornell Med Ctr 1975; **Fellow:** Pulmonary Disease, Montefiore Med Ctr 1977; **Fac Appt:** Prof Med, Cornell Univ-Weill Med Coll

Strollo, Patrick J MD [Pul] - **Spec Exp:** Sleep Disorders/Apnea; **Hospital:** UPMC Montefiore, UPMC Presby, Pittsburgh; **Address:** Montefiore Univ Hospital, 3459 5th Ave, Ste S639.11, Pittsburgh, PA 15213; **Phone:** 412-692-2880; **Board Cert:** Internal Medicine 1984; Pulmonary Disease 1988; **Med School:** Uniformed Srvs Univ, Bethesda 1981; **Resid:** Internal Medicine, Wilford Hall Med Ctr 1984; **Fellow:** Pulmonary Disease, Wilford Hall Med Ctr 1987; **Fac Appt:** Assoc Prof Med, Univ Pittsburgh

Teirstein, Alvin MD [Pul] - **Spec Exp:** Sarcoidosis; Interstitial Lung Disease; Lung Cancer; **Hospital:** Mount Sinai Med Ctr, VA Med Ctr - Bronx; **Address:** Mount Sinai Med Ctr, 1 Gustave Levy Pl, Box 1232, New York, NY 10029; **Phone:** 212-241-5656; **Board Cert:** Internal Medicine 1961; Pulmonary Disease 1969; **Med School:** SUNY Downstate 1953; **Resid:** Internal Medicine, Mt Sinai Med Ctr 1957; **Fellow:** Pulmonary Disease, Mt Sinai Med Ctr 1954; Pulmonary Disease, VA Med Ctr 1956; **Fac Appt:** Prof Med, Mount Sinai Sch Med

Terry, Peter Browne MD [Pul] - **Hospital:** Johns Hopkins Hosp - Baltimore (page 61); **Address:** 1830 E Monument St Fl 5, Baltimore, MD 21205; **Phone:** 410-955-3467; **Board Cert:** Internal Medicine 1973; Pulmonary Disease 1976; **Med School:** St Louis Univ 1968; **Resid:** Internal Medicine, Univ Conn Hlth Ctr 1970; Internal Medicine, Johns Hopkins Hosp 1973; **Fellow:** Pulmonary Disease, Johns Hopkins Hosp 1974; Pulmonary Disease, Mayo Clinic 1975; **Fac Appt:** Prof Med, Johns Hopkins Univ

Thomashow, Byron MD [Pul] - **Spec Exp:** Emphysema; Asthma; Respiratory Failure; Chronic Obstructive Lung Disease (COPD); **Hospital:** NY-Presby Hosp/Columbia (page 66); **Address:** 161 Fort Washington Ave, rm 311, New York, NY 10032; **Phone:** 212-305-5261; **Board Cert:** Internal Medicine 1977; Pulmonary Disease 1980; **Med School:** Columbia P&S 1974; **Resid:** Internal Medicine, Roosevelt Hosp 1977; Pulmonary Disease, Roosevelt Hosp 1978; **Fellow:** Pulmonary Disease, Harlem Hosp Ctr 1979; **Fac Appt:** Clin Prof Med, Columbia P&S

Pulmonary Disease

Tino, Gregory MD [Pul] - **Spec Exp:** Emphysema-Lung Volume Reduction; Interstitial Lung Disease; Bronchiectasis; Chronic Obstructive Lung Disease (COPD); **Hospital:** Hosp Univ Penn - UPHS (page 72); **Address:** Hosp Univ Penn, Div Pulmonary & Critical Care, 3400 Spruce St Radvin Bldg Fl 3 - Ste F, Philadelphia, PA 19104; **Phone:** 215-349-5303; **Board Cert:** Internal Medicine 1989; **Med School:** Mount Sinai Sch Med 1986; **Resid:** Internal Medicine, Hosp Univ Penn 1989; **Fellow:** Pulmonary Disease, Hosp Univ Penn 1992; **Fac Appt:** Assoc Prof Med, Univ Pennsylvania

Unger, Michael MD [Pul] - **Spec Exp:** Lung Cancer; Bronchoscopy; Cancer Prevention; **Hospital:** Fox Chase Cancer Ctr (page 59); **Address:** Fox Chase Cancer Center, 7701 Burholme Ave, Philadelphia, PA 19111; **Phone:** 215-728-6900; **Board Cert:** Internal Medicine 1977; Pulmonary Disease 1978; **Med School:** France 1971; **Resid:** Internal Medicine, Mt Sinai Hosp 1974; **Fellow:** Pulmonary Disease, New York Hosp-Cornell 1976; **Fac Appt:** Clin Prof Med, Thomas Jefferson Univ

Wenzel, Sally E MD [Pul] - **Spec Exp:** Asthma; Bronchiolitis Obliterans; Allergy; **Hospital:** UPMC Presby, Pittsburgh; **Address:** UPMC, NW 628 Montefiore, 36013459 Fifth Ave, Pittsburgh, PA 15213; **Phone:** 412-648-6859; **Board Cert:** Internal Medicine 1984; Pulmonary Disease 1986; **Med School:** Univ Fla Coll Med 1981; **Resid:** Internal Medicine, NC Baptist Hosp 1984; **Fellow:** Pulmonary Disease, Med Coll VA Hosp 1986; **Fac Appt:** Prof Med, Univ Colorado

White, Dorothy MD [Pul] - **Spec Exp:** Lung Cancer; AIDS/HIV; AIDS Related Cancers; **Hospital:** Meml Sloan Kettering Cancer Ctr; **Address:** 1275 York Ave, rm H803, Box 13, New York, NY 10021; **Phone:** 212-639-8022; **Board Cert:** Internal Medicine 1980; Pulmonary Disease 1984; **Med School:** SUNY Hlth Sci Ctr 1977; **Resid:** Internal Medicine, New York Hosp 1980; Internal Medicine, Meml Sloan Kettering Inst 1981; **Fellow:** Pulmonary Disease, Yale-New Haven Hosp 1984; **Fac Appt:** Prof Med, Cornell Univ-Weill Med Coll

Southeast

Alberts, W Michael MD [Pul] - **Spec Exp:** Lung Cancer; **Hospital:** H Lee Moffitt Cancer Ctr & Research Inst; **Address:** H Lee Moffitt Cancer Ctr, Thoracic Onc, 12902 Magnolia Drive, Tampa, FL 33612; **Phone:** 813-903-4679; **Board Cert:** Internal Medicine 1980; Pulmonary Disease 1982; **Med School:** Univ IL Coll Med 1977; **Resid:** Internal Medicine, Ohio State Univ Hosp 1980; **Fellow:** Pulmonary Critical Care Medicine, UCSD Med Ctr 1983; **Fac Appt:** Prof Med, Univ S Fla Coll Med

Antony, Veena B MD [Pul] - **Spec Exp:** Pleural Disease; **Hospital:** Shands Hlthcre at Univ of FL; **Address:** Shands at the Univ of Florida, 1600 SW Archer Rd, Box 100225, Gainesville, FL 32610-0225; **Phone:** 352-392-2666; **Board Cert:** Internal Medicine 1979; Pulmonary Disease 1982; **Med School:** India 1974; **Resid:** Internal Medicine, Kingsbrook Jewish Med Ctr; **Fellow:** Pulmonary Disease, Univ Co Hlth Sci Ctr; Pulmonary Disease, Natl Jewish Hosp-Asthma Ctr

Bayly, Timothy C MD [Pul] - **Spec Exp:** Critical Care; Sleep Disorders/Apnea; **Hospital:** Inova Fairfax Hosp, Potomac Hosp; **Address:** 5510 Alma Ln, Ste 300, Springfield, VA 22151; **Phone:** 703-642-5990; **Board Cert:** Internal Medicine 1975; Pulmonary Disease 1976; **Med School:** Georgetown Univ 1972; **Resid:** Internal Medicine, Cornell Univ Med Coll 1975; **Fellow:** Pulmonary Disease, Georgetown Univ Hosp 1976; **Fac Appt:** Asst Clin Prof Med, Georgetown Univ

Brooks, Stuart M MD [Pul] - **Spec Exp:** Occupational Lung Disease; Asthma; Lung Injuries-Inhalation Induced; **Hospital:** Tampa Genl Hosp, H Lee Moffitt Cancer Ctr & Research Inst; **Address:** USF College of Public Health, 12901 Bruce B Downs Blvd, Box 56 MDC, Tampa, FL 33612-3805; **Phone:** 813-974-7545; **Board Cert:** Internal Medicine 1977; Pulmonary Disease 1969; Occupational Medicine 1987; **Med School:** Univ Cincinnati 1962; **Resid:** Internal Medicine, Boston City Hosp 1967; **Fellow:** Pulmonary Disease, Boston City Hosp 1969; **Fac Appt:** Prof Med, Univ S Fla Coll Med

Campbell, G Douglas MD [Pul] - **Spec Exp:** Infectious Disease-Lung; **Hospital:** Univ Hosps & Clins - Jackson, VA Med Ctr; **Address:** Univ Mississippi Med Ctr, Div Pulm, 2500 N State St, Jackson, MS 39216-4505; **Phone:** 601-984-5650; **Board Cert:** Internal Medicine 1979; Pulmonary Disease 1986; **Med School:** Univ Miss 1976; **Resid:** Internal Medicine, Univ Miss Hosp 1979; **Fellow:** Pulmonary Disease, Univ Tex Hlth Sci Ctr 1983; Infectious Disease, Univ Calgary HSC 1985; **Fac Appt:** Prof Med, Univ Miss

Christman, Brian W MD [Pul] - **Spec Exp:** Chronic Obstructive Lung Disease (COPD); Sepsis; Critical Care; **Hospital:** VA Med Ctr - Nashville, Vanderbilt Univ Med Ctr; **Address:** VA Tennessee Valley Hlth Care System, 1310 24th Ave S, MC 111, Nashville, TN 37212; **Phone:** 615-327-4751 x5349; **Board Cert:** Internal Medicine 1984; Pulmonary Disease 1986; Critical Care Medicine 1999; **Med School:** Univ Okla Coll Med 1981; **Resid:** Internal Medicine, Vanderbilt Univ Med Ctr 1984; **Fellow:** Pulmonary Disease, Vanderbilt Univ Med Ctr 1987

Cooper, John Allen D MD [Pul] - **Spec Exp:** Drug Induced Lung Disease; Chronic Obstructive Lung Disease (COPD); **Hospital:** Univ of Ala Hosp at Birmingham, VA Med Ctr; **Address:** 215 Tinsley Harrison Tower, 1900 University Blvd, Birmingham, AL 35294; **Phone:** 205-934-7941; **Board Cert:** Internal Medicine 1981; Pulmonary Disease 1984; **Med School:** Duke Univ 1978; **Resid:** Internal Medicine, Univ Virginia Hosp 1981; **Fellow:** Pulmonary Disease, Yale Univ 1985; **Fac Appt:** Prof Med, Univ Ala

Cooper, William R MD [Pul] - **Spec Exp:** Critical Care; Asthma; Chronic Obstructive Lung Disease (COPD); **Hospital:** Sentara VA Beach Genl Hosp; **Address:** 1008 First Colonial Rd, Ste 103, Virginia Beach, VA 23454-3071; **Phone:** 757-481-2515; **Board Cert:** Internal Medicine 1972; Pulmonary Disease 1974; Critical Care Medicine 1999; **Med School:** Univ VA Sch Med 1969; **Resid:** Internal Medicine, Cleveland Metro Genl Hosp 1971; Pulmonary Disease, Univ Va Hosp 1973; **Fellow:** Pulmonary Disease, Mount Sinai Med Ctr 1974

Doherty, Dennis E MD [Pul] - **Spec Exp:** Asthma; Chronic Obstructive Lung Disease (COPD); Interstitial Lung Disease; **Hospital:** Univ of Kentucky Chandler Hosp, VA Med Ctr - Lexington; **Address:** Univ Kentucky Med Ctr, Div Pulm & Crit Care, 740 S Limestone, rm K-528, Lexington, KY 40536-0284; **Phone:** 859-323-5045; **Board Cert:** Internal Medicine 1985; Pulmonary Disease 1988; **Med School:** Ohio State Univ 1980; **Resid:** Internal Medicine, Ohio State Univ Hosp 1983; **Fellow:** Pulmonary Disease, Univ Colorado Hlth Sci Ctr 1986; **Fac Appt:** Prof Med, Univ KY Coll Med

Donohue, James MD [Pul] - **Spec Exp:** Asthma; Chronic Obstructive Lung Disease (COPD); Sarcoidosis; **Hospital:** Univ NC Hosps; **Address:** Univ NC, Div Pulmonary Disease, 4125 Bio-informatics Bldg. CB 7020, Chapel Hill, NC 27599-7020; **Phone:** 919-966-2531; **Board Cert:** Internal Medicine 1975; Pulmonary Disease 1976; **Med School:** UMDNJ-NJ Med Sch, Newark 1969; **Resid:** Internal Medicine, UMDNJ-Newark 1971; Internal Medicine, NC Meml Hosp 1974; **Fellow:** Pulmonary Disease, Univ North Carolina 1976; **Fac Appt:** Prof Med, Univ NC Sch Med

Pulmonary Disease

Downie, Gordon H MD/PhD [Pul] - **Spec Exp:** Lung Cancer; Photodynamic Therapy; Asthma; Clinical Trials; **Hospital:** Pitt Cty Mem Hosp - Univ Med Ctr East Carolina; **Address:** The Brody School of Medicine, Ste 3E-149, Greenville, NC 27858-4354; **Phone:** 252-744-4653; **Board Cert:** Pulmonary Disease 2004; **Med School:** Northwestern Univ 1986; **Resid:** Internal Medicine, Univ North Carolina 1989; **Fellow:** Pulmonary Intensive Care, Univ North Carolina 1992; **Fac Appt:** Assoc Prof Med, E Carolina Univ

Dunlap, Nancy E MD/PhD [Pul] - **Spec Exp:** Critical Care; **Hospital:** Univ of Ala Hosp at Birmingham; **Address:** 2000 6th Ave S Fl 3/Admin, Birmingham, AL 35233; **Phone:** 205-801-7900; **Board Cert:** Internal Medicine 1984; Pulmonary Disease 1988; Critical Care Medicine 1999; **Med School:** Duke Univ 1981; **Resid:** Internal Medicine, Univ Alabama Med Ctr 1984; **Fellow:** Pulmonary Disease, Univ Alabama 1987; **Fac Appt:** Prof Med, Univ Ala

Fulkerson Jr, William J MD [Pul] - **Spec Exp:** Respiratory Failure; Thromboembolic Disorders; Asthma; **Hospital:** Duke Univ Med Ctr; **Address:** Duke Univ Med Ctr, Trent Drive, Box 3708, Durham, NC 27710; **Phone:** 919-684-8076; **Board Cert:** Internal Medicine 1981; Pulmonary Disease 1984; Critical Care Medicine 1996; **Med School:** Univ NC Sch Med 1977; **Resid:** Internal Medicine, Vanderbilt Univ Hosp 1980; **Fellow:** Pulmonary Disease, Vanderbilt Univ Hosp 1983; **Fac Appt:** Prof Med, Duke Univ

Goldman, Allan L MD [Pul] - **Spec Exp:** Occupational Lung Disease; Airway Disorders; Lung Cancer; **Hospital:** Tampa Genl Hosp, James A Haley VA Hosp; **Address:** USF Coll Med, Dept Internal Medicine, 12901 Bruce B Downs Blvd, Box MDC19, Tampa, FL 33612-4742; **Phone:** 813-974-2271; **Board Cert:** Internal Medicine 1972; Pulmonary Disease 1972; **Med School:** Univ Minn 1968; **Resid:** Internal Medicine, Brooke Army Hosp 1970; **Fellow:** Pulmonary Disease, Walter Reed Army Hosp 1972; **Fac Appt:** Prof Med, Univ S Fla Coll Med

Harman, Eloise M MD [Pul] - **Hospital:** Shands Hlthcre at Univ of FL; **Address:** Shands at Univ of Florida, 1600 SW Archer Rd, Box 100225, Gainesville, FL 32610-0225; **Phone:** 352-392-2666; **Board Cert:** Internal Medicine 1973; Pulmonary Disease 1976; Critical Care Medicine 1997; **Med School:** Johns Hopkins Univ 1970; **Resid:** Internal Medicine, Johns Hopkins Hosp 1972; **Fellow:** Pulmonary Disease, NY Hosp-Cornell Med Ctr 1974; **Fac Appt:** Prof Med, Univ Fla Coll Med

Haynes, Johnson MD [Pul] - **Spec Exp:** Sickle Cell Disease-Lung; Chronic Obstructive Lung Disease (COPD); **Hospital:** Univ of S AL Med Ctr; **Address:** Univ S Alabama Medical Ctr, 2451 Fillingim St, Ste 10G, Mobile, AL 36617; **Phone:** 251-471-7847; **Board Cert:** Internal Medicine 1983; Pulmonary Disease 1986; **Med School:** Univ S Ala Coll Med 1980; **Resid:** Internal Medicine, Univ S Alabama Med Ctr 1983; **Fellow:** Pulmonary Disease, Univ S Alabama Med Ctr 1986; **Fac Appt:** Prof Med, Univ S Ala Coll Med

Henke, David Carroll MD [Pul] - **Spec Exp:** Asthma; Chronic Obstructive Lung Disease (COPD); Vasculitis; **Hospital:** Univ NC Hosps; **Address:** Univ NC Med Sch, Div Pulm Dis & Crit Care Med, 130 Mason Farm Rd, Box 7020, Chapel Hill, NC 27599-7020; **Phone:** 919-966-6838; **Board Cert:** Internal Medicine 1980; Dermatology 1983; Pulmonary Disease 1988; **Med School:** Univ NC Sch Med 1977; **Resid:** Internal Medicine, NC Memorial Hosp 1980; Dermatology, NC Meml NIEHS 1984; **Fellow:** Pulmonary Disease, NC Memorial Hosp 1987; **Fac Appt:** Assoc Prof Med, Univ NC Sch Med

Johnson, Bruce Ellsworth MD [Pul] - **Spec Exp:** Sleep Disorders/Apnea; **Hospital:** Sentara VA Beach Genl Hosp; **Address:** 1008 First Colonial Rd, Ste 103, Virginia Beach, VA 23454-3002; **Phone:** 757-481-2515; **Board Cert:** Internal Medicine 1981; Pulmonary Disease 1986; Critical Care Medicine 2001; **Med School:** Med Coll GA 1978; **Resid:** Internal Medicine, Univ VA Med Ctr 1981; **Fellow:** Pulmonary Disease, Univ VA Med Ctr 1983

Koenig, Steven Michael MD [Pul] - **Spec Exp:** Sleep Disorders/Apnea; Occupational Lung Disease; Asthma; **Hospital:** Univ Virginia Med Ctr; **Address:** Univ Va Hlth System, Dept Med, Pulmonary Div, Box 800546, Charlottesville, VA 22908-0546; **Phone:** 434-243-9212; **Board Cert:** Internal Medicine 1987; Pulmonary Disease 2000; Critical Care Medicine 2001; **Med School:** Univ Pennsylvania 1984; **Resid:** Internal Medicine, Univ Chicago Hosps 1987; **Fellow:** Pulmonary Critical Care Medicine, Univ Chicago 1990; Sleep Medicine, Deaconess Hosp 1994; **Fac Appt:** Prof Med, Univ VA Sch Med

Light, Richard W MD [Pul] - **Spec Exp:** Pleural Disease; **Hospital:** Vanderbilt Univ Med Ctr; **Address:** Vanderbilt Univ Med Ctr-Pulmonary Medicine, 1161 21st Ave S, T1218 MCN, Nashville, TN 37232-2650; **Phone:** 615-322-3412; **Board Cert:** Internal Medicine 1972; Pulmonary Disease 1974; **Med School:** Johns Hopkins Univ 1968; **Resid:** Internal Medicine, Johns Hopkins Hosp 1970; **Fellow:** Pulmonary Disease, Johns Hopkins Hosp 1972; **Fac Appt:** Prof Med, Vanderbilt Univ

LoRusso, Thomas J MD [Pul] - **Spec Exp:** Critical Care; **Hospital:** Inova Fairfax Hosp; **Address:** 1800 Town Ctr Drive, Ste 419, Reston, VA 20190; **Phone:** 703-620-3926; **Board Cert:** Internal Medicine 2003; Pulmonary Disease 2002; Critical Care Medicine 2001; **Med School:** SUNY Upstate Med Univ 1987; **Resid:** Internal Medicine, Univ Hosp-SUNY 1990; **Fellow:** Pulmonary Disease, Cedars Sinai Med Ctr 1993

Loyd, James E MD [Pul] - **Spec Exp:** Pulmonary Fibrosis; Interstitial Lung Disease; Transplant Medicine-Lung; **Hospital:** Vanderbilt Univ Med Ctr; **Address:** Vanderbilt Univ Med Ctr, Div Pulmonary Medicine, Medical Ctr North, rm T-1218, Nashville, TN 37232; **Phone:** 615-936-0393; **Board Cert:** Internal Medicine 1978; Pulmonary Disease 1984; Critical Care Medicine 1997; **Med School:** W VA Univ 1973; **Resid:** Internal Medicine, Vanderbilt Univ Hosp 1976; **Fellow:** Pulmonary Disease, Vanderbilt Univ Hosp 1978; **Fac Appt:** Prof Med, Vanderbilt Univ

Sahn, Steven A MD [Pul] - **Spec Exp:** Pleural Disease; Interstitial Lung Disease; Chronic Obstructive Lung Disease (COPD); Pulmonary Fibrosis; **Hospital:** MUSC Med Ctr; **Address:** MUSC, Div Pulm & Crit Care Med, 96 Jonathan Lucas St, Box 250630, Charleston, SC 29425-8900; **Phone:** 843-792-3167; **Board Cert:** Internal Medicine 1974; Pulmonary Disease 1974; **Med School:** Univ Louisville Sch Med 1968; **Resid:** Internal Medicine, Univ Iowa Hosp 1971; **Fellow:** Pulmonary Disease, Univ CO Hlth Sci Ctr 1973; **Fac Appt:** Prof Med, Med Univ SC

Schwartz, David A MD [Pul] - **Spec Exp:** Occupational Lung Disease; Pulmonary Fibrosis; Asthma; **Hospital:** Duke Univ Med Ctr; **Address:** Natl Inst Environmental Hlth Scis, Box 12233, Research Triangle Park, NC 27709; **Phone:** 919-541-3201; **Board Cert:** Internal Medicine 1984; Occupational Medicine 1987; Pulmonary Disease 1988; **Med School:** UCSD 1979; **Resid:** Internal Medicine, Boston City Hosp 1984; Preventive Medicine, Harvard Sch Public Health 1986; **Fellow:** Pulmonary Disease, Univ Seattle Medical Ctr 1988; **Fac Appt:** Prof Med, Duke Univ

Pulmonary Disease

Tapson, Victor MD [Pul] - **Spec Exp:** Pulmonary Hypertension; Transplant Medicine-Lung; Chronic Obstructive Lung Disease (COPD); Emphysema; **Hospital:** Duke Univ Med Ctr; **Address:** Duke Univ Med Ctr, Dept Pulm Critical Care Med, Box 31175, Durham, NC 27710; **Phone:** 919-684-6237; **Board Cert:** Internal Medicine 1986; Pulmonary Disease 2000; **Med School:** Hahnemann Univ 1982; **Resid:** Internal Medicine, Duke Univ Med Ctr 1986; **Fellow:** Pulmonary Disease, Boston Univ 1989; **Fac Appt:** Prof Med, Duke Univ

Vaughey, Ellen MD [Pul] - **Spec Exp:** Critical Care; **Hospital:** Inova Fairfax Hosp, Virginia Hosp Ctr - Arlington; **Address:** 3289 Woodburn Rd, Ste 350, Annandale, VA 22003; **Phone:** 703-641-8616; **Board Cert:** Internal Medicine 2001; Pulmonary Disease 2002; Critical Care Medicine 2003; **Med School:** Georgetown Univ 1987; **Resid:** Internal Medicine, Thomas Jefferson Univ 1990; **Fellow:** Pulmonary Disease, Roger Williams Hosp-Brown Univ 1993

Wanner, Adam MD [Pul] - **Spec Exp:** Asthma; **Hospital:** Jackson Meml Hosp; **Address:** Univ Miami Sch Med, Div Pulm & Crit Care, Box 016960 (R-47), Miami, FL 33101; **Phone:** 305-243-3045; **Board Cert:** Internal Medicine 1973; Pulmonary Disease 1974; **Med School:** Switzerland 1966; **Resid:** Internal Medicine, Kantonsspital Aarau 1970; **Fellow:** Pulmonary Disease, Mt Sinai Med Ctr 1972; **Fac Appt:** Prof Med, Univ Miami Sch Med

Wheeler, Arthur P MD [Pul] - **Spec Exp:** Critical Care; Sepsis; Respiratory Distress Syndrome (ARDS); **Hospital:** Vanderbilt Univ Med Ctr; **Address:** Vanderbilt Univ Medical Ctr, 1161 21st Ave S, rm T-1217 MCN, Nashville, TN 37232-2650; **Phone:** 615-322-3412; **Board Cert:** Internal Medicine 1985; Pulmonary Disease 1988; Critical Care Medicine 1999; **Med School:** Univ MD Sch Med 1982; **Resid:** Internal Medicine, Vanderbilt Univ Med Ctr 1985; **Fellow:** Pulmonary Disease, Vanderbilt Univ Med Ctr 1986; **Fac Appt:** Assoc Prof Med, Vanderbilt Univ

Young Jr, K Randall MD [Pul] - **Spec Exp:** Transplant Medicine-Lung; Cystic Fibrosis; **Hospital:** Univ of Ala Hosp at Birmingham; **Address:** 215 Tinsley Harrison Tower, 1900 University Blvd, Birmingham, AL 35294; **Phone:** 205-934-5400; **Board Cert:** Internal Medicine 1982; Pulmonary Disease 1986; Allergy & Immunology 1987; **Med School:** Jefferson Med Coll 1978; **Resid:** Internal Medicine, Yale-New Haven Hosp 1982; Pulmonary Critical Care Medicine, Yale-New Haven Hosp 1985; **Fellow:** Allergy & Immunology, Nat Inst Hlth 1988; **Fac Appt:** Prof Med, Univ Ala

Midwest

Balk, Robert A MD [Pul] - **Spec Exp:** Asthma; Cystic Fibrosis; Respiratory Failure; **Hospital:** Rush Univ Med Ctr, Rush Oak Park Hosp; **Address:** 1725 W Harrison St, Ste 054, Chicago, IL 60612; **Phone:** 312-942-6744; **Board Cert:** Internal Medicine 1981; Pulmonary Disease 1986; Critical Care Medicine 1997; **Med School:** Univ MO-Kansas City 1978; **Resid:** Internal Medicine, Univ MO-Kansas City Affil Hosps 1981; **Fellow:** Pulmonary Critical Care Medicine, Univ Ark Hosp 1983; **Fac Appt:** Prof Med, Rush Med Coll

Cromydas, George MD [Pul] - **Spec Exp:** Emphysema; Lung Disease; **Hospital:** Northwest Comm Hosp; **Address:** 1614 W Central Rd, Ste 107, Arlington Heights, IL 60005; **Phone:** 847-818-1184; **Board Cert:** Internal Medicine 1980; Pulmonary Disease 1984; Critical Care Medicine 1999; **Med School:** Univ IL Coll Med 1977; **Resid:** Internal Medicine, Univ Illinois Hosp & Clin 1980; **Fellow:** Pulmonary Critical Care Medicine, Univ Illinois Hosp & Clin 1982

Fahey, Patrick J MD [Pul] - **Hospital:** Loyola Univ Med Ctr, Hines VA Hosp; **Address:** Loyola Univ Med Ctr, 2160 1st Ave Bldg 102 - rm 7606, Maywood, IL 60153-3304; **Phone:** 708-216-3300; **Board Cert:** Internal Medicine 1976; Pulmonary Disease 1978; **Med School:** Univ Wisc 1973; **Resid:** Internal Medicine, St Elizabeth's Hosp 1976; **Fellow:** Pulmonary Disease, Strong Meml Hosp 1980; **Fac Appt:** Prof Med, Loyola Univ-Stritch Sch Med

Fletcher, Eugene MD [Pul] - **Spec Exp:** Chronic Obstructive Lung Disease (COPD); Sleep Disorders/Apnea; **Hospital:** Floyd Meml Hosp & Hlth Svcs; **Address:** 428 Vincennes, New Albany, IN 47150; **Phone:** 812-948-5841; **Board Cert:** Internal Medicine 1974; Pulmonary Disease 1980; **Med School:** Temple Univ 1971; **Resid:** Internal Medicine, Univ Colo Affil Hosp 1973; Internal Medicine, Fitzsimons Army Med Ctr 1974; **Fellow:** Pulmonary Disease, Univ Okla Hlth Scis Ctr 1974

Garrity Jr, Edward MD [Pul] - **Spec Exp:** Transplant Medicine-Lung; Pulmonary Vascular Disease; Asthma; Cystic Fibrosis; **Hospital:** Univ of Chicago Hosps; **Address:** Univ of Chicago Hospitals, 5841 S Maryland Ave, MC 0999, Chicago, IL 60637; **Phone:** 773-702-9660; **Board Cert:** Internal Medicine 1979; Pulmonary Disease 1998; Critical Care Medicine 1998; **Med School:** Loyola Univ-Stritch Sch Med 1976; **Resid:** Internal Medicine, Loyola Univ Med Ctr 1979; **Fellow:** Pulmonary Disease, Univ Chicago 1983; **Fac Appt:** Prof Med, Univ Chicago-Pritzker Sch Med

Gracey, Douglas Robert MD [Pul] - **Spec Exp:** Respiratory Failure; Chronic Obstructive Lung Disease (COPD); **Hospital:** Mayo Med Ctr & Clin - Rochester; **Address:** Mayo Clinic, 200 First St SW, Rochester, MN 55905-0001; **Phone:** 507-284-4348; **Board Cert:** Internal Medicine 1969; Pulmonary Disease 1970; **Med School:** Northwestern Univ 1962; **Resid:** Internal Medicine, Mayo Grad Sch Med 1966; **Fellow:** Pulmonary Disease, Mayo Grad Sch Med 1969; **Fac Appt:** Prof Med, Mayo Med Sch

Grum, Cyril M MD [Pul] - **Spec Exp:** Asthma; Cystic Fibrosis; **Hospital:** Univ Michigan Hlth Sys; **Address:** Univ Mich, Div Pulm & Crit Care Med, 1500 E Med Ctr Drive, rm 3110, Taubman Ctr, Ann Arbor, MI 48109-0368; **Phone:** 734-647-9342; **Board Cert:** Internal Medicine 1980; Pulmonary Disease 1982; **Med School:** Med Coll Wisc 1977; **Resid:** Internal Medicine, Cleveland Clinic; **Fellow:** Pulmonary Disease, Univ Mich Hosps; **Fac Appt:** Prof Med, Univ Mich Med Sch

Hall, Jesse MD [Pul] - **Spec Exp:** Respiratory Failure; Critical Care; Sleep Disorders/Apnea; **Hospital:** Univ of Chicago Hosps; **Address:** 5841 S Maryland Ave, MC 6026, Chicago, IL 60637; **Phone:** 773-702-1454; **Board Cert:** Internal Medicine 1980; Critical Care Medicine 1998; **Med School:** Univ Chicago-Pritzker Sch Med 1977; **Resid:** Internal Medicine, Univ Chicago Hosps 1982; **Fac Appt:** Prof Med, Univ Chicago-Pritzker Sch Med

Hertz, Marshall MD [Pul] - **Spec Exp:** Transplant Medicine-Lung; Transplant Medicine-Heart & Lung; Pulmonary Hypertension; **Hospital:** Univ Minn Med Ctr, Fairview - Univ Campus; **Address:** Pulmonary, Allergy & Critical Care Med, 420 Delaware St SE, MMC 276, Minneapolis, MN 55455; **Phone:** 612-624-0999; **Board Cert:** Internal Medicine 1981; Pulmonary Disease 1987; **Med School:** Univ Mich Med Sch 1978; **Resid:** Internal Medicine, Univ Minn Med Ctr 1982; **Fellow:** Pulmonary Critical Care Medicine, Univ Minn Med Ctr 1984; **Fac Appt:** Prof Med, Univ Minn

Pulmonary Disease

Hunninghake, Gary MD [Pul] - **Spec Exp:** Sarcoidosis; Interstitial Lung Disease; **Hospital:** Univ Iowa Hosp & Clinics; **Address:** Univ Iowa, Div Pulmonary Disease, 200 Hawkins Drive C33GH, Iowa City, IA 52242-1081; **Phone:** 319-356-4187; **Board Cert:** Internal Medicine 1975; Pulmonary Disease 1980; Allergy & Immunology 1977; **Med School:** Univ Kans 1972; **Resid:** Internal Medicine, Univ Kansas Med Ctr 1974; Pulmonary Disease, Natl Inst Hlth 1976; **Fac Appt:** Prof Med, Univ Iowa Coll Med

Hyers, Thomas M MD [Pul] - **Spec Exp:** Thromboembolic Disorders; Chronic Obstructive Lung Disease (COPD); Occupational Medicine; **Hospital:** SSM St Joseph Hosp of Kirkwood; **Address:** 533 Couch Ave, Ste 140, St Louis, MO 63122; **Phone:** 314-909-9779; **Board Cert:** Internal Medicine 1974; Pulmonary Disease 1980; Critical Care Medicine 1999; **Med School:** Duke Univ 1968; **Resid:** Internal Medicine, Univ Wash Med Ctr 1975; Pulmonary Disease, Univ Colorado Hosp 1977; **Fellow:** Pulmonary Disease, Natl Inst Hlth 1972; **Fac Appt:** Clin Prof Med, St Louis Univ

Jett, James R MD [Pul] - **Spec Exp:** Lung Cancer; Mesothelioma; Thymoma; **Hospital:** Mayo Med Ctr & Clin - Rochester; **Address:** Mayo Clinic, Thoracic Diseases, 200 First St SW, Rochester, MN 55905; **Phone:** 507-284-3764; **Board Cert:** Internal Medicine 1976; Pulmonary Disease 1978; **Med School:** Univ MO-Columbia Sch Med 1973; **Resid:** Internal Medicine, Mayo Clinic 1976; **Fellow:** Pulmonary Disease, Mayo Clinic 1978; **Fac Appt:** Prof Med, Mayo Med Sch

Kaye, Mitchell MD [Pul] - **Spec Exp:** Chronic Obstructive Lung Disease (COPD); Asthma; Sleep Disorders/Apnea; **Hospital:** Univ Minn Med Ctr, Fairview - Univ Campus; **Address:** Minn Lung Ctr, 920 E 28th St, Ste 700, Minneapolis, MN 55407; **Phone:** 612-863-3750; **Board Cert:** Internal Medicine 1987; Pulmonary Disease 2000; Critical Care Medicine 2001; **Med School:** Univ Minn 1984; **Resid:** Internal Medicine, Univ Ill Hosps & Clins 1987; **Fellow:** Pulmonary Disease, Northwestern Univ Med Sch 1989

Kovitz, Kevin L MD [Pul] - **Spec Exp:** Interventional Pulmonology; **Hospital:** St Alexius Med Ctr; **Address:** Suburban Lung Associates, 800 Biesterfield Rd, Ste 510, Elk Grove Village, IL 60007; **Phone:** 847-981-3660; **Board Cert:** Internal Medicine 1988; Pulmonary Disease 1992; Critical Care Medicine 1995; **Med School:** Israel 1985; **Resid:** Internal Medicine, Univ Maryland Hosps 1988; **Fellow:** Pulmonary Disease, Johns Hopkins Hosp 1992; Interventional Pulmonology, Sainte Marguerite Hosp 1993

Krowka, Michael J MD [Pul] - **Spec Exp:** Hepatopulmonary Syndrome; Pulmonary Hypertension; Chronic Obstructive Lung Disease (COPD); **Hospital:** Mayo Med Ctr & Clin - Rochester; **Address:** Mayo Clinic, Div Pulm & Crit Care Med, 200 First St SW, Rochester, MN 55905; **Phone:** 507-284-2921; **Board Cert:** Internal Medicine 1983; Pulmonary Disease 1986; **Med School:** Univ Nevada 1980; **Resid:** Internal Medicine, Evanston Hosp 1983; **Fellow:** Pulmonary Disease, Mayo Clinic 1986; **Fac Appt:** Prof Med, Mayo Med Sch

Lefrak, Stephen MD [Pul] - **Spec Exp:** Emphysema-Lung Volume Reduction; Critical Care; **Hospital:** Barnes-Jewish Hosp; **Address:** Wash Univ Sch Med, Div Pulm & Crit Care Med, 660 S Euclid Ave, Box 8052, St Louis, MO 63110; **Phone:** 314-362-6044; **Board Cert:** Internal Medicine 1972; Pulmonary Disease 1972; **Med School:** SUNY Downstate 1965; **Resid:** Internal Medicine, Boston Univ Hosp 1968; Pulmonary Disease, Kings Co Hosp Ctr 1969; **Fellow:** Cardiopulmonary Disease, Columbia-Presby Hosp 1970; **Fac Appt:** Prof Med, Washington Univ, St Louis

Lem, Vincent M MD [Pul] - **Spec Exp:** Asthma; **Hospital:** St Luke's Hosp of Kansas City; **Address:** 4321 Washington St, Ste 5100, Kansas City, MO 64111; **Phone:** 816-756-2255; **Board Cert:** Internal Medicine 1982; Pulmonary Disease 1984; **Med School:** Univ Kans 1978; **Resid:** Internal Medicine, St Luke's Hosp 1982; **Fellow:** Pulmonary Disease, Univ Texas Hlth Sci Ctr 1984; **Fac Appt:** Assoc Clin Prof Med, Univ MO-Kansas City

Marini, John Joseph MD [Pul] - **Spec Exp:** Critical Care; Mechanical Ventilation; Chronic Obstructive Lung Disease (COPD); **Hospital:** Regions Hosp - St Paul; **Address:** 640 Jackson St, MS 11203B, St Paul, MN 55101; **Phone:** 651-254-3456; **Board Cert:** Internal Medicine 2004; Pulmonary Disease 2003; Critical Care Medicine 2002; **Med School:** Johns Hopkins Univ 1973; **Resid:** Internal Medicine, Univ Washington Med Ctr 1976; **Fellow:** Pulmonary Disease, Univ Washington Med Ctr 1978; **Fac Appt:** Prof Med, Univ Minn

Martinez, Fernando J MD [Pul] - **Spec Exp:** Lung Disease; Critical Care; **Hospital:** Univ Michigan Hlth Sys; **Address:** 1500 E Med Ctr Dr Taubman Bldg - rm 3110, Ann Arbor, MI 48109-0360; **Phone:** 734-763-7668; **Board Cert:** Internal Medicine 1986; Pulmonary Disease 1988; Critical Care Medicine 2000; **Med School:** Univ Fla Coll Med 1983; **Resid:** Internal Medicine, Beth Israel Hosp 1986; **Fellow:** Pulmonary Disease, Boston Univ 1989; **Fac Appt:** Prof Med, Univ Mich Med Sch

Mehta, Atul Chandrakant MD [Pul] - **Spec Exp:** Transplant Medicine-Lung; Emphysema-Lung Volume Reduction; Interventional Pulmonology; **Hospital:** Cleveland Clin Fdn (page 57); **Address:** Cleveland Clin Fdn, 9500 Euclid Ave, Ste A-90, Cleveland, OH 44195-0001; **Phone:** 216-444-2911; **Board Cert:** Internal Medicine 1981; Pulmonary Disease 1984; **Med School:** India 1976; **Resid:** Internal Medicine, St Francis Med Ctr 1980; Internal Medicine, Easton Hosp 1981; **Fellow:** Pulmonary Disease, Cleveland Clin 1983

Popovich Jr, John MD [Pul] - **Spec Exp:** Lung Disease; Pulmonary Embolism; Interstitial Lung Disease; Critical Care; **Hospital:** Henry Ford Hosp; **Address:** Henry Ford Hosp, Dept Int Med, 2799 W Grand Blvd, Detroit, MI 48202; **Phone:** 313-916-1828; **Board Cert:** Internal Medicine 1978; Pulmonary Disease 1980; Critical Care Medicine 1996; **Med School:** Univ Mich Med Sch 1975; **Resid:** Internal Medicine, Henry Ford Hosp 1978; **Fellow:** Pulmonary Disease, Henry Ford Hosp 1980; **Fac Appt:** Prof Med, Wayne State Univ

Prakash, Udaya MD [Pul] - **Spec Exp:** Bronchoscopy; **Hospital:** Mayo Med Ctr & Clin - Rochester; **Address:** Mayo Clinic, Div Pulm & Crit Care Med, 200 First St SW, Rochester, MN 55905; **Phone:** 507-284-4162; **Board Cert:** Internal Medicine 1987; Pulmonary Disease 1976; **Med School:** India 1969; **Resid:** Internal Medicine, Mayo Clinic 1973; **Fellow:** Pulmonary Disease, Mayo Clinic 1976; **Fac Appt:** Prof Med, Mayo Med Sch

Shore, Bernard L MD [Pul] - **Spec Exp:** Lung Disease; Palliative Care; Pain Management; **Hospital:** Barnes-Jewish Hosp; **Address:** 4652 Maryland Ave, St Louis, MO 63108-1913; **Phone:** 314-367-3113; **Board Cert:** Internal Medicine 1980; Pulmonary Disease 1982; **Med School:** Washington Univ, St Louis 1977; **Resid:** Internal Medicine, Barnes Hosp 1980; **Fellow:** Pulmonary Disease, Wash Univ Med Ctr 1982; **Fac Appt:** Assoc Clin Prof Med, Washington Univ, St Louis

Silver, Michael R MD [Pul] - **Spec Exp:** Chronic Obstructive Lung Disease (COPD); Lung Cancer; Asthma; **Hospital:** Rush Univ Med Ctr, Rush Oak Park Hosp; **Address:** 1725 W Harrison St, Prof Bldg 3, Ste 054, Chicago, IL 60612; **Phone:** 312-942-6744; **Board Cert:** Internal Medicine 1984; Pulmonary Disease 1988; Critical Care Medicine 1999; **Med School:** Albany Med Coll 1981; **Resid:** Internal Medicine, Rush-Presby-St Luke's Med Ctr 1985; **Fellow:** Pulmonary Critical Care Medicine, Rush-Presby-St Luke's Med Ctr 1987; **Fac Appt:** Assoc Prof Med, Rush Med Coll

Pulmonary Disease

Stoller, James MD [Pul] - **Spec Exp:** Emphysema/Alpha-1 Antitrypsin Deficiency; **Hospital:** Cleveland Clin Fdn (page 57); **Address:** Cleveland Clinic Fdn, Div Pulmonary Med, 9500 Euclid Ave, Desk A90, Cleveland, OH 44195; **Phone:** 216-444-1960; **Board Cert:** Internal Medicine 1982; Pulmonary Disease 1984; **Med School:** Yale Univ 1979; **Resid:** Internal Medicine, Peter Bent Brigham Hosp 1982; **Fellow:** Pulmonary Disease, Brigham & Women's Hosp 1983; Critical Care Medicine, Mass Genl Hosp 1985; **Fac Appt:** Prof Med, Cleveland Cl Coll Med/Case West Res

Tobin, Martin MD [Pul] - **Spec Exp:** Mechanical Ventilation; Chronic Obstructive Lung Disease (COPD); **Hospital:** Loyola Univ Med Ctr, Hines VA Hosp; **Address:** Hines VA Hosp (111N), Fifth Ave and Roosevelt Rd, Bldg 1 - rm E438, Hines, IL 60141; **Phone:** 708-202-2705; **Board Cert:** Internal Medicine 1983; Pulmonary Disease 1984; **Med School:** Ireland 1975; **Resid:** Internal Medicine, Trinity Coll Hosps 1979; Pulmonary Disease, Kings Coll Hosp 1980; **Fellow:** Pulmonary Critical Care Medicine, Mount Sinai Hosp 1983; Pulmonary Critical Care Medicine, Univ Pittsburgh 1983; **Fac Appt:** Prof Med, Loyola Univ-Stritch Sch Med

Trulock, Elbert MD [Pul] - **Spec Exp:** Transplant Medicine-Lung; Emphysema-Lung Volume Reduction; Pulmonary Hypertension; Cystic Fibrosis; **Hospital:** Barnes-Jewish Hosp; **Address:** Wash Univ Sch Med, Dept Pulm, 660 S Euclid Ave, Box 8052, St Louis, MO 63110; **Phone:** 314-454-8766; **Board Cert:** Internal Medicine 1981; Pulmonary Disease 1984; **Med School:** Emory Univ 1978; **Resid:** Internal Medicine, Barnes Hosp 1981; **Fellow:** Pulmonary Disease, Wash Univ Med Ctr 1983; **Fac Appt:** Prof Med, Washington Univ, St Louis

Wiedemann, Herbert P MD [Pul] - **Spec Exp:** Respiratory Distress Syndrome (ARDS); Asthma; Emphysema; **Hospital:** Cleveland Clin Fdn (page 57); **Address:** Cleveland Clinic-Pulmonary & Allergy, 9500 Euclid Ave, Desk A90, Cleveland, OH 44195; **Phone:** 216-444-8335; **Board Cert:** Internal Medicine 1980; Pulmonary Disease 1984; Critical Care Medicine 1997; **Med School:** Cornell Univ-Weill Med Coll 1977; **Resid:** Internal Medicine, Univ Wash Hosps 1980; Internal Medicine, Harborview Hosp 1981; **Fellow:** Pulmonary Disease, Yale Univ 1984

Wunderink, Richard MD [Pul] - **Spec Exp:** Infectious Disease-Lung; Pneumonia; Sepsis; **Hospital:** Northwestern Meml Hosp; **Address:** 675 N St Clair, Galter 18-250, Chicago, IL 60611; **Phone:** 312-695-1800; **Board Cert:** Internal Medicine 1983; Pulmonary Disease 1986; Critical Care Medicine 1997; **Med School:** Indiana Univ 1980; **Resid:** Internal Medicine, Butterworth Hosp 1983; **Fellow:** Pulmonary Disease, Henry Ford Hosp 1985; **Fac Appt:** Prof Med, Northwestern Univ

Great Plains and Mountains

Brown, Kevin K MD [Pul] - **Spec Exp:** Pulmonary Fibrosis; Interstitial Lung Disease; Autoimmune Lung Disease; **Hospital:** Natl Jewish Med & Rsch Ctr, Univ Colorado Hosp; **Address:** Natl Jewish Med & Rsch Ctr, 1400 Jackson St, Denver, CO 80206-2762; **Phone:** 303-398-1621; **Board Cert:** Internal Medicine 1989; Pulmonary Disease 2005; **Med School:** Univ Minn 1984; **Resid:** Internal Medicine, Providence Med Ctr 1989; **Fellow:** Pulmonary Disease, Maine Med Ctr 1992; Pulmonary Disease, Univ Colo Hlth Scis Ctr 1994; **Fac Appt:** Assoc Prof Med, Univ Colorado

Elliott, C Gregory MD [Pul] - **Spec Exp:** Pulmonary Hypertension; Thromboembolic Disorders; **Hospital:** LDS Hosp; **Address:** Department of Medicine, LDS Hosp, Pulmonary Div, 8th Ave & C St, Salt Lake City, UT 84143; **Phone:** 801-408-1875; **Board Cert:** Internal Medicine 1976; Pulmonary Disease 1978; **Med School:** Univ MD Sch Med 1973; **Resid:** Internal Medicine, Univ Maryland Hosp 1976; **Fellow:** Pulmonary Disease, Univ Utah 1978; **Fac Appt:** Prof Med, Univ Utah

Iseman, Michael MD [Pul] - **Spec Exp:** Tuberculosis; Mycobacterial Infections; **Hospital:** Natl Jewish Med & Rsch Ctr; **Address:** Natl Jewish Med & Rsch Ctr, 1400 Jackson St, rm J223, Denver, CO 80206; **Phone:** 303-398-1667; **Board Cert:** Internal Medicine 1972; Pulmonary Disease 1976; **Med School:** Columbia P&S 1965; **Resid:** Internal Medicine, Bellevue Hosp 1967; Internal Medicine, Harlem Hosp 1970; **Fellow:** Pulmonary Disease, Harlem Hosp 1972; **Fac Appt:** Prof Med, Univ Colorado

Kaplan, James MD [Pul] - **Spec Exp:** Critical Care; Sleep Disorders/Apnea; **Hospital:** Overland Pk Regl Med Ctr, Providence Med Ctr; **Address:** 10550 Quivira , Ste 480, Overland Park, KS 66215-2304; **Phone:** 913-599-3800; **Board Cert:** Internal Medicine 1987; Pulmonary Disease 2000; Critical Care Medicine 2003; **Med School:** Univ MO-Kansas City 1984; **Resid:** Internal Medicine, Barnes Hosp 1987; **Fellow:** Pulmonary Disease, Barnes Hosp-Wash Univ 1987

Make, Barry J MD [Pul] - **Spec Exp:** Chronic Obstructive Lung Disease (COPD); Emphysema; Asthma; **Hospital:** Natl Jewish Med & Rsch Ctr, Rose Med Ctr; **Address:** Natl Jewish Med & Rsch Ctr, 1400 Jackson St, rm J211, Denver, CO 80206-2762; **Phone:** 303-398-1703; **Board Cert:** Internal Medicine 1973; **Med School:** Jefferson Med Coll 1970; **Resid:** Internal Medicine, Univ Michigan Med Ctr 1973; **Fellow:** Pulmonary Disease, West Virginia Med Ctr 1974; Pulmonary Disease, Boston Univ Med Ctr 1976; **Fac Appt:** Prof Med, Univ Colorado

Martin, Richard Jay MD [Pul] - **Spec Exp:** Asthma; Vocal Cord Disorders; Chronic Obstructive Lung Disease (COPD); **Hospital:** Natl Jewish Med & Rsch Ctr, Univ Colorado Hosp; **Address:** Natl Jewish Med & Research Ctr, 1400 Jackson St, Denver, CO 80206-2762; **Phone:** 303-398-1847; **Board Cert:** Internal Medicine 1976; Pulmonary Disease 1978; **Med School:** Univ Mich Med Sch 1971; **Resid:** Internal Medicine, Tulane Univ Affil Hosp 1976; **Fellow:** Pulmonary Disease, Univ Oklahoma 1978; **Fac Appt:** Prof Med, Univ Colorado

Newman, Lee MD [Pul] - **Spec Exp:** Occupational Lung Disease; Sarcoidosis; Lung Disease; **Hospital:** Univ Colorado Hosp; **Address:** Univ Colorado Hlth Science Ctr, 4200 E 9th Ave, rm B-164, Denver, CO 80262; **Phone:** 303-315-7601; **Board Cert:** Internal Medicine 1983; Pulmonary Disease 1986; **Med School:** Vanderbilt Univ 1980; **Resid:** Internal Medicine, Emory Univ Affil Prgm 1984; **Fellow:** Pulmonary Disease, Univ Colorado 1987; **Fac Appt:** Prof Med, Univ Colorado

Pingleton, Susan MD [Pul] - **Spec Exp:** Critical Care; Hospital Acquired Infections; **Hospital:** Univ of Kansas Hosp; **Address:** 3901 Rainbow Blvd, MS 1022, Kansas City, KS 66160; **Phone:** 913-588-6000; **Board Cert:** Internal Medicine 1977; Pulmonary Disease 1978; Critical Care Medicine 1991; **Med School:** Univ Kans 1972; **Resid:** Internal Medicine, Univ Kansas Med Ctr 1975; **Fac Appt:** Prof Med, Univ Kans

Rennard, Stephen I MD [Pul] - **Spec Exp:** Chronic Obstructive Lung Disease (COPD); Emphysema; **Hospital:** Nebraska Med Ctr; **Address:** University of Nebraska Medical Ctr, 985885 Nebrasaka Medical Center, Omaha, NE 68198-5885; **Phone:** 402-559-7313; **Board Cert:** Internal Medicine 1978; Pulmonary Disease 1982; **Med School:** Baylor Coll Med 1975; **Resid:** Internal Medicine, Barnes Hosp-Washington Univ 1977; **Fac Appt:** Prof Med, Univ Nebr Coll Med

Rose, Cecile MD [Pul] - **Spec Exp:** Occupational Lung Disease; Sarcoidosis; Pneumonia; **Hospital:** Natl Jewish Med & Rsch Ctr; **Address:** 1400 Jackson St, rm G-211, Denver, CO 80206-2761; **Phone:** 303-398-1520; **Board Cert:** Internal Medicine 1983; Pulmonary Disease 1986; Occupational Medicine 1987; **Med School:** Univ IL Coll Med 1980; **Resid:** Internal Medicine, Med Coll Virginia Hosp 1983; **Fellow:** Pulmonary Disease, Med Coll Virginia Hosp 1985; **Fac Appt:** Assoc Prof Med, Univ Colorado

Pulmonary Disease

Schwarz, Marvin I MD [Pul] - **Spec Exp:** Interstitial Lung Disease; Pulmonary Vascular Disease; Lung Hemorrhage; **Hospital:** Univ Colorado Hosp, Natl Jewish Med & Rsch Ctr; **Address:** Div Pulmonary Science & Critical Care, 4200 Ninth Ave, Denver, CO 80262-0001; **Phone:** 303-315-4211; **Board Cert:** Internal Medicine 1970; Pulmonary Disease 1971; **Med School:** Tulane Univ 1964; **Resid:** Internal Medicine, Charity Hosp 1967; **Fellow:** Pulmonary Disease, Charity Hosp/Tulane Univ 1969; **Fac Appt:** Prof Med, Univ Colorado

Voelkel, Norbert F MD [Pul] - **Spec Exp:** Pulmonary Hypertension; Asthma; Emphysema; **Hospital:** Univ Colorado Hosp, Natl Jewish Med & Rsch Ctr; **Address:** Univ Colorado Hlth Sci Ctr, 4200 E 9th Ave, Box C272, Denver, CO 80262-0001; **Phone:** 303-315-7047; **Med School:** Germany 1972; **Resid:** Internal Medicine, Univ Hamburg 1977; **Fellow:** Research, Univ Colorado 1978; Pulmonary Disease, Univ Colorado 1981; **Fac Appt:** Prof Med, Univ Colorado

Southwest

Arroliga, Alejandro C MD [Pul] - **Spec Exp:** Pulmonary Hypertension; Respiratory Distress Syndrome (ARDS); Critical Care; **Hospital:** Scott & White Mem Hosp; **Address:** 2401 S 31st St, Temple, TX 76508; **Phone:** 254-724-9887; **Board Cert:** Internal Medicine 2000; Pulmonary Disease 2000; Critical Care Medicine 2003; **Med School:** Mexico 1984; **Resid:** Internal Medicine, Coney Island Hosp 1990; **Fellow:** Pulmonary Critical Care Medicine, Yale-New Haven Hosp 1993; **Fac Appt:** Prof Med, Cleveland Cl Coll Med/Case West Res

Guidry, George Gary MD [Pul] - **Spec Exp:** Chronic Obstructive Lung Disease (COPD); Asthma; Pneumonia; Lung Cancer; **Hospital:** Lafayette Genl Med Ctr, Our Lady of Lourdes Reg Med Ctr - Lafayette; **Address:** 155 Hospital Drive, Ste 206, Lafayette, LA 70503-2852; **Phone:** 337-234-3204; **Board Cert:** Internal Medicine 1988; Pulmonary Disease 1999; **Med School:** Louisiana State Univ 1985; **Resid:** Internal Medicine, LSU Med Ctr 1988; **Fellow:** Pulmonary Disease, LSU Med Ctr; **Fac Appt:** Assoc Clin Prof Med, Louisiana State Univ

Jenkinson, Stephen George MD [Pul] - **Spec Exp:** Lung Cancer; Chronic Obstructive Lung Disease (COPD); Asthma; **Hospital:** Audie L Murphy Meml Vets Hosp, Univ Hlth Sys - Univ Hosp; **Address:** Audie Murphy VA Hosp, Dept Pulm Dis, 7400 Merton Minter Blvd, MC 111E, San Antonio, TX 78229; **Phone:** 210-617-5256; **Board Cert:** Internal Medicine 1976; Pulmonary Disease 1978; **Med School:** Louisiana State Univ 1973; **Resid:** Internal Medicine, LSU Med Ctr 1976; **Fellow:** Pulmonary Disease, LSU Med Ctr 1978; **Fac Appt:** Prof Med, Univ Tex, San Antonio

Levin, David C MD [Pul] - **Spec Exp:** Critical Care; **Hospital:** OU Med Ctr, VA Med Ctr - Oklahoma City; **Address:** OU Physicians Building, 825 NE 10th St, Ste 2500, Oklahoma City, OK 73104; **Phone:** 405-271-7001; **Board Cert:** Internal Medicine 1973; Pulmonary Disease 1976; **Med School:** Case West Res Univ 1970; **Resid:** Internal Medicine, Univ Colorado Hlth Sci Ctr 1974; **Fellow:** Pulmonary Disease, Univ Colorado Hlth Sci Ctr 1975; **Fac Appt:** Prof Med, Univ Okla Coll Med

Perret, Philip S MD [Pul] - **Spec Exp:** Chronic Obstructive Lung Disease (COPD); **Hospital:** Our Lady of Lourdes Reg Med Ctr - Lafayette; **Address:** 614 W St Mary Blvd, Lafayette, LA 70506; **Phone:** 337-232-6435; **Board Cert:** Internal Medicine 1978; Pulmonary Disease 1980; Critical Care Medicine 1997; **Med School:** Emory Univ 1974; **Resid:** Internal Medicine, Emory Univ Hosp 1977; **Fellow:** Pulmonary Disease, Emory Univ Hosp 1979

Shellito, Judd E MD [Pul] - **Spec Exp:** Pulmonary Infections; Occupational Lung Disease; **Hospital:** L Boggs Med Ctr; **Address:** 3600 Prytania St, Ste 35, New Orleans, LA 70115; **Phone:** 504-895-5748; **Board Cert:** Internal Medicine 1977; Pulmonary Disease 1980; **Med School:** Tulane Univ 1974; **Resid:** Internal Medicine, Evanston Hosp 1978; **Fellow:** Pulmonary Critical Care Medicine, Univ New Mexico Hosp 1980; **Fac Appt:** Prof Med, Louisiana State Univ

Summer, Warren MD [Pul] - **Spec Exp:** Chronic Obstructive Lung Disease (COPD); Asthma; Respiratory Distress Syndrome (ARDS); **Hospital:** L Boggs Med Ctr; **Address:** 3600 Prytania St, Ste 35, New Orleans, LA 70115; **Phone:** 504-895-5748; **Board Cert:** Internal Medicine 1972; Pulmonary Disease 1972; **Med School:** Georgetown Univ 1965; **Resid:** Internal Medicine, Maimonides Med Ctr 1968; **Fellow:** Pulmonary Disease, Georgetown Univ Hosp 1969; **Fac Appt:** Prof Med, Louisiana State Univ

Weissler, Jonathan C MD [Pul] - **Spec Exp:** Interstitial Lung Disease; Asthma; **Hospital:** UT Southwestern Med Ctr - Dallas, Parkland Meml Hosp - Dallas; **Address:** 5323 Harry Hines Blvd, Dallas, TX 75390-9034; **Phone:** 214-645-1825; **Board Cert:** Internal Medicine 1982; Pulmonary Disease 1984; Critical Care Medicine 1997; **Med School:** NYU Sch Med 1979; **Resid:** Internal Medicine, Univ Texas Hlth Sci Ctr 1982; **Fellow:** Pulmonary Disease, Univ Texas HlthSci Ctr 1985; **Fac Appt:** Prof Med, Univ Tex SW, Dallas

West Coast and Pacific

Albertson, Timothy MD/PhD [Pul] - **Spec Exp:** Critical Care; Transplant Medicine-Lung; **Hospital:** UC Davis Med Ctr; **Address:** UC Davis, Div Pulm Crit Care, 4150 V St, Ste 3400, Patient Support Svcs Bldg, Sacramento, CA 95817-9002; **Phone:** 916-734-3564; **Board Cert:** Pulmonary Disease 1984; Critical Care Medicine 1996; Emergency Medicine 1997; Medical Toxicology 2005; **Med School:** UC Davis 1977; **Resid:** Internal Medicine, Univ Arizona 1980; Internal Medicine, UC Davis Med Ctr 1981; **Fellow:** Pulmonary Critical Care Medicine, UC Davis Med Ctr 1983; **Fac Appt:** Prof Med, UC Davis

Balmes, John Randolph MD [Pul] - **Spec Exp:** Occupational Lung Disease; **Hospital:** San Francisco Genl Hosp, UCSF Med Ctr; **Address:** UCSF, Division Occup & Envr Med, Campus Box 0843, San Francisco, CA 94143-0843; **Phone:** 415-206-8314; **Board Cert:** Internal Medicine 1979; Pulmonary Disease 1984; **Med School:** Mount Sinai Sch Med 1976; **Resid:** Internal Medicine, Mount Sinai Hosp 1979; **Fellow:** Pulmonary Disease, Yale-New Haven Hosp 1981; **Fac Appt:** Prof Med, UCSF

Bellamy, Paul E MD [Pul] - **Spec Exp:** Critical Care; **Hospital:** KFH Woodland Hills Med Ctr; **Address:** Kaiser Woodland Hills Med Ctr, Pulm Div, 5601 De Soto Ave, Med Office Twr, Fl 4, Woodland Hills, CA 91367; **Phone:** 818-719-3530; **Board Cert:** Internal Medicine 1978; Pulmonary Disease 1980; Critical Care Medicine 1997; **Med School:** SUNY Buffalo 1975; **Resid:** Internal Medicine, Univ Hosps-Case West Res 1978; **Fellow:** Pulmonary Disease, UCLA Med Ctr 1980; **Fac Appt:** Clin Prof Med, UCLA

Boushey Jr, Homer A MD [Pul] - **Spec Exp:** Asthma; **Hospital:** UCSF Med Ctr; **Address:** UCSF Med Ctr, Dept Med, 400 Parnassus Ave, Box 0359, San Francisco, CA 94143; **Phone:** 415-353-2961; **Board Cert:** Internal Medicine 1972; Pulmonary Disease 1974; **Med School:** UCSF 1968; **Resid:** Internal Medicine, UCSF Med Ctr 1970; Internal Medicine, Beth Israel Hosp 1971; **Fellow:** Pulmonary Disease, Oxford Univ 1972; Pulmonary Disease, UCSF Hosp 1973; **Fac Appt:** Prof Med, UCSF

Pulmonary Disease

Catanzaro, Antonino MD [Pul] - **Spec Exp:** Tuberculosis; Coccidioidomycosis; Mycobacterial Infections; **Hospital:** UCSD Med Ctr; **Address:** 200 W Arbor Drive, rm 8374, San Diego, CA 92103-8374; **Phone:** 619-543-5550; **Board Cert:** Internal Medicine 1972; Pulmonary Disease 1976; **Med School:** SUNY Buffalo 1965; **Resid:** Internal Medicine, Georgetown Univ Hosp 1970; **Fellow:** Pulmonary Critical Care Medicine, UCSD Med Ctr 1972; Research, Scripps Clin Rsch Fdn 1972; **Fac Appt:** Prof Med, UCSD

Gong Jr, Henry MD [Pul] - **Spec Exp:** Lung Disease; Environmental Diseases; **Hospital:** Rancho Los Amigos Natl Rehab Ctr; **Address:** Rancho Los Amigos Natl Rehab Ctr, 7601 E Imperial Hwy, rm HB-145, Downey, CA 90242; **Phone:** 562-401-7611; **Board Cert:** Internal Medicine 1977; Pulmonary Disease 1980; **Med School:** UC Davis 1973; **Resid:** Internal Medicine, Boston Hosp 1975; **Fellow:** Pulmonary Disease, UCLA Med Ctr 1977; **Fac Appt:** Prof Med, USC Sch Med

Heffner, John E MD [Pul] - **Spec Exp:** Critical Care; Respiratory Failure; **Hospital:** Providence Portland Med Ctr; **Address:** 5050 NE Hoyt St, Ste 540, Portland, OR 97213; **Phone:** 503-215-6600; **Board Cert:** Internal Medicine 1977; Pulmonary Disease 1982; Critical Care Medicine 1987; **Med School:** UCLA 1974; **Resid:** Internal Medicine, Univ Colo Med Ctr 1978; **Fac Appt:** Prof Med, Med Univ SC

Hopewell, Philip MD [Pul] - **Spec Exp:** AIDS/HIV; Tuberculosis; Infectious Disease-Lung; **Hospital:** San Francisco Genl Hosp; **Address:** 1001 Potrero Ave, Ste 5K1, San Francisco, CA 94110; **Phone:** 415-206-8313; **Board Cert:** Internal Medicine 1973; Pulmonary Disease 1974; **Med School:** W VA Univ 1965; **Resid:** Internal Medicine, UCSF Med Ctr 1971; **Fellow:** Pulmonary Disease, UCSF Med Ctr 1973; **Fac Appt:** Prof Med, UCSF

Huang, Laurence MD [Pul] - **Spec Exp:** AIDS/HIV; Pneumocystis Carinii Pneumonia (PCP); **Hospital:** San Francisco Genl Hosp; **Address:** UCSF Positive Health Program - SFGH, 995 Potrero Ave, Bldg 80-Ward 84, San Francisco, CA 94110; **Phone:** 415-206-2400; **Board Cert:** Internal Medicine 1993; Pulmonary Disease 1996; Critical Care Medicine 1997; **Med School:** Columbia P&S 1989; **Resid:** Internal Medicine, Columbia-Presby Hosp 1992; Pulmonary Critical Care Medicine, UCSF Med Ctr 1995; **Fac Appt:** Assoc Clin Prof Med, UCSF

Hudson, Leonard MD [Pul] - **Spec Exp:** Critical Care; Lung Injury/ARDS; Respiratory Failure; **Hospital:** Harborview Med Ctr; **Address:** Harborview Medical Ctr, 325 9th Ave, Box 359762, Seattle, WA 98104; **Phone:** 206-731-3123; **Board Cert:** Internal Medicine 1973; Pulmonary Disease 1974; **Med School:** Univ Wash 1964; **Resid:** Internal Medicine, New York Hosp 1966; Internal Medicine, Univ Wash Hosps 1969; **Fellow:** Pulmonary Disease, Univ Colo Med Ctr 1971; **Fac Appt:** Prof Med, Univ Wash

Jacoby, David MD [Pul] - **Hospital:** OR Hlth & Sci Univ; **Address:** 3181 SW Sam Jackson Park Rd, MC UHN67, Dept Pulmonary/Crit Care, Portland, OR 97239; **Phone:** 503-494-6158; **Board Cert:** Internal Medicine 1983; Pulmonary Disease 1986; **Med School:** NY Med Coll 1980; **Resid:** Internal Medicine, Temple Univ Hosp 1983; **Fellow:** Pulmonary Critical Care Medicine, UCSF Hosp 1987; **Fac Appt:** Prof Med, Oregon Hlth Sci Univ

King Jr, Talmadge E MD [Pul] - **Spec Exp:** Interstitial Lung Disease; Sarcoidosis; Asthma; **Hospital:** San Francisco Genl Hosp, UCSF Med Ctr; **Address:** 1001 Potrero Ave, Ste 5H22, San Francisco, CA 94110; **Phone:** 415-206-3465; **Board Cert:** Internal Medicine 1977; Pulmonary Disease 1982; **Med School:** Harvard Med Sch 1974; **Resid:** Internal Medicine, Grady-Emory Univ Affil Hosp 1977; **Fellow:** Pulmonary Critical Care Medicine, Univ Colo Hlth Sci Ctr 1979; **Fac Appt:** Prof Med, UCSF

Lynch, Joseph P MD [Pul] - **Spec Exp:** Transplant Medicine-Lung; Interstitial Lung Disease; Pulmonary Fibrosis; **Hospital:** UCLA Med Ctr; **Address:** UCLA - Div Pulmonary Med, 200 UCLA Med Plaza, Ste 365-B2, Los Angeles, CA 90095; **Phone:** 310-825-8599; **Board Cert:** Internal Medicine 1976; Pulmonary Disease 1980; **Med School:** Harvard Med Sch 1973; **Resid:** Internal Medicine, Univ Mich Med Ctr 1976; **Fellow:** Pulmonary Disease, Univ Mich Med Ctr 1978; **Fac Appt:** Prof Med, UCLA

Martin, Thomas R MD [Pul] - **Spec Exp:** Respiratory Distress Syndrome (ARDS); Critical Care; **Hospital:** VA Puget Sound Hlth Care Sys; **Address:** Seattle VA Hosp - Pulmonary Rsch 151L, 1660 S Columbian Way, Seattle, WA 98108; **Phone:** 206-764-2219; **Board Cert:** Internal Medicine 1976; Pulmonary Disease 1980; **Med School:** Univ Pennsylvania 1973; **Resid:** Internal Medicine, Univ Washington Med Ctr 1977; **Fellow:** Pulmonary Disease, Univ Washington 1980; **Fac Appt:** Prof Med, Univ Wash

Matthay, Michael Anthony MD [Pul] - **Spec Exp:** Critical Care; Respiratory Distress Syndrome (ARDS); **Hospital:** UCSF Med Ctr; **Address:** UCSF Med Ctr, 505 Parnasas Ave, rm M-917, San Francisco, CA 94143-0624; **Phone:** 415-353-1206; **Board Cert:** Internal Medicine 1976; Pulmonary Disease 1980; Critical Care Medicine 1987; **Med School:** Univ Pennsylvania 1973; **Resid:** Internal Medicine, Univ Colo Med Ctr 1976; **Fellow:** Surgery, UCLA Med Ctr 1979; **Fac Appt:** Prof Med, UCSF

Mosenifar, Zab MD [Pul] - **Spec Exp:** Chronic Obstructive Lung Disease (COPD); Interstitial Lung Disease; Asthma; Pulmonary Hypertension; **Hospital:** Cedars-Sinai Med Ctr; **Address:** Cedars-Sinai Med Ctr, Div Pulmonary Med, 8700 Beverly Blvd, rm 6732 South Twr, Los Angeles, CA 90048-1804; **Phone:** 310-423-4685; **Board Cert:** Internal Medicine 1978; Pulmonary Disease 1980; **Med School:** Iran 1973; **Resid:** Internal Medicine, Thomas Jefferson Univ Hosp; Internal Medicine, UCLA Med Ctr; **Fellow:** Pulmonary Disease, UCLA Med Ctr; **Fac Appt:** Prof Med, UCLA

Patterson, James R MD [Pul] - **Spec Exp:** Chronic Obstructive Lung Disease (COPD); **Hospital:** Providence Portland Med Ctr; **Address:** 1111 NE 99th Ave, Ste 200, Portland, OR 97220; **Phone:** 503-963-3030; **Board Cert:** Internal Medicine 1972; Pulmonary Disease 2001; **Med School:** Columbia P&S 1968; **Resid:** Internal Medicine, Columbia-Presby Med Ctr 1970; **Fellow:** Pulmonary Disease, Fitzsimons Army Med Ctr 1973; **Fac Appt:** Clin Prof Med, Oregon Hlth Sci Univ

Raghu, Ganesh MD [Pul] - **Spec Exp:** Interstitial Lung Disease; Pulmonary Fibrosis; Sarcoidosis; Transplant-Lung; **Hospital:** Univ Wash Med Ctr; **Address:** 1959 NE Pacific St, Box 356166, Seattle, WA 98195; **Phone:** 206-598-4615; **Board Cert:** Internal Medicine 1982; **Med School:** India 1974; **Resid:** Internal Medicine, Univ Rochester-Strong Meml Hosp 1978; Internal Medicine, SUNY Buffalo Med Ctr 1981; **Fellow:** Pulmonary Critical Care Medicine, Univ Washington 1984; **Fac Appt:** Prof Med, Univ Wash

Ries, Andrew MD [Pul] - **Spec Exp:** Chronic Obstructive Lung Disease (COPD); Pulmonary Rehabilitation; **Hospital:** UCSD Med Ctr; **Address:** UCSD Med Ctr, 200 W Arbor Dr, San Diego, CA 92103-8377; **Phone:** 619-543-7350; **Board Cert:** Internal Medicine 1977; Pulmonary Disease 1980; **Med School:** Yale Univ 1974; **Resid:** Internal Medicine, Bellevue Hosp Ctr 1977; **Fellow:** Pulmonary Disease, UCSD Med Ctr 1981; **Fac Appt:** Prof Med, UCSD

Rizk, Norman W MD [Pul] - **Spec Exp:** Critical Care; Asthma; **Hospital:** Stanford Univ Med Ctr; **Address:** 300 Pasteur Drive, Ste H3142, Stanford, CA 94305-5236; **Phone:** 650-725-7061; **Board Cert:** Internal Medicine 1979; Pulmonary Disease 1984; Critical Care Medicine 1996; **Med School:** Yale Univ 1976; **Resid:** Internal Medicine, San Fran Genl Hosp 1980; **Fellow:** Pulmonary Disease, Moffitt Hosp-UCSF 1983; **Fac Appt:** Prof Med, Stanford Univ

Rubin, Lewis MD [Pul] - **Spec Exp:** Pulmonary Hypertension; Pulmonary Vascular Disease; **Hospital:** UCSD Med Ctr; **Address:** UCSD Med Ctr, Pulmonary & Critical Care, 9300 Campus Point Drive, MC 7381, La Jolla, CA 92037-7381; **Phone:** 858-657-8700; **Board Cert:** Internal Medicine 1978; Pulmonary Disease 1980; **Med School:** Albert Einstein Coll Med 1975; **Resid:** Internal Medicine, Duke Univ Med Ctr 1978; **Fellow:** Pulmonary Disease, Duke Univ Med Ctr 1979; **Fac Appt:** Prof Med, UCSD

Sharma, Om Prakash MD [Pul] - **Spec Exp:** Sarcoidosis; Interstitial Lung Disease; Hypersensitivity Pneumonitis; **Hospital:** LAC & USC Med Ctr, USC Univ Hosp - R K Eamer Med Plz; **Address:** 1200 N State St, Bldg GNH 11900, Los Angeles, CA 90033; **Phone:** 323-226-7923; **Board Cert:** Internal Medicine 1987; **Med School:** India 1959; **Resid:** Internal Medicine, Norwalk Hosp 1963; Internal Medicine, Einstein Med Coll Hosp 1965; **Fellow:** Pulmonary Disease, Einstein Med Coll Hosp 1966; Research, Royal Coll Physicians 1969; **Fac Appt:** Prof Med, USC Sch Med

Tharratt, Robert S MD [Pul] - **Spec Exp:** Bioterrorism Preparedness; Toxicology; **Hospital:** UC Davis Med Ctr; **Address:** UC Davis Med Ctr, Div Pulm Crit Care, 4150 V St, Ste 3400-Pt Support Services Bldg, Sacramento, CA 95817-2214; **Phone:** 916-734-3564; **Board Cert:** Pulmonary Disease 1988; Critical Care Medicine 1999; Medical Toxicology 2004; Emergency Medicine 1997; **Med School:** UCLA 1983; **Resid:** Internal Medicine, UC Davis Med Ctr 1986; **Fellow:** Pulmonary Critical Care Medicine, UC Davis Med Ctr 1989; **Fac Appt:** Prof Med, UC Davis

Wallace, Jeanne Marie MD [Pul] - **Spec Exp:** Pulmonary Infections; Sleep Disorders/Apnea; Asthma; **Hospital:** Olive View Med Ctr; **Address:** Olive View UCLA Med Ctr, 14445 Olive View Dr, Sylmar, CA 91342-1437; **Phone:** 818-364-3205; **Board Cert:** Internal Medicine 1977; Pulmonary Disease 1980; **Med School:** UCLA 1974; **Resid:** Internal Medicine, UCSF Med Ctr 1977; **Fellow:** Pulmonary Disease, UCSD Med Ctr 1980; **Fac Appt:** Assoc Prof Med, UCLA

Cleveland Clinic

Pulmonary, Allergy and Critical Care Medicine

Individuals with all types of acute or chronic lung diseases, as well as sleep disordered breathing (sleep apnea), can access specialty care at Cleveland Clinic. In 2006, physicians in the Department of Pulmonary, Allergy and Critical Care Medicine provided over 54,000 outpatient visits and cared for more than 1,400 hospital admissions.

Lung Transplantation

Cleveland Clinic's Lung Transplant Program is the largest in Ohio and among the largest in the United States. Since the program began, it has grown to include dozens of single lung, double lung, and heart/lung transplants every year. The average wait time for a lung transplantation at Cleveland Clinic is significantly lower than the national average.

Sarcoidosis Center of Excellence

In January 2003, Cleveland Clinic was awarded a $2 million grant from the Department of Health and Human Services to establish a Sarcoidosis Center of Excellence. The only such center in Northeastern Ohio, the center aims to raise awareness of pulmonary sarcoidosis, improve the quality of sarcoidosis care and minimize the degree to which it can affect quality of life.

Areas of Expertise

Acute respiratory distress syndrome (ARDS), Allergy rhinitis, Allergies (drug and food; latex), Aspirin desensitization, Asthma, Beryllium-induced lung disease, Chronic obstructive pulmonary disease (COPD), Including alpha-1 antitrypsin deficiency, Interstitial lung disease, Interventional bronchology, Lung cancer, Lymphangioleiomyomatosis (LAM), Pulmonary alveolar proteinosis (PAP), Pulmonary vascular disease, Sarcoidosis, Sepsis, Sleep-disordered breathing, Urticaria, Weaning from mechanical ventilation

To schedule an appointment or for more information about the Cleveland Clinic Department of Pulmonary, Allergy and Critical Care Medicine call 800.890.2467 or visit www.clevelandclinic.org/pulmonarytopdocs.

Department of Pulmonary, Allergy and Critical Care Medicine
9500 Euclid Avenue / W14 | Cleveland OH 44195

In collaboration with thoracic surgery colleagues, we evaluate patients for:

- Lung transplantation
- Lung-volume reduction surgery (LVRS) for emphysema
- Pulmonary thomboednarterectomy (for chronic pulmonary hypertension secondary to thromboemboli)

Second Opinion-Online

Use e-Cleveland Clinic's convenient, online second opinion service without leaving home. Call 800.223.2273, ext 43223, or visit www.eclevelandclinic.org.

Assistance for Out-of-Town and International Patients

Get complimentary help scheduling medical appointments and arranging for hotels and transportation. For out-of-town patients call 800.223.2273, ext. 55580, or visit www.clevelandclinic.org/services. For International patients call 216.444.6404 or visit www.clevelandclinic.org/ic.

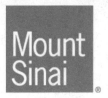

THE MOUNT SINAI MEDICAL CENTER
PULMONARY MEDICINE

One Gustave L. Levy Place (Fifth Avenue and 100th Street)
New York, NY 10029-6574
Physician Referral: 1-800-MD-SINAI (637-4624)
www.mountsinai.org

Patients at Mount Sinai have access to a number of special programs and services designed by our specialists in Pulmonary Medicine, including:

- *Asthma Program*, which uses a multidisciplinary team approach, focusing on patient education and skill-building to foster self management;
- *Chronic Obstructive Pulmonary Disease (COPD) Program*, offering —for one of the nation's most underdiagnosed conditions—a coordinated approach of exercise, treatment, and education that improves quality of life and clinical outlook;
- *Critical Care Medicine Program*, featuring state-of-the-art medical intensive care and respiratory care units;
- *Interventional Pulmonary Service*, which performs diagnostic and therapeutic procedures for patients with advanced pulmonary diseases;
- *Lung Transplant Program,* for patients with advanced lung disease that has progressed despite optimal medical therapy;
- *Occupational Lung Disorders Program*, specializing in diagnosis and management of occupational lung disorders, such as occupational asthma and bronchitis, asbestosis, silicosis, and heavy metal lung injury;
- *Pulmonary Fibrosis/Interstitial Lung Disease Program*, which treats patients with chronic inflammatory and scarring disorders of the lungs, including collagen vascular associated pulmonary diseases;
- *Pulmonary Physiology Laboratory*, a service that has recently doubled in capacity and that performs the full range of physiological testing for lung disease;
- *Pulmonary Vascular Program*, offering diagnosis and management of pulmonary hypertension;
- *Pulmonary Rehabilitation Program,* which provides occupational, physical, and cardiopulmonary rehabilitation programs for patients with disabling lung disorders, as well as pre- and post-operative consultation and therapy;
- *Respiratory Care Unit*, recently opened for chronic ventilator-dependent patients and those with advanced lung disease;
- *Thoracic Oncology Service*, which provides multidisciplinary medical care for lung cancer, as a joint effort with the Department of Cardiothoracic Surgery.

THE MOUNT SINAI MEDICAL CENTER

Mount Sinai's Sarcoidosis Service, the largest service of its kind in the world, is an NIH Center of Excellence for research in sarcoidosis. It is the only site that performs the diagnostic Kveim-Siltzbach skin test for sarcoidosis, which eliminates the need for more invasive, uncomfortable, and expensive procedures.

Through its Pulmonary Physiology Laboratory, Mount Sinai has been instrumental in establishing normal values for various pulmonary function tests and is currently conducting clinical studies of new tests for sarcoidosis, asthma, and lung cancer. Other pulmonary specialists at Mount Sinai are performing studies of asthma and emphysema, lung cancer, sarcoidosis, collagen vascular diseases, pulmonary infections, occupational lung diseases, and critical care outcomes.

625

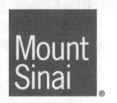

THE MOUNT SINAI MEDICAL CENTER
SLEEP MEDICINE

One Gustave L. Levy Place (Fifth Avenue and 100th Street)
New York, NY 10029-6574
Physician Referral: 1-800-MD-SINAI (637-4624)
www.mountsinai.org

Mount Sinai's recently expanded Center for Sleep Medicine is a full-service program that specializes in the comprehensive, compassionate, personalized care of individuals with sleep disorders. This is the first truly multidisciplinary sleep center in New York City.

We use state-of-the-art equipment to diagnose and treat all aspects of sleep pathology, including breathing-related disorders, insomnia, restless leg syndrome, periodic limb movements, and narcolepsy. An initial consultation includes a medical and surgical history, and physical examination. In some cases, the diagnosis and treatment plan can be completed in a single visit. In other cases, the evaluation requires a sleep study (typically over one or two nights) or other tests. As overnight tests are completed by 8 am, it is usually not necessary to miss a day of work. In rare instances, daytime studies are recommended, as well.

Services available at the Center for Sleep Medicine, include:

• Consultations with board-certified sleep specialists;

• Overnight sleep testing and daytime testing, provided by experienced physicians and technicians. During a sleep study, the patient is monitored by painless, noninvasive technology (PSG) that records breathing, heart rate, brain waves, oxygen levels, and eye and leg movement;

• Treatment for a sleep disorder, which may include a device to aid the patient's breathing while sleeping (called CPAP or BiPAP), medication, or light therapy as well as neuropsychiatric interventions, including biofeedback. If indicated, consultations with other specialists are available to aid in diagnosis and therapy;

• Mechanical, behavioral, surgical, dental, and pharmacological therapies, as required. Consultations can also be arranged with pulmonologists, ENT surgeons, bariatric surgeons, dentists, and psychiatrists.

THE MOUNT SINAI MEDICAL CENTER

Approximately 20 million Americans suffer from Obstructive sleep apnea (OSA), which occurs when muscles of the back of the mouth and the throat relax during sleep, causing a complete (apnea) or partial (hypopnea) blockage of the airway. Each time that happens, the oxygen level may fall, causing the heart to work harder. When untreated, this disorder can lead to hypertension, heart failure and stroke, as well as to bouts of daytime sleepiness that increase the risk of motor vehicle and industrial accidents. In seniors, sleepiness is often misperceived as a natural consequence of aging.
If you are concerned that you might have OSA, take the Epworth Sleepiness Test, a simple questionnaire available on the Mount Sinai Center for Sleep Medicine Website, www.nysleep.com. If you score higher than 10 on the Epworth Sleepiness Test or if you are overweight and snore, you may have sleep apnea or another sleep disorder.

626

NYU Medical Center

550 First Avenue (at 31st Street)
New York, NY 10016
Physician Referral:
(888)7-NYU-MED (888-769-8633)
www.nyumc.org

PULMONOLOGY

The Pulmonary and Critical Care Medicine Division at NYU Medical Center is characterized by its commitment to clinical excellence, teaching and clinical and basic science research.

PULMONOLOGY AND CRITICAL CARE MEDICINE

The NYU Medical Center Pulmonology and Critial Care Medicine section has a full continuum of services available for diagnosis, treatment and research of both the inpatient and ambulatory patient. Available services include a state-of-the-art Pulmonary Function Laboratory (see right), a specialized inpatient pulmonary unit with a dedicated respiratory care unit, a specialized medical critical care unit staffed with dedicated pulmonary/critical care physicians and a multidisciplinary interventional bronchoscopy program integrated with thoracic radiology.

In addition to the clinical services, active research is being conducted at the clinical and basic science levels in the areas of asthma and chronic obstructive pulmonary diseases, lung physiology and sleep disorders, interventional bronchoscopy, lung cancer screening and treatment, environmental and occupational lung diseases, pulmonary fibrosis, tuberculosis, and sepsis.

LUNG SURGERY AT NYU MEDICAL CENTER

The department of cardiothoracic surgery provides complete adult and pediatric general surgical and thoracic services, including surgery for congenital and acquired problems, tumor surgery, surgery on the lungs, esophageal surgery, and repair of chest wall deformities. We have over a decade of experience in using minimally invasive techniques to treat these problems. By using state-of-the-art instruments and techniques, often we can perform these procedures with minimal discomfort, little scarring and limited hospitalization.

PULMONARY REHABILITATION

Housed in the Joan and Joel Smilow *Cardiac Rehabilitation and Prevention Center of the Rusk Institute of Rehabilitation Medicine*, the cardiopulmonary rehabilitation unit is fully staff and equipped to handle both the inpatient and outpatient needs of the respiratory patient. The unit has dedicated inpatient beds for the hospitalized patients staffed by a Pulmonary Rehabilitation Team, comprised of pulmonologists, cardiologists, nurses, physical therapists, occupational therapists, psychologists, nutritionists, and social workers. Our exercise gym is equipped with exercise, monitoring, and resuscitation equipment for the safe and comprehensive delivery of services.

NYU MEDICAL CENTER

The Pulmonary Function Laboratory at NYU Medical Center offers several standard and specialized pulmonary tests, including:

· Spirometry (timed vital capacity, FEV1/FVC)

· Bronchodilator responsiveness (spirometry before and after bronchodilator administration)

· Flow volume loop

· Lung volumes (helium dilution and/or plethysmography)

· Maximum voluntary ventilation

· Diffusing capacity (single-breath carbon monoxide)

· Arterial and capillary blood gas analysis

· Pulse oximetry

· Airway resistance

· Maximal inspiratory and expiratory pressures

· Airway hyperactivity evaluation

· Oxygen dosage determinations

Radiation Oncology

a subspecialty of Radiology

A radiologist who deals with the therapeutic applications of radiant energy and its modifiers and the study and management of disease, especially malignant tumors.

Radiology: A radiologist utilizes radiologic methodologies to diagnose and treat disease. Physicians practicing in the field of radiology most often specialize in radiology, diagnostic radiology, radiation oncology or radiological physics.

Training Required: Four years in radiology *plus* additional training and examination.

Radiation Oncology

New England

Choi, Noah C MD [RadRO] - **Spec Exp:** Lung Cancer; Esophageal Cancer; **Hospital:** Mass Genl Hosp; **Address:** Mass Genl Hosp, Dept Rad Oncology, 100 Blossom St, Cox 307, Boston, MA 02114; **Phone:** 617-726-6050; **Board Cert:** Therapeutic Radiology 1970; **Med School:** South Korea 1963; **Resid:** Radiation Oncology, Princess Margaret Hosp 1970; **Fac Appt:** Assoc Prof, Harvard Med Sch

D'Amico, Anthony V MD/PhD [RadRO] - **Spec Exp:** Prostate Cancer; Brachytherapy; **Hospital:** Brigham & Women's Hosp, Dana-Farber Cancer Inst; **Address:** Brigham & Women's Hosp, Dept Rad Onc, 75 Francis St, Ste L2, Boston, MA 02115; **Phone:** 617-732-7936; **Board Cert:** Radiation Oncology 1999; **Med School:** Univ Pennsylvania 1990; **Resid:** Radiation Oncology, Hosp Univ Penn 1994; **Fac Appt:** Prof RadRO, Harvard Med Sch

DeLaney, Thomas Francis MD [RadRO] - **Spec Exp:** Sarcoma; Proton Beam Therapy; **Hospital:** Mass Genl Hosp; **Address:** Francis H. Burr Proton Therapy Ctr, 30 Fruit St, Bosont, MA 02114; **Phone:** 617-726-6876; **Board Cert:** Therapeutic Radiology 1986; Radiation Oncology 1999; **Med School:** Harvard Med Sch 1982; **Resid:** Therapeutic Radiology, Mass Gen Hosp 1986; **Fac Appt:** Assoc Prof RadRO, Harvard Med Sch

Harris, Jay R MD [RadRO] - **Spec Exp:** Breast Cancer; **Hospital:** Brigham & Women's Hosp, Dana-Farber Cancer Inst; **Address:** Dana Farber Cancer Inst, 44 Binney St, rm 1622, Boston, MA 02115; **Phone:** 617-632-2291; **Board Cert:** Therapeutic Radiology 1999; **Med School:** Stanford Univ 1970; **Resid:** Radiation Oncology, Joint Ctr Rad Ther 1976; **Fellow:** Radiation Therapy, Harvard Med Sch 1977; **Fac Appt:** Prof RadRO, Harvard Med Sch

Knisely, Jonathan MD [RadRO] - **Spec Exp:** Brain Tumors; Stereotactic Radiosurgery; Gastrointestinal Cancer; **Hospital:** Yale - New Haven Hosp; **Address:** Yale Univ Sch Med, Dept Therapeutic Radiology, 15 York St Bldg Hunter - Ste HRT 1, New Haven, CT 06520-8040; **Phone:** 203-785-2960; **Board Cert:** Internal Medicine 1989; Radiation Oncology 1993; **Med School:** Univ Pennsylvania 1986; **Resid:** Internal Medicine, Michael Reese Hosp 1989; Radiation Oncology, Univ Toronto Med Ctr 1992; **Fac Appt:** Assoc Prof, Yale Univ

Loeffler, Jay S MD [RadRO] - **Spec Exp:** Stereotactic Radiosurgery; Brain Tumors-Benign; **Hospital:** Mass Genl Hosp; **Address:** Mass General Hosp, Radiation Oncology, 100 Blossom St, Boston, MA 02114; **Phone:** 617-724-1548; **Board Cert:** Therapeutic Radiology 1986; **Med School:** Brown Univ 1982; **Resid:** Radiation Oncology, Harvard Joint Ctr for Rad Ther 1986; **Fellow:** Cancer Biology, Harvard Sch Pub Hlth 1985; **Fac Appt:** Prof RadRO, Harvard Med Sch

Mauch, Peter M MD [RadRO] - **Spec Exp:** Lymphoma; Hodgkin's Disease; **Hospital:** Dana-Farber Cancer Inst; **Address:** Dana Farber Cancer Inst, 75 Francis St, Ste RadOnc L2, Boston, MA 02115; **Phone:** 617-632-4116; **Board Cert:** Therapeutic Radiology 1978; **Med School:** St Louis Univ 1974; **Resid:** Radiation Therapy, Harvard Joint Ctr 1978; **Fac Appt:** Prof, Harvard Med Sch

Peschel, Richard E MD [RadRO] - **Spec Exp:** Prostate Cancer; **Hospital:** Yale - New Haven Hosp; **Address:** Yale-New Haven Hosp, Dept Radiology, 15 York St, rm HRT 142, New Haven, CT 06510; **Phone:** 203-785-2958; **Board Cert:** Therapeutic Radiology 1982; **Med School:** Yale Univ 1977; **Resid:** Radiation Oncology, Yale-New Haven Hosp 1981; **Fac Appt:** Prof RadRO, Yale Univ

Recht, Abram MD [RadRO] - **Spec Exp:** Breast Cancer; Gastrointestinal Cancer; Gynecologic Cancer; **Hospital:** Beth Israel Deaconess Med Ctr - Boston; **Address:** Beth Israel Deaconess Med Ctr, 330 Brookline Ave, Boston, MA 02215; **Phone:** 617-667-2345; **Board Cert:** Therapeutic Radiology 1984; **Med School:** Johns Hopkins Univ 1980; **Resid:** Radiation Oncology, Joint Ctr RadiationTherapy 1984; **Fac Appt:** Assoc Prof RadRO, Harvard Med Sch

Shipley, William U MD [RadRO] - **Spec Exp:** Bladder Cancer; Prostate Cancer; **Hospital:** Mass Genl Hosp; **Address:** Mass Genl Hosp, Dept Rad Oncology, 100 Blossom St, Cox 347, Boston, MA 02114; **Phone:** 617-726-8146; **Board Cert:** Therapeutic Radiology 1975; **Med School:** Harvard Med Sch 1966; **Resid:** Surgery, Mass Genl Hosp 1971; Radiation Therapy, Harvard Joint Ctr Rad Therapy 1973; **Fellow:** Radiation Therapy, Royal Marsden Hosp 1974; **Fac Appt:** Prof RadRO, Harvard Med Sch

Wazer, David E MD [RadRO] - **Spec Exp:** Breast Cancer; Melanoma; **Hospital:** Rhode Island Hosp, Tufts-New England Med Ctr; **Address:** 593 Eddy St, Providence, RI 02903; **Phone:** 401-444-8311; **Board Cert:** Radiation Oncology 1988; **Med School:** NYU Sch Med 1982; **Resid:** Radiation Oncology, Tufts New England Med Ctr 1988; **Fellow:** Neurological Chemistry, NYU Med Ctr 1984; **Fac Appt:** Prof RadRO, Tufts Univ

Wilson, Lynn D MD [RadRO] - **Spec Exp:** Lymphoma, Cutaneous T Cell (CTCL); Lymphoma, Cutaneous B Cell (CBCL); Lung Cancer; Head & Neck Cancer; **Hospital:** Yale - New Haven Hosp; **Address:** Yale Univ Sch Med, Dept Therapeutic Rad, PO Box 208040, New Haven, CT 06520-8040; **Phone:** 203-688-1861; **Board Cert:** Radiation Oncology 2004; **Med School:** Geo Wash Univ 1990; **Resid:** Therapeutic Radiology, Yale-New Haven Hosp 1994; **Fac Appt:** Prof RadRO, Yale Univ

Zietman, Anthony L MD [RadRO] - **Spec Exp:** Prostate Cancer; Urologic Cancer; **Hospital:** Mass Genl Hosp; **Address:** Mass Genl Hosp Cancer Ctr, Dept Radiation Oncology, 55 Fruit St, Boston, MA 02114; **Phone:** 617-724-4000; **Board Cert:** Radiation Oncology 1994; **Med School:** England 1983; **Resid:** Internal Medicine, St Stephens & Westminster Hosp 1986; Radiation Oncology, Mass Genl Hosp 1989; **Fellow:** Radiation Oncology, Middlesex/Mt Vernon Hosps 1991; **Fac Appt:** Prof RadRO, Harvard Med Sch

Mid Atlantic

Berg, Christine D MD [RadRO] - **Spec Exp:** Breast Cancer; **Hospital:** Natl Inst of Hlth - Clin Ctr; **Address:** 6130 Executive Blvd, Bethesda, MD 20892-7346; **Phone:** 301-496-8544; **Board Cert:** Internal Medicine 1980; Medical Oncology 1983; Therapeutic Radiology 1999; **Med School:** Northwestern Univ 1977; **Resid:** Internal Medicine, Northwestern Meml Hosp 1981; Radiation Oncology, Georgetown Univ Hosp 1986; **Fellow:** Medical Oncology, Natl Cancer Inst-NIH 1984

Coia, Lawrence R MD [RadRO] - **Spec Exp:** Gastrointestinal Cancer; Prostate Cancer; Breast Cancer; Brachytherapy; **Hospital:** Comm Med Ctr - Toms River (page 59), Southern Ocean County Hosp; **Address:** Community Medical Center, Dept Rad Oncology, 99 Route 37 W, Toms River, NJ 08755-6498; **Phone:** 732-557-8148; **Board Cert:** Therapeutic Radiology 1982; **Med School:** Temple Univ 1976; **Resid:** Radiation Oncology, Thos Jefferson Univ Hosp 1981; **Fac Appt:** Assoc Clin Prof, Univ Pennsylvania

Radiation Oncology

Curran Jr, Walter J MD [RadRO] - **Spec Exp:** Lung Cancer; Brain Tumors; Gastrointestinal Cancer; Esophageal Cancer; **Hospital:** Thomas Jefferson Univ Hosp; **Address:** Thomas Jefferson Univ Hosp, Dept Rad Onc, 111 S 11th St, Bodine Ctr, Philadelphia, PA 19107; **Phone:** 215-955-6701; **Board Cert:** Therapeutic Radiology 1986; **Med School:** Med Coll GA 1982; **Resid:** Radiation Therapy, Hosp Univ Penn 1986; **Fac Appt:** Prof RadRO, Jefferson Med Coll

Ennis, Ronald D MD [RadRO] - **Spec Exp:** Prostate Cancer; Brachytherapy; Gynecologic Cancer; **Hospital:** St Luke's - Roosevelt Hosp Ctr - Roosevelt Div, Beth Israel Med Ctr - Petrie Division; **Address:** St Luke's Roosevelt Hosp, Dept Rad Oncol, 1000 10th Ave, Lower Level, New York, NY 10019; **Phone:** 212-523-7165; **Board Cert:** Radiation Oncology 2005; **Med School:** Yale Univ 1990; **Resid:** Therapeutic Radiology, Yale-New Haven Hosp 1994

Flickinger, John C MD [RadRO] - **Spec Exp:** Neuro-Oncology; Brain & Spinal Tumors; **Hospital:** UPMC Presby, Pittsburgh; **Address:** UPMC Cancer Ctr, Radiation Oncology, 200 Lothrop St, Ste B 300, Pittsburgh, PA 15213; **Phone:** 412-647-3600; **Board Cert:** Therapeutic Radiology 1985; **Med School:** Univ Chicago-Pritzker Sch Med 1981; **Resid:** Radiation Therapy, Mass General Hosp 1985; **Fac Appt:** Prof RadRO, Univ Pittsburgh

Formenti, Silvia C MD [RadRO] - **Spec Exp:** Breast Cancer; Prostate Cancer; Chemo-Radiation Combined Therapy; **Hospital:** NYU Med Ctr (page 67); **Address:** NYU Med Ctr, Dept Radiation Oncology, 160 E 34th St, New York, NY 10016; **Phone:** 212-263-2601; **Board Cert:** Radiation Oncology 1991; **Med School:** Italy 1980; **Resid:** Internal Medicine, San Carlo Borromeo Hosp 1983; Medical Oncology, Univ of Pavia Med Ctr 1985; **Fellow:** Radiation Oncology, USC Med Ctr 1990; **Fac Appt:** Asst Prof RadRO, NYU Sch Med

Glatstein, Eli MD [RadRO] - **Spec Exp:** Lymphoma; Lung Cancer; Photodynamic Therapy; Sarcoma; **Hospital:** Hosp Univ Penn - UPHS (page 72); **Address:** Hosp Univ Penn, Dept Rad Oncology, 3400 Spruce St, Donner Bldg Fl 2, Philadelphia, PA 19104; **Phone:** 215-662-3383; **Board Cert:** Therapeutic Radiology 1972; **Med School:** Stanford Univ 1964; **Resid:** Radiation Therapy, Stanford Med Ctr 1970; **Fellow:** Radiological Biology, Hammersmith Hosp 1972; **Fac Appt:** Prof RadRO, Univ Pennsylvania

Goodman, Robert L MD [RadRO] - **Spec Exp:** Breast Cancer; Lymphoma; Prostate Cancer; **Hospital:** St Barnabas Med Ctr; **Address:** St Barnabas Med Ctr, Dept Rad Oncology, 94 Old Short Hills Rd, Livingston, NJ 07039; **Phone:** 973-322-5133; **Board Cert:** Internal Medicine 1971; Therapeutic Radiology 1974; Medical Oncology 1975; **Med School:** Columbia P&S 1966; **Resid:** Internal Medicine, Beth Israel Hosp 1970; Radiation Therapy, Harvard Joint Ctr Rad Therapy 1974; **Fellow:** Hematology, Presby Hosp 1969

Haffty, Bruce MD [RadRO] - **Spec Exp:** Breast Cancer; Head & Neck Cancer; Lung Cancer; **Hospital:** Robert Wood Johnson Univ Hosp - New Brunswick, Robert Wood Johnson Univ Hosp Hamilton; **Address:** The Cancer Institute of New Jersey, 195 Little Albany St, New Brunswick, NJ 08903; **Phone:** 732-253-3939; **Board Cert:** Radiation Oncology 1988; **Med School:** Yale Univ 1984; **Resid:** Radiation Oncology, Yale-New Haven Hosp 1988; **Fac Appt:** Prof RadRO, Robert W Johnson Med Sch

Hahn, Stephen M MD [RadRO] - **Spec Exp:** Lung Cancer; Prostate Cancer; Sarcoma; **Hospital:** Hosp Univ Penn - UPHS (page 72), Penn Presby Med Ctr - UPHS (page 72); **Address:** Hosp of the Univ of Penn, 3400 Spruce St 2 Donner Bldg, Philadelphia, PA 19104; **Phone:** 215-662-7296; **Board Cert:** Radiation Oncology 2004; Internal Medicine 1987; Medical Oncology 2001; **Med School:** Temple Univ 1984; **Resid:** Internal Medicine, UCSF Med Ctr 1988; Medical Oncology, Natl Inst Hlth 1991; **Fellow:** Radiation Oncology, Natl Inst Hlth 1994; **Fac Appt:** Prof RadRO, Univ Pennsylvania

Harrison, Louis MD [RadRO] - **Spec Exp:** Brachytherapy; Head & Neck Cancer; Radiation Therapy-Intraoperative; **Hospital:** Beth Israel Med Ctr - Petrie Division, St Luke's - Roosevelt Hosp Ctr - Roosevelt Div; **Address:** Beth Israel Med Ctr, Dept Rad Onc, 10 Union Square East, Ste 4G, New York, NY 10003-3314; **Phone:** 212-844-8087; **Board Cert:** Therapeutic Radiology 1986; **Med School:** SUNY Downstate 1982; **Resid:** Therapeutic Radiology, Yale-New Haven Hosp 1986; **Fac Appt:** Prof RadRO, Albert Einstein Coll Med

Horwitz, Eric MD [RadRO] - **Spec Exp:** Prostate Cancer; Intensity Modulated Radiotherapy (IMRT); Brachytherapy; **Hospital:** Fox Chase Cancer Ctr (page 59); **Address:** Fox Chase Cancer Ctr, Dept Radiation Oncology, 333 Cottman Ave, Philadelphia, PA 19111; **Phone:** 215-728-2995; **Board Cert:** Radiation Oncology 1999; **Med School:** Albany Med Coll 1992; **Resid:** Radiation Oncology, William Beaumont Hosp 1997

Isaacson, Steven MD [RadRO] - **Spec Exp:** Brain Tumors; Neuro-Oncology; **Hospital:** NY-Presby Hosp/Columbia (page 66); **Address:** Columbia Presby Med Ctr, Dept Rad Oncol, 622 W 168th St BHN Bldg - rm B11, New York, NY 10032-3720; **Phone:** 212-305-2611; **Board Cert:** Radiation Oncology 1988; Otolaryngology 1978; **Med School:** Jefferson Med Coll 1973; **Resid:** Otolaryngology, Hosp Univ Penn 1978; Radiation Oncology, SUNY Hlth Sci Ctr 1988; **Fac Appt:** Clin Prof RadRO, Columbia P&S

Kleinberg, Lawrence MD [RadRO] - **Spec Exp:** Brain & Spinal Cord Tumors; Brain Tumors-Metastatic; Stereotactic Radiosurgery; Esophageal Cancer; **Hospital:** Johns Hopkins Hosp - Baltimore (page 61); **Address:** Johns Hopkins Univ, Dept of Radiation Oncology, 401 N Broadway Weinberg Bldg - Ste 1440, Baltimore, MD 21231; **Phone:** 410-614-2597; **Board Cert:** Radiation Oncology 1994; **Med School:** Yale Univ 1989; **Resid:** Radiation Oncology, Meml Sloan-Kettering Canc Ctr 1993; **Fac Appt:** Assoc Prof RadRO, Johns Hopkins Univ

Lepanto, Philip B MD [RadRO] - **Hospital:** St Mary's Med Ctr - Huntington, Cabell Huntington Hosp; **Address:** St Mary's Med Ctr, Dept Radiation Oncology, 2900 First Ave, Huntington, WV 25702; **Phone:** 304-526-1143; **Board Cert:** Therapeutic Radiology 1975; **Med School:** Univ Louisville Sch Med 1970; **Resid:** Diagnostic Radiology, Graduate Hosp 1972; Radiation Therapy, Hosp Univ Penn 1975; **Fac Appt:** Clin Prof Rad, Marshall Univ

McCormick, Beryl MD [RadRO] - **Spec Exp:** Breast Cancer; Eye Tumors/Cancer; **Hospital:** Meml Sloan Kettering Cancer Ctr, NY-Presby Hosp/Weill Cornell (page 66); **Address:** Meml Sloan Kettering - Radiation Oncology, 1275 York Ave, rm SM 04, New York, NY 10021-6007; **Phone:** 212-639-6828; **Board Cert:** Therapeutic Radiology 1977; **Med School:** UMDNJ-NJ Med Sch, Newark 1973; **Resid:** Therapeutic Radiology, Meml Sloan Kettering Cancer Ctr 1977; **Fac Appt:** Prof RadRO, Cornell Univ-Weill Med Coll

Nori, Dattatreyudu MD [RadRO] - **Spec Exp:** Breast Cancer; Prostate Cancer; Gynecologic Cancer; **Hospital:** NY-Presby Hosp/Weill Cornell (page 66), NY Hosp Queens; **Address:** 525 E 68th St, Box 575, New York, NY 10021-4870; **Phone:** 212-746-3679; **Board Cert:** Therapeutic Radiology 1979; **Med School:** India 1970; **Resid:** Radiation Oncology, Meml Sloan Kettering Cancer Ctr 1975; **Fellow:** Radiation Oncology, Meml Sloan Kettering Cancer Ctr 1978; **Fac Appt:** Prof RadRO, Cornell Univ-Weill Med Coll

Pollack, Alan MD/PhD [RadRO] - **Spec Exp:** Prostate Cancer; Genitourinary Cancer; Sarcoma; **Hospital:** Fox Chase Cancer Ctr (page 59); **Address:** Fox Chase Cancer Ctr, Dept Rad Oncol, 333 Cottman Ave, Philadelphia, PA 19111; **Phone:** 215-728-2940; **Board Cert:** Radiation Oncology 1993; **Med School:** Univ Miami Sch Med 1987; **Resid:** Radiation Oncology, MD Anderson Cancer Ctr 1992; **Fac Appt:** Prof RadRO, Temple Univ

Rotman, Marvin MD [RadRO] - **Spec Exp:** Bladder Cancer; Gynecologic Cancer; Breast Cancer; Prostate Cancer; **Hospital:** SUNY Downstate Med Ctr, Long Island Coll Hosp; **Address:** 450 Clarkson Ave, Box 1211, Brooklyn, NY 11203-2056; **Phone:** 718-270-2181; **Board Cert:** Diagnostic Radiology 1966; Radiation Oncology 1999; **Med School:** Jefferson Med Coll 1958; **Resid:** Internal Medicine, Albert Einstein Med Ctr 1960; Radiation Oncology, Montefiore Hosp Med Ctr 1965; **Fac Appt:** Prof RadRO, SUNY Downstate

Schiff, Peter B MD/PhD [RadRO] - **Spec Exp:** Prostate Cancer; Gynecologic Cancer; Breast Cancer; **Hospital:** NY-Presby Hosp/Columbia (page 66); **Address:** Columbia Univ Med Ctr, Dept Rad Oncology, 622 W 168th St, New York, NY 10032-3720; **Phone:** 212-305-2991; **Board Cert:** Radiation Oncology 1990; **Med School:** Albert Einstein Coll Med 1984; **Resid:** Radiation Oncology, Meml Sloan Kettering Cancer Ctr 1988; **Fac Appt:** Prof RadRO, Columbia P&S

Solin, Lawrence J MD [RadRO] - **Spec Exp:** Breast Cancer; **Hospital:** Hosp Univ Penn - UPHS (page 72); **Address:** Univ Penn Med Ctr, Dept Rad Oncology, 3400 Spruce St, 2 Donner Bldg, Philadelphia, PA 19104; **Phone:** 215-662-7267; **Board Cert:** Radiation Oncology 1999; **Med School:** Brown Univ 1978; **Resid:** Surgery, Jefferson Univ Hosp 1981; Radiation Oncology, Jefferson Univ Hosp/Hosp Univ Penn 1984; **Fac Appt:** Prof RadRO, Univ Pennsylvania

Stock, Richard MD [RadRO] - **Spec Exp:** Prostate Cancer; **Hospital:** Mount Sinai Med Ctr; **Address:** 1184 5th Ave Fl 1 - rm PA-34, New York, NY 10029; **Phone:** 212-241-7502; **Board Cert:** Radiation Oncology 1993; **Med School:** Mount Sinai Sch Med 1988; **Resid:** Radiation Oncology, Meml Sloan Kettering Cancer Ctr 1992; **Fac Appt:** Prof RadRO, Mount Sinai Sch Med

Wharam Jr, Moody D MD [RadRO] - **Spec Exp:** Pediatric Cancers; Brain Tumors; Sarcoma-Soft Tissue; **Hospital:** Johns Hopkins Hosp - Baltimore (page 61); **Address:** Kimmel Cancer Ctr, Dept Rad Oncology, 401 N Broadway St, Ste 1440, Baltimore, MD 21231-1146; **Phone:** 410-955-7312; **Board Cert:** Therapeutic Radiology 1974; **Med School:** Univ VA Sch Med 1969; **Resid:** Radiation Oncology, UCSF Medical Ctr 1973; **Fac Appt:** Prof RadRO, Johns Hopkins Univ

Zelefsky, Michael J MD [RadRO] - **Spec Exp:** Prostate Cancer; Brachytherapy; Genitourinary Cancer; **Hospital:** Meml Sloan Kettering Cancer Ctr; **Address:** Meml Sloan-Kettering Cancer Ctr, 1275 York Ave, New York, NY 10021-6094; **Phone:** 212-639-6802; **Board Cert:** Radiation Oncology 1991; **Med School:** Albert Einstein Coll Med 1986; **Resid:** Radiation Oncology, Meml Sloan Kettering Cancer Ctr 1990; **Fac Appt:** Prof RadRO, Cornell Univ-Weill Med Coll

Southeast

Anscher, Mitchell MD [RadRO] - **Spec Exp:** Prostate Cancer; Brachytherapy; **Hospital:** Med Coll of VA Hosp, Henrico Doctors Hosp; **Address:** Virginia Commonwealth Univ, Department of Radiation Oncology, Box 980058, Richmond, VA 23298-0058; **Phone:** 804-828-7238; **Board Cert:** Radiation Oncology 1987; Internal Medicine 1984; **Med School:** Med Coll VA 1981; **Resid:** Internal Medicine, St Marys Hosp 1984; Radiation Oncology, Duke Univ Med Ctr 1987; **Fac Appt:** Prof RadRO, Duke Univ

Brizel, David M MD [RadRO] - **Spec Exp:** Head & Neck Cancer; Sarcoma; Lymphoma; **Hospital:** Duke Univ Med Ctr; **Address:** Duke Univ Med Ctr, Dept Rad Onc, Box 3085, Durham, NC 27710-0001; **Phone:** 919-668-5637; **Board Cert:** Radiation Oncology 1987; **Med School:** Northwestern Univ 1983; **Resid:** Radiation Oncology, Harvard Joint Center 1987; **Fac Appt:** Prof RadRO, Duke Univ

Crocker, Ian MD [RadRO] - **Spec Exp:** Brain Tumors; Eye Tumors/Cancer; Vascular Brachytherapy; **Hospital:** Emory Univ Hosp, Crawford Long Hosp of Emory Univ; **Address:** Emory Univ Hosp - Dept Radiation Oncology, 1365 Clifton Rd NE, T Ste 104, Atlanta, GA 30322; **Phone:** 404-778-3473; **Board Cert:** Therapeutic Radiology 1999; Internal Medicine 1980; **Med School:** Univ Saskatchewan 1976; **Resid:** Internal Medicine, Univ Hosp-Univ West Ontario 1980; **Fellow:** Radiation Oncology, Princess Margaret Hosp-Univ Toronto 1983; **Fac Appt:** Prof RadRO, Emory Univ

Halle, Jan MD [RadRO] - **Spec Exp:** Breast Cancer; Lung Cancer; **Hospital:** Univ NC Hosps; **Address:** Univ North Carolina Sch Med, Dept Rad Onc, CB 7512, 101 Manning Drive, Chapel Hill, NC 27599; **Phone:** 919-966-7700; **Board Cert:** Therapeutic Radiology 1982; **Med School:** Tufts Univ 1975; **Resid:** Radiation Oncology, North Carolina Meml Hosp 1981; **Fac Appt:** Assoc Prof RadRO, Univ NC Sch Med

Lewin, Alan A MD [RadRO] - **Spec Exp:** Breast Cancer; Lung Cancer; Brain & Spinal Cord Tumors; **Hospital:** Baptist Hosp of Miami; **Address:** Baptist Hosp Cancer Treatment Ctr, Dept Rad Onc, 8900 N Kendall Drive, Miami, FL 33176-2118; **Phone:** 786-596-6566; **Board Cert:** Therapeutic Radiology 1982; Medical Oncology 1981; Hematology 1978; Internal Medicine 1976; **Med School:** Geo Wash Univ 1973; **Resid:** Internal Medicine, Mt Sinai Hosp 1976; **Fellow:** Hematology & Oncology, Beth Israel Med Ctr 1978; Radiation Oncology, Joint Ctr Radiation Therapy 1980; **Fac Appt:** Clin Prof RadRO, Univ Miami Sch Med

Marcus Jr, Robert B MD [RadRO] - **Spec Exp:** Pediatric Cancers; Sarcoma; Bone Cancer; Brain Tumors; **Hospital:** Emory Univ Hosp; **Address:** Emory Clinic, Dept Rad Oncology, 1365 Clifton Rd NE, Ste A1300, Atlanta, GA 30322; **Phone:** 404-778-5751; **Board Cert:** Therapeutic Radiology 1980; **Med School:** Univ Fla Coll Med 1975; **Resid:** Radiation Oncology, Shands Hosp 1979; **Fac Appt:** Prof RadRO, Emory Univ

Marks, Lawrence MD [RadRO] - **Spec Exp:** Breast Cancer; Lung Cancer; **Hospital:** Duke Univ Med Ctr; **Address:** Duke Univ Med Ctr, Box 3085, Durham, NC 27710; **Phone:** 919-668-5640; **Board Cert:** Radiation Oncology 1989; **Med School:** Univ Rochester 1985; **Resid:** Radiation Oncology, Mass Genl Hosp 1989; **Fac Appt:** Prof RadRO, Duke Univ

Mendenhall, Nancy P MD [RadRO] - **Spec Exp:** Breast Cancer; Lymphoma; Hodgkin's Disease; **Hospital:** Shands Hlthcre at Univ of FL; **Address:** Univ Florida, Dept Radiation Oncology, Box 100385, Gainesville, FL 32610-0385; **Phone:** 352-265-0287; **Board Cert:** Therapeutic Radiology 1985; **Med School:** Univ Fla Coll Med 1980; **Resid:** Diagnostic Radiology, Shands-Univ of Florida 1984; **Fac Appt:** Prof RadRO, Univ Fla Coll Med

Mendenhall, William M MD [RadRO] - **Spec Exp:** Head & Neck Cancer; Stereotactic Radiosurgery; Colon Cancer; **Hospital:** Shands Hlthcre at Univ of FL; **Address:** Univ Florida, Dept Radiation Oncology, Box 100385, Gainesville, FL 32610-0385; **Phone:** 352-265-0287; **Board Cert:** Therapeutic Radiology 1983; **Med School:** Univ S Fla Coll Med 1978; **Resid:** Radiation Oncology, University of Florida 1983; **Fac Appt:** Prof RadRO, Univ Fla Coll Med

Prosnitz, Leonard MD [RadRO] - **Spec Exp:** Lymphoma; Breast Cancer; Hyperthermia Treatment of Cancer; Sarcoma; **Hospital:** Duke Univ Med Ctr; **Address:** Duke Univ Med Ctr, Dept Rad Onc, Box 3085, Durham, NC 27710; **Phone:** 919-668-5637; **Board Cert:** Therapeutic Radiology 1970; **Med School:** SUNY Downstate 1961; **Resid:** Internal Medicine, Dartmouth Affil Hosps 1963; Radiation Oncology, Yale-New Haven Hosp 1969; **Fellow:** Hematology & Oncology, Yale-New Haven Hosp 1967; **Fac Appt:** Prof RadRO, Duke Univ

Rich, Tyvin Andrew MD [RadRO] - **Spec Exp:** Colon & Rectal Cancer; Chemo-Radiation Combined Therapy; Esophageal Cancer; **Hospital:** Univ Virginia Med Ctr; **Address:** Univ Va Hlth Sys, Dept Rad Onc, Box 800383, Charlottesville, VA 22908-0383; **Phone:** 434-924-5191; **Board Cert:** Radiation Oncology 1978; **Med School:** Univ VA Sch Med 1973; **Resid:** Mass Genl Hosp 1978; **Fellow:** Radiation Oncology, Mt Vernon Hosp/Gray Lab; **Fac Appt:** Prof RadRO, Univ VA Sch Med

Rosenman, Julian MD [RadRO] - **Spec Exp:** Lung Cancer; Breast Cancer; Prostate Cancer; **Hospital:** Univ NC Hosps; **Address:** Univ North Carolina, Dept Rad Onc, CB 7512, 101 Manning Drive, Chapel Hill, NC 27599-7512; **Phone:** 919-966-7700; **Board Cert:** Therapeutic Radiology 1981; **Med School:** Univ Tex SW, Dallas 1977; **Resid:** Therapeutic Radiology, Mass Genl Hosp 1981; **Fac Appt:** Prof RadRO, Univ NC Sch Med

Sailer, Scott MD [RadRO] - **Spec Exp:** Head & Neck Cancer; Genitourinary Cancer; Pediatric Cancers; Pediatric Radiology; **Hospital:** WakeMed Cary, WakeMed New Bern; **Address:** 300 Ashville Ave, Ste 110, Cary, NC 27511; **Phone:** 919-854-4588; **Board Cert:** Radiation Oncology 1988; **Med School:** Harvard Med Sch 1984; **Resid:** Radiation Therapy, Mass Genl Hosp 1988

Shaw, Edward G MD [RadRO] - **Spec Exp:** Stereotactic Radiosurgery; Brain Tumors; **Hospital:** Wake Forest Univ Baptist Med Ctr (page 73); **Address:** Wake Forest Med Ctr, Dept Rad Onc, Medical Center Blvd, Comp Cancer Ctr, Winston Salem, NC 27157-1029; **Phone:** 336-713-6506; **Board Cert:** Radiation Oncology 1987; **Med School:** Rush Med Coll 1983; **Resid:** Radiation Oncology, Mayo Grad Sch Med 1987; **Fac Appt:** Prof RadRO, Wake Forest Univ

Tepper, Joel MD [RadRO] - **Spec Exp:** Gastrointestinal Cancer; Sarcoma; Rectal Cancer; **Hospital:** Univ NC Hosps; **Address:** North Carolina Clin Cancer Ctr, Dept Rad Onc - CB#7512, Chapel Hill, NC 27599-7512; **Phone:** 919-966-0400; **Board Cert:** Therapeutic Radiology 1976; **Med School:** Washington Univ, St Louis 1972; **Resid:** Therapeutic Radiology, Mass Genl Hosp 1976; **Fellow:** Therapeutic Radiology, Mass Genl Hosp 1977; **Fac Appt:** Prof RadRO, Univ NC Sch Med

Willett, Christopher MD [RadRO] - **Spec Exp:** Gastrointestinal Cancer; Clinical Trials; **Hospital:** Duke Univ Med Ctr; **Address:** Duke Univ Med Ctr, PO Box 3085, Durham, NC 27710; **Phone:** 919-668-5640; **Board Cert:** Therapeutic Radiology 1985; **Med School:** Tufts Univ 1981; **Resid:** Radiation Oncology, Mass Genl Hosp 1986; **Fac Appt:** Prof, Duke Univ

Midwest

Abrams, Ross A MD [RadRO] - **Spec Exp:** Gastrointestinal Cancer; Lymphoma; **Hospital:** Rush Univ Med Ctr; **Address:** Rush Univ Med Ctr, Dept Radiation Oncology, 1653 W Congress Pkwy Atrium Bldg, Chicago, IL 60612; **Phone:** 312-942-5751; **Board Cert:** Internal Medicine 1976; Medical Oncology 1979; Hematology 1982; Radiation Oncology 1987; **Med School:** Univ Pennsylvania 1973; **Resid:** Internal Medicine, Pennsylvania Hosp 1975; Hematology & Oncology, Hosp Univ Penn 1976; **Fellow:** Hematology & Oncology, Natl Cancer Inst 1978; Radiation Oncology, Med Coll Wisconsin 1987; **Fac Appt:** Prof RadRO, Rush Med Coll

Ben-Josef, Edgar MD [RadRO] - **Spec Exp:** Bone Cancer; Gastrointestinal Cancer; Pancreatic Cancer; Intensity Modulated Radiotherapy (IMRT); **Hospital:** Univ Michigan Hlth Sys; **Address:** University Hospital, 1500 E Medical Ctr Drive, rm UH B2C490, Ann Arbor, MI 48109-0010; **Phone:** 734-936-8207; **Board Cert:** Radiation Oncology 1994; **Med School:** Israel 1986; **Resid:** Radiation Oncology, Wayne State Univ Hosp 1994; **Fellow:** Cancer Biology, Wayne State Univ Hosp 1995; **Fac Appt:** Assoc Prof RadRO, Univ Mich Med Sch

Charboneau, J William MD [RadRO] - **Spec Exp:** Radiofrequency Tumor Ablation; Liver Cancer; Thyroid Cancer; **Hospital:** Mayo Med Ctr & Clin - Rochester; **Address:** 200 First St SW, Mayo Clinic, Rochester, MN 55905-0002; **Phone:** 507-284-2097; **Board Cert:** Diagnostic Radiology 1980; **Med School:** Univ Wisc 1976; **Resid:** Diagnostic Radiology, Mayo Clinic 1980; **Fac Appt:** Prof, Mayo Med Sch

Emami, Bahman MD [RadRO] - **Spec Exp:** Head & Neck Cancer; Lung Cancer; **Hospital:** Loyola Univ Med Ctr, Hines VA Hosp; **Address:** Loyola Univ Med Ctr, Dept Rad Onc, 2160 S First Ave Bldg 105 - rm 2932, Maywood, IL 60153-3328; **Phone:** 708-216-2729; **Board Cert:** Therapeutic Radiology 1976; **Med School:** Iran 1968; **Resid:** Radiation Therapy, Tufts Univ-New Eng Med Ctr 1976; **Fellow:** Radiation Therapy, Tufts Univ-New Eng Med Ctr 1977; **Fac Appt:** Prof RadRO, Loyola Univ-Stritch Sch Med

Forman, Jeffrey D MD [RadRO] - **Spec Exp:** Neutron Therapy for Advanced Cancer; Genitourinary Cancer; Prostate Cancer; **Hospital:** Karmanos Cancer Inst; **Address:** BA Karmanos Cancer Institute, 31995 Northwestern Hwy, Farmington Hills, MI 48334; **Phone:** 248-538-6545; **Board Cert:** Radiation Oncology 1986; **Med School:** NYU Sch Med 1982; **Resid:** Radiation Oncology, Johns Hopkins Hosp 1986; **Fellow:** Therapeutic Radiology, Johns Hopkins Hosp 1987; **Fac Appt:** Prof RadRO, Wayne State Univ

Halpern, Howard MD/PhD [RadRO] - **Spec Exp:** Breast Cancer; Esophageal Cancer; Gynecologic Cancer; **Hospital:** Univ of Chicago Hosps, Univ of IL Med Ctr at Chicago; **Address:** 1801 W Taylor St, rm C400, MC-933, Chicago, IL 60612; **Phone:** 312-996-3630; **Board Cert:** Therapeutic Radiology 1984; **Med School:** Univ Miami Sch Med 1980; **Resid:** Therapeutic Radiology, Jnt Ctr Rad Ther Harvard 1984; **Fellow:** Therapeutic Radiology, Jnt Ctr Rad Ther Harvard 1985; **Fac Appt:** Prof DR, Univ Chicago-Pritzker Sch Med

Hayman, James A MD [RadRO] - **Spec Exp:** Breast Cancer; Stomach Cancer; Lung Cancer; Brain Tumors; **Hospital:** Univ Michigan Hlth Sys; **Address:** University Hospital, 1500 E Medical Ctr Drive, rm UH B2C490, Ann Arbor, MI 48109-0010; **Phone:** 734-936-4288; **Board Cert:** Radiation Oncology 2004; **Med School:** Univ Chicago-Pritzker Sch Med 1991; **Resid:** Radiation Therapy, Joint Ctr for Radiation Therapy 1996; **Fac Appt:** Assoc Prof RadRO, Univ Mich Med Sch

Kiel, Krystyna D MD [RadRO] - **Spec Exp:** Breast Cancer; Sarcoma; Gastrointestinal Cancer; Colon & Rectal Cancer; **Hospital:** Northwestern Meml Hosp; **Address:** Northwestern Meml Hosp, Radiation Oncology, 251 E Huron St Galter Bldg - Ste L178, Chicago, IL 60611-2914; **Phone:** 312-926-2520; **Board Cert:** Therapeutic Radiology 2000; **Med School:** Univ Mass Sch Med 1977; **Resid:** Radiation Oncology, Mass Genl Hosp 1982; **Fac Appt:** Assoc Prof DR, Northwestern Univ

Kinsella, Timothy J MD [RadRO] - **Spec Exp:** Brain Tumors; Sarcoma; Gastrointestinal Cancer; **Hospital:** Univ Hosps Case Med Ctr; **Address:** Univ Hosps - Dept Radiation Oncology, 11100 Euclid Ave Fl BSMT - rm B181, MC LT6068, Cleveland, OH 44106-6068; **Phone:** 216-844-2530; **Board Cert:** Internal Medicine 1977; Medical Oncology 1979; Therapeutic Radiology 1980; **Med School:** Univ Rochester 1974; **Resid:** Internal Medicine, Mayo Clinic 1976; Radiation Oncology, Joint Ctr for Rad Therapy 1980; **Fellow:** Medical Oncology, Dana Farber Cancer Ctr 1977; **Fac Appt:** Prof RadRO, Case West Res Univ

Lawrence, Theodore S MD/PhD [RadRO] - **Spec Exp:** Gastrointestinal Cancer; Liver Cancer; Pancreatic Cancer; **Hospital:** Univ Michigan Hlth Sys; **Address:** Univ Hosp, Dept Radiation Oncology, 1500 E Med Ctr Dr, B2C502, Box 0010, Ann Arbor, MI 48109-0010; **Phone:** 734-936-4300; **Board Cert:** Internal Medicine 1983; Medical Oncology 1985; Radiation Oncology 1987; **Med School:** Cornell Univ-Weill Med Coll 1980; **Resid:** Internal Medicine, Stanford Univ Hosp 1983; Radiation Oncology, Natl Cancer Inst 1987; **Fellow:** Medical Oncology, Natl Cancer Inst 1986; **Fac Appt:** Prof RadRO, Univ Mich Med Sch

Macklis, Roger M MD [RadRO] - **Spec Exp:** Radioimmunotherapy of Cancer; Breast Cancer; Lymphoma; **Hospital:** Cleveland Clin Fdn (page 57); **Address:** Cleveland Cin Fdn, Dept Rad Onc T18, 9500 Euclid Ave, Cleveland, OH 44195; **Phone:** 216-444-5576; **Board Cert:** Radiation Oncology 1989; **Med School:** Harvard Med Sch 1983; **Resid:** Radiation Oncology, Joint Ctr Radiotherapy Inst 1987; **Fellow:** Research, Dana Farber Cancer Inst 1987; **Fac Appt:** Prof RadRO, Case West Res Univ

Martenson Jr, James A MD [RadRO] - **Spec Exp:** Mucositis; Esophageal Cancer; **Hospital:** Mayo Med Ctr & Clin - Rochester; **Address:** Mayo Clinic, Dept Rad/Onc, 200 First St SW, Rochester, MN 55905; **Phone:** 507-284-4561; **Board Cert:** Therapeutic Radiology 1985; **Med School:** Univ Wash 1981; **Resid:** Radiation Oncology, Mayo Clinic 1985; **Fac Appt:** Assoc Prof, Mayo Med Sch

Michalski, Jeff M MD [RadRO] - **Spec Exp:** Prostate Cancer; Sarcoma; Pediatric Cancers; **Hospital:** Barnes-Jewish Hosp, St Louis Chldns Hosp; **Address:** Washington Univ Sch Med, Dept Rad Oncology, 4921 Parkview Place, Lower Level, Box 8224, St Louis, MO 63110; **Phone:** 314-362-8566; **Board Cert:** Radiation Oncology 1991; **Med School:** Med Coll Wisc 1986; **Resid:** Radiation Oncology, Columbia Presbyterian Med Ctr 1988; Radiation Oncology, Mallinckrodt Inst of Radiology 1990; **Fellow:** Radiation Oncology, Mallinckrodt Inst of Radiology 1991; **Fac Appt:** Assoc Prof RadRO, Washington Univ, St Louis

Myerson, Robert J MD [RadRO] - **Spec Exp:** Gastrointestinal Cancer; Breast Cancer; Hyperthermia Treatment of Cancer; **Hospital:** Barnes-Jewish Hosp; **Address:** Ctr for Advanced Med-Siteman Cancer Ctr, 4921 Parkview Pl, Box 9038635, St Louis, MO 63110; **Phone:** 314-747-7236; **Board Cert:** Therapeutic Radiology 1985; **Med School:** Univ Miami Sch Med 1980; **Resid:** Radiation Therapy, Hosp Univ Penn 1984; **Fac Appt:** Prof RadRO, Washington Univ, St Louis

Pierce, Lori J MD [RadRO] - **Spec Exp:** Breast Cancer; **Hospital:** Univ Michigan Hlth Sys; **Address:** Univ Hosp, Dept Rad Onc, 1500 E Med Ctr Dr, rm B2C440, Box 0010, Ann Arbor, MI 48109-0999; **Phone:** 734-936-4300; **Board Cert:** Radiation Oncology 1989; **Med School:** Duke Univ 1985; **Resid:** Radiation Oncology, Hosp Univ Penn 1989; **Fac Appt:** Prof RadRO, Univ Mich Med Sch

Sandler, Howard M MD [RadRO] - **Spec Exp:** Prostate Cancer; Genitourinary Cancer; Brain Tumors; **Hospital:** Univ Michigan Hlth Sys; **Address:** Univ Michigan Med Ctr, Dept Rad Onc, 1500 E Medical Ctr Dr. UH B2C502, Box 0010, Ann Arbor, MI 48109-0010; **Phone:** 734-936-9338; **Board Cert:** Radiation Oncology 1989; **Med School:** Univ Conn 1985; **Resid:** Radiation Oncology, Hosp Univ Penn 1989; **Fac Appt:** Prof RadRO, Univ Mich Med Sch

Taylor, Marie E MD [RadRO] - **Spec Exp:** Breast Cancer; **Hospital:** Barnes-Jewish Hosp, Barnes-Jewish West County Hosp; **Address:** Center for Advanced Med-Siteman Cancer Ctr, 4921 Parkview Pl, Box 9038635, St Louis, MO 63110; **Phone:** 314-747-7236; **Board Cert:** Radiation Oncology 1987; **Med School:** Univ Wash 1982; **Resid:** Radiation Oncology, Univ Wash Med Ctr 1986

Vicini, Frank A MD [RadRO] - **Spec Exp:** Breast Cancer; Prostate Cancer; Brachytherapy; **Hospital:** William Beaumont Hosp; **Address:** William Beaumont Hospital, 3601 W 13 Mile Rd, Royal Oak, MI 48073; **Phone:** 248-551-1219; **Board Cert:** Radiation Oncology 1999; **Med School:** Wayne State Univ 1985; **Resid:** Radiation Oncology, William Beaumont Hosp 1989; **Fellow:** Radiation Oncology, Harvard Med Sch/Joint Ctr for Rad Ther 1990; **Fac Appt:** Clin Prof RadRO, Univ Mich Med Sch

Weichselbaum, Ralph R MD [RadRO] - **Spec Exp:** Gene Targeted Radiotherapy; Head & Neck Cancer; Esophageal Cancer; **Hospital:** Univ of Chicago Hosps; **Address:** Univ Chicago, Dept Rad Onc, 5758 S Maryland Ave, MC-9006-DCAM-1D, Chicago, IL 60637; **Phone:** 773-702-0817; **Board Cert:** Therapeutic Radiology 1975; **Med School:** Univ IL Coll Med 1971; **Resid:** Therapeutic Radiology, Harvard Jt Ctr Rad Therapy 1975; **Fellow:** Diagnostic Radiology, Harvard Med Sch 1976; **Fac Appt:** Prof DR, Univ Chicago-Pritzker Sch Med

Wilson, J Frank MD [RadRO] - **Spec Exp:** Breast Cancer; Skin Cancer; **Hospital:** Froedtert Meml Lutheran Hosp; **Address:** Dept Radiation Oncology, 9200 W Wisconsin Ave, Milwaukee, WI 53226; **Phone:** 414-805-4400; **Board Cert:** Therapeutic Radiology 1971; **Med School:** Univ MO-Columbia Sch Med 1965; **Resid:** Radiation Oncology, Penrose Cancer Hosp 1969; **Fellow:** Radiation Oncology, Natl Cancer Inst/NIH 1971; **Fac Appt:** Prof RadRO, Med Coll Wisc

Great Plains and Mountains

Smalley, Stephen R MD [RadRO] - **Spec Exp:** Colon Cancer; Gastrointestinal Cancer; **Hospital:** Olathe Med Ctr; **Address:** Olathe Med Ctr, 20375 W 151st St, Doctors Bldg, Ste 180, Olathe, KS 66061-4575; **Phone:** 913-768-7200; **Board Cert:** Internal Medicine 1982; Radiation Oncology 1987; Medical Oncology 1985; **Med School:** Univ MO-Kansas City 1979; **Resid:** Internal Medicine, Mayo Clinic 1982; Radiation Oncology, Mayo Clinic 1986; **Fellow:** Medical Oncology, Mayo Clinic 1984; **Fac Appt:** Prof RadRO, Univ Kans

Radiation Oncology

Southwest

Ang, Kie-Kian MD/PhD [RadRO] - **Spec Exp:** Head & Neck Cancer; **Hospital:** UT MD Anderson Cancer Ctr (page 71); **Address:** UT MD Anderson Cancer Ctr, 1515 Holcombe Blvd, Box 97, Houston, TX 77030; **Phone:** 713-563-8400; **Board Cert:** Radiation Oncology 1987; **Med School:** Belgium 1975; **Resid:** Radiation Oncology, Univ Hosp Louvian 1980; **Fac Appt:** Prof, Univ Tex, Houston

Buchholz, Thomas A MD [RadRO] - **Spec Exp:** Breast Cancer; **Hospital:** UT MD Anderson Cancer Ctr (page 71); **Address:** Univ Texas MD Anderson Cancer Ctr, 1515 Holcombe Blvd, Unit 1202, Houston, TX 77030; **Phone:** 713-794-4892; **Board Cert:** Radiation Oncology 1993; **Med School:** Tufts Univ 1988; **Resid:** Radiation Oncology, Univ Washington Med Ctr 1993; **Fellow:** Research, Univ Washington Med Ctr 1994; **Fac Appt:** Prof RadRO, Univ Tex, Houston

Cox, James D MD [RadRO] - **Spec Exp:** Lymphoma; Lung Cancer; Gynecologic Cancer; **Hospital:** UT MD Anderson Cancer Ctr (page 71); **Address:** Univ Tex MD Anderson Cancer Ctr, 1515 Holcombe Blvd, Unit 97, Houston, TX 77030; **Phone:** 713-563-2316; **Board Cert:** Radiation Oncology 1999; **Med School:** Univ Rochester 1965; **Resid:** Diagnostic Radiology, Penrose Cancer Hosp 1969; **Fellow:** Therapeutic Radiology, Inst Gustave-Roussy 1970; **Fac Appt:** Prof RadRO, Univ Tex, Houston

Eifel, Patricia J MD [RadRO] - **Spec Exp:** Cervical Cancer; Uterine Cancer; Vulvar Disease/Cancer; Vaginal Cancer; **Hospital:** UT MD Anderson Cancer Ctr (page 71); **Address:** MD Anderson Cancer Ctr, Dept Rad Onc, 1515 Holcombe Blvd, Unit 1202, Houston, TX 77030-4009; **Phone:** 713-563-6830; **Board Cert:** Therapeutic Radiology 1983; **Med School:** Stanford Univ 1977; **Resid:** Radiation Oncology, Stanford Univ Med Ctr 1981; **Fellow:** Therapeutic Radiology, Stanford Univ Med Ctr 1982

Grado, Gordon L MD [RadRO] - **Spec Exp:** Prostate Cancer; Brachytherapy; **Hospital:** Scottsdale Hlthcare - Shea; **Address:** 2926 N Civic Center Plaza, Scottsdale, AZ 85251; **Phone:** 480-614-6300; **Board Cert:** Therapeutic Radiology 1981; Radiation Oncology 1999; **Med School:** Southern IL Univ 1977; **Resid:** Therapeutic Radiology, Mayo Clinic 1981

Gunderson, Leonard MD [RadRO] - **Spec Exp:** Gastrointestinal Cancer; Brachytherapy; Sarcoma; **Hospital:** Mayo Clin Hosp - Scottsdale; **Address:** Mayo Clinic, Dept Radiation Oncol, 13400 E Shea Blvd, Scottsdale, AZ 85259-5404; **Phone:** 480-342-1262; **Board Cert:** Therapeutic Radiology 1975; **Med School:** Univ KY Coll Med 1969; **Resid:** Radiation Oncology, Latter Day Saints Hosp 1974; **Fac Appt:** Prof RadRO, Mayo Med Sch

Herman, Terence Spencer MD [RadRO] - **Spec Exp:** Breast Cancer; Sarcoma; Brain Tumors; **Hospital:** OU Med Ctr; **Address:** Oklahoma Univ Health Sci Ctr, 825 NE 10th St, OUPB 1430, Oklahoma City, OK 73104-5417; **Phone:** 405-271-5641; **Board Cert:** Internal Medicine 1975; Medical Oncology 1977; Therapeutic Radiology 1985; **Med School:** Univ Conn 1972; **Resid:** Internal Medicine, Univ Arizona 1975; Radiation Oncology, Stanford Univ 1985; **Fellow:** Medical Oncology, Univ Arizona 1977; **Fac Appt:** Prof RadRO, Univ Okla Coll Med

Janjan, Nora Anita MD [RadRO] - **Spec Exp:** Gastrointestinal Cancer; Palliative Care; **Hospital:** UT MD Anderson Cancer Ctr (page 71); **Address:** Univ TX MD Anderson Cancer Ctr, 1515 Holcombe Blvd, Box 97, Houston, TX 77030; **Phone:** 713-563-2326; **Board Cert:** Radiation Oncology 2000; **Med School:** Univ Ariz Coll Med 1979; **Resid:** Internal Medicine, Baylor Affil Hosps 1981; Radiation Oncology, Baylor Affil Hosps 1984; **Fac Appt:** Prof RadRO, Univ Tex, Houston

Komaki, Ritsuko MD [RadRO] - **Spec Exp:** Lung Cancer; Thymoma; Esophageal Cancer; **Hospital:** UT MD Anderson Cancer Ctr (page 71); **Address:** UT-MD Anderson Cancer Ctr, Dept Rad Onc, 1515 Holcombe Blvd, Unit 97, Houston, TX 77030; **Phone:** 713-563-2300; **Board Cert:** Therapeutic Radiology 1977; Radiation Oncology 2001; **Med School:** Japan 1969; **Resid:** Radiation Oncology, Med Coll Wisc 1978; **Fac Appt:** Prof RadRO, Univ Tex, Houston

Kuske, Robert R MD [RadRO] - **Spec Exp:** Breast Cancer; **Hospital:** Scottsdale Hlthcare - Shea; **Address:** 8994 E Desert Cove Ave, Ste 100, Scottsdale, AZ 85260; **Phone:** 602-274-4484; **Board Cert:** Therapeutic Radiology 1985; **Med School:** Univ Cincinnati 1980; **Resid:** Radiation Oncology, Univ Cincinnati Med Ctr 1984

Medbery, Clinton A MD [RadRO] - **Spec Exp:** Breast Cancer; Gynecologic Cancer; **Hospital:** St Anthony Hosp; **Address:** Frank C Love Cancer Institute, 1000 N Lee St, Oklahoma City, OK 73102; **Phone:** 405-272-7311; **Board Cert:** Internal Medicine 1980; Medical Oncology 1983; Radiation Oncology 1987; **Med School:** Med Univ SC 1976; **Resid:** Internal Medicine, Naval Hosp 1980; Radiation Oncology, Natl Cancer Inst 1987; **Fellow:** Medical Oncology, Naval Hosp 1982

Pistenmaa, David A MD/PhD [RadRO] - **Spec Exp:** Stereotactic Radiosurgery; Prostate Cancer; Breast Cancer; **Hospital:** UT Southwestern Med Ctr - Dallas, Parkland Meml Hosp - Dallas; **Address:** UTSW Med Ctr, Dept Rad Oncology, 5801 Forest Park Rd, Dallas, TX 75390; **Phone:** 214-645-8525; **Board Cert:** Therapeutic Radiology 1974; **Med School:** Stanford Univ 1969; **Resid:** Radiation Oncology, Stanford Univ Med Ctr 1973; **Fac Appt:** Prof RadRO, Univ Tex SW, Dallas

Senzer, Neil N MD [RadRO] - **Spec Exp:** Clinical Trials; Gene Targeted Radiotherapy; Gene Therapy; **Hospital:** Baylor Univ Medical Ctr; **Address:** Morg Crowley Medical Research Ctr, 3535 Worth St, Ste 302, Dallas, TX 75246-2044; **Phone:** 214-370-1400; **Board Cert:** Pediatrics 1976; Pediatric Hematology-Oncology 1978; Therapeutic Radiology 1985; **Med School:** SUNY Buffalo 1971; **Resid:** Pediatrics, Johns Hopkins Hosp 1974; Radiation Oncology, St Barnabas Med Ctr 1985; **Fellow:** Pediatric Hematology-Oncology, St Jude Chldns Rsch Hosp 1978

Shina, Donald C MD [RadRO] - **Spec Exp:** Breast Cancer; **Hospital:** St Vincent Hosp - Santa Fe; **Address:** Santa Fe Cancer Ctr at St Vincent Hosp, 455 Saint Michael's Drive, Santa Fe, NM 87505; **Phone:** 505-820-5233; **Board Cert:** Internal Medicine 1977; Medical Oncology 1979; Therapeutic Radiology 1981; **Med School:** Case West Res Univ 1974; **Resid:** Internal Medicine, Univ Hosps 1977; **Fellow:** Radiation Oncology, Univ Hosps 1980; Medical Oncology, Univ Hosps 1980

Stea, Baldassarre MD/PhD [RadRO] - **Spec Exp:** Brain Tumors; Stereotactic Radiosurgery; Pediatric Cancers; **Hospital:** Univ Med Ctr - Tucson, Tucson Med Ctr; **Address:** Univ Hlth Scis Ctr, Dept Rad Onc, 1501 N Campbell Ave, Tucson, AZ 85724-0001; **Phone:** 520-626-6724; **Board Cert:** Radiation Oncology 1987; **Med School:** Geo Wash Univ 1983; **Resid:** Radiation Oncology, Natl Cancer Inst 1987; **Fac Appt:** Prof RadRO, Univ Ariz Coll Med

Radiation Oncology

West Coast and Pacific

Blasko, John C MD [RadRO] - **Spec Exp:** Prostate Cancer; **Hospital:** Swedish Med Ctr - Seattle; **Address:** 1101 Madison, Ste 1101, Seattle, WA 98104; **Phone:** 206-215-2480; **Board Cert:** Therapeutic Radiology 1976; **Med School:** Univ MD Sch Med 1969; **Resid:** Diagnostic Radiology, Maine Med Ctr 1974; Radiation Therapy, Univ Washington 1976; **Fac Appt:** Prof, Univ Wash

Donaldson, Sarah S MD [RadRO] - **Spec Exp:** Pediatric Cancers; Hodgkin's Disease; **Hospital:** Stanford Univ Med Ctr; **Address:** 875 Blake Wilbur Drive, CC Bldg Fl G - rm 226, MC 5847, Stanford, CA 94305-5847; **Phone:** 650-723-6195; **Board Cert:** Therapeutic Radiology 1974; **Med School:** Harvard Med Sch 1968; **Resid:** Radiation Oncology, Stanford Univ Med Ctr 1972; **Fellow:** Pediatric Hematology-Oncology, Inst Gustave-Roussy 1973; Pediatric Hematology-Oncology, MD Anderson Cancer Ctr 1971; **Fac Appt:** Prof RadRO, Stanford Univ

Halberg, Francine MD [RadRO] - **Spec Exp:** Breast Cancer; **Hospital:** Marin Genl Hosp, UCSF Med Ctr; **Address:** Marin Cancer Inst-Dept of Rad.Oncology, 1350 S Eliseo Drive, Ste 100, Greenbrae, CA 94904; **Phone:** 415-925-7326; **Board Cert:** Internal Medicine 1981; Therapeutic Radiology 1984; **Med School:** Cornell Univ-Weill Med Coll 1978; **Resid:** Internal Medicine, USPHS Hosp 1981; **Fellow:** Radiation Oncology, Stanford Univ Med Ctr 1984; **Fac Appt:** Assoc Prof RadRO, UCSF

Hoppe, Richard T MD [RadRO] - **Spec Exp:** Lymphoma; Hodgkin's Disease; **Hospital:** Stanford Univ Med Ctr; **Address:** Stanford Med Ctr, Dept Rad Onc, 875 Blake Wilbur, MC 5847, Stanford, CA 94305-5847; **Phone:** 650-723-5510; **Board Cert:** Therapeutic Radiology 1976; **Med School:** Cornell Univ-Weill Med Coll 1971; **Resid:** Radiation Therapy, Stanford Univ Med Ctr 1976; **Fac Appt:** Prof DR, Stanford Univ

Koh, Wui-Jin MD [RadRO] - **Spec Exp:** Gynecologic Cancer; Brachytherapy; Clinical Trials; **Hospital:** Univ Wash Med Ctr; **Address:** Univ Washington Med Ctr, Dept of Radiation Oncology, Box 356043, Seattle, WA 98195; **Phone:** 206-598-4121; **Board Cert:** Radiation Oncology 1988; **Med School:** Loma Linda Univ 1984; **Resid:** Radiation Oncology, Univ Washington Med Ctr 1988; **Fellow:** Tumor Imaging, Univ Washington Med Ctr 1988; **Fac Appt:** Prof RadRO, Univ Wash

Laramore, George E MD [RadRO] - **Spec Exp:** Neutron Therapy for Advanced Cancer; Salivary Gland Tumors; Head & Neck Cancer; Skin Cancer; **Hospital:** Univ Wash Med Ctr; **Address:** Univ Washington Med Ctr, Dept Rad Onc Box 356043, Seattle, WA 98195; **Phone:** 206-598-4110; **Board Cert:** Therapeutic Radiology 1980; Radiation Oncology 2000; **Med School:** Univ Miami Sch Med 1976; **Resid:** Radiation Oncology, Univ Washington 1980; **Fac Appt:** Prof RadRO, Univ Wash

Larson, David Andrew MD/PhD [RadRO] - **Spec Exp:** Neuro-Oncology; Brain Tumors; Stereotactic Radiosurgery; **Hospital:** UCSF Med Ctr; **Address:** UCSF Med Ctr, Dept Rad Onc, 505 Parnassus Ave, rm L-75, San Francisco, CA 94143-0226; **Phone:** 415-353-8900; **Board Cert:** Therapeutic Radiology 1986; **Med School:** Univ Miami Sch Med 1981; **Resid:** Radiation Therapy, Joint Ctr RadTherapy 1985; **Fac Appt:** Prof RadRO, UCSF

Le, Quynh-Thu Xuan MD [RadRO] - **Spec Exp:** Head & Neck Cancer; Lung Cancer; Thoracic Cancers; Clinical Trials; **Hospital:** Stanford Univ Med Ctr; **Address:** Stanford Univ, Dept Rad Oncology, 875 Blake Wilbur Drive, MC 5847, Stanford, CA 94305; **Phone:** 650-498-5032; **Board Cert:** Radiation Oncology 1998; **Med School:** UCSF 1993; **Resid:** Radiation Oncology, UCSF Med Ctr 1997; **Fac Appt:** Assoc Prof RadRO, Stanford Univ

Leibel, Steven A MD [RadRO] - **Spec Exp:** Prostate Cancer; **Hospital:** Stanford Univ Med Ctr; **Address:** Stanford Univ Med Ctr, 875 Blake Wilber Dr, MC5827, Stanford, CA 94305-5827; **Phone:** 650-723-4250; **Board Cert:** Therapeutic Radiology 1976; Radiation Oncology 1999; **Med School:** UCSF 1972; **Resid:** Radiation Oncology, UCSF Med Ctr 1976; **Fac Appt:** Prof RadRO, Stanford Univ

Mundt, Arno J MD [RadRO] - **Spec Exp:** Gynecologic Cancer; Intensity Modulated Radiotherapy (IMRT); **Hospital:** UCSD Med Ctr; **Address:** Moores UCSD Cancer Center, 3855 Health Sciences Drive, MC 0843, La Jolla, CA 92093; **Phone:** 858-822-6040; **Board Cert:** Radiation Oncology 1994; **Med School:** Univ Mich Med Sch 1987; **Resid:** Physical Medicine & Rehabilitation, George Washington Univ Hosp 1990; Radiation Oncology, Univ Chicago Hosps 1993; **Fac Appt:** Assoc Prof RadRO, Univ Chicago-Pritzker Sch Med

Quivey, Jeanne Marie MD [RadRO] - **Spec Exp:** Head & Neck Cancer; Breast Cancer; Eye Tumors/Cancer; Intensity Modulated Radiotherapy (IMRT); **Hospital:** UCSF Med Ctr; **Address:** 1600 Divisadero St, Ste H1031, San Francisco, CA 94115-3010; **Phone:** 415-353-7175; **Board Cert:** Therapeutic Radiology 1974; **Med School:** UCSF 1970; **Resid:** Radiation Therapy, UCSF Med Ctr 1974; **Fac Appt:** Prof RadRO, UCSF

Roach III, Mack MD [RadRO] - **Spec Exp:** Prostate Cancer; Genitourinary Cancer; Lung Cancer; **Hospital:** UCSF - Mt Zion Med Ctr, UCSF Med Ctr; **Address:** UCSF Mt Zion Cancer Ctr, Div Rad Oncol, 1600 Divisadero St, Ste H1031, San Francisco, CA 94115; **Phone:** 415-353-7175; **Board Cert:** Medical Oncology 1985; Radiation Oncology 1987; Internal Medicine 1984; **Med School:** Stanford Univ 1979; **Resid:** Internal Medicine, ML King Genl Hosp 1981; Radiation Oncology, Stanford Univ Med Ctr 1987; **Fellow:** Medical Oncology, UCSF Med Ctr 1983; **Fac Appt:** Prof RadRO, UCSF

Rose, Christopher M MD [RadRO] - **Spec Exp:** Prostate Cancer; Breast Cancer; Intensity Modulated Radiotherapy (IMRT); **Address:** Santa Fe Radiation Therapy, 9229 Wilshire Blvd, Beverly Hills, CA 90210; **Phone:** 310-205-5700; **Board Cert:** Radiation Oncology 1999; **Med School:** Harvard Med Sch 1974; **Resid:** Internal Medicine, Beth Israel Deaconess 1976; Radiation Oncology, Joint Ctr Rad Therapy 1979; **Fellow:** Research, British Inst Cancer Rsch 1979; **Fac Appt:** Assoc Clin Prof RadRO, UCLA

Streeter Jr, Oscar E MD [RadRO] - **Spec Exp:** Lung Cancer; Head & Neck Cancer; **Hospital:** USC Norris Comp Cancer Ctr, USC Univ Hosp - R K Eamer Med Plz; **Address:** Norris Comp Cancer Ctr-Dept Rad Onc, 1441 Eastlake Ave Fl Ground, Los Angeles, CA 90033; **Phone:** 323-865-3051; **Board Cert:** Radiation Oncology 1989; **Med School:** Howard Univ 1982; **Resid:** Radiation Oncology, Howard Univ 1986; **Fac Appt:** Assoc Prof RadRO, USC Sch Med

Tripuraneni, Prabhakar MD [RadRO] - **Spec Exp:** Prostate Cancer; Head & Neck Cancer; Lymphoma; **Hospital:** Scripps Green Hosp, Scripps Meml Hosp - La Jolla; **Address:** Scripps Clinic, Div Radiation Oncology, 10666 N Torrey Pines Rd, MSB 1, La Jolla, CA 92037; **Phone:** 858-554-2000; **Board Cert:** Therapeutic Radiology 1983; **Med School:** India 1976; **Resid:** Radiation Oncology, Univ Alberta 1981; Radiation Oncology, UCSF Med Ctr 1983; **Fac Appt:** Clin Prof DR, UCSD

Wong, Jeffrey Y C MD [RadRO] - **Spec Exp:** Radioimmunotherapy of Cancer; Prostate Cancer; **Hospital:** City of Hope Natl Med Ctr & Beckman Rsch; **Address:** City of Hope Med Ctr-Dept Radiation Onc, 1500 E Duarte Rd, Duarte, CA 91768-3000; **Phone:** 626-359-8111 x62969; **Board Cert:** Therapeutic Radiology 1985; **Med School:** Johns Hopkins Univ 1981; **Resid:** Radiation Oncology, UCSF Med Ctr 1985; **Fac Appt:** Clin Prof, UC Irvine

Cleveland Clinic

Radiation Oncology

The Department of Radiation Oncology at the Cleveland Clinic Taussig Cancer Center is one of the busiest and most technologically advanced clinical radiotherapy programs in the country. Our specialists provide care at eight additional facilities in Northeast Ohio and one in Florida.

Technology: Cleveland Clinic offers a full range of advanced technology equipment, including two simulators, six linear accelerators, two- and three-dimensional treatment planning computers, a high-dose-rate brachytherapy unit, an orthovoltage unit and a contact unit for early-stage rectal lesions. In addition, Cleveland Clinic is one of the few hospitals to offer treatment of intracranial and extracranial tumors using the Gamma Knife and Novalis platforms.

Innovation: Cleveland Clinic has one of the most active brachytherapy programs in the U.S. In addition to intracavitary and intraluminal treatments, Cleveland Clinic has developed many novel approaches to brachytherapy, especially with prostate cancer. Cleveland Clinic Radiation Oncology was also one of the first programs to implement intensity-modulated radiation therapy (IMRT), image-guided radiation therapy (IGRT) and radioimmunotherapy (RIT).

Patient Services: Cleveland Clinic offers free round trip transportation for patients who have difficulty getting to daily treatments from their homes. In addition, our free wellness program, Reflections, offers a variety of complementary and aesthetic therapies, which allow patients the opportunity to be pampered, to regain a sense of control and to take some time for themselves. The treatments are designed to reduce anxiety, and include healing therapies such as Reiki, reflexology, guided imagery, facials, makeovers and massotherapy.

Research: Cleveland Clinic is active in a number of in-house, pharmaceutical and cooperative group trials. We have been one of the leading enrollers in many national studies and are a leader in combining novel agents such as radiation sensitizers with radiation therapy. In addition, our Department of Radiation Oncology houses one of the largest prostate cancer databases in the nation.

To schedule an appointment or for more information about the Cleveland Clinic Department of Radiation Oncology call 800.890.2467 or visit www.clevelandclinic.org/radonctopdocs.

Department of Radiation Oncology | 9500 Euclid Avenue / W14 | Cleveland OH 44195

How do you measure quality?

Visit clevelandclinic.org/quality for information on the criteria most often used to measure quality in health care; data on how Cleveland Clinic compares with other health care centers; patient satisfaction data; and quality measures for numerous specific diseases and conditions, including cancer.

Special Service for Out-of-State Patients

Global Patient Services provides personalized concierge programs and services to welcome patients and add to their comfort before, during and after their stay. Call 800.223.2273, ext. 55580, or send an e-mail to medicalconcierge@ccf.org.

FOX CHASE
CANCER CENTER

333 Cottman Avenue
Philadelphia, PA 19111-2497
Phone: 1-888-FOX CHASE • Fax: 215-728-2702
www.fccc.edu

RADIATION ONCOLOGY

Fox Chase Cancer Center has one of the country's largest, most experienced programs in radiation oncology. Recognized as international leaders in developing the most advanced treatment technologies, our radiation oncologists include nationally and internationally known experts in prostate, breast, lung and gastrointestinal cancers. Other major treatment interests include central nervous system and head and neck cancers and sarcomas.

We treat patients with radiation therapy alone, in combination with surgery and/or chemotherapy and through Fox Chase and national clinical trials offering the newest treatments. We also conduct research in medical physics and radiation biology to enhance the effectiveness of therapy.

- Fox Chase physicians are among the nation's most experienced in treating patients with intensity-modulated radiation therapy (IMRT) and are developing the image-guided radiation therapies of the future.
- Advances in brachytherapy such as real-time intraoperative planning mean our patients receive the most precise prostate implants, either permanent low-dose-rate or temporary high-dose-rate.
- Stereotactic radiosurgery and radiation therapy permits sub-millimeter precision for brain and lung cancers.

We offer treatment with radiation alone, as part of a multidisciplinary regimen or through clinical trials to determine the most effective approaches for specific cancers. Fox Chase uses sophisticated imaging tools during treatment planning and daily treatment sessions to target the cancer better and spare any healthy surrounding tissue undue exposure to radiation.

Because of our outstanding reputation as a leader in cancer therapy, we frequently work with the world's foremost makers of medical equipment to test prototypes and develop the best applications—long before they are available elsewhere.

For example, Fox Chase has the first high-intensity focused ultrasound (HIFU) dedicated for cancer treatment in North America. This allows us to deliver hyperthermia treatment in conjunction with radiation to treat patients with certain primary and recurrent tumors.

The Most Precise Treatment
- Fox Chase has been first in the region to offer these advanced tools for the most targeted radiation therapy.
- The Calypso 4-D Localization System is brand-new four-dimensional monitoring technology to localize and track the prostate throughout treatment for more accurate radiation delivery.
- Magnetic resonance spectroscopy (MRS, or functional MRI) aids treatment planning to tailor radiation therapy for some prostate and brain cancers by identifying the metabolic activity of the tumor.
- The Trilogy Stereotactic System for image-guided radiation therapy and stereotactic radiosurgery is the world's premier image-guided system for delivering all forms of external radiation. It automatically adjusts the treatment table position as needed and tailors treatment to phases in the patient's breathing cycle.
- A 4-D CT treatment simulator helps doctors plan treatment to correlate with patient motion such as breathing-especially important for patients with lung, breast or some gastrointestinal cancers.

For more about Fox Chase physicians and services, visit our web site, www.fccc.edu, or call 1-888-FOX CHASE.

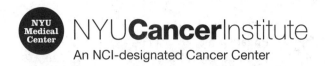
NYU**Cancer**Institute
An NCI-designated Cancer Center

NYU Clinical Cancer Center
160 East 34th Street
New York, New York 10016
www.nyuci.org/atcd

NYU Medical Center
550 First Avenue (at 31st Street)
New York, New York 10016
www.nyumc.org/atcd

A Collaborative Approach
The NYU Cancer Institute, an NCI designated center, is a "matrix cancer center" without walls operating within the larger NYU Medical Center. With over 250 members and a research funding base of over $80 million, this structure strengthens our capabilities to forge collaborations across medical and scientific disciplines, which translates to comprehensive care for our patients and discoveries that will influence the future of this disease.

Renowned Expertise
NYU Medical Center's Cancer Program has been recognized as one of the top programs nationwide according to the 2005 *U.S. News & World Report's* Best Hospitals Survey. Our highly skilled Magnet™ nursing team not only plays a pivotal role in coordinating direct patient care, but is also a source of invaluable patient education. Team members' compassion and expertise help patients better manage the symptoms of their disease as well as their special needs.

A Patient-Focused Setting
The NYU Clinical Cancer Center, with over 60 faculty members from various disciplines at the New York University School of Medicine, is the principal outpatient facility of the Cancer Institute and serves as home for our patients and their caregivers. The center and its multidisciplinary team of experts provide access to the latest treatment options and clinical trials along with a variety of programs in cancer prevention, screening, diagnostics, genetic counseling, and supportive services. Our affiliation with Bellevue Hospital, the oldest public hospital in the country, affords clinically distinctive opportunities to learn and care for patients with cancer by observing its presentation and behavior in a variety of patient groups.

RADIATION ONCOLOGY

The Radiation Treatment Center at M. D. Anderson is the most comprehensive facility of its kind in the world. We offer the latest, most advanced technology, and provide the broadest range of radiation treatment options available anywhere. We hold ourselves to quality standards that are higher than the industry requires, and provide a rare breadth of technology, expertise, and experience, all which translate into personalized care and the best outcomes for the over 5,000 new patients we treat a year.

M. D. Anderson radiation oncologists are specially trained, board-certified, and skilled in both standard and unique radiation therapies. We are constantly seeking innovative ways to use existing technology, and developing new therapies to help our patients have the best outcomes possible.

PROTON THERAPY

M. D. Anderson's Proton Therapy Center opened in May 2006 as the largest and most sophisticated center of its type. Proton therapy allows for the most aggressive cancer therapy possible, deriving its advantage over traditional forms of radiation treatment from its ability to deliver targeted radiation doses to the tumor with remarkable precision. Proton therapy radiation avoids the surrounding tissue, generates fewer side effects, and improves tumor control. It is used to treat cancers of the prostate, lung, brain and skull base, head and neck, eye, and various forms of pediatric cancer.

Combined with M. D. Anderson's more than 60 years of expertise and pioneering research in radiation therapy, the Proton Therapy Center is the premier destination for cancer patients seeking the best treatment by the most experienced radiation oncologists.

MORE INFORMATION

For more information or to make an appointment, call 877-MDA-6789, or visit us online at http://www.mdanderson.org.

At M. D. Anderson Cancer Center, our mission is simple – to eliminate cancer. Achieving that goal begins with integrated programs in cancer treatment, clinical trials, education programs and cancer prevention.

We focus exclusively on cancer and have seen cases of every kind. That means you receive expert care no matter what your diagnosis.

Choosing the right partner for cancer care really does make a difference. The fact is, people who choose M. D. Anderson over other hospitals and clinics often have better results. That is how we've been making cancer history for over sixty years.

841

Radiology

A radiologist utilizes radiologic methodologies to diagnose and treat disease. Physicians practicing in the field of radiology most often specialize in radiology, diagnostic radiology, radiation oncology or radiological physics.

Diagnostic Radiology: A radiologist who utilizes X-ray, radionuclides, ultrasound and electromagnetic radiation to diagnose and treat disease.

Training Required: Four years

Radiation Oncology: A radiologist who deals with the therapeutic applications of radiant energy and its modifiers and the study and management of disease, especially malignant tumors.

Certification in one of the following subspecialties requires additional training and examination.

Neuroradiology: A radiologist who diagnoses and treats diseases utilizing imaging procedures as they relate to the brain, spine and spinal cord, head, neck and organs of special sense in adults and children.

Pediatric Radiology: A radiologist who is proficient in all forms of diagnostic imaging as it pertains to the treatment of diseases in the newborn, infant, child and adolescent. This specialist has knowledge of both imaging and interventional procedures related to the care and management of diseases of children. A pediatric radiologist must be highly knowledgeable of all organ systems as they relate to growth and development, congenital malformations, diseases peculiar to infants and children and diseases that begin in childhood but cause substantial residual impairment in adulthood.

(continued on next page)

Vascular and Interventional Radiology: A radiologist who diagnoses and treats diseases by various radiologic imaging modalities. These include fluoroscopy, digital radiography, computed tomography, sonography and magnetic resonance imaging.

Diagnostic Radiology

New England

Benson, Carol MD [DR] - **Spec Exp:** Obstetric Ultrasound; Thyroid Ultrasound; Fetal Surgical Imaging; **Hospital:** Brigham & Women's Hosp; **Address:** Brigham & Women's Hospital, Dept Radiology, 75 Francis St, Boston, MA 02115; **Phone:** 617-732-6280; **Board Cert:** Diagnostic Radiology 1984; **Med School:** Univ Pennsylvania 1980; **Resid:** Diagnostic Radiology, New York Hosp-Cornell 1984; **Fellow:** Ultrasound, Brigham & Womens Hosp 1985; **Fac Appt:** Prof, Harvard Med Sch

Black, William C MD [DR] - **Spec Exp:** Chest Radiology; Lung Cancer; CT Chest Scan; **Hospital:** Dartmouth - Hitchcock Med Ctr; **Address:** Dartmouth Hitchcock Med Ctr, Dept Radiology, 1 Medical Center Drive, Lebanon, NH 03756; **Phone:** 603-650-7443; **Board Cert:** Diagnostic Radiology 1983; **Med School:** Med Coll VA 1979; **Resid:** Diagnostic Radiology, Univ Virginia Hosp 1983; **Fellow:** Ultrasound/CT, Univ Virginia Hosp 1984; **Fac Appt:** Prof Rad, Dartmouth Med Sch

Kopans, Daniel B MD [DR] - **Spec Exp:** Breast Imaging; **Hospital:** Mass Genl Hosp; **Address:** Mass Genl Hosp - Avon Comprehensive Breast Ctr, 15 Parkman St, WAC 240, Boston, MA 02114-3117; **Phone:** 617-724-9729; **Board Cert:** Diagnostic Radiology 1977; **Med School:** Harvard Med Sch 1973; **Resid:** Diagnostic Radiology, Mass Genl Hosp 1977; **Fac Appt:** Prof, Harvard Med Sch

McCarthy, Shirley M MD/PhD [DR] - **Spec Exp:** Gynecologic Cancer; Pelvic Imaging; **Hospital:** Yale - New Haven Hosp; **Address:** Yale-New Haven Hosp, 333 Cedar St, Ste TE2, New Haven, CT 06520; **Phone:** 203-785-2384; **Board Cert:** Diagnostic Radiology 1983; **Med School:** Yale Univ 1979; **Resid:** Diagnostic Radiology, Yale-New Haven Hosp 1983; **Fellow:** Cross Sectional Imaging, UCSF Med Ctr 1984; **Fac Appt:** Prof Rad, Yale Univ

Schepps, Barbara MD [DR] - **Spec Exp:** Breast Imaging; **Hospital:** Rhode Island Hosp; **Address:** Anne C Pappas Breast Imaging Ctr, 2 Dudley St, Ste G85, Providence, RI 02903; **Phone:** 401-444-6266; **Board Cert:** Diagnostic Radiology 1973; **Med School:** Hahnemann Univ 1968; **Resid:** Diagnostic Radiology, Boston City Hosp 1972; **Fac Appt:** Clin Prof, Brown Univ

Weinreb, Jeffrey C MD [DR] - **Spec Exp:** MRI; Breast Cancer; Abdominal Imaging; Prostate Cancer; **Hospital:** Yale - New Haven Hosp; **Address:** Yale Univ Sch Medicine, Dept Radiology, 333 Cedar St, rm MRC147, Box 208042, New Haven, CT 06520-8042; **Phone:** 203-785-5913; **Board Cert:** Diagnostic Radiology 1983; **Med School:** Mount Sinai Sch Med 1978; **Resid:** Diagnostic Radiology, LI Jewish Med Ctr 1982; **Fellow:** Ultrasound/CT, Hosp Univ Penn 1983; **Fac Appt:** Prof Rad, Yale Univ

Mid Atlantic

Adler, Ronald S MD/PhD [DR] - **Spec Exp:** Musculoskeletal Imaging; Ultrasound; Power Doppler Imaging; **Hospital:** Hosp For Special Surgery (page 60), NY-Presby Hosp/Weill Cornell (page 66); **Address:** Hospital for Special Surgery, 535 E 70th St, New York, NY 10021; **Phone:** 212-606-1635; **Board Cert:** Diagnostic Radiology 1988; **Med School:** Wayne State Univ 1984; **Resid:** Diagnostic Radiology, Univ Mich Med Ctr 1988; **Fellow:** Ultrasound/CT/MRI, Univ Mich Med Ctr 1989; **Fac Appt:** Prof Rad, Cornell Univ-Weill Med Coll

Diagnostic Radiology

Austin, John H M MD [DR] - **Spec Exp:** Lung Cancer; **Hospital:** NY-Presby Hosp/Columbia (page 66); **Address:** Columbia Presby Hosp, Dept Radiology, 622 W 168th St, MHB 3-202C, New York, NY 10032-3784; **Phone:** 212-305-2986; **Board Cert:** Diagnostic Radiology 1970; **Med School:** Yale Univ 1965; **Resid:** Diagnostic Radiology, UCSF Med Ctr 1968; **Fellow:** Diagnostic Radiology, UCSF Med Ctr 1970; **Fac Appt:** Prof Rad, Columbia P&S

Berg, Wendie A MD/PhD [DR] - **Spec Exp:** Breast Imaging; Breast Cancer; **Hospital:** Johns Hopkins Hosp - Baltimore (page 61); **Address:** Johns Hopkins - Greenspring Station Breast Ctr, 10755 Falls Rd, Pav 1, Ste 440, Lutherville, MD 21093; **Phone:** 410-583-2888; **Board Cert:** Diagnostic Radiology 1992; **Med School:** Johns Hopkins Univ 1987; **Resid:** Diagnostic Radiology, Johns Hopkins Hosp 1992; **Fellow:** Abdominal Imaging, Johns Hopkins Univ 1992

Bluemke, David A MD/PhD [DR] - **Spec Exp:** Cardiac Imaging; **Hospital:** Johns Hopkins Hosp - Baltimore (page 61); **Address:** Johns Hopkins Hospital, Dept Radiology, 600 N Wolfe St MRI Bldg - rm 143, Baltimore, MD 21287; **Phone:** 410-955-4062; **Board Cert:** Diagnostic Radiology 1993; **Med School:** Univ Chicago-Pritzker Sch Med 1989; **Resid:** Diagnostic Radiology, Johns Hopkins Hosp 1993; **Fellow:** Diagnostic Imaging, Johns Hopkins Hosp 1994; **Fac Appt:** Assoc Prof, Johns Hopkins Univ

Brem, Rachel F MD [DR] - **Spec Exp:** Breast Imaging; **Hospital:** G Washington Univ Hosp; **Address:** GW Medical Faculty Assocs, 2150 Pennsylvania Ave NW, DC Level, Washington, DC 20037; **Phone:** 202-741-3036; **Board Cert:** Diagnostic Radiology 1990; **Med School:** Columbia P&S 1984; **Resid:** Diagnostic Radiology, Johns Hopkins Hosp 1989; **Fellow:** Mammography, Johns Hopkins Hosp 1990; **Fac Appt:** Prof, Geo Wash Univ

Cohen, Harris L MD [DR] - **Spec Exp:** Pediatric Ultrasound/Imaging; Pediatric Radiology; Fetal Ultrasound/Obstetrical Imaging; Obstetric Ultrasound; **Hospital:** Stony Brook Univ Med Ctr; **Address:** Stony Brook Univ Hosp, Dept Radiology, HCS level 4, rm 120, Stony Brook, NY 11794-8460; **Phone:** 631-444-8193; **Board Cert:** Diagnostic Radiology 1980; Pediatric Radiology 2005; **Med School:** SUNY Downstate 1976; **Resid:** Internal Medicine, Nassau County Med Ctr 1977; Diagnostic Radiology, Univ Hosp 1980; **Fellow:** Pediatric Radiology, Children's Hosp 1981; **Fac Appt:** Prof Rad, SUNY Stony Brook

Dalinka, Murray MD [DR] - **Spec Exp:** Bone Disorders-Metabolic; Musculoskeletal Disorders; Musculoskeletal Imaging; MRI; **Hospital:** Hosp Univ Penn - UPHS (page 72); **Address:** Hosp Univ Penn, Dept Radiology, 3400 Spruce St, Philadelphia, PA 19104; **Phone:** 215-662-3019; **Board Cert:** Diagnostic Radiology 1969; **Med School:** Univ Mich Med Sch 1964; **Resid:** Diagnostic Radiology, Montefiore Med Ctr 1968; **Fac Appt:** Prof Rad, Univ Pennsylvania

Dershaw, D David MD [DR] - **Spec Exp:** Breast Imaging; Breast Cancer; **Hospital:** Meml Sloan Kettering Cancer Ctr; **Address:** 1275 York Ave, New York, NY 10021-6007; **Phone:** 212-639-7295; **Board Cert:** Diagnostic Radiology 1978; **Med School:** Jefferson Med Coll 1974; **Resid:** Diagnostic Radiology, New York Hosp 1978; **Fellow:** Ultrasound, Thos Jefferson Univ Hosp 1979; **Fac Appt:** Prof Rad, Cornell Univ-Weill Med Coll

Edelstein, Barbara A MD [DR] - **Spec Exp:** Breast Cancer; Women's Imaging; **Address:** 1045 Park Ave, New York, NY 10028; **Phone:** 212-860-7700; **Board Cert:** Diagnostic Radiology 1983; **Med School:** NY Med Coll 1977; **Resid:** Diagnostic Radiology, Montefiore Hosp 1982

Fishman, Elliot MD [DR] - **Spec Exp:** CT Body Scan; Abdominal Imaging; CT Cardiac Scan; Cardiac Imaging; **Hospital:** Johns Hopkins Hosp - Baltimore (page 61); **Address:** Johns Hopkins Hosp, Dept Radiology, 601 N Caroline St, JHOC 3254, Baltimore, MD 21287-0006; **Phone:** 410-955-5173; **Board Cert:** Diagnostic Radiology 1981; **Med School:** Univ MD Sch Med 1977; **Resid:** Diagnostic Radiology, Sinai Hosp 1980; **Fellow:** Computerized Tomography, Johns Hopkins Hosp 1981; **Fac Appt:** Prof Rad, Johns Hopkins Univ

Fuhrman, Carl R MD [DR] - **Spec Exp:** Thoracic Imaging; **Hospital:** UPMC Presby, Pittsburgh; **Address:** UPMC-Dept Radiology, 200 Lothrop St, Ste E177 PUH, Pittsburgh, PA 15213; **Phone:** 412-647-7288; **Board Cert:** Diagnostic Radiology 1983; **Med School:** Univ Pittsburgh 1979; **Resid:** Diagnostic Radiology, Presbyterian Univ Hosp 1983; **Fac Appt:** Prof, Univ Pittsburgh

Gefter, Warren B MD [DR] - **Spec Exp:** Thoracic Imaging; **Hospital:** Hosp Univ Penn - UPHS (page 72); **Address:** Hospital Univ of Pennsylvania, 1 Silverstein, 3400 Spruce St, Philadelphia, PA 19104; **Phone:** 215-662-6724; **Board Cert:** Diagnostic Radiology 1978; **Med School:** Univ Pennsylvania 1974; **Resid:** Diagnostic Radiology, Hosp U Penn 1978; **Fac Appt:** Prof Rad, Univ Pennsylvania

Hann, Lucy MD [DR] - **Spec Exp:** Liver & Biliary Cancer Ultrasound; Ovarian Cancer Ultrasound Diagnosis; Thyroid Ultrasound; **Hospital:** Meml Sloan Kettering Cancer Ctr; **Address:** Memorial Sloan-Kettering Cancer Ctr, 1275 York Ave, rm C278, New York, NY 10021; **Phone:** 212-639-2179; **Board Cert:** Diagnostic Radiology 1977; **Med School:** Harvard Med Sch 1971; **Resid:** Diagnostic Radiology, Hosp Univ Penn 1974; Diagnostic Radiology, Mass General Hosp 1977; **Fellow:** Body Imaging, Mass General Hosp 1978; **Fac Appt:** Prof Rad, Cornell Univ-Weill Med Coll

Henschke, Claudia L MD/PhD [DR] - **Spec Exp:** Lung Cancer; Lung Disease Imaging; Thoracic Imaging; **Hospital:** NY-Presby Hosp/Weill Cornell (page 66); **Address:** NY Weill Medical College, Dept Radiology, 525 E 68th St, Box 586, New York, NY 10021; **Phone:** 212-746-1325; **Board Cert:** Diagnostic Radiology 1981; **Med School:** Howard Univ 1977; **Resid:** Diagnostic Radiology, Brigham & Womens Hosp 1983; **Fac Appt:** Prof, Cornell Univ-Weill Med Coll

Hricak, Hedvig MD/PhD [DR] - **Spec Exp:** Prostate Cancer-MR Spectroscopy (MRSI); Breast Imaging; Breast Cancer; **Hospital:** Meml Sloan Kettering Cancer Ctr; **Address:** Meml Sloan Kettering Cancer Ctr, Dept Radiology, 1275 York Ave, New York, NY 10021-6007; **Phone:** 212-639-7284; **Board Cert:** Diagnostic Radiology 1978; **Med School:** Yugoslavia 1970; **Resid:** Diagnostic Radiology, St Joseph Mercy Hosp 1977; **Fellow:** Ultrasound/CT, Henry Ford Hosp 1978; **Fac Appt:** Prof Rad, Cornell Univ-Weill Med Coll

Jaramillo, Diego MD [DR] - **Spec Exp:** Pediatric Radiology; **Hospital:** Chldns Hosp of Philadelphia, The; **Address:** Children's Hosp of Philadelphia, Radiology, 34th & Civic Center Blvd, rm 3184, Philadelphia, PA 19104; **Phone:** 215-590-4842; **Board Cert:** Diagnostic Radiology 1987; Pediatric Radiology 2005; **Med School:** Colombia 1981; **Resid:** Diagnostic Radiology, U Texas 1987; **Fellow:** Pediatric Radiology, Children's Hosp 1989; **Fac Appt:** Assoc Prof Rad, Univ Pennsylvania

Kanal, Emanuel MD [DR] - **Spec Exp:** Neuroradiology; MRI; **Hospital:** UPMC Presby, Pittsburgh; **Address:** Univ Pittsburgh Med Ctr, Dept Radiology, 200 Lothrop St, rm D132, Pittsburgh, PA 15213-2582; **Phone:** 412-647-3540; **Board Cert:** Diagnostic Radiology 1985; Neuroradiology 1997; **Med School:** Univ Pittsburgh 1981; **Resid:** Diagnostic Radiology, U Pittsburgh Med Ctr 1985; **Fellow:** Magnetic Resonance Imaging, Pittsburgh NMR Inst 1986; Neurological Radiology, U Pittsburgh Med Ctr 1993; **Fac Appt:** Prof, Univ Pittsburgh

Diagnostic Radiology

Kurtz, Alfred B MD [DR] - **Spec Exp:** Obstetric Ultrasound; **Hospital:** Thomas Jefferson Univ Hosp; **Address:** Thomas Jefferson Univ Hosp, Dept Radiology, 111 S 11th St, Ste 3350A-B, Philadelphia, PA 19107; **Phone:** 215-955-6343; **Board Cert:** Diagnostic Radiology 1977; **Med School:** Stanford Univ 1972; **Resid:** Internal Medicine, Montefiore Med Ctr 1974; Diagnostic Radiology, Montefiore Med Ctr 1977; **Fellow:** Ultrasound, Thomas Jefferson Univ Hosp 1978; **Fac Appt:** Prof Rad, Jefferson Med Coll

Levy, Angela D MD [DR] - **Spec Exp:** Gastrointestinal Cancer; **Hospital:** Unif Serv Univ of the Hlth Sci, Armed Forces Inst of Path; **Address:** Uniformed Services Univ of the Hlth Scis, Dept Radiology, 4301 Jones Bridge Rd, Bethesda, MD 20814; **Phone:** 301-295-3145; **Board Cert:** Diagnostic Radiology 1993; **Med School:** Uniformed Srvs Univ, Bethesda 1988; **Resid:** Diagnostic Radiology, Walter Reed Army Hosp 1992; **Fac Appt:** Assoc Prof Rad, Uniformed Srvs Univ, Bethesda

Mirvis, Stuart E MD [DR] - **Spec Exp:** Trauma Radiology; **Hospital:** Univ of MD Med Sys; **Address:** Univ Maryland Med Ctr, Dept Radiology, 22 S Greene St, Baltimore, MD 21201; **Phone:** 410-328-8845; **Board Cert:** Diagnostic Radiology 1984; **Med School:** Johns Hopkins Univ 1979; **Resid:** Diagnostic Radiology, Univ Maryland Med Ctr 1984; **Fellow:** Trauma Radiology, Univ Maryland Med Ctr 1985; **Fac Appt:** Prof, Univ MD Sch Med

Mitnick, Julie MD [DR] - **Spec Exp:** Mammography; Breast Cancer; **Address:** 650 1st Ave, New York, NY 10016; **Phone:** 212-686-4440; **Board Cert:** Diagnostic Radiology 1977; **Med School:** NYU Sch Med 1973; **Resid:** Diagnostic Radiology, NYU Med Ctr 1977; **Fellow:** Pediatric Radiology, NYU Med Ctr 1978; **Fac Appt:** Assoc Clin Prof Rad, NYU Sch Med

Norton, Karen MD [DR] - **Spec Exp:** Pediatric Radiology; **Hospital:** Newark Beth Israel Med Ctr; **Address:** 201 Lyons Ave, Newark, NJ 07112; **Phone:** 973-926-7689; **Board Cert:** Diagnostic Radiology 1984; Pediatric Radiology 2005; **Med School:** Mount Sinai Sch Med 1980; **Resid:** Pediatrics, NYU Med Ctr 1981; Diagnostic Radiology, Mount Sinai Hosp 1984; **Fellow:** Pediatric Radiology, Mount Sinai Hosp 1985; **Fac Appt:** Prof Rad, Mount Sinai Sch Med

Panicek, David MD [DR] - **Spec Exp:** Bone Cancer; Soft Tissue Tumors; **Hospital:** Meml Sloan Kettering Cancer Ctr; **Address:** Memorial Hosp - Dept Radiology, 1275 York Ave, rm C276G, New York, NY 10021; **Phone:** 212-639-5825; **Board Cert:** Diagnostic Radiology 1984; **Med School:** Cornell Univ-Weill Med Coll 1980; **Resid:** Diagnostic Radiology, New York Hosp-Cornell 1984; **Fac Appt:** Prof Rad, Cornell Univ-Weill Med Coll

Potter, Hollis J MD [DR] - **Spec Exp:** Musculoskeletal Imaging; Cartilage Damage; Arthroplasty Imaging; **Hospital:** Hosp For Special Surgery (page 60); **Address:** Hosp for Special Surgery, MRI-basement, 535 E 70th St, New York, NY 10021-4892; **Phone:** 212-606-1882; **Board Cert:** Diagnostic Radiology 1990; **Med School:** NY Med Coll 1985; **Resid:** Diagnostic Radiology, North Shore Univ Hosp 1990; **Fellow:** Diagnostic Radiology, Hosp Special Surgery 1991; **Fac Appt:** Prof Rad, Cornell Univ-Weill Med Coll

Rao, Vijay M MD [DR] - **Spec Exp:** Head & Neck Tumors Imaging; TMJ Imaging; Ear Nose & Throat Imaging; **Hospital:** Thomas Jefferson Univ Hosp; **Address:** 132 S 10th St, 1087, Main Bldg, Philadelphia, PA 19107-4824; **Phone:** 215-955-4804; **Board Cert:** Diagnostic Radiology 1978; Neuroradiology 1997; **Med School:** India 1973; **Resid:** Diagnostic Radiology, Thomas Jefferson Univ Hosp 1978; **Fac Appt:** Prof Rad, Thomas Jefferson Univ

Teal, James S MD [DR] - **Spec Exp:** Interventional Radiology; **Hospital:** Howard Univ Hosp; **Address:** Howard Univ Hosp, Dept Radiology, 2041 Georgia Ave NW, Washington, DC 20060-0001; **Phone:** 202-865-1571; **Board Cert:** Diagnostic Radiology 1970; **Med School:** Univ Tex Med Br, Galveston 1965; **Resid:** Diagnostic Radiology, Mt Zion Hosp 1969; **Fellow:** Neurology, LAC-USC Med Ctr 1970; **Fac Appt:** Prof, Howard Univ

White, Charles S MD [DR] - **Spec Exp:** Thoracic Imaging; **Hospital:** Univ of MD Med Sys; **Address:** Univ Maryland Med Ctr, Dept Radiology, 22 S Greene St, Baltimore, MD 21201; **Phone:** 410-328-5700; **Board Cert:** Diagnostic Radiology 1991; Internal Medicine 1987; **Med School:** SUNY Buffalo 1984; **Resid:** Internal Medicine, Columbia-Presby Hosp 1987; Diagnostic Radiology, Columbia-Presby Hosp 1991; **Fellow:** Thoracic Radiology, Columbia-Presby Med Ctr; **Fac Appt:** Prof, Univ MD Sch Med

Southeast

Abbitt, Patricia L MD [DR] - **Spec Exp:** Ultrasound; Interventional Radiology; Breast Imaging; Breast Cancer; **Hospital:** Shands Hlthcre at Univ of FL; **Address:** Shands Healthcare, Dept Radiology, 1600 SW Archer Rd, PO Box 100374, Gainesville, FL 32610; **Phone:** 352-265-0291; **Board Cert:** Diagnostic Radiology 1986; **Med School:** Tufts Univ 1981; **Resid:** Diagnostic Radiology, Univ VA Med Ctr 1986; **Fellow:** Breast Imaging, Univ VA Med Ctr 1987; **Fac Appt:** Prof DR, Univ Fla Coll Med

Berland, Lincoln L MD [DR] - **Spec Exp:** Abdominal Imaging; Gastrointestinal Imaging; **Hospital:** Univ of Ala Hosp at Birmingham; **Address:** Univ of Alabama Hosp, Jefferson Twr Bldg, 619 S 19th St, rm N348, Birmingham, AL 35249; **Phone:** 205-934-7978; **Board Cert:** Diagnostic Radiology 1980; **Med School:** Washington Univ, St Louis 1975; **Resid:** Diagnostic Radiology, Med Coll Wisconsin Hosps 1979; **Fellow:** Ultrasound/CT, Med Coll Wisconsin Hosps 1980; **Fac Appt:** Prof, Univ Ala

Mancuso, Anthony MD [DR] - **Spec Exp:** Head & Neck Imaging; Neuroradiology; **Hospital:** Shands Hlthcre at Univ of FL; **Address:** Shands Hosp, Univ Florida, Dept Rad, 1600 SW Archer Rd, Gainesville, FL 32610; **Phone:** 352-265-0296; **Board Cert:** Diagnostic Radiology 1978; **Med School:** Univ Miami Sch Med 1973; **Resid:** Diagnostic Radiology, UCLA Med Ctr 1977; **Fellow:** Neuroradiology, UCLA Med Ctr 1978; **Fac Appt:** Prof, Univ Fla Coll Med

Partain, C Leon MD/PhD [DR] - **Spec Exp:** MRI; Nuclear Radiology; **Hospital:** Vanderbilt Univ Med Ctr; **Address:** Vanderbilt Univ Med Ctr, Dept Radiology, 1161 21st Ave S, rm RR1223 MCN, Nashville, TN 37232-2675; **Phone:** 615-343-3588; **Board Cert:** Nuclear Medicine 1979; Diagnostic Radiology 1980; Nuclear Radiology 1981; **Med School:** Washington Univ, St Louis 1975; **Resid:** Diagnostic Radiology, Univ North Carolina 1979; Nuclear Medicine, Univ North Carolina 1979; **Fac Appt:** Prof, Vanderbilt Univ

Pisano, Etta D MD [DR] - **Spec Exp:** Breast Imaging; **Hospital:** Univ NC Hosps; **Address:** UNC Health Care, 101 Manning Dr, Box 7510, Chapel Hill, NC 27299-7510; **Phone:** 919-966-1081; **Board Cert:** Diagnostic Radiology 1988; **Med School:** Duke Univ 1983; **Resid:** Diagnostic Radiology, Beth Israel Hosp 1988; **Fac Appt:** Prof, Univ NC Sch Med

White, Richard D MD [DR] - **Spec Exp:** Cardiovascular Imaging; **Hospital:** Shands Jacksonville; **Address:** Univ Florida Coll of Med, Radiology, 655 W 8th St Fl 2, Jacksonville, FL 32209; **Phone:** 904-244-4224; **Board Cert:** Diagnostic Radiology 1986; **Med School:** Duke Univ 1981; **Resid:** Diagnostic Radiology, UCSF Med Ctr 1985; **Fellow:** Cardiovascular Radiology, UCSF Med Ctr 1987; **Fac Appt:** Prof, Univ Fla Coll Med

Yoon, Sydney MD [DR] - **Spec Exp:** MRI; CT Body Scan; Uterine Fibroid Embolization; Interventional Radiology; **Hospital:** Osceola Regional Med Ctr; **Address:** Osceola Regl Med Ctr, Dept Radiology, 700 W Oak St, Kissimmee, FL 34741; **Phone:** 407-518-3770; **Board Cert:** Internal Medicine 1989; Diagnostic Radiology 1993; Vascular & Interventional Radiology 1998; Neuroradiology 2006; **Med School:** Univ Chicago-Pritzker Sch Med 1986; **Resid:** Internal Medicine, Johns Hopkins Hosp 1989; Diagnostic Radiology, UCLA Med Ctr 1993; **Fellow:** Neuroradiology, Columbia Presby Med Ctr 1995; Vascular & Interventional Radiology, UCLA Med Ctr 1997

Midwest

Flamm, Scott D MD [DR] - **Spec Exp:** Cardiac MRI; Cardiovascular Imaging; Congenital Heart Disease; **Hospital:** Cleveland Clin Fdn (page 57); **Address:** Cleveland Clinic, 9500 Euclid Ave, MC Hb6, Cleveland, OH 44195; **Phone:** 216-444-2750; **Board Cert:** Diagnostic Radiology 1993; **Med School:** Geo Wash Univ 1988; **Resid:** Diagnostic Radiology, UCLA Med Ctr 1992; **Fellow:** Cardiovascular Disease, UCSF Med Ctr 1994; **Fac Appt:** Assoc Prof Rad, Case West Res Univ

Goodman, Lawrence R MD [DR] - **Spec Exp:** Thoracic Imaging; Pulmonary Embolism; Lung Disease Imaging; **Hospital:** Froedtert Meml Lutheran Hosp; **Address:** Froedtert Meml Lutheran Hosp, Dept Radiology, 9200 West Wisconsin Avenue, Milwaukee, WI 53226; **Phone:** 414-805-3120; **Board Cert:** Diagnostic Radiology 1973; **Med School:** SUNY Downstate 1968; **Resid:** Diagnostic Radiology, Boston Univ/City Hosp 1972; **Fellow:** Thoracic Radiology, UCSF Med Ctr 1973; **Fac Appt:** Prof Rad, Med Coll Wisc

McAlister, William MD [DR] - **Spec Exp:** Pediatric Radiology; **Hospital:** St Louis Chldns Hosp; **Address:** 510 S Kingshighway Blvd, Box 8131, Saint Louis, MO 63110; **Phone:** 314-454-6229; **Board Cert:** Diagnostic Radiology 1961; Pediatric Radiology 2003; **Med School:** Wayne State Univ 1954; **Resid:** Diagnostic Radiology, Cincinnati Genl Hosp 1960; **Fac Appt:** Prof, Washington Univ, St Louis

Monsees, Barbara MD [DR] - **Spec Exp:** Mammography; Breast Cancer; **Hospital:** Barnes-Jewish Hosp; **Address:** Ctr for Advanced Med, Campus Box 8131, 510 S Kingshighway Blvd, St Louis, MO 63110; **Phone:** 314-454-7500; **Board Cert:** Diagnostic Radiology 1980; **Med School:** Washington Univ, St Louis 1975; **Resid:** Pediatrics, St Louis Chldns Hosp 1977; Diagnostic Radiology, Mallinckrodt Inst Radiology 1980; **Fac Appt:** Prof DR, Washington Univ, St Louis

Sagel, Stuart S MD [DR] - **Spec Exp:** Lung Cancer; Occupational Lung Disease; Pulmonary Embolism; **Hospital:** Barnes-Jewish Hosp; **Address:** Mallinckrodt Inst Rad-Barnes Hosp, 510 S Kingshighway Blvd, Box 8131, St Louis, MO 63110-1016; **Phone:** 314-362-2927; **Board Cert:** Diagnostic Radiology 1970; **Med School:** Temple Univ 1965; **Resid:** Diagnostic Radiology, Yale New Haven Hosp 1968; Diagnostic Radiology, UCSF Med Ctr 1970; **Fac Appt:** Prof, Washington Univ, St Louis

Sivit, Carlos MD [DR] - **Spec Exp:** Pediatric Radiology; Abdominal Imaging; **Hospital:** Rainbow Babies & Chldns Hosp; **Address:** Univ Hosps Cleveland, Dept Radiology, 11100 Euclid Ave, Cleveland, OH 44106-1736; **Phone:** 216-844-1172; **Board Cert:** Pediatrics 1987; Diagnostic Radiology 1987; Pediatric Radiology 1995; **Med School:** Univ VA Sch Med 1981; **Resid:** Pediatrics, Vanderbilt Univ Hosp 1984; Diagnostic Radiology, George Washington Univ Hosp 1987; **Fellow:** Pediatric Radiology, Chldns Natl Med Ctr 1989; **Fac Appt:** Prof Rad, Case West Res Univ

Strife, Janet L MD [DR] - **Spec Exp:** Pediatric Radiology; Cardiac Imaging; **Hospital:** Cincinnati Chldns Hosp Med Ctr; **Address:** Children's Hospital, Dept Radiology, 3333 Burnet Ave, MC 5031, Cincinnati, OH 45229; **Phone:** 513-636-7535; **Board Cert:** Diagnostic Radiology 1974; Pediatric Radiology 2004; **Med School:** UMDNJ-NJ Med Sch, Newark 1968; **Resid:** Diagnostic Radiology, Univ Cincinnati Med Ctr 1971; Diagnostic Radiology, Johns Hopkins Hosp 1973; **Fellow:** Pediatrics, Johns Hopkins Hosp; **Fac Appt:** Prof, Univ Cincinnati

Swensen, Stephen J MD [DR] - **Spec Exp:** Lung Cancer; Lung Disease Imaging; **Hospital:** Mayo Med Ctr & Clin - Rochester; **Address:** Mayo Clinic - Diagnostic Radiology, 200 1st St SW, Rochester, MN 55905; **Phone:** 507-538-3270; **Board Cert:** Diagnostic Radiology 1986; **Med School:** Univ Wisc 1981; **Resid:** Diagnostic Radiology, Mayo Clinic 1986; **Fellow:** Pulmonary Radiology, Brigham & Womens Hosp 1987; **Fac Appt:** Prof Rad, Mayo Med Sch

Southwest

Dodd III, Gerald Dewey MD [DR] - **Spec Exp:** Ultrasound; **Hospital:** Univ Hlth Sys - Univ Hosp; **Address:** 7703 Floyd Curl Dr, MC-7800, San Antonio, TX 78229-3900; **Phone:** 210-567-5558; **Board Cert:** Diagnostic Radiology 1987; **Med School:** Univ Tex, Houston 1983; **Resid:** Diagnostic Radiology, Univ Hosp 1987; **Fellow:** Abdominal Imaging & Angio-Interventional, Univ Hosp 1988; **Fac Appt:** Prof, Univ Tex, San Antonio

Huynh, Phan Tuong MD [DR] - **Spec Exp:** Mammography; Breast Cancer; **Hospital:** St Luke's Episcopal Hosp - Houston; **Address:** 6624 Fannin St, St Luke's Tower, Women's Ctr Fl 10, Houston, TX 77030; **Phone:** 832-355-8130; **Board Cert:** Diagnostic Radiology 1994; **Med School:** Univ VA Sch Med 1989; **Resid:** Diagnostic Radiology, Univ Virginia Med Ctr 1994; **Fellow:** Mammography, Univ Virginia 1995; **Fac Appt:** Assoc Clin Prof Rad, Baylor Coll Med

Otto, Pamela MD [DR] - **Spec Exp:** Breast Imaging; **Hospital:** Univ Hlth Sys - Univ Hosp, Audie L Murphy Meml Vets Hosp; **Address:** 7703 Floyd Curl Drive, MC 7800, San Antonio, TX 78229-3900; **Phone:** 210-567-3448; **Board Cert:** Diagnostic Radiology 1993; **Med School:** Univ MO-Columbia Sch Med 1988; **Resid:** Diagnostic Radiology, Univ Texas Hlth Sci Ctr 1993; **Fellow:** Breast Imaging, Univ Texas Hlth Sci Ctr 1993; **Fac Appt:** Assoc Prof Rad, Univ Tex, San Antonio

West Coast and Pacific

Bassett, Lawrence W MD [DR] - **Spec Exp:** Breast Imaging; **Hospital:** UCLA Med Ctr; **Address:** 200 UCLA Med Plaza, rm 165-47, Los Angeles, CA 90095; **Phone:** 310-206-9608; **Board Cert:** Diagnostic Radiology 1975; **Med School:** UC Irvine 1968; **Resid:** Diagnostic Radiology, UCLA Med Ctr 1972; **Fac Appt:** Prof DR, UCLA

Filly, Roy A MD [DR] - **Spec Exp:** Obstetric Ultrasound; **Hospital:** UCSF Med Ctr; **Address:** UCSF Med Ctr, Dept Diagnostic Radiology, 505 Parnassus Ave, Box 0628, San Francisco, CA 94143-0628; **Phone:** 415-353-1628; **Board Cert:** Diagnostic Radiology 1974; **Med School:** Ohio State Univ 1970; **Resid:** Diagnostic Radiology, Stanford Univ Med Ctr 1974; **Fac Appt:** Prof, UCSF

Diagnostic Radiology

Gilsanz, Vicente MD [DR] - **Spec Exp:** Pediatric Radiology; Bone Disorders-Metabolic; **Hospital:** Chldns Hosp - Los Angeles (page 56); **Address:** Children's Hospital, LA, 4650 Sunset Blvd, MS 81, Los Angeles, CA 90027; **Phone:** 323-669-4571; **Board Cert:** Internal Medicine 1973; Diagnostic Radiology 1976; Pediatric Radiology 2004; **Med School:** Spain 1969; **Resid:** Internal Medicine, Mayo Clinic 1973; Diagnostic Radiology, Mt Sinai Hosp 1976; **Fellow:** Pediatric Radiology, Childrens Hosp 1978; **Fac Appt:** Prof, USC Sch Med

Rubin, Geoffrey D MD [DR] - **Spec Exp:** Cardiovascular Imaging; Cardiac Imaging; Thoracic Imaging; **Hospital:** Stanford Univ Med Ctr; **Address:** Stanford Univ Med Ctr, 300 Pasteur Drive, rm S 072, MC 510, Stanford, CA 94305-5105; **Phone:** 650-723-7647; **Board Cert:** Diagnostic Radiology 1992; **Med School:** UCSD 1987; **Resid:** Diagnostic Radiology, Stanford Univ Med Ctr 1992; **Fellow:** Body Imaging, Stanford Univ Med Ctr 1993; **Fac Appt:** Prof Rad, Stanford Univ

Thurmond, Amy S MD [DR] - **Spec Exp:** Women's Imaging; Infertility-Fallopian Tube Intervention; Women's Gynecological Health; **Hospital:** Legacy Meridian Park Hosp, OR Hlth & Sci Univ; **Address:** 8950 SW Nimbus Ave, Beaverton, OR 97008; **Phone:** 503-643-7226; **Board Cert:** Diagnostic Radiology 1987; **Med School:** UCLA 1982; **Resid:** Cardiovascular Disease, St Vincent Hosp Med Ctr 1984; Diagnostic Radiology, Oreg Hlth Scis Univ 1987; **Fellow:** Vascular & Interventional Radiology, Oreg Hlth Scis Univ 1988; **Fac Appt:** Assoc Prof, Oregon Hlth Sci Univ

Wood, Beverly MD/PhD [DR] - **Spec Exp:** Pediatric Radiology; **Hospital:** LAC & USC Med Ctr, Loma Linda Chldns Hosp; **Address:** Loma Linda Chldns Hosp, 11234 Anderson St, Loma Linda, CA 90033; **Phone:** 909-558-4281; **Board Cert:** Diagnostic Radiology 1972; Pediatric Radiology 2003; **Med School:** Univ Rochester 1965; **Resid:** Diagnostic Radiology, Strong Meml Hosp 1971; **Fellow:** Pediatric Radiology, Strong Meml Hosp 1972; **Fac Appt:** Prof, USC Sch Med

Neuroradiology

New England

Curtin, Hugh D MD [NRad] - **Spec Exp:** Head & Neck Radiology; Neuroradiology; **Hospital:** Mass Eye & Ear Infirmary; **Address:** Mass Eye & Ear Infirmary, Dept Radiology, 243 Charles St Fl 6, Boston, MA 02114; **Phone:** 617-573-3563 x4; **Board Cert:** Diagnostic Radiology 1976; Neuroradiology 1999; **Med School:** SUNY Upstate Med Univ 1972; **Resid:** Diagnostic Radiology, Presbyterian Univ Hosp 1976; **Fellow:** Neuroradiology, Foundation Rothschild; **Fac Appt:** Prof, Harvard Med Sch

Hackney, David B MD [NRad] - **Hospital:** Beth Israel Deaconess Med Ctr - Boston; **Address:** BIDMC, Dept Radiology, 330 Brookline Ave, Boston, MA 02215; **Phone:** 617-754-2009; **Board Cert:** Diagnostic Radiology 1984; Neuroradiology 2005; **Med School:** Harvard Med Sch 1980; **Resid:** Diagnostic Radiology, UCSD Med Ctr 1983; **Fellow:** Neurological Radiology, Mass Genl Hosp 1985; **Fac Appt:** Prof, Harvard Med Sch

Hirsch, Joshua A MD [NRad] - **Spec Exp:** Interventional Neuroradiology; Endovascular Surgery; Minimally Invasive Spinal Surgery; Osteoporosis Spine-Vertebroplasty; **Hospital:** Mass Genl Hosp; **Address:** Mass Genl Hospital, Interventional Neuroradiology, 55 Fruit St Gray Bldg - rm 241, Boston, MA 02114; **Phone:** 617-726-1767; **Board Cert:** Diagnostic Radiology 1996; **Med School:** Univ Pennsylvania 1991; **Resid:** Diagnostic Radiology, Hosp Univ Penn 1996; **Fellow:** Neuroradiology, Hosp Univ Penn 1995; Interventional Neuroradiology, Lahey Clinic 1998; **Fac Appt:** Asst Prof Rad, Harvard Med Sch

Norbash, Alexander M MD [NRad] - **Spec Exp:** Interventional Neuroradiology; Aneurysm-Cerebral; Osteoporosis Spine-Kyphoplasty; **Hospital:** Boston Med Ctr; **Address:** BMC, Dept Radiology, 88 E Newton St Fl 2, Boston, MA 02118; **Phone:** 617-638-6661; **Board Cert:** Diagnostic Radiology 1991; Neuroradiology 2004; **Med School:** Univ MO-Kansas City 1986; **Resid:** Diagnostic Radiology, St Francis Hosp 1990; Diagnostic Radiology, Presby Univ Hosp 1991; **Fellow:** Neurological Radiology, Stanford Univ Hosp 1993; Interventional Radiology, Stanford Univ Hosp 1994; **Fac Appt:** Prof, Boston Univ

Mid Atlantic

Berenstein, Alejandro MD [NRad] - **Spec Exp:** Interventional Neuroradiology; Aneurysm-Cerebral; Endovascular Surgery; **Hospital:** St Luke's - Roosevelt Hosp Ctr - St Luke's Hosp; **Address:** Hyman-Newman Inst Neurolgy & Neuro Surg, 1000 10th Ave, rm GG16, New York, NY 10019; **Phone:** 212-636-3400; **Board Cert:** Diagnostic Radiology 1976; **Med School:** Mexico 1970; **Resid:** Diagnostic Radiology, Mount Sinai Med Ctr 1976; **Fellow:** Neuroradiology, NYU Med Ctr 1978; **Fac Appt:** Prof Rad, NYU Sch Med

Drayer, Burton P MD [NRad] - **Spec Exp:** Stroke; Parkinson's Disease/Aging Brain; MRI & CT of Brain & Spine; **Hospital:** Mount Sinai Med Ctr; **Address:** 1 Gustave Levy Pl, Box 1234, New York, NY 10029; **Phone:** 212-241-6403; **Board Cert:** Neurology 1976; Diagnostic Radiology 1978; Neuroradiology 2006; **Med School:** Ros Franklin Univ/Chicago Med Sch 1971; **Resid:** Neurology, Univ Vt Med Ctr 1975; Diagnostic Radiology, Univ Pitt Hlth Ctr 1977; **Fellow:** Neuroradiology, Univ Pitt Hlth Ctr 1978; **Fac Appt:** Prof Rad, Mount Sinai Sch Med

Grossman, Robert I MD [NRad] - **Spec Exp:** Multiple Sclerosis Imaging; Brain Injury; MRI; **Hospital:** NYU Med Ctr (page 67), Bellevue Hosp Ctr; **Address:** NYU Med Ctr, Dept Radiology, 560 First Ave, RUSK 229, New York, NY 10016; **Phone:** 212-263-3269; **Board Cert:** Diagnostic Radiology 1979; Neuroradiology 2005; **Med School:** Univ Pennsylvania 1973; **Resid:** Neurological Surgery, Hosp Univ Penn 1976; Diagnostic Radiology, Hosp Univ Penn 1979; **Fellow:** Neuroradiology, Mass Genl Hosp 1981; **Fac Appt:** Prof Rad, NYU Sch Med

Hurst, Robert W MD [NRad] - **Spec Exp:** Interventional Neuroradiology; Stroke; Carotid Artery Stent Placement; Intracranial Angioplasty & Stent; **Hospital:** Hosp Univ Penn - UPHS (page 72); **Address:** Dept Radiology/Neuroradiology, HUP, 3400 Spruce St, Ground FL, Founders Bldg, Philadelphia, PA 19104; **Phone:** 215-662-3572; **Board Cert:** Neurology 1986; Diagnostic Radiology 1989; Neuroradiology 2005; **Med School:** Univ Tex, Houston 1981; **Resid:** Neurology, Univ Virginia Hosp 1985; Diagnostic Radiology, Univ Virginia Hosp 1989; **Fellow:** Neurological Radiology, Hosp Univ Penn 1990; Interventional Radiology, NYU Med Ctr 1991; **Fac Appt:** Prof Rad, Univ Pennsylvania

Khandji, Alexander G MD [NRad] - **Spec Exp:** Pituitary Disorders; Spinal Diseases; MRI; **Hospital:** NY-Presby Hosp/Columbia (page 66); **Address:** 177 Ft Washington Ave, Ste 4-156, New York, NY 10032-3173; **Phone:** 212-305-7669; **Board Cert:** Diagnostic Radiology 1985; Neuroradiology 2006; **Med School:** SUNY Downstate 1980; **Resid:** Surgery, MS Hershey Med Ctr 1982; Diagnostic Radiology, Columbia-Presby Med Ctr 1985; **Fellow:** Neuroradiology, Columbia-Presby Med Ctr 1987; **Fac Appt:** Clin Prof Rad, Columbia P&S

Litt, Andrew W MD [NRad] - **Spec Exp:** Vascular Lesions of the CNS; Cerebrovascular Disease; Stroke; **Hospital:** NYU Med Ctr (page 67); **Address:** NYU Medical Ctr, Dept Radiology, 560 1st Ave, IRM 232, New York, NY 10016-6402; **Phone:** 212-263-8121; **Board Cert:** Diagnostic Radiology 1988; Neuroradiology 2005; **Med School:** NYU Sch Med 1983; **Resid:** Diagnostic Radiology, NYU Med Ctr 1987; **Fellow:** Neuroradiology, NYU Med Ctr 1988; **Fac Appt:** Prof Rad, NYU Sch Med

Neuroradiology

Pile-Spellman, John MD [NRad] - **Spec Exp:** Interventional Neuroradiology; Cerebrovascular Disease; Aneurysm; Arteriovenous Malformations; **Hospital:** NY-Presby Hosp/Columbia (page 66); **Address:** 177 Fort Washington Ave, MHB 8SK, New York, NY 10032-3713; **Phone:** 212-305-6515; **Board Cert:** Diagnostic Radiology 1984; **Med School:** Tufts Univ 1978; **Resid:** Neurological Surgery, New England Med Ctr 1981; Neurological Radiology, Mass Genl Hosp 1984; **Fellow:** Interventional Neuroradiology, NYU Med Ctr 1986; **Fac Appt:** Prof Rad, Columbia P&S

Tenner, Michael MD [NRad] - **Spec Exp:** Stroke; Aneurysm-Cerebral; Arteriovenous Malformations; Carotid Artery Stent Placement; **Hospital:** Westchester Med Ctr; **Address:** NY Med Coll, Dept Radiology, Route 100, Valhalla, NY 10595; **Phone:** 914-493-8158; **Board Cert:** Diagnostic Radiology 1967; **Med School:** Univ MD Sch Med 1960; **Resid:** Diagnostic Radiology, Univ Maryland Hosp 1962; Diagnostic Radiology, Univ Maryland Hosp 1966; **Fellow:** Neuroradiology, Neurological Inst-Columbia Presby 1968; **Fac Appt:** Prof Rad, NY Med Coll

Vezina, L Gilbert MD [NRad] - **Spec Exp:** Pediatric Neuroradiology; Brain Tumors; Neurofibromatosis; **Hospital:** Chldns Natl Med Ctr; **Address:** Chldns Natl Med Ctr, Dept Radiology, 111 Michigan Ave NW, Washington, DC 20010-2970; **Phone:** 202-884-3651; **Board Cert:** Diagnostic Radiology 1987; Neuroradiology 1998; **Med School:** McGill Univ 1983; **Resid:** Diagnostic Radiology, Mass Genl Hosp 1987; **Fellow:** Neurological Radiology, Mass Genl Hosp 1989; Pediatric Neuroradiology, Chldns Natl Med Ctr 1991; **Fac Appt:** Prof, Geo Wash Univ

Yousem, David M MD [NRad] - **Hospital:** Johns Hopkins Hosp - Baltimore (page 61); **Address:** Johns Hopkins Hosp, Div Neuroradiology, 600 N Wolfe St Phipps Bldg - rm B-100, Baltimore, MD 21287; **Phone:** 410-955-2353; **Board Cert:** Diagnostic Radiology 1987; Neuroradiology 2005; **Med School:** Univ Mich Med Sch 1983; **Resid:** Diagnostic Radiology, Johns Hopkins Hosp 1987; **Fellow:** Neuroradiology, Hosp Univ Penn 1990; **Fac Appt:** Prof, Johns Hopkins Univ

Zimmerman, Robert A MD [NRad] - **Spec Exp:** Pediatric Neuroradiology; **Hospital:** Chldns Hosp of Philadelphia, The; **Address:** Childrens Hosp Philadelphia, Radiology, 34th St & Civic Center Blvd, Philadelphia, PA 19104; **Phone:** 215-590-2569; **Board Cert:** Diagnostic Radiology 1970; Neuroradiology 1995; **Med School:** Georgetown Univ 1964; **Resid:** Diagnostic Radiology, Hosp Univ Penn 1969; **Fac Appt:** Prof Rad, Univ Pennsylvania

Zinreich, S James MD [NRad] - **Spec Exp:** Head & Neck Radiology; **Hospital:** Johns Hopkins Hosp - Baltimore (page 61); **Address:** Johns Hopkins Hospital, 600 N Wolfe St Phipps Bldg - rm B-100, Baltimore, MD 21287; **Phone:** 410-614-3020; **Board Cert:** Diagnostic Radiology 1982; **Med School:** Belgium 1976; **Resid:** Diagnostic Radiology, Sinai Hosp; **Fac Appt:** Prof Oto, Johns Hopkins Univ

Southeast

Dion, Jacques MD [NRad] - **Spec Exp:** Stroke; Intracranial Angioplasty & Stent; Aneurysm-Cerebral; Osteoporosis Spine-Vertebroplasty; **Hospital:** Emory Univ Hosp; **Address:** Emory Univ Hosp, Dept Neuroradiology, 1364 Clifton Rd NE, rm A121, Atlanta, GA 30322; **Phone:** 404-712-4991; **Board Cert:** Diagnostic Radiology 1982; Neuroradiology 1998; **Med School:** Univ Ottawa 1978; **Resid:** Diagnostic Radiology, Harbor-UCLA Med Ctr 1981; Diagnostic Radiology, Notre Dame Hosp 1983; **Fellow:** Neuroradiology, Univ Hospital 1985; **Fac Appt:** Prof, Emory Univ

Jensen, Mary E MD [NRad] - **Spec Exp:** Interventional Neuroradiology; Osteoporosis Spine-Vertebroplasty; Aneurysm-Cerebral; **Hospital:** Univ Virginia Med Ctr; **Address:** Univ of Virginia Med Ctr, Dept Radiology, Box 800170, Charlottsville, VA 22908; **Phone:** 434-924-9719; **Board Cert:** Diagnostic Radiology 1987; **Med School:** Med Coll VA 1982; **Resid:** Diagnostic Radiology, Univ Virginia Med Ctr 1991; **Fellow:** Interventional Neuroradiology, UCLA Med Ctr 1992; **Fac Appt:** Assoc Prof, Univ VA Sch Med

Joseph, Gregory J MD [NRad] - **Spec Exp:** Stroke; Aneurysm-Cerebral; Intracranial Angioplasty & Stent; **Hospital:** Presby Hosp - Charlotte; **Address:** Presbyterian Hosp, Dept Radiology, 200 Hawthorne Ln, Charlotte, NC 28233; **Phone:** 704-384-4057; **Board Cert:** Diagnostic Radiology 1989; **Med School:** Georgetown Univ 1984; **Resid:** Diagnostic Radiology, Georgetown Univ Hosp 1989; Vascular & Interventional Radiology, Emory Univ Hosp 1990; **Fellow:** Neuroradiology, Emory Univ Hosp 1991

Provenzale, James M MD [NRad] - **Spec Exp:** Brain Tumor Imaging; Multiple Sclerosis Imaging; Brain Imaging-Pediatric; **Hospital:** Duke Univ Med Ctr; **Address:** Duke University Medical Ctr, Dept Radiology, Box 3808, Durham, NC 27710; **Phone:** 919-684-7218; **Board Cert:** Neurology 1988; Diagnostic Radiology 1991; Neuroradiology 2001; **Med School:** Albany Med Coll 1983; **Resid:** Neurology, NC Memorial Hosp 1987; Diagnostic Radiology, Mass General Hosp 1991; **Fellow:** Neuroradiology, Mass General Hosp 1992; **Fac Appt:** Prof DR, Duke Univ

Quencer, Robert MD [NRad] - **Spec Exp:** Spinal Cord Injury; **Hospital:** Jackson Meml Hosp, Univ of Miami Hosp & Clins/Sylvester Comp Canc Ctr; **Address:** Univ Miami, Dept Radiology, 1150 NW 14th St, Ste 511, M828, Miami, FL 33136-2116; **Phone:** 305-243-4701; **Board Cert:** Diagnostic Radiology 1972; Neuroradiology 1995; **Med School:** SUNY Upstate Med Univ 1967; **Resid:** Diagnostic Radiology, Columbia-Presbyterian Med Ctr 1971; **Fellow:** Neuroradiology, Neurological Inst 1972; **Fac Appt:** Prof, Univ Miami Sch Med

Midwest

Ball Jr, William S MD [NRad] - **Spec Exp:** Pediatric Neuroradiology; **Hospital:** Cincinnati Chldns Hosp Med Ctr; **Address:** Cincinnati Chldns Hosp, Dept Neuroradiology, 3333 Burnet Ave, ML 5031, Cincinnati, OH 45229-3039; **Phone:** 513-636-8574; **Board Cert:** Diagnostic Radiology 1982; Pediatrics 1982; Neuroradiology 1999; **Med School:** Tulane Univ 1974; **Resid:** Pediatrics, Oschner Fdn Hosp 1977; Diagnostic Radiology, Univ New Mexico 1978; **Fellow:** Pediatric Radiology, Chldns Hosp Med Ctr 1981; Neuroradiology, Univ New Mexico Med Ctr 1979; **Fac Appt:** Prof, Univ Cincinnati

Cross III, DeWitte T MD [NRad] - **Spec Exp:** Interventional Neuroradiology; Aneurysm-Cerebral; Stroke; **Hospital:** Barnes-Jewish Hosp, St Louis Chldns Hosp; **Address:** Wash Univ, Dept Radiology, 510 S Kingshighway Blvd , Box 8131, St Louis, MO 63110-1016; **Phone:** 314-362-5580; **Board Cert:** Diagnostic Radiology 1985; Neuroradiology 2006; **Med School:** Univ Ala 1980; **Resid:** Diagnostic Radiology, Naval Hosp 1985; **Fellow:** Neuroradiology, NY Med Coll 1988; Neuroradiology, Columbia Univ 1989; **Fac Appt:** Assoc Prof Rad, Washington Univ, St Louis

Haughton III, Victor M MD [NRad] - **Spec Exp:** Spinal Imaging; **Hospital:** Univ WI Hosp & Clins; **Address:** Univ WI Hosps & Clins, Dept Radiology, 600 Highland Ave, MC 3252, Madison, WI 53792; **Phone:** 608-263-9179; **Board Cert:** Diagnostic Radiology 1974; Neuroradiology 1995; **Med School:** Yale Univ 1967; **Resid:** Diagnostic Radiology, Peter Bent Brigham Hosp 1973; **Fellow:** Neurological Radiology, Peter Bent Brigham Hosp 1974; **Fac Appt:** Prof Rad, Univ Wisc

Kallmes, David F MD [NRad] - **Spec Exp:** Aneurysm-Cerebral; Stroke; Osteoporosis Spine-Vertebroplasty; **Hospital:** Mayo Med Ctr & Clin - Rochester; **Address:** Mayo Clinic, Old Marion Hall, 200 First St SW, Rochester, MN 55905; **Phone:** 507-255-5032; **Board Cert:** Diagnostic Radiology 1994; Neuroradiology 1998; **Med School:** Univ Mass Sch Med 1989; **Resid:** Diagnostic Radiology, Duke Univ Med Ctr 1993; **Fellow:** Neuroradiology, Univ Virginia Med Ctr 1995; **Fac Appt:** Assoc Prof, Mayo Med Sch

Koeller, Kelly K MD [NRad] - **Spec Exp:** Brain Tumor Imaging; Head & Neck Tumors; Spinal Tumor Imaging; **Hospital:** Mayo Med Ctr & Clin - Rochester; **Address:** Mayo Clinic, 200 First St SW Charlton Bldg - rm 2-290, Rochester, MN 55905; **Phone:** 507-266-3412; **Board Cert:** Diagnostic Radiology 1990; Neuroradiology 2004; **Med School:** Univ Tenn Coll Med, Memphis 1982; **Resid:** Diagnostic Radiology, Naval Hosp 1990; **Fellow:** Neuroradiology, UCSF Med Ctr 1992

Masaryk, Thomas MD [NRad] - **Spec Exp:** Cerebrovascular Disease; Aneurysm-Cerebral; Vascular Lesions of the CNS; Carotid Artery Stent Placement; **Hospital:** Cleveland Clin Fdn (page 57); **Address:** Cleveland Clinic, Dept Radiology, 9500 Euclid Ave, MC L10, Cleveland, OH 44195; **Phone:** 216-444-6653; **Board Cert:** Diagnostic Radiology 1985; Neuroradiology 2005; **Med School:** Med Coll OH 1981; **Resid:** Diagnostic Radiology, Cleveland Clinic 1984; **Fellow:** Neurological Radiology, Cleveland Clinic 1985

Modic, Michael MD [NRad] - **Spec Exp:** MRI; Spinal Imaging; **Hospital:** Cleveland Clin Fdn (page 57); **Address:** 9500 Euclid Ave, Desk P34, Cleveland, OH 44195; **Phone:** 216-444-9308; **Board Cert:** Diagnostic Radiology 1979; Neuroradiology 2003; **Med School:** Case West Res Univ 1975; **Resid:** Diagnostic Radiology, Cleveland Clinic 1978; **Fellow:** Neuroradiology, Cleveland Clinic 1979; **Fac Appt:** Prof, Ohio State Univ

Moran, Christopher J MD [NRad] - **Spec Exp:** Aneurysm-Cerebral; Cerebrovascular Disease/Stroke; Carotid Artery Stent Placement; Interventional Neuroradiology; **Hospital:** Barnes-Jewish Hosp; **Address:** Wash Univ Sch Med, Campus Box 8131, 510 S Kings Highway Blvd, St Louis, MO 63110; **Phone:** 314-362-5949; **Board Cert:** Diagnostic Radiology 1978; Neuroradiology 2004; **Med School:** St Louis Univ 1974; **Resid:** Diagnostic Radiology, Mallinckrodt Inst Rad/Wash U 1978; **Fellow:** Neuroradiology, Mallinckrodt Inst Rad/Wash U 1979; **Fac Appt:** Prof, Washington Univ, St Louis

Mukherji, Suresh K MD [NRad] - **Spec Exp:** Head & Neck Imaging; Head & Neck Tumors Imaging; **Hospital:** Univ Michigan Hlth Sys; **Address:** Univ of Michigan-Dept Radiology, 1500 E Medical Ctr Drive, A209B, Ann Arbor, MI 48109-0030; **Phone:** 734-936-8865; **Board Cert:** Diagnostic Radiology 1992; **Med School:** Georgetown Univ 1987; **Resid:** Diagnostic Radiology, Brigham & Women's Hosp 1992; **Fellow:** Neuroradiology, Univ of Florida 1994; **Fac Appt:** Prof Oto, Univ Mich Med Sch

Rowley, Howard A MD [NRad] - **Spec Exp:** Epilepsy; Cerebrovascular Disease/Stroke; **Hospital:** Univ WI Hosp & Clins; **Address:** Univ WI Hosp & Clins, Dept Rad, 600 Highland Ave, MC 3252, Madison, WI 53792; **Phone:** 608-263-9179; **Board Cert:** Neurology 1991; Diagnostic Radiology 1993; Neuroradiology 1997; **Med School:** Washington Univ, St Louis 1985; **Resid:** Neurology, UCSF Med Ctr 1989; Diagnostic Radiology, UCSF Med Ctr 1991; **Fellow:** Neurological Radiology, UCSF Med Ctr; **Fac Appt:** Prof, Univ Wisc

Great Plains and Mountains

Osborn, Anne G MD [NRad] - **Spec Exp:** Spinal Imaging; Brain Imaging; Head & Neck Radiology; **Hospital:** Univ Utah Hosps and Clins; **Address:** Univ Utah Med Ctr, Dept Radiology, 30 N 1900 E, rm 1A71, Salt Lake City, UT 84132-2140; **Phone:** 801-581-7553; **Board Cert:** Diagnostic Radiology 1974; Neuroradiology 2004; **Med School:** Stanford Univ 1970; **Resid:** Diagnostic Radiology, Stanford Univ Hosp 1974; **Fellow:** Diagnostic Radiology, Univ Utah Hosp 1977; **Fac Appt:** Prof, Univ Utah

Southwest

Hunter, Jill V MD [NRad] - **Spec Exp:** Pediatric Neuroradiology; Brain Injury-Pediatric; **Hospital:** Texas Chldns Hosp - Houston; **Address:** 6621 Fannin, West Twr, Ste B120, MC 2-2521, Houston, TX 77030; **Phone:** 832-824-5324; **Board Cert:** Diagnostic Radiology 1997; Neuroradiology 1998; **Med School:** England 1975; **Resid:** Diagnostic Radiology, Baylor Coll Med 1978; **Fellow:** Neuroradiology, Queen Square Hosp 1992; **Fac Appt:** Assoc Prof Rad, Baylor Coll Med

Mawad, Michel E MD [NRad] - **Spec Exp:** Interventional Neuroradiology; **Hospital:** St Luke's Episcopal Hosp - Houston; **Address:** Baylor Coll Med, Dept Rad, 1 Baylor Plaza, rm 165-B, Houston, TX 77030; **Phone:** 713-798-2200; **Board Cert:** Diagnostic Radiology 1980; Neuroradiology 1995; **Med School:** Lebanon 1976; **Resid:** Diagnostic Radiology, St Luke's-Roosevelt Hosp 1979; **Fellow:** Neurological Radiology, Columbia-Presby Med Ctr 1980; **Fac Appt:** Prof, Baylor Coll Med

West Coast and Pacific

Atlas, Scott W MD [NRad] - **Spec Exp:** Stroke; MRI; Brain Tumors; **Hospital:** Stanford Univ Med Ctr; **Address:** Stanford Univ Med Ctr, Dept Rad, 300 Pasteur Drive, rm S-047, Stanford, CA 94304-2204; **Phone:** 650-498-7152; **Board Cert:** Diagnostic Radiology 1985; Neuroradiology 2005; **Med School:** Univ Chicago-Pritzker Sch Med 1981; **Resid:** Diagnostic Radiology, Northwestern Univ Med Ctr 1985; **Fellow:** Neuroradiology, Hosp U Penn 1987; **Fac Appt:** Prof, Stanford Univ

Barkovich, A James MD [NRad] - **Spec Exp:** Pediatric Neuroradiology; MRI; Brain Development Abnormalities; **Hospital:** UCSF Med Ctr; **Address:** UCSF Med Ctr, Dept Neuroradiology, 505 Parnassus Ave, rm L361, Box 0628, San Francisco, CA 94143-0628; **Phone:** 415-353-1655; **Board Cert:** Diagnostic Radiology 1984; Neuroradiology 1996; **Med School:** Geo Wash Univ 1980; **Resid:** Diagnostic Radiology, Letterman AMC 1984; **Fellow:** Neuroradiology, Walter Reed AMC 1986; **Fac Appt:** Prof Rad, UCSF

Barnes, Patrick D MD [NRad] - **Spec Exp:** Pediatric Neuroradiology; Brain Injury-Pediatric; Brain Development Abnormalities; Fetal Neuroradiology; **Hospital:** Lucile Packard Chldns Hosp/Stanford Univ Med Ctr; **Address:** Lucile Packard Chldns Hosp, Pediatric Neuroradiology, 725 Welch Rd, Palo Alto, CA 94304; **Phone:** 650-497-8376; **Board Cert:** Diagnostic Radiology 1977; **Med School:** Univ Okla Coll Med 1973; **Resid:** Diagnostic Radiology, Univ Okla Coll Med 1976; **Fellow:** Pediatric Neuroradiology, Chldns Hosp/Harvard Med Sch 1977; **Fac Appt:** Assoc Prof, Stanford Univ

Dillon, William P MD [NRad] - **Spec Exp:** Brain Tumors; **Hospital:** UCSF Med Ctr; **Address:** 505 Parnassus Ave, rm L 371, San Francisco, CA 94143-0628; **Phone:** 415-353-1668; **Board Cert:** Diagnostic Radiology 1982; Neuroradiology 1996; **Med School:** Loyola Univ-Stritch Sch Med 1978; **Resid:** Diagnostic Radiology, Univ Utah Hosp 1982; **Fellow:** Neuroradiology, UCSF Med Ctr 1983; **Fac Appt:** Prof, UCSF

Neuroradiology

Higashida, Randall T MD [NRad] - **Spec Exp:** Aneurysm-Cerebral; Stroke; Intracranial Angioplasty & Stent; **Hospital:** UCSF Med Ctr; **Address:** UCSF Med Ctr, Dept Interven Neurorad, 505 Parnassus Ave, rm L352, San Francisco, CA 94143-0628; **Phone:** 415-353-1863; **Board Cert:** Diagnostic Radiology 1984; **Med School:** Tulane Univ 1980; **Resid:** Diagnostic Radiology, UCLA Med Ctr 1984; **Fellow:** Neuroradiology, UCLA Med Ctr 1985; **Fac Appt:** Clin Prof, UCSF

Norman, David MD [NRad] - **Hospital:** UCSF Med Ctr; **Address:** UCSF Med Ctr, Dept Rad, 505 Parnassus Ave, rm L358, Box 0628, San Francisco, CA 94143-0628; **Phone:** 415-353-1668; **Board Cert:** Diagnostic Radiology 1972; **Med School:** Univ Pennsylvania 1967; **Resid:** Diagnostic Radiology, Columbia-Presby Hosp 1971; **Fellow:** Neuroradiology, UCSF Med Ctr 1975; **Fac Appt:** Prof, UCSF

Teitelbaum, George P MD [NRad] - **Spec Exp:** Interventional Neuroradiology; Aneurysm-Cerebral; Carotid Artery Stent Placement; **Hospital:** USC Univ Hosp - R K Eamer Med Plz; **Address:** USC Healthcare Consultation Center II, 1520 San Pablo St, Ste 3800, Los Angeles, CA 90033; **Phone:** 626-351-3369; **Board Cert:** Diagnostic Radiology 1984; **Med School:** UCSD 1980; **Resid:** Diagnostic Radiology, UC Irvine Med Ctr 1984; Interventional Radiology, George Washington 1985; **Fellow:** Magnetic Resonance Imaging, Huntington Med Research Inst 1988; UCSF Med Ctr 1994; **Fac Appt:** Prof NS, USC Sch Med

Vinuela, Fernando MD [NRad] - **Spec Exp:** Stroke; Intracranial Angioplasty & Stent; Aneurysm-Cerebral; **Hospital:** UCLA Med Ctr; **Address:** UCLA Med Ctr, Dept Rad, 10833 Le Conte Ave, Box 951721, Los Angeles, CA 90095-1721; **Phone:** 310-825-6576; **Board Cert:** Diagnostic Radiology 1979; **Med School:** Uruguay 1970; **Resid:** Diagnostic Radiology, Westminster Hosp 1975; Diagnostic Radiology, Victoria Hosp 1977; **Fellow:** Neuroradiology, Univ Hosp 1979; **Fac Appt:** Prof, UCLA

Vascular & Interventional Radiology

New England

Hallisey, Michael J MD [VIR] - **Spec Exp:** Uterine Fibroid Embolization; Liver Cancer/Chemoembolization; **Hospital:** Hartford Hosp; **Address:** 85 Seymour St, Ste 200, Hartford, CT 06106; **Phone:** 860-246-6589; **Board Cert:** Diagnostic Radiology 1991; Vascular & Interventional Radiology 1998; **Med School:** Univ Conn 1987; **Resid:** Diagnostic Radiology, Hospital of St Raphael 1991

Kandarpa, Krishna MD/PhD [VIR] - **Spec Exp:** Thrombolytic Therapy; **Hospital:** UMass Meml - Univ Campus; **Address:** UMASS, Dept Radiology, 55 Lake Ave N, rm S2824, Worcester, MA 01655; **Phone:** 508-856-3253; **Board Cert:** Diagnostic Radiology 1984; **Med School:** Univ Miami Sch Med 1980; **Resid:** Diagnostic Radiology, Brigham & Women's-Harvard 1984; **Fellow:** Vascular & Interventional Radiology, Brigham & Women's-Harvard 1986; **Fac Appt:** Prof, Univ Mass Sch Med

Murphy, Timothy P MD [VIR] - **Spec Exp:** Uterine Fibroid Embolization; Aneurysm-Aortic; Hypertension-Renovascular; **Hospital:** Rhode Island Hosp; **Address:** Rhode Island Hospital, Dept Radiology, 593 Eddy Street, Providence, RI 02903-4970; **Phone:** 401-444-5194; **Board Cert:** Diagnostic Radiology 1992; Vascular & Interventional Radiology 2005; **Med School:** Boston Univ 1987; **Resid:** Diagnostic Radiology, Rhode Island Hosp 1992; Vascular & Interventional Radiology, Rhode Island Hosp 1993; **Fac Appt:** Asst Clin Prof, Brown Univ

White, Robert I MD [VIR] - **Spec Exp:** Uterine Fibroid Embolization; Pelvic Congestion Syndrome; Varicocele Embolization; Vascular Malformations; **Hospital:** Yale - New Haven Hosp; **Address:** Yale Univ Sch Med, Vasc & Interventional Rad, PO Box 208042, New Haven, CT 06520-8042; **Phone:** 203-737-5395; **Board Cert:** Diagnostic Radiology 1970; Vascular & Interventional Radiology 1994; **Med School:** Baylor Coll Med 1963; **Resid:** Diagnostic Radiology, Johns Hopkins Hosp 1969; **Fellow:** Cardiovascular Disease, Johns Hopkins Hospital 1958; Cardiovascular Radiology, Univ Minn Medical Ctr 1971; **Fac Appt:** Prof Rad, Yale Univ

Mid Atlantic

Geschwind, Jean Francois H MD [VIR] - **Spec Exp:** Liver Cancer/Chemoembolization; Cancer Chemoembolization; Cancer Radiotherapy; **Hospital:** Johns Hopkins Hosp - Baltimore (page 61); **Address:** Interventional Radiology, 600 N Wolfe St Blalock Bldg - rm 545, Baltimore, MD 21287; **Phone:** 410-955-6358; **Board Cert:** Diagnostic Radiology 1998; **Med School:** Boston Univ 1991; **Resid:** Diagnostic Radiology, UCSF Med Ctr 1996; **Fellow:** Interventional Radiology, Johns Hopkins Hosp 1998; **Fac Appt:** Assoc Prof DR, Johns Hopkins Univ

Haskal, Ziv MD [VIR] - **Spec Exp:** Uterine Fibroid Embolization; Vascular Malformations; Liver Cancer/Chemoembolization; **Hospital:** NY-Presby Hosp/Columbia (page 66); **Address:** Director, Div Interventional Radiology, 177 Fort Washington Ave, Ste MHB 4-100, New York, NY 10032; **Phone:** 212-305-8070; **Board Cert:** Diagnostic Radiology 1991; Vascular & Interventional Radiology 1999; **Med School:** Boston Univ 1986; **Resid:** Diagnostic Radiology, UCSF Med Ctr 1991; **Fellow:** Vascular & Interventional Radiology, UCSF Med Ctr 1992; **Fac Appt:** Prof Rad, Columbia P&S

McLean, Gordon K MD [VIR] - **Spec Exp:** Uterine Fibroid Embolization; **Hospital:** Western Penn Hosp; **Address:** Western Pennsylvania Hosp, Dept Radiology, 4800 Friendship Ave, Pittsburgh, PA 15224-1722; **Phone:** 412-578-1787; **Board Cert:** Diagnostic Radiology 1979; Vascular & Interventional Radiology 2005; **Med School:** Dartmouth Med Sch 1975; **Resid:** Diagnostic Radiology, Hosp Univ Penn 1979; **Fellow:** Angiography, Hosp Univ Penn 1980; **Fac Appt:** Prof, Univ Pennsylvania

Shlansky-Goldberg, Richard MD [VIR] - **Spec Exp:** Uterine Fibroid Embolization; Varicocele Embolization; Pelvic Congestion Syndrome; **Hospital:** Hosp Univ Penn - UPHS (page 72); **Address:** Hosp U Penn, Dept Radiology, 3400 Spruce St, 1 Silverstein Bldg, Philadelphia, PA 19104; **Phone:** 215-615-3541; **Board Cert:** Diagnostic Radiology 1989; Vascular & Interventional Radiology 1997; **Med School:** Univ Rochester 1984; **Resid:** Diagnostic Radiology, Thomas Jefferson Univ Hosp 1988; **Fac Appt:** Assoc Prof Rad, Univ Pennsylvania

Soulen, Michael C MD [VIR] - **Spec Exp:** Liver Cancer/Chemoembolization; Kidney Cancer; Radiofrequency Tumor Ablation; **Hospital:** Hosp Univ Penn - UPHS (page 72); **Address:** Hosp U Penn, Interventional Radiology, 3400 Spruce St, Philadelphia, PA 19104; **Phone:** 215-662-6839; **Board Cert:** Diagnostic Radiology 1989; Vascular & Interventional Radiology 1995; **Med School:** Univ Pennsylvania 1984; **Resid:** Diagnostic Radiology, Johns Hopkins Med Inst 1989; **Fellow:** Vascular & Interventional Radiology, Thomas Jefferson Univ Hosp 1991; **Fac Appt:** Prof Rad, Univ Pennsylvania

Vascular & Interventional Radiology

Trerotola, Scott O MD [VIR] - **Spec Exp:** Uterine Fibroid Embolization; Hereditary Hemorrhagic Telangiectasia; Varicocele Embolization; **Hospital:** Hosp Univ Penn - UPHS (page 72), Penn Presby Med Ctr - UPHS (page 72); **Address:** Hosp Univ Penn, Div Interventional Rad, 3400 Spruce St, 1 Silverstein, Philadelphia, PA 19104; **Phone:** 215-615-3540; **Board Cert:** Diagnostic Radiology 1991; Vascular & Interventional Radiology 2005; **Med School:** Univ Pennsylvania 1986; **Resid:** Diagnostic Radiology, Johns Hopkins Hosp 1991; **Fellow:** Vascular & Interventional Radiology, Johns Hopkins Hosp 1992; **Fac Appt:** Prof Rad, Univ Pennsylvania

Wood, Bradford J MD [VIR] - **Spec Exp:** Radiofrequency Tumor Ablation; Liver Cancer; Kidney Cancer; Gene Therapy Delivery Systems; **Hospital:** Natl Inst of Hlth - Clin Ctr; **Address:** National Inst Health, Bldg D, 9000 Rockville Pike, rm 1C-660, Bethesda, MD 20892; **Phone:** 301-594-4511; **Board Cert:** Diagnostic Radiology 1996; Vascular & Interventional Radiology 2000; **Med School:** Univ VA Sch Med 1991; **Resid:** Diagnostic Radiology, Georgetown Univ Med Ctr 1996; **Fellow:** Abdominal/Interventional Radiology, Mass General Hosp 1997; **Fac Appt:** Asst Clin Prof, Georgetown Univ

Southeast

Benenati, James F MD [VIR] - **Spec Exp:** Uterine Fibroid Embolization; Aneurysm-Abdominal Aortic; Peripheral Vascular Disease; **Hospital:** Baptist Hosp of Miami; **Address:** 8900 N Kendall Drive Fl 3, MC BCBI, Miami, FL 33176; **Phone:** 305-598-5990; **Board Cert:** Diagnostic Radiology 1988; Vascular & Interventional Radiology 2005; **Med School:** Univ S Fla Coll Med 1984; **Resid:** Diagnostic Radiology, Indiana Univ Hosp 1988; **Fellow:** Vascular & Interventional Radiology, Johns Hopkins Hosp 1989; **Fac Appt:** Prof Rad, Univ S Fla Coll Med

Bettmann, Michael A MD [VIR] - **Spec Exp:** Uterine Fibroid Embolization; Chemoembolization & Tumor Ablation; Carotid Artery Stent Placement; **Hospital:** Wake Forest Univ Baptist Med Ctr (page 73), Davis Reg Med Ctr; **Address:** Wake Forest Univ Sch Md - Radiology, Medical Center Blvd, Winston-Salem, NC 27157; **Phone:** 336-716-2463; **Board Cert:** Diagnostic Radiology 1975; Vascular & Interventional Radiology 2005; **Med School:** Albert Einstein Coll Med 1969; **Resid:** Diagnostic Radiology, Beth Israel Med Ctr-Harvard 1975; **Fellow:** Cardiovascular Radiology, Peter Bent Brigham Hosp-Harvard 1977; **Fac Appt:** Prof Rad, Wake Forest Univ

Dake, Michael David MD [VIR] - **Spec Exp:** Aortic Stent Grafts; Endovascular Stent Grafts; Vascular Disease; Aneurysm; **Hospital:** Univ Virginia Med Ctr; **Address:** Univ of VA Med Ctr, Dept Rad, Lee St, rm 1076, Box 800170, Charlottesville, VA 22908; **Phone:** 434-982-0211; **Board Cert:** Internal Medicine 1981; Pulmonary Disease 1986; Diagnostic Radiology 1986; Vascular & Interventional Radiology 2006; **Med School:** Baylor Coll Med 1978; **Resid:** Internal Medicine, Baylor Hosp 1982; Diagnostic Radiology, UCSF Med Ctr 1986; **Fellow:** Pulmonary Disease, UCSF Med Ctr 1983; Interventional Radiology, UCSF Med Ctr 1987; **Fac Appt:** Assoc Prof, Stanford Univ

Hawkins Jr, Irvin MD [VIR] - **Hospital:** Shands Hlthcre at Univ of FL; **Address:** Shands at Univ of Florida, 1600 SW Archer Rd, Box 100374, Gainesville, FL 32610; **Phone:** 352-265-0116; **Board Cert:** Diagnostic Radiology 1969; **Med School:** Univ MD Sch Med 1962; **Resid:** Diagnostic Radiology, Ohio State Univ 1968; **Fellow:** Cardiovascular Radiology, Shands Tchg Hosps 1970; **Fac Appt:** Prof, Univ Fla Coll Med

Katzen, Barry T MD [VIR] - **Spec Exp:** Peripheral Vascular Disease; Aneurysm-Aortic; Carotid Artery Disease; **Hospital:** Baptist Hosp of Miami; **Address:** Baptist Cardiac & Vascular Inst, 8900 N Kendall Drive, Miami, FL 33176-2118; **Phone:** 786-596-5990; **Board Cert:** Diagnostic Radiology 1974; Vascular & Interventional Radiology 2004; **Med School:** Univ Miami Sch Med 1970; **Resid:** Diagnostic Radiology, New York Hosp-Cornell Med Ctr 1974

Lewis, Curtis A MD [VIR] - **Hospital:** Grady Hlth Sys, Emory Univ Hosp; **Address:** Grady Meml Hosp, Dept Rad, 56 Butler St SE, PO Box 26010, Atlanta, GA 30335; **Phone:** 404-616-6753; **Board Cert:** Diagnostic Radiology 1991; **Med School:** Emory Univ 1986; **Resid:** Diagnostic Radiology, Emory Univ Affil Hosps 1991; **Fellow:** Interventional Radiology, Emory Univ Affil Hosps 1992; **Fac Appt:** Asst Prof Rad, Emory Univ

Mauro, Matthew MD [VIR] - **Spec Exp:** Cancer Chemoembolization; Cancer Radiotherapy; Gastrointestinal Cancer; **Hospital:** Univ NC Hosps; **Address:** University NC Hosps, Dept Radiology, CB 7510, 2006 Old Clinic Bldg, Chapel Hill, NC 27514; **Phone:** 919-966-4400; **Board Cert:** Diagnostic Radiology 1981; Vascular & Interventional Radiology 2003; **Med School:** Cornell Univ-Weill Med Coll 1977; **Resid:** Diagnostic Radiology, Univ NC Hosps 1981; **Fellow:** Interventional Radiology, Mallinckrodt Inst 1982; **Fac Appt:** Prof, Univ NC Sch Med

Midwest

Cho, Kyung J MD [VIR] - **Spec Exp:** Chemoembolization & Tumor Ablation; Vascular Malformations; Peripheral Vascular Disease; **Hospital:** Univ Michigan Hlth Sys; **Address:** Univ Michigan Med Ctr, Dept Radiology, 1500 E Med Ctr Drive, Rm BID 530, Box 0030, Ann Arbor, MI 48109; **Phone:** 734-936-4466; **Board Cert:** Diagnostic Radiology 1974; Vascular & Interventional Radiology 2005; **Med School:** Korea 1966; **Resid:** Diagnostic Radiology, Wayne Med Ctr 1973; **Fellow:** Cardiovascular Radiology, Univ Michigan 1975; **Fac Appt:** Prof, Univ Mich Med Sch

Cragg, Andrew H MD [VIR] - **Spec Exp:** Uterine Fibroid Embolization; Aortic Stent Grafts; Endovascular Stent Grafts; **Hospital:** Univ Minn Med Ctr, Fairview - Riverside Campus, Fairview Southdale Hosp; **Address:** Minneapolis Vascular Clinic, 6405 France Ave S, Ste W440, Edina, MN 55435; **Phone:** 952-345-4179; **Board Cert:** Diagnostic Radiology 1986; Vascular & Interventional Radiology 1990; **Med School:** Univ Minn 1982; **Resid:** Diagnostic Radiology, Univ Minn Hosp 1986; **Fellow:** Interventional Radiology, Univ Minn Hosp 1987; **Fac Appt:** Prof, Univ Minn

Darcy, Michael MD [VIR] - **Spec Exp:** Portal Hypertension; Chemoembolization & Tumor Ablation; **Hospital:** Barnes-Jewish Hosp; **Address:** Washington Univ, Mallinckrodt Inst Radiology, 510 S Kingshighway Blvd, St Louis, MO 63110; **Phone:** 314-362-2900; **Board Cert:** Diagnostic Radiology 1985; Vascular & Interventional Radiology 2004; **Med School:** Ohio State Univ 1979; **Resid:** Surgery, Univ Minn Hosps 1982; Diagnostic Radiology, Univ Minn Hosps 1985; **Fellow:** Interventional Radiology, Univ Minn Hosps 1987; **Fac Appt:** Prof, Washington Univ, St Louis

Hovsepian, David M MD [VIR] - **Spec Exp:** Uterine Fibroid Embolization; Aneurysm-Aortic; Vascular Malformations-Pediatric; **Hospital:** Barnes-Jewish Hosp; **Address:** Mallinckrodt Inst Radiology, 510 S Kings Highway Blvd, Box 8131, Saint Louis, MO 63110; **Phone:** 314-362-2900; **Board Cert:** Diagnostic Radiology 1991; Vascular & Interventional Radiology 2006; **Med School:** Columbia P&S 1986; **Resid:** Diagnostic Radiology, Columbia Presby Hosp 1991; **Fellow:** Interventional Radiology, Thomas Jefferson Univ Med Ctr 1993; **Fac Appt:** Assoc Prof, Washington Univ, St Louis

Vascular & Interventional Radiology

Johnson, Matthew S MD [VIR] - **Spec Exp:** Vascular Disease; Uterine Fibroid Embolization; **Hospital:** Indiana Univ Hosp; **Address:** Indiana U Hospital, 550 N University Blvd, rm 0279, Indianapolis, IN 46202-5253; **Phone:** 317-278-7785; **Board Cert:** Diagnostic Radiology 1992; Vascular & Interventional Radiology 2005; **Med School:** Univ Mich Med Sch 1986; **Resid:** Surgery, Loyola Univ 1988; Diagnostic Radiology, Loyola Univ 1992; **Fellow:** Interventional Radiology, Johns Hopkins 1994; **Fac Appt:** Assoc Prof, Indiana Univ

Ketcham, Douglas B MD [VIR] - **Spec Exp:** Uterine Fibroid Embolization; Varicocele Embolization; Osteoporosis Spine-Vertebroplasty; **Hospital:** United Hosp, Regions Hosp - St Paul; **Address:** United Hospital, Dept Radiology, 333 N Smith Ave, St Paul, MN 55102; **Phone:** 651-241-8404; **Board Cert:** Diagnostic Radiology 1972; Vascular & Interventional Radiology 1995; **Med School:** Univ Wisc 1965; **Resid:** Diagnostic Radiology, Univ Minn Hosp 1971; **Fellow:** Neuroradiology, Univ Minn Hosp 1972

Nemcek, Albert MD [VIR] - **Spec Exp:** Uterine Fibroid Embolization; Vascular Disease; **Hospital:** Northwestern Meml Hosp; **Address:** Northwestern Meml Hosp, 676 N St Clair St, Ste 800, Chicago, IL 60611; **Phone:** 312-926-5302; **Board Cert:** Diagnostic Radiology 1986; Vascular & Interventional Radiology 2005; **Med School:** UCSD 1982; **Resid:** Diagnostic Radiology, UCSD Med Ctr 1986; **Fellow:** Interventional Radiology, Northwestern Meml Hosp 1987; **Fac Appt:** Assoc Prof, Northwestern Univ

Rilling, William S MD [VIR] - **Spec Exp:** Liver Cancer/Chemoembolization; Arteriovenous Malformations; Uterine Fibroid Embolization; **Hospital:** Froedtert Meml Lutheran Hosp; **Address:** Froedtert & Med Coll Clinics, Interventional Radiology, 9200 W Wisconsin Ave, Milwaukee, WI 53226; **Phone:** 414-805-3028; **Board Cert:** Diagnostic Radiology 1995; Vascular & Interventional Radiology 1997; **Med School:** Univ Wisc 1990; **Resid:** Diagnostic Radiology, Univ Wisc Affil Hosps 1995; **Fellow:** Vascular & Interventional Radiology, Northwestern Meml Hosp 1996; **Fac Appt:** Assoc Prof DR, Univ Wisc

Salem, Riad MD [VIR] - **Spec Exp:** Cancer Radiotherapy; Cancer Chemoembolization; Liver Cancer/Chemoembolization; **Hospital:** Northwestern Meml Hosp; **Address:** Northwestern Univ Med Sch - Dept Radiology, 676 N St Clair St, Ste 800, Chicago, IL 60611; **Phone:** 312-695-0517; **Board Cert:** Diagnostic Radiology 1997; Vascular & Interventional Radiology 1999; **Med School:** McGill Univ 1993; **Resid:** Diagnostic Radiology, Geo Washington Univ Hosp 1997; **Fellow:** Interventional Radiology, Childrens Hosp 1998; Interventional Radiology, Hosp Univ Penn 1998; **Fac Appt:** Asst Prof, Northwestern Univ

Smith, Steven J MD [VIR] - **Spec Exp:** Angioplasty-Peripheral; Uterine Fibroid Embolization; Varicocele Embolization; **Hospital:** La Grange Meml Hosp; **Address:** LaGrange Meml Hosp, Dept Radiology, 5101 S Willow Springs Rd, La Grange, IL 60525; **Phone:** 708-352-1200 x4562; **Board Cert:** Diagnostic Radiology 1983; **Med School:** Wayne State Univ 1979; **Resid:** Diagnostic Radiology, Henry Ford Hosp 1983; **Fellow:** Vascular & Interventional Radiology, Northwestern Univ 1984; **Fac Appt:** Assoc Clin Prof Rad, Northwestern Univ

Vogelzang, Robert MD [VIR] - **Spec Exp:** Uterine Fibroid Embolization; Varicocele Embolization; Vascular Malformations; **Hospital:** Northwestern Meml Hosp; **Address:** Northwestern Meml Hosp, Dept Rad, 676 N St Clair St, Ste 800, Chicago, IL 60611; **Phone:** 312-926-5113; **Board Cert:** Diagnostic Radiology 1981; Vascular & Interventional Radiology 2005; **Med School:** Ros Franklin Univ/Chicago Med Sch 1977; **Resid:** Diagnostic Radiology, Northwestern Meml Hosp 1982; **Fellow:** Interventional Radiology, Northwestern Meml Hosp; **Fac Appt:** Prof, Northwestern Univ

Great Plains and Mountains

Durham, Janette D MD [VIR] - **Spec Exp:** Uterine Fibroid Embolization; Peripheral Vascular Disease; **Hospital:** Univ Colorado Hosp; **Address:** Univ Hosp, Dept Radiology, 4200 E Ninth Ave, Box A030, Denver, CO 80262; **Phone:** 303-372-6141; **Board Cert:** Diagnostic Radiology 1987; Vascular & Interventional Radiology 1996; **Med School:** Indiana Univ 1983; **Resid:** Diagnostic Radiology, Indiana Univ Hosp 1987; **Fellow:** Vascular & Interventional Radiology, Mass General Hosp 1988; **Fac Appt:** Assoc Prof, Univ Colorado

Kumpe, David A MD [VIR] - **Spec Exp:** Aneurysm-Cerebral; Stroke; Arterial & Venous Stents; Interventional Neuroradiology; **Hospital:** Univ Colorado Hosp; **Address:** Univ Hosp, Dept Radiology, 4200 E 9th Ave, Box A030, Denver, CO 80262; **Phone:** 303-372-6141; **Board Cert:** Diagnostic Radiology 1972; Vascular & Interventional Radiology 2005; **Med School:** Harvard Med Sch 1967; **Resid:** Diagnostic Radiology, Mass Genl Hosp 1971; **Fellow:** Neurological Radiology, Kantonsspital 1975; Angiography, Kantonsspital 1976; **Fac Appt:** Prof, Univ Colorado

Yakes, Wayne MD [VIR] - **Spec Exp:** Vascular Malformations; Interventional Neuroradiology; **Hospital:** Swedish Med Ctr - Englewood; **Address:** CNI, Vasc Malformation Ctr, 501 E Hampden Ave, Ste 4600, Englewood, CO 80113; **Phone:** 303-788-4280; **Board Cert:** Diagnostic Radiology 1983; Vascular & Interventional Radiology 1998; Neuroradiology 1999; **Med School:** Creighton Univ 1979; **Resid:** Diagnostic Radiology, Fitzsimons Med Ctr 1983; **Fellow:** Angiography, Walter Reed Med Ctr 1984; Interventional Neuroradiology, Baptist Hosp 1992; **Fac Appt:** Clin Prof, Univ Colorado

Southwest

Becker, Gary J MD [VIR] - **Spec Exp:** Endovascular Stent Grafts; Aneurysm-Abdominal & Thoracic Aortic; **Hospital:** Univ Med Ctr - Tucson; **Address:** Arizona Hlth Sciences Ctr, Dept Radiology, 1501 N Campbell Ave, rm 1363, Tucson, AZ 85724; **Phone:** 520-694-8888; **Board Cert:** Diagnostic Radiology 1981; Vascular & Interventional Radiology 2004; **Med School:** Indiana Univ 1977; **Resid:** Diagnostic Radiology, Ind Univ Med Ctr Hosp 1981; **Fac Appt:** Prof, Univ Ariz Coll Med

Kay, Dennis MD [VIR] - **Spec Exp:** Diagnostic Radiology; **Hospital:** Ochsner Fdn Hosp; **Address:** Ochsner Clin, Dept Interventional Radiology, 1514 Jefferson Hwy, New Orleans, LA 70121-2429; **Phone:** 504-842-3470; **Board Cert:** Diagnostic Radiology 1986; Vascular & Interventional Radiology 2004; **Med School:** Tulane Univ 1981; **Resid:** Diagnostic Radiology, Ochsner Fdn Hosp 1985; **Fellow:** Vascular & Interventional Radiology, Beth Israel Hosp 1986; **Fac Appt:** Assoc Clin Prof, Tulane Univ

Rivera, Frank James MD [VIR] - **Hospital:** Harris Methodist Hosp - Fort Worth; **Address:** 1301 Pennsylvania Ave, Fort Worth, TX 76104; **Phone:** 817-250-3566; **Board Cert:** Diagnostic Radiology 1989; Vascular & Interventional Radiology 1998; **Med School:** Univ Tex, San Antonio 1982; **Resid:** Diagnostic Radiology, SUNY Hlth Sci Ctr 1989; **Fellow:** Vascular & Interventional Radiology, SUNY Hlth Sci Ctr 1989; **Fac Appt:** Asst Prof, Univ Tex SW, Dallas

Vascular & Interventional Radiology

West Coast and Pacific

Gomes, Antoinette S MD [VIR] - **Spec Exp:** Cardiovascular Interventional Radiology; **Hospital:** UCLA Med Ctr; **Address:** UCLA Med Ctr, Dept Rad - rmBL-141 CHS, 10833 Le Conte Ave, Los Angeles, CA 90095-1721; **Phone:** 310-206-8909; **Board Cert:** Diagnostic Radiology 1975; Vascular & Interventional Radiology 2004; **Med School:** Med Coll PA Hahnemann 1969; **Resid:** Internal Medicine, LAC-USC MC 1972; Diagnostic Radiology, Stanford Univ Med Ctr 1975; **Fellow:** Cardiovascular Radiology, UCLA Med Ctr 1976; Cardiovascular Radiology, Univ Minn 1978; **Fac Appt:** Prof Rad, UCLA

Goodwin, Scott C MD [VIR] - **Spec Exp:** Uterine Fibroid Embolization; Liver Cancer/Chemoembolization; **Hospital:** VA Med Ctr - W Los Angeles; **Address:** VA Hosp-Dept Radiology, 11301 Wilshire Blvd, MC 114, Los Angeles, CA 90073; **Phone:** 310-268-3478; **Board Cert:** Diagnostic Radiology 1989; Vascular & Interventional Radiology 1996; **Med School:** Harvard Med Sch 1984; **Resid:** Diagnostic Radiology, UCLA Medical Ctr 1988; **Fellow:** Vascular & Interventional Radiology, UCLA Medical Ctr 1989; **Fac Appt:** Prof DR, UCLA

Kaufman, John MD [VIR] - **Spec Exp:** Uterine Fibroid Embolization; Angioplasty & Stent Placement; **Hospital:** Dotter Institute - OHSU; **Address:** Dotter Interven Inst-OHSU Hosps & Clins, 3181 SW Sam Jackson Park Rd, MC L 605, Portland, OR 97239; **Phone:** 503-494-7660; **Board Cert:** Diagnostic Radiology 1990; Vascular & Interventional Radiology 2005; **Med School:** Boston Univ 1982; **Resid:** Diagnostic Radiology, Boston Univ Med Ctr 1990; **Fellow:** Vascular & Interventional Radiology, Boston Univ Med Ctr 1991; **Fac Appt:** Prof, Oregon Hlth Sci Univ

Keller, Frederick S MD [VIR] - **Spec Exp:** Uterine Fibroid Embolization; Arterial & Venous Stents; Urinary Tract Interventions; **Hospital:** OR Hlth & Sci Univ; **Address:** Dotter Interventional Inst, L-605, 3181 SW Sam Jackson Park Rd, Portland, OR 97239; **Phone:** 503-494-7660; **Board Cert:** Diagnostic Radiology 1977; Vascular & Interventional Radiology 2003; **Med School:** Univ Pennsylvania 1968; **Resid:** Diagnostic Radiology, Univ Oreg Hlth Scis Ctr 1977; **Fac Appt:** Prof, Oregon Hlth Sci Univ

McGahan, John P MD [VIR] - **Spec Exp:** Radiofrequency Tumor Ablation; Liver Cancer; Kidney Cancer; **Hospital:** UC Davis Med Ctr; **Address:** UC Davis Medical Ctr, Dept Radiology, 4860 Y St, Ste 3100, Sacramento, CA 95817; **Phone:** 916-734-3606; **Board Cert:** Diagnostic Radiology 1979; Vascular & Interventional Radiology 1995; **Med School:** Oregon Hlth Sci Univ 1974; **Resid:** Surgery, UC Davis Med Ctr 1976; Diagnostic Radiology, UC Davis Med Ctr 1979; **Fac Appt:** Prof DR, UC Davis

Miller, Franklin MD [VIR] - **Spec Exp:** Hereditary Hemorrhagic Telangiectasia; Varicocele Embolization; Vascular Malformations; **Hospital:** UCSD Med Ctr; **Address:** 200 W Arbor Drive, San Diego, CA 92103-8756; **Phone:** 619-543-7965; **Board Cert:** Diagnostic Radiology 1973; **Med School:** Temple Univ 1966; **Resid:** Diagnostic Radiology, Johns Hopkins Hosp 1972; **Fellow:** Vascular & Interventional Radiology, Johns Hopkins Hosp 1973; **Fac Appt:** Prof, UCSD

Valji, Karim MD [VIR] - **Spec Exp:** Dialysis Access; **Hospital:** UCSD Med Ctr; **Address:** UCSD Med Ctr, 200 W Arbor Drive, San Diego, CA 92103-8756; **Phone:** 619-543-6607; **Board Cert:** Diagnostic Radiology 1989; Vascular & Interventional Radiology 1998; **Med School:** Harvard Med Sch 1982; **Resid:** Internal Medicine, UCSF Med Ctr 1984; Diagnostic Radiology, UCSD Med Ctr 1988; **Fellow:** Angiography, UCSD Med Ctr 1989; **Fac Appt:** Prof, Univ SD Sch Med

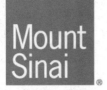

Mount Sinai offers patients one of the world's most comprehensive and sophisticated arrays of diagnostic and interventional radiology. Our imaging system is now based on filmless, digital technology that spans magnetic resonance imaging (MRI), multi-slice computed tomography (CT), positron emission tomography CT (PET-CT), single photon tomography CT (SPECT-CT), advanced ultrasound, and digital mammography. The Department of Radiology is utilizing state-of-the-art Picture Archiving Communication System (PACS) technology.

COMPREHENSIVE DIAGNOSTIC SERVICES

Mount Sinai offers the entire range of diagnostic radiology services, in a patient-friendly environment for the diagnosis of degenerative, infectious, vascular, neoplastic, genetic, traumatic, and toxic metabolic disorders of the brain, spine, bones and joints, heart, lungs, abdomen, pelvis, breast, and blood vessels.

EARLY DETECTION PROGRAMS

With funding from the Sharp Foundation, we are developing special screening approaches for early disease detection. Radiological screenings for colon cancer and Alzheimer's disease are joining those already in place for breast and lung cancer, and atherosclerosis. The early detection programs use a variety of imaging techniques (e.g., CT and MRI for atherosclerosis, CT for colon cancer, PET for oncology, and digital mammography, MRI, and computer-aided diagnosis for breast cancer).

MINIMALLY INVASIVE PROCEDURES

Radiology at Mount Sinai has moved beyond diagnosis to therapeutic intervention. Interventional radiologists at Mount Sinai perform biopsies, vascular therapies, uterine artery embolization for fibroids (an alternative to hysterectomy), as well as treatments for aneurysms, atherosclerosis, and some types of cancer.

Developing New Diagnostic Tools

Radiology at Mount Sinai is an active center of imaging research and development. Mount Sinai physicians and scientists developed a special form of MRI to non-invasively diagnose heart disease and atherosclerosis and thereby identify patients at greatest risk for stroke and heart attack.

We actively collaborate with other disciplines to develop and refine imaging tools that will make prevention, diagnosis, and prognosis increasingly effective. That is the case, for example, in neuroscience, where the work encompasses neurodegenerative conditions such as Parkinson's disease, as well as multiple sclerosis, stroke and brain tumors; and cardiovascular disease, where studies are underway for the peripheral, renal, abdominal, pulmonary, and coronary arteries; and liver disease, where Radiology and the transplant team work closely together.

617

NYU Medical Center

550 First Avenue (at 31st Street)
New York, NY 10016
Physician Referral:
(888)7-NYU-MED (888-769-8633)
www.nyumc.org

Radiology:
The Diagnostic Core of Modern Medicine

LEADING EDGE TECHNOLOGY

The Department of Radiology at NYU Medical Center is at the forefront of academic medicine and has some of the most advanced imaging equipment in the world, including:

-Dual source, dual energy multi-detector 64 slice CT
-Coronary Artery Disease and Virtual Colonoscopy screening programs
-Multi-channel MRI technology including two advanced state-of-the-art multi-channel 1.5 Tesla clinical scanners, two clinical/research 3--Tesla scanners and one 7-Tesla research scanner
-Advanced breast MR imaging
-High resolution / high sensitivity PET-CT
-Digital radiography
-Digital fluoroscopy
-Digital mammography
-Sterotactic biopsy capability
-Advanced digital subtraction angiography with 3D capability
-Minimally invasive techniques including radiofrequency ablation and chemoembolization
-State-of-the-art SPECT CT and SPECT gamma cameras
-Radioimmunotherapy
-Bone densitometry
-Cutting edge Medical Imaging Informatics and Radiology Information Systems

ON THE HORIZON

NYU Radiology is a leader in clinical care, research and education. Among Radiology Departments within Medical Schools, NYU is the 10th largest recipient of NIH research funding in the U.S. and first in New York.

Reproductive Endocrinology
a subspecialty of Obstetrics & Gynecology

An obstetrician/gynecologist who is capable of managing complex problems relating to reproductive endocrinology and infertility.

Training Required: Four years *plus* two years in clinical practice before certification in obstetrics and gynecology is complete *plus* additional training and examination in reproductive endocrinology.

Reproductive Endocrinology

New England

Carson, Sandra A MD [RE] - **Spec Exp:** Infertility-IVF; Laparoscopic Surgery; Endometriosis; Sexual Dysfunction; **Hospital:** Women & Infants Hosp - Rhode Island; **Address:** 101 Dudley St Fl 1, Providence, RI 02905; **Phone:** 401-274-1122; **Board Cert:** Obstetrics & Gynecology 2004; Reproductive Endocrinology 2004; **Med School:** Northwestern Univ 1977; **Resid:** Obstetrics & Gynecology, Prentice Womens Hosp. 1981; **Fellow:** Reproductive Endocrinology, Michael Reese Hosp. 1983; **Fac Appt:** Prof ObG, Baylor Coll Med

Crowley, William F MD [RE] - **Spec Exp:** Pituitary Disorders; Kallmann's Syndrome; Fertility Preservation in Cancer; **Hospital:** Mass Genl Hosp; **Address:** Mass Genl Hosp, Reproductive Science Ctr, 55 Fruit St, Bartlett Hall-Extension 5, Boston, MA 02114; **Phone:** 617-726-5390; **Board Cert:** Internal Medicine 1974; Endocrinology 1977; **Med School:** Tufts Univ 1969; **Resid:** Internal Medicine, Mass Genl Hosp 1971; Internal Medicine, Mass Genl Hosp 1974; **Fellow:** Endocrinology, Mass Genl Hosp 1976; **Fac Appt:** Prof Med, Harvard Med Sch

Hill III, Joseph A MD [RE] - **Spec Exp:** Miscarriage-Recurrent; Infertility-Female; Gynecology; **Hospital:** Portsmouth Regl Hosp, Winchester Hosp; **Address:** Fertility Ctr of New England, 330 Borthwick Ave, Ste 201, Portsmouth, NH 03801; **Phone:** 781-942-7000 x601; **Board Cert:** Obstetrics & Gynecology 2005; Reproductive Endocrinology 2005; **Med School:** Med Coll GA 1981; **Resid:** Obstetrics & Gynecology, Med Coll Ga 1985; **Fellow:** Reproductive Endocrinology, Brigham-Womens Hosp/Harvard 1987; Reproductive Immunology, Brigham-Womens Hosp/Harvard 1988; **Fac Appt:** Prof ObG, Harvard Med Sch

Isaacson, Keith B MD [RE] - **Spec Exp:** Infertility; Endometriosis; Minimally Invasive Surgery; **Hospital:** Newton - Wellesley Hosp, Mass Genl Hosp; **Address:** 2014 Washington St Fl 2 West, Newton, MA 02462; **Phone:** 617-243-5205; **Board Cert:** Obstetrics & Gynecology 2001; Reproductive Endocrinology 2001; **Med School:** Med Coll GA 1983; **Resid:** Obstetrics & Gynecology, Ochsner Fdn Hosp 1987; **Fellow:** Reproductive Endocrinology, Hosp Univ Penn 1989; **Fac Appt:** Assoc Prof ObG, Harvard Med Sch

Luciano, Anthony A MD [RE] - **Spec Exp:** Infertility; Endometriosis; Menopause Problems; Osteoporosis; **Hospital:** Hosp Central CT, Hartford Hosp; **Address:** 100 Grand St, Ste E3, New Britain, CT 06050; **Phone:** 860-224-5467; **Board Cert:** Obstetrics & Gynecology 1980; Reproductive Endocrinology 1981; **Med School:** Univ Conn 1973; **Resid:** Obstetrics & Gynecology, Univ Connecticut Hosp 1977; **Fellow:** Reproductive Endocrinology, Univ Connecticut Hosp 1979; **Fac Appt:** Prof ObG, Univ Conn

Manganiello, Paul D MD [RE] - **Spec Exp:** Infertility; Menopause Problems; **Hospital:** Dartmouth - Hitchcock Med Ctr; **Address:** Dartmouth-Hitchcock Med Ctr, Dept Ob/Gyn, One Medical Center Drive, Lebanon, NH 03756; **Phone:** 603-653-9240; **Board Cert:** Obstetrics & Gynecology 1980; Reproductive Endocrinology 1984; **Med School:** Jefferson Med Coll 1973; **Resid:** Obstetrics & Gynecology, Thomas Jefferson Univ Hosp 1977; **Fellow:** Reproductive Endocrinology, Med Coll Ga Hosp 1979; **Fac Appt:** Assoc Prof ObG, Dartmouth Med Sch

Patrizio, Pasquale MD [RE] - **Spec Exp:** Infertility-IVF; Fertility Preservation in Cancer; **Hospital:** Yale - New Haven Hosp; **Address:** Yale Fertility Ctr, Dept OB/GYN, 150 Sargent Drive, New Haven, CT 06511; **Phone:** 203-785-4708; **Board Cert:** Obstetrics & Gynecology 1997; Reproductive Endocrinology 1999; **Med School:** Italy 1983; **Resid:** Obstetrics & Gynecology, Univ Naples 1987; Reproductive Endocrinology, Univ Pisa 1990; **Fellow:** Infertility, UC Irvine 1995; **Fac Appt:** Prof ObG, Yale Univ

Schiff, Isaac MD [RE] - **Spec Exp:** Menopause Problems; Infertility-Female; **Hospital:** Mass Genl Hosp; **Address:** Mass Genl Hosp, Dept Ob/Gyn, 55 Fruit St, VBK 113, Boston, MA 02114; **Phone:** 617-726-3001; **Board Cert:** Obstetrics & Gynecology 1999; Reproductive Endocrinology 1999; **Med School:** McGill Univ 1968; **Resid:** Obstetrics & Gynecology, Boston Hosp Women 1973; Surgery, New England Med Ctr 1974; **Fellow:** Reproductive Endocrinology, Boston Hosp Women 1976; **Fac Appt:** Prof ObG, Harvard Med Sch

Mid Atlantic

Berkeley, Alan S MD [RE] - **Spec Exp:** Infertility-IVF; Reproductive Surgery; Uterine Fibroids; **Hospital:** NYU Med Ctr (page 67); **Address:** NYU Fertility Ctr, 660 First Ave, Fl 5, New York, NY 10016-3295; **Phone:** 212-263-7629; **Board Cert:** Obstetrics & Gynecology 1980; **Med School:** NY Med Coll 1973; **Resid:** Obstetrics & Gynecology, Yale-New Haven Hosp 1977; **Fellow:** Gynecologic Oncology, Yale-New Haven Hosp 1979; Infertility, Yale-New Haven Hosp 1979; **Fac Appt:** Prof ObG, NYU Sch Med

Bieber, Eric J MD [RE] - **Spec Exp:** Uterine Fibroids; Infertility; Endometriosis; **Hospital:** Geisinger-Wyoming Med Ctr (page 59), Geisinger Med Ctr (page 59); **Address:** 1000 E Mountain Drive, MC 34-66, Wilkes-Barre, PA 18711; **Phone:** 570-826-7893; **Board Cert:** Obstetrics & Gynecology 2005; Reproductive Endocrinology 2005; **Med School:** Loyola Univ-Stritch Sch Med 1986; **Resid:** Obstetrics & Gynecology, Rush Presby-St Lukes Med Ctr 1990; **Fellow:** Reproductive Endocrinology, Univ Chicago 1993

Copperman, Alan B MD [RE] - **Spec Exp:** Infertility-IVF; Endometriosis; Laparoscopic Surgery; Hysteroscopic Surgery; **Hospital:** Mount Sinai Med Ctr; **Address:** 635 Madison Ave Fl 10, New York, NY 10022; **Phone:** 212-756-5777; **Board Cert:** Obstetrics & Gynecology 1996; Reproductive Endocrinology 1999; **Med School:** NY Med Coll 1989; **Resid:** Obstetrics & Gynecology, Yale-New Haven Hosp 1993; **Fellow:** Reproductive Endocrinology, Mount Sinai Med Ctr 1995; **Fac Appt:** Assoc Clin Prof ObG, Mount Sinai Sch Med

Coutifaris, Christos MD/PhD [RE] - **Spec Exp:** Infertility-IVF; Fertility Preservation in Cancer; Polycystic Ovarian Syndrome; **Hospital:** Hosp Univ Penn - UPHS (page 72); **Address:** 3701 Market St Fl 8 - Ste 800, Philadelphia, PA 19104; **Phone:** 215-662-6100; **Board Cert:** Obstetrics & Gynecology 1998; Reproductive Endocrinology 1998; **Med School:** Univ Pennsylvania 1982; **Resid:** Obstetrics & Gynecology, Hosp Univ Penn 1986; **Fellow:** Reproductive Endocrinology, Univ Penn 1987; **Fac Appt:** Prof ObG, Univ Pennsylvania

Damewood, Marian D MD [RE] - **Spec Exp:** Infertility-IVF; **Hospital:** York Hosp, Hosp Univ Penn - UPHS (page 72); **Address:** York Hosp, Ob/Gyn Div, 1001 S George St, York, PA 17403; **Phone:** 717-851-2349; **Board Cert:** Obstetrics & Gynecology 1985; Reproductive Endocrinology 1987; **Med School:** Johns Hopkins Univ 1978; **Resid:** Obstetrics & Gynecology, Johns Hopkins Med Ctr 1982; **Fellow:** Reproductive Endocrinology, Johns Hopkins Med Ctr 1984; **Fac Appt:** Clin Prof ObG, Univ Pennsylvania

Grifo, James A MD/PhD [RE] - **Spec Exp:** Infertility-IVF; Prenatal Genetic Diagnosis; **Hospital:** NYU Med Ctr (page 67), Bellevue Hosp Ctr; **Address:** 660 1st Ave Fl 5, New York, NY 10016; **Phone:** 212-263-7978; **Board Cert:** Obstetrics & Gynecology 2005; Reproductive Endocrinology 2005; **Med School:** Case West Res Univ 1984; **Resid:** Obstetrics & Gynecology, NY Hosp-Cornell Med Ctr 1988; **Fellow:** Reproductive Endocrinology, Yale-New Haven Hosp 1990; **Fac Appt:** Prof ObG, NYU Sch Med

Grunfeld, Lawrence MD [RE] - **Spec Exp:** Infertility-IVF; Hysteroscopic Surgery; Laparoscopic Surgery; **Hospital:** Mount Sinai Med Ctr, Lenox Hill Hosp (page 62); **Address:** 635 Madison Ave Fl 10, New York, NY 10022-1009; **Phone:** 212-756-5777; **Board Cert:** Obstetrics & Gynecology 1997; Reproductive Endocrinology 1997; **Med School:** Mount Sinai Sch Med 1979; **Resid:** Obstetrics & Gynecology, Montefiore Med Ctr 1984; **Fellow:** Reproductive Endocrinology, Montefiore Med Ctr 1987; **Fac Appt:** Assoc Clin Prof ObG, Mount Sinai Sch Med

Legro, Richard S MD [RE] - **Spec Exp:** Ovarian Failure; Polycystic Ovarian Syndrome; Infertility-IVF; **Hospital:** Penn State Milton S Hershey Med Ctr; **Address:** Hershey Med Ctr, 500 University Drive, PO Box 850, MC H10, Hershey, PA 17033; **Phone:** 717-531-8478; **Board Cert:** Obstetrics & Gynecology 2003; Reproductive Endocrinology 2003; **Med School:** Mount Sinai Sch Med 1987; **Resid:** Obstetrics & Gynecology, Univ Pittsburgh/Magee Women's Hosp 1991; **Fellow:** Reproductive Endocrinology, USC/Women's Hosp 1993; **Fac Appt:** Prof ObG, Penn State Univ-Hershey Med Ctr

McClamrock, Howard D MD [RE] - **Spec Exp:** Infertility-IVF; Prenatal Genetic Diagnosis; **Hospital:** Univ of MD Med Sys, St Joseph Med Ctr; **Address:** Univ Maryland, Dept OB/GYN, 405 W Redwood St Fl 3, Baltimore, MD 21201; **Phone:** 410-328-2304; **Board Cert:** Obstetrics & Gynecology 1998; Reproductive Endocrinology 1998; **Med School:** Univ NC Sch Med 1981; **Resid:** Obstetrics & Gynecology, Univ Maryland Hosp 1986; **Fellow:** Reproductive Endocrinology, Univ Maryland 1988; **Fac Appt:** Assoc Prof ObG, Univ MD Sch Med

Pfeifer, Samantha MD [RE] - **Spec Exp:** Infertility-Female; Endometriosis; Turner Syndrome; **Hospital:** Hosp Univ Penn - UPHS (page 72); **Address:** Penn Health for Women, 250 King of Prussia Rd, Radnor, PA 19087; **Phone:** 610-902-2500; **Board Cert:** Obstetrics & Gynecology 1994; Reproductive Endocrinology 1997; **Med School:** Univ Pennsylvania 1986; **Resid:** Obstetrics & Gynecology, Hosp Univ Penn 1990; **Fellow:** Reproductive Endocrinology, Hosp Univ Penn 1993; **Fac Appt:** Asst Prof ObG, Univ Pennsylvania

Rosenwaks, Zev MD [RE] - **Spec Exp:** Infertility-IVF; Genetic Disorders; Fertility Preservation in Cancer; **Hospital:** NY-Presby Hosp/Weill Cornell (page 66); **Address:** Ctr For Reproductive Medicine & Infertility, 505 E 70th St, Ste 340, New York, NY 10021-4872; **Phone:** 212-746-1743; **Board Cert:** Obstetrics & Gynecology 1978; Reproductive Endocrinology 1981; **Med School:** SUNY Downstate 1972; **Resid:** Obstetrics & Gynecology, LI Jewish Med Ctr 1976; **Fellow:** Reproductive Endocrinology, Johns Hopkins Hosp 1978; **Fac Appt:** Prof ObG, Cornell Univ-Weill Med Coll

Sanfilippo, Joseph MD [RE] - **Spec Exp:** Adolescent Gynecology; Infertility; Minimally Invasive Surgery; Menopause Problems; **Hospital:** Magee-Womens Hosp - UPMC; **Address:** Ctr for Fertility & Repro Endo-Magee Hosp, 300 Halket St, Ste 2309, Pittsburgh, PA 15213; **Phone:** 412-641-1204; **Board Cert:** Obstetrics & Gynecology 2001; Reproductive Endocrinology 2001; **Med School:** Ros Franklin Univ/Chicago Med Sch 1973; **Resid:** Obstetrics & Gynecology, SUNY Upstate 1977; **Fellow:** Reproductive Endocrinology, Univ of Louisville 1979; **Fac Appt:** Prof ObG, Univ Pittsburgh

Sauer, Mark MD [RE] - **Spec Exp:** Infertility-IVF; **Hospital:** NY-Presby Hosp/Columbia (page 66); **Address:** 1790 Broadway Fl 2, New York, NY 10019; **Phone:** 646-756-8282; **Board Cert:** Obstetrics & Gynecology 1996; Reproductive Endocrinology 1996; **Med School:** Univ IL Coll Med 1980; **Resid:** Obstetrics & Gynecology, Univ Illinois Med Ctr 1984; **Fellow:** Reproductive Endocrinology, Harbor-UCLA Med Ctr 1986; **Fac Appt:** Prof ObG, Columbia P&S

Seifer, David B MD [RE] - **Spec Exp:** Infertility; Infertility-Advanced Maternal Age; Fertility Preservation in Cancer; **Hospital:** Maimonides Med Ctr (page 63); **Address:** 1355 84th St, Brooklyn, NY 11228; **Phone:** 718-283-8600; **Board Cert:** Obstetrics & Gynecology 1998; Reproductive Endocrinology 1998; **Med School:** Univ IL Coll Med 1981; **Resid:** Obstetrics & Gynecology, Stanford Univ Hosp 1985; **Fellow:** Reproductive Endocrinology, Yale-New Haven Hosp 1991; **Fac Appt:** Prof ObG, Mount Sinai Sch Med

Simon, James A MD [RE] - **Spec Exp:** Infertility; Menopause Problems; Osteoporosis; **Hospital:** G Washington Univ Hosp, Sibley Mem Hosp; **Address:** 1850 M St NW, Ste 450, Washington, DC 20036; **Phone:** 202-293-1000; **Board Cert:** Obstetrics & Gynecology 1998; Reproductive Endocrinology 1998; **Med School:** Rush Med Coll 1978; **Resid:** Obstetrics & Gynecology, George Washington Univ Hosp 1982; **Fellow:** Reproductive Endocrinology, Harbor-UCLA Medical Ctr 1985; **Fac Appt:** Clin Prof ObG, Geo Wash Univ

Sondheimer, Steven MD [RE] - **Spec Exp:** Infertility; **Hospital:** Hosp Univ Penn - UPHS (page 72); **Address:** Penn Fertility Care, 3701 Market St, Ste 800, Philadelphia, PA 19104; **Phone:** 215-662-6100; **Board Cert:** Obstetrics & Gynecology 1994; Reproductive Endocrinology 1982; **Med School:** Univ Pennsylvania 1974; **Resid:** Obstetrics & Gynecology, Hosp Univ Penn 1978; **Fellow:** Endocrinology, Hosp Univ Penn 1980; **Fac Appt:** Prof ObG, Univ Pennsylvania

Wallach, Edward E MD [RE] - **Spec Exp:** Uterine Fibroids; Infertility-IVF; **Hospital:** Johns Hopkins Hosp - Baltimore (page 61); **Address:** Johns Hopkins at Greenspring Station, 2330 W Joppa Rd, Ste 301, Lutherville, MD 21093; **Phone:** 410-583-2751; **Board Cert:** Obstetrics & Gynecology 1979; Reproductive Endocrinology 1975; **Med School:** Cornell Univ-Weill Med Coll 1958; **Resid:** Obstetrics & Gynecology, Kings Co Hosp 1963; **Fellow:** Reproductive Endocrinology, Worcester Fdn Exper Biol 1962; **Fac Appt:** Prof ObG, Johns Hopkins Univ

Weiss, Gerson MD [RE] - **Spec Exp:** Infertility; Menopause Problems; **Hospital:** Hackensack Univ Med Ctr, UMDNJ-Univ Hosp-Newark; **Address:** 214 Terrace Ave, Hasbrouck Heights, NJ 07604-1815; **Phone:** 201-288-6330; **Board Cert:** Obstetrics & Gynecology 1993; Reproductive Endocrinology 1974; **Med School:** NYU Sch Med 1964; **Resid:** Obstetrics & Gynecology, Bellevue Hosp Ctr 1969; **Fellow:** Reproductive Endocrinology, Univ Pittsburgh 1973; **Fac Appt:** Prof ObG, UMDNJ-NJ Med Sch, Newark

Zacur, Howard A MD/PhD [RE] - **Spec Exp:** Prolactin Disorders; Uterine Fibroids; Hormonal Disorders; **Hospital:** Johns Hopkins Hosp - Baltimore (page 61); **Address:** Johns Hopkins at Green Spring Station, 10755 Falls Rd, Pavilion 2, Ste 335, Lutherville, MD 21093; **Phone:** 410-616-7140; **Board Cert:** Obstetrics & Gynecology 1994; Reproductive Endocrinology 1984; **Med School:** Univ Miami Sch Med 1973; **Resid:** Obstetrics & Gynecology, Johns Hopkins Hosp 1980; **Fellow:** Reproductive Endocrinology, Johns Hopkins Hosp 1982; **Fac Appt:** Prof ObG, Johns Hopkins Univ

Reproductive Endocrinology

Southeast

Berga, Sarah L MD [RE] - **Spec Exp:** Infertility-IVF; Hormonal Disorders; Menstrual Disorders; **Hospital:** Emory Univ Hosp, Crawford Long Hosp of Emory Univ; **Address:** Dept Gynecology & Obstetrics, 1639 Pierce Drive, rm 4208-WMB, Atlanta, GA 30322; **Phone:** 404-727-8600; **Board Cert:** Obstetrics & Gynecology 1998; Reproductive Endocrinology 1998; **Med School:** Univ VA Sch Med 1980; **Resid:** Obstetrics & Gynecology, Mass Genl Hosp 1984; **Fellow:** Reproductive Endocrinology, UCSD Med Ctr 1986; **Fac Appt:** Prof ObG, Emory Univ

Blackwell, Richard MD/PhD [RE] - **Spec Exp:** Infertility-Female; Reproductive Medicine; Women's Health; **Hospital:** Univ of Ala Hosp at Birmingham, St Vincent's Hosp - Birmingham; **Address:** 618 S 20th St, Birmingham, AL 35294; **Phone:** 205-934-6090; **Board Cert:** Obstetrics & Gynecology 1982; Reproductive Endocrinology 1987; **Med School:** Baylor Coll Med 1975; **Resid:** Obstetrics & Gynecology, Univ Alabama Hosp 1979; **Fellow:** Reproductive Endocrinology, Univ Alabama Hosp 1981; Reproductive Endocrinology, The Salk Institute 1982; **Fac Appt:** Prof ObG, Univ Ala

Cowan, Bryan D MD [RE] - **Spec Exp:** Infertility-IVF; **Hospital:** Univ Hosps & Clins - Jackson; **Address:** University Hosp & Clinics, Dept Ob/Gyn, 2500 N State St, Jackson, MS 39216; **Phone:** 601-984-5300; **Board Cert:** Obstetrics & Gynecology 2005; Reproductive Endocrinology 2005; **Med School:** Univ Colorado 1975; **Resid:** Obstetrics & Gynecology, Portsmouth Naval Hosp 1979; **Fellow:** Reproductive Endocrinology, WRAH/NIH 1981; **Fac Appt:** Prof ObG, Univ Miss

DeVane, Gary W MD [RE] - **Spec Exp:** Infertility-IVF; Miscarriage-Recurrent; Endometriosis; **Hospital:** Florida Hosp - Orlando, Arnold Palmer Hosp for Chldn; **Address:** 3435 Pinehurst Ave, Orlando, FL 32804-4049; **Phone:** 407-740-0909; **Board Cert:** Obstetrics & Gynecology 1977; Reproductive Endocrinology 1982; **Med School:** Baylor Coll Med 1971; **Resid:** Obstetrics & Gynecology, UCSD Hosp 1975; **Fellow:** Reproductive Endocrinology, Univ Texas SW Hosp 1980

Fritz, Marc A MD [RE] - **Spec Exp:** Infertility; Menopause Problems; Menstrual Disorders; **Hospital:** Univ NC Hosps; **Address:** Univ NC Sch Med, Dept Ob/Gyn, CB 7570, 4001 Old Clinic, Chapel Hill, NC 27599-7570; **Phone:** 919-966-5283; **Board Cert:** Obstetrics & Gynecology 1996; Reproductive Endocrinology 1996; **Med School:** Tulane Univ 1977; **Resid:** Obstetrics & Gynecology, Wright State Univ 1981; **Fellow:** Reproductive Endocrinology, Oregon Hlth Sci Univ 1983; **Fac Appt:** Prof ObG, Univ NC Sch Med

Goodman, Neil MD [RE] - **Spec Exp:** Polycystic Ovarian Syndrome; Hormonal Disorders; Infertility; **Hospital:** Baptist Hosp of Miami, South Miami Hosp; **Address:** 9150 SW 87th Ave, Ste 210, Miami, FL 33176-2313; **Phone:** 305-595-6855; **Board Cert:** Internal Medicine 1973; Endocrinology, Diabetes & Metabolism 1975; **Med School:** Columbia P&S 1970; **Resid:** Internal Medicine, Beth Israel Hosp 1972; **Fellow:** Endocrinology, Mass Genl Hosp 1974; **Fac Appt:** Clin Prof Med, Univ Miami Sch Med

Hammond, Charles B MD [RE] - **Spec Exp:** Menopause Problems; Trophoblastic Disease; **Hospital:** Duke Univ Med Ctr; **Address:** Duke Univ Med Ctr, Box 3853, Durham, NC 27710-0001; **Phone:** 919-684-3008; **Board Cert:** Obstetrics & Gynecology 1972; Reproductive Endocrinology 1974; **Med School:** Duke Univ 1961; **Resid:** Obstetrics & Gynecology, Duke Med Ctr 1968; Obstetrics & Gynecology, Duke Med Ctr 1963; **Fellow:** Gynecology, Duke Med Ctr 1964; Reproductive Endocrinology, Natl Inst Hlth 1966; **Fac Appt:** Prof ObG, Duke Univ

Keefe, David Lawrence MD [RE] - **Spec Exp:** Infertility-IVF; Reproduction in Advanced Maternal Age; **Hospital:** Univ of S FL - Tampa; **Address:** 4 Columbia Drive, Ste 529, Tampa, FL 33606; **Phone:** 813-259-8500; **Board Cert:** Obstetrics & Gynecology 1993; Reproductive Endocrinology 1995; **Med School:** Georgetown Univ 1980; **Resid:** Psychiatry, Harvard Psych Srv/Camb Hosp 1983; Obstetrics & Gynecology, Yale New Haven Hosp 1989; **Fellow:** Psychiatry, Univ Chicago Hosp & Clins 1985; Reproductive Endocrinology, Yale New Haven Hosp 1991; **Fac Appt:** Prof ObG, Univ S Fla Coll Med

Murphy, Ana A MD [RE] - **Spec Exp:** Infertility; Endometriosis; Pelvic Surgery; **Hospital:** Med Coll of GA Hosp and Clin; **Address:** Med Coll Ga - Dept Ob/Gyn, BA-7313, 1120 15th St, Agusta, GA 30912; **Phone:** 706-722-4434; **Board Cert:** Obstetrics & Gynecology 2004; Reproductive Endocrinology 2004; **Med School:** Univ Mich Med Sch 1980; **Resid:** Obstetrics & Gynecology, Johns Hopkins Univ 1984; **Fellow:** Reproductive Endocrinology, Johns Hopkins Univ 1986; **Fac Appt:** Prof ObG, Med Coll GA

Ory, Steven MD [RE] - **Spec Exp:** Infertility; Hormonal Disorders; Endometriosis; **Hospital:** Northwest Med Ctr, Meml Regl Hosp - Hollywood; **Address:** 2960 N State Road 7, Ste 300, Margate, FL 33063-5737; **Phone:** 954-247-6200; **Board Cert:** Obstetrics & Gynecology 2005; Reproductive Endocrinology 2005; **Med School:** Baylor Coll Med 1976; **Resid:** Obstetrics & Gynecology, Mayo Clinic 1980; **Fellow:** Reproductive Endocrinology, Duke Univ 1982; **Fac Appt:** Assoc Clin Prof ObG, Univ Miami Sch Med

Rock, John A MD [RE] - **Spec Exp:** Infertility-Female; Endometriosis; Vaginal/Uterine Abnormalities; Pelvic Reconstruction; **Address:** Florida Intl Univ, Univ Park, HLS 2 69, 11200 SW 8th St, Miami, FL 33146; **Phone:** 305-348-0283; **Board Cert:** Obstetrics & Gynecology 2005; Reproductive Endocrinology 2005; **Med School:** Louisiana State Univ 1972; **Resid:** Obstetrics & Gynecology, Duke Univ Med Ctr 1976; **Fellow:** Reproductive Endocrinology, Johns Hopkins Hosp 1978

Session, Donna R MD [RE] - **Spec Exp:** Ultrasound Guided Surgery; Infertility-Female; **Hospital:** Emory Univ Hosp; **Address:** Emory Reproductive Endocrinology, 550 Peachtree St, Ste 1800 MOT, Atlanta, GA 30308; **Phone:** 404-778-3401; **Board Cert:** Obstetrics & Gynecology 2004; Reproductive Endocrinology 2004; **Med School:** Eastern VA Med Sch 1986; **Resid:** Obstetrics & Gynecology, Winthrop Hosp 1990; **Fellow:** Reproductive Endocrinology, Columbia Presby Med Ctr 1993

Steinkampf, Michael MD [RE] - **Spec Exp:** Infertility; **Hospital:** Brookwood Med Ctr, St Vincent Med Ctr; **Address:** 2700 Highway 280, Ste 370 East, East Birmingham, AL 35223; **Phone:** 205-874-0000; **Board Cert:** Obstetrics & Gynecology 1997; Reproductive Endocrinology 1997; **Med School:** Louisiana State Univ 1981; **Resid:** Obstetrics & Gynecology, Parkland Meml Hosp 1985; **Fellow:** Reproductive Endocrinology, Univ Texas SW Med Ctr 1987; **Fac Appt:** Prof ObG, Univ Ala

Walmer, David K MD/PhD [RE] - **Spec Exp:** Infertility; Miscarriage-Recurrent; DES-Exposed Females; Endometriosis; **Hospital:** Duke Univ Med Ctr; **Address:** 6704 Fayetteville Rd, Durham, NC 27713; **Phone:** 919-572-4673; **Board Cert:** Obstetrics & Gynecology 2004; Reproductive Endocrinology 2004; **Med School:** Univ NC Sch Med 1982; **Resid:** Obstetrics & Gynecology, Univ Texas Health Sci Ctr 1987; **Fellow:** Reproductive Endocrinology, Duke Univ Med Ctr 1989; **Fac Appt:** Assoc Prof ObG, Duke Univ

Reproductive Endocrinology

Midwest

Barnes, Randall B MD [RE] - **Spec Exp:** Infertility-IVF; Polycystic Ovarian Syndrome; Miscarriage-Recurrent; **Hospital:** Northwestern Meml Hosp; **Address:** 675 N St Clair St, Ste 14-200, Chicago, IL 60611; **Phone:** 312-695-7269; **Board Cert:** Obstetrics & Gynecology 1994; **Med School:** Johns Hopkins Univ 1979; **Resid:** Obstetrics & Gynecology, LAC-USC Med Ctr 1983; **Fellow:** Reproductive Endocrinology, LAC-USC Med Ctr 1985; **Fac Appt:** Assoc Prof ObG, Northwestern Univ

Christman, Gregory MD [RE] - **Spec Exp:** Infertility-IVF; Uterine Fibroids; **Hospital:** Univ Michigan Hlth Sys; **Address:** Univ Mich, Med Science Bldg I, 1301 Catherine St, rm 6428, Box 0617, Ann Arbor, MI 48109-0617; **Phone:** 734-763-4323; **Board Cert:** Obstetrics & Gynecology 2002; Reproductive Endocrinology 2002; **Med School:** Univ Wisc 1983; **Resid:** Obstetrics & Gynecology, Univ Wisconsin Med Sch 1987; **Fellow:** Reproductive Endocrinology, Univ North Carolina 1992; **Fac Appt:** Assoc Prof ObG, Univ Mich Med Sch

Diamond, Michael P MD [RE] - **Spec Exp:** Infertility-IVF; Infertility-Female; Polycystic Ovarian Syndrome; **Hospital:** Hutzel Hosp - Detroit, Harper Univ Hosp; **Address:** Univ Ctr for Women's Medicine, 26400 W 12 Mile Rd, Southfield, MI 48034; **Phone:** 248-352-8200; **Board Cert:** Obstetrics & Gynecology 1997; Reproductive Endocrinology 1997; **Med School:** Vanderbilt Univ 1981; **Resid:** Obstetrics & Gynecology, Vanderbilt Univ Med Ctr 1985; Reproductive Endocrinology, Yale-New Haven Hosp 1987; **Fac Appt:** Prof ObG, Wayne State Univ

Dodds, William G MD [RE] - **Spec Exp:** Infertility; Endometriosis; Infertility-IVF; **Hospital:** Spectrum Hlth Butterworth Campus, Bronson Meth Hosp; **Address:** 630 Kenmore Ave SE, Ste 100, Grand Rapids, MI 49546-8826; **Phone:** 616-988-2229; **Board Cert:** Obstetrics & Gynecology 2003; Reproductive Endocrinology 2003; **Med School:** Ohio State Univ 1982; **Resid:** Obstetrics & Gynecology, Ohio State Univ Med Ctr 1986; **Fellow:** Reproductive Endocrinology, Ohio State Univ 1988; **Fac Appt:** Assoc Prof ObG, Univ Mich Med Sch

Dumesic, Daniel Anthony MD [RE] - **Spec Exp:** Infertility-Female; Hormonal Disorders; Endometriosis; **Address:** Reproductive Med & Infertility Assocs, 2101 Woodwinds Drive, Ste 100, Woodbury, MN 55125; **Phone:** 651-222-6050; **Board Cert:** Obstetrics & Gynecology 1995; Reproductive Endocrinology 1995; **Med School:** Univ Wisc 1978; **Resid:** Obstetrics & Gynecology, UCSF Med Ctr 1982; **Fellow:** Reproductive Endocrinology, UCSF Med Ctr 1987

Falcone, Tommaso MD [RE] - **Spec Exp:** Minimally Invasive Surgery; Infertility; **Hospital:** Cleveland Clin Fdn (page 57); **Address:** Cleveland Clin, Dept Ob/Gyn, 9500 Euclid Ave, Desk A81, Cleveland, OH 44195-0001; **Phone:** 216-444-1758; **Board Cert:** Obstetrics & Gynecology 1998; Reproductive Endocrinology 1998; **Med School:** McGill Univ 1981; **Resid:** Obstetrics & Gynecology, McGill Univ 1986; **Fellow:** Reproductive Endocrinology, McGill Univ 1989

Haney, Arthur F MD [RE] - **Spec Exp:** Infertility-Female; DES-Exposed Females; **Hospital:** Univ of Chicago Hosps; **Address:** 5841 S Maryland Ave, MC 2050, Chicago, IL 60637; **Phone:** 773-702-6127; **Board Cert:** Obstetrics & Gynecology 2003; Reproductive Endocrinology 2003; **Med School:** Univ Ariz Coll Med 1972; **Resid:** Obstetrics & Gynecology, Duke Univ Med Ctr 1976; **Fellow:** Reproductive Endocrinology, Duke Univ Med Ctr 1978; **Fac Appt:** Prof ObG, Univ Chicago-Pritzker Sch Med

Jacobs, Laurence A MD [RE] - **Spec Exp:** Infertility-IVF; Polycystic Ovarian Syndrome; Endometriosis; **Hospital:** Adv Luth Genl Hosp, Northwest Comm Hosp; **Address:** 135 N Arlington Hts Rd, Ste 195, Buffalo Grove, IL 60089; **Phone:** 847-215-8899; **Board Cert:** Obstetrics & Gynecology 1981; **Med School:** Northwestern Univ 1975; **Resid:** Obstetrics & Gynecology, Northwestern Meml Hosp 1979; **Fellow:** Reproductive Endocrinology, Mayo Clinic 1988

Kazer, Ralph MD [RE] - **Spec Exp:** Polycystic Ovarian Syndrome; Infertility-IVF; **Hospital:** Northwestern Meml Hosp; **Address:** 675 N St Clair St Fl 14 - Ste 200, Chicago, IL 60611; **Phone:** 312-695-7269; **Board Cert:** Obstetrics & Gynecology 1996; Reproductive Endocrinology 1996; **Med School:** Tufts Univ 1979; **Resid:** Obstetrics & Gynecology, Tufts Univ Med Ctr 1983; **Fellow:** Reproductive Endocrinology, UC San Diego 1986; **Fac Appt:** Assoc Prof ObG, Northwestern Univ

Milad, Magdy P MD [RE] - **Spec Exp:** Reproductive Surgery; Infertility; Uterine Fibroids; **Hospital:** Northwestern Meml Hosp, Children's Mem Hosp; **Address:** Northwestern Med Fac Fdn, 675 North St Clair, Fl 14 - Ste 200, Chicago, IL 60611-5975; **Phone:** 312-695-7269; **Board Cert:** Obstetrics & Gynecology 1994; Reproductive Endocrinology 1996; **Med School:** Wayne State Univ 1987; **Resid:** Obstetrics & Gynecology, William Beaumont Hosp 1991; **Fellow:** Reproductive Endocrinology, Mayo Clinic 1993; **Fac Appt:** Prof ObG, Northwestern Univ

Molo, Mary Wood MD [RE] - **Spec Exp:** Infertility-IVF; Uterine Fibroids; Fertility Preservation in Cancer; **Hospital:** Rush Univ Med Ctr; **Address:** 1725 W Harrison St, 408E, Chicago, IL 60612; **Phone:** 312-997-2229; **Board Cert:** Obstetrics & Gynecology 2004; Reproductive Endocrinology 2004; **Med School:** Southern IL Univ 1982; **Resid:** Obstetrics & Gynecology, Southern Illinois Affil Hosps 1984; Obstetrics & Gynecology, Rush Presby St Lukes Hosp 1987; **Fellow:** Reproductive Endocrinology, Rush Presby St Lukes Hosp 1989; **Fac Appt:** Asst Prof ObG, Rush Med Coll

Nagel, Theodore C MD [RE] - **Spec Exp:** Infertility-IVF; Hysteroscopic Surgery; Vaginal/Uterine Abnormalities; Laparoscopic Surgery; **Hospital:** Univ Minn Med Ctr, Fairview - Riverside Campus; **Address:** Reproductive Med Ctr, Univ Minnesota, 606 24th Ave S, Ste 500, Minnneapolis, MN 55454; **Phone:** 612-627-4564; **Board Cert:** Internal Medicine 1970; Endocrinology 1975; Obstetrics & Gynecology 1981; Reproductive Endocrinology 1983; **Med School:** Cornell Univ-Weill Med Coll 1963; **Resid:** Internal Medicine, Bellevue Hosp Ctr 1968; Obstetrics & Gynecology, Univ Minn Hosps 1977; **Fellow:** Endocrinology, Diabetes & Metabolism, Northwestern Univ Med Sch 1972; Reproductive Endocrinology, Univ Minnesota 1980; **Fac Appt:** Assoc Clin Prof ObG, Univ Minn

Odem, Randall R MD [RE] - **Spec Exp:** Infertility; Reproductive Surgery; Miscarriage-Recurrent; **Hospital:** Barnes-Jewish Hosp; **Address:** 4444 Forest Park Ave, Ste 3100, St Louis, MO 63108-2212; **Phone:** 314-286-2421; **Board Cert:** Obstetrics & Gynecology 1996; Reproductive Endocrinology 1996; **Med School:** Univ Iowa Coll Med 1981; **Resid:** Obstetrics & Gynecology, Univ Illinois Hosps 1985; **Fellow:** Reproductive Endocrinology, Wash Univ Sch Med 1987; **Fac Appt:** Prof ObG, Washington Univ, St Louis

Ratts, Valerie S MD [RE] - **Spec Exp:** Polycystic Ovarian Syndrome; Uterine Fibroids; **Hospital:** Barnes-Jewish Hosp; **Address:** Washington Univ, Ctr for Reproductive Endo/Infertility, 4444 Forest Park Ave, Ste 3100, St Louis, MO 63110; **Phone:** 314-286-2400; **Board Cert:** Obstetrics & Gynecology 1995; Reproductive Endocrinology 1997; **Med School:** Johns Hopkins Univ 1987; **Resid:** Obstetrics & Gynecology, Johns Hopkins Hosp 1991; **Fellow:** Reproductive Endocrinology, Johns Hopkins Hosp 1993; **Fac Appt:** Asst Prof ObG, Washington Univ, St Louis

Reproductive Endocrinology

Smith, Yolanda MD [RE] - **Spec Exp:** Infertility; **Hospital:** Univ Michigan Hlth Sys; **Address:** Women's Hospital, 1500 E Med Ctr Drive, rm L4000, Box 0276, Ann Arbor, MI 48109-0276; **Phone:** 734-763-4323; **Board Cert:** Obstetrics & Gynecology 2005; Reproductive Endocrinology 2005; **Med School:** Wake Forest Univ 1989; **Resid:** Obstetrics & Gynecology, Univ Mich Hosp 1993; **Fellow:** Reproductive Endocrinology, Johns Hopkins Hosp 1995; **Fac Appt:** Assoc Prof ObG, Univ Mich Med Sch

Zinaman, Michael J MD [RE] - **Spec Exp:** Endometriosis; Infertility; Uterine Fibroids; **Hospital:** Loyola Univ Med Ctr, Elmhurst Meml Hosp; **Address:** Loyola Univ Med Ctr, Dept ObGyn, 2160 S First Ave Bldg 103 - Ste 1030, Maywood, IL 60153; **Phone:** 708-216-8563; **Board Cert:** Obstetrics & Gynecology 1996; Reproductive Endocrinology 1996; **Med School:** SUNY Downstate 1981; **Resid:** Obstetrics & Gynecology, Univ Chicago Hosps 1985; **Fellow:** Reproductive Endocrinology, Georgetown Univ 1987; **Fac Appt:** Prof ObG, Loyola Univ-Stritch Sch Med

Great Plains and Mountains

Richardson, Marilyn MD [RE] - **Spec Exp:** Menopause Problems; Infertility; Polycystic Ovarian Syndrome; **Hospital:** Univ of Kansas Hosp; **Address:** 12616 W 62nd Terr, Ste 111, Shawnee, KS 66216; **Phone:** 913-631-0277; **Board Cert:** Obstetrics & Gynecology 1995; **Med School:** Univ Kans 1979; **Resid:** Obstetrics & Gynecology, Truman Med Ctr 1983; **Fellow:** Reproductive Endocrinology, Univ Texas Hlth Scis Ctr 1985; **Fac Appt:** Asst Clin Prof ObG, Univ Kans

Schlaff, William D MD [RE] - **Spec Exp:** Infertility; Endometriosis; Vaginal/Uterine Abnormalities; **Hospital:** Univ Colorado Hosp, Rose Med Ctr; **Address:** Univ Colo Hlth Scis Ctr, AOP Bldg, 1635 N Ursula St, rm 3403, Box 6510, MS F701, Aurora, CO 80045; **Phone:** 720-848-1690; **Board Cert:** Obstetrics & Gynecology 1995; Reproductive Endocrinology 1995; **Med School:** Univ Mich Med Sch 1977; **Resid:** Obstetrics & Gynecology, Univ Mich Hosps 1981; **Fellow:** Reproductive Endocrinology, Johns Hopkins Med Ctr 1985; **Fac Appt:** Prof ObG, Univ Colorado

Surrey, Eric S MD [RE] - **Spec Exp:** Infertility-IVF; Endometriosis; **Hospital:** Swedish Med Ctr - Englewood, Sky Ridge Med Ctr; **Address:** 799 E Hamden Ave, Ste 300, Englewood, CO 80110; **Phone:** 303-788-8300; **Board Cert:** Obstetrics & Gynecology 1998; Reproductive Endocrinology 1998; **Med School:** Univ Pennsylvania 1981; **Resid:** Obstetrics & Gynecology, UCLA Med Ctr 1986; **Fellow:** Reproductive Endocrinology, UCLA Med Ctr 1988

Southwest

Schenken, Robert S MD [RE] - **Spec Exp:** Infertility-Female; Endometriosis; **Hospital:** Univ Hlth Sys - Univ Hosp, Baptist Hlth Sys; **Address:** Univ Texas Med Sch, Dept OB/GYN, 7703 Floyd Curl Dr, MSC 7836, San Antonio, TX 78229-3900; **Phone:** 210-567-4950; **Board Cert:** Obstetrics & Gynecology 1995; Reproductive Endocrinology 1995; **Med School:** Baylor Coll Med 1977; **Resid:** Obstetrics & Gynecology, Bexar Co Hosp 1981; **Fellow:** Reproductive Endocrinology, Natl Inst Hlth 1982; Reproductive Endocrinology, Univ Tex Hlth Sci Ctr 1983; **Fac Appt:** Prof ObG, Univ Tex, San Antonio

West Coast and Pacific

Adamson, G David MD [RE] - **Spec Exp:** Infertility-Female; Endometriosis; Infertility-IVF; **Hospital:** Good Samaritan Hosp - San Jose, Stanford Univ Med Ctr; **Address:** 540 University Ave, Ste 200, Palo Alto, CA 94301; **Phone:** 650-322-1900; **Board Cert:** Obstetrics & Gynecology 1980; Reproductive Endocrinology 1982; **Med School:** Univ Toronto 1973; **Resid:** Obstetrics & Gynecology, Toronto Genl Hosp 1977; **Fellow:** Obstetrics & Gynecology, Toronto Genl Hosp 1978; Reproductive Endocrinology, Stanford Univ Hosp 1980; **Fac Appt:** Clin Prof ObG, Stanford Univ

Azziz, Ricardo MD [RE] - **Spec Exp:** Infertility-Female; Reproductive Surgery; Polycystic Ovarian Syndrome; **Hospital:** Cedars-Sinai Med Ctr; **Address:** Cedars Sinai Med Ctr, Dept Ob/Gyn, 8700 Beverly Blvd, Ste 3611, Los Angeles, CA 90048; **Phone:** 310-423-9964; **Board Cert:** Obstetrics & Gynecology 1996; Reproductive Endocrinology 1996; **Med School:** Penn State Univ-Hershey Med Ctr 1981; **Resid:** Obstetrics & Gynecology, Georgetown Univ Hosp 1985; **Fellow:** Reproductive Endocrinology, Johns Hopkins Hosp 1987; **Fac Appt:** Prof ObG, UCLA

Burry, Kenneth Arnold MD [RE] - **Spec Exp:** Infertility-IVF; Menopause Problems; **Hospital:** OR Hlth & Sci Univ; **Address:** 3303 SW Bond Ave Fl 10th, MC CH10F, Portland, OR 97239-4501; **Phone:** 503-418-3700; **Board Cert:** Obstetrics & Gynecology 1977; Reproductive Endocrinology 1981; **Med School:** UC Irvine 1968; **Resid:** Obstetrics & Gynecology, Oreg Hlth Sci Univ & Clinics 1974; **Fellow:** Reproductive Endocrinology, Univ Wash Hosp 1976; **Fac Appt:** Prof ObG, Oregon Hlth Sci Univ

Marrs, Richard P MD [RE] - **Spec Exp:** Infertility-Female; Endometriosis; Uterine Fibroids; **Hospital:** Santa Monica - UCLA Med Ctr; **Address:** 11818 Wilshire Blvd, Ste 300, Los Angeles, CA 90025; **Phone:** 310-828-4008; **Board Cert:** Obstetrics & Gynecology 1980; Reproductive Endocrinology 1983; **Med School:** Univ Tex Med Br, Galveston 1974; **Resid:** Obstetrics & Gynecology, Univ Tex Hosps 1977; **Fellow:** Reproductive Endocrinology, USC Med Ctr 1979

Paulson, Richard John MD [RE] - **Spec Exp:** Infertility-IVF; Women of Advanced Reproductive Age; Infertility-Advanced Maternal Age; **Hospital:** LAC & USC Med Ctr, Good Samaritan Hosp - Los Angeles; **Address:** USC Rep Endocrinology & Infertility, 1127 Wilshire Blvd, Ste 1400, Los Angeles, CA 90017; **Phone:** 213-975-9990; **Board Cert:** Obstetrics & Gynecology 1997; Reproductive Endocrinology 1997; **Med School:** UCLA 1980; **Resid:** Obstetrics & Gynecology, Harbor-UCLA Med Ctr 1984; **Fellow:** Reproductive Endocrinology, LAC-USC Med Ctr 1986; **Fac Appt:** Prof ObG, USC Sch Med

Soules, Michael Roy MD [RE] - **Spec Exp:** Reproductive Medicine; Infertility-Female; **Hospital:** Northwest Hosp; **Address:** 1505 Westlake Ave N, Ste 400, Seattle, WA 98109; **Phone:** 206-301-5000; **Board Cert:** Obstetrics & Gynecology 2002; Reproductive Endocrinology 2002; **Med School:** UCLA 1972; **Resid:** Obstetrics & Gynecology, Univ Colorado Med Ctr 1976; **Fellow:** Reproductive Endocrinology, Duke Univ Hosp 1978; **Fac Appt:** Clin Prof ObG, Univ Wash

Winer, Sharon A MD [RE] - **Spec Exp:** Hormonal Disorders; Infertility-Female; Vaginitis; Gynecology; **Hospital:** Cedars-Sinai Med Ctr, USC Univ Hosp - R K Eamer Med Plz; **Address:** 9400 Brighton Way, Ste 206, Beverly Hills, CA 90210-4709; **Phone:** 310-274-9100; **Board Cert:** Obstetrics & Gynecology 2005; Reproductive Endocrinology 2005; **Med School:** USC Sch Med 1978; **Resid:** Obstetrics & Gynecology, LAC-USC Med Ctr 1982; **Fellow:** Microsurgery, Hammersmith Hosp 1983; Reproductive Endocrinology, LAC-USC Med Ctr 1985; **Fac Appt:** Clin Prof ObG, USC Sch Med

Yee, Billy MD [RE] - **Spec Exp:** Infertility-IVF; **Hospital:** Long Beach Meml Med Ctr, Little Company of Mary Hosp; **Address:** 13950 Milton Ave, Ste 101, Westminster, CA 92683; **Phone:** 714-702-3001; **Board Cert:** Obstetrics & Gynecology 2006; Reproductive Endocrinology 2006; **Med School:** UC Davis 1978; **Resid:** Obstetrics & Gynecology, LAC-USC Med Ctr 1982; **Fellow:** Reproductive Endocrinology, LAC-USC Med Ctr 1985; **Fac Appt:** Assoc Clin Prof ObG, UC Irvine

NYU Medical Center

550 First Avenue (at 31st Street)
New York, NY 10016
Physician Referral:
(888)7-NYU-MED (888-769-8633)
www.nyumc.org

NYU Fertility Center

Today, thanks to promising new options in the treatment of infertility, specialists at NYU Medical Center can help more patients realize their dreams of parenthood. With unique expertise in all aspects of reproductive endocrinology, including the diagnosis and treatment of endometriosis, fibroids, problems with ovulation or sperm function, and recurrent pregnancy loss, NYU Medical Center uses the most advanced technology to assist infertile women and men who wish to conceive children.

From the initial diagnosis through all stages of treatment, couples receive state-of-the-art compassionate care based on their specific needs. After a comprehensive evaluation to determine the cause of infertility, couples are counseled on whether assisted reproduction is necessary. (Often, surgery can correct disorders that lead to infertility, like fibroids or endometriosis. Similarly, stimulation of a woman's ovaries with medication often results in pregnancy.) When the physician and couple agree that assisted reproduction is appropriate, the program offers:

• In Vitro Fertilization and Egg Freezing for fertility preservation

• Donor Oocyte (Egg) and Sperm Services

• Intracytoplasmic Sperm Injection (injection of a single sperm directly into an egg)

• Assisted Hatching (creating an entry point in oocytes surrounded by tough tissue to assist sperm penetration)

• Preimplantation Genetic Diagnosis (for couples with a high risk of bearing children with specific genetic disorders)

• Cyropreservation (freezing eggs and embryos in liquid nitrogen to preserve them for future use)

• Comprehensive evaluation of sperm health and fertility

• Testicular Biopsy

• Vasectomy Reversal

• Epididymal Repair (surgery to clear sperm pathways within penis)

• Microsurgical Sperm Aspiration (retrieval of sperm from inside the testes, when it is not present in the semen)

• Variocele Repair (surgical reduction of enlarged veins around penis to reduce high temperature in groin area, which adversely impacts on fertility)

The Reproductive Endocrinologists at NYU Medical Center are dedicated not only to treating infertility, but also to researching its causes. Because of this first-hand knowledge of the latest breakthroughs in fertility treatment, our programs are among the most successful in the country. Among their achievements are:

• the first ICSI pregnancy
• the first Assisted Hatching pregnancy
• the first epididymal sperm retrieval and
• the first embryo biopsy in the world.

Physician Referral
(888) 7-NYU-MED
(888-769-8633)
www.med.nyu.edu

692

Rheumatology
a subspecialty of Internal Medicine

An internist who treats diseases of joints, muscle, bones and tendons. This specialist diagnoses and treats arthritis, back pain, muscle strains, common athletic injuries and "collagen" diseases.

Training Required: Three years in internal medicine *plus* additional training and examination for certification in rheumatology.

Rheumatology

Albert, Daniel A MD [Rhu] - **Spec Exp:** Juvenile Arthritis; Rheumatology-Adult & Pediatric; **Hospital:** Dartmouth - Hitchcock Med Ctr; **Address:** Dartmouth-Hitchcock Med Ctr Rheumatology, One Medical Center Drive, Lebanon, NH 03756; **Phone:** 603-650-8622; **Board Cert:** Internal Medicine 1977; Rheumatology 1980; **Med School:** NYU Sch Med 1974; **Resid:** Internal Medicine, NC Meml Hosp 1977; **Fellow:** Rheumatology, UCSD 1981; **Fac Appt:** Prof Med, Univ Pennsylvania

Brenner, Michael B MD [Rhu] - **Spec Exp:** Gout; Rheumatoid Arthritis; Lupus/SLE; **Hospital:** Brigham & Women's Hosp; **Address:** Div Rheumatology, Smith bldg, rm 552, 1 Jimmy Fund Way, Boston, MA 02115; **Phone:** 617-525-1000; **Board Cert:** Internal Medicine 1978; Rheumatology 1982; **Med School:** Vanderbilt Univ 1975; **Resid:** Internal Medicine, Vanderbilt Univ Hosp 1979; **Fellow:** Rheumatology, UCLA Med Ctr 1981; **Fac Appt:** Prof Med, Harvard Med Sch

Kay, Jonathan MD [Rhu] - **Spec Exp:** Rheumatoid Arthritis; Psoriatic Arthritis; Ankylosing Spondylitis; Nephrogenic Fibrosing Dermopathy; **Hospital:** Mass Genl Hosp; **Address:** Rheumatology Assocs-MGH,, 55 Fruit St Yawkey Bldg - Ste 2C, Boston, MA 02114; **Phone:** 617-726-7938; **Board Cert:** Internal Medicine 1986; Rheumatology 1988; **Med School:** UCSF 1983; **Resid:** Internal Medicine, Hosp Univ Penn 1986; **Fellow:** Rheumatology/Immunology, Brigham & Womens Hosp 1989; **Fac Appt:** Assoc Clin Prof Med, Harvard Med Sch

Merkel, Peter MD [Rhu] - **Spec Exp:** Vasculitis; Scleroderma; **Hospital:** Boston Med Ctr; **Address:** Boston Univ Vasculitis Ctr, 715 Albany St, E 533, Boston, MA 02118; **Phone:** 617-414-2500; **Board Cert:** Internal Medicine 2000; Rheumatology 2000; **Med School:** Yale Univ 1988; **Resid:** Internal Medicine, Hosp Univ Penn 1991; **Fellow:** Rheumatology, Mass General Hosp 1994

Polisson, Richard Paul MD [Rhu] - **Spec Exp:** Rheumatoid Arthritis; Lupus/SLE; **Hospital:** Mass Genl Hosp; **Address:** 55 Fruit St Yawkey Bldg - Ste 2C, Boston, MA 02114; **Phone:** 617-726-7938; **Board Cert:** Internal Medicine 1979; Rheumatology 1984; **Med School:** Duke Univ 1976; **Resid:** Internal Medicine, Duke Univ Med Ctr 1978; Natl Inst Hlth/NCI 1980; **Fellow:** Rheumatology, Mass Genl Hosp 1982; **Fac Appt:** Assoc Prof Med, Harvard Med Sch

Robinson, Dwight R MD [Rhu] - **Spec Exp:** Arthritis; **Hospital:** Mass Genl Hosp; **Address:** Mass Genl Hosp, Rheum Assocs, 55 Fruit St, Ste 2C, Boston, MA 02114; **Phone:** 617-726-7938; **Board Cert:** Internal Medicine 1968; **Med School:** Columbia P&S 1957; **Resid:** Surgery, Mass Genl Hosp 1959; Internal Medicine, Mass Genl Hosp 1961; **Fellow:** Research, Mass Genl Hosp 1960; Biochemistry, Brandeis Univ 1964; **Fac Appt:** Prof Med, Harvard Med Sch

Schoen, Robert T MD [Rhu] - **Spec Exp:** Rheumatoid Arthritis; Lyme Disease; Osteoporosis; **Hospital:** Yale - New Haven Hosp, Hosp of St Raphael; **Address:** 60 Temple St, Ste 6A, New Haven, CT 06510-2716; **Phone:** 203-789-2255; **Board Cert:** Internal Medicine 1979; Rheumatology 1982; **Med School:** Columbia P&S 1976; **Resid:** Internal Medicine, Yale New Haven Hosp 1979; **Fellow:** Rheumatology, Brigham & Womens Hosp 1981; **Fac Appt:** Clin Prof Med, Yale Univ

Shadick, Nancy A MD [Rhu] - **Spec Exp:** Lupus/SLE; Rheumatoid Arthritis; Osteoarthritis; **Hospital:** Brigham & Women's Hosp; **Address:** Brigham & Women's Hosp, Arthritis Ctr, 45 Francis St, Boston, MA 02115-6105; **Phone:** 617-732-5266; **Board Cert:** Internal Medicine 1989; Rheumatology 2002; **Med School:** NYU Sch Med 1986; **Resid:** Internal Medicine, Columbia-Presby Hosp 1989; **Fellow:** Rheumatology, Brigham & Womens Hosp 1992; **Fac Appt:** Asst Prof Med, Harvard Med Sch

Simms, Robert W MD [Rhu] - **Spec Exp:** Rheumatoid Arthritis; Fibromyalgia; Lyme Disease; **Hospital:** Boston Med Ctr; **Address:** Boston Univ Sch Med, Arthritis Ctr, 715 Albany St, Evans-501, Boston, MA 02118; **Phone:** 617-638-4312; **Board Cert:** Internal Medicine 1985; Rheumatology 1988; **Med School:** Univ Rochester 1980; **Resid:** Internal Medicine, North Shore Hosp 1982; Internal Medicine, Brigham & Women's Hosp 1985; **Fellow:** Rheumatology, Boston Univ Med Ctr 1987; **Fac Appt:** Prof Med, Boston Univ

Weinblatt, Michael Eliot MD [Rhu] - **Spec Exp:** Rheumatoid Arthritis; **Hospital:** Brigham & Women's Hosp; **Address:** Brigham & Womens Hosp, Arthritis Ctr, 45 Francis St, Boston, MA 02115-6110; **Phone:** 617-732-5331; **Board Cert:** Internal Medicine 1978; Rheumatology 1980; **Med School:** Univ MD Sch Med 1975; **Resid:** Internal Medicine, Univ Maryland Hosp 1978; **Fellow:** Rheumatology, Peter Bent Brigham Hosp 1980; **Fac Appt:** Prof Med, Harvard Med Sch

Mid Atlantic

Abramson, Steven B MD [Rhu] - **Spec Exp:** Arthritis; Inflammatory Muscle Disease; **Hospital:** Hosp For Joint Diseases (page 68), NYU Med Ctr (page 67); **Address:** Hosp for Joint Diseases, 301 E 17th St, rm 1410, New York, NY 10003; **Phone:** 212-598-6110; **Board Cert:** Internal Medicine 1977; Rheumatology 1980; **Med School:** Harvard Med Sch 1974; **Resid:** Internal Medicine, Bellevue Hosp/NYU Med Ctr 1978; **Fellow:** Rheumatology, Bellevue Hosp/NYU Med Ctr 1983; **Fac Appt:** Prof Med, NYU Sch Med

Belmont, Howard Michael MD [Rhu] - **Spec Exp:** Lupus/SLE; Rheumatoid Arthritis; Scleroderma; **Hospital:** Hosp For Joint Diseases (page 68), NYU Med Ctr (page 67); **Address:** 305 2nd Ave, Ste 16, New York, NY 10003-2739; **Phone:** 212-598-6516; **Board Cert:** Internal Medicine 1983; Rheumatology 1986; **Med School:** Univ Pittsburgh 1980; **Resid:** Internal Medicine, Mt Sinai Hosp 1983; **Fellow:** Rheumatology, NYU/Bellevue Hosp 1985; **Fac Appt:** Assoc Prof Med, NYU Sch Med

Blume, Ralph S MD [Rhu] - **Spec Exp:** Vasculitis; Lupus/SLE; Rheumatoid Arthritis; **Hospital:** NY-Presby Hosp/Columbia (page 66); **Address:** 161 Fort Washington Ave, Ste 537, New York, NY 10032-3713; **Phone:** 212-305-5512; **Board Cert:** Internal Medicine 1972; Rheumatology 1974; **Med School:** Columbia P&S 1964; **Resid:** Internal Medicine, Columbia-Presby Med Ctr 1968; **Fellow:** Rheumatology, Columbia-Presby Med Ctr 1970; **Fac Appt:** Clin Prof Med, Columbia P&S

Bunning, Robert D MD [Rhu] - **Spec Exp:** Exercise Therapy; Rheumatoid Arthritis; Musculoskeletal Disorders; **Hospital:** Natl Rehab Hosp; **Address:** National Rehab Hosp, 102 Irving St NW Fl 2, Washington, DC 20010; **Phone:** 202-877-1660; **Board Cert:** Internal Medicine 1984; Rheumatology 1986; **Med School:** Univ Cincinnati 1979; **Resid:** Internal Medicine, Wash Hosp Ctr 1984; **Fellow:** Rheumatology, Wash Hosp Ctr 1983; **Fac Appt:** Asst Clin Prof Med, Geo Wash Univ

Buyon, Jill P MD [Rhu] - **Spec Exp:** Lupus/SLE in Pregnancy; Lupus/SLE in Menopause; **Hospital:** Hosp For Joint Diseases (page 68), NYU Med Ctr (page 67); **Address:** 246 E 20th St, New York, NY 10003; **Phone:** 646-356-9400; **Board Cert:** Internal Medicine 1981; Rheumatology 1984; **Med School:** Albert Einstein Coll Med 1978; **Resid:** Internal Medicine, Albert Einstein 1981; **Fellow:** Rheumatology, NYU Med Ctr 1983; **Fac Appt:** Prof Med, NYU Sch Med

Cupps, Thomas R MD [Rhu] - **Spec Exp:** Vasculitis; Hepatitis B-Immune Response; **Hospital:** Georgetown Univ Hosp; **Address:** 3800 Resevoir Rd NW, GUMC - Lower Level, Kober Cogan Bldg, Ste B100, Washington, DC 20007; **Phone:** 202-687-8233; **Board Cert:** Internal Medicine 1978; Allergy & Immunology 1981; **Med School:** Stanford Univ 1975; **Resid:** Internal Medicine, Strong Meml Hosp 1978; **Fellow:** Allergy & Immunology, Natl Inst Allergy & Inf Dis 1980; **Fac Appt:** Assoc Prof Med, Georgetown Univ

Farber, Martin Stuart MD/PhD [Rhu] - **Hospital:** Sunnyview Hosp; **Address:** Sunnyview Hospital, 124 Rosa Rd, Schenectady, NY 12308-2198; **Phone:** 518-386-3644; **Board Cert:** Internal Medicine 1982; Rheumatology 1984; **Med School:** Albert Einstein Coll Med 1979; **Resid:** Internal Medicine, Boston City Hosp 1982; **Fellow:** Rheumatology, Boston Univ Sch Med 1984; **Fac Appt:** Asst Clin Prof Med, Albany Med Coll

Ginzler, Ellen MD [Rhu] - **Spec Exp:** Lupus/SLE; **Hospital:** SUNY Downstate Med Ctr, Kings County Hosp Ctr; **Address:** SUNY Downstate, Dept Rheumatology, 450 Clarkson Ave, Box 42, Brooklyn, NY 11203-0042; **Phone:** 718-270-1662; **Board Cert:** Internal Medicine 1972; Rheumatology 1974; **Med School:** Case West Res Univ 1969; **Resid:** Internal Medicine, Kings Co Hosp 1971; Internal Medicine, Bellevue Hosp 1972; **Fellow:** Rheumatology, Univ Hosp 1974; **Fac Appt:** Prof Med, SUNY Downstate

Gorevic, Peter D MD [Rhu] - **Spec Exp:** Autoimmune Disease; Amyloidosis/Joint Disease; Cryoglobulinemia; **Hospital:** Mount Sinai Med Ctr; **Address:** Mount Sinai Medical Ctr, 1 Gustave L Levy Pl, New York, NY 10029; **Phone:** 212-241-1671; **Board Cert:** Allergy & Immunology 1977; Rheumatology 1976; Diagnostic Lab Immunology 1986; Geriatric Medicine 1996; **Med School:** NYU Sch Med 1970; **Resid:** Internal Medicine, NYU Med Ctr 1974; **Fellow:** Rheumatology, NYU Med Ctr 1976; Allergy & Immunology, NYU Med Ctr 1977; **Fac Appt:** Prof Med, Mount Sinai Sch Med

Gourley, Mark MD [Rhu] - **Spec Exp:** Autoimmune Disease; Lupus/SLE; **Hospital:** Natl Inst of Hlth - Clin Ctr; **Address:** Natl Inst Hlth, 10 Center Drive Bldg 10 - rm 6C432D, Bethesda, MD 20892-1627; **Phone:** 301-451-6269; **Board Cert:** Internal Medicine 1988; Rheumatology 2002; **Med School:** Tulane Univ 1985; **Resid:** Internal Medicine, Univ Wisconsin Hosps 1988; **Fellow:** Rheumatology, Natl Inst Hlth 1996

Hochberg, Marc C MD [Rhu] - **Spec Exp:** Osteoporosis; Osteoarthritis; Rheumatoid Arthritis; **Hospital:** Univ of MD Med Sys; **Address:** Univ MD Sch Med, Div Rheum, 10 S Pine St, MSTF 8-34, Baltimore, MD 21201; **Phone:** 410-706-6474; **Board Cert:** Internal Medicine 1976; Rheumatology 1978; **Med School:** Johns Hopkins Univ 1973; **Resid:** Internal Medicine, Johns Hopkins Hosp 1975; **Fellow:** Rheumatology, Johns Hopkins Hosp 1977; **Fac Appt:** Prof Med, Univ MD Sch Med

Katz, Warren A MD [Rhu] - **Spec Exp:** Fibromyalgia; Pain-Musculoskeletal; **Address:** Rothman Institute, 170 N Henderson Rd, Ste 100, King of Prussia, PA 19406; **Phone:** 267-339-3500; **Board Cert:** Internal Medicine 1969; Rheumatology 1974; **Med School:** Jefferson Med Coll 1961; **Resid:** Internal Medicine, Boston City Hosp 1963; Internal Medicine, Mt Sinai Hosp 1965; **Fellow:** Rheumatology, NYU Med Ctr 1966

Kremer, Joel M MD [Rhu] - **Spec Exp:** Rheumatoid Arthritis; **Hospital:** Albany Med Ctr, St Peter's Hosp - Albany; **Address:** Center for Rheumatology, 1367 Washington Ave, Ste 101, Albany, NY 12206; **Phone:** 518-489-4471; **Board Cert:** Rheumatology 1980; Internal Medicine 1977; **Med School:** Temple Univ 1974; **Resid:** Internal Medicine, Albany Medical Ctr 1977; **Fellow:** Rheumatology, Albany Medical Ctr 1979; **Fac Appt:** Prof Med, Albany Med Coll

Lahita, Robert G MD/PhD [Rhu] - **Spec Exp:** Lupus/SLE; Endocrinology & Joint Disorders; Immunodeficiency Disorders; **Hospital:** Jersey City Med Ctr, St Vincent Cath Med Ctrs - Manhattan; **Address:** 610 Washington Blvd, Jersey City, NJ 07310; **Phone:** 201-222-1266; **Board Cert:** Internal Medicine 2004; Rheumatology 1997; **Med School:** Jefferson Med Coll 1973; **Resid:** Internal Medicine, New York Hosp-Cornell 1976; **Fellow:** Rheumatology, Rockefeller Hosp 1978; **Fac Appt:** Prof Med, Mount Sinai Sch Med

Lockshin, Michael D MD [Rhu] - **Spec Exp:** Lupus/SLE; Antiphospholipid Syndrome (APS); Pregnancy & Rheumatic Disease; Lupus/SLE in Pregnancy; **Hospital:** Hosp For Special Surgery (page 60), NY-Presby Hosp/Weill Cornell (page 66); **Address:** 535 E 70th St, rm 661, New York, NY 10021-4872; **Phone:** 212-606-1461; **Board Cert:** Internal Medicine 1969; Rheumatology 1972; **Med School:** Harvard Med Sch 1963; **Resid:** Internal Medicine, Bellevue Hosp 1968; **Fellow:** Rheumatology, Columbia-Presby Hosp 1970; **Fac Appt:** Prof Med, Cornell Univ-Weill Med Coll

Medsger Jr, Thomas A MD [Rhu] - **Spec Exp:** Scleroderma; Raynaud's Disease; Polymyositis; Dermatomyositis; **Hospital:** UPMC Presby, Pittsburgh; **Address:** Arthritis & Autoimmunity Ctr, 3601 Fifth Ave, 3B Falk Med Bldg, Pittsburgh, PA 15213; **Phone:** 412-647-6700; **Board Cert:** Internal Medicine 1972; Rheumatology 1972; **Med School:** Univ Pennsylvania 1962; **Resid:** Internal Medicine, Univ Pittsburgh 1968; **Fellow:** Rheumatology, Univ Pittsburgh 1966; Rheumatology, Univ Tenn Coll Med 1969; **Fac Appt:** Prof Med, Univ Pittsburgh

Mitnick, Hal J MD [Rhu] - **Spec Exp:** Rheumatoid Arthritis; Psoriatic Arthritis; Osteoporosis; **Hospital:** NYU Med Ctr (page 67); **Address:** 333 E 34th St, Ste 1C, New York, NY 10016-4956; **Phone:** 212-889-7217; **Board Cert:** Internal Medicine 1976; Rheumatology 1978; **Med School:** NYU Sch Med 1972; **Resid:** Internal Medicine, Bellevue Hosp 1976; **Fellow:** Rheumatology, NYU Med Ctr 1978; **Fac Appt:** Clin Prof Med, NYU Sch Med

Oddis, Chester MD [Rhu] - **Spec Exp:** Polymyositis; Dermatomyositis; Connective Tissue Disorders; **Hospital:** UPMC Presby, Pittsburgh, Penn State Milton S Hershey Med Ctr; **Address:** Univ Pittsburgh-Div Rheumatology, 3500 Terrace St, S 703 BST, Pittsburgh, PA 15261; **Phone:** 412-647-6700; **Board Cert:** Internal Medicine 1983; Rheumatology 1986; **Med School:** Penn State Univ-Hershey Med Ctr 1980; **Resid:** Internal Medicine, Hershey Med Ctr 1984; **Fellow:** Rheumatology, Univ Pittsburgh 1986; **Fac Appt:** Prof Med, Univ Pittsburgh

Paget, Stephen MD [Rhu] - **Spec Exp:** Rheumatoid Arthritis; Lupus/SLE; **Hospital:** Hosp For Special Surgery (page 60); **Address:** 535 E 70th St, rm 721 West, New York, NY 10021; **Phone:** 212-606-1845; **Board Cert:** Internal Medicine 1974; Rheumatology 1976; **Med School:** SUNY Downstate 1971; **Resid:** Internal Medicine, Johns Hopkins Hosp 1973; **Fellow:** Rheumatology, Hosp Special Surg 1975; **Fac Appt:** Clin Prof Med, Cornell Univ-Weill Med Coll

Rheumatology

Petri, Michelle A MD [Rhu] - **Spec Exp:** Lupus/SLE; Antiphospholipid Syndrome (APS); **Hospital:** Johns Hopkins Hosp - Baltimore (page 61); **Address:** Div of Rheumatology, 1830 E Monument St, Ste 7500, Baltimore, MD 21205-2100; **Phone:** 410-955-9114; **Board Cert:** Internal Medicine 1983; Allergy & Immunology 1985; Rheumatology 1986; **Med School:** Harvard Med Sch 1980; **Resid:** Internal Medicine, Mass Genl Hosp 1983; **Fellow:** Allergy & Immunology, UCSF Med Ctr 1985; Rheumatology, UCSF Med Ctr 1986; **Fac Appt:** Prof Med, Johns Hopkins Univ

Plotz, Paul MD [Rhu] - **Hospital:** Natl Inst of Hlth - Clin Ctr; **Address:** NIH Clin Ctr Bldg 10 - rm 9N-244, 10 Center Drive, MC 1820, Bethesda, MD 20892-1820; **Phone:** 301-496-9904; **Board Cert:** Internal Medicine 1970; **Med School:** Harvard Med Sch 1963; **Resid:** Internal Medicine, Beth Israel Hosp 1965; **Fellow:** Rheumatology, Clin Ctr- NIH 1968

Rosen, Antony MD [Rhu] - **Spec Exp:** Arthritis; Myositis; Vasculitis; **Hospital:** Johns Hopkins Hosp - Baltimore (page 61); **Address:** Johns Hopkins School of Medicine, Mason Lord Bldg, Center Toweer, 5200 Eastern Ave, rm 412, Baltimore, MD 21224; **Phone:** 410-550-1894; **Board Cert:** Internal Medicine 2003; Rheumatology 1996; **Med School:** South Africa 1984; **Resid:** Internal Medicine, Johns Hopkins Hosp 1992; **Fellow:** Rheumatology, Johns Hopkins Hosp 1994; Immunological Biology, Rockefeller Inst 1990; **Fac Appt:** Prof Med, Johns Hopkins Univ

Rothenberg, Russell R MD [Rhu] - **Spec Exp:** Fibromyalgia; Lupus/SLE; Rheumatoid Arthritis; **Hospital:** G Washington Univ Hosp; **Address:** 2141 K St NW, Ste 606, Washington, DC 20037; **Phone:** 202-223-2282; **Board Cert:** Internal Medicine 1980; Rheumatology 1982; **Med School:** Albany Med Coll 1977; **Resid:** Internal Medicine, LIJ Medical Ctr 1980; **Fellow:** Rheumatology, Mt Sinai Medical Ctr 1982; **Fac Appt:** Assoc Prof Med, Geo Wash Univ

Solomon, Gary MD [Rhu] - **Spec Exp:** Psoriatic Arthritis; Rheumatoid Arthritis; Autoimmune Disease; **Hospital:** Hosp For Joint Diseases (page 68), NYU Med Ctr (page 67); **Address:** Hosp Joint Diseases, Dept Rheumatology, 305 2nd Ave, Ste 16, New York, NY 10003; **Phone:** 212-598-6516; **Board Cert:** Internal Medicine 1980; Rheumatology 1982; **Med School:** Mount Sinai Sch Med 1977; **Resid:** Internal Medicine, Mount Sinai Med Ctr 1980; **Fellow:** Rheumatology, Montefiore Med Ctr 1982; **Fac Appt:** Assoc Clin Prof Med, NYU Sch Med

Spiera, Harry MD [Rhu] - **Spec Exp:** Lupus/SLE; Scleroderma; Vasculitis; **Hospital:** Mount Sinai Med Ctr, NY-Presby Hosp/Weill Cornell (page 66); **Address:** 1088 Park Ave, New York, NY 10128-1132; **Phone:** 212-860-4000 x36; **Board Cert:** Internal Medicine 1965; Rheumatology 1972; **Med School:** NYU Sch Med 1958; **Resid:** Internal Medicine, VA Med Ctr 1960; Internal Medicine, Mount Sinai Hosp 1961; **Fellow:** Rheumatology, Columbia-Presby Med Ctr 1963; **Fac Appt:** Clin Prof Med, Mount Sinai Sch Med

Starz, Terence W MD [Rhu] - **Spec Exp:** Arthritis; **Hospital:** UPMC St Margaret; **Address:** Arthritis & Int Medicine Assocs-UPMC, 3500 Fifth Ave Hieber Bldg Fl 4, Pittsburgh, PA 15213; **Phone:** 412-682-2434; **Board Cert:** Internal Medicine 1975; Rheumatology 1978; **Med School:** Jefferson Med Coll 1971; **Resid:** Internal Medicine, Presby-Univ Hosp 1975; **Fellow:** Rheumatology, Presby-Univ Hosp 1977; **Fac Appt:** Clin Prof Med, Univ Pittsburgh

Steen, Virginia MD [Rhu] - **Spec Exp:** Scleroderma; Lupus/SLE; Polymyositis; **Hospital:** Georgetown Univ Hosp; **Address:** 3800 Reservoir Rd, LL - Kober Cogan Bldg - Ste B100, Washington, DC 20007; **Phone:** 202-267-8233; **Board Cert:** Internal Medicine 1978; Rheumatology 1980; **Med School:** Univ Pittsburgh 1975; **Resid:** Internal Medicine, Hosp Univ Penn 1978; **Fellow:** Rheumatology, Presby Hosp 1980; **Fac Appt:** Prof Med, Georgetown Univ

Vivino, Frederick B MD [Rhu] - **Spec Exp:** Sjogren's Syndrome; **Hospital:** Penn Presby Med Ctr - UPHS (page 72); **Address:** Presbyterian Medical Ctr, 39th & Filberts Sts, PHI-2B, Philadelphia, PA 19104; **Phone:** 215-662-8233; **Board Cert:** Internal Medicine 1986; Rheumatology 1988; **Med School:** Temple Univ 1983; **Resid:** Internal Medicine, Hosp U Penn 1986; **Fellow:** Rheumatology, Hosp U Penn 1989; **Fac Appt:** Asst Clin Prof Med, Univ Pennsylvania

Weinstein, Arthur MD [Rhu] - **Spec Exp:** Lyme Disease; Lupus/SLE; **Hospital:** Washington Hosp Ctr, Georgetown Univ Hosp; **Address:** Washington Hosp Ctr, Div Rheumatology, 110 Irving St NW, rm 2A-66, Washington, DC 20010; **Phone:** 202-877-6274; **Board Cert:** Rheumatology 1976; Diagnostic Lab Immunology 1986; **Med School:** Univ Toronto 1967; **Resid:** Internal Medicine, Toronto Wellesley Hosp 1972; Rheumatology, Hammersmith Hosp 1971; **Fellow:** Rheumatology, Toronto Wellesley Hosp 1973; **Fac Appt:** Prof Med, Georgetown Univ

Wigley, Frederick M MD [Rhu] - **Spec Exp:** Scleroderma; Raynaud's Disease; **Hospital:** Johns Hopkins Bayview Med Ctr (page 61), Johns Hopkins Hosp - Baltimore (page 61); **Address:** 5501 Hopkins Bayview Cir, Ste 1B32, Baltimore, MD 21224; **Phone:** 410-550-7715; **Board Cert:** Internal Medicine 1975; Rheumatology 1980; **Med School:** Univ Fla Coll Med 1972; **Resid:** Internal Medicine, Johns Hopkins Hosp 1975; **Fellow:** Rheumatology, Johns Hopkins Hosp 1979; **Fac Appt:** Prof Med, Johns Hopkins Univ

Southeast

Allen, Nancy B MD [Rhu] - **Spec Exp:** Vasculitis; Wegener's Granulomatosis; Lupus/SLE; **Hospital:** Duke Univ Med Ctr; **Address:** Duke Univ Med Ctr, Box 3440, Durham, NC 27710; **Phone:** 919-684-2965; **Board Cert:** Internal Medicine 1981; Rheumatology 1984; **Med School:** Tufts Univ 1978; **Resid:** Internal Medicine, Duke Univ Med Ctr 1981; **Fellow:** Rheumatology, Duke Univ Med Ctr 1983; **Fac Appt:** Prof Med, Duke Univ

Chatham, Walter W MD [Rhu] - **Spec Exp:** Lupus/SLE; Connective Tissue Disorders; Rheumatoid Arthritis; **Hospital:** Univ of Ala Hosp at Birmingham; **Address:** Univ Alabama Birmingham Med Ctr, FOT 802, 1530 3rd Ave S, Birmingham, AL 35294-3408; **Phone:** 205-934-4212; **Board Cert:** Internal Medicine 1983; Rheumatology 1988; **Med School:** Vanderbilt Univ 1980; **Resid:** Internal Medicine, North Carolina Meml Hosp 1983; **Fellow:** Rheumatology, Univ Alabama Birmingham 1988; **Fac Appt:** Assoc Prof Med, Univ Ala

Crofford, Leslie MD [Rhu] - **Spec Exp:** Fibromyalgia; Rheumatoid Arthritis; Lupus/SLE; **Hospital:** Univ of Kentucky Chandler Hosp; **Address:** 740 S Limestone St, rm J509, Lexington, KY 40536-0284; **Phone:** 859-323-4939; **Board Cert:** Internal Medicine 1987; Rheumatology 2003; **Med School:** Univ Tenn Coll Med, Memphis 1984; **Resid:** Internal Medicine, Barnes/Wash Univ 1987; **Fellow:** Rheumatology, Natl Inst Hlth Clin Ctr 1992; **Fac Appt:** Prof Med, Univ KY Coll Med

Hadler, Nortin MD [Rhu] - **Spec Exp:** Occupational Musculoskeletal Disorders; Musculoskeletal Disorders; Spondylitis-Back Pain; **Hospital:** Univ NC Hosps; **Address:** Univ North Carolina, Dept Medicine, 3300 Thurston Building, Box 7280, Chapel Hill, NC 27599-7280; **Phone:** 919-966-0566; **Board Cert:** Rheumatology 1974; Allergy & Immunology 1975; Internal Medicine 1987; **Med School:** Harvard Med Sch 1968; **Resid:** Internal Medicine, Mass Genl Hosp 1973; **Fellow:** Rheumatology, Natl Inst Hlth 1972; Allergy & Immunology, Clin Res Ctr 1974; **Fac Appt:** Prof Med, Univ NC Sch Med

Heck, Louis W MD [Rhu] - **Spec Exp:** Lupus/SLE; Rheumatoid Arthritis; **Hospital:** Univ of Ala Hosp at Birmingham; **Address:** 1530 3rd Ave S, Faculty Office Tower - 858, Birmingham, AL 35294; **Phone:** 205-934-6485; **Board Cert:** Internal Medicine 1974; Rheumatology 1988; **Med School:** Indiana Univ 1970; **Resid:** Internal Medicine, Indiana Univ 1972; **Fellow:** Allergy & Immunology, Natl Inst Allergy & Inf Dis 1975; Rheumatology, Robert Bronton Hosp 1979; **Fac Appt:** Assoc Prof Med, Univ Ala

Kaplan, Stanley B MD [Rhu] - **Spec Exp:** Rheumatoid Arthritis; Lupus/SLE; Gout; **Hospital:** Methodist Univ Hosp - Memphis, Baptist Memorial Hospital - Memphis; **Address:** Univ Tenn Med Group, 7945 Wolf River Blvd, Ste 120, Germantown, TN 38138; **Phone:** 901-448-7260; **Board Cert:** Internal Medicine 1965; **Med School:** Univ Tenn Coll Med, Memphis 1954; **Resid:** Internal Medicine, Univ Tenn Hosps 1960; **Fellow:** Rheumatology, Univ Tenn Hosps 1962; **Fac Appt:** Prof Med, Univ Tenn Coll Med, Memphis

Moore, Walter J MD [Rhu] - **Spec Exp:** Rheumatoid Arthritis; Lupus/SLE; **Hospital:** Med Coll of GA Hosp and Clin; **Address:** Medical College of Georgia, 1120 15th St, rm BI 5083, Augusta, GA 30912; **Phone:** 706-721-2981; **Board Cert:** Internal Medicine 1980; Rheumatology 1984; **Med School:** Georgetown Univ 1977; **Resid:** Internal Medicine, Walter Reed AMC 1980; **Fellow:** Rheumatology, Walter Reed AMC 1983; **Fac Appt:** Assoc Prof Med, Med Coll GA

Sergent, John S MD [Rhu] - **Spec Exp:** Vasculitis; **Hospital:** Vanderbilt Univ Med Ctr; **Address:** Vanderbilt Univ Med Ctr - Dept Medicine, D3100 Medical Ctr North, Nashville, TN 37232-2358; **Phone:** 615-322-4752; **Board Cert:** Internal Medicine 1972; Rheumatology 1974; **Med School:** Vanderbilt Univ 1966; **Resid:** Internal Medicine, Johns Hopkins Hosp 1968; Internal Medicine, Vanderbilt Univ Hosp 1972; **Fellow:** Rheumatology, Hosp Special Surgery 1974; **Fac Appt:** Prof Med, Vanderbilt Univ

Silver, Richard MD [Rhu] - **Spec Exp:** Scleroderma & Lung Disease; Rheumatoid Arthritis; Pediatric Rheumatology; Connective Tissue Disorders; **Hospital:** MUSC Med Ctr; **Address:** MUSC Med Ctr, PO Box 250623, 96 Jonathan Lucas St, Ste 912, Charleston, SC 29425; **Phone:** 843-876-0500; **Board Cert:** Internal Medicine 1978; Rheumatology 1982; **Med School:** Vanderbilt Univ 1975; **Resid:** Internal Medicine, Univ NC Hosps 1978; **Fellow:** Rheumatology, UCSD Med Ctr 1981; **Fac Appt:** Prof Med, Med Univ SC

Sundy, John Sargent MD/PhD [Rhu] - **Spec Exp:** Rheumatoid Arthritis; Gout; Lupus/SLE; **Hospital:** Duke Univ Med Ctr, Durham Regional Hosp; **Address:** Duke Univ Med Ctr, Box 3278, Durham, NC 27710; **Phone:** 919-668-2169; **Board Cert:** Internal Medicine 1994; Rheumatology 1998; Allergy & Immunology 1999; **Med School:** Hahnemann Univ 1991; **Resid:** Internal Medicine, Duke Univ Med Ctr 1993; **Fellow:** Rheumatology, Duke Univ Med Ctr 1996; Allergy & Immunology, Duke Univ Med Ctr 1998; **Fac Appt:** Asst Prof Med, Duke Univ

Wise, Christopher M MD [Rhu] - **Spec Exp:** Gout; Sjogren's Syndrome; Rheumatoid Arthritis; **Hospital:** Med Coll of VA Hosp; **Address:** Virginia Commonwealth Univ/MCV Campus, Box 980647, Richmond, VA 23298; **Phone:** 804-828-9341; **Board Cert:** Internal Medicine 1980; Rheumatology 1982; **Med School:** Univ NC Sch Med 1977; **Resid:** Internal Medicine, Med Coll Virginia Hosp 1980; **Fellow:** Rheumatology, Med Coll Virginia Hosp 1982; **Fac Appt:** Prof Med, Va Commonwealth Univ

Midwest

Adams, Elaine MD [Rhu] - **Spec Exp:** Rheumatoid Arthritis; Lupus/SLE; Spondyloarthropathies; **Hospital:** Loyola Univ Med Ctr, Hines VA Hosp; **Address:** Loyola Univ Med Ctr, Dept Rheumatology, 2160 S 1st Ave, Bldg 54 - rm 121, Maywood, IL 60153-5590; **Phone:** 708-216-8563; **Board Cert:** Internal Medicine 1981; Rheumatology 1984; **Med School:** Loyola Univ-Stritch Sch Med 1978; **Resid:** Internal Medicine, Loyola Univ Med Ctr 1981; **Fellow:** Rheumatology, Univ Wisconsin Med Ctr 1983; **Fac Appt:** Assoc Prof Med, Loyola Univ-Stritch Sch Med

Ashman, Robert F MD [Rhu] - **Spec Exp:** Lupus/SLE; Rheumatoid Arthritis; Inflammatory Muscle Disease; **Hospital:** Univ Iowa Hosp & Clinics; **Address:** Univ Iowa Hosp & Clinics, Div Rheumatology, 200 Hawkins Drive, rm C31-P GH, Iowa City, IA 52242-1081; **Phone:** 319-356-2287; **Board Cert:** Internal Medicine 1974; Rheumatology 1976; **Med School:** Columbia P&S 1966; **Resid:** Internal Medicine, Peter Bent Brigham Hosp 1970; **Fellow:** Rheumatology, UCLA Med Ctr 1973; **Fac Appt:** Prof Med, Univ Iowa Coll Med

Barr, Walter Gerard MD [Rhu] - **Spec Exp:** Scleroderma; Vasculitis; Stem Cell Transplant/Autoimmune Disease; **Hospital:** Northwestern Meml Hosp; **Address:** 675 N St Clair St, Ste 14-100, Chicago, IL 60611-5972; **Phone:** 312-695-8628; **Board Cert:** Internal Medicine 1978; Rheumatology 1982; **Med School:** Loyola Univ-Stritch Sch Med 1975; **Resid:** Internal Medicine, Loyola Univ Med Ctr 1978; **Fellow:** Rheumatology, Loyola Univ Med Ctr 1979; Rheumatology, Mayo Clinic 1982; **Fac Appt:** Assoc Prof Med, Northwestern Univ

Brasington, Richard MD [Rhu] - **Hospital:** Barnes-Jewish Hosp; **Address:** 4921 Parkview Pl Fl 5CAM - Ste C, Rheumatology CB 8045, St Louis, MO 63110; **Phone:** 314-286-2635; **Board Cert:** Internal Medicine 1985; Rheumatology 1986; **Med School:** Duke Univ 1980; **Resid:** Internal Medicine, Univ Iowa 1982; Internal Medicine, Univ Iowa 1985; **Fellow:** Rheumatology, Univ Iowa 1986; **Fac Appt:** Assoc Prof Med, Washington Univ, St Louis

Chang, Rowland W MD [Rhu] - **Spec Exp:** Rheumatoid Arthritis; Arthritis; Ankylosing Spondylitis; **Hospital:** Northwestern Meml Hosp, Rehab Inst - Chicago; **Address:** Rehab Inst of Chicago Arthritis Ctr, 345 E Superior St Fl 9, Chicago, IL 60611-2654; **Phone:** 312-238-2784; **Board Cert:** Internal Medicine 1979; Rheumatology 1982; **Med School:** Tufts Univ 1976; **Resid:** Internal Medicine, Mt Auburn Hosp 1979; **Fellow:** Rheumatology, Hammersmith Hosp 1980; Rheumatology, Brigham & Womens Hosp 1982; **Fac Appt:** Prof Med, Northwestern Univ

Curran, James Joseph MD [Rhu] - **Spec Exp:** Rheumatoid Arthritis; Lupus/SLE; Sjogren's Syndrome; Polymyositis; **Hospital:** Univ of Chicago Hosps; **Address:** 5841 S Maryland Ave, MC-0930, Chicago, IL 60637-1463; **Phone:** 773-702-1232; **Board Cert:** Internal Medicine 1980; Rheumatology 1982; **Med School:** Univ IL Coll Med 1976; **Resid:** Internal Medicine, Bethesda Naval Hosp 1980; **Fellow:** Rheumatology, Univ Chicago Hosps 1982; **Fac Appt:** Prof Med, Univ Chicago-Pritzker Sch Med

Ellman, Michael H MD [Rhu] - **Spec Exp:** Scleroderma; Lupus/SLE; Rheumatoid Arthritis; **Hospital:** Univ of Chicago Hosps; **Address:** Univ Chicago-Pritzker Sch Med, 5841 S Maryland Ave, MC-0930, Chicago, IL 60637-1463; **Phone:** 773-702-1226; **Board Cert:** Internal Medicine 1972; Rheumatology 1972; **Med School:** Univ IL Coll Med 1964; **Resid:** Internal Medicine, Michael Reese Hosp 1970; **Fellow:** Rheumatology, Univ Chicago Hosps 1972; **Fac Appt:** Prof Med, Univ Chicago-Pritzker Sch Med

Fischbein, Lewis C MD [Rhu] - **Spec Exp:** Rheumatoid Arthritis; Lupus/SLE; Hypertension; **Hospital:** Barnes-Jewish Hosp; **Address:** One Barnes-Jewish Hospital Plaza, East Pavilion, Ste 16422, St. Louis, MO 63110; **Phone:** 314-367-9595; **Board Cert:** Internal Medicine 1977; Rheumatology 1980; **Med School:** Washington Univ, St Louis 1974; **Resid:** Internal Medicine, Barnes Jewish Hosp 1977; **Fellow:** Rheumatology, Barnes Jewish Hosp 1979; **Fac Appt:** Assoc Prof Med, Washington Univ, St Louis

Hoffman, Gary S MD [Rhu] - **Spec Exp:** Vasculitis; Wegener's Granulomatosis; **Hospital:** Cleveland Clin Fdn (page 57); **Address:** Gary S Hoffman, MD, 9500 Euclid Ave, Ste Desk A50, Cleveland, OH 44195; **Phone:** 216-445-6996; **Board Cert:** Internal Medicine 1976; Rheumatology 1978; **Med School:** Med Coll VA 1971; **Resid:** Internal Medicine, Dartmouth-Hitchcock Med Ctr 1973; **Fellow:** Rheumatology, Dartmouth-Hitchcock Med Ctr 1974; **Fac Appt:** Prof Med, Ohio State Univ

Houk, John L MD [Rhu] - **Hospital:** Univ Hosp - Cincinnati, Christ Hospital; **Address:** Christ Hosp Office Bldg, 2123 Auburn Ave, Ste 630, Cincinnati, OH 45219; **Phone:** 513-585-1970; **Board Cert:** Internal Medicine 1972; **Med School:** Univ Cincinnati 1965; **Resid:** Internal Medicine, Univ Hosp 1971; **Fellow:** Rheumatology, Univ Hosp 1973; **Fac Appt:** Prof Med, Univ Cincinnati

Katz, Robert S MD [Rhu] - **Spec Exp:** Rheumatoid Arthritis; Lupus/SLE; Fibromyalgia; **Hospital:** Rush Univ Med Ctr; **Address:** 1725 W Harrison St, Ste 1039, Chicago, IL 60612-3841; **Phone:** 312-942-2159; **Board Cert:** Internal Medicine 1975; Rheumatology 1976; **Med School:** Univ MD Sch Med 1970; **Resid:** Internal Medicine, Washington Univ Med Ctr 1972; **Fellow:** Rheumatology, Johns Hopkins Hosp 1976; **Fac Appt:** Assoc Prof Med, Rush Med Coll

Klearman, Micki MD [Rhu] - **Spec Exp:** Arthritis; Lupus/SLE; Vasculitis; **Hospital:** Barnes-Jewish Hosp; **Address:** One Barnes-Jewish Hospital Plaza, East Pavilion, Ste 16422, St Louis, MO 63110; **Phone:** 314-367-9595; **Board Cert:** Internal Medicine 1985; Rheumatology 1988; **Med School:** Washington Univ, St Louis 1981; **Resid:** Internal Medicine, Jewish Hosp 1985; **Fellow:** Rheumatology, Wash Univ 1987; **Fac Appt:** Assoc Clin Prof Med, Washington Univ, St Louis

Lawry, George V MD [Rhu] - **Hospital:** Univ Iowa Hosp & Clinics; **Address:** Univ Iowa Hosp & Clins, Dept Rheumatology, 200 Hawkins Drive, rm C31-GGH, Iowa City, IA 52242-1009; **Phone:** 319-356-1777; **Board Cert:** Internal Medicine 1978; Rheumatology 1982; **Med School:** Johns Hopkins Univ 1975; **Resid:** Internal Medicine, Mass Genl Hosp 1977; Internal Medicine, Stanford Hosp 1978; **Fellow:** Rheumatology, Wadsworth VA-UCLA Med Ctr 1981; **Fac Appt:** Clin Prof Med, Univ Iowa Coll Med

Luggen, Michael MD [Rhu] - **Hospital:** Univ Hosp - Cincinnati, Christ Hospital; **Address:** Christ Hosp Office Bldg, 2123 Auburn Ave, Ste 630, Cincinnati, OH 45219; **Phone:** 513-585-1970; **Board Cert:** Internal Medicine 1978; Rheumatology 1982; **Med School:** Columbia P&S 1974; **Resid:** Internal Medicine, Cinn Genl Hosp 1977; **Fellow:** Rheumatology, Univ Cincinnati 1982; **Fac Appt:** Prof Med, Univ Cincinnati

Luthra, Harvinder Singh MD [Rhu] - **Spec Exp:** Rheumatoid Arthritis; Ankylosing Spondylitis; Relapsing Polychondritis; **Hospital:** St Mary's Hosp - Rochester, Rochester Meth Hosp; **Address:** Mayo Clinic, 200 First St SW, Rochester, MN 55905-0002; **Phone:** 507-266-4439; **Board Cert:** Internal Medicine 1973; Rheumatology 2002; **Med School:** India 1967; **Resid:** Ophthalmology, Christian Med Coll; Internal Medicine, Mount Sinai Hosp 1972; **Fellow:** Rheumatology, Mayo Grad Sch 1974; **Fac Appt:** Prof Med, Mayo Med Sch

McCune, W Joseph MD [Rhu] - **Spec Exp:** Lupus/SLE; Rheumatoid Arthritis; **Hospital:** Univ Michigan Hlth Sys; **Address:** Univ Mich, Dept Rheum, 1500 E Med Ctr, rm 3918 Taubman Ctr, Ann Arbor, MI 48109-0358; **Phone:** 734-647-5900; **Board Cert:** Internal Medicine 1978; Rheumatology 1982; **Med School:** Univ Cincinnati 1975; **Resid:** Internal Medicine, Univ Mich Hosps 1976; Rheumatology, Brigham Womens Hosp 1978; **Fellow:** Rheumatology, Brigham Womens Hosp 1981; **Fac Appt:** Prof Med, Univ Mich Med Sch

Michalska, Margaret MD [Rhu] - **Spec Exp:** Rheumatoid Arthritis; Connective Tissue Disorders; Osteoporosis; **Hospital:** Rush Univ Med Ctr; **Address:** 1725 W Harrison St, Ste 1017, Chicago, IL 60612-3841; **Phone:** 312-563-2800; **Board Cert:** Internal Medicine 1988; Rheumatology 2000; **Med School:** Poland 1979; **Resid:** Internal Medicine, Hines VA Hosp 1988; **Fellow:** Biochemistry, Nortwestern Univ 1985; Rheumatology, Rush-Presby-St Lukes Med Ctr 1990; **Fac Appt:** Assoc Prof Med, Rush Med Coll

Moder, Kevin G MD [Rhu] - **Spec Exp:** Rheumatoid Arthritis; Lupus/SLE; **Hospital:** Mayo Med Ctr & Clin - Rochester; **Address:** Mayo Clinic, Div Rheumatology, 200 First St SW, Rochester, MN 55905-0002; **Phone:** 507-284-4550; **Board Cert:** Internal Medicine 2000; Rheumatology 2000; **Med School:** Univ MO-Columbia Sch Med 1987; **Resid:** Internal Medicine, Mayo Clinic 1990; **Fellow:** Rheumatology, Mayo Clinic 1993; **Fac Appt:** Asst Prof Med, Mayo Med Sch

Moskowitz, Roland MD [Rhu] - **Spec Exp:** Osteoarthritis; Connective Tissue Disorders; **Hospital:** Univ Hosps Case Med Ctr; **Address:** Parkway Med Ctr, 3609 Park East Drive, Ste 307N, Beachwod, OH 44122; **Phone:** 216-591-1443; **Board Cert:** Internal Medicine 1961; Rheumatology 1974; **Med School:** Temple Univ 1953; **Resid:** Internal Medicine, Mayo Clinic 1955; **Fellow:** Internal Medicine, Mayo Clinic 1960; **Fac Appt:** Prof Med, Case West Res Univ

Pope, Richard M MD [Rhu] - **Spec Exp:** Rheumatoid Arthritis; Sjogren's Syndrome; Psoriatic Arthritis; **Hospital:** Northwestern Meml Hosp; **Address:** 675 N St Clair, Ste 14-100, Chicago, IL 60611-5966; **Phone:** 312-695-8628; **Board Cert:** Internal Medicine 1973; Rheumatology 1976; Clinical & Laboratory Immunology 1986; **Med School:** Loyola Univ-Stritch Sch Med 1970; **Resid:** Internal Medicine, Michael Reese Hosp 1972; **Fellow:** Rheumatology, Univ Wash Med Ctr 1974; **Fac Appt:** Prof Med, Northwestern Univ

Warner, Ann E MD [Rhu] - **Hospital:** St Luke's Hosp of Kansas City; **Address:** 4330 Wornall St, Ste 40, Kansas City, MO 64111-3210; **Phone:** 816-531-0930; **Board Cert:** Internal Medicine 1986; Rheumatology 1988; Allergy & Immunology 1999; **Med School:** Univ Kans 1983; **Resid:** Internal Medicine, St Luke's Hosp 1986; **Fellow:** Rheumatology, Univ Kansas Med Ctr 1989; **Fac Appt:** Asst Clin Prof Med, Univ MO-Kansas City

Rheumatology

Great Plains and Mountains

Arend, William P MD [Rhu] - **Spec Exp:** Arthritis; Rheumatoid Arthritis; **Hospital:** Univ Colorado Hosp; **Address:** Outpatient Pavilion, 1635 N Ursula St, Aurora, CO 80010; **Phone:** 720-848-1940; **Board Cert:** Internal Medicine 1971; Rheumatology 1980; **Med School:** Columbia P&S 1964; **Resid:** Internal Medicine, Univ Washington Hosp 1969; **Fellow:** Rheumatology, Univ Washington Hosp 1971; **Fac Appt:** Prof Med, Univ Colorado

O'Dell, James R MD [Rhu] - **Spec Exp:** Osteoarthritis; Rheumatoid Arthritis; **Hospital:** Nebraska Med Ctr; **Address:** 983025 Nebraska Med Ctr, Omaha, NE 68198-3025; **Phone:** 402-559-4015; **Board Cert:** Internal Medicine 1980; Rheumatology 1984; **Med School:** Univ Nebr Coll Med 1977; **Resid:** Internal Medicine, Univ Nebraska Med Ctr 1981; **Fellow:** Rheumatology, Univ Colorado 1984; **Fac Appt:** Prof Med, Univ Nebr Coll Med

West, Sterling MD [Rhu] - **Spec Exp:** Lupus/SLE; Vasculitis; Osteoporosis; **Hospital:** Univ Colorado Hosp; **Address:** Univ Colo Hlth Sci Ctr, 4200 E Ninth Ave, Box B 115, Denver, CO 80262-0001; **Phone:** 303-724-7610; **Board Cert:** Internal Medicine 1979; Rheumatology 1982; **Med School:** Emory Univ 1976; **Resid:** Internal Medicine, Fitzsimons Army Med Ctr 1979; **Fellow:** Rheumatology, Walter Reed Army Med Ctr 1981; **Fac Appt:** Prof Med, Univ Colorado

Southwest

Arnett Jr, Frank C MD [Rhu] - **Spec Exp:** Reiter's Syndrome; Spondylitis; Scleroderma; **Hospital:** Meml Hermann Hosp - Houston; **Address:** Hermann Prof Bldg, 6410 Fannin St, Ste 1100, Houston, TX 77030-5302; **Phone:** 832-325-7191; **Board Cert:** Internal Medicine 1972; Rheumatology 1976; Clinical & Laboratory Immunology 1990; **Med School:** Univ Cincinnati 1968; **Resid:** Internal Medicine, Johns Hopkins Hosp 1970; **Fellow:** Rheumatology, Johns Hopkins Hosp 1972; **Fac Appt:** Prof Med, Univ Tex, Houston

Chang-Miller, April MD [Rhu] - **Spec Exp:** Connective Tissue Disorders; Spondyloarthropathies; **Hospital:** Mayo Clin Hosp - Scottsdale; **Address:** Mayo Clinic, Div Rheumatology, 13400 E Shea Blvd, Scottsdale, AZ 85259; **Phone:** 480-301-4342; **Board Cert:** Internal Medicine 1986; Rheumatology 2000; **Med School:** Yale Univ 1983; **Resid:** Internal Medicine, Mayo Clinic 1985; **Fellow:** Rheumatology, Mayo Clinic 1989; Biochemical and Molecular Biology, Mayo Clinic 1990; **Fac Appt:** Asst Prof Med, Mayo Med Sch

Davis, William Eugene MD [Rhu] - **Spec Exp:** Lupus/SLE; Rheumatoid Arthritis; Gout; **Hospital:** Ochsner Fdn Hosp; **Address:** Ochsner Clinic, Rheum, 1514 Jefferson Hwy, CA5, New Orleans, LA 70121-2483; **Phone:** 504-842-3920; **Board Cert:** Internal Medicine 1987; Rheumatology 1988; **Med School:** Louisiana State Univ 1983; **Resid:** Internal Medicine, Ochsner Fdn Hosp 1986; **Fellow:** Rheumatology, Univ Michigan 1988

Lindsey, Stephen M MD [Rhu] - **Spec Exp:** Osteoporosis; Lupus/SLE; **Hospital:** Baton Rouge Gen Med Ctr; **Address:** 9001 Summa Ave, Baton Rouge, LA 70809; **Phone:** 225-761-5500; **Board Cert:** Internal Medicine 1975; Rheumatology 1980; **Med School:** Louisiana State Univ 1972; **Resid:** Internal Medicine, Letterman AMC 1975; **Fellow:** Rheumatology, Walter Reed AMC 1979

Lipstate, James M MD [Rhu] - **Spec Exp:** Arthritis; Osteoporosis; **Hospital:** Our Lady of Lourdes Reg Med Ctr - Lafayette, Lafayette Genl Med Ctr; **Address:** 401 Audubon Blvd, Ste 102B, Lafayette, LA 70503; **Phone:** 337-237-7801; **Board Cert:** Internal Medicine 1983; Rheumatology 1986; **Med School:** Tulane Univ 1980; **Resid:** Internal Medicine, Univ Alabama Hosp 1983; **Fellow:** Rheumatology, Univ Alabama Hosp 1986; **Fac Appt:** Asst Clin Prof Med, Louisiana State Univ

Mayes, Maureen D MD/PhD [Rhu] - **Spec Exp:** Scleroderma; **Hospital:** Meml Hermann Hosp - Houston, LBJ General Hosp; **Address:** Univ Tex Hlth Sci Ctr, Div Rheum, 6431 Fannin, rm 5.270, Houston, TX 77030-1501; **Phone:** 832-325-7191; **Board Cert:** Internal Medicine 1980; Rheumatology 1982; **Med School:** Eastern VA Med Sch 1976; **Resid:** Internal Medicine, Cleveland Clinic Fnd 1979; **Fellow:** Rheumatology, Cleveland Clinic Fnd 1981; **Fac Appt:** Prof Med, Univ Tex, Houston

Sessoms, Sandra Lee MD [Rhu] - **Spec Exp:** Arthritis; Lupus/SLE; Autoimmune Disease; **Hospital:** Methodist Hosp - Houston, St Luke's Episcopal Hosp - Houston; **Address:** Meth Hosp, Div Rheum, 6560 Fannin St, Smith Twr, Ste 2500, Houston, TX 77030; **Phone:** 713-441-9000; **Board Cert:** Internal Medicine 1981; Rheumatology 1984; **Med School:** Baylor Coll Med 1978; **Resid:** Internal Medicine, Baylor Coll Med 1979; **Fellow:** Rheumatology, Baylor Coll Med 1983; **Fac Appt:** Assoc Prof Med, Baylor Coll Med

West Coast and Pacific

Bobrove, Arthur M MD [Rhu] - **Spec Exp:** Psoriatic Arthritis; Ankylosing Spondylitis; Sjogren's Syndrome; **Hospital:** Stanford Univ Med Ctr; **Address:** 795 El Camino Real, Palo Alto, CA 94301-2302; **Phone:** 650-853-2972; **Board Cert:** Internal Medicine 1972; Rheumatology 1976; **Med School:** Temple Univ 1967; **Resid:** Internal Medicine, Univ Mich Hosp 1969; Internal Medicine, Univ Mich Hosp 1972; **Fellow:** Immunology, Stanford Univ Hosp 1974; **Fac Appt:** Clin Prof Med, Stanford Univ

Clements, Philip J MD [Rhu] - **Spec Exp:** Scleroderma; Raynaud's Disease; **Hospital:** UCLA Med Ctr; **Address:** UCLA Sch Med, Rehab 32-59, 1000 Veteran Ave, Los Angeles, CA 90095-1670; **Phone:** 310-825-8414; **Board Cert:** Internal Medicine 1972; Rheumatology 1974; **Med School:** Indiana Univ 1965; **Resid:** Internal Medicine, Cedars-Sinai Med Ctr 1971; **Fellow:** Rheumatology, UCLA Med Ctr 1974; **Fac Appt:** Prof Med, UCLA

Ehresmann, Glenn Richard MD [Rhu] - **Hospital:** USC Univ Hosp - R K Eamer Med Plz; **Address:** 1520 San Pablo St, Ste 1000, Los Angeles, CA 90033; **Phone:** 323-442-5100; **Board Cert:** Internal Medicine 1977; Rheumatology 1978; **Med School:** UC Irvine 1973; **Resid:** Internal Medicine, LAC-USC Med Ctr 1978; **Fellow:** Rheumatology, LAC-USC Med Ctr 1978

Gardner, Gregory MD [Rhu] - **Hospital:** Univ Wash Med Ctr; **Address:** Univ Washington Med Ctr, Div Rheumatology, 1959 NE Pacific St, Box 356166, Seattle, WA 98195; **Phone:** 206-598-4615; **Board Cert:** Internal Medicine 1987; Rheumatology 2001; **Med School:** Baylor Coll Med 1984; **Resid:** Internal Medicine, North Carolina Meml Hosp 1987; **Fellow:** Rheumatology, UCSD Med Ctr 1989

Gershwin, Merrill Eric MD [Rhu] - **Spec Exp:** Allergy; Rheumatoid Arthritis; **Hospital:** UC Davis Med Ctr; **Address:** UC Davis Sch Med, Div Rheum, 451 E Health Sciences Drive, Ste 6510, Davis, CA 95616; **Phone:** 530-752-2884; **Board Cert:** Internal Medicine 1974; Rheumatology 1976; Allergy & Immunology 1979; **Med School:** Stanford Univ 1971; **Resid:** Internal Medicine, Tufts-New Eng Med Ctr 1972; Allergy & Immunology, Tufts-New Eng Med Ctr 1973; **Fellow:** Rheumatology, Natl Inst Hlth 1975; Allergy & Immunology, Natl Inst Hlth 1977; **Fac Appt:** Prof Med, UC Davis

Hahn, Bevra H MD [Rhu] - **Spec Exp:** Lupus/SLE; Vasculitis; **Hospital:** UCLA Med Ctr; **Address:** 1000 Veteran Ave, rm 31-81, Los Angeles, CA 90095-0001; **Phone:** 310-825-2448; **Board Cert:** Internal Medicine 1970; Rheumatology 1972; **Med School:** Johns Hopkins Univ 1964; **Resid:** Internal Medicine, Washington Univ-Barnes Hosp 1966; **Fellow:** Rheumatology, Johns Hopkins Hosp 1969; **Fac Appt:** Prof Med, UCLA

Mease, Philip J MD [Rhu] - **Spec Exp:** Arthritis; Autoimmune Disease; Fibromyalgia; **Hospital:** Swedish Med Ctr - Seattle, Swedish Med Ctr Providence Campus; **Address:** 1101 Madison Ave Fl 10, Seattle, WA 98104; **Phone:** 206-386-2000; **Board Cert:** Internal Medicine 1980; Rheumatology 1982; **Med School:** Stanford Univ 1977; **Resid:** Internal Medicine, Univ Wash Med Ctr 1981; **Fellow:** Rheumatology, Univ Wash Med Ctr 1982; **Fac Appt:** Assoc Clin Prof Med, Univ Wash

Sack, Kenneth Edward MD [Rhu] - **Hospital:** UCSF Med Ctr; **Address:** 533 Parnassus Ave, Box 0326, San Francisco, CA 94143-0326; **Phone:** 415-353-2497; **Board Cert:** Internal Medicine 1973; Rheumatology 1978; **Med School:** Tufts Univ 1968; **Resid:** Internal Medicine, Rhode Island Hosp 1970; Internal Medicine, Univ Mich Hosp 1974; **Fellow:** Rheumatology, Univ Ala Hosp 1978; **Fac Appt:** Clin Prof Med, UCSF

Wallace, Daniel J MD [Rhu] - **Spec Exp:** Lupus/SLE; Rheumatoid Arthritis; Scleroderma; **Hospital:** Cedars-Sinai Med Ctr, UCLA Med Ctr; **Address:** 8737 Beverly Blvd, Ste 302, Los Angeles, CA 90048-1828; **Phone:** 310-652-0920; **Board Cert:** Internal Medicine 1978; Rheumatology 1982; **Med School:** USC Sch Med 1974; **Resid:** Internal Medicine, Cedars-Sinai Med Ctr 1977; **Fellow:** Rheumatology, UCLA Med Ctr 1979; **Fac Appt:** Clin Prof Med, UCLA

Wener, Mark MD [Rhu] - **Spec Exp:** Lupus/SLE; Vasculitis; Immunodeficiency Disorders; **Hospital:** Univ Wash Med Ctr; **Address:** Univ Washington Med Ctr, Div Rheumatology, 1959 NE Pacific St, Box 356166, Seattle, WA 98195; **Phone:** 206-598-4615; **Board Cert:** Internal Medicine 1978; Rheumatology 1980; Clinical & Laboratory Immunology 1986; **Med School:** Washington Univ, St Louis 1974; **Resid:** Internal Medicine, Univ Iowa Hosps 1978; **Fellow:** Rheumatology, Univ Iowa Hosp 1980; Immunology, Univ Wash 1981; **Fac Appt:** Assoc Prof Med, Univ Wash

Wofsy, David MD [Rhu] - **Spec Exp:** Lupus/SLE; **Hospital:** UCSF Med Ctr, VA Med Ctr - San Francisco; **Address:** 533 Parnassus Ave, Box 0633, San Francisco, CA 94143; **Phone:** 415-750-2104; **Board Cert:** Internal Medicine 1977; Rheumatology 1980; **Med School:** UCSD 1974; **Resid:** Internal Medicine, UCSF Hosps 1977; **Fellow:** Rheumatology, UCSF 1979; **Fac Appt:** Prof Med, UCSF

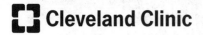
Rheumatic and Immunologic Diseases

Cleveland Clinic's Department of Rheumatic and Immunologic Diseases has a long-standing commitment to excellence and innovation in the research and care of patients with illnesses such as arthritis, osteoporosis and vasculitis. For the past several years, *U.S.News & World Report* has consistently ranked it among the nation's top five rheumatology programs.

Arthritis

Arthritis is a general term which describes inflammation in joints, characterized by redness, warmth, swelling and pain. Arthritis is a general term for more than 100 diseases. Some of the most common treated at the Department of Rheumatic and Immunologic Diseases include rheumatoid arthritis and osteoarthritis.

Osteoporosis

Cleveland Clinic's Center for Osteoporosis and Metabolic Bone Diseases is devoted to the evaluation and treatment of patients with osteoporosis and other forms of diseases that affect bones. The Center's goal is to evaluate patients at an early stage to prevent the complications of osteoporosis as well as additional disease manifestations.

Vasculitis

Cleveland Clinic's Center for Vasculitis Care and Research aims to ensure the best possible care for patients with vasculitis, discover the causes of these diseases and identify improved therapies. The department faculty has special expertise in vasculitis and established extensive collaborations with other departments of Cleveland Clinic to bring complementary skills to both service and research.

Autoimmune Disease

The Department of Rheumatic and Immunologic Diseases also provides expert care for a variety of illnesses for which arthritis may not be a major feature. These include conditions for which the body's immune defense system, in part, turns on itself and damages one's own body, thus the term autoimmune. Examples of such disorders include systemic lupus, scleroderma, myositis, polychondritis and vasculitis.

To schedule an appointment or for more information about the Cleveland Clinic Department of Rheumatic and Immunologic Diseases, call 800.890.2467 or visit www.clevelandclinic.org/arthritistopdocs.

Department of Rheumatic and Immunologic Diseases
9500 Euclid Avenue / W14 | Cleveland OH 44195

Special Service for Out-of-State Patients

Global Patient Services is a full-service department dedicated to meeting the needs and requirements of both out-of-state and international patients who receive their care at Cleveland Clinic. The National Center and the International Center, which make up global Patient Services, provide personalized concierge programs and services to welcome patients and add to their comfort before, during and after their stay. Call 800.223.2273, ext. 55580, or send an e-mail to medicalconcierge@ccf.org.

HOSPITAL
FOR
**SPECIAL
SURGERY**

HOSPITAL FOR SPECIAL SURGERY

Rheumatology

535 East 70th Street • New York, NY 10021
Physician Referral: 800.854.0071 • www.HSS.edu

FIRST IN ITS FIELD
Founded in 1863, Hospital for Special Surgery is the nation's largest specialty hospital for orthopedics and rheumatology.

GLOBAL LEADERS IN RHEUMATOLOGY
HSS Rheumatologists are international authorities and pioneering researchers in every known rheumatological and autoimmune condition and treatment. They are noted experts in correct diagnosis and innovative treatment of all autoimmune and inflammatory diseases including osteoarthritis, lupus, rheumatoid arthritis, scleroderma, gout, and pediatric rheumatoid arthritis.

MARY KIRKLAND CENTER FOR LUPUS RESEARCH
This world renowned center at HSS is dedicated to achieving new understanding of the molecular and cellular basis of systemic lupus erythematosus, develop new therapies, and improve patients' lives. Center sponsored research has led to landmark discoveries of the connection between lupus and heart disease as well as how pregnancy is affected by autoimmune disease.

THE BARBARA VOLCKER CENTER FOR WOMEN AND RHEUMATIC DISEASES
The first umbrella treatment center of its kind brings together doctors and scientists to focus on key issues such as mobility, chronic pain, pregnancy, and bone issues in women with rheumatic diseases, including rheumatoid arthritis, systemic lupus erythematosus, osteoporosis, and scleroderma.

GOSDEN ROBINSON EARLY ARTHRITIS CENTER
New York's first Early Arthritis Center provides treatment plans and education on the disease modifying importance of early intervention in rheumatoid arthritis for patients and primary care physicians.

SCLERODERMA CENTER
Teams of clinical and basic researchers seek molecular clues leading to new treatments for the connective tissue disorder.

OSTEOPOROSIS PREVENTION CENTER
The first center of its kind in the nation, providing prevention, diagnosis and personalized treatment plans.

Top Ranked in Rheumatology & Orthopedics in the Northeast by
U.S. News & World Report
for 16 Years in a Row

A National Institutes of Health Core Center for Musculoskeletal Repair and Regeneration

Two-Time Winner of Nursing's Highest Honor: Magnet Status for Nursing Excellence

Winner of NY's First Patient Safety Award

#1 Knee-Hip Orthopedic Hospital in AARP *Modern Maturity*

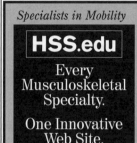

Specialists in Mobility

HSS.edu
Every Musculoskeletal Specialty.
One Innovative Web Site.

Conditions, Treatments, & Services:

- **Osteoarthritis**
- **Lupus**
- **Rheumatoid Arthritis**
- **Pediatric Rheumatoid Arthritis**
- **Scleroderma**
- **Osteoporosis**
- **Gout**
- **Early Detection of Autoimmune Disease & Cartilage Deterioration by Diagnostic Imaging**
- **Ankylosing Spondylitis**
- **Antiphospholipid Syndrome**
- **Childhood/Teenage Arthritis**
- **Bursitis**
- **Crohn's Disease**
- **Undifferentiated Connective Tissue Disease**
- **Lyme Disease**
- **Myositis**
- **Paget's Disease**
- **Sjogren's Syndrome**
- **Tendonitis**
- **Vasculitis**
- **Integrative Care Center with Acupuncture, Yoga, Massage & Pilates**
- **For more visit HSS.edu**

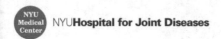

NYU**Hospital for Joint Diseases**

550 First Avenue (at 31st Street)
New York, NY 10016
Physician Referral:
(888)7-NYU-MED (888-769-8633
www.nyumc.org

301 East 17th Street (at 2nd Ave.)
New York, NY 10003
Physician Referral:
(888) HJD-D OCS (888-453-3627)
www.nyuhjd.org

RHEUMATOLOGY

The Division of Rheumatology at NYU Hospital for Joint Diseases (NYUHJD) is dedicated to the diagnosis and treatment of patients with rheumatic diseases and also focuses on autoimmune diseases. The department accomplishes its mission through a balanced combination of education, research, and clinical activities. The NYUHJD Division of Rheumatology is recognized by *U.S. News and World Report* as one of the top ten rheumatology programs in the country.

Patients receive care at the following centers:
Center for Arthritis and Autoimmunity
Staffed by a select group of leading academic researchers and physicians, it provides a comprehensive program for the prevention, diagnosis, and treatment of all rheumatologic conditions. The Center integrates patient care across a variety of disciplines. Patients receive complete rheumatologic evaluations, orthopaedic and neurological consultative services, sophisticated diagnostic testing, physiotherapy, and complementary medicine.
Osteoporosis Center
The Osteoporosis Center offers comprehensive care for the prevention, evaluation and treatment of osteoporosis. The Center includes a state-of-the-art bone densitometer which affords patients all-inclusive care for this condition.
Psoriatic Arthritis Center
The Psoriatic Arthritis Center is a collaborative effort with the Department of Dermatology at NYU. Patients are seen at the NYU Skin and Cancer Center for two half-day sessions on Monday and Wednesday and in the presence of both a rheumatologist and dermatologist with particular expertise in psoriatic arthritis.
Lupus Clinic
The Lupus Clinic is devoted solely to the treatment of patients with this multifaceted disease. Patients are seen regularly by rheumatologists, and have ready access to specialists in dermatology, nephrology, orthopaedics, and neurology, all of whom have expertise in systemic lupus erythematosus. Also offers expertise in pregnancy and hormonal issues.
Behcet's and Vasculitis Center
In close collaboration with the American Behcet's Disease Association, the only North American Behcet's Center was established for research and the evaluation and treatment of patients with Behcet's Syndrome and ANCA-assocciated vasculitis.
NYUHJD Infusion Center
Biological treatments for inflammatory arthritis and osteoporosis are administered in a dedicated unit where each patient has a personalized LCD television and support of a hospital based pharmacy.

Clinical Research Center

Basic science and medicine converge at the Peter D. Seligman Center for Advanced Therapeutics. The Center was established to promote new initiatives in clinical and translational investigation, focusing on developing improved treatments for rheumatic diseases. Researchers conduct protocols using a wide variety of new medications for the treatment of rheumatoid arthritis, osteoarthritis, systemic lupus erythematosus, and osteoporosis. The Seligman Center is a satellite of the NYU Department of Medicine NIH-funded General Clinical Research Center (GCRC).

Sports Medicine

a subspecialty of Internal Medicine, Family Practice, Pediatrics, or Orthopaedics

A specialist trained to be responsible for continuous care in the field of sports medicine, not only for the enhancement of health and fitness, but also for the prevention of injury and illness. A sports medicine physician must have knowledge and experience in the promotion of wellness and the prevention of injury. Knowledge about special areas of medicine such as exercise physiology, biomechanics, nutrition, psychology, physical rehabilitation, epidemiology, physical evaluation, injuries (treatment and prevention and referral practice) and the role of exercise in promoting a healthy life style are essential to the practice of sports medicine. The sports medicine physician requires special education to provide the knowledge to improve the healthcare of the individual engaged in physical exercise (sports) whether as an individual or in team participation.

Training Required: Three years in internal medicine, family practice, or pediatrics or seven years in orthopaedics *plus* additional training and examination for certification in sports medicine.

For more information about the main specialties of these physicians, see **Internal Medicine, Family Practice, Pediatrics, Orthopaedics** section(s).

Sports Medicine

Micheli, Lyle J MD [SM] - **Spec Exp:** Pediatric Sports Medicine; Dance/Ballet Injuries; **Hospital:** Beth Israel Deaconess Med Ctr - Boston, Children's Hospital - Boston; **Address:** Chldns Hosp, Div Sports Medicine, 300 Longwood Ave, Boston, MA 02115-5737; **Phone:** 617-355-6028; **Board Cert:** Orthopaedic Surgery 1973; **Med School:** Harvard Med Sch 1966; **Resid:** Surgery, Univ Hosps 1968; Orthopaedic Surgery, Mass Genl Hosp/Chldns Hosp 1972; **Fellow:** Pediatric Orthopaedic Surgery, Orth Rsch Soc-Traveling Fell 1973; **Fac Appt:** Assoc Clin Prof OrS, Harvard Med Sch

Scheller, Arnold D MD [SM] - **Spec Exp:** Sports Injuries; Ankle & Knee Surgery; Shoulder Surgery; Joint Replacement; **Hospital:** New England Bapt Hosp; **Address:** 235 Cypress St, Ste 300, Brookline, MA 02445; **Phone:** 617-738-8642; **Board Cert:** Orthopaedic Surgery 1980; **Med School:** Rush Med Coll 1980; **Resid:** Orthopaedic Surgery, New England Hosp 1983; **Fac Appt:** Asst Clin Prof OrS, Tufts Univ

Mid Atlantic

Altchek, David MD [SM] - **Spec Exp:** Shoulder Surgery; Elbow Surgery; Knee Surgery; Arthroscopic Surgery; **Hospital:** Hosp For Special Surgery (page 60), NY-Presby Hosp/Weill Cornell (page 66); **Address:** Hospital for Special Surgery, 535 E 70th St, New York, NY 10021; **Phone:** 212-606-1909; **Board Cert:** Orthopaedic Surgery 2001; **Med School:** Cornell Univ-Weill Med Coll 1982; **Resid:** Orthopaedic Surgery, Hosp for Special Surg 1987; **Fellow:** Sports Medicine, Hosp for Special Surg 1988; **Fac Appt:** Assoc Prof OrS, Cornell Univ-Weill Med Coll

Hershman, Elliott MD [SM] - **Spec Exp:** Knee Injuries; Knee Surgery; Arthroscopic Surgery; **Hospital:** Lenox Hill Hosp (page 62); **Address:** 130 E 77th St Fl 7, New York, NY 10021-1851; **Phone:** 212-744-8114; **Board Cert:** Orthopaedic Surgery 1998; **Med School:** Univ Rochester 1979; **Resid:** Orthopaedic Surgery, Lenox Hill Hosp 1984; **Fellow:** Sports Medicine, Cleveland Clinic 1985

Levine, William MD [SM] - **Spec Exp:** Arthroscopic Surgery; Shoulder & Knee Injuries; **Hospital:** NY-Presby Hosp/Columbia (page 66); **Address:** 622 W 168th St Fl PH-11, New York, NY 10032; **Phone:** 212-305-0762; **Board Cert:** Orthopaedic Surgery 1999; **Med School:** Case West Res Univ 1990; **Resid:** Surgery, Beth Israel Hosp 1991; Orthopaedic Surgery, New Eng Med Ctr Hosps 1995; **Fellow:** Shoulder Surgery, Columbia-Presby Med Ctr 1996; Sports Medicine, Univ MD Med Ctr 1998; **Fac Appt:** Assoc Prof OrS, Columbia P&S

Maharam, Lewis G MD [SM] - **Spec Exp:** Running Injuries; Primary Care Sports Medicine; Knee Injuries; Shoulder Injuries; **Hospital:** Hosp For Joint Diseases (page 68), NYU Med Ctr (page 67); **Address:** 24 W 57th St, New York, NY 10019-3918; **Phone:** 212-765-5763; **Med School:** Emory Univ 1985; **Resid:** Internal Medicine, Danbury Hosp 1987; Internal Medicine, NY Infirm/Beekman Downtown 1989; **Fellow:** Sports Medicine, Pascack Valley Hosp 1990; **Fac Appt:** Asst Clin Prof OrS, NYU Sch Med

Metzl, Jordan D MD [SM] - **Spec Exp:** Adolescent Sports Medicine; Running Injuries; **Hospital:** Hosp For Special Surgery (page 60); **Address:** Hospital for Special Surgery, Sports Med, 535 E 70 St, New York, NY 10021-4872; **Phone:** 212-606-1678; **Board Cert:** Sports Medicine 2001; **Med School:** Univ MO-Columbia Sch Med 1993; **Resid:** Pediatrics, New England Med Ctr 1996; **Fellow:** Sports Medicine, Vanderbilt Univ Med Ctr 1996; Sports Medicine, Hosp Special Surgery 1997; **Fac Appt:** Asst Prof Ped, Cornell Univ-Weill Med Coll

Nisonson, Barton MD [SM] - **Spec Exp:** Knee Injuries; Shoulder & Knee Surgery; Sports Medicine; **Hospital:** Lenox Hill Hosp (page 62); **Address:** 130 E 77th St, New York, NY 10021-1851; **Phone:** 212-570-9120; **Board Cert:** Orthopaedic Surgery 1974; **Med School:** Columbia P&S 1966; **Resid:** Surgery, Columbia-Presby Med Ctr 1968; Orthopaedic Surgery, Columbia-Presby Med Ctr 1973

Plancher, Kevin D MD [SM] - **Spec Exp:** Shoulder Surgery; Elbow Surgery; Cartilage Damage & Transplant; Shoulder Replacement; **Hospital:** Beth Israel Med Ctr - Petrie Division, NY Westchester Sq Med Ctr; **Address:** 1160 Park Ave, New York, NY 10128; **Phone:** 212-876-5200; **Board Cert:** Orthopaedic Surgery 2004; Hand Surgery 2005; **Med School:** Georgetown Univ 1986; **Resid:** Orthopaedic Surgery, Mass Genl Hosp/Brigham & Womens Hosp 1991; **Fellow:** Hand Surgery, Indiana Hand Ctr 1993; Sports Medicine, Steadman-Hawkins Clinic 1994; **Fac Appt:** Assoc Clin Prof OrS, Albert Einstein Coll Med

Rodeo, Scott A MD [SM] - **Spec Exp:** Knee Injuries; Cartilage Damage; **Hospital:** Hosp For Special Surgery (page 60); **Address:** Hospital for Special Surgery, 535 E 70th St, New York, NY 10021; **Phone:** 212-606-1513; **Board Cert:** Orthopaedic Surgery 1998; **Med School:** Cornell Univ-Weill Med Coll 1989; **Resid:** Orthopaedic Surgery, Hosp Special Surgery 1994; **Fellow:** Sports Medicine, Hosp Special Surgery 1996; **Fac Appt:** Assoc Clin Prof OrS, Cornell Univ-Weill Med Coll

Southeast

Andrews, James R MD [SM] - **Spec Exp:** Shoulder Surgery; Elbow Surgery; Knee Surgery; **Hospital:** St Vincent's Hosp - Birmingham; **Address:** 806 St Vincents Drive, Women & Childrens Ctr, Ste 415, Birmingham, AL 35205; **Phone:** 205-939-3000; **Board Cert:** Orthopaedic Surgery 1974; **Med School:** Louisiana State Univ 1967; **Resid:** Orthopaedic Surgery, USPHS Hosp 1969; Orthopaedic Surgery, Touro Infirm-Tulane 1970; **Fellow:** Hand Surgery, VA Med Ctr; **Fac Appt:** Clin Prof OrS, Univ Ala

Garth Jr, William P MD [SM] - **Spec Exp:** Knee Ligament Reconstruction; Shoulder Reconstruction; **Hospital:** Univ of Ala Hosp at Birmingham, Children's Hospital - Birmingham; **Address:** Univ Alabama Birmingham - Sports Medicine, 1600 7th Ave S, Birmingham, AL 35233-1711; **Phone:** 205-934-1041; **Board Cert:** Orthopaedic Surgery 1980; **Med School:** Tulane Univ 1973; **Resid:** Surgery, Duke Univ Hosp 1975; Orthopaedic Surgery, Campbell Clinic 1979; **Fellow:** Sports Medicine, Sports Med Clinic 1984; **Fac Appt:** Prof OrS, Univ Ala

Speer, Kevin MD [SM] - **Spec Exp:** Shoulder Surgery; **Hospital:** Duke Health Raleigh; **Address:** 3404 Wake Forest Rd, Ste 201, Raleigh, NC 27609; **Phone:** 919-256-1511; **Board Cert:** Orthopaedic Surgery 2005; **Med School:** Johns Hopkins Univ 1985; **Resid:** Orthopaedic Surgery, Duke Univ Med Ctr 1991; **Fellow:** Sports Medicine, Hosp Special Surgery 1992; **Fac Appt:** Assoc Prof OrS, Duke Univ

Sports Medicine

Midwest

Cole, Brian J MD [SM] - **Spec Exp:** Cartilage Damage; Shoulder & Elbow Injuries; Knee Injuries; **Hospital:** Rush Univ Med Ctr; **Address:** 1725 W Harrison St, Ste 1063, Chicago, IL 60612-3841; **Phone:** 312-432-2381; **Board Cert:** Orthopaedic Surgery 1999; **Med School:** Univ Chicago-Pritzker Sch Med 1990; **Resid:** Orthopaedic Surgery, Hosp for Special Surgery 1996; **Fellow:** Sports Medicine, Univ Pittsburgh Med Ctr 1997; **Fac Appt:** Prof OrS, Rush Med Coll

Dimeff, Robert J MD [SM] - **Spec Exp:** Primary Care Sports Medicine; Nutrition; **Hospital:** Cleveland Clin Fdn (page 57); **Address:** Cleveland Clinic Fdn, 9500 Euclid Ave, Desk A41, Cleveland, OH 44195; **Phone:** 216-444-2185; **Board Cert:** Family Medicine 2003; Sports Medicine 2003; **Med School:** NE Ohio Univ 1985; **Resid:** Family Medicine, Presbyterian-St Lukes Med Ctr 1989; **Fellow:** Sports Medicine, Cleveland Clinic 1990; **Fac Appt:** Assoc Prof FMed, Ohio State Univ

Ho, Sherwin MD [SM] - **Spec Exp:** Shoulder & Knee Injuries; Arthroscopic Surgery; Cartilage Damage; **Hospital:** Univ of Chicago Hosps; **Address:** Univ Chicago, Dept Surgery, 5841 S Maryland Ave, MS 3079, Chicago, IL 60637-3079; **Phone:** 773-702-5978; **Board Cert:** Orthopaedic Surgery 1994; **Med School:** Univ Hawaii JA Burns Sch Med 1985; **Resid:** Orthopaedic Surgery, Univ Hawaii 1991; **Fellow:** Sports Medicine, Univ Chicago 1992; **Fac Appt:** Assoc Prof OrS, Univ Chicago-Pritzker Sch Med

McKeag, Douglas B MD [SM] - **Spec Exp:** Sports Medicine; Adolescent Sports Medicine; Preventive Medicine; **Hospital:** Indiana Univ Hosp, Methodist Hosp - Indianapolis; **Address:** Indiana Univ Sch Med, Dept Fam Med, 1110 W Michigan St, Ste 200, Indianapolis, IN 46202; **Phone:** 317-278-0360; **Board Cert:** Family Medicine 1996; Sports Medicine 1993; **Med School:** Mich State Univ 1973; **Resid:** Family Medicine, Grand Rapids Area Med Ctr 1976; **Fellow:** Family Medicine, Michigan St Univ 1977; Adolescent Medicine, Michigan St Univ 1977; **Fac Appt:** Prof FMed, Indiana Univ

Miniaci, Anthony MD [SM] - **Spec Exp:** Shoulder Reconstruction; Knee Reconstruction; Cartilage Damage; Knee Resurfacing; **Hospital:** Cleveland Clin Fdn (page 57); **Address:** Cleveland Clinic, 9500 Euclid Ave, MC A41, Cleveland, OH 44195; **Phone:** 216-444-2625; **Med School:** Univ Western Ontario 1982; **Resid:** Orthopaedic Surgery, Univ Western Ontario 1987; **Fellow:** Sports Medicine, Kerlan-Jobe Orthopaedic Clin 1989; Orthopaedic Research, Univ Calgary 1990

Noyes, Frank MD [SM] - **Spec Exp:** Knee Reconstruction; Knee Ligament/Meniscus Transplants; Knee Replacement; **Hospital:** Health Alliance of Greater Cincinnati, Deaconess Hosp - Cincinnati; **Address:** 10663 Montgomery Rd, Cincinnati, OH 45242-4469; **Phone:** 513-891-3200; **Board Cert:** Orthopaedic Surgery 1972; **Med School:** Geo Wash Univ 1966; **Resid:** Orthopaedic Surgery, Univ Mich Med Ctr 1971; **Fellow:** Biomedical Engineering, Aerospace Med Rsch Lab 1975; **Fac Appt:** Clin Prof OrS, Univ Cincinnati

Paletta, George A MD [SM] - **Spec Exp:** Ankle Surgery; Knee Surgery; **Hospital:** Barnes-Jewish West County Hosp; **Address:** The Orthopaedic Ctr of St Louis, 14825 N Outer Forty Rd, Chesterfield, MO 63017; **Phone:** 314-336-2555; **Board Cert:** Orthopaedic Surgery 1998; **Med School:** Johns Hopkins Univ 1988; **Resid:** Orthopaedic Surgery, Cornell Univ Med Ctr 1994; **Fellow:** Orthopaedic Surgery, Cleveland Clin Fnd 1995; **Fac Appt:** Assoc Prof OrS, Washington Univ, St Louis

Reider, Bruce MD [SM] - **Spec Exp:** Foot & Ankle Surgery; Shoulder Injuries; **Hospital:** Univ of Chicago Hosps; **Address:** Univ Chicago Sports Med, 5841 S Maryland Ave, MS 3079, Chicago, IL 60637; **Phone:** 773-702-6346; **Board Cert:** Orthopaedic Surgery 1992; **Med School:** Harvard Med Sch 1975; **Resid:** Orthopaedic Surgery, Hosp Special Surg 1980; Sports Medicine, Univ Wisc Med Ctr 1981; **Fellow:** Knee Surgery, Kantonsspital Bruderholz 1982; **Fac Appt:** Prof OrS, Univ Chicago-Pritzker Sch Med

Schwenk, Thomas L MD [SM] - **Spec Exp:** Primary Care Sports Medicine; **Hospital:** Univ Michigan Hlth Sys; **Address:** Womens Hosp, Dept of Family Med, 1500 E Med Ctr Drive, Ste L2003, Box 0239, Ann Arbor, MI 48109; **Phone:** 734-615-2688; **Board Cert:** Family Medicine 2003; Sports Medicine 2002; **Med School:** Univ Mich Med Sch 1975; **Resid:** Family Medicine, Univ Utah Affil Hosps 1978; **Fellow:** Family Medicine, Univ Utah Affil Hosps 1982; **Fac Appt:** Prof FMed, Univ Mich Med Sch

Shively, Robert A MD [SM] - **Spec Exp:** Ankle & Knee Surgery; Knee Replacement; Shoulder Surgery; **Hospital:** Barnes-Jewish Hosp, Barnes-Jewish West County Hosp; **Address:** Wash Univ Sch Med, Dept Orth Surg, 1020 N Mason Rd, St Louis, MO 63141; **Phone:** 314-996-8550; **Board Cert:** Orthopaedic Surgery 1981; **Med School:** Univ IL Coll Med 1969; **Resid:** Surgery, Carolinas Med Ctr Prgm 1971; Orthopaedic Surgery, St Louis Univ Sch Med 1979; **Fellow:** Sports Medicine, Univ Okla Hlth Scis Ctr-Presby Hosp 1980; **Fac Appt:** Asst Prof OrS, Washington Univ, St Louis

Southwest

Calmbach, Walter L MD [SM] - **Spec Exp:** Primary Care Sports Medicine; **Hospital:** Univ Hlth Sys - Univ Hosp; **Address:** Univ Texas Hlth Sci Ctr, 7703 Floyd Curl Drive, MSC-7795, San Antonio, TX 78229; **Phone:** 210-358-3930; **Board Cert:** Family Medicine 2005; Sports Medicine 2005; **Med School:** Univ Tex, San Antonio 1979; **Resid:** Family Medicine, Univ Hosp, S Texas Med Ctr 1983; **Fac Appt:** Assoc Prof FMed, Univ Tex, San Antonio

West Coast and Pacific

Fronek, Jan MD [SM] - **Spec Exp:** Knee Injuries; Shoulder Injuries; Arthroscopic Surgery; Rotator Cuff Surgery; **Hospital:** Scripps Meml Hosp - La Jolla; **Address:** Scripps Clinic, 10666 N Torrey Pines Rd, MS B4, La Jolla, CA 92037; **Phone:** 858-554-9753; **Board Cert:** Orthopaedic Surgery 1999; **Med School:** Univ Rochester 1978; **Resid:** Orthopaedic Surgery, UCSD Med Ctr 1984; **Fellow:** Sports Medicine, Hosp Special Surgery 1985

Gambardella, Ralph A MD [SM] - **Spec Exp:** Cartilage Restoration; Shoulder & Elbow Surgery; Knee Surgery; **Hospital:** Centinela Freeman Reg Med Ctr-Centinela, USC Univ Hosp - R K Eamer Med Plz; **Address:** Kerlan-Jobe Clinic, 6801 Park Terr, Ste 400, Los Angeles, CA 90045; **Phone:** 310-665-7200; **Board Cert:** Orthopaedic Surgery 1985; **Med School:** USC Sch Med 1977; **Resid:** Orthopaedic Surgery, USC Med Ctr 1982; **Fellow:** Sports Medicine, Southwestern Ortho Grp 1983; **Fac Appt:** Assoc Clin Prof S, USC Sch Med

Jobe, Frank Wilson MD [SM] - **Spec Exp:** Shoulder Surgery; Elbow Surgery; **Hospital:** Centinela Freeman Reg Med Ctr-Centinela; **Address:** 6801 Park Terr, Ste 400, Los Angeles, CA 90045; **Phone:** 310-665-7206; **Board Cert:** Orthopaedic Surgery 1968; **Med School:** Loma Linda Univ 1956; **Resid:** Orthopaedic Surgery, LAC Genl Hosp 1964; **Fac Appt:** Clin Prof OrS, USC Sch Med

Sports Medicine

Mirzayan, Raffy MD [SM] - **Spec Exp:** Fractures-Non Union; Cartilage Damage; Knee Injuries; **Hospital:** Kaiser Permanente Baldwin Pk Med Ctr; **Address:** Kaiser Permanente Med Ctr, Orthopaedics, 1011 Baldwin Park Blvd, Baldwin Park, CA 91706; **Phone:** 626-851-5256; **Board Cert:** Orthopaedic Surgery 2003; **Med School:** USC Sch Med 1995; **Resid:** Orthopaedic Surgery, LAC/USC Med Ctr 2000; **Fellow:** Sports Medicine, Kerlan Jobe Ortho Clinic 2001

Schechter, David L MD [SM] - **Spec Exp:** Pain-Back; Sports Injuries; Muscle Pain-Stress Related; **Hospital:** Cedars-Sinai Med Ctr, Olympia Med Ctr; **Address:** 8530 Wilshire Blvd, Ste 250, Beverly Hills, CA 90211; **Phone:** 310-657-0366; **Board Cert:** Sports Medicine 2003; Family Medicine 2001; **Med School:** NYU Sch Med 1984; **Resid:** Family Medicine, UCLA/Santa Monica Hosp 1987; **Fac Appt:** Assoc Clin Prof FMed, USC Sch Med

Cleveland Clinic

Sports Health

Cleveland Clinic Sports Health brings together top orthopaedic surgeons, primary care sports physicians, physician assistants, nurses, physical therapists, athletic trainers, exercise physiologists, and strength and conditioning specialists to get athletes back in the game. Leaders in their specialties, our physicians work to diagnose, treat and rehabilitate injuries so athletes can perform at their best.

Cleveland Clinic Sports Health treats athletes of all sports, ages and skill levels. We have been chosen to care for the major professional sports teams in Cleveland because of our care and treatment that is focused, one-on-one and state-of-the-art. This involves conditioning to become stronger and faster, maximizing abilities, preventing and treating injuries, and improving future performance.

As one of the largest sports health practices in the nation, Cleveland Clinic Sports Health provides a host of services to many of the world's top professional and amateur athletes.

We've provided the physicians for Cleveland's professional teams for more than 25 years. Currently, we are the team physicians for the Cleveland Browns, Cleveland Cavaliers and Cleveland Indians. Our experienced staff has treated athletes from the AHL, EPL (English Premier League), NBA, NCAA, NFL, NHL, MLB, MLS, PBA, U.S.A. Boxing, U.S.A. Hockey, U.S. Olympic Team and WNBA.

Our world-renowned team of physicians is trained in diagnosing and treating the unique problems associated with a high-performance athlete. They are involved in research every day to improve patient care and bring new treatments to the clinical setting.

Cleveland Clinic Sports Health offers specialized programs that focus on rehab, injury evaluation, injury prevention and strength and conditioning tailored to your sport. These programs include:

- Golf Performance Plus – designed for golfers of all ages and skill levels
- Jump Right – an eight week program designed to teach proper jumping and landing mechanics to help reduce the risk of serious knee injury.
- Optimal Runners Performance Program – Gait analysis, body comp testing, strength and flexibility testing, VO2 analysis, injury assessment, conditioning program
- Soccer Performance Program – conditioning programs, injury assessment and prevention
- Throw Right – A specialized baseball program designed to meet the needs of baseball athletes.

To schedule an appointment or for more information about Cleveland Clinic Sports Health call 800.890.2467 or visit www.clevelandclinic.org/sportstopdocs

Sports Health | 9500 Euclid Avenue / W14 | Cleveland OH 44195

Surgery

A surgeon manages a broad spectrum of surgical conditions affecting almost any area of the body. The surgeon establishes the diagnosis and provides the preoperative, operative and postoperative care to surgical patients and is usually responsible for the comprehensive management of the trauma victim and the critically ill surgical patient.

The surgeon uses a variety of diagnostic techniques, including endoscopy, for observing internal structures and may use specialized instruments during operative procedures. A general surgeon is expected to be familiar with the salient features of other surgical specialties in order to recognize problems in those areas and to know when to refer a patient to another specialist.

Training Required: Five years

For a description of the subspecialty **Hand Surgery**, **Pediatric Surgery** and **Vascular Surgery** see the corresponding section(s).

Surgery

New England

Baker, Christopher C MD [S] - **Spec Exp:** Trauma/Critical Care; Colon & Rectal Surgery; Hernia; **Hospital:** Beth Israel Deaconess Med Ctr - Boston; **Address:** Beth Israel Deaconess Med Ctr, Dept Surg, 110 Francis St, Ste 2G, Boston, MA 02215; **Phone:** 617-632-9929; **Board Cert:** Surgery 2002; Surgical Critical Care 1996; **Med School:** Harvard Med Sch 1974; **Resid:** Surgery, UCSF Med Ctr 1981; **Fellow:** Trauma, San Francisco Genl Hosp 1979; **Fac Appt:** Prof S, Harvard Med Sch

Becker, James MD [S] - **Spec Exp:** Inflammatory Bowel Disease; Gastrointestinal Cancer; Gastrointestinal Surgery; **Hospital:** Boston Med Ctr, Qunicy Med Ctr; **Address:** Boston Med Ctr, Dept Surg, 88 E Newton St, rm C500, Boston, MA 02118-2393; **Phone:** 617-638-8600; **Board Cert:** Surgery 1999; **Med School:** Case West Res Univ 1975; **Resid:** Surgery, Univ Utah Med Ctr 1980; **Fellow:** Research, Mayo Clinic 1982; **Fac Appt:** Prof S, Boston Univ

Brooks, David C MD [S] - **Spec Exp:** Gastrointestinal Surgery; **Hospital:** Brigham & Women's Hosp; **Address:** Brigham & Women's Hospital, Dept Surgery, 75 Francis St, ASB II Fl 3, Boston, MA 02115; **Phone:** 617-732-6337; **Board Cert:** Surgery 2003; **Med School:** Brown Univ 1976; **Resid:** Surgery, Brigham & Women's Hosp 1983; **Fac Appt:** Assoc Prof S, Harvard Med Sch

Cady, Blake MD [S] - **Spec Exp:** Breast Cancer; Thyroid Cancer; **Hospital:** Rhode Island Hosp, Women & Infants Hosp - Rhode Island; **Address:** 503 Eddy St, APC 435, Providence, RI 02903; **Phone:** 401-444-6158; **Board Cert:** Surgery 1966; **Med School:** Cornell Univ-Weill Med Coll 1957; **Resid:** Surgery, Boston City Hosp/Tufts 1959; Surgery, Boston City Hosp/Harvard 1965; **Fellow:** Surgery, NY Meml Cancer Hosp 1967; **Fac Appt:** Prof S, Brown Univ

Cioffi, William MD [S] - **Spec Exp:** Trauma; Cancer Surgery; **Hospital:** Rhode Island Hosp; **Address:** Rhode Island Hosp, Dept Surg, 2 Dudley St, Ste 470, Providence, RI 02905; **Phone:** 401-553-8348; **Board Cert:** Surgery 1995; Surgical Critical Care 1997; **Med School:** Univ VT Coll Med 1981; **Resid:** Surgery, Med Ctr Hosp VT 1986; **Fac Appt:** Prof S, Brown Univ

Eisenberg, Burton L MD [S] - **Spec Exp:** Breast Cancer; Melanoma; Sarcoma; **Hospital:** Dartmouth - Hitchcock Med Ctr; **Address:** Dartmouth-Hitchcock Med Ctr, Dept Surgery, One Medical Center Drive, Lebanon, NH 03756; **Phone:** 603-650-9479; **Board Cert:** Surgery 1999; **Med School:** Univ Tenn Coll Med, Memphis 1974; **Resid:** Surgery, Wilford Hall USAF Med Ctr 1979; **Fellow:** Surgical Oncology, Meml Sloan-Kettering Cancer Ctr 1981; **Fac Appt:** Prof S, Dartmouth Med Sch

Hebert, James C MD [S] - **Spec Exp:** Biliary Surgery; Colon & Rectal Surgery; **Hospital:** FAHC - Med Ctr Campus; **Address:** Fletcher Allen Hlth Care, 111 Colchester Ave, Burlington, VT 05401; **Phone:** 802-847-3344; **Board Cert:** Surgery 2000; **Med School:** Univ VT Coll Med 1977; **Resid:** Surgery, Med Ctr Hosp 1982; **Fac Appt:** Prof S, Univ VT Coll Med

Hughes, Kevin S MD [S] - **Spec Exp:** Breast Cancer; Ovarian Cancer; **Hospital:** Mass Genl Hosp; **Address:** Massachusetts General Hosp, Dept Surgery, Wang Bldg Fl 2 - rm 240, Boston, MA 02114; **Phone:** 617-724-4800; **Board Cert:** Surgery 1993; **Med School:** Dartmouth Med Sch 1979; **Resid:** Surgery, Mercy Hosp 1984; **Fellow:** Surgical Oncology, National Cancer Inst 1985; **Fac Appt:** Assoc Prof S, Harvard Med Sch

Iglehart, J Dirk MD [S] - **Spec Exp:** Breast Cancer; **Hospital:** Brigham & Women's Hosp, Dana-Farber Cancer Inst; **Address:** Brigham & Women's Hospital, 75 Francis St, Surgical Oncology, Smith 822, Boston, MA 02115; **Phone:** 617-632-5178; **Board Cert:** Surgery 2005; **Med School:** Harvard Med Sch 1975; **Resid:** Surgery, Duke Univ Med Ctr 1981; Thoracic Surgery, Duke Univ Med Ctr 1984; **Fac Appt:** Prof S, Harvard Med Sch

Jenkins, Roger L MD [S] - **Spec Exp:** Transplant-Liver; Liver & Biliary Cancer; Biliary Surgery; **Hospital:** Lahey Clin, Children's Hospital - Boston; **Address:** Lahey Clin, Dept Hepatobiliary Surg, 41 Mall Rd, Burlington, MA 01805; **Phone:** 781-744-2500; **Board Cert:** Surgery 2005; **Med School:** Univ VT Coll Med 1977; **Resid:** Surgery, New Eng Deaconess Hosp 1982; **Fellow:** Cardiovascular Surgery, Deaconess Hosp 1983; Transplant Surgery, Univ Pittsburgh Hosp 1983; **Fac Appt:** Prof S, Tufts Univ

Krag, David MD [S] - **Spec Exp:** Sentinel Node Surgery; Breast Cancer; **Hospital:** FAHC - UHC Campus; **Address:** Univ Vermont Coll Med, Dept Surgery, 89 Beaumont Ave, Given Bldg - E309C, Burlington, VT 05405; **Phone:** 802-656-5830; **Board Cert:** Surgery 1996; **Med School:** Loyola Univ-Stritch Sch Med 1980; **Resid:** Surgery, UC Davis Med Ctr 1983; **Fellow:** Surgical Oncology, UCLA Med Ctr 1984; **Fac Appt:** Assoc Prof S, Univ VT Coll Med

Lipkowitz, George S MD [S] - **Spec Exp:** Transplant-Kidney; **Hospital:** Baystate Med Ctr; **Address:** 208 Ashley Ave, West Springfield, MA 01089; **Phone:** 413-747-4170 x151; **Board Cert:** Surgery 1996; **Med School:** SUNY Downstate 1980; **Resid:** Surgery, SUNY Kings Co Hosp 1985; **Fellow:** Transplant Surgery, SUNY Hlth Scis Ctr 1986; **Fac Appt:** Assoc Prof S, Tufts Univ

Ryan, Colleen MD [S] - **Spec Exp:** Burn Care; Toxic Epidermal Neurolysis; Wound Healing/Care; **Hospital:** Mass Genl Hosp, Boston Shriners Hosp; **Address:** Burns & Surg Crit Care, 55 Fruit St GRB Bldg - Ste 1303, Boston, MA 02114-2621; **Phone:** 617-726-3712; **Board Cert:** Surgery 1999; Surgical Critical Care 2003; **Med School:** Georgetown Univ 1982; **Resid:** Surgery, NE Deaconess Hosp 1988; **Fellow:** Hepatology, Hammersmith Hosp 1986; Burn Surgery, Mass Genl Hosp 1989; **Fac Appt:** Assoc Prof S, Harvard Med Sch

Salem, Ronald R MD [S] - **Spec Exp:** Cancer Surgery; Liver & Biliary Surgery; Gastrointestinal Cancer; **Hospital:** Yale - New Haven Hosp; **Address:** Yale Univ Sch Med, Dept Surg, 330 Cedar St, TMP 202, New Haven, CT 06520-8062; **Phone:** 203-785-3577; **Board Cert:** Surgery 2000; **Med School:** Zimbabwe 1978; **Resid:** Surgery, Hammersmith Hosp 1985; Surgery, New England Deaconess Hosp 1989; **Fac Appt:** Assoc Prof S, Yale Univ

Shikora, Scott A MD [S] - **Spec Exp:** Obesity/Bariatric Surgery; Laparoscopic Abdominal Surgery; Minimally Invasive Bariatric Surgery; **Hospital:** Tufts-New England Med Ctr; **Address:** New England Medical Ctr, 750 Washington St, Box NEMC 900, Boston, MA 02111; **Phone:** 617-636-6093; **Board Cert:** Surgery 2001; **Med School:** Columbia P&S 1985; **Resid:** Surgery, New England Deaconess Hosp 1991; **Fellow:** Nutrition & Metabolism, New England Deaconess Hos 1989; **Fac Appt:** Prof S, Tufts Univ

Smith, Barbara Lynn MD/PhD [S] - **Spec Exp:** Breast Cancer; **Hospital:** Mass Genl Hosp; **Address:** Mass Genl Hosp, 55 Fruit St, Yawkey - 9A, Boston, MA 02114; **Phone:** 617-724-4800; **Board Cert:** Surgery 2000; **Med School:** Harvard Med Sch 1983; **Resid:** Surgery, Brigham & Women's Hosp 1989; **Fac Appt:** Asst Prof S, Harvard Med Sch

Sutton, John E MD [S] - **Spec Exp:** Esophageal Cancer; Liver & Biliary Surgery; Pancreatic Cancer; **Hospital:** Dartmouth - Hitchcock Med Ctr; **Address:** One Medical Center Drive, Lebanon, NH 03756; **Phone:** 603-650-8022; **Board Cert:** Surgery 2001; Surgical Critical Care 1995; **Med School:** Georgetown Univ 1974; **Resid:** Surgery, Dartmouth-Hitchcock Med Ctr 1981; **Fellow:** Surgical Critical Care, Dartmouth-Hitchcock Med Ctr 1983; **Fac Appt:** Prof S, Dartmouth Med Sch

Tanabe, Kenneth K MD [S] - **Spec Exp:** Liver Cancer; Colon & Rectal Cancer; Melanoma; **Hospital:** Mass Genl Hosp, Newton - Wellesley Hosp; **Address:** Mass General Hosp, Div Surgical Oncology, 55 Fruit St, Yawkey 7.924, Boston, MA 02114; **Phone:** 617-724-3868; **Board Cert:** Surgery 2000; **Med School:** UCSD 1985; **Resid:** Surgery, New York Hosp-Cornell 1990; **Fellow:** Surgical Oncology, MD Anderson Cancer Ctr 1993; **Fac Appt:** Assoc Prof S, Harvard Med Sch

Udelsman, Robert MD [S] - **Spec Exp:** Parathyroid Cancer; Adrenal Tumors; Thyroid Cancer; **Hospital:** Yale - New Haven Hosp; **Address:** Yale School Medicine, Chair of Surgery, 789 Howard Ave FMB Bldg - rm 102, New Haven, CT 06511; **Phone:** 203-785-2697; **Board Cert:** Surgery 1999; **Med School:** Geo Wash Univ 1981; **Resid:** Surgery, Natl Inst Hlth 1986; Surgery, Johns Hopkins Hosp 1989; **Fellow:** Gastrointestinal Surgery, Johns Hopkins Hosp 1990; **Fac Appt:** Prof S, Yale Univ

Ward, Barbara MD [S] - **Spec Exp:** Breast Cancer; Breast Disease; **Hospital:** Greenwich Hosp; **Address:** 77 Lafayette Pl, Ste 301, Greenwich, CT 06830-5426; **Phone:** 203-863-4250; **Board Cert:** Surgery 2002; **Med School:** Temple Univ 1983; **Resid:** Surgery, Yale-New Haven Hosp 1990; **Fellow:** Surgical Oncology, Natl Cancer Inst 1987; **Fac Appt:** Assoc Clin Prof S, Yale Univ

Warshaw, Andrew L MD [S] - **Spec Exp:** Pancreatic Cancer; Pancreatic Surgery; Liver Cancer; **Hospital:** Mass Genl Hosp; **Address:** Mass Genl Hosp, Dept Surg, 55 Fruit St, WHT 506, Boston, MA 02114-2696; **Phone:** 617-726-8254; **Board Cert:** Surgery 1971; **Med School:** Harvard Med Sch 1963; **Resid:** Surgery, Mass Genl Hosp 1971; **Fellow:** Internal Medicine, Mass Genl Hosp 1970; **Fac Appt:** Prof S, Harvard Med Sch

Zinner, Michael MD [S] - **Spec Exp:** Colon & Rectal Cancer; Gastrointestinal Surgery; Pancreatic Cancer; **Hospital:** Brigham & Women's Hosp, Dana-Farber Cancer Inst; **Address:** Brigham & Women's Hosp, Dept Surg, 75 Francis St, Twr 1, Ste 220, Boston, MA 02115; **Phone:** 617-732-8181; **Board Cert:** Surgery 2000; **Med School:** Univ Fla Coll Med 1971; **Resid:** Surgery, Johns Hopkins Hosp 1974; Surgery, Johns Hopkins Hosp 1979; **Fac Appt:** Prof S, Harvard Med Sch

Mid Atlantic

Alfonso, Antonio MD [S] - **Spec Exp:** Breast Cancer; Head & Neck Surgery; Thyroid Cancer; **Hospital:** Long Island Coll Hosp, SUNY Downstate Med Ctr; **Address:** Long Island Coll Hosp, 339 Hicks St, Brooklyn, NY 11201; **Phone:** 718-875-3244; **Board Cert:** Surgery 1973; **Med School:** Philippines 1968; **Resid:** Surgery, Temple Univ Hosp 1972; **Fellow:** Surgical Oncology, Meml Sloan Kettering Cancer Ctr 1974; **Fac Appt:** Prof S, SUNY Downstate

August, David MD [S] - **Spec Exp:** Cancer Surgery; Gastrointestinal Cancer; Breast Cancer; Sarcoma-Soft Tissue; **Hospital:** Robert Wood Johnson Univ Hosp - New Brunswick; **Address:** Canc Inst NJ, 195 Little Albany St, New Brunswick, NJ 08903-1914; **Phone:** 732-235-7701; **Board Cert:** Surgery 2005; **Med School:** Yale Univ 1980; **Resid:** Surgery, Yale-New Haven Hosp 1986; **Fellow:** Surgical Oncology, Natl Cancer Inst 1984; **Fac Appt:** Prof S, UMDNJ-RW Johnson Med Sch

Axelrod, Deborah MD [S] - **Spec Exp:** Breast Cancer; Breast Disease; **Hospital:** NYU Med Ctr (page 67), St Vincent Cath Med Ctrs - Manhattan; **Address:** NYU Clinical Cancer Ctr, 160 E 34th St, New York, NY 10016; **Phone:** 212-731-5366; **Board Cert:** Surgery 1998; **Med School:** Israel 1982; **Resid:** Surgery, Beth Israel Med Ctr 1988; **Fellow:** Surgical Oncology, Meml Sloan Kettering Cancer Ctr 1986; **Fac Appt:** Assoc Prof S, NYU Sch Med

Balch, Charles MD [S] - **Spec Exp:** Sentinel Node Surgery; Melanoma; Cancer Surgery; **Hospital:** Johns Hopkins Hosp - Baltimore (page 61); **Address:** 600 N Wolfe St Osler Bldg - Ste 624, Baltimore, MD 21287; **Phone:** 410-502-5977; **Board Cert:** Surgery 1997; **Med School:** Columbia P&S 1967; **Resid:** Surgery, Univ Alabama Med Ctr 1971; Surgery, Univ Alabama Med Ctr 1975; **Fellow:** Immunology, Scripps Clin-Rsch Fdn 1973; **Fac Appt:** Prof Surg & Onc, Johns Hopkins Univ

Ballantyne, Garth MD [S] - **Spec Exp:** Laparoscopic Surgery; Gastroesophageal Reflux Disease (GERD); Colon Cancer; **Hospital:** Hackensack Univ Med Ctr; **Address:** 20 Prospect Ave, Ste 901, Hackensack, NJ 07601-1974; **Phone:** 201-996-2959; **Board Cert:** Surgery 1984; Colon & Rectal Surgery 1985; **Med School:** Columbia P&S 1977; **Resid:** Surgery, UCLA Med Ctr 1980; Surgery, Northwestern Univ 1982; **Fellow:** Colon & Rectal Surgery, Mayo Clinic 1984; **Fac Appt:** Prof S, UMDNJ-NJ Med Sch, Newark

Bartlett, David L MD [S] - **Spec Exp:** Peritoneal Carcinomatosis; Pancreatic Cancer; Liver Cancer; Appendix Cancer; **Hospital:** UPMC Shadyside; **Address:** UPMC Cancer Ctr, 5150 Centre Ave Fl 4 - rm 415, Pittsburgh, PA 15232; **Phone:** 412-692-2852; **Board Cert:** Surgery 2004; **Med School:** Univ Tex, Houston 1987; **Resid:** Surgery, Hosp Univ Penn 1993; **Fellow:** Surgical Oncology, Meml Sloan-Kettering Cancer Ctr 1995; **Fac Appt:** Assoc Prof S, Univ Pittsburgh

Bartlett, Stephen T MD [S] - **Spec Exp:** Transplant-Pancreas; Transplant-Kidney; **Hospital:** Univ of MD Med Sys; **Address:** 22 S Greene St, rm N4E40, Baltimore, MD 21201; **Phone:** 410-328-8407; **Board Cert:** Surgery 2004; Vascular Surgery 1996; **Med School:** Univ Chicago-Pritzker Sch Med 1979; **Resid:** Surgery, Hosp Univ Penn 1985; **Fellow:** Vascular Surgery, Northwestern Univ 1986; **Fac Appt:** Prof S, Univ MD Sch Med

Bauer, Joel MD [S] - **Spec Exp:** Colon & Rectal Surgery; Inflammatory Bowel Disease; Laparoscopic Surgery; **Hospital:** Mount Sinai Med Ctr; **Address:** 25 E 69th St, New York, NY 10021-4925; **Phone:** 212-517-8600; **Board Cert:** Surgery 1974; **Med School:** NYU Sch Med 1967; **Resid:** Surgery, Mount Sinai Hosp 1973; **Fac Appt:** Clin Prof S, Mount Sinai Sch Med

Bessler, Marc MD [S] - **Spec Exp:** Obesity/Bariatric Surgery; Laparoscopic Surgery; **Hospital:** NY-Presby Hosp/Columbia (page 66); **Address:** NY Presby Med Ctr, Dept of Surgery, 161 Fort Washington Ave, rm 620, New York, NY 10032; **Phone:** 212-305-9506; **Board Cert:** Surgery 1997; **Med School:** NYU Sch Med 1989; **Resid:** Surgery, Columbia Presby Med Ctr 1995; **Fac Appt:** Assoc Prof S, Columbia P&S

Borgen, Patrick I MD [S] - **Spec Exp:** Breast Cancer; **Hospital:** Maimonides Med Ctr (page 63); **Address:** Maimonides Cancer Ctr, 6300 8th Ave, Brooklyn, NY 11220; **Phone:** 718-765-2570; **Board Cert:** Surgery 1991; **Med School:** Louisiana State Univ 1984; **Resid:** Surgery, Ochsner Fdn Hosp 1989; **Fellow:** Surgical Oncology, Meml Sloan Kettering Canc Ctr 1990; **Fac Appt:** Prof S, Cornell Univ-Weill Med Coll

Surgery

Brennan, Murray MD [S] - **Spec Exp:** Sarcoma; Pancreatic Cancer; Cancer Surgery; **Hospital:** Meml Sloan Kettering Cancer Ctr; **Address:** 1275 York Ave, rm H1203, New York, NY 10021; **Phone:** 212-639-6586; **Board Cert:** Surgery 1975; **Med School:** New Zealand 1964; **Resid:** Surgery, Univ Otago Hosp 1969; **Fellow:** Surgery, Harvard Med Sch 1972; Surgery, Peter Bent Brigham Hosp 1975; **Fac Appt:** Prof S, Cornell Univ-Weill Med Coll

Brody, Fredrick J MD [S] - **Spec Exp:** Gastrointestinal Surgery; Laparoscopic Surgery; Hernia; **Hospital:** G Washington Univ Hosp; **Address:** George Washington Univ Dept Surgery, 2150 Pennsylvania Ave, Ste 6B, Washington, DC 20037; **Phone:** 202-741-2587; **Board Cert:** Surgery 1998; **Med School:** Univ NC Sch Med 1991; **Resid:** Surgery, G Washington Univ Med Ctr 1997; **Fellow:** Laparoscopic Surgery, Duke Univ Med Ctr 1998; **Fac Appt:** Assoc Prof S, Geo Wash Univ

Bromberg, Jonathan S MD/PhD [S] - **Spec Exp:** Transplant-Kidney; Transplant-Pancreas; **Hospital:** Mount Sinai Med Ctr; **Address:** Mount Sinai Medical Ctr, One Gustave Levy Pl, Box 1104, New York, NY 10029-6500; **Phone:** 212-659-8008; **Board Cert:** Surgery 1997; Surgical Critical Care 1993; **Med School:** Harvard Med Sch 1983; **Resid:** Surgery, Univ Washington Med Ctr 1988; **Fellow:** Transplant Surgery, Hosp U Penn 1990; **Fac Appt:** Prof S, Mount Sinai Sch Med

Buyske, Jo MD [S] - **Spec Exp:** Gastrointestinal Surgery; Laparoscopic Surgery; **Hospital:** Penn Presby Med Ctr - UPHS (page 72); **Address:** Presbyterian Medical Ctr, Wright Saunders Bldg, 39th and Market Sts, rm 266, Philadelphia, PA 19104; **Phone:** 215-662-9711; **Board Cert:** Surgery 2003; **Med School:** Columbia P&S 1987; **Resid:** Surgery, Mass General Hosp 1993; **Fac Appt:** Assoc Prof S, Univ Pennsylvania

Cameron, John MD [S] - **Spec Exp:** Pancreatic Cancer; Pancreatic Surgery; Biliary Cancer; **Hospital:** Johns Hopkins Hosp - Baltimore (page 61); **Address:** 600 N Wolfe St Blalock Bldg - Ste 679, Baltimore, MD 21287; **Phone:** 410-955-5166; **Board Cert:** Surgery 1970; Thoracic Surgery 1971; **Med School:** Johns Hopkins Univ 1962; **Resid:** Surgery, Johns Hopkins Hosp 1970; **Fellow:** Thoracic Surgery, Johns Hopkins Hosp 1971; **Fac Appt:** Prof S, Johns Hopkins Univ

Chabot, John A MD [S] - **Spec Exp:** Liver & Biliary Surgery; Pancreatic Cancer; Thyroid & Parathyroid Surgery; **Hospital:** NY-Presby Hosp/Columbia (page 66), Lawrence Hosp Ctr; **Address:** 161 Ft Washington Ave, Fl 8, New York, NY 10032; **Phone:** 212-305-9468; **Board Cert:** Surgery 2000; **Med School:** Dartmouth Med Sch 1983; **Resid:** Surgery, Columbia-Presby Med Ctr 1990; **Fac Appt:** Assoc Prof S, Columbia P&S

Choti, Michael A MD [S] - **Spec Exp:** Gastrointestinal Cancer; Colon & Rectal Cancer; Carcinoid Tumors; Palliative Care; **Hospital:** Johns Hopkins Hosp - Baltimore (page 61); **Address:** Johns Hopkins Hosp., 600 N Wolfe St Blalock Bldg - rm 665, Baltimore, MD 21287; **Phone:** 410-955-7113; **Board Cert:** Surgery 1991; **Med School:** Yale Univ 1983; **Resid:** Surgery, Hosp Univ Penn 1990; **Fellow:** Surgical Oncology, Meml Sloan-Kettering Canc Ctr 1992; **Fac Appt:** Prof S, Johns Hopkins Univ

Coit, Daniel G MD [S] - **Spec Exp:** Melanoma; Pancreatic Cancer; Stomach Cancer; **Hospital:** Meml Sloan Kettering Cancer Ctr; **Address:** 1275 York Ave, New York, NY 10021-6007; **Phone:** 212-639-8411; **Board Cert:** Surgery 2004; **Med School:** Univ Cincinnati 1976; **Resid:** Internal Medicine, New England Deaconess Hosp 1978; Surgery, New England Deaconess Hosp 1983; **Fellow:** Surgical Oncology, Meml Sloan Kettering Canc Ctr 1985; **Fac Appt:** Assoc Prof S, Cornell Univ-Weill Med Coll

Conti, David J MD [S] - **Spec Exp:** Transplant-Kidney; **Hospital:** Albany Med Ctr; **Address:** Albany Medical Center, 47 New Scotland Ave, MC 61GE, Albany, NY 12208; **Phone:** 518-262-5614; **Board Cert:** Surgery 1998; **Med School:** Northwestern Univ 1981; **Resid:** Surgery, Northwestern Meml Hosp 1987; **Fellow:** Transplant Surgery, Mass Genl Hosp 1989; **Fac Appt:** Prof S, Albany Med Coll

Cornwell III, Edward E MD [S] - **Spec Exp:** Trauma; **Hospital:** Johns Hopkins Hosp - Baltimore (page 61); **Address:** Johns Hopkins Hospital, 600 N Wolfe St Blalock Bldg - rm 688, Baltimore, MD 21287-5675; **Phone:** 410-955-2244; **Board Cert:** Surgery 1996; Surgical Critical Care 1998; **Med School:** Howard Univ 1982; **Resid:** Surgery, LAC-USC Med Ctr 1987; **Fellow:** Trauma, Emer/Med Svcs System 1989; **Fac Appt:** Assoc Prof S, Johns Hopkins Univ

Deitch, Edwin MD [S] - **Spec Exp:** Critical Care; Trauma; Burn Care; **Hospital:** UMDNJ-Univ Hosp-Newark; **Address:** 185 S Orange Ave, MSB, rm G506, Newark, NJ 07103; **Phone:** 973-972-5045; **Board Cert:** Surgery 1997; Surgical Critical Care 1995; **Med School:** Univ MD Sch Med 1973; **Resid:** Surgery, US Public Hlth Svc Hosp 1976; Surgery, US Public Hlth Svc Hosp 1978; **Fac Appt:** Prof S, UMDNJ-NJ Med Sch, Newark

Dempsey, Daniel MD [S] - **Spec Exp:** Gastrointestinal & Esophageal Surgery; Laparoscopic Surgery; Gastroesophageal Reflux Disease (GERD); **Hospital:** Temple Univ Hosp; **Address:** Temple Univ Hosp - Dept Surgery, 3401 N Broad St, 400 Parkinson Pavilion, Philadelphia, PA 19140; **Phone:** 215-707-5080; **Board Cert:** Surgery 1996; **Med School:** Univ Rochester 1979; **Resid:** Surgery, Hosp U Penn 1986; **Fac Appt:** Prof S, Temple Univ

Drebin, Jeffrey A MD/PhD [S] - **Spec Exp:** Pancreatic Cancer; Liver Cancer; Biliary Cancer; Stomach Cancer; **Hospital:** Hosp Univ Penn - UPHS (page 72); **Address:** Hosp Univ of Pennsylvania, 3400 Spruce St, 4 Silverstein Pavilion, Fl 4, Philadelphia, PA 19104; **Phone:** 215-662-2165; **Board Cert:** Surgery 2004; **Med School:** Harvard Med Sch 1987; **Resid:** Surgery, Johns Hopkins Hosp 1994; **Fellow:** Medical Oncology, Johns Hopkins Hosp 1991; Surgical Oncology, Johns Hopkins Hosp 1995; **Fac Appt:** Prof S, Univ Pennsylvania

Edge, Stephen B MD [S] - **Spec Exp:** Breast Cancer; **Hospital:** Roswell Park Cancer Inst; **Address:** Roswell Park Cancer Inst, Dept Surg Onc, Elm & Carlton Streets, Buffalo, NY 14263; **Phone:** 716-845-5789; **Board Cert:** Surgery 1996; **Med School:** Case West Res Univ 1979; **Resid:** Surgery, Univ Hosp 1986; **Fellow:** Surgical Oncology, Natl Cancer Inst 1984; **Fac Appt:** Prof S, SUNY Buffalo

Edington, Howard D MD [S] - **Spec Exp:** Breast Cancer; Melanoma; Reconstructive Surgery; **Hospital:** UPMC Presby, Pittsburgh, Magee-Womens Hosp - UPMC; **Address:** Magee-Women's Hospital, Dept Surgery, 300 Halket St, rm 2502, Pittsburgh, PA 15213; **Phone:** 412-641-1342; **Board Cert:** Surgery 1998; Plastic Surgery 1993; **Med School:** Temple Univ 1983; **Resid:** Surgery, Univ Pittsburgh Med Ctr 1989; Plastic Surgery, Univ Pittsburgh Med Ctr 1990; **Fellow:** Hand Surgery, Univ Pittsburgh Med Ctr 1991; Surgical Oncology, National Cancer Inst 1993; **Fac Appt:** Assoc Prof S, Univ Pittsburgh

Edye, Michael MD [S] - **Spec Exp:** Laparoscopic Abdominal Surgery; Colon Cancer; Diverticulitis; Obesity/Bariatric Surgery; **Hospital:** Mount Sinai Med Ctr, Westchester Med Ctr; **Address:** 1060 Fifth Ave, New York, NY 10128; **Phone:** 212-426-9614; **Med School:** Australia 1977; **Resid:** Surgery, St Vincents Hosp 1980; Surgery, Royal N Shore Hosp 1984; **Fellow:** Laparoscopic Surgery, Univ Bordeaux 1992; **Fac Appt:** Assoc Clin Prof S, Mount Sinai Sch Med

Emond, Jean C MD [S] - **Spec Exp:** Transplant-Liver; Liver Cancer; **Hospital:** NY-Presby Hosp/Columbia (page 66); **Address:** 622 W 168th St, PH - Fl 14, New York, NY 10032; **Phone:** 212-305-0914; **Board Cert:** Surgery 1994; **Med School:** Univ Chicago-Pritzker Sch Med 1979; **Resid:** Surgery, Cook Cty Hosp 1984; **Fellow:** Surgery, Hopital P Brousse/Univ de Paris Sud 1985; Transplant Surgery, Univ Chicago Hosps 1987; **Fac Appt:** Prof S, Columbia P&S

Emre, Sukru MD [S] - **Spec Exp:** Transplant-Liver-Adult & Pediatric; Hepatobiliary Surgery; Portal Hypertension; **Hospital:** Mount Sinai Med Ctr; **Address:** Mount Sinai Medical Ctr, 19 E 98 St, Box 1104, New York, NY 10029-6501; **Phone:** 212-241-6766; **Med School:** Turkey 1977; **Resid:** Surgery, Univ Istanbul 1982; **Fellow:** Hepatobiliary Surgery, Univ Istanbul 1988; Transplant Surgery, Mount Sinai Med Ctr 1994; **Fac Appt:** Prof S, Mount Sinai Sch Med

Eng, Kenneth MD [S] - **Spec Exp:** Colon & Rectal Cancer & Surgery; Pancreatic Cancer; Inflammatory Bowel Disease; **Hospital:** NYU Med Ctr (page 67); **Address:** 530 1st Ave, Ste 6B, New York, NY 10016-6402; **Phone:** 212-263-7301; **Board Cert:** Surgery 1982; **Med School:** NYU Sch Med 1967; **Resid:** Surgery, NYU Med Ctr 1972; **Fac Appt:** Prof S, NYU Sch Med

Estabrook, Alison MD [S] - **Spec Exp:** Breast Cancer; Breast Disease; Breast Cancer-High Risk Women; **Hospital:** St Luke's - Roosevelt Hosp Ctr - Roosevelt Div; **Address:** 425 W 59th St, Ste 7A, New York, NY 10019-1104; **Phone:** 212-523-7500; **Board Cert:** Surgery 2004; **Med School:** NYU Sch Med 1978; **Resid:** Surgery, Columbia Presby Med Ctr 1984; **Fellow:** Surgical Oncology, Columbia Presby Med Ctr 1982; **Fac Appt:** Prof S, Columbia P&S

Fahey III, Thomas J MD [S] - **Spec Exp:** Endocrine Surgery; Pheochromocytoma; Pancreatic Cancer; **Hospital:** NY-Presby Hosp/Weill Cornell (page 66), Meml Sloan Kettering Cancer Ctr; **Address:** NY Presby Cornell Med Ctr, Dept Surgery, 525 E 68 St, rm F2024, Box 249, New York, NY 10021; **Phone:** 212-746-5130; **Board Cert:** Surgery 2002; **Med School:** Cornell Univ-Weill Med Coll 1986; **Resid:** Surgery, New York Hosp 1992; **Fellow:** Surgery, Royal North Shore Hosp 1993; **Fac Appt:** Assoc Prof S, Cornell Univ-Weill Med Coll

Ferzli, George MD [S] - **Spec Exp:** Laparoscopic Surgery; Obesity/Bariatric Surgery; Endocrine Surgery; **Hospital:** Lutheran Med Ctr - Brooklyn, Staten Island Univ Hosp-North Site; **Address:** 65 Cromwell Ave, Staten Island, NY 10304-3944; **Phone:** 718-667-8100; **Board Cert:** Surgery 2003; Surgical Critical Care 2006; **Med School:** Lebanon 1979; **Resid:** Surgery, Staten Island Univ Hosp 1984; **Fac Appt:** Prof S, SUNY Downstate

Fong, Yuman MD [S] - **Spec Exp:** Pancreatic Cancer; Liver & Biliary Cancer; Stomach Cancer; **Hospital:** Meml Sloan Kettering Cancer Ctr, NY-Presby Hosp/Weill Cornell (page 66); **Address:** Memorial Sloan-Kettering Cancer Ctr, 1275 York Ave, New York, NY 10021; **Phone:** 212-639-2016; **Board Cert:** Surgery 2002; **Med School:** Cornell Univ-Weill Med Coll 1986; **Resid:** Surgery, New York Hosp-Cornell Med Ctr 1992; **Fellow:** Surgical Oncology, Meml Sloan-Kettering Cancer Ctr 1994; **Fac Appt:** Prof S, Cornell Univ-Weill Med Coll

Fowler, Dennis MD [S] - **Spec Exp:** Minimally Invasive Surgery; **Hospital:** NY-Presby Hosp/Columbia (page 66); **Address:** 622 W 168th St Fl PH 12 - rm 126, New York, NY 10032; **Phone:** 212-305-0577; **Board Cert:** Surgery 1998; **Med School:** Univ Kans 1973; **Resid:** Surgery, St Lukes Hosp 1979; **Fellow:** Endoscopy, Mass Genl Hosp 1980; **Fac Appt:** Prof S, Columbia P&S

Fraker, Douglas L MD [S] - **Spec Exp:** Melanoma; Endocrine Tumors; Liver Cancer; Sarcoma; **Hospital:** Hosp Univ Penn - UPHS (page 72); **Address:** Hosp Univ Penn, Dept Surgery, 3400 Spruce St, 4 Silverstein Pavilion, Philadelphia, PA 19104; **Phone:** 215-662-7866; **Board Cert:** Surgery 2002; **Med School:** Harvard Med Sch 1983; **Resid:** Surgery, UCSF Med Ctr 1986; Surgery, UCSF Med Ctr 1991; **Fellow:** Surgical Oncology, National Cancer Inst 1989; **Fac Appt:** Prof S, Univ Pennsylvania

Gagner, Michel MD [S] - **Spec Exp:** Obesity/Bariatric Surgery; Adrenal Surgery; Pancreatic Surgery; **Hospital:** NY-Presby Hosp/Weill Cornell (page 66); **Address:** NY Presby-NY Weill Cornell Med Ctr, 525 E 68th St, Box 294, New York, NY 10021; **Phone:** 212-746-5294; **Board Cert:** Surgery 2003; **Med School:** Canada 1982; **Resid:** Surgery, Royal Victoria Hosp/McGill 1988; **Fellow:** Hepatobiliary Surgery, Hosp Paul-Brousse 1989; Hepatobiliary Surgery, Lahey Clinic 1990; **Fac Appt:** Prof S, Cornell Univ-Weill Med Coll

Gibbs, John F MD [S] - **Spec Exp:** Liver Cancer; Liver & Biliary Surgery; Pancreatic Cancer; **Hospital:** Roswell Park Cancer Inst; **Address:** Roswell Park Cancer Inst, Dept Surg Onc, Elm & Carlton Sts, Buffalo, NY 14263-0001; **Phone:** 716-845-5807; **Board Cert:** Surgery 2000; **Med School:** UCSD 1985; **Resid:** Surgery, Rush Presby-St Luke's Med Ctr 1990; **Fellow:** Transplant Surgery, Baylor Univ Med Ctr 1992; Surgical Oncology, Roswell Park Cancer Inst 1996; **Fac Appt:** Assoc Prof S, SUNY Buffalo

Hardy, Mark MD [S] - **Spec Exp:** Transplant-Kidney; Parathyroid Surgery; Islet Cell Transplant; Immunotherapy; **Hospital:** NY-Presby Hosp/Columbia (page 66); **Address:** 177 Fort Washington Ave, New York, NY 10032; **Phone:** 212-305-5502; **Board Cert:** Surgery 1972; **Med School:** Albert Einstein Coll Med 1962; **Resid:** Surgery, Strong Meml Hosp 1964; Surgery, Bronx Muni Hosp Ctr/Einstein 1971; **Fellow:** Transplant Surgery, Harvard Med Sch 1969; **Fac Appt:** Prof S, Columbia P&S

Hoffman, John P MD [S] - **Spec Exp:** Pancreatic Cancer; Gastrointestinal Cancer; Breast Cancer; Pancreatic Surgery; **Hospital:** Fox Chase Cancer Ctr (page 59); **Address:** Fox Chase Cancer Ctr, 333 Cottman Ave, Philadelphia, PA 19111-2497; **Phone:** 215-728-3518; **Board Cert:** Surgery 1998; **Med School:** Case West Res Univ 1970; **Resid:** Surgery, Virginia Mason Hosp 1977; **Fellow:** Surgical Oncology, Meml Sloan Kettering Cancer Ctr 1980; **Fac Appt:** Prof S, Temple Univ

Hofstetter, Steven MD [S] - **Spec Exp:** Laparoscopic Abdominal Surgery; Gastrointestinal Cancer; Hernia; **Hospital:** NYU Med Ctr (page 67); **Address:** 530 1st Ave, Ste 6C, New York, NY 10016-6402; **Phone:** 212-263-7302; **Board Cert:** Surgery 2000; **Med School:** SUNY Hlth Sci Ctr 1971; **Resid:** Surgery, Bellevue Hosp/NYU Med Ctr 1976; **Fac Appt:** Assoc Prof S, NYU Sch Med

Johnson, Ronald R MD [S] - **Spec Exp:** Breast Cancer; **Hospital:** Magee-Womens Hosp - UPMC; **Address:** Magee-Womens Hosp - UPMC, 300 Halket St, Ste 2601, Pittsburgh, PA 15213; **Phone:** 412-641-1225; **Board Cert:** Surgery 1999; **Med School:** Univ Pittsburgh 1983; **Resid:** Surgery, Univ Pittsburgh Med Ctr 1989; **Fac Appt:** Asst Prof S, Univ Pittsburgh

Karpeh Jr, Martin S MD [S] - **Spec Exp:** Gastrointestinal Cancer; Esophageal Cancer; Colon & Rectal Cancer; **Hospital:** Stony Brook Univ Med Ctr; **Address:** Stony Brook Univ Hosp, Hlth Science Ctr, Fl 18 - rm 060, Stony Brook, NY 11794-8191; **Phone:** 631-444-1793; **Board Cert:** Surgery 1998; **Med School:** Penn State Univ-Hershey Med Ctr 1983; **Resid:** Surgery, Hosp Univ Penn 1989; **Fellow:** Surgical Oncology, Memorial Sloan Kettering Cancer Ctr 1991; **Fac Appt:** Prof S, SUNY Stony Brook

Surgery

Kaufman, Howard L MD [S] - **Spec Exp:** Cancer Surgery; Vaccine Therapy; Melanoma; Immunotherapy; **Hospital:** NY-Presby Hosp/Columbia (page 66); **Address:** Columbia University, MHB-7SK, 177 Fort Washington Ave, New York, NY 10032-3733; **Phone:** 212-342-6042; **Board Cert:** Surgery 1996; **Med School:** Loyola Univ-Stritch Sch Med 1986; **Resid:** Surgery, Boston Univ Hosp 1995; **Fellow:** Surgical Oncology, Natl Cancer Inst 1996; **Fac Appt:** Assoc Prof S, Columbia P&S

Lentz, Christopher MD [S] - **Spec Exp:** Burn Care; Trauma; Critical Care; Wound Healing/Care; **Hospital:** Univ of Rochester Strong Meml Hosp; **Address:** Univ Rochester, Surgery Dept, 601 Elmwood Ave, Box SURG, Rochester, NY 14642; **Phone:** 585-275-2876; **Board Cert:** Surgery 1995; Surgical Critical Care 1996; **Med School:** Wayne State Univ 1988; **Resid:** Surgery, Med Coll Wisc 1994; **Fellow:** Surgical Critical Care, Shriners Burns Inst 1991; Burn Surgery, Univ N Carolina Med Ctr 1996; **Fac Appt:** Assoc Prof S, Univ Rochester

Lotze, Michael T MD/PhD [S] - **Spec Exp:** Melanoma; Gene Therapy; Immunotherapy; **Hospital:** UPMC Presby, Pittsburgh; **Address:** Hillman Cancer Ctr, Research Pavilion Fl 1 - Ste G21, 5117 Center Ave, Pittsburgh, PA 15213; **Phone:** 412-623-7732; **Board Cert:** Surgery 1983; **Med School:** Northwestern Univ 1974; **Resid:** Surgery, Strong Meml Hosp 1977; **Fellow:** Surgical Oncology, Natl Cancer Institute 1980; **Fac Appt:** Prof S, Univ Pittsburgh

Manzarbeitia, Cosme Y MD [S] - **Spec Exp:** Transplant-Liver; Hepatobiliary Surgery; **Hospital:** Albert Einstein Med Ctr; **Address:** Albert Einstein Med Ctr, 5401 Old York Rd, Klein, Ste 509, Philadelphia, PA 19141; **Phone:** 215-456-4985; **Board Cert:** Surgery 1998; **Med School:** Spain 1982; **Resid:** Surgery, North Genl Hosp 1989; **Fellow:** Transplant Surgery, Mt Sinai Hosp 1991

Markmann, James F MD [S] - **Spec Exp:** Transplant-Pancreas; Transplant-Liver; Liver & Biliary Surgery; Liver & Biliary Cancer; **Hospital:** Hosp Univ Penn - UPHS (page 72), Children's Inst - Pittsburgh; **Address:** Hospital of U Pennsylvania, Surgery, 3400 Spruce St Silverstein Bldg Fl 4, Philadelphia, PA 19104; **Phone:** 215-662-7367; **Board Cert:** Surgery 1997; **Med School:** Univ Pennsylvania 1986; **Resid:** Surgery, Hosp U Penn 1992; **Fellow:** Transplant Surgery, UCLA Med Ctr 1994; **Fac Appt:** Assoc Prof S, Univ Pennsylvania

Marsh Jr, James W MD [S] - **Spec Exp:** Transplant-Liver; Liver Cancer; **Hospital:** UPMC Presby, Pittsburgh; **Address:** UPMC, Starzl Transplant Inst, 3459 Fifth Ave 7 South, Pittsburgh, PA 15213; **Phone:** 412-692-2001; **Board Cert:** Surgery 2003; **Med School:** Univ Ark 1979; **Resid:** Surgery, St Paul Hosp 1984; **Fellow:** Transplant Surgery, Mayo Clinic 1985; Transplant Surgery, Univ Pittsburgh Hosps 1986; **Fac Appt:** Assoc Prof S, Univ Pittsburgh

Michelassi, Fabrizio MD [S] - **Spec Exp:** Gastrointestinal Cancer; Inflammatory Bowel Disease/Crohn's; Pancreatic Cancer; Ulcerative Colitis; **Hospital:** NY-Presby Hosp/Weill Cornell (page 66); **Address:** Weill Med College, Dept Surgery, 525 E 68th St, rm F-739, New York, NY 10021; **Phone:** 212-746-6006; **Board Cert:** Surgery 2002; **Med School:** Italy 1975; **Resid:** Surgery, NYU Med Ctr 1981; **Fellow:** Research, Mass Genl Hosp 1983; **Fac Appt:** Prof S, Cornell Univ-Weill Med Coll

Montgomery, Robert A MD/PhD [S] - **Spec Exp:** Transplant-Kidney; **Hospital:** Johns Hopkins Hosp - Baltimore (page 61); **Address:** Johns Hopkins Hosp, Transplant Surgery, 720 Rutland Ave Ross Bldg - Ste 765, Baltimore, MD 21205; **Phone:** 410-614-8297; **Board Cert:** Surgery 1997; **Med School:** Univ Rochester 1987; **Resid:** Surgery, Johns Hopkins Hosp 1995; **Fellow:** Transplant Surgery, Johns Hopkins Hosp 1997; **Fac Appt:** Assoc Prof S, Johns Hopkins Univ

Morrow, Monica MD [S] - **Spec Exp:** Breast Cancer; **Hospital:** Fox Chase Cancer Ctr (page 59); **Address:** Fox Chase Cancer Ctr, Div Surg Oncology, 333 Cottman Ave, rm C 302, Philadelphia, PA 19111-2497; **Phone:** 215-728-3096; **Board Cert:** Surgery 2001; **Med School:** Jefferson Med Coll 1976; **Resid:** Surgery, Med Ctr Hosp Vermont 1981; **Fellow:** Surgical Oncology, Meml Sloan Kettering Cancer Ctr 1983; **Fac Appt:** Prof S, Temple Univ

Nava-Villarreal, Hector MD [S] - **Spec Exp:** Esophageal Cancer; Stomach Cancer; Barrett's Esophagus; **Hospital:** Roswell Park Cancer Inst; **Address:** Roswell Park Cancer Inst, Elm & Carlton Sts, Buffalo, NY 14263; **Phone:** 716-845-5915; **Board Cert:** Surgery 2001; **Med School:** Mexico 1967; **Resid:** Surgery, Buffalo Genl Hosp 1974; **Fellow:** Surgical Oncology, Roswell Park Cancer Inst 1976; **Fac Appt:** Assoc Prof S, SUNY Buffalo

Niederhuber, John E MD [S] - **Spec Exp:** Breast Cancer; Liver Cancer; Esophageal Cancer; Pancreatic Cancer; **Hospital:** Natl Inst of Hlth - Clin Ctr; **Address:** Natl Cancer Institute, 31 Center Drive Bldg 31, rm 11A48, MS 2590, Bethesda, MD 20892-2590; **Phone:** 301-594-6369; **Board Cert:** Surgery 1974; **Med School:** Ohio State Univ 1964; **Resid:** Surgery, Univ Mich Hosp 1973; **Fellow:** Immunology, Karolinska Inst 1971

Nowak, Eugene MD [S] - **Spec Exp:** Breast Cancer; Hernia; Gastrointestinal Disorders; **Hospital:** NY-Presby Hosp/Weill Cornell (page 66); **Address:** 325 E 79th St, New York, NY 10021-0954; **Phone:** 212-517-6693; **Board Cert:** Surgery 2003; **Med School:** UMDNJ-NJ Med Sch, Newark 1975; **Resid:** Surgery, New York Hosp- Cornell Med Ctr 1980; **Fac Appt:** Assoc Prof S, Cornell Univ-Weill Med Coll

Olthoff, Kim M MD [S] - **Spec Exp:** Transplant-Liver-Adult & Pediatric; Liver & Biliary Surgery; Liver Cancer; **Hospital:** Hosp Univ Penn - UPHS (page 72), Chldns Hosp of Philadelphia, The; **Address:** Hosp Univ Penn - Dept Surgery, 3400 Spruce St Dulles Bldg Fl 2, Philadelphia, PA 19104; **Phone:** 215-662-6136; **Board Cert:** Surgery 2003; **Med School:** Univ Chicago-Pritzker Sch Med 1986; **Resid:** Surgery, UCLA Med Ctr 1990; **Fellow:** Transplant Surgery, UCLA Med Ctr; **Fac Appt:** Assoc Prof S, Univ Pennsylvania

Osborne, Michael P MD [S] - **Spec Exp:** Breast Cancer; Breast Cancer-High Risk Women; Breast Disease; **Hospital:** NY-Presby Hosp/Weill Cornell (page 66); **Address:** 425 E 61 St Fl 8, New York, NY 10021-8722; **Phone:** 212-821-0828; **Med School:** England 1970; **Resid:** Surgery, Charing Cross Hosp 1977; Surgery, Royal Marsden Hosp 1980; **Fellow:** Surgical Oncology, Meml Sloan-Kettering Canc Ctr 1981; **Fac Appt:** Prof S, Cornell Univ-Weill Med Coll

Pachter, H Leon MD [S] - **Spec Exp:** Laparoscopic Surgery-Adrenal; Gastrointestinal Surgery; Pancreatic Cancer; **Hospital:** NYU Med Ctr (page 67), Bellevue Hosp Ctr; **Address:** 530 1st Ave, Ste 6C, New York, NY 10016; **Phone:** 212-263-7302; **Board Cert:** Surgery 2000; **Med School:** NYU Sch Med 1971; **Resid:** Surgery, NYU Med Ctr 1976; **Fac Appt:** Prof S, NYU Sch Med

Park, Adrian E MD [S] - **Spec Exp:** Minimally Invasive Surgery; Gastrointestinal Surgery; Laparoscopic Surgery; **Hospital:** Univ of MD Med Sys; **Address:** Univ Maryland Dept Surgery, 22 S Greene St, S4B14, Baltimore, MD 21201; **Phone:** 410-328-7994; **Board Cert:** Surgery 2005; **Med School:** McMaster Univ 1987; **Resid:** Surgery, MC Master Univ 1992; **Fellow:** Laparoscopic Surgery, Hotel Dieu de Montreal 1993; **Fac Appt:** Prof S, Univ MD Sch Med

Paty, Philip B MD [S] - **Spec Exp:** Colon & Rectal Cancer; Pelvic Tumors; Appendix Cancer; **Hospital:** Meml Sloan Kettering Cancer Ctr; **Address:** Memorial Sloan Kettering Cancer Ctr, 1275 York Ave, rm C1081, New York, NY 10021; **Phone:** 212-639-6703; **Board Cert:** Surgery 2001; **Med School:** Stanford Univ 1983; **Resid:** Surgery, UCSF Med Ctr 1990; **Fellow:** Surgical Oncology, Memorial Sloan Kettering Cancer Ctr 1992; **Fac Appt:** Prof S, Cornell Univ-Weill Med Coll

Peitzman, Andrew B MD [S] - **Spec Exp:** Trauma; Gastrointestinal Surgery; Critical Care; **Hospital:** UPMC Presby, Pittsburgh, UPMC Shadyside; **Address:** Presbyterian Univ Hosp, Dept Surg - F 1281, 200 Lothrop St, Pittsburgh, PA 15213; **Phone:** 412-647-0635; **Board Cert:** Surgery 2004; Surgical Critical Care 1997; **Med School:** Univ Pittsburgh 1976; **Resid:** Surgery, Univ Pittsburgh Med Ctr 1979; Surgery, Univ Pittsburgh Med Ctr 1984; **Fellow:** Surgery, New York Hosp-Cornell Univ 1981; **Fac Appt:** Prof S, Univ Pittsburgh

Peters, Jeffrey H MD [S] - **Spec Exp:** Esophageal Surgery; Gastroesophageal Reflux Disease (GERD); **Hospital:** Univ of Rochester Strong Meml Hosp; **Address:** 601 Elmwood Ave, Box SURG, Rochester, NY 14642-8410; **Phone:** 585-275-2725; **Board Cert:** Surgery 1998; **Med School:** Ohio State Univ 1981; **Resid:** Surgery, Johns Hopkins Hosp 1988; **Fellow:** Allergy & Immunology, Johns Hopkins Hosp 1985; Esophageal Surgery, Creighton Univ; **Fac Appt:** Prof S, Univ Rochester

Ramanathan, Ramesh Chandran MD [S] - **Spec Exp:** Obesity/Bariatric Surgery; Minimally Invasive Surgery; Colon Cancer; Clinical Trials; **Hospital:** Magee-Womens Hosp - UPMC, UPMC Presby, Pittsburgh; **Address:** 3380 Boulevard of the Allies, Ste 390, Pittsburgh, PA 15213; **Phone:** 412-641-3668; **Board Cert:** Surgery 2004; **Med School:** India 1988; **Resid:** Surgery, Univ Hlth Ctr Univ Pitt Med Ctr 2003; **Fellow:** Surgical Oncology, Univ Pitt Med Ctr 1999; Minimally Invasive Surgery, Univ Pitt Med Ctr 2000; **Fac Appt:** Asst Prof S, Univ Pittsburgh

Reiner, Mark MD [S] - **Spec Exp:** Laparoscopic Surgery; Hernia; Esophageal Surgery; Pancreatic Surgery; **Hospital:** Mount Sinai Med Ctr, Lenox Hill Hosp (page 62); **Address:** 1010 5th Ave, New York, NY 10028-0130; **Phone:** 212-879-6677; **Board Cert:** Surgery 2001; **Med School:** SUNY Downstate 1974; **Resid:** Surgery, Mount Sinai Hosp 1979; **Fac Appt:** Clin Prof S, Mount Sinai Sch Med

Ridge, John A MD/PhD [S] - **Spec Exp:** Head & Neck Cancer & Surgery; Thyroid Cancer & Surgery; Laryngeal Cancer; **Hospital:** Fox Chase Cancer Ctr (page 59); **Address:** Fox Chase Cancer Ctr, Dept Surgical Oncology, 333 Cottman Ave, Philadelphia, PA 19111; **Phone:** 215-728-3517; **Board Cert:** Surgery 1997; **Med School:** Stanford Univ 1981; **Resid:** Surgery, Univ Colorado Med Ctr 1987; **Fellow:** Surgical Oncology, Meml Sloan-Kettering Cancer Ctr 1989

Roh, Mark S MD [S] - **Spec Exp:** Liver Cancer; Cancer Surgery; **Hospital:** Allegheny General Hosp; **Address:** Allegheny General Hospital, Dept Surgery, 320 E North Ave, Pittsburgh, PA 15212; **Phone:** 412-359-6738; **Board Cert:** Surgery 1996; **Med School:** Ohio State Univ 1979; **Resid:** Surgery, Univ Pittsburgh Med Ctr 1982; Surgery, Univ Pittsburgh Med Ctr 1986; **Fellow:** Surgical Oncology, Meml Sloan-Kettering Cancer Ctr 1984; Surgical Oncology, Meml Sloan-Kettering Cancer Ctr 1987; **Fac Appt:** Prof S, Drexel Univ Coll Med

Rosato, Ernest F MD [S] - **Spec Exp:** Gastrointestinal Cancer & Surgery; Esophageal Cancer; Pancreatic Cancer; **Hospital:** Hosp Univ Penn - UPHS (page 72); **Address:** Hosp Univ Penn, Dept Surg, 3400 Spruce St, 4 Silverstein, Philadelphia, PA 19104; **Phone:** 215-662-2033; **Board Cert:** Surgery 1969; **Med School:** Univ Pennsylvania 1962; **Resid:** Surgery, Hosp Univ Penn 1968; **Fac Appt:** Prof S, Univ Pennsylvania

Rosenberg, Steven MD [S] - **Spec Exp:** Melanoma; Kidney Cancer; **Hospital:** Natl Inst of Hlth - Clin Ctr; **Address:** National Cancer Institute, 9000 Rockville Pike CRC Bldg, rm 3W-3940, Bethesda, MD 20892; **Phone:** 301-496-4164; **Board Cert:** Surgery 1975; **Med School:** Johns Hopkins Univ 1964; **Resid:** Surgery, Peter Bent Brigham Hosp 1974

Roses, Daniel F MD [S] - **Spec Exp:** Breast Cancer; Melanoma; Thyroid Cancer; Parathyroid Surgery; **Hospital:** NYU Med Ctr (page 67); **Address:** 530 First Ave, Ste 6E, New York, NY 10016-6402; **Phone:** 212-263-7329; **Board Cert:** Surgery 1975; **Med School:** NYU Sch Med 1969; **Resid:** Surgery, NYU-Bellevue Hosp 1974; **Fellow:** Surgical Oncology, NYU-Bellevue Hosp 1978; **Fac Appt:** Prof Surg & Onc, NYU Sch Med

Salky, Barry A MD [S] - **Spec Exp:** Laparoscopic Surgery; Gastroesophageal Reflux Disease (GERD); Pancreatic Surgery; **Hospital:** Mount Sinai Med Ctr; **Address:** Mt Sinai Medical Center, Div of Laparoscopic Surgery, 5 E 98th St, Box 1259, New York, NY 10029; **Phone:** 212-241-6156; **Board Cert:** Surgery 1998; **Med School:** Univ Tenn Coll Med, Memphis 1970; **Resid:** Surgery, Mount Sinai Hosp 1973; Surgery, Mount Sinai Hosp 1978; **Fac Appt:** Prof S, Mount Sinai Sch Med

Schnabel, Freya MD [S] - **Spec Exp:** Breast Cancer; Breast Cancer-High Risk Women; **Hospital:** NYU Med Ctr (page 67); **Address:** 160 E 34th St Fl 3, New York, NY 10016; **Phone:** 212-731-5367; **Board Cert:** Surgery 1998; **Med School:** NYU Sch Med 1982; **Resid:** Surgery, NYU Med Ctr 1987; **Fellow:** Research, SUNY Hlth Sci Ctr 1988

Schraut, Wolfgang H MD [S] - **Spec Exp:** Inflammatory Bowel Disease; Gastrointestinal Surgery; Colon & Rectal Cancer & Surgery; Laparoscopic Surgery; **Hospital:** UPMC Presby, Pittsburgh, Magee-Womens Hosp - UPMC; **Address:** Univ Pittsburgh Med Ctr, Dept Surgery, 497 Scaife Hall, 3550 Terrace St, Pittsburgh, PA 15261; **Phone:** 412-647-0311; **Board Cert:** Surgery 1999; **Med School:** Germany 1970; **Resid:** Surgery, Univ Chicago Hosps 1978; **Fac Appt:** Prof S, Univ Pittsburgh

Schwartz, Gordon F MD [S] - **Spec Exp:** Breast Cancer; Breast Disease; **Hospital:** Thomas Jefferson Univ Hosp, Pennsylvania Hosp (page 72); **Address:** 1015 Chestnut St, Ste 510, Philadelphia, PA 19107-4305; **Phone:** 215-627-8487; **Board Cert:** Surgery 1970; **Med School:** Harvard Med Sch 1960; **Resid:** Surgery, Columbia-Presby Med Ctr 1968; **Fellow:** Oncology, Univ Penn 1969; **Fac Appt:** Prof S, Jefferson Med Coll

Shah, Jatin P MD [S] - **Spec Exp:** Head & Neck Cancer; Thyroid Cancer; Skull Base Tumors; **Hospital:** Meml Sloan Kettering Cancer Ctr; **Address:** 1275 York Ave, Ste C1061, New York, NY 10021-6007; **Phone:** 212-639-7604; **Board Cert:** Surgery 1975; **Med School:** India 1964; **Resid:** Surgery, SSG Hosp 1967; Surgery, New York Infirm 1974; **Fellow:** Head & Neck Surgical Oncology, Meml Sloan-Kettering Hosp 1972 **Fac Appt:** Prof S, Cornell Univ-Weill Med Coll

Shaha, Ashok MD [S] - **Spec Exp:** Head & Neck Cancer; Thyroid Cancer; Parathyroid Cancer; **Hospital:** Meml Sloan Kettering Cancer Ctr; **Address:** 1275 York Ave, Dept of Head & Neck Surgery, New York, NY 10021-6007; **Phone:** 212-639-7649; **Board Cert:** Surgery 1992; **Med School:** India 1970; **Resid:** Surgery, Downstate Med Ctr 1981; **Fellow:** Surgical Oncology, Meml Sloan Kettering Cancer Ctr 1976; Head and Neck Surgery, Meml Sloan Kettering Cancer Ctr 1982; **Fac Appt:** Prof S, Cornell Univ-Weill Med Coll

Shapiro, Ron MD [S] - **Spec Exp:** Transplant-Kidney; Transplant-Pancreas; Islet Cell Transplant; **Hospital:** UPMC Presby, Pittsburgh, Chldns Hosp of Pittsburgh - UPMC; **Address:** Starzl Transplantation Inst, UPMC_Montefiore - 7 South, 3459 Fifth Ave, Pittsburgh, PA 15213-2582; **Phone:** 412-647-5800; **Board Cert:** Surgery 1996; **Med School:** Stanford Univ 1980; **Resid:** Surgery, Mt Sinai Hosp 1986; **Fellow:** Transplant Surgery, Univ Pittsburgh 1988; **Fac Appt:** Prof S, Univ Pittsburgh

Sigurdson, Elin R MD [S] - **Spec Exp:** Breast Cancer; Colon & Rectal Cancer; Melanoma; Gastrointestinal Cancer; **Hospital:** Fox Chase Cancer Ctr (page 59); **Address:** 333 Cottman Ave, Philadelphia, PA 19111-2412; **Phone:** 215-728-3519; **Board Cert:** Surgery 1997; **Med School:** Canada 1980; **Resid:** Surgery, Univ Toronto Med Ctr 1984; **Fellow:** Surgical Oncology, Meml Sloan-Kettering Cancer Ctr 1987; **Fac Appt:** Assoc Prof S

Singer, Samuel MD [S] - **Spec Exp:** Sarcoma-Soft Tissue; **Hospital:** Meml Sloan Kettering Cancer Ctr; **Address:** Meml Sloan Kettering Cancer Ctr, 1275 York Ave, rm 1210, New York, NY 10021; **Phone:** 212-639-2940; **Board Cert:** Surgery 1998; **Med School:** Harvard Med Sch 1982; **Resid:** Surgery, Brigham & Women's Hosp 1988; **Fellow:** Surgical Oncology, Dana Farber Cancer Inst 1990; **Fac Appt:** Assoc Prof S, Cornell Univ-Weill Med Coll

Skinner, Kristin A MD [S] - **Spec Exp:** Breast Cancer; Gastrointestinal Cancer; Melanoma; **Hospital:** Univ of Rochester Strong Meml Hosp; **Address:** Univ Rochester Med Ctr, 601 Elmwood Ave, Box SURG, Rochester, NY 14642; **Phone:** 585-276-3332; **Board Cert:** Surgery 1996; **Med School:** Johns Hopkins Univ 1988; **Resid:** Surgery, UCLA Med Ctr 1995; **Fellow:** Surgical Oncology, UCLA Med Ctr 1994; **Fac Appt:** Assoc Prof S, Univ Rochester

Sugarbaker, Paul H MD [S] - **Spec Exp:** Peritoneal Carcinomatosis; Cystadenocarcinoma; Ovarian Cancer; Appendix Cancer; **Hospital:** Washington Hosp Ctr; **Address:** Washington Hosp Ctr, 106 Irving St NW, Ste 3900N, Washington, DC 20010; **Phone:** 202-877-3908; **Board Cert:** Surgery 1973; **Med School:** Cornell Univ-Weill Med Coll 1967; **Resid:** Surgery, Peter Bent Brigham Hosp 1973; **Fellow:** Surgical Oncology, Mass Genl Hosp 1976; **Fac Appt:** Prof S, Univ Wash

Swistel, Alexander MD [S] - **Spec Exp:** Breast Cancer; Breast Disease; Sentinel Node Surgery; **Hospital:** NY-Presby Hosp/Weill Cornell (page 66), St Luke's - Roosevelt Hosp Ctr - Roosevelt Div; **Address:** 425 E 61st St Fl 8, New York, NY 10021; **Phone:** 212-821-0602; **Board Cert:** Surgery 2005; **Med School:** Brown Univ 1975; **Resid:** Surgery, St Luke's Roosevelt Hosp Ctr 1981; **Fellow:** Surgical Oncology, Meml Sloan Kettering Canc Ctr 1983; **Fac Appt:** Asst Prof S, Cornell Univ-Weill Med Coll

Tartter, Paul MD [S] - **Spec Exp:** Breast Cancer; Breast Cancer in Elderly; Sentinel Node Surgery; **Hospital:** St Luke's - Roosevelt Hosp Ctr - Roosevelt Div, Mount Sinai Med Ctr; **Address:** 425 W 59th St, Ste 7A, New York, NY 10019; **Phone:** 212-523-7500; **Board Cert:** Surgery 2003; **Med School:** Brown Univ 1977; **Resid:** Surgery, Mount Sinai Hosp 1982; **Fac Appt:** Assoc Prof S, Columbia P&S

Teperman, Lewis W MD [S] - **Spec Exp:** Transplant-Liver; Transplant-Kidney; Liver Tumors; **Hospital:** NYU Med Ctr (page 67); **Address:** 403 E 34th St Fl 3, New York, NY 10016; **Phone:** 212-263-8134; **Board Cert:** Surgery 1997; **Med School:** Mount Sinai Sch Med 1981; **Resid:** Surgery, Columbia Presby Med Ctr 1984; Surgery, LI Jewish Med Ctr 1986; **Fellow:** Transplant Surgery, Univ Pittsburgh 1988; **Fac Appt:** Assoc Prof S, NYU Sch Med

Tsangaris, Theodore N MD [S] - **Spec Exp:** Breast Cancer; **Hospital:** Johns Hopkins Hosp - Baltimore (page 61); **Address:** Johns Hopkins Hospital, 600 N Wolfe St, Carnegie 686, Baltimore, MD 21287; **Phone:** 410-955-2615; **Board Cert:** Surgery 2005; **Med School:** Geo Wash Univ 1983; **Resid:** Surgery, Geo Washington Univ Med Ctr 1989; **Fellow:** Surgical Oncology, Baylor Univ Med Ctr 1990; **Fac Appt:** Assoc Prof S, Johns Hopkins Univ

Yeo, Charles MD [S] - **Spec Exp:** Pancreatic Cancer; **Hospital:** Thomas Jefferson Univ Hosp; **Address:** 1015 Walnut St, Ste 620, Philadelphia, PA 19107; **Phone:** 215-955-9402; **Board Cert:** Surgery 2005; **Med School:** Johns Hopkins Univ 1979; **Resid:** Surgery, Johns Hopkins Hosp 1985; **Fellow:** Research, SUNY Downstate 1982; **Fac Appt:** Prof S, Thomas Jefferson Univ

Yurt, Roger W MD [S] - **Spec Exp:** Burn Care; Wound Healing/Care; Hyperbaric Medicine; **Hospital:** NY-Presby Hosp/Weill Cornell (page 66); **Address:** 525 E 68th St, rm L706, New York, NY 10021-4885; **Phone:** 212-746-5410; **Board Cert:** Surgery 1999; **Med School:** Univ Miami Sch Med 1972; **Resid:** Surgery, Parkland Meml Hosp 1974; Surgery, New York Hosp-Cornell Med Ctr 1980; **Fellow:** Internal Medicine, Brigham & Womens Hosp 1978; **Fac Appt:** Prof S, Cornell Univ-Weill Med Coll

Southeast

Albertson, David A MD [S] - **Spec Exp:** Endocrine Surgery; **Hospital:** Wake Forest Univ Baptist Med Ctr (page 73); **Address:** Wake Forest Univ Sch Med, Dept Surgery, Medical Center Blvd, Winston-Salem, NC 27157-1095; **Phone:** 336-716-0664; **Board Cert:** Surgery 1998; **Med School:** Univ VA Sch Med 1972; **Resid:** Surgery, NC Bapt Hosp 1977; **Fellow:** Endocrine Surgery, Boston Univ 1978; **Fac Appt:** Assoc Prof S, Wake Forest Univ

Beauchamp, Robert Daniel MD [S] - **Spec Exp:** Breast Cancer; Colon & Rectal Cancer; Pancreatic Cancer; Cancer Surgery; **Hospital:** Vanderbilt Univ Med Ctr; **Address:** Medical Center North, rm D4316, 1161 21st Ave S, Nashville, TN 37232; **Phone:** 615-322-2363; **Board Cert:** Surgery 1997; **Med School:** Univ Tex Med Br, Galveston 1982; **Resid:** Surgery, Univ Tex Med Br 1987; **Fellow:** Cellular Molecular Biology, Vanderbilt Univ 1989; **Fac Appt:** Prof S, Vanderbilt Univ

Behrns, Kevin E MD [S] - **Spec Exp:** Pancreatic Cancer; Gastrointestinal Cancer & Surgery; **Hospital:** Shands Hlthcre at Univ of FL; **Address:** Shands Healthcare at Univ Florida, PO Box 100286, Gainesville, FL 32610-0286; **Phone:** 352-265-0761; **Board Cert:** Surgery 2005; **Med School:** Mayo Med Sch 1988; **Resid:** Surgery, Mayo Clinic 1995; **Fac Appt:** Prof S, Univ Fla Coll Med

Bland, Kirby MD [S] - **Spec Exp:** Breast Cancer; Colon Cancer; Thyroid & Parathyroid Cancer & Surgery; **Hospital:** Univ of Ala Hosp at Birmingham; **Address:** University of Alabama, Dept Surgery, 1530 3rd Ave S, BDB 502, Birmingham, AL 35294-0002; **Phone:** 205-975-2193; **Board Cert:** Surgery 2000; **Med School:** Univ Ala 1968; **Resid:** Surgery, Univ Fla Hosp 1970; Surgery, Univ Fla Hosp 1976; **Fellow:** Surgical Oncology, MD Anderson Cancer Ctr 1977; **Fac Appt:** Prof S, Univ Ala

Britt, L D MD [S] - **Spec Exp:** Trauma; Head Injury; **Hospital:** Sentara Norfolk Genl Hosp; **Address:** Eastren Virginia Med Sch, Dept Surgery, 825 Fairfax Ave, Ste 610, Norfolk, VA 23507; **Phone:** 757-446-8950; **Board Cert:** Surgery 2003; Surgical Critical Care 1997; **Med School:** Harvard Med Sch 1977; **Resid:** Surgery, Barnes Hosp-Wash Univ 1979; Surgery, Univ Illinois Chicago Med Ctr 1984; **Fellow:** Trauma, Md Inst Emer Med Serv Sys 1986; **Fac Appt:** Prof S, Eastern VA Med Sch

Cance, William George MD [S] - **Spec Exp:** Pancreatic Cancer; Colon & Rectal Cancer; Endocrine Cancers; **Hospital:** Shands Hlthcre at Univ of FL, VA Med Ctr - Gainesville; **Address:** Shands at Univ Florida-Dept Surgery, 1600 SW Archer Rd, PO Box 100286, Gainesville, FL 32610-0286; **Phone:** 352-265-0622; **Board Cert:** Surgery 1998; **Med School:** Duke Univ 1982; **Resid:** Surgery, Barnes Hosp-Wash Univ 1988; **Fellow:** Surgical Oncology, Meml Sloan Kettering Canc Ctr 1990; **Fac Appt:** Prof S, Univ Fla Coll Med

Cole, David J MD [S] - **Spec Exp:** Breast Brachytherapy; Gastrointestinal Cancer; Vaccine Therapy; Gene Therapy; **Hospital:** MUSC Med Ctr; **Address:** 96 Jonathan Lucas St, PO BOX 250613, Charleston, SC 29425; **Phone:** 843-792-4638; **Board Cert:** Surgery 2000; **Med School:** Cornell Univ-Weill Med Coll 1986; **Resid:** Surgery, Emory Univ School Med 1991; **Fellow:** Surgical Oncology, Natl Cancer Institute 1994; **Fac Appt:** Prof S, Med Univ SC

Copeland III, Edward M MD [S] - **Spec Exp:** Breast Cancer; Colon & Rectal Cancer; Melanoma; **Hospital:** Shands Hlthcre at Univ of FL; **Address:** Univ Florida Coll Medicine, Dept Surgery, 1600 SW Archer Rd, Box 100286, Gainesville, FL 32610; **Phone:** 352-265-0169; **Board Cert:** Surgery 1971; **Med School:** Cornell Univ-Weill Med Coll 1963; **Resid:** Surgery, Hosp Univ Penn 1969; Surgical Oncology, Univ TX MD Anderson Cancer Ctr 1972; **Fellow:** Research, Hosp Univ Penn 1967; **Fac Appt:** Prof S, Univ Fla Coll Med

Dilawari, Raza A MD [S] - **Spec Exp:** Skin Cancer; Melanoma; Breast Cancer; Ovarian Cancer; **Hospital:** Methodist Univ Hosp - Memphis, St Francis Hosp - Memphis; **Address:** Methodist Univ Hosp, 1325 Eastmoreland Ave, Ste 410, Memphis, TN 38104; **Phone:** 901-767-7204; **Board Cert:** Surgery 1975; **Med School:** Pakistan 1968; **Resid:** Surgery, SUNY-Upstate Med Ctr 1974; **Fellow:** Surgical Oncology, Roswell Park Meml Hosp 1976; **Fac Appt:** Prof S, Univ Tenn Coll Med, Memphis

Eckhoff, Devin E MD [S] - **Spec Exp:** Transplant-Liver; Hepatobiliary Surgery; Transplant-Kidney; Hepatitis C; **Hospital:** Univ of Ala Hosp at Birmingham; **Address:** University of Alabama School of Medicine, 701 19th St S, LHRB Bldg - rm 710, Birmingham, AL 35294-0007; **Phone:** 205-975-7622; **Board Cert:** Surgery 2000; Surgical Critical Care 2001; **Med School:** Univ Minn 1986; **Resid:** Surgery, Univ Wisconsin Med Ctr 1992; **Fellow:** Transplant Surgery, Univ Wisconsin Med Ctr 1994; **Fac Appt:** Prof S, Univ Ala

Feliciano, David V MD [S] - **Spec Exp:** Vascular Surgery; Trauma; **Hospital:** Grady Hlth Sys; **Address:** Grady Memorial Hosp, Glenn Meml Bldg, 69 Jesse Hill Jr Dr SE, rm 304, Atlanta, GA 30303; **Phone:** 404-616-5456; **Board Cert:** Surgery 1998; Surgical Critical Care 1998; **Med School:** Georgetown Univ 1970; **Resid:** Surgery, Mayo Clinic 1977; **Fellow:** Cardiovascular Surgery, Texas Med Ctr/Baylor 1978; **Fac Appt:** Prof S, Emory Univ

Flint Jr, Lewis M MD [S] - **Spec Exp:** Trauma; Critical Care; Gastrointestinal Surgery; **Hospital:** Tampa Genl Hosp; **Address:** Tampa Genl Hosp, Trauma Ctr, Box 1289, Ste G417, Tampa, FL 33601-1289; **Phone:** 813-844-7968; **Board Cert:** Surgery 1987; Surgical Critical Care 2004; **Med School:** Duke Univ 1965; **Resid:** Surgery, Duke Univ Hosp 1967; Surgery, Univ SC Med Ctr 1974; **Fellow:** Trauma, Univ Tex SW 1975; **Fac Appt:** Prof S, Univ Fla Coll Med

Flynn, Michael B MD [S] - **Spec Exp:** Head & Neck Cancer; Head & Neck Surgery; **Hospital:** Univ of Louisville Hosp, Norton Hosp; **Address:** 601 S Floyd St, Ste 700, Louisville, KY 40202; **Phone:** 502-583-8303; **Board Cert:** Surgery 1972; **Med School:** Ireland 1962; **Resid:** Surgery, Univ Maryland Hosp 1969; **Fellow:** Surgical Oncology, MD Anderson Hosp 1971; **Fac Appt:** Prof S, Univ Louisville Sch Med

Gabram, Sheryl MD [S] - **Spec Exp:** Breast Cancer; Breast Disease; **Hospital:** Emory Univ Hosp, Grady Hlth Sys; **Address:** Winship Cancer Institute, 1365 Clifton Rd NE C Bldg Fl 2, Atlanta, GA 30322; **Phone:** 404-778-1230; **Board Cert:** Surgery 1996; **Med School:** Georgetown Univ 1982; **Resid:** Surgery, Washington Hosp Ctr 1987; **Fellow:** Trauma, Hartford Hosp 1988; **Fac Appt:** Prof S, Emory Univ

Goldstein, Richard E MD/PhD [S] - **Spec Exp:** Endocrine Tumors; Thyroid Cancer & Surgery; Parathyroid Cancer; Parathyroid Surgery; **Hospital:** Univ of Louisville Hosp; **Address:** University Surgical Assocs, 601 S Floyd St, Ste 700, Louisville, KY 40202; **Phone:** 502-583-8303; **Board Cert:** Surgery 1999; **Med School:** Jefferson Med Coll 1982; **Resid:** Surgery, Vanderbilt Univ Hosp 1990; **Fac Appt:** Prof S, Univ Louisville Sch Med

Greene, Frederick L MD [S] - **Spec Exp:** Gastrointestinal Surgery; Gastrointestinal Cancer; Hernia; **Hospital:** Carolinas Med Ctr; **Address:** Carolinas Medical Ctr, 1025 Morehead Medical Drive, Ste 275, Charlotte, NC 28203; **Phone:** 704-355-1813; **Board Cert:** Surgery 1998; **Med School:** Univ VA Sch Med 1970; **Resid:** Surgery, Yale-New Haven Hosp 1976; **Fellow:** Surgical Oncology, Yale-New Haven Hosp 1973; **Fac Appt:** Prof S, Univ NC Sch Med

Hanks, John B MD [S] - **Spec Exp:** Endocrine Cancers; Breast Cancer; Thyroid Cancer & Surgery; Endocrine Surgery; **Hospital:** Univ Virginia Med Ctr; **Address:** Univ VA Hlth Sys, Dept Surg, PO Box 800709, Charlottesville, VA 22908-0709; **Phone:** 434-924-0376; **Board Cert:** Surgery 2001; **Med School:** Univ Rochester 1973; **Resid:** Surgery, Duke Univ Med Ctr 1982; **Fac Appt:** Prof S, Univ VA Sch Med

Hemming, Alan W MD [S] - **Spec Exp:** Liver Cancer; Transplant-Liver; Hepatobiliary Surgery; Pancreatic Cancer; **Hospital:** Shands Hlthcre at Univ of FL; **Address:** University of Florida, Dept Surgery, 1600 SW Archer Rd, rm 6142, Box 100286, Gainsville, FL 32610-3003; **Phone:** 352-265-0606; **Board Cert:** Surgery 2005; **Med School:** Canada 1987; **Resid:** Surgery, Univ British Columbia Med Ctr 1993; **Fellow:** Transplant Surgery, Univ Toronto/Hosp for Sick Children 1995; Hepatobiliary Surgery, Univ Toronto 1996; **Fac Appt:** Prof S, Univ Fla Coll Med

Herrmann, Virginia M MD [S] - **Spec Exp:** Breast Cancer; Nutrition & Cancer Prevention/Control; **Hospital:** Meml Hlth Univ Med Ctr - Savannah; **Address:** Center for Breast Care, 4700 Waters Ave, Ste 405, Savannah, GA 31404; **Phone:** 912-350-2700; **Board Cert:** Surgery 2000; **Med School:** St Louis Univ 1974; **Resid:** Surgery, St Louis Univ Hosps 1979; **Fellow:** Surgery, Brigham & Women's Hosp/Harvard 1980; **Fac Appt:** Prof S, Mercer Univ Sch Med

Howard, Richard J MD [S] - **Spec Exp:** Endocrine Surgery; Transplant-Kidney; Gastrointestinal Surgery; **Hospital:** Shands Hlthcre at Univ of FL; **Address:** Shands Healthcare Transplant Surgery, 1600 SW Archer Rd, Ste 6142, Gainesville, FL 32610; **Phone:** 352-265-0606; **Board Cert:** Surgery 2004; **Med School:** Yale Univ 1966; **Resid:** Surgery, Univ Minn Hosp 1975; **Fac Appt:** Prof S, Univ Fla Coll Med

Israel, Philip Z MD [S] - **Spec Exp:** Breast Cancer; **Hospital:** WellStar Kennestone Hosp; **Address:** 702 Canton Rd, Marietta, GA 30060; **Phone:** 770-428-4486; **Board Cert:** Surgery 1967; **Med School:** Emory Univ 1961; **Resid:** Surgery, Emory Univ Hosp 1966; **Fac Appt:** Prof S, Univ Tenn Coll Med,Chattanooga

Koruda, Mark Joseph MD [S] - **Spec Exp:** Gastrointestinal Surgery; Minimally Invasive Surgery; Inflammatory Bowel Disease; **Hospital:** Univ NC Hosps; **Address:** Univ NC Chapel Hill, Div Gastrointestinal Surgery, 320 Med Wing E, Campus Box 7081, Chapel Hill, NC 27599; **Phone:** 919-966-8436; **Board Cert:** Surgery 1999; **Med School:** Yale Univ 1981; **Resid:** Surgery, Hosp Univ Penn 1988; **Fac Appt:** Prof S, Univ NC Sch Med

Leight, George MD [S] - **Spec Exp:** Breast Cancer; Thyroid Cancer; Parathyroid Cancer; **Hospital:** Duke Univ Med Ctr; **Address:** Duke Univ Med Ctr, Dept Surgery, DUMC Box 3513, Durham, NC 27710; **Phone:** 919-684-6849; **Board Cert:** Surgery 1999; **Med School:** Duke Univ 1972; **Resid:** Surgery, Duke Univ Med Ctr 1978; **Fac Appt:** Prof S, Duke Univ

Levine, Edward A MD [S] - **Spec Exp:** Breast Cancer; Esophageal Cancer; Peritoneal Carcinomatosis; **Hospital:** Wake Forest Univ Baptist Med Ctr (page 73); **Address:** Wake Forest Univ Baptist Med Ctr, Dept of Surgery, Medical Center Blvd, Winston-Salem, NC 27157; **Phone:** 336-716-4276; **Board Cert:** Surgery 1999; **Med School:** Ros Franklin Univ/Chicago Med Sch 1985; **Resid:** Surgery, Michael Reese Hosp 1990; **Fellow:** Surgical Oncology, Univ Illinois 1992; **Fac Appt:** Prof S, Wake Forest Univ

Lind, David Scott MD [S] - **Spec Exp:** Breast Cancer; Melanoma; Sarcoma; **Hospital:** Med Coll of GA Hosp and Clin; **Address:** MCG Health System-Dept Hem Onc, 1120 15th St, Augusta, GA 30912; **Phone:** 706-721-6744; **Board Cert:** Surgery 2000; **Med School:** Eastern VA Med Sch 1984; **Resid:** Surgery, Univ Texas 1989; **Fellow:** Medical Oncology, Med Coll Virginia 1992; **Fac Appt:** Prof Surg & Onc, Med Coll GA

Livingstone, Alan S MD [S] - **Spec Exp:** Liver & Biliary Cancer; Stomach Cancer; Pancreatic Cancer; Esophageal Cancer; **Hospital:** Jackson Meml Hosp, Univ of Miami Hosp & Clins/Sylvester Comp Canc Ctr; **Address:** Sylvester Comp Cancer Ctr, Dept Surgery (310T), 1475 NW 12th Ave, rm 3550, Miami, FL 33136; **Phone:** 305-243-4902; **Board Cert:** Surgery 1995; **Med School:** McGill Univ 1971; **Resid:** Surgery, Montreal Genl Hosp 1976; Surgery, Jackson Meml Hosp 1975; **Fac Appt:** Prof S, Univ Miami Sch Med

Luterman, Arnold MD [S] - **Spec Exp:** Burn Care; Wound Healing/Care; Critical Care; **Hospital:** Univ of S AL Med Ctr; **Address:** Univ of S Alabama Med Ctr, Mastin Bldg, 2451 Fillingim St, rm 719, Mobile, AL 36617; **Phone:** 251-470-5827; **Board Cert:** Surgery 1996; Surgical Critical Care 1996; **Med School:** McGill Univ 1970; **Resid:** Surgery, Sinai Hospital 1973; Surgery, Jewish Gen Hosp. McGill U 1976; **Fellow:** Burn Surgery, Univ Washington Medical Ctr 1976; **Fac Appt:** Prof S, Univ S Ala Coll Med

Lyerly, H Kim MD [S] - **Spec Exp:** Breast Cancer; Immunotherapy; **Hospital:** Duke Univ Med Ctr, Durham Regional Hosp; **Address:** Duke Univ Med Ctr, Dept Surg, DUMC Box 2714, Durham, NC 27710; **Phone:** 919-684-5613; **Board Cert:** Surgery 2001; **Med School:** UCLA 1983; **Resid:** Surgery, Duke Univ Med Ctr 1990; **Fac Appt:** Prof S, Duke Univ

MacDonald Jr, Kenneth G MD [S] - **Spec Exp:** Gastrointestinal Surgery; Obesity/Bariatric Surgery; Pancreatic Surgery; **Hospital:** Pitt Cty Mem Hosp - Univ Med Ctr East Carolina; **Address:** Southern Surgical Assoc, PA, 2455 Emerald Pl, Greenville, NC 27834; **Phone:** 252-758-2224; **Board Cert:** Surgery 1998; **Med School:** W VA Univ 1981; **Resid:** Surgery, NC Baptist Hosp 1984; Surgery, Univ Med Ctr of E Carolina 1987; **Fac Appt:** Prof S, E Carolina Univ

MacFadyen, Bruce MD [S] - **Spec Exp:** Laparoscopic Surgery; Gastrointestinal Surgery; Endoscopy; **Hospital:** Med Coll of GA Hosp and Clin; **Address:** Medical College GA, Dept Surgery, 1120 15th St, Ste 4076, Augusta, GA 30912; **Phone:** 706-721-1066; **Board Cert:** Surgery 1975; **Med School:** Hahnemann Univ 1968; **Resid:** Surgery, Hosp Univ Penn 1972; Surgery, Hermann Hosp 1974; **Fellow:** MD Anderson Cancer Ctr 1978; **Fac Appt:** Prof S, Med Coll GA

McGrath, Patrick C MD [S] - **Spec Exp:** Breast Cancer; Cancer Surgery; **Hospital:** Univ of Kentucky Chandler Hosp; **Address:** Univ Kentucky Med Ctr, Dept Genl Surgery, 800 Rose St, rm C224, Lexington, KY 40536-0293; **Phone:** 859-323-6346 x233; **Board Cert:** Surgery 1996; **Med School:** Univ IL Coll Med 1980; **Resid:** Surgery, Med Coll Virginia Hosp 1986; **Fellow:** Surgical Oncology, Med Coll Virginia Hosp 1988; **Fac Appt:** Prof S, Univ KY Coll Med

Meyer, Anthony A MD [S] - **Spec Exp:** Trauma/Critical Care; Burn Care; **Hospital:** Univ NC Hosps; **Address:** Univ NC-Sch Med, Dept Surgery, 4041 Burnett-Womack Bldg, CB7050, Chapel Hill, NC 27599-7050; **Phone:** 919-966-4321; **Board Cert:** Surgery 2001; Surgical Critical Care 1994; **Med School:** Univ Chicago-Pritzker Sch Med 1977; **Resid:** Surgery, UCSF Med Ctr 1982; **Fac Appt:** Prof S, Univ NC Sch Med

Newell, Kenneth MD/PhD [S] - **Spec Exp:** Transplant-Kidney; Transplant-Pancreas; Transplant-Liver; **Hospital:** Emory Univ Hosp; **Address:** Emory Transplant Ctr, 101 Woodruff Cir, rm 5105 WMB, Atlanta, GA 30322; **Phone:** 404-727-2489; **Board Cert:** Surgery 1999; **Med School:** Univ Mich Med Sch 1984; **Resid:** Surgery, Loyola Univ Med Ctr 1989; **Fellow:** Transplant Surgery, Univ Chicago 1994; **Fac Appt:** Assoc Prof S, Emory Univ

Pappas, Theodore N MD [S] - **Spec Exp:** Pancreatic Surgery; Laparoscopic Surgery; **Hospital:** Duke Univ Med Ctr; **Address:** Duke Univ Med Ctr, Dept Surgery, DUMC Box 3479, Durham, NC 27710-0001; **Phone:** 919-681-3442; **Board Cert:** Surgery 1997; **Med School:** Ohio State Univ 1981; **Resid:** Surgery, Brigham & Womens Hosp 1988; **Fellow:** Research, Wadworth VA Med Ctr 1985; **Fac Appt:** Prof S, Duke Univ

Pinson, C Wright MD [S] - **Spec Exp:** Transplant-Liver; Liver & Biliary Cancer; Pancreatic Cancer; Liver & Biliary Surgery; **Hospital:** Vanderbilt Univ Med Ctr; **Address:** Vanderbilt Transplant Ctr, TVC 3810A, 1301 21st Ave S, Nashville, TN 37232-5545; **Phone:** 615-343-9324; **Board Cert:** Surgery 1996; Surgical Critical Care 1997; **Med School:** Vanderbilt Univ 1980; **Resid:** Surgery, Oregon Health Sci Ctr 1986; **Fellow:** Gastrointestinal Surgery, Lahey Clinic 1987; Transplant Surgery, Deaconess Hosp 1988; **Fac Appt:** Prof S, Vanderbilt Univ

Polk Jr, Hiram C MD [S] - **Spec Exp:** Melanoma; Colon Cancer; **Hospital:** Univ of Louisville Hosp, Norton Hosp; **Address:** 601 S Floyd St, Ste 700, Louisville, KY 40292; **Phone:** 502-583-8303; **Board Cert:** Surgery 1966; **Med School:** Harvard Med Sch 1960; **Resid:** Surgery, Barnes Hosp 1965; **Fac Appt:** Prof S, Univ Louisville Sch Med

Reintgen, Douglas Scott MD [S] - **Spec Exp:** Melanoma; Breast Cancer; Cancer Surgery; **Hospital:** Lakeland Regl Med Ctr; **Address:** 3525 Lakeland Hills Blvd, Lakeland, FL 33805-1965; **Phone:** 863-603-6565; **Board Cert:** Surgery 1997; **Med School:** Duke Univ 1979; **Resid:** Surgery, Duke Univ Med Ctr 1987; **Fac Appt:** Prof S, Univ S Fla Coll Med

Scantlebury, Velma P MD [S] - **Spec Exp:** Transplant-Kidney; Kidney Disease; **Hospital:** Univ of S AL Med Ctr, Mobile Infirmary Med Ctr; **Address:** Univ of S Alabama, Div Transplantation, 2451 Fillingim St Fl 10 - Ste F, Mobile, AL 36617-2293; **Phone:** 251-471-7542; **Board Cert:** Surgery 2001; **Med School:** Columbia P&S 1981; **Resid:** Surgery, Harlem Hosp 1986; **Fellow:** Transplant Surgery, Univ Pittsburgh Med Ctr 1988; **Fac Appt:** Prof S, Univ S Ala Coll Med

Schirmer, Bruce D MD [S] - **Spec Exp:** Laparoscopic Surgery; Gastrointestinal Surgery; Pancreatic Surgery; Liver Surgery; **Hospital:** Univ Virginia Med Ctr; **Address:** Univ VA Hlth Sys, Dept Surgery, PO Box 800709, Charlottesville, VA 22908; **Phone:** 434-924-2104; **Board Cert:** Surgery 2005; **Med School:** Duke Univ 1978; **Resid:** Surgery, Duke Med Ctr 1985; **Fac Appt:** Prof S, Univ VA Sch Med

Sharp, Kenneth MD [S] - **Spec Exp:** Gastrointestinal Surgery; Esophageal Disorders; Laparoscopic Surgery; Pancreatic Surgery; **Hospital:** Vanderbilt Univ Med Ctr; **Address:** Vanderbilt Univ Med Ctr, Dept Surgery, D-5203 Medical Center North, Nashville, TN 37232-2577; **Phone:** 615-322-0259; **Board Cert:** Surgery 2003; **Med School:** Johns Hopkins Univ 1977; **Resid:** Surgery, Johns Hopkins Univ Med Ctr 1984; **Fellow:** Hepatobiliary Surgery, Loch Raven VA Hosp 1981; Surgery, John Radcliffe Hosp 1982; **Fac Appt:** Prof S, Vanderbilt Univ

Sondak, Vernon K MD [S] - **Spec Exp:** Cancer Surgery; Melanoma; Sarcoma; **Hospital:** H Lee Moffitt Cancer Ctr & Research Inst; **Address:** H Lee Moffitt Cancer Ctr-Cutaneous Program, 12902 Magnolia Drive, Tampa, FL 33612; **Phone:** 813-745-1968; **Board Cert:** Surgery 1996; **Med School:** Boston Univ 1980; **Resid:** Surgery, UCLA Med Ctr 1987; **Fellow:** Surgical Oncology, UCLA Med Ctr 1984; **Fac Appt:** Prof S, Univ S Fla Coll Med

Stratta, Robert MD [S] - **Spec Exp:** Transplant-Pancreas; Transplant-Kidney; Gastrointestinal Surgery; **Hospital:** Wake Forest Univ Baptist Med Ctr (page 73); **Address:** Wake Forest Univ Baptist Med Ctr, Dept Surgery, Medical Center Blvd, Winston-Salem, NC 27157-1095; **Phone:** 336-716-6371; **Board Cert:** Surgery 1996; **Med School:** Univ Chicago-Pritzker Sch Med 1980; **Resid:** Surgery, Univ Utah Med Ctr 1986; **Fellow:** Transplant Surgery, Univ Wisc Hosps & Clins 1988; **Fac Appt:** Prof S, Wake Forest Univ

Tyler, Douglas S MD [S] - **Spec Exp:** Pancreatic Cancer; Colon & Rectal Cancer; Rectal Cancer/Sphincter Preservation; Melanoma; **Hospital:** Duke Univ Med Ctr; **Address:** Duke University Med Ctr, Box 3118, Durham, NC 27710; **Phone:** 919-684-6858; **Board Cert:** Surgery 2000; **Med School:** Dartmouth Med Sch 1985; **Resid:** Surgery, Duke Univ Med Ctr 1992; **Fellow:** Surgical Oncology, MD Anderson Cancer Ctr 1994; **Fac Appt:** Prof S, Duke Univ

Tzakis, Andreas MD [S] - **Spec Exp:** Transplant-Liver; Transplant-Bowel; **Hospital:** Jackson Meml Hosp; **Address:** 1801 NW 9th Ave, Ste 511, Miami, FL 33136; **Phone:** 305-355-5011; **Board Cert:** Surgery 2003; **Med School:** Greece 1974; **Resid:** Surgery, Mt Sinai Hosp 1979; Surgery, SUNY Stony Brook 1983; **Fellow:** Transplant Surgery, Univ Pittsburgh Med Ctr 1985; **Fac Appt:** Prof S, Univ Miami Sch Med

Urist, Marshall M MD [S] - **Spec Exp:** Cancer Surgery; Breast Cancer; Melanoma; **Hospital:** Univ of Ala Hosp at Birmingham; **Address:** Univ Alabama Sch Med, Dept Surgery, 1922 7th Ave S, Kracke Bldg, Ste 321, Birmingham, AL 35294; **Phone:** 205-934-3065; **Board Cert:** Surgery 2000; **Med School:** Univ Chicago-Pritzker Sch Med 1971; **Resid:** Surgery, Johns Hopkins Hosp 1978; **Fellow:** Surgical Oncology, UCLA Med Ctr 1976; **Fac Appt:** Prof S, Univ Ala

Vogel, Stephen Burton MD [S] - **Spec Exp:** Esophageal Cancer; Liver Cancer; **Hospital:** Shands Hlthcre at Univ of FL; **Address:** University of Florida, Dept Surgery, PO Box 100286, Gainesville, FL 32610-0286; **Phone:** 352-265-0604; **Board Cert:** Surgery 1976; **Med School:** Univ Fla Coll Med 1967; **Resid:** Surgery, Univ Minn Hosp 1975; **Fac Appt:** Prof S, Univ Fla Coll Med

White Jr, Richard L MD [S] - **Spec Exp:** Breast Cancer; Melanoma; Sarcoma; Immunotherapy; **Hospital:** Carolinas Med Ctr; **Address:** Carolinas Medical Center, 1000 Blythe Blvd, Box 32861, Charlotte, NC 28203; **Phone:** 704-355-2884; **Board Cert:** Surgery 2002; **Med School:** Columbia P&S 1986; **Resid:** Surgery, Georgetown Univ Hosp 1992; **Fellow:** Surgical Oncology, NIH- Natl Cancer Inst 1995; **Fac Appt:** Assoc Clin Prof S, Univ NC Sch Med

Willis, Irvin MD [S] - **Spec Exp:** Pancreatic Surgery; Cancer Surgery; Laparoscopic Surgery; **Hospital:** Mount Sinai Med Ctr - Miami; **Address:** 4302 Alton Rd, Ste 630, Miami Beach, FL 33140-2876; **Phone:** 305-534-6050; **Board Cert:** Surgery 1970; **Med School:** Univ Cincinnati 1964; **Resid:** Surgery, Univ Miami-Jackson Meml 1969

Wood, William C MD [S] - **Spec Exp:** Breast Cancer; **Hospital:** Emory Univ Hosp; **Address:** Emory Univ Hosp, Dept Surgery, 1364 Clifton Rd NE, Ste B206, Atlanta, GA 30322; **Phone:** 404-727-5800; **Board Cert:** Surgery 1974; **Med School:** Harvard Med Sch 1966; **Resid:** Surgery, Mass Genl Hosp 1968; Surgery, Mass Genl Hosp 1974; **Fac Appt:** Prof S, Emory Univ

Midwest

Angelos, Peter MD/PhD [S] - **Spec Exp:** Endocrine Tumors; Pheochromocytoma; Carcinoid Tumors; Islet Cell Tumors; **Hospital:** Univ of Chicago Hosps; **Address:** Bernard A. Mitchell Hospital, 5841 S Maryland Ave, MC 5031, Chicago, IL 60637; **Phone:** 773-702-4429; **Board Cert:** Surgery 2004; **Med School:** Boston Univ 1989; **Resid:** Surgery, Northwestern Univ 1995; **Fellow:** Medical Ethics, Univ of Chicago-Pritzker Sch Med 1992; Endocrine Surgery, Univ of Michigan Med Sch 1996; **Fac Appt:** Prof S, Univ Chicago-Pritzker Sch Med

Benedetti, Enrico MD [S] - **Spec Exp:** Transplant-Liver; Transplant-Pancreas; Transplant-Kidney; Transplant-Bowel; **Hospital:** Univ of IL Med Ctr at Chicago; **Address:** Univ Illinois, Dept Surgery/Transplant, 840 S Wood St, rm 402, Chicago, IL 60612; **Phone:** 312-996-6771; **Board Cert:** Surgery 2003; **Med School:** Italy 1985; **Resid:** Surgery, Univ IL at Chicago Med Ctr 1993; **Fellow:** Transplant Surgery, Univ Minn 1994; **Fac Appt:** Prof S, Univ IL Coll Med

Brems, John MD [S] - **Spec Exp:** Transplant-Liver; Pancreatic Cancer; Liver Cancer; **Hospital:** Loyola Univ Med Ctr; **Address:** 2160 S 1st Ave, MC-EMS-3268, Maywood, IL 60153-3304; **Phone:** 708-327-2539; **Board Cert:** Surgery 2004; Surgical Critical Care 2000; **Med School:** St Louis Univ 1981; **Resid:** Surgery, St Louis Univ 1986; **Fellow:** Transplant Surgery, UCLA Med Ctr 1987; **Fac Appt:** Prof S, Loyola Univ-Stritch Sch Med

Brunt, L Michael MD [S] - **Spec Exp:** Minimally Invasive Surgery; Adrenal Tumors; Hernia; **Hospital:** Barnes-Jewish Hosp; **Address:** Washington Univ Sch Medicine, Dept Surg, 660 S Euclid Ave, Box 8109, St Louis, MO 63110; **Phone:** 314-454-7194; **Board Cert:** Surgery 1996; **Med School:** Johns Hopkins Univ 1980; **Resid:** Surgery, Barnes Jewish Hosp 1987; **Fellow:** Surgery, Barnes Jewish Hosp 1984; **Fac Appt:** Prof S, Washington Univ, St Louis

Chang, Alfred E MD [S] - **Spec Exp:** Breast Cancer; Gastrointestinal Cancer; Melanoma; Sarcoma; **Hospital:** Univ Michigan Hlth Sys; **Address:** Univ Mich Comp Cancer Ctr/Geriatric Ctr, 1500 E Med Ctr Dr 3302 CGC, Ann Arbor, MI 48109-0932; **Phone:** 734-936-4392; **Board Cert:** Surgery 2001; **Med School:** Harvard Med Sch 1974; **Resid:** Surgery, Duke Univ Med Ctr 1976; Surgery, Hosp Univ Penn 1982; **Fellow:** Surgical Oncology, Natl Cancer Inst 1979; **Fac Appt:** Prof S, Univ Mich Med Sch

Chapman, William C MD [S] - **Spec Exp:** Transplant-Liver-Adult & Pediatric; Liver Cancer; Liver & Biliary Surgery; **Hospital:** Barnes-Jewish Hosp, St Louis Chldns Hosp; **Address:** Washington Univ Sch Med, 660 S Euclid Ave, Box 8604, St Louis, MO 63110; **Phone:** 314-362-7792; **Board Cert:** Surgery 2001; Surgical Critical Care 2001; **Med School:** Med Univ SC 1984; **Resid:** Surgery, Vanderbilt Univ Med Ctr 1991; **Fellow:** Hepatobiliary Surgery, Kings College Hosp 1992; **Fac Appt:** Prof S, Washington Univ, St Louis

Crowe Jr, Joseph P MD [S] - **Spec Exp:** Breast Cancer; Tumor Surgery; **Hospital:** Cleveland Clin Fdn (page 57); **Address:** Cleveland Clinic Fdn, Dept Surg, 9500 Euclid Ave, Desk A10, Cleveland, OH 44195; **Phone:** 216-444-3024; **Board Cert:** Surgery 2004; **Med School:** Case West Res Univ 1978; **Resid:** Surgery, Univ Hosp-Case West Reserve 1983; **Fellow:** Surgical Oncology, Meml Sloan Kettering Cancer Ctr 1985

Deziel, Daniel J MD [S] - **Spec Exp:** Hepatobiliary Surgery; Pancreatic Surgery; Laparoscopic Surgery; **Hospital:** Rush Univ Med Ctr; **Address:** 1725 W Harrison, Ste 810, Chicago, IL 60612-3828; **Phone:** 312-942-6500; **Board Cert:** Surgery 2003; **Med School:** Univ Minn 1979; **Resid:** Surgery, Rush-Presby-St Luke's Med Ctr 1984; **Fellow:** Gastrointestinal Surgery, Lahey Clinic 1985; **Fac Appt:** Prof S, Rush Med Coll

Doherty, Gerard M MD [S] - **Spec Exp:** Endocrine Surgery; Adrenal Surgery; Laparoscopic Surgery; **Hospital:** Univ Michigan Hlth Sys; **Address:** A Taubman Hlth Care Center, 1500 E Medical Center Drive, rm 2920, Ann Arbor, MI 48109-0331; **Phone:** 734-615-4741; **Board Cert:** Surgery 2003; **Med School:** Yale Univ 1986; **Resid:** Surgery, UCSF Med Ctr 1993; **Fellow:** Medical Oncology, Natl Cancer Inst 1991; **Fac Appt:** Prof S, Univ Mich Med Sch

Donohue, John H MD [S] - **Spec Exp:** Gastrointestinal Cancer; Breast Cancer; Stomach Cancer; **Hospital:** Mayo Med Ctr & Clin - Rochester; **Address:** Mayo Clinic, Dept Surgery, 200 First St SW, Rochester, MN 55905; **Phone:** 507-284-0362; **Board Cert:** Surgery 2005; **Med School:** Harvard Med Sch 1978; **Resid:** Surgery, UCSF Med Ctr 1981; Surgery, UCSF Med Ctr 1985; **Fellow:** Surgery, Natl Inst Hlth 1983; Surgical Oncology, Meml Sloan-Kettering Canc Ctr 1987; **Fac Appt:** Prof S, Mayo Med Sch

Eberlein, Timothy J MD [S] - **Spec Exp:** Breast Cancer; Melanoma; Immunotherapy; **Hospital:** Barnes-Jewish Hosp, St Louis Chldns Hosp; **Address:** Wash Univ School of Med, Dept Surgery, 660 S Euclid Ave, Box 8109, St Louis, MO 63110-1093; **Phone:** 314-362-8020; **Board Cert:** Surgery 1995; **Med School:** Univ Pittsburgh 1977; **Resid:** Surgery, Peter Bent Brigham Hosp 1979; Surgery, Brigham-Womens Hosp 1985; **Fellow:** Allergy & Immunology, Natl Inst Hlth 1982; **Fac Appt:** Prof S, Washington Univ, St Louis

Ellison, E Christopher MD [S] - **Spec Exp:** Biliary Surgery; Biliary Cancer; Pancreatic Cancer; **Hospital:** Ohio St Univ Med Ctr; **Address:** 1654 Upham Drive, Ste 327 Means Hall, Columbus, OH 43210-1236; **Phone:** 614-293-9722; **Board Cert:** Surgery 2001; **Med School:** Univ Wisc 1975; **Resid:** Surgery, Ohio State Univ 1981; **Fac Appt:** Prof S, Ohio State Univ

Farley, David R MD [S] - **Spec Exp:** Endocrine Surgery; Hepatobiliary Surgery; Laparoscopic Surgery; Hernia; **Hospital:** Mayo Med Ctr & Clin - Rochester; **Address:** Mayo Clinic, 200 First St SW, Mayo West 12, ATTN: Dr. Farley, Rochester, MN 55905; **Phone:** 507-284-2644; **Board Cert:** Surgery 2002; **Med School:** Univ Wisc 1988; **Resid:** Surgery, Mayo Clinic 1994; **Fellow:** Endocrinology, Mayo Clinic 1995; **Fac Appt:** Assoc Prof S, Mayo Med Sch

Farrar, William B MD [S] - **Spec Exp:** Breast Cancer; Thyroid Cancer; **Hospital:** Arthur G James Cancer Hosp & Research Inst, Ohio St Univ Med Ctr; **Address:** 410 W 10th Ave, N924 Doan Hall, Columbus, OH 43210-1240; **Phone:** 614-293-8890; **Board Cert:** Surgery 2000; **Med School:** Univ VA Sch Med 1975; **Resid:** Surgery, Ohio State Univ Hosps 1980; **Fellow:** Surgical Oncology, Meml Sloan-Kettering Cancer Ctr 1982; **Fac Appt:** Prof S, Ohio State Univ

Ferguson, Ronald MD [S] - **Spec Exp:** Transplant-Kidney; **Hospital:** Ohio St Univ Med Ctr; **Address:** 1654 Upham Drive, Ste 363 Means, Columbus, OH 43210-1250; **Phone:** 614-293-6724; **Board Cert:** Surgery 2002; **Med School:** Washington Univ, St Louis 1971; **Resid:** Surgery, Univ Minn Hosp 1979; **Fellow:** Immunology, Univ Minn Hosp 1980; **Fac Appt:** Prof S, Ohio State Univ

Fung, John J MD/PhD [S] - **Spec Exp:** Transplant-Liver; Transplant-Kidney; Liver & Biliary Cancer; **Hospital:** Cleveland Clin Fdn (page 57), Euclid Hosp (page 57); **Address:** Cleveland Clinic, Dept Surgery, Desk A80, 9500 Euclid Ave, Cleveland, OH 44195-0001; **Phone:** 216-444-3776; **Board Cert:** Surgery 1997; **Med School:** Univ Chicago-Pritzker Sch Med 1982; **Resid:** Surgery, Strong Memorial Hosp 1988; **Fellow:** Transplant Surgery, Univ Pittsburgh 1986; **Fac Appt:** Prof S, Cleveland Cl Coll Med/Case West Res

Gamelli, Richard L MD [S] - **Spec Exp:** Burn Care; Trauma/Critical Care; **Hospital:** Loyola Univ Med Ctr; **Address:** 2160 S First Ave EMS Bldg - rm 3244, Maywood, IL 60153; **Phone:** 708-216-8563; **Board Cert:** Surgery 1989; **Med School:** Univ VT Coll Med 1974; **Resid:** Surgery, Vermont Med Ctr Hosp 1979; **Fac Appt:** Prof S, Loyola Univ-Stritch Sch Med

Goulet Jr, Robert J MD [S] - **Spec Exp:** Breast Cancer; **Hospital:** Indiana Univ Hosp; **Address:** Indiana Univ Hosp, Cancer Pavilion, 535 Barnhill Drive, Ste 431, Indianapolis, IN 46202-5112; **Phone:** 317-274-9800; **Board Cert:** Surgery 1995; **Med School:** SUNY Downstate 1979; **Resid:** Surgery, SUNY-Downstate Med Ctr 1986; **Fellow:** Surgical Research, SUNY-Downstate Med Ctr 1983; **Fac Appt:** Assoc Prof S, Indiana Univ

Grant, Clive S MD [S] - **Spec Exp:** Thyroid & Parathyroid Cancer & Surgery; Adrenal Tumors; Breast Cancer; **Hospital:** Mayo Med Ctr & Clin - Rochester; **Address:** Mayo Clinic, Dept Surgery, 200 First St SW, Rochester, MN 55905-0001; **Phone:** 507-284-2644; **Board Cert:** Surgery 2001; **Med School:** Univ Colorado 1975; **Resid:** Surgery, Mayo Clinic 1980; **Fac Appt:** Prof S, Mayo Med Sch

Gruber, Scott MD/PhD [S] - **Spec Exp:** Transplant-Kidney; Transplant-Pancreas; **Hospital:** Detroit Med Ctr, Harper Univ Hosp; **Address:** Harper Professional Bldg, 4160 John R, Ste 400, Detroit, MI 48201; **Phone:** 313-745-7319; **Board Cert:** Surgery 2001; **Med School:** SUNY Downstate 1983; **Resid:** Surgery, Univ Minnesota Med Ctr 1986; **Fellow:** Surgery, Univ Minnesota Med Ctr 1989; Transplant Surgery, Univ Minnesota Med Ctr 1993; **Fac Appt:** Prof S, Wayne State Univ

Hansen, Nora Marie MD [S] - **Spec Exp:** Sentinel Node Surgery; Breast Cancer-High Risk Women; Endocrine Surgery; **Hospital:** St John's Hlth Ctr, Santa Monica; **Address:** 675 N St Clair, Galter, Ste 13-174, Chicago, IL 60611; **Phone:** 312-926-9039; **Board Cert:** Surgery 1996; **Med School:** NY Med Coll 1988; **Resid:** Surgery, Univ Chicago Hosps 1995; **Fellow:** Surgical Oncology, Univ Chicago 1996; **Fac Appt:** Assoc Prof S, Northwestern Univ

Harkema, James M MD [S] - **Spec Exp:** Breast Cancer; Thyroid Cancer; Parathyroid Cancer; **Hospital:** Mich State Univ-Sparrow Hos, Ingham Regl Med Ctr- Greenlawn Campus; **Address:** Sparrow Professional Bldg, 1200 E Michigan Ave, Ste 655, Lansing, MI 48912; **Phone:** 517-267-2461; **Board Cert:** Surgery 1975; **Med School:** Univ Mich Med Sch 1968; **Resid:** Surgery, Univ Mich Hosp 1974; **Fac Appt:** Prof S, Mich State Univ

Kagan, Richard J MD [S] - **Spec Exp:** Burn Care; **Hospital:** Cincinnati Shriners Hosp, Univ Hosp - Cincinnati; **Address:** Cincinnati Shriners Hosp, 3229 Burnet Ave, Cincinnati, OH 45229; **Phone:** 513-872-6210; **Board Cert:** Surgery 1997; **Med School:** St Louis Univ 1974; **Resid:** Surgery, Univ IL Hosp 1980; **Fac Appt:** Prof S, Univ Cincinnati

Kim, Julian A MD [S] - **Spec Exp:** Melanoma; Breast Cancer; Gastrointestinal Cancer; Immunotherapy; **Hospital:** Univ Hosps Case Med Ctr; **Address:** Univ Hosps of Cleveland, LKS 5047, 11100 Euclid Ave, Cleveland, OH 44106; **Phone:** 216-844-8247; **Board Cert:** Surgery 2002; **Med School:** Med Univ Ohio at Toledo 1986; **Resid:** Surgery, Univ Maryland Hosps 1991; **Fellow:** Surgical Oncology, Arthur James Cancer Hosp & Rsch Inst 1993; Immunotherapy, Ohio State Univ Comp Cancer Ctr 1994; **Fac Appt:** Assoc Prof S, Case West Res Univ

Kraybill Jr, William G MD [S] - **Spec Exp:** Sarcoma-Soft Tissue; Melanoma; Skin Cancer-Advanced; **Hospital:** St Luke's Hosp of Kansas City; **Address:** Medical Director of Surgical Services, St Luke's Cancer Inst, 4320 Wornall Rd, Ste 420, Kansas City, MO 64111; **Phone:** 816-932-1601; **Board Cert:** Surgery 2005; **Med School:** Univ Cincinnati 1969; **Resid:** Surgery, Univ Oregon Hlth Sci Ctr 1978; **Fellow:** Surgical Oncology, Meml Sloan Kettering Cancer Ctr 1980; **Fac Appt:** Prof S, Univ MO-Kansas City

Lillemoe, Keith D MD [S] - **Spec Exp:** Pancreatic Cancer; Colon Cancer; Pancreatic & Biliary Surgery; **Hospital:** Indiana Univ Hosp; **Address:** Indiana Univ, Dept Surgery, 545 Barnhill Drive, EH 203, Indianapolis, IN 46202-5112; **Phone:** 317-274-5707; **Board Cert:** Surgery 1995; **Med School:** Johns Hopkins Univ 1978; **Resid:** Surgery, Johns Hopkins Hosp 1985; **Fac Appt:** Prof S, Indiana Univ

Matas, Arthur J MD [S] - **Spec Exp:** Transplant-Kidney; **Hospital:** Univ Minn Med Ctr, Fairview - Univ Campus; **Address:** Dept Surgery, 420 Delaware St SE, MMC 328, Minneapolis, MN 55455; **Phone:** 612-625-6460; **Board Cert:** Surgery 1989; **Med School:** Univ Manitoba 1972; **Resid:** Surgery, Univ Minnesota Hosps 1979; **Fellow:** Transplant Surgery, Univ Minnesota Hosps 1980; **Fac Appt:** Prof S, Univ Minn

McHenry, Christopher R MD [S] - **Spec Exp:** Adrenal Surgery; Thyroid Surgery; Parathyroid Surgery; **Hospital:** MetroHealth Med Ctr; **Address:** MetroHealth Medical Ctr, Dept Surgery, 2500 Metro Health Drive, H917, Cleveland, OH 44109-1998; **Phone:** 216-778-4753; **Board Cert:** Surgery 1997; **Med School:** NE Ohio Univ 1984; **Resid:** Surgery, Loyola Univ Med Ctr 1989; **Fellow:** Endocrinology, Univ Toronto Med Ctr 1990; Head and Neck Surgery, Univ Toronto Med Ctr 1990; **Fac Appt:** Prof S, Case West Res Univ

Melvin, W Scott MD [S] - **Spec Exp:** Liver & Biliary Surgery; Pancreatic Cancer; Laparoscopic Surgery; **Hospital:** Ohio St Univ Med Ctr; **Address:** 410 W 10th Ave, Ste N729 Doan Hall, Columbus, OH 43210; **Phone:** 614-293-4499; **Board Cert:** Surgery 1993; **Med School:** Med Coll OH 1987; **Resid:** Surgery, Univ Maryland 1992; **Fellow:** Gastrointestinal Surgery, Grant Med Ctr 1993; **Fac Appt:** Prof S, Ohio State Univ

Merrick III, Hollis W MD [S] - **Spec Exp:** Cancer Surgery; **Hospital:** Univ of Toledo Med Ctr; **Address:** 3065 Arlington Ave, Toledo, OH 43614-2570; **Phone:** 419-383-4421; **Board Cert:** Surgery 1997; **Med School:** McGill Univ 1964; **Resid:** Surgery, Royal Victoria Hosp 1972; **Fac Appt:** Prof S, Med Coll OH

Millis, J Michael MD [S] - **Spec Exp:** Transplant-Liver-Adult & Pediatric; Liver Cancer; Transplant-Pancreas; **Hospital:** Univ of Chicago Hosps; **Address:** Univ Chicago, Dept Surgery, 5841 S Maryland Ave, MC 5027, Chiciago, IL 60637; **Phone:** 773-702-6319; **Board Cert:** Surgery 2001; Surgical Critical Care 2001; **Med School:** Univ Tenn Coll Med, Memphis 1985; **Resid:** Surgery, UCLA Med Ctr 1992; **Fellow:** Transplant Surgery, UCLA Med Ctr 1994; **Fac Appt:** Prof S, Univ Chicago-Pritzker Sch Med

Moley, Jeffrey F MD [S] - **Spec Exp:** Thyroid Cancer & Surgery; Endocrine Cancers; Melanoma; **Hospital:** Barnes-Jewish Hosp; **Address:** Washington Univ School Med, Dept Surgery, 660 S Euclid Ave, Box 8109, St. Louis, MO 63110; **Phone:** 314-362-2280; **Board Cert:** Surgery 1998; **Med School:** Columbia P&S 1980; **Resid:** Surgery, Yale-New Haven Hosp 1985; **Fellow:** Surgical Oncology, National Cancer Inst 1987; **Fac Appt:** Prof S, Washington Univ, St Louis

Nagorney, David M MD [S] - **Spec Exp:** Pancreatic Cancer; Hepatobiliary Surgery; Gastrointestinal Cancer; **Hospital:** Mayo Med Ctr & Clin - Rochester; **Address:** Mayo Clinic, Dept Surgery, 200 1st St SW, Mayo E12, Rochester, MN 55905; **Phone:** 507-284-2644; **Board Cert:** Surgery 2001; **Med School:** Univ Kans 1975; **Resid:** Surgery, Mayo Clinic 1982; **Fellow:** Hepatobiliary Surgery, Hammersmith Hosp 1985; **Fac Appt:** Prof S, Mayo Med Sch

Nathanson, S David MD [S] - **Spec Exp:** Breast Cancer; Breast Cancer Risk Assessment; Melanoma; Sarcoma; **Hospital:** Henry Ford Hosp; **Address:** 2799 W Grand Blvd, Detroit, MI 48202; **Phone:** 313-916-2917; **Board Cert:** Surgery 2002; **Med School:** South Africa 1966; **Resid:** Surgery, Univ Witwaterstrand 1974; Surgical Oncology, UCLA Med Ctr 1980; **Fellow:** Surgery, UC Davis 1982; **Fac Appt:** Prof S, Case West Res Univ

Onders, Raymond P MD [S] - **Spec Exp:** Laparoscopic Surgery; Diaphragm Pacing via Laparoscopy; Gastrointestinal Cancer; **Hospital:** Univ Hosps Case Med Ctr; **Address:** University Hosps Cleveland, 11100 Euclid Ave, LKS 5047, Cleveland, OH 44106; **Phone:** 216-844-5797; **Board Cert:** Surgery 2001; **Med School:** NE Ohio Univ 1988; **Resid:** Surgery, Case Western Reserve Univ 1993; **Fac Appt:** Asst Prof S, Case West Res Univ

Ponsky, Jeffrey L MD [S] - **Spec Exp:** Minimally Invasive Surgery; Gastrointestinal Surgery; Endoscopy; **Hospital:** Univ Hosps Case Med Ctr; **Address:** Univ Hosps Cleveland, Dept Surgery, 11100 Euclid Ave, Cleveland, OH 44106; **Phone:** 216-844-3209; **Board Cert:** Surgery 1997; **Med School:** Case West Res Univ 1971; **Resid:** Surgery, Univ Hosps 1976; **Fac Appt:** Prof S, Case West Res Univ

Posner, Mitchell C MD [S] - Spec Exp: Pancreatic Cancer; Gastrointestinal Cancer; Esophageal Cancer; **Hospital:** Univ of Chicago Hosps; **Address:** Univ of Chicago Hospitals, 5841 S Maryland Ave, Ste G209, MC 5094, Chicago, IL 60637; **Phone:** 773-834-0156; **Board Cert:** Surgery 1997; **Med School:** SUNY Buffalo 1981; **Resid:** Surgery, Univ Colorado Sch Med 1986; **Fellow:** Surgical Oncology, Meml Sloan Kettering 1988; **Fac Appt:** Prof S, Univ Chicago-Pritzker Sch Med

Prinz, Richard A MD [S] - Spec Exp: Adrenal Surgery; Thyroid & Parathyroid Surgery; Pancreatic & Biliary Surgery; **Hospital:** Rush Univ Med Ctr, Rush Oak Park Hosp; **Address:** 1725 W Harrison, Ste 818, Chicago, IL 60612-3841; **Phone:** 312-942-6511; **Board Cert:** Surgery 1994; **Med School:** Loyola Univ-Stritch Sch Med 1972; **Resid:** Surgery, Barnes Hosp 1974; Surgery, Loyola Univ Hosp 1977; **Fellow:** Endocrinology, Diabetes & Metabolism, Hammersmith Hosp 1980; **Fac Appt:** Prof S, Rush Med Coll

Rikkers, Layton F MD [S] - Spec Exp: Liver & Biliary Surgery; Pancreatic Cancer; Liver & Biliary Cancer; **Hospital:** Univ WI Hosp & Clins; **Address:** 600 Highland Ave, rm H4-710D, Madison, WI 53792; **Phone:** 608-265-8854; **Board Cert:** Surgery 1996; **Med School:** Stanford Univ 1970; **Resid:** Surgery, Univ Utah Hosp 1973; Surgery, Univ Utah Hosp 1976; **Fellow:** Hepatology, Royal Free Hosp 1974; **Fac Appt:** Prof S, Univ Wisc

Rosen, Charles B MD [S] - Spec Exp: Transplant-Liver; Transplant-Bile Duct; **Hospital:** Mayo Med Ctr & Clin - Rochester; **Address:** Dept Surg-Div Transplantation, 200 First St SW, Charlton 10A, Rochester, MN 55905-0001; **Phone:** 507-266-6640; **Board Cert:** Surgery 1999; **Med School:** Mayo Med Sch 1984; **Resid:** Surgery, Mayo Clinic 1989; **Fellow:** Transplant Surgery, Mayo Clinic 1991; **Fac Appt:** Assoc Prof S, Mayo Med Sch

Saha, Sukamal MD [S] - Spec Exp: Sentinel Node Surgery; Colon Cancer; Head & Neck Cancer & Surgery; **Hospital:** McLaren Reg Med Ctr, Genesys Reg Med Ctr - St Joseph Campus; **Address:** 3500 Calkins Rd, Ste A, Flint, MI 48532; **Phone:** 810-230-9600 x500; **Board Cert:** Surgery 2000; **Med School:** India 1977; **Resid:** Surgery, Hahnemann Univ Hosp 1985; Surgery, Easton Hosp 1987; **Fellow:** Surgical Oncology, Tulane Univ Med Ctr 1989; Head and Neck Surgery, Roswell Park Meml Hosp; **Fac Appt:** Asst Prof S, Mich State Univ

Sarr, Michael G MD [S] - Spec Exp: Pancreatic Cancer; Gastrointestinal Cancer; Obesity/Bariatric Surgery; Gastrointestinal Motility Disorders; **Hospital:** Mayo Med Ctr & Clin - Rochester; **Address:** Mayo Clinic, Dept Surg, Desk West 6, Rochester, MN 55905; **Phone:** 507-284-2644; **Board Cert:** Surgery 2001; **Med School:** Johns Hopkins Univ 1976; **Resid:** Surgery, Johns Hopkins Hosp 1982; **Fellow:** Surgery, Mayo Clinic 1984; Surgery, Johns Hopkins Hosp 1985; **Fac Appt:** Prof S, Mayo Med Sch

Schreiber, Helmut MD [S] - Spec Exp: Obesity/Bariatric Surgery; **Hospital:** St Vincent Charity Hosp; **Address:** St Vincent Charity Hosp, Cleveland Ctr for Bariatric Surg, 2322 E 22nd St, Ste 210, Cleveland, OH 44115; **Phone:** 216-363-2588; **Board Cert:** Surgery 1997; **Med School:** Ohio State Univ 1970; **Resid:** Surgery, Case West Res Affil Hosps 1975; **Fac Appt:** Assoc Clin Prof S, Case West Res Univ

Schulak, James A MD [S] - Spec Exp: Transplant-Kidney-Adult & Pediatric; Transplant-Pancreas & Liver; Pancreatic Surgery; **Hospital:** Univ Hosps Case Med Ctr; **Address:** Univ Hosps of Cleveland, Dept Surgery, 11100 Euclid Ave, MS 5047, Cleveland, OH 44106-5407; **Phone:** 216-844-3020; **Board Cert:** Surgery 2000; **Med School:** Univ Chicago-Pritzker Sch Med 1974; **Resid:** Surgery, Univ Chicago Hosp 1980; **Fellow:** Transplant Surgery, Univ Chicago Hosp 1981; **Fac Appt:** Prof S, Case West Res Univ

Schwartzentruber, Douglas J MD [S] - **Spec Exp:** Cancer Surgery; Melanoma; Kidney Cancer; **Hospital:** Goshen Genl Hosp; **Address:** Cancer Ctr at Goshen Health System, 200 High Park Ave, Goshen, IN 46526; **Phone:** 574-535-2888; **Board Cert:** Surgery 1997; **Med School:** Indiana Univ 1982; **Resid:** Surgery, Indiana Univ Med Ctr 1987; **Fellow:** Surgical Oncology, Natl Cancer Inst 1990; **Fac Appt:** Assoc Clin Prof S, Indiana Univ

Scott-Conner, Carol E.H. MD/PhD [S] - **Spec Exp:** Breast Cancer; Cancer Surgery; Laparoscopic Surgery; **Hospital:** Univ Iowa Hosp & Clinics, VA Med Ctr - Iowa City; **Address:** Univ Iowa, Dept Surg, 200 Hawkins Drive, rm 4601-JCP, Iowa City, IA 52242-1086; **Phone:** 319-356-0330; **Board Cert:** Surgery 2000; Surgical Critical Care 1998; **Med School:** NYU Sch Med 1976; **Resid:** Surgery, NYU Med Ctr 1981; **Fac Appt:** Prof S, Univ Iowa Coll Med

Sielaff, Timothy D MD/PhD [S] - **Spec Exp:** Liver Cancer; Pancreatic Cancer; Gallbladder & Biliary Cancer; **Hospital:** Abbott - Northwestern Hosp; **Address:** Virginia Piper Cancer Inst, Liver and Pancreas Clinic, 800 E 28th St, Minneapolis, MN 55407; **Phone:** 612-863-7553; **Board Cert:** Surgery 1998; **Med School:** Med Coll VA 1989; **Resid:** Surgery, Univ Minn Hosps 1997; **Fellow:** Transplant Surgery, Univ Toronto 1998; **Fac Appt:** Assoc Prof S, Univ Minn

Siperstein, Allan E MD [S] - **Spec Exp:** Laparoscopic Surgery; Endocrine Tumors; Thyroid & Parathyroid Cancer & Surgery; **Hospital:** Cleveland Clin Fdn (page 57); **Address:** Cleveland Clinic Fdn, Dept Genl Surg, 9500 Euclid Ave, Desk A80, Cleveland, OH 44195; **Phone:** 216-444-5664; **Board Cert:** Surgery 1997; **Med School:** Univ Tex SW, Dallas 1983; **Resid:** Surgery, UCSF Med Ctr 1990; **Fellow:** Research, UCSF Med Ctr 1988

Sollinger, Hans W MD/PhD [S] - **Spec Exp:** Transplant-Kidney; Transplant-Pancreas; **Hospital:** Univ WI Hosp & Clins; **Address:** 600 Highland Ave, rm H5-701, Madison, WI 53792; **Phone:** 608-262-8360; **Board Cert:** Surgery 1996; **Med School:** Germany 1974; **Resid:** Surgery, Univ Wisc Hosp 1980; **Fellow:** Immunological Biology, Univ Wisc Hosp 1977; **Fac Appt:** Prof S, Univ Wisc

Soper, Nathaniel MD [S] - **Spec Exp:** Laparoscopic Surgery; Gastroesophageal Reflux Disease (GERD); Biliary Surgery; **Hospital:** Northwestern Meml Hosp; **Address:** Northwestern Meml Hosp, Dept Surg, 251 E Huron St, Galter 3-150, Chicago, IL 60611; **Phone:** 312-926-4962; **Board Cert:** Surgery 1996; **Med School:** Univ Iowa Coll Med 1980; **Resid:** Surgery, Univ Utah Hosps 1986; **Fellow:** Digestive Dis, Mayo Clinic 1988; **Fac Appt:** Prof S, Northwestern Univ

Stahl, Donna L MD [S] - **Spec Exp:** Breast Cancer; Breast Surgery; **Hospital:** Good Samaritan Hosp - Cincinnati; **Address:** Donna Stahl & Assocs, 4850 Red Bank Expwy Fl 3, Cincinnati, OH 45227; **Phone:** 513-221-2544; **Board Cert:** Surgery 2000; **Med School:** Univ Iowa Coll Med 1971; **Resid:** Surgery, Univ Cincinnati Hosps 1978

Strasberg, Steven M MD [S] - **Spec Exp:** Liver & Biliary Cancer; Pancreatic Cancer; Gastrointestinal Cancer; **Hospital:** Barnes-Jewish Hosp; **Address:** Washington University School of Medicine, Dept Surgery, 660 S Euclid Ave, Box 8109, Saint Louis, MO 63110; **Phone:** 314-362-7147; **Board Cert:** Surgery 2005; **Med School:** Canada 1963; **Resid:** Surgery, Toronto General Hosp 1969; **Fellow:** Surgical Research, Toronto General Hosp 1971; **Fac Appt:** Prof S, Washington Univ, St Louis

Sutherland, David E MD/PhD [S] - **Spec Exp:** Transplant-Pancreas; Transplant-Kidney; Immunotherapy; **Hospital:** Univ Minn Med Ctr, Fairview - Univ Campus; **Address:** 420 Delaware St SE, MMC 280, Minneapolis, MN 55455-0341; **Phone:** 612-625-7600; **Board Cert:** Surgery 1995; **Med School:** Univ Minn 1966; **Resid:** Surgery, West Virginia Univ Hosp 1968; **Fellow:** Transplant Surgery, Univ Minn Hosps 1975; **Fac Appt:** Prof S, Univ Minn

Talamonti, Mark S MD [S] - **Spec Exp:** Pancreatic Cancer; Liver Cancer; Gastrointestinal Cancer & Surgery; Melanoma; **Hospital:** Northwestern Meml Hosp; **Address:** Northwestern University Hosp, 675 N St Clair Fl 21, Chicago, IL 60611; **Phone:** 312-695-0990; **Board Cert:** Surgery 1999; **Med School:** Northwestern Univ 1983; **Resid:** Surgery, Northwestern Meml Hosp 1989; **Fellow:** Surgical Oncology, MD Anderson Cancer Ctr 1991; **Fac Appt:** Assoc Prof S, Northwestern Univ

Thistlethwaite, J Richard MD/PhD [S] - **Spec Exp:** Transplant-Kidney; Transplant-Pancreas; Transplant-Liver; Pediatric Transplant Surgery; **Hospital:** Univ of Chicago Hosps; **Address:** 5841 S Maryland Ave, rm J-517, MC 5026, Chicago, IL 60637; **Phone:** 773-702-6104; **Board Cert:** Surgery 1996; **Med School:** Duke Univ 1977; **Resid:** Surgery, Mass Genl Hosp 1983; **Fellow:** Surgical Oncology, Natl Inst Hlth 1981; Transplant Surgery, Mass Genl Hosp 1984; **Fac Appt:** Prof S, Univ Chicago-Pritzker Sch Med

Tuttle, Todd M MD [S] - **Spec Exp:** Breast Cancer; Minimally Invasive Surgery; Cancer Surgery; **Hospital:** Univ Minn Med Ctr, Fairview - Univ Campus, Univ Minn Med Ctr, Fairview - Riverside Campus; **Address:** Univ Minn, Dept Surgery, 420 Delaware St SE, MMC 195, Minneapolis, MN 55455; **Phone:** 612-625-2991; **Board Cert:** Surgery 1995; **Med School:** Johns Hopkins Univ 1988; **Resid:** Surgery, Med Coll Virginia Hosps 1994; **Fellow:** Surgical Oncology, MD Anderson Cancer Ctr 1996; **Fac Appt:** Assoc Prof S

Vickers, Selwyn M MD [S] - **Spec Exp:** Pancreatic Cancer; Liver Tumors; Gastrointestinal Surgery; **Hospital:** Univ Minn Med Ctr, Fairview - Univ Campus; **Address:** University of Minnesota, 420 Delaware St SE, Phillips Wangensteen Bldg, MMC 195, Minneapolis, MN 55455; **Phone:** 612-625-5411; **Board Cert:** Surgery 2003; **Med School:** Johns Hopkins Univ 1986; **Resid:** Surgery, Johns Hopkins Hosp 1992; **Fac Appt:** Prof S, Johns Hopkins Univ

Wakefield, Thomas MD [S] - **Spec Exp:** Thrombotic Disorders; Bleeding/Coagulation Disorders; Pulmonary Embolism; **Hospital:** Univ Michigan Hlth Sys, VA Med Ctr - Ann Arbor; **Address:** Univ Mich, Dept Surg, Div Vasc Surg, 1500 E Medical Ctr Drive, 2210 Taubaum, Ann Arbor, MI 48109-0329; **Phone:** 734-936-5820; **Board Cert:** Surgery 2002; Vascular Surgery 2005; Surgical Critical Care 2000; **Med School:** Med Coll OH 1978; **Resid:** Surgery, Univ Mich Med Ctr 1984; **Fellow:** Peripheral Vascular Surgery, Univ Mich Med Ctr 1986; **Fac Appt:** Prof S, Univ Mich Med Sch

Walker, Alonzo P MD [S] - **Spec Exp:** Breast Cancer; **Hospital:** Froedtert Meml Lutheran Hosp; **Address:** Dept Surgery, 9200 W Wisconsin Ave, Milwaukee, WI 53226-3522; **Phone:** 414-805-5737; **Board Cert:** Surgery 2004; **Med School:** Univ Fla Coll Med 1976; **Resid:** Surgery, Univ Maryland Hosps 1983; **Fac Appt:** Prof S, Med Coll Wisc

Walsh, R Matthew MD [S] - **Spec Exp:** Pancreatic Cancer; Gastrointestinal Surgery; Hepatobiliary Surgery; **Hospital:** Cleveland Clin Fdn (page 57); **Address:** Cleveland Clinic, Dept Surgery, Desk A80, 9500 Euclid Ave, Cleveland, OH 44195; **Phone:** 216-445-7576; **Board Cert:** Surgery 1999; **Med School:** Med Coll Wisc 1985; **Resid:** Surgery, Loyola Univ Hosp 1990; **Fellow:** Endoscopy, Mass General Hosp 1991; Hepatopancreatobiliary Surgery, Cleveland Clinic; **Fac Appt:** Assoc Prof S, Cleveland Cl Coll Med/Case West Res

Great Plains and Mountains

Edney, James A MD [S] - **Spec Exp:** Breast Cancer; Thyroid & Parathyroid Cancer & Surgery; Cancer Surgery; **Hospital:** Nebraska Med Ctr; **Address:** Univ Nebraska Med Ctr, Dept Surgery, 984030 Nebraska Medical Ctr, Omaha, NE 68198-4030; **Phone:** 402-559-7272; **Board Cert:** Surgery 2001; **Med School:** Univ Nebr Coll Med 1975; **Resid:** Surgery, Univ Nebraska Med Ctr 1980; **Fellow:** Surgical Oncology, Univ Colorado Med Ctr 1981; **Fac Appt:** Prof S, Univ Nebr Coll Med

Filipi, Charles J MD [S] - **Spec Exp:** Laparoscopic Surgery; Gastroesophageal Reflux Disease (GERD); Esophageal Surgery; **Hospital:** Creighton Univ Med Ctr; **Address:** Creighton Univ Med Ctr, Dept Surgery, 601 N 30th St, Ste 3700, Omaha, NE 68131; **Phone:** 402-280-4213; **Board Cert:** Surgery 1973; **Med School:** Univ Iowa Coll Med 1967; **Resid:** Surgery, Geo Washington Univ Hosp 1972; **Fac Appt:** Prof S, Creighton Univ

Fitzgibbons Jr, Robert J MD [S] - **Spec Exp:** Hernia; Minimally Invasive Surgery; Gastrointestinal Surgery; **Hospital:** Creighton Univ Med Ctr, Archbishop Bergen Mercy Med Ctr; **Address:** Creighton Univ, Dept Surgery, 601 N 30th St, Ste 3700, Omaha, NE 68131-2100; **Phone:** 402-280-4503; **Board Cert:** Surgery 2002; **Med School:** Creighton Univ 1974; **Resid:** Surgery, Charity Hosp/LA State Univ 1979; **Fellow:** Surgery, Lahey Clinic 1980; **Fac Appt:** Prof S, Creighton Univ

Moore, Ernest E MD [S] - **Spec Exp:** Liver Trauma; Aortic Injuries; **Hospital:** Denver Health Med Ctr, Vail Valley Med Ctr; **Address:** Denver Hlth Med Ctr, 777 Bannock St, MC 0206, Denver, CO 80204-4597; **Phone:** 303-436-6558; **Board Cert:** Surgery 1996; Surgical Critical Care 1996; **Med School:** Univ Pittsburgh 1972; **Resid:** Surgery, Univ Vt Med Ctr 1976; **Fac Appt:** Prof S, Univ Colorado

Mulvihill, Sean J MD [S] - **Spec Exp:** Gastrointestinal Surgery; Liver & Biliary Cancer; Pancreatic Cancer; **Hospital:** Univ Utah Hosps and Clins; **Address:** Univ Utah, Dept Surgery, 30 N 1900 E, rm 3B110, Salt Lake City, UT 84132; **Phone:** 801-581-7304; **Board Cert:** Surgery 1999; **Med School:** USC Sch Med 1981; **Resid:** Surgery, UCLA Med Ctr 1987; **Fac Appt:** Prof S, Univ Utah

Nelson, Edward W MD [S] - **Spec Exp:** Breast Cancer; **Hospital:** Univ Utah Hosps and Clins; **Address:** University Utah Medical Ctr, Dept Surgery, 50 N Medical Drive, Salt Lake City, UT 84132; **Phone:** 801-581-7738; **Board Cert:** Surgery 1999; **Med School:** Univ Utah 1974; **Resid:** Surgery, Univ Utah Medical Ctr 1979; **Fac Appt:** Prof S, Univ Utah

Petelin, Joseph B MD [S] - **Spec Exp:** Laparoscopic Abdominal Surgery; **Hospital:** Shawnee Mission Med Ctr; **Address:** 9119 W 74th St, Ste 255, Shawnee Mission, KS 66204; **Phone:** 913-432-5420; **Board Cert:** Surgery 1990; **Med School:** Univ Kans 1976; **Resid:** Surgery, Univ Kansas 1981; **Fac Appt:** Assoc Clin Prof S, Univ Kans

Surgery

Saffle, Jeffrey MD [S] - **Spec Exp:** Burn Care; Wound Healing/Care; **Hospital:** Univ Utah Hosps and Clins; **Address:** Univ Utah, Dept Surgery, 30 N 1900 E, rm 3B306, Salt Lake City, UT 84132; **Phone:** 801-581-3595; **Board Cert:** Surgery 2002; Surgical Critical Care 1998; **Med School:** Univ Chicago-Pritzker Sch Med 1976; **Resid:** Surgery, Univ Utah Med Ctr 1982; **Fellow:** Burn Surgery, Univ Utah Med Ctr 1980; **Fac Appt:** Prof S, Univ Utah

Shaw Jr, Byers W MD [S] - **Spec Exp:** Transplant-Liver; Hepatobiliary Surgery; Liver Tumors; **Hospital:** Nebraska Med Ctr; **Address:** 983285 Nebraska Med Ctr, Omaha, NE 68198-3285; **Phone:** 402-559-4076; **Board Cert:** Surgery 2003; Surgical Critical Care 1996; **Med School:** Case West Res Univ 1976; **Resid:** Surgery, Univ Utah Med Ctr 1981; **Fellow:** Transplant Surgery, Univ Pittsburgh 1983; **Fac Appt:** Prof S, Univ Nebr Coll Med

Southwest

Beitsch, Peter D MD [S] - **Spec Exp:** Breast Cancer; **Hospital:** Med City Dallas Hosp, Presby Hosp of Dallas; **Address:** 5920 Forrest Park Rd, Ste 500, Dallas, TX 75235; **Phone:** 214-956-6802; **Board Cert:** Surgery 2002; **Med School:** Univ Tex SW, Dallas 1986; **Resid:** Surgery, Univ TX SW Med Ctr 1993; **Fellow:** Surgical Oncology, MD Anderson Cancer Ctr 1990; Surgical Oncology, John Wayne Cancer Inst 1994

Bentley, Frederick R MD [S] - **Spec Exp:** Transplant Surgery; Transplant-Kidney; Transplant-Pancreas; **Hospital:** UAMS Med Ctr; **Address:** 4301 W Markham St, Slot 520, Little Rock, AR 72205; **Phone:** 501-686-8211; **Board Cert:** Surgery 1996; **Med School:** Louisiana State Univ 1977; **Resid:** Surgery, LSU Med Ctr 1983; **Fellow:** Research, Univ Minnesota 1982; Transplant Surgery, Univ Minnesota 1984; **Fac Appt:** Assoc Prof S, Univ Louisville Sch Med

Brunicardi, F Charles MD [S] - **Spec Exp:** Islet Cell Transplant; Pancreatic Cancer; Gastroesophageal Reflux Disease (GERD); **Hospital:** St Luke's Episcopal Hosp - Houston; **Address:** 1709 Dryden, Ste 1500, Houston, TX 77030; **Phone:** 713-798-8070; **Board Cert:** Surgery 1998; **Med School:** UMDNJ-Rutgers Med Sch 1980; **Resid:** Surgery, SUNY Brooklyn Hlth Sci Ctr 1989; **Fellow:** Pancreatic Physiology, SUNY Brooklyn Hlth Sci Ctr 1986; **Fac Appt:** Prof S, Baylor Coll Med

Curley, Steven A MD [S] - **Spec Exp:** Colon & Rectal Cancer; Liver Cancer; Hepatobiliary Surgery; **Hospital:** UT MD Anderson Cancer Ctr (page 71); **Address:** MD Anderson Cancer Ctr, Dept Surg Oncology, Unit 444, PO Box 301402, Houston, TX 77230-1402; **Phone:** 713-794-4957; **Board Cert:** Surgery 1997; **Med School:** Univ Tex, Houston 1982; **Resid:** Surgery, Univ New Mexico Hosps 1988; **Fellow:** Surgical Oncology, MD Anderson Cancer Ctr 1990; **Fac Appt:** Prof S, Univ Tex, Houston

Demarest III, Gerald B MD [S] - **Spec Exp:** Trauma; Burn Care; **Hospital:** Univ NM Hlth & Sci Ctr; **Address:** U New Mexico Health Science Ctr, 1 University New Mexico, MS 10-5610, Albuquerque, NM 83131-0001; **Phone:** 505-272-6441; **Board Cert:** Surgery 1999; Surgical Critical Care 2005; **Med School:** Columbia P&S 1973; **Resid:** Surgery, Univ Washington Med Ctr 1978; **Fellow:** Burn Surgery, Harborview Med Ctr 1979; Harborview Med Ctr 1980; **Fac Appt:** Assoc Prof S, Univ New Mexico

Dooley, William C MD [S] - **Spec Exp:** Breast Cancer; Tumors-Rare & Multiple; **Hospital:** OU Med Ctr, VA Med Ctr - Oklahoma City; **Address:** 825 NE 10th St, Ste 5200, Oklahoma City, OK 73104; **Phone:** 405-271-7867; **Board Cert:** Surgery 1997; **Med School:** Vanderbilt Univ 1982; **Resid:** Surgical Oncology, Oxford Univ 1986; Surgery, Johns Hopkins Hosp 1987; **Fellow:** Surgical Oncology, Johns Hopkins 1988; **Fac Appt:** Prof S, Univ Okla Coll Med

Edwards, Michael J MD [S] - **Spec Exp:** Breast Cancer; Melanoma; **Hospital:** UAMS Med Ctr; **Address:** 4301 W Markham St Slot 520, Shorey Bldg - Ste S706, Little Rock, AR 72205; **Phone:** 501-686-7874; **Board Cert:** Surgery 1996; **Med School:** Emory Univ 1981; **Resid:** Surgery, Univ Louisville Hosp 1986; **Fellow:** Surgical Oncology, MD Anderson Cancer Ctr 1987; **Fac Appt:** Prof S, Univ Ark

Ellis, Lee M MD [S] - **Spec Exp:** Liver Cancer; Colon & Rectal Cancer; Metastatic Cancer; **Hospital:** UT MD Anderson Cancer Ctr (page 71); **Address:** MD Anderson Cancer Ctr, Dept Surgery, 1515 Holcombe Blvd, Box 444, Houston, TX 77030; **Phone:** 713-792-6926; **Board Cert:** Surgery 1999; **Med School:** Univ VA Sch Med 1983; **Resid:** Surgery, Univ Fla-Shands Hosp 1990; **Fellow:** Surgical Oncology, MD Anderson Cancer Ctr 1992; **Fac Appt:** Prof S, Univ Tex, Houston

Euhus, David M MD [S] - **Spec Exp:** Breast Cancer; **Hospital:** UT Southwestern Med Ctr - Dallas; **Address:** Univ Texas SW Med Ctr - Div Surg Oncology, 5323 Harry Hines Blvd, Dallas, TX 75390-9155; **Phone:** 214-648-6467; **Board Cert:** Surgery 2001; **Med School:** St Louis Univ 1984; **Resid:** Surgery, UCLA Med Ctr 1991; **Fellow:** Surgical Oncology, UCLA Med Ctr 1988; Breast Disease, Queens Med Ctr 1990; **Fac Appt:** Assoc Prof S, Univ Tex SW, Dallas

Evans, Douglas B MD [S] - **Spec Exp:** Pancreatic Cancer; Thyroid Cancer; Endocrine Cancers; **Hospital:** UT MD Anderson Cancer Ctr (page 71); **Address:** Dept Surgery/Oncology, Unit 444, P.O. Box 301402, Houston, TX 77030-4095; **Phone:** 713-794-4324; **Board Cert:** Surgery 1996; **Med School:** Boston Univ 1983; **Resid:** Surgery, Dartmouth-Hitchcock Med Ctr 1988; **Fellow:** Surgical Oncology, MD Anderson Cancer Ctr 1990; **Fac Appt:** Prof S, Univ Tex, Houston

Feig, Barry W MD [S] - **Spec Exp:** Gastrointestinal Cancer; Sarcoma; Breast Cancer; **Hospital:** UT MD Anderson Cancer Ctr (page 71); **Address:** UT MD Anderson Cancer Ctr, Dept Surg Onc, Unit 444, PO Box 301402, Houston, TX 77230-1402; **Phone:** 713-794-1002; **Board Cert:** Surgery 1998; Surgical Critical Care 1996; **Med School:** SUNY Upstate Med Univ 1984; **Resid:** Surgery, Northwestern Univ Med Ctr 1990; **Fellow:** Trauma, Univ Minnesota 1991; Surgical Oncology, UT MD Anderson Cancer Ctr 1994; **Fac Appt:** Prof S, Univ Tex, Houston

Franklin, Morris E MD [S] - **Spec Exp:** Laparoscopic Abdominal Surgery; Colon & Rectal Surgery; **Hospital:** Southeast Baptist Hosp, Baptist Med Ctr - San Antonio; **Address:** 4242 E Southcross Blvd, Ste 1, San Antonio, TX 78222; **Phone:** 210-333-7510; **Board Cert:** Surgery 1973; **Med School:** Univ Tex SW, Dallas 1967; **Resid:** Surgery, Bexar Co Hosp 1972; **Fac Appt:** Clin Prof S, Univ Tex, San Antonio

Griswold, John A MD [S] - **Spec Exp:** Burn Care; **Hospital:** Univ Med Ctr - Lubbock; **Address:** Texas Tech Univ Hlth Scis Ctr, Dept Surg, 3601 4th St, MS 8312, Lubbock, TX 79430; **Phone:** 806-743-2373; **Board Cert:** Surgery 1999; Surgical Critical Care 2000; **Med School:** Creighton Univ 1981; **Resid:** Surgery, Texas Tech Univ Hlth Scis Ctr 1986; **Fellow:** Burn Surgery, Univ Washington 1988

Halff, Glenn A MD [S] - **Spec Exp:** Transplant-Liver; Liver Surgery; **Hospital:** Univ Hlth Sys - Univ Hosp, Christus Santa Rosa Children's Hosp; **Address:** Univ TX Hlth Sci Ctr-Transplantation Ctr, 7703 Floyd Curl Drive, MC 785, San Antonio, TX 78229; **Phone:** 210-567-5777; **Board Cert:** Surgery 1998; Surgical Critical Care 2000; **Med School:** Univ Tex, Houston 1983; **Resid:** Surgery, NYU Med Ctr 1987; **Fellow:** Transplant Surgery, Univ Pittsburgh 1989; **Fac Appt:** Assoc Prof S, Univ Tex, San Antonio

Jackson, Gilchrist MD [S] - **Spec Exp:** Thyroid & Parathyroid Surgery; Head & Neck Cancer & Surgery; Endocrine Tumors; Gastrointestinal Cancer & Surgery; **Hospital:** St Luke's Episcopal Hosp - Houston, Woman's Hosp TX, The; **Address:** 2727 W Holcombe Blvd, MC 3, Houston, TX 77025; **Phone:** 713-442-1132; **Board Cert:** Surgery 1998; **Med School:** Univ Louisville Sch Med 1974; **Resid:** Surgery, Parkland Hosp 1979; **Fellow:** Surgical Oncology, MD Anderson Hosp 1980; **Fac Appt:** Assoc Clin Prof S, Baylor Coll Med

Kahan, Barry MD [S] - **Spec Exp:** Transplant-Kidney; **Hospital:** Meml Hermann Hosp - Houston; **Address:** 6431 Fannin St, rm 6-240, Houston, TX 77030-1501; **Phone:** 713-500-7400; **Board Cert:** Surgery 1973; **Med School:** Univ Chicago-Pritzker Sch Med 1965; **Resid:** Surgery, Mass Genl Hosp 1972; **Fac Appt:** Prof S, Univ Tex, Houston

Klimberg, Vicki Suzanne MD [S] - **Spec Exp:** Breast Cancer; Radiofrequency Tumor Ablation; **Hospital:** UAMS Med Ctr; **Address:** Univ Arkansas Medical Sciences, 4301 W Markham, MS 721-7, Little Rock, AR 72205; **Phone:** 501-686-5669; **Board Cert:** Surgery 1999; **Med School:** Univ Fla Coll Med 1984; **Resid:** Surgery, Univ Fla 1990; **Fellow:** Clinical Oncology, Univ Fla 1991; Breast Disease, Univ Arkansas for Med Scis 1991; **Fac Appt:** Prof S, Univ Ark

Kuhn, Joseph A MD [S] - **Spec Exp:** Liver Cancer; Peritoneal Carcinomatosis; Melanoma; **Hospital:** Baylor Univ Medical Ctr; **Address:** 3409 Worth St, Ste 420, Sammons Tower, Dallas, TX 75246; **Phone:** 214-824-9963; **Board Cert:** Surgery 1999; Surgical Critical Care 1993; **Med School:** Univ Tex Med Br, Galveston 1984; **Resid:** Surgery, Baylor Univ Med Ctr 1989; **Fellow:** Surgical Oncology, City Hosp Natl Med Ctr 1992

Lee, Jeffrey E MD [S] - **Spec Exp:** Melanoma; Pancreatic Cancer; Endocrine Tumors; **Hospital:** UT MD Anderson Cancer Ctr (page 71); **Address:** UT MD Anderson Cancer Ctr, 1400 Holcombe Blvd, Unit 444 Fl 12, Houston, TX 77030-4009; **Phone:** 713-792-7218; **Board Cert:** Surgery 1999; **Med School:** Stanford Univ 1984; **Resid:** Surgery, Stanford Univ Hosp 1987; Surgery, Stanford Univ Hosp 1991; **Fellow:** Immunology, Stanford Univ Sch Med 1989; Surgical Oncology, Univ Tex-MD Anderson Cancer Ctr 1993; **Fac Appt:** Prof S, Univ Tex, Houston

Livingston, Edward H MD [S] - **Spec Exp:** Gastrointestinal Surgery; Endocrine Surgery; Obesity/Bariatric Surgery; **Hospital:** UT Southwestern Med Ctr - Dallas; **Address:** UT Southwestern Medical Ctr, 5323 Harry Hines Blvd, MC 9156, Dallas, TX 75390-9156; **Phone:** 214-648-7956; **Board Cert:** Surgery 2003; **Med School:** UCLA 1985; **Resid:** Surgery, UCLA Med Ctr 1992; **Fac Appt:** Prof S, Univ Tex SW, Dallas

Pollock, Raphael E MD/PhD [S] - **Spec Exp:** Sarcoma; **Hospital:** UT MD Anderson Cancer Ctr (page 71); **Address:** MD Anderson Cancer Ctr, Dept Surg Oncology, 1515 Holcombe Blvd, Unit 345, Houston, TX 77230; **Phone:** 713-792-8850; **Board Cert:** Surgery 2003; **Med School:** St Louis Univ 1977; **Resid:** Surgery, Univ Chicago 1979; Surgery, Rush Presby-St Lukes Hosp 1982; **Fellow:** Surgical Oncology, MD Anderson Cancer Ctr 1984; **Fac Appt:** Prof S, Univ Tex, Houston

Postier, Russell MD [S] - **Spec Exp:** Pancreatic Cancer; Biliary Surgery; **Hospital:** OU Med Ctr; **Address:** Univ Oklahoma Dept Surgery, PO Box 26901, WP-2140, Oklahoma City, OK 73190; **Phone:** 405-271-3445; **Board Cert:** Surgery 2000; **Med School:** Univ Okla Coll Med 1975; **Resid:** Surgery, Johns Hopkins Hosp 1981; **Fac Appt:** Prof S, Univ Okla Coll Med

Ross, Merrick I MD [S] - **Spec Exp:** Sentinel Node Surgery; Breast Cancer; Melanoma; **Hospital:** UT MD Anderson Cancer Ctr (page 71); **Address:** UT MD Anderson Cancer Ctr, Dept Surg Onc, PO Box 301402, Unit 444, Houston, TX 77230-1402; **Phone:** 713-792-7217; **Board Cert:** Surgery 1997; **Med School:** Univ IL Coll Med 1980; **Resid:** Surgery, Univ Illinois Hosp & Clin 1982; Surgery, Univ Illinois Hosp & Clin 1987; **Fellow:** Research, Scripps Clin & Rsch 1984; Surgical Oncology, Univ TX-MD Anderson Cancer Ctr 1989; **Fac Appt:** Prof S, Univ Tex, Houston

Schlinkert, Richard T MD [S] - **Spec Exp:** Endocrine Surgery; Laparoscopic Surgery; Gastrointestinal Surgery; Adrenal Surgery; **Hospital:** Mayo Clin Hosp - Scottsdale; **Address:** Mayo Clinic, Dept Surgery, 13400 E Shea Blvd, Scottsdale, AZ 85259-5404; **Phone:** 480-342-1051; **Board Cert:** Surgery 1996; **Med School:** Med Coll OH 1981; **Resid:** Surgery, Mayo Clinic 1986; **Fellow:** Hepatobiliary Surgery, Royal Infirmary 1987; **Fac Appt:** Prof S, Mayo Med Sch

Singletary, Sonja Eva MD [S] - **Spec Exp:** Breast Cancer; **Hospital:** UT MD Anderson Cancer Ctr (page 71); **Address:** Univ Tex MD Anderson Cancer Ctr, 1515 Holcombe Blvd, Box 444, Houston, TX 77030-4009; **Phone:** 713-792-6937; **Board Cert:** Surgery 2003; **Med School:** Med Univ SC 1977; **Resid:** Surgery, Shands Hosp-Univ Florida 1983; **Fellow:** Surgery, MD Anderson Hosp 1985; **Fac Appt:** Prof S, Univ Tex, Houston

Stewart, Ronald M MD [S] - **Spec Exp:** Trauma; **Hospital:** Univ Hlth Sys - Univ Hosp; **Address:** Univ Tex Hlth Sci Ctr, Dept Surg-Trauma, 7703 Floyd Curl Drive, MC 7740, San Antonio, TX 78229-3900; **Phone:** 210-567-3623; **Board Cert:** Surgery 2000; Surgical Critical Care 2002; **Med School:** Univ Tex, San Antonio 1985; **Resid:** Surgery, Univ Tex Hlth Sci Ctr 1991; **Fellow:** Trauma, Univ Tenn Coll Med 1993; **Fac Appt:** Assoc Prof S, Univ Tex, San Antonio

Stolier, Alan J MD [S] - **Spec Exp:** Breast Cancer; **Hospital:** Ochsner Baptist Med Ctr, Louisiana State Univ Hosp; **Address:** 2525 Severn Ave, Metairie, LA 70001; **Phone:** 504-832-4200; **Board Cert:** Surgery 1994; **Med School:** Louisiana State Univ 1970; **Resid:** Surgery, Charity Hosp 1974; **Fellow:** Surgical Oncology, MD Anderson Hosp 1976

Wood, R Patrick MD [S] - **Spec Exp:** Transplant-Liver; Liver Cancer; Liver Surgery; **Hospital:** St Luke's Episcopal Hosp - Houston; **Address:** 6624 Fannin St, Ste 1200, Houston, TX 77030; **Phone:** 713-795-8994; **Board Cert:** Surgery 2004; **Med School:** Univ Rochester 1979; **Resid:** Surgery, NYU/Bellevue Hosp Ctr 1984; **Fellow:** Transplant Surgery, Univ Pittsburgh 1985; **Fac Appt:** Clin Prof S, Univ Tex, Houston

West Coast and Pacific

Anderson, Benjamin O MD [S] - **Spec Exp:** Breast Cancer; International Breast Healthcare; **Hospital:** Univ Wash Med Ctr; **Address:** Univ Washington Dept Surgery, 1959 NE Pacific St, Box 356410, Seattle, WA 98195-6410; **Phone:** 206-598-5500; **Board Cert:** Surgery 2002; **Med School:** Albert Einstein Coll Med 1985; **Resid:** Surgery, Univ Colorado 1992; **Fellow:** Surgical Oncology, Meml Sloan Kettering Cancer Ctr 1994; **Fac Appt:** Prof S, Univ Wash

Surgery

Ascher, Nancy L MD/PhD [S] - **Spec Exp:** Transplant-Liver; Transplant-Kidney; **Hospital:** UCSF Med Ctr; **Address:** 513 Parnassus Ave, Box 0104, San Francisco, CA 94143-0104; **Phone:** 415-476-1236; **Board Cert:** Surgery 2002; **Med School:** Univ Mich Med Sch 1974; **Resid:** Surgery, Univ Minn Hosp 1981; **Fellow:** Transplant Surgery, Univ Minn Hosp 1982; **Fac Appt:** Prof S, UCSF

Bilchik, Anton J MD [S] - **Spec Exp:** Gastrointestinal Cancer; Laparoscopic Surgery; **Hospital:** St John's Hlth Ctr, Santa Monica, Cedars-Sinai Med Ctr; **Address:** John Wayne Cancer Institute, 2200 Santa Monica Blvd, Santa Monica, CA 90404; **Phone:** 310-449-5206; **Board Cert:** Surgery 1997; **Med School:** South Africa 1985; **Resid:** Surgery, UCLA Med Ctr 1996; **Fellow:** John Wayne Cancer Inst. 1998; **Fac Appt:** Asst Clin Prof S, UCLA

Brunson, Mathew E MD [S] - **Spec Exp:** Obesity/Bariatric Surgery; **Hospital:** Scripps Green Hosp; **Address:** Scripps Clinic & Rsch Fdn, Div Surgery, 10666 N Torrey Pines Rd, La Jolla, CA 92037; **Phone:** 858-554-8984; **Board Cert:** Surgery 2005; **Med School:** Univ Fla Coll Med 1981; **Resid:** Surgery, Univ Florida-Shands Hosp 1987; **Fellow:** Transplant Surgery, Univ Cincinnati 1989

Busuttil, Ronald W MD/PhD [S] - **Spec Exp:** Transplant-Liver; **Hospital:** UCLA Med Ctr; **Address:** UCLA Dept Surg, Transplant, 77-120 CHS Box 957054, Los Angeles, CA 90095-7054; **Phone:** 310-825-5318; **Board Cert:** Surgery 1997; **Med School:** Tulane Univ 1971; **Resid:** Surgery, UCLA Med Ctr 1976; **Fellow:** Surgery, UCLA Med Ctr 1975; **Fac Appt:** Prof S, UCLA

Butler, John A MD [S] - **Spec Exp:** Breast Cancer; Thyroid Cancer; Adrenal Tumors; Small Bowel Cancer; **Hospital:** UC Irvine Med Ctr; **Address:** UCI Medical Ctr, 101 City Drive S, Bldg 56 Office 252 Rt 81, Orange, CA 92868-3298; **Phone:** 714-456-8030; **Board Cert:** Surgery 2003; **Med School:** Loyola Univ-Stritch Sch Med 1976; **Resid:** Surgery, LAC-USC Med Ctr 1982; Surgery, Harbor-UCLA Med Ctr 1982; **Fellow:** Surgical Oncology, Meml Sloan-Kettering Cancer Ctr 1984; **Fac Appt:** Assoc Prof S, UC Irvine

Byrd, David MD [S] - **Spec Exp:** Tumor Surgery; Breast Cancer; Melanoma; **Hospital:** Univ Wash Med Ctr; **Address:** Univ Washington Med Ctr, Dept Surgical Specialites Center, 1959 NE Pacific St, Box 356165, Seattle, WA 98195; **Phone:** 206-598-4477; **Board Cert:** Surgery 1998; **Med School:** Tulane Univ 1982; **Resid:** Surgery, Univ Wash Med Ctr 1987; **Fellow:** Surgical Oncology, Univ Tex-MD Anderson Cancer Ctr 1992; **Fac Appt:** Assoc Prof S, Univ Wash

Chang, Helena MD [S] - **Spec Exp:** Breast Cancer; Cancer Surgery; **Hospital:** UCLA Med Ctr; **Address:** 200 UCLA Medical Plaza, Ste B265-1, Revlon Breast Clinic, Los Angeles, CA 90095-8344; **Phone:** 310-825-2144; **Board Cert:** Surgery 1997; **Med School:** Temple Univ 1981; **Resid:** Surgery, Episcopal Hosp 1986; **Fellow:** Cellular Molecular Biology, Temple Univ 1977; Surgical Oncology, Meml Sloan-Kettering Cancer Ctr 1988; **Fac Appt:** Prof S, UCLA

Clark, Orlo H MD [S] - **Spec Exp:** Thyroid Cancer & Surgery; Neuroendocrine Tumors; Parathyroid Cancer; **Hospital:** UCSF - Mt Zion Med Ctr, UCSF Med Ctr; **Address:** UCSF Mt Zion Med Ctr, 1600 Divisadero St Fl 3, Box 1674, San Francisco, CA 94115-1926; **Phone:** 415-353-7687; **Board Cert:** Surgery 1974; **Med School:** Cornell Univ-Weill Med Coll 1967; **Resid:** Surgery, UCSF Med Ctr 1970; Surgery, UCSF Med Ctr 1973; **Fellow:** Surgery, Royal Med Sch London 1971; **Fac Appt:** Prof S, UCSF

Castle Connolly America's Top Doctors® 7th Edition

Curet, Myriam MD [S] - **Spec Exp:** Obesity/Bariatric Surgery; Robotic Surgery; Minimally Invasive Surgery; **Hospital:** Stanford Univ Med Ctr; **Address:** 300 Pasteur Drive, rm H3680, Stanford, CA 94305-5655; **Phone:** 650-498-5308; **Board Cert:** Surgery 1997; **Med School:** Harvard Med Sch 1982; **Resid:** Surgery, Univ Chicago Hosps 1989; **Fellow:** Univ New Mexico 1994; **Fac Appt:** Prof S, Stanford Univ

Eilber, Frederick R MD [S] - **Spec Exp:** Tumor Surgery; Sarcoma; **Hospital:** UCLA Med Ctr; **Address:** 200 UCLA Medical Plaza, Ste 120, Los Angeles, CA 90095-1718; **Phone:** 310-825-7086; **Board Cert:** Surgery 1973; **Med School:** Univ Mich Med Sch 1965; **Resid:** Surgery, Univ Maryland Hosp 1972; **Fellow:** Surgery, Univ Tex-MD Anderson Hosp 1973; **Fac Appt:** Prof S, UCLA

Esquivel, Carlos Orlando MD [S] - **Spec Exp:** Transplant-Liver; **Hospital:** Stanford Univ Med Ctr, Lucile Packard Chldns Hosp/Stanford Univ Med Ctr; **Address:** 750 Welch Rd, Ste 319, Palo Alto, CA 94304; **Phone:** 650-498-5689; **Board Cert:** Surgery 2003; Surgical Critical Care 1999; **Med School:** Costa Rica 1975; **Resid:** Surgery, UC- Davis Med Ctr 1984; **Fellow:** Transplant Surgery, Univ Hlth Ctr Pittsburgh 1985; **Fac Appt:** Prof S, Stanford Univ

Esserman, Laura J MD [S] - **Spec Exp:** Breast Cancer; **Hospital:** UCSF - Mt Zion Med Ctr, UCSF Med Ctr; **Address:** UCSF-Mt Zion Hosp, Clin Cancer Ctr, 1600 Divisadero St Fl 2, San Francisco, CA 94115; **Phone:** 415-353-7070; **Board Cert:** Surgery 2001; **Med School:** Stanford Univ 1983; **Resid:** Surgery, Stanford Univ Med Ctr 1991; **Fellow:** Oncology, Stanford Univ Med Ctr 1988; **Fac Appt:** Assoc Prof S, UCSF

Essner, Richard MD [S] - **Spec Exp:** Sentinel Node Surgery; Melanoma; Gastrointestinal Surgery; **Hospital:** St John's Hlth Ctr, Santa Monica, Century City Hosp; **Address:** John Wayne Cancer Inst, 2200 Santa Monica Blvd, Santa Monica, CA 90404-2302; **Phone:** 310-998-3906; **Board Cert:** Surgery 1994; **Med School:** Emory Univ 1985; **Resid:** Surgery, Univ NC Hosps 1992; **Fac Appt:** Asst Clin Prof S, USC Sch Med

Giuliano, Armando E MD [S] - **Spec Exp:** Breast Cancer; Thyroid & Parathyroid Surgery; **Hospital:** St John's Hlth Ctr, Santa Monica, UCLA Med Ctr; **Address:** John Wayne Cancer Inst, 2200 Santa Monica Blvd, Santa Monica, CA 90404; **Phone:** 310-829-8089; **Board Cert:** Surgery 1999; **Med School:** Univ Chicago-Pritzker Sch Med 1973; **Resid:** Surgery, UCSF Med Ctr 1980; **Fellow:** Surgical Oncology, UCLA Med Ctr 1978; **Fac Appt:** Prof S, UCLA

Goodson III, William H MD [S] - **Spec Exp:** Breast Cancer; Breast Disease; **Hospital:** CA Pacific Med Ctr - Pacific Campus, UCSF - Mt Zion Med Ctr; **Address:** 2100 Webster St, Ste 401, San Francisco, CA 94115; **Phone:** 415-923-3925; **Board Cert:** Surgery 1996; **Med School:** Harvard Med Sch 1971; **Resid:** Surgery, Univ Hosps 1976; Surgery, Children's Hosp 1977

Gower, Roland E MD [S] - **Spec Exp:** Breast Surgery; Biliary Surgery; Thyroid Surgery; **Hospital:** Providence Alaska Med Ctr, Alaska Regl Hosp; **Address:** 2841 De Barr Rd, Ste 41, Anchorage, AK 99508-2973; **Phone:** 907-279-3564; **Board Cert:** Surgery 1997; **Med School:** Vanderbilt Univ 1971; **Resid:** Surgery, Kansas Med Ctr 1975

Greenhalgh, David MD [S] - **Spec Exp:** Burn Care; Nutrition; Wound Healing/Care; **Hospital:** Northern CA Shriners Hosp; **Address:** Shriners Hosp Chldn, 2425 Stockton Blvd, Sacramento, CA 95817; **Phone:** 916-453-2050; **Board Cert:** Surgery 2005; Surgical Critical Care 1998; **Med School:** SUNY Upstate Med Univ 1981; **Resid:** Surgery, MC Hosp of VT 1986; **Fellow:** Burn Surgery, Univ Wash Hosp 1989; **Fac Appt:** Prof S, UC Davis

Surgery

Hoyt, David MD [S] - **Spec Exp:** Trauma; Critical Care; Burn Care; **Hospital:** UC Irvine Med Ctr; **Address:** Univ California, Irvine-Dept Surgery, 333 City Blvd West, City Twr, Ste 700, Orange, CA 92868; **Phone:** 714-456-6262; **Board Cert:** Surgery 1994; Surgical Critical Care 1997; **Med School:** Case West Res Univ 1976; **Resid:** Surgery, UCSD Med Ctr 1979; Surgery, UCSD Med Ctr 1984; **Fellow:** Research, UCSD Med Ctr 1980; Immunopathology, Scripps Clin 1982; **Fac Appt:** Prof S, UC Irvine

Hunter, John G MD [S] - **Spec Exp:** Gastrointestinal & Esophageal Surgery; Laparoscopic Abdominal Surgery; Gastroesophageal Reflux Disease (GERD); **Hospital:** OR Hlth & Sci Univ; **Address:** Oregon Hlth & Sci Univ, Dept Surgery, 3181 SW Sam Jackson Park Rd, MC L223, Portland, OR 97239-3098; **Phone:** 503-494-4373; **Board Cert:** Surgery 1997; **Med School:** Univ Pennsylvania 1981; **Resid:** Surgery, Univ Utah Med Ctr 1987; **Fellow:** Gastrointestinal Surgery, Mass Genl Hosp 1988; Endoscopy, Univ West Ontario 1989; **Fac Appt:** Assoc Prof S, Oregon Hlth Sci Univ

Klein, Andrew S MD [S] - **Spec Exp:** Transplant-Liver; Liver Cancer; Liver Failure; **Hospital:** Cedars-Sinai Med Ctr; **Address:** Cedars-Sinai Medical Center, 8635 W Third St, Ste 590W, Los Angeles, CA 90048; **Phone:** 310-423-2641; **Board Cert:** Surgery 1996; **Med School:** Johns Hopkins Univ 1979; **Resid:** Surgery, Johns Hopkins Hosp 1982; Surgery, Johns Hopkins Hosp 1986; **Fellow:** Transplant Surgery, UCLA-CHS 1988; **Fac Appt:** Clin Prof S, UCLA

Knudson, Mary Margaret MD [S] - **Spec Exp:** Breast Cancer; Trauma; **Hospital:** UCSF Med Ctr, San Francisco Genl Hosp; **Address:** 1001 Potrero Ave, Ste 3A, San Francisco, CA 94110; **Phone:** 415-206-8814; **Board Cert:** Surgery 1992; Surgical Critical Care 1998; **Med School:** Univ Mich Med Sch 1976; **Resid:** Surgery, Beth Israel Hosp 1979; Surgery, Univ Mich Med Ctr 1982; **Fellow:** Pediatric Surgery, Stanford Univ Hosps; **Fac Appt:** Assoc Prof S, UCSF

Moossa, AR MD [S] - **Spec Exp:** Pancreatic Cancer; Gastrointestinal Cancer; Hepatobiliary Surgery; **Hospital:** UCSD Med Ctr; **Address:** 9300 Campus Point Drive, MC 7212, La Jolla, CA 92037; **Phone:** 858-657-6113; **Med School:** England 1965; **Resid:** Surgery, Liverpool Univ Hosps 1970; **Fellow:** Surgical Oncology, Johns Hopkins Hosp 1972; **Fac Appt:** Prof S, UCSD

Nguyen, Ninh T MD [S] - **Spec Exp:** Laparoscopic Surgery; Obesity/Bariatric Surgery; Gastrointestinal Cancer & Surgery; **Hospital:** UC Irvine Med Ctr; **Address:** Div Gastrointestinal Surgery, 333 City Blvd W, Ste 850, Orange, CA 92868; **Phone:** 714-456-8598; **Board Cert:** Surgery 1996; **Med School:** Univ Tex, San Antonio 1990; **Resid:** Surgery, Mt Sinai Med Ctr 1995; **Fellow:** Surgical Oncology, Univ Pittsburgh Med Ctr 1997; Laparoscopic Surgery, Univ Pittsburgh Med Ctr 1998; **Fac Appt:** Assoc Prof S, UC Irvine

Norton, Jeffrey A MD [S] - **Spec Exp:** Pancreatic Cancer; Gastrointestinal Cancer & Surgery; Endocrine Surgery; **Hospital:** Stanford Univ Med Ctr; **Address:** 875 Blake Wilbur Drive, Clinic F, Stanford, CA 94305; **Phone:** 650-723-5461; **Board Cert:** Surgery 2001; **Med School:** SUNY Upstate Med Univ 1973; **Resid:** Surgery, Duke Univ Med Ctr 1978; **Fellow:** Research, Natl Cancer Inst 1982; **Fac Appt:** Prof S, Stanford Univ

Pellegrini, Carlos MD [S] - **Spec Exp:** Esophageal Cancer; Esophageal Surgery; Barrett's Esophagus; Gastrointestinal Cancer & Surgery; **Hospital:** Univ Wash Med Ctr; **Address:** Univ Washington Medical Ctr, Dept Surgery, 1959 NE Pacific St, Box 356410, Seattle, WA 98195; **Phone:** 206-543-3106; **Board Cert:** Surgery 1998; **Med School:** Argentina 1971; **Resid:** Surgery, Granadero Hosp 1975; Surgery, Univ Chicago Hosps 1979; **Fac Appt:** Prof S, Univ Wash

Perkins, James D MD [S] - **Spec Exp:** Transplant-Pancreas; Transplant-Liver; Transplant-Kidney; **Hospital:** Univ Wash Med Ctr, Chldns Hosp and Regl Med Ctr - Seattle; **Address:** Univ Wash Med Ctr, Dept Surg, 1959 NE Pacific St, Box 356410, Seattle, WA 98195; **Phone:** 206-543-3825; **Board Cert:** Surgery 2004; **Med School:** Univ Ark 1979; **Resid:** Surgery, St Francis Regl Med Ctr 1984; **Fellow:** Transplant Surgery, Mayo Grad Sch; **Fac Appt:** Prof S, Univ Wash

Phillips, Edward Harvey MD [S] - **Spec Exp:** Laparoscopic Surgery; Obesity/Bariatric Surgery; **Hospital:** Cedars-Sinai Med Ctr; **Address:** 8635 W 3rd St, Ste 795W, Los Angeles, CA 90048-6101; **Phone:** 310-423-8350; **Board Cert:** Surgery 1998; **Med School:** USC Sch Med 1973; **Resid:** Surgery, USC Medical Ctr 1978; Vascular Surgery, Los Angeles Co-USC Medical Ctr 1979; **Fac Appt:** Assoc Clin Prof S, USC Sch Med

Rassman, William R MD [S] - **Spec Exp:** Hair Restoration/Transplant; **Address:** 9911 W Pico Blvd, Ste 301, Los Angeles, CA 90035; **Phone:** 310-553-9113; **Board Cert:** Surgery 1975; **Med School:** Med Coll VA 1966; **Resid:** Surgery, New York Hos -Cornell 1969; Surgery, Dartmouth Med Ctr 1973

Reber, Howard A MD [S] - **Spec Exp:** Pancreatic Cancer; Pancreatic Surgery; Gastrointestinal Cancer; **Hospital:** UCLA Med Ctr; **Address:** UCLA Medical Ctr, Dept Surgery, 10833 Le Conte Ave, Los Angeles, CA 90095-6904; **Phone:** 310-825-4976; **Board Cert:** Surgery 1971; **Med School:** Univ Pennsylvania 1964; **Resid:** Surgery, Hosp Univ Penn 1970; **Fac Appt:** Prof S, UCLA

Roberts, John P MD [S] - **Spec Exp:** Transplant-Liver; **Hospital:** UCSF Med Ctr, CA Pacific Med Ctr - Pacific Campus; **Address:** UCSF Medical Ctr, Div Transplant Surgery, 505 Parnassus Ave, rm M896, Box 0780, San Francisco, CA 94143-0780; **Phone:** 415-353-1888; **Board Cert:** Surgery 1997; **Med School:** UCSD 1980; **Resid:** Surgery, Univ Wash 1983; Surgery, Univ Wash 1987; **Fellow:** Surgery, Cornell-New York Hosp 1986; Transplant Surgery, Univ Minn Med Ctr 1988; **Fac Appt:** Prof S, UCSF

Satava, Richard M MD [S] - **Spec Exp:** Laparoscopic Abdominal Surgery; Gastrointestinal Surgery; **Hospital:** Univ Wash Med Ctr; **Address:** Univ Washington Med Ctr, Dept Surgery, 1959 NE Pacific St, Box 356410, Seattle, WA 98195; **Phone:** 206-685-0052; **Board Cert:** Surgery 2000; **Med School:** Hahnemann Univ 1968; **Resid:** Surgery, Mayo Clinic 1974; **Fellow:** Research, Mayo Clinic 1972

Selby, Robert Rick MD [S] - **Spec Exp:** Transplant-Liver; Transplant-Kidney; Transfusion Free Surgery; **Hospital:** USC Univ Hosp - R K Eamer Med Plz; **Address:** USC Univ Hosp, Organ Transplant, 1510 San Pablo St, Ste 200, Los Angeles, CA 90033-4612; **Phone:** 323-442-5908; **Board Cert:** Surgery 1999; Surgical Critical Care 2001; **Med School:** Univ MO-Columbia Sch Med 1979; **Resid:** Internal Medicine, Good Samaritan Hosp 1981; Surgery, Good Samaritan Hosp 1986; **Fellow:** Transplant Surgery, Presby Univ Hosp 1988; **Fac Appt:** Prof S, USC Sch Med

Silverstein, Melvin J MD [S] - **Spec Exp:** Breast Cancer; **Hospital:** USC Norris Comp Cancer Ctr; **Address:** USC Norris Cancer Center, 1441 Eastlake Ave, rm 7415, Los Angeles, CA 90033; **Phone:** 323-865-3535; **Board Cert:** Surgery 1971; **Med School:** Albany Med Coll 1965; **Resid:** Surgery, Boston City Hosp-Tufts Univ 1970; **Fellow:** Surgical Oncology, UCLA Med Ctr 1975; **Fac Appt:** Prof S, USC Sch Med

Sinanan, Mika N MD [S] - **Spec Exp:** Gastrointestinal Surgery; Gastrointestinal Cancer; Liver & Biliary Cancer; Laparoscopic Surgery; **Hospital:** Univ Wash Med Ctr; **Address:** Univ Washington, Dept Surgery, 1959 NE Pacific St, Box 356410, Seattle, WA 98195-6410; **Phone:** 206-543-5511; **Board Cert:** Surgery 1998; **Med School:** Johns Hopkins Univ 1980; **Resid:** Surgery, Univ Washington Hosp 1988; **Fellow:** Gastrointestinal Surgery, Univ Brit Columbia Med Ctr 1986; **Fac Appt:** Prof S, Univ Wash

Smith, Craig Vernon MD [S] - **Spec Exp:** Islet Cell Transplant; Transplant-Pancreas; Transplant-Kidney; **Hospital:** City of Hope Natl Med Ctr & Beckman Rsch; **Address:** City of Hope Islet Rsch Prog, 1500 E Duarte Rd, Duarte, CA 90190; **Phone:** 626-359-8111 x65208; **Board Cert:** Surgery 1996; **Med School:** UCLA 1986; **Resid:** Surgery, Harbor-UCLA Med Ctr 1989; Surgery, Harbor-UCLA Med Ctr 1994; **Fellow:** Research, Mass Genl Hosp 1992; Transplant Surgery, Univ Pittsburgh Med Ctr 1996; **Fac Appt:** Assoc Prof S, UCLA

Sobel, Michael MD [S] - **Spec Exp:** Vein Disorders; **Hospital:** Univ Wash Med Ctr; **Address:** East Side Specialty Center, 1700 116th Ave NE, Bellevue, WA 98004; **Phone:** 425-646-7777; **Board Cert:** Surgery 1992; Vascular Surgery 1996; **Med School:** Albert Einstein Coll Med 1975; **Resid:** Surgery, Beth Israel Hosp 1982; **Fellow:** Vascular Surgery, NYU Med Ctr 1983; **Fac Appt:** Prof VascS, Univ Wash

Traverso, L William MD [S] - **Spec Exp:** Pancreatic Cancer; Laparoscopic Surgery; **Hospital:** Virginia Mason Med Ctr; **Address:** Virginia Mason Med Ctr, Dept Surg, 1100 9th Ave, Seattle, WA 98101; **Phone:** 206-223-8855; **Board Cert:** Surgery 1998; **Med School:** UCLA 1973; **Resid:** Surgery, UCLA Med Ctr 1978; **Fac Appt:** Clin Prof S, Univ Wash

Warren, Robert S MD [S] - **Spec Exp:** Liver Cancer; **Hospital:** UCSF Med Ctr; **Address:** UCSF Comprehensive Cancer Center, 1600 Divisadero St, rm A710, San Francisco, CA 94143-1932; **Phone:** 415-353-9846; **Board Cert:** Surgery 1998; **Med School:** Univ Minn 1980; **Resid:** Surgery, Univ Minn Hosps 1988; **Fellow:** Surgical Oncology, Meml Sloan-Kettering Cancer Ctr 1986; **Fac Appt:** Prof S, UCSF

Way, Lawrence W MD [S] - **Spec Exp:** Minimally Invasive Surgery; Liver Surgery; Pancreatic & Biliary Surgery; **Hospital:** UCSF Med Ctr; **Address:** 400 Parnassus Ave, Ste A655, Box 0338, San Francisco, CA 94143-0338; **Phone:** 415-353-2161; **Board Cert:** Surgery 1969; **Med School:** SUNY Buffalo 1959; **Resid:** Surgery, UCSF Med Ctr 1967; **Fellow:** Physiology, UCLA Med Ctr 1969; **Fac Appt:** Prof S, UCSF

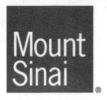

THE MOUNT SINAI MEDICAL CENTER
MINIMALLY INVASIVE SURGERY

One Gustave L. Levy Place (Fifth Avenue and 100th St)
New York, NY 10029-6574
Physician Referral: 1-800-MD-SINAI (637-4624)
www.mountsinai.org

The expert surgeons at Mount Sinai continue to be at the forefront of highly advanced minimally invasive surgery. Using the latest instrumentation, Mount Sinai surgeons have applied these techniques to a broad spectrum of general and vascular surgical procedures including aortic aneurysm repair, kidney transplantation, colon cancer resection, Crohn's disease surgery, robotic prostatectomy, and bariatric (weight loss) surgery.

Cardiac Surgeries
We perform many procedures using minimally invasive approaches, including aortic valve replacement, mitral valve replacement, mitral valve repair, and offpump coronary artery bypasses.

Weight Loss Surgeries
At Mount Sinai we use the latest minimally invasive techniques to perform laparoscopic gastric bypass, lap band placement, duodenal switch, and sleeve gastrectomy. A full multidisciplinary team follows all aspects of pre- and post-operative care.

Urologic Surgeries
We can perform most traditional open surgeries laparoscopically, including nephrectomy, nephroureterectomy, radical prostatectomy, and cystectomy.

Transplant Surgeries
With laparoscopic kidney donation, we can remove kidneys from living donors using laparoscopic techniques.

Vascular Surgeries
Our vascular surgeons provide minimally invasive durable treatments for vascular diseases such as aortic aneurysms, peripheral arterial occlusions, acute and chronic venous disease, vascular trauma and long-term vascular access for medical therapy or dialysis. Our surgeons were the first in the country to perform minimally invasive aortic aneurysm repairs and are among the most experienced physicians in the world using this technique.

Abdominal Surgeries
We offer minimally invasive approaches for the treatment of diseases of the alimentary tract (esophagus, stomach), gastrointestinal tract (small and large intestine, colon and rectum) as well as benign and malignant diseases of the hepatobiliary system.

Gynecologic Surgeries
We routinely treat endometriosis, uterine fibroids, ovarian cysts, and urinary incontinence laparoscopically. Surgeries for uterine, cervical, and ovarian cancers are also performed laparoscopically by our expert gynecologic oncologists.

ENT Surgeries
Top specialists in otolaryngologic surgery at Mount Sinai offer minimally invasive procedures and surgeries to treat many conditions involving the ear, nose and throat, including cranial based lesions, head and neck cancers, and nasal and sinus conditions.

THE MOUNT SINAI MEDICAL CENTER

In surveys of the area's top minimally invasive surgeons in a variety of specialties, Mount Sinai's physicians are consistently at the top of the lists, in areas including gynecologic oncology surgery, obstetrical surgery, colon and rectal surgery, liver and bilary surgery, thyroid surgery, hernia surgery, gastrointestinal surgery, thoracic surgery, and vascular surgery. Compared with traditional open surgery, minimally invasive procedures result in less tissue trauma, less scarring, and faster post-operative recovery time. Although the techniques vary from procedure to procedure and among different surgical subspecialties, minimally invasive surgical procedures typically employ video cameras and lens systems to provide anatomic visualization within a region of the body.

611

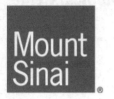

THE MOUNT SINAI MEDICAL CENTER
TRANSPLANTATION

One Gustave L. Levy Place (Fifth Avenue and 100th Street)
New York, NY 10029-6574
Physician Referral: 1-800-MD-SINAI (637-4624)
www.mountsinai.org

Technological advances, along with improved medical therapies, continue to make hopes of a normal life after organ transplantation a reality. Today, transplantation has become an accepted form of treatment for adults and children with a wide variety of diseases. Intensely committed to clinical and basic science research, members of Mount Sinai's Recanati/Miller Transplantation Institute investigate ways to improve organ preservation and reduce post-transplant complications and the side effects of immunosuppression. They also focus on the prevention of disease after a transplant, and overall quality of life after this relatively new medical miracle.

A HISTORY OF ACHIEVEMENT
Mount Sinai surgeons were the first in New York State to perform liver transplantation, and also the first in the state to perform living donor liver transplantation.

CONTINUING THE TRADITION OF EXCELLENCE
Mount Sinai is one of the few hospitals in the country with expertise in small intestine/small bowel transplantation. Working closely with each patient's referring physician, our transplant specialists perform state-of-the-art procedures are performed that profoundly affect patients' lives. Treatment at the Medical Center is not the end of the relationship. Caregivers at Mount Sinai continue to work with the referring physician to help maintain the patient's optimum health level.

A SAMPLING OF OUR INNOVATIVE PROGRAMS
The Kidney/Pancreas Transplant Program began over 30 years ago, making Mount Sinai one of the first kidney transplant programs in the region. Today, the Medical Center has performed over 1,000 kidney transplants and approximately 70 pancreas transplants or combination kidney/pancreas procedures, both for adults and children. Although pancreas transplantation has gained widespread acceptance in the United States, Mount Sinai is one of the few centers in the greater New York area that performs the operation, and is among the largest programs in the Northeast. Our Intestinal Transplant Program is one of the most established and respected in the country. We offer a comprehensive approach to intestinal failure, and have developed a team approach that includes specialists from different fields working together to achieve the best possible result for the patient.

THE MOUNT SINAI MEDICAL CENTER

The Recanati/Miller Transplantation Institute brings together clinical programs in adult and pediatric liver, kidney, pancreas, and intestine transplantation and includes major research initiatives. Meanwhile, within the Department of Cardiothoracic Surgery, heart and lung transplants are also offered. We are one of the largest transplant centers in the United States, performing over 350 procedures annually. Patients from around the world come to Mount Sinai for transplants, including living-donor and traditional surgeries. The total volume of organ transplants at Mount Sinai places the hospital among the top academic medical centers nationally in this field.

619

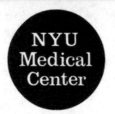

NYU Medical Center

550 First Avenue (at 31st Street)
New York, NY 10016
Physician Referral:
(888)7-NYU-MED (888-769-8633)
www.nyumc.org

MINIMALLY INVASIVE SURGERY

NYU Medical Center has been at the forefront of minimally invasive surgery for two decades, treating conditions from heart disease, to prostate cancer, to obesity, to fetal anomalies in utero. Today, more patients are opting for minimally invasive procedures, a decision resulting in less pain, scarring, and surgical trauma. Post-operative recovery is also significantly reduced, allowing patients to resume their normal activities much sooner than with traditional surgery.

In 1996, surgeons at NYU Medical Center performed the world's first minimally invasive valve repair and replacement, as well as the world's first triple cardiac bypass surgery. NYU vascular surgeons and radiologists helped pioneer minimally invasive aneurysm repair. In 1997, the Center installed the city's first Gamma Knife, a neurosurgical tool that allows surgeons to remove brain tumors that were once inoperable.

The Department of Surgery at New York University School of Medicine is a highly regarded and nationally recognized academic department. The department comprises divisions of:

- Cardiothoracic Surgery
- Minimally Invasive Surgery
- Pediatric Surgery
- Plastic Surgery (reconstructive and cosmetic)
- Surgical Oncology
- Transplantation Surgery
- Vascular Surgery
- Weight-Loss Surgery

Many faculty members receive national and international recognition for their work and hold leadership positions in both regional and national surgical societies. The department's goal is to develop leaders in clinical surgery and to provide the optimal academic surgical environment for patients, residents, and staff.

NYU MEDICAL CENTER

NYU is also taking the lead in noninvasive diagnostic procedures such as colonoscopy and bronchoscopy. MRI and CT scans have in many instances replaced the traditional angiogram to diagnose aortic aneurysm and vascular disease. For more information about these and other noninvasive tests, call 212-263-8904.

**Physician Referral
(888) 7-NYU-MED
(888-769-8633)
www.nyumc.org**

722

Thoracic Surgery

A thoracic surgeon provides the operative, perioperative care and critical care of patients with pathologic conditions within the chest. Included is the surgical care of coronary artery disease, cancers of the lung, esophagus and chest wall, abnormalities of the trachea, abnormalities of the great vessels and heart valves, congenital anomalies, tumors of the mediastinum and diseases of the diaphragm. The management of the airway and injuries of the chest is within the scope of the specialty.

Thoracic surgeons have the knowledge, experience and technical skills to accurately diagnose, operate upon safely and effectively manage patients with thoracic diseases of the chest. This requires substantial knowledge of cardiorespiratory physiology and oncology, as well as capability in the use of heart assist devices, management of abnormal heart rhythms and drainage of the chest cavity, respiratory support systems, endoscopy and invasive and noninvasive diagnostic techniques.

Training Required: Seven to eight years

Thoracic Surgery

New England

Akins, Cary W MD [TS] - **Spec Exp:** Heart Valve Surgery; Coronary Artery Surgery; Aneurysm-Thoracic Aortic; **Hospital:** Mass Genl Hosp; **Address:** Mass Genl Hosp Dept Surgery, Cardiac Surgery, Cox 648, Boston, MA 02114; **Phone:** 617-726-8218; **Board Cert:** Thoracic Surgery 2005; **Med School:** Harvard Med Sch 1970; **Resid:** Cardiovascular Surgery, Mass Genl Hosp 1975; **Fac Appt:** Clin Prof S, Harvard Med Sch

Bolman III, R Morton MD [TS] - **Spec Exp:** Transplant-Heart; Heart Failure & Ventricular Containment; Ventricular Assist Device (LVAD); Mitral Valve Surgery; **Hospital:** Brigham & Women's Hosp; **Address:** Brigham & Women's Hosp, Dept Cardiac Surg, 75 Francis St, rm CA211, Boston, MA 02115; **Phone:** 617-732-7678; **Board Cert:** Surgery 1991; Thoracic Surgery 2004; **Med School:** St Louis Univ 1973; **Resid:** Surgery, Duke Univ Med Ctr 1980; **Fellow:** Thoracic Surgery, Univ Minn Hosp 1982; **Fac Appt:** Prof S, Harvard Med Sch

Bueno, Raphael MD [TS] - **Spec Exp:** Lung Cancer; **Hospital:** Brigham & Women's Hosp; **Address:** Brigham and Women's Hospital, 75 Francis St, Boston, MA 02115; **Phone:** 617-732-6824; **Board Cert:** Thoracic Surgery 1997; Surgery 2002; Surgical Critical Care 2003; **Med School:** Harvard Med Sch 1985; **Resid:** Surgery, Brigham & Women's Hosp 1992; **Fellow:** Surgical Critical Care, Brigham & Women's Hosp 1993; Cardiothoracic Surgery, Mass Genl Hosp 1997; **Fac Appt:** Assoc Prof S, Harvard Med Sch

Cohn, Lawrence H MD [TS] - **Spec Exp:** Heart Valve Surgery; Congenital Heart Disease; Aneurysm-Aortic; **Hospital:** Brigham & Women's Hosp; **Address:** Brigham & Women's Hosp, Div Cardiac Surgery, 75 Francis St, Boston, MA 02115-6110; **Phone:** 617-732-7678; **Board Cert:** Surgery 1970; Thoracic Surgery 1971; **Med School:** Stanford Univ 1962; **Resid:** Surgery, UCSF Med Ctr 1969; Thoracic Surgery, Stanford Univ Med Ctr 1971; **Fac Appt:** Prof S, Harvard Med Sch

DeCamp Jr, Malcolm M MD [TS] - **Spec Exp:** Lung Surgery; Transplant-Lung; Esophageal Surgery; **Hospital:** Beth Israel Deaconess Med Ctr - Boston; **Address:** Beth Israel Deaconess Med Ctr, Thoracic Surgery, 110 Francis St, Ste 2a, Boston, MA 02215; **Phone:** 617-632-8383; **Board Cert:** Surgery 2001; Thoracic Surgery 2003; **Med School:** Univ Louisville Sch Med 1983; **Resid:** Surgery, Brighams & Womens Hosp 1986; Surgery, Brighams & Womens Hosp 1990; **Fellow:** Cardiac Surgery, Brighams & Womens Hosp 1993; **Fac Appt:** Assoc Prof S, Harvard Med Sch

Elefteriades, John MD [TS] - **Spec Exp:** Aneurysm-Thoracic Aortic; Transplant-Heart; Ventricular Assist Device (LVAD); **Hospital:** Yale - New Haven Hosp; **Address:** Yale Sch of Medicine, Dept Cardiothoracic Surgery, PO Box 208039, New Haven, CT 06520; **Phone:** 203-785-2705; **Board Cert:** Thoracic Surgery 2004; **Med School:** Yale Univ 1976; **Resid:** Surgery, Yale-New Haven Hosp 1981; Cardiothoracic Surgery, Yale-New Haven Hosp 1983; **Fellow:** Cardiothoracic Surgery, Yale-New Haven Hosp 1983; **Fac Appt:** Prof S, Yale Univ

Gaissert, Henning A MD [TS] - **Spec Exp:** Esophageal Cancer; Tracheal Surgery; Lung Cancer; **Hospital:** Mass Genl Hosp; **Address:** Division of Thoracic Surgery, 55 Fruit St, BLK 1570, Boston, MA 02114; **Phone:** 617-726-5341; **Board Cert:** Surgery 2001; Thoracic Surgery 2004; **Med School:** Germany 1984; **Resid:** Surgery, Mass Genl Hosp 1989; Surgery, Barnes Jewish Hosp 1991; **Fellow:** Research, Harvard Med Sch 1993; Cardiothoracic Surgery, Barnes Jewish Hosp 1996; **Fac Appt:** Assoc Prof S, Harvard Med Sch

Kopf, Gary S MD [TS] - **Spec Exp:** Cardiac Surgery; Pediatric Cardiothoracic Surgery; Congenital Heart Disease; **Hospital:** Yale - New Haven Hosp; **Address:** Yale University School of Medicine, Dept of Surgery, 333 Cedar St, FMB-121, Box 208039, New Haven, CT 06520-8039; **Phone:** 203-785-2702; **Board Cert:** Thoracic Surgery 2000; **Med School:** Harvard Med Sch 1970; **Resid:** Surgery, Peter Bent Brigham Hosp 1977; Cardiothoracic Surgery, Chldns Hosp Med Ctr 1980; **Fellow:** Cardiothoracic Surgery, Peter Bent Brigham Hosp 1980; **Fac Appt:** Prof S, Yale Univ

Mathisen, Douglas MD [TS] - **Spec Exp:** Tracheal Surgery; Lung Cancer; Esophageal Cancer; **Hospital:** Mass Genl Hosp, Newton - Wellesley Hosp; **Address:** Mass Genl Hosp, Dept Thor Surg, 55 Fruit St, Blake 1570, Boston, MA 02114; **Phone:** 617-726-6826; **Board Cert:** Thoracic Surgery 2002; **Med School:** Univ IL Coll Med 1974; **Resid:** Surgery, Mass Genl Hosp 1981; Thoracic Surgery, Mass Genl Hosp 1982; **Fellow:** Surgical Oncology, Natl Cancer Inst 1979; **Fac Appt:** Prof S, Harvard Med Sch

Nugent, William MD [TS] - **Spec Exp:** Thoracic Cancers; **Hospital:** Dartmouth - Hitchcock Med Ctr; **Address:** Dept Cardiothoracic Surgery, 1 Medical Center Drive, Lebanon, NH 03756-1000; **Phone:** 603-650-8572; **Board Cert:** Thoracic Surgery 2002; **Med School:** Albany Med Coll 1975; **Resid:** Surgery, Beth Israel Hosp 1980; Thoracic Surgery, Univ Michigan 1983; **Fellow:** Cardiothoracic Surgery, Mass Genl Hosp 1981; **Fac Appt:** Prof S, Dartmouth Med Sch

Sellke, Frank W MD [TS] - **Spec Exp:** Heart Valve Surgery; Angiogenesis; Coronary Artery Surgery; **Hospital:** Beth Israel Deaconess Med Ctr - Boston, Landmark Med Ctr; **Address:** Beth Israel Deaconess Med Ctr - Cardiac Surgery, 110 Francis St, Ste 2A, Boston, MA 02215; **Phone:** 617-632-8383; **Board Cert:** Surgery 2006; Thoracic Surgery 1999; **Med School:** Indiana Univ 1981; **Resid:** Surgery, Akron City Hosp 1987; Cardiothoracic Surgery, Univ Iowa Hosps & Clinics 1990; **Fac Appt:** Prof S, Harvard Med Sch

Singh, Arun K MD [TS] - **Spec Exp:** Cardiac Surgery; **Hospital:** Rhode Island Hosp; **Address:** CVT Surgical Group, 2 Dudley St, Ste 470, Providence, RI 02905-3248; **Phone:** 401-274-7546; **Board Cert:** Surgery 1973; Thoracic Surgery 1975; **Med School:** India 1967; **Resid:** Surgery, Columbia Presbyterian Med Ctr 1972; Cardiothoracic Surgery, Rhode Island Hosp 1974; **Fellow:** Cardiac Surgery, Hosp Sick Children 1975; **Fac Appt:** Clin Prof S, Brown Univ

Sugarbaker, David J MD [TS] - **Spec Exp:** Mesothelioma; Transplant-Lung; Esophageal Cancer; **Hospital:** Brigham & Women's Hosp, Dana-Farber Cancer Inst; **Address:** Brigham & Women's Hosp, Div Thoracic Surg, 75 Francis St, Boston, MA 02115-6110; **Phone:** 617-732-6824; **Board Cert:** Surgery 1987; Thoracic Surgery 1999; **Med School:** Cornell Univ-Weill Med Coll 1979; **Resid:** Surgery, Brigham & Women's Hosp 1982; Surgery, Brigham & Women's Hosp 1986; **Fellow:** Thoracic Surgery, Toronto Genl Hosp 1988; **Fac Appt:** Prof S, Harvard Med Sch

Vander Salm, Thomas MD [TS] - **Spec Exp:** Heart Valve Surgery-Mitral; Cardiovascular Surgery; **Hospital:** N Shore Med Ctr - Salem Hosp; **Address:** Salem Hosp, Div Cardiac Surgery, 81 Highland Ave, Salem, MA 01970; **Phone:** 978-354-2500; **Board Cert:** Surgery 1974; **Med School:** Johns Hopkins Univ 1966; **Resid:** Surgery, Mass Genl Hosp 1968; Surgery, Johns Hopkins Hosp; **Fac Appt:** Prof S, Univ Mass Sch Med

Thoracic Surgery

Wain, John MD [TS] - **Spec Exp:** Transplant-Lung; Lung Cancer; Esophageal Cancer; **Hospital:** Mass Genl Hosp; **Address:** Mass Genl Hosp, Dept Thoracic Surg, 55 Fruit St, Blake 1570, Boston, MA 02114; **Phone:** 617-726-5200; **Board Cert:** Thoracic Surgery 2000; **Med School:** Jefferson Med Coll 1980; **Resid:** Surgery, Mass Genl Hosp 1985; **Fellow:** Cardiothoracic Surgery, Mass Genl Hosp 1988; **Fac Appt:** Asst Prof TS, Harvard Med Sch

Wright, Cameron D MD [TS] - **Spec Exp:** Lung Cancer; Esophageal Cancer; Tracheal Surgery; **Hospital:** Mass Genl Hosp; **Address:** Division of Surgery, 55 Fruit St, Blake 1570, Boston, MA 02114-2696; **Phone:** 617-726-5801; **Board Cert:** Surgery 1995; Thoracic Surgery 1997; **Med School:** Univ Mich Med Sch 1980; **Resid:** Surgery, Mass Genl Hosp 1986; Thoracic Surgery, Mass Genl Hosp 1988; **Fac Appt:** Assoc Prof S, Harvard Med Sch

Mid Atlantic

Acker, Michael A MD [TS] - **Spec Exp:** Transplant-Heart; Ventricular Assist Device (LVAD); Coronary Artery Surgery; Heart Valve Surgery; **Hospital:** Hosp Univ Penn - UPHS (page 72); **Address:** 3400 Spruce St, 4 Silverstein Pavillion, Philadelphia, PA 19104-4227; **Phone:** 215-349-8305; **Board Cert:** Surgery 2001; Thoracic Surgery 2001; **Med School:** Brown Univ 1981; **Resid:** Surgery, Hosp Univ Penn 1988; Cardiothoracic Surgery, Johns Hopkins Hosp 1991; **Fac Appt:** Assoc Prof S, Univ Pennsylvania

Adams, David H MD [TS] - **Spec Exp:** Mitral Valve Surgery; Heart Valve Surgery; **Hospital:** Mount Sinai Med Ctr; **Address:** Mt Sinai Hosp, Cardiac & Thoracic Surg, Box 1028, 1190 Fifth Ave, New York, NY 10029; **Phone:** 212-659-6820; **Board Cert:** Thoracic Surgery 2003; **Med School:** Duke Univ 1983; **Resid:** Surgery, Brigham & Women's Hosp 1988; Thoracic Surgery, Brigham & Women's Hosp 1990; **Fac Appt:** Prof TS, Mount Sinai Sch Med

Altorki, Nasser MD [TS] - **Spec Exp:** Esophageal Cancer; Lung Cancer; Gastroesophageal Reflux Disease (GERD); Thoracic Cancers; **Hospital:** NY-Presby Hosp/Weill Cornell (page 66); **Address:** 525 E 68th St, New York, NY 10021-4870; **Phone:** 212-746-5156; **Board Cert:** Surgery 1996; Thoracic Surgery 1998; **Med School:** Egypt 1978; **Resid:** Surgery, Univ Chicago Hosps 1985; **Fellow:** Cardiothoracic Surgery, Univ Chicago Hosps 1987; **Fac Appt:** Prof S, Cornell Univ-Weill Med Coll

Argenziano, Michael MD [TS] - **Spec Exp:** Robotic Heart Surgery; Coronary Artery Robotic Surgery; Maze Procedure for Atrial Fibrillation; **Hospital:** NY-Presby Hosp/Columbia (page 66); **Address:** Columbia Presby Med Ctr, Milstein Bldg, 177 Fort Washington Ave, rm 7-435, New York, NY 10032; **Phone:** 212-305-5888; **Board Cert:** Surgery 1999; Thoracic Surgery 2002; **Med School:** Columbia P&S 1992; **Resid:** Surgery, Columbia Presby Med Ctr 1998; **Fellow:** Cardiothoracic Surgery, Columbia Presby Med Ctr 1999; **Fac Appt:** Asst Prof S, Columbia P&S

Bains, Manjit MD [TS] - **Spec Exp:** Cardiothoracic Surgery; Esophageal Cancer; Lung Cancer; **Hospital:** Meml Sloan Kettering Cancer Ctr; **Address:** 1275 York Ave, rm C-861, New York, NY 10021; **Phone:** 212-639-7450; **Board Cert:** Surgery 1971; Thoracic Surgery 1972; **Med School:** India 1963; **Resid:** Surgery, Rochester Genl Hosp 1970; **Fellow:** Thoracic Surgery, Sloan Kettering Cancer Ctr 1972; **Fac Appt:** Clin Prof S, Cornell Univ-Weill Med Coll

Baumgartner, William MD [TS] - **Spec Exp:** Cardiac Surgery; **Hospital:** Johns Hopkins Hosp - Baltimore (page 61); **Address:** 600 N Wolfe St, Blalock Bldg, Ste 618, Baltimore, MD 21287; **Phone:** 410-955-5248; **Board Cert:** Thoracic Surgery 2001; **Med School:** Univ KY Coll Med 1973; **Resid:** Surgery, Stanford Univ Med Ctr 1975; Thoracic Surgery, Stanford Univ Med Ctr 1976; **Fac Appt:** Prof S, Johns Hopkins Univ

Bavaria, Joseph E MD [TS] - **Spec Exp:** Aortic Surgery; Transplant-Lung; Heart Valve Surgery; **Hospital:** Hosp Univ Penn - UPHS (page 72); **Address:** Hosp Univ Pennsylvania, 3400 Spruce St, 4 Silverstein, Philadelphia, PA 19104; **Phone:** 215-662-2017; **Board Cert:** Thoracic Surgery 2001; **Med School:** Tulane Univ 1983; **Resid:** Surgery, Hosp U Penn 1990; Cardiothoracic Surgery, Hosp U Penn/Children's Hosp 1992; **Fac Appt:** Prof S, Univ Pennsylvania

Colvin, Stephen MD [TS] - **Spec Exp:** Minimally Invasive Cardiac Surgery; Robotic Heart Surgery; Heart Valve Surgery; **Hospital:** NYU Med Ctr (page 67), Bellevue Hosp Ctr; **Address:** 530 1st Ave, Ste 9V, New York, NY 10016; **Phone:** 212-263-6384; **Board Cert:** Thoracic Surgery 2002; **Med School:** Albert Einstein Coll Med 1969; **Resid:** Surgery, NYU/Bellevue Hosp 1971; Thoracic Surgery, NYU/Bellevue Hosp 1978; **Fellow:** Cardiothoracic Surgery, Natl Heart & Lung Inst 1973; **Fac Appt:** Assoc Clin Prof S, NYU Sch Med

Conte Jr, John V MD [TS] - **Spec Exp:** Transplant-Heart; Transplant-Lung; Cardiac Surgery-Adult; **Hospital:** Johns Hopkins Hosp - Baltimore (page 61); **Address:** 600 N Wolfe St, Blalock 618, Baltimore, MD 21287-4618; **Phone:** 410-955-1753; **Board Cert:** Thoracic Surgery 1997; **Med School:** Georgetown Univ 1986; **Resid:** Surgery, Georgetown Univ Med Ctr 1992; Stanford Univ Med Ctr 1995

Cooper, Joel D MD [TS] - **Spec Exp:** Transplant-Lung; Emphysema-Lung Volume Reduction; **Hospital:** Hosp Univ Penn - UPHS (page 72); **Address:** Hosp Univ Penn, 3400 Spruce St, 4 Silverstein, Philadelphia, PA 19104; **Phone:** 215-662-2005; **Board Cert:** Surgery 1971; Thoracic Surgery 1972; **Med School:** Harvard Med Sch 1964; **Resid:** Surgery, Mass Genl Hosp 1968; Thoracic Surgery, Frenchay Hosp; **Fellow:** Research, Hammersmith Hosp; Thoracic Surgery, Mass Genl Hosp; **Fac Appt:** Prof S, Univ Pennsylvania

Demmy, Todd L MD [TS] - **Spec Exp:** Lung Cancer; Thoracic Cancers; Esophageal Cancer; **Hospital:** Roswell Park Cancer Inst, Buffalo General Hosp; **Address:** Roswell Park Cancer Inst, Carlton Bldg, Elm & Carlton Sts, rm 243, Buffalo, NY 14263; **Phone:** 716-845-5873; **Board Cert:** Surgical Critical Care 1992; Surgery 1997; Thoracic Surgery 2000; **Med School:** Jefferson Med Coll 1983; **Resid:** Surgery, Baylor Univ Medical Ctr 1988; Thoracic Surgery, Allegheny Genl Hosp 1991; **Fac Appt:** Assoc Prof S, SUNY Buffalo

Diehl, James T MD [TS] - **Spec Exp:** Cardiac Surgery-Adult; Aortic Surgery; **Hospital:** Thomas Jefferson Univ Hosp, Albert Einstein Med Ctr; **Address:** 1025 Walnut St, Ste 607, Philadelphia, PA 19107; **Phone:** 215-955-5654; **Board Cert:** Thoracic Surgery 2004; **Med School:** Albert Einstein Coll Med 1978; **Resid:** Surgery, Cleveland Clinic 1984; Cardiothoracic Surgery, Univ Toronto Med Ctr 1986; **Fac Appt:** Prof S, Thomas Jefferson Univ

Friedberg, Joseph MD [TS] - **Spec Exp:** Lung Cancer; Mesothelioma; Pleural Disease; Photodynamic Therapy; **Hospital:** Penn Presby Med Ctr - UPHS (page 72), Hosp Univ Penn - UPHS (page 72); **Address:** Penn-Presbyterian Medical Ctr, 51 N 39th St, rm W250, Philadelphia, PA 19104; **Phone:** 215-662-9195; **Board Cert:** Surgery 1996; Thoracic Surgery 1997; **Med School:** Harvard Med Sch 1986; **Resid:** Surgery, Mass General Hosp 1994; **Fellow:** Cardiothoracic Surgery, Brigham & Womens Hosp 1996

Furukawa, Satoshi MD [TS] - **Spec Exp:** Transplant-Heart & Lung; Cardiac Surgery-High Risk; Heart Valve Surgery; Minimally Invasive Surgery; **Hospital:** Temple Univ Hosp; **Address:** 3401 N Broad St, Ste 300, Philadelphia, PA 19140; **Phone:** 215-707-3601; **Board Cert:** Surgery 2003; Thoracic Surgery 2005; **Med School:** Univ Pennsylvania 1984; **Resid:** Surgery, Hosp Univ Penn 1991; Thoracic Surgery, Hosp Univ Penn 1993; **Fac Appt:** Prof TS, Temple Univ

Galloway, Aubrey MD [TS] - **Spec Exp:** Minimally Invasive Heart Valve Surgery; Coronary Artery Surgery; Aneurysm-Thoracic Aortic; **Hospital:** NYU Med Ctr (page 67), Bellevue Hosp Ctr; **Address:** 530 1st Ave, Ste 9V, New York, NY 10016-6402; **Phone:** 212-263-7185; **Board Cert:** Thoracic Surgery 1996; **Med School:** Tulane Univ 1978; **Resid:** Surgery, Univ Colo Hlth Sci Ctr 1983; Cardiovascular Surgery, NYU Med Ctr 1985; **Fellow:** Research, Boston Children's Hosp 1981; Cardiothoracic Surgery, NYU Med Ctr 1985; **Fac Appt:** Prof TS, NYU Sch Med

Gharagozloo, Farid MD [TS] - **Spec Exp:** Video Assisted Thoracic Surgery (VATS); Lung Cancer; **Hospital:** G Washington Univ Hosp, Harbor Hosp Ctr; **Address:** 2175 K St NW, Ste 300, Washington, DC 20037; **Phone:** 202-775-8600; **Board Cert:** Surgery 1990; Thoracic Surgery 1993; **Med School:** Johns Hopkins Univ 1983; **Resid:** Surgery, Mayo Clinic 1989; Research, Harvard Med Sch 1986; **Fellow:** Cardiothoracic Surgery, Mayo Clinic 1992; **Fac Appt:** Prof S

Girardi Jr, Leonard N MD [TS] - **Spec Exp:** Aneurysm-Aortic; Cardiac Surgery; Marfan's Syndrome; **Hospital:** NY-Presby Hosp/Weill Cornell (page 66); **Address:** 525 E 68th St, M404, New York, NY 10021; **Phone:** 212-746-5194; **Board Cert:** Surgery 2005; Thoracic Surgery 1998; **Med School:** Cornell Univ-Weill Med Coll 1989; **Resid:** Surgery, NY Presby Hosp 1994; **Fellow:** Cardiac Surgery, NY Presby Hosp 1996; Cardiovascular Surgery, Baylor Coll Med 1997; **Fac Appt:** Assoc Prof TS, Cornell Univ-Weill Med Coll

Goldberg, Melvyn MD [TS] - **Spec Exp:** Lung Cancer; Esophageal Cancer; Barrett's Esophagus; **Hospital:** Fox Chase Cancer Ctr (page 59); **Address:** Fox Chase Cancer Center, 7701 Burholme Ave, Philadelphia, PA 19111; **Phone:** 215-728-2654; **Board Cert:** Surgery 1971; Thoracic Surgery 1977; **Med School:** Canada 1965; **Resid:** Surgery, Toronto General Hosp 1971; **Fellow:** Cardiothoracic Surgery, The London Chest Hosp 1973; **Fac Appt:** Prof S, Temple Univ

Graver, L Michael MD [TS] - **Spec Exp:** Heart Valve Surgery-Aortic; Coronary Artery Surgery; Atrial Fibrillation; **Hospital:** Long Island Jewish Med Ctr, N Shore Univ Hosp at Manhasset; **Address:** 270-05 76th Ave, New Hyde Park, NY 11040-1433; **Phone:** 718-470-7460; **Board Cert:** Surgery 1993; Thoracic Surgery 1995; **Med School:** Albany Med Coll 1977; **Resid:** Surgery, St Luke's-Roosevelt Hosp Ctr 1982; Cardiovascular Surgery, Deaconness Hosp 1983; **Fellow:** Cardiovascular Pathology, NY Hosp-Cornell Med Ctr 1985; **Fac Appt:** Prof TS, Albert Einstein Coll Med

Griepp, Randall MD [TS] - **Spec Exp:** Aneurysm-Abdominal Aortic; Aneurysm-Thoracic Aortic; Endovascular Surgery; **Hospital:** Mount Sinai Med Ctr; **Address:** Mt Sinai Med Ctr, Dept Cardiothoracic Surg, 1190 5th Ave, New York, NY 10029; **Phone:** 212-659-9495; **Board Cert:** Thoracic Surgery 1997; **Med School:** Stanford Univ 1967; **Resid:** Surgery, Stanford Univ Hosp 1973; **Fellow:** Cardiothoracic Surgery, Stanford Univ Hosp 1972; **Fac Appt:** Prof TS, Mount Sinai Sch Med

Griffith, Bartley MD [TS] - **Spec Exp:** Transplant-Heart & Lung; Heart Valve Surgery; Aneurysm-Aortic; **Hospital:** Univ of MD Med Sys; **Address:** Univ Maryland, Div Cardiac Surg, N4W94, 22 S Greene St, Baltimore, MD 21201; **Phone:** 410-328-3822; **Board Cert:** Thoracic Surgery 2001; **Med School:** Jefferson Med Coll 1974; **Resid:** Surgery, Univ Hlth Ctr Hosps 1979; Thoracic Surgery, Univ Hlth Ctr Hosps 1981; **Fellow:** Research, Univ Hlth Ctr Hosps 1978; **Fac Appt:** Prof S, Univ MD Sch Med

Grossi, Eugene A MD [TS] - **Spec Exp:** Minimally Invasive Cardiac Surgery; Mitral Valve Surgery; Cardiac Tumors, Myxomas; **Hospital:** NYU Med Ctr (page 67); **Address:** NYU Med Ctr, 530 1st Ave, Ste 9V, New York, NY 10016-6402; **Phone:** 212-263-7452; **Board Cert:** Thoracic Surgery 2002; **Med School:** Columbia P&S 1981; **Resid:** Surgery, NYU Med Ctr 1987; Thoracic Surgery, NYU Med Ctr 1991; **Fac Appt:** Assoc Prof S, NYU Sch Med

Hargrove III, W Clark MD [TS] - **Spec Exp:** Mitral Valve Robotic Surgery; Heart Valve Surgery; **Hospital:** Penn Presby Med Ctr - UPHS (page 72); **Address:** Philadelphia Heart Inst, 51 N 39th St, Ste 2D, Philadelphia, PA 19104; **Phone:** 215-662-9595; **Board Cert:** Thoracic Surgery 1994; **Med School:** Wake Forest Univ 1973; **Resid:** Surgery, Hosp U Penn 1979; Cardiothoracic Surgery, Hosp U Penn 1984; **Fellow:** Vascular Surgery, Hosp U Penn 1981; **Fac Appt:** Clin Prof S, Univ Pennsylvania

Heitmiller, Richard F MD [TS] - **Spec Exp:** Esophageal Surgery; Esophageal Cancer; Lung Cancer; **Hospital:** Union Meml Hosp - Baltimore; **Address:** 3333 N Calvert St, Ste 610, Baltimore, MD 21218; **Phone:** 410-554-2063; **Board Cert:** Surgery 1997; Thoracic Surgery 1999; **Med School:** Johns Hopkins Univ 1979; **Resid:** Surgery, Mass Genl Hosp 1985; **Fellow:** Thoracic Surgery, Mass Genl Hosp 1987; **Fac Appt:** Assoc Prof Surg & Onc, Johns Hopkins Univ

Isom, O Wayne MD [TS] - **Spec Exp:** Cardiac Surgery; Coronary Artery Surgery; Heart Valve Surgery; **Hospital:** NY-Presby Hosp/Weill Cornell (page 66), NY Hosp Queens; **Address:** 525 E 68th St, rm M-404, New York, NY 10021; **Phone:** 212-746-5151; **Board Cert:** Surgery 1971; Thoracic Surgery 1972; **Med School:** Univ Tex, Houston 1965; **Resid:** Surgery, Parkland Meml Hosp 1970; **Fellow:** Thoracic Surgery, NYU Med Ctr 1972; **Fac Appt:** Prof TS, Cornell Univ-Weill Med Coll

Jonas, Richard A MD [TS] - **Spec Exp:** Pediatric Cardiothoracic Surgery; Congenital Heart Surgery; **Hospital:** Chldns Natl Med Ctr, Georgetown Univ Hosp; **Address:** 111 Michigan Ave NW, Washington, DC 20010; **Phone:** 202-884-2811; **Med School:** Australia 1974; **Resid:** Surgery, Royal Melbourne Hosp 1979; Thoracic Surgery, Green Lane Hosp 1982; **Fellow:** Thoracic Surgery, Brigham & Women's Hosp 1984

Kaiser, Larry R MD [TS] - **Spec Exp:** Lung Cancer; Esophageal Cancer; Mediastinal Tumors; **Hospital:** Hosp Univ Penn - UPHS (page 72), Pennsylvania Hosp (page 72); **Address:** Hosp Univ Pennsylvania, Dept Surgery, 3400 Spruce St, 4 Silverstein, Philadelphia, PA 19104-4219; **Phone:** 215-662-7538; **Board Cert:** Surgery 2005; Thoracic Surgery 1996; **Med School:** Tulane Univ 1977; **Resid:** Surgery, UCLA Med Ctr 1983; Cardiothoracic Surgery, Univ Toronto Hosps 1985; **Fellow:** Surgical Oncology, UCLA Med Ctr 1981; **Fac Appt:** Prof S, Univ Pennsylvania

Kanda, Louis T MD [TS] - **Spec Exp:** Heart Valve Surgery; **Hospital:** Washington Hosp Ctr; **Address:** Washington Regl Cardiac Surg, 110 Irving St NW, Ste 1E3, Washington, DC 20010; **Phone:** 202-291-1430; **Board Cert:** Thoracic Surgery 1991; **Med School:** Geo Wash Univ 1970; **Resid:** Surgery, Washington Hosp Ctr 1975; **Fellow:** Cardiothoracic Surgery, Cleveland Clin Fdn 1980; **Fac Appt:** Asst Prof S, Howard Univ

Katz, Nevin M MD [TS] - **Spec Exp:** Coronary Artery Surgery; Heart Valve Surgery; Critical Care; **Hospital:** G Washington Univ Hosp; **Address:** 2175 K St NW, Ste 300, Washington, DC 20037; **Phone:** 202-775-8600; **Board Cert:** Thoracic Surgery 2000; **Med School:** Case West Res Univ 1971; **Resid:** Surgery, Mass Genl Hosp 1976; Cardiothoracic Surgery, Univ Alabama Hosp 1980; **Fellow:** Cardiovascular Surgery, Univ Alabama 1978; **Fac Appt:** Clin Prof S, Geo Wash Univ

Keenan, Robert J MD [TS] - **Spec Exp:** Lung Cancer; Esophageal Cancer; Mediastinal Tumors; **Hospital:** Allegheny General Hosp, Westmoreland Regl Hosp; **Address:** Allegheny Genl Hosp, 14th Fl, 320 E North Ave, Pittsburgh, PA 15212; **Phone:** 412-359-6137; **Board Cert:** Surgery 2000; **Med School:** Canada 1984; **Resid:** Surgery, Univ Toronto Med Ctr 1989; **Fellow:** Thoracic Surgery, Univ Pittsburgh Med Ctr 1990; Thoracic Surgery, Univ Toronto Med Ctr 1991; **Fac Appt:** Prof TS, Drexel Univ Coll Med

Keller, Steven M MD [TS] - **Spec Exp:** Lung Cancer; Esophageal Cancer; Palmar Hyperhidrosis; **Hospital:** Montefiore Med Ctr; **Address:** Greene Medical Arts Pavilion, 3400 Bainbridge Ave, Ste 5B, Bronx, NY 10467-2404; **Phone:** 718-920-7580; **Board Cert:** Surgery 1996; Thoracic Surgery 1996; **Med School:** Albany Med Coll 1977; **Resid:** Surgery, Mount Sinai Hosp 1985; Thoracic Surgery, Mem Sloan Kettering Cancer Ctr 1987; **Fellow:** Surgical Oncology, NIH/National Cancer Inst 1983; **Fac Appt:** Prof TS, Albert Einstein Coll Med

Kormos, Robert MD [TS] - **Spec Exp:** Transplant-Heart; Heart-Artificial; **Hospital:** UPMC Presby, Pittsburgh; **Address:** UPMC Presbyterian Hosp, 200 Lothrop St, Ste C700, Pittsburgh, PA 15213; **Phone:** 412-648-6259; **Med School:** Univ Western Ontario 1976; **Resid:** Surgery, Toronto Western Hosp 1978; Cardiothoracic Surgery, Toronto Genl Hosp/Hosp for Sick Chldn 1982; **Fellow:** Transplant Surgery, Univ Pittsburgh Med Ctr 1987; **Fac Appt:** Prof S, Univ Pittsburgh

Krasna, Mark MD [TS] - **Spec Exp:** Esophageal Cancer; Lung Cancer; Mesothelioma; **Hospital:** St Joseph Med Ctr, Univ of MD Med Sys; **Address:** 7505 Osler Drive Odea Bldg - Ste 303, Towson, MD 21204; **Phone:** 410-427-2220; **Board Cert:** Thoracic Surgery 2000; **Med School:** Israel 1982; **Resid:** Surgery, CMDNJ-Rutgers Med Sch 1988; **Fellow:** Cardiothoracic Surgery, New England Deaconess-Harvard 1990; **Fac Appt:** Prof S, Univ MD Sch Med

Krellenstein, Daniel J MD [TS] - **Spec Exp:** Lung Cancer; Minimally Invasive Thoracic Surgery; **Hospital:** Mount Sinai Med Ctr, Lenox Hill Hosp (page 62); **Address:** 16 E 98th St, Ste 1F, New York, NY 10029-6545; **Phone:** 212-423-9311; **Board Cert:** Surgery 1974; Thoracic Surgery 1977; **Med School:** SUNY Buffalo 1964; **Resid:** Surgery, SUNY Downstate Med Ctr 1972; **Fac Appt:** Assoc Clin Prof TS, Mount Sinai Sch Med

Krieger, Karl H MD [TS] - **Spec Exp:** Heart Valve Surgery; Coronary Artery Surgery; Cardiac Surgery-Adult; **Hospital:** NY-Presby Hosp/Weill Cornell (page 66), NY Hosp Queens; **Address:** Cardiothoracic Surgery Dept, 525 E 68th St, Ste M404, New York, NY 10021-4873; **Phone:** 212-746-5152; **Board Cert:** Thoracic Surgery 1994; **Med School:** Johns Hopkins Univ 1975; **Resid:** Surgery, Johns Hopkins 1976; Bellevue Hosp 1979; **Fellow:** Thoracic Surgery, NYU Med Ctr 1981; **Fac Appt:** Prof S, Cornell Univ-Weill Med Coll

Lang, Samuel MD [TS] - **Spec Exp:** Minimally Invasive Cardiac Surgery; Heart Valve Surgery; **Hospital:** St Vincent Cath Med Ctrs - Manhattan; **Address:** 170 W 12th St, Spellman-6, New York, NY 10011; **Phone:** 212-604-2488; **Board Cert:** Thoracic Surgery 1996; **Med School:** Univ Ala 1978; **Resid:** Surgery, UCLA Med Ctr 1982; Thoracic Surgery, NYU Med Ctr 1983; **Fellow:** Cardiothoracic Surgery, UCLA Med Ctr 1985; Pediatric Cardiac Surgery, Hosp for Sick Chldn 1986

Loulmet, Didier MD [TS] - **Spec Exp:** Heart Valve Surgery; Robotic Heart Surgery; Minimally Invasive Cardiac Surgery; **Hospital:** Lenox Hill Hosp (page 62); **Address:** Lenox Hill Hosp, William Black Hall, 130 E 77th St, Fl 4, New York, NY 10021; **Phone:** 212-434-3000; **Med School:** France 1984; **Resid:** Cardiothoracic Surgery, Paris Univ Hosp 1990; Cardiothoracic Surgery, Brigham & Women's Hosp 1991; **Fellow:** Pediatric Cardiac Surgery, Chldn's Hosp, Harvard Univ 1992

Magovern Jr, George J MD [TS] - **Spec Exp:** Cardiothoracic Surgery; Ventricular Assist Device (LVAD); **Hospital:** Allegheny General Hosp; **Address:** Cardiovascular Surgery Ctr, CVI-1, 320 E North Ave, NW Wing-Snyder Pavilion, Pittsburgh, PA 15212; **Phone:** 412-359-8820; **Board Cert:** Surgery 1993; Thoracic Surgery 1996; **Med School:** Univ Pittsburgh 1978; **Resid:** Surgery, Johns Hopkins Hosp 1981; Cardiovascular Surgery, Johns Hopkins Hosp 1985; **Fac Appt:** Prof S, Drexel Univ Coll Med

Michler, Robert MD [TS] - **Spec Exp:** Heart Valve Surgery; Coronary Artery Surgery; Heart Failure; Pediatric Cardiothoracic Surgery; **Hospital:** Montefiore Med Ctr - Weiler-Einstein Div; **Address:** Dept Cardiothoracic Surg, 3400 Bainbridge Ave Fl 5, Bronx, NY 10467; **Phone:** 718-920-2100; **Board Cert:** Surgery 1990; Thoracic Surgery 2000; **Med School:** Dartmouth Med Sch 1981; **Resid:** Surgery, Columbia Presby Med Ctr 1987; **Fellow:** Cardiothoracic Surgery, Columbia Presby Med Ctr 1989; Pediatric Surgery, Boston Children's Hosp 1990; **Fac Appt:** Prof S, Albert Einstein Coll Med

Morris, Rohinton J MD [TS] - **Spec Exp:** Transplant-Heart; Ventricular Assist Device (LVAD); **Hospital:** Hosp Univ Penn - UPHS (page 72), Penn Presby Med Ctr - UPHS (page 72); **Address:** Philadelphia Heart Inst, 51 N 39th St, Ste 2D, Philadelphia, PA 19104-4227; **Phone:** 215-349-8419; **Board Cert:** Thoracic Surgery 2003; **Med School:** Hahnemann Univ 1984; **Resid:** Surgery, Hahnemann Univ Hosp 1989; Thoracic Surgery, Hahnemann Univ Hosp 1992; **Fac Appt:** Assoc Clin Prof TS, Univ Pennsylvania

Naka, Yoshifumi MD/PhD [TS] - **Spec Exp:** Transplant-Heart & Lung; Ventricular Assist Device (LVAD); Heart Failure & Ventricular Containment; Mitral Valve Surgery; **Hospital:** NY-Presby Hosp/Columbia (page 66); **Address:** 177 Fort Washington Ave, MHB 7-435, New York, NY 10032; **Phone:** 212-305-0828; **Med School:** Japan 1984; **Resid:** Surgery, Osaka Police Hosp 1991; **Fellow:** Cardiovascular Surgery, Osaka Police Hosp 1993; Cardiothoracic Surgery, Columbia Univ 1998; **Fac Appt:** Asst Prof S, Columbia P&S

Oz, Mehmet C MD [TS] - **Spec Exp:** Transplant-Heart; Heart Valve Surgery; Minimally Invasive Cardiac Surgery; **Hospital:** NY-Presby Hosp/Columbia (page 66); **Address:** NY Presby Hosp, Dept Cardiothoracic Surg, 177 Ft Washington Ave, MHB- Rm 7, GN435, New York, NY 10032; **Phone:** 212-305-4434; **Board Cert:** Thoracic Surgery 2003; **Med School:** Univ Pennsylvania 1986; **Resid:** Surgery, Columbia Presby Med Ctr 1991; **Fellow:** Cardiothoracic Surgery, Columbia Presby Med Ctr 1993; **Fac Appt:** Prof S, Columbia P&S

Pass, Harvey MD [TS] - **Spec Exp:** Lung Cancer; Mesothelioma; Clinical Trials; **Hospital:** NYU Med Ctr (page 67); **Address:** NYU Cancer Ctr, 160 E 34th St Fl 8, New York, NY 10016; **Phone:** 212-731-5414; **Board Cert:** Thoracic Surgery 2001; **Med School:** Duke Univ 1973; **Resid:** Surgery, Duke Univ Med Ctr 1975; Surgery, Univ Miss Med Ctr 1980; **Fellow:** Cardiothoracic Surgery, MUSC Med Ctr 1982; **Fac Appt:** Prof S, NYU Sch Med

Pierson III, Richard N MD [TS] - **Spec Exp:** Transplant-Lung; Lung Cancer; Transplant-Heart; **Hospital:** Univ of MD Med Sys; **Address:** Univ MD Med Ctr, Dept Cardiothoracic Surg, 22 S Greene St, rm N4W94, Baltimore, MD 21201; **Phone:** 410-328-5842; **Board Cert:** Surgery 2000; Thoracic Surgery 2002; **Med School:** Columbia P&S 1983; **Resid:** Surgery, Univ Mich Med Ctr 1990; **Fellow:** Cardiothoracic Surgery, Mass General Hosp 1992; **Fac Appt:** Assoc Prof TS, Univ MD Sch Med

Pochettino, Alberto MD [TS] - **Spec Exp:** Aneyrysm-Thoracic Aortic; Transplant-Lung; Left Ventricular Assist Device (LVAD); Heart Valve Disease; **Hospital:** Hosp Univ Penn - UPHS (page 72), Penn Presby Med Ctr - UPHS (page 72); **Address:** Hosp U Penn, 6 Silverstein Bldg, 3400 Spruce St, Philadelphia, PA 19104; **Phone:** 215-662-2957; **Board Cert:** Thoracic Surgery 2005; Surgery 2005; **Med School:** Northwestern Univ 1987; **Resid:** Surgery, SUNY-Upstate Med Ctr 1992; Thoracic Surgery, Hosp U Penn 1994; **Fac Appt:** Assoc Prof TS, Univ Pennsylvania

Rosengart, Todd MD [TS] - **Spec Exp:** Transfusion Free Surgery; Gene Therapy-Cardiac Angiogenesis; Minimally Invasive Surgery; Cardiac Surgery; **Hospital:** Stony Brook Univ Med Ctr; **Address:** Stonybrook Univ Hosp, Health Sci Ctr, Cardiothoracic Surgery, HSC-T19, rm 080, Stonybrook, NY 11794-8191; **Phone:** 631-444-1820; **Board Cert:** Surgery 1999; Thoracic Surgery 2002; **Med School:** Northwestern Univ 1983; **Resid:** Surgery, NYU Med Ctr 1985; Surgery, NYU Med Ctr 1989; **Fellow:** Thoracic Surgery, Natl Inst Hlth 1987; Cardiothoracic Surgery, NY-Cornell Med Ctr 1991; **Fac Appt:** Prof S, SUNY Stony Brook

Samuels, Louis MD [TS] - **Spec Exp:** Transplant-Heart; Artificial Heart Devices; Ventricular Assist Device (LVAD); **Hospital:** Lankenau Hosp; **Address:** 100 Lancaster Ave, 280 Lankenau Medical Science Bldg, Wynnwood, PA 19096; **Phone:** 610-896-9255; **Board Cert:** Surgery 1994; Thoracic Surgery 1996; **Med School:** Hahnemann Univ 1987; **Resid:** Surgery, Hahnemann Hosp 1992; Thoracic Surgery, Hahnemann Hosp 1995; **Fac Appt:** Prof S, Hahnemann Univ

Shrager, Joseph B MD [TS] - **Spec Exp:** Emphysema-Lung Volume Reduction; Tracheal Surgery; Lung Cancer; **Hospital:** Hosp Univ Penn - UPHS (page 72), Pennsylvania Hosp (page 72); **Address:** Hosp Univ Penn, Div Thoracic Surg, 3400 Spruce St, 4 Silverstein Bldg, Philadelphia, PA 19104; **Phone:** 215-662-4767; **Board Cert:** Thoracic Surgery 1999; Surgery 1996; **Med School:** Harvard Med Sch 1988; **Resid:** Surgery, Hosp U Penn 1995; Cardiothoracic Surgery, Mass General Hosp 1997; **Fac Appt:** Assoc Prof S, Univ Pennsylvania

Smith, Craig R MD [TS] - **Spec Exp:** Mitral Valve Surgery; Transplant-Heart; Minimally Invasive Cardiac Surgery; Robotic Heart Surgery; **Hospital:** NY-Presby Hosp/Columbia (page 66); **Address:** Columbia Presbyterian Med Ctr, 177 Fort Washington Ave, Ste 7-435, New York, NY 10032; **Phone:** 212-305-8312; **Board Cert:** Thoracic Surgery 2004; **Med School:** Case West Res Univ 1977; **Resid:** Surgery, Strong Meml Hosp 1982; **Fellow:** Cardiothoracic Surgery, Columbia Presby Med Ctr 1984; **Fac Appt:** Prof S, Columbia P&S

Sonett, Joshua R MD [TS] - **Spec Exp:** Minimally Invasive Thoracic Surgery; Transplant-Lung; Thoracic Cancers; **Hospital:** NY-Presby Hosp/Columbia (page 66); **Address:** 161 Fort Washington Ave, New York, NY 10032; **Phone:** 212-305-8086; **Board Cert:** Surgery 1994; Thoracic Surgery 1997; **Med School:** E Carolina Univ 1988; **Resid:** Surgery, Univ Mass Med Ctr 1993; **Fellow:** Cardiothoracic Surgery, Univ Pittsburgh Med Ctr 1994; Thoracic Surgery, Meml Sloan Kettering Cancer Ctr; **Fac Appt:** Assoc Prof S, Columbia P&S

Strong III, Michael D MD [TS] - **Spec Exp:** Coronary Artery Surgery; Heart Valve Surgery; Thoracic Aortic Surgery; **Hospital:** Hahnemann Univ Hosp; **Address:** Hahnemann Univ Hosp, Cardiothoracic Surg, 245 N 15th St, 744 N Tower, Philadelphia, PA 19102; **Phone:** 215-762-7802; **Board Cert:** Surgery 1974; **Med School:** Jefferson Med Coll 1966; **Resid:** Surgery, Jefferson Hosp 1973; Thoracic Surgery, Temple Univ Hosp 1975; **Fac Appt:** Assoc Prof TS, Drexel Univ Coll Med

Subramanian, Valavanur MD [TS] - **Spec Exp:** Minimally Invasive Cardiac Surgery; Coronary Artery Robotic Surgery; Cardiothoracic Surgery; **Hospital:** Lenox Hill Hosp (page 62); **Address:** 130 E 77th St, Fl 4, New York, NY 10021; **Phone:** 212-434-3000; **Board Cert:** Surgery 1972; Thoracic Surgery 1974; **Med School:** India 1962; **Resid:** Surgery, NY Hosp-Cornell 1972

Swanson, Scott J MD [TS] - **Spec Exp:** Lung Cancer; Video Assisted Thoracic Surgery (VATS); Esophageal Cancer; **Hospital:** Mount Sinai Med Ctr; **Address:** 1190 5th Ave, Box 1028, New York, NY 10029; **Phone:** 212-659-6815; **Board Cert:** Surgery 1991; Thoracic Surgery 1996; **Med School:** Harvard Med Sch 1985; **Resid:** Surgery, Brigham & Womens Hosp 1990; **Fellow:** Cardiothoracic Surgery, Brigham & Womens Hosp 1994

Tranbaugh, Robert MD [TS] - **Spec Exp:** Coronary Artery Surgery; Heart Valve Surgery; Aneurysm; **Hospital:** Beth Israel Med Ctr - Petrie Division; **Address:** 317 E 17th St Fl 11, New York, NY 10003; **Phone:** 212-420-2584; **Board Cert:** Thoracic Surgery 2005; **Med School:** Univ Pennsylvania 1976; **Resid:** Surgery, UCSF Med Ctr 1983; Cardiothoracic Surgery, UCSF Med Ctr 1985; **Fac Appt:** Assoc Prof TS, Albert Einstein Coll Med

Yang, Stephen C MD [TS] - **Spec Exp:** Mesothelioma; Lung Cancer; Esophageal Cancer; **Hospital:** Johns Hopkins Hosp - Baltimore (page 61), Johns Hopkins Bayview Med Ctr (page 61); **Address:** Johns Hopkins Hosp, 600 N Wolfe St Blalock Bldg - rm 240, Baltimore, MD 21287-5674; **Phone:** 410-614-3891; **Board Cert:** Surgery 2004; Thoracic Surgery 2006; **Med School:** Med Coll VA 1984; **Resid:** Surgery, Univ Tex Hlth Sci Ctr 1990; **Fellow:** Thoracic Surgery, MD Anderson Cancer Ctr 1992; Cardiothoracic Surgery, Med Coll Virginia 1994; **Fac Appt:** Assoc Prof TS, Johns Hopkins Univ

Southeast

Boyd, W Douglas MD [TS] - **Spec Exp:** Robotic Heart Surgery; Ventricular Assist Device (LVAD); Minimally Invasive Cardiac Surgery; **Hospital:** Cleveland Clin - Weston (page 57); **Address:** Cleveland Clinic, Cardiothoracic Surgery, 2950 Cleveland Clinic Blvd, Weston, FL 33331; **Phone:** 954-659-5320; **Med School:** Univ Ottawa 1984; **Resid:** Surgery, Ottawa Civic Hospital 1990; Ottawa Civic Hospital 1992; **Fellow:** Transplantation/Mechanical Assist Devices, Ottawa Heart Inst 1995; **Fac Appt:** Assoc Prof S, Univ S Fla Coll Med

Brunsting III, Louis A MD [TS] - **Spec Exp:** Coronary Artery Robotic Surgery; **Hospital:** Centennial Med Ctr, Baptist Hosp - Nashville; **Address:** Cardiothoracic Surgery Associates, 2400 Patterson St, Ste 223, Nashville, TN 37203; **Phone:** 615-329-1122; **Board Cert:** Thoracic Surgery 2001; **Med School:** UCSD 1983; **Resid:** Surgery, Univ Rochester 1985; Surgery, Univ Rochester 1989; **Fellow:** Surgery, Duke Univ 1987; Thoracic Surgery, Duke Univ 1991

Cerfolio, Robert J MD [TS] - **Spec Exp:** Lung Cancer; Tracheal Surgery; Chest Wall Tumors; Esophageal Cancer; **Hospital:** Univ of Ala Hosp at Birmingham; **Address:** 703 S 19th St, Ste 739, Birmingham, AL 35294; **Phone:** 205-934-5937; **Board Cert:** Thoracic Surgery 1997; Surgery 2003; **Med School:** Univ Rochester 1988; **Resid:** Surgery, Cornell-NY Hosp 1990; Surgery, Mayo Clinic 1993; **Fellow:** Cardiothoracic Surgery, Mayo Clinic 1996; **Fac Appt:** Prof TS, Univ Ala

Chitwood Jr, W Randolph MD [TS] - **Spec Exp:** Robotic Heart Surgery; Minimally Invasive Cardiac Surgery; Heart Valve Surgery; Mitral Valve Surgery; **Hospital:** Pitt Cty Mem Hosp - Univ Med Ctr East Carolina; **Address:** ECU Dept Surgery, 600 Moye Blvd, PCMH Teaching Annex, rm 277, Greenville, NC 27834; **Phone:** 252-744-4536; **Board Cert:** Surgery 1993; Thoracic Surgery 1994; **Med School:** Univ VA Sch Med 1974; **Resid:** Surgery, Duke Univ Med Ctr 1983; **Fellow:** Cardiovascular Surgery, Duke Univ Med Ctr 1984; **Fac Appt:** Prof S, E Carolina Univ

Christian, Karla G MD [TS] - **Spec Exp:** Congenital Heart Surgery; Transplant-Heart-Adult & Pediatric; Cardiac Surgery-Adult & Pediatric; **Hospital:** Vanderbilt Children's Hosp, Vanderbilt Univ Med Ctr; **Address:** Vanderbilt Chldns Hosp, Cardiac Surgery, 2200 Childrens Way, 5247 DOT, Nashville, TN 37232-9292; **Phone:** 615-936-5500; **Board Cert:** Surgery 2001; Thoracic Surgery 2003; **Med School:** Univ Wash 1985; **Resid:** Surgery, Univ Washington Med Ctr 1987; Surgery, Vanderbilt Univ Med Ctr 1991; **Fellow:** Cardiothoracic Surgery, Vanderbilt Univ Med Ctr 1994; **Fac Appt:** Assoc Prof S, Vanderbilt Univ

Dowling, Robert MD [TS] - **Spec Exp:** Cardiac Surgery; Transplant-Heart; **Hospital:** Jewish Hosp HlthCre Svcs Inc; **Address:** 201 Abraham Flexner Way, Ste 1200, Louisville, KY 40202; **Phone:** 502-583-8383; **Board Cert:** Surgery 1992; Thoracic Surgery 1995; **Med School:** Univ Pittsburgh 1985; **Resid:** Surgery, Presbyterian Hosp; **Fellow:** Thoracic Surgery, Univ Pittsburgh Med Ctr; **Fac Appt:** Prof S, Univ Louisville Sch Med

Drinkwater Jr, Davis C MD [TS] - **Spec Exp:** Transplant-Heart & Lung; Cardiac Surgery-Adult & Pediatric; **Hospital:** Centennial Med Ctr; **Address:** 2400 Patterson St, Ste 400, Nashville, TN 37203; **Phone:** 615-342-5812; **Board Cert:** Surgery 1997; Thoracic Surgery 2005; **Med School:** Univ VT Coll Med 1976; **Resid:** Surgery, McGill Univ 1981; Cardiothoracic Surgery, McGill Univ 1983; **Fellow:** Cardiothoracic Surgery, Childrens Hosp 1984

Egan, Thomas MD [TS] - **Spec Exp:** Transplant-Lung; Thoracic Cancers; **Hospital:** Univ NC Hosps; **Address:** Univ N Carolina Hosps, 3040 Burnett, CB7065, Womack Bldg, Chapel Hill, NC 27599-7065; **Phone:** 919-966-3381; **Board Cert:** Thoracic Surgery 1999; **Med School:** Univ Toronto 1976; **Resid:** Surgery, Univ Toronto 1986; Thoracic Surgery, Univ Toronto 1988; **Fellow:** Transplant Surgery, Washington Univ 1989; **Fac Appt:** Prof S, Univ NC Sch Med

Glassford Jr, David M MD [TS] - **Spec Exp:** Cardiothoracic Surgery; **Hospital:** Saint Thomas Hosp - Nashville; **Address:** Cardiovascular Surgery Assocs, 4230 Harding Rd, Ste 450, Nashville, TN 37205; **Phone:** 615-385-4781; **Board Cert:** Surgery 1998; Thoracic Surgery 1997; Surgical Critical Care 1999; **Med School:** Univ Tex Med Br, Galveston 1970; **Resid:** Surgery, Univ Texas Med Br 1975; Thoracic Surgery, Ochsner Clinic 1977; **Fac Appt:** Asst Clin Prof TS, Vanderbilt Univ

Hammon, John W MD [TS] - **Spec Exp:** Cardiac Surgery; Thoracic Surgery; **Hospital:** Wake Forest Univ Baptist Med Ctr (page 73); **Address:** Wake Forest Univ Sch Med, Medical Center Blvd, Winston Salem, NC 27157-1096; **Phone:** 336-716-6002; **Board Cert:** Thoracic Surgery 1997; **Med School:** Tulane Univ 1968; **Resid:** Thoracic Surgery, Duke Univ Med Ctr 1978; **Fac Appt:** Prof TS, Wake Forest Univ

Harpole Jr, David H MD [TS] - **Spec Exp:** Lung Cancer; Mesothelioma; Esophageal Cancer; **Hospital:** Duke Univ Med Ctr; **Address:** Duke Univ Med Ctr-Thoracic Surgery, 2424 Erwin Rd, Ste 403 - rm 4071, Durham, NC 27705; **Phone:** 919-668-8413; **Board Cert:** Surgery 2002; Thoracic Surgery 2003; **Med School:** Univ VA Sch Med 1984; **Resid:** Surgery, Duke Univ Med Ctr 1991; **Fellow:** Thoracic Surgery, Duke Univ Med Ctr 1993; **Fac Appt:** Prof S, Duke Univ

Heidary, Dariush H MD [TS] - **Spec Exp:** Cardiothoracic Surgery; Cardiovascular Surgery; **Hospital:** Meml Hlth Univ Med Ctr - Savannah, St Joseph's-Candler Hosp; **Address:** Memorial Hlth Univ Med Ctr, 4700 Waters Ave, Ste 403, Savannah, GA 31404-6220; **Phone:** 912-354-7188; **Board Cert:** Thoracic Surgery 1997; **Med School:** Iran 1967; **Resid:** Surgery, Albert Einstein Medical Ctr 1974; Cardiothoracic Surgery, Albert Einstein Medical Ctr 1975; **Fellow:** Cardiothoracic Surgery, Med Coll Georgia 1977

Jones, David R MD [TS] - **Spec Exp:** Lung Cancer; Esophageal Cancer; Minimally Invasive Thoracic Surgery; **Hospital:** Univ Virginia Med Ctr; **Address:** Department of Surgery, Box 800679, Charlottesville, VA 22901; **Phone:** 434-243-6443; **Board Cert:** Surgery 1996; Thoracic Surgery 1999; **Med School:** W VA Univ 1989; **Resid:** Surgery, West Va Univ 1995; **Fellow:** Thoracic Surgery, Univ North Carolina 1998; **Fac Appt:** Assoc Prof S, Univ VA Sch Med

Kiernan, Paul D MD [TS] - **Spec Exp:** Lung Cancer; Esophageal Cancer; Mediastinal Tumors; **Hospital:** Inova Fairfax Hosp, Inova Alexandria Hosp; **Address:** 2921 Telestar Court, Falls Church, VA 22042; **Phone:** 703-280-5858; **Board Cert:** Thoracic Surgery 2002; **Med School:** Georgetown Univ 1974; **Resid:** Surgery, Mayo Clinic 1979; Cardiothoracic Surgery, Mayo Clinic 1981; **Fellow:** Vascular Surgery, Mayo Clinic 1982; **Fac Appt:** Assoc Clin Prof S, Georgetown Univ

Kiev, Jonathan MD [TS] - **Spec Exp:** Chest Wall Tumors; **Hospital:** Med Coll of VA Hosp; **Address:** 1250 E Marshall St, PO Box 980068, Richmond, VA 23298; **Phone:** 804-828-2775; **Board Cert:** Surgery 1996; Thoracic Surgery 2002; **Med School:** Tulane Univ 1989; **Resid:** Surgery, Hahnemann Univ 1994; **Fellow:** Thoracic Surgery, Univ Pittsburgh 2001; Thoracic Surgery, Mayo Clinic 2001; **Fac Appt:** Prof S, Va Commonwealth Univ

Kirklin, James MD [TS] - **Spec Exp:** Transplant-Heart-Adult & Pediatric; Cardiac Surgery-Adult & Pediatric; **Hospital:** Univ of Ala Hosp at Birmingham; **Address:** Univ Alabama Med Ctr, THT 760, 1900 University Blvd, Birmingham, AL 35294; **Phone:** 205-934-3368; **Board Cert:** Thoracic Surgery 2000; **Med School:** Harvard Med Sch 1973; **Resid:** Surgery, Mass Genl Hosp 1977; Cardiothoracic Surgery, Mass Genl Hosp 1979; **Fellow:** Cardiothoracic Surgery, Chidren's Hosp Med Ctr 1979; **Fac Appt:** Prof S, Univ Ala

Kron, Irving L MD [TS] - **Spec Exp:** Coronary Artery Surgery; Transplant-Heart; **Hospital:** Univ Virginia Med Ctr; **Address:** Univ VA Hlth Sys, Div Cardiovascular Surg, PO Box 800679, Charlottesville, VA 22908; **Phone:** 434-924-2158; **Board Cert:** Surgery 1999; Thoracic Surgery 2001; Surgical Critical Care 1996; Vascular Surgery 1995; **Med School:** Med Coll Wisc 1975; **Resid:** Surgery, Maine Med Ctr 1980; **Fellow:** Cardiothoracic Surgery, Univ Virginia Med Ctr 1982; **Fac Appt:** Prof S, Univ VA Sch Med

Martin, Tomas D MD [TS] - **Spec Exp:** Cardiothoracic Surgery; Aortic Surgery; Aneurysm-Abdominal Aortic; **Hospital:** Shands Hlthcre at Univ of FL; **Address:** 1600 SW Archer Rd, Box 100286, Gainesville, FL 32610-0286; **Phone:** 352-273-5470; **Board Cert:** Thoracic Surgery 1999; **Med School:** Univ Tex, Houston 1981; **Resid:** Surgery, Baylor Coll Med 1986; Vascular Surgery, Baylor Coll Med 1987; **Fellow:** Cardiothoracic Surgery, Shands/Univ Florida 1989; **Fac Appt:** Assoc Prof S, Univ Fla Coll Med

Miller, Daniel L MD [TS] - **Spec Exp:** Esophageal Cancer; Lung Cancer; Mesothelioma; Emphysema-Lung Volume Reduction; **Hospital:** Emory Univ Hosp; **Address:** Emory Clinic, 1365 Clifton Rd NE, Atlanta, GA 30322; **Phone:** 404-778-3755; **Board Cert:** Thoracic Surgery 2005; Surgery 2001; **Med School:** Univ KY Coll Med 1985; **Resid:** Surgery, Georgetown Univ Hosp 1991; **Fellow:** Cardiothoracic Surgery, Mayo Clinic 1994; **Fac Appt:** Assoc Prof S, Emory Univ

Miller, Joseph MD [TS] - **Spec Exp:** Lung Cancer; **Hospital:** Emory Univ Hosp, Crawford Long Hosp of Emory Univ; **Address:** 550 Peachtree St NE, MOT-6th Fl, Atlanta, GA 30308; **Phone:** 404-686-2515; **Board Cert:** Surgery 1973; Thoracic Surgery 1975; **Med School:** Emory Univ 1965; **Resid:** Surgery, Mayo Clin 1972; Thoracic Surgery, Emory Univ Hosp 1974; **Fac Appt:** Prof S, Emory Univ

Mullett, Timothy W MD [TS] - **Spec Exp:** Lung Cancer; Transplant-Heart & Lung; Cardiac Surgery-Adult & Pediatric; Esophageal Surgery; **Hospital:** Univ of Kentucky Chandler Hosp; **Address:** 900 S Limestone St, Lexington, KY 40536; **Phone:** 859-323-6494; **Board Cert:** Thoracic Surgery 1997; Surgery 2005; **Med School:** Univ Fla Coll Med 1987; **Resid:** Surgery, Shands/Univ of FL 1993; **Fellow:** Pediatric Surgery, Shands/Univ of FL 1994; Cardiothoracic Surgery, Shands/Univ of FL 1995; **Fac Appt:** Assoc Prof S, Univ KY Coll Med

Murphy, Douglas A MD [TS] - **Spec Exp:** Mitral Valve Robotic Surgery; **Hospital:** St Joseph's Hosp - Atlanta; **Address:** 5665 Peachtree Dunwoody Rd NE, Ste 150, Atlanta, GA 30342; **Phone:** 404-252-6104; **Board Cert:** Internal Medicine 1978; Thoracic Surgery 2004; **Med School:** Univ Pennsylvania 1975; **Resid:** Internal Medicine, Mass Genl Hosp 1977; Surgery, Mass Genl Hosp 1981; **Fellow:** Thoracic Surgery, Emory Univ Affil Hosp 1983

Nesbitt, Jonathan C MD [TS] - **Spec Exp:** Lung Cancer; Esophageal Cancer; Chest Diseases-Benign; **Hospital:** Saint Thomas Hosp - Nashville; **Address:** The Surgical Clinic, St Thomas Med Bldg, 4230 Harding Rd, Ste 525, Nashville, TN 37205; **Phone:** 615-385-1547; **Board Cert:** Surgery 1998; Thoracic Surgery 1998; **Med School:** Georgetown Univ 1981; **Resid:** Surgery, Vanderbilt Univ Medical Ctr 1987; Thoracic Surgery, Albany Medical Ctr 1989; **Fac Appt:** Asst Clin Prof S, Vanderbilt Univ

Ninan, Mathew MD [TS] - **Spec Exp:** Lung Cancer; Transplant-Lung; Esophageal Cancer; **Hospital:** Baptist Memorial Hospital - Memphis, Methodist LeBonheur Germantown Hosp; **Address:** Cardiovascular Surgery Clinic, LLC, 6029 Walnut Grove Rd, Ste 401, East Office, Memphis, TN 38120; **Phone:** 901-747-3066; **Med School:** India 1988; **Resid:** Surgery, University of London 1994; **Fellow:** Cardiothoracic Surgery, Univ Pittsburgh 1998; **Fac Appt:** Asst Prof TS, Vanderbilt Univ

Perryman, Richard A MD [TS] - **Spec Exp:** Pediatric Cardiothoracic Surgery; Congenital Heart Disease-Adult; Ross Procedure for Aortic Valve Disease; **Hospital:** Joe Di Maggio Chldns Hosp, Meml Regl Hosp - Hollywood; **Address:** Joe DiMaggio Cardiac Surg Ctr, 1150 N 35th Ave, Ste 575, Hollywood, FL 33021; **Phone:** 954-985-6939; **Board Cert:** Thoracic Surgery 2002; **Med School:** England 1967; **Resid:** Thoracic Surgery, Duke Univ Med Ctr 1977; Cardiothoracic Surgery, Univ Florida 1981; **Fellow:** Cardiovascular Disease, Duke Univ Med Ctr 1971; **Fac Appt:** Prof TS, Univ Miami Sch Med

Putnam Jr, Joe B MD [TS] - **Spec Exp:** Lung Cancer; Esophageal Cancer; Sarcoma-Soft Tissue; **Hospital:** Vanderbilt Univ Med Ctr, VA Med Ctr - Nashville; **Address:** Vanderbilt Univ Med Ctr - Thoracic Surgery, 1301 Medical Center Drive, 2971 TVC, Nashville, TN 37232-5734; **Phone:** 615-343-9202; **Board Cert:** Thoracic Surgery 1997; **Med School:** Univ NC Sch Med 1979; **Resid:** Surgery, Univ Rochester 1986; Thoracic Surgery, Univ Mich Med Ctr 1988; **Fellow:** Surgical Oncology, NCI/NIH-Surg Branch 1984; **Fac Appt:** Prof TS, Vanderbilt Univ

Quintessenza, James A MD [TS] - **Spec Exp:** Transplant-Heart; Coronary Artery Surgery; Cardiovascular Surgery; **Hospital:** All Children's Hosp; **Address:** 603 7th St S, Ste 450, St Petersburg, FL 33701-4734; **Phone:** 727-822-6666; **Board Cert:** Thoracic Surgery 1999; **Med School:** Univ Fla Coll Med 1981; **Resid:** Surgery, Univ Florida Hosps 1986; **Fellow:** Thoracic Surgery, UCSD Medical Ctr 1988; **Fac Appt:** Asst Clin Prof S, Univ S Fla Coll Med

Reed, Carolyn E MD [TS] - **Spec Exp:** Esophageal Cancer; Lung Cancer; **Hospital:** MUSC Med Ctr; **Address:** Med Univ S Carolina, Hollings Cancer Ctr, 96 Jonathan Lucas St, Ste 418, Charleston, SC 29425; **Phone:** 843-792-3362; **Board Cert:** Thoracic Surgery 2006; **Med School:** Univ Rochester 1977; **Resid:** Surgery, New York Hosp 1982; Thoracic Surgery, New York Hosp 1985; **Fellow:** Surgical Oncology, Meml Sloan Kettering Cancer Ctr 1983; **Fac Appt:** Prof S, Med Univ SC

Smith, Peter K MD [TS] - **Spec Exp:** Coronary Artery Surgery; Heart Valve Surgery; **Hospital:** Duke Univ Med Ctr, VA Med Ctr - Durham; **Address:** Duke Univ Med Ctr, Cardiothoracic Surg, Box 3442, Durham, NC 27710; **Phone:** 919-684-2890; **Board Cert:** Surgery 1995; Thoracic Surgery 1998; **Med School:** Duke Univ 1977; **Resid:** Surgery, Duke Univ Med Ctr 1984; Thoracic Surgery, Duke Univ Med Ctr 1987; **Fac Appt:** Prof S, Duke Univ

Staples, Edward D MD [TS] - **Spec Exp:** Transplant-Heart & Lung; Ventricular Assist Device (LVAD); **Hospital:** Shands Hlthcre at Univ of FL; **Address:** Shands Hlthcre, Dept Cardiothoracic Surg, 1600 SW Archer Rd, Box 100286, Gainesville, FL 32610-0268; **Phone:** 352-273-5509; **Board Cert:** Thoracic Surgery 2004; Surgical Critical Care 2002; **Med School:** Univ S Fla Coll Med 1977; **Resid:** Surgery, Med Coll Va 1979; Surgery, Univ Hosp 1982; **Fellow:** Cardiothoracic Surgery, Univ Florida 1984; **Fac Appt:** Assoc Prof S, Univ Fla Coll Med

Tedder, Mark MD [TS] - **Spec Exp:** Transplant-Heart; Cardiac Surgery; Artificial Heart Devices; **Hospital:** Saint Thomas Hosp - Nashville; **Address:** 4230 Harding Rd, Ste 450, Nashville, TN 37205; **Phone:** 615-385-4781; **Board Cert:** Surgery 1996; Thoracic Surgery 1998; **Med School:** Duke Univ 1988; **Resid:** Surgery, Duke Univ Med Ctr 1995; Cardiothoracic Surgery, Duke Univ Med Ctr 1997

Williams, Donald B MD [TS] - **Spec Exp:** Cardiac Surgery; **Hospital:** Mount Sinai Med Ctr - Miami; **Address:** Mount Sinai Medical Ctr, 4300 Alton Rd, Ste 2110, Miami Beach, FL 33140-2800; **Phone:** 305-674-2780; **Board Cert:** Thoracic Surgery 2000; **Med School:** Jefferson Med Coll 1974; **Resid:** Surgery, Dartmouth-Hitchcock Med Ctr 1979; **Fellow:** Thoracic Surgery, Mayo Clinic 1981

Midwest

Alexander Jr, John C MD [TS] - **Spec Exp:** Minimally Invasive Cardiac Surgery; Robotic Heart Surgery; Mitral Valve Surgery; Arrhythmias; **Hospital:** Evanston Hosp; **Address:** Evanston Hosp, Cardiothoracic Surgery, 2650 Ridge Ave Walgreens Bldg - Ste 3507, Chicago, IL 60201; **Phone:** 847-570-2868; **Board Cert:** Thoracic Surgery 2001; **Med School:** Duke Univ 1972; **Resid:** Surgery, Duke Univ Med Ctr 1979; **Fellow:** Cardiothoracic Surgery, Duke Univ Med Ctr 1980; **Fac Appt:** Prof S, UMDNJ-NJ Med Sch, Newark

Bakhos, Mamdouh MD [TS] - **Spec Exp:** Mitral Valve Surgery; Minimally Invasive Cardiac Surgery; Transplant-Heart & Lung; **Hospital:** Loyola Univ Med Ctr, Adv Good Samaritan Hosp; **Address:** Loyola Univ, Dept Cardiothoracic Surgery, 2160 S First Ave, Bldg 110 - rm 6240, Maywood, IL 60153; **Phone:** 708-327-2503; **Board Cert:** Thoracic Surgery 1998; **Med School:** Syria 1971; **Resid:** Surgery, Huron Road Hosp 1976; **Fellow:** Thoracic Surgery, Loyola Univ Med Ctr 1978; **Fac Appt:** Prof TS, Loyola Univ-Stritch Sch Med

Bassett, Joseph MD [TS] - **Spec Exp:** Heart Valve Surgery; Coronary Artery Surgery; **Hospital:** William Beaumont Hosp; **Address:** 1663 W Big Beaver Rd, Troy, MI 48084; **Phone:** 248-643-8633; **Board Cert:** Surgery 1967; Thoracic Surgery 1969; **Med School:** Wayne State Univ 1961; **Resid:** Surgery, Wayne State Univ Affil Hosp 1966; Thoracic Surgery, Wayne State Univ Affil Hosp 1968; **Fac Appt:** Assoc Clin Prof S, Wayne State Univ

Behrendt, Douglas M MD [TS] - **Spec Exp:** Congenital Heart Disease; Transplant-Heart; **Hospital:** Univ Iowa Hosp & Clinics; **Address:** Univ Iowa Hosp & Clins, Dept Surg, 200 Hawkins Drive, Colloton Pavilion, rm 1622, Iowa City, IA 52242; **Phone:** 319-356-2761; **Board Cert:** Surgery 1972; Thoracic Surgery 1972; **Med School:** Harvard Med Sch 1963; **Resid:** Surgery, Mass Genl Hosp 1971; Cardiothoracic Surgery, Natl Inst Hlth 1968; **Fellow:** Pediatric Cardiac Surgery, Hosp Sick Chldn 1970; **Fac Appt:** Prof TS, Univ Iowa Coll Med

Brown, John W MD [TS] - **Spec Exp:** Cardiac Surgery-Neonatal & Pediatric; Transplant-Heart; Heart Valve Surgery; **Hospital:** Riley Hosp for Children, Methodist Hosp - Indianapolis; **Address:** 545 Barnhill Drive, EH215, Indianapolis, IN 46202-5112; **Phone:** 317-274-7150; **Board Cert:** Thoracic Surgery 1998; **Med School:** Indiana Univ 1970; **Resid:** Surgery, Univ Mich Med Ctr 1976; Univ Mich Med Ctr 1978; **Fellow:** Cardiovascular Surgery, Natl Heart Lung-Blood Inst 1974; **Fac Appt:** Prof S, Indiana Univ

Damiano Jr, Ralph J MD [TS] - **Spec Exp:** Minimally Invasive Cardiac Surgery; Robotic Cardiac Surgery; **Hospital:** Barnes-Jewish Hosp; **Address:** 660 S Euclid Ave, Campus Box 8234, St. Louis, MO 63110; **Phone:** 314-362-7327; **Board Cert:** Thoracic Surgery 2002; **Med School:** Duke Univ 1980; **Resid:** Surgery, Duke Univ Med Ctr 1988; **Fellow:** Cardiothoracic Surgery, Duke Univ Med Ctr 1989; **Fac Appt:** Prof S, Washington Univ, St Louis

Deschamps, Claude MD [TS] - **Spec Exp:** Gastroesophageal Reflux Disease (GERD); Esophageal Cancer; Lung Cancer; **Hospital:** St Mary's Hosp - Rochester; **Address:** Mayo Clinic, Div Thoracic Surgery, 200 First St SW, Rochester, MN 55905; **Phone:** 507-284-8462; **Board Cert:** Surgery 1994; **Med School:** Univ Montreal 1979; **Resid:** Surgery, Univ Montreal Hosps 1984; Thoracic Surgery, Univ Montreal Hosp 1985; **Fellow:** Thoracic Surgery, Mayo Clinic 1987; **Fac Appt:** Prof S, Mayo Med Sch

Durham, Samuel J MD [TS] - **Spec Exp:** Cardiothoracic Surgery; **Hospital:** Univ of Toledo Med Ctr; **Address:** Univ of Toledo Med Ctr, Dowling Hall, 3065 Arlington Ave, Ste 2261, Toledo, OH 43614; **Phone:** 419-383-5150; **Board Cert:** Surgery 2001; Thoracic Surgery 2003; **Med School:** Harvard Med Sch 1983; **Resid:** Surgery, Univ Pittsburgh Med Ctr 1987; Thoracic Surgery, Univ Pittsburgh Med Ctr 1988; **Fellow:** Pediatric Surgery, Chlidren's Hosp 1993; **Fac Appt:** Prof S, Ohio State Univ

Faber, L Penfield MD [TS] - **Spec Exp:** Lung Cancer; Esophageal Cancer; Thoracic Cancers; **Hospital:** Rush Univ Med Ctr; **Address:** 1725 W Harrison St, Ste 774, Chicago, IL 60612-3817; **Phone:** 312-738-3732; **Board Cert:** Surgery 1962; Thoracic Surgery 1963; **Med School:** Northwestern Univ 1956; **Resid:** Surgery, Presby-St Luke's Hosp 1961; Thoracic Surgery, Hines VA Hosp 1963; **Fac Appt:** Prof TS, Rush Med Coll

Ferguson, Mark MD [TS] - **Spec Exp:** Barrett's Esophagus; Esophageal Cancer; Lung Cancer; **Hospital:** Univ of Chicago Hosps; **Address:** 5841 S Maryland Ave, MC 5035, Univ of Chicago Hospitals, Chicago, IL 60637-1470; **Phone:** 773-702-3551; **Board Cert:** Surgery 1993; Thoracic Surgery 2003; **Med School:** Univ Chicago-Pritzker Sch Med 1977; **Resid:** Surgery, Univ Chicago Hosps 1982; **Fellow:** Cardiothoracic Surgery, Univ Chicago Hosps 1984; **Fac Appt:** Prof S, Univ Chicago-Pritzker Sch Med

Frederiksen, James W MD [TS] - **Spec Exp:** Cardiothoracic Surgery; **Hospital:** Northwestern Meml Hosp; **Address:** 201 E Huron St, Ste 11-140, Chicago, IL 60611; **Phone:** 312-695-3121; **Board Cert:** Thoracic Surgery 2000; **Med School:** Harvard Med Sch 1972; **Resid:** Surgery, Peter Bent Brigham Hosp 1974; Northwestern Meml Hosp 1978; **Fellow:** Cardiothoracic Surgery, Johns Hopkins Hosp 1976; **Fac Appt:** Assoc Prof S, Northwestern Univ

Howington, John A MD [TS] - **Spec Exp:** Lung Cancer; **Hospital:** Evanston NW Hlthcare; **Address:** Evanston Northwestern Hospital, 2650 Ridge Ave, Walgreen Bldg - Ste 3507, Evanston, IL 60201; **Phone:** 847-570-2868; **Board Cert:** Thoracic Surgery 1998; Surgery 1998; **Med School:** Univ Tenn Coll Med, Memphis 1989; **Resid:** Surgery, Truman Med Ctr/U Missouri 1994; Cardiothoracic Surgery, Vanderbilt Univ Med Ctr 1997; **Fac Appt:** Assoc Prof S, Northwestern Univ

Huddleston, Charles B MD [TS] - **Spec Exp:** Transplant-Lung-Pediatric; Transplant-Heart-Pediatric; **Hospital:** St Louis Chldns Hosp; **Address:** St Louis Children's Hospital, One Children's Pl, Ste 5 South 50, St Louis, MO 63110; **Phone:** 314-454-6165; **Board Cert:** Thoracic Surgery 1997; **Med School:** Vanderbilt Univ 1978; **Resid:** Surgery, Vanderbilt Univ Hosp 1986; Cardiothoracic Surgery, Vanderbilt Univ Hosp 1988; **Fellow:** Pediatric Cardiothoracic Surgery, Hosp for Sick Children 1989; **Fac Appt:** Prof S, Washington Univ, St Louis

Iannettoni, Mark D MD [TS] - **Spec Exp:** Transplant-Lung; Lung Cancer; Esophageal Disorders; **Hospital:** Univ Iowa Hosp & Clinics; **Address:** Univ Iowa Hosp & Clinics, 200 Hawkins Drive, rm SE514GH, Iowa City, IA 52242; **Phone:** 319-356-1133; **Board Cert:** Surgery 2002; Thoracic Surgery 2002; **Med School:** SUNY Upstate Med Univ 1985; **Resid:** Surgery, SUNY Upstate Med Ctr 1991; Thoracic Surgery, Univ Mich Med Ctr 1993; **Fellow:** Thoracic Surgery, Univ Mich Med Sch 1994

Jeevanandam, Valluvan MD [TS] - **Spec Exp:** Minimally Invasive Heart Valve Surgery; Transplant-Heart; Artificial Heart Devices; **Hospital:** Univ of Chicago Hosps; **Address:** 5841 S Maryland Ave, Ste E500, MC 5040, Chicago, IL 60637-1483; **Phone:** 773-702-2500; **Board Cert:** Surgery 1990; Thoracic Surgery 2002; **Med School:** Columbia P&S 1984; **Resid:** Surgery, Columbia-Presby Med Ctr 1989; **Fellow:** Cardiothoracic Surgery, Columbia-Presby Med Ctr 1991; **Fac Appt:** Prof S, Univ Chicago-Pritzker Sch Med

Kouchoukos, Nicholas T MD [TS] - **Spec Exp:** Cardiac Surgery; Heart Valve Surgery; Aortic Surgery; **Hospital:** Missouri Baptist Med Ctr; **Address:** Missouri Baptist Hospital, 3009 N Ballas Rd C Bldg - Ste 360, St. Louis, MO 63131-2322; **Phone:** 314-996-5287; **Board Cert:** Surgery 1967; Thoracic Surgery 1970; **Med School:** Washington Univ, St Louis 1961; **Resid:** Surgery, Barnes Hosp-Wash Univ 1967; Thoracic Surgery, Univ Alabama Hosps 1970; **Fellow:** Univ Alabama Hosps 1968; **Fac Appt:** Prof S, Washington Univ, St Louis

Little, Alex G MD [TS] - **Hospital:** Wright State Univ, Miami Valley Hosp; **Address:** 30 E Apple St, Ste 5253, Dayton, OH 45409; **Phone:** 937-208-2552; **Board Cert:** Surgery 1998; Thoracic Surgery 1990; **Med School:** Johns Hopkins Univ 1974; **Resid:** Surgery, Univ Chicago Hosp 1979; Thoracic Surgery, Univ Chicago Hosp 1981; **Fac Appt:** Prof TS, Wright State Univ

Lytle, Bruce W MD [TS] - **Spec Exp:** Heart Valve Surgery; Coronary Artery Surgery; Aortic Surgery; **Hospital:** Cleveland Clin Fdn (page 57); **Address:** Cleveland Clinic, Dept Thoracic Surgery, 9500 Euclid Ave, Desk F24, Cleveland, OH 44195; **Phone:** 216-444-6962; **Board Cert:** Thoracic Surgery 1998; **Med School:** Harvard Med Sch 1971; **Resid:** Surgery, Mass Genl Hsop 1975; Surgery, Shotley Bridge Hosp 1976; **Fellow:** Thoracic Surgery, Mass Genl Hosp 1979; **Fac Appt:** Prof TS, Cleveland Cl Coll Med/Case West Res

McCarthy, Patrick M MD [TS] - **Spec Exp:** Heart Valve Surgery; Coronary Artery Surgery; Ventricular Assist Device (LVAD); **Hospital:** Northwestern Meml Hosp; **Address:** Northwestern Med Faculty Fdn, 201 E Huron St, Ste 11-140, Chicago, IL 60611-2968; **Phone:** 312-695-6984; **Board Cert:** Thoracic Surgery 1998; **Med School:** Loyola Univ-Stritch Sch Med 1980; **Resid:** Surgery, Mayo Clinic 1985; Thoracic Surgery, Mayo Clinic 1988; **Fellow:** Cardiopulmonary Transplant Surgery, Stanford Univ 1989; **Fac Appt:** Prof S, Northwestern Univ

McGregor, Christopher MD [TS] - **Spec Exp:** Transplant-Heart & Lung; Cardiac Surgery; **Hospital:** Mayo Med Ctr & Clin - Rochester, St Mary's Hosp - Rochester; **Address:** Mayo Clinic - St Mary's Hospital, 200 First St SW, rm Joseph 5-200, Rochester, MN 55905; **Phone:** 507-255-6038; **Med School:** Scotland 1972; **Resid:** Surgery, Edinburgh Royal Infirm 1978; Surgery, Glasgow Royal Infirm 1981; **Fellow:** Cardiothoracic Transplant Surg, Stanford Univ Hosp 1984; **Fac Appt:** Prof S, Mayo Med Sch

Merrill, Walter H MD [TS] - **Spec Exp:** Cardiothoracic Surgery; Cardiac Surgery-Adult & Pediatric; Transplant-Heart; **Hospital:** Univ Hosp - Cincinnati, VA Med Ctr; **Address:** Univ Cincinnati, Sect Cardiothoracic Surg, 231 Albert Sabin Way, ML 0588, Cincinnati, OH 45267-0001; **Phone:** 513-584-3278; **Board Cert:** Surgery 2000; Thoracic Surgery 2001; Surgical Critical Care 1999; **Med School:** Johns Hopkins Univ 1974; **Resid:** Thoracic Surgery, Natl Inst Hlth 1978; Thoracic Surgery, Johns Hopkins Hosp 1982; **Fellow:** Pediatric Surgery, Hosp for Sick Chldn 1983; **Fac Appt:** Prof S, Univ Cincinnati

Meyers, Bryan MD [TS] - **Spec Exp:** Lung Cancer; Esophageal Cancer; Transplant-Lung; **Hospital:** Barnes-Jewish Hosp, Barnes-Jewish West County Hosp; **Address:** 4921 Parkview Pl, Ste 8B, St Louis, MO 63110; **Phone:** 314-362-8598; **Board Cert:** Surgery 1998; Thoracic Surgery 1999; **Med School:** Univ Chicago-Pritzker Sch Med 1986; **Resid:** Surgery, Mass Genl Hosp 1996; **Fellow:** Cardiothoracic Surgery, Barnes Hosp-Wash Univ 1998; **Fac Appt:** Assoc Prof S, Washington Univ, St Louis

Naunheim, Keith S MD [TS] - **Spec Exp:** Lung Cancer; Esophageal Cancer; Chest Wall Tumors; Video Assisted Thoracic Surgery (VATS); **Hospital:** St Louis Univ Hosp; **Address:** St Lous Univ Med Ctr, Dept Surgery, 3635 Vista Ave, St Louis, MO 63110-0250; **Phone:** 314-577-8360; **Board Cert:** Thoracic Surgery 2004; **Med School:** Univ Chicago-Pritzker Sch Med 1978; **Resid:** Surgery, Univ Chicago Hosp 1983; **Fellow:** Cardiothoracic Surgery, Univ Chicago Hosp 1985; **Fac Appt:** Prof S, St Louis Univ

Orringer, Mark B MD [TS] - **Spec Exp:** Esophageal Cancer; Lung Cancer; Mediastinal Tumors; Lung Cancer; **Hospital:** Univ Michigan Hlth Sys; **Address:** Univ Mich, Taubman Ctr, 1500 E Med Ctr Drive, rm TC 2120, Box 0344, Ann Arbor, MI 48109-0344; **Phone:** 734-936-4975; **Board Cert:** Surgery 1973; Thoracic Surgery 1974; **Med School:** Univ Pittsburgh 1967; **Resid:** Thoracic Surgery, Johns Hopkins Hosp 1973; **Fac Appt:** Prof S, Univ Mich Med Sch

Pagani, Francis Domenic MD [TS] - **Spec Exp:** Transplant-Heart; Coronary Artery Surgery; **Hospital:** Univ Michigan Hlth Sys; **Address:** Univ Mich Med Ctr, Sect Cardiac Surg, 1500 E Med Ctr Drive, rm 2120 Taubm, Ann Arbor, MI 48109-0348; **Phone:** 734-647-2894; **Board Cert:** Surgery 2002; Thoracic Surgery 2004; **Med School:** Georgetown Univ 1986; **Resid:** Surgery, Georgetown Univ Med Ctr 1993; Thoracic Surgery, Univ Mich Hosp 1995; **Fellow:** Research, Univ Mass Med Ctr 1990; **Fac Appt:** Assoc Prof S, Univ Mich Med Sch

Patterson, G Alexander MD [TS] - **Spec Exp:** Lung Cancer; Esophageal Cancer; Transplant-Lung; Transplant-Heart & Lung; **Hospital:** Barnes-Jewish Hosp; **Address:** 660 S Euclid Ave, Box 8234, St Louis, MO 63110; **Phone:** 314-362-6025; **Board Cert:** Surgery 1978; Thoracic Surgery 1981; Vascular Surgery 1982; **Med School:** Canada 1974; **Resid:** Surgery, Queens Univ Med Ctr 1978; Vascular Surgery, Univ Toronto Med Ctr 1979; **Fellow:** Research, Toronto Genl Hosp 1981; Surgical Critical Care, Johns Hopkins Hosp 1982; **Fac Appt:** Prof S, Washington Univ, St Louis

Piccione, William MD [TS] - **Spec Exp:** Transplant-Heart; Vein Disorders; Artificial Heart Devices; Heart Valve Surgery; **Hospital:** Rush Oak Park Hosp; **Address:** 610 S Maple, Ste 2800, Oak Park, IL 60304; **Phone:** 312-563-4120; **Board Cert:** Surgery 1997; Thoracic Surgery 1999; **Med School:** Univ Rochester 1980; **Resid:** Surgery, Harvard/New England Deaconess Hosp 1986; **Fellow:** Cardiothoracic Surgery, Rush Presby-St Lukes Med Ctr 1988; Thoracic Surgery, Meml Sloan Kettering Cancer Ctr 1988; **Fac Appt:** Assoc Prof TS, Rush Med Coll

Raman, Jai MD/PhD [TS] - **Spec Exp:** Robotic Heart Surgery; Heart Failure & Ventricular Containment; Transplant-Heart; Atrial Fibrillation; **Hospital:** Univ of Chicago Hosps; **Address:** University of Chicago Hosps, 5841 S Maryland Ave, Ste E500, MC 5040, Chicago, IL 60637; **Phone:** 773-702-2500; **Med School:** India 1990; **Resid:** Cardiothoracic Surgery, St Vincent's Hosp 1991; Cardiothoracic Surgery, Austin Hospital 1995; **Fellow:** Thoracic Surgery, Austin Hosp 1994; Pediatric Cardiac Surgery, Royal Children's Hosp 1996; **Fac Appt:** Assoc Prof S, Univ Chicago-Pritzker Sch Med

Rice, Thomas W MD [TS] - **Spec Exp:** Esophageal Surgery; Minimally Invasive Thoracic Surgery; Transplant-Lung; **Hospital:** Cleveland Clin Fdn (page 57); **Address:** Cleveland Clinic, 9500 Euclid Ave, Desk F-24, Cleveland, OH 44195; **Phone:** 216-444-1921; **Board Cert:** Surgery 2002; Thoracic Surgery 2005; **Med School:** Univ Toronto 1978; **Resid:** Surgery, Univ Toronto Med Ctr 1983; Thoracic Surgery, Univ Toronto Med Ctr 1986; **Fellow:** Pulmonary Disease, UCSF Med Ctr 1984; **Fac Appt:** Prof S, Cleveland Cl Coll Med/Case West Res

Schaff, Hartzell MD [TS] - **Spec Exp:** Heart Valve Surgery; Congenital Heart Disease; Maze Procedure for Atrial Fibrillation; **Hospital:** St Mary's Hosp - Rochester; **Address:** Mayo Clin, Div Cardiovasc Surg, 200 First St SW, Rochester, MN 55905-0001; **Phone:** 507-255-7068; **Board Cert:** Thoracic Surgery 2001; **Med School:** Univ Okla Coll Med 1973; **Resid:** Surgery, Johns Hopkins Hosp 1978; Thoracic Surgery, Johns Hopkins Hosp 1980; **Fellow:** Surgery, Johns Hopkins Hosp 1976; **Fac Appt:** Prof S, Mayo Med Sch

Silverman, Norman A MD [TS] - **Spec Exp:** Heart Valve Surgery; Aortic Surgery; Transplant-Heart; **Hospital:** Henry Ford Hosp; **Address:** Henry Ford Hosp, Div Cardiothoracic Surg, 2799 W Grand Blvd, Detroit, MI 48202-2608; **Phone:** 313-916-2695; **Board Cert:** Surgery 1989; Thoracic Surgery 2001; **Med School:** Boston Univ 1971; **Resid:** Surgery, Duke Univ Med Ctr 1973; Thoracic Surgery, Duke Univ Med Ctr 1980; **Fac Appt:** Prof S, Case West Res Univ

Smedira, Nicholas MD [TS] - **Spec Exp:** Transplant-Heart; Transplant-Lung; Ventricular Assist Device (LVAD); Aortic Surgery; **Hospital:** Cleveland Clin Fdn (page 57); **Address:** Cleveland Clin, Dept Cardiothoracic Surg, 9500 Euclid Ave, Desk F24, Cleveland, OH 44195; **Phone:** 216-445-7052; **Board Cert:** Thoracic Surgery 2003; **Med School:** Univ Rochester 1984; **Resid:** Surgery, UCSF Med Ctr 1991; Thoracic Surgery, UCSF Med Ctr 1994; **Fellow:** Cardiothoracic Surgery, UCSF Med Ctr 1994

Smith, John Michael MD [TS] - **Spec Exp:** Mitral Valve Robotic Surgery; **Hospital:** Good Samaritan Hosp - Cincinnati; **Address:** 4030 Smith Rd, Ste 300, Cincinnati, OH 45209; **Phone:** 513-421-3494; **Board Cert:** Surgery 2003; Thoracic Surgery 1997; **Med School:** Univ Louisville Sch Med 1989; **Resid:** Surgery, Good Samaritan Hosp 1994; **Fellow:** Cardiothoracic Surgery, Yale Univ Hosp 1996

Stuart, Richard Scott MD [TS] - **Spec Exp:** Cardiac Surgery; Thoracic Surgery; Robotic Cardiac Surgery; **Hospital:** St Luke's Hosp of Kansas City, N Kansas City Hosp; **Address:** 4320 Wornall Rd Bldg 2 - Ste 50, Kansas City, MO 64111; **Phone:** 816-931-3312; **Board Cert:** Thoracic Surgery 1999; Surgical Critical Care 1993; **Med School:** Johns Hopkins Univ 1981; **Resid:** Surgery, Johns Hopkins Hosp 1986; **Fellow:** Cardiothoracic Surgery, Johns Hopkins Hosp 1989; **Fac Appt:** Clin Prof TS, Univ MO-Kansas City

Sundt III, Thoralf Mauritz MD [TS] - **Spec Exp:** Heart Valve Surgery; Aneurysm-Thoracic Aortic; Pulmonary Embolism; **Hospital:** Mayo Med Ctr & Clin - Rochester; **Address:** Mayo Clinic, 200 First St SW, Rochester, MN 55905-0002; **Phone:** 507-255-7064; **Board Cert:** Surgery 2000; Thoracic Surgery 2004; **Med School:** Johns Hopkins Univ 1984; **Resid:** Surgery, Mass Genl Hosp 1991; Cardiothoracic Surgery, Wash Univ Sch Med 1993; **Fellow:** Cardiothoracic Surgery, Harefield Hosp 1994; **Fac Appt:** Prof S, Mayo Med Sch

Turrentine, Mark W MD [TS] - **Spec Exp:** Cardiac Surgery-Pediatric; Transplant-Heart; Transplant-Lung; **Hospital:** Riley Hosp for Children, Methodist Hosp - Indianapolis; **Address:** 545 Barnhill Dr, Emerson Hall, Ste 215, Indianapolis, IN 46202; **Phone:** 317-274-1121; **Board Cert:** Thoracic Surgery 2002; **Med School:** Univ Kans 1983; **Resid:** Surgery, Univ Kansas Med Ctr 1988; Cardiothoracic Surgery, Indiana Univ Med Ctr 1991; **Fellow:** Cardiothoracic Surgery, Texas Heart Inst 1986; Transplant Surgery, Indiana Univ Med Ctr 1989; **Fac Appt:** Prof S, Indiana Univ

Wolf, Randall K MD [TS] - **Spec Exp:** Robotic Heart Surgery; Minimally Invasive Cardiac Surgery; **Hospital:** Univ Hosp - Cincinnati; **Address:** Univ Cincinnati, Sect Cardiothoracic Surg, 231 Albert Sabin Way, ML 0558, Cincinnati, OH 45267; **Phone:** 513-584-3278; **Board Cert:** Thoracic Surgery 1998; **Med School:** Indiana Univ 1979; **Resid:** Surgery, Roanoke Meml Hosps 1984; Vascular Surgery, Jewish Hosp 1986; **Fellow:** Thoracic Surgery, Univ Cincinnati Med Ctr 1989; **Fac Appt:** Prof TS, Univ Cincinnati

Great Plains and Mountains

Bull, David A MD [TS] - **Spec Exp:** Cardiothoracic Surgery; Esophageal Cancer; **Hospital:** Univ Utah Hosps and Clins; **Address:** Univ Utah, Dept Cardiothoracic Surgery, 30 N 1900 East, rm 3C127, Salt Lake City, UT 84132; **Phone:** 801-581-5311; **Board Cert:** Thoracic Surgery 2004; Vascular Surgery 2003; Surgery 1999; Surgical Critical Care 1999; **Med School:** UCSF 1985; **Resid:** Surgery, UCSF Medical Ctr 1987; Surgery, Univ Arizona Hosps 1990; **Fellow:** Vascular Surgery, Univ Arizona Hosps 1992; Cardiothoracic Surgery, Univ Arizona Hosps 1994; **Fac Appt:** Assoc Prof TS, Univ Utah

Campbell, David N MD [TS] - **Spec Exp:** Pediatric Cardiothoracic Surgery; Transplant-Heart-Pediatric; Transplant-Lung; **Hospital:** Chldn's Hosp - Denver, The, Univ Colorado Hosp; **Address:** 1056 E 19th Ave, Ste B-200, Denver, CO 80218; **Phone:** 303-861-6660; **Board Cert:** Surgery 1999; Thoracic Surgery 2000; Surgical Critical Care 2000; **Med School:** Rush Med Coll 1974; **Resid:** Surgery, Univ Colo Med Ctr 1980; Cardiothoracic Surgery, Univ Colo Med Ctr 1979; **Fellow:** Cardiovascular Surgery, Boston Chldns Hosp 1980; **Fac Appt:** Prof S, Univ Colorado

Doty, Donald B MD [TS] - **Spec Exp:** Cardiac Surgery-Adult; **Hospital:** LDS Hosp; **Address:** 324 10th Ave, Ste 154, Salt Lake City, UT 84103; **Phone:** 801-408-8666; **Board Cert:** Surgery 1968; Thoracic Surgery 1971; **Med School:** Stanford Univ 1962; **Resid:** Surgery, Los Angeles Co Hosp 1967; **Fellow:** Thoracic Surgery, Univ Ala Med Ctr 1971; **Fac Appt:** Clin Prof TS, Univ Utah

Fullerton, David A MD [TS] - **Spec Exp:** Maze Procedure for Atrial Fibrillation; Ross Procedure for Aortic Valve Disease; Mitral Valve Surgery; Transplant-Heart & Lung; **Hospital:** Univ Colorado Hosp, VA Med Ctr; **Address:** Univ of Colorado, Cardiothoracic Surgery, 12631 E 17th Ave, L15, RM 6602, MSC310, PO Box 6511, Aurora, CO 80045; **Phone:** 303-724-2798; **Board Cert:** Surgery 1997; Surgical Critical Care 2001; Thoracic Surgery 2001; **Med School:** Univ MO-Columbia Sch Med 1981; **Resid:** Surgery, Univ Wash Med Ctr 1987; Thoracic Surgery, Univ Colorado Hosp 1990; **Fac Appt:** Prof S, Univ Colorado

Karwande, Shreekanth V MD [TS] - **Spec Exp:** Thoracic Cancers; Lung Cancer; **Hospital:** Univ Utah Hosps and Clins; **Address:** Univ Utah Med Ctr, Cardiothoracic Surg, 30 N 1900 E, Ste 3C127, Salt Lake City, UT 84132; **Phone:** 801-581-5311; **Board Cert:** Thoracic Surgery 2003; **Med School:** India 1973; **Resid:** Surgery, Erie Co Med Ctr 1981; Cardiothoracic Surgery, New York Hosp 1985; **Fellow:** Cardiothoracic Surgery, Meml Sloan Kettering Cancer Ctr; **Fac Appt:** Prof S, Univ Utah

Pomerantz, Marvin MD [TS] - **Spec Exp:** Mycobacterial Pulmonary Surgery; Lung Infections; Tuberculosis; **Hospital:** Univ Colorado Hosp, VA Med Ctr; **Address:** 4200 E Ninth Ave, Box C 310, Denver, CO 80262; **Phone:** 303-315-8527; **Board Cert:** Surgery 1968; Thoracic Surgery 1968; **Med School:** Univ Rochester 1959; **Resid:** Surgery, Duke Univ Med Ctr 1963; Thoracic Surgery, Duke Univ Med Ctr 1967; **Fac Appt:** Prof S, Univ Colorado

Southwest

Aklog, Lishan MD [TS] - **Spec Exp:** Mitral Valve Surgery; Minimally Invasive Cardiac Surgery; Coronary Artery Surgery; **Hospital:** St Joseph's Hosp & Med Ctr - Phoenix; **Address:** Heart and Lung Inst, St Joseph's Hosp Med Ctr, 500 W Thomas Rd, Phoenix, AZ 85013-4224; **Phone:** 602-406-2996; **Board Cert:** Surgery 1997; Thoracic Surgery 2000; **Med School:** Harvard Med Sch 1989; **Resid:** Surgery, Brigham & Women's Hosp 1996; **Fellow:** Cardiothoracic Surgery, Brigham & Women's Hosp 1998; Cardiac Surgery, Harefield Hosp 1999

Antakli, Tamim MD [TS] - **Spec Exp:** Heart Valve Surgery; Arrhythmias; Esophageal Surgery; **Hospital:** UAMS Med Ctr, Cent Ark Vet Hlthcare Sys; **Address:** UAMS, Div Cardiothoracic Surg, 4301 W Markham St, Slot 713, Little Rock, AR 72205; **Phone:** 501-686-7884; **Board Cert:** Surgery 2005; Thoracic Surgery 1997; **Med School:** Syria 1983; **Resid:** Surgery, Meth Hosp 1993; Thoracic Surgery, Univ Arkansas Med Ctr 1996; **Fac Appt:** Assoc Prof S, Univ Ark

Calhoon, John H MD [TS] - **Spec Exp:** Transplant-Heart & Lung; Congenital Heart Surgery; Cardiac Surgery-Adult & Pediatric; **Hospital:** Univ Hlth Sys - Univ Hosp, Christus Santa Rosa Children's Hosp; **Address:** UTHSCSA, Dept Thoracic Surg, 7703 Floyd Curl Drive, MC 7841, San Antonio, TX 78229-3901; **Phone:** 210-567-6863; **Board Cert:** Surgery 1996; Thoracic Surgery 1997; **Med School:** Baylor Coll Med 1981; **Resid:** Surgery, Univ Hosp/Univ Texas HSC 1986; Univ Hosp/Univ Texas HSC 1988; **Fellow:** Pediatric Cardiac Surgery, Chldns Hosp/Harvard 1989; **Fac Appt:** Prof TS, Univ Tex, San Antonio

Copeland III, Jack G MD [TS] - **Spec Exp:** Transplant-Heart; Transplant-Heart & Lung; Artificial Heart Devices; **Hospital:** Univ Med Ctr - Tucson, VA Medical Center - Tucson; **Address:** Univ Ariz Hlth Sci Ctr, 1501 N Campbell Rd, rm 4402, Box 245071, Tucson, AZ 85724-5071; **Phone:** 520-626-6339; **Board Cert:** Thoracic Surgery 1997; **Med School:** Stanford Univ 1969; **Resid:** Surgery, UCSD Med Ctr 1971; Cardiovascular Surgery, Natl Inst Hlth 1973; **Fellow:** Cardiothoracic Surgery, Stanford Univ 1977; **Fac Appt:** Prof TS, Univ Ariz Coll Med

Coselli, Joseph S MD [TS] - **Spec Exp:** Aneurysm-Abdominal & Thoracic Aortic; Marfan's Syndrome; Aortic Surgery; **Hospital:** St Luke's Episcopal Hosp - Houston; **Address:** 6770 Bertner Ave, Ste C350, MC 1-103, Houston, TX 77030; **Phone:** 832-355-9910; **Board Cert:** Thoracic Surgery 2004; **Med School:** Univ Tex Med Br, Galveston 1977; **Resid:** Surgery, Baylor Coll Med 1982; Thoracic Surgery, Baylor Coll Med 1984; **Fac Appt:** Assoc Prof S, Baylor Coll Med

Diethrich, Edward B MD [TS] - **Spec Exp:** Vascular Surgery; Endovascular Surgery; Cardiovascular Surgery; **Hospital:** Arizona Heart Hosp; **Address:** Arizona Heart Inst, 2632 N 20th St, Phoenix, AZ 85006-1339; **Phone:** 602-240-6165; **Board Cert:** Thoracic Surgery 1967; Surgery 1966; **Med School:** Univ Mich Med Sch 1960; **Resid:** Surgery, St Joseph Mercy Hosp 1964; **Fellow:** Cardiothoracic Surgery, Baylor Coll Med 1966; **Fac Appt:** Prof TS, Univ Ariz Coll Med

Forbess, Joseph MD [TS] - **Spec Exp:** Pediatric Cardiothoracic Surgery; Heart Valve Surgery-Pediatric; **Hospital:** Chldns Med Ctr of Dallas, UT Southwestern Med Ctr - Dallas; **Address:** Univ Texas SW Med Ctr, Div Ped Cardiothor Surg, 1935 Motor St, Ste E03.320.Z, MC 8835, Dallas, TX 75235; **Phone:** 214-456-5000; **Board Cert:** Surgery 2000; Thoracic Surgery 1998; **Med School:** Harvard Med Sch 1990; **Resid:** Surgery, Duke Univ Med Ctr 1997; Cardiothoracic Surgery, Duke Univ Med Ctr 1999; **Fellow:** Cardiac Surgery, Childrens Hosp 1994; **Fac Appt:** Assoc Prof TS, Univ Tex SW, Dallas

Fraser, Charles D MD [TS] - **Spec Exp:** Pediatric Cardiothoracic Surgery; Congenital Heart Surgery; **Hospital:** Texas Chldns Hosp - Houston; **Address:** Texas Chldns Hosp-Heart Ctr, 6621 Fannin St, MC WT 19-345H, Houston, TX 77030-2399; **Phone:** 832-826-2030; **Board Cert:** Surgery 2000; Thoracic Surgery 1994; **Med School:** Univ Tex Med Br, Galveston 1984; **Resid:** Surgery, Johns Hopkins Hosp 1990; Johns Hopkins Hosp 1993; **Fac Appt:** Prof S, Baylor Coll Med

Frazier, Oscar Howard MD [TS] - **Spec Exp:** Transplant-Heart; Lung Surgery; Artificial Heart Devices; **Hospital:** St Luke's Episcopal Hosp - Houston; **Address:** Surgical Assocs - Texas Heart Institute, 6770 Bertner, Ste C355, Houston, TX 77030; **Phone:** 832-355-4900; **Board Cert:** Surgery 1975; Thoracic Surgery 1997; **Med School:** Baylor Coll Med 1967; **Resid:** Surgery, Baylor Affil Hosp 1974; Thoracic Surgery, Texas Heart Inst 1976; **Fac Appt:** Prof S, Univ Tex, Houston

Harrell Jr, James E MD [TS] - **Spec Exp:** Transplant-Heart; Cardiac Surgery-Pediatric; **Hospital:** Covenant Children's Med Ctr; **Address:** 3606 21st St, Ste 103, Lubbock, TX 79410; **Phone:** 806-725-4425; **Board Cert:** Surgery 1995; Thoracic Surgery 1996; **Med School:** Baylor Coll Med 1978; **Resid:** Surgery, Univ Tex Hlth Scis Ctr 1984; Thoracic Surgery, Baylor Coll Med 1986; **Fellow:** Cardiovascular Surgery, Hosp Sick Chldn 1987

Noon, George P MD [TS] - **Spec Exp:** Transplant-Heart; Transplant-Lung; Artificial Heart Devices; **Hospital:** Methodist Hosp - Houston; **Address:** 6560 Fannin St, Scurlock Twr, Ste 1860, Houston, TX 77030; **Phone:** 713-790-3155; **Board Cert:** Surgery 1966; Thoracic Surgery 1966; **Med School:** Baylor Coll Med 1960; **Resid:** Surgery, Baylor Coll Med 1966; Surgery, Ben Taub Genl Hosp 1966; **Fac Appt:** Prof S, Baylor Coll Med

Ott, David A MD [TS] - **Spec Exp:** Heart Valve Surgery; Coronary Artery Surgery; Aneurysm-Abdominal Aortic; **Hospital:** St Luke's Episcopal Hosp - Houston; **Address:** 1101 Bates St, Ste P-514, Houston, TX 77030-2607; **Phone:** 832-355-4900; **Board Cert:** Thoracic Surgery 1997; Vascular Surgery 1995; **Med School:** Baylor Coll Med 1972; **Resid:** Surgery, Baylor Coll Med 1976; Cardiothoracic Surgery, Tex Heart Inst 1978; **Fac Appt:** Clin Prof S, Baylor Coll Med

Reardon, Michael J MD [TS] - **Spec Exp:** Cardiac Tumors/Cancer; Heart Valve Surgery-Aortic; **Hospital:** Methodist Hosp - Houston, UT MD Anderson Cancer Ctr (page 71); **Address:** 6560 Fannin St, Ste 1002, Houston, TX 77030; **Phone:** 713-793-7409; **Board Cert:** Thoracic Surgery 2006; **Med School:** Baylor Coll Med 1978; **Resid:** Surgery, Baylor Affil Hosps 1983; Thoracic Surgery, Texas Heart Inst 1985; **Fac Appt:** Clin Prof S, Baylor Coll Med

Reul, George J MD [TS] - **Spec Exp:** Coronary Artery Surgery; Heart Valve Surgery; Vascular Surgery; **Hospital:** St Luke's Episcopal Hosp - Houston, Texas Chldns Hosp - Houston; **Address:** Surg Assocs of Tex - Tex Heart Inst, 1101 Bates St, Ste P514, Houston, TX 77030-2607; **Phone:** 832-355-4929; **Board Cert:** Surgery 1971; Thoracic Surgery 1971; Vascular Surgery 1984; **Med School:** Med Coll Wisc 1962; **Resid:** Surgery, Marquette Sch Med 1969; Thoracic Surgery, Baylor Coll Med 1971; **Fac Appt:** Clin Prof S, Univ Tex, Houston

Ring, William Steves MD [TS] - **Spec Exp:** Cardiac Surgery-Adult & Pediatric; Transplant-Heart & Lung; Congenital Heart Surgery; Coronary Revascularization; **Hospital:** Parkland Meml Hosp - Dallas, Chldns Med Ctr of Dallas; **Address:** 5323 Harry Hines Blvd, MC 8879, Dallas, TX 75390-8879; **Phone:** 214-645-7706; **Board Cert:** Surgery 1999; Thoracic Surgery 2004; **Med School:** Harvard Med Sch 1971; **Resid:** Surgery, Duke Univ Med Ctr 1977; Surgery, Univ Minn Hosps 1980; **Fellow:** Thoracic Surgery, Univ Minn Hosps 1982; **Fac Appt:** Prof TS, Univ Tex SW, Dallas

Thoracic Surgery

Safi, Hazim Jawad MD [TS] - **Spec Exp:** Aneurysm-Abdominal Aortic; **Hospital:** Meml Hermann Hosp - Houston; **Address:** UT, Dept Cardiothoracic & Vascular Surg, 6410 Fannin St, Ste 450, Houston, TX 77030; **Phone:** 713-500-5304; **Board Cert:** Surgery 1994; Thoracic Surgery 1997; **Med School:** Iraq 1970; **Resid:** Surgery, Baylor Coll Med 1980; Radiation Oncology, Baylor Coll Med 1981; **Fellow:** Thoracic Surgery, Baylor Coll Med 1983; **Fac Appt:** Assoc Prof S, Univ Tex, Houston

Srivastava, Sudhir Prem MD [TS] - **Spec Exp:** Coronary Artery Robotic Surgery; **Hospital:** Alliance Hosp; **Address:** 710 E 6th St, Odessa, TX 79761; **Phone:** 432-332-4044; **Board Cert:** Thoracic Surgery 1999; **Med School:** India 1970; **Resid:** Vascular Surgery, Vancouver Genl Hosp 1977; Thoracic Surgery, Vancouver Genl Hosp 1978; **Fellow:** Surgery, Vancouver Genl Hosp 1979

Turner, William F MD [TS] - **Spec Exp:** Coronary Artery Surgery; Cardiac Surgery; **Hospital:** E TX Med Ctr, Trinity Mother Frances Hlth Sys; **Address:** 1100 E Lake St, Ste 210, Tyler, TX 75701; **Phone:** 903-593-0900; **Board Cert:** Surgery 1997; Thoracic Surgery 1998; **Med School:** Baylor Coll Med 1981; **Resid:** Surgery, Baylor Coll Med 1987; Thoracic Surgery, Baylor Coll Med 1989

West Coast and Pacific

Bailey, Leonard L MD [TS] - **Spec Exp:** Cardiac Surgery-Pediatric; Congenital Heart Surgery; Transplant-Heart-Pediatric; **Hospital:** Loma Linda Chldns Hosp, Loma Linda Univ Med Ctr; **Address:** Dept Surgery, 11175 Campus St, Ste 21120, Loma Linda, CA 92354; **Phone:** 909-558-4200; **Board Cert:** Surgery 1975; Thoracic Surgery 1998; **Med School:** Loma Linda Univ 1969; **Resid:** Surgery, Loma Linda Univ Med Ctr 1973; Thoracic Surgery, Loma Linda Univ Med Ctr 1974; **Fellow:** Cardiovascular Surgery, Hosp Sick Chldn 1975; **Fac Appt:** Prof S, Loma Linda Univ

Cannon, Walter Bradford MD [TS] - **Spec Exp:** Chest Wall Tumors; **Hospital:** Stanford Univ Med Ctr, VA Hlth Care Sys - Palo Alto; **Address:** Stanford Univ Med Ctr, Dept Cardiothoracic Surgery, 300 Pasteur Dr, Falk Bldg CVRB, Stanford, CA 94305-5407; **Phone:** 650-736-7191; **Board Cert:** Thoracic Surgery 1996; Surgery 1996; **Med School:** Harvard Med Sch 1969; **Resid:** Thoracic Surgery, Stanford Univ Hosp 1975; **Fac Appt:** Clin Prof S, Stanford Univ

Cohen, Robbin G MD [TS] - **Spec Exp:** Minimally Invasive Surgery; Heart Valve Surgery; Thoracic Aortic Surgery; **Hospital:** USC Univ Hosp - R K Eamer Med Plz, Huntington Memorial Hosp; **Address:** 1520 San Pueblo St, Ste 4300, Los Angeles, CA 90033; **Phone:** 323-442-5850; **Board Cert:** Thoracic Surgery 1999; **Med School:** Univ Colorado 1980; **Resid:** Surgery, Stanford Univ Med Ctr 1986; **Fellow:** Cardiothoracic Surgery, Stanford Univ Med Ctr 1989; **Fac Appt:** Assoc Prof TS, USC Sch Med

Dang, Michael H MD [TS] - **Spec Exp:** Cardiac Surgery; Peripheral Vascular Disease; Transplant-Heart; **Hospital:** Queen's Med Ctr - Honolulu; **Address:** Queens Heart Physicians Practice, 550 S Beretania St, Ste 30-D, Honolulu, HI 96813; **Phone:** 808-545-8400; **Board Cert:** Thoracic Surgery 2002; **Med School:** Univ Colorado 1968; **Resid:** Surgery, Baylor Univ Med Ctr 1976; Thoracic Surgery, Baylor Univ Med Ctr 1978

De Meester, Tom R MD [TS] - **Spec Exp:** Stomach Cancer; Esophageal Cancer; Lung Cancer; Tracheal Surgery; **Hospital:** USC Univ Hosp - R K Eamer Med Plz; **Address:** 1510 San Pablo St, Ste 514, Los Angeles, CA 90033; **Phone:** 323-442-5925; **Board Cert:** Surgery 1971; Thoracic Surgery 1971; **Med School:** Univ Mich Med Sch 1963; **Resid:** Surgery, Johns Hopkins Hosp 1966; **Fellow:** Thoracic Surgery, Johns Hopkins Hosp 1968; **Fac Appt:** Prof S, USC Sch Med

Flachsbart, Keith D MD [TS] - **Spec Exp:** Cardiac Surgery; **Hospital:** Kaiser Permanente South San Francisco Med Ctr; **Address:** 2350 Geary Blvd Fl 1, San Francisco, CA 94115; **Phone:** 415-833-3800; **Board Cert:** Thoracic Surgery 2000; **Med School:** Univ Nebr Coll Med 1971; **Resid:** Surgery, Rush-Presby St Lukes Hosp 1978; Thoracic Surgery, Hosp Good Samaritan 1980

Fontana, Gregory MD [TS] - **Spec Exp:** Minimally Invasive Surgery; Cardiac Surgery-Pediatric; Mitral Valve Surgery; **Hospital:** Cedars-Sinai Med Ctr; **Address:** 8700 Beverly Blvd, North Twr, rm 6215, Los Angeles, CA 90048-1804; **Phone:** 310-423-3851; **Board Cert:** Surgery 1993; Thoracic Surgery 1994; **Med School:** UCLA 1984; **Resid:** Surgery, Duke Univ Med Ctr 1990; Thoracic Surgery, Duke Univ Med Ctr 1993; **Fellow:** Pediatric Cardiac Surgery, UCLA Med Ctr; Pediatric Cardiac Surgery, Chldns Hosp; **Fac Appt:** Assoc Clin Prof S, UCLA

Gundry, Steven MD [TS] - **Spec Exp:** Cardiac Surgery-Adult & Pediatric; Cardiac Surgery-High Risk; Nutrition in Heart Disease; **Hospital:** Desert Regl Med Ctr; **Address:** International Heart & Lung Inst, 555 Tachevah Drive, 3W - Ste 103, Palm Springs, CA 92262; **Phone:** 760-323-5553; **Board Cert:** Thoracic Surgery 2005; **Med School:** Med Coll GA 1977; **Resid:** Surgery, Univ Michigan Hosps 1983; Thoracic Surgery, Univ Michigan Hosps 1985; **Fellow:** Pediatric Cardiac Surgery, Hosp-Sick Chldn 1986; **Fac Appt:** Clin Prof S, Loma Linda Univ

Handy Jr, John R MD [TS] - **Spec Exp:** Lung Cancer; Esophageal Cancer; Mesothelioma; Chest Wall Tumors; **Hospital:** Providence Portland Med Ctr; **Address:** Oregon Clinic-Cardiothoracic Surgery, 1111 NE 99th Ave, Ste 201, Portland, OR 97213; **Phone:** 503-215-2300; **Board Cert:** Thoracic Surgery 2001; Surgery 1999; **Med School:** Duke Univ 1983; **Resid:** Surgery, Brown Univ Hosp 1990; **Fellow:** Cardiothoracic Surgery, MUSC Med Ctr 1993

Hanley, Frank L MD [TS] - **Spec Exp:** Pediatric Thoracic Surgery; **Hospital:** Lucile Packard Chldns Hosp/Stanford Univ Med Ctr, Chldns Hosp - Oakland; **Address:** 300 Pasteur Drive, FALK CVRB, Stanford, CA 94305-5407; **Phone:** 650-723-0190; **Board Cert:** Thoracic Surgery 2002; **Med School:** Tufts Univ 1978; **Resid:** Surgery, UCSF Med Ctr 1981; Cardiothoracic Surgery, UCSF Med Ctr 1988; **Fellow:** Research, UCSF Sch Med 1984; **Fac Appt:** Prof S, UCSF

Jamieson, Stuart W MD [TS] - **Spec Exp:** Pulmonary Embolism; Transplant-Heart & Lung; **Hospital:** UCSD Med Ctr; **Address:** UCSD Med Ctr, Div CTS, 200 W Arbor Drive, MC 8892, San Diego, CA 92103; **Phone:** 619-543-7777; **Med School:** England 1971; **Resid:** Surgery 1975; **Fellow:** Cardiothoracic Surgery 1977; Cardiothoracic Surgery, Stanford Univ/American Heart Assoc 1980; **Fac Appt:** Prof S, UCSD

Kernstine, Kemp H MD/PhD [TS] - **Spec Exp:** Lung Cancer; Esophageal Cancer; Tracheal Surgery; Esophageal Surgery; **Hospital:** City of Hope Natl Med Ctr & Beckman Rsch; **Address:** City of Hope Comprehensive Cancer Ctr, 1500 E Duarte Rd, Duarte, CA 91010; **Phone:** 626-359-8111 x68845; **Board Cert:** Thoracic Surgery 1996; Surgery 2001; **Med School:** Duke Univ 1982; **Resid:** Surgery, Univ Minn Med Ctr 1988; **Fellow:** Cardiothoracic Surgery, Brigham & Women's Hosp 1994; **Fac Appt:** Assoc Prof S, Univ Iowa Coll Med

Laks, Hillel MD [TS] - **Spec Exp:** Congenital Heart Disease; Transplant-Heart; **Hospital:** UCLA Med Ctr; **Address:** UCLA Med Ctr, Dept Surg-Cardio Thoracic, 10833 Le Conte Ave, rm 62-182A CHS, Los Angeles, CA 90095-1741; **Phone:** 310-206-8232; **Board Cert:** Surgery 1975; **Med School:** Africa 1965; **Resid:** Surgery, Peter Bent Brigham Hosp 1969; Thoracic Surgery, Peter Bent Brigham Hosp 1973; **Fac Appt:** Prof S, UCLA

Lamberti Jr, John J MD [TS] - **Spec Exp:** Pediatric Cardiac Surgery; Heart Valve Surgery; Congenital Heart Surgery; **Hospital:** Rady Children's Hosp - San Diego, UCSD Med Ctr; **Address:** Chldns Hosp, 3030 Children's Way, Ste 202, San Diego, CA 92123-4227; **Phone:** 858-966-8030; **Board Cert:** Surgery 1973; Thoracic Surgery 1975; **Med School:** Univ Pittsburgh 1967; **Resid:** Surgery, Peter Bent Brigham Hosp 1972; Thoracic Surgery, Peter Bent Brigham Hosp 1973; **Fellow:** Pediatric Cardiac Surgery, Chldns Hosp 1974; **Fac Appt:** Prof S, UCSD

McKenna Jr, Robert J MD [TS] - **Spec Exp:** Lung Cancer; Gastroesophageal Reflux Disease (GERD); Video Assisted Thoracic Surgery (VATS); **Hospital:** Cedars-Sinai Med Ctr; **Address:** 8635 W 3rd St, Ste 975 West Twr, Los Angeles, CA 90048-6101; **Phone:** 310-652-0530; **Board Cert:** Thoracic Surgery 1997; **Med School:** USC Sch Med 1977; **Resid:** Surgery, Stanford Univ Hosp 1982; Cardiothoracic Surgery, Good Samaritan Hosp 1987; **Fellow:** Thoracic Surgery, MD Anderson Tumor Inst 1983; **Fac Appt:** Clin Prof TS, UCLA

Merrick, Scot H MD [TS] - **Spec Exp:** Cardiac Surgery-Adult; Heart Valve Surgery; Coronary Revascularization; **Hospital:** UCSF Med Ctr; **Address:** UCSF Med Ctr, Div Cardiothoracic Surg, 500 Parnassus Ave, San Francisco, CA 94143-0118; **Phone:** 415-353-1606; **Board Cert:** Surgery 1995; Thoracic Surgery 1997; **Med School:** Univ Wash 1980; **Resid:** Surgery, UCSF Med Ctr 1985; **Fellow:** Cardiothoracic Surgery, UCSF Med Ctr 1987; **Fac Appt:** Assoc Prof S, UCSF

Miller, David Craig MD [TS] - **Spec Exp:** Thoracic Aortic Surgery; Heart Valve Surgery; Endovascular Stent Grafts; **Hospital:** Stanford Univ Med Ctr; **Address:** Stanford Univ Sch Medicine, Div Cardiothoracic Surgery, 300 Pasteur Drive Falk Rsch Bldg, Stanford, CA 94305-5407; **Phone:** 650-725-3826; **Board Cert:** Thoracic Surgery 1988; **Med School:** Stanford Univ 1972; **Resid:** Thoracic Surgery, Standford Univ Med Ctr 1978; **Fac Appt:** Prof TS, Stanford Univ

Reitz, Bruce A MD [TS] - **Spec Exp:** Transplant-Heart & Lung; Heart Valve Surgery; Congenital Heart Surgery; **Hospital:** Stanford Univ Med Ctr, El Camino Hosp/Camino Hlthcare Sys; **Address:** Stanford Univ Sch Med, Dept Cardiothoracic Surgery, 300 Pasteur Drive, Stanford, CA 94305-5407; **Phone:** 650-725-4497; **Board Cert:** Thoracic Surgery 1999; **Med School:** Yale Univ 1970; **Resid:** Cardiovascular Surgery, Stanford Univ Hosp 1972; Thoracic Surgery, Stanford Univ Hosp 1978; **Fellow:** Cardiac Surgery, Natl Heart Inst 1974; **Fac Appt:** Prof TS, Stanford Univ

Robbins, Robert C MD [TS] - **Spec Exp:** Transplant-Heart; Transplant-Lung; **Hospital:** Stanford Univ Med Ctr; **Address:** Cardiovascular Rsch Bldg, Fl 2, 300 Pasteur Drive, Stanford, CA 94305-2200; **Phone:** 650-725-3828; **Board Cert:** Thoracic Surgery 2002; Surgery 2002; **Med School:** Univ Miss 1983; **Resid:** Surgery, Univ Miss Med Ctr 1988; **Fellow:** Thoracic Surgery, Stanford Univ Med Ctr 1991; **Fac Appt:** Asst Prof TS, Stanford Univ

Shemin, Richard MD [TS] - **Spec Exp:** Minimally Invasive Cardiac Surgery; Heart Valve Surgery; Aneurysm-Thoracic Aortic; **Hospital:** UCLA Med Ctr; **Address:** UCLA-David Geffen School Medicine, 10833 Le Conte Ave, Los Angeles, CA 90095; **Phone:** 310-206-8232; **Board Cert:** Thoracic Surgery 2002; **Med School:** Boston Univ 1974; **Resid:** Surgery, PB Brigham Hosp 1980; NYU Med Ctr 1982; **Fellow:** Cardiac Surgery, Natl Inst Hlth 1978; **Fac Appt:** Prof TS, UCLA-David Geffen Sch Med

Starnes, Vaughn A MD [TS] - **Spec Exp:** Transplant-Heart & Lung; Heart Valve Surgery; Ross Procedure for Aortic Valve Disease; Robotic Heart Surgery; **Hospital:** USC Univ Hosp - R K Eamer Med Plz, Huntington Memorial Hosp; **Address:** USC Cardiothoracic Surgery, 1520 San Pablo St, Ste 4300, Los Angeles, CA 90033; **Phone:** 323-442-5849; **Board Cert:** Thoracic Surgery 1998; **Med School:** Univ NC Sch Med 1977; **Resid:** Surgery, Vanderbilt Univ Hosp 1984; Cardiovascular Surgery, Stanford Unv Hosp 1986; **Fellow:** Cardiothoracic Transplant Surg, Stanford Unv Hosp 1987; Pediatric Cardiac Surgery, Univ NC Hosp; **Fac Appt:** Prof TS, USC Sch Med

Thistlethwaite, Patricia A MD/PhD [TS] - **Spec Exp:** Cardiac Surgery; Lung Cancer; **Hospital:** UCSD Med Ctr; **Address:** UCSD Med Ctr, Div CTS, 200 W Arbor Drive, MC 8892, San Diego, CA 92103; **Phone:** 619-543-7777; **Board Cert:** Surgery 1995; Thoracic Surgery 1998; **Med School:** Harvard Med Sch 1989; **Resid:** Surgery, Mass Genl Hosp 1994; **Fellow:** Cardiothoracic Surgery, Univ Pittsburgh 1997; **Fac Appt:** Assoc Prof S, UCSD

Trento, Alfredo MD [TS] - **Spec Exp:** Transplant-Heart; Cardiac Surgery; Pediatric Cardiac Surgery; **Hospital:** Cedars-Sinai Med Ctr; **Address:** Cedars-Sinai Med Ctr, Dept Thoracic Surg, 8700 Beverly Blvd, North Tower - rm 6215, Los Angeles, CA 90048; **Phone:** 310-423-3851; **Board Cert:** Thoracic Surgery 2005; **Med School:** Italy 1975; **Resid:** Surgery, Univ Mass Med Ctr 1982; Thoracic Surgery, Univ Pittsburgh Med Ctr 1985; **Fellow:** Cardiothoracic Surgery, Univ Mass; **Fac Appt:** Prof S, UCLA

Ungerleider, Ross M MD [TS] - **Spec Exp:** Congenital Heart Disease; Cardiac Surgery; Pediatric Cardiac Surgery; **Hospital:** Doernbecher Chldns Hosp/OHSU; **Address:** Oregon Health Science Univ, Dept Cardiothoracic Surgery, 3181 SW Sam Jackson Park Rd, L353 Rd, Portland, OR 97239; **Phone:** 503-418-5443; **Board Cert:** Thoracic Surgery 1997; **Med School:** Rush Med Coll 1977; **Resid:** Surgery, Duke Univ Med Ctr 1987; **Fellow:** Cardiothoracic Surgery, Duke Univ Med Ctr 1989; Pediatric Cardiac Surgery, UCSF; **Fac Appt:** Prof S, Oregon Hlth Sci Univ

Verrier, Edward D MD [TS] - **Spec Exp:** Coronary Artery Surgery; Heart Valve Surgery; **Hospital:** Univ Wash Med Ctr, Northwest Hosp; **Address:** University Washington Medical Ctr, 1959 NE Pacific St, Ste AA115, Box 356310, Seattle, WA 98195-6310; **Phone:** 206-598-3636; **Board Cert:** Surgery 1992; Thoracic Surgery 1993; **Med School:** Tufts Univ 1974; **Resid:** Surgery, UCSF Med Ctr 1982; Thoracic Surgery, UCSF Med Ctr 1984; **Fellow:** Cardiac Surgery, UCSF Med Ctr 1980; **Fac Appt:** Prof TS, Univ Wash

Wells, Winfield J MD [TS] - **Spec Exp:** Tracheal Surgery-Pediatric; Congenital Heart Surgery; **Hospital:** Chldns Hosp - Los Angeles (page 56); **Address:** Chlds Hosp, Div Cardiothoracic Surgery, 4650 Sunset Blvd, MS 66, Los Angeles, CA 90027; **Phone:** 323-669-4148; **Board Cert:** Thoracic Surgery 1997; **Med School:** USC Sch Med 1970; **Resid:** Surgery, Columbia-Presby Med Ctr 1976; **Fac Appt:** Assoc Prof S, USC Sch Med

Whyte, Richard MD [TS] - **Spec Exp:** Lung Cancer; Esophageal Cancer; **Hospital:** Stanford Univ Med Ctr; **Address:** Stanford Univ Sch Med, Div Thor Surg, 300 Pasteur Dr, Bldg CVRB - rm 205, Stanford, CA 94305-5407; **Phone:** 650-723-6649; **Board Cert:** Surgery 1991; Thoracic Surgery 1993; **Med School:** Univ Pittsburgh 1983; **Resid:** Surgery, Mass Genl Hosp 1990; Thoracic Surgery, Univ Michigan Hosp 1992; **Fac Appt:** Assoc Prof TS, Stanford Univ

Wood, Douglas E MD [TS] - **Spec Exp:** Lung Cancer; Esophageal Cancer; Tracheal Surgery; Mesothelioma; **Hospital:** Univ Wash Med Ctr, Northwest Hosp; **Address:** Univ Washington, Div Cardiothoracic Surg, 1959 NE Pacific St, AA Bldg - rm 115, Box 356310, Seattle, WA 98195-6310; **Phone:** 206-685-3228; **Board Cert:** Surgery 1999; Thoracic Surgery 2001; Surgical Critical Care 1993; **Med School:** Harvard Med Sch 1983; **Resid:** Surgery, Mass Genl Hosp 1989; Thoracic Surgery, Mass Genl Hosp 1991; **Fellow:** Surgical Critical Care, Mass Genl Hosp 1991; **Fac Appt:** Prof S, Univ Wash

THE MOUNT SINAI MEDICAL CENTER
CARDIOTHORACIC SURGERY

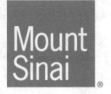

One Gustave L. Levy Place (Fifth Avenue and 100th Street)
New York, NY 10029-6574
Physician Referral: 1-800-MD-SINAI (637-4624)
www.mountsinai.org

The Department of Cardiothoracic Surgery at Mount Sinai is one of the country's most prestigious programs. Cardiothoracic surgical patients benefit from an integrated and personalized care plan designed in coordination with expert cardiologists, anesthesiologists, perfusionists, and intensive care physicians. Mount Sinai is a quaternary referral center, meaning we often operate on the sickest and most complicated patients.

THE HEART VALVE CENTER

The Mitral Valve Repair Program at Mount Sinai is one of the largest and most advanced in the country. The superiority of mitral valve repair, instead of replacement with a mechanical or bioprosthetic valve, is now well-established. The Mitral Valve Repair Program at Mount Sinai—directed by Dr. David Adams—offers patients one of the highest percentages of successful valve repair anywhere in the world. For example, in patients with mitral valve prolapse, our success rate in avoiding valve replacement approaches 100 percent. Our physicians are also experts in mitral valve repair for patients with advanced cardiomyopathy. If patients have associated atrial fibrillation, we offer the latest in concomitant arrhythmia surgery, including the MAZE procedure. We can also perform mitral valve repair with minimally invasive approaches, when appropriate.

The Aortic Valve Repair Program offers patients with aortic valve disease an alternative to replacement of their aortic valve and the freedom from taking blood-thining medications. Our surgeons are completely versed in nonthrombogenic alternatives to mechanical valve replacement, including valve sparring procedures such as the David and Yacoub procedures. Mount Sinai's Dr. Paul Stelzer is one of the most experienced surgeons in the country using the Ross procedure, in which the diseased aortic valve is replaced with the patient's own pulmonary valve. This technique has improved durability over other replacement options, particularly in younger patients.

The Thoracic Aortic Surgery Program is internationally renowned for its leadership role in surgical therapy of complex aortic disease. This program specializes in the operative management of all diseases of the ascending aorta, arch, and descending thoracic aorta. Ascending aortic replacement, trifurcation-graft arch replacement, acute aortic dissection repair, and thoraco-abdominal aortic surgery are all commonly performed procedures at Mount Sinai. Special emphasis is placed on cerebral and spinal protection, where we also have a significant clinical and scientific research interest led by our pioneering director, Dr. Randall Griepp. Our surgeons have also been involved in the early development of minimally invasive aortic stent grafting.

The Cardiac Transplant and Assist Program, one of the largest in the United States, is now under the direction of Dr. Anelchi Anyanwu. We have been involved in the field of mechanical cardiac assistance from its inception and have experience with most of the currently available FDA-approved devices. We have also played an active role in multi-institutional studies exploring permanent mechanical heart support.

THE MOUNT SINAI MEDICAL CENTER

The Department of Cardiothoracic Surgery at Mount Sinai is chaired by David Adams, MD, the Marie-Josée and Henry R. Kravis Professor.

Randall Griepp, MD, Professor of Cardiothoracic Surgery, is a world-renowned leader in thoracic aortic surgery, and Paul Stelzer, MD, is a specialist in aortic root surgery. His experience with the Ross procedure exceeds 20 years and 415 cases, the largest and longest in the word.

These leaders of cardiothoracic surgery work in concert with other members of Mount Sinai Heart, which is under the direction of worldrenowned cardiologist Valentin Fuster, MD, PhD, to deliver unparalleled possibilities for patients with cardiovascular disease.

622

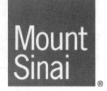

THE MOUNT SINAI MEDICAL CENTER
THORACIC SURGERY

One Gustave L. Levy Place (Fifth Avenue and 100th Street)
New York, NY 10029-6574
Physician Referral: 1-800-MD-SINAI (637-4624)
www.mountsinai.org

Comprehensive Care

Thoracic Surgery at Mount Sinai is world renowned for its state-of-the-art surgery, protocol-driven, multidisciplinary team approach to treatment, and commitment to compassionate patient care.

Surgical Treatment for Benign and Malignant Diseases of Lung and Esophagus

Our team of dedicated thoracic surgeons is expert in the treatment of all primary cancers of the chest, lung, esophagus, mediastinum and airway, and all metastatic tumors of the chest. We also diagnose and treat patients who are affected by GERD, achalasia, and motility disorders.

State-of-the-Art Technology

Mount Sinai is a leader in the development and implementation of the latest technologies and treatment options for disorders of the lung and esophagus, including the following:

Video-assisted thoracic surgery
VATS lobotomy
Minimally invasive esophagectomy
Robotic surgery
Stent and laser treatment of the airway and esophagus
Radiofrequency ablation of lung tumors
Stereotactic radiosurgery of the lung
Navigational bronchoscopy—a new, innovative, non-invasive method via bronchoscopy to perform biopsies on small lung lesions, including those in subpleural locations
Lung volume reduction surgery

Protocol-Driven Therapy

Mount Sinai patients are given access to many clinical trials.

Transplant Program

One of two accredited programs in the tri-state area dedicated to lung transplantation for a wide variety of conditions.

Translational Research

State-of-the-art translational thoracic research including genomic analysis of tumors to better understand and predict behavior in order to develop more directed, personalized therapeutic approaches to treatment.

Screening and Diagnosis

Mount Sinai offers comprehensive screening and diagnostic tests, including CT scans for early detection, advanced endoscopic techniques to detect early lesions and recurrence, PET scans, and innovative MRI technology with ultrasensitive resolution. Our developing program for the screening and detection of esophageal cancer is the first of its kind in New York City.

Mount Sinai....Taking Care of One Patient at a Time

Here at Mount Sinai we believe in personalized care. Each patient benefits from a team approach to medical care, including thoracic surgeons, anesthesiologists, medical oncologists, radiation oncologists, and oncology-dedicated nurses. Coordinating information among team members to ensure seamless delivery of care is one the Program's highest priorities.

627

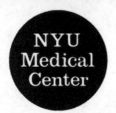

NYU Hospital Center Thoracic Surgery: Aggressive use of the Newest Technologies and Laboratory Discovery to Treat Thoracic Diseases

The Division of Thoracic Surgery of the NYU Hospital Center is a leader in diagnosing and treating both benign and malignant neoplasms (tissue growths), as well as providing management of other disorders of the lungs, esophagus, mediastinum and the chest wall.

The NYU Thoracic Oncology Program's multidisciplinary approach unites the disciplines of medical oncology, surgery, radiation therapy, pulmonary medicine, radiology and pathology. We use evidence-based discussion and multifaceted expert opinions to tailor care to individual patients' needs. Weekly discussions of new and existing patients are held to decide the appropriate management, and see if patients are eligible to participate in new clinical trials.

The involvement of multiple sites at the Manhatten VA, Bellevue Hospital and Tisch Hospital allows us to provide the greatest number of patients with the newest developments in treatment available through NYU Medical Center.

Our minimally invasive surgery program incorporates video-assisted and "open chest" techniques along with new methods for post-operative pain relief. Procedures include:

- video-assisted thoracoscopy for the chest
- video-assisted laparoscopy for the abdomen
- video-assisted procedures on benign lesions of the esophagus and lungs
- minimally invasive esophagectomy and pulmonary resection

We also place a unique emphasis on the treatment of pleural mesothelioma using a multimodal approach.

A key part of providing compassionate clinical care is research. That's why NYU Thoracic Surgery is committed to state-of-the-art surgical management and to developing novel treatment strategies using clinical trials. We also use the resources at the New York Thoracic Surgery Laboratory housed at Bellevue Hospital to launch investigations at the gene or protein level. Through studies like these we make clinically relevant "bench to bedside" discoveries in early detection and develop targeted therapies.

We also provide the newest in pioneering treatments, including:

- early detection of airway malignancies with fluorescence bronchoscopy
- novel diagnostic and staging modalities including endobronchial ultrasound
- novel endobronchial treatment strategies including photodynamic therapy
- investigation of non-surgical techniques selectively used for destruction of lung cancer nodules, including radiofrequency ablation and stereotactic radiation
- use of stents to relieve blockages of the windpipe and esophagus
- investigation of the use of replaceable stents in the windpipe and esophagus

685

Urology

A urologist manages benign and malignant medical and surgical disorders of the genitourinary system and the adrenal gland. This specialist has comprehensive knowledge of, and skills in, endoscopic, percutaneous and open surgery of congenital and acquired conditions of the urinary and reproductive systems and their contiguous structures.

Training Required: Five years

Urology

New England

Caldamone, Anthony A MD [U] - **Spec Exp:** Pediatric Urology; **Hospital:** Rhode Island Hosp; **Address:** 2 Dudley St, Ste 185, Providence, RI 02905; **Phone:** 401-421-0710; **Board Cert:** Urology 1983; **Med School:** Brown Univ 1975; **Resid:** Urology, Strong Meml Hosp 1981; **Fellow:** Pediatric Urology, Childrens Hosp 1982; **Fac Appt:** Prof U, Brown Univ

Gomery, Pablo MD [U] - **Spec Exp:** Neuro-Urology; Erectile Dysfunction; Voiding Dysfunction; Infertility-Male; **Hospital:** Mass Genl Hosp, Spaulding Rehab Hosp; **Address:** Mass General Hospital, Dept Urology, 55 Fruit St, GRB 1102, Boston, MA 02114; **Phone:** 617-726-8482; **Board Cert:** Urology 2000; **Med School:** Albert Einstein Coll Med 1974; **Resid:** Surgery, New England Deaconess Hosp 1977; Urology, Mass General Hosp 1980

Heney, Niall M MD [U] - **Spec Exp:** Urologic Cancer; **Hospital:** Mass Genl Hosp; **Address:** Mass Genl Hosp, Dept Urol, 55 Fruit St, GRB 1102, Boston, MA 02114; **Phone:** 617-726-3011; **Board Cert:** Urology 1977; **Med School:** Ireland 1965; **Resid:** Urology, Regional Hosp 1972; Urology, Mass Genl Hosp 1976; **Fac Appt:** Prof Med, Harvard Med Sch

Libertino, John A MD [U] - **Spec Exp:** Kidney Cancer; Prostate Cancer; Adrenal Tumors; **Hospital:** Lahey Clin; **Address:** Lahey Clinic, Dept Urology, 41 Mall Rd, Burlington, MA 01805; **Phone:** 781-744-2511; **Board Cert:** Urology 1973; **Med School:** Georgetown Univ 1965; **Resid:** Urology, Univ Rochester-Strong Meml Hosp 1967; Urology, Yale-New Haven Hosp 1970; **Fellow:** Surgery, Yale-New Haven Hosp 1968; **Fac Appt:** Assoc Clin Prof S, Harvard Med Sch

Loughlin, Kevin R MD [U] - **Spec Exp:** Prostate Cancer; Genitourinary Cancer; Incontinence; **Hospital:** Brigham & Women's Hosp, Dana-Farber Cancer Inst; **Address:** Brigham & Women's Hosp, Div Urology, 45 Francis St, ASBII-3, Boston, MA 02115; **Phone:** 617-732-6325; **Board Cert:** Urology 2004; **Med School:** NY Med Coll 1975; **Resid:** Pediatrics, New York Hosp-Cornell 1978; Surgery, Bellevue Hosp Ctr-NYU 1979; **Fellow:** Urology, Brigham & Women's Hosp 1983; Urologic Oncology, Meml Sloan Kettering Cancer Ctr; **Fac Appt:** Prof S, Harvard Med Sch

McDougal, W Scott MD [U] - **Spec Exp:** Penile Cancer; Prostate Cancer; Urologic Cancer; **Hospital:** Mass Genl Hosp; **Address:** Mass Genl Hosp, 55 Fruit St, Bldg GRB - rm 1102, Boston, MA 02114; **Phone:** 617-726-3010; **Board Cert:** Surgery 1975; Urology 2004; **Med School:** Cornell Univ-Weill Med Coll 1968; **Resid:** Surgery, Univ Hosps Cleveland 1975; Urology, Univ Hosps Cleveland 1975; **Fellow:** Physiology, Yale Med Sch 1972; **Fac Appt:** Prof U, Harvard Med Sch

McGovern, Francis MD [U] - **Spec Exp:** Prostate Cancer; **Hospital:** Mass Genl Hosp; **Address:** One Hawthorne Pl, Ste 109, Boston, MA 02114; **Phone:** 617-726-3574; **Board Cert:** Urology 1999; **Med School:** Case West Res Univ 1983; **Resid:** Urology, Mass Genl Hosp 1989

O'Leary, Michael P MD [U] - **Spec Exp:** Sexual Dysfunction; Kidney Stones; Prostate Disease; **Hospital:** Brigham & Women's Hosp, Dana-Farber Cancer Inst; **Address:** Brigham & Women's Hosp, Div Urology, 45 Francis St, ASBIII-3, Boston, MA 02155; **Phone:** 617-732-6325; **Board Cert:** Urology 2000; **Med School:** Geo Wash Univ 1980; **Resid:** Urology, Tufts New Eng Med Ctr 1982; Urology, Mass Genl Hosp 1986; **Fellow:** Urology, UCSF Med Ctr 1989; **Fac Appt:** Assoc Prof S, Harvard Med Sch

Oates, Robert Davis MD [U] - **Spec Exp:** Infertility-Male; Vasectomy Reversal; Reproductive Genetics; **Hospital:** Boston Med Ctr; **Address:** Boston Univ Med Ctr, Dept Urology, 720 Harrison Ave, Ste 606, Boston, MA 02118-2334; **Phone:** 617-638-8485; **Board Cert:** Urology 2000; **Med School:** Boston Univ 1982; **Resid:** Surgery, Boston Univ Hosp 1984; Urology, Boston Univ Hosp 1987; **Fellow:** Reproductive Medicine, Baylor Coll Med 1988; **Fac Appt:** Prof U, Boston Univ

Retik, Alan MD [U] - **Spec Exp:** Pediatric Urology; Urinary Reconstruction-Pediatric; **Hospital:** Children's Hospital - Boston; **Address:** Chldns Hosp, Dept Urology, 300 Longwood Ave Honnewell Bldg Fl 3, Boston, MA 02115-5724; **Phone:** 617-355-3339; **Board Cert:** Urology 1969; **Med School:** Cornell Univ-Weill Med Coll 1957; **Resid:** Surgery, Strong Meml Hosp 1961; Urology, Peter Bent Brigham Hosp 1965; **Fellow:** Pediatric Urology, Hosp Sich Chldn 1967; **Fac Appt:** Prof U, Harvard Med Sch

Richie, Jerome MD [U] - **Spec Exp:** Prostate Cancer; Testicular Cancer; Kidney Cancer; **Hospital:** Brigham & Women's Hosp, Dana-Farber Cancer Inst; **Address:** Brigham & Womens Hosp, 75 Francis St, Ste ASB2, Boston, MA 02115; **Phone:** 617-732-6325; **Board Cert:** Urology 1992; **Med School:** Univ Tex Med Br, Galveston 1969; **Resid:** Surgery, UCLA Med Ctr 1971; Urology, UCLA Med Ctr 1975; **Fac Appt:** Prof U, Harvard Med Sch

Sigman, Mark MD [U] - **Spec Exp:** Infertility-Male; Vasectomy Reversal; **Hospital:** Rhode Island Hosp; **Address:** 2 Dudley St, Ste 175, Providence, RI 02905-3247; **Phone:** 401-421-0710; **Board Cert:** Urology 2000; **Med School:** Univ Conn 1981; **Resid:** Urology, Univ VA 1987; Surgery, Univ VA 1983; **Fellow:** Male Reproduction, Baylor Coll Med 1989; **Fac Appt:** Assoc Prof U, Brown Univ

Weiss, Robert M MD [U] - **Spec Exp:** Pediatric Urology; **Hospital:** Yale - New Haven Hosp; **Address:** Yale Univ Sch Med, Dept Urology, 800 Howard Ave, Box 208041, New Haven, CT 06520-8041; **Phone:** 203-785-2815; **Board Cert:** Urology 1999; **Med School:** SUNY Downstate 1960; **Resid:** Surgery, Beth Israel Hosp 1962; Urology, Columbia Presby Hosp 1967; **Fellow:** Pharmacology, Columbia Presby Hosp 1965; **Fac Appt:** Prof U, Yale Univ

Mid Atlantic

Alexander, Richard B MD [U] - **Spec Exp:** Prostate Disease; **Hospital:** Univ of MD Med Sys; **Address:** 419 W Redwood St, Ste 320, Baltimore, MD 21201; **Phone:** 410-328-5109; **Board Cert:** Urology 1999; **Med School:** Johns Hopkins Univ 1981; **Resid:** Surgery, Vanderbilt Univ Affl Hosps 1983; Urology, Johns Hopkins Hosp 1988; **Fellow:** Cancer Immunology, Natl Cancer Inst 1989; **Fac Appt:** Assoc Prof U, Univ MD Sch Med

Bagley, Demetrius H MD [U] - **Spec Exp:** Endourology; Kidney Stones; Kidney Cancer; **Hospital:** Thomas Jefferson Univ Hosp; **Address:** 833 Chestnut St E, Ste 703, Philadelphia, PA 19107; **Phone:** 215-955-1000; **Board Cert:** Urology 1981; **Med School:** Johns Hopkins Univ 1970; **Resid:** Surgery, Yale-New Haven Hosp 1972; Urology, Yale-New Haven Hosp 1979; **Fellow:** Surgery, NCI-USPHS 1975; **Fac Appt:** Prof U, Thomas Jefferson Univ

Bar-Chama, Natan MD [U] - **Spec Exp:** Infertility-Male; Erectile Dysfunction; Microsurgery; **Hospital:** Mount Sinai Med Ctr; **Address:** 5 E 98th St, Box 1272, New York, NY 10029-6501; **Phone:** 212-241-4812; **Board Cert:** Urology 1996; **Med School:** Albert Einstein Coll Med 1987; **Resid:** Urology, Montefiore/Albert Einstein 1993; **Fellow:** Urology, Baylor Coll Med 1994; **Fac Appt:** Assoc Prof U, Mount Sinai Sch Med

Belman, A Barry MD [U] - **Spec Exp:** Pediatric Urology; Hypospadias; **Hospital:** Chldns Natl Med Ctr; **Address:** Chldns Natl Med Ctr, 111 Michigan Ave NW, Washington, DC 20010-2978; **Phone:** 202-884-5042; **Board Cert:** Urology 1973; **Med School:** Northwestern Univ 1964; **Resid:** Urology, Northwestern Univ Med Ctr 1970; **Fac Appt:** Prof U, Geo Wash Univ

Benson, Mitchell C MD [U] - **Spec Exp:** Prostate Cancer/Robotic Surgery; Bladder Cancer; Kidney Cancer; Continent Urinary Diversions; **Hospital:** NY-Presby Hosp/Columbia (page 66); **Address:** NY Presby Hosp-Columbia, Dept Urology, 161 Ft Washington Ave Fl 11 - rm 1102, New York, NY 10032-3713; **Phone:** 212-305-5201; **Board Cert:** Urology 1984; **Med School:** Columbia P&S 1977; **Resid:** Surgery, Mount Sinai Med Ctr 1979; Urology, Columbia-Presby Hosp 1982; **Fellow:** Oncology, Johns Hopkins Hosp 1984; **Fac Appt:** Prof U, Columbia P&S

Blaivas, Jerry G MD [U] - **Spec Exp:** Uro-Gynecology; Urology-Female; Neurogenic Bladder; Incontinence after Prostate Cancer; **Hospital:** NY-Presby Hosp/Weill Cornell (page 66), Lenox Hill Hosp (page 62); **Address:** 445 E 77th St, New York, NY 10021; **Phone:** 212-772-3900; **Board Cert:** Urology 1978; **Med School:** Tufts Univ 1964; **Resid:** Surgery, Boston Med Ctr 1971; Urology, New England Med Ctr 1976; **Fac Appt:** Clin Prof U, Cornell Univ-Weill Med Coll

Burnett II, Arthur L MD [U] - **Spec Exp:** Prostate Cancer; Erectile Dysfunction; **Hospital:** Johns Hopkins Hosp - Baltimore (page 61); **Address:** 600 N Wolfe St, Marburg Bldg, Ste 407, Baltimore, MD 21287; **Phone:** 410-614-3986; **Board Cert:** Urology 1998; **Med School:** Johns Hopkins Univ 1988; **Resid:** Urology, Johns Hopkins Hosp 1994; Surgery, Johns Hopkins Hosp 1990; **Fac Appt:** Prof U, Johns Hopkins Univ

Canning, Douglas MD [U] - **Spec Exp:** Pediatric Urology; Hypospadias; Bladder Exstrophy; **Hospital:** Chldns Hosp of Philadelphia, The; **Address:** Childrens Hosp, Div Urology, 34th St & Civic Center Blvd, Wood Bldg, 3rd Fl, Philadelphia, PA 19104; **Phone:** 215-590-2754; **Board Cert:** Urology 2000; **Med School:** Dartmouth Med Sch 1982; **Resid:** Urology, Naval Hosp 1987; **Fellow:** Pediatric Urology, Johns Hopkins Hosp 1988; **Fac Appt:** Assoc Prof U, Univ Pennsylvania

Carter, H Ballentine MD [U] - **Spec Exp:** Prostate Cancer; **Hospital:** Johns Hopkins Hosp - Baltimore (page 61); **Address:** Brady Urological Inst, Johns Hopkins Hosp, 600 N Wolfe St Marburg Bldg - rm 145, Baltimore, MD 21287-2101; **Phone:** 410-955-6100; **Board Cert:** Urology 1999; **Med School:** Med Univ SC 1981; **Resid:** Surgery, New York Hosp 1983; Urology, New York Hosp 1987; **Fellow:** Research, Johns Hopkins Hosp 1989; **Fac Appt:** Prof U, Johns Hopkins Univ

Chancellor, Michael B MD [U] - **Spec Exp:** Incontinence-Female; Urology-Female; Neuro-Urology; **Hospital:** UPMC Presby, Pittsburgh; **Address:** 3471 Fifth Ave, Kaufmann Bldg, rm 700, Pittsburgh, PA 15213; **Phone:** 412-692-4096; **Board Cert:** Urology 2000; **Med School:** Med Coll Wisc 1983; **Resid:** Surgery, Univ Mich 1985; Urology, Univ Mich 1988; **Fellow:** Neurourology, Columbia-Presby Med Ctr 1990; **Fac Appt:** Prof U, Univ Pittsburgh

Droller, Michael J MD [U] - **Spec Exp:** Urologic Cancer; Bladder Cancer; Prostate Cancer; Kidney Cancer; **Hospital:** Mount Sinai Med Ctr; **Address:** 5 E 98th St Fl 6th, Box 1272, New York, NY 10029-6501; **Phone:** 212-241-3868; **Board Cert:** Urology 2001; **Med School:** Harvard Med Sch 1968; **Resid:** Surgery, Peter Bent Brigham Hosp 1970; Urology, Stanford Univ Med Ctr 1976; **Fellow:** Immunology, Univ Stockholm 1977; **Fac Appt:** Prof U, Mount Sinai Sch Med

Eid, Jean Francois MD [U] - **Spec Exp:** Erectile Dysfunction; Urological Prostheses; Incontinence; Peyronie's Disease; **Hospital:** NY-Presby Hosp/Weill Cornell (page 66); **Address:** 50 E 69th St, New York, NY 10021; **Phone:** 212-535-6690; **Board Cert:** Urology 1999; **Med School:** Cornell Univ-Weill Med Coll 1982; **Resid:** Surgery, New York Hosp-Cornell Med Ctr 1984; Urology, New York Hosp-Cornell Med Ctr 1988; **Fac Appt:** Assoc Clin Prof U, Cornell Univ-Weill Med Coll

Fisch, Harry MD [U] - **Spec Exp:** Infertility-Male; Microsurgery; Vasectomy Reversal; **Hospital:** NY-Presby Hosp/Columbia (page 66), Lenox Hill Hosp (page 62); **Address:** 944 Park Ave, Ste 1C, New York, NY 10028; **Phone:** 212-879-0800; **Board Cert:** Urology 1999; **Med School:** Mount Sinai Sch Med 1983; **Resid:** Surgery, Montefiore Hosp Med Ctr 1985; Urology, Montefiore Hosp Med Ctr 1989; **Fac Appt:** Prof U, Columbia P&S

Gearhart, John P MD [U] - **Spec Exp:** Pediatric Urology; Bladder Exstrophy; **Hospital:** Johns Hopkins Hosp - Baltimore (page 61); **Address:** Johns Hopkins Hospital, Brady Urological Institute, 600 N Wolfe St Marburg Bldg - Ste 146, Baltimore, MD 21287-2101; **Phone:** 410-955-5358; **Board Cert:** Urology 1982; **Med School:** Univ Louisville Sch Med 1975; **Resid:** Urology, Med Coll Georgia Hosp 1980; **Fellow:** Pediatric Urology, Alder Hey Chldns Hosp 1981; Pediatric Urology, Johns Hopkins Hosp 1985; **Fac Appt:** Prof U, Johns Hopkins Univ

Glassberg, Kenneth MD [U] - **Spec Exp:** Pediatric Urology; Genital Reconstruction; Varicocele In Adolescents; **Hospital:** NYPresby-Morgan Stanley Children's Hosp; **Address:** Morgan Stanley Chlds Hosp of NY-Presby, 3959 Broadway, BHN 1116, New York, NY 10032; **Phone:** 212-305-9918; **Board Cert:** Urology 1977; **Med School:** SUNY Downstate 1968; **Resid:** Surgery, Montefiore Hosp Med Ctr 1972; Urology, Univ Hosp 1975; **Fellow:** Pediatric Urology, Adler Hey Chldns Hosp 1976; Pediatric Urology, Hosp For Sick Chldn 1976; **Fac Appt:** Prof U, Columbia P&S

Goldstein, Marc MD [U] - **Spec Exp:** Infertility-Male; Vasectomy Reversal; Varicocele Microsurgery; Vasectomy-Scalpelless; **Hospital:** NY-Presby Hosp/Weill Cornell (page 66); **Address:** Cornell Inst for Reproductive Med, 525 E 68th St, Box 580, New York, NY 10021; **Phone:** 212-746-5470; **Board Cert:** Urology 1982; **Med School:** SUNY Downstate 1972; **Resid:** Surgery, Columbia-Presby Med Ctr 1974; Urology, SUNY Downstate Med Ctr 1980; **Fellow:** Microsurgery, Rockefeller Univ 1982; **Fac Appt:** Prof U, Cornell Univ-Weill Med Coll

Gomella, Leonard G MD [U] - **Spec Exp:** Prostate Cancer; Laparoscopic Surgery; Urologic Cancer; **Hospital:** Thomas Jefferson Univ Hosp; **Address:** Thomas Jefferson Univ, 1015 Walnut St Fl 11 - Ste 1112, Philadelphia, PA 19107-5001; **Phone:** 215-955-1000; **Board Cert:** Urology 1998; **Med School:** Univ KY Coll Med 1980; **Resid:** Surgery, Univ Kentucky Med Ctr 1982; Urology, Univ Kentucky Med Ctr 1986; **Fellow:** Urologic Oncology, Natl Cancer Inst 1988; **Fac Appt:** Prof U, Jefferson Med Coll

Grasso, Michael MD [U] - **Spec Exp:** Urologic Cancer; Laparoscopic Surgery; Kidney Stones; **Hospital:** St Vincent Cath Med Ctrs - Manhattan; **Address:** 170 W 12th St, Ste 205, Dept Urology - Cronin 205, New York, NY 10011; **Phone:** 212-604-1270; **Board Cert:** Urology 2002; **Med School:** Jefferson Med Coll 1986; **Resid:** Surgery, Jefferson Univ Hosp 1988; Urology, Jefferson Univ Hosp 1992; **Fac Appt:** Prof U, NY Med Coll

Greenberg, Richard E MD [U] - **Spec Exp:** Prostate Cancer; Bladder Cancer; Kidney Cancer; **Hospital:** Fox Chase Cancer Ctr (page 59), Abington Mem Hosp; **Address:** Fox Chase Cancer Ctr, Div Urol-Dept Surg, 333 Cottman Ave, Ste H3 - rm H3-116, Philadelphia, PA 19111; **Phone:** 215-728-5341; **Board Cert:** Urology 2005; **Med School:** Cornell Univ-Weill Med Coll 1976; **Resid:** Surgery, New York Hosp 1979; Urology, New York Hosp 1983; **Fac Appt:** Prof U, Temple Univ

Gribetz, Michael MD [U] - **Spec Exp:** Prostate Disease; Urology-Female; Sexual Dysfunction; Kidney Stones; **Hospital:** Mount Sinai Med Ctr; **Address:** 1155 Park Ave, New York, NY 10128-1209; **Phone:** 212-831-1300; **Board Cert:** Urology 1980; **Med School:** Albert Einstein Coll Med 1973; **Resid:** Surgery, Montefiore Hosp Med Ctr 1975; Urology, Mount Sinai Hosp 1978; **Fac Appt:** Asst Clin Prof U, Mount Sinai Sch Med

Hensle, Terry MD [U] - **Spec Exp:** Pediatric Urology; **Hospital:** NYPresby-Morgan Stanley Children's Hosp, Hackensack Univ Med Ctr; **Address:** Morgan Stanley Chldns Hosp of NY-Presby, 3959 Broadway, Ste 219N, New York, NY 10032; **Phone:** 212-305-8510; **Board Cert:** Urology 1978; **Med School:** Cornell Univ-Weill Med Coll 1968; **Resid:** Surgery, Boston City Hosp 1973; Urology, Mass Genl Hosp 1976; **Fellow:** Pediatric Urology, Mass Genl Hosp 1977; Pediatric Urology, Great Ormond St Hosp 1978; **Fac Appt:** Prof U, Columbia P&S

Herr, Harry W MD [U] - **Spec Exp:** Bladder Cancer; Prostate Cancer; Testicular Cancer; **Hospital:** Meml Sloan Kettering Cancer Ctr, NY-Presby Hosp/Weill Cornell (page 66); **Address:** Meml Sloan Kettering Canc Ctr, Dept Urol, 1275 York Ave, New York, NY 10021; **Phone:** 646-422-4411; **Board Cert:** Urology 1976; **Med School:** UCSF 1969; **Resid:** Urology, UC Irvine Med Ctr 1974; **Fellow:** Urology, Meml Sloan Kettering Cancer Ctr 1976; **Fac Appt:** Assoc Prof S, Cornell Univ-Weill Med Coll

Huben, Robert P MD [U] - **Spec Exp:** Prostate Cancer; Kidney Cancer; Urologic Cancer; **Hospital:** Roswell Park Cancer Inst; **Address:** Roswell Park Cancer Inst, Elm & Carlton Sts, Buffalo, NY 14263-0001; **Phone:** 716-845-3389; **Board Cert:** Urology 1983; **Med School:** Cornell Univ-Weill Med Coll 1976; **Resid:** Urology, East Virginia Med Ctr 1981; **Fellow:** Urologic Oncology, Roswell Park Meml Inst 1982

Jarow, Jonathan P MD [U] - **Spec Exp:** Infertility-Male; Prostate Cancer; Erectile Dysfunction; Incontinence after Prostate Cancer; **Hospital:** Johns Hopkins Hosp - Baltimore (page 61); **Address:** Johns Hopkins Outpatient Ctr-Urology, 601 N Caroline St, Fl 4, Baltimore, MD 21287; **Phone:** 410-955-3617; **Board Cert:** Urology 1999; **Med School:** Northwestern Univ 1980; **Resid:** Surgery, Johns Hopkins Hosp 1982; Urology, Johns Hopkins Hosp 1986; **Fellow:** Andrology, Baylor Univ 1989; **Fac Appt:** Assoc Prof U, Johns Hopkins Univ

Kaplan, Steven A MD [U] - **Spec Exp:** Urodynamics; Voiding Dysfunction; Incontinence after Prostate Cancer; Incontinence; **Hospital:** NY-Presby Hosp/Weill Cornell (page 66); **Address:** NY Presbyterian-Weill Cornell Medical Ctr, 525 E 68th St, rm F9West, New York, NY 10021; **Phone:** 212-746-4811; **Board Cert:** Urology 2001; **Med School:** Mount Sinai Sch Med 1982; **Resid:** Surgery, Mount Sinai Hosp 1984; Urology, Columbia Presby Med Ctr 1988; **Fellow:** Urology, Columbia Presby Med Ctr 1990; **Fac Appt:** Prof U, Cornell Univ-Weill Med Coll

Katz, Aaron E MD [U] - **Spec Exp:** Prostate Cancer-Cryosurgery; Kidney Cancer-Cryosurgery; Complementary Medicine; **Hospital:** NY-Presby Hosp/Columbia (page 66); **Address:** NY Presby Med Ctr, Herbert Irving Pav, 161 Ft Washington Ave Fl 11, New York, NY 10032; **Phone:** 212-305-6408; **Board Cert:** Urology 2006; **Med School:** NY Med Coll 1986; **Resid:** Urology, Maimonides Med Ctr 1992; **Fellow:** Urologic Oncology, Columbia Presby Med Ctr 1993; **Fac Appt:** Assoc Clin Prof U, Columbia P&S

Kavoussi, Louis R MD [U] - **Spec Exp:** Laparoscopic Surgery; Endourology; Kidney Stones; **Hospital:** Long Island Jewish Med Ctr; **Address:** 450 Lakeville Rd, Ste M-41, New Hyde Park, NY 11040; **Phone:** 516-562-2880; **Board Cert:** Urology 1999; **Med School:** SUNY Buffalo 1983; **Resid:** Surgery, Barnes Jewish Hosp 1985; Urology, Barnes Jewish Hosp 1989; **Fac Appt:** Prof U, NYU Sch Med

Kirschenbaum, Alexander M MD [U] - **Spec Exp:** Prostate Cancer; Bladder Cancer; Kidney Cancer; **Hospital:** Mount Sinai Med Ctr; **Address:** 58A E 79th St, New York, NY 10021; **Phone:** 646-422-0926; **Board Cert:** Urology 2005; **Med School:** Mount Sinai Sch Med 1980; **Resid:** Surgery, Mount Sinai Hosp 1982; Urology, Mount Sinai Hosp 1985; **Fellow:** Urologic Oncology, Mount Sinai Hosp 1987; **Fac Appt:** Assoc Prof U, Mount Sinai Sch Med

Lepor, Herbert MD [U] - **Spec Exp:** Prostate Cancer; **Hospital:** NYU Med Ctr (page 67); **Address:** 150 E 32nd St Fl 2, New York, NY 10016; **Phone:** 646-825-6327; **Board Cert:** Urology 2005; **Med School:** Johns Hopkins Univ 1975; **Resid:** Urology, Johns Hopkins Hosp 1986; **Fac Appt:** Prof U, NYU Sch Med

Lowe, Franklin MD [U] - **Spec Exp:** Prostate Disease; Complementary Medicine; Prostate Cancer; **Hospital:** St Luke's - Roosevelt Hosp Ctr - Roosevelt Div, NY-Presby Hosp/Columbia (page 66); **Address:** 425 W 59th St, Ste 3A, New York, NY 10019; **Phone:** 212-523-7790; **Board Cert:** Urology 2006; **Med School:** Columbia P&S 1979; **Resid:** Surgery, Johns Hopkins Hosp 1981; Urology, Johns Hopkins Hosp 1984; **Fac Appt:** Clin Prof U, Columbia P&S

Macchia, Richard MD [U] - **Spec Exp:** Prostate Disease; Prostate Cancer; Voiding Dysfunction; **Hospital:** SUNY Downstate Med Ctr, Kings County Hosp Ctr; **Address:** SUNY Downstate Med School, Dept Urology, 445 Lenox Rd, Box 79, Brooklyn, NY 11203-2098; **Phone:** 718-270-2554; **Board Cert:** Urology 1977; **Med School:** NY Med Coll 1969; **Resid:** Surgery, St Vincent's Hosp 1971; Urology, SUNY Downstate Med Ctr 1974; **Fellow:** Urologic Oncology, Meml Sloan Kettering Cancer Ctr 1976; **Fac Appt:** Prof U, SUNY Downstate

Malkowicz, S Bruce MD [U] - **Spec Exp:** Urologic Cancer; **Hospital:** Hosp Univ Penn - UPHS (page 72); **Address:** Hosp Univ Penn, Dept Urology, 3400 Spruce St, 9 Penn Tower, Philadelphia, PA 19104; **Phone:** 215-662-2891; **Board Cert:** Urology 2000; **Med School:** Univ Pennsylvania 1981; **Resid:** Surgery, Hosp Univ Penn 1983; Urology, Hosp Univ Penn 1987; **Fellow:** Urologic Oncology, USC Med Ctr 1998; Urologic Oncology, Hosp Univ Penn/Wistar Inst 1990; **Fac Appt:** Assoc Prof U, Univ Pennsylvania

Melman, Arnold MD [U] - **Spec Exp:** Erectile Dysfunction; Prostate Disease (Thermodilation); Prostate Cancer; **Hospital:** Montefiore Med Ctr; **Address:** 969 Park Ave, New York, NY 10028; **Phone:** 212-639-1561; **Board Cert:** Urology 1976; **Med School:** Univ Rochester 1966; **Resid:** Urology, Strong Meml Hosp 1968; Urology, UCLA Med Ctr 1974; **Fellow:** Nephrology, Cedars-Sinai Med Ctr 1972; **Fac Appt:** Prof U, Albert Einstein Coll Med

Mostwin, Jacek L MD/PhD [U] - **Spec Exp:** Prostate Cancer; **Hospital:** Johns Hopkins Hosp - Baltimore (page 61); **Address:** Johns Hopkins Hosp, 600 N Wolfe St, Marburg-401C, Baltimore, MD 21287; **Phone:** 410-955-4461; **Board Cert:** Urology 1997; **Med School:** Univ MD Sch Med 1975; **Resid:** Surgery, Univ Michigan Med Ctr 1978; Urology, Johns Hopkins Hosp 1983; **Fac Appt:** Prof U, Johns Hopkins Univ

Mulhall, John P MD [U] - **Spec Exp:** Erectile Dysfunction; Peyronie's Disease; Penile Prostheses; Infertility-Male; **Hospital:** NY-Presby Hosp/Columbia (page 66), Meml Sloan Kettering Cancer Ctr; **Address:** Weill Cornell Medical Ctr, 525 E 68th St, Box 94, New York, NY 10021; **Phone:** 212-746-5653; **Board Cert:** Urology 1999; **Med School:** Ireland 1985; **Resid:** Urology, Univ Conn Health Ctr 1995; **Fellow:** Urology, Boston Univ Med Ctr 1996; **Fac Appt:** Assoc Prof U, Cornell Univ-Weill Med Coll

Nagler, Harris M MD [U] - **Spec Exp:** Vasectomy Reversal; Infertility-Male; Varicocele Microsurgery; Erectile Dysfunction; **Hospital:** Beth Israel Med Ctr - Petrie Division; **Address:** Beth Israel Med Ctr, Dept Urology, 10 Union Square E, Ste 3A, New York, NY 10003; **Phone:** 212-844-8700; **Board Cert:** Urology 1982; **Med School:** Temple Univ 1975; **Resid:** Urology, Columbia Presby Hosp 1980; **Fellow:** Reproductive Medicine, Columbia Presby Hosp 1981; **Fac Appt:** Prof U, Albert Einstein Coll Med

Naslund, Michael MD [U] - **Spec Exp:** Prostate Cancer; Prostate Disease; **Hospital:** Univ of MD Med Sys; **Address:** Maryland Prostate Ctr, 419 W Redwood St, Ste 320, Baltimore, MD 21201; **Phone:** 410-328-0800; **Board Cert:** Urology 2000; **Med School:** Johns Hopkins Univ 1981; **Resid:** Surgery, Johns Hopkins Hosp 1983; Urology, Johns Hopkins Hosp 1987; **Fac Appt:** Prof U, Univ MD Sch Med

Nelson, Joel B MD [U] - **Spec Exp:** Prostate Cancer; **Hospital:** UPMC Shadyside; **Address:** UPMC Shadyside Med Ctr, 5200 Centre Ave, Ste 209, Pittsburgh, PA 15232; **Phone:** 412-605-3013; **Board Cert:** Urology 1998; **Med School:** Northwestern Univ 1988; **Resid:** Surgery, Northwestern Meml Hosp 1990; Urology, Northwestern Meml Hosp 1994; **Fellow:** Urology, Johns Hopkins Hosp; **Fac Appt:** Prof U, Univ Pittsburgh

Nitti, Victor MD [U] - **Spec Exp:** Urology-Female; Incontinence-Male & Female; Urodynamics; Voiding Dysfunction; **Hospital:** NYU Med Ctr (page 67); **Address:** 150 E 32nd St, Ste 200, New York, NY 10016; **Phone:** 646-825-6324; **Board Cert:** Urology 2002; **Med School:** UMDNJ-NJ Med Sch, Newark 1985; **Resid:** Surgery, Univ Hosp 1987; Urology, Univ Hosp 1991; **Fellow:** Urology, UCLA Med Ctr 1992; **Fac Appt:** Assoc Prof U, NYU Sch Med

Partin, Alan W MD/PhD [U] - **Spec Exp:** Prostate Cancer; Prostate Disease; **Hospital:** Johns Hopkins Hosp - Baltimore (page 61); **Address:** Johns Hopkins Hosp, 600 N Wolfe St Marburg Bldg - rm 134, Baltimore, MD 21287; **Phone:** 410-614-4876; **Board Cert:** Urology 1998; **Med School:** Johns Hopkins Univ 1989; **Resid:** Surgery, Johns Hopkins Hosp 1991; Urology, Johns Hopkins Hosp 1994; **Fac Appt:** Prof U, Johns Hopkins Univ

Poppas, Dix P MD [U] - **Spec Exp:** Genital Reconstruction-Pediatric; Robotic Surgery-Pediatric; Minimally Invasive Surgery-Pediatric; **Hospital:** NY-Presby Hosp/Weill Cornell (page 66); **Address:** Inst for Pediatric Urology, NY Presby Hosp-Weill Cornell, 525 E 68th St, Box 94, New York, NY 10021-4870; **Phone:** 212-746-5337; **Board Cert:** Urology 1999; **Med School:** Eastern VA Med Sch 1988; **Resid:** Urology, New York Hosp-Cornell Med Ctr 1994; **Fellow:** Pediatric Urology, Children's Hosp 1996; **Fac Appt:** Assoc Prof U, Cornell Univ-Weill Med Coll

Rushton, H Gil MD [U] - **Spec Exp:** Pediatric Urology; Fetal Urology; Hypospadias; **Hospital:** Chldns Natl Med Ctr; **Address:** Chldns Natl Med Ctr, Dept Urology, 111 Michigan Ave NW, Washington, DC 20010; **Phone:** 202-884-5042; **Board Cert:** Urology 2004; **Med School:** Univ SC Sch Med 1978; **Resid:** Urology, Univ SC Medical Ctr 1983; **Fellow:** Pediatric Urology, Hosp Sick Children 1984; Pediatric Urology, Emory/Egleston Childrens Hosp 1986; **Fac Appt:** Prof U, Geo Wash Univ

Sawczuk, Ihor S MD [U] - **Spec Exp:** Kidney Cancer; Bladder Cancer; Prostate Cancer/Robotic Surgery; **Hospital:** Hackensack Univ Med Ctr, NY-Presby Hosp/Columbia (page 66); **Address:** Hackensack Univ Med Ctr, 360 Essex St, Hackensack, NJ 07601; **Phone:** 201-336-8090; **Board Cert:** Urology 1996; **Med School:** Med Coll PA Hahnemann 1979; **Resid:** Surgery, St Vincent's Hosp & Med Ctr 1981; Urology, Columbia-Presby Med Ctr 1984; **Fellow:** Urologic Oncology, Columbia-Presby Med Ctr 1986; **Fac Appt:** Prof U, Columbia P&S

Scardino, Peter T MD [U] - **Spec Exp:** Prostate Cancer; **Hospital:** Meml Sloan Kettering Cancer Ctr; **Address:** 1275 York Ave, Box 27, New York, NY 10021; **Phone:** 646-422-4329; **Board Cert:** Urology 1981; **Med School:** Duke Univ 1971; **Resid:** Surgery, Mass Genl Hosp 1973; Urology, UCLA Med Ctr 1979; **Fellow:** Urology, Natl Cancer Inst 1976; **Fac Appt:** Prof U, Cornell Univ-Weill Med Coll

Schlegel, Peter MD [U] - **Spec Exp:** Prostate Cancer; Infertility-Male; Fertility Preservation in Cancer; Erectile Dysfunction; **Hospital:** NY-Presby Hosp/Weill Cornell (page 66); **Address:** 525 E 68th St, Starr 900, New York, NY 10021-4870; **Phone:** 212-746-5491; **Board Cert:** Urology 2007; **Med School:** Univ Mass Sch Med 1983; **Resid:** Surgery, Johns Hopkins Hosp 1985; Urology, Johns Hopkins Hosp 1989; **Fellow:** Medical Oncology, Johns Hopkins Hosp 1987; Male Reproduction, NY Hosp-Cornell Med Ctr 1991; **Fac Appt:** Prof U, Cornell Univ-Weill Med Coll

Sheinfeld, Joel MD [U] - **Spec Exp:** Testicular Cancer; Bladder Cancer; Fertility Preservation in Cancer; **Hospital:** Meml Sloan Kettering Cancer Ctr; **Address:** Meml Sloan Kettering Canc Ctr-Kimmel Ctr, 353 E 68th St, New York, NY 10021; **Phone:** 646-422-4311; **Board Cert:** Urology 2000; **Med School:** Univ Fla Coll Med 1981; **Resid:** Urology, Strong Meml Hosp 1986; **Fellow:** Urologic Oncology, Meml Sloan Kettering Cancer Ctr 1989; **Fac Appt:** Assoc Prof U, Cornell Univ-Weill Med Coll

Snyder III, Howard M MD [U] - **Spec Exp:** Pediatric Urology; Genital Reconstruction; Reconstructive Urologic Surgery; **Hospital:** Chldns Hosp of Philadelphia, The, Hosp Univ Penn - UPHS (page 72); **Address:** Chldrns Hosp, Dept Ped Urology, 34th St & Civic Ctr Blvd, Wood Bldg, Fl 3, Philadelphia, PA 19104; **Phone:** 215-590-2767; **Board Cert:** Surgery 1995; Urology 1982; Pediatric Surgery 1995; **Med School:** Harvard Med Sch 1969; **Resid:** Surgery, Peter Bent Brigham Hosp 1973; Pediatric Surgery, Boston Chldns Hosp Med Ctr 1974; **Fellow:** Urology, Peter Bent Brigham Hosp 1980; **Fac Appt:** Prof U, Univ Pennsylvania

Sosa, R Ernest MD [U] - **Spec Exp:** Kidney Stones; Laparoscopic Surgery; Adrenal Surgery; **Hospital:** NY-Presby Hosp/Weill Cornell (page 66), Lenox Hill Hosp (page 62); **Address:** 880 5th Ave, New York, NY 10021; **Phone:** 212-570-6800; **Board Cert:** Urology 2006; **Med School:** Cornell Univ-Weill Med Coll 1978; **Resid:** Surgery, New York Hosp-Cornell 1980; Urology, New York Hosp-Cornell 1984; **Fellow:** Renal Physiology, New York Hosp-Cornell 1986; **Fac Appt:** Assoc Clin Prof U, Cornell Univ-Weill Med Coll

Taneja, Samir S MD [U] - **Spec Exp:** Kidney Cancer; Prostate Cancer; Bladder Cancer; **Hospital:** NYU Med Ctr (page 67); **Address:** 150 E 32nd St, Ste 200, New York, NY 10016; **Phone:** 646-825-6321; **Board Cert:** Urology 1999; **Med School:** Northwestern Univ 1990; **Resid:** Urology, UCLA Med Ctr 1996; **Fac Appt:** Assoc Prof U, NYU Sch Med

Tarry, William F MD [U] - **Spec Exp:** Pediatric Urology; **Hospital:** WV Univ Hosp - Ruby Memorial; **Address:** W VA Univ Hlth Sci Ctr, Div Urology, Box 9238, Morgantown, WV 26506-9251; **Phone:** 304-293-2706; **Board Cert:** Urology 1995; **Med School:** Penn State Univ-Hershey Med Ctr 1977; **Resid:** Surgery, W Va U Hosp 1979; Urology, W Va U Hosp 1982; **Fellow:** Pediatric Urology, Children's Hosp 1984; **Fac Appt:** Assoc Prof U, W VA Univ

Tewari, Ashutosh MD [U] - **Spec Exp:** Prostate Cancer/Robotic Surgery; **Hospital:** NY-Presby Hosp/Weill Cornell (page 66); **Address:** Weill Cornell Brady Urologic Health Ct, 525 E 68th St, Starr 916, New York, NY 10021; **Phone:** 212-746-5638; **Med School:** India 1983; **Resid:** Surgery, GSVM Medical College 1990; Urology, Henry Ford Hosp 2003; **Fellow:** Transplant Surgery, Liverpool 1993; Urologic Oncology, Shands Healthcare 1995; **Fac Appt:** Assoc Prof U, Cornell Univ-Weill Med Coll

Uzzo, Robert MD [U] - **Spec Exp:** Kidney Cancer; Bladder Cancer; Prostate Cancer; Testicular Cancer; **Hospital:** Fox Chase Cancer Ctr (page 59); **Address:** 333 Cottman Ave, rm H3116, Philadelphia, PA 19111; **Phone:** 215-728-3501; **Board Cert:** Urology 2001; **Med School:** Cornell Univ-Weill Med Coll 1991; **Resid:** Surgery, New York Hosp-Cornell Med Ctr 1993; Urology, New York Hosp-Cornell Med Ctr 1997; **Fellow:** Urologic Oncology, Cleveland Clinic 1999; Renal Transplant, Cleveland Clinic 2000; **Fac Appt:** Assoc Prof S, Temple Univ

Van Arsdalen, Keith N MD [U] - **Spec Exp:** Infertility-Male; Varicocele Microsurgery; Urologic Cancer; Vasectomy Reversal; **Hospital:** Hosp Univ Penn - UPHS (page 72), Chldns Hosp of Philadelphia, The; **Address:** Hosp Univ Penn, Div Urol, 3400 Spruce St, 9 Penn Tower, Philadelphia, PA 19104-4283; **Phone:** 215-662-2891; **Board Cert:** Urology 1984; **Med School:** Med Coll VA 1977; **Resid:** Surgery, Univ Maryland Hosp 1979; Urology, Med Coll Virginia 1982; **Fellow:** Urodynamics, Hosp Univ Penn 1983; **Fac Appt:** Prof U, Univ Pennsylvania

Vapnek, Jonathan M MD [U] - **Spec Exp:** Incontinence; Urology-Female; Neurogenic Bladder; **Hospital:** Mount Sinai Med Ctr; **Address:** 229 E 79th St, New York, NY 10021; **Phone:** 212-717-9500; **Board Cert:** Urology 2005; **Med School:** UCSD 1986; **Resid:** Surgery, UCSD Med Ctr 1988; Urology, UCSF Med Ctr 1992; **Fellow:** Urology, UC Davis Med Ctr 1993; **Fac Appt:** Assoc Clin Prof U, Mount Sinai Sch Med

Vaughan, Edwin D MD [U] - **Spec Exp:** Urologic Cancer; Adrenal Tumors; Prostate Disease; **Hospital:** NY-Presby Hosp/Weill Cornell (page 66), Meml Sloan Kettering Cancer Ctr; **Address:** New York Presby Hosp, Dept Urology, 525 E 68th St, Starr 900, Box 94, New York, NY 10021-4870; **Phone:** 212-746-5480; **Board Cert:** Urology 1986; **Med School:** Univ VA Sch Med 1965; **Resid:** Surgery, Vanderbilt Univ Med Ctr 1967; Urology, Univ Virginia Hosp 1971; **Fellow:** Internal Medicine, Columbia Univ 1973; **Fac Appt:** Prof U, Cornell Univ-Weill Med Coll

Waldbaum, Robert MD [U] - **Spec Exp:** Prostate Cancer; Prostate Disease; Urologic Cancer; **Hospital:** N Shore Univ Hosp at Manhasset, St Francis Hosp - The Heart Ctr (page 70); **Address:** 535 Plandome Rd, Ste 3, Manhasset, NY 11030-1961; **Phone:** 516-627-6188; **Board Cert:** Urology 1973; **Med School:** Columbia P&S 1962; **Resid:** Surgery, Columbia Presby Med Ctr 1966; Urology, New York Hosp-Cornell 1970; **Fac Appt:** Clin Prof U, Cornell Univ-Weill Med Coll

Walsh, Patrick MD [U] - **Spec Exp:** Prostate Cancer; Urologic Cancer; **Hospital:** Johns Hopkins Hosp - Baltimore (page 61); **Address:** Brady Urological Inst, 600 N Wolfe St, Phipps 554A, Baltimore, MD 21287-2101; **Phone:** 410-955-6100; **Board Cert:** Urology 1975; **Med School:** Case West Res Univ 1964; **Resid:** Surgery, Peter Bent Brigham Hosp/Childrens Hosp 1967; Urology, UCLA Med Ctr 1971; **Fellow:** Endocrinology, Harbor Genl Hosp 1970; **Fac Appt:** Prof U, Johns Hopkins Univ

Wein, Alan J MD [U] - **Spec Exp:** Neuro-Urology; Prostate Cancer; Testicular Cancer; Urologic Cancer; **Hospital:** Hosp Univ Penn - UPHS (page 72), Pennsylvania Hosp (page 72); **Address:** Univ Penn Hlth System, Div Urology, 3400 Spruce St, 9 Penn Tower, Philadelphia, PA 19104-4283; **Phone:** 215-662-2891; **Board Cert:** Urology 1995; **Med School:** Univ Pennsylvania 1966; **Resid:** Surgery, Hosp Univ Penn 1968; Urology, Hosp Univ Penn 1972; **Fellow:** Urology, Hosp Univ Penn 1969; **Fac Appt:** Prof U, Univ Pennsylvania

Yu, George W MD [U] - **Spec Exp:** Urologic Cancer; Nutrition & Disease Prevention/Control; Nutrition & Cancer Prevention/Control; **Hospital:** G Washington Univ Hosp, Anne Arundel Med Ctr; **Address:** 116 Defense Hwy, Ste 200, Annapolis, MD 21401; **Phone:** 410-897-0540; **Board Cert:** Urology 1983; **Med School:** Tufts Univ 1973; **Resid:** Surgery, Brigham & Women's Hosp 1976; Urology, Johns Hopkins Hosp 1981; **Fac Appt:** Prof U, Geo Wash Univ

Southeast

Abramson, Edward G MD [U] - **Hospital:** Inova Alexandria Hosp; **Address:** 1707 Osage St, Ste 301, Alexandria, VA 22302; **Phone:** 703-836-8010; **Board Cert:** Urology 1977; **Med School:** Univ VA Sch Med 1967; **Resid:** Surgery, George Washington Univ Hosp 1969; Urology, George Washington Univ Hosp 1972; **Fac Appt:** Asst Clin Prof U, Geo Wash Univ

Albala, David Mois MD [U] - **Spec Exp:** Laparoscopic Surgery; Kidney Stones; Prostate Cancer/Robotic Surgery; **Hospital:** Duke Univ Med Ctr, VA Med Ctr - Durham; **Address:** Duke Univ Med Ctr, Green Zone, Trent Drive, Box 3457, Durham, NC 27710; **Phone:** 919-668-6401; **Board Cert:** Urology 2002; **Med School:** Mich State Univ 1983; **Resid:** Surgery, Dartmouth-Hitchcock Med Ctr 1985; Urology, Dartmouth-Hitchcock Med Ctr 1990; **Fellow:** Endourology, Wash Univ Med Ctr 1991; **Fac Appt:** Prof U, Duke Univ

Amling, Christopher L MD [U] - **Spec Exp:** Urologic Cancer; Prostate Cancer/Robotic Surgery; Kidney Cancer; Bladder Cancer; **Hospital:** Univ of Ala Hosp at Birmingham; **Address:** 1530 3rd Ave S, Ste FOT-1105, Birmingham, AL 35294; **Phone:** 205-975-0088; **Board Cert:** Urology 1999; **Med School:** Oregon Hlth Sci Univ 1985; **Resid:** Urology, Duke Univ Med Ctr 1996; **Fellow:** Urologic Oncology, Mayo Clinic 1997; **Fac Appt:** Prof U, Univ Ala

Assimos, Dean George MD [U] - **Spec Exp:** Kidney Stones; Reconstructive Urologic Surgery; **Hospital:** Wake Forest Univ Baptist Med Ctr (page 73); **Address:** WFU Baptist Med Ctr, Dept Urology, Reynolds Tower Fl Main, Medical Center Blvd, Winston-Salem, NC 27157; **Phone:** 336-716-4131; **Board Cert:** Urology 2003; **Med School:** Loyola Univ-Stritch Sch Med 1977; **Resid:** Surgery, Northwestern Univ Hosp 1979; Urology, Northwestern Univ Hosp 1983; **Fellow:** Urology, Bowman Gray Sch Med 1986; **Fac Appt:** Prof S, Wake Forest Univ

Atala, Anthony MD [U] - **Spec Exp:** Pediatric Urology; Reconstructive Surgery; Hernia; Microsurgery; **Hospital:** Wake Forest Univ Baptist Med Ctr (page 73); **Address:** Wake Forest Univ-Baptist, MC, Dept Urology, Medical Center Blvd, Winston-Salem, NC 27157; **Phone:** 336-716-4131; **Board Cert:** Urology 2004; **Med School:** Univ Louisville Sch Med 1985; **Resid:** Surgery, Univ Louisville Hosp 1987; Urology, Univ Louisville Hosp 1990; **Fellow:** Research, Childrens Hosp/Harvard 1991; Pediatric Urology, Childrens Hosp/Harvard 1992; **Fac Appt:** Prof U, Wake Forest Univ

Beall, Michael E MD [U] - **Spec Exp:** Prostate Cancer; Testicular Cancer; Vasectomy Reversal; **Hospital:** Inova Fairfax Hosp, Reston Hosp Ctr; **Address:** 8503 Arlington Blvd, Ste 310, Fairfax, VA 22030; **Phone:** 703-208-4200; **Board Cert:** Urology 1979; **Med School:** Geo Wash Univ 1972; **Resid:** Surgery, Geo Wash Univ Hosp 1974; Urology, Geo Wash Univ Hosp 1977; **Fac Appt:** Assoc Clin Prof U, Geo Wash Univ

Brock III, John W MD [U] - **Spec Exp:** Pediatric Urology; **Hospital:** Vanderbilt Children's Hosp; **Address:** Vanderbilt Chldns Hosp, Div Ped Urology, 2200 Childrens Way, Ste 4102 DOT, Nashville, TN 37232; **Phone:** 615-936-1060; **Board Cert:** Urology 2004; **Med School:** Med Coll GA 1978; **Resid:** Urology, Vanderbilt Univ Med Ctr 1983; **Fac Appt:** Prof U, Vanderbilt Univ

Broderick, Gregory MD [U] - **Spec Exp:** Erectile Dysfunction; Voiding Dysfunction; Peyronie's Disease; **Hospital:** St Luke's Hosp - Jacksonville; **Address:** Mayo Clinic, Dept Urology, 4500 San Pablo Rd, Jacksonville, FL 32224; **Phone:** 904-953-7330; **Board Cert:** Urology 2002; **Med School:** UCSF 1983; **Resid:** Surgery, UCSF Med Ctr 1985; Urology, UCSF Med Ctr 1988; **Fellow:** Neurourology, UC Davis Med Ctr 1990; **Fac Appt:** Prof U, Mayo Med Sch

Carson, Culley MD [U] - **Spec Exp:** Erectile Dysfunction; Kidney Stones; Peyronie's Disease; **Hospital:** Univ NC Hosps; **Address:** Univ North Carolina, Dept Urol, 2140 Bioinformatics Bldg, Chapel Hill, NC 27599-7235; **Phone:** 919-966-2571; **Board Cert:** Urology 1980; **Med School:** Geo Wash Univ 1971; **Resid:** Surgery, Dartmouth-Hitchcock Med Ctr 1973; Urology, Mayo Clinic 1978; **Fac Appt:** Prof U, Univ NC Sch Med

El-Galley, Rizk MD [U] - **Spec Exp:** Urologic Cancer; Laparoscopic Surgery; Bladder Cancer; Hydrocele; **Hospital:** Univ of Ala Hosp at Birmingham; **Address:** UAB Hosp FOT-1105, 1530 3rd Ave S, Birmingham, AL 35294-3411; **Phone:** 205-996-8765; **Board Cert:** Urology 2003; **Med School:** Egypt 1983; **Resid:** Urology, Emory Univ Hosp 1999; **Fac Appt:** Asst Prof U, Univ Ala

Fraser, Lionel B MD [U] - **Spec Exp:** Prostate Cancer; Incontinence after Prostate Cancer; Erectile Dysfunction; **Hospital:** Baptist Hosp - Jackson; **Address:** Metropolitan Urology-St Dominic East Med Tower, 971 Lakeland Drive, Ste 315, Jackson, MS 39216; **Phone:** 601-982-0982; **Board Cert:** Urology 2005; **Med School:** Univ Mich Med Sch 1977; **Resid:** Surgery, New England Deaconness Hosp 1979; **Fellow:** Urology, Brigham & Womens Hosp 1983

Harty, James MD [U] - **Spec Exp:** Urologic Cancer; **Hospital:** Norton Hosp, Jewish Hosp HlthCre Svcs Inc; **Address:** 210 E Gray St, Ste 1000, Louisville, KY 40202; **Phone:** 502-629-5904; **Board Cert:** Urology 1979; **Med School:** Ireland 1969; **Resid:** Surgery, Johns Hopkins Hosp 1973; Urology, Johns Hopkins Hosp 1977; **Fac Appt:** Prof S, Univ Louisville Sch Med

Howards, Stuart S MD [U] - **Spec Exp:** Infertility-Male; Pediatric Urology; **Hospital:** Univ Virginia Med Ctr; **Address:** Univ Virginia Hosp, Dept Urology, PO Box 800422, Charlottesville, VA 22908; **Phone:** 434-924-9559; **Board Cert:** Urology 1975; **Med School:** Columbia P&S 1963; **Resid:** Surgery, Chldns Hosp 1965; Urology, Peter Bent Brigham Hosp 1971; **Fellow:** Renal Physiology, Natl Inst Hlth 1968; **Fac Appt:** Prof U, Univ VA Sch Med

Irby III, Pierce B MD [U] - **Spec Exp:** Kidney Stones; Minimally Invasive Surgery; Vasectomy & Vasectomy Reversal; **Hospital:** Carolinas Med Ctr, Presby Hosp - Charlotte; **Address:** McKay Urology, 1023 Edgehill Rd S, Charlotte, NC 28207; **Phone:** 704-355-8686; **Board Cert:** Urology 2003; **Med School:** Uniformed Srvs Univ, Bethesda 1983; **Resid:** Urology, Letterman Army Med Ctr 1990; **Fellow:** Endourology, UCSF Med Ctr 1992; **Fac Appt:** Asst Clin Prof U, Univ NC Sch Med

Jordan, Gerald H MD [U] - **Spec Exp:** Incontinence; Urinary Reconstruction; Prostate Cancer; **Hospital:** Sentara Norfolk Genl Hosp; **Address:** 400 W Brambleton Ave, Ste 100, Norfolk, VA 23510; **Phone:** 757-457-5100; **Board Cert:** Urology 1984; **Med School:** Univ Tex, San Antonio 1977; **Resid:** Urology, Naval Reg Med Ctr 1978; **Fellow:** Reconstructive Surgery, Eastern Va Med Sch 1984; **Fac Appt:** Prof U, Eastern VA Med Sch

Joseph, David B MD [U] - **Spec Exp:** Pediatric Urology; Urodynamics; **Hospital:** Children's Hospital - Birmingham; **Address:** Childrens Hospital, Dept Urology, 1600 7th Ave S, Ste ACC-318, Birmingham, AL 35233; **Phone:** 205-934-6149; **Board Cert:** Urology 1997; **Med School:** Univ Wisc 1980; **Resid:** Urology, Univ Wisconsin Med Ctr 1985; **Fellow:** Pediatric Urology, Boston Childrens Hosp 1986; **Fac Appt:** Prof U, Univ Ala

Keane, Thomas E MD [U] - **Spec Exp:** Urologic Cancer; Genitourinary Cancer; Prostate Cancer; Clinical Trials; **Hospital:** MUSC Med Ctr; **Address:** MUSC-Urology Dept, 96 Jonathan Lucas St, Ste CSB644, Charleston, SC 29425; **Phone:** 843-792-1666; **Board Cert:** Urology 2003; **Med School:** Ireland 1981; **Resid:** Urology, St Vincents Hosp 1986; Urology, N Tees Gen Hosp 1988; **Fellow:** Urology, Duke Univ Med Ctr 1993; **Fac Appt:** Prof U, Univ SC Sch Med

Kennelly, Michael J MD [U] - **Spec Exp:** Incontinence; Voiding Dysfunction; Pelvic Organ Prolapse Repair; Neurogenic Bladder; **Hospital:** Carolinas Med Ctr, Presby Hosp - Charlotte; **Address:** 1023 Edgehill Rd S, Charlotte, NC 28207; **Phone:** 704-355-8686; **Board Cert:** Urology 2005; **Med School:** Univ Cincinnati 1989; **Resid:** Urology, Univ Mich Med Ctr 1994; **Fellow:** Neurology, Univ Tex Hlth Sci Ctr 1995; **Fac Appt:** Clin Prof U, Univ NC Sch Med

Kim, Edward D MD [U] - **Spec Exp:** Infertility-Male; Prostate Cancer; Bladder Cancer; **Hospital:** Univ of Tennesee Mem Hosp; **Address:** University Urology, 1928 Alcoa Hwy, Med Office B-Bldg-Ste 222, Knoxville, TN 37920; **Phone:** 865-544-9254; **Board Cert:** Urology 1998; **Med School:** Northwestern Univ 1989; **Resid:** Urology, Northwestern Meml Hosp 1995; **Fellow:** Baylor Coll Med 1996; **Fac Appt:** Assoc Prof U, Univ Tenn Coll Med, Memphis

Lloyd, Lewis Keith MD [U] - **Spec Exp:** Erectile Dysfunction; Incontinence; Interstitial Cystitis; Voiding Dysfunction; **Hospital:** Univ of Ala Hosp at Birmingham; **Address:** FOT 1120, 510 20th St S, Birmingham, AL 35294-3411; **Phone:** 205-975-0088; **Board Cert:** Urology 1976; **Med School:** Tulane Univ 1966; **Resid:** Urology, Tulane Univ Hosp 1974; **Fac Appt:** Prof U, Univ Ala

Lockhart, Jorge L MD [U] - **Spec Exp:** Voiding Dysfunction; Urologic Cancer; **Hospital:** H Lee Moffitt Cancer Ctr & Research Inst, Tampa Genl Hosp; **Address:** H Lee Moffitt Cancer Ctr, Dept Urology, 12902 Magnolia Drive, Tampa, FL 33612; **Phone:** 813-745-6033; **Board Cert:** Urology 1980; **Med School:** Uruguay 1973; **Resid:** Urology, Duke Univ Med Ctr 1977; **Fellow:** Urodynamics, Duke Univ Med Ctr 1978; **Fac Appt:** Prof S, Univ S Fla Coll Med

Lynne, Charles M MD [U] - **Spec Exp:** Infertility-Male in Spinal Cord Injury; Voiding Dysfunction/Spinal Cord Injury; Urodynamics; **Hospital:** Jackson Meml Hosp, Cedars Med Ctr - Miami; **Address:** Univ Miami, Dept Urology 814, PO Box 016960, Miami, FL 33101; **Phone:** 305-243-6590; **Board Cert:** Urology 1974; **Med School:** Univ Miami Sch Med 1964; **Resid:** Urology, Univ Miami Affil Hosps 1971; **Fac Appt:** Prof U, Univ Miami Sch Med

Marshall, Fray F MD [U] - **Spec Exp:** Urologic Cancer; Prostate Cancer; Kidney Cancer; **Hospital:** Emory Univ Hosp; **Address:** Emory Clinic, Dept Urology, 1365 Clifton Rd NE B Bldg - Ste 1400, Atlanta, GA 30322; **Phone:** 404-778-4898; **Board Cert:** Urology 1977; **Med School:** Univ VA Sch Med 1969; **Resid:** Surgery, Univ Mich Hosps 1972; Urology, Mass Genl Hosp 1975; **Fac Appt:** Prof U, Emory Univ

Milam, Douglas F MD [U] - **Spec Exp:** Urodynamics; Voiding Dysfunction; **Hospital:** Vanderbilt Univ Med Ctr; **Address:** Vanderbilt Univ Med Ctr North, Dept Urol, rm A-1302, Nashville, TN 37232-2765; **Phone:** 615-322-2880; **Board Cert:** Urology 2003; **Med School:** W VA Univ 1986; **Resid:** Surgery, Univ Utah Hosps 1988; Urology, Univ Utah Hosps 1991; **Fac Appt:** Assoc Prof U, Vanderbilt Univ

Moul, Judd W MD [U] - **Spec Exp:** Prostate Cancer; Testicular Cancer; **Hospital:** Duke Univ Med Ctr, Durham Regional Hosp; **Address:** Duke Univ Med Ctr, Div Urologic Surgery, Box 3707, Durham, NC 27710; **Phone:** 919-684-2446; **Board Cert:** Urology 1999; **Med School:** Jefferson Med Coll 1982; **Resid:** Urology, Walter Reed Army Med Ctr 1987; **Fellow:** Urologic Oncology, Duke Univ Med Ctr 1989; **Fac Appt:** Prof S, Duke Univ

Patterson, Anthony L MD [U] - **Spec Exp:** Laparoscopic Surgery; Kidney Stones; **Hospital:** Univ of Tennesee Mem Hosp; **Address:** UT Medical Group, 7945 Wolf River Blvd, Ste 350, Germantown, TN 38138-1733; **Phone:** 901-347-8350; **Board Cert:** Urology 1999; **Med School:** Univ Tenn Coll Med, Memphis 1982; **Resid:** Surgery, Univ Tenn Med Ctr 1984; Urology, Univ Tenn Med Ctr 1987; **Fac Appt:** Assoc Prof U, Univ Tenn Coll Med, Memphis

Preminger, Glenn M MD [U] - **Spec Exp:** Kidney Stones; **Hospital:** Duke Univ Med Ctr; **Address:** Duke Univ Med Ctr, Div Urologic Surgery, rm 1587, Box 3167, White Zone Duke S, Durham, NC 27710; **Phone:** 919-684-4226; **Board Cert:** Urology 2003; **Med School:** NY Med Coll 1977; **Resid:** Surgery, N Carolina Meml Hosp 1979; Urology, N Carolina Meml Hosp 1983; **Fellow:** Urology, Univ Texas SW Med Ctr 1985; **Fac Appt:** Prof U, Duke Univ

Robertson, Cary N MD [U] - **Spec Exp:** Prostate Cancer; Kidney Cancer; High Intensity Focused Ultrasound(HIFU); Testicular Cancer; **Hospital:** Duke Univ Med Ctr; **Address:** Duke Univ Med Ctr, Trent Drive, Box 3833, Durham, NC 27710; **Phone:** 919-681-6768; **Board Cert:** Urology 2005; **Med School:** Tulane Univ 1977; **Resid:** Urology, Duke Univ Med Ctr 1985; **Fellow:** Urologic Oncology, Natl Inst Hlth 1987; **Fac Appt:** Assoc Prof U, Duke Univ

Rowland, Randall MD [U] - **Spec Exp:** Urologic Cancer; **Hospital:** Univ of Kentucky Chandler Hosp; **Address:** Univ Kentucky Med Ctr, Div Urology, 800 Rose St, rm MS283, Lexington, KY 40536-0298; **Phone:** 859-323-6677; **Board Cert:** Urology 1980; **Med School:** Northwestern Univ 1972; **Resid:** Urology, Northwestern Meml Hosp 1978; **Fac Appt:** Prof U, Univ KY Coll Med

Sanders, William H MD [U] - **Spec Exp:** Prostate Cancer; Kidney Stones; Kidney Cancer; **Hospital:** St Joseph's Hosp - Atlanta, Northside Hosp; **Address:** 5673 Peachtree Dunwoody Rd, Ste 910, Atlanta, GA 30342-1767; **Phone:** 404-255-3822; **Board Cert:** Urology 2006; **Med School:** Emory Univ 1988; **Resid:** Urology, Yale-New Haven Hosp 1993

Schellhammer, Paul MD [U] - **Spec Exp:** Prostate Cancer; Urologic Cancer; **Hospital:** Sentara Norfolk Genl Hosp; **Address:** 6333 Center Drive Bldg 16, Norfolk, VA 23502; **Phone:** 757-457-5100; **Board Cert:** Urology 1999; **Med School:** Cornell Univ-Weill Med Coll 1966; **Resid:** Surgery, Univ Hosps 1968; Urology, Med Coll Va Hosp 1973; **Fellow:** Urology, Memorial Hosp 1974; **Fac Appt:** Prof U, Eastern VA Med Sch

Shaban, Stephen F MD [U] - **Spec Exp:** Infertility-Male; **Hospital:** Rex HlthCare, WakeMed New Bern; **Address:** 3320 Wake Forest Rd, Ste 320, Raleigh, NC 27609; **Phone:** 919-790-5500; **Board Cert:** Urology 2004; **Med School:** Mount Sinai Sch Med 1982; **Resid:** Urology, Univ S Fla 1987; **Fellow:** Male Reproduction, Baylor Coll Med 1988; **Fac Appt:** Prof U, Univ NC Sch Med

Smith, Joseph A MD [U] - **Spec Exp:** Prostate Cancer/Robotic Surgery; Bladder Cancer; Kidney Cancer; **Hospital:** Vanderbilt Univ Med Ctr; **Address:** Vanderbilt Univ Med Ctr, Dept Urology, A-1302 MCN, Nashville, TN 37232-2765; **Phone:** 615-343-0234; **Board Cert:** Urology 2000; **Med School:** Univ Tenn Coll Med, Memphis 1974; **Resid:** Surgery, Parkland Meml Hosp 1976; Urology, Univ Utah 1979; **Fellow:** Urologic Oncology, Meml Sloan Kettering Cancer Ctr 1980; **Fac Appt:** Prof U, Vanderbilt Univ

Soloway, Mark S MD [U] - **Spec Exp:** Bladder Cancer; Kidney Cancer; Prostate Cancer; **Hospital:** Jackson Meml Hosp, Cedars Med Ctr - Miami; **Address:** 1150 NW 14th St, Ste 309, Miami, FL 33136; **Phone:** 305-243-6596; **Board Cert:** Urology 1977; **Med School:** Case West Res Univ 1968; **Resid:** Surgery, Univ Hosps 1970; Urology, Univ Hosps 1975; **Fellow:** Surgery, Natl Cancer Inst 1972; **Fac Appt:** Prof U, Univ Miami Sch Med

Steers, William D MD [U] - **Spec Exp:** Incontinence; Erectile Dysfunction; Robotic Surgery; **Hospital:** Univ Virginia Med Ctr; **Address:** UVA Hlth System, Dept Urology, PO Box 800422, Charlottesville, VA 22908-0422; **Phone:** 434-924-9107; **Board Cert:** Urology 1999; **Med School:** Med Coll OH 1980; **Resid:** Urology, Univ Tex Hlth Sci Ctr 1986; **Fellow:** Neurology, Univ Pittsburgh Med Ctr 1988; **Fac Appt:** Prof U, Univ VA Sch Med

Teigland, Chris M MD [U] - **Spec Exp:** Prostate Cancer/Robotic Surgery; Kidney Cancer; **Hospital:** Carolinas Med Ctr; **Address:** Mckay Urology, 1023 Edgehill Rd S, Charlotte, NC 28207; **Phone:** 704-355-8686; **Board Cert:** Urology 1999; **Med School:** Duke Univ 1980; **Resid:** Surgery, Univ Utah Affil Hosps 1982; Urology, Univ Texas SW Med Ctr 1987; **Fac Appt:** Clin Prof S, Univ NC Sch Med

Terris, Martha K MD [U] - **Spec Exp:** Prostate Cancer; Brachytherapy; Urologic Cancer; Bladder Cancer; **Hospital:** VA Medical Ctr - Augusta, Med Coll of GA Hosp and Clin; **Address:** Augusta VA Administration Hosp, 1 Freedom Way, Augusta, GA 30904; **Phone:** 706-733-0188; **Board Cert:** Urology 1998; **Med School:** Univ Miss 1986; **Resid:** Surgery, Duke Univ Med Ctr 1988; Urology, Stanford Univ Med Ctr 1995; **Fellow:** Ultrasound, Stanford Univ Med Ctr 1991; **Fac Appt:** Prof S, Med Coll GA

Webster, George D MD [U] - **Spec Exp:** Reconstructive Urologic Surgery; Urology-Female; Urodynamics; **Hospital:** Duke Univ Med Ctr; **Address:** Duke Univ Medical Ctr -Dept Urolology, Box 3146, Durham, NC 27710; **Phone:** 919-684-2516; **Board Cert:** Urology 1981; **Med School:** England 1968; **Resid:** Surgery, Harare Hosp 1972; Urology, Inst Urology 1974; **Fellow:** Urology, Duke Univ Med Ctr 1978; **Fac Appt:** Prof U, Duke Univ

Midwest

Andriole, Gerald L MD [U] - **Spec Exp:** Urologic Cancer; Prostate Cancer; Laparoscopic Surgery; **Hospital:** Barnes-Jewish Hosp; **Address:** 4960 Children's Place, Campus Box 8242, St Louis, MO 63110; **Phone:** 314-362-8212; **Board Cert:** Urology 2003; **Med School:** Jefferson Med Coll 1978; **Resid:** Surgery, Strong Meml Hosp 1980; Urology, Brigham & Womens Hosp 1983; **Fellow:** Urologic Oncology, NCI/NIH 1985; **Fac Appt:** Prof U, Washington Univ, St Louis

Bahnson, Robert MD [U] - **Spec Exp:** Prostate Cancer; Bladder Cancer; Continent Urinary Diversions; **Hospital:** Ohio St Univ Med Ctr, Arthur G James Cancer Hosp & Research Inst; **Address:** 456 West 10th Avenue, Dept of Urology, 4980 Cramblett Med Ctr, Columbus, OH 43210-1240; **Phone:** 614-293-8155; **Board Cert:** Urology 2006; **Med School:** Tufts Univ 1979; **Resid:** Surgery, Northwestern Univ 1981; Urology, Northwestern Univ 1985; **Fellow:** Urology, Northwestern Univ 1984; Research, Univ Pittsburgh 1991; **Fac Appt:** Prof U, Ohio State Univ

Bloom, David A MD [U] - **Spec Exp:** Pediatric Urology; Voiding Dysfunction; Genitourinary Reconstruction; **Hospital:** Univ Michigan Hlth Sys; **Address:** Univ Mich, Dept Ped Urology, 1500 E Med Ctr Dr, F-7805 Mott, Ann Arbor, MI 48109-0330; **Phone:** 734-615-0200; **Board Cert:** Urology 1982; **Med School:** SUNY Buffalo 1971; **Resid:** Urology, UCLA Med Ctr 1980; Surgery, UCLA Med Ctr 1976; **Fellow:** Pediatric Urology, Inst Urol-St Peters Hosp 1978; **Fac Appt:** Prof U, Univ Mich Med Sch

Brendler, Charles B MD [U] - **Spec Exp:** Prostate Cancer; **Hospital:** Evanston NW Hlthcare; **Address:** Evanston Northwestern Hosp, 2650 Ridge Ave Walgreen Bldg - Ste 2507, Evanston, IL 60201; **Phone:** 847-547-1090; **Board Cert:** Urology 1981; **Med School:** Univ VA Sch Med 1974; **Resid:** Surgery, Duke Univ Med Ctr 1976; Urology, Duke Univ Med Ctr 1979; **Fellow:** Urologic Oncology, Univ Hosp Wales 1980; Urologic Oncology, Johns Hopkins Hosp 1982; **Fac Appt:** Prof U, Univ Chicago-Pritzker Sch Med

Bruskewitz, Reginald C MD [U] - **Spec Exp:** Urologic Cancer; Prostate Disease; **Hospital:** Univ WI Hosp & Clins; **Address:** Univ Wisconsin Hosp, Urology, 600 Highland Ave, C-52, Madison, WI 53792; **Phone:** 608-263-4757; **Board Cert:** Urology 1981; **Med School:** Univ Wisc 1973; **Resid:** Urology, Univ Wisconsin Hosp 1978; **Fellow:** Urodynamics, UCLA Med Ctr 1979; **Fac Appt:** Assoc Prof S, Univ Wisc

Bushman, Wade MD [U] - **Spec Exp:** Neuro-Urology; Urodynamics; Urology-Female; **Hospital:** Univ WI Hosp & Clins; **Address:** Univ Wisconsin, C5/350 Clin Sci Ctr, 600 Highland Ave, Madison, WI 53792-3236; **Phone:** 608-263-4757; **Board Cert:** Urology 1997; **Med School:** Univ Chicago-Pritzker Sch Med 1986; **Resid:** Urology, Univ VA Med Ctr 1992; **Fac Appt:** Assoc Prof U, Univ Wisc

Campbell, Steven C MD/PhD [U] - **Spec Exp:** Kidney Cancer; Prostate Cancer; Bladder Cancer; **Hospital:** Cleveland Clin Fdn (page 57); **Address:** Cleveland Clinic/Glickman Urological Inst, 9500 Euclid Ave, Desk A100, Cleveland, OH 44195; **Phone:** 216-444-5595; **Board Cert:** Urology 1999; **Med School:** Univ Chicago-Pritzker Sch Med 1989; **Resid:** Urology, Cleveland Clinic 1995; **Fellow:** Urology, Meml Sloan Kettering Cancer Ctr 1996; **Fac Appt:** Prof S, Cleveland Cl Coll Med/Case West Res

Catalona, William J MD [U] - **Spec Exp:** Urologic Cancer; Prostate Cancer; Prostate Disease; **Hospital:** Northwestern Meml Hosp; **Address:** Northwestern Med Faculty Foundation, 675 N St Clair St, Ste 20-150, Chicago, IL 60611; **Phone:** 312-695-6126; **Board Cert:** Urology 1978; **Med School:** Yale Univ 1968; **Resid:** Surgery, UCSF Med Ctr 1970; Urology, Johns Hopkins Hosp 1976; **Fellow:** Surgical Oncology, Natl Cancer Inst 1972; **Fac Appt:** Prof U, Northwestern Univ

Chodak, Gerald MD [U] - **Spec Exp:** Prostate Cancer; Prostate Disease; **Hospital:** Weiss Meml Hosp; **Address:** 4646 N Marine Drive, Ste A5500, Chicago, IL 60640-5759; **Phone:** 773-564-5006; **Board Cert:** Urology 1984; **Med School:** SUNY Buffalo 1975; **Resid:** Surgery, UCLA Med Ctr 1977; Urology, Brigham & Womens Hosp 1979; **Fellow:** Research, Univ Chicago 1981; Research, Harvard/Chldns Hosp 1982

Coplen, Douglas E MD [U] - **Spec Exp:** Pediatric Urology; Urologic Cancer-Pediatric; Testicular Cancer-Pediatric; Fetal Urology; **Hospital:** St Louis Chldns Hosp; **Address:** St. Louis Children's Hosp, 4990 Children's Pl, Ste 1120, St Louis, MO 63110; **Phone:** 314-454-6034; **Board Cert:** Urology 1996; **Med School:** Indiana Univ 1985; **Resid:** Urology, Barnes Jewish Hosp 1992; **Fellow:** Pediatric Urology, Children's Hosp 1994; **Fac Appt:** Asst Prof S, Washington Univ, St Louis

Donovan Jr, James F MD [U] - **Spec Exp:** Prostate Cancer/Robotic Surgery; Urologic Surgery; Kidney Cancer; Adrenal Tumors; **Hospital:** Univ Hosp - Cincinnati, Christ Hospital; **Address:** Univ Cincinnati Med Ctr, Medical Arts Bldg, 222 Piedmont Ave, Ste 7000, Cincinnati, OH 45219; **Phone:** 513-475-8787; **Board Cert:** Surgery 1997; Urology 1999; **Med School:** Northwestern Univ 1978; **Resid:** Surgery, Northwestern Meml Hosp 1982; Urology, Northwestern Meml Hosp 1986; **Fellow:** Male Infertility, Baylor Coll Med 1986; **Fac Appt:** Prof U, Univ Cincinnati

Elder, Jack S MD [U] - **Spec Exp:** Pediatric Urology; Hypospadias; Urinary Reconstruction; **Hospital:** Rainbow Babies & Chldns Hosp, MetroHealth Med Ctr; **Address:** Rainbow Babies & Children's Hosp, Dept Pediatric Urology, 11100 Euclid Ave, Ste 2311, Cleveland, OH 44106-6011; **Phone:** 216-844-8455; **Board Cert:** Urology 1984; **Med School:** Univ Okla Coll Med 1976; **Resid:** Surgery, Yale-New Haven Hosp 1978; Urology, Johns Hopkins Hosp 1982; **Fellow:** Pediatric Urology, Johns Hopkins Hosp 1982; Pediatric Urology, Children's Hosp 1986; **Fac Appt:** Prof U, Case West Res Univ

Firlit, Casimir MD/PhD [U] - **Spec Exp:** Pediatric Urology; Genitourinary Reconstruction; Transplant-Kidney-Pediatric; **Hospital:** Cardinal Glennon Mem Children's Hosp; **Address:** Cardinal Glennon Chlds Hosp, 1465 S Grand Blvd Fl 5, Glennon Hall, St Louis, MO 63104; **Phone:** 314-577-5334; **Board Cert:** Urology 1975; **Med School:** Loyola Univ-Stritch Sch Med 1965; **Resid:** Surgery, Hines VA Hosp 1970; Urology, Hines VA Hosp 1973; **Fellow:** Pediatric Urology, Chldns Meml Hosp 1974; **Fac Appt:** Prof U, Univ MO-Columbia Sch Med

Flanigan, Robert C MD [U] - **Spec Exp:** Prostate Cancer; Bladder Cancer; Transplant-Kidney; Kidney Cancer; **Hospital:** Loyola Univ Med Ctr, Hines VA Hosp; **Address:** Loyola Univ Med-Fahey Bldg 54, 2160 S First Ave, rm 267, Maywood, IL 60153; **Phone:** 708-216-5100; **Board Cert:** Surgery 1998; Urology 2001; **Med School:** Case West Res Univ 1972; **Resid:** Surgery, Case West Univ Med Ctr 1978; Urology, Case West Univ Med Ctr 1978; **Fac Appt:** Prof U, Loyola Univ-Stritch Sch Med

Foster, Richard S MD [U] - **Spec Exp:** Testicular Cancer; **Hospital:** Indiana Univ Hosp; **Address:** 535 N Barnhill Drive, Ste 420, Indianapolis, IN 46202; **Phone:** 317-274-3458; **Board Cert:** Urology 1998; **Med School:** Indiana Univ 1980; **Resid:** Urology, Indiana Univ Hosp 1986; **Fac Appt:** Prof U, Indiana Univ

Gill, Inderbir Singh MD [U] - **Spec Exp:** Prostate Cancer; Kidney Cancer; Urologic Cancer; Laparoscopic Surgery; **Hospital:** Cleveland Clin Fdn (page 57); **Address:** Cleveland Clinic Urological Inst, 9500 Euclid Ave, Ste A100, Cleveland, OH 44195; **Phone:** 216-445-1530; **Board Cert:** Urology 1997; **Med School:** India 1980; **Resid:** Surgery, Dayanand Med Coll & Hosp; Urology, Univ Kentucky Hosp 1993; **Fellow:** Cleveland Clinic

Gluckman, Gordon MD [U] - **Spec Exp:** Prostate Cancer; Kidney Cancer; Minimally Invasive Urologic Surgery; **Hospital:** Adv Luth Genl Hosp, Resurrection Med Ctr; **Address:** Parkside Center, 1875 Dempster St, Ste 506, Park Ridge, IL 60068; **Phone:** 847-823-4700; **Board Cert:** Urology 2005; **Med School:** Northwestern Univ 1989; **Resid:** Surgery, UCSF Med Ctr 1991; Urology, UCSF Med Ctr 1995

Gujral, Saroj K MD [U] - **Spec Exp:** Urologic Cancer; Urology-Female; **Hospital:** Albert Lea Med Ctr-Mayo Hlth Sys; **Address:** 404 W Fountain St, Albert Lea, MN 56007; **Phone:** 507-379-2130; **Board Cert:** Urology 1979; **Med School:** India 1970; **Resid:** Urology, Suburban Hosp 1978; Urology, Dalhousie Univ Med Ctrs

Kass, Evan MD [U] - **Spec Exp:** Pediatric Urology; **Hospital:** William Beaumont Hosp; **Address:** 2221 Livernois, Ste 103, Troy, MI 48084; **Phone:** 248-519-0305; **Board Cert:** Urology 1978; **Med School:** SUNY Downstate 1968; **Resid:** Urology, Univ Mich Hosp 1976; **Fellow:** Pediatric Urology, Hosp for Sick Chldn 1978; **Fac Appt:** Assoc Prof U, Wayne State Univ

Klein, Eric A MD [U] - **Spec Exp:** Prostate Cancer; Testicular Cancer; Urologic Cancer; **Hospital:** Cleveland Clin Fdn (page 57); **Address:** Cleveland Clinic Fdn, Dept Urol, Sect Urol-Onc, 9500 Euclid Ave, Fl A100, Cleveland, OH 44195-0001; **Phone:** 216-444-5591; **Board Cert:** Urology 1999; **Med School:** Univ Pittsburgh 1981; **Resid:** Urology, Cleveland Clinic Fdn 1986; **Fellow:** Urologic Oncology, Meml Sloan Kettering Canc Ctr 1989; **Fac Appt:** Prof S, Cleveland Cl Coll Med/Case West Res

Klutke, Carl G MD [U] - **Spec Exp:** Urology-Female; Incontinence; Urodynamics; **Hospital:** Barnes-Jewish Hosp; **Address:** 1040 N Mason Rd, Ste 122, St Louis, MO 63141; **Phone:** 314-996-8060; **Board Cert:** Urology 2000; **Med School:** Univ Mich Med Sch 1983; **Resid:** Surgery, Henry Ford Hosp 1985; Urology, Henry Ford Hosp 1988; **Fellow:** Female Urology, UCLA Med Ctr 1989; **Fac Appt:** Assoc Prof S, Washington Univ, St Louis

Koff, Stephen A MD [U] - **Spec Exp:** Pediatric Urology; **Hospital:** Chldn's Hosp - Columbus; **Address:** Chldns Hosp, Dept Urology, 555 S 18th St, Ste 6D, Columbus, OH 43205; **Phone:** 614-722-3114; **Board Cert:** Urology 1978; **Med School:** Duke Univ 1969; **Resid:** Internal Medicine, NY Hosp-Cornell 1971; Urology, Univ Mich Med Ctr 1975; **Fellow:** Pediatric Urology, Alder Hey Chldns Hosp 1977; **Fac Appt:** Prof U, Ohio State Univ

Kozlowski, James M MD [U] - **Spec Exp:** Prostate Cancer; Continent Urinary Diversions; Laparoscopic Surgery; **Hospital:** Northwestern Meml Hosp, Jesse A Brown VA Med Ctr; **Address:** 675 N St Clair St, Galter Bldg Fl 20 - Ste 150, Chicago, IL 60611; **Phone:** 312-695-8146; **Board Cert:** Surgery 1993; Urology 1983; **Med School:** Northwestern Univ 1975; **Resid:** Surgery, Northwestern Univ-McGaw 1979; Urology, Northwestern Univ-McGaw 1981; **Fellow:** Research, NCI-Frederick Cancer Rsch 1984; **Fac Appt:** Assoc Prof U, Northwestern Univ

Levine, Laurence Adan MD [U] - **Spec Exp:** Erectile Dysfunction; Infertility-Male; Peyronie's Disease; Prostate Cancer; **Hospital:** Rush Univ Med Ctr; **Address:** 1725 W Harrison St, Ste 352, Chicago, IL 60612; **Phone:** 312-563-5000; **Board Cert:** Urology 1999; **Med School:** Univ Colorado 1980; **Resid:** Surgery, Tufts-New England Med Ctr 1982; Urology, Brigham & Women's Hosp/Harvard 1987; **Fac Appt:** Prof U, Rush Med Coll

McGuire, Edward J MD [U] - **Spec Exp:** Incontinence; Urology-Female; Neurogenic Bladder; **Hospital:** Univ Michigan Hlth Sys; **Address:** Univ Mich Med Ctr, Dept Urology, 1500 E Med Ctr Drive, rm 3888, 2916 Taubman Ctr, Box 2918B, Ann Arbor, MI 48109-0330; **Phone:** 734-936-7030; **Board Cert:** Urology 1975; **Med School:** Wayne State Univ 1965; **Resid:** Surgery, Yale-New Haven Hosp 1969; Urology, Yale-New Haven Hosp 1972; **Fac Appt:** Prof U, Univ Mich Med Sch

McVary, Kevin MD [U] - **Spec Exp:** Prostate Cancer; Erectile Dysfunction; Prostate Disease; **Hospital:** Northwestern Meml Hosp; **Address:** 675 N St Clair St, Galter Bldg Fl 20 - Ste 150, Chicago, IL 60611-4813; **Phone:** 312-695-8146; **Board Cert:** Urology 2000; **Med School:** Northwestern Univ 1983; **Resid:** Surgery, Northwestern Meml Hosp 1985; Urology, Northwestern Meml Hosp 1988; **Fellow:** Research, Northwestern Meml Hosp; **Fac Appt:** Prof U, Northwestern Univ

Menon, Mani MD [U] - **Spec Exp:** Prostate Cancer/Robotic Surgery; Transplant-Kidney; Urologic Cancer; **Hospital:** Henry Ford Hosp; **Address:** Henry Ford Hosp - Vattikuti Urology Inst, 2799 W Grand Bvd, Clinic Bldg - #K-9, Detroit, MI 48202; **Phone:** 313-916-2062; **Board Cert:** Urology 1982; **Med School:** India 1969; **Resid:** Urology, Bryn Mawr Hosp 1974; Urology, Johns Hopkins Hosp 1980; **Fellow:** Transplant Surgery, Johns Hopkins Univ 1977; **Fac Appt:** Prof S, Univ Mass Sch Med

Mesrobian, Hrair-George O MD [U] - **Spec Exp:** Pediatric Urology; **Hospital:** Chldns Hosp - Wisconsin; **Address:** 999 N 92nd St, Ste 330, Milwaukee, WI 53226; **Phone:** 414-266-3794; **Board Cert:** Urology 2005; **Med School:** Lebanon 1978; **Resid:** Surgery, SUNY Upstate Med Ctr 1980; Urology, UCSF Med Ctr 1983; **Fellow:** Pediatric Urology, Mayo Clinic 1984; **Fac Appt:** Prof U, Med Coll Wisc

Mitchell, Michael E MD [U] - **Spec Exp:** Genitourinary Congenital Abnormality; Pediatric Urology; Bladder reconstruction; **Hospital:** Chldns Hosp - Wisconsin; **Address:** Children's Hospital of Wisconsin, 999 N 92nd St, Ste 330, Milwaukee, WI 53226; **Phone:** 414-266-3794; **Board Cert:** Urology 2000; **Med School:** Harvard Med Sch 1969; **Resid:** Surgery, Peter Bent Brigham Hosp 1974; Urology, Mass Genl Hosp 1977; **Fellow:** Pediatric Urology, Mass Genl Hosp 1978; **Fac Appt:** Prof U, Univ Wisc

Montague, Drogo K MD [U] - **Spec Exp:** Erectile Dysfunction; Genitourinary Prosthetics; Incontinence; **Hospital:** Cleveland Clin Fdn (page 57); **Address:** Cleveland Clinic Foundation-Urological Inst, 9500 Euclid Ave, Ste A100, Cleveland, OH 44195-5041; **Phone:** 216-444-5590; **Board Cert:** Urology 1975; **Med School:** Univ Mich Med Sch 1968; **Resid:** Surgery, Cleveland Clinic 1970; Urology, Cleveland Clinic 1973; **Fac Appt:** Prof U, Cleveland Cl Coll Med/Case West Res

Montie, James MD [U] - **Spec Exp:** Bladder Cancer; Prostate Cancer; Genitourinary Cancer; **Hospital:** Univ Michigan Hlth Sys; **Address:** 1500 E Medical Ctr Dr, Dept Urology, Taubman Hlth Care Ctr, rm 3876, Box 0330, Ann Arbor, MI 48109-0330; **Phone:** 734-647-8903; **Board Cert:** Urology 1978; **Med School:** Univ Mich Med Sch 1971; **Resid:** Urology, Cleveland Clinic Fdn 1976; **Fellow:** Urologic Oncology, Meml Sloan-Kettering Cancer Ctr 1979; **Fac Appt:** Prof U, Univ Mich Med Sch

Myers, Robert P MD [U] - **Spec Exp:** Prostate Cancer; **Hospital:** Mayo Med Ctr & Clin - Rochester, Rochester Meth Hosp; **Address:** Mayo Clinic, Dept Urology, 200 First St SW, Rochester, MN 55905; **Phone:** 507-284-3077; **Board Cert:** Urology 1976; **Med School:** Columbia P&S 1967; **Resid:** Urology, Mayo Clinic 1972; **Fac Appt:** Prof U, Mayo Med Sch

Novick, Andrew MD [U] - **Spec Exp:** Transplant-Kidney; Kidney Cancer; Urologic Cancer; **Hospital:** Cleveland Clin Fdn (page 57); **Address:** Cleveland Clinic-Urological Inst, 9500 Euclid Ave, Desk A100, Cleveland, OH 44195; **Phone:** 216-444-5600; **Board Cert:** Urology 1996; **Med School:** McGill Univ 1972; **Resid:** Surgery, Royal Victoria Hosp 1974; Urology, Cleveland Clinic 1977; **Fac Appt:** Prof S, Cleveland Cl Coll Med/Case West Res

O'Donnell, Michael A MD [U] - **Spec Exp:** Bladder Cancer; Immunotherapy; Urologic Cancer; **Hospital:** Univ Iowa Hosp & Clinics; **Address:** Univ Iowa Hosp & Clins, Dept Urology, 200 Hawkins Drive, 3RCP, Iowa City, IA 52242-1089; **Phone:** 319-384-6040; **Board Cert:** Urology 2005; **Med School:** Duke Univ 1984; **Resid:** Surgery, Brigham & Womens Hosp 1987; Urology, Brigham & Womens Hosp 1991; **Fellow:** Urology, Brigham & Womens Hosp 1993; **Fac Appt:** Prof U, Univ Iowa Coll Med

Ohl, Dana Alan MD [U] - **Spec Exp:** Infertility-Male; Erectile Dysfunction; **Hospital:** Univ Michigan Hlth Sys; **Address:** Michigan Urology Ctr, 1500 E Med Ctr Drive, Ann Arbor, MI 48109-0330; **Phone:** 734-936-7030; **Board Cert:** Urology 1999; **Med School:** Univ Mich Med Sch 1982; **Resid:** Urology, Univ Mich Hosps 1987; **Fac Appt:** Prof U, Univ Mich Med Sch

Rink, Richard C MD [U] - **Spec Exp:** Pediatric Urology; Reconstructive Urologic Surgery; Genital Reconstruction; **Hospital:** Riley Hosp for Children, Indiana Univ Hosp; **Address:** Indiana Univ Med Ctr, 702 Barnhill Drive, Ste 4230, Indianapolis, IN 46202-5128; **Phone:** 317-274-7472; **Board Cert:** Urology 2004; **Med School:** Indiana Univ 1978; **Resid:** Surgery, Emory Univ Med Ctr 1980; Urology, Indiana Univ Med Ctr 1984; **Fellow:** Pediatrics, Chldns Hosp-Harvard 1985; **Fac Appt:** Prof U, Indiana Univ

Ross, Lawrence S MD [U] - **Spec Exp:** Infertility-Male; Erectile Dysfunction; Prostate Disease; **Hospital:** Univ of IL Med Ctr at Chicago; **Address:** 60 E Delaware Ave, Ste 1420, Chicago, IL 60611; **Phone:** 312-440-5127; **Board Cert:** Urology 1974; **Med School:** Univ Chicago-Pritzker Sch Med 1965; **Resid:** Urology, Michael Reese Hosp 1970; **Fac Appt:** Prof U, Univ IL Coll Med

Sandlow, Jay MD [U] - **Spec Exp:** Infertility-Male; Varicocele Microsurgery; Vasectomy & Vasectomy Reversal; **Hospital:** Froedtert Meml Lutheran Hosp; **Address:** Med Coll of WI, Urology Dept, 9200 W Wisconsin Ave, Milwakee, WI 53226-3522; **Phone:** 414-456-6977; **Board Cert:** Urology 2005; **Med School:** Rush Med Coll 1987; **Resid:** Surgery, Univ Iowa Hosps 1993; **Fellow:** Infertility, Univ Iowa Hosps 1995; **Fac Appt:** Assoc Prof U, Med Coll Wisc

Schaeffer, Anthony MD [U] - **Spec Exp:** Interstitial Cystitis; Incontinence after Prostate Cancer; Urology-Female; **Hospital:** Northwestern Meml Hosp; **Address:** 675 N St Clair, Galter Bldg Fl 20 - Ste 150, Chicago, IL 60611; **Phone:** 312-695-8146; **Board Cert:** Urology 1978; **Med School:** Northwestern Univ 1968; **Resid:** Surgery, Northwestern Meml Hosp 1970; Urology, Stanford Med Ctr 1976; **Fac Appt:** Prof U, Northwestern Univ

See, William MD [U] - **Spec Exp:** Prostate Cancer; Bladder Cancer; Testicular Cancer; **Hospital:** Froedtert Meml Lutheran Hosp; **Address:** Med Coll Wisconsin, Dept Urology, 9200 W Wisconsin Ave, Milwaukee, WI 53226; **Phone:** 414-456-6950; **Board Cert:** Urology 2000; **Med School:** Univ Chicago-Pritzker Sch Med 1982; **Resid:** Urology, Univ Washington 1988; **Fellow:** Research, Natl Kidney Fdn/Univ Wash 1986; Research, Amer Fdn for Urol Dis/Univ Iowa 1990; **Fac Appt:** Prof U, Med Coll Wisc

Seftel, Allen D MD [U] - **Spec Exp:** Sexual Dysfunction-Male & Female; Infertility-Male; Prostate Disease; **Hospital:** Univ Hosps Case Med Ctr; **Address:** Univ Hosp-Cleveland, 11100 Euclid Ave, MS 5046, Cleveland, OH 44106-1736; **Phone:** 216-844-3009; **Board Cert:** Urology 2003; **Med School:** SUNY Downstate 1984; **Resid:** Urology, SUNY Downstate Med Ctr 1987; Urology, Univ Hosps-Case West Res 1990; **Fellow:** Reproductive Medicine, Boston Univ Med Ctr 1992; **Fac Appt:** Prof U, Case West Res Univ

Silber, Sherman J MD [U] - **Spec Exp:** Infertility-Male; Vasectomy Reversal; Infertility-IVF; Transplant-Ovarian Tissue; **Hospital:** St Luke's Hosp - Chesterfield, MO; **Address:** 224 S Woods Mill Rd, Ste 730, St Louis, MO 63017-3451; **Phone:** 314-576-1400; **Board Cert:** Urology 1977; **Med School:** Univ Mich Med Sch 1966; **Resid:** Internal Medicine, PH Service Comm Corps 1969; Urology, Univ Michigan 1973; **Fellow:** Microsurgery, Univ Melbourne 1974

Steinberg, Gary D MD [U] - **Spec Exp:** Bladder Cancer; Kidney Cancer; Prostate Cancer; **Hospital:** Univ of Chicago Hosps; **Address:** 5841 S Maryland Ave, rm J653, MC 6038, Chicago, IL 60637; **Phone:** 773-702-3080; **Board Cert:** Urology 2003; **Med School:** Univ Chicago-Pritzker Sch Med 1985; **Resid:** Surgery, Johns Hopkins Hosp 1987; Urology, Brady Urol Inst/Johns Hopkins 1991; **Fellow:** Oncology, Johns Hopkins Hosp 1989; **Fac Appt:** Assoc Prof U, Univ Chicago-Pritzker Sch Med

Thomas Jr, Anthony J MD [U] - **Spec Exp:** Infertility-Male; Vasectomy Reversal; Fertility Preservation in Cancer; **Hospital:** Cleveland Clin Fdn (page 57); **Address:** Cleveland Clinic-Urological Inst, 9500 Euclid Ave, Desk A100, Cleveland, OH 44195; **Phone:** 216-444-5600; **Board Cert:** Urology 1978; **Med School:** Univ Cincinnati 1969; **Resid:** Surgery, Wayne State Univ Affil Hosp 1971; Urology, Wayne State Univ Affil Hosp 1976

Williams, Richard D MD [U] - **Spec Exp:** Kidney Cancer; Bladder Cancer; Prostate Cancer; **Hospital:** Univ Iowa Hosp & Clinics; **Address:** Univ Iowa Hosp, Dept Urology, 200 Hawkins Dr, rm 3251 RCP, Iowa City, IA 52242-1089; **Phone:** 319-356-0760; **Board Cert:** Urology 1979; **Med School:** Univ Kans 1970; **Resid:** Surgery, Univ Minn Hosp 1972; Urology, Univ Minn Hosp 1976; **Fellow:** Urologic Oncology, Univ Minn Hosp 1979; **Fac Appt:** Prof U, Univ Iowa Coll Med

Winfield, Howard N MD [U] - **Spec Exp:** Kidney Stones; Laparoscopic Surgery; Robotic Surgery; **Hospital:** Univ Iowa Hosp & Clinics; **Address:** Univ Iowa - Dept Urology, 200 Hawkins Drive, 3235 RCP, Iowa Ctiy, IA 52242-1089; **Phone:** 319-384-9183; **Board Cert:** Urology 1999; **Med School:** McGill Univ 1978; **Resid:** Urology, McGill Univ Tchg Hosp 1984; **Fellow:** Urology, Washington Univ 1985; Urology, UCLA 1986; **Fac Appt:** Prof U, Univ Iowa Coll Med

Wood, David P MD [U] - **Spec Exp:** Genitourinary Cancer; Bladder Cancer; Prostate Cancer; **Hospital:** Univ Michigan Hlth Sys; **Address:** Univ Mich, Dept Urology, 3875 Taubman Cancer Ctr, 1500 E Medical Center Drive, Ann Arbor, MI 48109-0999; **Phone:** 734-763-9269; **Board Cert:** Urology 2002; **Med School:** Univ Mich Med Sch 1983; **Resid:** Urology, Cleveland Clinic 1988; **Fellow:** Urologic Oncology, Meml Sloan-Kettering Cancer Ctr 1991; **Fac Appt:** Prof U, Univ Mich Med Sch

Zippe, Craig D MD [U] - **Spec Exp:** Prostate Cancer; Bladder Cancer; Incontinence after Prostate Cancer; **Hospital:** Cleveland Clin Fdn (page 57); **Address:** 12000 McCracken Rd, Ste 451, Garfield Heights, OH 44125; **Phone:** 216-587-4370; **Board Cert:** Urology 1997; **Med School:** Rush Med Coll 1980; **Resid:** Urology, Columbia Presby Med Ctr 1989; **Fellow:** Urologic Oncology, Meml Sloan Kettering Cancer Ctr 1992

Great Plains and Mountains

Cartwright, Patrick MD [U] - **Spec Exp:** Pediatric Urology; **Hospital:** Primary Children's Med Ctr, Univ Utah Hosps and Clins; **Address:** Pediatric Urology, 100 N Medical Dr, Ste 2200, Salt Lake City, UT 84113-1100; **Phone:** 801-662-5555; **Board Cert:** Urology 2001; **Med School:** Univ Tex SW, Dallas 1984; **Resid:** Urology, Univ Utah Affil Hosp 1989; **Fellow:** Pediatric Urology, Childrens Hosp 1990; **Fac Appt:** Assoc Prof S, Univ Utah

Childs, Stacy J MD [U] - **Spec Exp:** Voiding Dysfunction; Erectile Dysfunction; Prostate Cancer; Bladder Cancer; **Hospital:** Yampa Valley Med Ctr, Memorial Hosp - Craig; **Address:** 501 Anglers Drive, Ste 202, Steamboat Springs, CO 80487-8841; **Phone:** 970-871-9710; **Board Cert:** Urology 1979; **Med School:** Louisiana State Univ 1972; **Resid:** Urology, Carraway Meth Med Ctr 1977; **Fac Appt:** Clin Prof U, Univ Colorado

Crawford, E David MD [U] - **Spec Exp:** Prostate Cancer; Testicular Cancer; Bladder Cancer; **Hospital:** Univ Colorado Hosp; **Address:** Urologic Oncology, MS F710, 1665 N Ursula St, rm 1004, Box 6510, Aurora, CO 80045; **Phone:** 720-848-0170; **Board Cert:** Urology 1980; **Med School:** Univ Cincinnati 1973; **Resid:** Urology, Good Samaritan Hosp 1977; **Fellow:** Genitourinary Surgery, UCLA Med Ctr 1978; **Fac Appt:** Prof U, Univ Colorado

Davis, Bradley E MD [U] - **Spec Exp:** Urologic Cancer; Bladder Cancer; Reconstructive Surgery; Prostate Cancer; **Hospital:** Overland Pk Regl Med Ctr, St Luke's Hosp of Kansas City; **Address:** Urologic Surgical Associates, 10550 Quivira Rd, Ste 105, Overland Park, KS 66215; **Phone:** 913-438-3833; **Board Cert:** Urology 2004; **Med School:** Univ Kans 1986; **Resid:** Surgery, St Lukes Hosp 1991; Urology, Univ Kansas Med Ctr 1991; **Fellow:** Urologic Oncology, Meml Sloan-Kettering Cancer Ctr 1993; **Fac Appt:** Asst Clin Prof U, Univ Kans

Koyle, Martin A MD [U] - **Spec Exp:** Pediatric Urology; Genitourinary Reconstruction; Transplant-Kidney-Pediatric; **Hospital:** Chldn's Hosp - Denver, The, Univ Colorado Hosp; **Address:** Childrens Hosp, 1056 E 19th Ave, rm B-463, Denver, CO 80218-1007; **Phone:** 303-861-3926; **Board Cert:** Urology 2004; **Med School:** Canada 1976; **Resid:** Surgery, Hlth Scis Ctr 1978; Urology, Brigham & Womens Hosp 1984; **Fellow:** Transplant Surgery, Pacific Med Ctr 1982; **Fac Appt:** Prof U, Univ Colorado

Lugg, James A MD [U] - **Spec Exp:** Prostate Cancer; Laparoscopic Surgery; Incontinence after Prostate Cancer; **Hospital:** Cheyenne Regl Med Ctr, Univ Colorado Hosp; **Address:** 2301 House Ave, Ste 502, Cheyenne, WY 82001; **Phone:** 307-635-4131; **Board Cert:** Urology 1998; **Med School:** Northwestern Univ 1990; **Resid:** Urology, UCLA Med Ctr 1995; **Fac Appt:** Asst Prof U, Univ Colorado

Middleton, Richard MD [U] - **Spec Exp:** Urologic Cancer; Reconstructive Urologic Surgery; Infertility; **Hospital:** Univ Utah Hosps and Clins, VA Medical Center - Salt Lake City; **Address:** University of Utah Medical Ctr, 50 N Medical Drive, Salt Lake City, UT 84132; **Phone:** 801-587-4888; **Board Cert:** Urology 1970; **Med School:** Cornell Univ-Weill Med Coll 1958; **Resid:** Surgery, New York Hosp-Cornell Med Ctr 1961; Urology, New York Hosp-Cornell Med Ctr 1967; **Fac Appt:** Prof U, Univ Utah

Southwest

Appell, Rodney A MD [U] - **Spec Exp:** Voiding Dysfunction; Urology-Female; Uro-Gynecology; **Hospital:** Methodist Hosp - Houston; **Address:** 6560 Fannin St, Ste 2100, Houston, TX 77030; **Phone:** 713-798-6115; **Board Cert:** Urology 1981; **Med School:** Jefferson Med Coll 1973; **Resid:** Surgery, George Wash Univ Med Ctr 1975; **Fellow:** Urology, Yale Univ Sch Med 1979; **Fac Appt:** Prof U, Baylor Coll Med

Babaian, Richard MD [U] - **Spec Exp:** Prostate Cancer; **Hospital:** UT MD Anderson Cancer Ctr (page 71); **Address:** MD Anderson Cancer Ctr, 1515 Holcombe Blvd, Unit 1373, Houston, TX 77030; **Phone:** 713-792-3250; **Board Cert:** Urology 1980; **Med School:** Georgetown Univ 1972; **Resid:** Surgery, Univ Wisconsin 1974; Urology, Univ NC Hosp 1977; **Fellow:** Urologic Oncology, MD Anderson Cancer Ctr 1979; Immunology, Univ NC Hosps 1978; **Fac Appt:** Prof U, Univ Tex, Houston

Bans, Larry L MD [U] - **Spec Exp:** Prostate Cancer; Prostate Disease; **Hospital:** Banner Good Samaritan Regl Med Ctr - Phoenix; **Address:** Prostate Solutions of Arizona, 2525 E Arizona Biltmore Cir, Ste C236, Phoenix, AZ 85016; **Phone:** 602-426-9772; **Board Cert:** Urology 2004; **Med School:** Cornell Univ-Weill Med Coll 1978; **Resid:** Urology, Ind Univ Med Ctr 1983

Bardot, Stephen F MD [U] - **Spec Exp:** Urologic Cancer; Prostate Cancer; **Hospital:** Ochsner Fdn Hosp, Summit Hosp-Baton Rouge; **Address:** Ochsner Clinic, 1514 Jefferson Hwy Fl 4, Atrium 4 West, Dept of Urology, New Orleans, LA 70121-2483; **Phone:** 504-842-4083; **Board Cert:** Urology 1993; **Med School:** Univ Kans 1985; **Resid:** Surgery, St Luke's Hosp 1987; Urology, Kansas City Univ Med Ctr 1990; **Fellow:** Urologic Oncology, Cleveland Clinic 1991

Basler, Joseph W MD [U] - **Spec Exp:** Prostate Cancer; Urologic Cancer; Kidney Stones; **Hospital:** Audie L Murphy Meml Vets Hosp, Santa Rosa Hlth care Corp; **Address:** 7703 Floyd Curl Dr, MC-7845, San Antonio, TX 78229-3900; **Phone:** 210-567-5640; **Board Cert:** Urology 1992; **Med School:** Univ MO-Columbia Sch Med 1984; **Resid:** Surgery, Univ Missouri 1986; Urology, Barnes Hosp/Wash Univ 1990; **Fac Appt:** Prof U, Univ Tex, San Antonio

Boone, Timothy B MD/PhD [U] - **Spec Exp:** Neuro-Urology; Urinary Reconstruction; Incontinence; **Hospital:** Methodist Hosp - Houston, St Luke's Episcopal Hosp - Houston; **Address:** Scurlock Tower, 6560 Fannin, Ste 2100, Houston, TX 77030-2769; **Phone:** 713-798-4001; **Board Cert:** Urology 1995; **Med School:** Univ Tex, Houston 1985; **Resid:** Surgery, Univ Tex SW Med Ctr 1987; Urology, Univ Tex SW Med Ctr 1991; **Fac Appt:** Prof U, Baylor Coll Med

Buch, Jeffrey Phillip MD [U] - **Spec Exp:** Infertility-Male; Sexual Dysfunction; Vasectomy Reversal; **Hospital:** Med Ctr of Plano; **Address:** 1600 Coit Rd, Ste 408, Male Fertility Specialists, Plano, TX 75075; **Phone:** 972-612-7131; **Board Cert:** Urology 2005; **Med School:** Univ Mich Med Sch 1980; **Resid:** Surgery, Albany Med Ctr 1982; Urology, Albany Med Ctr 1985; **Fellow:** Male Infertility, Baylor Coll Med 1987; Microsurgery, Baylor Coll Med 1987

Culkin, Daniel J MD [U] - **Spec Exp:** Voiding Dysfunction; Interstitial Cystitis; **Hospital:** OU Med Ctr, VA Med Ctr - Oklahoma City; **Address:** Oklahoma Univ HSC, Div Urology, 920 Stanton L Young Blvd, Ste WP 3150, Oklahoma City, OK 73104; **Phone:** 405-271-6900; **Board Cert:** Urology 1997; **Med School:** Creighton Univ 1979; **Resid:** Surgery, Loyola Univ Med Ctr 1981; Urology, Loyola Univ Med Ctr 1983; **Fellow:** Neurourology, Loyola Univ Med Ctr 1984; **Fac Appt:** Prof U, Univ Okla Coll Med

Ewalt, David H MD [U] - **Spec Exp:** Pediatric Urology; Hypospadias; Urinary Reconstruction; Neurogenic Bladder; **Hospital:** Chldns Med Ctr of Dallas, Med City Dallas Hosp; **Address:** 8315 Walnut Hill Lane, Ste 205, Dallas, TX 75231; **Phone:** 214-750-0808; **Board Cert:** Urology 2003; **Med School:** Univ Tex SW, Dallas 1984; **Resid:** Urology, Univ Texas SW Affil Hosps 1990; **Fellow:** Pediatric Urology, Chldns Hosp 1992

Fuselier Jr, Harold A MD [U] - **Spec Exp:** Kidney Stones; Prostate Disease; Erectile Dysfunction; **Hospital:** Ochsner Fdn Hosp; **Address:** Ochsner Clinic, Dept Urology, 1514 Jefferson Hwy Fl 4W, New Orleans, LA 70121-2483; **Phone:** 504-842-4083; **Board Cert:** Urology 1976; **Med School:** Louisiana State Univ 1967; **Resid:** Urology, Alton Ochsner Med Fdn 1973; Urology, Mobile Genl Hosp 1974; **Fac Appt:** Prof U, Louisiana State Univ

Gonzales, Edmond MD [U] - **Spec Exp:** Pediatric Urology; **Hospital:** Texas Chldns Hosp - Houston; **Address:** Clinical Care Center, Ste 660, 6701 Fannin St, Houston, TX 77030; **Phone:** 832-822-3160; **Board Cert:** Urology 1975; **Med School:** Tulane Univ 1965; **Resid:** Surgery, Duke Univ Med Ctr 1968; Urology, Duke Univ Med Ctr 1972; **Fellow:** Pediatric Urology, Childrens Hosp; **Fac Appt:** Prof U, Baylor Coll Med

Greene, Graham MD [U] - **Spec Exp:** Urologic Cancer; **Hospital:** UAMS Med Ctr, Arkansas Chldns Hosp; **Address:** 4301 W Markham, Slot 774, Little Rock, AR 72205; **Phone:** 501-296-1545; **Board Cert:** Urology 1999; **Med School:** Dalhousie Univ 1989; **Resid:** Urology, Victoria Genl 1994; **Fellow:** Urologic Oncology, M.D. Anderson Cancer Ctr 1997; **Fac Appt:** Assoc Prof U, Univ Ark

Lerner, Seth P MD [U] - **Spec Exp:** Bladder Cancer; Testicular Cancer; Urinary Reconstruction; **Hospital:** St Luke's Episcopal Hosp - Houston, Methodist Hosp - Houston; **Address:** 6560 Fannin St, Ste 2100, Houston, TX 77030; **Phone:** 713-798-6841; **Board Cert:** Urology 1994; **Med School:** Baylor Coll Med 1984; **Resid:** Surgery, Virginia Mason Hosp 1986; Urology, Baylor Coll Med 1990; **Fellow:** Urologic Oncology, LAC-USC Med Ctr 1992; **Fac Appt:** Prof U, Baylor Coll Med

Lipshultz, Larry MD [U] - **Spec Exp:** Infertility-Male; Microsurgery; Erectile Dysfunction; **Hospital:** St Luke's Episcopal Hosp - Houston, Methodist Hosp - Houston; **Address:** 6560 Fannin St, Scurlock Twr, Ste 2100, Houston, TX 77030-2706; **Phone:** 713-798-4001; **Board Cert:** Urology 1977; **Med School:** Univ Pennsylvania 1968; **Resid:** Urology, Hosp Univ Penn 1971; **Fellow:** Reproductive Medicine, Univ Tex Med Sch 1971; **Fac Appt:** Prof U, Baylor Coll Med

McConnell, John D MD [U] - **Spec Exp:** Prostate Cancer; **Hospital:** UT Southwestern Med Ctr - Dallas, Chldns Med Ctr of Dallas; **Address:** Univ Texas SW Med Ctr, 5323 Harry Hines Blvd, Dallas, TX 75390-9131; **Phone:** 214-648-5630; **Board Cert:** Urology 2004; **Med School:** Loyola Univ-Stritch Sch Med 1978; **Resid:** Surgery, Univ Tex Hlth Sci Ctr-Parkland 1980; Urology, Univ Tex Hlth Sci Ctr-Parkland 1984; **Fac Appt:** Prof U, Univ Tex SW, Dallas

Miles, Brian J MD [U] - **Spec Exp:** Prostate Cancer; Urologic Cancer; Gene Therapy; **Hospital:** Methodist Hosp - Houston, St Luke's Episcopal Hosp - Houston; **Address:** Dept Urology, Scurlock Tower, 6560 Fannin St, Ste 2100, Houston, TX 77030-2769; **Phone:** 713-798-4001; **Board Cert:** Urology 1984; **Med School:** Univ Mich Med Sch 1974; **Resid:** Urology, Walter Reed Army Med Ctr 1982; **Fac Appt:** Prof U, Baylor Coll Med

Pisters, Louis L MD [U] - **Spec Exp:** Prostate Cancer; Bladder Cancer; Genitourinary Cancer; Prostate Cancer/Robotic Surgery; **Hospital:** UT MD Anderson Cancer Ctr (page 71); **Address:** MD Anderson Cancer Ctr, 1515 Holcombe Blvd, Unit 1373, Houston, TX 77030; **Phone:** 713-792-3250; **Board Cert:** Urology 2003; **Med School:** Univ Western Ontario 1986; **Resid:** Urology, Shands Hosp/UNIV Florida 1991; **Fellow:** Urologic Oncology, MD Anderson Cancer Ctr 1993; **Fac Appt:** Assoc Prof U, Univ Tex, Houston

Roehrborn, Claus MD [U] - **Spec Exp:** Prostate Disease; Prostate Cancer; **Hospital:** UT Southwestern Med Ctr - Dallas, Parkland Meml Hosp - Dallas; **Address:** UT Southwestern Med Ctr, Dept Urology, 5323 Harry Hines Blvd, J8-148, Dallas, TX 75390-9110; **Phone:** 214-645-8765; **Board Cert:** Urology 2004; **Med School:** Germany 1980; **Resid:** Surgery, W Germany Army Hosp 1982; Urology, UT SW Med Ctr 1989; **Fellow:** Urology, Am Fdn Urol Dis 1991; **Fac Appt:** Prof U, Univ Tex SW, Dallas

Sagalowsky, Arthur I MD [U] - **Spec Exp:** Urologic Cancer; Transplant-Kidney; Testicular Cancer; **Hospital:** UT Southwestern Med Ctr - Dallas; **Address:** UT SW Med Ctr, Dept Urology, 5323 Harry Hines Blvd, J8.114, Dallas, TX 75390-9110; **Phone:** 214-648-3976; **Board Cert:** Urology 1980; **Med School:** Indiana Univ 1973; **Resid:** Surgery, Indiana Univ Hosps 1975; Urology, Indiana Univ Hosps 1978; **Fellow:** Clinical Pharmacology, Univ Tex SW Med Ctr 1980; **Fac Appt:** Prof U, Univ Tex SW, Dallas

Strand, William MD [U] - **Spec Exp:** Pediatric Urology; Laparoscopic Surgery; Hypospadias; Reconstructive Surgery; **Hospital:** Chldns Med Ctr of Dallas; **Address:** 4001 W 15th St Bldg 3 - Ste 300, Plano, TX 75093; **Phone:** 214-750-0808; **Board Cert:** Urology 2001; **Med School:** Mayo Med Sch 1983; **Resid:** Surgery, Naval Med Ctr 1984; Urology, Natl Naval Med Ctr 1988; **Fac Appt:** Assoc Prof U, Univ Tex SW, Dallas

Swanson, David A MD [U] - **Spec Exp:** Kidney Cancer; Prostate Cancer; Testicular Cancer; **Hospital:** UT MD Anderson Cancer Ctr (page 71); **Address:** UT MD Anderson Canc Ctr, Dept Urol, 1515 Holcombe Blvd, Unit 1373, Houston, TX 77030-4009; **Phone:** 713-792-3250; **Board Cert:** Urology 1977; **Med School:** Univ Pennsylvania 1967; **Resid:** Surgery, Harbor Genl Hosp 1969; Urology, UC Davis Med Ctr 1975; **Fellow:** Urologic Oncology, Univ Tex-MD Anderson Hosp 1978

Thompson Jr, Ian M MD [U] - **Spec Exp:** Prostate Cancer; Prostate Disease; **Hospital:** Univ Hlth Sys - Univ Hosp; **Address:** Univ Tex Hlth Scis Ctr, Dept Urol, 7703 Floyd Curl Drive, rm 216L, MC 7845, San Antonio, TX 78229-3900; **Phone:** 210-567-5643; **Board Cert:** Urology 2005; **Med School:** Tulane Univ 1980; **Resid:** Urology, Brooke Army Med Ctr 1985; **Fellow:** Medical Oncology, Meml Sloan-Kettering Canc Ctr 1988; **Fac Appt:** Prof S, Univ Tex, San Antonio

Winters, Jack C MD [U] - **Spec Exp:** Voiding Dysfunction; Urology-Female; Urinary Reconstruction; **Hospital:** Ochsner Fdn Hosp; **Address:** Ochsner Clinic, Dept Urology, 1514 Jefferson Hwy Fl 4W, New Orleans, LA 70121; **Phone:** 504-842-4083; **Board Cert:** Urology 1997; **Med School:** Louisiana State Univ 1988; **Resid:** Surgery, Ochsner Fdn Hosp 1990; Urology, Ochsner Fdn Hosp 1994; **Fellow:** Female Urology, Cleveland Clinic Fdn 1995

Urology

West Coast and Pacific

Baskin, Laurence S MD [U] - **Spec Exp:** Pediatric Urology; Hypospadias; **Hospital:** UCSF Med Ctr, CA Pacific Med Ctr - Pacific Campus; **Address:** Urology Faculty Practice, 400 Parnassus Ave, Ste 610A, Box 0330, San Francisco, CA 94143-0330; **Phone:** 415-353-2200; **Board Cert:** Urology 2004; **Med School:** UCLA 1986; **Resid:** Urology, UCSF Med Ctr 1991; **Fellow:** Pediatric Urology, Childrens Hosp 1993; **Fac Appt:** Assoc Prof U, UCSF

Berger, Richard E MD [U] - **Spec Exp:** Infertility-Male; Infectious Disease; Urologic Surgery; **Hospital:** Univ Wash Med Ctr; **Address:** Univ Washington, Dept Urology, 1959 NE Pacific St, Box 356510, Seattle, WA 98195-6510; **Phone:** 206-598-4294; **Board Cert:** Urology 1981; **Med School:** Univ Chicago-Pritzker Sch Med 1973; **Resid:** Surgery, Univ Colo Hlth Sci Ctr 1975; Urology, Univ Wash Med Ctr 1979; **Fellow:** Infectious Disease, Univ Wash Med Ctr 1977; **Fac Appt:** Prof U, Univ Wash

Boyd, Stuart D MD [U] - **Spec Exp:** Incontinence; Erectile Dysfunction; Urologic Cancer; **Hospital:** USC Norris Comp Cancer Ctr, USC Univ Hosp - R K Eamer Med Plz; **Address:** 1441 Eastlake Ave, Ste 7416, Los Angeles, CA 90089-9178; **Phone:** 323-865-3704; **Board Cert:** Urology 1984; **Med School:** UCLA 1975; **Resid:** Urology, UCLA Med Ctr 1982; **Fac Appt:** Prof U, USC Sch Med

Carroll, Peter R MD [U] - **Spec Exp:** Testicular Cancer; Prostate Cancer; Bladder Cancer; Bladder reconstruction; **Hospital:** UCSF - Mt Zion Med Ctr; **Address:** UCSF Urologic Oncology Practice, Box 1711, San Francisco, CA 94143-1711; **Phone:** 415-353-7171; **Board Cert:** Urology 1998; **Med School:** Georgetown Univ 1979; **Resid:** Surgery, UCSF Med Ctr 1984; **Fellow:** Urology, Meml Sloan Kettering Cancer Ctr 1986; **Fac Appt:** Prof U, UCSF

Clayman, Ralph V MD [U] - **Spec Exp:** Kidney Stones; Kidney Cancer; Laparoscopic Surgery; **Hospital:** UC Irvine Med Ctr; **Address:** UCI Med Ctr, Dept Urology, 101 The City Drive, Bldg 55, Route 81, Orange, CA 92868; **Phone:** 714-456-3330; **Board Cert:** Urology 1981; **Med School:** UCSD 1973; **Resid:** Urology, Univ Minn Med Ctr 1979; **Fac Appt:** Prof U, UC Irvine

Danoff, Dudley S MD [U] - **Spec Exp:** Prostate Cancer; Bladder Cancer; Erectile Dysfunction; **Hospital:** Cedars-Sinai Med Ctr; **Address:** 8635 W 3rd St, Ste 1 West, Los Angeles, CA 90048; **Phone:** 310-854-9898; **Board Cert:** Urology 1974; **Med School:** Yale Univ 1963; **Resid:** Urology, Yale-New Haven Hosp 1965; Urology, Columbia-Presby Med Ctr 1969

de Kernion, Jean B MD [U] - **Spec Exp:** Urologic Cancer; Kidney Cancer; Prostate Cancer; Prostate Disease; **Hospital:** UCLA Med Ctr; **Address:** UCLA-Geffen Sch Med, Dept Urology, rm 66-133CHS, Box 951738, Los Angeles, CA 90095-1738; **Phone:** 310-206-6453; **Board Cert:** Surgery 1973; Urology 1975; **Med School:** Louisiana State Univ 1965; **Resid:** Surgery, Univ Hosps-Case West Res 1967; Urology, Univ Hosps-Case West Res 1973; **Fellow:** Urologic Oncology, Natl Cancer Inst 1969; **Fac Appt:** Prof U, UCLA

Fuchs, Eugene F MD [U] - **Spec Exp:** Infertility-Male; Kidney Stones; Vasectomy Reversal; **Hospital:** OR Hlth & Sci Univ, Legacy Emanuel Hospitals; **Address:** 1750 SW Harbor Way, Ste 230, Portland, OR 97201; **Phone:** 503-418-9033; **Board Cert:** Urology 1977; **Med School:** Univ VT Coll Med 1970; **Resid:** Urology, Univ Oregon Hosp 1975; **Fac Appt:** Prof U, Oregon Hlth Sci Univ

Gill, Harcharan Singh MD [U] - **Spec Exp:** Urologic Cancer; Prostate Cancer; Prostate Disease; **Hospital:** Stanford Univ Med Ctr; **Address:** 875 Blake Wilbur Drive, Stanford, CA 94305-5826; **Phone:** 650-725-5544; **Board Cert:** Urology 1995; **Med School:** Kenya 1977; **Resid:** Urology, Inst of Urol; Urology, Univ Penn 1991; **Fellow:** Urology, Univ Penn 1986; **Fac Appt:** Prof U, Stanford Univ

Ginsberg, David A MD [U] - **Spec Exp:** Incontinence; Urinary Reconstruction; Neuro-Urology; **Hospital:** USC Univ Hosp - R K Eamer Med Plz; **Address:** USC-Norris Cancer Ctr, 1441 Eastlake Ave, Ste 7416, Los Angeles, CA 90033; **Phone:** 323-865-3703; **Board Cert:** Urology 1999; **Med School:** USC Sch Med 1990; **Resid:** Surgery, LAC-USC Med Ctr 1992; Urology, LAc-USC Med Ctr 1996; **Fellow:** Reconstructive Surgery, UCLA 1997; **Fac Appt:** Assoc Clin Prof U, USC-Keck School of Medicine

Holden, Stuart MD [U] - **Spec Exp:** Kidney Cancer; **Hospital:** Cedars-Sinai Med Ctr; **Address:** 8635 W 3rd St, Ste 1 West, Los Angeles, CA 90048; **Phone:** 310-854-9898; **Board Cert:** Urology 1977; **Med School:** Cornell Univ-Weill Med Coll 1968; **Resid:** Surgery, NY Hosp-Cornell 1970; Urology, Emory Univ Hosp 1975; **Fellow:** Urology, Meml Sloan Kettering Cancer Ctr 1978

Huffman, Jeffry L MD [U] - **Spec Exp:** Kidney Stones; Kidney Cancer; Bladder Cancer; Prostate Cancer; **Hospital:** USC Univ Hosp - R K Eamer Med Plz, USC Norris Comp Cancer Ctr; **Address:** 1975 Zonal Ave, rm 512, Los Angeles, CA 90033; **Phone:** 323-442-6284; **Board Cert:** Urology 2005; **Med School:** Loyola Univ-Stritch Sch Med 1978; **Resid:** Surgery, St Francis Hosp 1980; Urology, Univ Chicago Hosps 1983; **Fellow:** Urologic Oncology, Meml Sloan Kettering Cancer Ctr 1985; **Fac Appt:** Prof U, USC-Keck School of Medicine

Kawachi, Mark H MD [U] - **Spec Exp:** Prostate Cancer/Robotic Surgery; Minimally Invasive Urologic Surgery; **Hospital:** City of Hope Natl Med Ctr & Beckman Rsch; **Address:** City of Hope Natl Med Ctr, Div Urologic Onc, 1500 E Duarte Rd, Duarte, CA 91010-3012; **Phone:** 626-359-8111 x62655; **Board Cert:** Urology 2004; **Med School:** USC Sch Med 1979; **Resid:** Urology, USC Med Ctr 1984

Lieskovsky, Gary MD [U] - **Spec Exp:** Prostate Cancer; **Hospital:** USC Norris Comp Cancer Ctr, USC Univ Hosp - R K Eamer Med Plz; **Address:** 1441 Eastlake Ave, Ste 7416, Los Angeles, CA 90089-0112; **Phone:** 323-865-3702; **Board Cert:** Urology 1980; **Med School:** Canada 1973; **Resid:** Urology, Univ Alberta Hosp 1978; **Fellow:** Urology, UCLA Med Ctr 1980; **Fac Appt:** Prof U, USC Sch Med

Marsh, Christopher L MD [U] - **Spec Exp:** Transplant-Kidney; Transplant-Pancreas; Islet Cell Transplant; Adrenal Surgery; **Hospital:** Scripps Green Hosp; **Address:** Scripps Green Hospital, 10666 N Torrey Pines Rd, MC 200N, La Jolla, CA 92037; **Phone:** 858-554-4310; **Board Cert:** Urology 2006; **Med School:** Loma Linda Univ 1980; **Resid:** Urology, Loma Linda U Med Ctr 1986; **Fellow:** Transplant Surgery, Mayo Clinic 1987

McAninch, Jack W MD [U] - **Spec Exp:** Genitourinary Trauma; Genitourinary Reconstruction; **Hospital:** UCSF Med Ctr, San Francisco Genl Hosp; **Address:** San Francisco Genl Hosp, Dept Urology, 1001 Potrero Ave, Ste 3A20, San Francisco, CA 94110; **Phone:** 415-476-3372; **Board Cert:** Urology 1995; **Med School:** Univ Tex Med Br, Galveston 1964; **Resid:** Surgery, Darnall Army Hosp 1966; Urology, Letterman AMC 1969; **Fac Appt:** Prof U, UCSF

McClure, Robert D MD [U] - **Spec Exp:** Infertility-Male; **Hospital:** Virginia Mason Med Ctr; **Address:** Virginia Mason Med Ctr, 1100 9th Ave, Seattle, WA 98101; **Phone:** 206-223-6179; **Board Cert:** Urology 1979; **Med School:** Canada 1968; **Resid:** Urology, McGill Univ Hosp 1975; **Fellow:** Endocrinology, Univ Washington Med Ctr 1977

Padma-Nathan, Harin MD [U] - **Spec Exp:** Erectile Dysfunction; **Hospital:** USC Norris Comp Cancer Ctr; **Address:** 9100 Wilshire Blvd, East Tower, Ste 350, Beverly Hills, CA 90212; **Phone:** 310-858-4455; **Med School:** Dalhousie Univ 1980; **Resid:** Urology, Dalhoise Univ 1985; **Fellow:** Urology, Boston Univ Med Ctr 1988; **Fac Appt:** Clin Prof U, USC Sch Med

Payne, Christopher K MD [U] - **Spec Exp:** Interstitial Cystitis; Pelvic Organ Prolapse Repair; Incontinence; **Hospital:** Stanford Univ Med Ctr; **Address:** Stanford Univ, Dept Urology, 300 Pasteur Drive, rm S-287, Stanford, CA 94305-5118; **Phone:** 650-723-3391; **Board Cert:** Urology 2004; **Med School:** Vanderbilt Univ 1986; **Resid:** Urology, Univ Penn 1992; **Fellow:** Urology, UCLA Med Ctr 1993; **Fac Appt:** Assoc Prof U, Stanford Univ

Perkash, Inder MD [U] - **Spec Exp:** Neurogenic Bladder; Laser Surgery; Neuro-Urology; Spinal Cord Injury; **Hospital:** VA Hlth Care Sys - Palo Alto, Stanford Univ Med Ctr; **Address:** VA Med Ctr - Spinal Cord Injury Service, Surgical Service (112), 3801 Miranda Ave, Palo Alto, CA 94304-1207; **Phone:** 650-858-3984; **Board Cert:** Physical Medicine & Rehabilitation 1977; Spinal Cord Injury Medicine 2001; **Med School:** India 1957; **Resid:** Urology, Hammersmith Hosp 1963; Physical Medicine & Rehabilitation, Baylor Affil Hosp 1973; **Fellow:** Urology, Stanford Univ Med Ctr 1965; **Fac Appt:** Prof U, Stanford Univ

Presti Jr, Joseph C MD [U] - **Spec Exp:** Prostate Cancer; Bladder Cancer; Kidney Cancer; **Hospital:** Stanford Univ Med Ctr; **Address:** Stanford Univ Sch Med-Dept Urology, 875 Blake Wilbur Dr MC 5826, Stanford, CA 94305; **Phone:** 650-725-5544; **Board Cert:** Urology 2002; **Med School:** UC Irvine 1984; **Resid:** Surgery, UCSF Med Ctr 1986; Urology, UCSF Med Ctr 1989; **Fellow:** Urologic Oncology, Meml Sloan-Kettering Cancer Ctr 1992; **Fac Appt:** Prof U, Stanford Univ

Rajfer, Jacob MD [U] - **Spec Exp:** Erectile Dysfunction; Prostate Disease; Infertility-Male; **Hospital:** LAC - Harbor - UCLA Med Ctr; **Address:** 1000 W Carson St, Box 5, Torrance, CA 90509-2004; **Phone:** 310-222-2727; **Board Cert:** Urology 1980; **Med School:** Northwestern Univ 1972; **Resid:** Surgery, St Josephs Hosp 1974; Urology, Johns Hopkins Hosp 1978; **Fellow:** Research, Johns Hopkins Hosp 1976; **Fac Appt:** Prof U, UCLA

Raz, Shlomo MD [U] - **Spec Exp:** Incontinence-Female; Urology-Female; **Hospital:** UCLA Med Ctr; **Address:** UCLA Urology, 924 Westwood Blvd, Ste 520, Los Angeles, CA 90024-1738; **Phone:** 310-794-0206; **Board Cert:** Urology 1979; **Med School:** Uruguay 1962; **Resid:** Surgery, Hadassah Univ Hosp 1973; **Fellow:** Urology, UCLA Med Ctr 1975; **Fac Appt:** Prof U, UCLA

Schmidt, Joseph MD [U] - **Spec Exp:** Prostate Cancer; Clinical Trials; **Hospital:** UCSD Med Ctr; **Address:** 200 W Arbor Drive, San Diego, CA 92103-8897; **Phone:** 619-543-5904; **Board Cert:** Urology 1971; **Med School:** Univ IL Coll Med 1961; **Resid:** Surgery, Rush-Presby-St Lukes Hosp 1963; Urology, Johns Hopkins Hosp 1967; **Fellow:** Urology, Johns Hopkins Sch Med 1967; **Fac Appt:** Prof U, UCSD

Sharlip, Ira D MD [U] - **Spec Exp:** Vasectomy Reversal; Erectile Dysfunction; Infertility-Male; **Hospital:** CA Pacific Med Ctr - Pacific Campus, UCSF Med Ctr; **Address:** 2100 Webster St, Ste 222, San Francisco, CA 94115-2376; **Phone:** 415-202-0250; **Board Cert:** Internal Medicine 1972; Urology 1977; **Med School:** Univ Pennsylvania 1965; **Resid:** Internal Medicine, Hosp Univ Penn 1967; Urology, UCSF Medical Center 1975; **Fellow:** Urology, Middlesex Hosp 1976; **Fac Appt:** Clin Prof U, UCSF

Shortliffe, Linda MD [U] - **Spec Exp:** Pediatric Urology; Hypospadias; Kidney Disease; **Hospital:** Lucile Packard Chldns Hosp/Stanford Univ Med Ctr, Stanford Univ Med Ctr; **Address:** 300 Pasteur Drive, rm S287, Stanford, CA 94305-5118; **Phone:** 650-724-7608; **Board Cert:** Urology 2001; **Med School:** Stanford Univ 1975; **Resid:** Surgery, Tufts-New England Med Ctr 1977; Urology, Stanford Univ Med Ctr 1981; **Fac Appt:** Prof U, Stanford Univ

Skinner, Donald G MD [U] - **Spec Exp:** Bladder Cancer; Testicular Cancer; Prostate Cancer; **Hospital:** USC Norris Comp Cancer Ctr, USC Univ Hosp - R K Eamer Med Plz; **Address:** 1441 Eastlake Ave, Ste 7416, Los Angeles, CA 90089-9178; **Phone:** 323-865-3707; **Board Cert:** Urology 1974; **Med School:** Yale Univ 1964; **Resid:** Surgery, Mass Genl Hosp 1966; Urology, Mass Genl Hosp 1971; **Fac Appt:** Prof U, USC Sch Med

Skinner, Eila C MD [U] - **Spec Exp:** Urologic Cancer; Genitourinary Disorders-Geriatric; Urinary Reconstruction; **Hospital:** USC Norris Comp Cancer Ctr, USC Univ Hosp - R K Eamer Med Plz; **Address:** USC-Keck Sch Med, Dept Urology, 1441 Eastlake Ave, Ste 7416, Los Angeles, CA 90089; **Phone:** 323-865-3700; **Board Cert:** Urology 2001; **Med School:** USC Sch Med 1983; **Resid:** Urology, LAC-USC Med Ctr 1988; **Fellow:** Urologic Oncology, LAC-USC Med Ctr 1990; **Fac Appt:** Assoc Prof U, USC Sch Med

Smith, Robert B MD [U] - **Spec Exp:** Urologic Cancer; **Hospital:** UCLA Med Ctr; **Address:** UCLA-Geffen Sch Med, Dept Urology, Box 951738, Los Angeles, CA 90095-1738; **Phone:** 310-825-9273; **Board Cert:** Urology 1972; **Med School:** UCLA 1963; **Resid:** Surgery, UCLA Med Ctr 1965; Urology, UCLA Med Ctr 1969; **Fac Appt:** Prof S, UCLA

Stein, John P MD [U] - **Spec Exp:** Bladder Cancer; Prostate Cancer; Testicular Cancer; **Hospital:** USC Norris Comp Cancer Ctr; **Address:** 1441 Eastlake Ave, Ste 7416, Los Angeles, CA 90089; **Phone:** 323-865-3709; **Board Cert:** Urology 1999; **Med School:** Loyola Univ-Stritch Sch Med 1989; **Resid:** Surgery, LAC-USC Med Ctr 1991; Urology, LAC-USC Med Ctr 1993; **Fellow:** Urologic Oncology, LAC-USC Med Ctr 1997; **Fac Appt:** Assoc Prof U, USC Sch Med

Stoller, Marshall L MD [U] - **Spec Exp:** Laparoscopic Surgery; Kidney Stones; **Hospital:** UCSF Med Ctr; **Address:** 400 Panassus Ave Fl 6, San Francisco, CA 94143; **Phone:** 415-353-2200; **Board Cert:** Urology 1999; **Med School:** Baylor Coll Med 1981; **Resid:** Surgery, UCSF Med Ctr 1983; Urology, UCSF Med Ctr 1987; **Fellow:** Urology, Prince Henry Hosptial 1986; **Fac Appt:** Prof U, UCSF

Stone, Anthony MD [U] - **Spec Exp:** Urology-Female; Voiding Dysfunction; **Hospital:** UC Davis Med Ctr; **Address:** 4860 Y St, Ste 3500, Sacramento, CA 95817-2214; **Phone:** 916-734-2222; **Board Cert:** Urology 1997; **Med School:** Scotland 1972; **Resid:** Western Genl Hosp 1980; Urology, Cardiff Royal Infirm 1983; **Fellow:** Urodynamics, Duke Univ Med Ctr 1986; **Fac Appt:** Prof U, UC Davis

Tomera, Kevin M MD [U] - **Spec Exp:** Urologic Cancer; Voiding Dysfunction; **Hospital:** Alaska Regl Hosp, Providence Alaska Med Ctr; **Address:** 1200 Airport Heights Drive, Ste 101, Anchorage, AK 99508-2944; **Phone:** 907-276-2803; **Board Cert:** Urology 1995; **Med School:** Northwestern Univ 1978; **Resid:** Urology, Mayo Clinic 1983

Wilson, Timothy G MD [U] - **Spec Exp:** Prostate Cancer/Robotic Surgery; Minimally Invasive Urologic Surgery; Urinary Reconstruction; **Hospital:** City of Hope Natl Med Ctr & Beckman Rsch; **Address:** City of Hope Natl Med Ctr, Div Urologic Onc, 1500 E Duarte Rd, Duarte, CA 91010; **Phone:** 626-359-8111 x62655; **Board Cert:** Urology 2001; **Med School:** Oregon Hlth Sci Univ 1984; **Resid:** Urology, USC Med Ctr 1990; **Fellow:** Urologic Oncology, City Hosp Natl Med Ctr 1991; **Fac Appt:** Assoc Clin Prof U, USC Sch Med

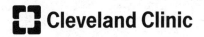 **Cleveland Clinic**

Glickman Urological and Kidney Institute

One of the Best

With 65 physicians and scientists, the Cleveland Clinic Glickman Urological and Kidney Institute is the largest and most comprehensive urological group in the world. Many procedures have been developed or perfected here and adopted around the world. These include laparoscopic urological surgery, female incontinence procedures, kidney-sparing surgery for kidney cancer, kidney artery reconstruction and kidney transplantation. The Institute also offers innovative treatment for sexual dysfunction, male infertility and testicular and bladder cancer. The latest and most effective treatments are provided for every urological disorder in adults and children. Because of its clinical and academic achievements, the Glickman Urological and Kidney Institute has consistently received national and international recognition. *U.S.News & World Report* ranks the Cleveland Clinic Glickman Urological and Kidney Institute one of the top two urological groups in the United States.

A National Leader in Urology

The Glickman Urological and Kidney Institute provides the highest quality of care for adult and pediatric patients with routine or complex disorders. Successful results in the practice and science of urology have won the Institute international acclaim as one of the most progressive and accomplished urologic groups in the country.

Innovative Care

In the treatment of kidney disease, the Cleveland Clinic Gilckman Urological and Kidney Institute has made numerous pioneering contributions including the development of "bench surgery," a technique designed to repair the kidney outside the body and then transplant it back into the patient.

The Cleveland Clinic Glickman Urological Institute is also a recognized leader in partial nephrectomies, or kidney-sparing surgery, for the treatment of kidney cancer. More than 800 laparoscopic, or minimally invasive kidney-sparing procedures, have been performed here, representing the largest experience in the world. Another treatment option pioneered at Cleveland Clinic for kidney cancer is cryoablation, a minimally invasive treatment that uses a freezing probe to destroy the cancerous portion of the kidney. An Institute urologist performed the world's first laparoscopic cryoablation.

Defining State of the Art

The Cleveland Clinic Glickman Urological and Kidney Institute has been instrumental in perfecting and refining many laparoscopic techniques that may offer patients improved outcomes. These techniques are now routinely used for many urological diseases and conditions including prostate cancer, kidney and bladder cancer, urinary incontinence and in removing and transplanting kidneys in live-donor transplants. As one of the first centers in the country to begin using the latest versions of robotic surgery systems for prostate cancer, the Cleveland Clinic Glickman Urological and Kidney Institute is leading the way in minimally invasive urologic surgery.

To schedule an appointment or for more information about the Cleveland Clinic Glickman Urological Institute call 800.890.2467 or visit www.cancer.org/urologytopdocs.

Glickman Urological Institute | 9500 Euclid Avenue / W14 | Cleveland OH 44195

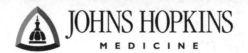

NYU Medical Center

550 First Avenue (at 31st Street)
New York, NY 10016
Physician Referral:
(888)7-NYU-MED (888-769-8633)
www.nyumc.org

UROLOGY

NYU Medical Center's urologists are internationally renowned specialists who have pioneered numerous advances in the surgical and pharmacological treatment of urological disease. They are an interdisciplinary team of physicians, nurses, and allied health professionals dedicated to providing the highest-quality state-of-the-art care. All of our doctors are also faculty at NYU School of Medicine who specialize in all aspects of urological disease. Our programs include:

Urologic Oncology – aggressively treating and curing urologic cancers while maintaining the highest quality of life. Cancers of the prostate, kidney, bladder, and testes are the most common malignancies treated in this program. Since treating cancer often requires a multidisciplinary approach, urologists work closely with NYU's medical and radiation oncologists to tailor treatment to each patient's priorities and objectives.

Minimally Invasive Surgery – committed to developing new technologies to treat even the most complex disorders more effectively and less invasively, so patients experience less pain and a quicker recovery.

Male Fertility and Sexual Health – collaborating closely with the world-renowned NYU In Vitro Fertilization Program, the fertility treatment program uses state-of-the-art technology and a multidisciplinary approach to diagnose and treat the underlying causes of both male and female sexual dysfunction.

Benign Prostatic Diseases – developing innovative medical and surgical therapies for benign prostatic diseases, such as benign prostatic hyperplasia (BPH, or enlarged prostate) and prostatitis (infection in the prostate).

Female Urology and Incontinence –expertise in the many urological problems unique to women, including recurrent urinary tract infections, pelvic pain, prolapse, and sexual dysfunction.

Pediatric Urology and Reconstructive Surgery – treating urologic diseases in children.

NYU MEDICAL CENTER

National Institutes for Health funding for NYU urological research is among the highest for a Urology department in the nation. To assure the continued cross-fertilization of research and patient care, basic scientists with primary academic appointments work closely with the NYU Medical Center urologists on research, leading to a superior understanding of clinical problems.

**Physician Referral
(888) 7-NYU-MED
(888-769-8633)
www.nyumc.org**

723

Vascular Surgery

a subspecialty of Surgery

A surgeon with expertise in the management of surgical disorders of the blood vessels, excluding the intercranial vessels or the heart.

Training Required: Five years in surgery *plus* additional training and examination.

Vascular Surgery

New England

Belkin, Michael MD [VascS] - **Spec Exp:** Aneurysm; Arterial Bypass Surgery; Carotid Artery Surgery; **Hospital:** Brigham & Women's Hosp, Faulkner Hosp; **Address:** Brigham & Women's Hosp, Dept Vasc Surg, 75 Francis St, Boston, MA 02115; **Phone:** 617-732-6816; **Board Cert:** Surgery 1997; Vascular Surgery 1998; **Med School:** Univ Conn 1982; **Resid:** Surgery, Hartford Hosp 1987; **Fellow:** Vascular Surgery, Boston Univ/Brigham-Womens Hosp 1989; **Fac Appt:** Assoc Prof S, Harvard Med Sch

Brewster, David C MD [VascS] - **Spec Exp:** Aneurysm-Abdominal Aortic; Endovascular Surgery; Angioplasty & Stent Placement; **Hospital:** Mass Genl Hosp, Newton - Wellesley Hosp; **Address:** One Hawthorne Pl, Ste 111, Boston, MA 02114; **Phone:** 617-726-3567; **Board Cert:** Surgery 1975; Vascular Surgery 2003; **Med School:** Columbia P&S 1967; **Resid:** Surgery, Mass Genl Hosp 1975; **Fellow:** Vascular Surgery, Mass Genl Hosp 1976; **Fac Appt:** Clin Prof S, Harvard Med Sch

Cambria, Richard P MD [VascS] - **Spec Exp:** Aneurysm-Abdominal Aortic; Cerebrovascular Disease; Renovascular Disease; Aortic Reconstruction; **Hospital:** Mass Genl Hosp; **Address:** Mass Genl Hosp, Dept Vascular Surgery, 15 Parkman St, WAC 336, Boston, MA 02114-3117; **Phone:** 617-726-8278; **Board Cert:** Vascular Surgery 1994; **Med School:** Columbia P&S 1977; **Resid:** Surgery, Mass Genl Hosp 1978; **Fellow:** Vascular Surgery, Mass Genl Hosp 1984; **Fac Appt:** Prof S, Harvard Med Sch

Cronenwett, Jack MD [VascS] - **Spec Exp:** Peripheral Vascular Surgery; Aneurysm-Abdominal Aortic; Carotid Artery Surgery; **Hospital:** Dartmouth - Hitchcock Med Ctr, Mary Hitchcock Mem Hosp; **Address:** Dartmouth Hitchcock Med Ctr, Sect Vasc Surg, 1 Med Ctr Drive, Lebanon, NH 03756; **Phone:** 603-650-8670; **Board Cert:** Vascular Surgery 2003; **Med School:** Stanford Univ 1973; **Resid:** Surgery, Univ Mich Hosp 1979; **Fellow:** Vascular Surgery, Univ Tenn Hosp 1980; **Fac Appt:** Prof S, Dartmouth Med Sch

Gibbons, Gary William MD [VascS] - **Spec Exp:** Diabetic Vascular Disease; Diabetic Leg/Foot; **Hospital:** Boston Med Ctr, Quncity Med Ctr; **Address:** 732 Harrison Ave Preston Bldg - Ste 219, Boston, MA 02118; **Phone:** 617-414-6840; **Board Cert:** Vascular Surgery 1992; **Med School:** Univ Cincinnati 1971; **Resid:** Surgery, New England Deaconess Hosp 1976; **Fellow:** Nutrition, New England Deaconess Hosp; **Fac Appt:** Prof S, Boston Univ

Kwolek, Christopher J MD [VascS] - **Spec Exp:** Aneurysm-Abdominal & Thoracic Aortic; Endovascular Surgery; Carotid Artery Stent Placement; **Hospital:** Mass Genl Hosp, Newton - Wellesley Hosp; **Address:** 15 Parkman St, Wang Bldg Fl 4, Boston, MA 02114; **Phone:** 617-724-6101; **Board Cert:** Surgery 2003; Vascular Surgery 1997; **Med School:** UCSF 1987; **Resid:** Surgery, New England Deaconess Hosp 1993; Vascular Surgery, Mass Genl Hosp 1995; **Fellow:** Endovascular Surgery, Arizona Heart Inst 1999; **Fac Appt:** Assoc Prof VascS, Harvard Med Sch

LaMuraglia, Glenn M MD [VascS] - **Spec Exp:** Percutaneous Vascular Interventions; Angioplasty & Stent Placement-Legs; Carotid Body Tumors; **Hospital:** Mass Genl Hosp; **Address:** Mass General Hospital, Vascular Surgery, 55 Fruit St, Boston, MA 02114; **Phone:** 617-726-6997; **Board Cert:** Surgery 2004; Vascular Surgery 1997; **Med School:** Harvard Med Sch 1979; **Resid:** Surgery, Mass General Hosp 1985; Vascular Surgery, Mass General Hosp 1986; **Fac Appt:** Assoc Prof S, Harvard Med Sch

Mackey, William C MD [VascS] - **Spec Exp:** Carotid Artery Surgery; Aneurysm-Abdominal Aortic; Lower Limb Arterial Disease; **Hospital:** Tufts-New England Med Ctr; **Address:** 750 Washington St, Ste 1035, Boston, MA 02111-1526; **Phone:** 617-636-5927; **Board Cert:** Surgery 2002; Vascular Surgery 2004; Surgical Critical Care 1997; **Med School:** Duke Univ 1977; **Resid:** Surgery, New York Hosp 1982; **Fellow:** Vascular Surgery, Tufts-New Eng Med Ctr 1984; **Fac Appt:** Prof S, Tufts Univ

Sumpio, Bauer E MD/PhD [VascS] - **Spec Exp:** Diabetic Leg/Foot; Endovascular Surgery; **Hospital:** Yale - New Haven Hosp; **Address:** Yale Univ School Medicine, Dept Surgery, 333 Cedar St, rm FMB137, Box 208062, New Haven, CT 06520; **Phone:** 203-785-6217; **Board Cert:** Vascular Surgery 1997; Surgery 1998; **Med School:** Cornell Univ-Weill Med Coll 1980; **Resid:** Surgery, Yale-New Haven Hosp 1986; **Fellow:** Vascular Surgery, Unic N Carolina Hosp 1987; **Fac Appt:** Prof S, Yale Univ

Whittemore, Anthony D MD [VascS] - **Spec Exp:** Carotid Artery Surgery; Aortic Surgery; Aneurysm-Abdominal Aortic; **Hospital:** Brigham & Women's Hosp; **Address:** Brigham & Women's Hosp, 75 Francis St, Boston, MA 02115; **Phone:** 617-732-8515; **Board Cert:** Vascular Surgery 2002; **Med School:** Columbia P&S 1970; **Resid:** Surgery, Columbia-Presby Med Ctr 1976; **Fellow:** Vascular Surgery, Peter Bent Brigham Hosp 1977; **Fac Appt:** Prof S, Harvard Med Sch

Mid Atlantic

Adelman, Mark MD [VascS] - **Spec Exp:** Carotid Artery Surgery; Aneurysm-Abdominal Aortic; Vein Disorders; Endovascular Surgery; **Hospital:** NYU Med Ctr (page 67), Bellevue Hosp Ctr; **Address:** 530 1st Ave, Ste 6F, New York, NY 10016-6402; **Phone:** 212-263-7311; **Board Cert:** Surgery 1999; Vascular Surgery 2001; **Med School:** NYU Sch Med 1985; **Resid:** Surgery, NYU Med Ctr 1990; **Fellow:** Vascular Surgery, NYU Med Ctr 1991; **Fac Appt:** Prof VascS, NYU Sch Med

Ascher, Enrico MD [VascS] - **Spec Exp:** Endovascular Surgery; Carotid Artery Surgery; Limb Sparing Surgery; Aneurysm; **Hospital:** Maimonides Med Ctr (page 63), Mount Sinai Med Ctr; **Address:** Maimonides Med Ctr, Dept Vascular Surg, 4802 10th Ave Fl 4, Brooklyn, NY 11219-2844; **Phone:** 718-283-7957; **Board Cert:** Vascular Surgery 2004; **Med School:** Brazil 1974; **Resid:** Surgery, NY Med Coll 1981; **Fellow:** Vascular Surgery, Montefiore Hosp Med Ctr 1982; **Fac Appt:** Prof S, SUNY Downstate

Atnip, Robert G MD [VascS] - **Spec Exp:** Aneurysm-Abdominal Aortic; Peripheral Vascular Disease; Carotid Artery Disease; **Hospital:** Penn State Milton S Hershey Med Ctr; **Address:** Hershey Med Ctr, rm C 4632, 500 University Dr, Box 850, MC HO5, Hershey, PA 17033; **Phone:** 717-531-8888; **Board Cert:** Surgery 1995; Vascular Surgery 1997; Surgical Critical Care 2000; **Med School:** Univ Ala 1978; **Resid:** Surgery, Mass Genl Hosp 1984; **Fellow:** Vascular Surgery, Mass Genl Hosp 1985; **Fac Appt:** Prof S, Penn State Univ-Hershey Med Ctr

Benvenisty, Alan I MD [VascS] - **Spec Exp:** Peripheral Vascular Surgery; Endovascular Surgery; Transplant-Kidney; **Hospital:** St Luke's - Roosevelt Hosp Ctr - St Luke's Hosp, St Luke's - Roosevelt Hosp Ctr - Roosevelt Div; **Address:** 1090 Amsterdam Ave Fl 12, New York, NY 10025; **Phone:** 212-523-4706; **Board Cert:** Surgery 2004; Vascular Surgery 1999; **Med School:** Columbia P&S 1978; **Resid:** Surgery, Columbia-Presby Med Ctr 1983; **Fellow:** Vascular Surgery, Columbia-Presby Med Ctr 1984; Transplant Surgery, Columbia-Presby Med Ctr 1984; **Fac Appt:** Clin Prof S, Columbia P&S

Brener, Bruce J MD [VascS] - **Spec Exp:** Endovascular Surgery; Minimally Invasive Vascular Surgery; Carotid Artery Surgery; **Hospital:** Newark Beth Israel Med Ctr, St Barnabas Med Ctr; **Address:** 200 South Orange Ave, Livingston, NJ 07039; **Phone:** 973-322-7233; **Board Cert:** Surgery 1972; Vascular Surgery 2005; **Med School:** Harvard Med Sch 1966; **Resid:** Surgery, Chldns Hosp Med Ctr 1968; Surgery, Peter Bent Brigham Hosp 1972; **Fellow:** Vascular Surgery, Mass Genl Hosp 1973; **Fac Appt:** Assoc Clin Prof S, Columbia P&S

Calligaro, Keith D MD [VascS] - **Spec Exp:** Aneurysm-Abdominal & Thoracic Aortic; Carotid Artery Disease; **Hospital:** Pennsylvania Hosp (page 72), Lankenau Hosp; **Address:** 700 Spruce St, Ste 101, Philadelphia, PA 19106; **Phone:** 215-829-5000; **Board Cert:** Surgery 1997; Vascular Surgery 1999; **Med School:** UMDNJ-Rutgers Med Sch 1982; **Resid:** Surgery, St Barnabas Med Ctr 1984; Surgery, Univ Hlth Scis/Chicago Med Sch 1987; **Fellow:** Vascular Surgery, Montefiore Med Ctr 1989; **Fac Appt:** Assoc Clin Prof S, Univ Pennsylvania

Carabasi III, R Anthony MD [VascS] - **Spec Exp:** Carotid Artery Disease; Vein Disorders; **Hospital:** Thomas Jefferson Univ Hosp; **Address:** Advanced Vein and Vascular Center, 744 W Lancaster Ave, Devon Square 11, Ste 225, Wayne, PA 19087; **Phone:** 610-687-5347; **Board Cert:** Vascular Surgery 1998; **Med School:** Thomas Jefferson Univ 1977; **Resid:** Surgery, Thomas Jefferson Univ Hosp 1982; **Fellow:** Vascular Surgery, Pennsylvania Hosp 1983; **Fac Appt:** Prof S, Jefferson Med Coll

Carpenter, Jeffrey P MD [VascS] - **Spec Exp:** Aneurysm-Abdominal & Thoracic Aortic; Carotid Artery Surgery; Peripheral Vascular Disease; **Hospital:** Hosp Univ Penn - UPHS (page 72); **Address:** Hospital U Penn, 4 Silverstein Pavilion, 3400 Spruce St, Philadelphia, PA 19104; **Phone:** 215-662-2029; **Board Cert:** Surgery 2001; Vascular Surgery 2001; **Med School:** Yale Univ 1986; **Resid:** Surgery, Hosp Univ Penn 1991; **Fellow:** Vascular Surgery, Hosp Univ Penn 1992; **Fac Appt:** Prof S, Univ Pennsylvania

Criado, Frank J MD [VascS] - **Spec Exp:** Endovascular Surgery; Aneurysm-Abdominal & Thoracic Aortic; Carotid Artery Stent Placement; **Hospital:** Union Meml Hosp - Baltimore; **Address:** 3333 N Calvert St, Ste 570, Baltimore, MD 21218; **Phone:** 410-554-6400; **Board Cert:** Surgery 1989; Vascular Surgery 1997; **Med School:** Uruguay 1974; **Resid:** Surgery, Union Memorial Hosp 1980; Vascular Surgery, Union Memorial Hosp 1985; **Fellow:** Cardiovascular Surgery, Baylor Univ Med Ctr 1981

Darling III, R Clement MD [VascS] - **Spec Exp:** Aneurysm-Abdominal & Thoracic Aortic; Arterial Bypass Surgery; Carotid Artery Surgery; **Hospital:** Albany Med Ctr, St Peter's Hosp - Albany; **Address:** Albany Med Ctr, Vascular Inst, 43 New Scotland Ave, MC 157, Albany, NY 12208; **Phone:** 518-262-5640; **Board Cert:** Surgery 1999; Vascular Surgery 2002; **Med School:** Univ Cincinnati 1984; **Resid:** Surgery, Beth Israel Deaconess Hosp 1989; **Fellow:** Vascular Surgery, Albany Med Ctr 1991; **Fac Appt:** Prof S, Albany Med Coll

Fairman, Ronald M MD [VascS] - **Spec Exp:** Aneurysm-Aortic; Peripheral Vascular Disease; Carotid Artery Surgery; **Hospital:** Hosp Univ Penn - UPHS (page 72); **Address:** Hosp Univ Penn, 4 Silverstein Pavilion, 3400 Spruce St, Philadelphia, PA 19104; **Phone:** 215-662-2050; **Board Cert:** Surgery 1996; Vascular Surgery 2000; **Med School:** Thomas Jefferson Univ 1977; **Resid:** Surgery, Hosp U Penn 1983; **Fellow:** Vascular Surgery, Hosp U Penn 1984; **Fac Appt:** Assoc Prof S, Univ Pennsylvania

Fantini, Gary A MD [VascS] - **Spec Exp:** Spinal Access Surgery; Vein Disorders; Wound Healing/Care; **Hospital:** Hosp For Special Surgery (page 60), NY-Presby Hosp/Weill Cornell (page 66); **Address:** 635 Madison Ave Fl 7, New York, NY 10022; **Phone:** 212-317-4550; **Board Cert:** Surgery 1999; Vascular Surgery 2000; **Med School:** Albert Einstein Coll Med 1983; **Resid:** Surgery, New York Hosp-Cornell Med Ctr 1989; **Fellow:** Vascular Surgery, UCSF Med Ctr 1990; **Fac Appt:** Assoc Prof S, Cornell Univ-Weill Med Coll

Freischlag, Julie A MD [VascS] - **Spec Exp:** Aneurysm-Aortic; Carotid Artery Disease; Thoracic Outlet Syndrome; **Hospital:** Johns Hopkins Hosp - Baltimore (page 61); **Address:** Johns Hopkins Hosp, Dept Surg, 720 Rutland Ave, Ross Bldg-759, Baltimore, MD 21205; **Phone:** 443-287-3497; **Board Cert:** Surgery 1995; Vascular Surgery 1995; **Med School:** Rush Med Coll 1980; **Resid:** Surgery, UCLA Medical Ctr 1986; **Fellow:** Vascular Surgery, UCLA Medical Ctr 1987; **Fac Appt:** Prof S, Johns Hopkins Univ

Giangola, Gary MD [VascS] - **Spec Exp:** Carotid Artery Surgery; Aneurysm-Aortic; Diabetic Leg/Foot; **Hospital:** Lenox Hill Hosp (page 62); **Address:** Dept Vascular Surg, 130 E 77th St, Black Hall Fl 13, New York, NY 10021; **Phone:** 212-434-4230; **Board Cert:** Surgery 1996; Vascular Surgery 1998; **Med School:** NYU Sch Med 1980; **Resid:** Surgery, NYU Med Ctr 1985; **Fellow:** Vascular Surgery, NYU Med Ctr 1986; **Fac Appt:** Assoc Clin Prof S, Columbia P&S

Green, Richard M MD [VascS] - **Spec Exp:** Aneurysm-Abdominal Aortic; Carotid Artery Surgery; Percutaneous Vascular Interventions; **Hospital:** Lenox Hill Hosp (page 62); **Address:** 130 E 77th St Fl 13, New York, NY 10021; **Phone:** 212-434-3420; **Board Cert:** Vascular Surgery 2003; **Med School:** Univ Rochester 1970; **Resid:** Surgery, Strong Meml Hosp 1976

Harrington, Elizabeth MD [VascS] - **Spec Exp:** Carotid Artery Surgery; Aneurysm-Aortic; Arterial Bypass Surgery-Leg; **Hospital:** Mount Sinai Med Ctr, Lenox Hill Hosp (page 62); **Address:** 1225 Park Ave, Ste 1D, New York, NY 10128-1758; **Phone:** 212-876-7400; **Board Cert:** Surgery 1999; Vascular Surgery 1997; **Med School:** NY Med Coll 1975; **Resid:** Surgery, Mount Sinai Hosp 1980; **Fellow:** Vascular Surgery, Mount Sinai Hosp 1981; **Fac Appt:** Assoc Prof VascS, Mount Sinai Sch Med

Hobson II, Robert Wayne MD [VascS] - **Spec Exp:** Carotid Artery Surgery; Carotid Artery Stent Placement; Endovascular Stent Grafts; Aneurysm-Abdominal Aortic; **Hospital:** UMDNJ-Univ Hosp-Newark, St Clare's Hosp - Denville; **Address:** UMDNJ-New Jersey Med Sch, 30 Bergen St, Bldg 6, rm 620, Newark, NJ 07101; **Phone:** 973-972-6633; **Board Cert:** Surgery 1972; Vascular Surgery 2003; **Med School:** Geo Wash Univ 1963; **Resid:** Surgery, Walter Reed AMC 1971; **Fellow:** Vascular Surgery, Walter Reed AMC 1973; **Fac Appt:** Prof S, UMDNJ-NJ Med Sch, Newark

Kent, K Craig MD [VascS] - **Spec Exp:** Carotid Artery Surgery; Aneurysm-Abdominal Aortic; Lower Limb Arterial Disease; **Hospital:** NY-Presby Hosp/Columbia (page 66); **Address:** 525 E 68th St, rm 107, New York, NY 10021-9800; **Phone:** 212-746-5192; **Board Cert:** Surgery 1997; Vascular Surgery 1998; **Med School:** UCSF 1981; **Resid:** Surgery, UCSF Med Ctr 1986; **Fellow:** Vascular Surgery, Brigham & Women's Hosp 1988; **Fac Appt:** Prof S, Cornell Univ-Weill Med Coll

Makaroun, Michel MD [VascS] - **Spec Exp:** Endovascular Surgery; Aneurysm; Carotid Artery Disease; **Hospital:** UPMC Presby, Pittsburgh, UPMC Shadyside; **Address:** Presby-Univ Hosp, A-1011, Pittsburgh, PA 15213; **Phone:** 412-802-3028; **Board Cert:** Surgery 2004; Vascular Surgery 1998; **Med School:** Lebanon 1978; **Resid:** Surgery, American Univ Hosp 1980; Surgery, Univ Pittsburgh Med Ctr 1985; **Fac Appt:** Prof S, Univ Pittsburgh

Marin, Michael L MD [VascS] - **Spec Exp:** Aneurysm-Aortic; Carotid Artery Surgery; Limb Sparing Surgery; Endovascular Surgery; **Hospital:** Mount Sinai Med Ctr; **Address:** Mount Sinai Medical Ctr, 5 E 98th St, Box 1273, New York, NY 10029; **Phone:** 212-241-5392; **Board Cert:** Surgery 1999; **Med School:** Mount Sinai Sch Med 1984; **Resid:** Surgery, Columbia-Presby Med Ctr 1990; **Fellow:** Transplant Surgery, Columbia-Presby Med Ctr 1988; Vascular Surgery, Montefiore Med Ctr 1992; **Fac Appt:** Prof S, Mount Sinai Sch Med

Vascular Surgery

Perler, Bruce MD [VascS] - **Spec Exp:** Carotid Artery Surgery; Aneurysm; Arterial Bypass Surgery-Leg; **Hospital:** Johns Hopkins Hosp - Baltimore (page 61); **Address:** Johns Hopkins Hosp-Surg, 600 N Wolfe St Bldg Harvey - Ste 611, Baltimore, MD 21287-8611; **Phone:** 410-955-2618; **Board Cert:** Vascular Surgery 1997; **Med School:** Duke Univ 1976; **Resid:** Surgery, Mass Genl Hosp 1981; **Fellow:** Vascular Surgery, Mass Genl Hosp 1982; **Fac Appt:** Prof S, Johns Hopkins Univ

Ricotta, John MD [VascS] - **Spec Exp:** Aneurysm; Carotid Artery Surgery; Vein Disorders; **Hospital:** Stony Brook Univ Med Ctr; **Address:** SUNY HSC, Dept Surgery, HSC T19, rm 020, Stony Brook, NY 11794-8191; **Phone:** 631-444-7875; **Board Cert:** Surgery 2000; Vascular Surgery 1995; **Med School:** Johns Hopkins Univ 1973; **Resid:** Surgery, Johns Hopkins Hosp 1977; **Fellow:** Vascular Surgery, Johns Hopkins Hosp 1979; **Fac Appt:** Prof S, Johns Hopkins Univ

Riles, Thomas MD [VascS] - **Spec Exp:** Aneurysm-Abdominal Aortic; Carotid Artery Surgery; **Hospital:** NYU Med Ctr (page 67); **Address:** NYU Med Ctr, Univ Vascular Assoc, 530 1st Ave, HCC-6D, New York, NY 10016; **Phone:** 212-263-6360; **Board Cert:** Vascular Surgery 2003; **Med School:** Baylor Coll Med 1969; **Resid:** Surgery, NYU Med Ctr 1976; **Fellow:** Vascular Surgery, NYU Med Ctr 1977; **Fac Appt:** Prof S, NYU Sch Med

Steed, David L MD [VascS] - **Spec Exp:** Wound Healing/Care; **Hospital:** UPMC Presby, Pittsburgh; **Address:** UPMC Presbyterian Hosp, 200 Lothrop St, Ste A-1011, Pittsburgh, PA 15213; **Phone:** 412-802-3333; **Board Cert:** Surgery 1999; Vascular Surgery 1997; Surgical Critical Care 1995; **Med School:** Univ Pittsburgh 1973; **Resid:** Surgery, Univ Pittsburgh Med Ctr 1980; **Fellow:** Thoracic Surgery, UCLA Med Ctr 1977; **Fac Appt:** Prof S, Univ Pittsburgh

Todd, George MD [VascS] - **Spec Exp:** Minimally Invasive Vascular Surgery; Aneurysm-Abdominal Aortic; Carotid Artery Surgery; **Hospital:** St Luke's - Roosevelt Hosp Ctr - Roosevelt Div; **Address:** St Luke's-Roosevelt Hosp Ctr, Dept Surg, 1000 10th Ave, rm 5G77, New York, NY 10019; **Phone:** 212-523-7481; **Board Cert:** Surgery 2000; **Med School:** Penn State Univ-Hershey Med Ctr 1974; **Resid:** Surgery, Columbia-Presby Med Ctr 1979; **Fellow:** Vascular Surgery, Columbia-Presby Med Ctr 1980; **Fac Appt:** Prof S, Columbia P&S

Southeast

Bandyk, Dennis MD [VascS] - **Spec Exp:** Endovascular Stent Grafts; Lower Limb Arterial Disease; Thoracic Outlet Syndrome; **Hospital:** Tampa Genl Hosp, Univ of S FL - Tampa; **Address:** Harborside Med Tower, 4 Columbia Dr, Ste 650, Tampa, FL 33606; **Phone:** 813-259-0921; **Board Cert:** Vascular Surgery 2001; Surgery 2000; **Med School:** Univ Mich Med Sch 1975; **Resid:** Surgery, Univ Wash Hosp 1980; **Fellow:** Vascular Surgery, Univ Wash Hosp 1981; **Fac Appt:** Prof S, Univ S Fla Coll Med

Chaikof, Elliot L MD/PhD [VascS] - **Spec Exp:** Aneurysm-Aortic; Carotid Artery Disease; Limb Sparing Surgery; **Hospital:** Emory Univ Hosp, Chldns Hlthcare Atlanta - Egleston; **Address:** Emory Vascular Surgery, 101 Woodruff Cir, Ste 5501 WMB, Atlanta, GA 30322; **Phone:** 404-778-5451; **Board Cert:** Surgery 2002; Vascular Surgery 2003; **Med School:** Johns Hopkins Univ 1982; **Resid:** Surgery, Mass Genl Hosp 1985; Surgery, Mass Genl Hosp 1991; **Fellow:** Vascular Surgery, Emory Univ Hosp 1992; **Fac Appt:** Prof S, Emory Univ

Cherry Jr, Kenneth J MD [VascS] - **Spec Exp:** Vascular Reconstruction; Aortic Graft Infections; **Hospital:** Univ Virginia Med Ctr; **Address:** Univ Virginia Health System, PO Box 800679, Charlottsville, VA 22908-0679; **Phone:** 434-243-7052; **Board Cert:** Vascular Surgery 2004; **Med School:** Univ VA Sch Med 1974; **Resid:** Surgery, Univ Virginia Hosp 1980; Vascular Surgery, UCSF Med Ctr 1981; **Fac Appt:** Prof S, Univ VA Sch Med

Flynn, Timothy C MD [VascS] - **Spec Exp:** Peripheral Vascular Disease; Aortic Graft Infections; **Hospital:** Shands Hlthcre at Univ of FL; **Address:** Shands Hlthcare Univ Florida, PO Box 100321, Gainesville, FL 32610-0286; **Phone:** 352-265-0152; **Board Cert:** Surgery 1999; Vascular Surgery 1994; Surgical Critical Care 1998; **Med School:** Baylor Coll Med 1974; **Resid:** Surgery, Univ Texas 1980; **Fac Appt:** Prof S, Univ Fla Coll Med

Hakaim, Albert G MD [VascS] - **Spec Exp:** Aneurysm-Abdominal Aortic; Endovascular Surgery; **Hospital:** Mayo - Jacksonville; **Address:** Mayo Clinic, Dept Vascular Surgery, 323N, 4500 San Pablo Rd, Jacksonville, FL 32224; **Phone:** 904-953-2077; **Board Cert:** Surgery 2002; Vascular Surgery 2003; **Med School:** Ohio State Univ 1984; **Resid:** Surgery, Cleveland Clinic 1989; **Fellow:** Transplant Surgery, Boston Univ Hosp 1991; Vascular Surgery, Cleveland Clinic 1992; **Fac Appt:** Assoc Prof S, Mayo Med Sch

Hallett Jr, John MD [VascS] - **Spec Exp:** Aneurysm-Abdominal Aortic; Carotid Artery Surgery; Thoracic Outlet Syndrome; **Hospital:** Roper Hosp; **Address:** Roper St Francis Heart & Vascular Ctr, 316 Calhoun St, Charleston, SC 29401; **Phone:** 843-720-8347; **Board Cert:** Surgery 1999; Vascular Surgery 2003; **Med School:** Duke Univ 1973; **Resid:** Surgery, Wilford Hall USAF Med Ctr 1978; **Fellow:** Vascular Surgery, Mass Genl Hosp-Harvard Med Sch 1979; **Fac Appt:** Assoc Clin Prof VascS, Med Univ SC

Hansen, Kimberley J MD [VascS] - **Spec Exp:** Aortic & Visceral Artery Surgery; Renovascular Disease; Carotid Artery Surgery; **Hospital:** Wake Forest Univ Baptist Med Ctr (page 73), Forsyth Med Ctr; **Address:** Wake Forest Univ Sch Med, Dept Surg, Medical Center Blvd, Winston-Salem, NC 27157-1095; **Phone:** 336-716-4151; **Board Cert:** Surgery 1997; Vascular Surgery 1998; Surgical Critical Care 2001; **Med School:** Univ Ala 1980; **Resid:** Surgery, NC Baptist Hosp/WFU Sch MEd 1986; **Fellow:** Vascular Surgery, Univ California 1987; **Fac Appt:** Prof S, Wake Forest Univ

Keagy, Blair A MD [VascS] - **Hospital:** Univ NC Hosps; **Address:** UNC-Chapel Hill, Div Vascular Surgery, 3024 Burnett-Womack Bldg, CB 7212, Chapel Hill, NC 27599; **Phone:** 919-966-3391; **Board Cert:** Vascular Surgery 1998; **Med School:** Univ Pittsburgh 1970; **Resid:** Surgery, Univ North Carolina 1977; **Fellow:** Vascular Surgery, Univ North Carolina 1978; **Fac Appt:** Prof TS, Univ NC Sch Med

McCann, Richard L MD [VascS] - **Spec Exp:** Endovascular Surgery; **Hospital:** Duke Univ Med Ctr; **Address:** Duke Univ Med Ctr, Box 2990, Durham, NC 27710; **Phone:** 919-684-2620; **Board Cert:** Surgery 2003; Vascular Surgery 1996; **Med School:** Cornell Univ-Weill Med Coll 1974; **Resid:** Surgery, Duke Univ Med Ctr 1983; **Fac Appt:** Prof S, Duke Univ

Parodi, Juan Carlos MD [VascS] - **Spec Exp:** Aneurysm-Abdominal & Thoracic Aortic; Peripheral Vascular Disease; Endovascular Stent Grafts; **Hospital:** Univ of Miami Hosp & Clins/Sylvester Comp Canc Ctr; **Address:** 1611 NW 12th St, Ste 3016, Miami, FL 33136; **Phone:** 314-747-8272; **Med School:** Argentina 1966; **Resid:** Surgery, University Med Ctr 1972; Surgery, Univ Chicago Hosps 1974; **Fellow:** Vascular Surgery, Cleveland Clinic 1976; **Fac Appt:** Prof S, Washington Univ, St Louis

Vascular Surgery

Rosenthal, David MD [VascS] - **Spec Exp:** Stroke; Aneurysm; Endovascular Surgery; **Hospital:** Atlanta Med Ctr; **Address:** 315 Blvd NE, Ste 412, Atlanta, GA 30312; **Phone:** 404-524-0095; **Board Cert:** Vascular Surgery 2003; **Med School:** SUNY Downstate 1973; **Resid:** Surgery, Tufts-New Eng Med Ctr 1977; **Fellow:** Vascular Surgery, Tufts-New Eng Med Ctr 1978; **Fac Appt:** Clin Prof S, Med Coll GA

Seeger, James M MD [VascS] - **Spec Exp:** Lower Limb Arterial Disease; Aneurysm-Aortic; Kidney & Bowel Arterial Disease; **Hospital:** Shands Hlthcre at Univ of FL; **Address:** Univ Florida, Dept Vascular Surgery, 1600 SW Archer Rd, JHMHC Bldg-rm NG-45, Box 100286, Gainesville, FL 32610-0286; **Phone:** 352-273-5484; **Board Cert:** Surgery 2000; Vascular Surgery 1992; **Med School:** Med Coll GA 1973; **Resid:** Surgery, Univ Utah Med Ctr 1980; **Fellow:** Vascular Surgery, Eastern VA Med Sch 1981; **Fac Appt:** Prof S, Univ Fla Coll Med

Sivina, Manuel MD [VascS] - **Hospital:** Mount Sinai Med Ctr - Miami; **Address:** Mount Sinai Med Ctr, 4300 Alton Rd, Ste 2240, Miami Beach, FL 33140-2800; **Phone:** 305-674-2760; **Board Cert:** Surgery 2000; **Med School:** Peru 1969; **Resid:** Surgery, Mt Sinai Med Ctr 1975; **Fellow:** Vascular Surgery, Mt Sinai Med Ctr 1976

Midwest

Alexander, J Jeffrey MD [VascS] - **Hospital:** MetroHealth Med Ctr; **Address:** Metrohealth Med Ctr, Heart & Vascular Dept, 2500 Metrohealth Drive, Cleveland, OH 44109; **Phone:** 216-778-4811; **Board Cert:** Vascular Surgery 1995; Surgery 2002; **Med School:** Univ Pittsburgh 1978; **Resid:** Surgery, Univ Chicago Hosps 1983; **Fellow:** Vascular Surgery, Univ Chicago Hosps 1984; **Fac Appt:** Assoc Prof S, Case West Res Univ

Berguer, Ramon MD/PhD [VascS] - **Spec Exp:** Cerebrovascular Disease; Aortic & Visceral Artery Surgery; **Hospital:** Univ Michigan Hlth Sys; **Address:** Univ Michigan Hlth Sys, 1500 E Medical Ctr Dr TC 22-10, Box 0329, Ann Arbor, MI 48109; **Phone:** 734-936-8247; **Board Cert:** Surgery 1970; Vascular Surgery 2003; **Med School:** Spain 1963; **Resid:** Surgery, Henry Ford Hosp 1969; **Fellow:** Vascular Surgery, Henry Ford Hosp 1970; Vascular Surgery, Kings College Hosp; **Fac Appt:** Prof S, Univ Mich Med Sch

Clair, Daniel G MD [VascS] - **Spec Exp:** Carotid Artery Surgery; Aneurysm-Abdominal & Thoracic Aortic; Peripheral Vascular Surgery; Endovascular Stent Grafts; **Hospital:** Cleveland Clin Fdn (page 57); **Address:** Cleveland Clinic, Dept Vascular Surgery, 9500 Euclid Ave, MC S40, Cleveland, OH 44195; **Phone:** 216-444-3857; **Board Cert:** Surgery 2003; Vascular Surgery 2004; **Med School:** Univ VA Sch Med 1986; **Resid:** Surgery, Brigham & Women's Hosp 1987; **Fellow:** Vascular Surgery, Brigham & Women's Hosp 1994

Comerota, Anthony J MD [VascS] - **Spec Exp:** Carotid Artery Disease; Gene Therapy; Aneurysm-Aortic; **Hospital:** Toledo Hosp; **Address:** Jobst Vascular Ctr, 2109 Hughes Drive, Ste 400, Toledo, OH 43606; **Phone:** 419-291-2088; **Board Cert:** Surgery 1999; Vascular Surgery 2003; **Med School:** Temple Univ 1974; **Resid:** Surgery, Temple Univ Hosp 1978; **Fellow:** Vascular Surgery, Good Samaritan Hosp 1981; **Fac Appt:** Clin Prof S, Univ Mich Med Sch

Gloviczki, Peter MD [VascS] - **Spec Exp:** Aneurysm-Abdominal Aortic; Lower Limb Arterial Disease; Vein Disorders; **Hospital:** Mayo Med Ctr & Clin - Rochester; **Address:** Mayo Clinic, Div Vasc Surg, 200 First St SW, Rochester, MN 55905-0001; **Phone:** 507-284-4652; **Board Cert:** Surgery 1998; Vascular Surgery 1998; **Med School:** Hungary 1972; **Resid:** Vascular Surgery, Semmelweis Med Sch 1980; Surgery, Mayo Clin 1987; **Fellow:** Vascular Surgery, Mayo Clin 1983; **Fac Appt:** Prof S, Mayo Med Sch

Greisler, Howard MD [VascS] - **Spec Exp:** Peripheral Vascular Surgery; Aneurysm; Carotid Artery Disease; **Hospital:** Loyola Univ Med Ctr, Hines VA Hosp; **Address:** Loyola Univ Med Ctr, Dept Surgery, 2160 S 1st Ave, rm 3218, Maywood, IL 60153-5590; **Phone:** 708-216-8541; **Board Cert:** Vascular Surgery 2003; **Med School:** Penn State Univ-Hershey Med Ctr 1975; **Resid:** Surgery, Columbia Presby Med Ctr 1980; **Fellow:** Vascular Surgery, Columbia Presby Med Ctr 1981; **Fac Appt:** Prof S, Loyola Univ-Stritch Sch Med

Hodgson, Kim John MD [VascS] - **Spec Exp:** Aneurysm; Carotid Artery Surgery; Endovascular Surgery; **Hospital:** St John's Hosp - Springfield, Memorial Med Ctr - Springfield; **Address:** PO Box 19638, Springfield, IL 62794-9638; **Phone:** 217-545-5555; **Board Cert:** Surgery 1995; Vascular Surgery 2005; **Med School:** Univ Pennsylvania 1981; **Resid:** Surgery, Albany Med Ctr 1986; **Fellow:** Vascular Surgery, Southern Ill Univ 1987; **Fac Appt:** Prof VascS, Southern IL Univ

Pearce, William MD [VascS] - **Spec Exp:** Aneurysm-Abdominal Aortic; Stroke; Peripheral Vascular Disease; **Hospital:** Northwestern Meml Hosp; **Address:** Northwestern Meml Hosp - Galter Pavilion, 675 N St Clair St, Ste 19-100, Chicago, IL 60611-2647; **Phone:** 312-695-2714; **Board Cert:** Surgery 2001; Vascular Surgery 2003; Surgical Critical Care 1999; **Med School:** Univ Colorado 1975; **Resid:** Surgery, Univ Co Hlth Sci Ctr 1981; **Fellow:** Cardiovascular Disease, Northwestern Meml Hosp 1982; **Fac Appt:** Prof S, Northwestern Univ

Reddy, Daniel MD [VascS] - **Spec Exp:** Aneurysm-Aortic; Carotid Artery Surgery; **Hospital:** Henry Ford Hosp; **Address:** Henry Ford Hosp, Dept Vascular Surgery, 2799 W Grand Blvd, Detroit, MI 48202-2608; **Phone:** 313-916-3156; **Board Cert:** Surgery 1998; Vascular Surgery 2002; **Med School:** Univ Mich Med Sch 1973; **Resid:** Surgery, Wayne State Univ 1978; **Fellow:** Vascular Surgery, Wayne State Univ 1979

Sanchez, Luis A MD [VascS] - **Spec Exp:** Aneurysm-Abdominal & Thoracic Aortic; Endovascular Stent Grafts; Peripheral Vascular Disease; **Hospital:** Barnes-Jewish Hosp; **Address:** Washington Univ School Medicine, 660 S Euclid Ave, Box 8109-Surgery, Saint Louis, MO 63110; **Phone:** 314-362-7408; **Board Cert:** Surgery 2004; Vascular Surgery 2003; **Med School:** Harvard Med Sch 1987; **Resid:** Surgery, Montefiore Med Ctr 1992; **Fellow:** Vascular Surgery, Montefiore Med Ctr 1994; **Fac Appt:** Prof VascS, Washington Univ, St Louis

Shepard, Alexander D MD [VascS] - **Spec Exp:** Aneurysm-Aortic; Aortic Reconstruction; Vascular Surgery-Secondary; **Hospital:** Henry Ford Hosp; **Address:** 2799 W Grand Blvd, Detroit, MI 48202-2608; **Phone:** 313-916-3155; **Board Cert:** Surgery 2001; Vascular Surgery 1994; **Med School:** Johns Hopkins Univ 1976; **Resid:** Surgery, Johns Hopkins Hosp 1982; **Fellow:** Vascular Surgery, New England Med Ctr 1985

Sicard, Gregorio A MD [VascS] - **Spec Exp:** Aneurysm-Abdominal Aortic; **Hospital:** Barnes-Jewish Hosp; **Address:** Wash Univ Med Sch, Dept Surg, 660 S Euclid Ave, Box 8109, St Louis, MO 63110; **Phone:** 314-362-7841; **Board Cert:** Surgery 1996; Vascular Surgery 1992; **Med School:** Univ Puerto Rico 1972; **Resid:** Surgery, Barnes Hosp 1977; **Fellow:** Transplant Surgery, Wash Univ Hosp 1978; **Fac Appt:** Prof S, Washington Univ, St Louis

Stanley, James C MD [VascS] - **Spec Exp:** Peripheral Vascular Surgery; Renovascular Disease; Aneurysm; **Hospital:** Univ Michigan Hlth Sys; **Address:** Univ Mich, Dept Vascular Surgery, 1500 E Med Ctr Drive, rm 2210B, Taubman Ctr, Ann Arbor, MI 48109-0329; **Phone:** 734-936-5786; **Board Cert:** Surgery 1973; Vascular Surgery 2001; **Med School:** Univ Mich Med Sch 1964; **Resid:** Surgery, Univ Mich Med Ctr 1972; **Fac Appt:** Prof S, Univ Mich Med Sch

Vascular Surgery

Towne, Jonathan MD [VascS] - **Spec Exp:** Peripheral Vascular Surgery; Thoracic Outlet Syndrome; Aneurysm-Abdominal Aortic; **Hospital:** Froedtert Meml Lutheran Hosp; **Address:** Med Coll Wisconsin, 9200 W Wisconsin Ave, Milwaukee, WI 53226; **Phone:** 414-805-6633; **Board Cert:** Surgery 2003; Vascular Surgery 2002; **Med School:** Univ Rochester 1967; **Resid:** Surgery, Univ Mich Med Ctr 1969; Surgery, Univ Nebraska Coll Med 1972; **Fellow:** Vascular Surgery, Baylor Coll Med 1975; **Fac Appt:** Prof VascS, Med Coll Wisc

Great Plains and Mountains

Annest, Stephen J MD [VascS] - **Spec Exp:** Thoracic Outlet Syndrome; **Hospital:** Presby - St Luke's Med Ctr, Exempla Saint Jos. Hosp. - Denver; **Address:** The Vascular Institute of the Rockies, 1601 E 19th Ave, Ste 3950, Denver, CO 80218; **Phone:** 303-539-0736; **Board Cert:** Surgery 2000; Vascular Surgery 2005; **Med School:** Univ Wash 1975; **Resid:** Surgery, Albany Med Ctr 1981; **Fellow:** Trauma, Albany Med Ctr 1980; Vascular Surgery, Baylor Univ Med Ctr 1982; **Fac Appt:** Asst Clin Prof S, Hahnemann Univ

Howard, Thomas C MD [VascS] - **Spec Exp:** Aortic Surgery; Aneurysm-Aortic; Carotid Artery Surgery; Lower Limb Arterial Disease; **Hospital:** Nebraska Med Ctr, Immanuel Med Ctr; **Address:** Surgery Ctr of the Heartland, 4239 Farnam St, Ste 823, Omaha, NE 68131; **Phone:** 402-552-3015; **Board Cert:** Surgery 1975; Vascular Surgery 2002; **Med School:** Yale Univ 1969; **Resid:** Surgery, Yale-New Haven Hosp 1974; **Fac Appt:** Assoc Prof S, Univ Nebr Coll Med

Southwest

Clagett, George Patrick MD [VascS] - **Spec Exp:** Aneurysm-Abdominal Aortic; **Hospital:** Parkland Meml Hosp - Dallas, UT Southwestern Med Ctr - Dallas; **Address:** Univ Tex SW Med Ctr, 5909 Harry Hines Blvd, HA8.130, Dallas, TX 75390-9157; **Phone:** 214-645-0548; **Board Cert:** Surgery 1996; Vascular Surgery 2004; **Med School:** Univ VA Sch Med 1968; **Resid:** Surgery, Univ Mich Med Ctr 1972; Surgery, Univ Mich Med Ctr 1976; **Fellow:** Research, Beth Israel-Harvard 1974; Vascular Surgery, Walter Reed Army Med Ctr 1979; **Fac Appt:** Prof S, Univ Tex SW, Dallas

Corson, John MD [VascS] - **Spec Exp:** Carotid Artery Surgery; Vascular Disease in the Elderly; Limb Sparing Surgery; **Hospital:** VA Med Ctr; **Address:** VA Medical Ctr, 1501 San Pedro SE, MS 112, Albequerque, NM 87108; **Phone:** 505-265-1711 x2385; **Board Cert:** Surgery 2002; Vascular Surgery 2001; **Med School:** Scotland 1968; **Resid:** Surgery, Univ Hosp Wales 1975; Surgery, Boston Univ Med Ctr 1980; **Fellow:** Research, Boston Univ Med Ctr 1977; Vascular Surgery, Mass Genl Hosp/Harvard 1981; **Fac Appt:** Prof S, Univ New Mexico

Eidt, John MD [VascS] - **Spec Exp:** Aneurysm-Abdominal Aortic; Carotid Artery Stent Placement; Endovascular Surgery; Peripheral Vascular Disease; **Hospital:** UAMS Med Ctr, John L McClellan VA Med Ctr; **Address:** 4301 W Markham St, Slot 520-2, Little Rock, AR 72205; **Phone:** 501-686-6176; **Board Cert:** Vascular Surgery 1996; Surgical Critical Care 2004; **Med School:** Univ Tex SW, Dallas 1981; **Resid:** Surgery, Brigham-Womens Hosp 1986; **Fellow:** Vascular Surgery, Univ Tex SW Med Ctr; **Fac Appt:** Prof S, Univ Ark

Fowl, Richard J MD [VascS] - **Spec Exp:** Aneurysm-Aortic; Carotid Artery Surgery; Arterial Bypass Surgery-Leg; **Hospital:** Mayo Clin Hosp - Scottsdale; **Address:** Mayo Clinic, Dept Vascular Surgery, 5777 E Mayo Blvd, Phoenix, AZ 85054; **Phone:** 480-342-2868; **Board Cert:** Surgery 2002; Vascular Surgery 2004; **Med School:** Rush Med Coll 1978; **Resid:** Surgery, Med Coll Virginia 1980; Surgery, Univ Iowa Med Ctr 1983; **Fellow:** Vascular Surgery, Mayo Clinic 1985; **Fac Appt:** Prof S, Mayo Med Sch

Hollier, Larry H MD [VascS] - **Spec Exp:** Aortic Surgery; Carotid Artery Surgery; Endovascular Surgery; **Hospital:** Ochsner Baptist Med Ctr, Med Ctr LA @ New Orleans (Univ Hosp); **Address:** 433 Bolivar St, Ste 815, New Orleans, LA 70112; **Phone:** 504-568-4800; **Board Cert:** Surgery 1995; Vascular Surgery 2001; **Med School:** Louisiana State Univ 1968; **Resid:** Surgery, Charity Hosp 1973; **Fellow:** Vascular Surgery, Baylor Med Ctr 1974; **Fac Appt:** Prof S, Louisiana State Univ

Lumsden, Alan B MD [VascS] - **Spec Exp:** Aortic Stent Grafts; Minimally Invasive Surgery; Vein Disorders; **Hospital:** Methodist Hosp - Houston, St Luke's Episcopal Hosp - Houston; **Address:** 1709 Dryden, Ste 1500, Houston, TX 77030; **Phone:** 713-798-5700; **Board Cert:** Vascular Surgery 2002; **Med School:** Scotland 1981; **Resid:** Surgery, Emory Univ Hosp 1989; **Fellow:** Vascular Surgery, Emory Univ Hosp; **Fac Appt:** Prof VascS, Baylor Coll Med

Money, Samuel R MD [VascS] - **Spec Exp:** Aneurysm-Abdominal Aortic; Arterial Bypass Surgery-Leg; Endovascular Surgery; **Hospital:** Mayo Clin Hosp - Scottsdale; **Address:** Mayo Clinic, Dept Surgery, 5777 E Mayo Blvd, Phoenix, AZ 85054; **Phone:** 480-342-2868; **Board Cert:** Surgery 2000; Vascular Surgery 2002; **Med School:** SUNY Downstate 1983; **Resid:** Surgery, Kings Co Med Ctr 1990; **Fellow:** Vascular Surgery, Ochsner Clinic 1993; **Fac Appt:** Prof S, Mayo Med Sch

West Coast and Pacific

Ahn, Sam S MD [VascS] - **Spec Exp:** Minimally Invasive Vascular Surgery; Endovascular Surgery; Thoracic Outlet Syndrome; Hyperhidrosis; **Hospital:** UCLA Med Ctr, St John's Hlth Ctr, Santa Monica; **Address:** 1082 Glendon Ave, Los Angeles, CA 90024; **Phone:** 310-209-2011; **Board Cert:** Surgery 2004; Vascular Surgery 1997; **Med School:** Univ Tex SW, Dallas 1978; **Resid:** Surgery, UCLA Med Ctr 1984; **Fellow:** Vascular Surgery, UCLA Med Ctr 1986; **Fac Appt:** Prof S, UCLA

Andros, George MD [VascS] - **Spec Exp:** Aneurysm-Aortic; Carotid Artery Surgery; **Hospital:** Providence St Joseph Med Ctr; **Address:** 16500 Ventura Blvd, Ste 360, Encino, CA 91436; **Phone:** 818-461-0040; **Board Cert:** Surgery 1970; **Med School:** Univ Chicago-Pritzker Sch Med 1960; **Resid:** Surgery, Mass Genl Hosp 1969

Dilley, Ralph B MD [VascS] - **Spec Exp:** Vascular Reconstruction; **Hospital:** Scripps Green Hosp; **Address:** Scripps Clinic-Torrey Pines, 10666 N Torrey Pines Rd, rm SW208, La Jolla, CA 92037; **Phone:** 858-554-8988; **Board Cert:** Surgery 1966; Thoracic Surgery 1966; Vascular Surgery 2002; **Med School:** Stanford Univ 1959; **Resid:** Surgery, UCLA Med Ctr 1965; Surgery, Johns Hopkins Hosp 1961; **Fellow:** Cardiovascular Surgery, UCSF Med Ctr 1970; **Fac Appt:** Clin Prof S, UCSD

Flanigan, D Preston MD [VascS] - **Spec Exp:** Carotid Artery Disease; Aneurysm; Vein Disorders; **Hospital:** St Joseph's Hosp - Orange; **Address:** 1140 W LaVeta Ave, Ste 850, Orange, CA 92868; **Phone:** 714-560-4450; **Board Cert:** Vascular Surgery 2002; **Med School:** Jefferson Med Coll 1972; **Resid:** Surgery, St Joseph-Mercy Hosp 1977; **Fellow:** Vascular Surgery, Northwest Med Ctr 1978; **Fac Appt:** Clin Prof S, UC Irvine

Gewertz, Bruce MD [VascS] - **Spec Exp:** Carotid Artery Surgery; Peripheral Vascular Disease; Aneurysm-Aortic; **Hospital:** Cedars-Sinai Med Ctr; **Address:** 8700 Beverly Blvd, N Tower, Ste 8215, Los Angeles, CA 90048; **Phone:** 310-423-5884; **Board Cert:** Vascular Surgery 2002; **Med School:** Jefferson Med Coll 1972; **Resid:** Surgery, Univ Mich Hosp 1977; **Fac Appt:** Prof S, UCLA

Vascular Surgery

Grey, Douglas P MD [VascS] - **Hospital:** KFH San Francisco Med Ctr; **Address:** 2238 Geary Blvd, Fl 2, San Francisco, CA 94115; **Phone:** 415-833-3383; **Board Cert:** Thoracic Surgery 2003; Vascular Surgery 2004; **Med School:** UC Irvine 1975; **Resid:** Surgery, Peter Bent Brigham Hosp 1980; Thoracic Surgery, Texas Heart Institute 1982; **Fac Appt:** Clin Prof S, UCSF

Moore, Wesley S MD [VascS] - **Spec Exp:** Aneurysm-Abdominal Aortic; Carotid Artery Surgery; Arterial Reconstruction; **Hospital:** UCLA Med Ctr; **Address:** UCLA Gonda Vascular Ctr, 200 UCLA Med Plaza, rm 510-6, Box 956908, Los Angeles, CA 90095-6908; **Phone:** 310-206-6294; **Board Cert:** Surgery 1966; Vascular Surgery 2003; **Med School:** UCSF 1959; **Resid:** Surgery, UCSF Med Ctr 1964; **Fellow:** Research, VA Hosp-Natl Inst Hlth 1967; **Fac Appt:** Prof S, UCLA

Pevec, William C MD [VascS] - **Spec Exp:** Vascular Disease; Angioplasty & Stent Placement; **Hospital:** UC Davis Med Ctr; **Address:** UC Davis Med Ctr, Dept Vascular Surgery, 4860 Y St, Ste 2100, Sacramento, CA 95817; **Phone:** 916-734-3524; **Board Cert:** Surgery 1999; Vascular Surgery 2001; **Med School:** Univ Cincinnati 1984; **Resid:** Surgery, U Pittsburgh Med Ctr 1990; **Fellow:** Vascular Surgery, Mass Genl Hosp 1992; **Fac Appt:** Assoc Prof VascS, UC Davis

White, Rodney Allen MD [VascS] - **Spec Exp:** Endovascular Surgery; Aneurysm; Carotid Artery Surgery; **Hospital:** LAC - Harbor - UCLA Med Ctr; **Address:** Harbor-UCLA Med Ctr, 1000 W Carson St, Box 11, Torrance, CA 90502; **Phone:** 310-222-2704; **Board Cert:** Surgery 1998; Vascular Surgery 1987; **Med School:** SUNY Upstate Med Univ 1974; **Resid:** Surgery, LAC-Harbor-UCLA Med Ctr 1979; **Fellow:** Vascular Surgery, LAC-Harbor-UCLA Med Ctr 1980; **Fac Appt:** Prof S, UCLA

Zarins, Christopher K MD [VascS] - **Spec Exp:** Carotid Artery Surgery; Aneurysm-Abdominal Aortic; Endovascular Surgery; **Hospital:** Stanford Univ Med Ctr, El Camino Hosp/Camino Hlthcare Sys; **Address:** Stanford Univ Med Ctr, Div Vascular Surg, 300 Pasteur Drive, rm H-3600, Stanford, CA 94305; **Phone:** 650-725-5227; **Board Cert:** Surgery 1975; Vascular Surgery 2002; **Med School:** Johns Hopkins Univ 1968; **Resid:** Surgery, Univ Michigan Hosp 1974; **Fellow:** Surgery, Johns Hopkins Hosp 1972; **Fac Appt:** Prof S, Stanford Univ

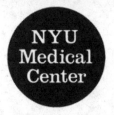

NYU Medical Center

550 First Avenue (at 31st Street)
New York, NY 10016
Physician Referral:
(888)7-NYU-MED (888-769-8633)
www.nyumc.org

VASCULAR SURGERY
A Kinder, Gentler Approach to Aneurysm Repair

When a patient has heart disease, aneurysms, or bulges in the aorta are often an unfortunate, potentially deadly symptom. Most aortic aneurysms occur in areas damaged by artherosclerosis, a condition in which the arteries become hardened from the buildup of cholesterol and other material over many years. It is estimated that one to five percent of people over the age of 65 have an aneurysm. There are usually few symptoms, although some people may feel deep back pain. Severe, excruciating pain is usually the first symptom of a rupture.

Ten years ago, a patient with an aortic aneurysm would have undergone an extensive operation to repair it. Today, NYU Medical Center is among a select group of institutions worldwide that offer minimally invasive surgical solutions to complex aortic problems.

The new, minimally invasive procedure involves making small incisions in the groin and inserting a stent graft, which the surgeon guides to the exact position in the artery needed to ease pressure and prevent rupture. Usually, patients require no blood transfusion and are able to leave the hospital just one or two days after surgery.

As the site of early FDA testing of one of the newest devices used in endovascular surgery, NYU Medical Center is leading the way in both clinical and scientific research in the burgeoning field of vascular surgery. It also is a major training center, where vascular surgeons learn and perfect the latest minimally invasive techniques. NYU's outstanding specialists continue to achieve high rates of success with the new stent graft procedure, even in patients over 75 years of age. Judging from the pace of research at NYU, it is extremely likely that the new techniques will be used to treat other types of conditions in the very near future.

NYU MEDICAL CENTER

At NYU Medical Center, we pride ourselves on delivering the highest quality care. Our emphasis on the newest surgical technologies is not an end in itself, but a way to ease pain and decrease recovery time, as well as achieve the best possible outcomes. In conventional aneurysm repair, the surgeon performs an open-chest procedure, involving blood transfusions, intensive care, and lengthy hospital stays. With the new devices and minimally invasive techniques, our patients not only get well – they return to normal activity and improved quality of life as soon as one week after surgery.

Physician Referral
(888) 7-NYU-MED
(888-769-8633)
www.mininvasive.med.nyu.edu

724

Appendices

APPENDIX A:
Medical Boards

Introduction to ABMS and Osteopathic Specialties

The following pages contain descriptions of the "official" medical specialties, approved by the American Board of Medical Specialists (for M.D.s) or by the American Osteopathic Association (for D.O.s). These are important because they are the only specialties recognized by the official governing boards. There may be physicians who call themselves one kind of specialist or another, but they may not be certified by the "official" boards. There are, in fact, over 100 such "self-designated" boards, some simply groups of physicians interested in a given area of medicine with no qualifications for membership to other groups with very specific qualifications for membership.

It is important for the medical consumer to seek out physicians certified by the ABMS or AOA to assure their doctor has had the appropriate training and passed the board certification exam.

ABMS

The ABMS is an organization of ABMS Approved medical specialty boards. The mission of the ABMS is to maintain and improve the quality of medical care by assisting the Member Boards in their efforts to develop and utilize professional and educational standards for the evaluation and certification of physician specialists. The intent of certification of physicians is to provide assurance to the public that a physician specialist certified by a Member Board of the ABMS has successfully completed an approved educational program and evaluation process which includes an examination designed to assess the knowledge, skills, and experience required to provide quality patient care in that specialty. The ABMS serves to coordinate the activities of its Member Boards and to provide information to the public, the government, the profession and its Members concerning issues involving specialization and certification in medicine.

Following is a list of the addresses of the various medical specialty boards approved by the ABMS. Note that there are 24 board organizations for 25 medical specialties. Psychiatry and Neurology share the same board.

To find out if a physician is certified, consumers can call the individual boards which may charge a fee for the information, or they can contact the ABMS at (866) 275-2267 (no fee) or www.abms.org.

American Board of Allergy and Immunology
510 Walnut Street, Suite 1701
Philadelphia, PA 19106-3699
(215) 592-9466, (866) 264-5568

General Certification in Allergy and Immunology. Certifications awarded since 1989 are valid for 10 years. For those certified prior to 1989 there is no recertification requirement.

American Board of Anesthesiology
4101 Lake Boone Trail
Raleigh, NC 27607-7506
(919) 881-2570

General Certification in Anesthesiology; with Special and Added Qualifications in Critical Care Medicine and Pain Management. Certifications awarded since 2000 are valid for 10 years.

American Board of Colon and Rectal Surgery
20600 Eureka Road, Suite 600
Taylor, MI 48180
(734) 282-9400

General Certification is in Colon and Rectal Surgery. Certifications awarded since 1990 are valid for 10 years.

American Board of Dermatology
Henry Ford Health System
Detriot, MI 48202-3450
(313) 874-1088

General Certification in Dermatology; with Special Qualifications in Clinical and Laboratory Dermatological Immunology, Dermatopathology, and Pediatric Dermatology. Certifications awarded since 1991 are valid for 10 years.

American Board of Emergency Medicine
3000 Coolidge Road
East Lansing, MI 48823-6319
(517) 332-4800

General Certification in Emergency Medicine; with Special and Added Qualifications in Medical Toxicology, Pediatric Emergency Medicine, Sports Medicine and Undersea and Hyperbaric Medicine. Certifications awarded since 1980 are valid for 10 years

American Board of Family Practice
2228 Young Drive
Lexington, KY 40505-4294
(859) 269-5626, (888) 995-5700

General Certification in Family Practice; with Added Qualifications in Adolescent
Medicine, Geriatric Medicine and Sports Medicine. Certifications awarded since 1970
are valid for 7 years.

American Board of Internal Medicine
510 Walnut Street, Suite 1700
Philadelphia, PA 19106-3699
(215) 446-3500, (800) 441-ABIM

General Certification in Internal Medicine; with Special Qualifications in Cardiovascular
Disease, Endocrinology, Diabetes and Metabolism, Gastroenterology, Hematology,
Infectious Disease, Medical Oncology, Nephrology, Pulmonary Disease, and
Rheumatology; and Added Qualifications in Adolescent Medicine, Clinical Cardiac
Electrophysiology, Critical Care Medicine, Geriatric Medicine, Interventional Cardiology,
Sleep Medicine, Sports Medicine and Transplant Hepatology. Certifications awarded
since 1990 are valid for 10 years.

American Board of Medical Genetics
9650 Rockville Pike
Bethesda, MD 20814-3998
(301) 634-7315

General Certification in Clinical Genetics (MD), PhD Medical Genetics, Clinical
Biochemical Genetics, Clinical Cytogenetics and Clinical Molecular Genetics; with
Added Qualifications in Molecular Genetic Pathology. Certifications awarded since 2002
are valid for 2 years.

American Board of Neurological Surgery
6550 Fannin Street, Suite 2139
Houston, TX 77030-2701
(713) 441-6015

General Certification in Neurological Surgery. Certifications awarded since 1999 are
valid for 10 years.

American Board of Nuclear Medicine
4555 Forest Park Boulevard, Suite 119
St. Louis, MO 63108
(314) 367-2225

General Certification in Nuclear Medicine. Certifications awarded since 1992 are valid for 10 years.

American Board of Obstetrics and Gynecology
2915 Vine Street, Suite 300
Dallas, TX 75204
(214) 871-1619

General Certification in Obstetrics and Gynecology; with Special Qualifications in Gynecologic Oncology, Maternal and Fetal Medicine, Reproductive Endocrinology; and Added Qualifications in Critical Care Medicine. Certifications awarded since 1986 are valid for 6 years.

American Board of Ophthalmology
111 Presidential Boulevard, Suite 241
Bala Cynwyd, PA 19004-1075
(610) 664-1175

Certifications Awarded since 1992 are valid for 10 years. For those certified priorto 1992, there is no recertification requirement.

American Board of Orthopaedic Surgery
400 Silver Cedar Court
Chapel Hill, NC 27514
(919) 929-7103

General Certification in Orthopaedic Surgery; with Added Qualification in Hand Surgery; with Added Qualifications in Hand Surgery and Orthopaedic Sports Medicine. Certifications awarded since 1986 are valid for 10 years.

American Board of Otolaryngology
5615 Kirby Drive, Suite 600
Houston, TX 77005
(713) 850-0399

General Certification in Otolaryngology; with Added Qualifications in Neurotology, Pediatric Otolaryngology and Plastic Surgery within the Head and Neck. Certifications awarded since 2002 are valid for10 years.

American Board of Pathology
P.O. Box 25915
Tampa, FL 33622-5915
(813) 286-2444

General Certification in Anatomic and Clinical Pathology, Anatomic Pathology and Clinical Pathology; with Special Qualifications in Blood Banking/Transfusion Medicine, Chemical Pathology, Dermatopathology, Forensic Pathology, Hematology, Medical Microbiology, Molecular Genetic Pathology, Neuropathology and Pediatric Pathology; and Added Qualifications in Cytopathology. Certifications awarded since 1997 are valid for 10 years.

American Board of Pediatrics
111 Silver Cedar Court
Chapel Hill, NC 27514-1651
(919) 929-0461

General Certification in Pediatrics; with Special Qualifications in Adolescent Medicine, Developmental-Behavioral Pediatrics, Neonatal-Perinatal Medicine, Pediatric Cardiology, Pediatric Critical Care Medicine, Pediatric Emergency Medicine, Pediatric Endocrinology, Pediatric Gastroenterology, Pediatric Hematology-Oncology, Pediatric Infectious Diseases, Pediatric Nephrology, Pediatric Pulmonology, and Pediatric Rheumatology; and Added Qualifications in Medical Toxicology, Neurodevelopmental Disabilities, Pediatric Transplant Hepatology and Sports Medicine. Certifications awarded since 1988 valid for 7 years.

American Board of Physical Medicine and Rehabilitation
3015 Allegro Park Lane, S.W.
Rochester, MN 55902-4139
(507) 282-1776

General Certification in Physical Medicine and Rehabilitation; with Special Qualifications in Pain Medicine, Pediatric Rehabilitation Medicine, and Spinal Cord Injury Medicine. Certifications awarded since 1993 are valid for 10 years.

American Board of Plastic Surgery
Seven Penn Center, Suite 400
Philadelphia, PA 19103-2204
(215) 587-9322

General Certification in Plastic Surgery; with Added Qualifications in Hand Surgery. Certifications awarded since 1995 are valid for a 10-year period.

American Board of Preventive Medicine
330 South Wells Street, Suite 1018
Chicago, IL 60606-7106
(312) 939-ABPM [2276]

General Certification in Aerospace Medicine, Occupational Medicine and Public Health
and General Preventive Medicine; with Added Qualifications in Undersea and
Hyperbaric Medicine and Medical Toxicology. Certifications awarded since 1997 are
valid for 10 years.

American Board of Psychiatry and Neurology
500 Lake Cook Road, Suite 335
Deerfield, IL 60015-5349
(847) 945-7900

General Certification in Psychiatry, Neurology and Neurology with Special Qualification
in Child Neurology; with Special Qualifications in Child and Adolescent Psychiatry, Pain
Medicine and Sleep Medicine; and Added Qualifications in Addiction Psychiatry,
Clinical Neurophysiology, Forensic Psychiatry, Geriatric Psychiatry, Neurodevelopmental
Disabilities, Psychosomatic Medicine and Vascular Neurology . Certifications awarded
since 1994 are valid for 10 years.

American Board of Radiology
5441 E. Williams Boulevard, Suite 200
Tucson, AZ 85711
(520) 790-2900

General Certification in Diagnostic Radiology or Radiation Oncology; with Special
Competency in Nuclear Radiology; and Added Qualifications in Neuroradiology,
Pediatric Radiology and Vascular and Interventional Radiology. Radiological Physics is a
non-clinical certification. Certificates are valid for 10 years.

American Board of Surgery
1617 John F. Kennedy Boulevard, Suite 860
Philadelphia, PA 19103-1847
(215) 568-4000

General Certification in Surgery and Vascular Surgery; with Special Qualifications in
Pediatric Surgery and Surgery of the Hand; and Added Qualifications in Surgical Critical
Care. Certifications awarded since 1976 are valid for 10 years.

American Board of Thoracic Surgery
  633 North St. Clair Street, Suite 2320
  Chicago, IL 60611
  (312 202-5900

  General Certification in Thoracic Surgery. Certifications awarded since 1976 are valid for 10 years.

American Board of Urology
  2216 Ivy Road, Suite 210
  Charlottesville, VA 22903
  (434) 979-0059

  General Certification in Urology. Certifications awarded as of 1985 are valid for 10 years.

Osteopathic

The American Osteopathic Association (AOA) is a member association representing more than 56,000 osteopathic physicians (D.O.s). The AOA serves as the primary certifying body for D.O.s, and is the accrediting agency for all osetopathic medical colleges and health care facilities. The AOA's mission is to advance the philosophy and practice of osteopathic medicine by promoting excellence in education, research, and the delivery of quality, cost-effective healthcare within a distinct, unified profession. American Osteopathic Association 142 E Ontario Street Chicago, IL 60611.

Consumers may call the American Osteopathic Association at (800) 621-1773 or visit the website, www.osteopathic.org, for general certification information.

American Osteopathic Board of Anesthesiology

  General certification in Anesthesiology; with Added Qualifications in Addiction Medicine, Critical Care Medicine, and Pain Management. Certifications awarded since 2004 are valid for 10 years. For those certified prior to 2004 there is no recertification requirement.

American Osteopathic Board of Dermatology

  General certification in Dermatology; with Added Qualifications in Dermatopathology and MOHS-Micrographic Surgery. Certifications awarded since 2004 are valid for 10 years.

American Osteopathic Board of Emergency Medicine

General certification in Emergency Medicine; with Added Qualifications in Emergency Medical Services, Medical Toxicology, and Sports Medicine. Certifications awarded since 1994 are valid for 10 years.

American Osteopathic Board of Family Physicians

General certification in Family Practice and Osteopathic Manipulative Treatment (OMT); with Added Qualifications in Geriatric Medicine and Sports Medicine. Certifications awarded since March 1,1997 are valid for 8 years.

American Osteopathic Board of Internal Medicine

General certification in Internal Medicine; with Special Qualifications in Allergy/Immunology, Cardiology, Endocrinology, Gastroenterology, Hematology, Infectious Disease, Nephrology, Oncology, Pulmonary Disease, Rheumatology; with Added Qualifications in Addiction Medicine, Critical Care Medicine, Clinical Cardiac Electrophysiology, Geriatric Medicine, Interventional Cardiology and Sports Medicine. Certifications awarded since 1993 are valid for 10 years.

American Osteopathic Board of Neurology and Psychiatry

General certification in Neurology and Psychiatry; with Special Qualifications in Child/Adolescent Psychiatry and Child/Adolescent Neurology; with Added Qualifications in Addiction Medicine, Neurophysiology, and Sports Medicine. Certifications awarded since 1995 are valid for 10 years.

American Osteopathic Board of Neuromusculoskeletal Medicine

(Formerly American Osteopathic Board of Special Proficiency in Osteopathic Manipulative Medicine)

General certification in Neuromusculoskeletal Medicine. Certifications awarded since 1995 are valid for 10 years. For those certified prior to 1995 there is no recertification requirement.

American Osteopathic Board of Nuclear Medicine

General certification in Nuclear Medicine. Certifications awarded since 1995 are valid for 10 years

American Osteopathic Board of Obstetrics and Gynecology

General certification in Obstetrics and Gynecology; with Special Qualifications in Gynecologic Oncology; Maternal and Fetal Medicine and Reproductive Endocrinology. Certifications awarded since June, 2002 are valid for 6 years.

American Osteopathic Board of Ophthalmology and Otolaryngology/Head and Neck Surgery

General certification in Ophthalmology, Otolaryngolgy, Facial Plastic Surgery and Otolaryngology/Facial Plastic Surgery; with Added Qualifications in Otolaryngic Allergy. Certifications awarded in Ophthalmology since 2000 are valid for 10 years. For those certified prior to 2000 there is no recertification requirement. Certifications awarded in Otolaryngology and/or Otolaryngology/Facial Plastic Surgery since 2002 are valid for 10 years.

American Osteopathic Board of Orthopaedic Surgery

General certification in Orthopaedic Surgery; with Added Qualifications in Hand Surgery. Certifications awarded since 1994 are valid for 10 years.

American Osteopathic Board of Pathology

General certification in Laboratory Medicine, Anatomic Pathology and Anatomic Pathology and Laboratory Medicine; with Special Qualifications in Forensic Pathology; and with Added Qualifications in Dermatopathology. Certifications awarded since 1995 are valid for 10 years.

American Osteopathic Board of Pediatrics

General certification in Pediatrics with Special Qualifications in Adolescent and Young Adult Medicine, Neonatology, Pediatric Allergy/Immunology and Pediatric Endocrinology; with Added Qualifications in Sports Medicine. Certifications awarded since 1995 are valid for 7 years.

American Osteopathic Board of Physical Medicine and Rehabilitation Medicine

General certification in Physical Medicine and Rehabilitation; with Added Qualifications in Sports Medicine. Certifications awarded since 2004 are valid for 10 years.

American Osteopathic Board of Preventive Medicine

General certification in Preventive Medicine/Aerospace Medicine, Preventive Medicine/Occupational-Environmental Medicine and Preventive Medicine/Public Health; with Added Qualifications in Occupational Medicine and Sports Medicine. Certifications awarded since 1994 are valid for 10 years.

American Osteopathic Board of Proctology

General certification in Proctology. Certifications awarded since 2004 are valid for 10 years.

Appendix A: Medical Boards

American Osteopathic Board of Radiology

General certification in Diagnostic Radiology and Radiation Oncology; with Added Qualifications in Body Imaging, Diagnostic Ultrasound, Neuroradiology, Pediatric Radiology and Vascular and Interventional Radiology. Certifications awarded since 2002 are valid for 10 years.

American Osteopathic Board of Surgery

General certification in Surgery, Neurological Surgery, Plastic and Reconstructive Surgery, Cardiothoracic Surgery, Urological Surgery and General Vascular Surgery; with Added Qualifications in Surgical Critical Care. Certifications awarded since 1997 are valid for 10 years.

Appendix B:
Self-Designated Medical Specialties

This list of self-designated medical specialty groups was obtained from the American Board of Medical Specialties. However, it is important to point out that these groups are not recognized by the ABMS, the governing board for the recognized twenty-four medical specialty boards (listed in Appendix A).

The organizations listed below range from highly organized groups that are attempting to formalize training and certification in their field to informal groups interested in a particular aspect of medicine.

If you wish to obtain information from any of these groups you will have to do some detective work. Because so many are informal, the location, phone and mailing addresses change frequently, depending upon the person who is functioning as secretary or administrator.

The best way to track down one of these groups is to consult the doctor listings to find a doctor who has expressed a special interest in that field, and call his or her office. You might also call a nearby academic health center in the area to see if they have a faculty or staff member known to be involved in that particular medical interest. If that fails, take the same approach with your community hospital.

A

Abdominal Surgeons
Acupuncture Medicine
Addiction Medicine
Addictionology
Adolescent Psychiatry
Aesthetic Plastic Surgery
Alcoholism and Other Drug
    Dependencies (AMSAODD)
Algology (Chronic Pain)
Alternative Medicine
Ambulatory Anesthesia
Ambulatory Foot Surgery
Anesthesia
Arthroscopic Surgery
Arthroscopy (Board of North America)

B

Bariatric Medicine
Bionic Psychology
Bloodless Medicine & Surgery

C

Chelation Therapy
Chemical Dependence
Clinical Chemistry
Clinical Ecology
Clinical Medicine and Surgery
Clinical Neurology
Clinical Neurophysiology
Clinical Neurosurgery
Clinical Nutrition
Clinical Orthopaedic Surgery
Clinical Pharmacology
Clinical Polysomnography
Clinical Psychiatry
Clinical Psychology
Clinical Toxicology
Cosmetic Plastic Surgery
Cosmetic Surgery
Council of Non-Board Certified Physicians
Critical Care in Medicine & Surgery

D

Disability Analysis
Disability Evaluating Physicians

E

Electrodiagnostic Medicine
Electroencephalography
Electromyography & Electrodiagnosis
Environmental Medicine
Epidemiology (College)
Eye Surgery

F

Facial Cosmetic Surgery
Facial Plastic & Reconstructive Surgery
Family Practice, Certification
Forensic Examiners
Forensic Psychiatry
Forensic Toxicology

H

Hand Surgery
Head, Facial & Neck Pain & TMJ Orthopaedics
Health Physics
Homeopathic Physicians
Homeotherapeutics
Hypnotic Anesthesiology, National Board for

I

Independent Medical Examiners
Industrial Medicine & Surgery
Insurance Medicine
International Cosmetic & Plastic
    Facial Reconstructive Standards
Interventional Radiology

L

Laser Surgery
Law in Medicine
Longevity Medicine/Surgery

M

Malpractice Physicians
Maxillofacial Surgeons
Medical Accreditation (American Federation for)
Medical Hypnosis
Medical Laboratory Immunology
Medical-Legal Analysis of Medicine & Surgery
Medical Legal & Workers
    Comp. Medicine & Surgery
Medical-Legal Consultants
Medical Management
Medical Microbiology
Medical Preventics (Academy)
Medical Psychotherapists
Medical Toxicology
Microbiology (Medical Microbiology)
Military Medicine
Mohs Micrographic Surgery &
    Cutaneous Oncology

N

Neuroimaging
Neurologic & Orthopaedic Dental
    Medicine and Surgery
Neurological & Orthopaedic Medicine
Neurological & Orthopaedic Surgery
Neurological Microsurgery
Neurology
Neuromuscular Thermography
Neuro-Orthopaedic Dental Medicine
Neuro-Orthopaedic Electrodiagnosis
Neuro-Orthopaedic Laser Surgery
Neuro-Orthopaedic Psychiatry
Neuro-Orthopaedic Thoracic Medicine
Neurorehabilitation
Nutrition

O

Orthopaedic Medicine
Orthopaedic Microneurosurgery
Otorhinolaryngology

P

Pain Management (American Academy of)
Pain Management Specialties
Pain Medicine
Palliative Medicine
Percutaneous Diskectomy
Plastic Esthetic Surgeons
Prison Medicine
Professional Disability Consultants Psychiatric
    Medicine
Psychiatry (American National Board of)
Psychoanalysis (American Examining
    Board in)
Psychological Medicine (International)

Q

Quality Assurance & Utilization Review

R

Radiology & Medical Imaging
Rheumatologic Surgery
Rheumatological & Reconstructive Medicine
Ringside Medicine & Surgery

S

Skin Specialists
Sleep Medicine (Polysomnography)
Spinal Cord Injury
Spinal Surgery
Sports Medicine
Sports Medicine/Surgery

T

Toxicology
Trauma Surgery
Traumatologic Medicine & Surgery
Tropical Medicine

U

Ultrasound Technology
Urologic Allied Health Professionals
Urological Surgery

W

Weight Reduction Medicine

APPENDIX C:
Hospital Listings

The following is an alphabetical listing of all hospitals that have at least one Castle Connolly Top Doctor in this guide. Institutions listed in **Bold** are profiled in this guide in association with Castle Connolly's *Partnership For Excellence* program. The abbreviations as they appear in the listings are in *italics* below. Due to the many changes taking place in the hospital industry the names on this list may have changed subsequent to publication of this guide.

Abbott - Northwestern Hospital		(612) 863-4000
Abbott - Northwestern Hosp		
800 E 28th St	Minneapolis, MN 55407	MIDWEST
Advocate Christ Medical Center		(708) 684-8000
Adv Christ Med Ctr		
4440 W 95th St	Oak Lawn, IL 60453	MIDWEST
Advocate Good Samaritan Hospital		(630) 275-5900
Adv Good Samaritan Hosp		
3815 Highland Ave	Downers Grove, IL 60515	MIDWEST
Advocate Illinois Masonic Medical Center		(773) 975-1600
Adv Illinois Masonic Med Ctr		
836 W Wellington Ave	Chicago, IL 60657-5147	MIDWEST
Advocate Lutheran General Hospital		(847) 723-2210
Adv Luth Genl Hosp		
1775 West Dempster St	Park Ridge, IL 60068	MIDWEST
Alaska Regional Hospital		(907) 276-1131
Alaska Regl Hosp		
2801 DeBarr Rd	Anchorage, AK 99508	WEST COAST AND PACIFIC
Albany Medical Center		(518) 262-3125
Albany Med Ctr		
43 New Scotland Ave	Albany, NY 12208	MID ATLANTIC
Albert Einstein Medical Center		(215) 456-7890
Albert Einstein Med Ctr		
5501 Old York Rd	Philadelphia, PA 19141	MID ATLANTIC
Albert Lea Medical Center-Mayo Health System		(507) 373-2384
Albert Lea Med Ctr-Mayo Hlth Sys		
404 W Fountain St	Albert Lea, MN 56007	MIDWEST

Alfred I duPont Hospital for Children		(302) 651-4000
Alfred I duPont Hosp for Children		
1600 Rockland Rd	Wilmington, DE 19803	MID ATLANTIC
All Children's Hospital		(727) 767-7451
All Children's Hosp		
801 Sixth Street South	St. Petersburg, FL 33701	SOUTHEAST
Allegheny General Hospital		(412) 359-3131
Allegheny General Hosp		
320 E. North Avenue	Pittsburgh, PA 15212	MID ATLANTIC
Alliance Hospital		(432) 550-1000
Alliance Hosp		
515 N Adams	Odessa, TX 79760	SOUTHWEST
Alta Bates Summit Medical Center		(510) 204-4444
Alta Bates Summit Med Ctr		
2450 Ashby Avenue	Berkeley, CA 94705	WEST COAST AND PACIFIC
Arizona Heart Hospital		(602) 532-1000
Arizona Heart Hosp		
1930 Thomas Rd	Phoenix, AZ 85016	SOUTHWEST
Arkansas Children's Hospital		(501) 364-1100
Arkansas Chldns Hosp		
800 Marshall St	Little Rock, AR 72202	SOUTHWEST
Arthur G. James Cancer Hospital & Research Institute		(614) 293-3300
Arthur G James Cancer Hosp & Research Inst		
300 West 10th Avenue	Columbus, OH 43210	MIDWEST
Atlanta Medical Center		(404) 265-4000
Atlanta Med Ctr		
303 Parkway Dr. NE	Atlanta, GA 30312	SOUTHEAST
Audie L Murphy Memorial Veterans Hospital		(210) 617-5300
Audie L Murphy Meml Vets Hosp		
7400 Merton Minter Blvd	San Antonio, TX 78229	SOUTHWEST
Austen Riggs Center		(413) 298-5511
Austen Riggs Ctr		
25 Main Street or PO Box 962	Stockbridge, MA 01262-0962	NEW ENGLAND
Banner Desert Medical Center		(480) 512-3000
Banner Desert Med Ctr		
1400 S Dobson Rd	Mesa, AZ 85202	SOUTHWEST

Banner Good Samaritan Regional Medical Center - Phoenix   (602) 239-2000
Banner Good Samaritan Regl Med Ctr - Phoenix
1111 E McDowell Rd   Phoenix, AZ 85060   SOUTHWEST

Baptist Hospital - Jackson   (601) 968-1000
Baptist Hosp - Jackson
1225 N State St   Jackson, MS 39202   SOUTHEAST

Baptist Hospital - Nashville   (615) 284-5555
Baptist Hosp - Nashville
2000 Church St   Nashville, TN 37236   SOUTHEAST

Baptist Hospital of Miami   (786) 596-1960
Baptist Hosp of Miami
8900 N Kendall Dr   Miami, FL 33176   SOUTHEAST

Baptist Medical Center - San Antonio   (210) 297-7000
Baptist Med Ctr - San Antonio
111 Dallas St   San Antonio, TX 78205   SOUTHWEST

Baptist Memorial Hospital - Memphis   (901) 226-5000
Baptist Memorial Hospital - Memphis
6019 Walnut Grove Rd   Memphis, TN 38120   SOUTHEAST

Barnes-Jewish Hospital   (314) 362-5000
Barnes-Jewish Hosp
One Barnes-Jewish Hospital Plaza   St. Louis, MO 63110   MIDWEST

Barnes-Jewish West County Hospital   (314) 996-8000
Barnes-Jewish West County Hosp
12634 Olive Blvd   St. Louis, MO 63141   MIDWEST

Bascom Palmer Eye Institute   (305) 326-6000
Bascom Palmer Eye Inst.
900 NW 17 St   Miami, FL 33136   SOUTHEAST

Baton Rouge General Medical Center   (225) 387-7000
Baton Rouge Gen Med Ctr
3600 Florida Boulevard   Baton Rouge, LA 70806   SOUTHWEST

Baylor University Medical Center   (214) 820-0111
Baylor Univ Medical Ctr
3500 Gaston Avenue   Dallas, TX 75246   SOUTHWEST

Baystate Medical Center   (413) 794-0000
Baystate Med Ctr
759 Chestnut Street   Springfield, MA 01199   NEW ENGLAND

Ben Taub General Hospital   (713) 873-2000
Ben Taub General Hosp
1504 Taub Loop   Houston, TX 77001   SOUTHWEST

Beth Israel Deaconess Medical Center - Boston   (617) 667-7000
Beth Israel Deaconess Med Ctr - Boston
330 Brookline Ave   Boston, MA 02215   NEW ENGLAND

Beth Israel Medical Center - Milton & Caroll Petrie Division   (212) 420-2000
Beth Israel Med Ctr - Petrie Division
First Avenue @ 16th Street   New York, NY 10003   MID ATLANTIC

Bethesda North Hospital   (513) 745-1111
Bethesda North Hosp
10500 Montgomery Rd   Cincinnati, OH 45242-4415   MIDWEST

Boca Raton Community Hosp   (561) 395-7100
Boca Raton Comm Hosp
800 Meadows Road   Boca Raton, FL 33486   SOUTHEAST

Boston Medical Center   (617) 638-8000
Boston Med Ctr
1 Boston Medical Center Pl   Boston, MA 02118   NEW ENGLAND

Boulder Community Hospital   (303) 440-2273
Boulder Community Hospital
1100 Balsam Ave, Box 9019   Boulder, CO 80301-9019   GREAT PLAINS AND MOUNTAINS

Boys Town National Research Hospital   (402) 498-6511
Boys Town Natl Rsch Hosp
555 N 30th St   Omaha, NE 68101   GREAT PLAINS AND MOUNTAINS

Brigham & Women's Hospital   (617) 732-5500
Brigham & Women's Hosp
75 Francis St   Boston, MA 02115   NEW ENGLAND

Brook Lane Health Services   (301) 733-0330
Brook Lane Hlth Services
13218 Brook Lane Dr, PO Box 1945   Hagerstown, MD 21742   MID ATLANTIC

Brooklyn Hospital Center-Downtown   (718) 250-8000
Brooklyn Hosp Ctr-Downtown
121 DeKalb Avenue   Brooklyn, NY 11201   MID ATLANTIC

Brookwood Medical Center   (205) 877-1000
Brookwood Med Ctr
2010 Brookwood Medical Ctr Drive   Birmingham, AL 35209-6804   SOUTHEAST

Broward General Medical Center   (954) 355-4400
Broward General Med Ctr
1600 S Andrews Ave   Fort Lauderdale, FL 33316   SOUTHEAST

Bryn Mawr Hospital   (610) 526-3000
Bryn Mawr Hosp
130 S Bryn Mawr Ave   Bryn Mawr, PA 19010-3143   MID ATLANTIC

Buffalo General Hospital   (716) 859-5600
Buffalo General Hosp
100 High Street   Buffalo, NY 14203   MID ATLANTIC

Burke Rehabilitation Hospital   (914) 597-2500
Burke Rehab Hosp
785 Mamaroneck Avenue   White Plains, NY 10605   MID ATLANTIC

Butler Hospital   (401) 455-6200
Butler Hosp
345 Blackstone Blvd   Providence, RI 02906   NEW ENGLAND

Cabrini Medical Center   (212) 995-6000
Cabrini Med Ctr
227 East 19th Street   New York, NY 10003   MID ATLANTIC

California Hospital Medical Center   (213) 748-2411
California Hosp Med Ctr
1401 S. Grand Avenue   Los Angeles, CA 90015   WEST COAST AND PACIFIC

California Pacific Medical Center   (415) 600-6000
CA Pacific Med Ctr
PO Box 7999   San Francisco, CA 94120   WEST COAST AND PACIFIC

California Pacific Medical Center - Pacific Campus   (415) 600-6000
CA Pacific Med Ctr - Pacific Campus
2333 Buchanan St   San Francisco, CA 94115   WEST COAST AND PACIFIC

Carilion Roanoke Memorial Hospital   (540) 224-4966
Carilion Roanoke Meml Hosp
Jefferson At Belleview SE   Roanoke, VA 24033   SOUTHEAST

Carolinas Medical Center   (704) 355-2000
Carolinas Med Ctr
1000 Blythe Blvd   Charlotte, NC 28203-5871   SOUTHEAST

Carolinas Medical Center-University   (704) 548-6000
Carolinas Med Ctr-Univ
PO Box 560727   Charlotte, NC 28256   SOUTHEAST

Cedars Medical Center - Miami		(305) 325-5511
Cedars Med Ctr - Miami		
1400 NW 12 Ave	Miami, FL 33136	SOUTHEAST
Cedars-Sinai Medical Center		(310) 423-3277
Cedars-Sinai Med Ctr		
8700 Beverly Boulevard	Los Angeles, CA 90048	WEST COAST AND PACIFIC
Centennial Medical Center		(615) 342-1000
Centennial Med Ctr		
2300 Patterson Street	Nashville, TN 37203	SOUTHEAST
Centinela Freeman Regional Medical Center-Centinela Campus		(310) 673-4660
Centinela Freeman Reg Med Ctr-Centinela		
555 East Hardy Street	Inglewood, CA 90301	WEST COAST AND PACIFIC
Central Baptist Hospital		(859) 260-6592
Central Baptist Hosp		
1740 Nicholasville Rd	Lexington, KY 40503-1499	SOUTHEAST
Chelsea Community Hospital		(734) 475-1311
Chelsea Comm Hosp		
775 S Main St	Chelsea, MI 48118	MIDWEST
Cheyenne Regional Medical Center		(307) 634-2273
Cheyenne Regl Med Ctr		
214 E 23rd St	Cheyenne, WY 82001	GREAT PLAINS AND MOUNTAINS
Children's Healthcare of Atlanta - Egleston		(404) 325-6000
Chldns Hlthcare Atlanta - Egleston		
1405 Clifton Rd NE	Atlanta, GA 30322	SOUTHEAST
Children's Healthcare of Atlanta - Scottish Rite		(404) 250-5437
Chldns Hlthcare Atlanta - Scottish Rite		
1001 Johnson Ferry Rd	Atlanta, GA 30342	SOUTHEAST
Children's Hospital - Boston		(617) 355-6000
Children's Hospital - Boston		
300 Longwood Avenue	Boston, MA 02115	NEW ENGLAND
Children's Hospital - Columbus, OH		(614) 722-2000
Chldn's Hosp - Columbus		
700 Children's Drive	Columbus, OH 43205	MIDWEST
Children's Hospital - Denver, The		(303) 861-8888
Chldn's Hosp - Denver, The		
1056 E 19th Ave	Denver, CO 80218-1088	GREAT PLAINS AND MOUNTAINS

Children's Hospital - Los Angeles (323) 660-2450
Chldns Hosp - Los Angeles
4650 Sunset Blvd   Los Angeles, CA 90027   WEST COAST AND PACIFIC

Children's Hospital - New Orleans (504) 899-9511
Children's Hospital - New Orleans
200 Henry Clay Ave   New Orleans, LA 70118   SOUTHWEST

Children's Hospital - Oakland (510) 428-3000
Chldns Hosp - Oakland
747 52nd St   Oakland, CA 94609   WEST COAST AND PACIFIC

Children's Hospital and Clinics - Minneapolis (612) 813-6111
Chldns Hosp and Clinics - Minneapolis
2525 Chicago Ave S   Minneapolis, MN 55404   MIDWEST

Children's Hospital and Regional Medical Center - Seattle (206) 987-2000
Chldns Hosp and Regl Med Ctr - Seattle
4800 Sand Point Way NE   Seattle, WA 98145   WEST COAST AND PACIFIC

Children's Hospital at OU Medical Center (405) 271-5437
Chldns Hosp OU Med Ctr
940 Northeast 13th St   Oklahoma City, OK 73104   SOUTHWEST

Children's Hospital Central California (559) 353-3000
Chldns Hosp Central California
9300 Valley Children's Pl   Madera, CA 93638   WEST COAST AND PACIFIC

Children's Hospital Medical Center - Akron (330) 379-8200
Children's Hosp & Med Ctr- Akron
One Perkins Square   Akron, OH 44308   MIDWEST

Children's Hospital of Alabama - Birmingham (205) 939-9100
Children's Hospital - Birmingham
1600 7th Ave South   Birmingham, AL 35233   SOUTHEAST

Children's Hospital of Michigan (313) 745-5437
Chldns Hosp of Michigan
3901 Beaubian Blvd   Detroit, MI 48201   MIDWEST

Children's Hospital of Philadelphia, The (215) 590-1000
Chldns Hosp of Philadelphia, The
34th St & Civic Center Blvd   Philadelphia, PA 19104   MID ATLANTIC

Children's Hospital of Pittsburgh - UPMC (412) 692-8583
Chldns Hosp of Pittsburgh - UPMC
3705 Fifth Avenue   Pittsburgh, PA 15213   MID ATLANTIC

Children's Hospital of the King's Daughters		(757) 668-7500
Chldns Hosp of King's Daughters		
601 Children's Ln	Norfolk, VA 23507	SOUTHEAST

Children's Hospital of Wisconsin		(414) 266-2000
Chldns Hosp - Wisconsin		
9000 W Wisconsin Ave	Milwaukee, WI 53201	MIDWEST

Children's Medical Center of Dallas		(214) 456-7000
Chldns Med Ctr of Dallas		
1935 Motor St	Dallas, TX 75235	SOUTHWEST

Children's Memorial Hospital		(773) 880-4000
Children's Mem Hosp		
2300 Children's Plaza	Chicago, IL 60614	MIDWEST

Children's Mercy Hospitals & Clinics		(816) 234-3000
Chldns Mercy Hosps & Clinics		
2401 Gilham Rd	Kansas City, MO 64108	MIDWEST

Children's National Medical Center - DC		(202) 884-5000
Chldns Natl Med Ctr		
111 Michigan Ave NW	Washington, DC 20010	MID ATLANTIC

Christ Hospital, The		(513) 585-2000
Christ Hospital		
2139 Auburn Ave	Cincinnati, OH 45219	MIDWEST

Christiana Hospital		(302) 733-1000
Christiana Hospital		
4755 Ogletown-Stanton Rd	Newark, DE 19718-0001	MID ATLANTIC

Christus Santa Rosa Children's Hospital		(512) 228-2011
Christus Santa Rosa Children's Hosp		
333 N Santa Rosa St	San Antonio, TX 78207	SOUTHWEST

Cincinnati Children's Hospital Medical Center		(800) 344-2462
Cincinnati Chldns Hosp Med Ctr		
3333 Burnet Ave	Cincinnati, OH 45229-3039	MIDWEST

Cincinnati Shriners Hospital		(513) 872-6000
Cincinnati Shriners Hosp		
3229 Burnet Ave	Cincinnati, OH 45229-3095	MIDWEST

City of Hope National Medical Center & Beckman Research		(626) 359-8111
City of Hope Natl Med Ctr & Beckman Rsch		
1500 E Duarte Rd	Duarte, CA 91010	WEST COAST AND PACIFIC

CJW Medical Center Johnston-Willis Campus (804) 330-2000
CJW Med Ctr
1401 Johnston-Willis Dr Richmond, VA 23235 SOUTHEAST

Cleveland Clinic Florida - Weston (954) 659-5000
Cleveland Clin - Weston
2950 Cleveland Clinic Blvd Weston, FL 33331 SOUTHEAST

Cleveland Clinic Foundation (800) 223-2273
Cleveland Clin Fdn
9500 Euclid Avenue Cleveland, OH 44195 MIDWEST

Columbus Hospital (973) 268-1400
Columbus Hosp
495 N 13th Street Newark, NJ 07107 MID ATLANTIC

Community Medical Center - Toms River (908) 240-8000
Comm Med Ctr - Toms River
99 Highway 37 W Toms River, NJ 08755 MID ATLANTIC

Concord Hospital (603) 225-2711
Concord Hospital
250 Pleasant St Concord, NH 03301-2598 NEW ENGLAND

Connecticut Children's Medical Center (860) 545-9000
CT Chldns Med Ctr
282 Washington St Hartford, CT 06106 NEW ENGLAND

Connecticut Mental Health Center (203) 789-7092
Connecticut Mental Hlth Ctr
34 Park St New Haven, CT 06508-1842 NEW ENGLAND

Cook Children's Medical Center (682) 885-4000
Cook Chldns Med Ctr
801 7th Ave Fort Worth, TX 76104-2796 SOUTHWEST

Cooper University Hospital (856) 342-2000
Cooper Univ Hosp
1 Cooper Plaza Camden, NJ 08103-1489 MID ATLANTIC

Covenant Children's Medical Center (806) 725-1011
Covenant Children's Med Ctr
3610 21st St Lubbock, TX 79410 SOUTHWEST

Craig Hospital (303) 789-8000
Craig Hosp
3425 S Clarkson Englewood, CO 80113 GREAT PLAINS AND MOUNTAINS

Crawford Long Hospital of Emory University (404) 686-4411
Crawford Long Hosp of Emory Univ
550 Peachtree St NE Atlanta, GA 30365 SOUTHEAST

Creighton University Medical Center (402) 449-4000
Creighton Univ Med Ctr
601 N 30th St Omaha, NE 68131-2197 GREAT PLAINS AND MOUNTAINS

Dana-Farber Cancer Institute (617) 632-3000
Dana-Farber Cancer Inst
44 Binney St Boston, MA 02115 NEW ENGLAND

Dartmouth - Hitchcock Medical Center (603) 650-5000
Dartmouth - Hitchcock Med Ctr
1 Medical Center Dr Lebanon, NH 03756-0002 NEW ENGLAND

Delnor - Community Hospital (630) 208-3000
Delnor - Comm Hosp
300 Randall Road Geneva, IL 60134 MIDWEST

Denver Health Medical Center (303) 436-6000
Denver Health Med Ctr
777 Bannock St Denver, CO 80204 GREAT PLAINS AND MOUNTAINS

Desert Regional Medical Center (760) 323-6511
Desert Regl Med Ctr
1150 N Indian Canyon Dr Palm Springs, CA 92262 WEST COAST AND PACIFIC

Detroit Medical Center (313) 578-3930
Detroit Med Ctr
3663 Woodward Ave, Ste 200 Detroit, MI 48201-2403 MIDWEST

DeVos Children's Hospital (616) 957-0866
DeVos Children's Hosp
1000 E Paris SE Grand Rapids, MI 49546 MIDWEST

Doctors Hospital (706) 651-3232
Doctors Hosp
3651 Wheeler Rd Augusta, GA 30909 SOUTHEAST

Doctors' Hospital (305) 666-2111
Doctors' Hosp
5000 University Dr Coral Gables, FL 33146 SOUTHEAST

Doernbecher Children's Hospital/Oregon Health Science University (503) 494-8811
Doernbecher Chldns Hosp/OHSU
3181 SW Sam Jackson Park Rd Portland, OR 97201-3098 WEST COAST AND PACIFIC

Dotter Interventional Institute - OHSU (503) 494-7660
Dotter Institute - OHSU
3181 SW Sam Jackson Park Rd   Portland, OR 97201   WEST COAST AND PACIFIC

Duke Health Raleigh Hospital (919) 954-3000
Duke Health Raleigh
3400 Wake Forest Rd   Raleigh, NC 27609   SOUTHEAST

Duke University Medical Center (919) 684-8111
Duke Univ Med Ctr
DUMC, Box 3708   Durham, NC 27710   SOUTHEAST

Durham Regional Hospital (919) 470-4000
Durham Regional Hosp
3643 N Roxboro Rd   Durham, NC 27704   SOUTHEAST

East Cooper Regional Medical Center (843) 881-0100
E Cooper Reg Med Ctr
1200 Johnnie Dodds Blvd   Mount Pleasant, SC 29464-3231   SOUTHEAST

East Jefferson General Hospital (504) 454-4000
E Jefferson Genl Hosp
4200 Houma Blvd   Metairie, LA 70006-2973   SOUTHWEST

East Texas Medical Center (903) 597-0351
E TX Med Ctr
1000 South Beckham Ave.   Tyler, TX 75701   SOUTHWEST

El Camino Hospital/Camino Healthcare System (650) 940-7000
El Camino Hosp/Camino Hlthcare Sys
2500 Grant Road   Mountain View, CA 94039   WEST COAST AND PACIFIC

Emory University Hospital (404) 712-2000
Emory Univ Hosp
1364 Clifton Rd NE   Atlanta, GA 30322   SOUTHEAST

Englewood Hospital & Medical Center (201) 894-3000
Englewood Hosp & Med Ctr
350 Engle Street   Englewood, NJ 07631   MID ATLANTIC

Evanston Hospital (847) 570-2000
Evanston Hosp
2650 Ridge Ave   Evanston, IL 60201   MIDWEST

Evanston Northwestern Healthcare (847) 570-2000
Evanston NW Hlthcare
1301 Central Ave   Evanston, IL 60201   MIDWEST

Evergreen Hospital Medical Center   (425) 899-1000
Evergreen Hosp Med Ctr
12040 NE 128th St   Kirkland, WA 98034-3013   WEST COAST AND PACIFIC

Fairview Southdale Hospital   (952) 924-5000
Fairview Southdale Hosp
6401 France Ave S   Edina, MN 55435-2199   MIDWEST

Fletcher Allen Health Care - Medical Center Campus   (802) 847-0000
FAHC - Med Ctr Campus
111 Colchester Ave (Burgess 1)   Burlington, VT 05401   NEW ENGLAND

Fletcher Allen Health Care - UHC Campus   (802) 847-0000
FAHC - UHC Campus
1 S Prospect St   Burlington, VT 05401   NEW ENGLAND

Florida Hospital - Celebration Health   (407) 764-4000
Florida Hosp Celebration Hlth
400 Celebration Pl   Celebration, FL 34747   SOUTHEAST

Florida Hospital - Orlando   (407) 303-5600
Florida Hosp - Orlando
601 E Rollins St   Orlando, FL 32803   SOUTHEAST

Floyd Memorial Hospital & Health Services   (812) 944-7701
Floyd Meml Hosp & Hlth Svcs
1850 State St   New Albany, IN 47150-4997   MIDWEST

Forsyth Medical Center   (336) 718-5000
Forsyth Med Ctr
3333 Silas Creek Pkwy   Winston-Salem, NC 27103   SOUTHEAST

Fort Sanders Regional Medical Center   (865) 541-1111
Fort Sanders Reg Med Ctr
1901 Clinch Ave SW   Knoxville, TN 37916-2398   SOUTHEAST

Four Winds Hospital   (914) 763-8151
Four Winds Hosp
800 Cross River Road   Katonah, NY 10536   MID ATLANTIC

Fox Chase Cancer Center   (215) 728-6900
Fox Chase Cancer Ctr
333 Cottman Avenue   Philadelphia, PA 19111   MID ATLANTIC

Franklin Square Hospital   (410) 682-7000
Franklin Square Hosp
9000 Franklin Square Drive   Baltimore, MD 21237   MID ATLANTIC

Froedtert Memorial Lutheran Hospital		(414) 805-6644
Froedtert Meml Lutheran Hosp		
9200 W Wisconsin Ave	Milwaukee, WI 53226	MIDWEST

Gaston Memorial Hospital		(704) 834-2000
Gaston Meml Hosp		
2525 Court Dr	Gastonia, NC 28054	SOUTHEAST

Geisinger-Wyoming Valley Medical Center		(570) 826-7300
Geisinger-Wyoming Med Ctr		
1000 E Mountain Blvd	Wilkes-Barre, PA 18711	MID ATLANTIC

George Washington University Hospital		(202) 715-4000
G Washington Univ Hosp		
900 23rd St NW	Washington, DC 20037	MID ATLANTIC

Georgetown University Hospital		(202) 444-2000
Georgetown Univ Hosp		
3800 Reservoir Rd NW	Washington, DC 20007	MID ATLANTIC

Glenbrook Hospital		(847) 657-5800
Glenbrook Hosp		
2100 Pfingsten Rd	Glenview, IL 60025	MIDWEST

Good Samaritan Hosp - Cincinnati		(513) 872-1400
Good Samaritan Hosp - Cincinnati		
375 Dixmyth Ave	Cincinnati, OH 45220	MIDWEST

Good Samaritan Hospital - Los Angeles		(213) 977-2121
Good Samaritan Hosp - Los Angeles		
1225 Wilshire Boulevard	Los Angeles, CA 90017	WEST COAST AND PACIFIC

Good Samaritan Hospital - San Jose		(408) 559-2011
Good Samaritan Hosp - San Jose		
2425 Samaritan Drive	San Jose, CA 95124	WEST COAST AND PACIFIC

Good Samaritan Medical Center - West Palm Beach		(561) 655-5511
Good Sam Med Ctr - W Palm Beach		
1309 N Flagler Dr	West Palm Beach, FL 33401	SOUTHEAST

Goshen General Hospital		(574) 533-2141
Goshen Genl Hosp		
200 High Park Ave	Goshen, IN 46526	MIDWEST

Gottlieb Memorial Hospital		(708) 681-3200
Gottlieb Meml Hosp		
701 W North Ave	Melrose Park, IL 60160	MIDWEST

Grady Health System		(404) 616-4307
Grady Hlth Sys		
80 Jesse Hill Jr Dr	Atlanta, GA 30303	SOUTHEAST
Greater Baltimore Medical Center		(443) 849-2000
Greater Baltimore Med Ctr		
6701 N Charles St	Baltimore, MD 21204	MID ATLANTIC
Greenwich Hospital		(203) 863-3000
Greenwich Hosp		
Five Perryridge Road	Greenwich, CT 06830	NEW ENGLAND
H Lee Moffitt Cancer Center & Research Institute		(813) 972-4673
H Lee Moffitt Cancer Ctr & Research Inst		
12902 Magnolia Drive	Tampa, FL 33612-9497	SOUTHEAST
Hackensack University Medical Center		(201) 996-2000
Hackensack Univ Med Ctr		
30 Prospect Avenue	Hackensack, NJ 07601	MID ATLANTIC
Hahnemann University Hospital		(215) 762-7000
Hahnemann Univ Hosp		
Broad & Vine St	Philadelphia, PA 19102	MID ATLANTIC
Hamot Medical Center		(814) 877-6000
Hamot Med Ctr		
201 State Street	Erie, PA 16550-0001	MID ATLANTIC
Harborview Medical Center		(206) 731-3000
Harborview Med Ctr		
325 9th Ave, Box 359717	Seattle, WA 98104	WEST COAST AND PACIFIC
Harlem Hospital Center		(212) 939-1000
Harlem Hosp Ctr		
506 Lenox Avenue	New York, NY 10037	MID ATLANTIC
Harper University Hospital		(313) 745-8040
Harper Univ Hosp		
3990 John R St	Detroit, MI 48201-2097	MIDWEST
Harris Methodist Hospital - Fort Worth		(817) 882-2000
Harris Methodist Hosp - Fort Worth		
1301 Pennsylvania Ave	Fort Worth, TX 76104	SOUTHWEST
Harrison Memorial Hospital		(360) 377-3911
Harrison Meml Hosp		
2520 Cherry Ave	Bremerton, WA 98310-4270	WEST COAST AND PACIFIC

Hartford Hospital	(860) 545-5000
Hartford Hosp	
80 Seymour St, Box 5037 Hartford, CT 06102-5037	NEW ENGLAND

Health Alliance of Greater Cincinnati	(513) 632-3700
Health Alliance of Greater Cincinnati	
2060 Reading Rd Cincinnati, OH 45202	MIDWEST

Healthsouth Medical Center - Birmingham	(205) 930-7000
Healthsouth Med Ctr - Birmingham	
1201 11th Ave S Birmingham, AL 35205-5299	SOUTHEAST

Hennepin County Medical Center	(612) 347-2121
Hennepin Cnty Med Ctr	
701 Park Ave S Minneapolis, MN 55415	MIDWEST

Henry Ford Hospital	(313) 916-2600
Henry Ford Hosp	
2799 W Grand Blvd Detroit, MI 48202	MIDWEST

Highland Park Hospital	(847) 432-8000
Highland Park Hosp	
718 Glenview Ave Highland Park, IL 60035	MIDWEST

Hillcrest Hospital Cleveland Clinic Health System	(440) 449-4500
Hillcrest Hosp-Mayfield Hts	
6780 Mayfield Rd Mayfield Heights, OH 44124	MIDWEST

Hinsdale Hospital	(630) 856-9000
Hinsdale Hosp	
120 N Oak St Hinsdale, IL 60521	MIDWEST

Hoag Memorial Hospital Presbyterian	(949) 645-8600
Hoag Meml Hosp Presby	
One Hoag Drive Newport Beach, CA 92663	WEST COAST AND PACIFIC

Holy Cross Hospital - Silver Spring	(301) 754-7000
Holy Cross Hospital - Silver Spring	
1500 Forest Glen Road Silver Spring, MD 20910	MID ATLANTIC

Hospital for Joint Diseases	(212) 598-6000
Hosp For Joint Diseases	
301 East 17th Street New York, NY 10003	MID ATLANTIC

Hospital for Special Surgery	(212) 606-1000
Hosp For Special Surgery	
535 East 70th Street New York, NY 10021	MID ATLANTIC

Hospital of Central Connecticut		(860) 224-5011
Hosp Central CT		
100 Grand St	New Britain, CT 06050	NEW ENGLAND

Hospital of St Raphael		(203) 789-3000
Hosp of St Raphael		
1450 Chapel Street	New Haven, CT 06511	NEW ENGLAND

Hospital of the University of Pennsylvania - UPHS		(215) 662-4000
Hosp Univ Penn - UPHS		
3400 Spruce Street	Philadelphia, PA 19104	MID ATLANTIC

Howard University Hospital		(202) 865-6100
Howard Univ Hosp		
2041 Georgia Ave NW	Washington, DC 20060	MID ATLANTIC

Hunter Holmes McGuire Veterans Affairs Medical Center		(804) 675-5500
Hunter Holmes McGuire VA Med Ctr		
1201 Broad Rock Boulevard	Richmond, VA 23249	SOUTHEAST

Hutzel Women's Hospital - Detroit		(313) 745-7555
Hutzel Hosp - Detroit		
3980 John R. Blvd	Detroit, MI 48201-2018	MIDWEST

Imperial Point Medical Center		(954) 776-8500
Imperial Point Med Ctr		
6401 N Federal Hwy	Fort Lauderdale, FL 33308	SOUTHEAST

Indian River Memorial Hosp		(772) 567-4311
Indian River Mem Hosp		
1000 36th St	Vero Beach, FL 32960	SOUTHEAST

Indiana University Hospital		(317) 274-5000
Indiana Univ Hosp		
550 N University Blvd	Indianapolis, IN 46202	MIDWEST

Ingalls Memorial Hospital		(708) 333-2300
Ingalls Meml Hosp		
1 Ingalls Dr	Harvey, IL 60426	MIDWEST

Inova Alexandria Hospital		(703) 504-3000
Inova Alexandria Hosp		
4320 Seminary Rd	Alexandria, VA 22304	SOUTHEAST

Inova Fair Oaks Hospital		(703) 391-3600
Inova Fair Oaks Hosp		
3600 Joseph Siewick Dr	Fairfax, VA 22033	SOUTHEAST

Inova Fairfax Hospital		(703) 698-1110
Inova Fairfax Hosp		
3300 Gallows Road	Falls Church, VA 22042	SOUTHEAST

Intergris Baptist Medical Center - Oklahoma   (405) 949-3011
Intergris Baptist Med Ctr - OK
3300 NW Expressway   Oklahoma City, OK 73112-9028   SOUTHWEST

Iowa Methodist Medical Center   (515) 241-6212
Iowa Methodist Med Ctr
1200 Pleasant St   Des Moines, IA 50309   MIDWEST

Jackson Memorial Hospital   (305) 585-1111
Jackson Meml Hosp
1611 NW 12th Ave   Miami, FL 33136   SOUTHEAST

Jersey City Medical Center   (201) 915-2000
Jersey City Med Ctr
355 Grand Street   Jersey City, NJ 07302   MID ATLANTIC

Jewish Hospital HealthCare Services, Inc.   (502) 587-4011
Jewish Hosp HlthCre Svcs Inc
200 Abraham Slexner Way   Louisville, KY 40202   SOUTHEAST

JFK Medical Center - Atlantis   (561) 642-3791
JFK Med Ctr - Atlantis
5301 S Congress Ave   Atlantis, FL 33462   SOUTHEAST

JFK Medical Center - Edison   (732) 321-7000
JFK Med Ctr - Edison
65 James Street   Edison, NJ 08818   MID ATLANTIC

Joe Di Maggio Children's Hospital   (954) 987-2000
Joe Di Maggio Chldns Hosp
3501 Johnson St   Hollywood, FL 33021   SOUTHEAST

John L McClellan VA Medical Center   (501) 257-1000
John L McClellan VA Med Ctr
4300 W 7th St   Little Rock, AR 72205   SOUTHWEST

John Sealy Hospital - UTMB   (409) 747-1935
UTMB - John Sealy Hospital
301 University Blvd   Galveston, TX 77555   SOUTHWEST

Johns Hopkins Bayview Medical Center   (410) 550-0100
Johns Hopkins Bayview Med Ctr
4940 Eastern Avenue   Baltimore, MD 21224   MID ATLANTIC

Johns Hopkins Hospital - Baltimore, The   (410) 955-5000
Johns Hopkins Hosp - Baltimore
600 N Wolfe St   Baltimore, MD 21287   MID ATLANTIC

Kaiser Permanente Baldwin Park Medical Center   (626) 851-1011
Kaiser Permanente Baldwin Pk Med Ctr
1011 Baldwin Park Blvd   Baldwin Park, CA 91706   WEST COAST AND PACIFIC

Kaiser Permanente Oakland Medical Center   (510) 752-1000
Kaiser Permanente Oakland Med Ctr
280 West MacArthur Boulevard   Oakland, CA 94611   WEST COAST AND PACIFIC

Kaiser Permanente South San Francisco Medical Center   (650) 742-2000
Kaiser Permanente South San Francisco Med Ctr
1200 El Camino Real   South San Francisco, CA 94080   WEST COAST AND PACIFIC

Kapiolani Medical Center for Women & Children   (808) 983-6000
Kapiolani Med Ctr for Women & Chldn
1319 Punahou St   Honolulu, HI 96826   WEST COAST AND PACIFIC

Karmanos Cancer Institute   (800) 527-6266
Karmanos Cancer Inst
4100 John R   Detroit, MI 48201   MIDWEST

Kennedy Krieger Institute   (443) 923-9200
Kennedy Krieger Inst
707 N Broadway   Baltimore, MD 21205   MID ATLANTIC

Kessler Institute for Rehabilitation - West Orange   (973) 243-6800
Kessler Inst for Rehab - W Orange
1199 Pleasant Valley Way   West Orange, NJ 07052-1499   MID ATLANTIC

KFH San Francisco Medical Center   (415) 833-2000
KFH San Francisco Med Ctr
2425 Geary Blvd   San Francisco, CA 94115   WEST COAST AND PACIFIC

KFH Woodland Hills Medical Center   (818) 719-2000
KFH Woodland Hills Med Ctr
5601 DeSoto Avenue   Woodland Hills, CA 91365   WEST COAST AND PACIFIC

Kootenai Medical Center   (208) 666-2000
Kootenai Med Ctr
2003 Lincoln Way   Coeur d'Alene, ID 83814   GREAT PLAINS AND MOUNTAINS

Kosair Children's Hospital   (502) 629-6000
Kosair Chldn's Hosp
231 E Chestnut St   Louisville, KY 40202   SOUTHEAST

La Grange Memorial Hospital   (708) 352-1200
La Grange Meml Hosp
5101 S Willow Springs Rd   La Grange, IL 60525   MIDWEST

La Rabida Children's Hospital (773) 363-6700
La Rabida Chlds Hosp
E 65th at Lake Michigan Chicago, IL 60649 MIDWEST

LAC & USC Medical Center (323) 226-2622
LAC & USC Med Ctr
1200 N State St Los Angeles, CA 90033-4525 WEST COAST AND PACIFIC

LAC - Harbor - UCLA Medical Center (310) 222-2345
LAC - Harbor - UCLA Med Ctr
1000 W Carson St Torrance, CA 90509-2059 WEST COAST AND PACIFIC

LAC - King/Drew Medical Center (310) 668-4321
LAC - King/Drew Med Ctr
12021 South Wilmington Avenue Los Angeles, CA 90059 WEST COAST AND PACIFIC

Lafayette General Medical Center (337) 289-7991
Lafayette Genl Med Ctr
1214 Coolidge Blvd Lafayette, LA 70503 SOUTHWEST

Lahey Clinic (781) 744-5100
Lahey Clin
41 Mall Road Burlington, MA 01805 NEW ENGLAND

Lakeland Regional Medical Center (863) 687-1100
Lakeland Regl Med Ctr
1324 Lakeland Hills Blvd Lakeland, FL 33805 SOUTHEAST

Lankenau Hospital (610) 645-2000
Lankenau Hosp
100 Lancaster Ave Wynnewood, PA 19096-3498 MID ATLANTIC

Laureate Psychiatric Clinic & Hospital (918) 481-4000
Laureate Psyc Clinic & Hosp
6655 S Yale Ave, Box 470207 Tulsa, OK 74147 SOUTHWEST

LDS Hospital (801) 408-1100
LDS Hosp
8th Ave & C St Salt Lake City, UT 84143 GREAT PLAINS AND MOUNTAINS

Le Bonheur Children's Medical Center (901) 572-3000
Le Bonheur Chldns Med Ctr
50 N Dunlap Memphis, TN 38103-2893 SOUTHEAST

Legacy Good Samaritan Hospital and Medical Center (503) 413-7711
Legacy Good Samaritan Hosp and Med Ctr
1015 NW 22nd Ave Portland, OR 97210-3025 WEST COAST AND PACIFIC

Legacy Meridian Park Hospital   (503) 692-1212
Legacy Meridian Park Hosp
19300 SW 65th Ave   Tualatin, OR 97062   WEST COAST AND PACIFIC

Lenox Hill Hospital   (212) 434-2000
Lenox Hill Hosp
100 East 77th Street   New York, NY 10021   MID ATLANTIC

Lindy Boggs Medical Center   (504) 483-5000
L Boggs Med Ctr
301 N Jefferson Davis Pkwy   New Orleans, LA 70119   SOUTHWEST

Loma Linda Children's Hospital   (909) 558-8000
Loma Linda Chldns Hosp
11234 Anderson St   Loma Linda, CA 92354   WEST COAST AND PACIFIC

Loma Linda University Medical Center   (909) 558-4000
Loma Linda Univ Med Ctr
11234 Anderson St   Loma Linda, CA 92354   WEST COAST AND PACIFIC

Long Beach Memorial Medical Center   (562) 933-2000
Long Beach Meml Med Ctr
2801 Atlantic Ave   Long Beach, CA 90801   WEST COAST AND PACIFIC

Long Island College Hospital   (718) 780-1000
Long Island Coll Hosp
339 Hicks Street   Brooklyn, NY 11201   MID ATLANTIC

Long Island Jewish Medical Center   (516) 470-7000
Long Island Jewish Med Ctr
270-05 76th Avenue   New Hyde Park, NY 11040   MID ATLANTIC

Los Alamitos Medical Center   (562) 598-1311
Los Alamitos Med Ctr
3751 Katella Ave   Los Alamitos, CA 90720   WEST COAST AND PACIFIC

Louis A Weiss Memorial Hospital   (773) 878-8700
Weiss Meml Hosp
4646 N Marine Dr   Chicago, IL 60640   MIDWEST

Louisiana State University Hospital   (318) 675-4239
Louisiana State Univ Hosp
1501 Kings Highway P.O. Box 33932   Shreveport, LA 71130   SOUTHWEST

Lovelace Medical Center   (505) 262-7000
Lovelace Medical Center
5400 Gibson Blvd SE   Albuquerque, NM, NM 87106   SOUTHWEST

Loyola University Medical Center   (708) 216-9000
Loyola Univ Med Ctr
2160 S 1st Ave   Maywood, IL 60153   MIDWEST

Lucile Packard Children's Hospital/Stanford University Medical Center   (650) 497-8000
Lucile Packard Chldns Hosp/Stanford Univ Med Ctr
725 Welch Rd   Palo Alto, CA 94304   WEST COAST AND PACIFIC

Lutheran Medical Center - Brooklyn   (718) 630-7000
Lutheran Med Ctr - Brooklyn
150 55th Street   Brooklyn, NY 11220   MID ATLANTIC

Lynchburg General Hospital   (434) 947-3000
Lynchburg Genl Hosp
1901 Tate Springs Rd   Lynchburg, VA 24501-1167   SOUTHEAST

Magee Rehabilitation Hospital   (215) 587-3000
Magee Rehab Hosp
1513 Race St   Philadelphia, PA 19102-1177   MID ATLANTIC

Magee-Womens Hospital - UPMC   (412) 641-1000
Magee-Womens Hosp - UPMC
300 Halket Street   Pittsburgh, PA 15213   MID ATLANTIC

Maimonides Medical Center   (718) 283-6000
Maimonides Med Ctr
4802 Tenth Avenue   Brooklyn, NY 11219   MID ATLANTIC

Maine Medical Center   (207) 871-0111
Maine Med Ctr
22 Bramhall St   Portland, ME 04102   NEW ENGLAND

Manhattan Eye, Ear & Throat Hospital   (212) 838-9200
Manhattan Eye, Ear & Throat Hosp
210 East 64th Street   New York, NY 10021   MID ATLANTIC

Marin General Hospital   (415) 925-7000
Marin Genl Hosp
250 Bon Air Rd   Greenbrae, CA 94904   WEST COAST AND PACIFIC

Mary Shiels Hospital   (214) 443-3000
Mary Shiels Hosp
3515 Howell St   Dallas, TX 75204   SOUTHWEST

Maryland General Hospital   (410) 225-8000
Maryland Genl Hosp
827 Linden Ave   Baltimore, MD 21201   MID ATLANTIC

Massachusetts Eye and Ear Infirmary		(617) 523-7900
Mass Eye & Ear Infirmary		
243 Charles Street	Boston, MA 02114	NEW ENGLAND

Massachusetts General Hospital		(617) 726-2000
Mass Genl Hosp		
55 Fruit St	Boston, MA 02114	NEW ENGLAND

Massachusetts Mental Health Center		(617) 626-9300
MA Mental Hlth Ctr		
180 Morton St	Jamaica Plain, MA 02130	NEW ENGLAND

Mattel Children's Hospital at UCLA		(310) 825-9111
Mattel Chldns Hosp at UCLA		
10833 Le Conte Ave	Los Angeles, CA 90095-1752	WEST COAST AND PACIFIC

Mayo Clinic - Jacksonville, FL		(904) 953-2000
Mayo - Jacksonville		
4500 San Pablo Road	Jacksonville, FL 32224	SOUTHEAST

Mayo Clinic - Rochester, MN		(507) 284-2511
Mayo Med Ctr & Clin - Rochester		
200 First St SW	Rochester, MN 55905	MIDWEST

Mayo Clinic - Scottsdale		(480) 301-8000
Mayo Clin Hosp - Scottsdale		
13400 E Shea Blvd	Scottsdale, AZ 85259	SOUTHWEST

Mayo Clinic Hospital - Phoenix		(480) 515-6296
Mayo - Phoenix		
5777 E Mayo Blvd	Phoenix, AZ 85054	SOUTHWEST

McLaren Regional Medical Center		(810) 342-2000
McLaren Reg Med Ctr		
401 S. Ballenger Highway	Flint, MI 48532	MIDWEST

McLean Hospital		(617) 855-2000
McLean Hosp		
115 Mill St	Belmont, MA 02478	NEW ENGLAND

Medical Center of Central Georgia		(478) 633-1000
Med Ctr of Central GA		
777 Hemlock Street	Macon, GA 31201	SOUTHEAST

Medical Center of Louisiana @ New Orleans (University Hospital)		(504) 903-3000
Med Ctr LA @ New Orleans (Univ Hosp)		
2021 Perdido St	New Orleans, LA 70112	SOUTHWEST

Medical Center of Plano *Med Ctr of Plano* 3901 W 15th St	Plano, TX 75075-7799	(972) 596-6800 SOUTHWEST
Medical City Dallas Hospital *Med City Dallas Hosp* 7777 Forest Ln	Dallas, TX 75230-2594	(972) 566-7000 SOUTHWEST
Medical College of Georgia Hospital and Clinic *Med Coll of GA Hosp and Clin* 1120 15th Street	Augusta, GA 30912	(706) 721-6569 SOUTHEAST
Medical College of Virginia Hospitals *Med Coll of VA Hosp* 1250 E Marshall St, Box 980510	Richmond, VA 23219	(804) 828-9000 SOUTHEAST
Medical University of South Carolina Children's Hospital *MUSC Chldns Hosp* 169 Ashley Ave	Charleston, SC 29425	(843) 792-1414 SOUTHEAST
Medical University of South Carolina Medical Center *MUSC Med Ctr* 169 Ashley Ave	Charleston, SC 29425	(843) 792-2300 SOUTHEAST
Memorial Health University Medical Center - Savannah *Meml Hlth Univ Med Ctr - Savannah* 4700 Waters Ave	Savannah, GA 31404	(912) 350-8000 SOUTHEAST
Memorial Hermann Hospital - Houston *Meml Hermann Hosp - Houston* 6411 Fannin	Houston, TX 77030	(713) 704-4000 SOUTHWEST
Memorial Regional Hospital - Hollywood *Meml Regl Hosp - Hollywood* 3501 Johnson Street	Hollywood, FL 33021	(954) 987-2000 SOUTHEAST
Memorial Sloan-Kettering Cancer Center *Meml Sloan Kettering Cancer Ctr* 1275 York Avenue	New York, NY 10021	(212) 639-2000 MID ATLANTIC
Menninger Clinic *Menninger Clinic* PO Box 809045	Houston, TX 77280	(800) 351-9058 SOUTHWEST
Mercy General Hospital - Sacramento *Mercy General Hosp - Sacramento* 4001 J Street	Sacramento, CA 95819	(916) 453-4545 WEST COAST AND PACIFIC

Mercy Hospital - Coon Rapids		(763) 236-6000
Mercy Hosp - Coon Rapids		
4050 Coon Rapids Blvd	Coon Rapids, MN 55433-2522	MIDWEST
Mercy Hospital - Miami, FL		(305) 854-4400
Mercy Hosp - Miami		
3663 S Miami Ave	Miami, FL 33133	SOUTHEAST
Mercy Medical Center Inc		(410) 332-9000
Mercy Medical Center Inc		
301 St Paul Place	Baltimore, MD 21202	MID ATLANTIC
MeritCare Hospital		(701) 234-6000
MeritCare Hosp		
720 Fourth Street North	Fargo, ND 58122	GREAT PLAINS AND MOUNTAINS
Methodist Children's Hospital of South Texas		(210) 575-7105
Methodist Chldns Hosp of South Texas		
7700 Floyd Curl Dr	San Antonio, TX 78229-3311	SOUTHWEST
Methodist Hospital		(215) 952-9000
Methodist Hosp		
2301 S Broad St	Philadelphia, PA 19148-3594	MID ATLANTIC
Methodist Hospital - Houston		(713) 790-3311
Methodist Hosp - Houston		
6565 Fannin St, D200	Houston, TX 77030	SOUTHWEST
Methodist Hospital - Indianapolis		(317) 962-2000
Methodist Hosp - Indianapolis		
1701 N Senate Blvd	Indianapolis, IN 46202	MIDWEST
Methodist Hospital Healthsystem - Minnesota		(952) 993-5000
Methodist Hosp - Minnesota		
6500 Excelsior Blvd	Minneapolis, MN 55426-4700	MIDWEST
Methodist Specialty & Transplant Hospital - San Antonio, TX		(210) 575-8110
Methodist Spec & Transpl Hosp		
8026 Floyd Curl Dr	San Antonio, TX 78229	SOUTHWEST
Methodist University Hospital		(901) 516-7000
Methodist Univ Hosp - Memphis		
1265 Union Ave	Memphis, TN 38104	SOUTHEAST
MetroHealth Medical Center		(216) 778-7800
MetroHealth Med Ctr		
2500 MetroHealth Drive	Cleveland, OH 44109-1998	MIDWEST

Metropolitan Hospital Center - NY		(212) 423-6262
Metropolitan Hosp Ctr - NY		
1901 First Avenue	New York, NY 10029	MID ATLANTIC

Metropolitan Methodist Hospital		(210) 208-2200
Metro Methodist Hosp		
1310 McCullough Ave	San Antonio, TX 78212	SOUTHWEST

Miami Children's Hospital		(305) 666-6511
Miami Children's Hosp		
3100 SW 62nd Ave	Miami, FL 33155	SOUTHEAST

Michael E. DeBakey VA Medical Center		(713) 791-1414
DeBakey VA Med Ctr-Houston		
2002 Holcombe Blvd	Houston, TX 77030-1414	SOUTHWEST

Michael Reese Hospital & Medical Center		(312) 791-2000
Michael Reese Hosp & Med Ctr		
2929 S Ellis Ave	Chicago, IL 60616	MIDWEST

Michigan State University-Sparrow Hospital		(517) 364-1000
Mich State Univ-Sparrow Hos		
1215 E Michigan Ave, MS 0	Lansing, MI 48912	MIDWEST

Milford Hospital		(203) 876-4000
Milford Hosp		
300 Seaside Ave	Milford, CT 06460	NEW ENGLAND

Millard Fillmore Gates Circle Hospital		(716) 887-4600
Millard Fillmore Gates Cir Hosp		
3 Gates Cir	Buffalo, NY 14209	MID ATLANTIC

Mills - Peninsula Health Services		(650) 696-5400
Mills - Peninsula Hlth Svcs		
1783 El Camino Real	Burlingame, CA 94010	WEST COAST AND PACIFIC

Miriam Hospital		(401) 793-2500
Miriam Hosp		
164 Summit Avenue	Providence, RI 02906-2894	NEW ENGLAND

Missouri Baptist Medical Center		(314) 996-5000
Missouri Baptist Med Ctr		
3015 N Ballas Rd	St Louis, MO 63131	MIDWEST

Mobile Infirmary Medical Center		(334) 431-2400
Mobile Infirmary Med Ctr		
5 Mobile Infirmary Circle	Mobile, AL 36607-3513	SOUTHEAST

Montefiore Medical Center		(718) 920-4321
Montefiore Med Ctr		
111 East 210 Street	Bronx, NY 10467	MID ATLANTIC

Montefiore Medical Center - Weiler-Einstein Division		(718) 904-2000
Montefiore Med Ctr - Weiler-Einstein Div		
1825 Eastchester Road	Bronx, NY 10461	MID ATLANTIC

Morristown Memorial Hospital		(973) 971-5000
Morristown Mem Hosp		
100 Madison Avenue	Morristown, NJ 07960	MID ATLANTIC

MossRehab Hospital		(215) 663-6000
MossRehab Hosp		
60 E Township Line Rd	Elkins Park, PA 19027	MID ATLANTIC

Mott Children's Hospital		(734) 936-4000
Mott Chldns Hosp		
1500 E Medical Center Dr	Ann Arbor, MI 48109	MIDWEST

Mount Auburn Hospital		(617) 492-3500
Mount Auburn Hosp		
330 Mount Auburn St	Cambridge, MA 02238	NEW ENGLAND

Mount Sinai Medical Center		(212) 241-6500
Mount Sinai Med Ctr		
One Gustave L. Levy Pl	New York, NY 10029	MID ATLANTIC

Mount Sinai Medical Center - Miami		(305) 674-2121
Mount Sinai Med Ctr - Miami		
4300 Alton Rd	Miami Beach, FL 33140	SOUTHEAST

National Institutes of Health - Clinical Center		(301) 496-4000
Natl Inst of Hlth - Clin Ctr		
6100 Executive Blvd, rm 3C01, MS 7511		Bethesda, MD 20892-7511
MID ATLANTIC		

National Jewish Medical & Research Center		(303) 388-4461
Natl Jewish Med & Rsch Ctr		
1400 Jackson St	Denver, CO 80206-2762	GREAT PLAINS AND MOUNTAINS

National Rehabilitation Hospital		(202) 877-1000
Natl Rehab Hosp		
102 Irving St NW	Washington, DC 20010	MID ATLANTIC

Nebraska Medical Center		(402) 552-2000
Nebraska Med Ctr		
987400 Nebraska Med Ctr	Omaha, NE 68198-7400	GREAT PLAINS AND MOUNTAINS

Nebraska Methodist Hospital		(402) 354-4000
Nebraska Meth Hosp		
8303 Dodge St	Omaha, NE 68114	GREAT PLAINS AND MOUNTAINS

New England Baptist Hospital		(617) 754-5800
New England Bapt Hosp		
125 Parker Hill Ave	Boston, MA 02120	NEW ENGLAND

New Hanover Regional Medical Center		(910) 343-7000
New Hanover Reg Med Ctr		
2131 S 17th St	Wilmington, NC 28401	SOUTHEAST

New York Eye & Ear Infirmary		(212) 979-4000
New York Eye & Ear Infirm		
310 East 14th Street	New York, NY 10003	MID ATLANTIC

New York Hospital Queens		(718) 670-1231
NY Hosp Queens		
56-45 Main Street	Flushing, NY 11355	MID ATLANTIC

New York Methodist Hospital		(718) 780-3000
New York Methodist Hosp		
506 Sixth Street	Brooklyn, NY 11215	MID ATLANTIC

New York State Psychiatric Institute		(212) 543-5000
NY State Psychiatric Inst		
1051 Riverside Dr	New York, NY 10032	MID ATLANTIC

Newark Beth Israel Medical Center		(973) 926-7000
Newark Beth Israel Med Ctr		
201 Lyons Ave	Newark, NJ 07112	MID ATLANTIC

Newton - Wellesley Hospital		(617) 243-6000
Newton - Wellesley Hosp		
2014 Washington St	Newton, MA 02462	NEW ENGLAND

NewYork-Presbyterian Hospital/Columbia		(212) 305-2500
NY-Presby Hosp/Columbia		
622 W 168th St	New York, NY 10032	MID ATLANTIC

NewYork-Presbyterian Hospital/The Allen Pavilion		(212) 932-4000
NY-Presby Hosp/The Allen Pavilion		
5141 Broadway	New York, NY 10034	MID ATLANTIC

NewYork-Presbyterian Hospital/Weill Cornell		(212) 746-5454
NY-Presby Hosp/Weill Cornell		
525 E 68th St	New York, NY 10021	MID ATLANTIC

NewYork-Presbyterian/Morgan Stanley Children's Hospital (212) 305-2500
NYPresby-Morgan Stanley Children's Hosp
622 W 168th St | New York, NY 10032 | MID ATLANTIC

North Florida Regional Medical Center (352) 333-4000
North Florida Regl Med Ctr
6500 Newberry Rd | Gainesville, FL 32605 | SOUTHEAST

North Oaks Medical Center (985) 230-6601
North Oaks Med Ctr
15790 Paul Vega MD Dr | Hammond, LA 70403 | SOUTHWEST

North Shore Medical Center - Salem Hospital (978) 741-1215
N Shore Med Ctr - Salem Hosp
81 Highland Avenue | Salem, MA 01970 | NEW ENGLAND

North Shore University Hospital at Manhasset (516) 562-0100
N Shore Univ Hosp at Manhasset
300 Community Dr | Manhasset, NY 11030 | MID ATLANTIC

Northern California Shriners Hospital (916) 453-2000
Northern CA Shriners Hosp
2425 Stockton Blvd | Sacramento, CA 95817 | WEST COAST AND PACIFIC

Northern Memorial Health Care, Robbinsdale (763) 520-5200
Northern Meml Hlth Care
3300 Oakdale Ave N | Robbinsdale, MN 55422 | MIDWEST

Northern Westchester Hospital (914) 666-1200
Northern Westchester Hosp
400 East Main Street | Mount Kisco, NY 10549 | MID ATLANTIC

Northside Hospital - Atlanta (404) 851-8000
Northside Hosp
1000 Johnson Ferry Rd NE | Atlanta, GA 30342 | SOUTHEAST

Northwest Community Hospital (847) 618-1000
Northwest Comm Hosp
800 W Central Rd | Arlington Heights, IL 60005 | MIDWEST

Northwest Hospital (206) 364-0500
Northwest Hosp
1550 N 115th St | Seattle, WA 98133-0806 | WEST COAST AND PACIFIC

Northwest Medical Center (954) 974-0400
Northwest Med Ctr
2801 N State Rd 7 | Margate, FL 33063 | SOUTHEAST

Northwestern Memorial Hospital		(312) 926-2000
Northwestern Meml Hosp		
251 E Huron St	Chicago, IL 60611	MIDWEST
Norton Hospital		(502) 629-8000
Norton Hosp		
200 E Chestnut St	Louisville, KY 40202	SOUTHEAST
NYU Medical Center		(212) 263-7300
NYU Med Ctr		
550 First Avenue	New York, NY 10016	MID ATLANTIC
Ochsner Baptist Medical Center		(504) 899-9311
Ochsner Baptist Med Ctr		
2700 Napoleon Ave	New Orleans, LA 70115	SOUTHWEST
Ochsner Foundation Hospital		(504) 842-3000
Ochsner Fdn Hosp		
1516 Jefferson Hwy	New Orleans, LA 70121	SOUTHWEST
Ohio State University Medical Center		(614) 293-8000
Ohio St Univ Med Ctr		
410 W 10th Avenue	Columbus, OH 43210	MIDWEST
Olathe Medical Center		(913) 791-4200
Olathe Med Ctr		
20333 W 151st St	Olathe, KS 66061-5352	GREAT PLAINS AND MOUNTAINS
Olive View Medical Center		(818) 364-1555
Olive View Med Ctr		
14445 Olive View Dr	Sylmar, CA 91342	WEST COAST AND PACIFIC
Olympia Medical Center		(310) 657-5900
Olympia Med Ctr		
5900 W Olympic Blvd	Los Angeles, CA 90036	WEST COAST AND PACIFIC
Oregon Health & Science University		(503) 494-8311
OR Hlth & Sci Univ		
3181 SW Sam Jackson Park Rd	Portland, OR 97239-3098	WEST COAST AND PACIFIC
Orlando Regional Medical Center		(407) 841-5111
Orlando Regl Med Ctr		
1414 Kuhl Ave	Orlando, FL 32806	SOUTHEAST
Orthopaedic Hospital		(213) 742-1000
Orthopaedic Hosp		
2400 South Flower Street	Los Angeles, CA 90007	WEST COAST AND PACIFIC

Orthopedic Specialty Hospital, The (TOSH)   (801) 314-4100
Ortho Spec Hosp, The (TOSH)
5848 Fashion Blvd   Salt Lake City, UT 84107   GREAT PLAINS AND MOUNTAINS

Osceola Regional Medical Center   (407) 846-2266
Osceola Regional Med Ctr
700 West Oak St   Kissimmee, FL 37412   SOUTHEAST

OSF Saint Francis Medical Center   (309) 655-2000
OSF Saint Francis Med Ctr
530 NE Glen Oak Ave   Peoria, IL 61637   MIDWEST

OU Medical Center   (405) 271-4700
OU Med Ctr
1200 Everett Dr   Oklahoma City, OK 73104-5098   SOUTHWEST

Our Lady of Lourdes Regional Medical Center - Lafayette   (337) 289-2000
Our Lady of Lourdes Reg Med Ctr - Lafayette
611 St. Landry St   Lafayette, LA 70506-4697   SOUTHWEST

Our Lady of the Lake Regional Medical Center   (225) 765-6565
Our Lady of the Lake Regl Med Ctr
5000 Hennessy Blvd   Baton Rouge, LA 70808-4398   SOUTHWEST

Overlake Hospital Medical Center   (425) 688-5000
Overlake Hosp Med Ctr
1035 116th Ave NE   Bellevue, WA 98004-4687   WEST COAST AND PACIFIC

Overland Park Regional Medical Center   (913) 541-5000
Overland Pk Regl Med Ctr
10500 Quivira Rd   Overland Park, KS 66215   GREAT PLAINS AND MOUNTAINS

Park Plaza Hospital   (713) 527-5000
Park Plaza Hosp
1313 Herman Dr   Houston, TX 77004   SOUTHWEST

Park Ridge Hospital   (585) 723-7000
Park Ridge Hosp
1555 Long Pond Rd   Rochester, NY 14626-4182   MID ATLANTIC

Parkinson's Institute/Movement Disorders Treament Center, The   (408) 734-2800
Parkinson's Inst/Movement Disorders Trmt Ctr, The
1170 Morse Ave   Sunnyvale, CA 94089-1605   WEST COAST AND PACIFIC

Parkland Memorial Hospital - Dallas   (214) 590-8000
Parkland Meml Hosp - Dallas
5201 Harry Hines Blvd   Dallas, TX 75235   SOUTHWEST

Penn Presbyterian Medical Center - UPHS		(215) 662-8000
Penn Presby Med Ctr - UPHS		
51 N 39th St	Philadelphia, PA 19104	MID ATLANTIC

Penn State Milton S Hershey Medical Center		(717) 531-8521
Penn State Milton S Hershey Med Ctr		
500 University Drive	Hershey, PA 17033-0850	MID ATLANTIC

Pennsylvania Hospital		(215) 829-3000
Pennsylvania Hosp		
3600 Market St, Ste 240	Philadelphia, PA 19104	MID ATLANTIC

Philadelphia Shriners Hospital		(215) 430-4000
Philadelphia Shriners Hosp		
3351 N Broad St	Philadelphia, PA 19140	MID ATLANTIC

Phillips Eye Institute		(612) 775-8800
Phillips Eye Inst		
2215 Park Ave S	Minneapolis, MN 55404	MIDWEST

Phoenix Children's Hospital		(602) 546-1000
Phoenix Children's Hosp		
1919 E Thomas Rd	Phoenix, AZ 85106	SOUTHWEST

Physicians Regional Medical Center		(239) 348-4000
Physicians Regl Med Ctr		
6101 Pine Ridge Rd	Naples, FL 34119	SOUTHEAST

Piedmont Hospital		(404) 605-5000
Piedmont Hosp		
1968 Peachtree Rd NW	Atlanta, GA 30309	SOUTHEAST

Pitt County Memorial Hospital - Univ Health System East Carolina		(252) 847-4100
Pitt Cty Mem Hosp - Univ Med Ctr East Carolina		
2100 Stantonsburg Rd	Greenville, NC 27835-6028	SOUTHEAST

Portsmouth Regional Hospital		(603) 436-5110
Portsmouth Regl Hosp		
333 Borthwick Ave	NH 03801-7002	NEW ENGLAND

Presbyterian - St Luke's Medical Center		(303) 839-6000
Presby - St Luke's Med Ctr		
1719 E 19th Ave	Denver, CO 80218	GREAT PLAINS AND MOUNTAINS

Presbyterian Hospital - Albuquerque		(505) 841-1234
Presbyterian Hospital - Albuquerque		
1100 Central Ave SE	Albuquerque, NM 87106	SOUTHWEST

Presbyterian Hospital - Charlotte   (704) 384-4000
Presby Hosp - Charlotte
200 Hawthorne Ln   Charlotte, NC 28204-2528   SOUTHEAST

Presbyterian Hospital - Plano   (972) 608-8000
Presby Hosp - Plano
6200 West Parker Road   Plano, TX 75093   SOUTHWEST

Presbyterian Hospital of Dallas   (214) 345-6789
Presby Hosp of Dallas
8200 Walnut Hill Ln   Dallas, TX 75231   SOUTHWEST

Primary Children's Medical Center   (801) 588-2000
Primary Children's Med Ctr
100 N Medical Drive   Salt Lake City, UT 84113   GREAT PLAINS AND MOUNTAINS

Providence Alaska Medical Center   (907) 562-2211
Providence Alaska Med Ctr
3200 Providence Dr   Anchorage, AK 99508-4615   WEST COAST AND PACIFIC

Providence Hospital - Southfield   (248) 424-3000
Providence Hosp - Southfield
16001 W Nine Mile Rd   Southfield, MI 48075   MIDWEST

Providence Portland Medical Center   (503) 215-1111
Providence Portland Med Ctr
4805 NE Glisan   Portland, OR 97213-2967   WEST COAST AND PACIFIC

Providence Saint Joseph Medical Center   (818) 843-5111
Providence St Joseph Med Ctr
501 S Buena Vista St   Burbank, CA 91505   WEST COAST AND PACIFIC

Queen's Medical Center - Honolulu   (808) 538-9011
Queen's Med Ctr - Honolulu
1301 Punchbowl Street   Honolulu, HI 96813   WEST COAST AND PACIFIC

Rady Children's Hospital - San Diego   (858) 576-1700
Rady Children's Hosp - San Diego
3020 Children's Way   San Diego, CA 92123   WEST COAST AND PACIFIC

Rainbow Babies & Children's Hospital   (216) 844-1000
Rainbow Babies & Chldns Hosp
11100 Euclid Ave   Cleveland, OH 44106   MIDWEST

Rancho Los Amigos National Rehabilitation Center   (562) 401-7111
Rancho Los Amigos Natl Rehab Ctr
7601 East Imperial Highway   Downey, CA 90242   WEST COAST AND PACIFIC

Rapid City Regional Hospital
Rapid City Reg Hosp
353 Fairmount Blvd   Rapid City, SD 57701   (605) 719-1000
GREAT PLAINS AND MOUNTAINS

Regional Medical Center - Memphis
Regional Med Ctr - Memphis
877 Jefferson Avenue   Memphis, TN 38103   (901) 545-7100
SOUTHEAST

Regional West Medical Center
Regional West Med Ctr
4021 Ave B   Scottbluff, NE 69361   (308) 635-3711
GREAT PLAINS AND MOUNTAINS

Regions Hospital - St Paul
Regions Hosp - St Paul
640 Jackson Street   St Paul, MN 55101   (651) 254-3456
MIDWEST

Rehabilitation Institute - Chicago
Rehab Inst - Chicago
345 E. Superior Street   Chicago, IL 60611   (312) 238-1000
MIDWEST

Rehabilitation Institute of St. Louis
Rehab Inst St. Louis
4455 Duncan Ave   St. Louis, MO 63110   (314) 658-3800
MIDWEST

Rex HealthCare
Rex HlthCare
4420 Lake Boone Trail   Raleigh, NC 27607   (919) 784-3100
SOUTHEAST

Rhode Island Hospital
Rhode Island Hosp
593 Eddy Street   Providence, RI 02903   (401) 444-4000
NEW ENGLAND

Riddle Memorial Hospital
Riddle Meml Hosp
1068 W Baltimore Pike   Media, PA 19063   (610) 566-9400
MID ATLANTIC

Riley Hospital for Children
Riley Hosp for Children
702 Barnhill Drive   Indianapolis, IN 46202   (317) 274-5000
MIDWEST

Riverside Community Hospital
Riverside Comm Hosp
4445 Magnolia Avenue   Riverside, CA 92502   (951) 788-3000
WEST COAST AND PACIFIC

Riverview Medical Center
Riverview Med Ctr
1 Riverview Plaza   Red Bank, NJ 07701   (732) 741-2700
MID ATLANTIC

Robert Wood Johnson University Hospital - New Brunswick   (732) 828-3000
Robert Wood Johnson Univ Hosp - New Brunswick
1 Robert Wood Johnson Pl   New Brunswick, NJ 08901   MID ATLANTIC

Rochester Methodist Hospital   (507) 284-2511
Rochester Meth Hosp
201 W Center St   Rochester, MN 55905-3003   MIDWEST

Rockefeller University   (212) 327-8000
Rockefeller Univ
1230 York Avenue   New York, NY 10021   MID ATLANTIC

Roger Williams Hospital   (401) 456-2000
Roger Williams Hosp
825 Chalkstone Avenue   Providence, RI 02908   NEW ENGLAND

Roper Hospital   (843) 724-2000
Roper Hosp
316 Calhoun St   Charleston, SC 29401   SOUTHEAST

Rose Medical Center   (303) 320-2121
Rose Med Ctr
4567 E 9th Ave   Denver, CO 80220-3941   GREAT PLAINS AND MOUNTAINS

Roswell Park Cancer Institute   (716) 845-5770
Roswell Park Cancer Inst
Elm and Carlton Streets   Buffalo, NY 14263   MID ATLANTIC

Rush - Copley Medical Center   (630) 978-6200
Rush - Copley Med Ctr
2000 Ogden Ave   Aurora, IL 60504-4206   MIDWEST

Rush Oak Park Hospital   (708) 383-9300
Rush Oak Park Hosp
520 S Maple Ave   Oak Park, IL 60304   MIDWEST

Rush University Medical Center   (312) 942-5000
Rush Univ Med Ctr
1653 W Congress Pkwy   Chicago, IL 60612-3833   MIDWEST

Rusk Institute of Rehabilitation Medicine   (212) 263-2606
Rusk Inst of Rehab Med
400 East 34th Street   New York, NY 10016   MID ATLANTIC

Saint Francis Hospital - Memphis   (901) 765-1000
St Francis Hosp - Memphis
5959 Park Ave   Memphis, TN 38119   SOUTHEAST

Saint John's Health Center
St John's Hlth Ctr, Santa Monica
1328 22nd St   Santa Monica, CA 90404   (310) 829-5511
                                                                            WEST COAST AND PACIFIC

Saint Thomas Hospital - Nashville
Saint Thomas Hosp - Nashville
4220 Harding Road   Nashville, TN 37205   (615) 222-2111
                                                                            SOUTHEAST

Saint Vincent Catholic Medical Centers - St Vincent's Manhattan
St Vincent Cath Med Ctrs - Manhattan
170 West 12th Street   New York, NY 10011   (212) 604-7000
                                                                            MID ATLANTIC

Salt Lake Regional Medical Center
Salt Lake Regional Med Ctr
1050 E South Temple   Salt Lake City, UT 84102   (801) 350-4111
                                                                            GREAT PLAINS AND MOUNTAINS

San Francisco General Hospital
San Francisco Genl Hosp
1001 Potrero Avenue   San Francisco, CA 94110   (415) 206-8000
                                                                            WEST COAST AND PACIFIC

Santa Barbara Cottage Hospital
Santa Barbara Cottage Hosp
Pueblo at Bath St, PO Box 689   Santa Barbara, CA 93105   (805) 682-7111
                                                                            WEST COAST AND PACIFIC

Santa Clara Valley Medical Center
Santa Clara Vly Med Ctr
751 S Bascom Ave   San Jose, CA 95128   (408) 885-5000
                                                                            WEST COAST AND PACIFIC

Santa Monica - UCLA Medical Center
Santa Monica - UCLA Med Ctr
1250 16th St   Santa Monica, CA 90404   (310) 319-4000
                                                                            WEST COAST AND PACIFIC

Sarasota Memorial Hospital
Sarasota Meml Hosp
1700 S Tamiami Trail   Sarasota, FL 34239   (941) 917-9000
                                                                            SOUTHEAST

Schneider Children's Hospital
Schneider Chldn's Hosp
269-01 76th Ave   New Hyde Park, NY 11040   (718) 470-3000
                                                                            MID ATLANTIC

Schwab Rehabilitation Hospital
Schwab Rehab Hosp
1401 S. California Boulevard   Chicago, IL 60608   (773) 522-2010
                                                                            MIDWEST

Scott & White Memorial Hospital
Scott & White Mem Hosp
2401 South 31st Street   Temple, TX 76508-0001   (254) 724-2111
                                                                            SOUTHWEST

Scottsdale Healthcare - Osborn (480) 675-4000
Scottsdale Hlthcare - Osborn
7400 E Osborn Rd   Scottsdale, AZ 85251-6403   SOUTHWEST

Scottsdale Healthcare - Shea (480) 860-3000
Scottsdale Hlthcare - Shea
9000 E Shea Blvd   Scottsdale, AZ 85258-4514   SOUTHWEST

Scripps Green Hospital (858) 455-9100
Scripps Green Hosp
10666 N Torrey Pines Rd   La Jolla, CA 92037   WEST COAST AND PACIFIC

Scripps Memorial Hospital - La Jolla (858) 457-4123
Scripps Meml Hosp - La Jolla
9888 Genesee Ave   La Jolla, CA 92037   WEST COAST AND PACIFIC

Scripps Mercy Hospital & Medical Center (619) 294-8111
Scripps Mercy Hosp & Med Ctr
4077 Fifth Ave   San Diego, CA 92103   WEST COAST AND PACIFIC

Self Regional Healthcare (864) 227-4111
Self Regional Healthcare
1325 Spring St   Greenwood, SC 29646   SOUTHEAST

Sentara Leigh Hospital (757) 466-6000
Sentara Leigh Hosp
830 Kempsville Rd   Norfolk, VA 23502-3981   SOUTHEAST

Sentara Norfolk General Hospital (757) 668-3000
Sentara Norfolk Genl Hosp
600 Gresham Dr   Norfolk, VA 23507   SOUTHEAST

Sentara Virginia Beach General Hospital (757) 395-8000
Sentara VA Beach Genl Hosp
1060 First Colonial Rd   Virginia Beach, VA 23454   SOUTHEAST

Seton Medical Center (650) 992-4000
Seton Med Ctr
1900 Sullivan Avenue   Daly City, CA 94015   WEST COAST AND PACIFIC

Shady Grove Adventist Hospital (301) 279-6000
Shady Grove Adven Hosp
9901 Medical Center Drive   Rockville, MD 20850   MID ATLANTIC

Shands Healthcare at University of Florida (352) 265-0111
Shands Hlthcre at Univ of FL
1600 SW Archer Rd   Gainesville, FL 32610   SOUTHEAST

Shands Jacksonville
Shands Jacksonville
655 W 8th St   Jacksonville, FL 32209   (904) 244-0411

SOUTHEAST

Sharp Mary Birch Hospital for Women   (858) 939-3400
Sharp Mary Birch Hosp for Wmn
3003 Health Center Drive   San Diego, CA 92123-2700   WEST COAST AND PACIFIC

Sharp Memorial Hospital   (858) 541-3400
Sharp Meml Hosp
7901 Frost St   San Diego, CA 92123   WEST COAST AND PACIFIC

Shawnee Mission Medical Center   (913) 676-2000
Shawnee Mission Med Ctr
9100 W 74th St   Shawnee Mission, KS 66204   GREAT PLAINS AND MOUNTAINS

Sheppard Pratt Health System   (410) 938-3000
Sheppard Pratt Hlth Sys
6501 N Charles St   Baltimore, MD 21285-6815   MID ATLANTIC

Sibley Memorial Hospital   (202) 537-4000
Sibley Mem Hosp
5255 Loughboro Road NW   Washington, DC 20016   MID ATLANTIC

Silver Hill Hospital   (203) 966-3561
Silver Hill Hosp
208 Valley Rd   New Canaan, CT 06840-3899   NEW ENGLAND

Sinai Hospital - Baltimore   (410) 601-9000
Sinai Hosp - Baltimore
2401 W Belvedere Ave   Baltimore, MD 21215   MID ATLANTIC

Sinai-Grace Hospital - Detroit   (313) 966-3300
Sinai-Grace Hosp - Detroit
6071 W. Outer Drive   Detroit, MI 48235   MIDWEST

South Miami Hospital   (305) 661-4611
South Miami Hosp
6200 SW 73 St   South Miami, FL 33143   SOUTHEAST

Southeast Baptist Hospital   (210) 297-3000
Southeast Baptist Hosp
4214 E Southcross Blvd   San Antonio, TX 78222   SOUTHWEST

Southwest Florida Regional Medical Center   (239) 939-1147
Southwest Florida Regional Medical Center
2727 Winkler Ave.   Fort Myers, FL 33901   SOUTHEAST

Southwest Texas Methodist Hospital		(210) 575-4000
SW TX Meth Hosp		
7700 Floyd Curl Dr	San Antonio, TX 78229	SOUTHWEST

Spaulding Rehabilitation Hospital		(617) 720-6400
Spaulding Rehab Hosp		
125 Nashua Street	Boston, MA 02114	NEW ENGLAND

Spectrum Health - Blodgett Campus		(616) 774-7444
Spectrum Hlth Blodgett Campus		
1840 Wealthy St SE	Grand Rapids, MI 49506	MIDWEST

Spectrum Health Butterworth Campus		(616) 391-1774
Spectrum Hlth Butterworth Campus		
100 Michigan St NE	Grand Rapids, MI 49503	MIDWEST

SSM Cardinal Glennon Children's Hospital		(314) 577-5600
Cardinal Glennon Mem Children's Hosp		
1465 S Grand Blvd	St Louis, MO 63104	MIDWEST

SSM St Joseph Hospital of Kirkwood		(314) 966-1500
SSM St Joseph Hosp of Kirkwood		
525 Couch Ave	St Louis, MO 63122	MIDWEST

St Alexius Medical Center		(847) 843-2000
St Alexius Med Ctr		
1555 Barrington Rd	Hoffman Estates, IL 60194	MIDWEST

St Alphonsus Regional Medical Center		(208) 367-2121
St Alphonsus Regl Med Ctr		
1055 N Curtis Rd	Boise, ID 83706-1370	GREAT PLAINS AND MOUNTAINS

St Anthony Hospital		(405) 272-7000
St Anthony Hosp		
1000 N Lee St	Oklahoma City, OK 73102	SOUTHWEST

St Anthony's Hospital - St Petersburg		(727) 893-6814
St Anthony's Hosp - St Petersburg		
1200 7th Avenue North	St Petersburg, FL 33705	SOUTHEAST

St Barnabas Medical Center		(973) 322-5000
St Barnabas Med Ctr		
94 Old Short Hills Rd	Livingston, NJ 07039-5672	MID ATLANTIC

St Christopher's Hospital for Children		(215) 427-5000
St Christopher's Hosp for Chldn		
Erie Ave at Front St	Philadelphia, PA 19134	MID ATLANTIC

St Elizabeth Medical Center (South Unit)   (859) 344-2000
St Elizabeth Med Ctr (South Unit)
1 Medical Village Dr   Edgewood, KY 41017   SOUTHEAST

St Elizabeth's Medical Center   (617) 789-3000
St Elizabeth's Med Ctr
736 Cambridge St   Brighton, MA 02135   NEW ENGLAND

St Francis Hospital & Medical Center   (860) 714-4000
St Francis Hosp & Med Ctr
114 Woodland St   Hartford, CT 06105   NEW ENGLAND

St Francis Hospital - The Heart Center   (516) 562-6000
St Francis Hosp - The Heart Ctr
100 Port Washington Boulevard   Roslyn, NY 11576   MID ATLANTIC

St Francis Medical Center   (318) 362-4000
St Francis Med Ctr
309 Jackson St   Monroe, LA 71210-7498   SOUTHWEST

St John Hospital and Medical Center   (313) 343-4000
St John Hosp and Med Ctr
22101 Moross Road   Detroit, MI 48236-2172   MIDWEST

St John's Hospital - Springfield   (217) 544-6464
St John's Hosp - Springfield
800 E Carpenter St   Springfield, IL 62769   MIDWEST

St John's Mercy Medical Center - St Louis   (314) 569-6000
St John's Mercy Med Ctr - St Louis
615 S New Ballas Rd   St Louis, MO 63141   MIDWEST

St Joseph Hospital   (603) 882-3000
St Joseph Hosp
172 Kinsley St   Nashua, NH 03060   NEW ENGLAND

St Joseph Medical Center   (410) 337-1000
St Joseph Med Ctr
7601 Osler Drive   Baltimore, MD 21208   MID ATLANTIC

St Joseph Medical Center - Tacoma   (253) 627-4101
St Joseph Med Ctr - Tacoma
1717 South J St   Tacoma, WA 98401   WEST COAST AND PACIFIC

St Joseph Mercy Hospital - Ann Arbor   (734) 712-3456
St Joseph Mercy Hosp - Ann Arbor
5301 E Huron River Dr, Box 992   Ann Arbor, MI 48106   MIDWEST

St Joseph Mercy Oakland Hospital		(248) 858-3000
St Joseph Mercy Oakland Hosp		
44405 Woodward Ave	Pontiac, MI 48341	MIDWEST
St Joseph's Hospital & Medical Center - Phoenix		(602) 406-3000
St Joseph's Hosp & Med Ctr - Phoenix		
350 W Thomas Rd	Phoenix, AZ 85013-4496	SOUTHWEST
St Joseph's Hospital - Atlanta		(404) 851-7001
St Joseph's Hosp - Atlanta		
5665 Peachtree Dunwoody Rd NE	Atlanta, GA 30342	SOUTHEAST
St Joseph's Hospital - Orange		(714) 633-9111
St Joseph's Hosp - Orange		
1100 West Stewart Drive	Orange, CA 92868	WEST COAST AND PACIFIC
St Joseph's Hospital - Tampa		(813) 870-4000
St Joseph's Hosp - Tampa		
3001 W Martin Luther King Jr Blvd	Tampa, FL 33607	SOUTHEAST
St Joseph's Hospital - Tucson		(520) 296-3211
St Joseph's Hosp - Tucson		
350 N Wilmot Rd	Tucson, AZ 85711	SOUTHWEST
St Jude Children's Research Hospital		(901) 495-3300
St Jude Children's Research Hosp		
332 N Lauderdale St	Memphis, TN 38105	SOUTHEAST
St Louis Children's Hospital		(314) 454-6000
St Louis Chldns Hosp		
One Children's Pl	St Louis, MO 63110	MIDWEST
St Louis University Hospital		(314) 577-8000
St Louis Univ Hosp		
3635 Vista at Grand Blvd	St Louis, MO 63110	MIDWEST
St Luke's - Roosevelt Hospital Center - Roosevelt Division		(212) 523-4000
St Luke's - Roosevelt Hosp Ctr - Roosevelt Div		
1000 Tenth Avenue	New York, NY 10019	MID ATLANTIC
St Luke's - Roosevelt Hospital Center - St Luke's Hospital		(212) 523-4000
St Luke's - Roosevelt Hosp Ctr - St Luke's Hosp		
1111 Amsterdam Ave	New York, NY 10025	MID ATLANTIC
St Luke's Episcopal Hospital - Houston		(832) 355-1000
St Luke's Episcopal Hosp - Houston		
6720 Bertner Avenue	Houston, TX 77030	SOUTHWEST

St Luke's Hospital - Bethlehem   (610) 954-4000
St Luke's Hosp - Bethlehem
801 Ostrum Street   Bethlehem, PA 18015   MID ATLANTIC

St Luke's Hospital - Chesterfield, MO   (314) 434-1500
St Luke's Hosp - Chesterfield, MO
232 S Woods Mill Rd   Chesterfield, MO 63017   MIDWEST

St Luke's Hospital - Duluth   (218) 249-5555
St Luke's Hosp - Duluth
915 E 1st St   Duluth, MN 55805-2193   MIDWEST

St Luke's Hospital - Jacksonville   (904) 296-3700
St Luke's Hosp - Jacksonville
4201 Belfort Rd   Jacksonville, FL 32216   SOUTHEAST

St Luke's Hospital of Kansas City   (816) 932-2000
St Luke's Hosp of Kansas City
4401 Wornall Rd   Kansas City, MO 64111   MIDWEST

St Mary Medical Center - Long Beach, CA   (562) 491-9000
St Mary Med Ctr - Long Beach, CA
1050 Linden Ave   Long Beach, CA 90813   WEST COAST AND PACIFIC

St Mary's Hospital - Rochester, MN (Mayo Clinic)   (507) 255-5123
St Mary's Hosp - Rochester
1216 2nd St SW   Rochester, MN 55902   MIDWEST

St Mary's Hospital Medical Center   (608) 251-6100
St Mary's Hosp-Madison
707 S Mills St   Madison, WI 53715   MIDWEST

St Mary's Medical Center - Huntington   (304) 526-1234
St Mary's Med Ctr - Huntington
2900 First Ave   Huntington, WV 25702-1272   MID ATLANTIC

St Mary's Medical Center - West Palm Beach   (561) 844-6300
St Mary's Med Ctr - W Palm Bch
901 45th St   West Palm Beach, FL 33407   SOUTHEAST

St Peter's University Hospital   (732) 745-8600
St Peter's Univ Hosp
254 Easton Ave   New Brunswick, NJ 08901-1780   MID ATLANTIC

St Vincent Carmel Hospital   (317) 573-7000
St Vincent Carmel Hosp
13500 N Meridian St   Carmel, IN 46032-1496   MIDWEST

St Vincent Charity Hospital		(216) 861-6200
St Vincent Charity Hosp		
2351 E 22nd St	Cleveland, OH 44115-3197	MIDWEST

St Vincent Hospital & Health Services - Indianapolis		(317) 338-2345
St Vincent Hosp & Hlth Svcs - Indianapolis		
2001 W 86th St	Indianapolis, IN 46260-1991	MIDWEST

St Vincent Hospital - Green Bay		(920) 433-0111
St Vincent Hosp - Green Bay		
835 S Van Buren St, P.O. Box 13508	Green Bay, WI 54307-3508	MIDWEST

St Vincent Hospital - Santa Fe		(505) 983-3361
St Vincent Hosp - Santa Fe		
455 St Michaels Dr	Santa Fe, NM 87504-2107	SOUTHWEST

St Vincent's Hospital - Birmingham		(205) 939-7000
St Vincent's Hosp - Birmingham		
810 St. Vincent's Drive or PO Box 12407		
Birmingham, AL 35202-2407		SOUTHEAST

St Vincent's Medical Center - Jacksonville		(904) 308-7300
St Vincent's Med Ctr - Jacksonville		
1800 Barrs St	Jacksonville, FL 32204	SOUTHEAST

St Vincent's Medical Center - Los Angeles		(213) 484-7111
St Vincent's Med Ctr - Los Angeles		
2131 W 3rd St	Los Angeles, CA 90057	WEST COAST AND PACIFIC

St. Alexius Medical Center		(701) 530-7000
St. Alexius Med Ctr - Bismarck		
900 E Broadway Ave	Bismarck, ND 58501	GREAT PLAINS AND MOUNTAINS

St. Luke's Regional Medical Center		(208) 381-2222
St. Luke's Reg Med Ctr - Boise		
190 E Bannock St	Boise, ID 83712	GREAT PLAINS AND MOUNTAINS

Stanford University Medical Center		(650) 723-4000
Stanford Univ Med Ctr		
300 Pasteur Dr	Stanford, CA 94305	WEST COAST AND PACIFIC

Stony Brook University Medical Center		(631) 689-8333
Stony Brook Univ Med Ctr		
Nicolls Rd	Stony Brook, NY 11794-8410	MID ATLANTIC

Suburban Hospital Healthcare Systems		(301) 896-3100
Suburban Hosp - Bethesda		
8600 Old Georgetown Road	Bethesda, MD 20814	MID ATLANTIC

Sunnyview Hospital and Rehabilitation Center   (518) 382-4500
Sunnyview Hosp
1270 Belmont Ave   Schenectady, NY 12308-2198   MID ATLANTIC

Sunrise Hospital & Medical Center/Sunrise Children's Hospital   (702) 731-8000
Sunrise Hosp & Med Ctr/Sunrise Chldn's Hosp
3186 Maryland Pkwy   Las Vegas, NV 89109-2306   WEST COAST AND PACIFIC

SUNY Downstate Medical Center   (718) 270-1000
SUNY Downstate Med Ctr
450 Clarkson Ave   Brooklyn, NY 11203   MID ATLANTIC

Swedish Covenant Hospital   (773) 878-8200
Swedish Covenant Hosp
5145 N California Ave   Chicago, IL 60625   MIDWEST

Swedish Medical Center - Englewood   (303) 788-5000
Swedish Med Ctr - Englewood
501 E Hamden Ave   Englewood, CO 80110-2795   GREAT PLAINS AND MOUNTAINS

Swedish Medical Center - Seattle   (206) 386-6000
Swedish Med Ctr - Seattle
747 Broadway   Seattle, WA 98122   WEST COAST AND PACIFIC

Tacoma General Hospital   (253) 403-1000
Tacoma Genl Hosp
315 Martin Luther King Jr Way   Tacoma, WA 98405   WEST COAST AND PACIFIC

Tampa General Hospital   (813) 844-7000
Tampa Genl Hosp
PO BOX 1289   Tampa, FL 33601   SOUTHEAST

Temple University Hospital   (215) 707-2000
Temple Univ Hosp
3401 N Broad St   Philadelphia, PA 19140-5189   MID ATLANTIC

Texas Children's Hospital - Houston   (832) 824-1000
Texas Chldns Hosp - Houston
6621 Fannin St   Houston, TX 77030   SOUTHWEST

Texas Orthopedic Hospital   (713) 799-8600
Texas Ortho Hosp
7401 S Main   Houston, TX 77030   SOUTHWEST

Texas Scottish Rite Hospital for Children   (214) 559-5000
Texas Scottish Rite Hosp for Chldn
2222 Welborn St   Dallas, TX 75219   SOUTHWEST

Thomas Jefferson University Hospital   (215) 955-6000
Thomas Jefferson Univ Hosp
111 S 11th St   Philadelphia, PA 19107   MID ATLANTIC

TIRR		(713) 799-5000
TIRR		
1333 Moursund	Houston, TX 77030	SOUTHWEST

Toledo Hospital		(419) 291-4000
Toledo Hosp		
2142 N Cove Blvd	Toledo, OH 43606	MIDWEST

Tucson Medical Center		(520) 327-5461
Tucson Med Ctr		
5301 E Grant Rd	Tucson, AZ 85712-2874	SOUTHWEST

Tufts - New England Medical Center		(617) 636-5000
Tufts-New England Med Ctr		
750 Washington Street	Boston, MA 02111	NEW ENGLAND

Tulane University Hospital & Clinic		(504) 588-5263
Tulane Univ Hosp & Clin		
1415 Tulane Ave	New Orleans, LA 70112	SOUTHWEST

UCLA Medical Center		(310) 825-9111
UCLA Med Ctr		
10833 Le Conte Avenue	Los Angeles, CA 90095	WEST COAST AND PACIFIC

UCLA Neuropsychiatric Hospital		(310) 825-9989
UCLA Neuropsychiatric Hosp		
760 Westwood Plaza	Los Angeles, CA 90024	WEST COAST AND PACIFIC

UCSD Medical Center		(619) 543-6222
UCSD Med Ctr		
200 W Arbor Dr	San Diego, CA 92103	WEST COAST AND PACIFIC

UCSF - Mount Zion Medical Center		(415) 567-6600
UCSF - Mt Zion Med Ctr		
1600 Divisadero St	San Francisco, CA 94115	WEST COAST AND PACIFIC

UCSF Medical Center		(415) 476-1000
UCSF Med Ctr		
500 Parnassus Ave	San Francisco, CA 94143	WEST COAST AND PACIFIC

UMass Memorial - Memorial Campus		(508) 793-6611
UMass Meml - Meml Campus		
119 Belmont St	Worcester, MA 01605	NEW ENGLAND

UMass Memorial - University Campus		(508) 856-0011
UMass Meml - Univ Campus		
55 Lake Ave N	Worcester, MA 01655-0002	NEW ENGLAND

UMass Memorial Medical Center (508) 334-1000
UMass Memorial Med Ctr
55 Lake Ave N   Worcester, MA 01655   NEW ENGLAND

UMDNJ-University Hospital-Newark (973) 972-4300
UMDNJ-Univ Hosp-Newark
150 Bergen St   Newark, NJ 07103-2406   MID ATLANTIC

Uniformed Services University of the Health Sciences (301) 295-9390
Unif Serv Univ of the Hlth Sci
4301 Jones Bridge Rd   Bethesda, MD 20814-4799   MID ATLANTIC

Union Memorial Hospital - Baltimore (410) 554-2000
Union Meml Hosp - Baltimore
201 E University Pkwy   Baltimore, MD 21218   MID ATLANTIC

United Hospital (651) 241-8000
United Hosp
333 N Smith Ave   St Paul, MN 55102   MIDWEST

University Community Hospital (813) 971-6000
University Comm Hosp
3100 E Fletcher Avenue   Tampa, FL 33613   SOUTHEAST

University Health System - University Hospital (210) 358-4000
Univ Hlth Sys - Univ Hosp
4502 Medical Dr   San Antonio, TX 78229   SOUTHWEST

University Hospital & Clinics - Mississippi (601) 984-1000
Univ Hosps & Clins - Jackson
2500 N State St   Jackson, MS 39216   SOUTHEAST

University Hospital - Cincinnati (513) 584-1000
Univ Hosp - Cincinnati
234 Goodman St   Cincinnati, OH 45219   MIDWEST

University Hospital - SUNY Upstate Medical University (315) 464-5540
Univ. Hosp.- SUNY Upstate
750 E Adams Street   Syracuse, NY 13210   MID ATLANTIC

University Hospitals Case Medical Center (216) 844-1000
Univ Hosps Case Med Ctr
11100 Euclid Ave   Cleveland, OH 44106   MIDWEST

University Medical Center Health System (806) 775-8200
Univ Med Ctr - Lubbock
PO Box 5980   Lubbock, TX 79408   SOUTHWEST

University Medical Center of Southern Nevada - Las Vegas   (702) 383-2000
Univ Med Ctr - Las Vegas
1800 W Charleston Blvd   Las Vegas, NV 89102   WEST COAST AND PACIFIC

University Medical Center- Tucson   (520) 694-0111
Univ Med Ctr - Tucson
1501 N Campbell Ave   Tucson, AZ 85724-5128   SOUTHWEST

University New Mexico Health & Science Center   (505) 272-2111
Univ NM Hlth & Sci Ctr
2211 Lomas Blvd NE   Albuquerque, NM 87106   SOUTHWEST

University of Alabama Hospital at Birmingham   (205) 934-4011
Univ of Ala Hosp at Birmingham
619 South 19th Street   Birmingham, AL 35249-6544   SOUTHEAST

University of Arkansas for Medical Sciences Medical Center   (501) 686-7000
UAMS Med Ctr
4301 W Markham St   Little Rock, AR 72205   SOUTHWEST

University of California - Davis Medical Center   (916) 734-2011
UC Davis Med Ctr
2315 Stockton Blvd   Sacramento, CA 95817   WEST COAST AND PACIFIC

University of California - Irvine Medical Center   (714) 456-6011
UC Irvine Med Ctr
101 The City Dr   Orange, CA 92868   WEST COAST AND PACIFIC

University of Chicago Hospitals   (773) 702-1000
Univ of Chicago Hosps
5841 S Maryland Ave   Chicago, IL 60637   MIDWEST

University of Colorado Hospital   (303) 372-0000
Univ Colorado Hosp
4200 E 9th Ave   Denver, CO 80262   GREAT PLAINS AND MOUNTAINS

University of Connecticut Health Center, John Dempsey Hospital   (860) 679-2100
Univ of Conn Hlth Ctr, John Dempsey Hosp
263 Farmington Ave   Farmington, CT 06030   NEW ENGLAND

University of Illinois at Chicago Eye & Ear Infirmary   (312) 996-6500
Univ of IL at Chicago Eye & Ear Infirm
1855 W Taylor St   Chicago, IL 60612   MIDWEST

University of Illinois Medical Center at Chicago   (312) 996-7000
Univ of IL Med Ctr at Chicago
1740 W Taylor St   Chicago, IL 60612   MIDWEST

University of Iowa Hospitals and Clinics		(319) 356-1616
Univ Iowa Hosp & Clinics		
200 Hawkins Drive	Iowa City, IA 52242	MIDWEST

University of Kansas Hospital		(913) 588-5000
Univ of Kansas Hosp		
3901 Rainbow Blvd	Kansas City, KS 66160	GREAT PLAINS AND MOUNTAINS

University of Kentucky Chandler Hospital		(800) 333-8874
Univ of Kentucky Chandler Hosp		
800 Rose Street	Lexington, KY 40536	SOUTHEAST

University of Louisville Hospital		(502) 562-3000
Univ of Louisville Hosp		
530 S Jackson St	Louisville, KY 40202	SOUTHEAST

University of Maryland Medical System		(410) 328-8667
Univ of MD Med Sys		
22 S Greene St	Baltimore, MD 21201	MID ATLANTIC

University of Miami Hosp & Clinics/ Sylvester Comprehensive Cancer Cntr		(305) 243-1000
Univ of Miami Hosp & Clins/Sylvester Comp Canc Ctr		
1475 NW 12th Ave	Miami, FL 33136	SOUTHEAST

University of Michigan Health System		(734) 936-4000
Univ Michigan Hlth Sys		
1500 E Medical Center Dr	Ann Arbor, MI 48109	MIDWEST

University of Minnesota Medical Center, Fairview - Riverside Campus		(612) 672-6000
Univ Minn Med Ctr, Fairview - Riverside Campus		
2450 Riverside Ave S	Minneapolis, MN 55454	MIDWEST

University of Minnesota Medical Center, Fairview - University Campus		(612) 273-3000
Univ Minn Med Ctr, Fairview - Univ Campus		
420 Delaware St SE	Minneapolis, MN 55455	MIDWEST

University of Missouri Hospitals & Clinics		(573) 882-4141
Univ of Missouri Hosp & Clins		
1 Hospital Dr	Columbia, MO 65212	MIDWEST

University of North Carolina Hospitals		(919) 966-4131
Univ NC Hosps		
101 Manning Drive, Box 7600	Chapel Hill, NC 27514	SOUTHEAST

University of Rochester Strong Memorial Hospital		(585) 275-2121
Univ of Rochester Strong Meml Hosp		
601 Elmwood Ave	Rochester, NY 14642	MID ATLANTIC

University of South Alabama Medical Center		(251) 471-7000
Univ of S AL Med Ctr		
2451 Fillingim St	Mobile, AL 36617	SOUTHEAST

University of South Florida - Tampa		(813) 974-2011
Univ of S FL - Tampa		
4202 E Fowler Ave	Tampa, FL 33620	SOUTHEAST

University of Tennesee Memorial Hospital		(865) 544-9000
Univ of Tennesee Mem Hosp		
1924 Alcoa Hwy	Knoxville, TN 37920	SOUTHEAST

University of Texas Health Center at Tyler		(903) 877-3451
UT Hlth Ctr at Tyler		
11937 US Hwy 271	Tyler, TX 75708	SOUTHWEST

University of Texas MD Anderson Cancer Center		(713) 792-2121
UT MD Anderson Cancer Ctr		
1515 Holcombe Blvd	Houston, TX 77030-4095	SOUTHWEST

University of Texas Medical Branch Hospital at Galveston		(409) 772-1011
UT Med Br Hosp at Galveston		
301 University Blvd	Galveston, TX 77555	SOUTHWEST

University of Texas Southwestern Medical Center at Dallas, The		(214) 648-3111
UT Southwestern Med Ctr - Dallas		
5323 Harry Hines Blvd	Dallas, TX 75390	SOUTHWEST

University of Toledo Medical Center		(419) 383-4000
Univ of Toledo Med Ctr		
3000 Arlington Ave	Toledo, OH 43614	MIDWEST

University of Utah Hospitals and Clinics		(801) 581-2121
Univ Utah Hosps and Clins		
50 N Medical Dr	Salt Lake City, UT 84132	GREAT PLAINS AND MOUNTAINS

University of Virginia Medical Center		(434) 924-0211
Univ Virginia Med Ctr		
1215 Lee Street	Charlottesville, VA 22908-0001	SOUTHEAST

University of Washington Medical Center		(206) 598-3300
Univ Wash Med Ctr		
1959 NE Pacific St, Box 356355	Seattle, WA 98195	WEST COAST AND PACIFIC

University of Wisconsin Hospital & Clinics		(608) 263-6400
Univ WI Hosp & Clins		
600 Highland Avenue	Madison, WI 53792	MIDWEST

UPMC Montefiore
UPMC Montefiore
200 Lothrop St — Pittsburgh, PA 15213 — (412) 647-2345 — MID ATLANTIC

UPMC Passavant-Cranberry
UPMC Passavant-Cranberry
1 St Francis Way — Cranberry Township, PA 16066 — (724) 772-5300 — MID ATLANTIC

UPMC Presbyterian
UPMC Presby, Pittsburgh
200 Lothrop St — Pittsburgh, PA 15213 — (412) 647-2345 — MID ATLANTIC

UPMC Shadyside
UPMC Shadyside
5230 Centre Ave — Pittsburgh, PA 15232 — (412) 623-2121 — MID ATLANTIC

UPMC St Margaret
UPMC St Margaret
815 Freeport Rd — Pittsburgh, PA 15215-3301 — (412) 784-4000 — MID ATLANTIC

Upstate Medical University Hospital
Upstate Med Univ Hosp
750 E Adams St — Syracuse, NY 13210-2306 — (315) 464-5540 — MID ATLANTIC

USC Norris Comprehensive Cancer Center and Hospital
USC Norris Comp Cancer Ctr
1441 Eastlake Ave — Los Angeles, CA 90033 — (323) 865-3000 — WEST COAST AND PACIFIC

USC University Hospital - Richard K. Eamer Medical Plaza
USC Univ Hosp - R K Eamer Med Plz
1500 San Pablo St — Los Angeles, CA 90033 — (323) 442-8444 — WEST COAST AND PACIFIC

VA Connecticut Healthcare System
VA Conn Hlthcre Sys
950 Campbell Ave — West Haven, CT 06516 — (203) 932-5711 — NEW ENGLAND

VA Health Care System - Palo Alto
VA Hlth Care Sys - Palo Alto
3801 Miranda Ave — Palo Alto, CA 94304 — (650) 493-5000 — WEST COAST AND PACIFIC

VA Medical Center - Atlanta
VA Med Ctr - Atlanta
1670 Clairmont Rd — Decatur, GA 30033 — (404) 321-6111 — SOUTHEAST

VA Medical Center - Cleveland
VA Med Ctr - Cleveland
10701 East Blvd — Cleveland, OH 44106 — (216) 791-3800 — MIDWEST

VA Medical Center - Indianapolis		(317) 554-0000
VA Med Ctr - Indianapolis		
1481 W 10th St	Indianapolis, IN 46202	MIDWEST

VA Medical Center - Memphis		(901) 523-8990
VA Med Ctr - Memphis		
1030 Jefferson Ave	Memphis, TN 38104	SOUTHEAST

VA Medical Center - Nashville		(615) 327-4751
VA Med Ctr - Nashville		
1310 24th Ave S	Nashville, TN 37212	SOUTHEAST

VA Medical Center - San Francisco		(415) 221-4810
VA Med Ctr - San Francisco		
4150 Clement St	San Francisco, CA 94121	WEST COAST AND PACIFIC

VA Medical Center - Washington, DC		(202) 745-8000
VA Med Ctr - Washington		
50 Irving St NW	Washington, DC 20422	MID ATLANTIC

VA Medical Center - West Los Angeles		(310) 478-3711
VA Med Ctr - W Los Angeles		
11301 Wilshire Blvd	Los Angeles, CA 90073	WEST COAST AND PACIFIC

VA Medical Center North Texas Health System		(214) 742-8387
VA Med Ctr N TX Hlth Sys		
4500 S Lancaster Rd	Dallas, TX 75216	SOUTHWEST

VA Pittsburgh Health Care System		(412) 688-6000
VA Pittsburgh Hlth Care Sys		
University Drive	Pittsburgh, PA 15240	MID ATLANTIC

VA Puget Sound Health Care System		(206) 762-1010
VA Puget Sound Hlth Care Sys		
1660 S Columbian Way	Seattle, WA 98108	WEST COAST AND PACIFIC

VA San Diego Healthcare System		(858) 552-8585
VA San Diego Hlthcre Sys		
3350 La Jolla Village Drive	San Diego, CA 92161	WEST COAST AND PACIFIC

Vail Valley Medical Center		(970) 476-2451
Vail Valley Med Ctr		
181 W Meadow Dr	Vail, CO 81657-5058	GREAT PLAINS AND MOUNTAINS

Valley Hospital Medical Center		(702) 388-4000
Valley Hosp Med Ctr		
620 Shadow Ln	Las Vegas, NV 89106-4194	WEST COAST AND PACIFIC

Vanderbilt Children's Hospital		(615) 936-1000
Vanderbilt Children's Hosp		
2200 Children's Way	Nashville, TN 37232	SOUTHEAST
Vanderbilt University Medical Center		(615) 322-5000
Vanderbilt Univ Med Ctr		
1313 21st Avenue South	Nashville, TN 37232	SOUTHEAST
Veterans Affairs Medical Center - Albuquerque		(505) 265-1711
VA Med Ctr		
1501 San Pedro, SE	Albuquerque, NM 87108	SOUTHWEST
Veterans Affairs Medical Center - Augusta		(706) 733-0188
VA Medical Ctr - Augusta		
One Freedom Way	Augusta, GA 30904	SOUTHEAST
Veterans Affairs Medical Center - White River Junction		(802) 295-9363
VA Aff Med Ctr - White River Junction		
215 North Maine Street	White River Junction, VT 05009	NEW ENGLAND
Virginia Hospital Center - Arlington		(703) 558-5000
Virginia Hosp Ctr - Arlington		
1701 N George Mason Dr	Arlington, VA 22205-3698	SOUTHEAST
Virginia Mason Medical Center		(206) 223-6600
Virginia Mason Med Ctr		
1100 Ninth Ave, Box 900	Seattle, WA 98111	WEST COAST AND PACIFIC
Wake Forest University Baptist Medical Center		(336) 716-2011
Wake Forest Univ Baptist Med Ctr		
Medical Center Blvd	Winston-Salem, NC 27157-1015	SOUTHEAST
WakeMed Cary Hospital		(919) 350-2300
WakeMed Cary		
1900 Kildaire Farm Rd	Cary, NC 27511-6616	SOUTHEAST
WakeMed New Bern Avenue Campus		(919) 350-8000
WakeMed New Bern		
3000 New Bern Ave	Raleigh, NC 27610	SOUTHEAST
Walter Reed Army Medical Center		(202) 782-3501
W Reed Army Med Ctr		
6900 Georgia Ave NW	Washington, DC 20307-5001	MID ATLANTIC
Washington Hospital Center		(202) 877-7000
Washington Hosp Ctr		
110 Irving St NW	Washington, DC 20010	MID ATLANTIC

Washington University Medical Center		(314) 362-6828
Washington Univ Med Ctr		
4444 Forest Park Ave	St Louis, MO 63108	MIDWEST

WellStar Kennestone Hospital		(770) 793-5000
WellStar Kennestone Hosp		
677 Church Street	Marietta, GA 30060	SOUTHEAST

Wesley Woods Geriatric Hospital		(404) 728-6200
Wesley Woods Ger Hosp		
1821 Clifton Rd	Atlanta, GA 30329	SOUTHEAST

West Virginia University Hospital - Ruby Memorial		(304) 598-4000
WV Univ Hosp - Ruby Memorial		
1 Medical Center Drive	Morgantown, WV 26506	MID ATLANTIC

Westchester Medical Center		(914) 493-7000
Westchester Med Ctr		
95 Grasslands Road	Valhalla, NY 10595	MID ATLANTIC

Western Pennsylvania Hospital		(412) 578-5120
Western Penn Hosp		
4800 Friendship Avenue	Pittsburgh, PA 15224	MID ATLANTIC

Western Psychiatric Institute and Clinic - UPMC		(412) 624-2100
Western Psych Inst & Clin - UPMC		
3811 O'Hara St	Pittsburgh, PA 15213	MID ATLANTIC

Wheaton Franciscan Healthcare-St Joseph		(414) 447-2000
Wheaton Franciscan Hlthcare-St Joseph-Milwaukee		
5000 W. Chambers Street	Milwaukee, WI 53210	MIDWEST

William Beaumont Hospital		(248) 551-5000
William Beaumont Hosp		
3601 W 13 Mile Rd	Royal Oak, MI 48073	MIDWEST

William S Hall Psychiatric Institute		(803) 898-1693
William S Hall Psyc Inst		
1800 Colonial Dr, Box 202	Columbia, SC 29202-6827	SOUTHEAST

Wills Eye Hospital		(215) 928-3000
Wills Eye Hosp		
840 Walnut St	Philadelphia, PA 19107-5598	MID ATLANTIC

Winthrop - University Hospital		(516) 663-0333
Winthrop - Univ Hosp		
259 1st St	Mineola, NY 11501	MID ATLANTIC

Wishard Health Services   (317) 630-7592
Wishard Hlth Srvs
1001 West 10th Street   Indianapolis, IN 46202   MIDWEST

Wolfson Children's Hospital   (904) 202-8000
Wolfson Chldns Hosp
800 Prudential Dr   Jacksonville, FL 32207   SOUTHEAST

Woman's Hospital of Texas, The   (713) 790-1234
Woman's Hosp TX, The
7600 Fannin St   Houston, TX 77054   SOUTHWEST

Women & Children's Hospital - Los Angeles   (323) 226-3427
Women & Children's Hosp - LA
1240 North Mission Road   Los Angeles, CA 90033   WEST COAST AND PACIFIC

Women & Infants Hospital - Rhode Island   (401) 274-1100
Women & Infants Hosp - Rhode Island
101 Dudley Street   Providence, RI 02905   NEW ENGLAND

Women's and Children's Hospital of Buffalo, The   (716) 878-7000
Women's & Chldn's Hosp of Buffalo, The
219 Bryant St   Buffalo, NY 14222   MID ATLANTIC

Wright State University   (937) 775-2550
Wright State Univ
3640 Colonel Glenn Hwy   Dayton, OH 45435-0001   MIDWEST

Yale - New Haven Hospital   (203) 688-4242
Yale - New Haven Hosp
20 York St   New Haven, CT 06510   NEW ENGLAND

Yampa Valley Medical Center   (970) 879-1322
Yampa Valley Med Ctr
1024 Central Park Dr   Steamboat Springs, CO 80487   GREAT PLAINS AND MOUNTAINS

York Hospital   (717) 851-3500
York Hosp
1001 S George St   York, PA 17405-7198   MID ATLANTIC

Appendix D:
Selected Resources

GENERAL RESOURCES

AMERICAN AMBULANCE ASSOCIATION (AAA)

The American Ambulance Association represents emergency and non-emergency medical transportation providers, advocating high quality pre-hospital care and keeping these providers aware of legislation and news that may affect them.

8201 Greensboro Drive, Ste 300
McLean, VA 22102

800-523-4447
703-610-9018
fax 703-610-9005
www.the-aaa.org/

AMERICA'S HEALTH INSURANCE PLANS (AHIP)

America's Health Insurance Plans is a national trade association representing nearly 1,300 member companies providing health benefits to more than 200 million Americans.

601 Pennsylvania Ave, NW
South Building Suite 500
Washington, DC 20004

202-778-3200
fax: 202-331-7487
www.ahip.org/

AMERICAN BOARD OF MEDICAL SPECIALTIES (ABMS)

The ABMS is the authoritative body for the recognition of medical specialties, coordinating 24 medical specialty boards (including 25 medical specialties) and providing information on the board certification of doctors.

1007 Church Street, Suite 404
Evanston, Illinois 60201-5913

847-491-9091 or 866-ASK-ABMS
fax 847-328-3596
www.abms.org

AMERICAN HOSPITAL ASSOCIATION (AHA)

A national health advocacy organization, the AHA represents hospitals and healthcare networks in legislative and regulatory matters. In 1973 the AHA adopted the Patient Bill of Rights to help patients understand their rights and responsibilities.

1 North Franklin
Chicago, IL 60606

800-424-4301 or 312-422-3000
fax 312-422-4796
www.aha.org/

325 7th St. NW
Washington, DC 20004

800-424-4301 or 202-638-1100
fax 202-626-2345

American Medical Association (AMA)

The AMA is an association that maintains information on physicians practicing throughout the nation. Healthcare consumers can use their database to check the location, licensing, education and specialty of many doctors in the United States.

515 North State Street
Chicago, IL 60610

800-621-8335
www.ama-assn.org/

Center for Medical Consumers

Provides volume and outcome data on certain medical procedures performed in New York state.

239 Thompson St.
New York, NY 10012

212-674-7105
fax 212-674-7100
medconsumers@earthlink.net
www.medicalconsumers.org

Centers for Disease Control and Prevention (CDC)

Part of the Department of Health and Human Services, the CDC's mission is to prevent and manage diseases and illnesses. Its Web site contains information on a range of illnesses and the research being pursued to manage them. It also provides free faxed reports on disease risk and prevention in various parts of the world.

Public Inquiries/MASO
Mailstop E11
1600 Clifton Road
Atlanta, GA 30333

1-800-311-3435

toll free number for international travelers 877 FYI-TRIP or 404-639-3534
fax information service for international travelers 888-232-3299
www.cdc.gov/netinfo.htm

The CenterWatch Clinical Trials Listing Service

Profiles centers conducting clinical research by therapeutic area and geographic region, including more than 41,000 international industry and government-sponsored clinical trials and new FDA approved drug therapies, as well as 5,200 clinical trials that are actively recruiting patients.

22 Thomson Place, 47F1
Boston, MA 02210-1212

617-856-5900
fax 617-856-5901
www.centerwatch.com

Health Care Choices

Provides information on volume and outcomes of certain medical procedures performed in hospitals in various states throughout the country.

P.O. Box 21039
Columbus Circle Station
New York, NY 10023

212-724-9395
www.healthcarechoices.org
info@healthcarechoices.org

International Association for Medical Assistance To Travellers (IAMAT)

IAMAT is a non-profit organization that disseminates information on health and sanitary conditions worldwide. Membership is free but donations are appreciated. Members will receive a membership card making them eligible to access English speaking physicians all over the world. The organization also provides information on immunization requirements, malaria, and other tropical diseases, and sanitary and climactic conditions around the world. For information, send request in writing.

1623 Military Road #279   716-754-4883
Niagra Falls, New York 14304-1745   www.iamat.org

Joint Commission on Accreditation of Healthcare Organizations

The Joint Commission (JCAHO) is an independent, not-for-profit organization, which evaluates the quality and safety of care for nearly 17,000 health care organizations. To maintain and earn accreditation, organizations must have an extensive on-site review by a team of JCAHO health care professionals, at least once every three years. JCAHO is governed by a board that includes physicians, nurses, and consumers. JCAHO sets the standards by which health care quality is measured in America and around the world.

One Renaissance Boulevard   630-792-5000
Oakbrook Terrace, IL 60181   fax 630-792-5005
      www.jcaho.org

Medic Alert Foundation

The Medic Alert Foundation (a non-profit organization) provides an "ID tag" engraved with personal medical facts, as well as a 24-hour emergency response center which can release additional personal medical details. Membership is $20/year (waived for the first year) and members need to purchase the "ID tag" which sells for as low as $35.

2323 Colorado Avenue   888-633-4298
Turlock, CA 95382   Fax 209-669-2450
      www.medicalert.org

Medline

One Medline Place   1-800-MEDLINE (800-633-5463)
Mundelein, Illinois 60060   fax 1-800-351-1512
      www.medline.com

A medical database including millions of medical references and abstracts from thousands of scientific and medical journals.

The National Cancer Institute (NCI)

Part of the NIH, the NCI sponsors cancer clinical trials at more than 100 sites in the United States. Trials are carried out in major medical research centers, such as teaching hospitals, as well as in community hospitals, specialized medical clinics and even in doctors' offices.

Clinical Studies Support Center (CSSC)   800-4-CANCER (800-422-6237)
6116 Executive Boulevard   www.nci.nih.gov
Bethesda, MD 20892-8322   www.cancer.gov
      cancergovstaff@mail.nih.gov

National Center for Complementary and Alternative Medicine Clearinghouse (NCCAMC)

The NCCAMC facilitates the evaluation of alternative medical treatment modalities to help determine their effectiveness and bring alternative medicine into mainstream medicine. This agency does not provide referrals.

9000 Rockville Pike
Bethesda, MD 20892

888-644-6226
fax 866-464-3616
www.nccam.nih.gov
info@nccam.nih.gov

National Consumers League (NCL)

NCL is a private, nonprofit consumer advocacy organization. NCL strives to investigate, educate, and advocate on a variety of issues including healthcare. Membership is $20 annually, but individuals can also write to the organization for a list of publications that non-members can purchase.

1701 K Street, NW, Suite 1200
Washington, DC 20006

202-835-3323
fax 202-835-0747
www.nclnet.org
info@nclnet.org

The National Institutes of Health (NIH)

An organization operated by the U.S. government, the NIH operates its own hospital at which the care provided is usually related to clinical studies its researchers are undertaking. Information about the Warren G. Magnuson Clinical Center is also available.

Patient Recruitment Referral Center
9000 Rockville Pike
Bethesda, MD 20892

800-411-1222 or 301-496-4000
www.nih.gov
www.clinicaltrials.gov
nihinfo@od.nih.gov

National Insurance Information Institute

The National Insurance Information Institute Helpline advises consumers on how to choose an insurance company or broker. It also offers an analysis of life insurance and assists in insurance complaints.

110 William St
New York, NY 10038

800-942-4242 or 212-346-5500
www.iii.org

The Patient Advocate Foundation

A national non-profit organization that provides consultation, referrals and case management to patients to ensure that they are not denied access to healthcare, insurance coverage, employment and public assistance programs during an illness. In particular, the organization maintains comprehensive information on cancer treatment options that are available to consumers through a separate Web site: www.oncology.com.

700 Thimble Shoals Boulevard, Suite 200
Newport News, VA 23606

800-532-5274
fax 757-873-8999
www.patientadvocate.org/
help@patientadvocate.org

PEOPLE'S MEDICAL SOCIETY

The People's Medical Society, a nonprofit organization, is focused on educating the healthcare consumer about healthcare issues and medical rights. Their Web site provides information on useful books and publications as well as the latest healthcare developments.

P.O. Box 868
Allentown, PA 18105

610-770-1670
fax 610-770-0607
www.peoplesmed.org/index.html
cbi@peoplesmed.org

PERSONS UNITED LIMITING SUBSTANDARDS AND ERRORS IN HEALTHCARE (P.U.L.S.E.)

A support group for the survivors of medical malpractice and substandard healthcare, this nonprofit group also advocates patient education and patient-doctor communication.

PO Box 353
3300 Park Avenue
Wantagh NY 11793-0353

800-96-pulse (800-967-8573) or
516-579-4711
fax: 516-520-8105
www.PULSEamerica.org
www.PULSEofNY.com
pulse516@aol.com

Colorado Office

719-250-1286
PULSECOLO@YAHOO.COM

PUBLIC CITIZEN'S HEALTH AND RESEARCH GROUP

A non-profit organization, the Public Citizen's Group acts as a watchdog agency by advocating accountability and the open use of doctors' disciplinary backgrounds.

1600 20th Street NW
Washington, D.C. 20009

202-588-1000
www.citizen.org/hrg/

VERITAS MEDICINE

An organization that allows individuals to perform confidential, personalized searches of their clinical trials database and to access information on new treatment and drug options. The text is submitted by Harvard-affiliated doctors.

11 Cambridge Center
Cambridge, Massachusetts 02142

617-234-1500 or
877-5-TRIALS (877-587-4257)
fax 617-234-1555
www.veritasmedicine.com
info@veritasmedicine.com

Indices

Subject Index

A

B

C

D

Postgraduate Training 10
Prevention Trials 27
Primary Care 1, 4, 7, 8, 15, 18, 19, 31, 42, 43, 49
Private Insurance 29
Professional Reputation 13
Protocol 27, 28, 30

R

Recertification 12, 50
Referral 2, 8, 18, 35, 53
Residency 10, 11, 16, 17, 37, 49, 50

S

Second Opinions 17
Selection Process 2
Self-Designated Medical Specialties 12
Side Effects 26, 27, 32, 33
Special Resources 25, 26, 28, 30, 32, 34
Specialists 1, 3, 4, 5, 6, 7, 8, 9, 10, 12, 14, 15, 16, 18, 37, 41, 43, 49, 50, 51, 53
Specialties xxiii, 2, 3, 5, 6, 9, 10, 11, 12, 14, 24, 38, 41, 42, 43, 44, 45, 46, 47, 49, 50, 51, 53
Standard Therapies 25
Subspecialties 1, 5, 6, 10, 12, 13, 15, 41, 42, 49, 50, 53

T

Therapeutic Approaches 1, 6, 25
Treatment Plan 21, 30
Treatment Studies 25, 30
Trust 19

U

United States Department of Health 33
United States Medical Licensing Exam 9

V

Veritas Medicine 26

W

Warren Grant Magnuson Clinical Center 33, 34, 35

Special Expertise Index

This index lists the areas which the physicians listed in the Guide have identified as their "special expertise." These are not medical specialities. They are specific elements of disease, procedures, techniques and treatments for which these physicians are best known and are referred patients.

Special Expertise Index

Spec	Name	St	Pg
N	Farlow, M	IN	477
N	Feinberg, T	NY	465
N	Filley, C	CO	483
N	Fox, J	IL	477
N	Gilman, S	MI	477
N	Henderson, V	CA	488
N	Jordan, B	NY	466
N	Mesulam, M	IL	479
N	Morris, J	MO	479
N	Petersen, R	MN	480
N	Relkin, N	NY	470
N	Sadowsky, C	FL	475
N	Selkoe, D	MA	461
N	Zimmerman, E	NY	471
Psyc	Eisdorfer, C	FL	809
Psyc	Marin, D	NY	807
Psyc	Raskind, M	WA	816
Psyc	Weiner, M	TX	814

Amblyopia

Spec	Name	St	Pg
Oph	Diamond, G	PA	525
Oph	Gallin, P	NY	526
Oph	Miller, J	AZ	545
Oph	Tychsen, L	MO	543
Oph	Weiss, A	WA	552

Amblyopia & Vision Development

Spec	Name	St	Pg
Oph	Burke, M	OH	538
Oph	France, T	WI	539

Amniocentesis

Spec	Name	St	Pg
MF	McLaren, R	VA	389
MF	Philipson, E	OH	391
MF	Strassner, H	IL	391

Amniotic Membrane Transplant

Spec	Name	St	Pg
Oph	John, T	IL	539

Amputation Surgery

Spec	Name	St	Pg
OrS	Pinzur, M	IL	581
OrS	Polly, D	MN	581

Amputee Rehabilitation

Spec	Name	St	Pg
PMR	Dillingham, T	WI	760
PMR	Donovan, W	TX	763
PMR	Esquenazi, A	PA	757
PMR	Gitler, M	IL	761
PMR	Kuiken, T	IL	761
PMR	Leonard, J	MI	761
PMR	Munin, M	PA	758

Amyloidosis

Spec	Name	St	Pg
Hem	Gertz, M	MN	300
Onc	Vescio, R	CA	346

Amyloidosis/Joint Disease

Spec	Name	St	Pg
Rhu	Gorevic, P	NY	930

Amyotrophic Lateral Sclerosis (ALS)

Spec	Name	St	Pg
N	Armon, C	MA	460
N	Barohn, R	KS	482
N	Drachman, D	MD	464
N	Feldman, E	MI	477
N	Glass, J	GA	472
N	Graves, M	CA	488
N	Lacomis, D	PA	467
N	Mitsumoto, H	NY	468
N	Pascuzzi, R	IN	480

Spec	Name	St	Pg
N	Roos, R	IL	481
N	Siddique, T	IL	481
N	Valenstein, E	FL	475
N	Weiner, L	CA	490
N	Windebank, A	MN	482

Anal Cancer

Spec	Name	St	Pg
CRS	Gorfine, S	NY	165
CRS	Welton, M	CA	172

Anal Disorders & Reconstruction

Spec	Name	St	Pg
CRS	Gorfine, S	NY	165
CRS	Rafferty, J	OH	169
CRS	Wong, W	NY	166

Anal Sphincter Repair

Spec	Name	St	Pg
CRS	Coutsoftides, T	CA	171
CRS	Lowry, A	MN	168

Anal Surgery

Spec	Name	St	Pg
CRS	MacKeigan, J	MI	168

Anaphylaxis

Spec	Name	St	Pg
A&I	Greenberger, P	IL	86
A&I	Korenblat, P	MO	87
A&I	Lieberman, P	TN	85
A&I	Montanaro, A	OR	88
A&I	Reisman, R	NY	83
A&I	Sullivan, T	GA	85
PA&I	Ownby, D	GA	668
PA&I	Sampson, H	NY	667

Anemia

Spec	Name	St	Pg
Ger	Freedman, M	NY	249
Hem	Blinder, M	MO	300
Hem	Zalusky, R	NY	298
PHO	Salvi, S	IL	700

Anemia & Red Cell Disorders

Spec	Name	St	Pg
Hem	Telen, M	NC	299

Anemia-Aplastic

Spec	Name	St	Pg
Hem	Maciejewski, J	OH	302
PHO	Abella, E	AZ	701
PHO	Boxer, L	MI	698
PHO	Wang, W	TN	698

Anemia-Cancer Related

Spec	Name	St	Pg
Path	Rodgers, G	UT	653

Anemias & Red Cell Disorders

Spec	Name	St	Pg
Hem	Benz, E	MA	294
PHO	Boxer, L	MI	698

Aneurysm

Spec	Name	St	Pg
NRad	Pile-Spellman, J	NY	898
TS	Tranbaugh, R	NY	1007
VascS	Ascher, E	NY	1067
VascS	Belkin, M	MA	1066
VascS	Flanigan, D	CA	1075
VascS	Greisler, H	IL	1073
VascS	Hodgson, K	IL	1073
VascS	Makaroun, M	PA	1069
VascS	Perler, B	MD	1070
VascS	Ricotta, J	NY	1070
VascS	Rosenthal, D	GA	1072
VascS	Stanley, J	MI	1073
VascS	White, R	CA	1076

Spec	Name	St	Pg
VIR	Dake, M	VA	904

Aneurysm-Abdominal & Thoracic Aortic

Spec	Name	St	Pg
TS	Coselli, J	TX	1018
VascS	Calligaro, K	PA	1068
VascS	Carpenter, J	PA	1068
VascS	Clair, D	OH	1072
VascS	Criado, F	MD	1068
VascS	Darling, R	NY	1068
VascS	Kwolek, C	MA	1066
VascS	Parodi, J	FL	1071
VascS	Sanchez, L	MO	1073
VIR	Becker, G	AZ	907

Aneurysm-Abdominal Aortic

Spec	Name	St	Pg
TS	Griepp, R	NY	1002
TS	Martin, T	FL	1009
TS	Ott, D	TX	1019
TS	Safi, H	TX	1020
VascS	Adelman, M	NY	1067
VascS	Atnip, R	PA	1067
VascS	Brewster, D	MA	1066
VascS	Cambria, R	MA	1066
VascS	Clagett, G	TX	1074
VascS	Cronenwett, J	NH	1066
VascS	Eidt, J	AR	1074
VascS	Gloviczki, P	MN	1072
VascS	Green, R	NY	1069
VascS	Hakaim, A	FL	1071
VascS	Hallett, J	SC	1071
VascS	Hobson, R	NJ	1069
VascS	Kent, K	NY	1069
VascS	Mackey, W	MA	1067
VascS	Money, S	AZ	1075
VascS	Moore, W	CA	1076
VascS	Pearce, W	IL	1073
VascS	Riles, T	NY	1070
VascS	Sicard, G	MO	1073
VascS	Todd, G	NY	1070
VascS	Towne, J	WI	1074
VascS	Whittemore, A	MA	1067
VascS	Zarins, C	CA	1076
VIR	Benenati, J	FL	904

Aneurysm-Aortic

Spec	Name	St	Pg
TS	Cohn, L	MA	998
TS	Girardi, L	NY	1002
TS	Griffith, B	MD	1003
VascS	Andros, G	CA	1075
VascS	Chaikof, E	GA	1070
VascS	Comerota, A	OH	1072
VascS	Fairman, R	PA	1068
VascS	Fowl, R	AZ	1074
VascS	Freischlag, J	MD	1069
VascS	Gewertz, B	CA	1075
VascS	Giangola, G	NY	1069
VascS	Harrington, E	NY	1069
VascS	Howard, T	NE	1074
VascS	Marin, M	NY	1069
VascS	Reddy, D	MI	1073
VascS	Seeger, J	FL	1072
VascS	Shepard, A	MI	1073
VIR	Hovsepian, D	MO	905
VIR	Katzen, B	FL	905
VIR	Murphy, T	RI	902

Aneurysm-Cerebral

Spec	Name	St	Pg
N	Mohr, J	NY	469

Special Expertise Index

Special Expertise Index

Special Expertise Index

Spec	Name	St	Pg	Spec	Name	St	Pg	Spec	Name	St	Pg
Onc	Buys, S	UT	336	Onc	Robert, N	VA	325	RadRO	Recht, A	MA	869
Onc	Buzdar, A	TX	337	Onc	Romond, E	KY	326	RadRO	Rose, C	CA	881
Onc	Camoriano, J	AZ	337	Onc	Rosen, S	IL	333	RadRO	Rosenman, J	NC	874
Onc	Canellos, G	MA	307	Onc	Russell, C	CA	345	RadRO	Rotman, M	NY	872
Onc	Carlson, R	CA	342	Onc	Salem, P	TX	341	RadRO	Schiff, P	NY	872
Onc	Chap, L	CA	342	Onc	Schnipper, L	MA	309	RadRO	Shina, D	NM	879
Onc	Chitambar, C	WI	330	Onc	Schuchter, L	PA	320	RadRO	Solin, L	PA	872
Onc	Chlebowski, R	CA	342	Onc	Schwartz, B	MN	334	RadRO	Taylor, M	MO	877
Onc	Cobleigh, M	IL	330	Onc	Schwartz, M	FL	326	RadRO	Vicini, F	MI	877
Onc	Cohen, P	DC	311	Onc	Shapiro, C	OH	334	RadRO	Wazer, D	RI	869
Onc	Cohen, S	NY	311	Onc	Shulman, L	MA	309	RadRO	Wilson, J	WI	877
Onc	Come, S	MA	307	Onc	Sledge, G	IN	334	S	Alfonso, A	NY	956
Onc	Daly, M	PA	312	Onc	Smith, T	VA	327	S	Anderson, B	WA	985
Onc	Davidson, N	MD	312	Onc	Speyer, J	NY	320	S	August, D	NJ	956
Onc	Disis, M	WA	343	Onc	Stockdale, F	CA	346	S	Axelrod, D	NY	957
Onc	Doroshow, J	MD	312	Onc	Stone, J	FL	327	S	Beauchamp, R	TN	967
Onc	Dreicer, R	OH	330	Onc	Stopeck, A	AZ	341	S	Beitsch, P	TX	982
Onc	Ebbert, L	SD	336	Onc	Sutton, L	NC	327	S	Bland, K	AL	967
Onc	Ellis, G	WA	343	Onc	Urba, W	OR	346	S	Borgen, P	NY	957
Onc	Fabian, C	KS	336	Onc	Valero, V	TX	341	S	Butler, J	CA	986
Onc	Fox, K	PA	313	Onc	Vogel, V	PA	321	S	Byrd, D	WA	986
Onc	Fracasso, P	MO	330	Onc	Ward, J	UT	336	S	Cady, B	RI	954
Onc	Ganz, P	CA	343	Onc	Weisberg, T	ME	310	S	Chang, A	MI	974
Onc	Garber, J	MA	308	Onc	Wicha, M	MI	335	S	Chang, H	CA	986
Onc	Geyer, C	PA	314	Onc	Winer, E	MA	310	S	Copeland III, E	FL	968
Onc	Glaspy, J	CA	343	Path	Allred, D	MO	651	S	Crowe, J	OH	974
Onc	Glick, J	PA	314	Path	Connolly, J	MA	644	S	Dilawari, R	TN	968
Onc	Goldstein, L	PA	314	Path	Cote, R	CA	656	S	Donohue, J	MN	974
Onc	Graham, M	NC	323	Path	Dubeau, L	CA	656	S	Dooley, W	OK	983
Onc	Gralow, J	WA	344	Path	Masood, S	FL	656	S	Eberlein, T	MO	974
Onc	Grossbard, M	NY	314	Path	Mies, C	PA	647	S	Edge, S	NY	959
Onc	Hait, W	NJ	314	Path	Page, D	TN	651	S	Edington, H	PA	959
Onc	Hartmann, L	MN	331	Path	Patchefsky, A	PA	647	S	Edney, J	NE	981
Onc	Hayes, D	MI	331	Path	Rosen, P	NY	648	S	Edwards, M	AR	983
Onc	Herbst, R	TX	338	Path	Ross, J	NY	648	S	Eisenberg, B	NH	954
Onc	Holland, J	NY	315	Path	Sanchez, M	NJ	648	S	Esserman, L	CA	987
Onc	Hortobagyi, G	TX	338	Path	Schnitt, S	MA	645	S	Estabrook, A	NY	960
Onc	Hudis, C	NY	315	Path	Thor, A	CO	653	S	Euhus, D	TX	983
Onc	Hutchins, L	AR	338	Path	Tornos, C	NY	649	S	Farrar, W	OH	975
Onc	Ingle, J	MN	331	Path	Wilczynski, S	CA	658	S	Feig, B	TX	983
Onc	Isaacs, C	DC	315	Path	Young, R	MA	645	S	Gabram, S	GA	969
Onc	Johnson, D	TN	324	PIS	Collins, E	NH	770	S	Giuliano, A	CA	987
Onc	Jones, S	TX	338	RadRO	Berg, C	MD	869	S	Goodson, W	CA	987
Onc	Kaufman, P	NH	309	RadRO	Buchholz, T	TX	878	S	Goulet, R	IN	975
Onc	Kosova, L	IL	331	RadRO	Coia, L	NJ	869	S	Grant, C	MN	975
Onc	Legha, S	TX	339	RadRO	Formenti, S	NY	870	S	Hanks, J	VA	969
Onc	Levine, E	NY	316	RadRO	Goodman, R	NJ	870	S	Harkema, J	MI	976
Onc	Lippman, M	MI	331	RadRO	Haffty, B	NJ	870	S	Herrmann, V	SC	969
Onc	Livingston, R	AZ	339	RadRO	Halberg, F	CA	880	S	Hoffman, J	PA	961
Onc	Locker, G	IL	332	RadRO	Halle, J	NC	873	S	Hughes, K	MA	954
Onc	Loprinzi, C	MN	332	RadRO	Halpern, H	IL	875	S	Iglehart, J	MA	955
Onc	Lyman, G	NY	317	RadRO	Harris, J	MA	868	S	Israel, P	GA	969
Onc	Marcom, P	NC	325	RadRO	Hayman, J	MI	875	S	Johnson, R	PA	961
Onc	McGuire, W	MD	317	RadRO	Herman, T	OK	878	S	Kim, J	OH	976
Onc	Moore, A	NY	318	RadRO	Kiel, K	IL	876	S	Klimberg, V	AR	984
Onc	Mortimer, J	CA	344	RadRO	Kuske, R	AZ	879	S	Knudson, M	CA	988
Onc	Muss, H	VT	309	RadRO	Lewin, A	FL	873	S	Krag, D	VT	955
Onc	Nabell, L	AL	325	RadRO	Macklis, R	OH	876	S	Leight, G	NC	970
Onc	Nissenblatt, M	NJ	318	RadRO	Marks, L	NC	873	S	Levine, E	NC	970
Onc	Northfelt, D	AZ	340	RadRO	McCormick, B	NY	871	S	Lind, D	GA	970
Onc	Norton, L	NY	318	RadRO	Medbery, C	OK	879	S	Lyerly, H	NC	970
Onc	O'Shaughnessy, J	TX	340	RadRO	Mendenhall, N	FL	873	S	McGrath, P	KY	971
Onc	Offit, K	NY	318	RadRO	Myerson, R	MO	876	S	Morrow, M	PA	963
Onc	Olopade, O	IL	332	RadRO	Nori, D	NY	871	S	Nathanson, S	MI	977
Onc	Osborne, C	TX	340	RadRO	Pierce, L	MI	877	S	Nelson, J	UT	981
Onc	Oster, M	NY	319	RadRO	Pistenmaa, D	TX	879	S	Niederhuber, J	MD	963
Onc	Perez, E	FL	325	RadRO	Prosnitz, L	NC	874	S	Nowak, E	NY	963
Onc	Perry, M	MO	332	RadRO	Quivey, J	CA	881	S	Osborne, M	NY	963

Special Expertise Index

Special Expertise Index

Special Expertise Index

Special Expertise Index

Special Expertise Index

Special Expertise Index

Special Expertise Index

Spec	Name	St	Pg
Onc	Legha, S	TX	339
Path	Li Volsi, V	PA	647
S	Cance, W	FL	968
S	Evans, D	TX	983
S	Hanks, J	VA	969
S	Moley, J	MO	977

Endocrine Disorders

Spec	Name	St	Pg
EDM	Chopra, I	CA	209

Endocrine Pathology

Spec	Name	St	Pg
Path	DeLellis, R	RI	644
Path	Silverberg, S	MD	648

Endocrine Surgery

Spec	Name	St	Pg
S	Albertson, D	NC	967
S	Doherty, G	MI	974
S	Fahey, T	NY	960
S	Farley, D	MN	975
S	Ferzli, G	NY	960
S	Hanks, J	VA	969
S	Hansen, N	IL	976
S	Howard, R	FL	969
S	Livingston, E	TX	984
S	Norton, J	CA	988
S	Schlinkert, R	AZ	985

Endocrine Tumors

Spec	Name	St	Pg
Onc	Jahan, T	CA	344
S	Angelos, P	IL	973
S	Fraker, D	PA	961
S	Goldstein, R	KY	969
S	Jackson, G	TX	984
S	Lee, J	TX	984
S	Siperstein, A	OH	979

Endocrinology

Spec	Name	St	Pg
EDM	LeBoff, M	MA	197
EDM	Recker, R	NE	208
EDM	Semenkovich, C	MO	207
Ger	Abrass, I	WA	253
Ger	Gambert, S	MD	249
Ger	Halter, J	MI	251
Ger	Morley, J	MO	251
IM	Beaser, R	MA	378

Endocrinology & Joint Disorders

Spec	Name	St	Pg
Rhu	Lahita, R	NJ	931

Endocrinology & Thyroid Disease

Spec	Name	St	Pg
IM	Rivlin, R	NY	379

Endometriosis

Spec	Name	St	Pg
GO	Magrina, J	AZ	272
ObG	Filip, S	NC	510
ObG	Lauter, M	MA	508
ObG	Merritt, D	MO	512
ObG	Steege, J	NC	511
RE	Adamson, G	CA	923
RE	Bieber, E	PA	915
RE	Carson, S	RI	914
RE	Copperman, A	NY	915
RE	DeVane, G	FL	918
RE	Dodds, W	MI	920
RE	Dumesic, D	MN	920
RE	Isaacson, K	MA	914
RE	Jacobs, L	IL	921
RE	Luciano, A	CT	914
RE	Marrs, R	CA	923
RE	Murphy, A	GA	919
RE	Ory, S	FL	919
RE	Pfeifer, S	PA	916
RE	Rock, J	FL	919
RE	Schenken, R	TX	922
RE	Schlaff, W	CO	922
RE	Surrey, E	CO	922
RE	Walmer, D	NC	919
RE	Zinaman, M	IL	922

Endometriosis-Intestine

Spec	Name	St	Pg
CRS	Bailey, H	TX	170

Endoscopic Sinus Surgery

Spec	Name	St	Pg
Oto	Close, L	NY	603
Oto	Edelstein, D	NY	604
Oto	Fried, M	NY	604
Oto	Gold, S	NY	604
Oto	Josephson, J	NY	605
Oto	Kennedy, D	PA	606
Oto	Kuhn, F	GA	611
Oto	Schaefer, S	NY	608
Oto	Senders, C	CA	626
Oto	Stankiewicz, J	IL	619

Endoscopic Strip Craniectomy

Spec	Name	St	Pg
NS	Jimenez, D	TX	444

Endoscopic Surgery

Spec	Name	St	Pg
NS	Kassam, A	PA	429
Oto	Snyderman, C	PA	609
PS	Tracy, T	RI	725

Endoscopic Ultrasound

Spec	Name	St	Pg
Ge	Chang, K	CA	238
Ge	Das, A	AZ	236
Ge	Gerdes, H	NY	219
Ge	Ginsberg, G	PA	219
Ge	Greenwald, B	MD	220
Ge	Haluszka, O	PA	220
Ge	Hawes, R	SC	226
Ge	Hoffman, B	SC	226
Ge	Kantsevoy, S	MD	220
Ge	Kimmey, M	WA	239
Ge	Lambiase, L	FL	226
Ge	Lightdale, C	NY	222
Ge	Mertz, H	TN	226
Ge	Pochapin, M	NY	223
Ge	Rex, D	IN	232

Endoscopy

Spec	Name	St	Pg
Ge	Barkin, J	FL	224
Ge	Baron, T	MN	228
Ge	Bjorkman, D	UT	234
Ge	Carr-Locke, D	MA	216
Ge	Cello, J	CA	238
Ge	Das, A	AZ	236
Ge	Dieterich, D	NY	219
Ge	Edmundowicz, S	MO	229
Ge	Ellis, J	CA	238
Ge	Fang, J	UT	235
Ge	Gerdes, H	NY	219
Ge	Ginsberg, G	PA	219
Ge	Gostout, C	MN	230
Ge	Green, P	NY	219
Ge	Haluszka, O	PA	220
Ge	Hoops, T	PA	220
Ge	Kalloo, A	MD	220
Ge	Kimmey, M	WA	239
Ge	Kochman, M	PA	221
Ge	Konicek, F	IL	230
Ge	Kurtz, R	NY	221
Ge	Lebwohl, O	NY	221
Ge	Magun, A	NY	222
Ge	Markowitz, D	NY	222
Ge	Miskovitz, P	NY	223
Ge	Reichelderfer, M	WI	232
Ge	Rex, D	IN	232
Ge	Seidner, D	OH	233
Ge	Sherman, S	IN	233
Ge	Shike, M	NY	224
Ge	Waxman, I	IL	234
Ge	Waye, J	NY	224
Ge	Wilcox, C	AL	227
Oto	Aviv, J	NY	603
PGe	Schwarz, S	NY	688
S	MacFadyen, B	GA	971
S	Ponsky, J	OH	977

Endourology

Spec	Name	St	Pg
U	Bagley, D	PA	1031
U	Kavoussi, L	NY	1035

Endovascular Stent Grafts

Spec	Name	St	Pg
TS	Miller, D	CA	1022
VascS	Bandyk, D	FL	1070
VascS	Clair, D	OH	1072
VascS	Parodi, J	FL	1071
VascS	Sanchez, L	MO	1073
VIR	Becker, G	AZ	907
VIR	Cragg, A	MN	905
VIR	Dake, M	VA	904

Endovascular Surgery

Spec	Name	St	Pg
NRad	Berenstein, A	NY	897
NRad	Hirsch, J	MA	896
NS	Hopkins, L	NY	429
TS	Diethrich, E	AZ	1018
TS	Griepp, R	NY	1002
VascS	Adelman, M	NY	1067
VascS	Ahn, S	CA	1075
VascS	Ascher, E	NY	1067
VascS	Benvenisty, A	NY	1067
VascS	Brener, B	NJ	1068
VascS	Brewster, D	MA	1066
VascS	Criado, F	MD	1068
VascS	Eidt, J	AR	1074
VascS	Hakaim, A	FL	1071
VascS	Hobson, R	NJ	1069
VascS	Hodgson, K	IL	1073
VascS	Hollier, L	LA	1075
VascS	Kwolek, C	MA	1066
VascS	Makaroun, M	PA	1069
VascS	Marin, M	NY	1069
VascS	McCann, R	NC	1071
VascS	Money, S	AZ	1075
VascS	Rosenthal, D	GA	1072
VascS	Sumpio, B	CT	1067
VascS	White, R	CA	1076
VascS	Zarins, C	CA	1076

Environmental Diseases

Spec	Name	St	Pg
Pul	Bascom, R	PA	843
Pul	Gong, H	CA	858

Special Expertise Index

Special Expertise Index

Column 1

Spec	Name	St	Pg
TS	Acker, M	PA	1000
TS	Adams, D	NY	1000
TS	Akins, C	MA	998
TS	Antakli, T	AR	1018
TS	Bassett, J	MI	1012
TS	Bavaria, J	PA	1001
TS	Brown, J	IN	1012
TS	Chitwood, W	NC	1008
TS	Cohen, R	CA	1020
TS	Cohn, L	MA	998
TS	Colvin, S	NY	1001
TS	Furukawa, S	PA	1002
TS	Griffith, B	MD	1003
TS	Hargrove, W	PA	1003
TS	Isom, O	NY	1003
TS	Kanda, L	DC	1003
TS	Katz, N	DC	1004
TS	Kouchoukos, N	MO	1014
TS	Krieger, K	NY	1004
TS	Lamberti, J	CA	1022
TS	Lang, S	NY	1004
TS	Loulmet, D	NY	1005
TS	Lytle, B	OH	1014
TS	McCarthy, P	IL	1014
TS	Merrick, S	CA	1022
TS	Michler, R	NY	1005
TS	Miller, D	CA	1022
TS	Ott, D	TX	1019
TS	Oz, M	NY	1005
TS	Piccione, W	IL	1015
TS	Reitz, B	CA	1022
TS	Reul, G	TX	1019
TS	Schaff, H	MN	1015
TS	Sellke, F	MA	999
TS	Shemin, R	CA	1022
TS	Silverman, N	MI	1016
TS	Smith, P	NC	1011
TS	Starnes, V	CA	1023
TS	Strong, M	PA	1007
TS	Sundt, T	MN	1016
TS	Tranbaugh, R	NY	1007
TS	Verrier, E	WA	1023

Heart Valve Surgery-Aortic

Spec	Name	St	Pg
TS	Graver, L	NY	1002
TS	Reardon, M	TX	1019

Heart Valve Surgery-Mitral

Spec	Name	St	Pg
TS	Vander Salm, T	MA	999

Heart Valve Surgery-Pediatric

Spec	Name	St	Pg
TS	Forbess, J	TX	1018

Heart-Artificial

Spec	Name	St	Pg
TS	Kormos, R	PA	1004

Hemangiomas

Spec	Name	St	Pg
D	Burton, C	NC	182
D	Frieden, I	CA	189
PO	Cunningham, M	MA	713
PO	McGill, T	MA	713

Hemangiomas/Birthmarks

Spec	Name	St	Pg
D	Alster, T	DC	178
D	Orlow, S	NY	180
Oto	Waner, M	NY	609
PlS	Zide, B	NY	777

Column 2

Hematologic Malignancies

Spec	Name	St	Pg
Hem	Cheson, B	DC	295
Hem	Damon, L	CA	305
Hem	Feinstein, D	CA	305
Hem	Flynn, P	MN	300
Hem	Grever, M	OH	301
Hem	Kessler, C	DC	296
Hem	Kraut, E	OH	301
Hem	Lin, W	AL	298
Hem	Maciejewski, J	OH	302
Hem	Maddox, A	AR	305
Onc	Algazy, K	PA	310
Onc	Bolwell, B	OH	328
Onc	Deeg, H	WA	342
Onc	Di Persio, J	MO	330
Onc	Flinn, I	TN	323
Onc	Mitchell, B	CA	344
Onc	Rosen, S	IL	333
Onc	Schilder, R	PA	320
Onc	Smith, M	PA	320
PHO	Falletta, J	NC	697
PHO	Hord, J	OH	699

Hematopathology

Spec	Name	St	Pg
Path	Banks, P	NC	649
Path	Braylan, R	FL	650
Path	Chesney, C	TN	650
Path	Harris, N	MA	644
Path	Jaffe, E	MD	646
Path	Kinney, M	TX	654
Path	McCurley, T	TN	650
Path	Nathwani, B	CA	657
Path	Rodgers, G	UT	653
Path	Swerdlow, S	PA	649
Path	Warnke, R	CA	658
Path	Weisenburger, D	NE	653
Path	Weiss, L	CA	658

Hemolytic Uremic Syndrome

Spec	Name	St	Pg
PNep	Kaplan, B	PA	709
PNep	Watkins, S	WA	713

Hemophilia

Spec	Name	St	Pg
Hem	Kessler, C	DC	296
Hem	Ortel, T	NC	299
Hem	Palascak, J	OH	303
Onc	Romond, E	KY	326
Ped	Berman, B	OH	666
PHO	Buchanan, G	TX	702
PHO	Glader, B	CA	703
PHO	Hoots, W	TX	702
PHO	Manco-Johnson, M	CO	701
PHO	Shapiro, A	IN	700
PHO	Valentino, L	IL	701

Hemophilia Related Disease

Spec	Name	St	Pg
OrS	Luck, J	CA	587

Hemophilia-Adult

Spec	Name	St	Pg
Hem	Lutcher, C	GA	299

Hemorrhoids

Spec	Name	St	Pg
CRS	Golub, R	FL	167
CRS	Gorfine, S	NY	165

Hepatic Iron Metabolism

Spec	Name	St	Pg
Ge	Bacon, B	MO	228

Column 3

Hepatitis

Spec	Name	St	Pg
Ge	Bodenheimer, H	NY	218
Ge	Bonkovsky, H	CT	216
Ge	Boyer, T	AZ	236
Ge	Davis, G	TX	236
Ge	Di Bisceglie, A	MO	229
Ge	Dienstag, J	MA	216
Ge	Dieterich, D	NY	219
Ge	Everson, G	CO	235
Ge	Fitz, J	TX	236
Ge	Glombicki, A	TX	237
Ge	Hunter, E	ID	235
Ge	Jacobson, I	NY	220
Ge	Magun, A	NY	222
Ge	Martin, P	NY	222
Ge	Reddy, K	PA	223
Ge	Sorrell, M	NE	235
Ge	Van Thiel, D	IL	233
Ge	Vierling, J	TX	238
PGe	Suchy, F	NY	688

Hepatitis B & C

Spec	Name	St	Pg
Ge	Keeffe, E	CA	239
Ge	Kwo, P	IN	230
Ge	Maddrey, W	TX	237
Ge	Tobias, H	NY	224
Inf	Nahass, R	NJ	365
PGe	Schwarz, K	MD	688

Hepatitis B-Immune Response

Spec	Name	St	Pg
Rhu	Cupps, T	DC	930

Hepatitis C

Spec	Name	St	Pg
Ge	Bacon, B	MO	228
Ge	Balart, L	LA	235
Ge	Blei, A	IL	228
Ge	Brown, K	MI	228
Ge	Chung, R	MA	216
Ge	Di Bisceglie, A	MO	229
Ge	Fallon, M	AL	225
Ge	Galati, J	TX	237
Ge	Jensen, D	IL	230
Ge	Luxon, B	IA	231
Ge	Pimstone, N	CA	239
Ge	Schiff, E	FL	227
Ge	Scudera, P	VA	227
Ge	Shiffman, M	VA	227
Inf	Craven, D	MA	362
S	Eckhoff, D	AL	968

Hepatobiliary Surgery

Spec	Name	St	Pg
S	Curley, S	TX	982
S	Deziel, D	IL	974
S	Eckhoff, D	AL	968
S	Emre, S	NY	960
S	Farley, D	MN	975
S	Hemming, A	FL	969
S	Manzarbeitia, C	PA	962
S	Moossa, A	CA	988
S	Nagorney, D	MN	977
S	Shaw, B	NE	982
S	Walsh, R	OH	981

Hepatopulmonary Syndrome

Spec	Name	St	Pg
Pul	Krowka, M	MN	852

Special Expertise Index

Castle Connolly America's Top Doctors® 7th Edition

Special Expertise Index

L

Special Expertise Index

Special Expertise Index

Spec	Name	St	Pg
Lung Surgery			
TS	DeCamp, M	MA	998
TS	Frazier, O	TX	1019
Lupus Nephritis			
Nep	Appel, G	NY	411
Nep	Dosa, S	DC	411
Nep	Falk, R	NC	414
Nep	Hura, C	TX	416
Nep	Lewis, E	IL	416
Nep	Madaio, M	PA	412
Nep	Salant, D	MA	410
Nep	Suki, W	TX	418
Lupus/SLE			
D	Braverman, I	CT	176
D	Callen, J	KY	182
D	Fivenson, D	MI	185
D	Franks, A	NY	179
D	Sontheimer, R	OK	188
D	Werth, V	PA	181
D	Weston, W	CO	187
PNep	Bunchman, T	MI	711
PRhu	Bernstein, B	CA	724
PRhu	Finkel, T	PA	722
PRhu	Haines, K	NJ	722
PRhu	Ilowite, N	NY	722
PRhu	Lehman, T	NY	722
PRhu	McCarthy, P	CT	722
PRhu	Sandborg, C	CA	724
PRhu	Sherry, D	PA	723
PRhu	Sills, E	MD	723
PRhu	Wagner-Weiner, L	IL	723
PRhu	Warren, R	TX	724
PRhu	Wilking, A	TX	724
Pul	Matthay, R	CT	841
Rhu	Adams, E	IL	935
Rhu	Allen, N	NC	933
Rhu	Ashman, R	IA	935
Rhu	Belmont, H	NY	929
Rhu	Blume, R	NY	929
Rhu	Brenner, M	MA	928
Rhu	Chatham, W	AL	933
Rhu	Crofford, L	KY	933
Rhu	Curran, J	IL	935
Rhu	Davis, W	LA	938
Rhu	Ellman, M	IL	936
Rhu	Fischbein, L	MO	936
Rhu	Ginzler, E	NY	930
Rhu	Gourley, M	MD	930
Rhu	Hahn, B	CA	940
Rhu	Heck, L	AL	934
Rhu	Kaplan, S	TN	934
Rhu	Katz, R	IL	936
Rhu	Klearman, M	MO	936
Rhu	Lahita, R	NJ	931
Rhu	Lindsey, S	LA	938
Rhu	Lockshin, M	NY	931
Rhu	McCune, W	MI	937
Rhu	Moder, K	MN	937
Rhu	Moore, W	GA	934
Rhu	Paget, S	NY	931
Rhu	Petri, M	MD	932
Rhu	Polisson, R	MA	928
Rhu	Rothenberg, R	DC	932
Rhu	Sessoms, S	TX	939
Rhu	Shadick, N	MA	929

Spec	Name	St	Pg
Rhu	Spiera, H	NY	932
Rhu	Steen, V	DC	933
Rhu	Sundy, J	NC	934
Rhu	Wallace, D	CA	940
Rhu	Weinstein, A	DC	933
Rhu	Wener, M	WA	940
Rhu	West, S	CO	938
Rhu	Wofsy, D	CA	940
Lupus/SLE in Menopause			
Rhu	Buyon, J	NY	930
Lupus/SLE in Pregnancy			
MF	Druzin, M	CA	393
ObG	Muraskas, E	IL	512
ObG	Witter, F	MD	510
Rhu	Buyon, J	NY	930
Rhu	Lockshin, M	NY	931
Lyme Disease			
A&I	Dattwyler, R	NY	83
IM	Fisher, L	NY	378
Inf	Auwaerter, P	MD	362
Inf	Perlman, D	NY	365
Inf	Welch, P	NY	365
Inf	Wormser, G	NY	365
Inf	Yancovitz, S	NY	366
N	Coyle, P	NY	463
N	Logigian, E	NY	468
N	Petito, F	NY	469
PInf	Krilov, L	NY	705
PInf	Munoz, J	NY	705
PInf	Shapiro, E	CT	705
PRhu	Ilowite, N	NY	722
Rhu	Schoen, R	CT	928
Rhu	Simms, R	MA	929
Rhu	Weinstein, A	DC	933
Lymph Node Pathology			
Path	Arber, D	CA	655
Path	Cote, R	CA	656
Path	Foucar, M	NM	654
Path	Knowles, D	NY	646
Path	Kurtin, P	MN	652
Lymphatic Malformations-Head & Neck			
PO	Friedman, E	TX	717
PO	McGill, T	MA	713
PO	Richardson, M	OR	718
Lymphedema Imaging			
NuM	Kramer, E	NY	500
Lymphoma			
Hem	Baron, J	IL	300
Hem	Buadi, F	TN	298
Hem	Cooper, B	TX	304
Hem	Duffy, T	CT	294
Hem	Emerson, S	PA	295
Hem	Forman, S	CA	305
Hem	Gaynor, E	IL	300
Hem	Gregory, S	IL	301
Hem	Kempin, S	NY	296
Hem	Kuzel, T	IL	301
Hem	Rai, K	NY	296
Hem	Raphael, B	NY	297
Hem	Rosenblatt, J	FL	299
Hem	Savage, D	NY	297

Spec	Name	St	Pg
Hem	Saven, A	CA	306
Hem	Strauss, J	TX	305
Hem	Tallman, M	IL	303
Hem	van Besien, K	IL	303
Hem	Walters, T	ID	303
Hem	Wisch, N	NY	297
Hem	Zalusky, R	NY	298
Hem	Zuckerman, K	FL	300
NuM	Goldsmith, S	NY	500
NuM	Podoloff, D	TX	502
NuM	Silberstein, E	OH	502
Onc	Ambinder, R	MD	311
Onc	Armitage, J	NE	335
Onc	Bunn, P	CO	335
Onc	Camoriano, J	AZ	337
Onc	Canellos, G	MA	307
Onc	Chao, N	NC	322
Onc	Chitambar, C	WI	330
Onc	Coleman, M	NY	312
Onc	Fisher, R	NY	313
Onc	Flinn, I	TN	323
Onc	Glaspy, J	CA	343
Onc	Gockerman, J	NC	323
Onc	Grossbard, M	NY	314
Onc	Horning, S	CA	344
Onc	Jillella, A	GA	324
Onc	Kaminski, M	MI	331
Onc	Kaplan, L	CA	344
Onc	Kosova, L	IL	331
Onc	Kwak, L	TX	339
Onc	Lossos, I	FL	325
Onc	Maloney, D	WA	344
Onc	Marks, S	PA	317
Onc	Mitchell, B	CA	344
Onc	Nadler, L	MA	309
Onc	Nichols, C	OR	345
Onc	O'Brien, S	TX	340
Onc	Offit, K	NY	318
Onc	Press, O	WA	345
Onc	Rosen, S	IL	333
Onc	Salem, P	TX	341
Onc	Schiffer, C	MI	334
Onc	Schwartz, B	MN	334
Onc	Schwartz, M	FL	326
Onc	Serody, J	NC	326
Onc	Shea, T	NC	326
Onc	Shulman, L	MA	309
Onc	Smith, M	PA	320
Onc	Straus, D	NY	321
Onc	Williams, M	VA	328
Onc	Zelenetz, A	NY	321
Path	Banks, P	NC	649
Path	Braylan, R	FL	650
Path	Grogan, T	AZ	654
Path	Harris, N	MA	644
Path	Jaffe, E	MD	646
Path	Kinney, M	TX	654
Path	Knowles, D	NY	646
Path	Kurtin, P	MN	652
Path	Nathwani, B	CA	657
Path	Swerdlow, S	PA	649
Path	Warnke, R	CA	658
Path	Weisenburger, D	NE	653
Path	Weiss, L	CA	658
PHO	Andrews, R	WA	703
PHO	Brecher, M	NY	693
PHO	Cairo, M	NY	693
PHO	Fallon, R	IN	699

Special Expertise Index

Special Expertise Index

Special Expertise Index

Special Expertise Index

Spec	Name	St	Pg
NRad	Jensen, M	VA	899
NRad	Kallmes, D	MN	900
VIR	Ketcham, D	MN	906

Osteoporosis-Juvenile

Spec	Name	St	Pg
PEn	Key, L	SC	683
PNep	Langman, C	IL	712

Otology

Spec	Name	St	Pg
Oto	De la Cruz, A	CA	624
Oto	Farrior, J	FL	611
Oto	Macias, J	AZ	623
Oto	McKenna, M	MA	601
Oto	Tucci, D	NC	614
PO	Arnold, J	OH	715
PO	Bluestone, C	PA	714
PO	Darrow, D	VA	715
PO	Tunkel, D	MD	715

Otology & Neuro-Otology

Spec	Name	St	Pg
Oto	Beatty, C	MN	615
Oto	Bojrab, D	MI	615
Oto	McMenomey, S	OR	626

Otology & Neurotology

Spec	Name	St	Pg
Oto	Arriaga, M	PA	603
Oto	Goebel, J	MO	617

Otosclerosis/Stapedectomy

Spec	Name	St	Pg
Oto	De la Cruz, A	CA	624
Oto	Farrior, J	FL	611
Oto	Wiet, R	IL	620

Ovarian Cancer

Spec	Name	St	Pg
CG	Weitzel, J	CA	159
GO	Abu-Rustum, N	NY	263
GO	Alleyn, J	FL	265
GO	Alvarez, R	AL	265
GO	Barakat, R	NY	263
GO	Barter, J	MD	263
GO	Belinson, J	OH	268
GO	Berchuck, A	NC	266
GO	Berek, J	CA	272
GO	Bristow, R	MD	263
GO	Cain, J	OR	272
GO	Caputo, T	NY	263
GO	Carlson, J	NJ	264
GO	Chalas, E	NY	264
GO	Chambers, S	AZ	271
GO	Cohen, C	NY	264
GO	Copeland, L	OH	268
GO	Curtin, J	NY	264
GO	De Geest, K	IA	268
GO	Finan, M	AL	266
GO	Fishman, D	NY	264
GO	Goff, B	WA	272
GO	Herzog, T	NY	264
GO	Horowitz, I	GA	266
GO	Karlan, B	CA	273
GO	Kim, W	MI	269
GO	Lancaster, J	FL	267
GO	Look, K	IN	269
GO	Lurain, J	IL	269
GO	Muto, M	MA	262
GO	Partridge, E	AL	267
GO	Poliakoff, S	FL	267
GO	Potkul, R	IL	269
GO	Remmenga, S	NE	271

Spec	Name	St	Pg
GO	Rice, L	VA	267
GO	Rose, P	OH	270
GO	Rosenblum, N	PA	265
GO	Rotmensch, J	IL	270
GO	Rubin, S	PA	265
GO	Rutherford, T	CT	262
GO	Schink, J	IL	270
GO	Schwartz, P	CT	262
GO	Smith, D	IL	270
GO	Smith, H	NM	272
GO	Smith, L	CA	273
GO	Spann, C	GA	268
GO	Spirtos, N	NV	273
GO	Teng, N	CA	273
GO	Van Nagell, J	KY	268
GO	Waggoner, S	OH	270
GO	Wallach, R	NY	265
Onc	Disis, M	WA	343
Onc	Fracasso, P	MO	330
Onc	Hartmann, L	MN	331
Onc	Locker, G	IL	332
Onc	Markman, M	TX	339
Onc	McGuire, W	MD	317
Onc	Ozols, R	PA	319
Onc	Pasmantier, M	NY	319
Onc	Speyer, J	NY	320
Onc	Spriggs, D	NY	320
Onc	Verschraegen, C	NM	341
Path	Dubeau, L	CA	656
Path	Kurman, R	MD	647
Path	Tornos, C	NY	649
Path	Wilczynski, S	CA	658
Path	Young, R	MA	645
S	Dilawari, R	TN	968
S	Hughes, K	MA	954
S	Sugarbaker, P	DC	966

Ovarian Cancer & Borderline Tumors

Spec	Name	St	Pg
GO	Gershenson, D	TX	271

Ovarian Cancer Genetics

Spec	Name	St	Pg
ObG	Shulman, L	IL	513

Ovarian Cancer Risk Assessment

Spec	Name	St	Pg
Onc	Daly, M	PA	312

Ovarian Cancer Ultrasound Diagnosis

Spec	Name	St	Pg
DR	Hann, L	NY	891

Ovarian Cancer-Early Detection

Spec	Name	St	Pg
GO	Cain, J	OR	272
GO	DePriest, P	KY	266
GO	Fishman, D	NY	264
GO	Rutherford, T	CT	262

Ovarian Failure

Spec	Name	St	Pg
ObG	Simpson, J	FL	511
RE	Legro, R	PA	916

Oxalosis

Spec	Name	St	Pg
PNep	Langman, C	IL	712

P

Pacemakers

Spec	Name	St	Pg
CE	Callans, D	PA	118
CE	Chinitz, L	NY	119

Spec	Name	St	Pg
CE	Cohen, M	NY	119
CE	Curtis, A	FL	120
CE	DiMarco, J	VA	120
CE	Ellenbogen, K	VA	120
CE	Gomes, J	NY	119
CE	Hammill, S	MN	121
CE	Hayes, D	MN	121
CE	Kay, G	AL	120
CE	Levine, J	NY	119
CE	Marchlinski, F	PA	119
CE	Sorrentino, R	GA	121
Cv	Myerburg, R	FL	105
Cv	Naccarelli, G	PA	101
PCd	Fish, F	TN	674
PCd	Sodt, P	IL	677

Paget's Disease of Bone

Spec	Name	St	Pg
EDM	Econs, M	IN	204
EDM	Siris, E	NY	201
EDM	Watts, N	OH	207

Pain & Spasticity

Spec	Name	St	Pg
NS	Whiting, D	PA	432

Pain Management

Spec	Name	St	Pg
AdP	Howell, E	UT	819
Ger	Finucane, T	MD	248
IM	Billings, J	MA	378
N	Hiesiger, E	NY	466
N	Max, M	MD	460
NS	Berger, M	CA	446
NS	Burchiel, K	OR	446
NS	de Lotbiniere, A	NY	427
NS	Di Giacinto, G	NY	428
NS	Hassenbusch, S	TX	444
Onc	Levy, M	PA	316
PCCM	Anand, K	AR	680
Ped	Zeltzer, L	CA	667
PMR	Creamer, M	FL	759
PMR	Slipman, C	PA	758
Psyc	Ray, A	FL	810
Pul	Shore, B	MO	853

Pain Management-Pediatric

Spec	Name	St	Pg
PM	Anderson, C	WA	639
PM	Anghelescu, D	TN	636
PM	Berde, C	MA	634
PM	Weisman, S	WI	638

Pain-Abdominal Recurrent

Spec	Name	St	Pg
PGe	Gunasekaran, T	IL	689
PGe	Kirschner, B	IL	690

Pain-Abdominal/Functional

Spec	Name	St	Pg
Ge	Drossman, D	NC	225
Ge	Olden, K	AR	238

Pain-Acute

Spec	Name	St	Pg
PM	De Leon-Casasola, O	NY	634
PM	Lema, M	NY	635
PM	Rogers, J	TX	639
PM	Swarm, R	MO	638

Pain-after Spinal Intervention

Spec	Name	St	Pg
PM	Huntoon, M	MN	637
PM	Racz, G	TX	639
PM	Rosner, H	CA	640

Special Expertise Index

Special Expertise Index

Special Expertise Index

Spec	Name	St	Pg
EDM	Young, I	NY	202
NRad	Khandji, A	NY	897
Path	Scheithauer, B	MN	652
PEn	Levy, R	IL	684
PEn	Sklar, C	NY	682
RE	Crowley, W	MA	914

Pituitary Function/Hormones
EDM	Melmed, S	CA	210

Pituitary Surgery
NS	Atkinson, J	MN	436
NS	Black, K	CA	446
NS	Chandler, W	MI	437
NS	Laws, E	CA	447
NS	Mayberg, M	WA	448
NS	Selman, W	OH	441

Pituitary Tumors
EDM	Darwin, C	CA	209
EDM	Fitzgerald, P	CA	209
EDM	Hoffman, A	CA	210
EDM	Melmed, S	CA	210
EDM	Snyder, P	PA	201
NS	Berger, M	CA	446
NS	Black, P	MA	424
NS	Brem, H	MD	426
NS	Brem, S	FL	433
NS	Bruce, J	NY	426
NS	Couldwell, W	UT	443
NS	de Lotbiniere, A	NY	427
NS	Grady, M	PA	428
NS	Guthikonda, M	MI	439
NS	Harsh, G	CA	447
NS	Macdonald, R	IL	440
NS	Murali, R	NY	431
NS	Post, K	NY	431
NS	Shapiro, S	IN	442
NS	Tatter, S	NC	435
NS	Weiss, M	CA	449
Path	Scheithauer, B	MN	652

Plasma Cell Disorders
Hem	Barlogie, B	AR	304
Hem	Gertz, M	MN	300
Hem	Gregory, S	IL	301

Platelet Disorders
Hem	Kaushansky, K	CA	306
Hem	Lyons, R	TX	304
PHO	Olson, T	GA	697
PHO	Parker, R	NY	696

Pleural Disease
Pul	Antony, V	FL	846
Pul	Light, R	TN	849
Pul	Sahn, S	SC	849
TS	Friedberg, J	PA	1001

Pneumococcal Infections
PInf	Kaplan, S	TX	708

Pneumocystis Carinii Pneumonia (PCP)
Pul	Huang, L	CA	858

Pneumonia
Inf	Craven, D	MA	362
Inf	Cunha, B	NY	363

Spec	Name	St	Pg
Inf	Dismukes, W	AL	367
Inf	Quagliarello, V	CT	362
Inf	Yu, V	PA	366
PPul	Murphy, T	NC	719
Pul	Guidry, G	LA	856
Pul	Nash, T	NY	843
Pul	Niederman, M	NY	843
Pul	Rose, C	CO	855
Pul	Wunderink, R	IL	854

Poison Control
PrM	Hoffman, R	NY	797

Polio Rehabilitation
PMR	Esquenazi, A	PA	757
PMR	Silver, J	MA	756
PMR	Sliwa, J	IL	762

Polycystic Kidney Disease
Nep	Bennett, W	OR	418
Nep	Blumenfeld, J	NY	411
Nep	Perrone, R	MA	410
Nep	Rakowski, T	VA	414
Nep	Schrier, R	CO	417
Nep	Torres, V	MN	416
PNep	Avner, E	WI	711
PNep	Kaplan, B	PA	709

Polycystic Ovarian Syndrome
EDM	Ehrmann, D	IL	205
EDM	Korytkowski, M	PA	199
EDM	Marshall, J	VA	203
EDM	Nestler, J	VA	203
EDM	Ovalle, F	AL	203
PEn	Rosenfield, R	IL	685
RE	Azziz, R	CA	923
RE	Barnes, R	IL	920
RE	Coutifaris, C	PA	915
RE	Diamond, M	MI	920
RE	Goodman, N	FL	918
RE	Jacobs, L	IL	921
RE	Kazer, R	IL	921
RE	Legro, R	PA	916
RE	Rafts, V	MO	921
RE	Richardson, M	KS	922

Polycythemia Rubra Vera
Hem	Fruchtman, S	NY	295
Hem	Spivak, J	MD	297

Polymyositis
Rhu	Curran, J	IL	935
Rhu	Medsger, T	PA	931
Rhu	Oddis, C	PA	931
Rhu	Steen, V	DC	933

Polypharmacology (Excess Medications)
Ger	Carr, D	MO	251
Ger	Tenover, J	GA	251

Porphyria
CG	Desnick, R	NY	153
Ge	Anderson, K	TX	235
Ge	Bloomer, J	AL	224
Ge	Pimstone, N	CA	239
Hem	Solberg, L	FL	299
IM	Bissell, D	CA	381

Spec	Name	St	Pg
Portal Hypertension			
S	Emre, S	NY	960
VIR	Darcy, M	MO	905

Post Polio Syndrome (PPS)
PM	Walsh, N	TX	639

Post Traumatic Stress Disorder
ChAP	Abright, A	NY	822
Psyc	Eth, S	NY	806
Psyc	Friedman, M	VT	802
Psyc	Greiner, C	NE	812
Psyc	Manevitz, A	NY	807
Psyc	Marmar, C	CA	816
Psyc	Pitman, R	MA	803
Psyc	Pynoos, R	CA	816
Psyc	Raskind, M	WA	816
Psyc	Roy-Byrne, P	WA	817
Psyc	Spiegel, D	CA	817
Psyc	Stein, M	CA	817
Psyc	van der Kolk, B	MA	804
Psyc	Wait, S	MD	809

Postpartum Depression (PPD)
Psyc	Dell, D	NC	809

Power Doppler Imaging
DR	Adler, R	NY	889

Prader-Willi Syndrome
CG	Cassidy, S	CA	157
CG	Driscoll, D	FL	154

Praxis Functional Electrical Stim (FES)
OrS	Betz, R	PA	563

Pregnancy & Endocrine Disorders
EDM	Seely, E	MA	197

Pregnancy & Hematologic Abnormalities
Hem	Rand, J	NY	297
MF	Berkowitz, R	NY	387

Pregnancy & Mental Health Issues
Psyc	Dell, D	NC	809

Pregnancy & Rheumatic Disease
Rhu	Lockshin, M	NY	931

Pregnancy-Advanced Maternal Age
MF	Heffner, L	MA	386

Pregnancy-High Risk
MF	Acker, D	MA	386
MF	Bahado-Singh, R	MI	390
MF	Bardeguez, A	NJ	387
MF	Bartelsmeyer, J	MO	390
MF	Boehm, F	TN	388
MF	Chervenak, F	NY	389
MF	Chescheir, N	TN	389
MF	Copel, J	CT	386
MF	D'Alton, M	NY	387
MF	Dooley, S	IL	390
MF	Dugoff, L	CO	392
MF	Edersheim, T	NY	388
MF	Ferguson, J	KY	389
MF	Fox, H	MD	388
MF	Frigoletto, F	MA	386

Special Expertise Index

Special Expertise Index

Spec	Name	St	Pg
Rheumatologic Diseases of the Lung			
Pul	Steiger, D	NY	845
Rheumatology			
A&I	deShazo, R	MS	84
Ger	Cooney, L	CT	248
PMR	Lipkin, D	FL	760
Rheumatology-Adult & Pediatric			
Rhu	Albert, D	NH	928
Rhinitis			
A&I	Buchbinder, E	NY	82
A&I	Busse, W	WI	86
A&I	Freeman, T	TX	87
A&I	Kaiser, H	MN	86
A&I	Kaliner, M	MD	83
A&I	Lieberman, P	TN	85
A&I	Lockey, R	FL	85
A&I	Nelson, H	CO	87
A&I	Pacin, M	FL	85
A&I	Sanders, G	MI	87
A&I	Slankard, M	NY	84
A&I	Tamaroff, M	CA	88
A&I	Wasserman, S	CA	89
Oto	Lanza, D	FL	612
PA&I	Kelly, C	VA	668
PA&I	Skoner, D	PA	668
Rhinoplasty			
Oto	Denenberg, S	NE	621
Oto	Farrior, E	FL	611
Oto	Gliklich, R	MA	601
Oto	Kamer, F	CA	625
Oto	Kern, R	IL	617
Oto	Larrabee, W	WA	625
Oto	Papel, I	MD	607
Oto	Pastorek, N	NY	608
Oto	Quatela, V	NY	608
Oto	Setzen, M	NY	609
Oto	Szachowicz, E	MN	619
Oto	Toriumi, D	IL	620
PlS	Aston, S	NY	771
PlS	Baker, D	NY	772
PlS	Constantian, M	NH	770
PlS	Cutting, C	NY	773
PlS	Daniel, R	CA	788
PlS	Fisher, G	CA	788
PlS	Gunter, J	TX	786
PlS	Hamra, S	TX	786
PlS	Hidalgo, D	NY	773
PlS	Hurwitz, D	PA	774
PlS	Matarasso, A	NY	774
PlS	Mustoe, T	IL	782
PlS	Ristow, B	CA	791
PlS	Rohrich, R	TX	787
PlS	Romano, J	CA	791
PlS	Sullivan, P	RI	771
PlS	Tabbal, N	NY	777
PlS	Tebbetts, J	TX	787
Rhinoplasty & Ear Reshaping (Otoplasty)			
PlS	Bermant, M	VA	778
Rhinoplasty Revision			
Oto	Kuhn, F	GA	611
PlS	Constantian, M	NH	770

Spec	Name	St	Pg
PlS	Gunter, J	TX	786
Rhinosinusitis			
A&I	Fox, R	FL	84
A&I	Wong, J	MA	82
Oto	Stankiewicz, J	IL	619
Rhinosinusitis & Asthma			
A&I	Shepherd, G	NY	83
Rickettsial Diseases			
Inf	Westerman, E	TX	371
Robotic Cardiac Surgery			
TS	Damiano, R	MO	1012
TS	Stuart, R	MO	1016
Robotic Heart Surgery			
TS	Alexander, J	IL	1012
TS	Argenziano, M	NY	1000
TS	Boyd, W	FL	1007
TS	Chitwood, W	NC	1008
TS	Colvin, S	NY	1001
TS	Loulmet, D	NY	1005
TS	Raman, J	IL	1015
TS	Smith, C	NY	1006
TS	Starnes, V	CA	1023
TS	Wolf, R	OH	1016
Robotic Surgery			
GO	Magrina, J	AZ	272
PS	Glick, P	NY	726
PS	Jackson, R	AR	733
PS	Jennings, R	MA	724
PS	Krummel, T	CA	734
PS	Lobe, T	IA	731
PS	Shlasko, E	NY	727
S	Curet, M	CA	987
U	Winfield, H	IA	1049
Robotic Surgery-Pediatric			
U	Poppas, D	NY	1036
Rocky Mountain Spotted Fever			
PInf	Givner, L	NC	706
Rosacea			
D	James, W	PA	179
D	Shalita, A	NY	181
Ross Procedure for Aortic Valve Disease			
TS	Fullerton, D	CO	1017
TS	Perryman, R	FL	1010
TS	Starnes, V	CA	1023
Rotator Cuff Surgery			
OrS	Cofield, R	MN	578
OrS	Flatow, E	NY	565
OrS	Matsen, F	WA	588
OrS	Yamaguchi, K	MO	582
SM	Fronek, J	CA	949
Running Injuries			
SM	Maharam, L	NY	946
SM	Metzl, J	NY	947

S

Spec	Name	St	Pg
Sacral Stimulation/Fecal Incontinence			
CRS	Coller, J	MA	164
Salivary Gland Tumors			
RadRO	Laramore, G	WA	880
Salivary Gland Tumors & Surgery			
Oto	Clayman, G	TX	622
Oto	Deschler, D	MA	601
Oto	Eisele, D	CA	625
Oto	Olsen, K	MN	618
Oto	Osguthorpe, J	SC	612
Oto	Urken, M	NY	609
Oto	Weber, R	TX	624
Sarcoidosis			
Pul	Donohue, J	NC	847
Pul	Hunninghake, G	IA	852
Pul	King, T	CA	858
Pul	Newman, L	CO	855
Pul	Raghu, G	WA	859
Pul	Rose, C	CO	855
Pul	Rossman, M	PA	844
Pul	Sharma, O	CA	860
Pul	Teirstein, A	NY	845
Sarcoma			
Onc	Benjamin, R	TX	337
Onc	Borden, E	OH	329
Onc	Chow, W	CA	342
Onc	Demetri, G	MA	307
Onc	Ettinger, D	MD	313
Onc	Grosh, W	VA	324
Onc	Hande, K	TN	324
Onc	Jacobs, C	CA	344
Onc	Kraft, A	SC	324
Onc	Legha, S	TX	339
Onc	Samuels, B	ID	336
Onc	Saroja, A	IL	333
Onc	Stewart, F	WA	346
Onc	von-Mehren, M	PA	321
OrS	Biermann, J	MI	577
OrS	Conrad, E	WA	586
OrS	Lackman, R	PA	568
OrS	Malawer, M	DC	569
OrS	Scarborough, M	FL	576
OrS	Scully, S	FL	576
Path	Brooks, J	PA	645
Path	Fletcher, C	MA	644
Path	Goldblum, J	OH	652
Path	Patchefsky, A	PA	647
Path	Weiss, S	GA	651
PHO	Meyers, P	NY	695
PHO	Olson, T	GA	697
RadRO	Brizel, D	NC	873
RadRO	DeLaney, T	MA	868
RadRO	Glatstein, E	PA	870
RadRO	Gunderson, L	AZ	878
RadRO	Hahn, S	PA	870
RadRO	Herman, T	OK	878
RadRO	Kiel, K	IL	876
RadRO	Kinsella, T	OH	876
RadRO	Marcus, R	GA	873
RadRO	Michalski, J	MO	876
RadRO	Pollack, A	PA	872
RadRO	Prosnitz, L	NC	874
RadRO	Tepper, J	NC	874

Special Expertise Index

Special Expertise Index

Spec	Name	St	Pg
SM	Nisonson, B	NY	947

Sports Medicine Back Injuries

OrS	Spivak, J	NY	572

Sports Medicine-Hand

HS	Rosenwasser, M	NY	282

Sports Medicine-Women

OrS	Hannafin, J	NY	566

Sports Neurology

N	Jordan, B	NY	466

Staphylococcal Infections

Inf	Archer, G	VA	366
Inf	Westerman, E	TX	371
Inf	Yu, V	PA	366

Stem Cell Therapy in Heart Failure

Cv	Hare, J	FL	105
Cv	Willerson, J	TX	115
IC	Losordo, D	IL	127
IC	Perin, E	TX	128

Stem Cell Transplant

Hem	Buadi, F	TN	298
Hem	Champlin, R	TX	304
Hem	Damon, L	CA	305
Hem	Files, J	MS	298
Hem	Fruchtman, S	NY	295
Hem	Greer, J	TN	298
Hem	Lazarus, H	OH	302
Hem	Maciejewski, J	OH	302
Hem	Nimer, S	NY	296
Hem	Savage, D	NY	297
Hem	Schwartzberg, L	TN	299
Hem	van Besien, K	IL	303
Onc	Antin, J	MA	307
Onc	Flomenberg, N	PA	313
Onc	Gerson, S	OH	331
Onc	Pecora, A	NJ	319
Onc	Wicha, M	MI	335
PA&I	Kamani, N	DC	667
PHO	Davies, S	OH	698
PHO	Fallon, R	IN	699
PHO	Graham, M	AZ	702
PHO	Horn, B	CA	703
PHO	Link, M	CA	703
PHO	Lipton, J	NY	695
PHO	Sondel, P	WI	701

Stem Cell Transplant in Lupus/Crohn's

Onc	Burt, R	IL	329

Stem Cell Transplant in MS

Onc	Burt, R	IL	329

Stem Cell Transplant-Fetal

PA&I	Cowan, M	CA	670
PS	Flake, A	PA	726

Stem Cell Transplant/Autoimmune Disease

Rhu	Barr, W	IL	935

Stereotactic Radiosurgery

NS	Adler, J	CA	446
NS	Andrews, D	PA	426

Spec	Name	St	Pg
NS	Apuzzo, M	CA	446
NS	Barnett, G	OH	436
NS	Branch, C	NC	433
NS	Burchiel, K	OR	446
NS	Edwards, M	CA	447
NS	Guthrie, B	AL	434
NS	Hassenbusch, S	TX	444
NS	Kondziolka, D	PA	430
NS	Levy, R	IL	439
NS	Lunsford, L	PA	430
NS	McDermott, M	CA	448
NS	Nazzaro, J	KS	443
NS	Ott, K	CA	448
NS	Papadopoulos, S	AZ	445
NS	Penar, P	VT	425
NS	Rich, K	MO	441
NS	Swaid, S	AL	435
NS	Tatter, S	NC	435
NS	Young, A	KY	436
Oto	McMenomey, S	OR	626
RadRO	Kleinberg, L	MD	871
RadRO	Knisely, J	CT	868
RadRO	Larson, D	CA	880
RadRO	Loeffler, J	MA	868
RadRO	Mendenhall, W	FL	874
RadRO	Pistenmaa, D	TX	879
RadRO	Shaw, E	NC	874
RadRO	Stea, B	AZ	879

Stomach Cancer

Onc	Goldberg, R	NC	323
RadRO	Hayman, J	MI	875
S	Coit, D	NY	958
S	Donohue, J	MN	974
S	Drebin, J	PA	959
S	Fong, Y	NY	960
S	Livingstone, A	FL	970
S	Nava-Villarreal, H	NY	963
TS	De Meester, T	CA	1020

Strabismus

Oph	Bateman, J	CO	544
Oph	Buckley, E	NC	533
Oph	Capo, H	FL	533
Oph	Caputo, A	NJ	524
Oph	Day, S	CA	548
Oph	Demer, J	CA	548
Oph	Diamond, G	PA	525
Oph	Eggers, H	NY	525
Oph	Feldon, S	NY	525
Oph	Flynn, J	NY	526
Oph	Gallin, P	NY	526
Oph	Granet, D	CA	549
Oph	Guyton, D	MD	527
Oph	Hall, L	NY	527
Oph	Hess, J	FL	534
Oph	Hunter, D	MA	522
Oph	Isenberg, S	CA	549
Oph	Lambert, S	GA	535
Oph	Magramm, I	NY	529
Oph	Mets, M	IL	541
Oph	Miller, J	AZ	545
Oph	Mills, M	PA	529
Oph	Olitsky, S	MO	541
Oph	Palmer, E	OR	550
Oph	Paul, T	CA	551
Oph	Pollard, Z	GA	536
Oph	Price, R	OH	541

Spec	Name	St	Pg
Oph	Reynolds, J	NY	530
Oph	Robb, R	MA	523
Oph	Simon, J	NY	531
Oph	Tychsen, L	MO	543
Oph	Wang, F	NY	532
Oph	Weiss, A	WA	552

Strabismus-Adult

Oph	Del Monte, M	MI	538
Oph	Mazow, M	TX	545

Strabismus-Adult & Pediatric

Oph	France, T	WI	539
Oph	Jaafar, M	DC	528
Oph	Kushner, B	WI	540
Oph	McKeown, C	FL	535
Oph	Mims, J	TX	546
Oph	Raab, E	NY	530
Oph	Rogers, G	OH	542
Oph	Wright, K	CA	552

Strabismus-Pediatric

Oph	Freedman, S	NC	534
Oph	Wilson, M	SC	537

Streptococcal Infections

PInf	Baker, C	TX	707
PInf	Givner, L	NC	706
PInf	Shulman, S	IL	707

Stress Management

GerPsy	Stein, E	FL	830
Psyc	Ray, A	FL	810

Stroke

Cv	Huang, P	MA	94
N	Adams, H	IA	476
N	Adams, R	GA	472
N	Adornato, B	CA	486
N	Albers, G	CA	486
N	Bell, R	PA	462
N	Bernad, P	VA	472
N	Broderick, J	OH	476
N	Brust, J	NY	463
N	Caplan, L	MA	460
N	Charney, J	NY	463
N	Chui, H	CA	487
N	Couch, J	OK	484
N	Coull, B	AZ	484
N	Dobkin, B	CA	487
N	Easton, J	RI	460
N	Feldmann, E	RI	460
N	Fisher, M	CA	488
N	Furlan, A	OH	477
N	Goldstein, L	NC	473
N	Gress, D	VA	473
N	Grotta, J	TX	484
N	Haley, E	VA	473
N	Hart, R	TX	484
N	Hess, D	GA	473
N	Josephson, D	IN	478
N	Kase, C	MA	461
N	Kirshner, H	TN	473
N	Kistler, J	MA	461
N	Koroshetz, W	MD	466
N	Levine, D	NY	467
N	Levine, S	NY	467
N	Mohr, J	NY	469

Special Expertise Index

Special Expertise Index

Alphabetical Listing of Doctors

Alphabetical Listing of Doctors

Name	Specialty	Pg	Name	Specialty	Pg
Altchek, David (NY)	SM	946	Appen, Richard (WI)	Oph	537
Alter, Gary J (CA)	PlS	787	Applegate, Robert (NC)	IC	126
Altorki, Nasser (NY)	TS	1000	April, Max (NY)	PO	714
Alvarez, Ronald (AL)	GO	265	Apuzzo, Michael (CA)	NS	446
Alvarez-Elcoro, Salvador (FL)	Inf	366	Arber, Daniel (CA)	Path	655
Alward, Wallace (IA)	Oph	537	Arcasoy, Selim (NY)	Pul	842
Amato, Anthony (MA)	N	460	Arceci, Robert (MD)	PHO	693
Ambinder, Richard (MD)	Onc	311	Archer, Gordon (VA)	Inf	366
Aminoff, Michael (CA)	N	486	Archer, Steven (MI)	Oph	538
Amling, Christopher (AL)	U	1039	Arend, William (CO)	Rhu	938
Amonette, Rex A (TN)	D	182	Arensman, Robert (LA)	PS	732
Amstey, Marvin (NY)	ObG	508	Argenta, Louis Charles (NC)	PlS	777
Anand, Kanwaljeet (AR)	PCCM	680	Argenziano, Michael (NY)	TS	1000
Andersen, Arnold (IA)	Psyc	811	Ariagno, Ronald (CA)	NP	406
Andersen, James (CA)	PlS	787	Ariyan, Stephan (CT)	PlS	770
Anderson, Benjamin (WA)	S	985	Armitage, James (NE)	Onc	335
Anderson, Corrie (WA)	PM	639	Armon, Carmel (MA)	N	460
Anderson, Douglas (FL)	Oph	533	Armstrong, William (MI)	Cv	107
Anderson, Jeffrey (UT)	Cv	113	Arnason, Barry (IL)	N	476
Anderson, Joseph (MI)	Onc	328	Arndt, Kenneth (MA)	D	176
Anderson, Karl (TX)	Ge	235	Arnett, Frank (TX)	Rhu	938
Anderson, Kenneth (MA)	Onc	307	Arnold, Anthony (CA)	Oph	547
Anderson, Lesley (CA)	OrS	585	Arnold, James (OH)	PO	715
Anderson, Mark (IA)	CE	121	Aron, Alan (NY)	ChiN	143
Anderson, Martin (CA)	AM	79	Aronchick, Craig (PA)	Ge	218
Anderson, Richard (UT)	Oph	544	Aronson, James (AR)	OrS	584
Anderson, Richard (MA)	D	176	Aronson, Peter (CT)	Nep	410
Andiman, Warren (CT)	PInf	704	Arriaga, Moises Alberto (PA)	Oto	603
Andreoli, Sharon (IN)	PNep	711	Arroliga, Alejandro (TX)	Pul	856
Andrews, David (PA)	NS	426	Arslanian, Silva (PA)	PEn	681
Andrews, James (AL)	SM	947	Artman, Michael (IA)	PCd	675
Andrews, Robert (WA)	PHO	703	Arts, H Alexander (MI)	Oto	614
Andriole, Gerald (MO)	U	1044	Ascher, Enrico (NY)	VascS	1067
Andros, George (CA)	VascS	1075	Ascher, Nancy (CA)	S	986
Ang, Kie-Kian (TX)	RadRO	878	Aseff, John (DC)	PMR	756
Angelos, Peter (IL)	S	973	Ashman, Robert (IA)	Rhu	935
Anghelescu, Doralina (TN)	PM	636	Ashwal, Stephen (CA)	ChiN	147
Anhalt, Grant (MD)	D	178	Assimos, Dean (NC)	U	1039
Annest, Stephen (CO)	VascS	1074	Aston, Sherrell (NY)	PlS	771
Anscher, Mitchell (VA)	RadRO	873	Atala, Anthony (NC)	U	1040
Antakli, Tamim (AR)	TS	1018	Athanasian, Edward (NY)	HS	280
Antin, Joseph Harry (MA)	Onc	307	Atkins, Michael B (MA)	Onc	307
Anton, Raymond (SC)	AdP	819	Atkinson, James (CA)	PS	733
Antony, Veena (FL)	Pul	846	Atkinson, John (MN)	NS	436
Anyane-Yeboa, Kwame (NY)	CG	152	Atkinson, Robert (HI)	HS	288
Apatoff, Brian (NY)	N	462	Atlas, Scott (CA)	NRad	901
Apfelbaum, Ronald (UT)	NS	442	Atnip, Robert (PA)	VascS	1067
Appel, Gerald (NY)	Nep	411	Attinger, Christopher (DC)	PlS	772
Appelbaum, Frederick (WA)	Onc	342	August, David (NJ)	S	956
Appelbaum, Paul (NY)	Psyc	804	August, Phyllis (NY)	Nep	411
Appell, Rodney (TX)	U	1051	Austin, John (NY)	DR	890
Appelman, Henry (MI)	Path	651	Auwaerter, Paul (MD)	Inf	362

Name	Specialty	Pg
Avery, Eric (TX)	Psyc	813
Aviv, Jonathan (NY)	Oto	603
Avner, Ellis (WI)	PNep	711
Axelrod, Deborah (NY)	S	957
Axelrod, Lloyd (MA)	EDM	196
Azar, Dimitri (IL)	Oph	538
Azziz, Ricardo (CA)	RE	923

B

Name	Specialty	Pg
Babaian, Richard (TX)	U	1051
Bach, Bernard (IL)	OrS	577
Bach, John (NJ)	PMR	756
Bacon, Bruce (MO)	Ge	228
Baerveldt, George (CA)	Oph	547
Bagley, Demetrius (PA)	U	1031
Bahado-Singh, Ray (MI)	MF	390
Bahn, Rebecca (MN)	EDM	204
Bahna, Sami (LA)	PA&I	670
Bahnson, Robert (OH)	U	1044
Bailey, Harold (TX)	CRS	170
Bailey, Leonard (CA)	TS	1020
Bailey, Steven (TX)	IC	127
Bailin, Philip (OH)	D	184
Baim, Howard (IL)	Oto	614
Bains, Manjit (NY)	TS	1000
Bairey-Merz, C Noel (CA)	Cv	115
Bakay, Roy (IL)	NS	436
Baker, Carol (TX)	PInf	707
Baker, Christopher (MA)	S	954
Baker, Daniel (NY)	PlS	772
Baker, Emily (NH)	MF	386
Baker, James (MI)	A&I	86
Baker, John (MI)	Oph	538
Baker, Robert (NY)	PGe	686
Baker, Shan (MI)	Oto	615
Baker, Susan (NY)	PGe	686
Bakhos, Mamdouh (IL)	TS	1012
Bakken, Johan (MN)	Inf	369
Balady, Gary (MA)	Cv	94
Balart, Luis (LA)	Ge	235
Balch, Charles (MD)	S	957
Baldassano, Robert (PA)	PGe	687
Balderston, Richard (PA)	OrS	562
Baldessarini, Ross (MA)	Psyc	802
Balducci, Lodovico (FL)	Onc	322
Bale, James (UT)	ChiN	147
Balk, Robert (IL)	Pul	850
Balkany, Thomas (FL)	Oto	610
Ball, Edward D (CA)	Onc	342
Ball, William (OH)	NRad	899
Balla, Andre (IL)	Path	651

Name	Specialty	Pg
Ballantyne, Garth (NJ)	S	957
Ballard, Pamela (DC)	PMR	756
Ballon-Landa, Gonzalo (CA)	Inf	371
Balmes, John (CA)	Pul	857
Baltimore, Robert (CT)	PInf	705
Baltuch, Gordon (PA)	NS	426
Bancalari, Eduardo (FL)	NP	402
Bandyk, Dennis (FL)	VascS	1070
Banks, Peter (NC)	Path	649
Banks, Peter (MA)	Ge	216
Bans, Larry (AZ)	U	1051
Bar-Chama, Natan (NY)	U	1032
Barakat, Richard (NY)	GO	263
Baraniuk, James (DC)	A&I	82
Baranko, Paul (AZ)	PHO	702
Baratz, Mark (PA)	OrS	562
Barber, Douglas (TX)	PMR	763
Barcenas, Camilo (TX)	Nep	417
Bardeguez, Arlene (NJ)	MF	387
Bardot, Stephen (LA)	U	1051
Barkin, Jamie (FL)	Ge	224
Barkovich, A James (CA)	NRad	901
Barksdale, Edward (PA)	PS	725
Barlogie, Bart (AR)	Hem	304
Barnes, Patrick (CA)	NRad	901
Barnes, Randall (IL)	RE	920
Barnes, Willard (DC)	GO	263
Barnett, Gene (OH)	NS	436
Barohn, Richard (KS)	N	482
Baron, Joseph (IL)	Hem	300
Baron, Todd (MN)	Ge	228
Barone, Constance (TX)	PlS	785
Barr, Walter (IL)	Rhu	935
Barrett, Eugene (VA)	EDM	202
Barry, Michele (CT)	IM	378
Bartelsmeyer, James (MO)	MF	390
Barter, James (MD)	GO	263
Bartlett, David (PA)	S	957
Bartlett, John (MD)	Inf	363
Bartlett, Scott (PA)	PlS	772
Bartlett, Stephen (MD)	S	957
Bartolozzi, Arthur (PA)	OrS	562
Barton, Fritz (TX)	PlS	785
Basch, Samuel (NY)	Psyc	804
Bascom, Rebecca (PA)	Pul	843
Baser, Susan (PA)	N	462
Bashore, Thomas (NC)	Cv	103
Baskin, Laurence (CA)	U	1054
Basler, Joseph (TX)	U	1051
Bass, Theodore (FL)	Cv	103
Bassett, Joseph (MI)	TS	1012
Bassett, Lawrence (CA)	DR	895

Alphabetical Listing of Doctors

Name	Specialty	Pg	Name	Specialty	Pg
Bastian, Robert (IL)	Oto	615	Belsito, Donald (KS)	D	187
Bateman, J Bronwyn (CO)	Oph	544	Belsky, Mark (MA)	HS	280
Batjer, Hunt (IL)	NS	437	Ben-Josef, Edgar (MI)	RadRO	875
Batsford, William (CT)	CE	118	Benedetti, Enrico (IL)	S	973
Bauer, Bruce (IL)	PlS	781	Benedetti, Thomas (WA)	MF	393
Bauer, Jerry (IL)	NS	437	Benedetto, Pasquale (FL)	Onc	322
Bauer, Joel (NY)	S	957	Benenati, James (FL)	VIR	904
Baughman, Kenneth (MA)	Cv	94	Benenati, Susan (FL)	A&I	84
Bauman, Phillip (NY)	OrS	563	Benevenia, Joseph (NJ)	OrS	563
Baumann, Patricia (GA)	PM	636	Benjamin, Ivor (UT)	Cv	113
Baumgartner, William (MD)	TS	1001	Benjamin, Robert (TX)	Onc	337
Bavaria, Joseph (PA)	TS	1001	Benjamin, Vallo (NY)	NS	426
Baxi, Laxmi (NY)	ObG	508	Benkov, Keith (NY)	PGe	687
Bayer, Arnold (CA)	Inf	371	Bennett, David (IL)	N	476
Bayless, Theodore (MD)	Ge	218	Bennett, Richard (CA)	D	188
Baylis, Henry (CA)	Oph	547	Bennett, William (OR)	Nep	418
Bayly, Timothy (VA)	Pul	846	Benninger, Michael (MI)	Oto	615
Bazari, Hasan (MA)	Nep	410	Benson, Al (IL)	Onc	328
Beall, Michael (VA)	U	1040	Benson, Carol (MA)	DR	889
Beals, Stephen (AZ)	PlS	785	Benson, Mitchell (NY)	U	1032
Beamis, John (MA)	Pul	840	Bentley, Frederick (AR)	S	982
Beart, Robert (CA)	CRS	171	Bentz, Brandon (UT)	Oto	621
Beaser, Richard (MA)	IM	378	Bentz, Michael (WI)	PlS	781
Beasley, Michael (NC)	PlS	778	Benvenisty, Alan (NY)	VascS	1067
Beatty, Charles (MN)	Oto	615	Benz, Edward (MA)	Hem	294
Beaty, James H (TN)	OrS	574	Benzel, Edward (OH)	NS	437
Beauchamp, Robert (TN)	S	967	Benzon, Honorio (IL)	PM	637
Beaudet, Arthur (TX)	CG	156	Berchuck, Andrew (NC)	GO	266
Beck, David E (LA)	CRS	170	Berde, Charles (MA)	PM	634
Becker, Dorothy (PA)	PEn	681	Berek, Jonathan (CA)	GO	272
Becker, Ferdinand (FL)	Oto	610	Berenstein, Alejandro (NY)	NRad	897
Becker, Gary (AZ)	VIR	907	Berg, Christine (MD)	RadRO	869
Becker, James (MA)	S	954	Berg, Daniel (WA)	D	189
Becker, Kyra (WA)	N	486	Berg, Stacey (TX)	PHO	702
Beekman, Robert (OH)	PCd	675	Berg, Wendie A (MD)	DR	890
Beer, Tomasz (OR)	Onc	342	Berga, Sarah (GA)	RE	918
Beerman, Lee (PA)	PCd	671	Berger, Jerry (FL)	PM	636
Behrendt, Douglas (IA)	TS	1012	Berger, Joseph (KY)	N	472
Behrens, Myles (NY)	Oph	524	Berger, Melvin (OH)	A&I	86
Behrns, Kevin (FL)	S	967	Berger, Mitchel (CA)	NS	446
Beitsch, Peter (TX)	S	982	Berger, Richard (WA)	U	1054
Belani, Chandra (PA)	Onc	311	Bergey, Gregory (MD)	N	462
Belenky, Walter (MI)	PO	716	Bergfeld, John (OH)	OrS	577
Belinson, Jerome (OH)	GO	268	Bergman, Donald (NY)	EDM	198
Belkin, Michael (MA)	VascS	1066	Berguer, Ramon (MI)	VascS	1072
Bell, David (AL)	EDM	202	Berke, Gerald (CA)	Oto	624
Bell, Edward (IA)	NP	403	Berkeley, Alan (NY)	RE	915
Bell, Rodney (PA)	N	462	Berkowitz, Carol (CA)	Ped	666
Bellamy, Paul (CA)	Pul	857	Berkowitz, Leonard (NY)	Inf	363
Beller, George (VA)	Cv	103	Berkowitz, Richard (NY)	MF	387
Belman, A Barry (DC)	U	1032	Berkowitz, Ross (MA)	GO	262
Belmont, Howard (NY)	Rhu	929	Berkson, Richard (CA)	EDM	209

Alphabetical Listing of Doctors

Name	Specialty	Pg	Name	Specialty	Pg
Berl, Tomas (CO)	Nep	417	Bleiberg, Efrain (TX)	ChAP	827
Berland, Lincoln (AL)	DR	893	Blinder, Morey (MO)	Hem	300
Berlin, Cheston (PA)	Ped	664	Blitzer, Andrew (NY)	Oto	603
Berman, Brian (OH)	Ped	666	Block, Susan (MA)	Psyc	802
Berman, James (IL)	PGe	689	Bloom, David (MI)	U	1044
Berman, Michael (CA)	GO	272	Bloom, Patricia (NY)	Ger	248
Bermant, Michael (VA)	PlS	778	Bloomer, Joseph (AL)	Ge	224
Bermudez, Ovidio (OK)	AM	79	Bluemke, David (MD)	DR	890
Bernad, Peter (VA)	N	472	Bluestone, Charles (PA)	PO	714
Bernstein, Bram (CA)	PRhu	724	Blum, Conrad (NY)	EDM	198
Bernstein, Daniel (CA)	PCd	678	Blum, Paul (MN)	PA&I	669
Bernstein, Robert (NY)	D	178	Blumberg, Henry (GA)	Inf	366
Bessler, Marc (NY)	S	957	Blume, Ralph (NY)	Rhu	929
Bettmann, Michael (NC)	VIR	904	Blumenfeld, Hal (CT)	N	460
Betz, Randal (PA)	OrS	563	Blumenfeld, Jon (NY)	Nep	411
Bhan, Atul (MA)	Path	644	Blumenfield, Michael (NY)	Psyc	804
Bialer, Martin (NY)	CG	152	Blumenkranz, Mark (CA)	Oph	547
Biancaniello, Thomas (NY)	PCd	672	Blumenthal, David (NY)	Cv	97
Bianchi, Diana (MA)	CG	152	Blumenthal, Roger (MD)	Cv	98
Bieber, Eric (PA)	RE	915	Boachie-Adjei, Oheneba (NY)	OrS	563
Biederman, Joseph (MA)	ChAP	820	Bobrove, Arthur (CA)	Rhu	939
Bierbaum, Benjamin (MA)	OrS	560	Bock, S Allan (CO)	PA&I	669
Bierbrauer, Karin (OH)	NS	437	Bockenstedt, Paula (MI)	Hem	300
Bierman, Fredrick (NY)	PCd	672	Bockman, Richard (NY)	EDM	198
Biermann, J Sybil (MI)	OrS	577	Boden, Scott (GA)	OrS	574
Bigelow, Carolyn (MS)	Hem	298	Bodenheimer, Henry (NY)	Ge	218
Bigliani, Louis (NY)	OrS	563	Boehm, Frank (TN)	MF	388
Bilchik, Anton (CA)	S	986	Boggan, James (CA)	NS	446
Bilezikian, John (NY)	EDM	198	Bogrov, Michael (MD)	ChAP	822
Biller, Beverly (MA)	EDM	196	Bohlman, Henry (OH)	OrS	578
Billings, J Andrew (MA)	IM	378	Bojrab, Dennis (MI)	Oto	615
Billmire, David (OH)	PlS	781	Boles, Richard (CA)	CG	157
Bilsky, Mark (NY)	NS	426	Bolger, Graeme (AL)	Onc	322
Binder, Perry (CA)	Oph	547	Bolger, William (MD)	Oto	603
Bird, Hector (NY)	ChAP	822	Bollen, Andrew (CA)	Path	656
Bishop, Allen (MN)	HS	284	Bolman, R Morton (MA)	TS	998
Bissell, Dwight (CA)	IM	381	Bolton, W Kline (VA)	Nep	413
Bitan, Fabien (NY)	OrS	563	Bolwell, Brian (OH)	Onc	328
Bitran, Jacob (IL)	Onc	328	Bond, Sheldon (KY)	PS	728
Bjorkman, David (UT)	Ge	234	Bonkovsky, Herbert (CT)	Ge	216
Black, Keith (CA)	NS	446	Bonner, James (AL)	A&I	84
Black, Peter (MA)	NS	424	Bonomi, Philip (IL)	Onc	329
Black, William (NH)	DR	889	Bonow, Robert (IL)	Cv	107
Blackwell, Richard (AL)	RE	918	Boone, Timothy (TX)	U	1051
Blaha, John (MI)	OrS	578	Boop, Frederick (TN)	NS	433
Blaivas, Jerry (NY)	U	1032	Booth, Robert (PA)	OrS	563
Bland, Kirby (AL)	S	967	Borchert, Mark (CA)	Oph	547
Blaser, Martin (NY)	Inf	363	Borden, Ernest (OH)	Onc	329
Blasko, John C (WA)	RadRO	880	Borer, Jeffrey (NY)	Cv	98
Blazer, Dan (NC)	Psyc	809	Borgen, Patrick (NY)	S	957
Bleday, Ronald (MA)	CRS	164	Borges, Lawrence (MA)	NS	424
Blei, Andres (IL)	Ge	228	Borkowsky, William (NY)	PInf	705

Alphabetical Listing of Doctors

Name	Specialty	Pg	Name	Specialty	Pg
Boronow, John (MD)	Psyc	804	Brecher, Martin (NY)	PHO	693
Borowitz, Drucy (NY)	PPul	718	Breidenbach, Warren (KY)	HS	283
Borson, Soo (WA)	GerPsy	831	Breitbart, William (NY)	Psyc	805
Borum, Marie (DC)	Ge	218	Brem, Henry (MD)	NS	426
Borzak, Steven (FL)	Cv	104	Brem, Rachel (DC)	DR	890
Bosl, George (NY)	Onc	311	Brem, Steven (FL)	NS	433
Boston, Barry (TN)	Onc	322	Brems, John (IL)	S	973
Bostwick, David (VA)	Path	649	Brendler, Charles (IL)	U	1044
Boucek, Mark (FL)	PCd	673	Brener, Bruce (NJ)	VascS	1068
Boucek, Robert (WA)	PCd	678	Brennan, Daniel (MO)	Nep	415
Bourdette, Dennis (OR)	N	487	Brennan, Michael (MN)	EDM	204
Bourge, Robert (AL)	Cv	104	Brennan, Murray (NY)	S	958
Boushey, Homer (CA)	Pul	857	Brennan, Stephen (TX)	Nep	417
Bove, Alfred (PA)	Cv	98	Brenner, Barry (MA)	Nep	410
Bove, Edward (MI)	PS	730	Brenner, Joel (MD)	PCd	672
Bowden, Charles (TX)	Psyc	813	Brenner, Michael (MA)	Rhu	928
Bowen, James (WA)	N	487	Brent, Burton (CA)	PlS	788
Bower, Charles (AR)	PO	717	Brent, David (PA)	ChAP	822
Bowers, Malcolm (CT)	Psyc	802	Bresalier, Robert (TX)	Ge	236
Boxer, Gary (MO)	ChAP	825	Bressler, Neil (MD)	Oph	524
Boxer, Laurence (MI)	PHO	698	Bressman, Susan (NY)	N	462
Boxer Wachler, Brian (CA)	Oph	548	Brewster, David (MA)	VascS	1066
Boxrud, Cynthia (CA)	Oph	548	Bricker, John (KY)	PCd	673
Boyajian, Michael (DC)	PlS	772	Bricker, Leslie J (MI)	Onc	329
Boyce, H Worth (FL)	Ge	224	Bridwell, Keith (MO)	OrS	578
Boyd, Stuart (CA)	U	1054	Brill, Judith (CA)	PCCM	680
Boyd, W Douglas (FL)	TS	1007	Brindis, Ralph (CA)	Cv	115
Boyer, Thomas (AZ)	Ge	236	Brink, Robert (CA)	PlS	788
Boyle, Robert (VA)	NP	402	Bristow, Robert (MD)	GO	263
Brackmann, Derald (CA)	Oto	624	Britt, L D (VA)	S	967
Braddom, Randall (NJ)	PMR	756	Brizel, David (NC)	RadRO	873
Bradford, Carol (MI)	Oto	615	Brock, John (TN)	U	1040
Bradford, David (CA)	OrS	586	Broderick, Gregory (FL)	U	1040
Bradley, James P (PA)	OrS	564	Broderick, Joseph (OH)	N	476
Bradley, John (CA)	PInf	708	Brodeur, Garrett (PA)	PHO	693
Brady, Charles (TX)	Ge	236	Brodkin, Edward (PA)	Psyc	805
Brady, Kathleen (SC)	AdP	819	Brodman, Michael (NY)	ObG	509
Braman, Sidney (RI)	Pul	840	Brodsky, James (TX)	OrS	584
Branch, Charles (NC)	NS	433	Brody, Fred (DC)	S	958
Brandt, Fredric (FL)	D	182	Brody, Harold (GA)	D	182
Brandt, Harry (MD)	Psyc	805	Bromberg, Jonathan (NY)	S	958
Brandt, Keith (MO)	PlS	781	Bromberg, Mark B (UT)	N	482
Brandt, Lawrence (NY)	Ge	218	Bromfield, Edward (MA)	N	460
Brandt-Rauf, Paul (NY)	OM	796	Bronheim, Harold (NY)	Psyc	805
Branham, Gregory (MO)	Oto	615	Brooks, Benjamin (WI)	N	476
Brasington, Richard (MO)	Rhu	935	Brooks, David (MA)	S	954
Braunstein, Seth (PA)	IM	378	Brooks, John (PA)	Path	645
Brause, Barry (NY)	Inf	363	Brooks, Stuart (FL)	Pul	847
Braverman, Alan (MO)	Cv	107	Brown, Frederick (IL)	NS	437
Braverman, Irwin (CT)	D	176	Brown, Gary (PA)	Oph	524
Braylan, Raul (FL)	Path	650	Brown, John (IN)	TS	1012
Brazer, Scott (NC)	Ge	225	Brown, Kevin K (CO)	Pul	854

Alphabetical Listing of Doctors

Name	Specialty	Pg	Name	Specialty	Pg
Brown, Kimberly (MI)	Ge	228	Burns, Alton (TX)	PlS	785
Brown-Jackson, Amie (AL)	PMR	759	Burns, Richard (AZ)	N	483
Browner, Bruce (CT)	OrS	560	Burris, Howard A (TN)	Onc	322
Brozena, Susan (PA)	Cv	98	Burry, Kenneth (OR)	RE	923
Bruce, Jeffrey (NY)	NS	426	Burt, Randall (UT)	Ge	234
Brucker, Alexander (PA)	Oph	524	Burt, Richard (IL)	Onc	329
Bruner, Janet (TX)	Path	653	Burt, Vivien (CA)	Psyc	814
Bruner, Joseph (TN)	MF	389	Burton, Allen (TX)	PM	638
Brunicardi, F Charles (TX)	S	982	Burton, Claude (NC)	D	182
Brunson, Mathew (CA)	S	986	Burton, John (MD)	Ger	248
Brunsting, Louis (TN)	TS	1007	Bury, Robert (ND)	ObG	513
Brunstrom, Janice E (MO)	ChiN	145	Bushman, Wade (WI)	U	1044
Brunt, L Michael (MO)	S	973	Busse, William (WI)	A&I	86
Brushart, Thomas (MD)	OrS	564	Bussel, James (NY)	PHO	693
Bruskewitz, Reginald (WI)	U	1044	Busuttil, Ronald (CA)	S	986
Brust, John (NY)	N	463	Butler, David (TX)	D	187
Bryson, Yvonne (CA)	PInf	708	Butler, John (CA)	S	986
Buadi, Francis (TN)	Hem	298	Buxton, Alfred (RI)	CE	118
Bucciarelli, Richard (FL)	NP	403	Buyon, Jill (NY)	Rhu	930
Buch, Jeffrey (TX)	U	1051	Buys, Saundra (UT)	Onc	336
Buchanan, George (TX)	PHO	702	Buyske, Jo (PA)	S	958
Buchbinder, Ellen (NY)	A&I	82	Buzdar, Aman (TX)	Onc	337
Buchbinder, Maurice (CA)	IC	128	Byrd, Benjamin F (TN)	Cv	104
Buchholz, David (MD)	N	463	Byrd, David (WA)	S	986
Buchholz, Thomas (TX)	RadRO	878	Byrd, H Stephenson (TX)	PlS	785
Buchman, Steven (MI)	PlS	781	Byrd, John (OH)	Onc	329
Bucholz, Robert (TX)	OrS	584	Bystritsky, Alexander (CA)	Psyc	814
Buckley, Edward (NC)	Oph	533	Bystryn, Jean (NY)	D	178
Buckley, Rebecca (NC)	PA&I	668			
Buckwalter, Joseph (IA)	OrS	578	**C**		
Bucky, Louis (PA)	PlS	772	Cabin, Henry (CT)	Cv	94
Budd, George (OH)	Onc	329	Cady, Blake (RI)	S	954
Budenz, Donald (FL)	Oph	533	Cagle, Philip (TX)	Path	654
Budoff, Matthew (CA)	Cv	116	Cahill, John (NY)	PrM	797
Bueno, Raphael (MA)	TS	998	Cain, Joanna (OR)	GO	272
Bukowski, Ronald (OH)	Onc	329	Cairo, Mitchell (NY)	PHO	693
Bull, David (UT)	TS	1017	Calabrese, Joseph (OH)	Psyc	811
Bull, Marilyn (IN)	Ped	666	Caldamone, Anthony (RI)	U	1030
Buly, Robert (NY)	OrS	564	Caldarelli, David (IL)	Oto	615
Bumpous, Jeffrey (KY)	Oto	610	Caldwell, Randall (IN)	PCd	675
Bunchman, Timothy (MI)	PNep	711	Calhoon, John (TX)	TS	1018
Bunn, Paul (CO)	Onc	335	Callaghan, John (IA)	OrS	578
Bunning, Robert (DC)	Rhu	929	Callans, David (PA)	CE	118
Burchiel, Kim (OR)	NS	446	Callen, Jeffrey (KY)	D	182
Burger, Peter (MD)	Path	645	Calligaro, Keith (PA)	VascS	1068
Burgess, David (NJ)	Ped	664	Calmbach, Walter L (TX)	SM	949
Burke, Allan (IL)	N	476	Cambria, Richard (MA)	VascS	1066
Burke, Miles (OH)	Oph	538	Cameron, John (MD)	S	958
Burke, William (NE)	GerPsy	830	Camins, Martin (NY)	NS	427
Burket, Mark (OH)	Cv	108	Camisa, Charles (FL)	D	182
Burkey, Brian (TN)	Oto	610	Cammisa, Frank (NY)	OrS	564
Burnett, Arthur (MD)	U	1032			

Alphabetical Listing of Doctors

Name	Specialty	Pg	Name	Specialty	Pg
Camoriano, John (AZ)	Onc	337	Carter, John (TX)	N	483
Campbell, David (CO)	TS	1017	Carter, Keith (IA)	Oph	538
Campbell, G Douglas (MS)	Pul	847	Carter, William (AR)	Ger	253
Campbell, J William (MO)	Inf	369	Cartwright, Patrick (UT)	U	1050
Campbell, James (MD)	NS	427	Casella, Samuel (NH)	PEn	681
Campbell, Steven (OH)	U	1045	Cassidy, Suzanne (CA)	CG	157
Campo, John (OH)	ChAP	826	Cassisi, Nicholas (FL)	Oto	610
Campochiaro, Peter (MD)	Oph	524	Castell, Donald (SC)	Ge	225
Canady, John (IA)	PlS	781	Castle, Valerie (MI)	PHO	698
Cance, William (FL)	S	968	Catalona, William (IL)	U	1045
Cancio, Margarita (FL)	Inf	366	Catanzaro, Antonino (CA)	Pul	858
Canellos, George P (MA)	Onc	307	Cederbaum, Stephen (CA)	CG	157
Canning, Douglas (PA)	U	1032	Celli, Bartolome (MA)	Pul	840
Cannom, David (CA)	CE	123	Cello, John (CA)	Ge	238
Cannon, W Dilworth (CA)	OrS	586	Cerfolio, Robert (AL)	TS	1008
Cannon, Walter (CA)	TS	1020	Cerqueira, Manuel (OH)	Cv	108
Canterbury, Randolph (VA)	Psyc	809	Cetta, Frank (MN)	PCd	675
Caplan, Louis (MA)	N	460	Chabot, John (NY)	S	958
Capo, Hilda (FL)	Oph	533	Chaikof, Elliot (GA)	VascS	1070
Caprioli, Joseph (CA)	Oph	548	Chaisson, Richard (MD)	Inf	363
Caputo, Anthony (NJ)	Oph	524	Chait, Alan (WA)	EDM	209
Caputo, Thomas (NY)	GO	263	Chaitman, Bernard (MO)	Cv	108
Caputy, Anthony (DC)	NS	427	Chalas, Eva (NY)	GO	264
Carabasi, R Anthony (PA)	VascS	1068	Chalian, Ara (PA)	Oto	603
Carabello, Blase (TX)	Cv	114	Chambers, Richard (CA)	OrS	586
Carbone, David (TN)	Onc	322	Chambers, Setsuko (AZ)	GO	271
Cardenas, Diana (FL)	PMR	759	Champlin, Richard (TX)	Hem	304
Carey, John (UT)	CG	156	Chan, Kenny (CO)	PO	716
Carey, Timothy (NC)	IM	379	Chancellor, Michael (PA)	U	1032
Carlson, John (NJ)	GO	264	Chandar, Jayanthi (FL)	PNep	710
Carlson, Robert (CA)	Onc	342	Chandler, Michael (NY)	A&I	82
Carmel, Peter (NJ)	NS	427	Chandler, William F (MI)	NS	437
Carneiro, Ronaldo (FL)	HS	283	Chandrasoma, Parakrama (CA)	Path	656
Carney, John (AR)	D	187	Chang, Alfred (MI)	S	974
Caronna, John (NY)	N	463	Chang, Helena (CA)	S	986
Carpenter, Jeffrey (PA)	VascS	1068	Chang, Kenneth (CA)	Ge	238
Carr, Bruce (TX)	ObG	513	Chang, Rowland (IL)	Rhu	935
Carr, Daniel (MA)	PM	634	Chang, Stanley (NY)	Oph	524
Carr, David (MO)	Ger	251	Chang-Miller, April (AZ)	Rhu	938
Carr-Locke, David (MA)	Ge	216	Chao, Nelson (NC)	Onc	322
Carragee, Eugene (CA)	OrS	586	Chap, Linnea (CA)	Onc	342
Carrasquillo, Jorge (NY)	NuM	500	Chapman, Paul (MA)	NS	424
Carrau, Ricardo (PA)	Oto	603	Chapman, Paul (NY)	Onc	311
Carraway, James (VA)	PlS	778	Chapman, Stanley W (MS)	Inf	366
Carroll, Charles (IL)	HS	284	Chapman, William (MO)	S	974
Carroll, Peter (CA)	U	1054	Char, Devron (CA)	Oph	548
Carroll, William (NY)	PHO	693	Charboneau, J William (MN)	RadRO	875
Carson, Benjamin (MD)	NS	427	Chari, Suresh (MN)	Ge	228
Carson, Culley (NC)	U	1040	Charnas, Lawrence (MN)	ChiN	145
Carson, Sandra (RI)	RE	914	Charney, Jonathan (NY)	N	463
Carstens, Michael (CA)	PlS	788	Charrow, Joel (IL)	CG	155
Carter, H Ballentine (MD)	U	1032	Chatham, Walter (AL)	Rhu	933

Name	Specialty	Pg	Name	Specialty	Pg
Chatterjee, Kanu (CA)	Cv	116	Clements, Stephen (GA)	Cv	104
Chen, Allen (MD)	PHO	694	Clewell, William (AZ)	MF	392
Chen, Chun (NY)	NS	427	Cloherty, John (MA)	NP	400
Chen, David (IL)	PMR	760	Cloninger, C Robert (MO)	Psyc	811
Cherny, W Bruce (ID)	NS	442	Clore, John (VA)	EDM	202
Cherry, James (CA)	PInf	708	Close, Lanny (NY)	Oto	603
Cherry, Kenneth (VA)	VascS	1071	Cloughesy, Timothy (CA)	N	487
Chervenak, Francis (NY)	MF	387	Clouse, Ray (MO)	Ge	228
Chescheir, Nancy (TN)	MF	389	Clutter, William E (MO)	EDM	204
Chesney, Carolyn M (TN)	Path	650	Cobleigh, Melody (IL)	Onc	330
Cheson, Bruce (DC)	Hem	295	Cobos, Everardo (TX)	Hem	304
Childs, Stacy (CO)	U	1050	Coccia, Peter (NE)	PHO	701
Chinitz, Larry (NY)	CE	119	Cochran, Alistair (CA)	Path	656
Chiocca, E Antonio (OH)	NS	437	Cockerell, Clay (TX)	D	187
Chitambar, Christopher (WI)	Onc	330	Coe, Fredric (IL)	Nep	415
Chitwood, W Randolph (NC)	TS	1008	Coffey, Barbara (NY)	ChAP	822
Chiu, David (NY)	PlS	772	Coffman, Thomas M (NC)	Nep	413
Chlebowski, Rowan (CA)	Onc	342	Cofield, Robert (MN)	OrS	578
Cho, Kyung (MI)	VIR	905	Coggins, Cecil (MA)	Nep	410
Chodak, Gerald (IL)	U	1045	Cohen, Alan (OH)	NS	437
Choi, Noah (MA)	RadRO	868	Cohen, Bernard (FL)	D	183
Chopra, Inder (CA)	EDM	209	Cohen, Bruce (MA)	Psyc	802
Choti, Michael (MD)	S	958	Cohen, Carmel (NY)	GO	264
Chow, Warren (CA)	Onc	342	Cohen, David (NY)	Nep	411
Chowdhury, Khalid (CO)	Oto	621	Cohen, Harris (NY)	DR	890
Choy, Andrew (CA)	Oph	548	Cohen, Herbert (NY)	Ped	664
Christian, Karla (TN)	TS	1008	Cohen, Howard (NY)	Cv	98
Christiani, David (MA)	Pul	840	Cohen, Jeffrey (OH)	N	477
Christiansen, Thomas (MN)	Oto	616	Cohen, Jonathan (NY)	Ge	218
Christie, Dennis (WA)	PGe	691	Cohen, Lawrence (NY)	Ge	218
Christman, Brian (TN)	Pul	847	Cohen, Lawrence (CT)	Cv	94
Christman, Gregory (MI)	RE	920	Cohen, Mark (IL)	HS	284
Chui, Helena (CA)	N	487	Cohen, Martin (NY)	CE	119
Chung, Kevin (MI)	HS	284	Cohen, Michael (IA)	Path	651
Chung, Raymond (MA)	Ge	216	Cohen, Mitchell (OH)	PGe	689
Church, Joseph (CA)	PA&I	670	Cohen, Mitchell (PA)	Psyc	805
Chutorian, Abraham (NY)	ChiN	143	Cohen, Myron (NC)	Inf	367
Cilo, Mark (CO)	N	483	Cohen, Philip (DC)	Onc	311
Ciocon, Jerry (FL)	Ger	250	Cohen, Robbin (CA)	TS	1020
Cioffi, William (RI)	S	954	Cohen, Roger (PA)	Onc	311
Cionni, Robert (OH)	Oph	538	Cohen, Seymour (NY)	Onc	311
Cirigliano, Michael (PA)	IM	378	Cohen, Steven (CA)	PlS	788
Civin, Curt (MD)	PHO	694	Cohen, William (PA)	Ped	665
Clagett, George (TX)	VascS	1074	Cohn, David (CO)	Inf	370
Clair, Daniel (OH)	VascS	1072	Cohn, Lawrence (MA)	TS	998
Clairmont, Albert (OH)	PMR	760	Cohn, Richard (IL)	PNep	711
Clark, Orlo (CA)	S	986	Cohn, Susan (IL)	PHO	698
Clarke-Pearson, Daniel (NC)	GO	266	Coia, Lawrence (NJ)	RadRO	869
Clayman, Gary (TX)	Oto	622	Coit, Daniel (NY)	S	958
Clayman, Ralph (CA)	U	1054	Coker, Newton (TX)	Oto	622
Clements, Dennis (NC)	PInf	706	Colachis, Samuel (OH)	PMR	760
Clements, Philip (CA)	Rhu	939	Colby, Thomas (AZ)	Path	654

Alphabetical Listing of Doctors

Name	Specialty	Pg	Name	Specialty	Pg
Cole, Andrew (MA)	N	460	Corey, Lawrence (WA)	Inf	372
Cole, Brian (IL)	SM	948	Cornblath, David (MD)	N	463
Cole, Cynthia (MA)	NP	400	Cornelius, Lynn (MO)	D	184
Cole, David (SC)	S	968	Cornwell, Edward (MD)	S	959
Cole, Francis (MO)	NP	403	Corson, John (NM)	VascS	1074
Coleman, John (IN)	PlS	782	Coselli, Joseph (TX)	TS	1018
Coleman, Morton (NY)	Onc	312	Cosgrove, G Rees (MA)	NS	424
Coleman, Ralph E (NC)	NuM	502	Costantino, Peter (NY)	Oto	604
Collea, Joseph (DC)	MF	387	Cote, Richard (CA)	Path	656
Coller, Barry (NY)	Hem	295	Cotsarelis, George (PA)	D	178
Coller, John (MA)	CRS	164	Cotton, Peter (SC)	Ge	225
Collins, Eva (NH)	PlS	770	Cotton, Robin (OH)	PO	716
Colombani, Paul (MD)	PS	726	Couch, James (OK)	N	484
Colon, Gustavo (LA)	PlS	785	Coughlin, Michael (ID)	OrS	582
Colvin, Edward (AL)	PCd	673	Couldwell, William (UT)	NS	443
Colvin, Stephen (NY)	TS	1001	Coull, Bruce (AZ)	N	484
Come, Steven (MA)	Onc	307	Courey, Mark (CA)	Oto	624
Comerota, Anthony (OH)	VascS	1072	Coutifaris, Christos (PA)	RE	915
Comi, Richard (NH)	EDM	196	Coutsoftides, Theodore (CA)	CRS	171
Cominelli, Fabio (VA)	Ge	225	Covington, Edward (OH)	PM	637
Comis, Robert (PA)	Onc	312	Cowan, Bryan (MS)	RE	918
Conant, Marcus (CA)	D	189	Cowan, Morton (CA)	PA&I	670
Connolly, Heidi (MN)	Cv	108	Cox, James (TX)	RadRO	878
Connolly, James (MA)	Path	644	Coyle, Joseph (MA)	ChAP	820
Conrad, Ernest (WA)	OrS	586	Coyle, Patricia (NY)	N	463
Constantian, Mark B (NH)	PlS	770	Cragg, Andrew (MN)	VIR	905
Conte, John (MD)	TS	1001	Craig, Robert (IL)	Ge	229
Conti, Charles (FL)	Cv	104	Craigen, William (TX)	CG	156
Conti, David (NY)	S	959	Crandall, Alan (UT)	Oph	544
Cook, Stuart (NJ)	N	463	Craven, Donald (MA)	Inf	362
Cooney, Leo (CT)	Ger	248	Crawford, E David (CO)	U	1050
Cooper, Barry (TX)	Hem	304	Crawford, James (FL)	Path	650
Cooper, Christopher (OH)	Cv	108	Crawford, Jeffrey (NC)	Onc	323
Cooper, Daniel (TX)	OrS	584	Crawford, Thomas (MD)	ChiN	143
Cooper, David (MD)	EDM	198	Creamer, Michael (FL)	PMR	759
Cooper, Joel (PA)	TS	1001	Criado, Frank (MD)	VascS	1068
Cooper, John (AL)	Pul	847	Crippin, Jeffrey (MO)	Ge	229
Cooper, Rubin (NY)	PCd	672	Crocker, Ian (GA)	RadRO	873
Cooper, William (VA)	Pul	847	Crockett, Dennis (CA)	PO	717
Copel, Joshua (CT)	MF	386	Crofford, Leslie (KY)	Rhu	933
Copeland, Jack (AZ)	TS	1018	Crombleholme, Timothy (OH)	PS	730
Copeland, Larry J (OH)	GO	268	Cromydas, George (IL)	Pul	850
Copeland III, Edward (FL)	S	968	Cronenwett, Jack (NH)	VascS	1066
Coplen, Douglas (MO)	U	1045	Cross, DeWitte (MO)	NRad	899
Copp, Steven (CA)	OrS	586	Crossett, Lawrence (PA)	OrS	564
Copperman, Alan (NY)	RE	915	Crow, Scott (MN)	Psyc	811
Coppola, John (NY)	Cv	98	Crowe, Joseph (OH)	S	974
Corbett, Eugene (VA)	IM	379	Crowley, Thomas (CO)	AdP	819
Corbett, James (MS)	N	472	Crowley, William (MA)	RE	914
Cordeiro, Peter (NY)	PlS	772	Cruse, C Wayne (FL)	PlS	778
Corey, G Ralph (NC)	Inf	367	Cryer, Philip (MO)	EDM	204
Corey, Jacquelynne (IL)	Oto	616	Cuckler, John (AL)	OrS	574

Alphabetical Listing of Doctors

Name	Specialty	Pg	Name	Specialty	Pg
Culbertson, William (FL)	Oph	533	Darcy, Michael (MO)	VIR	905
Culkin, Daniel (OK)	U	1052	Darling, R Clement (NY)	VascS	1068
Cullen, Kevin (MD)	Onc	312	Darras, Basil (MA)	ChiN	142
Cullen, Mark (CT)	OM	796	Darrow, David (VA)	PO	715
Culp, Randall (PA)	HS	281	Darwin, Christine H (CA)	EDM	209
Cummings, Charles (MD)	Oto	604	Das, Ananya (AZ)	Ge	236
Cummings, Jeffrey (CA)	N	487	Daspit, C Phillip (AZ)	Oto	622
Cunha, Burke (NY)	Inf	363	Dattwyler, Raymond (NY)	A&I	83
Cunniff, Christopher (AZ)	CG	156	Daud, Adil (FL)	Onc	323
Cunningham, Glenn (TX)	EDM	208	David, Carlos (MA)	NS	424
Cunningham, John (AZ)	Ge	236	Davidoff, Andrew (TN)	PS	728
Cunningham, Michael (MA)	PO	713	Davidoff, Ravin (MA)	Cv	94
Cunningham-Rundles, Charlotte (NY)	A&I	82	Davidson, Bruce (DC)	Oto	604
Cupps, Thomas (DC)	Rhu	930	Davidson, Dennis (NY)	NP	400
Curet, Myriam (CA)	S	987	Davidson, Joyce (TX)	Psyc	813
Curl, Walton (NC)	OrS	574	Davidson, Nancy (MD)	Onc	312
Curley, Steven (TX)	S	982	Davidson, Richard (PA)	OrS	564
Curran, James (IL)	Rhu	935	Davidson, Susan (CO)	GO	271
Curran, Walter (PA)	RadRO	870	Davies, Stella (OH)	PHO	698
Currie, John (CT)	GO	262	Davies, Terry (NY)	EDM	198
Curry, Cynthia (CA)	CG	157	Davis, Bradley (KS)	U	1050
Curtin, Hugh (MA)	NRad	896	Davis, Gary (TX)	Ge	236
Curtin, John (NY)	GO	264	Davis, Ira (OH)	PNep	711
Curtis, Anne (FL)	CE	120	Davis, James (CA)	Ger	254
Cushman, William (TN)	IM	380	Davis, Jessica (NY)	CG	153
Cutrer, F Michael (MN)	N	477	Davis, Pamela (OH)	PPul	720
Cutting, Court (NY)	PlS	773	Davis, William (LA)	Rhu	938
			Day, Arthur L (MA)	NS	424

D

Name	Specialty	Pg	Name	Specialty	Pg
			Day, Susan (CA)	Oph	548
D'Alton, Mary (NY)	MF	387	Day, Terrence (SC)	Oto	611
D'Amico, Anthony (MA)	RadRO	868	De Angelis, Lisa (NY)	N	464
D'Amico, Donald (NY)	Oph	525	De Geest, Koen (IA)	GO	268
Daar, Eric (CA)	IM	381	De Juan, Eugene (CA)	Oph	548
Dabbagh, Shermine (DE)	PNep	709	de Kernion, Jean (CA)	U	1054
Dabezies, Eugene (TX)	OrS	584	De la Cruz, Antonio (CA)	Oto	624
Dacey, Ralph (MO)	NS	438	De Lateur, Barbara (MD)	PMR	757
Dae, Michael (CA)	NuM	503	De Leon-Casasola, Oscar (NY)	PM	634
Dagum, Alexander (NY)	PlS	773	De Lia, Julian (WI)	ObG	511
Dake, Michael (VA)	VIR	904	De Long, Mahlon (GA)	N	472
Dalakas, Marinos (PA)	N	463	de Lotbiniere, Alain (NY)	NS	427
Dale, Lowell (MN)	Ger	251	De Masters, Bette (CO)	Path	653
Dalinka, Murray (PA)	DR	890	De Meester, Tom (CA)	TS	1020
Dalkin, Alan (VA)	EDM	202	De Monte, Franco (TX)	NS	444
Daly, Mary (PA)	Onc	312	De Simone, Philip (KY)	Onc	323
Damewood, Marian (PA)	RE	915	De Vivo, Darryl (NY)	ChiN	143
Damiano, Ralph (MO)	TS	1012	Dean, Jonathan (UT)	PCCM	680
Damon, Lloyd E (CA)	Hem	305	Deas, Deborah (SC)	ChAP	825
Dang, Michael (HI)	TS	1020	DeBaun, Michael (MO)	PHO	699
Daniel, Rollin (CA)	PlS	788	DeCamp, Malcolm (MA)	TS	998
Daniels, Gilbert (MA)	EDM	196	DeCherney, Alan (MD)	ObG	509
Danoff, Dudley (CA)	U	1054	Deeg, H. Joachim (WA)	Onc	342
			DeGiorgio, Christopher (CA)	N	487

Alphabetical Listing of Doctors

Name	Specialty	Pg	Name	Specialty	Pg
Deitch, Edwin (NJ)	S	959	Diamond, Michael (MI)	RE	920
DeKosky, Steven (PA)	N	464	Diamond, Paul (VA)	PMR	759
Del Giudice, Stephen (NH)	D	176	Diaz, Angela (NY)	AM	78
Del Monte, Monte (MI)	Oph	538	Diaz, Fernando (MI)	NS	438
Del Negro, Albert (VA)	CE	120	Dichek, David (WA)	Cv	116
Del Priore, Lucian (NY)	Oph	525	Dichter, Marc (PA)	N	464
Delahay, John (DC)	OrS	564	Dick, Macdonald (MI)	PCd	676
Delamarter, Rick (CA)	OrS	586	Diehl, James (PA)	TS	1001
DeLancey, John (MI)	ObG	512	Dienstag, Jules (MA)	Ge	216
Deland, Jonathan (NY)	OrS	565	Dieterich, Douglas (NY)	Ge	219
Delaney, Conor (OH)	CRS	168	Diethrich, Edward (AZ)	TS	1018
Delaney, Thomas (MA)	RadRO	868	Dilawari, Raza (TN)	S	968
DeLellis, Ronald (RI)	Path	644	Dilley, Ralph (CA)	VascS	1075
Deleo, Vincent (NY)	D	178	Dillingham, Michael (CA)	OrS	586
Deleyiannis, Frederic (PA)	PlS	773	Dillingham, Timothy (WI)	PMR	760
Delivoria-Papadopoulos, Maria (PA)	NP	401	Dillon, William (CA)	NRad	901
Dell, Diana (NC)	Psyc	809	DiMarco, John (VA)	CE	120
Della Rocca, Robert (NY)	Oph	525	DiMarino, Anthony (PA)	Ge	219
Delmez, James (MO)	Nep	415	Dimeff, Robert (OH)	SM	948
Demarest, Gerald (NM)	S	982	Dines, David (NY)	OrS	565
Demer, Joseph (CA)	Oph	548	Dion, Jacques (GA)	NRad	898
Demetri, George D (MA)	Onc	307	Disis, Mary (WA)	Onc	343
Demetris, A Jake (PA)	Path	645	Dismukes, William (AL)	Inf	367
Demmy, Todd (NY)	TS	1001	Diuguid, David (NY)	Hem	295
Demopoulos, Laura (PA)	Cv	98	Diver, Daniel (CT)	IC	123
Dempsey, Daniel (PA)	S	959	Divon, Michael (NY)	ObG	509
Dempsey, Robert (WI)	NS	438	Dobkin, Bruce (CA)	N	487
Denenberg, Steven (NE)	Oto	621	Dobs, Adrian (MD)	EDM	198
Denson, Susan (TX)	NP	405	Dodd, Gerald (TX)	DR	895
DePaulo, J Raymond (MD)	Psyc	805	Dodds, William (MI)	RE	920
DePriest, Paul (KY)	GO	266	Dodick, David (AZ)	N	484
Deren, Julius (PA)	Ge	219	Doghramji, Karl (PA)	Psyc	805
Derman, Gordon (IL)	HS	284	Doherty, Dennis (KY)	Pul	847
Dershaw, D David (NY)	DR	890	Doherty, Gerard (MI)	S	974
DeSanctis, Roman (MA)	Cv	94	Dolgin, Stephen (NY)	PS	726
Deschamps, Claude (MN)	TS	1012	Dolitsky, Jay (NY)	PO	714
Deschler, Daniel (MA)	Oto	601	Donald, Paul (CA)	Oto	625
deShazo, Richard (MS)	A&I	84	Donaldson, Sarah (CA)	RadRO	880
Desnick, Robert (NY)	CG	153	Donaldson, William (PA)	OrS	565
Desposito, Franklin (NJ)	CG	153	Donehower, Ross (MD)	Onc	312
DeVane, Gary (FL)	RE	918	Donn, Steven (MI)	NP	404
DeVault, Kenneth (FL)	Ge	225	Donohue, James (NC)	Pul	847
Devereux, Richard (NY)	Cv	99	Donohue, John H (MN)	S	974
Devinsky, Orrin (NY)	N	464	Donovan, Donald (TX)	Oto	622
DeVita, Vincent (CT)	Onc	308	Donovan, James (OH)	U	1045
Dewberry, Robert (MD)	N	464	Donovan, William (TX)	PMR	763
Deziel, Daniel (IL)	S	974	Dooley, Sharon (IL)	MF	390
Di Bisceglie, Adrian (MO)	Ge	229	Dooley, William (OK)	S	983
Di Giacinto, George (NY)	NS	428	Dorfman, Howard (NY)	Path	645
Di Persio, John (MO)	Onc	330	Dormans, John (PA)	OrS	565
Diamond, Frank (FL)	PEn	683	Doroshow, James (MD)	Onc	312
Diamond, Gary (PA)	Oph	525	Dorr, Lawrence (CA)	OrS	587

Name	Specialty	Pg	Name	Specialty	Pg
Dosa, Stefan (DC)	Nep	411	Duthie, Edmund H (WI)	Ger	251
Dottino, Peter (NY)	GO	264	Dutton, Jonathan (NC)	Oph	533
Doty, Donald (UT)	TS	1017	Duvic, Madeleine (TX)	D	187
Douglas, John (GA)	Cv	104	Dyer, Carmel (TX)	Ger	253
Dover, Jeffrey (MA)	D	176	Dzau, Victor (NC)	Cv	104
Dowling, Robert (KY)	TS	1008	Dzubow, Leonard (PA)	D	178
Downie, Gordon (NC)	Pul	848			
Dozor, Allen (NY)	PPul	718			

E

Name	Specialty	Pg	Name	Specialty	Pg
Drachman, Daniel (MD)	N	464	Eagle, Kim (MI)	Cv	108
Drake, Amelia (NC)	PO	715	Eagle, Ralph (PA)	Oph	525
Drayer, Burton (NY)	NRad	897	Earp, H Shelton (NC)	EDM	202
Drebin, Jeffrey (PA)	S	959	Easton, J Donald (RI)	N	460
Dreicer, Robert (OH)	Onc	330	Eaton, James (DC)	Psyc	805
Dreyer, William (TX)	PCd	677	Eavey, Roland (MA)	PO	713
Driebe, William (FL)	Oph	533	Ebbert, Larry (SD)	Onc	336
Drinkwater, Davis (TN)	TS	1008	Eberlein, Timothy (MO)	S	974
Driscoll, Colin (MN)	Oto	616	Ebraheim, Nabil (OH)	OrS	578
Driscoll, Daniel (FL)	CG	154	Eckardt, Jeffrey (CA)	OrS	587
Driscoll, David (MN)	PCd	676	Eckel, Robert (CO)	EDM	208
Driscoll, Deborah (PA)	CG	153	Eckhardt, S (CO)	Onc	336
Driver, Larry (TX)	PM	638	Eckhoff, Devin (AL)	S	968
Droller, David (FL)	Inf	367	Econs, Michael (IN)	EDM	204
Droller, Michael (NY)	U	1033	Edelson, Richard (CT)	D	176
Dromerick, Alexander (DC)	N	464	Edelstein, Barbara (NY)	DR	890
Drossman, Douglas (NC)	Ge	225	Edelstein, David (NY)	Oto	604
Drucker, David (FL)	PS	728	Edersheim, Terri (NY)	MF	388
Druker, Brian (OR)	Onc	343	Edgar, Terence (WI)	ChiN	145
Druzin, Maurice (CA)	MF	393	Edge, Stephen (NY)	S	959
Du Pen, Stuart (WA)	PM	639	Edington, Howard (PA)	S	959
Dubeau, Louis (CA)	Path	656	Edmundowicz, Steven (MO)	Ge	229
Dubois, Michel (NY)	PM	634	Edney, James (NE)	S	981
Duff, W Patrick (FL)	ObG	510	Edwards, John (CA)	Inf	372
Duffner, Patricia (NY)	ChiN	144	Edwards, Kathryn (TN)	PInf	706
Duffy, Thomas (CT)	Hem	294	Edwards, Michael (AR)	S	983
Dufresne, Craig (MD)	PlS	773	Edwards, Michael S (CA)	NS	447
Dugoff, Lorraine (CO)	MF	392	Edye, Michael (NY)	S	959
Duhaime, Ann (NH)	NS	424	Efron, Jonathan (AZ)	CRS	171
Duker, Jay (MA)	Oph	522	Egan, James (MD)	ChAP	822
Dulcan, Mina (IL)	ChAP	826	Egan, Thomas (NC)	TS	1008
Dumesic, Daniel (MN)	RE	920	Eggers, Howard (NY)	Oph	525
Dumitru, Daniel (TX)	PMR	763	Ehrenkranz, Richard (CT)	NP	400
Duncan, Brian (OH)	PS	730	Ehresmann, Glenn (CA)	Rhu	939
Duncan, John (RI)	NS	425	Ehrlich, Michael (RI)	OrS	560
Duncan, Newton (TX)	PO	717	Ehrlich, Peter (MI)	PS	730
Dunlap, Nancy (AL)	Pul	848	Ehrmann, David (IL)	EDM	205
Dunn, Harold (UT)	OrS	583	Ehya, Hormoz (PA)	Path	645
DuPont, Herbert (TX)	Inf	370	Eichelberger, Martin (DC)	PS	726
Durbin, William (MA)	PInf	705	Eichenfield, Lawrence (CA)	D	189
Dure, Leon (AL)	N	472	Eichler, Craig (FL)	D	183
Durham, Janette (CO)	VIR	907	Eid, Jean (NY)	U	1033
Durham, Samuel (OH)	TS	1013	Eidt, John (AR)	VascS	1074
Durrie, Daniel (KS)	Oph	544			

Alphabetical Listing of Doctors

Name	Specialty	Pg	Name	Specialty	Pg
Eifel, Patricia (TX)	RadRO	878	Epstein, Leon (IL)	ChiN	145
Eilber, Frederick (CA)	S	987	Epstein, Michael (FL)	PCd	674
Einhorn, Lawrence (IN)	Onc	330	Epstein, Stuart (CA)	PA&I	670
Einhorn, Thomas (MA)	OrS	560	Eriksson, Elof (MA)	PlS	770
Eisdorfer, Carl (FL)	Psyc	809	Ernst, Armin (MA)	Pul	840
Eisele, David (CA)	Oto	625	Errico, Thomas (NY)	OrS	565
Eisen, Howard (PA)	Cv	99	Eschenbach, David (WA)	ObG	513
Eisenberg, Burton (NH)	S	954	Escobedo, Marilyn (OK)	NP	405
Eisenberg, Howard (MD)	NS	428	Esquenazi, Alberto (PA)	PMR	757
Eisenberger, Mario (MD)	Onc	313	Esquivel, Carlos Orlando (CA)	S	987
Eisendrath, Stuart (CA)	Psyc	815	Esserman, Laura (CA)	S	987
Eismont, Frank (FL)	OrS	574	Essner, Richard (CA)	S	987
El-Galley, Rizk (AL)	U	1040	Estabrook, Alison (NY)	S	960
El-Youssef, Mounif (MN)	PGe	689	Eth, Spencer (NY)	Psyc	806
Elder, Jack (OH)	U	1045	Ettenger, Robert (CA)	PNep	712
Elefteriades, John (CT)	TS	998	Ettinger, David (MD)	Onc	313
Elias, Jack (CT)	Pul	840	Eugster, Erica (IN)	PEn	684
Elias, Sherman (IL)	ObG	512	Euhus, David (TX)	S	983
Elias, Stanton (MI)	N	477	Eustis, Horatio (LA)	Oph	544
Elkayam, Uri (CA)	Cv	116	Evans, Douglas (TX)	S	983
Ellenbogen, Kenneth (VA)	CE	120	Evans, Mark (NY)	ObG	509
Ellenbogen, Richard (WA)	NS	447	Evans, Sarah (DC)	PMR	757
Elliott, C Gregory (UT)	Pul	854	Everson, Gregory (CO)	Ge	235
Elliott, David (IA)	Ge	229	Eviatar, Lydia (NY)	ChiN	144
Elliott, John (AZ)	MF	392	Ewalt, David (TX)	U	1052
Ellis, George S (LA)	Oph	544	Ezaki, Marybeth (TX)	HS	287
Ellis, Georgiana (WA)	Onc	343			
Ellis, Jonathan (CA)	Ge	238	**F**		
Ellis, Lee (TX)	S	983			
Ellis, Stephen (OH)	IC	126	Faber, L Penfield (IL)	TS	1013
Ellison, David (OR)	Nep	419	Fabian, Carol J (KS)	Onc	336
Ellison, E Christopher (OH)	S	974	Fahey, Patrick (IL)	Pul	851
Ellman, Michael (IL)	Rhu	936	Fahey, Thomas (NY)	S	960
Elmets, Craig (AL)	D	183	Fahn, Stanley (NY)	N	464
Elta, Grace (MI)	Ge	229	Failla, Joseph (MI)	HS	285
Emami, Bahman (IL)	RadRO	875	Fairman, Ronald (PA)	VascS	1068
Emans, Sarah (MA)	AM	78	Falanga, Vincent (RI)	D	176
Emanuele, Mary Ann (IL)	EDM	205	Falcone, Tommaso (OH)	RE	920
Emanuele, Nicholas (IL)	EDM	205	Falk, Rena (CA)	CG	157
Emerson, Stephen (PA)	Hem	295	Falk, Ronald (NC)	Nep	414
Emery, Helen (WA)	PRhu	724	Fallat, Mary (KY)	PS	728
Emmanuel, Patricia (FL)	PInf	706	Falletta, John (NC)	PHO	697
Emond, Jean (NY)	S	960	Fallon, Michael (AL)	Ge	225
Emre, Sukru (NY)	S	960	Fallon, Robert (IN)	PHO	699
Emslie, Graham (TX)	ChAP	827	Fan, Leland (TX)	PPul	721
Eng, Kenneth (NY)	S	960	Fang, John (UT)	Ge	235
Engel, William King (CA)	N	487	Fann, Jesse (WA)	Psyc	815
Engstrom, John (CA)	N	488	Fanous, Yvonne (CA)	PA&I	670
Ennis, Ronald (NY)	RadRO	870	Fanta, Christopher (MA)	Pul	841
Ensminger, William (MI)	Onc	330	Fantini, Gary (NY)	VascS	1068
Epstein, Andrew (AL)	CE	120	Farber, Martin (NY)	Rhu	930
Epstein, Jonathan (MD)	Path	646	Farcy, Jean (NY)	OrS	565

Name	Specialty	Pg	Name	Specialty	Pg
Farley, David (MN)	S	975	Fine, Perry (UT)	PM	638
Farlow, Martin (IN)	N	477	Fine, Robert (NY)	Onc	313
Farmer, Joseph (NC)	Oto	611	Finerman, Gerald (CA)	OrS	587
Farmer, Richard (NY)	Ge	219	Finger, Paul (NY)	Oph	525
Faro, Sebastian (TX)	ObG	513	Fink, Matthew (NY)	N	465
Farrar, William (OH)	S	975	Finkel, Michael (FL)	N	472
Farrior, Edward (FL)	Oto	611	Finkel, Terri (PA)	PRhu	722
Farrior, Joseph (FL)	Oto	611	Finucane, Thomas (MD)	Ger	248
Fasano, Alessio (MD)	PGe	687	Fiorica, James (FL)	GO	266
Fauci, Anthony (MD)	Inf	363	Firlit, Casimir (MO)	U	1045
Feder, Robert (IL)	Oph	538	First, Michael (NY)	Psyc	806
Fee, Willard (CA)	Oto	625	Fisch, Harry (NY)	U	1033
Feig, Barry (TX)	S	983	Fischbein, Lewis (MO)	Rhu	936
Fein, William (CA)	Oph	549	Fischer, Thomas (IN)	HS	285
Feinberg, Joseph (NY)	PMR	757	Fish, Frank (TN)	PCd	674
Feinberg, Todd (NY)	N	465	Fishbein, Daniel (WA)	Cv	116
Feinglos, Mark (NC)	EDM	202	Fishbein, Michael (CA)	Path	656
Feinstein, Donald I (CA)	Hem	305	Fisher, David (MA)	PHO	692
Feldman, David (NY)	OrS	565	Fisher, Garth (CA)	PlS	788
Feldman, Eva (MI)	N	477	Fisher, Laura (NY)	IM	378
Feldman, Joel (MA)	PlS	770	Fisher, Mark (CA)	N	488
Feldman, Kenneth (WA)	Ped	666	Fisher, Paul G (CA)	ChiN	148
Feldman, Mark (TX)	Ge	236	Fisher, Richard (NY)	Onc	313
Feldman, Ted (IL)	IC	126	Fisher, Robert (CA)	N	488
Feldmann, Edward (RI)	N	460	Fishman, David (NY)	GO	264
Feldon, Steven (NY)	Oph	525	Fishman, Elliot (MD)	DR	891
Feldstein, Neil (NY)	NS	428	Fishman, Marvin (TX)	ChiN	147
Feliciano, David (GA)	S	968	Fishman, Scott (CA)	PM	640
Felig, Philip (NY)	EDM	199	Fitz, J Gregory (TX)	Ge	236
Fenichel, Gerald (TN)	ChiN	144	Fitzgerald, Paul Anthony (CA)	EDM	209
Fennell, Robert (FL)	PNep	710	Fitzgibbon, Dermot (WA)	PM	640
Fennerty, Brian (OR)	Ge	239	Fitzgibbons, Robert (NE)	S	981
Fenske, Neil A (FL)	D	183	Fitzpatrick, Richard (CA)	D	189
Ferguson, James (KY)	MF	389	Fivenson, David (MI)	D	185
Ferguson, Mark (IL)	TS	1013	Fivush, Barbara (MD)	PNep	709
Ferguson, Ronald (OH)	S	975	Fix, R Jobe (AL)	PlS	778
Fernhoff, Paul (GA)	CG	154	Flachsbart, Keith (CA)	TS	1021
Ferrante, F Michael (CA)	PM	639	Flake, Alan (PA)	PS	726
Ferrara, James (MI)	PHO	699	Flamm, Eugene (NY)	NS	428
Ferrell, Linda (CA)	Path	656	Flamm, Scott (OH)	DR	894
Ferrendelli, James (TX)	N	484	Flanigan, D Preston (CA)	VascS	1075
Ferriero, Donna (CA)	ChiN	147	Flanigan, Robert (IL)	U	1046
Ferzli, George (NY)	S	960	Flanigan, Timothy (RI)	Inf	362
Fessler, Richard (IL)	NS	438	Flatow, Evan (NY)	OrS	565
Fewkes, Jessica (MA)	D	177	Fleischer, David (AZ)	Ge	237
Figlin, Robert (CA)	Onc	343	Fleischer, Norman (NY)	EDM	199
Files, Joe (MS)	Hem	298	Fleisher, Gary (MA)	PCCM	679
Filip, Stanley (NC)	ObG	510	Fleshman, James (MO)	CRS	168
Filipi, Charles (NE)	S	981	Fletcher, Christopher (MA)	Path	644
Filley, Christopher (CO)	N	483	Fletcher, Eugene (IN)	Pul	851
Filly, Roy (CA)	DR	895	Flickinger, John (PA)	RadRO	870
Finan, Michael (AL)	GO	266	Flinn, Ian (TN)	Onc	323

Alphabetical Listing of Doctors

Name	Specialty	Pg	Name	Specialty	Pg
Flint, Lewis (FL)	S	968	Francisco, Gerard (TX)	PMR	763
Flomenberg, Neal (PA)	Onc	313	Frank, Erica (GA)	PrM	797
Flowers, Franklin (FL)	D	183	Frank, Ian (PA)	Inf	363
Flowers, Robert (HI)	PlS	788	Franklin, Morris (TX)	S	983
Flynn, Harry (FL)	Oph	534	Franks, Andrew (NY)	D	179
Flynn, John (NY)	Oph	526	Fraser, Charles (TX)	TS	1018
Flynn, Joseph (WA)	PNep	712	Fraser, Lionel (MS)	U	1040
Flynn, Michael (KY)	S	968	Frassica, Frank J (MD)	OrS	566
Flynn, Patrick (MN)	Hem	300	Frazee, John (CA)	NS	447
Flynn, Timothy (FL)	VascS	1071	Frazier, Oscar (TX)	TS	1019
Fodor, Peter (CA)	PlS	788	Frederiksen, James (IL)	TS	1013
Foglia, Robert (TX)	PS	732	Freedman, Michael (NY)	Ger	249
Foley, Carmel (NY)	ChAP	823	Freedman, Robert (CO)	Psyc	812
Foley, Eugene (VA)	CRS	166	Freedman, Sharon (NC)	Oph	534
Foley, Kathleen (NY)	PM	635	Freeman, Gregory (TX)	Cv	114
Follansbee, William (PA)	Cv	99	Freeman, Leonard (NY)	NuM	500
Follen-Mitchell, Michele (TX)	GO	271	Freeman, Theodore (TX)	A&I	87
Fonarow, Gregg (CA)	Cv	116	Freeman, Thomas (FL)	NS	433
Fong, Yuman (NY)	S	960	Freemark, Michael (NC)	PEn	683
Fontana, Gregory (CA)	TS	1021	Freischlag, Julie (MD)	VascS	1069
Forastiere, Arlene (MD)	Onc	313	French, Jacqueline (PA)	N	465
Forbess, Joseph (TX)	TS	1018	Fricker, Frederick (FL)	PCd	674
Ford, Carol Ann (NC)	AM	78	Fried, Guy (PA)	PMR	757
Ford, Charles (WI)	Oto	616	Fried, Marvin P (NY)	Oto	604
Ford, Henri (CA)	PS	733	Friedberg, Joseph (PA)	TS	1001
Ford, James (CA)	Onc	343	Frieden, Ilona (CA)	D	189
Fordtran, John (TX)	Ge	237	Friedlaender, Gary (CT)	OrS	560
Forman, Jeffrey (MI)	RadRO	875	Friedland, Jack (AZ)	PlS	785
Forman, Stephen (CA)	Hem	305	Friedman, Aaron (RI)	PNep	709
Formenti, Silvia (NY)	RadRO	870	Friedman, Allan (NC)	NS	433
Fornari, Victor (NY)	ChAP	823	Friedman, Barry (CA)	Psyc	815
Forsmark, Christopher (FL)	Ge	226	Friedman, Ellen M (TX)	PO	717
Forster, Richard (FL)	Oph	534	Friedman, Henry S (NC)	PHO	697
Fortenberry, J Dennis (IN)	AM	78	Friedman, Lawrence (MA)	Ge	216
Fossella, Frank (TX)	Onc	337	Friedman, Lloyd (CT)	Pul	841
Fost, Norman (WI)	Ped	666	Friedman, Matthew (VT)	Psyc	802
Foster, Carol (UT)	PEn	685	Friedman, Michael (IL)	Oto	616
Foster, Charles (MA)	Oph	522	Friedman, Nancy (NC)	PEn	683
Foster, Richard (IN)	U	1046	Friedman, Richard (TX)	PCd	677
Foucar, M (NM)	Path	654	Friedman, Stuart (FL)	A&I	84
Fowl, Richard (AZ)	VascS	1074	Frigoletto, Fredric (MA)	MF	386
Fowler, Dennis (NY)	S	960	Frim, David M (IL)	NS	438
Fowler, Wesley (NC)	GO	266	Fritz, Gregory (RI)	ChAP	820
Fox, Harold (MD)	MF	388	Fritz, Marc (NC)	RE	918
Fox, Jacob (IL)	N	477	Fronek, Jan (CA)	SM	949
Fox, Kevin (PA)	Onc	313	Frontera, Walter (MA)	PMR	756
Fox, Peter (TX)	N	484	Frost, Frederick (OH)	PMR	761
Fox, Roger (FL)	A&I	84	Fruchtman, Steven M (NY)	Hem	295
Fracasso, Paula M (MO)	Onc	330	Fry, Robert (PA)	CRS	165
Fraker, Douglas (PA)	S	961	Fu, Freddie (PA)	OrS	566
France, Thomas (WI)	Oph	539	Fuchs, Eugene (OR)	U	1054
Frances, Richard (NY)	AdP	818	Fuchs, Wayne (NY)	Oph	526

Name	Specialty	Pg	Name	Specialty	Pg
Fuhrman, Bradley (NY)	PCCM	679	Garth, William (AL)	SM	947
Fuhrman, Carl (PA)	DR	891	Garvin, James (NY)	PHO	694
Fulkerson, William (NC)	Pul	848	Garvin, Kevin L (NE)	OrS	583
Fullerton, David (CO)	TS	1017	Gater, David (VA)	PMR	759
Fung, John (OH)	S	975	Gaynor, Ellen (IL)	Hem	300
Funk, Gerry (IA)	Oto	616	Gearhart, John (MD)	U	1033
Furlan, Anthony (OH)	N	477	Gebhardt, Mark (MA)	OrS	560
Furukawa, Satoshi (PA)	TS	1002	Geffner, Mitchell (CA)	PEn	686
Fuselier, Harold (LA)	U	1052	Gefter, Warren (PA)	DR	891
Fuster, Valentin (NY)	Cv	99	Gelberman, Richard (MO)	HS	285
			Gelenberg, Alan (AZ)	Psyc	813
			Gelfand, Erwin (CO)	PA&I	669

G

Name	Specialty	Pg	Name	Specialty	Pg
Gaasterland, Douglas (MD)	Oph	526	Geller, Kenneth (CA)	PO	717
Gabbard, Glen (TX)	Psyc	813	Gelmann, Edward P (DC)	Onc	314
Gabbe, Steven (TN)	MF	389	Geltman, Edward (MO)	Cv	109
Gabram, Sheryl (GA)	S	969	Gendelman, Seymour (NY)	N	465
Gabrilove, Janice (NY)	Onc	314	Genden, Eric (NY)	Oto	604
Gagel, Robert (TX)	EDM	208	Gentile, Ronald (NY)	Oph	526
Gagner, Michel (NY)	S	961	Georgeson, Keith (AL)	PS	728
Gaissert, Henning (MA)	TS	998	Georgiade, Gregory (NC)	PlS	778
Galandiuk, Susan (KY)	CRS	166	Gerdes, Hans (NY)	Ge	219
Galante, Jorge (IL)	OrS	578	Geronemus, Roy (NY)	D	179
Galanter, Marc (NY)	AdP	818	Gershenson, David (TX)	GO	271
Galati, Joseph (TX)	Ge	237	Gershwin, Merrill (CA)	Rhu	940
Galetta, Steven (PA)	N	465	Gerson, Stanton (OH)	Onc	331
Galland, Leopold (NY)	IM	378	Gertz, Morris (MN)	Hem	300
Gallico, G Gregory (MA)	PlS	770	Geschwind, Jean (MD)	VIR	903
Gallin, Pamela (NY)	Oph	526	Gewertz, Bruce (CA)	VascS	1075
Galloway, Aubrey (NY)	TS	1002	Gewirtz, Alan (PA)	Hem	295
Gambardella, Ralph (CA)	SM	949	Gewitz, Michael (NY)	PCd	672
Gambert, Steven (MD)	Ger	249	Gewolb, Ira (MI)	NP	404
Gambetti, Pierluigi (OH)	Path	652	Gewurz, Anita (IL)	A&I	86
Gamelli, Richard (IL)	S	975	Geyer, Charles (PA)	Onc	314
Gandara, David (CA)	Onc	343	Geyer, J Russell (WA)	PHO	703
Gandy, Winston (GA)	Cv	105	Gharagozloo, Farid (DC)	TS	1002
Gang, Eli (CA)	CE	123	Giangola, Gary (NY)	VascS	1069
Ganguli, Rohan (PA)	Psyc	806	Giannotta, Steven (CA)	NS	447
Gantz, Bruce (IA)	Oto	616	Gianoli, Gerard (LA)	Oto	622
Ganz, Patricia (CA)	Onc	343	Gianopoulos, John (IL)	MF	390
Garber, Judy E (MA)	Onc	308	Giardina, Patricia (NY)	PHO	694
Garcia-Prats, Joseph (TX)	NP	405	Gibbons, Gary (MA)	VascS	1066
Garden, Jerome (IL)	D	185	Gibbons, Raymond (MN)	Cv	109
Gardin, Julius (MI)	Cv	108	Gibbs, John (NY)	S	961
Gardner, Gregory (WA)	Rhu	939	Gibbs, Ronald (CO)	MF	392
Garfin, Steven (CA)	OrS	587	Gibralter, Richard (NY)	Oph	526
Garin, Eduardo (FL)	PNep	710	Gilbert, Mark (TX)	N	484
Garner, Warren (CA)	PlS	789	Gilchrest, Barbara (MA)	D	177
Garnick, Marc B (MA)	Onc	308	Gill, Harcharan (CA)	U	1055
Garrett, William (NC)	OrS	575	Gill, Inderbir (OH)	U	1046
Garrity, Edward (IL)	Pul	851	Gillette, Paul (TX)	PCd	677
Garst, Jennifer (NC)	Onc	323	Gilman, Sid (MI)	N	477
			Gilsanz, Vicente (CA)	DR	896

Alphabetical Listing of Doctors

Name	Specialty	Pg	Name	Specialty	Pg
Gingold, Bruce (NY)	CRS	165	Goldberg, Melvyn (PA)	TS	1002
Ginsberg, David (CA)	U	1055	Goldberg, Michael (IL)	Ge	229
Ginsberg, Gregory (PA)	Ge	219	Goldberg, Morton (MD)	Oph	526
Ginsburg, Howard (NY)	PS	726	Goldberg, Richard (NC)	Onc	323
Ginzler, Ellen (NY)	Rhu	930	Goldberg, Victor (OH)	OrS	579
Girardi, Leonard (NY)	TS	1002	Goldblum, John (OH)	Path	652
Gitlin, Michael (CA)	Psyc	815	Goldman, Allan (FL)	Pul	848
Gittes, George (PA)	PS	726	Goldner, Richard (NC)	OrS	575
Gittler, Michelle (IL)	PMR	761	Goldsmith, Ari (NY)	PO	714
Giuliano, Armando (CA)	S	987	Goldsmith, Stanley (NY)	NuM	500
Giustra, Lawrence (GA)	Psyc	810	Goldstein, Larry (NC)	N	473
Givner, Laurence (NC)	PInf	706	Goldstein, Lori (PA)	Onc	314
Gizzi, Martin (NJ)	N	465	Goldstein, Marc (NY)	U	1033
Glader, Bertil (CA)	PHO	703	Goldstein, Martin (NY)	ObG	509
Glaser, Joel (FL)	Oph	534	Goldstein, Richard (KY)	S	969
Glashow, Jonathan (NY)	OrS	566	Goldstein, Wayne (IL)	OrS	579
Glaspy, John (CA)	Onc	343	Golub, Richard (FL)	CRS	167
Glass, Jon (PA)	N	465	Gomella, Leonard (PA)	U	1033
Glass, Jonathan (GA)	N	472	Gomery, Pablo (MA)	U	1030
Glassberg, Kenneth (NY)	U	1033	Gomes, Antoinette (CA)	VIR	908
Glassford, David (TN)	TS	1008	Gomes, J Anthony (NY)	CE	119
Glatstein, Eli (PA)	RadRO	870	Gong, Henry (CA)	Pul	858
Glick, John (PA)	Onc	314	Gonik, Bernard (MI)	ObG	512
Glick, Philip (NY)	PS	726	Gonzales, Edmond (TX)	U	1052
Glickel, Steven (NY)	HS	281	Goodgold, Albert (NY)	N	466
Gliklich, Jerry (NY)	Cv	99	Goodin, Douglas (CA)	N	488
Gliklich, Richard (MA)	Oto	601	Goodman, Annekathryn (MA)	GO	262
Glisson, Bonnie (TX)	Onc	337	Goodman, Dennis (CA)	Cv	116
Glode, L (CO)	Onc	336	Goodman, Lawrence (WI)	DR	894
Glogau, Richard (CA)	D	189	Goodman, Neil (FL)	RE	918
Glombicki, Alan (TX)	Ge	237	Goodman, Robert (NJ)	RadRO	870
Gloviczki, Peter (MN)	VascS	1072	Goodman, Robert (NY)	NS	428
Gluck, Joan (FL)	A&I	85	Goodman, Stuart (CA)	OrS	587
Gluck, Paul (FL)	ObG	510	Goodrich, James (NY)	NS	428
Gluck, Stephen (CA)	Nep	419	Goodson, William (CA)	S	987
Gluckman, Gordon (IL)	U	1046	Goodwin, Scott (CA)	VIR	908
Gluckman, Jack (OH)	Oto	616	Goodwin, W Jarrard (FL)	Oto	611
Gochfeld, Michael (NJ)	OM	796	Gorbien, Martin (IL)	Ger	251
Gockerman, Jon (NC)	Onc	323	Gordon, Leo I (IL)	Hem	301
Godine, John (MA)	EDM	196	Gordon, Marsha (NY)	D	179
Godwin, John (IL)	Hem	301	Gorensek, Margaret (FL)	Inf	367
Godzik, Cathleen (CA)	HS	288	Gorevic, Peter (NY)	Rhu	930
Goebel, Joel (MO)	Oto	617	Gorfine, Stephen (NY)	CRS	165
Goetz, Christopher (IL)	N	478	Gorin, Michael (PA)	Oph	527
Goff, Barbara (WA)	GO	272	Gorovoy, Mark (FL)	Oph	534
Goff, Donald (MA)	Psyc	802	Gostout, Christopher (MN)	Ge	230
Goitz, Henry (MI)	OrS	579	Gottdiener, John (MD)	Cv	99
Golbe, Lawrence (NJ)	N	465	Gottlieb, Stephen (MD)	Cv	99
Gold, Alan (NY)	PlS	773	Gould, K Lance (TX)	Cv	114
Gold, Scott (NY)	Oto	604	Goulet, Robert (IN)	S	975
Goldberg, Jack (NJ)	Hem	296	Gourley, Mark (MD)	Rhu	930
Goldberg, James (CA)	MF	393	Govindarajan, Sugantha (CA)	Path	656

Name	Specialty	Pg	Name	Specialty	Pg
Gower, Roland (AK)	S	987	Gregory, Richard (FL)	PlS	778
Gracey, Douglas (MN)	Pul	851	Gregory, Stephanie (IL)	Hem	301
Grado, Gordon (AZ)	RadRO	878	Greiner, Carl (NE)	Psyc	812
Grady, M Sean (PA)	NS	428	Greipp, Philip R (MN)	Hem	301
Graf, Ben (WI)	OrS	579	Greisler, Howard (IL)	VascS	1073
Graham, John (CA)	CG	157	Grelsamer, Ronald (NY)	OrS	566
Graham, Mark (NC)	Onc	323	Gress, Daryl (VA)	N	473
Graham, Michael (AZ)	PHO	702	Grever, Michael (OH)	Hem	301
Graham, Thomas (MD)	HS	281	Grey, Douglas (CA)	VascS	1076
Graham-Pole, John (FL)	PHO	697	Gribetz, Michael (NY)	U	1034
Gralow, Julie (WA)	Onc	344	Griepp, Randall (NY)	TS	1002
Grammer, Leslie (IL)	A&I	86	Grier, Holcombe (MA)	PHO	692
Granet, David (CA)	Oph	549	Griffin, John (MD)	N	466
Granstein, Richard (NY)	D	179	Griffith, Bartley (MD)	TS	1003
Grant, Clive S (MN)	S	975	Grifo, James (NY)	RE	916
Grant, Richard (OH)	OrS	579	Grimes, Pearl (CA)	D	189
Grasso, Michael (NY)	U	1034	Griswold, John (TX)	S	983
Graver, L Michael (NY)	TS	1002	Grody, Wayne (CA)	CG	157
Graves, Michael (CA)	N	488	Groene, Linda (FL)	Ger	250
Gravett, Michael (WA)	MF	393	Grogan, Thomas (AZ)	Path	654
Greco, F Anthony (TN)	Onc	324	Groopman, Jerome E (MA)	Hem	294
Greden, John (MI)	Psyc	811	Grosfeld, Jay L (IN)	PS	730
Green, Barth (FL)	NS	433	Grosh, William (VA)	Onc	324
Green, Carmen R (MI)	PM	637	Gross, Charles (VA)	Oto	611
Green, Daniel (NY)	PHO	694	Gross, Ian (CT)	NP	400
Green, Howard (FL)	D	183	Grossbard, Michael (NY)	Onc	314
Green, Peter (NY)	Ge	219	Grossberg, George (MO)	GerPsy	830
Green, Richard (NY)	VascS	1069	Grossi, Eugene (NY)	TS	1003
Green, William (MD)	Oph	527	Grossman, John (CO)	PlS	784
Greenberg, Harly (NY)	Pul	843	Grossman, Melanie (NY)	D	179
Greenberg, Harry (MI)	N	478	Grossman, Robert (NY)	NRad	897
Greenberg, Mark (NY)	Cv	99	Grossman, Stuart (MD)	Onc	314
Greenberg, Richard (PA)	U	1034	Grossniklaus, Hans (GA)	Oph	534
Greenberger, Paul (IL)	A&I	86	Grotta, James (TX)	N	484
Greene, Clarence (MO)	NS	438	Grotting, James (AL)	PlS	778
Greene, Frederick (NC)	S	969	Grubb, Blair (OH)	Cv	109
Greene, Graham (AR)	U	1052	Grubb, Robert (MO)	NS	438
Greene, Loren (NY)	EDM	199	Gruber, Scott (MI)	S	975
Greene, Michael (MA)	MF	386	Gruchalla, Rebecca (TX)	A&I	88
Greene, Thomas (FL)	HS	283	Grum, Cyril (MI)	Pul	851
Greenhalgh, David (CA)	S	987	Grundfast, Kenneth (MA)	Oto	601
Greenson, Joel K (MI)	Path	652	Grunfeld, Lawrence (NY)	RE	916
Greenspan, Stanley (MD)	ChAP	823	Gruss, Joseph (WA)	PlS	789
Greenspan, Susan (PA)	EDM	199	Guerrant, Richard (VA)	Inf	367
Greenwald, Blaine (NY)	GerPsy	828	Gugenheim, Joseph (TX)	OrS	584
Greenwald, Bruce (MD)	Ge	220	Guidry, George (LA)	Pul	856
Greenwald, Mark (IL)	Oph	539	Guillem, Jose (NY)	CRS	165
Greenway, Hubert T (CA)	D	189	Guilleminault, Christian (CA)	Psyc	815
Greenwood, Robert (NC)	ChiN	144	Gujral, Saroj (MN)	U	1046
Greer, Benjamin (WA)	GO	273	Gumprecht, Jeffrey (NY)	Inf	364
Greer, John P (TN)	Hem	298	Gunasekaran, T S (IL)	PGe	689
Greganti, Mac Andrew (NC)	Ger	250	Gunderson, Leonard (AZ)	RadRO	878

Alphabetical Listing of Doctors

Name	Specialty	Pg	Name	Specialty	Pg
Gundry, Steven (CA)	TS	1021	Hammill, Stephen (MN)	CE	121
Gunter, Jack (TX)	PlS	786	Hammon, John (NC)	TS	1008
Gupta, Prabodh (PA)	Path	646	Hammond, Charles (NC)	RE	918
Gutai, James (MI)	PEn	684	Hammond, Dennis (MI)	PlS	782
Guthikonda, Murali (MI)	NS	439	Hamra, Sameer (TX)	PlS	786
Guthrie, Barton (AL)	NS	434	Hamvas, Aaron (MO)	NP	404
Gutierrez, Francisco (IL)	NS	439	Hanauer, Stephen (IL)	Ge	230
Gutin, Philip (NY)	NS	428	Handa, James (MD)	Oph	527
Guyton, David (MD)	Oph	527	Hande, Kenneth (TN)	Onc	324
			Handy, John (OR)	TS	1021

H

Name	Specialty	Pg	Name	Specialty	Pg
			Hanel, Douglas (WA)	HS	288
Haas, Richard (CA)	ChiN	148	Haney, Arthur (IL)	RE	920
Haas, Steven (NY)	OrS	566	Hanifin, Jon (OR)	D	189
Hackney, David (MA)	NRad	896	Hanke, C William (IN)	D	185
Haddad, Joseph (NY)	PO	714	Hankins, Gary (TX)	MF	393
Hadler, Nortin (NC)	Rhu	934	Hankinson, Hal (NM)	NS	444
Hadley, Mark (AL)	NS	434	Hanks, John (VA)	S	969
Haffty, Bruce (NJ)	RadRO	870	Hanley, Frank (CA)	TS	1021
Hafler, David (MA)	N	461	Hann, Lucy (NY)	DR	891
Hagan, Kevin (TN)	PlS	779	Hanna, Ehab (TX)	Oto	623
Hager, W David (KY)	ObG	510	Hannafin, Jo (NY)	OrS	566
Hahn, Bevra (CA)	Rhu	940	Hansen, Kimberley (NC)	VascS	1071
Hahn, Stephen (PA)	RadRO	870	Hansen, Nora (IL)	S	976
Haid, Regis (GA)	NS	434	Hansen, Ronald (AZ)	D	188
Haig, Andrew (MI)	PMR	761	Hansen, Sigvard (WA)	OrS	587
Haik, Barrett (TN)	Oph	534	Hansen-Flaschen, John (PA)	Pul	843
Hain, Timothy (IL)	N	478	Hanson, Laura (NC)	Ger	250
Haines, Kathleen (NJ)	PRhu	722	Haque, Waheedul (TX)	Psyc	814
Hait, William (NJ)	Onc	314	Har-El, Gady (NY)	Oto	605
Hakaim, Albert (FL)	VascS	1071	Harbaugh, Robert (PA)	NS	429
Halberg, Francine (CA)	RadRO	880	Harber, Philip (CA)	OM	796
Haley, Elliott (VA)	N	473	Harden, R Norman (IL)	PM	637
Halff, Glenn (TX)	S	984	Hardesty, Robert (CA)	PlS	789
Hall, Jesse (IL)	Pul	851	Hardy, Mark (NY)	S	961
Hall, Lisabeth (NY)	Oph	527	Hare, Joshua (FL)	Cv	105
Halle, Jan (NC)	RadRO	873	Hargrove, W Clark (PA)	TS	1003
Haller, Daniel (PA)	Onc	315	Harkema, James (MI)	S	976
Hallett, John (SC)	VascS	1071	Harman, Eloise (FL)	Pul	848
Hallisey, Michael (CT)	VIR	902	Harmon, William (MA)	PNep	709
Halmi, Katherine (NY)	Psyc	806	Harnsberger, Jeffrey (NH)	CRS	164
Halperin, Jonathan (NY)	Cv	100	Harper, Richard (TX)	NS	444
Halpern, Allan (NY)	D	179	Harpole, David (NC)	TS	1009
Halpern, Howard (IL)	RadRO	875	Harrell, James (TX)	TS	1019
Halter, Jeffrey (MI)	Ger	251	Harrington, Elizabeth (NY)	VascS	1069
Haluska, Frank (MA)	Onc	308	Harris, Jay (MA)	RadRO	868
Haluszka, Oleh (PA)	Ge	220	Harris, Jeffrey (CA)	Oto	625
Hamilton, Stanley (TX)	Path	654	Harris, Nancy (MA)	Path	644
Hamilton, William (NY)	OrS	566	Harrison, John (NC)	Cv	105
Hammar, Samuel (WA)	Path	657	Harrison, Louis (NY)	RadRO	871
Hammer, Glenn (NY)	Inf	364	Harrison, Michael (CA)	PS	733
Hammer, Scott (NY)	Inf	364	Harsh, Griffith (CA)	NS	447
			Hart, Robert (TX)	N	484

Name	Specialty	Pg	Name	Specialty	Pg
Hartman, Barry (NY)	Inf	364	Herbst, Roy (TX)	Onc	338
Hartmann, Lynn (MN)	Onc	331	Herling, Irving (PA)	Cv	100
Hartmann, Rene (FL)	CRS	167	Herman, John (MA)	Psyc	802
Harty, James (KY)	U	1040	Herman, Terence (OK)	RadRO	878
Haskal, Ziv (NY)	VIR	903	Herman, William (MI)	EDM	205
Hassenbusch, Samuel (TX)	NS	444	Heros, Roberto (FL)	NS	434
Hastings, Hill (IN)	HS	285	Heroux, Alain (IL)	Cv	109
Hatch, Kenneth (AZ)	GO	271	Herr, Harry (NY)	U	1034
Haughey, Bruce (MO)	Oto	617	Herring, Stanley (WA)	PMR	764
Haughton, Victor (WI)	NRad	899	Herrmann, Howard (PA)	IC	124
Hauser, Stephen (CA)	N	488	Herrmann, Virginia (SC)	S	969
Hausman, Michael (NY)	OrS	567	Hersh, Peter (NJ)	Oph	527
Hawes, Robert (SC)	Ge	226	Hershman, Elliott (NY)	SM	946
Hawkins, Irvin (FL)	VIR	904	Hertz, Marshall (MN)	Pul	851
Hayani, Ammar (IL)	PHO	699	Hertzig, Margaret (NY)	ChAP	823
Hayashi, Robert (MO)	PHO	699	Herzenberg, John (MD)	OrS	567
Hayden, Richard (AZ)	Oto	623	Herzog, David (MA)	ChAP	821
Hayes, Daniel (MI)	Onc	331	Herzog, Thomas (NY)	GO	264
Hayes, David (MN)	CE	121	Hess, David (GA)	N	473
Hayes, Sharonne (MN)	Cv	109	Hess, J Bruce (FL)	Oph	534
Hayman, James (MI)	RadRO	875	Hester, T Roderick (GA)	PlS	779
Haynes, Johnson (AL)	Pul	848	Heston, Jerry (TN)	ChAP	825
Healey, John (NY)	OrS	567	Heuer, Dale (WI)	Oph	539
Healy, Gerald (MA)	PO	713	Heyman, Melvin (CA)	PGe	691
Heber, David (CA)	EDM	210	Hibbard, Judith (IL)	MF	390
Hebert, James (VT)	S	954	Hicks, Wesley (NY)	Oto	605
Heck, Louis (AL)	Rhu	934	Hidalgo, David (NY)	PlS	773
Hecox, Kurt (WI)	N	478	Hiesiger, Emile (NY)	N	466
Hedges, Thomas (MA)	Oph	522	Higashida, Randall (CA)	NRad	902
Heffner, John (OR)	Pul	858	Hijazi, Ziyad (IL)	PCd	676
Heffner, Linda (MA)	MF	386	Hilden, Joanne (IN)	PHO	699
Heidary, Dariush (GA)	TS	1009	Hilfiker, Mary (CA)	PS	733
Heilman, Carl (MA)	NS	425	Hilger, Peter (MN)	Oto	617
Heilman, Kenneth (FL)	N	473	Hilibrand, Alan (PA)	OrS	567
Heimburger, Douglas (AL)	IM	380	Hill, Ivor (NC)	PGe	688
Heitmiller, Richard (MD)	TS	1003	Hill, Joseph (NH)	RE	914
Helderman, J Harold (TN)	Nep	414	Hillebrand, Donald (CA)	Ge	239
Helfet, David (NY)	OrS	567	Hillemeier, A Craig (PA)	PGe	687
Hellenbrand, William (NY)	PCd	672	Hirsch, Barry (PA)	Oto	605
Helman, Lee (MD)	PHO	694	Hirsch, Joshua (MA)	NRad	896
Hemming, Alan (FL)	S	969	Hirschfeld, Robert (TX)	Psyc	814
Henderson, Victor (CA)	N	488	Ho, Sherwin (IL)	SM	948
Hendricks-Munoz, Karen (NY)	NP	401	Hobel, Calvin (CA)	MF	393
Hendrickson, Michael (CA)	Path	657	Hobson, Robert (NJ)	VascS	1069
Heney, Niall (MA)	U	1030	Hochberg, Marc (MD)	Rhu	930
Henke, David Carroll (NC)	Pul	848	Hochman, Judith (NY)	Cv	100
Henry, Timothy (MN)	IC	127	Hochschuler, Stephen (TX)	OrS	584
Henschke, Claudia (NY)	DR	891	Hochster, Howard (NY)	Onc	315
Hensinger, Robert (MI)	OrS	579	Hodge, Charles (NY)	NS	429
Hensle, Terry (NY)	U	1034	Hodges, David (TX)	Ge	237
Hentz, Vincent (CA)	HS	288	Hodgson, Kim (IL)	VascS	1073
Heppell, Jacques (AZ)	CRS	171	Hoefflin, Steven (CA)	PlS	789

Alphabetical Listing of Doctors

I

Name	Specialty	Pg	Name	Specialty	Pg
Iliff, Nicholas Taylor (MD)	Oph	527	Janicak, Philip (IL)	Psyc	811
Ilowite, Norman (NY)	PRhu	722	Janjan, Nora (TX)	RadRO	878
Imber, Gerald (NY)	PlS	774	Jankovic, Joseph (TX)	N	485
Imbriglia, Joseph (PA)	HS	281	Jaramillo, Diego (PA)	DR	891
Infante, Ernesto (TX)	N	485	Jarow, Jonathan (MD)	U	1034
Ingle, James (MN)	Onc	331	Jeevanandam, Valluvan (IL)	TS	1013
Inglis, Andrew (WA)	PO	718	Jenike, Michael (MA)	Psyc	802
Ingram, David (NC)	PInf	706	Jenkins, Herman (CO)	Oto	621
Inra, Lawrence (NY)	Cv	100	Jenkins, Roger (MA)	S	955
Interian, Alberto (FL)	CE	120	Jenkinson, Stephen (TX)	Pul	856
Inzucchi, Silvio (CT)	EDM	196	Jennings, Russell (MA)	PS	724
Ipp, Eli (CA)	EDM	210	Jensen, Donald (IL)	Ge	230
Irby, Pierce (NC)	U	1041	Jensen, Mary (VA)	NRad	899
Irvine, John (CA)	Oph	549	Jensen, Michael (MN)	EDM	205
Irwin, Charles (CA)	AM	79	Jenson, Hal (MA)	PInf	705
Irwin, Richard (MA)	Pul	841	Jett, James (MN)	Pul	852
Isaacs, Claudine (DC)	Onc	315	Jewell, Mark (OR)	PlS	789
Isaacson, Keith (MA)	RE	914	Jho, Hae-Dong (PA)	NS	429
Isaacson, Steven (NY)	RadRO	871	Jillella, Anand (GA)	Onc	324
Iseman, Michael (CO)	Pul	855	Jimenez, David (TX)	NS	444
Isenberg, Sherwin (CA)	Oph	549	Jobe, Alan (OH)	NP	404
Iskandrian, Ami (AL)	Cv	105	Jobe, Frank (CA)	SM	949
Ismail, Mahmoud (IL)	MF	391	Jobst, Barbara (NH)	N	461
Isom, O Wayne (NY)	TS	1003	John, Thomas (IL)	Oph	539
Israel, Mark (NH)	PHO	692	Johnson, Allen (CA)	Cv	117
Israel, Philip (GA)	S	969	Johnson, Bruce (VA)	Pul	849
Ivanhoe, Cindy (TX)	PMR	763	Johnson, Bruce (MA)	Onc	308
Iwach, Andrew (CA)	Oph	549	Johnson, Calvin (LA)	Oto	623
			Johnson, Carl (MD)	OrS	568
			Johnson, Darren (KY)	OrS	575

J

Name	Specialty	Pg	Name	Specialty	Pg
			Johnson, David (TN)	Onc	324
Jaafar, Mohamad (DC)	Oph	528	Johnson, Jonas (PA)	Oto	605
Jackler, Robert (CA)	Oto	625	Johnson, Kenneth (MD)	N	466
Jackman, Warren (OK)	CE	123	Johnson, Maryl (WI)	Cv	109
Jackson, Gilchrist (TX)	S	984	Johnson, Matthew (IN)	VIR	906
Jackson, Richard (AR)	PS	733	Johnson, Paula (MA)	Cv	95
Jacob, Molly (IL)	Ped	666	Johnson, Ronald (PA)	S	961
Jacobs, Alice (MA)	IC	123	Johnson, Stephen (CO)	NS	443
Jacobs, Charlotte (CA)	Onc	344	Johnson, Timothy (MI)	MF	391
Jacobs, Laurence (IL)	RE	921	Johnson, Timothy (MI)	D	185
Jacobs, Richard (AR)	PInf	708	Johnson, Warren (NY)	Inf	364
Jacobs, Thomas (NY)	EDM	199	Johnston, Carolyn Marie (MI)	GO	269
Jacobson, Ira (NY)	Ge	220	Johnston, James (PA)	Nep	412
Jacoby, David (OR)	Pul	858	Johr, Robert (FL)	D	183
Jaffe, Allan (MN)	Cv	109	Jokl, Peter (CT)	OrS	560
Jaffe, Elaine (MD)	Path	646	Jonas, Adam (CA)	CG	158
Jaffe, Kenneth (WA)	PMR	764	Jonas, Richard (DC)	TS	1003
Jahan, Thierry (CA)	Onc	344	Jones, David (VA)	TS	1009
Jahrsdoerfer, Robert (VA)	PO	715	Jones, Howard (TN)	GO	267
Jain, Subhash (NY)	PM	635	Jones, Jacqueline (NY)	PO	714
James, William (PA)	D	179	Jones, Kenneth (CA)	Ped	667
Jamieson, Stuart (CA)	TS	1021	Jones, Marilyn (CA)	CG	158

Alphabetical Listing of Doctors

Name	Specialty	Pg	Name	Specialty	Pg
Jones, Neil (CA)	HS	288	Kaplan, Lawrence (CA)	Onc	344
Jones, Paul (IL)	Oto	617	Kaplan, Sheldon (TX)	PInf	708
Jones, Stephen (TX)	Onc	338	Kaplan, Stanley (TN)	Rhu	934
Jordan, Barry (NY)	N	466	Kaplan, Steven (NY)	U	1034
Jordan, Gerald (VA)	U	1041	Kappy, Michael (CO)	PEn	685
Jordan, Stanley (CA)	PNep	712	Karas, Spero (GA)	OrS	575
Jorizzo, Joseph (NC)	D	183	Karlan, Beth Young (CA)	GO	273
Joseph, David (AL)	U	1041	Karp, Daniel (TX)	Onc	338
Joseph, Gregory (NC)	NRad	899	Karp, Judith (MD)	Onc	315
Josephson, David (IN)	N	478	Karpeh, Martin (NY)	S	961
Josephson, Jordan (NY)	Oto	605	Karram, Mickey (OH)	ObG	512
Josephson, Mark (MA)	Cv	95	Karrer, Frederick (CO)	PS	732
Josephson, Michelle (IL)	Nep	415	Kartush, Jack (MI)	Oto	617
Joyce, Michael (OH)	OrS	580	Karwande, Shreekanth (UT)	TS	1017
Judelson, Debra (CA)	Cv	117	Kase, Carlos (MA)	N	461
Judy, Kevin (PA)	NS	429	Kashtan, Clifford (MN)	PNep	711
Jupiter, Jesse (MA)	OrS	561	Kasinath, Balakuntalam (TX)	Nep	418
			Kasiske, Bertram (MN)	Nep	415

K

Name	Specialty	Pg	Name	Specialty	Pg
			Kass, Evan (MI)	U	1046
Kadota, Richard (CA)	PHO	703	Kassam, Amin (PA)	NS	429
Kaelin, William (MA)	Onc	308	Kasser, James (MA)	OrS	561
Kagan, Richard (OH)	S	976	Katner, Harold (GA)	Inf	367
Kahan, Barry (TX)	S	984	Katowitz, James (PA)	Oph	528
Kahn, Leonard (NY)	Path	646	Kattan, Meyer (NY)	PPul	718
Kahrilas, Peter (IL)	Ge	230	Kattwinkel, John (VA)	NP	403
Kaiser, Harold (MN)	A&I	86	Katz, Aaron (NY)	U	1035
Kaiser, Larry (PA)	TS	1003	Katz, Nevin (DC)	TS	1004
Kalaycio, Matt (OH)	Onc	331	Katz, Philip (PA)	Ge	220
Kaliner, Michael (MD)	A&I	83	Katz, Robert (IL)	Rhu	936
Kallmes, David (MN)	NRad	900	Katz, Robert L (OH)	PO	716
Kalloo, Anthony (MD)	Ge	220	Katz, Stephen (MD)	D	179
Kamani, Naynesh (DC)	PA&I	667	Katz, Warren (PA)	Rhu	930
Kamdar, Vikram (CA)	EDM	210	Katzen, Barry (FL)	VIR	905
Kamen, Barton A (NJ)	PHO	694	Katzenstein, Anna-Luise (NY)	Path	646
Kamer, Frank (CA)	Oto	625	Kaufman, Bruce (WI)	NS	439
Kamholz, Stephan (NY)	Pul	843	Kaufman, Francine (CA)	PEn	686
Kaminski, Mark (MI)	Onc	331	Kaufman, Herbert (LA)	Oph	545
Kampman, Kyle (PA)	AdP	818	Kaufman, Howard (NY)	S	962
Kanal, Emanuel (PA)	DR	891	Kaufman, John (OR)	VIR	908
Kanda, Louis (DC)	TS	1003	Kaufman, Paul (WI)	Oph	539
Kandarpa, Krishna (MA)	VIR	902	Kaufman, Peter (NH)	Onc	309
Kane, Alex (MO)	PlS	782	Kaul, Sanjiv (OR)	Cv	117
Kanel, Gary (CA)	Path	657	Kaushansky, Kenneth (CA)	Hem	306
Kantarjian, Hagop (TX)	Hem	304	Kavey, Neil (NY)	Psyc	806
Kantoff, Philip (MA)	Onc	308	Kavoussi, Louis (NY)	U	1035
Kantsevoy, Sergey (MD)	Ge	220	Kawachi, Mark (CA)	U	1055
Kaplan, Allen (SC)	A&I	85	Kawamoto, Henry (CA)	PlS	789
Kaplan, Bernard (PA)	PNep	709	Kay, Dennis (LA)	VIR	907
Kaplan, David (CO)	AM	79	Kay, G Neal (AL)	CE	120
Kaplan, Frederick (PA)	OrS	568	Kay, Jonathan (MA)	Rhu	928
Kaplan, James (KS)	Pul	855	Kaye, Mitchell (MN)	Pul	852
			Kaysen, George (CA)	Nep	419

Alphabetical Listing of Doctors

Name	Specialty	Pg	Name	Specialty	Pg
Klotman, Mary (NY)	Inf	364	Kotagal, Suresh (MN)	ChiN	145
Klotman, Paul (NY)	Nep	412	Kotler, Donald (NY)	Ge	221
Klutke, Carl (MO)	U	1046	Kouchoukos, Nicholas (MO)	TS	1014
Kneisl, Jeffrey (NC)	OrS	575	Koufman, Jamie (NY)	Oto	606
Knisely, Jonathan (CT)	RadRO	868	Kovac, S Robert (GA)	ObG	510
Knize, David (CO)	PlS	784	Kovitz, Kevin (IL)	Pul	852
Knoefel, Janice (NM)	N	485	Kovnar, Edward (WI)	ChiN	146
Knowles, Daniel (NY)	Path	646	Koyle, Martin (CO)	U	1050
Knudson, Mary (CA)	S	988	Kozarek, Richard (WA)	Ge	239
Kobashigawa, Jon (CA)	Cv	117	Kozin, Scott (PA)	HS	281
Kobrin, Sidney (PA)	Nep	412	Kozlowski, James (IL)	U	1047
Kobrine, Arthur (DC)	NS	430	Krachmer, Jay (MN)	Oph	539
Koch, Douglas (TX)	Oph	545	Krackow, Kenneth (NY)	OrS	568
Koch, Wayne (MD)	Oto	606	Kraft, Andrew (SC)	Onc	324
Kocher, Mininder (MA)	OrS	561	Kraft, George (WA)	PMR	764
Kochman, Michael (PA)	Ge	221	Krag, David (VT)	S	955
Kodner, Ira (MO)	CRS	168	Krajcer, Zvonimir (TX)	Cv	114
Koeller, Kelly (MN)	NRad	900	Kramer, Barry (CA)	GerPsy	831
Koenig, Steven Michael (VA)	Pul	849	Kramer, Elissa (NY)	NuM	500
Koff, Stephen (OH)	U	1046	Kranzler, Leonard (IL)	NS	439
Koh, Wui-Jin (WA)	RadRO	880	Krasna, Mark (MD)	TS	1004
Kohler, Matthew (SC)	GO	267	Kraus, Dennis (NY)	Oto	606
Kokotailo, Patricia (WI)	AM	79	Krauss, Gregory (MD)	N	467
Koller, Harold (PA)	Oph	528	Kraut, Eric H (OH)	Hem	301
Kolodny, Edwin (NY)	N	466	Krauth, Lee (NE)	NS	443
Komaki, Ritsuko (TX)	RadRO	879	Kraybill, William (MO)	S	976
Koman, L Andrew (NC)	HS	284	Krebs, Nancy (CO)	PGe	691
Kondziolka, Douglas (PA)	NS	430	Kreitzer, Joel (NY)	PM	635
Konicek, Frank (IL)	Ge	230	Krellenstein, Daniel (NY)	TS	1004
Konstam, Marvin (MA)	Cv	95	Kremer, Joel (NY)	Rhu	931
Konstan, Michael (OH)	PPul	720	Krespi, Yosef (NY)	Oto	606
Koo, John (CA)	D	190	Kriegel, David (NY)	D	180
Koos, Brian (CA)	MF	394	Krieger, Karl (NY)	TS	1004
Kopans, Daniel (MA)	DR	889	Krilov, Leonard (NY)	PInf	705
Kopf, Gary (CT)	TS	999	Kris, Mark (NY)	Onc	316
Koplewicz, Harold (NY)	ChAP	823	Kron, Irving (VA)	TS	1009
Koplin, Lawrence (CA)	PlS	790	Krowka, Michael (MN)	Pul	852
Kopp, Peter (IL)	EDM	206	Krueger, Gerald (UT)	D	187
Koran, Lorrin (CA)	Psyc	815	Krueger, Ronald (OH)	Oph	539
Korelitz, Burton (NY)	Ge	221	Krumholz, Allan (MD)	N	467
Korenblat, Phillip (MO)	A&I	87	Krummel, Thomas (CA)	PS	734
Korf, Bruce (AL)	CG	154	Kuhn, Frederick (GA)	Oto	611
Kormos, Robert (PA)	TS	1004	Kuhn, Joseph (TX)	S	984
Kornmehl, Ernest (MA)	Oph	522	Kuiken, Todd (IL)	PMR	761
Koroshetz, Walter (MD)	N	466	Kula, Roger (NY)	N	467
Korsten, Mark (NY)	Ge	221	Kulick, Roy (NY)	HS	281
Koruda, Mark (NC)	S	970	Kumpe, David (CO)	VIR	907
Korytkowski, Mary (PA)	EDM	199	Kunkel, Elisabeth (PA)	Psyc	806
Kosova, Leonard (IL)	Onc	331	Kupersmith, Mark (NY)	Oph	528
Koss, Michael (CA)	Path	657	Kupfer, David (PA)	Psyc	807
Kosten, Thomas (TX)	AdP	820	Kurachek, Stephen (MN)	PPul	720
Kostis, John (NJ)	Cv	100	Kurman, Robert (MD)	Path	647

Name	Specialty	Pg
Kurtin, Paul (MN)	Path	652
Kurtz, Alfred (PA)	DR	892
Kurtz, Robert (NY)	Ge	221
Kurtzke, Robert (VA)	N	473
Kushner, Brian (NY)	PHO	695
Kushner, Burton (WI)	Oph	540
Kuske, Robert (AZ)	RadRO	879
Kuttesch, John F (TN)	PHO	697
Kuzel, Timothy (IL)	Hem	301
Kuzniecky, Ruben (NY)	N	467
Kuzon, William (MI)	PlS	782
Kveton, John (CT)	Oto	601
Kvols, Larry (FL)	Onc	324
Kwak, Larry (TX)	Onc	339
Kwo, Paul (IN)	Ge	230
Kwolek, Christopher (MA)	VascS	1066

L

Name	Specialty	Pg
La Ban, Myron (MI)	PMR	761
La Gamma, Edmund (NY)	NP	401
La Quaglia, Michael (NY)	PS	727
La Russo, Nicholas (MN)	Ge	230
Labiner, David (AZ)	N	485
Lachs, Mark (NY)	Ger	249
Lackman, Richard (PA)	OrS	568
Lacomis, David (PA)	N	467
Ladenson, Paul (MD)	EDM	200
Laham, Roger (MA)	IC	124
Lahita, Robert (NJ)	Rhu	931
Laks, Hillel (CA)	TS	1021
Lambert, George (NJ)	NP	401
Lambert, H Michael (TX)	Oph	545
Lambert, Paul (SC)	Oto	612
Lambert, Scott (GA)	Oph	535
Lamberti, John (CA)	TS	1022
Lambiase, Louis (FL)	Ge	226
Lammertse, Daniel (CO)	PMR	762
LaMuraglia, Glenn M (MA)	VascS	1066
Lancaster, Johnathan (FL)	GO	267
Landefeld, Charles (CA)	Ger	254
Landers, Daniel (CA)	MF	394
Landrigan, Philip (NY)	OM	796
Landy, Helain (DC)	MF	388
Lane, Dorothy S (NY)	PrM	797
Lane, Joseph (NY)	OrS	568
Lane, Lewis (NY)	HS	281
Lane, Stephen (MN)	Oph	540
Lang, Frederick (TX)	NS	444
Lang, Samuel (NY)	TS	1004
Lange, Beverly (PA)	PHO	695
Langer, Corey (PA)	Onc	316

Name	Specialty	Pg
Langman, Craig (IL)	PNep	712
Langston, J William (CA)	N	488
Lantos, John (IL)	Ped	666
Lanza, Donald (FL)	Oto	612
Lanzkowsky, Philip (NY)	PHO	695
Lapey, Allen (MA)	PPul	718
Laramore, George (WA)	RadRO	880
Larrabee, Wayne (WA)	Oto	625
Larsen, Gary (CO)	PPul	721
Larson, David Andrew (CA)	RadRO	880
Larson, Richard (IL)	Hem	302
Larson, Steven (NY)	NuM	500
Lashner, Bret (OH)	Ge	231
Lask, Gary (CA)	D	190
Latchaw, Laurie (NH)	PS	724
Latson, Larry (OH)	PCd	676
Lauerman, William (DC)	OrS	569
Laufer, Marc (MA)	ObG	508
Laurencin, Cato (VA)	OrS	575
Lavertu, Pierre (OH)	Oto	617
Lavery, Ian (OH)	CRS	168
Lavis, Victor (TX)	EDM	208
Lavyne, Michael (NY)	NS	430
Lawrence, Theodore S (MI)	RadRO	876
Lawry, George (IA)	Rhu	936
Laws, Edward (CA)	NS	447
Lawson, Edward (MD)	NP	401
Lawson, William (NY)	Oto	606
Lawson, William (DC)	Psyc	807
Lazarus, Hillard (OH)	Hem	302
Le, Quynh-Thu Xuan (CA)	RadRO	880
Le Boit, Philip (CA)	Path	657
Leaf, Norman (CA)	PlS	790
LeBoff, Meryl (MA)	EDM	197
Lebwohl, Mark (NY)	D	180
Lebwohl, Oscar (NY)	Ge	221
Lechan, Ronald (MA)	EDM	197
Leckman, James (CT)	ChAP	821
Ledford, Dennis (FL)	A&I	85
Lee, Andrew G (IA)	Oph	540
Lee, Jeffrey (TX)	S	984
Lee, Paul (NC)	Oph	535
Lee, W P Andrew (PA)	HS	282
Leffell, David (CT)	D	177
Lefrak, Stephen (MO)	Pul	852
Legato, Marianne (NY)	IM	379
Legha, Sewa (TX)	Onc	339
Legro, Richard (PA)	RE	916
Lehman, Thomas (NY)	PRhu	722
Lehman, Wallace (NY)	OrS	569
Leibel, Steven A (CA)	RadRO	881
Leight, George (NC)	S	970

Alphabetical Listing of Doctors

Name	Specialty	Pg	Name	Specialty	Pg
Leipziger, Lyle (NY)	PlS	774	Levy, Steven (GA)	Psyc	810
Lem, Vincent (MO)	Pul	853	Lewin, Alan A (FL)	RadRO	873
Lema, Mark (NY)	PM	635	Lewis, Curtis (GA)	VIR	905
Lemanske, Robert (WI)	PA&I	669	Lewis, Edmund (IL)	Nep	416
Lemons, James (IN)	NP	404	Lewis, Hilel (OH)	Oph	540
Lenke, Lawrence (MO)	OrS	580	Lewis, John (AZ)	A&I	88
Lentz, Christopher (NY)	S	962	Lewis, Richard (TX)	Oph	545
Leon, Martin (NY)	IC	124	Lewis, Sandra (OR)	Cv	117
Leonard, Henrietta (RI)	ChAP	821	Lewkowiez, Laurent (CO)	CE	122
Leonard, James (MI)	PMR	761	Li Volsi, Virginia (PA)	Path	647
Leonetti, John (IL)	Oto	617	Liang, Bruce (CT)	Cv	95
Leopold, Donald (NE)	Oto	622	Libby, Daniel (NY)	Pul	843
Lepanto, Philip (WV)	RadRO	871	Libby, Peter (MA)	Cv	95
Lepor, Herbert (NY)	U	1035	Liberman, Robert (CA)	Psyc	815
Lerman, Bruce (NY)	CE	119	Libertino, John (MA)	U	1030
Lerner, Seth (TX)	U	1052	Libow, Leslie (NY)	Ger	249
Lesavoy, Malcolm (CA)	PlS	790	Licata, Angelo (OH)	EDM	206
Leshin, Barry (NC)	D	184	Lichtenstein, Gary (PA)	Ge	221
Leslie, Kevin O (AZ)	Path	654	Lichter, Paul (MI)	Oph	540
Lessin, Stuart (PA)	D	180	Liddle, Rodger Alan (NC)	Ge	226
Leuchter, Andrew (CA)	Psyc	815	Lieberman, Phillip (TN)	A&I	85
Leung, Donald (CO)	PA&I	670	Liebmann, Jeffrey (NY)	Oph	528
Leung, Lawrence (CA)	Hem	306	Liem, Pham (AR)	Ger	253
Leventhal, Bennett (IL)	ChAP	826	Lieskovsky, Gary (CA)	U	1055
Levin, Bernard (TX)	Ge	237	Light, Richard (TN)	Pul	849
Levin, David (OK)	Pul	856	Light, Terry (IL)	HS	285
Levin, L Scott (NC)	PlS	779	Lightdale, Charles (NY)	Ge	222
Levin, Victor (TX)	N	485	Lillemoe, Keith (IN)	S	976
Levine, Alexandra (CA)	Hem	306	Lim, Henry (MI)	D	185
Levine, David (NY)	N	467	Lin, Weei-Chin (AL)	Hem	298
Levine, Edward (NC)	S	970	Lind, Christopher (TN)	Ge	226
Levine, Elliot (IL)	ObG	512	Lind, David (GA)	S	970
Levine, Ellis (NY)	Onc	316	Lindenfeld, JoAnn (CO)	Cv	113
Levine, Joel (CT)	Ge	216	Lindor, Keith (MN)	Ge	231
Levine, Joseph (NY)	CE	119	Lindsay, Bruce D (MO)	CE	121
Levine, Laurence (IL)	U	1047	Lindsey, Stephen (LA)	Rhu	938
Levine, Melvin (NC)	Ped	665	Lindstrom, Richard (MN)	Oph	540
Levine, Paul A (VA)	Oto	612	Linenberger, Michael (WA)	Hem	306
Levine, Robert (NH)	EDM	197	Link, Michael (MN)	NS	439
Levine, Stephen (OH)	Psyc	811	Link, Michael (CA)	PHO	703
Levine, Steven (NY)	N	467	Linker, Charles (CA)	Hem	306
Levine, William (NY)	SM	946	Linstrom, Christopher (NY)	Oto	606
Levinson, Arnold (PA)	A&I	83	Linton, MacRae F (TN)	Cv	105
Levitan, Ruven (IL)	Ge	231	Lipkin, David (FL)	PMR	760
Levitsky, Lynne (MA)	PEn	681	Lipkowitz, George (MA)	S	955
Levy, Angela (MD)	DR	892	Liporace, Joyce (PA)	N	467
Levy, Joseph (NY)	PGe	687	Lippman, Marc (MI)	Onc	331
Levy, Michael (PA)	Onc	316	Lippman, Scott (TX)	Onc	339
Levy, Moise (TX)	D	188	Lipschitz, David (AR)	Ger	253
Levy, Philip (AZ)	EDM	208	Lipscomb, Gary (TN)	ObG	511
Levy, Richard (IL)	PEn	684	Lipshultz, Larry (TX)	U	1052
Levy, Robert (IL)	NS	439	Lipshutz, William (PA)	Ge	222

Name	Specialty	Pg	Name	Specialty	Pg
Lipsitz, Lewis (MA)	Ger	248	Lowry, Ann (MN)	CRS	168
Lipstate, James (LA)	Rhu	939	Loyd, James (TN)	Pul	849
Lipton, Jeffrey (NY)	PHO	695	Lubahn, John (PA)	HS	282
Lipton, Richard (NY)	N	468	Lublin, Fred (NY)	N	468
Lisak, Robert (MI)	N	478	Luby, James (TX)	Inf	371
Lisman, Richard (NY)	Oph	528	Luby, Joan (MO)	ChAP	826
List, Alan F (FL)	Hem	298	Lucente, Vincent R (PA)	ObG	509
Litt, Andrew (NY)	NRad	897	Lucey, Michael (WI)	Ge	231
Little, Alex G (OH)	TS	1014	Luchins, Daniel (IL)	GerPsy	830
Little, John (DC)	PlS	774	Luciano, Anthony (CT)	RE	914
Litzow, Mark (MN)	Hem	302	Luck, James (CA)	OrS	587
Liu, Grant (PA)	N	468	Lucky, Anne (OH)	D	185
Livingston, Edward (TX)	S	984	Luders, Hans (OH)	N	479
Livingston, Philip (NY)	Onc	317	Ludwig, David (MA)	PEn	681
Livingston, Robert B (AZ)	Onc	339	Ludwig, Kirk (NC)	CRS	167
Livingstone, Alan (FL)	S	970	Ludwig, Stephen (PA)	Ped	665
Lloyd, Lewis (AL)	U	1041	Lueder, Gregg (MO)	Oph	540
Lobe, Thom (IA)	PS	731	Luerssen, Thomas (TX)	NS	445
Locala, Joseph (OH)	Psyc	811	Lugg, James (WY)	U	1050
Lock, James (MA)	PCd	671	Luggen, Michael (OH)	Rhu	936
Lock, Terrence (MI)	OrS	580	Luken, Martin (IL)	NS	439
Locker, Gershon (IL)	Onc	332	Lumsden, Alan (TX)	VascS	1075
Lockey, Richard (FL)	A&I	85	Lunsford, L Dade (PA)	NS	430
Lockhart, Jorge (FL)	U	1042	Lurain, John (IL)	GO	269
Lockshin, Michael (NY)	Rhu	931	Lusher, Jeanne (MI)	PHO	700
Lockwood, Charles (CT)	MF	387	Lusk, Rodney (NE)	PO	717
Loder, Elizabeth (MA)	PM	634	Lutcher, Charles (GA)	Hem	299
Loeffler, Jay S (MA)	RadRO	868	Luterman, Arnold (AL)	S	970
Loehrer, Patrick (IN)	Onc	332	Luthra, Harvinder (MN)	Rhu	937
Loewenstein, Richard (MD)	Psyc	807	Lutsep, Helmi (OR)	N	489
Loftus, Christopher (PA)	NS	430	Lutz, Gregory (NY)	PMR	757
Logan, William (MO)	N	478	Luxon, Bruce (IA)	Ge	231
Logigian, Eric (NY)	N	468	Lyckholm, Laurel (VA)	Onc	325
Logothetis, Christopher (TX)	Onc	339	Lyerly, H Kim (NC)	S	970
Long, Donlin (MD)	NS	430	Lyketsos, Constantine (MD)	GerPsy	829
Long, Sarah (PA)	PInf	705	Lyles, Kenneth (NC)	Ger	250
Longo, Walter (CT)	CRS	164	Lyman, Gary H (NY)	Onc	317
Longworth, David (MA)	Inf	362	Lynch, Joseph (CA)	Pul	859
Look, Katherine (IN)	GO	269	Lynch, Thomas (MA)	Onc	309
Loprinzi, Charles (MN)	Onc	332	Lynne, Charles (FL)	U	1042
LoRusso, Thomas (VA)	Pul	849	Lyons, Roger (TX)	Hem	304
Loscalzo, Joseph (MA)	Cv	96	Lytle, Bruce (OH)	TS	1014
Losordo, Douglas (IL)	IC	127			
Lossos, Izidore (FL)	Onc	325			
Lott, Ira (CA)	ChiN	148	**M**		
Lotze, Michael (PA)	S	962			
Loughlin, Gerald (NY)	PPul	719	Ma, Dong (NY)	PMR	758
Loughlin, Kevin (MA)	U	1030	Mabrey, Jay (TX)	OrS	585
Louis, Dean (MI)	HS	286	Macchia, Richard (NY)	U	1035
Loulmet, Didier (NY)	TS	1005	Macdonald, John (NY)	Onc	317
Lowe, Franklin (NY)	U	1035	MacDonald, Kenneth (NC)	S	970
Lowenberg, David (CA)	OrS	587	Macdonald, R Loch (IL)	NS	440
			MacFadyen, Bruce (GA)	S	971

Alphabetical Listing of Doctors

Name	Specialty	Pg	Name	Specialty	Pg
Macias, John (AZ)	Oto	623	Manske, Paul (MO)	HS	286
Maciejewski, Jaroslow (OH)	Hem	302	Manson, Paul (MD)	PlS	774
MacKeigan, John (MI)	CRS	168	Manzarbeitia, Cosme (PA)	S	962
MacKenzie, Richard (CA)	AM	79	Mapstone, Timothy (OK)	NS	445
Mackey, William (MA)	VascS	1067	Marcet, Jorge (FL)	CRS	167
MacKinnon, Susan (MO)	PlS	782	March, John (NC)	ChAP	825
Macklis, Roger (OH)	RadRO	876	Marchlinski, Francis (PA)	CE	119
Mackool, Richard (NY)	Oph	528	Marcom, Paul (NC)	Onc	325
MacLean, James A (MA)	A&I	82	Marcus, Carole (PA)	PPul	719
Macones, George (MO)	MF	391	Marcus, Robert (GA)	RadRO	873
Madaio, Michael (PA)	Nep	412	Marder, Stephen (CA)	Psyc	816
Maddox, Anne (AR)	Hem	305	Marentette, Lawrence (MI)	Oto	618
Maddrey, Willis (TX)	Ge	237	Margolis, James (FL)	IC	126
Madoff, Robert D (MN)	CRS	169	Marin, Deborah (NY)	Psyc	807
Madsen, Joseph (MA)	NS	425	Marin, Michael (NY)	VascS	1069
Magovern, George (PA)	TS	1005	Marini, John (MN)	Pul	853
Magramm, Irene (NY)	Oph	529	Marino, Ralph (PA)	PMR	758
Magrina, Javier (AZ)	GO	272	Marion, Robert (NY)	CG	153
Maguire, Leo (MN)	Oph	540	Mark, Eugene (MA)	Path	644
Magun, Arthur (NY)	Ge	222	Markman, Maurie (TX)	Onc	339
Maharam, Lewis (NY)	SM	946	Markmann, James (PA)	S	962
Mahler, Donald (NH)	Pul	841	Markowitz, Bernard (CA)	PlS	790
Mahler, Richard (NY)	EDM	200	Markowitz, David (NY)	Ge	222
Mahon, Kathleen (NV)	Oph	549	Markowitz, Sanford (OH)	Onc	332
Mahoney, Maurice (CT)	CG	152	Marks, Lawrence (NC)	RadRO	873
Mahony, Lynn (TX)	PCd	677	Marks, Stanley (PA)	Onc	317
Mahowald, Mark (MN)	N	479	Marmar, Charles (CA)	Psyc	816
Majd, Massoud (DC)	NuM	500	Marmor, Michael (CA)	Oph	550
Makaroun, Michel (PA)	VascS	1069	Maroon, Joseph (PA)	NS	430
Make, Barry (CO)	Pul	855	Marrs, Richard (CA)	RE	923
Maki, Dennis (WI)	Inf	369	Marsh, Christopher (CA)	U	1055
Malawer, Martin (DC)	OrS	569	Marsh, James (PA)	S	962
Malik, Ghaus (MI)	NS	440	Marsh, James (CT)	OrS	561
Malkowicz, S Bruce (PA)	U	1035	Marsh, Jeffrey L (MO)	PlS	782
Malloy, Michael (TX)	NP	406	Marshall, Fray (GA)	U	1042
Maloney, David (WA)	Onc	344	Marshall, John (VA)	EDM	203
Maloney, Mary (MA)	D	177	Marshall, John (DC)	Onc	317
Maloney, Robert (CA)	Oph	549	Marshall, Lawrence (CA)	NS	447
Mamelak, Adam (CA)	NS	447	Martell, John (IL)	OrS	580
Manche, Edward (CA)	Oph	549	Marten, Timothy (CA)	PlS	790
Manco-Johnson, Marilyn (CO)	PHO	701	Martenson, James (MN)	RadRO	876
Mancuso, Anthony (FL)	DR	893	Martin, Neil (CA)	NS	448
Mandel, Eric (NY)	Oph	529	Martin, Paul (NY)	Ge	222
Mandel, Susan (PA)	EDM	200	Martin, Richard (OH)	NP	404
Mandelbaum, David E (RI)	ChiN	142	Martin, Richard Jay (CO)	Pul	855
Manders, Ernest (PA)	PlS	774	Martin, Rick (MO)	CG	155
Manevitz, Alan (NY)	Psyc	807	Martin, Thomas (WA)	Pul	859
Manganiello, Paul (NH)	RE	914	Martin, Tomas (FL)	TS	1009
Mangat, Devinder (KY)	Oto	612	Martinez, Fernando (MI)	Pul	853
Manning, Warren (MA)	Cv	96	Martuza, Robert L (MA)	NS	425
Mannis, Mark (CA)	Oph	550	Masaryk, Thomas (OH)	NRad	900
Manoli, Arthur (MI)	OrS	580	Masket, Samuel (CA)	Oph	550

Name	Specialty	Pg	Name	Specialty	Pg
Mason, Joel (MA)	Ge	217	McCarthy, Shirley (CT)	DR	889
Mason, Kristin (CO)	PMR	762	McClamrock, Howard (MD)	RE	916
Mason, Wilbert (CA)	PInf	708	McClure, Robert (WA)	U	1055
Masood, Shahla (FL)	Path	650	McConnell, John (TX)	U	1052
Mass, Daniel (IL)	HS	286	McConnell, Robert (NY)	EDM	200
Massagli, Teresa (WA)	PMR	764	McCord, Clinton (GA)	Oph	535
Massin, Edward Krauss (TX)	Cv	114	McCormick, Beryl (NY)	RadRO	871
Mast, Bruce (FL)	PlS	779	McCormick, Paul C (NY)	NS	431
Masters, Gregory (DE)	Onc	317	McCormick, Steven (NY)	Path	647
Masur, Henry (MD)	Inf	364	McCormick, Wayne (WA)	Ger	254
Matar, Fadi (FL)	IC	126	McCracken, George (TX)	PInf	708
Matarasso, Alan (NY)	PlS	774	McCracken, James (CA)	ChAP	828
Matas, Arthur (MN)	S	976	McCraw, John (MS)	PlS	780
Mathisen, Douglas (MA)	TS	999	McCulley, James (TX)	Oph	545
Matsen, Frederick (WA)	OrS	588	McCune, W Joseph (MI)	Rhu	937
Matthay, Katherine (CA)	PHO	704	McCurley, Thomas (TN)	Path	650
Matthay, Michael (CA)	Pul	859	McDermott, Michael (CA)	NS	448
Matthay, Richard (CT)	Pul	841	McDiarmid, Suzanne (CA)	PGe	691
Matthews, David (NC)	PlS	779	McDonald, Charles (RI)	D	177
Matthews, Dennis (CO)	PMR	763	McDonald, Douglas (MO)	OrS	580
Mattox, Douglas (GA)	Oto	612	McDonald, John (MD)	N	468
Mauch, Peter (MA)	RadRO	868	McDonald, Ruth (WA)	PNep	713
Maurer, William (IL)	PEn	684	McDougal, W Scott (MA)	U	1030
Mauro, Matthew (NC)	VIR	905	McDougle, Christopher (IN)	ChAP	826
Mavroudis, Constantine (IL)	PS	731	McFarland, Edward (MD)	OrS	569
Mawad, Michel (TX)	NRad	901	McGahan, John (CA)	VIR	908
Max, Mitchell (MD)	N	468	McGill, Janet (MO)	EDM	206
Maxwell, G Patrick (TN)	PlS	779	McGill, Trevor (MA)	PO	713
May, James (MA)	PlS	770	McGlashan, Thomas (CT)	Psyc	803
Mayberg, Marc (WA)	NS	448	McGlave, Philip (MN)	Hem	302
Mayer, John (MA)	PS	725	McGovern, Francis (MA)	U	1030
Mayer, Lloyd (NY)	Ge	222	McGrath, Patrick (KY)	S	971
Mayer, Nathaniel (PA)	PMR	758	McGregor, Christopher (MN)	TS	1014
Mayer, Robert J (MA)	Onc	309	McGuire, Edward (MI)	U	1047
Mayes, Maureen (TX)	Rhu	939	McGuire, William (MD)	Onc	317
Maytal, Joseph (NY)	ChiN	144	McHenry, Christopher (OH)	S	976
Mazow, Malcolm L (TX)	Oph	545	McHugh, Paul (MD)	Psyc	807
Mazza, David (NY)	A&I	83	McKeag, Douglas (IN)	SM	948
Mazzone, Theodore (IL)	EDM	206	McKelvey, Robert (OR)	ChAP	828
McAfee, Paul (MD)	OrS	569	McKenna, Michael (MA)	Oto	601
McAlister, William (MO)	DR	894	McKenna, Robert J (CA)	TS	1022
McAninch, Jack (CA)	U	1055	McKeown, Craig (FL)	Oph	535
McArthur, Justin (MD)	N	468	McKinney, Ross (NC)	PInf	707
McCall, William (NC)	Psyc	810	McLaren, Rodney (VA)	MF	389
McCallum, Kimberli (MO)	Psyc	812	McLean, Gordon (PA)	VIR	903
McCance-Katz, Elinore (VA)	AdP	819	McMahon, M Molly (MN)	EDM	206
McCann, Merle (MD)	Psyc	807	McMenomey, Sean O (OR)	Oto	626
McCann, Peter (NY)	OrS	569	McNutt, N Scott (NY)	Path	647
McCann, Richard (NC)	VascS	1071	McPherson, David (TX)	Cv	114
McCarthy, Joseph (NY)	PlS	775	McVary, Kevin (IL)	U	1047
McCarthy, Patrick (IL)	TS	1014	Meacham, Lillian (GA)	PEn	683
McCarthy, Paul (CT)	PRhu	722	Meadow, William (IL)	NP	404

Alphabetical Listing of Doctors

Name	Specialty	Pg	Name	Specialty	Pg
Meals, Roy (CA)	HS	288	Meyers, Paul (NY)	PHO	695
Meara, John (MA)	PlS	771	Meyers, Rebecka (UT)	PS	732
Mease, Philip (WA)	Rhu	940	Michalska, Margaret (IL)	Rhu	937
Medbery, Clinton (OK)	RadRO	879	Michalski, Jeff M (MO)	RadRO	876
Medich, David (PA)	CRS	165	Michelassi, Fabrizio (NY)	S	962
Medina, Jesus (OK)	Oto	623	Micheli, Lyle (MA)	SM	946
Medow, Norman (NY)	Oph	529	Michler, Robert (NY)	TS	1005
Medsger, Thomas (PA)	Rhu	931	Mickey, Bruce (TX)	NS	445
Meek, Rita (DE)	PHO	695	Middleton, Richard (UT)	U	1051
Mehler, Philip (CO)	IM	380	Mieler, William (IL)	Oph	541
Mehlman, David (IL)	Cv	110	Mies, Carolyn (PA)	Path	647
Mehta, Atul (OH)	Pul	853	Mih, Alexander (IN)	HS	286
Meier, Diane (NY)	Ger	249	Mihm, Martin (MA)	D	177
Meiselman, Mick (IL)	Ge	231	Mikkelsen, Tommy (MI)	N	479
Meller, Jose (NY)	Cv	100	Milad, Magdy (IL)	RE	921
Mellow, Alan (MI)	GerPsy	830	Milam, Douglas (TN)	U	1042
Melman, Arnold (NY)	U	1035	Mildvan, Donna (NY)	Inf	364
Melmed, Shlomo (CA)	EDM	210	Miles, Brian (TX)	U	1053
Melone, Charles (NY)	HS	282	Milhorat, Thomas (NY)	NS	431
Meltzer, Eli (CA)	A&I	88	Millenson, Michael (PA)	Hem	296
Meltzer, Toby (AZ)	PlS	786	Miller, Carol (CA)	Ped	667
Melvin, W Scott (OH)	S	977	Miller, D Douglas (GA)	Cv	105
Mendell, Jerry (OH)	N	479	Miller, Daniel (GA)	TS	1010
Mendelsohn, Janis (IL)	Ped	666	Miller, David (CA)	TS	1022
Mendenhall, Nancy (FL)	RadRO	873	Miller, Franklin (KY)	MF	389
Mendenhall, William (FL)	RadRO	874	Miller, Franklin (CA)	VIR	908
Mendley, Susan (MD)	PNep	709	Miller, Joan (MA)	Oph	522
Menezes, Arnold (IA)	NS	440	Miller, Joseph (AZ)	Oph	545
Menick, Frederick (AZ)	PlS	786	Miller, Joseph (GA)	TS	1010
Menon, Mani (MI)	U	1047	Miller, Kenneth (MA)	Hem	294
Menon, Ram (MI)	PEn	684	Miller, Neil (MD)	Oph	529
Menter, M Alan (TX)	D	188	Miller, Robert (IL)	PO	716
Meredith, Travis (NC)	Oph	535	Miller, Sheldon (IL)	AdP	819
Merkel, Peter (MA)	Rhu	928	Miller, Stanley (MD)	D	180
Meropol, Neal (PA)	Onc	318	Miller, Timothy (CA)	PlS	790
Merrick, Hollis (OH)	S	977	Millett, Peter (CO)	OrS	583
Merrick, Scot (CA)	TS	1022	Milley, J Ross (UT)	NP	405
Merrill, Walter (OH)	TS	1014	Millikan, Randall (TX)	Onc	339
Merritt, Diane (MO)	ObG	512	Millis, J Michael (IL)	S	977
Mersey, James (MD)	EDM	200	Millman, Richard (RI)	Pul	841
Mertz, Howard (TN)	Ge	226	Mills, Monte (PA)	Oph	529
Mesrobian, Hrair-George (WI)	U	1047	Mills, Stacey (VA)	Path	650
Messer, Joseph (IL)	Cv	110	Milsom, Jeffrey (NY)	CRS	165
Mesulam, Marel (IL)	N	479	Mims, James (TX)	Oph	546
Metcalfe, Dean (MD)	A&I	83	Minaker, Kenneth (MA)	Ger	248
Metersky, Mark (CT)	Pul	841	Minckler, Donald (CA)	Oph	550
Mets, Marilyn (IL)	Oph	541	Miniaci, Anthony (OH)	SM	948
Metson, Ralph (MA)	Oto	601	Minich, Lois (UT)	PCd	677
Metz, David (PA)	Ge	222	Minkoff, Howard (NY)	ObG	509
Metzl, Jordan (NY)	SM	947	Minor, Lloyd (MD)	Oto	607
Meyer, Anthony (NC)	S	971	Miro-Quesada, Miguel (TX)	Hem	305
Meyers, Bryan (MO)	TS	1014	Mirvis, Stuart (MD)	DR	892

Name	Specialty	Pg	Name	Specialty	Pg
Mirzayan, Raffy (CA)	SM	950	Morris, Colleen (NV)	CG	158
Miskovitz, Paul (NY)	Ge	223	Morris, Douglas (GA)	IC	126
Mitch, William (TX)	Nep	418	Morris, John (MO)	N	479
Mitchell, Beverly (CA)	Onc	344	Morris, Robert E (CA)	AM	79
Mitchell, Charles (FL)	PInf	707	Morris, Rohinton (PA)	TS	1005
Mitchell, James (ND)	Psyc	813	Morrison, Glenn (FL)	NS	434
Mitchell, Michael (WI)	U	1047	Morrow, Monica (PA)	S	963
Mitchell, Paul (CT)	Oph	523	Mortimer, Joanne (CA)	Onc	344
Mitchell, Wendy (CA)	ChiN	148	Mosca, Lori (NY)	Cv	101
Mitnick, Hal (NY)	Rhu	931	Moscatello, Augustine (NY)	Oto	607
Mitnick, Julie (NY)	DR	892	Mosenifar, Zab (CA)	Pul	859
Mitros, Frank (IA)	Path	652	Moses, Jeffrey (NY)	IC	124
Mitsumoto, Hiroshi (NY)	N	468	Moshang, Thomas (PA)	PEn	682
Miyamoto, Richard (IN)	Oto	618	Mosher, Deane (WI)	Hem	302
Mobley, William (CA)	ChiN	148	Moskowitz, Roland (OH)	Rhu	937
Moder, Kevin (MN)	Rhu	937	Moskowitz, William (VA)	PCd	674
Modic, Michael (OH)	NRad	900	Moss, R Lawrence (CT)	PS	725
Mohammad, Yousef (OH)	N	479	Mostwin, Jacek (MD)	U	1036
Mohl, Paul (TX)	Psyc	814	Motzer, Robert (NY)	Onc	318
Mohr, Jay (NY)	N	469	Moul, Judd (NC)	U	1042
Moley, Jeffrey (MO)	S	977	Mountz, James (PA)	NuM	501
Molleston, Jean (IN)	PGe	690	Mukherji, Suresh (MI)	NRad	900
Molnar, Joseph (NC)	PlS	780	Muldoon, Thomas (NY)	Oph	529
Molo, Mary (IL)	RE	921	Mulhall, John (NY)	U	1036
Mondino, Bartly (CA)	Oph	550	Mullett, Timothy (KY)	TS	1010
Moneim, Moheb (NM)	HS	287	Mulliken, John (MA)	PlS	771
Money, Samuel (AZ)	VascS	1075	Mulvihill, John (OK)	CG	156
Monsees, Barbara (MO)	DR	894	Mulvihill, Sean (UT)	S	981
Montague, Drogo (OH)	U	1047	Mundt, Arno J (CA)	RadRO	881
Montanaro, Anthony (OR)	A&I	88	Munin, Michael (PA)	PMR	758
Montgomery, Elizabeth (MD)	Path	647	Munoz, Jose (NY)	PInf	705
Montgomery, Erwin (WI)	N	479	Murali, Raj (NY)	NS	431
Montgomery, Robert (MD)	S	962	Muraskas, Erik (IL)	ObG	512
Montie, James (MI)	U	1048	Muraskas, Jonathan (IL)	NP	404
Moodie, Douglas (LA)	PCd	678	Murphree, A Linn (CA)	Oph	550
Moore, Anne (NY)	Onc	318	Murphy, Ana (GA)	RE	919
Moore, Ernest (CO)	S	981	Murphy, Douglas (GA)	TS	1010
Moore, Thomas (CA)	MF	394	Murphy, Sharon (TX)	PHO	702
Moore, Walter (GA)	Rhu	934	Murphy, Thomas (NC)	PPul	719
Moore, Wesley (CA)	VascS	1076	Murphy, Timothy (RI)	VIR	902
Moossa, AR (CA)	S	988	Murray, Joseph (MN)	Ge	231
Morady, Fred (MI)	CE	121	Murray, Pamela (PA)	AM	78
Moran, Cesar (TX)	Path	654	Muschler, George (OH)	OrS	580
Moran, Christopher (MO)	NRad	900	Muss, Hyman B (VT)	Onc	309
Moran, John (IL)	Cv	110	Mustoe, Thomas (IL)	PlS	782
Morgan, Linda (FL)	ObG	511	Mutch, David (MO)	GO	269
Morgan, Mark (PA)	GO	265	Muto, Michael (MA)	GO	262
Morgan, Raymond (VA)	PlS	780	Myer, Charles (OH)	PO	716
Morgan, Wayne J (AZ)	PPul	721	Myerburg, Robert (FL)	Cv	105
Morgenlander, Joel (NC)	N	474	Myers, Eugene (PA)	Oto	607
Morley, John (MO)	Ger	251	Myers, Jeffrey (MI)	Path	652
Morrell, Martha (CA)	N	489	Myers, Jeffrey (TX)	Oto	623

Alphabetical Listing of Doctors

Name	Specialty	Pg	Name	Specialty	Pg
Myers, Lawrence (CA)	N	489	Neppe, Vernon (WA)	Psyc	816
Myers, Robert P (MN)	U	1048	Nerad, Jeffrey (IA)	Oph	541
Myers, Stanley (NY)	PMR	758	Nesbitt, Jonathan C (TN)	TS	1010
Myerson, Mark (MD)	OrS	569	Nesburn, Anthony (CA)	Oph	550
Myerson, Robert (MO)	RadRO	876	Nestler, John (VA)	EDM	203
Myones, Barry (TX)	PRhu	723	Netterville, James (TN)	Oto	612
Mysiw, W Jerry (OH)	PMR	761	Neu, Josef (FL)	NP	403
			Neuburg, Marcelle (WI)	D	186

N

Name	Specialty	Pg	Name	Specialty	Pg
			Neumann, Donald (OH)	NuM	502
Nabell, Lisle (AL)	Onc	325	Neumann, Ronald (MD)	NuM	501
Naccarelli, Gerald (PA)	Cv	101	Neuwirth, Michael (NY)	OrS	569
Nachman, James (IL)	PHO	700	Nevins, Thomas (MN)	PNep	712
Naclerio, Robert (IL)	Oto	618	New, Maria (NY)	PEn	682
Nadler, Lee M (MA)	Onc	309	Newburger, Jane (MA)	PCd	671
Nadol, Joseph (MA)	Oto	601	Newell, Kenneth (GA)	S	971
Nagel, Theodore (MN)	RE	921	Newman, Lawrence (NY)	N	469
Nagib, Mahmoud (MN)	NS	440	Newman, Lee (CO)	Pul	855
Nagle, Daniel (IL)	HS	286	Newman, Leonard (NY)	PGe	687
Nagle, Deborah (MA)	CRS	164	Newman, Nancy (GA)	N	474
Nagler, Harris (NY)	U	1036	Ngeow, Jeffrey (NY)	PM	635
Nagorney, David (MN)	S	977	Nguyen, Ninh (CA)	S	988
Nahai, Foad (GA)	PlS	780	Nicholas, Stephen (NY)	OrS	570
Nahass, Ronald (NJ)	Inf	365	Nicholl, Jeffrey (LA)	N	485
Naka, Yoshifumi (NY)	TS	1005	Nichols, Craig (OR)	Onc	345
Nakayama, Don (NC)	PS	728	Nichols, David (MD)	PCCM	679
Nand, Sucha (IL)	Hem	302	Nicholson, Henry (OR)	PHO	704
Napoli, Joseph (DE)	PlS	775	Nichter, Larry (CA)	PlS	790
Nardell, Edward (MA)	Pul	842	Niederhuber, John (MD)	S	963
Nash, David (PA)	IM	379	Niederman, Michael (NY)	Pul	843
Nash, Martin (NY)	PNep	710	Nigra, Thomas (DC)	D	180
Nash, Thomas (NY)	Pul	843	Nimer, Stephen (NY)	Hem	296
Naslund, Michael (MD)	U	1036	Ninan, Mathew (TN)	TS	1010
Natale, Andrea (OH)	CE	121	Niparko, John (MD)	Oto	607
Natale, Ronald (CA)	Onc	345	Nishimura, Rick (MN)	Cv	110
Nath, Rahul (TX)	PlS	786	Nisonson, Barton (NY)	SM	947
Nathanson, S David (MI)	S	977	Nissen, Steven (OH)	Cv	111
Nathwani, Bharat (CA)	Path	657	Nissenblatt, Michael (NJ)	Onc	318
Naunheim, Keith (MO)	TS	1014	Nitti, Victor (NY)	U	1036
Nava-Villarreal, Hector (NY)	S	963	Nobunaga, Austin (OH)	PMR	761
Nazzaro, Jules (KS)	NS	443	Nocero, Michael (FL)	Cv	106
Neglia, Joseph (MN)	PHO	700	Noetzel, Michael (MO)	ChiN	146
Negrin, Robert (CA)	Hem	306	Nogee, Lawrence (MD)	NP	402
Neiberger, Richard (FL)	PNep	710	Nogueras, Juan (FL)	CRS	167
Nelson, Edward (UT)	S	981	Nolan, Bruce (FL)	N	474
Nelson, Harold (CO)	A&I	87	Noller, Kenneth (MA)	ObG	508
Nelson, Heidi (MN)	CRS	169	Noon, George P (TX)	TS	1019
Nelson, J Craig (CA)	Psyc	816	Noone, R Barrett (PA)	PlS	775
Nelson, Joel (PA)	U	1036	Norbash, Alexander (MA)	NRad	897
Nelson, Maureen (NC)	PMR	760	Nordli, Douglas (IL)	ChiN	146
Nemcek, Albert (IL)	VIR	906	Norenberg, Michael (FL)	Path	650
Nemickas, Rimgaudas (IL)	Cv	110	Nori, Dattatreyudu (NY)	RadRO	871
			Norman, David (CA)	NRad	902

Name	Specialty	Pg	Name	Specialty	Pg
Norman, Kim (CA)	Psyc	816	Oeffinger, Kevin (NY)	Ped	665
Northfelt, Donald (AZ)	Onc	340	Offit, Kenneth (NY)	Onc	318
Northrup, Hope (TX)	CG	156	Offit, Paul (PA)	Ped	665
Norton, Jeffrey (CA)	S	988	Oh, Shin (AL)	N	474
Norton, Karen (NJ)	DR	892	Ohl, Dana (MI)	U	1048
Norton, Larry (NY)	Onc	318	Okusa, Mark (VA)	Nep	414
Nour, Nawal (MA)	ObG	508	Olanow, C Warren (NY)	N	469
Novak, Donald (FL)	PGe	689	Olden, Kevin (AR)	Ge	238
Novick, Andrew (OH)	U	1048	Oldham, Keith (WI)	PS	731
Novotny, Edward (CT)	ChiN	142	Olitsky, Scott (MO)	Oph	541
Nowak, Eugene (NY)	S	963	Oliva-Hemker, Maria (MD)	PGe	687
Noyes, Frank (OH)	SM	948	Olivero, Juan (TX)	Nep	418
Nuber, Gordon (IL)	OrS	581	Olopade, Olufunmilayo (IL)	Onc	332
Nuchtern, Jed (TX)	PS	733	Olsen, Elise A (NC)	D	184
Nugent, William (NH)	TS	999	Olsen, Kerry (MN)	Oto	618
Nunery, William (KY)	Oph	535	Olson, Jack (IL)	Ger	252
Nunley, James (NC)	OrS	575	Olson, Thomas (GA)	PHO	697
Nurnberger, John (IN)	Psyc	812	Olthoff, Kim (PA)	S	963
Nuss, Daniel (LA)	Oto	623	Onders, Raymond (OH)	S	977
Nuss, Donald (VA)	PS	729	Ondra, Stephen (IL)	NS	440
Nussbaum, Julian (GA)	Oph	535	Ontjes, David (NC)	EDM	203
Nussbaum, Robert (CA)	CG	158	Oommen, Kalarickal (OK)	N	485
Nutt, John (OR)	N	489	Oparil, Suzanne (AL)	Cv	106
			Orenstein, Jan (DC)	Path	647
			Orgill, Dennis (MA)	PlS	771

O

Name	Specialty	Pg	Name	Specialty	Pg
			Origitano, Thomas (IL)	NS	440
O'Brien, John (NE)	Ge	235	Orlow, Seth (NY)	D	180
O'Brien, Susan (TX)	Onc	340	Orlowski, Robert (NC)	Onc	325
O'Day, Steven (CA)	Onc	345	Orobello, Peter (FL)	PO	715
O'Dell, James R (NE)	Rhu	938	Orringer, Mark B (MI)	TS	1015
O'Donnell, Michael (IA)	U	1048	Ortel, Thomas (NC)	Hem	299
O'Donnell, Richard (CA)	OrS	588	Orwoll, Eric (OR)	EDM	210
O'Gara, Patrick (MA)	Cv	96	Ory, Steven (FL)	RE	919
O'Keefe, Regis (NY)	OrS	570	Osborn, Anne (UT)	NRad	901
O'Laughlin, Martin (MO)	PCd	676	Osborne, Charles (TX)	Onc	340
O'Leary, Michael P (MA)	U	1031	Osborne, Michael (NY)	S	963
O'Leary, Patrick (NY)	OrS	570	Osguthorpe, John (SC)	Oto	612
O'Malley, Bert (PA)	Oto	607	Osher, Robert (OH)	Oph	541
O'Neill, William (FL)	Cv	106	Oster, Martin (NY)	Onc	319
O'Reilly, Eileen (NY)	Onc	318	Osterman, A Lee (PA)	HS	282
O'Reilly, Richard (NY)	PHO	695	Ostrer, Harry (NY)	CG	153
O'Rourke, Donald (PA)	NS	431	Ostroff, James Warren (CA)	Ge	239
O'Shaughnessy, Joyce (TX)	Onc	340	Ostrom, Nancy (CA)	A&I	88
Oakes, W Jerry (AL)	NS	434	Ott, David (TX)	TS	1019
Oates, Robert (MA)	U	1031	Ott, Kenneth (CA)	NS	448
Oberfield, Sharon (NY)	PEn	682	Otto, Pamela (TX)	DR	895
Oddis, Chester (PA)	Rhu	931	Otto, Randal (TX)	Oto	624
Odel, Jeffrey (NY)	Oph	529	Ouslander, Joseph (GA)	Ger	250
Odem, Randall (MO)	RE	921	Ovalle, Fernando (AL)	EDM	203
Odom, Lorrie (CO)	PHO	701	Ownby, Dennis (GA)	PA&I	668
Odom, Michael (TX)	NP	406	Owyang, Chung (MI)	Ge	232
Odze, Robert D (MA)	Path	644	Oz, Mehmet (NY)	TS	1005

Alphabetical Listing of Doctors

Name	Specialty	Pg	Name	Specialty	Pg
Ozols, Robert (PA)	Onc	319	Passo, Murray (OH)	PRhu	723
			Pastorek, Norman (NY)	Oto	608
P			Patchefsky, Arthur (PA)	Path	647
			Patchell, Roy (KY)	N	474
Pachter, H Leon (NY)	S	963	Patel, Mukund (NY)	HS	282
Pacin, Michael (FL)	A&I	85	Patel, Sunil (SC)	NS	434
Pack, Allan (PA)	Pul	844	Patrizio, Pasquale (CT)	RE	915
Packer, Milton (TX)	Cv	114	Patt, Yehuda (NM)	Onc	340
Packer, Roger (DC)	ChiN	144	Patterson, Anthony (TN)	U	1042
Padma-Nathan, Harin (CA)	U	1056	Patterson, G Alexander (MO)	TS	1015
Pagani, Francis (MI)	TS	1015	Patterson, James (OR)	Pul	859
Paganini, Emil (OH)	Nep	416	Patterson, Jan E Evans (TX)	Inf	371
Page, David L (TN)	Path	651	Patterson, Marc (MN)	ChiN	146
Paget, Stephen (NY)	Rhu	931	Patterson, Thomas (TX)	Inf	371
Pagon, Roberta (WA)	CG	158	Paty, Philip (NY)	S	964
Paidas, Charles (FL)	PS	729	Patzakis, Michael (CA)	OrS	588
Palacios, Igor (MA)	Cv	96	Paul, Malcolm (CA)	PlS	791
Palascak, Joseph (OH)	Hem	303	Paul, T Otis (CA)	Oph	551
Paletta, George (MO)	SM	948	Paulos, Leon (TX)	OrS	585
Palevsky, Harold (PA)	Pul	844	Paulson, Richard (CA)	RE	923
Paley, Dror (MD)	OrS	570	Payne, Christopher (CA)	U	1056
Palfrey, Judith (MA)	Ped	664	Payne, Richard (NC)	PM	636
Paller, Amy (IL)	D	186	Pearce, William (IL)	VascS	1073
Palmberg, Paul (FL)	Oph	536	Pearson, Richard (VA)	Inf	368
Palmer, Andrew (NY)	OrS	570	Pearson, Thomas (NY)	PrM	797
Palmer, Earl (OR)	Oph	550	Pecora, Andrew (NJ)	Onc	319
Palmer, Robert (OH)	Ger	252	Pedley, Timothy (NY)	N	469
Panicek, David (NY)	DR	892	Pegram, Paul (NC)	Inf	368
Pantell, Robert (CA)	Ped	667	Peitzman, Andrew (PA)	S	964
Papadopoulos, Nicholas (TX)	Onc	340	Pellegrini, Carlos (WA)	S	988
Papadopoulos, Stephen (AZ)	NS	445	Pellicci, Paul (NY)	OrS	570
Paparella, Michael (MN)	Oto	618	Pelzer, Harold (IL)	Oto	618
Papel, Ira (MD)	Oto	607	Pemberton, John (MN)	CRS	169
Pappas, Theodore N (NC)	S	971	Pena, Alberto (OH)	PS	731
Parisier, Simon (NY)	Oto	607	Penalver, Manuel A (FL)	GO	267
Park, Adrian (MD)	S	963	Penar, Paul (VT)	NS	425
Park, Tae Sung (MO)	NS	440	Pensak, Myles (OH)	Oto	618
Parker, Robert (NY)	PHO	696	Pepine, Carl (FL)	Cv	106
Parmacek, Michael (PA)	Cv	101	Pepose, Jay (MO)	Oph	541
Parness, Ira (NY)	PCd	672	Peppercorn, Mark (MA)	Ge	217
Parodi, Juan (FL)	VascS	1071	Perez, Edith (FL)	Onc	325
Parrillo, Joseph (NJ)	Cv	101	Perez Fontan, J Julio (TX)	PCCM	680
Parrish, Richard (FL)	Oph	536	Pergament, Eugene (IL)	CG	155
Parsons, Polly (VT)	Pul	842	Perin, Emerson (TX)	IC	128
Partain, C Leon (TN)	DR	893	Perkash, Inder (CA)	U	1056
Partin, Alan (MD)	U	1036	Perkins, James (WA)	S	989
Partridge, Edward (AL)	GO	267	Perler, Bruce (MD)	VascS	1070
Pascuzzi, Robert (IN)	N	480	Perlman, David (NY)	Inf	365
Pasmantier, Mark (NY)	Onc	319	Perlman, Jeffrey (NY)	NP	402
Pasquariello, Patrick (PA)	Ped	665	Perlmutter, Joel (MO)	N	480
Pasricha, Pankaj (TX)	Ge	238	Perret, Philip (LA)	Pul	856
Pass, Harvey (NY)	TS	1005	Perrone, Ronald (MA)	Nep	410

Name	Specialty	Pg	Name	Specialty	Pg
Perry, Michael (MO)	Onc	332	Piraino, Beth (PA)	Nep	412
Perry, Stanton (CA)	PCd	678	Pisano, Etta (NC)	DR	893
Perryman, Richard (FL)	TS	1010	Pistenmaa, David (TX)	RadRO	879
Persky, Mark (NY)	Oto	608	Pisters, Katherine (TX)	Onc	340
Peschel, Richard (CT)	RadRO	869	Pisters, Louis (TX)	U	1053
Pestronk, Alan (MO)	N	480	Pitman, Gerald (NY)	PlS	775
Petelin, Joseph (KS)	S	981	Pitman, Karen (MS)	Oto	613
Peters, Charles (MO)	PHO	700	Pitman, Roger (MA)	Psyc	803
Peters, Glenn (AL)	Oto	613	Pitt, Bertram (MI)	IC	127
Peters, Jeffrey (NY)	S	964	Pitts, Lawrence (CA)	NS	448
Petersen, Robert (MA)	Oph	523	Plancher, Kevin (NY)	SM	947
Petersen, Ronald (MN)	N	480	Platt, Lawrence (CA)	MF	394
Peterson, Davis (AK)	OrS	588	Platzker, Arnold (CA)	PPul	721
Petito, Carol (FL)	Path	651	Plehn, Jonathan (DC)	Cv	101
Petito, Frank (NY)	N	469	Plotnick, Leslie (MD)	PEn	682
Petras, Robert (OH)	Path	652	Plotz, Paul (MD)	Rhu	932
Petri, Michelle (MD)	Rhu	932	Pochapin, Mark (NY)	Ge	223
Petru, Ann (CA)	PInf	709	Pochettino, Alberto (PA)	TS	1006
Petruzzelli, Guy (IL)	Oto	619	Podoloff, Donald (TX)	NuM	502
Petrylak, Daniel (NY)	Onc	319	Podolsky, Daniel (MA)	Ge	217
Pettrone, Frank (VA)	OrS	575	Podos, Steven (NY)	Oph	529
Pevec, William (CA)	VascS	1076	Podratz, Karl (MN)	GO	269
Pfeffer, Marc (MA)	Cv	96	Poe, Dennis (MA)	Oto	602
Pfeifer, Samantha (PA)	RE	916	Poehling, Gary (NC)	OrS	576
Pflugfelder, Stephen (TX)	Oph	546	Pohl, Marc (OH)	Nep	416
Philipson, Elliot (OH)	MF	391	Poliakoff, Steven (FL)	GO	267
Phillips, Edward (CA)	S	989	Polin, Richard (NY)	NP	402
Phillips, Harry (NC)	Cv	106	Polisson, Richard (MA)	Rhu	928
Phillips, Katharine (RI)	Psyc	803	Polk, Hiram C (KY)	S	971
Phillips, Peter (PA)	ChiN	144	Pollack, Alan (PA)	RadRO	872
Phillips, Robert (MA)	Cv	96	Pollack, Ian (PA)	NS	431
Phuphanich, Surasak (GA)	N	474	Pollard, Zane (GA)	Oph	536
Pi, Edmond (CA)	Psyc	816	Polley, John (IL)	PlS	783
Piccione, William (IL)	TS	1015	Pollock, Raphael (TX)	S	984
Piccirillo, Jay (MO)	Oto	619	Polly, David (MN)	OrS	581
Piccoli, David (PA)	PGe	687	Polonsky, Kenneth (MO)	EDM	206
Pichard, Augusto (DC)	IC	124	Polsky, Bruce (NY)	Inf	365
Picken, Catherine (DC)	Oto	608	Pomerantz, Marvin (CO)	TS	1017
Picozzi, Vincent (WA)	Onc	345	Pomeroy, John (NY)	ChAP	823
Pienta, Kenneth (MI)	Onc	332	Pomeroy, Scott (MA)	ChiN	142
Piepgras, David (MN)	NS	441	Pongracic, Jacqueline (IL)	PA&I	669
Piepmeier, Joseph (CT)	NS	425	Ponsky, Jeffrey (OH)	S	977
Pierce, Lori (MI)	RadRO	877	Ponton, Lynn (CA)	ChAP	828
Pierson, Richard (MD)	TS	1006	Poole, Michael (GA)	Oto	613
Piest, Kenneth (TX)	Oph	546	Poon, Michael (NY)	Cv	101
Pile-Spellman, John (NY)	NRad	898	Pope, Harrison (MA)	Psyc	803
Pillsbury, Harold (NC)	Oto	613	Pope, Richard (IL)	Rhu	937
Pimstone, Neville (CA)	Ge	239	Popovich, John (MI)	Pul	853
Pinckert, Thomas (MD)	MF	388	Poppas, Dix (NY)	U	1036
Pingleton, Susan (KS)	Pul	855	Portenoy, Russell (NY)	PM	635
Pinson, C Wright (TN)	S	971	Porter, Co-burn (MN)	PCd	676
Pinzur, Michael (IL)	OrS	581	Porter, David (PA)	Hem	296

Alphabetical Listing of Doctors

Name	Specialty	Pg	Name	Specialty	Pg
Posner, Jerome (NY)	N	469	Quintessenza, James (FL)	TS	1011
Posner, Mitchell (IL)	S	978	Quittell, Lynne (NY)	PPul	719
Posnick, Jeffrey (MD)	PlS	775	Quivey, Jeanne Marie (CA)	RadRO	881
Post, Kalmon (NY)	NS	431			
Postier, Russell (OK)	S	985			
Postma, Gregory (GA)	Oto	613	**R**		
Potkul, Ronald (IL)	GO	269			
Potsic, William (PA)	PO	714	Raab, Edward (NY)	Oph	530
Potter, Hollis (NY)	DR	892	Racz, Gabor (TX)	PM	639
Powell, Bayard (NC)	Hem	299	Rader, Daniel (PA)	IM	379
Powell, Catherine (CA)	GO	273	Radtke, Wolfgang (DE)	PCd	673
Powell, Nelson (CA)	Oto	626	Raffel, Corey (MN)	NS	441
Powers, Alvin (TN)	EDM	203	Rafferty, Janice (OH)	CRS	169
Powers, Eric (SC)	Cv	106	Raghavan, Derek (OH)	Onc	333
Powers, Pauline (FL)	Psyc	810	Raghu, Ganesh (WA)	Pul	859
Prados, Michael (CA)	Onc	345	Ragnarsson, Kristjan (NY)	PMR	758
Prager, Joshua (CA)	PM	640	Rahal, James (NY)	Inf	365
Prakash, Udaya (MN)	Pul	853	Rahko, Peter (WI)	Cv	111
Preminger, Glenn (NC)	U	1042	Rai, Kanti (NY)	Hem	296
Prensky, Arthur (MO)	ChiN	146	Raiford, David (TN)	Ge	227
Present, Daniel (NY)	Ge	223	Raja, Srinivasa (MD)	PM	635
Press, Joel (IL)	PMR	762	Rajfer, Jacob (CA)	U	1056
Press, Oliver W (WA)	Onc	345	Rakowski, Thomas (VA)	Nep	414
Presti, Joseph C (CA)	U	1056	Ramamurthy, Somayaji (TX)	PM	639
Price, Lawrence (RI)	Psyc	803	Raman, Jai (IL)	TS	1015
Price, Ronald (OH)	Oph	541	Ramanathan, Ramesh (PA)	S	964
Prieto, Victor (TX)	Path	655	Ramee, Stephen (LA)	Cv	115
Prinz, Richard (IL)	S	978	Ramirez, Oscar (MD)	PlS	775
Prosnitz, Leonard (NC)	RadRO	874	Ramsay, David (NY)	D	180
Provenzale, James (NC)	NRad	899	Ramsey, Bonnie (WA)	PPul	721
Pruitt, David (MD)	ChAP	824	Ramsey, Matthew (PA)	OrS	570
Prystowsky, Eric (IN)	CE	122	Ranawat, Chitranjan (NY)	OrS	571
Puccetti, Diane (WI)	PHO	700	Rand, Jacob (NY)	Hem	297
Puckett, Charles (MO)	PlS	783	Rand, Richard (WA)	PlS	791
Pui, Ching (TN)	PHO	697	Randall, R Lor (UT)	OrS	583
Pula, Thaddeus (MD)	N	469	Randolph, Gregory (MA)	Oto	602
Puliafito, Carmen (FL)	Oph	536	Randolph, Linda (CA)	CG	159
Putnam, Joe (TN)	TS	1011	Rao, Nalini (PA)	Inf	365
Putnam, Matthew (MN)	HS	286	Rao, Narsing (CA)	Oph	551
Putterman, Allen (IL)	Oph	541	Rao, Satish (IA)	Ge	232
Pyeritz, Reed (PA)	CG	153	Rao, Vijay (PA)	DR	892
Pynoos, Robert (CA)	Psyc	816	Raphael, Bruce (NY)	Hem	297
			Rapoport, Judith (MD)	ChAP	824
Q			Rappaport, Leonard (MA)	Ped	664
			Rashid, Asif (TX)	Path	655
			Raskin, Keith (NY)	HS	282
Quaegebeur, Jan (NY)	PS	727	Raskin, Philip (TX)	EDM	209
Quagliarello, Vincent (CT)	Inf	362	Raskind, Murray (WA)	Psyc	816
Quatela, Vito (NY)	Oto	608	Rasmussen, Steven (RI)	Psyc	803
Quencer, Robert (FL)	NRad	899	Rassman, William (CA)	S	989
Quigley, Harry (MD)	Oph	530	Ratain, Mark J (IL)	Onc	333
Quinn, Graham (PA)	Oph	530	Ratner, Robert (DC)	EDM	200
Quinn, Suzanne (FL)	EDM	203	Ratts, Valerie (MO)	RE	921

Alphabetical Listing of Doctors

Name	Specialty	Pg	Name	Specialty	Pg
Ratzan, Kenneth (FL)	Inf	368	Retik, Alan (MA)	U	1031
Rauch, Steven (MA)	Oto	602	Reuben, David (CA)	Ger	254
Rauck, Richard (NC)	PM	637	Reul, George (TX)	TS	1019
Rausen, Aaron (NY)	PHO	696	Reus, Victor (CA)	Psyc	817
Ravich, William (MD)	Ge	223	Rex, Douglas (IN)	Ge	232
Ray, Albert (FL)	Psyc	810	Reynolds, James (NY)	Oph	530
Rayan, Ghazi (OK)	HS	287	Reynolds, Marleta (IL)	PS	731
Raz, Shlomo (CA)	U	1056	Reynolds, R Kevin (MI)	GO	270
Ready, John (MA)	OrS	561	Rezai, Ali (OH)	NS	441
Ready, L Brian (WA)	PM	640	Rheingold, Susan R (PA)	PHO	696
Reaman, Gregory (DC)	PHO	696	Rhoads, J Marc (TX)	PGe	691
Reardon, Michael (TX)	TS	1019	Rice, Dale (CA)	Oto	626
Reasner, Charles A (TX)	EDM	209	Rice, Henry (NC)	PS	729
Reber, Howard (CA)	S	989	Rice, Laurel (VA)	GO	267
Recht, Abram (MA)	RadRO	869	Rice, Thomas (OH)	TS	1015
Rechtine, Glenn (NY)	OrS	571	Rich, Keith (MO)	NS	441
Recker, Robert (NE)	EDM	208	Rich, Stuart (IL)	Cv	111
Redberg, Rita (CA)	Cv	117	Rich, Tyvin (VA)	RadRO	874
Redding, Gregory (WA)	PPul	722	Richard, James (OK)	Oph	546
Reddy, Daniel (MI)	VascS	1073	Richards, Jon (IL)	Onc	333
Reddy, K Rajender (PA)	Ge	223	Richardson, Marilyn (KS)	RE	922
Reder, Anthony (IL)	N	480	Richardson, Mark (OR)	PO	718
Redlich, Carrie (CT)	Pul	842	Richardson, William (NC)	OrS	576
Reed, Carolyn (SC)	TS	1011	Richie, Jerome (MA)	U	1031
Reed, Kathryn (AZ)	MF	393	Richman, Douglas (CA)	Inf	372
Reed, Robert (OH)	N	480	Richter, Joel (PA)	Ge	223
Rees, Riley (MI)	PlS	783	Ricketts, Richard (GA)	PS	729
Regillo, Carl D (PA)	Oph	530	Ricotta, John (NY)	VascS	1070
Reich, Stephen (MD)	N	469	Riddle, Mark (MD)	ChAP	824
Reichelderfer, Mark (WI)	Ge	232	Riddle, Matthew (OR)	EDM	211
Reichman, Lee (NJ)	Pul	844	Ridge, John A (PA)	S	964
Reider, Bruce (IL)	SM	949	Ridgway, E (CO)	EDM	208
Reilly, Donald (MA)	OrS	561	Ridker, Paul (MA)	Cv	96
Reilly, John (MA)	Pul	842	Ries, Andrew (CA)	Pul	859
Reilly, Raymond (MA)	ObG	508	Riew, K Daniel (MO)	OrS	581
Rein, Michael (VA)	Inf	368	Rigamonti, Daniele (MD)	NS	431
Reiner, Jonathan (DC)	IC	125	Rigel, Darrell (NY)	D	180
Reiner, Mark (NY)	S	964	Rikkers, Layton (WI)	S	978
Reinisch, John (CA)	PlS	791	Riles, Thomas (NY)	VascS	1070
Reintgen, Douglas (FL)	S	971	Riley, Laura (MA)	MF	387
Reis, Steven (PA)	Cv	101	Rilling, William (WI)	VIR	906
Reisberg, Barry (NY)	GerPsy	829	Rimoin, David L (CA)	CG	159
Reisman, Robert (NY)	A&I	83	Ring, William (TX)	TS	1019
Reiss, Craig (MO)	Cv	111	Ringel, Steven (CO)	N	483
Reitz, Bruce (CA)	TS	1022	Rink, Richard (IN)	U	1048
Relkin, Norman (NY)	N	470	Riordan, John (CA)	Nep	419
Remmenga, Steven (NE)	GO	271	Ristow, Brunno (CA)	PlS	791
Rennard, Stephen (NE)	Pul	855	Ritch, Robert (NY)	Oph	530
Rennke, Helmut (MA)	Path	644	Ritchey, Arthur (PA)	PHO	696
Renshaw, Domeena (IL)	Psyc	812	Rivera, Frank (TX)	VIR	907
Resar, Jon (MD)	IC	125	Riviello, James (MA)	ChiN	142
Resnick, Neil (PA)	Ger	249	Rivlin, Richard (NY)	IM	379

Alphabetical Listing of Doctors

Name	Specialty	Pg	Name	Specialty	Pg
Rizk, Norman (CA)	Pul	860	Rosen, Charles (MN)	S	978
Rizza, Robert (MN)	EDM	207	Rosen, Clark A (PA)	Oto	608
Roach, Mack (CA)	RadRO	881	Rosen, Jules (PA)	GerPsy	829
Robb, Geoffrey (TX)	PlS	786	Rosen, Paul (NY)	Path	648
Robb, Richard (MA)	Oph	523	Rosen, Steven (IL)	Onc	333
Robbins, Lawrence (IL)	PM	637	Rosenbaum, Jerrold (MA)	Psyc	803
Robbins, Robert (CA)	TS	1022	Rosenbaum, Kenneth (DC)	CG	154
Robert, Nicholas (VA)	Onc	325	Rosenbaum, Richard (OR)	N	489
Roberts, Barbara (RI)	Cv	97	Rosenberg, Aaron (IL)	OrS	581
Roberts, John (CA)	S	989	Rosenberg, Howard (CA)	PlS	791
Roberts, Patricia L (MA)	CRS	164	Rosenberg, Michael (IL)	Oph	542
Roberts, William (TX)	Path	655	Rosenberg, Steven (MD)	S	965
Robertson, Cary N (NC)	U	1042	Rosenberg, Thomas (UT)	OrS	583
Robins, Perry (NY)	D	180	Rosenblatt, Joseph (FL)	Hem	299
Robinson, Dwight (MA)	Rhu	928	Rosenblum, Marc (NY)	Path	648
Robinson, Lawrence (WA)	PMR	764	Rosenblum, Mark (MI)	NS	441
Rocchini, Albert (MI)	PCd	676	Rosenblum, Norman (PA)	GO	265
Roche, James (VA)	Ge	227	Rosenbush, Stuart (IL)	Cv	111
Rochester, Carolyn (CT)	Pul	842	Rosenfeld, Myrna (PA)	N	470
Rock, John (FL)	RE	919	Rosenfeld, Philip (FL)	Oph	536
Roddy, Sarah (CA)	ChiN	148	Rosenfeld, Richard (NY)	PO	714
Rodeo, Scott (NY)	SM	947	Rosenfeld, Steven (NY)	N	470
Rodgers, Bradley (VA)	PS	729	Rosenfield, Robert (Il)	PEn	685
Rodgers, George (UT)	Path	653	Rosengart, Todd (NY)	TS	1006
Rodts, Gerald (GA)	NS	435	Rosenman, Julian (NC)	RadRO	874
Roehrborn, Claus (TX)	U	1053	Rosenquist, Richard (IA)	PM	638
Rogers, Douglas (OH)	PEn	684	Rosenthal, Amnon (MI)	PCd	677
Rogers, Gary (OH)	Oph	542	Rosenthal, David (GA)	VascS	1072
Rogers, James (TX)	PM	639	Rosenthal, Joseph (CA)	PHO	704
Rogers, James (TX)	PCd	678	Rosenthal, Perry (MA)	Oph	523
Rogers, Joseph (NC)	Cv	106	Rosenwaks, Zev (NY)	RE	916
Rogers, Lisa (MI)	N	480	Rosenwasser, Lanny (MO)	A&I	87
Rogers, Robert (PA)	Pul	844	Rosenwasser, Melvin (NY)	HS	282
Roh, Mark (PA)	S	964	Rosenwasser, Robert (PA)	NS	432
Rohrich, Rod (TX)	PlS	787	Roses, Daniel (NY)	S	965
Rokito, Andrew (NY)	OrS	571	Rosier, Randy (NY)	OrS	571
Roman-Lopez, Juan J (AR)	GO	272	Roskes, Saul (MD)	PNep	710
Romano, James (CA)	PlS	791	Rosner, Howard (CA)	PM	640
Rombeau, John (PA)	CRS	166	Rosoff, Phillip (NC)	PHO	698
Romond, Edward H (KY)	Onc	326	Ross, Helen (OR)	Onc	345
Roodman, G David (PA)	Hem	297	Ross, Jeffrey (NY)	Path	648
Rook, Alain (PA)	D	181	Ross, Lawrence (IL)	U	1048
Roos, Karen (IN)	N	480	Ross, Merrick (TX)	S	985
Roos, Raymond (IL)	N	481	Rosse, Richard (DC)	Psyc	808
Roose, Steven (NY)	Psyc	807	Rosser, Tena (CA)	ChiN	148
Ropper, Allan (MA)	N	461	Rossman, Milton (PA)	Pul	844
Rosato, Ernest (PA)	S	964	Rostain, Anthony (PA)	ChAP	824
Rosbe, Kristina (CA)	PO	718	Roth, Bennett (CA)	Ge	239
Rose, Cecile (CO)	Pul	855	Roth, Bruce (TN)	Onc	326
Rose, Christopher (CA)	RadRO	881	Roth, David (FL)	Nep	414
Rose, Peter (OH)	GO	270	Roth, Elliot (IL)	PMR	762
Rosen, Antony (MD)	Rhu	932	Rothbaum, Robert (MO)	PGe	690

Name	Specialty	Pg
Rothenberg, Mace (TN)	Onc	326
Rothenberg, Russell (DC)	Rhu	932
Rothenberger, David (MN)	CRS	169
Rothman, Richard (PA)	OrS	571
Rothrock, John (AL)	N	474
Rothstein, Richard (NH)	Ge	217
Rotman, Marvin (NY)	RadRO	872
Rotmensch, Jacob (IL)	GO	270
Roubin, Gary (NY)	IC	125
Rovner, Barry (PA)	GerPsy	829
Rowbotham, Michael (CA)	PM	640
Rowland, Randall (KY)	U	1043
Rowley, Howard (WI)	NRad	900
Roy-Byrne, Peter (WA)	Psyc	817
Roye, David (NY)	OrS	571
Rozbruch, S Robert (NY)	OrS	571
Rubin, Geoffrey (CA)	DR	896
Rubin, Lewis (CA)	Pul	860
Rubin, Mark (CA)	D	190
Rubin, Peter (MA)	Oph	523
Rubin, Robert (MA)	Inf	362
Rubin, Stephen (PA)	GO	265
Rubin, Susan (IL)	N	481
Ruckdeschel, John C (MI)	Onc	333
Rudnick, Michael (PA)	Nep	412
Rudolph, Colin (WI)	PGe	690
Ruff, Robert L (OH)	N	481
Ruge, John (IL)	NS	441
Rushton, H Gil (DC)	U	1037
Ruskin, Jeremy (MA)	CE	118
Russell, Andrew (CA)	ChAP	828
Russell, Christy (CA)	Onc	345
Rutherford, Thomas (CT)	GO	262
Ryan, Colleen (MA)	S	955
Ryan, Neal (PA)	ChAP	824
Ryken, Timothy (IA)	NS	441

S

Name	Specialty	Pg
Saag, Michael (AL)	Inf	368
Saal, Howard (OH)	CG	155
Saal, Jeffrey (CA)	PMR	764
Sacchi, Terrence (NY)	Cv	102
Sacco, Ralph (FL)	N	474
Sachar, David (NY)	Ge	223
Sachs, Greg (IL)	Ger	252
Sack, Kenneth (CA)	Rhu	940
Saclarides, Theodore (IL)	CRS	169
Sadock, Virginia (NY)	Psyc	808
Sadowsky, Carl (FL)	N	475
Safai, Bijan (NY)	D	181
Saffle, Jeffrey (UT)	S	982

Name	Specialty	Pg
Safi, Hazim (TX)	TS	1020
Safian, Robert (MI)	Cv	111
Sagalowsky, Arthur (TX)	U	1053
Sagar, Stephen (OH)	N	481
Sage, Jacob (NJ)	N	470
Sagel, Stuart (MO)	DR	894
Saha, Sukamal (MI)	S	978
Sahn, Steven (SC)	Pul	849
Saiki, John (NM)	Onc	340
Sailer, Scott (NC)	RadRO	874
Saiman, Lisa (NY)	PInf	706
Sakamoto, Kathleen (CA)	PHO	704
Salant, David (MA)	Nep	410
Salem, Philip (TX)	Onc	341
Salem, Riad (IL)	VIR	906
Salem, Ronald (CT)	S	955
Salgia, Ravi (IL)	Onc	333
Salky, Barry (NY)	S	965
Sallan, Stephen (MA)	Ped	664
Sallent, Jorge (FL)	PPul	719
Saltz, Leonard B (NY)	Onc	319
Saltzman, Charles (UT)	OrS	583
Salvati, Eduardo A (NY)	OrS	571
Salvi, Sharad (IL)	PHO	700
Salz, James (CA)	Oph	551
Salzman, Carl (MA)	Psyc	803
Samberg, Eslee (NY)	Psyc	808
Sampson, Christian (MA)	HS	280
Sampson, Hugh (NY)	PA&I	667
Samson, Duke (TX)	NS	445
Samuels, Brian L (ID)	Onc	336
Samuels, Louis (PA)	TS	1006
Samuels, Martin (MA)	N	461
Samuelson, Thomas (MN)	Oph	542
Sanborn, Timothy (IL)	Cv	111
Sanchez, Luis (MO)	VascS	1073
Sanchez, Miguel (NJ)	Path	648
Sandborg, Christy (CA)	PRhu	724
Sandborn, William (MN)	Ge	232
Sanders, Georgiana (MI)	A&I	87
Sanders, William (GA)	U	1043
Sandhu, Harvinder (NY)	OrS	572
Sandler, Howard (MI)	RadRO	877
Sandler, Martin (TN)	NuM	502
Sandlow, Jay (WI)	U	1048
Sanfilippo, Joseph (PA)	RE	916
Sanford, Robert A (TN)	NS	435
Sangeorzan, Bruce (WA)	OrS	588
Sanger, James (WI)	PlS	783
Sankar, Raman (CA)	ChiN	148
Sanz, Luis (VA)	ObG	511
Saper, Joel (MI)	N	481

Alphabetical Listing of Doctors

Name	Specialty	Pg	Name	Specialty	Pg
Sargent, A John (TX)	ChAP	827	Schiff, Isaac (MA)	RE	915
Sarnaik, Ashok (MI)	PCCM	679	Schiff, Peter (NY)	RadRO	872
Sarno, John (NY)	PM	636	Schiff, William (NY)	Oph	531
Saroja, Kurubarahalli (IL)	Onc	333	Schiffer, Charles (MI)	Onc	334
Sarosi, George (IN)	IM	380	Schilder, Russell (PA)	Onc	320
Sarr, Michael (MN)	S	978	Schiller, Alan (NY)	Path	648
Sartor, R Balfour (NC)	Ge	227	Schiller, Gary J (CA)	Hem	306
Sasaki, Clarence (CT)	Oto	602	Schiller, Joan (TX)	Onc	341
Sataloff, Robert (PA)	Oto	608	Schilsky, Richard (IL)	Onc	334
Satava, Richard (WA)	S	989	Schink, Julian C (IL)	GO	270
Sato, Thomas (WI)	PS	731	Schirmer, Bruce (VA)	S	972
Saudek, Christopher (MD)	EDM	200	Schlaepfer, William (PA)	Path	648
Sauer, Mark (NY)	RE	917	Schlaff, William (CO)	RE	922
Saul, Robert (SC)	CG	155	Schlegel, Peter (NY)	U	1037
Saunders, Elijah (MD)	Cv	102	Schley, W Shain (NY)	Oto	608
Savage, David (NY)	Hem	297	Schlinkert, Richard (AZ)	S	985
Saven, Alan (CA)	Hem	306	Schluger, Neil (NY)	Pul	844
Savino, Peter (PA)	Oph	530	Schmalzried, Thomas (CA)	OrS	588
Sawaya, Raymond (TX)	NS	445	Schmidt, Joseph (CA)	U	1056
Sawczuk, Ihor (NJ)	U	1037	Schmidt, Warren (IA)	Ge	232
Sawin, Robert (WA)	PS	734	Schnabel, Freya (NY)	S	965
Sax, Paul (MA)	Inf	362	Schnipper, Lowell (MA)	Onc	309
Scandling, John (CA)	Nep	419	Schnitt, Stuart (MA)	Path	645
Scantlebury, Velma (AL)	S	972	Schnittger, Ingela (CA)	Cv	118
Scarborough, Mark (FL)	OrS	576	Schoen, Robert (CT)	Rhu	928
Scardino, Peter (NY)	U	1037	Schoetz, David (MA)	CRS	164
Schachat, Andrew (OH)	Oph	542	Schold, S Clifford (FL)	N	475
Schaefer, Steven (NY)	Oto	608	Schooley, Robert (CA)	Inf	372
Schaeffer, Anthony (IL)	U	1049	Schottenfeld, Richard (CT)	AdP	818
Schafer, Michael (IL)	OrS	581	Schraut, Wolfgang (PA)	S	965
Schaff, Hartzell (MN)	TS	1015	Schreiber, Helmut (OH)	S	978
Schanberg, Laura (NC)	PRhu	723	Schreiber, James (MO)	ObG	513
Schapiro, Randall (MN)	N	481	Schreiber, Theodore (MI)	IC	127
Schatz, Norman (FL)	N	475	Schrier, Robert (CO)	Nep	417
Schatzberg, Alan (CA)	Psyc	817	Schubert, Mark (AZ)	A&I	88
Schechter, David (CA)	SM	950	Schuberth, Kenneth (MD)	PA&I	668
Scheel, Paul (MD)	Nep	412	Schuchter, Lynn (PA)	Onc	320
Scheff, Alice M (CA)	NuM	503	Schuckit, Marc (CA)	AdP	820
Schein, Oliver (MD)	Oph	530	Schuger, Claudio (MI)	CE	122
Scheinberg, David (NY)	Onc	319	Schulak, James (OH)	S	978
Scheinman, Steven (NY)	Nep	412	Schuller, David (OH)	Oto	619
Scheithauer, Bernd (MN)	Path	652	Schulman, Steven (MD)	Cv	102
Schelbert, Heinrich (CA)	NuM	503	Schulze, Konrad (IA)	Ge	232
Scheld, William (VA)	Inf	368	Schuman, Joel (PA)	Oph	531
Scheller, Arnold (MA)	SM	946	Schurman, David (CA)	OrS	588
Schellhammer, Paul (VA)	U	1043	Schuster, Michael (NY)	Hem	297
Schenck, Robert (IL)	HS	286	Schusterman, Mark (TX)	PlS	787
Schenken, Robert (TX)	RE	922	Schwab, Richard (PA)	Pul	844
Schepps, Barbara (RI)	DR	889	Schwartz, Allan (NY)	Cv	102
Scher, Charles (LA)	PHO	702	Schwartz, Burton (MN)	Onc	334
Scher, Howard (NY)	Onc	320	Schwartz, Cindy (RI)	PHO	692
Schiff, Eugene (FL)	Ge	227	Schwartz, David (NC)	Pul	849

Castle Connolly America's Top Doctors® 7th Edition

Alphabetical Listing of Doctors

Name	Specialty	Pg	Name	Specialty	Pg
Sherman, David (TX)	N	486	Silver, Julie (MA)	PMR	756
Sherman, James (VA)	PPul	719	Silver, Michael (IL)	Pul	853
Sherman, Orrin (NY)	OrS	572	Silver, Richard (SC)	Rhu	934
Sherman, Randolph (CA)	PlS	791	Silverberg, Steven (MD)	Path	648
Sherman, Stuart (IN)	Ge	233	Silverman, Norman (MI)	TS	1016
Sherry, David (PA)	PRhu	723	Silverman, William (IA)	Ge	233
Sherwin, Robert (CT)	EDM	197	Silverstein, Herbert (FL)	Oto	613
Sherwood, Mark (FL)	Oph	536	Silverstein, Janet (FL)	PEn	683
Shields, Carol (PA)	Oph	531	Silverstein, Melvin (CA)	S	989
Shields, Jerry (PA)	Oph	531	Silverstein, Roy (OH)	Hem	303
Shields, William (CA)	ChiN	149	Simmons, James (TX)	OrS	585
Shiffman, Mitchell (VA)	Ge	227	Simms, Robert (MA)	Rhu	929
Shike, Moshe (NY)	Ge	224	Simon, James (DC)	RE	917
Shikora, Scott (MA)	S	955	Simon, John (NY)	Oph	531
Shin, Dong Moon (GA)	Onc	327	Simon, Michael (IL)	OrS	582
Shina, Donald (NM)	RadRO	879	Simon, Robert (MD)	Psyc	808
Shipley, William U (MA)	RadRO	869	Simons, Michael (NH)	Cv	97
Shively, Robert (MO)	SM	949	Simpson, Joe Leigh (FL)	ObG	511
Shlansky-Goldberg, Richard (PA)	VIR	903	Sinanan, Mika (WA)	S	990
Shlasko, Edward (NY)	PS	727	Sinatra, Frank (CA)	PGe	692
Shlofmitz, Richard (NY)	Cv	102	Singer, Daniel (HI)	OrS	588
Shochat, Stephen J (TN)	PS	729	Singer, Peter (CA)	EDM	211
Shore, Bernard (MO)	Pul	853	Singer, Robert (CA)	PlS	792
Shorofsky, Stephen (MD)	IC	125	Singer, Samuel (NY)	S	966
Shortliffe, Linda (CA)	U	1057	Singh, Arun (RI)	TS	999
Shoulson, Ira (NY)	N	470	Singh, Nalini (DC)	PInf	706
Shrager, Joseph (PA)	TS	1006	Singletary, Sonja (TX)	S	985
Shuer, Lawrence (CA)	NS	448	Sinha, Uttam (CA)	Oto	626
Shuldiner, Alan (MD)	EDM	201	Siperstein, Allan (OH)	S	979
Shulman, Lawrence (MA)	Onc	309	Sirdofsky, Michael (DC)	N	470
Shulman, Lee (IL)	ObG	513	Siris, Ethel (NY)	EDM	201
Shulman, Stanford (IL)	PInf	707	Sison, Joseph (NJ)	NP	402
Shupack, Jerome L (NY)	D	181	Sisung, Charles (IL)	PMR	762
Siatkowski, R Michael (OK)	Oph	546	Sivina, Manuel (FL)	VascS	1072
Sibley, Richard (CA)	Path	657	Sivit, Carlos (OH)	DR	894
Sicard, Gregorio (MO)	VascS	1073	Skinner, Donald G (CA)	U	1057
Siddique, Teepu (IL)	N	481	Skinner, Eila (CA)	U	1057
Sidransky, David (MD)	Onc	320	Skinner, Kristin (NY)	S	966
Siebert, John (NY)	PlS	776	Sklar, Charles (NY)	PEn	682
Siegel, Barry (MO)	NuM	502	Sklar, Frederick (TX)	NS	445
Siegel, Gordon (IL)	Oto	619	Skoner, David (PA)	PA&I	668
Siegel, Stuart (CA)	PHO	704	Skyler, Jay (FL)	EDM	203
Sielaff, Timothy (MN)	S	979	Slama, Thomas (IN)	Inf	369
Siemionow, Maria (OH)	PlS	783	Slankard, Marjorie (NY)	A&I	84
Sigman, Mark (RI)	U	1031	Slap, Gail (PA)	AM	78
Sigurdson, Elin (PA)	S	966	Slatkin, Neal (CA)	PM	640
Silber, Sherman (MO)	U	1049	Sleasman, John (FL)	PRhu	723
Silberstein, Edward (OH)	NuM	502	Sledge, George (IN)	Onc	334
Silberstein, Stephen (PA)	N	470	Slezak, Sheri (MD)	PlS	776
Sillers, Michael (AL)	Oto	613	Slipman, Curtis (PA)	PMR	758
Sills, Edward (MD)	PRhu	723	Sliwa, James (IL)	PMR	762
Silva, Elvio (TX)	Path	655	Slomowitz, Marcia (IL)	ChAP	826

Name	Specialty	Pg	Name	Specialty	Pg
Sly, R Michael (DC)	PA&I	668	Sonett, Joshua (NY)	TS	1006
Small, Eric (CA)	Onc	346	Sonnenblick, Edmund (NY)	Cv	102
Small, Gary (CA)	GerPsy	831	Sonntag, Volker (AZ)	NS	445
Smalley, Stephen (KS)	RadRO	877	Sontheimer, Richard (OK)	D	188
Smalling, Richard (TX)	IC	128	Sood, Rajiv (IN)	PlS	783
Smart, Frank (NJ)	Cv	102	Soparkar, Charles (TX)	Oph	546
Smedira, Nicholas (OH)	TS	1016	Soper, John (NC)	GO	268
Smith, Barbara (MA)	S	955	Soper, Nathaniel (IL)	S	979
Smith, Craig (NY)	TS	1006	Sorrell, Michael (NE)	Ge	235
Smith, Craig (CA)	S	990	Sorrentino, Robert (GA)	CE	121
Smith, David (FL)	PlS	780	Sosa, R Ernest (NY)	U	1037
Smith, Donna (IL)	GO	270	Soter, Nicholas (NY)	D	181
Smith, Harriet (NM)	GO	272	Soulen, Michael (PA)	VIR	903
Smith, Joanne (IL)	PMR	762	Soules, Michael (WA)	RE	923
Smith, John (OH)	TS	1016	Souryal, Tarek (TX)	OrS	585
Smith, Joseph A (TN)	U	1043	Sowers, James (MO)	EDM	207
Smith, Lee (DC)	CRS	166	Spann, Cyril (GA)	GO	268
Smith, Lloyd (CA)	GO	273	Sparling, P Frederick (NC)	Inf	368
Smith, Mitchell (PA)	Onc	320	Spear, Scott (DC)	PlS	776
Smith, Peter (NC)	TS	1011	Speeg, Kermit V (TX)	Ge	238
Smith, Robert (CA)	U	1057	Speer, Kevin (NC)	SM	947
Smith, Ronald (CA)	Oph	551	Spence, Alexander (WA)	N	489
Smith, Sidney (NC)	Cv	107	Spence, Robert (MD)	PlS	776
Smith, Steven (IL)	VIR	906	Spencer, Dennis (CT)	NS	425
Smith, Thomas (VA)	Onc	327	Spencer, Susan (CT)	N	461
Smith, Wade (CA)	N	489	Spencer, Thomas (MA)	ChAP	821
Smith, Yolanda (MI)	RE	922	Spengler, Dan (TN)	OrS	576
Snustad, Diane (VA)	Ger	250	Sperling, Mark (PA)	PEn	682
Snyder, Howard (PA)	U	1037	Sperling, Michael (PA)	N	470
Snyder, Peter (PA)	EDM	201	Spetzler, Robert (AZ)	NS	446
Snyderman, Carl (PA)	Oto	609	Speyer, James (NY)	Onc	320
Sobel, Jack (MI)	Inf	369	Spiegel, David (CA)	Psyc	817
Sobel, Michael (WA)	S	990	Spiera, Harry (NY)	Rhu	932
Sobel, Stuart (FL)	D	184	Spindler, Kurt (TN)	OrS	576
Sober, Arthur (MA)	D	177	Spinelli, Henry (NY)	PlS	776
Socinski, Mark (NC)	Onc	327	Spirtos, Nicola (NV)	GO	273
Socol, Michael (IL)	MF	391	Spitzer, Thomas (MA)	Hem	294
Sodt, Peter (IL)	PCd	677	Spivak, Jeffrey (NY)	OrS	572
Soisson, Andrew (UT)	GO	271	Spivak, Jerry (MD)	Hem	297
Sokol, Mae (NE)	ChAP	827	Spivak, William (NY)	PGe	688
Sokoloff, Daniel (FL)	D	184	Sponseller, Paul (MD)	OrS	572
Sola, Augusto (NJ)	NP	402	Spray, Thomas (PA)	PS	727
Solberg, Lawrence (FL)	Hem	299	Spriggs, David (NY)	Onc	320
Solin, Lawrence (PA)	RadRO	872	Springfield, Dempsey (MA)	OrS	561
Sollinger, Hans (WI)	S	979	Squires, Robert (PA)	PGe	688
Solomon, Gary (NY)	Rhu	932	Srivastava, Sudhir Prem (TX)	TS	1020
Solomon, Robert (NY)	NS	432	Staats, Peter (NJ)	PM	636
Soloway, Mark (FL)	U	1043	Stadelmann, Wayne (NH)	PlS	771
Somerville, James (MN)	Nep	416	Stadler, Walter (IL)	Onc	334
Sondak, Vernon K (FL)	S	972	Stadtmauer, Edward (PA)	Onc	321
Sondel, Paul (WI)	PHO	701	Staffenberg, David (NY)	PlS	776
Sondheimer, Steven (PA)	RE	917	Stahl, Donna (OH)	S	979

Alphabetical Listing of Doctors

Name	Specialty	Pg	Name	Specialty	Pg
Stahl, Richard (CT)	PlS	771	Stieg, Philip E (NY)	NS	432
Stal, Samuel (TX)	PlS	787	Stiehm, E Richard (CA)	PA&I	671
Stamos, Michael (CA)	CRS	171	Stiff, Patrick (IL)	Hem	303
Stankiewicz, James (IL)	Oto	619	Stiles, Alan (NC)	NP	403
Stanley, Charles (PA)	PEn	682	Stock, Richard (NY)	RadRO	872
Stanley, James (MI)	VascS	1073	Stockdale, Frank (CA)	Onc	346
Stanley, John (PA)	D	181	Stolar, Charles (NY)	PS	727
Staples, Edward (FL)	TS	1011	Stolier, Alan (LA)	S	985
Stapleton, F Bruder (WA)	PNep	713	Stoller, James (OH)	Pul	854
Stark, Walter (MD)	Oph	532	Stoller, Marshall (CA)	U	1057
Starnes, Vaughn (CA)	TS	1023	Stone, Anthony (CA)	U	1057
Starr, Arnold (CA)	N	489	Stone, Edwin (IA)	Oph	542
Starz, Terence (PA)	Rhu	932	Stone, Gregg (NY)	IC	125
Stea, Baldassarre (AZ)	RadRO	879	Stone, Joel (FL)	Onc	327
Steadman, J Richard (CO)	OrS	583	Stone, Michael (NY)	Psyc	808
Steed, David (PA)	VascS	1070	Stone, Richard (MA)	Hem	294
Steege, John (NC)	ObG	511	Stoopler, Mark (NY)	Onc	321
Steen, Virginia (DC)	Rhu	933	Stopeck, Alison (AZ)	Onc	341
Steers, William (VA)	U	1043	Stout, John (OR)	Oph	552
Stehman, Frederick (IN)	GO	270	Stover-Pepe, Diane (NY)	Pul	845
Steichen, James (IN)	HS	287	Strain, Eric (MD)	AdP	819
Steiger, David (NY)	Pul	845	Strakowski, Stephen (OH)	Psyc	812
Stein, Elliott (FL)	GerPsy	830	Strand, William (TX)	U	1053
Stein, James (CA)	PS	734	Strasberg, Steven M (MO)	S	979
Stein, James (WI)	Cv	112	Strashun, Arnold (NY)	NuM	501
Stein, John (CA)	U	1057	Strassner, Howard (IL)	MF	391
Stein, Mark (FL)	A&I	85	Stratta, Robert (NC)	S	972
Stein, Murray (CA)	Psyc	817	Strauch, Robert (NY)	HS	283
Steinberg, Gary (IL)	U	1049	Straus, David (NY)	Onc	321
Steinberg, Gary (CA)	NS	448	Strauss, H William (NY)	NuM	501
Steinberg, Harry (NY)	Pul	845	Strauss, James (TX)	Hem	305
Steiner, Hans (CA)	ChAP	828	Streeter, Oscar (CA)	RadRO	881
Steinert, Roger (CA)	Oph	551	Streim, Joel (PA)	GerPsy	829
Steingart, Richard (NY)	Cv	103	Strife, Janet (OH)	DR	895
Steinhagen, Randolph (NY)	CRS	166	Stringer, Scott (MS)	Oto	613
Steinherz, Peter (NY)	PHO	696	Strober, Warren (MD)	A&I	84
Steinhorn, Robin (IL)	NP	405	Strollo, Patrick (PA)	Pul	845
Steinkampf, Michael (AL)	RE	919	Strome, Marshall (OH)	Oto	619
Stern, Jeffrey (CA)	GO	273	Strome, Scott (MD)	Oto	609
Stern, Matthew (PA)	N	471	Strong, Michael (PA)	TS	1007
Stern, Peter (OH)	HS	287	Strongwater, Allan (NY)	OrS	572
Stern, Robert (OH)	PPul	720	Strouse, Thomas (CA)	Psyc	817
Sternberg, Paul (TN)	Oph	536	Strunk, Robert (MO)	PA&I	669
Stevenson, David (CA)	NP	406	Stryker, Steven (IL)	CRS	170
Stevenson, Lynne (MA)	Cv	97	Stuart, Richard (MO)	TS	1016
Stevenson, Roger (SC)	CG	155	Stubblefield, Michael (NY)	PMR	759
Stevenson, Thomas (CA)	PlS	792	Stuchin, Steven (NY)	OrS	573
Stevenson, William (MA)	CE	118	Studenski, Stephanie (PA)	Ger	249
Stewart, Forrest (WA)	Onc	346	Stulberg, S David (IL)	OrS	582
Stewart, Michael (NY)	Oto	609	Stulting, R Doyle (GA)	Oph	536
Stewart, Ronald (TX)	S	985	Stuzin, James (FL)	PlS	780
Stewart, William (OH)	Cv	112	Stylianos, Steven (FL)	PS	729

Name	Specialty	Pg	Name	Specialty	Pg
Subramanian, Valavanur (NY)	TS	1007	Takahashi, Masato (CA)	PCd	678
Suchy, Frederick (NY)	PGe	688	Takimoto, Chris (TX)	Onc	341
Suen, James Y (AR)	Oto	624	Talamonti, Mark (IL)	S	980
Sugarbaker, David (MA)	TS	999	Tallman, Martin (IL)	Hem	303
Sugarbaker, Paul (DC)	S	966	Tamargo, Rafael (MD)	NS	432
Suki, Wadi (TX)	Nep	418	Tamaroff, Marc (CA)	A&I	88
Sullivan, Mark (WA)	Psyc	817	Tamborlane, William (CT)	PEn	681
Sullivan, Patrick (RI)	PlS	771	Tamer, Dolores (FL)	PCd	674
Sullivan, Timothy (GA)	A&I	85	Tanabe, Kenneth (MA)	S	956
Sultan, Mark (NY)	PlS	776	Taneja, Samir (NY)	U	1037
Summer, Warren (LA)	Pul	857	Tanner, Caroline (CA)	N	490
Summers, C Gail (MN)	Oph	542	Tapson, Victor (NC)	Pul	850
Sumpio, Bauer (CT)	VascS	1067	Tardo, Carmela (LA)	ChiN	147
Sundt, Thoralf (MN)	TS	1016	Targan, Stephan (CA)	Ge	240
Sundy, John (NC)	Rhu	934	Tarraza, Hector (ME)	GO	263
Supiano, Mark (UT)	Ger	252	Tarry, William (WV)	U	1038
Surawicz, Christina (WA)	Ge	240	Tartter, Paul (NY)	S	966
Surks, Martin (NY)	EDM	201	Tatter, Stephen (NC)	NS	435
Surrey, Eric (CO)	RE	922	Taylor, Frederick (MN)	N	482
Sussman, Norman (NY)	Psyc	808	Taylor, Marie (MO)	RadRO	877
Suster, Saul (OH)	Path	653	Taylor, Peyton (VA)	GO	268
Suter, Cary (NM)	N	486	Taylor, R Stan (TX)	D	188
Sutherland, David (MN)	S	980	Taylor, Richard (TX)	PCCM	680
Sutton, John (NH)	S	956	Tchou, Patrick (OH)	CE	122
Sutton, Leslie (PA)	NS	432	Teal, James (DC)	DR	893
Sutton, Linda (NC)	Onc	327	Tebbetts, John (TX)	PlS	787
Swaid, Swaid (AL)	NS	435	Tedder, Mark (TN)	TS	1011
Swanson, David (TX)	U	1053	Teigland, Chris (NC)	U	1043
Swanson, Jerry (MN)	N	481	Teirstein, Alvin (NY)	Pul	845
Swanson, Neil (OR)	D	190	Teirstein, Paul (CA)	IC	128
Swanson, Scott (NY)	TS	1007	Teitel, David (CA)	PCd	679
Swarm, Robert (MO)	PM	638	Teitelbaum, George (CA)	NRad	902
Swartz, Richard (MI)	Nep	416	Teknos, Theodoros (MI)	Oto	620
Sweet, Richard (CA)	ObG	514	Telen, Marilyn (NC)	Hem	299
Swensen, Stephen (MN)	DR	895	Telian, Steven (MI)	Oto	620
Swerdloff, Ronald (CA)	EDM	211	Tempero, Margaret (CA)	Onc	346
Swerdlow, Charles (CA)	CE	123	Ten, Rosa Maria (IN)	A&I	87
Swerdlow, Michael (NY)	N	471	Tenenbaum, Joseph (NY)	Cv	103
Swerdlow, Steven (PA)	Path	649	Teng, Nelson (CA)	GO	273
Swetter, Susan (CA)	D	190	Tenner, Michael (NY)	NRad	898
Swiontkowski, Marc (MN)	OrS	582	Tenover, Joyce (GA)	Ger	251
Swistel, Alexander (NY)	S	966	Teperman, Lewis (NY)	S	966
Szabo, Robert (CA)	HS	288	Tepper, Joel (NC)	RadRO	874
Szachowicz, Edward (MN)	Oto	619	Terr, Lenore (CA)	ChAP	828
			Terris, David (GA)	Oto	614
T			Terris, Martha (GA)	U	1043
			Terry, Peter (MD)	Pul	845
Tabak, Brian (CA)	D	190	Tetrud, James (CA)	N	490
Tabbal, Nicolas (NY)	PlS	777	Tewari, Ashutosh (NY)	U	1038
Tabsh, Khalil (CA)	MF	394	Textor, Stephen (MN)	Nep	416
Taft, Timothy (NC)	OrS	576	Thalgott, John (NV)	OrS	589
Tajik, A Jamil (AZ)	Cv	115	Thames, Marc (AZ)	Cv	115

Alphabetical Listing of Doctors

Name	Specialty	Pg	Name	Specialty	Pg
Tharratt, Robert (CA)	Pul	860	Treem, William (NY)	PGe	688
Thase, Michael (PA)	Psyc	808	Tremaine, William (MN)	Ge	233
Thiers, Bruce H (SC)	D	184	Trenholme, Gordon (IL)	Inf	370
Thistlethwaite, J Richard (IL)	S	980	Trento, Alfredo (CA)	TS	1023
Thistlethwaite, Patricia (CA)	TS	1023	Treon, Steven (MA)	Onc	310
Thomas, Anthony (OH)	U	1049	Trerotola, Scott (PA)	VIR	904
Thomas, James (TX)	PCCM	680	Trese, Michael (MI)	Oph	543
Thomashow, Byron (NY)	Pul	845	Trick, Lorence (TX)	OrS	585
Thompson, Ann Ellen (PA)	PCCM	679	Tripuraneni, Prabhakar (CA)	RadRO	881
Thompson, B Gregory (MI)	NS	442	Trivedi, Madhukar H (TX)	Psyc	814
Thompson, Ian (TX)	U	1053	Trobe, Jonathan (MI)	Oph	543
Thompson, John (FL)	PGe	689	Troner, Michael (FL)	Onc	327
Thor, Ann (CO)	Path	653	True, Lawrence D (WA)	Path	658
Thorne, Charles (NY)	PlS	777	Trulock, Elbert (MO)	Pul	854
Thornhill, Thomas (MA)	OrS	562	Trumble, Thomas (WA)	HS	289
Thorp, John M (NC)	MF	389	Tsai, James (CT)	Oph	523
Thorson, Alan (NE)	CRS	170	Tsai, Tsu (KY)	HS	284
Thurmond, Amy (OR)	DR	896	Tsangaris, Theodore (MD)	S	967
Tiel, Robert (MS)	NS	435	Tse, David (FL)	Oph	537
Tinetti, Mary (CT)	Ger	248	Tucci, Debara (NC)	Oto	614
Tino, Gregory (PA)	Pul	846	Tulipan, Noel (TN)	NS	435
Tischler, Henry (NY)	OrS	573	Tune, Larry (GA)	GerPsy	830
Tobias, Hillel (NY)	Ge	224	Tunkel, David (MD)	PO	715
Tobin, Gordon (KY)	PlS	780	Turecki, Stanley (NY)	ChAP	824
Tobin, Martin (IL)	Pul	854	Turk, William (FL)	ChiN	145
Todd, George (NY)	VascS	1070	Turner, William (TX)	TS	1020
Todd, Richard (MO)	ChAP	826	Turrentine, Mark (IN)	TS	1016
Todd, Robert (MI)	Onc	334	Tuttle, Robert (NY)	EDM	201
Toledano, Stuart R (FL)	PHO	698	Tuttle, Todd (MN)	S	980
Tolkoff-Rubin, Nina (MA)	Nep	411	Tychsen, Lawrence (MO)	Oph	543
Tolo, Vernon (CA)	OrS	589	Tyler, Douglas (NC)	S	972
Tomaszewski, John (PA)	Path	649	Tyson, Jon (TX)	NP	406
Tomera, Kevin (AK)	U	1057	Tzakis, Andreas (FL)	S	972

U

Name	Specialty	Pg
Tomich, Paul (NE)	MF	392
Tomita, Tadanori (IL)	NS	442
Toriumi, Dean (IL)	Oto	620
Tornos, Carmen (NY)	Path	649
Torres, Vicente (MN)	Nep	416
Torti, Frank (NC)	Onc	327
Toskes, Phillip (FL)	Ge	227
Toto, Robert (TX)	Nep	418
Towne, Jonathan (WI)	VascS	1074
Townsend, Raymond (PA)	Nep	413
Traboulsi, Elias (OH)	Oph	542
Tracy, Thomas (RI)	PS	725
Tranbaugh, Robert (NY)	TS	1007
Trauner, Doris (CA)	ChiN	149
Traverso, L William (WA)	S	990
Travis, William (NY)	Path	649
Traynelis, Vincent (IA)	NS	442
Treadwell, Marjorie (MI)	MF	391
Treadwell, Patricia (IN)	D	186

Name	Specialty	Pg
Udelsman, Robert (CT)	S	956
Uhde, Thomas (PA)	Psyc	809
Ulbright, Thomas M (IN)	Path	653
Ulshen, Martin (NC)	PGe	689
Umans, Jason (DC)	Nep	413
Umetsu, Dale (MA)	A&I	82
Underwood, Paul (SC)	ObG	511
Unger, Michael (PA)	Pul	846
Ungerleider, Ross (OR)	TS	1023
Urba, Susan (MI)	Onc	334
Urba, Walter (OR)	Onc	346
Uribe, John (FL)	OrS	577
Urist, Marshall M (AL)	S	972
Urken, Mark (NY)	Oto	609
Uzzo, Robert (PA)	U	1038

Alphabetical Listing of Doctors

Name	Specialty	Pg	Name	Specialty	Pg
Wallach, Robert (NY)	GO	265	Wazen, Jack (FL)	Oto	614
Walmer, David (NC)	RE	919	Wazer, David E (RI)	RadRO	869
Walsh, B Timothy (NY)	Psyc	809	Weaver, David (IN)	CG	155
Walsh, Christine (NY)	PCd	673	Weaver, W Douglas (MI)	Cv	113
Walsh, Edward (MA)	PCd	671	Webb, Lawrence (NC)	OrS	577
Walsh, John (LA)	NS	446	Weber, Randal (TX)	Oto	624
Walsh, Joseph (NY)	Oph	532	Weber, Thomas (NY)	PS	728
Walsh, Mary (IN)	Cv	112	Webster, George (NC)	U	1044
Walsh, Nicolas (TX)	PM	639	Wechsler, Lawrence (PA)	N	471
Walsh, Patrick (MD)	U	1039	Weder, Alan (MI)	IM	380
Walsh, R Matthew (OH)	S	981	Wei, Jeanne (AR)	Ger	253
Walters, Mark (OH)	ObG	513	Weichselbaum, Ralph R (IL)	RadRO	877
Walters, Theodore (ID)	Hem	303	Weiland, Andrew (NY)	HS	283
Walton, David (MA)	Oph	523	Wein, Alan (PA)	U	1039
Walton, Robert (IL)	PlS	783	Weinberg, Harold (NY)	N	471
Waner, Milton (NY)	Oto	609	Weinberg, Paul (PA)	PCd	673
Wang, Frederick (NY)	Oph	532	Weinberger, Malvin (FL)	PS	730
Wang, Ming (TN)	Oph	537	Weinberger, Michael (NY)	PM	636
Wang, Winfred (TN)	PHO	698	Weinblatt, Michael (MA)	Rhu	929
Wanner, Adam (FL)	Pul	850	Weiner, Howard (MA)	N	462
Wapner, Keith (PA)	OrS	573	Weiner, I David (FL)	Nep	415
Wapner, Ronald (PA)	MF	388	Weiner, Kenneth (CO)	Psyc	813
Wara, Diane (CA)	PA&I	671	Weiner, Leslie (CA)	N	490
Warady, Bradley (MO)	PNep	712	Weiner, Louis M (PA)	Onc	321
Ward, Barbara (CT)	S	956	Weiner, Michael (NY)	PHO	696
Ward, John H (UT)	Onc	336	Weiner, Myron (TX)	Psyc	814
Ward, Robert (NY)	PO	715	Weiner, Richard (NC)	Psyc	810
Ward, William (NC)	OrS	577	Weiner, Richard (FL)	OrS	577
Waring, George (GA)	Oph	537	Weiner, William (MD)	N	471
Warner, Ann (MO)	Rhu	937	Weingeist, Thomas (IA)	Oph	543
Warner, Brad (OH)	PS	732	Weinreb, Jeffrey (CT)	DR	889
Warnick, Ronald (OH)	NS	442	Weinstein, Arthur (DC)	Rhu	933
Warnke, Roger A (CA)	Path	658	Weinstein, Gregory (PA)	Oto	609
Warnock, David (AL)	Nep	414	Weinstein, Howard J (MA)	PHO	692
Warren, Robert (TX)	PRhu	724	Weinstein, James (NH)	OrS	562
Warren, Robert (AR)	PPul	721	Weinstein, Stuart (IA)	OrS	582
Warren, Robert (CA)	S	990	Weinstock, Robert (CA)	Psyc	817
Warren, Russell (NY)	OrS	573	Weisberg, Tracey (ME)	Onc	310
Warshaw, Andrew L (MA)	S	956	Weisenburger, Dennis (NE)	Path	653
Wartofsky, Leonard (DC)	EDM	201	Weisler, Richard (NC)	Psyc	810
Wasserman, Stephen (CA)	A&I	89	Weisman, Robert (CA)	Oto	626
Waters, Peter (MA)	HS	280	Weisman, Steven (WI)	PM	638
Watkins, Robert (CA)	OrS	589	Weiss, Arnold (RI)	HS	280
Watkins, Sandra (WA)	PNep	713	Weiss, Avery (WA)	Oph	552
Watts, Nelson (OH)	EDM	207	Weiss, Geoffrey R (VA)	Onc	327
Watts, Ray (AL)	N	475	Weiss, Gerson (NJ)	RE	917
Wax, Mark (OR)	Oto	626	Weiss, Lawrence M (CA)	Path	658
Waxman, Alan (CA)	NuM	503	Weiss, Martin (CA)	NS	449
Waxman, Harvey (PA)	Cv	103	Weiss, Robert (CT)	U	1031
Waxman, Irving (IL)	Ge	234	Weiss, Sharon (GA)	Path	651
Way, Lawrence (CA)	S	990	Weiss, Stanley H (NJ)	PrM	797
Waye, Jerome (NY)	Ge	224	Weissler, Jonathan (TX)	Pul	857

Alphabetical Listing of Doctors

Name	Specialty	Pg	Name	Specialty	Pg
Wityk, Robert (MD)	N	471	Yamaguchi, Ken (MO)	OrS	582
Wiviott, Lory (CA)	Inf	372	Yan, Albert (PA)	D	182
Wixson, Richard (IL)	OrS	582	Yancovitz, Stanley (NY)	Inf	366
Wiznitzer, Max (OH)	ChiN	146	Yang, Stephen C (MD)	TS	1007
Woeber, Kenneth (CA)	EDM	211	Yannuzzi, Lawrence (NY)	Oph	532
Wofsy, David (CA)	Rhu	940	Yeager, Andrew (AZ)	Hem	305
Wolf, Gregory (MI)	Oto	620	Yee, Billy (CA)	RE	924
Wolf, Randall (OH)	TS	1016	Yen, Yun (CA)	Onc	347
Wolf, Raoul (IL)	PA&I	669	Yeo, Charles (PA)	S	967
Wolfe, M Michael (MA)	Ge	217	Yetman, Randall (OH)	PlS	784
Wolfe, S Anthony (FL)	PlS	781	Yeung, Alan (CA)	IC	128
Wolfe, Scott (NY)	HS	283	Yonkers, Kimberly (CT)	Psyc	804
Wolff, Bruce (MN)	CRS	170	Yoo, Jung (OR)	OrS	589
Wolff, Grace (FL)	PCd	674	Yoon, Sydney (FL)	DR	894
Wolff, Robert (TX)	IM	380	Yoshikawa, Thomas (CA)	Inf	372
Wolinsky, Jerry (TX)	N	486	Yoshizumi, Marc (CA)	Oph	552
Wong, Jeffrey (CA)	RadRO	881	Young, A Byron (KY)	NS	436
Wong, Johnson (MA)	A&I	82	Young, Anne (MA)	N	462
Wong, Ronald (HI)	CRS	172	Young, Bruce (NY)	ObG	510
Wong, W Douglas (NY)	CRS	166	Young, Iven (NY)	EDM	202
Woo, Peak (NY)	Oto	610	Young, James (OH)	Cv	113
Wood, Beverly (CA)	DR	896	Young, K Randall (AL)	Pul	850
Wood, Bradford (MD)	VIR	904	Young, Ming-Lon (FL)	PCd	674
Wood, David (MI)	U	1050	Young, Nancy (IL)	Oto	621
Wood, Douglas (WA)	TS	1024	Young, Robert (MA)	Path	645
Wood, Gary (WI)	D	186	Young, Vernon (MO)	PlS	784
Wood, John (MO)	A&I	87	Younge, Brian (MN)	Oph	543
Wood, R Patrick (TX)	S	985	Yousem, David (MD)	NRad	898
Wood, Robert (MD)	PA&I	668	Yousem, Samuel (PA)	Path	649
Wood, William (GA)	S	973	Yu, George (MD)	U	1039
Woodson, B Tucker (WI)	Oto	621	Yu, John S (CA)	NS	449
Woodson, Gayle (IL)	Oto	621	Yu, Victor (PA)	Inf	366
Wooten, George (VA)	N	475	Yuen, James (AR)	PlS	787
Wooten, Virgil (OH)	Psyc	812	Yurt, Roger (NY)	S	967
Wormser, Gary (NY)	Inf	365			
Worsey, M Jonathan (CA)	CRS	172	**Z**		
Wright, Cameron (MA)	TS	1000			
Wright, Harry (SC)	ChAP	825	Zackai, Elaine (PA)	CG	154
Wright, Jackson (OH)	IM	380	Zacur, Howard (MD)	RE	917
Wright, Kenneth (CA)	Oph	552	Zafonte, Ross (PA)	PMR	759
Wright, Robert (IL)	N	482	Zahn, Evan (FL)	PCd	675
Wunderink, Richard (IL)	Pul	854	Zaidman, Gerald (NY)	Oph	532
Wyatt, Robert (TN)	PNep	710	Zalusky, Ralph (NY)	Hem	298
Wyllie, Elaine (OH)	ChiN	146	Zalzal, George (DC)	Oto	610
Wyllie, Robert (OH)	PGe	690	Zaret, Barry (CT)	Cv	97
Y			Zarins, Bertram (MA)	OrS	562
			Zarins, Christopher (CA)	VascS	1076
			Zdeblick, Thomas (WI)	OrS	582
Yaddanapudi, Ravindranath (MI)	PHO	701	Zeanah, Charles (LA)	ChAP	827
Yaffe, Bruce (NY)	IM	379	Zeitels, Steven (MA)	Oto	602
Yager, Joel (NM)	Psyc	814	Zeitlin, Pamela (MD)	PPul	719
Yakes, Wayne (CO)	VIR	907	Zelefsky, Michael (NY)	RadRO	872

Castle Connolly America's Top Doctors® 7th Edition

Acknowledgments

The publishers would like to thank the entire staff for their many hours and days of intense and precise work on this guide in order to further its goal of assisting consumers in making the best healthcare choices.

Castle Connolly Executive Management:

Chairman	John K. Castle
President & CEO	John J. Connolly, Ed.D.
Vice President, Chief Medical & Research Officer	Jean Morgan, M.D.
Vice President, Chief Strategy & Operations Officer	William Liss-Levinson, Ph.D.
Marketing & Public Relations Coordinator	Terese Cecilia

We also would like to extend our gratitude to the American Board of Medical Specialties (ABMS) for allowing us to use excerpts, especially the descriptions of medical specialties and subspecialties, from the text of their publication "Which Medical Specialist for You?"

We wish to thank our research coordinators Maryann Hynd, RN, Sara Belly and Naomi Valensi with additional thanks to our layout/Editorial staff: Stephenie Galvan, Tara Rolandelli, Krista Feierabend, Russell Hodgson and Matt Pretka

Other Publications from Castle Connolly Medical Ltd.:
*America's Top Doctors for Cancer; Top Doctors: New York Metro Area; Top Doctors: Chicago Metro Area; Cancer Made Easier: New York Metro Area,*and others...
Order online at http://www.castleconnolly.com/books

Doctor-Patient Advisor

Doctor-Patient Advisor is a Castle Connolly Medical Ltd., service providing one-on-one consultations with a physician or nurse to individuals who have serious or complex medical problems or to anyone who feels he/she needs assistance finding the right physician for any purpose. Each client will receive personalized assistance in identifying the appropriate specialists for his/her condition, utilizing the Castle Connolly Medical Ltd. database of physicians and hospitals, as well as individual searches, to locate the best resources to meet the client's needs.

Fee: $275. For further information call (212) 367-8400 x 16.

National Physician of the Year Awards

Castle Connolly Medical Ltd. proudly hosted our second annual National Physician of the Year Awards on March 13, 2007 at the elegant Pierre Hotel in Manhattan, New York. It was a spectacular evening which allowed us to recognize both the outstanding honorees and the excellence of the many thousands of physicians throughout the nation.

The Genesis of the National Physician of the Year Award

Each year we receive thousands of nominations from physicians and the medical leadership of major medical centers, specialty hospitals, teaching hospitals and regional and community medical centers across the U.S. as an integral part of our research, screening and selection process to identify *America's Top Doctors®*. The selected physicians, while spread across all fifty states and involved in more than 70 medical specialties and subspecialties, all share one distinguishing professional attribute: an unwavering dedication to their patients and to medicine as a whole. Each and every one of these outstanding medical professionals is a symbol of the clinical excellence that characterizes American medicine. In honor of these exemplary physicians, Castle Connolly Medical Ltd. has created the National Physician of the Year Awards to recognize the thousands of excellent, dedicated physicians across the United States. Our Medical Advisory Board selected the three honorees from the hundreds nominated in a special nomination process conducted months before the event.

Our three honorees, Drs. Delos M. Cosgrove, Joseph G. McCarthy and Patrick C. Walsh, are shining examples of excellence in clinical medical practice. In addition to these awards, Castle Connolly Medical Ltd. honored Dr. Maria Delivoria-Papadopoulos for her lifetime achievement in the medical community. Her career in neonatology has spanned almost fifty years and she has contributed countless revolutionary procedures and instruments to the specialty, making her the ideal honoree for the Lifetime Achievement Award. The Honorable Nancy G. Brinker, a tireless fundraiser for the Susan G. Komen for the Cure, was an exemplary recipient of our second National Health Leadership Award. Her fundraising efforts have helped extend the

Susan G. Komen for the Cure's many programs and services, reaching millions of people devastated by this disease, providing both education and hope. Neither the medical community nor the public would ever have reaped the benefits of years of research and medical breakthroughs if not for the gallant and tireless efforts of individuals such as Dr. Maria Delivoria-Papadopoulos and the Honorable Nancy G. Brinker.

Each honoree received Imagination, a beautiful and distinctive porcelain figurine from the world renowned Lladro. Portraying an angel with soaring wings, this statue represents the hope and comfort all five honorees have brought to the world through their devotion to their patients and their profession.

National Physician of the Year Awards Honorees

For Clinical Excellence

Delos M. Cosgrove, M.D.
Board of Governors, Chief Executive Officer & President
The Cleveland Clinic Health System

Joseph G. McCarthy, M.D.
Lawrence D. Bell Professor of Plastic Surgery,
Director, Institute of Reconstructive Surgery
NYU Medical Center

Patrick C. Walsh, M.D.
Professor and Director,
The Brady Urological Institute at The John Hopkins Hospital

For Lifetime Achievement

Maria Delivoria-Papadopoulos, M.D.
Professor, Pediatrics, Physiology and Obstetrics/Gynecology
Drexel University College of Medicine
Director, Neonatal Intensive Care Unit, St. Christoper's Hospital for Children

For National Health Leadership

The Honorable Nancy G. Brinker
Former U.S. Ambassador to Republic of Hungary
Founder, Susan G. Komen for the Cure